DATE			

PHYSICAL REHABILITATION

Evidence-Based Examination,
Evaluation, and Intervention

PHYSICAL REHABILITATION

Evidence-Based Examination, Evaluation, and Intervention

Edited by

Michelle H. Cameron, MD, PT, OCS
Oregon Health Sciences University
Portland, Oregon

Linda G. Monroe, MPT, OCS
Lafayette, California

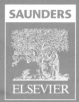

SAUNDERS

ELSEVIER

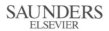

SAUNDERS
ELSEVIER

11830 Westline Industrial Drive
St. Louis, Missouri 63146

Library of Congress Control Number 2007920424

Publishing Director: Linda Duncan
Editor: Kathy Falk
Developmental Editor: Megan Fennell
Publishing Services Manager: Melissa Lastarria
Senior Project Manager: Joy Moore
Senior Designer: Jyotika Shroff

Printed in Canada

Last digit is the print number: 9 8 7 6 5 4 3 2 1

Contributors

DIANE D. ALLEN, PhD, PT

Adjunct Assistant Professor
Department of Physical Therapy
Samuel Merritt College
Oakland, California

NANCEY A. BOOKSTEIN, EdD, PT

Associate Professor, Director of Physical Therapy
   Admissions
Physical Therapy Program
School of Medicine
Senior Instructor
Cellular and Developmental Biology
University of Colorado at Denver, Health Sciences
   Center
Denver, Colorado

LAWRENCE P. CAHALIN, MA, PT, CCS

Clinical Professor
Department of Physical Therapy
Northeastern University
Boston, Massachusetts

CYNTHIA CHIARELLO, PhD, MPT

Associate Director
Physical Therapy Program
Columbia University
New York, New York

DEBRA CLAYTON-KRASINSKI, PhD, PT

Assistant Professor, Clinical Physical Therapy
Program in Physical Therapy
Columbia University
New York, New York

VANINA DAL BELLO-HAAS, PhD, PT

Associate Professor
School of Physical Therapy
University of Saskatchewan
Saskatoon, Canada

JENNIFER DEKERLEGAND, MPT

Heart Failure Coordinator, Research Team Leader
Hospital of the University of Pennsylvania
Division of Occupational and Physical Therapy
Philadelphia, Pennsylvania

ROBERT L. DEKERLEGAND, PT, MPT, CCS

Assistant Professor
Department of Developmental and Rehabilitative
   Services
School of Health Related Professions
University of Medicine and Dentistry of New Jersey
Stratford, New Jersey

**CHRISTOPHER J. DURALL, DPT, PT, MS, SCS,
LAT, CSCS**

Graduate Faculty
Director of Physical Therapy
Student Health Center
University of Wisconsin-LaCrosse
LaCrosse, Wisconsin

LISA L. DUTTON, PhD, PT

Associate Professor, Dean
College of Health Professions
The University of Findlay
Findlay, Ohio

JOAN E. EDELSTEIN, MA, PT, FISPO

Special Lecturer
Program in Physical Therapy
Columbia University
New York, New York

AHMED SAMIR ELOKDA, PhD, PT, CLT-LANA

Associate Professor, Director
Department of Physical Therapy
New York Institute of Technology
New York, New York

DONNA K. EVERIX, MPA, PT

Physician Services Manager
Mills-Peninsula Health Services
Burlingame, California

LINDA FIEBACK, MS, MA

Professional Associate
Mercy College
Dobbs Ferry, New York

GINNY GIBSON, MS, OTR/L, CHT

Assistant Professor
Department of Occupational Therapy
Samuel Merritt College
Oakland, California

SUSAN GRIEVE, MPT, MS
Senior Physical Therapist
Department of Rehabilitation Services
Kaiser Permanente
Richmond, California

ROSE LITTLE HAMM, DPT, PT, CWS, FCCWS
Assistant Professor of Clinical Physical Therapy
Department of Biokinesiology and Physical Therapy
University of Southern California
Los Angeles, California

KEVIN HELGESON, DHSc, PT, SCS
Assistant Professor
Department of Physical and Occupational Therapy
Idaho State University
Pocatello, Idaho

MOHAMED IBRAHIM, DSc, PT, MS, NCS
Physical Therapy Program
State University of New York, Downstate
Brooklyn, New York

DEBRA H. IWASAKI, MSPT, SCS, ATC, CSCS
Associate Head Athletic Trainer and Rehabilitation
    Coordinator
Department of Intercollegiate Athletics
University of California, Los Angeles
Los Angeles, California

SUSAN KLEPPER, PhD, PT
Assistant Professor of Clinical Physical Therapy
Department of Rehabilitation Medicine
Columbia University
New York, New York

L. VINCE LEPAK III, DPT, PT, MPH, CWS
Assistant Professor
Department of Physical Therapy
The University of Oklahoma
Tulsa, Oklahoma

ROBERT C. MANSKE, DPT, PT, MEd, SCS, ATC, CSCS
Assistant Professor
Department of Physical Therapy
Wichita State University
Teaching Associate
Department of Family Medicine
Via Christi Sports Medicine Fellowship Residency
    Program
Staff Physical Therapist
Via Christi Sports and Orthopedic Physical Therapy
Wichita, Kansas

VICTORIA MERRELL, MPT
Boise, Idaho

TOM METS, PT, MPT
Manager of Outpatient Services
San Joaquin Valley Rehabilitation
Fresno, California

MARTHA PATERSON, OTR/L, CHT
Owner
Artistic Advantage
Burbank, California

CHRISTIANE PERME, PT, CCS
Senior Physical Therapist
Department of Physical Therapy and Occupational
    Therapy
The Methodist Hospital
Houston, Texas

BRIAN K. PETERSON, MPT, MA
Jefferson County Hospital
Fairfield, Iowa

JULIE A. PRYDE, MS, PT, OCS, SCS, PA-C, ATC
Adjunct Assistant Professor
Samuel Merritt College
Oakland, California
Physician Assistant
Muir Orthopedic Specialists
Walnut Creek, California

LORI QUINN, EdD, PT
Clinical Faculty Associate
Program in Physical Therapy
New York Medical College
Valhalla, New York

MICHAEL P. REIMAN, PT, MEd, ATC, CSCS
Assistant Professor
Department of Physical Therapy
Wichita State University
Wichita, Kansas

PAMELA SCARBOROUGH, PT, MS, CDE, CWS, FCCWS
Director of Education
PARKS Institute
Wimberley, Texas

AMY SELINGER, PT, MS, OCS
Assistant Clinical Professor
Graduate Program in Physical Therapy
University of California San Francisco, San Francisco
    State University Joint Program in Physical Therapy
Owner, Chief Physical Therapist
Back to Life
San Francisco, California

LYNDA L. SPANGLER, MS, PT
Assistant Professor
Department of Physical Therapy
The College of St. Scholastica
Duluth, Minnesota

BONNIE J. SPARKS-DEFRIESE
Wound Ostomy Continence Nurse Clinician/
Instructor
Wound Ostomy Continence Nursing Educational
Center
School of Medicine
Emory University
Atlanta, Georgia

JAN STEPHEN TECKLIN, MS, PT
Professor
Department of Physical Therapy
Arcadia University
Glenside, Pennsylvania

TONI TYNER, MHSL, BS
Assistant Professor
Department of Physical Therapy
California State University, Fresno
Fresno, California

R. SCOTT WARD, PhD, PT
Professor, Chair
Division of Physical Therapy
The University of Utah
Salt Lake City, Utah

ROBERT WELLMON, PhD, PT, NCS
Assistant Professor
Institute for Physical Therapy Education
Widener University
Chester, Pennsylvania

Preface

The inspiration for writing this text came when editing the second edition of Michelle Cameron's book *Physical Agents in Rehabilitation.* As we updated that book so that it was consistent with the terminology presented in the *Guide to Physical Therapist Practice (Guide),* we realized that, although the *Guide* provides a framework for describing and implementing physical therapy, it does not evaluate the evidence for specific management approaches or make specific recommendations for patient care in physical rehabilitation. Furthermore, no other book met the need for a broad-based, entry-level textbook that used the structure and language of the *Guide* to present evidence-based patient management recommendations across the breadth of physical rehabilitation.

This text, and its ancillaries, provides rehabilitation students and practicing clinicians with clear recommendations for evidence-based physical rehabilitation examination, evaluation, and interventions for a wide range of patients. It provides information for the generalist and will guide the specialist in providing care beyond his or her area of expertise. The case studies provided in each chapter and on the accompanying CD demonstrate the application of the presented information within a clinical context.

The book starts with a chapter that more fully describes the rest of the chapters and the concepts presented. This is followed by an introduction to evidence-based practice. Thereafter, the book has one chapter for each preferred practice pattern (physical therapy diagnosis) presented in the *Guide* and four additional chapters that describe interventions, such as assistive devices and environmental adaptations that are common to various preferred practice patterns. The structure, sequence, language, and concepts presented in this book are based on those of the *Guide.*

The first four parts of the book are the same as the *Guide's* categories of preferred practice patterns. In addition, each chapter in these parts of the book covers pathology, examination, evaluation, and interventions related to the preferred practice pattern. Part Five of the book covers interventions that overlap many practice patterns and are therefore more effectively discussed together. All of the chapters have a consistent style and format to make information clear and readily accessible and to promote learning and recall. In addition, all chapters are thoroughly referenced with up-to-date primary research, and all have information about additional resources regarding the specific area of practice and have a complete glossary of useful terms and concepts.

The CD that comes with this book enhances the information in the text. The CD includes additional case studies for all chapters; direct electronic links to clinically useful resources online and to all listed references; printable, modifiable forms related to the content of the chapter; boards-style multiple-choice study questions; vocabulary-building exercises based on the glossaries; animations that demonstrate procedures or body processes; and a variety of other useful tools and information.

In addition, instructors using this book will have online access to all of the previously mentioned student resources along with lab activities for each chapter and an electronic image collection.

We hope this text provides you with the most clearly written, up-to-date, evidence-based information and recommendations you need for patient management in rehabilitation. Your feedback is welcome and will make future editions of this text even better for students.

Acknowledgments

We wish to thank the many people without whom this project would not have been possible.

First, we want to thank each of the chapter contributors who gave so willingly of their knowledge and expertise. Thank you all for sharing your knowledge to improve therapy and to better the lives of patients beyond those you treat yourselves. We know that for many it was easy to say "yes" when asked, "Would you be willing to write a chapter about . . . ?" But it was so much harder to follow through with the details, especially with so many deadlines. We thank you all for your hard work, dedication, discipline, and productivity. We owe extra special thanks to Joan Edelstein, who was not only the primary contributor for three chapters but also composed all the lab activities for the instructor's manual. Joan consistently volunteered to take on more work and responsibility when asked and always delivered what we wanted when we wanted. Thank you, Joan.

Thank you also to the Elsevier team who supported us and led us through the publication process, had faith in us, and reassured us that this really would all come together. Marion Waldman helped this vision get off the ground and take shape. We thank Kathy Falk, senior editor, for taking this project on as her own late in the process, reining it in and putting together a great team to take this project through to production. We especially thank Megan Fennell, associate developmental editor, who was endlessly patient with us and our contributors and who kept track of and took care of all the details calmly and efficiently. Thank you, Megan.

We also acknowledge the support of the manufacturers and other outside sources who provided us with illustrations and permission to use their images, questionnaires, forms, and other materials. All these components add to the richness of this resource.

We also gratefully acknowledge the support of our partners and friends. We know you are relieved that this project is complete, and we thank you for patiently, or not so patiently, supporting us through the ups and downs and the endless "it's almost done." We really would rather spend our time with you and should have a few more "free" evenings and weekends now . . . until the next edition.

Finally, we recognize and appreciate the endurance of our friendship. It is a testament to the strength of that bond that we never once became impatient with each other and that somehow one of us was always strong and ready to take the lead when the other needed to rest or divert.

Michelle H. Cameron
Linda G. Monroe

Contents

PART 5: INTERVENTIONS COMMON TO MANY CONDITIONS REQUIRING REHABILITATION

Introduction

Michelle H. Cameron

OBJECTIVES

After reading this chapter, the reader will be able to:
1. Describe physical rehabilitation and the roles of those involved in providing physical rehabilitation.
2. Understand the Nagi and World Health Organization disablement models.
3. Understand the role of the *Guide to Physical Therapist Practice*.
4. Easily access information in this book regarding pathology, examination, evaluation, diagnosis, prognosis, and interventions for patients involved in physical rehabilitation.
5. Access the ancillaries provided with this book, including useful printable forms, practice boards–style test questions, and electronic links to references and resources.

This textbook provides clear explanations of the concepts essential for safe, effective evidence-based physical rehabilitation *assessment* and *interventions* for a wide range of patients. It is intended to be read and used by physical *rehabilitation* students and clinicians, including those in *physical therapy, occupational therapy,* physiatry, and other professions. This introductory chapter briefly describes what rehabilitation is and who does it. It also provides an overview of the special features of this book, particularly its adherence to the *Guide to Physical Therapist Practice* (the *Guide*),[1] the consistent structure of each chapter, and features in and accompanying each chapter. This chapter concludes with a summary and glossary of terms used.

By reading and applying the information presented in this book, in conjunction with participating in didactic teaching and hands-on practice, the reader will learn to provide physical rehabilitation care at the level expected from a graduate of a professional training program. This is a broad-based, entry-level textbook that provides sufficient information for the generalist to provide care in many areas. It can also guide the specialist in providing care beyond his or her area of expertise. It is not intended as a specialty text for any single area of physical rehabilitation. This book will be valuable to students during their professional training and will continue to prove its value to practicing rehabilitation professionals throughout their career.

PHYSICAL REHABILITATION

Rehabilitation is a goal oriented *treatment* process intended to maximize independence in individuals with compromised *function* that results from primary pathological processes and resultant *impairments*. Rehabilitation generally addresses the sequelae of *pathology* rather than the pathology itself. Physical rehabilitation focuses particularly on sequelae that impact physical functioning and activity and uses interventions that are noninvasive and physical in nature to promote progress toward functional *goals*. For example, physical rehabilitation may focus on impairments in mobility and *functional limitations* associated with musculoskeletal and neurological *diseases* or injuries, such as fractures or strokes, and treating them with exercises and hands-on mobilization techniques. Rehabilitation is not directed at curing disease, and physical rehabilitation, in the context of this book, does not include the use of medications or surgery as therapeutic interventions.

PHYSICAL REHABILITATION PROVIDERS

A wide range of professionals are involved in providing physical rehabilitation services. These include physicians, licensed and certified allied health care professionals, and assistants. *Physiatrists* are physicians who specialize in physical medicine and rehabilitation. Physiatrists often oversee the care of patients requiring rehabilitation, referring them to various other physicians and allied health care professionals and following up on the outcome of these referrals. Physiatrists may also provide direct patient care, including *examination*, specialized testing, and a variety of medical interventions, particularly medications. *Physical therapists* (PTs) and *occupational therapists* (OTs) and their assistants, physical therapist assistants (PTAs) and certified occupational therapist assistants (COTAs), are the allied health professionals who specialize in providing physical rehabilitation.

According to the *Guide,* PTs "diagnose and manage movement *dysfunction* and enhance physical and functional abilities."[1] They "restore, maintain, and promote not only optimal physical function but optimal wellness and fitness and optimal quality of life as it relates to movement and health." They also "prevent the onset, *symptoms* and progression of impairments, functional limitations, and disabilities that may result from diseases, *disorders,* conditions, or injuries."[1]

According to the American Occupational Therapy Association, OTs "prevent the onset, symptoms, and progression of impairments, functional limitations, and disabilities that may result from diseases, disorders, conditions, or injuries."[2]

In addition to these physical rehabilitation specialists, patients involved in physical rehabilitation may be also be cared for by nurses, speech-language pathologists, and neuropsychologists.

Patients with a wide range of needs and problems typically receive physical rehabilitation. Most have a disease, disorder, condition, or injury with consequent impairments, functional limitations, and disabilities. The conditions underlying these limitations may involve any physical system, including the musculoskeletal, neuromuscular, cardiopulmonary, and integumentary systems. For example, patients with fractures, stroke, heart failure, or pressure ulcers commonly receive physical rehabilitation services. Physical rehabilitation may also be provided preventively in patients at risk for developing impairments, functional limitations, and disabilities. For example, clients with osteoporosis may receive physical therapy to reduce their risk of fractures and falls.

GOALS OF PHYSICAL REHABILITATION

The goals of physical rehabilitation are to optimize patient function at home, in the community, and at work. Although these outcomes are commonly measured in terms of impairments, ideally they should be focused on changes in functional limitations and disabilities and centered on the patient's own goals for functional improvement.[3] A wide range of outcome measures may be used to assess a patient's progression toward these goals.

DISABLEMENT MODELS

Two related conceptual frameworks that help guide examination, *evaluation,* and interventions for patients in rehabilitation are disablement models, particularly the Nagi and World Health Organization (WHO) models, and the *Guide to Physical Therapist Practice* (the *Guide*). These conceptual frameworks are described in the following sections.

Disablement models are approaches to thinking about the impacts or sequelae of disease on human functioning. A number of classification schemes have been proposed to categorize these sequelae. In 1980, WHO published the first classification scheme, the International Classification of Impairments, Disabilities, and Handicaps (ICIDH).[4-6] This scheme, based primarily on the work of Wood, classified the sequelae of pathology as impairments, disabilities, and handicaps.[7,8] Shortly thereafter, Nagi published a similar model that used the classifications of impairments, functional limitations, and disabilities.[9] In 1993, the National Center for Medical Rehabilitation Research (NCMRR) published a classification scheme that combined concepts from the Nagi model with the original ICIDH model.[10] Most recently, in 2001, WHO revised their classification scheme to produce the International Classification of Functioning, Disability, and Health-2 (ICF) scheme.[11]

Disablement model revisions are intended to reflect and create changes in perceptions of people with disabilities and meet the needs of more involved groups of people. The original models were intended to differentiate disease and pathology from the limitations they produced and were developed primarily for use by rehabilitation professionals. The newly expanded models try to have a more positive perspective on the changes resulting from pathology and disease and are intended for use by a wide range of people, including community, national, and global institutions that create policy and allocate resources for persons with disabilities. Specifically, the NCMRR model added a category of societal limitations to the functional problems associated with *disability* and abandoned the previous linear modeling approach to reflect the frequently nonsequential nature of the relationships between categories. The ICF has tried to change the perspective of disability from the negative focus of "consequences of disease" used in the 1980 model to a more positive focus on "components of health." Thus, while the first ICIDH model used categories of impairments, disabilities and handicaps to describe sequelae of pathology, ICF uses categories of health conditions, body functions, activities, and participation to focus on abilities rather than on restrictions and limitations. More detailed information on the WHO disablement models is available on the ICF web site at www.who.int/classification/icf/en.

This book uses a scheme consistent with the terminology and framework of the *Guide,*[1] which is based on the Nagi disablement model (Fig. 1-1). The *Guide* adopts Nagi's disablement model, stating that this "disablement model typifies physical therapist practice and is the model for understanding and organizing practice." The *Guide's* preferred practice patterns are based on the pathologies of four systems and their related impairments.[1]

THE NAGI MODEL

According to the Nagi model and the *Guide,* the sequelae of pathology are classified as impairments, functional

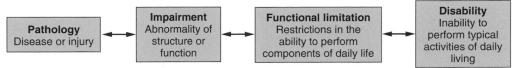

FIG. 1-1 The Nagi model of disablement. *Data from Nagi S: Disability concepts revisited. In Pope AM, Tarlov AR (eds):* Disability in America: Toward a National Agenda for Prevention, *Washington, DC, 1991, National Academy Press.*

limitations, and disabilities.[1,4,9] Pathology refers to the alteration of anatomy or physiology that is due to disease or injury and describes a specific disease process or *diagnosis*. The *Guide* defines pathology as "an abnormality characterized by a particular cluster of *signs* and symptoms and recognized by either the patient or practitioner as abnormal. Pathology is primarily identified at the cellular level." Examples of pathology, as described by the Nagi model, include the diagnoses of cerebral vascular accident or stroke, lumbar disc herniation, or joint inflammation.

Knowledge of pathology does not provide sufficient information to guide either examination or procedural interventions in rehabilitation. For example, different individuals with a stroke may have wide-ranging alterations of motor and cognitive performance resulting in the need for different levels, approaches, and focus of both examination and interventions. Variation in the etiology, severity, and location of a stroke, as well as variation in other aspects of the patient's biopsychosocial health, may result in a range of impairments, functional limitations, and disabilities from undetectable change from baseline to extreme change in all functional abilities and tremendous disability.

Impairments are defined by the Nagi model as disruptions in anatomical, physiological, or psychological structures or functions as the result of some underlying pathology,[6,11] and by the *Guide* as "a loss or abnormality of anatomical, physiological, mental, or psychological structure or function."[1] An impairment is a measure at the organ or organ system level and is equivalent to a sign or an objective measure. For example, decreased cervical flexibility, diminished deep tendon reflexes, reduced force production or endurance, and absent sensation are all impairments.

Impairments may lead to functional limitations. A functional limitation, as defined by the Nagi model, is a restriction in the ability to perform an activity in an efficient, typically expected, or competent manner, or as stated in the *Guide*, "the restriction of the ability to perform, at the level of the whole person, a physical action, task, or activity in an efficient, typically expected, or competent manner."[1] Examples of functional limitations are an inability to lift more than 20 lb or a limitation in sitting tolerance. Although functional limitations and impairments are related, it is not uncommon that an impairment does not, at least initially, result in any functional limitation. For example, patients may have the impairment of reduced vital capacity when tested but never demand enough of their respiratory system to encounter a functional limitation from this impairment.

The Nagi model then defines a disability as the inability to perform activities required for self-care, home, work, or community roles. Disability takes into account the barriers presented by society to performing expected roles in the face of functional limitations.[9] The *Guide* defines disability as "the inability to perform or a limitation in the performance of actions, tasks, and activities usually expected in specific social roles that are customary for the individual or expected for the person's status or role in a specific sociocultural context and physical environment."[1] In the *Guide*, the categories of required roles are self-care, home management, work (job/school/play), and community/leisure. Examples of disability according to the Nagi model are the inability to lift one's child or walk to the store.

Medical treatment is generally directed at the underlying pathology or disease, whereas rehabilitation focuses primarily on reversing or minimizing associated impairments, functional limitations, and disabilities. It is therefore essential that rehabilitation professionals assess and set goals not only at the level of impairment, such as pain, decreased range of motion, or hypertonicity, but also at the level of functional limitation and disability as they relate to the specific patient's goals.

Improvements in functional limitations along with disabilities will be most important to patients and to other individuals involved with their care. The therapist should identify the functional limitations that are the most important to the patient and that can be addressed by the therapist. Once the patient and therapist agree on the most important functional limitations, the therapist can begin to rank impairments found in the examination according to the degree to which they relate to the prioritized functional limitations. The therapist may then focus interventions both directly on the functional limitations and the related impairments to optimize the achievement of the patient's functional goals.

Using the Nagi model of disablement to guide the examination ensures that all aspects of the person are considered when making clinical decisions. The Nagi model of disablement is used throughout this book to guide and structure the examination, evaluation, and intervention strategies.

During all components of the patient examination, including the patient *history*, the *systems review*, and *tests and measures*, the clinician should gather data to gain understanding of the patient's impairments, functional limitations, and disabilities. This information can then be used to evaluate the patient and determine a diagnosis, *prognosis*, and *plan of care*; identify key outcomes; and select appropriate interventions.

THE *GUIDE TO PHYSICAL THERAPIST PRACTICE*

The *Guide,* the second edition of which was published in 2001, was developed by the American Physical Therapy Association (APTA) "to encourage a uniform approach to physical therapist practice and to explain to the world the nature of that practice."[1] This document took close to a decade to develop and forms a framework for describing the scope and content of physical therapist practice using standardized terms and a standardized practice model. Its consistent conceptual approach to patient care is intended to improve communication among clinicians and to those outside of rehabilitation.

The *Guide* is divided into two parts. Part 1 delineates the physical therapist's scope of practice and describes patient management by PTs, and Part 2 describes each of the diagnostic preferred practice patterns of patients typically treated by PTs.

According to the *Guide,* patient management by PTs involves examination, evaluation, diagnosis, prognosis, and intervention.

EXAMINATION

Examination is "a comprehensive *screening* and specific testing process leading to diagnostic classification or, as appropriate, to a referral to another practitioner." The examination's three components are the patient history, the systems review, and tests and measures.

Patient History. The patient history is a systematically gathered collection of information focused on why the patient is seeking care, as well as past and current functional status and activity level. The patient history may also include information about the patient's general demographics, social history, employment or work, growth and development, living environment, general health status, social and health habits, family history, medical and surgical history, medications, and results of previously performed clinical tests. This information may be collected through interviewing the patient, caretakers, or family members and by a thorough review of prior medical records. The patient history, particularly the pattern of symptoms, will give the clinician an idea of the nature of the patient's problem and indicate the most efficient course for the rest of the examination. In addition, the therapist can build rapport with the patient during this initial component of the examination.

A combination of open- and close-ended questions is recommended for obtaining the patient history. Initial questions regarding patient history should be open-ended to allow the patient to fully describe their concerns and problems. Later, questions may be focused to ensure that the clinician's concerns are addressed, although leading questions should be avoided. Close-ended questions such as "Where do you have pain?" assure that specific necessary information is obtained. Open-ended questions such as "Tell me about the problem that brings you here today" may reveal information about areas beyond those considered by the examiner and give the examiner a more accurate understanding of the patient's priorities and primary concerns.[12] In general, the history should start with broader questions and proceed toward more specific details. For example, if the patient reports numbness, the clinician can follow with "Where is the numbness?" If symptoms are present in more than one location, the therapist should determine if the nature of the symptoms is the same in all areas, if they occur in all areas concurrently, or if they are temporally related, with symptoms in one area typically preceding those in another area. In addition to the location of symptoms, their nature and severity and easing or aggravating factors should be ascertained. Once the nature of the current concerns has been determined, the therapist should then ascertain how the symptoms developed, including prior similar symptoms and their evolution, any precipitating event(s), and the duration and evolution of the current symptoms.

To obtain information about the functional impact of a patient's problem, one may ask how symptoms affect daytime activities, including those at work and at home, and how they affect the patient's sleep.

The patient history should end with questions about "red flags" and an open-ended question to check if the patient has any other concerns. Red flags are issues that may indicate the need for further work-up and should prompt referral to a physician. Red flags include a dramatic worsening of symptoms, unintentional weight change, changes in bowel or bladder function (incontinence or retention), and fever.

Systems Review. The systems review is the first "hands-on" component of the examination. It involves a "brief or limited examination of the status of the cardiovascular/pulmonary, integumentary, musculoskeletal and neuromuscular systems and the communication ability, affect, cognition, language, and learning style of the patient."[1] This brief review is used to target areas requiring further examination and define areas that may cause complications or indicate a need for precautions during the examination and intervention processes.

A limited examination of the cardiovascular and pulmonary systems would generally include measurement of heart rate, respiratory rate and pattern, and blood pressure (see Chapter 22). A limited examination of the integumentary system should include observation of the skin in the involved area, particularly looking for areas of breakdown or scar formation, rash, or color changes, and palpation of the area to assess for gross changes in surface temperature. A musculoskeletal scanning examination should include gross tests of range of motion and strength and observation of body size, proportion, and symmetry. The review of the neuromuscular systems may include gross examination of coordination, balance, locomotion, reflexes, sensation, and orientation to person, place, and time. Communication, affect, cognition, language, and learning style are generally grossly evaluated through attention to how the patient communicates the patient history. While obtaining the patient history, the therapist can generally assess the patient's ability to understand, communicate, and make their needs known, as well as determine the level of consciousness and orientation. The therapist can also gain an understanding of the patient's overall current psychological and emotional state.

Tests and Measures. The patient history and systems review are used to generate diagnostic hypotheses. Specific tests and measures of the musculoskeletal, neuromuscular, cardiopulmonary, and integumentary systems, as well as tests of patient function, are then selected to rule in or rule out causes of impairment and functional limitations. The results of these tests are used to establish a diagnosis, prognosis, and plan of care and to direct selection of interventions.

EVALUATION, DIAGNOSIS, AND PROGNOSIS

Evaluations are clinical judgments based on the data gathered during the examination. The evaluation involves synthesizing the findings from all of the components of the examination to establish the patient's diagnosis and prognosis. According to the *Guide,* PTs use diagnostic labels that "identify the impact of a condition on function at the level of the system (especially the movement system) and at the level of the whole person."[1] PTs assign a diagnostic label by classifying patients or clients within a specified preferred practice pattern.

According to the *Guide,* the prognosis is the "determination of the predicted optimal level of improvement in function and the amount of time needed to reach that level, and also may include a prediction of the improvement that may be reached at various intervals during the course of therapy." The prognosis should also include a plan of care that specifies "anticipated goals and expected outcomes, predicted level of optimal improvement, specific interventions to be used, and proposed duration and frequency of the interventions that are required to reach the anticipated goals and expected outcomes."

INTERVENTION

Interventions are "the purposeful interaction of the physical therapist with the patient using various physical therapy procedures and techniques to produce changes in the condition that are consistent with the diagnosis and prognosis."[1] Interventions may include coordination, communication, and documentation; patient/client-related instructions; and procedural interventions such as therapeutic exercise and physical agents.

Part 2 of the *Guide* includes sections on each of the diagnostic preferred practice patterns. These practice patterns are divided into four categories of conditions: musculoskeletal, neuromuscular, cardiovascular/pulmonary, and integumentary, with a number of preferred practice patterns within each of these categories. For each preferred practice pattern the *Guide* provides inclusion and exclusion criteria for the diagnostic classification, ICD-9-CM codes that may relate to the practice pattern, and descriptions of the examination, evaluation, diagnosis, prognosis, and interventions related to the management of patients within this preferred practice pattern.

STRUCTURE OF THIS BOOK

This textbook is structured around concepts presented in the *Guide.*[1] By adopting the structure of the *Guide,* this book promotes clinical integration of the *Guide's* concepts.

This book is divided into five parts. The first four parts are the same as the Guide's categories of preferred practice patterns: musculoskeletal, neuromuscular, cardiovascular/pulmonary, and integumentary (Table 1-1). As noted, these patterns reflect physical therapy diagnostic labels and "identify the impact of a condition on function at the level of the system (especially the movement system) and at the level of the whole person."[1] These practice patterns contrast with a physician's diagnosis that typically identifies diseases, disorders, or conditions at the level of the cell, tissue, organ, or system. Most of the chapters within the first three parts of this book parallel the preferred practice patterns presented in the *Guide.* However, Part 4, preferred practice patterns related to the integumentary system, is organized according to wound etiology, which is more commonly done in clinical practice and research, rather than according to wound depth as in the *Guide.* Part 5 covers interventions that overlap many practice patterns and are therefore most effectively discussed together rather than repetitively in many other chapters.

In addition to the parts and chapters of this book paralleling the structure of the *Guide,* the chapters also follow the recommendations of the *Guide,* describing patient management in terms of examination, including history, systems review, and tests and measures; evaluation, diagnosis, and prognosis; and interventions. This book also uses the language and concepts of the *Guide.* For example, the activities of physical rehabilitation are described using the terms tests and measures and interventions rather than the more traditional terms objective examination and treatment, respectively. This is intended to help meet one of the stated purposes of the *Guide:* "standardizing terminology used in and related to physical therapy practice."[1] Additionally, the practice of physical rehabilitation is described using the Nagi disablement model.

As with the *Guide,* the purposes of this book include improving quality of care, enhancing positive outcomes from physical rehabilitation interventions, enhancing patient satisfaction, and increasing the consistency, efficiency, and cost-effectiveness of health care.

STRUCTURE OF CHAPTERS

To facilitate learning of the presented ideas and their application in clinical practice, each chapter has a similar consistent structure (Box 1-1). This structure parallels recommendations of the *Guide,* makes information clear and readily accessible, and promotes learning and recall for the student and quick access to specific information for the experienced clinician.

EVIDENCE-BASED EXAMINATION, EVALUATION, DIAGNOSIS, PROGNOSIS, AND INTERVENTION

Although the *Guide* forms a framework for describing and implementing clinical practice, it does not evaluate or recommend specific approaches for patient management. In contrast, this book gives specific, detailed, evidence-based information on the pathology, etiology, examination, evaluation, diagnosis, prognosis, and intervention for patients involved in physical rehabilitation.

TABLE 1-1	Comparison of Preferred Practice Patterns from the *Guide to Physical Therapist Practice* with Chapters in This Book

Preferred Practice Patterns in the *Guide to Physical Therapist Practice*	Chapters in *Physical Rehabilitation: Evidence-Based Examination, Evaluation, and Intervention*
CATEGORY **PATTERN NUMBER: TITLE**	**PART: TITLE** **CHAPTER: TITLE**
Musculoskeletal	**1: Musculoskeletal System**
4A: Primary prevention/risk reduction for skeletal demineralization	3: Skeletal Demineralization
4B: Impaired posture	4: Posture
4C: Impaired muscle performance	5: Muscle Weakness
4D: Impaired joint mobility, motor function, muscle performance, and range of motion associated with connective tissue dysfunction	6: Connective Tissue Dysfunction
4E: Impaired joint mobility, motor function, muscle performance, and range of motion associated with localized inflammation	7: Localized Inflammation
4F: Impaired joint mobility, motor function, muscle performance, range of motion and reflex integrity associated with spinal disorders	8: Spinal Disorders
4G: Impaired joint mobility, muscle performance, and range of motion associated with fracture	9: Fractures
4H: Impaired joint mobility, motor function, muscle performance, and range of motion associated with joint arthroplasty	10: Joint Arthroplasty
4I: Impaired joint mobility, motor function, muscle performance, and range of motion associated with bony or soft tissue surgery	11: Soft Tissue Surgery
4J: Impaired motor function, muscle performance, range of motion, gait, locomotion and balance associated with amputation	12: Amputations and Prostheses
Neuromuscular	**2: Neuromuscular System**
5A: Primary prevention/risk reduction for loss of balance and falling	13: Balance and Fall Risk
5B: Impaired neuromotor development	14: Impaired Neuromotor Development
5C/5D: Impaired motor function and sensory integrity associated with nonprogressive disorders of the central nervous system—congenital origin or acquired in infancy or childhood	15: Pediatric Nonprogressive Central Nervous System Disorders
5D: Impaired motor function and sensory integrity associated with nonprogressive disorders of the central nervous system—acquired in adolescence or adulthood	16: Adult Nonprogressive Central Nervous System Disorders
5E: Impaired motor function and sensory integrity associated with progressive disorders of the central nervous system	17: Progressive Central Nervous System Disorders
5F: Impaired peripheral nerve integrity and muscle performance associated with peripheral nerve injury	18: Peripheral Nerve Injuries
5G: Impaired motor function and sensory integrity associated with acute or chronic polyneuropathies	19: Polyneuropathies
5H: Impaired motor function, peripheral nerve integrity, and sensory integrity associated with nonprogressive disorders of the spinal cord	20: Nonprogressive Spinal Cord Disorders
5I: Impaired arousal, range of motion, and motor control associated with coma, near coma, and vegetative state	21: Coma, Vegetative State, and Minimally Conscious State
	22: Vital Signs
Cardiovascular/Pulmonary	**3: Cardiopulmonary System**
6B: Impaired aerobic capacity/endurance associated with deconditioning	23: Deconditioning
6C: Impaired ventilation, respiration/gas exchange, and aerobic capacity/endurance associated with airway clearance dysfunction	24: Airway Clearance Dysfunction
6D: Impaired aerobic capacity/endurance associated with cardiovascular pump dysfunction or failure	25: Congestive Heart Failure
6E: Impaired ventilation and respiration/gas exchange associated with ventilatory pump dysfunction or failure	26: Respiratory Failure
6F: Impaired ventilation and respiration/gas exchange associated with respiratory failure	
6H: Impaired circulation and anthropometric dimensions associated with lymphatic system disorders	27: Lymphatic System Disorders
Integumentary	**4: Integumentary System**
7B: Impaired integumentary integrity associated with superficial skin involvement	28: Tissue Healing and Pressure Ulcers
7C: Impaired integumentary integrity associated with partial-thickness skin involvement and scar formation	29: Vascular Ulcers 30: Neuropathic Ulcers
7D: Impaired integumentary integrity associated with full-thickness skin involvement and scar formation	31: Burns
	5: Interventions Common to Many Conditions Requiring Rehabilitation
	32: Gait Assessment and Training
	33: Assistive Devices for Mobility
	34: Orthotics
	35: Environmental Assessment: Home, Community, and Work

The examination section of each chapter includes recommendations for a focused patient history, as well as appropriate tests and measures for each preferred practice pattern. Since the systems review is essentially similar for all patients, this is not discussed further within the individual chapters. The tests and measures are presented in categories, as recommended by the *Guide*. However, their selection and sequencing differs from the *Guide*. The *Guide* lists 24 categories of tests and measures, in alphabetical order, for all preferred practice patterns. Although these same categories of tests and measures are presented in this book, only those categories relevant to the particular preferred practice pattern are included, and for all patterns, the categories are presented in a systems-based sequence (Table 1-2). This systems-based approach promotes concurrent performance of physiologically related tests and measures and a clearer picture of relationships between related examination findings. Documentation of the examination in this order also promotes clear communication with other clinicians and will help the reader develop appropriate diagnoses and prognoses and select effective and efficient patient interventions.

The sections on intervention within each chapter include rationales for selection of interventions and in many cases explanations of how and when to apply recommended interventions. Where possible within the context of such a broad text, sufficient detail is provided to allow the reader to develop and execute an effective plan of care. Where such detail cannot be provided, the reader is directed to other specific sources for more detailed descriptions of how to apply the recommended methods and techniques. For all aspects of patient management, the research-based evidence regarding the approach is presented.

BOX 1-1   Standard Chapter Outline

Objectives
Pathology
Examination
    Patient History
    Systems Review
    Tests and Measures
Evaluation, Diagnosis, and Prognosis
Intervention
Case Study
Chapter Summary
Additional Resources
Glossary
References

TABLE 1-2   Comparison of the Sequence of Examination in the *Guide to Physical Therapist Practice* with the Examination Sequence

EXAMINATION SEQUENCE IN THE *GUIDE TO PHYSICAL THERAPIST PRACTICE* (ALPHABETICAL)	EXAMINATION SEQUENCE: A SYSTEMS-BASED APPROACH
Aerobic capacity and endurance	*Musculoskeletal*
Anthropometric characteristics	Posture
Arousal, attention, cognition	Anthropometric characteristics
Assistive & adaptive devices	Range of motion
Circulation	Muscle performance
Cranial and peripheral nerve integrity	Joint integrity and mobility
Environmental barriers	*Neuromuscular*
Ergonomics & body mechanics	Arousal, attention, and cognition
Gait, locomotion & balance	Pain
Integumentary integrity	Cranial nerve integrity
Joint integrity and mobility	Peripheral nerve integrity
Motor function—control & learning	Reflex integrity
Muscle performance—strength, power, endurance	Sensory integrity
Neuromotor development & sensory integration	Motor function—control and learning
Orthotic, protective & support devices	Neuromotor development and sensory integration
Pain	*Cardiovascular/pulmonary*
Posture	Circulation
Prosthetic requirements	Ventilation and respiration/gas exchange
Range of motion	Aerobic capacity and endurance
Reflex integrity	*Integumentary*
Self-care & home management	Integumentary integrity
Sensory integrity	*Function*
Ventilation & respiration/gas exchange	Gait, locomotion, and balance
Work, community & leisure integration	Assistive and adaptive devices
	Orthotic, protective, and supportive devices
	Prosthetic requirements
	Ergonomics and body mechanics
	Environmental barriers
	Self-care and home management
	Work, community, and leisure integration

CASE STUDIES, ADDITIONAL RESOURCES, AND GLOSSARY

This book includes a number of special features with all chapters. Each chapter includes a case study demonstrating the application of the principles and techniques described and a glossary of important terms. Each chapter also includes recommendations of other books, web sites, and organizations for further information. The book is thoroughly referenced throughout with citations of up-to-date research to facilitate evidence-based practice.

The CD that comes with this book includes additional case studies, direct electronic online links to useful resources and all listed references, printable forms related to the chapter, vocabulary-building exercises, and boards-style examination questions. Instructors using this text may also obtain online access to electronic versions of all figures in the text and to lab activities that complement the concepts described in each chapter. In addition, they may request a hard copy manual of all the lab activities.

CHAPTER SUMMARY

This text is intended for a wide range of rehabilitation students and clinicians and covers the breadth of physical rehabilitation. It applies the Nagi disablement model and concepts from the *Guide to Physical Therapist Practice*, in conjunction with evaluation of the current evidence, to derive recommendations for patient examination, evaluation, and intervention. These recommendations for each preferred practice pattern are presented in a clear and consistent manner in each chapter. Each chapter also has a number of special features including a case study, clinically useful resources, a glossary of terms used, and extensive references. The CD provides additional case studies, study questions, printable forms for clinic use, and direct online links to listed references and resources.

ADDITIONAL RESOURCES

Web Sites

International Classification of Functioning, Disability and Health (ICF) web site: www.who.int/classification/icf/en
American Physical Therapy Association web site: www.APTA.org

GLOSSARY

The definitions given in this glossary and throughout this book are consistent with definitions given in other rehabilitation documents. Definitions for terms vary among sources, including other textbooks, medical and general dictionaries, and the *Guide*. These differences are likely a result of differences in audience with respect to level of detail and complexity, as well as focus. General dictionaries avoid technical medical terms, whereas medical texts and dictionaries refer to other medical concepts in their definitions. Rehabilitation-oriented documents, including this textbook, use definitions that focus on functional abilities and physical interventions.

Assessment: The measurement or quantification of a variable or the placement of a value on something. Assessment should not be confused with examination or evaluation.

Diagnosis: A process and a label. The diagnostic process includes integrating and evaluating the data obtained during the examination to describe the patient condition in terms that will guide the prognosis, the plan of care, and intervention strategies. Diagnosis as a label denotes the disease or syndrome a person has or is believed to have and the use of scientific or clinical methods to establish the cause and nature of a person's illness.[13] PTs use diagnostic labels that identify the impact of a condition on function at the level of the system (especially the movement system) and at the level of the whole person.[1]

Disability: The inability to perform or a limitation in the performance of actions, tasks, and activities usually expected in specific social roles that are customary for the individual or expected for the person's status or role in a specific sociocultural context and physical environment. In the *Guide*, the categories of required roles are self-care, home management, work (job/school/play), and community/leisure.[1]

Disease: A pathological condition or abnormal entity with a characteristic group of signs and symptoms affecting the body and with known or unknown etiology.[1] A condition marked by subjective complaints, a specific history, and clinical signs, symptoms, and laboratory or radiographic findings.[13]

Disorder: Derangement or abnormality of function (anatomical or physiological); pathology.

Dysfunction: Disturbance, impairment, or abnormality of function of an organ.

Evaluation: A dynamic process in which the clinician makes clinical judgments based on data gathered during the examination.

Examination: A comprehensive screening and specific testing process. The examination has three components: Patient history, systems review, and tests and measures.

Function: Those activities identified by an individual as essential to support physical, social, and psychological well-being and create a personal sense of meaningful living.

Functional limitation: The restriction of the ability to perform, at the level of the whole person, a physical action, task, or activity in an efficient, typically expected, or competent manner.

Goals: The intended results of patient management. Goals indicate changes in impairment, functional limitations, and disabilities and changes in health, wellness, and fitness needs that are expected as a result of implementing the plan of care. Goals should be measurable and time limited. (If required, goals may be expressed as short- and long-term.)

History: A component of the examination. A systematic gathering of data—from both the past and the present—related to why the patient is seeking rehabilitation services. The data that are obtained (through interview, review of the patient record, or from other sources) include demographic information, social history, employment and work (job/school/play), growth and development, living environments, general health status, social and health habits (past and current), family history, medical/surgical history, current conditions or chief complaints, functional status and activity level, medications, and other clinical tests. While taking the history, the clinician also identifies health restoration and prevention needs and coexisting health problems that may have implications for intervention.

Impairment: A loss or abnormality of anatomical, physiological, mental, or psychological structure or function.

Intervention: The purposeful interaction of the clinician with the patient and when appropriate, with other individuals involved in patient care, using various procedures and techniques to produce change in the condition.

Occupational therapy: Therapeutic activities used to develop, regain, or maintain the skills necessary for health, productivity, and independence in everyday life. It may include the use of assistive technologies or orthotics to enhance function or prevent disability. Therapy by means of activity; especially creative activity prescribed for its effect in promoting recovery or rehabilitation.[14]

Occupational therapist: A person trained in or engaged in the practice of occupational therapy.[14]

Pathology/Pathophysiology: An abnormality characterized by a particular cluster of signs and symptoms and recognized by either the patient or practitioner as abnormal. Pathology is primarily identified at the cellular level.

Physiatrist: A physician who specializes in physical medicine.[14]

Physical therapist (PT): A person who is a graduate of an accredited physical therapist education program and is licensed to practice physical therapy. The terms *physical therapist* and *physiotherapist* are synonymous.[1]

Physical therapy: Examination, evaluation, diagnosis, prognosis, and intervention provided by a physical therapist.[1] The treatment of disease and movement-related dysfunction by physical and mechanical means such as massage, regulated exercise, water, light, heat, and electricity.[14]

Plan of care: Statements that specify the anticipated goals and expected outcomes, predicted level of optimal improvement, specific interventions to be used, and proposed duration and frequency of the interventions required to reach the goals and outcomes. The plan of care includes anticipated discharge plans.

Prognosis: The determination of the predicted optimal level of improvement in function and the amount of time needed to reach that level.[1] The act or art of foretelling the course of a disease or the prospect of survival and recovery from a disease as anticipated by the usual course of that disease or indicated by special features of the case.[14] The possible outcomes of a condition and the frequency with which they can be expected to occur.[15]

Rehabilitation: A set of actions designed to restore, following disease or injury, the ability to function in a normal or near-normal manner.[15] Rehabilitation is a goal-oriented treatment process that is intended to maximize independence in individuals with compromised function due to primary pathological processes and resultant impairments.

Screening: Determining the need for further examination or consultation.

Signs: Objective evidence of physical abnormality.

Symptoms: Subjective evidence of physical abnormality.

Systems review: A component of the examination. The systems review is a brief and gross examination, or "quick check," to identify information not presented in the patient history and to identify if other health problems should be considered in the diagnosis, prognosis, and plan of care or indicate the need for referral to another health provider.

Tests and measures: A component of the examination. Specific standardized methods and techniques used to gather data about the patient after the history and systems review have been performed.

Treatment: The sum of all interventions provided by a clinician during an episode of care.

References

1. American Physical Therapy Association: *Guide to Physical Therapist Practice*, ed 2, Alexandria, Va, 2001, The Association.
2. American Occupational Therapy Association Assembly of Representatives: May 2004, www.aota.org.
3. Randall KE, McEwen IR: Writing patient centered functional goals, *Phys Ther* 80(12):1197-1203, 2000.
4. Melvin JL, Nagi SZ: Factors in behavioral response to impairments, *Arch Phys Med Rehabil* 51:532-537, 1970.
5. Schenkman M, Butler RB: A model for multisystem evaluation, interpretation, and treatment of individuals with neurologic dysfunction, *Phys Ther* 69(7):538-547, 1989.
6. World Health Organization: *International Classification of Impairments, Disabilities and Handicaps (ICIDH)*, Geneva, 1980, WHO.
7. Wood PHN: The language of disablement: A glossary relating to disease and its consequences, *Int Rehab Med* 2:86-92, 1980.
8. Wagstaff S: The use of the International Classification of Impairments, Disabilities and Handicaps in rehabilitation, *Physiotherapy* 68:548-553, 1982.
9. Nagi S: Disability concepts revisited. In Pope AM, Tarlov AR (eds): *Disability in America: Toward a National Agenda for Prevention*, Washington, DC, 1991, National Academy Press.
10. National Institutes of Health: *Research Plan for the National Center for Medical Rehabilitation Research*, Bethesda, Md, 1993, The Institutes.
11. World Health Organization: *International Classification of Functioning, Disability and Health (ICFDH-2)*, Geneva, 2001, WHO.
12. Hertling D, Kessler RM: *Management of Common Musculoskeletal Disorders*, ed 3, Philadelphia, 1996, Lippincott-Raven.
13. *Taber's Cyclopedic Medical Dictionary*, ed 20, Philadelphia, 2005, FA Davis.
14. *Merriam-Webster Medical Dictionary*, Springfield, Mass, 1995, Merriam-Webster.
15. Guyatt G, Rennie D: *Users' Guides to the Medical Literature: A Manual for Evidence-Based Clinical Practice*, Chicago, 2001, AMA Press.

Chapter 2

Evidence-Based Practice

Michelle H. Cameron

OBJECTIVES

After reading this chapter, the reader will be able to:
1. Define evidence-based practice.
2. Describe the advantages and limitations of evidence-based practice.
3. Apply the concepts of evidence-based practice to the clinical practice of rehabilitation.
4. Locate and identify high quality evidence for the clinical practice of rehabilitation.

DEFINING EVIDENCE-BASED PRACTICE

Evidence-based practice (EBP) is defined by Sackett, the originator of the term, as "the conscientious, explicit, and judicious use of current best evidence in making decisions about the care of individual patients."[1,2] EBP is based on the application of the scientific method to clinical practice. EBP requires that clinical practice decisions be guided by the best available relevant clinical research data in conjunction with the clinician's experience, while also taking into account what is known about the pathophysiology of the patient's condition, the individual patient's values and preferences, and what is available in the clinical practice setting.

The goal of EBP is to identify and provide the best possible patient care. The best care is the care with the greatest likelihood of producing the best outcome for the patient. Although this may appear to be a simple and implicit goal of all patient care, it is actually complex, can be difficult to achieve, and requires integration of information from multiple sources. The best outcome requires consideration of the values of each patient within the context of their society and an ability to assess the outcome. Good outcome measures are needed to determine if an outcome has been achieved. These measures must be valid (measure what they claim to measure) and reliable (produce the same result each time they are applied) and quantify and communicate changes in patients that may result from clinical interventions. Once the clinician has identified goals and measures for *outcomes,* to apply EBP, the clinician must also know what is most likely to produce the best outcomes. This requires evidence, which is described in detail in the next sections.

TRADITIONAL APPROACHES

Traditionally, a number of other approaches based on logical, rational thinking and clinician experience have been used to direct clinical practice and make clinical decisions. One example is "experience-based practice." If most of a clinician's patients with low back pain and weak abdominal muscles had less pain a few weeks after being instructed in abdominal strengthening exercises, then the clinician would continue to apply this approach. Although this approach is appealing, it is limited. The patient's goals and expectations are not assessed, and the natural history of the pathology is not distinguished from the effects of interventions. Do we know if these patients get better because of the exercises or just because most back pain resolves spontaneously over time? This approach also fails to distinguish luck from probable outcome; for example, did these few patients just happen to respond well to this intervention when most would not have?

Another traditional approach to clinical practice in medicine and rehabilitation may be called "eminence-based practice." According to this approach, if a famous, respected, and renowned person said so, then it is so. For

TABLE 2-1	Evidence-Based Practice and Some of Its Alternatives	
Basis for Clinical Decisions	**Marker**	**Ideal Measuring Device**
Evidence	Randomized control trial	Meta-analysis
Experience	Repeat referrals	Patient satisfaction survey
Eminence	Radiance of white hair	Luminometer
Vehemence	Level of stridency	Audiometer
Eloquence	Smoothness of tongue or nap of suit	Teflometer
Nervousness	Litigation phobia level	Every conceivable test

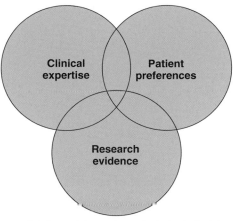

FIG. 2-1 Model for evidence-based clinical decision making.

example, if a well-known instructor at a course last weekend recommended strengthening the abdominal muscles in people with low back pain, then this is what should be done. Eminence-based practice also may be reinforced by publishing. If a recommendation is written by an authority in the field and appears in many places in print, it must be true. This use of expert opinion is common in clinical practice because evidence is frequently lacking.

Other alternatives to EBP, including "vehemence-based practice" (how loudly a perspective is supported), "eloquence-based practice" (how eloquently a perspective is presented), and "nervousness-based practice" (the anxiety level of the practitioner), have also been described (Table 2-1).[3]

ORIGIN OF EVIDENCE-BASED PRACTICE

In contrast to prior methods, EBP uses the best evidence in conjunction with clinical expertise and patient values to make clinical decisions (Fig. 2-1). Decisions may be made about examination, diagnosis, and *prognosis,* as well as preventive and treatment interventions. The ideas of EBP originated in mid-nineteenth century Paris but did not rise to the fore until the 1980s when they were reintroduced, primarily in Canada by Dr. David Sackett and in the United Kingdom by Dr. Archie Cochrane. EBP has continued to gain popularity over the last 2 decades, although not without resistance. EBP addresses the desire of patients and payers for the most up-to-date therapies while taking into account the need for cost containment. EBP takes advantage of the growing mass of research data, including outcomes data, and improved access to this data through advances in information systems to closely monitor and analyze research studies, practice patterns, and clinical outcomes. The American Physical Therapy Association, the American Occupational Therapy Association, and the American Medical Association, as well as many other groups, support the principles of EBP. Although EBP is still in its infancy in the rehabilitation professional's culture, its application can guide practitioners to the most efficient, effective, consistent, and highest quality clinical practice.

EBP requires a clinician's expertise and the best external clinical evidence. Although evidence derived from clinical research is a crucial component, *patient preferences,*

clinical circumstances, and the clinician's experience and judgment are also essential to clinical decision making. Clinical expertise is the proficiency and judgment that each clinician acquires through experience and practice. Those with greater expertise may demonstrate better practice in many ways, including, most often, more effective and efficient diagnosis and more thoughtful identification and effective integration of individual patients' predicaments, rights, and preferences in making clinical decisions about their care. However, clinicians with more experience may also practice more poorly by allowing their own personal experience to inappropriately outweigh high quality evidence.

The best external clinical evidence is clinically relevant, unbiased research. Although this research may be basic science, the most useful research for EBP comes from patient-centered clinical studies evaluating the validity and reliability of clinical tests and measures, the power of prognostic markers, and the efficacy and safety of therapeutic or preventive interventions. External clinical evidence can invalidate previously accepted measures or interventions and can replace them with those found to be more reliable, accurate, safe, and effective. Although EBP may seem to clearly be the best approach to patient care and decision making, a number of arguments both for and against the use of EBP have been proposed.

ARGUMENTS FOR EVIDENCE-BASED PRACTICE

EBP is considered to be less *biased* than its alternatives and overcomes differences in expert opinions to produce recommendations most likely to be effective. When evidence is not used, practice combines one's best logical guess from what is known with one's own limited personal experience. This reinforces the perception that *correlation* equals *causation.* In addition, personal experience is often biased toward current experience: If my last patient got better after I did *x,* then *x* made them better, and conversely, if they got worse after I did *y,* then *y* made them worse, so I should treat my next patient with a similar presentation with x and not y. Experts may then recommend this approach to others. For example, when asked for a recommendation, the response may be, "I usually find *x* works" or better yet, "this expert told me *x* works." EBP replaces these personal and chronological biases with data on the actual *probability* of producing a certain outcome with a certain intervention. Ideally, evidence-based recommendations are based on equally weighted, unbiased information from large numbers of patients, controlling for all potential confounding variables.

Another argument for EBP is that current practice varies according to geography and clinician experience without a basis for variation in the patient presentation. EBP recommends standardizing examination and interventions so they are based on the best available evidence. This standardization will not only improve patient outcomes but also help contain costs by reducing the use of ineffective treatments and accelerating achievement of the patient's goals.

New evidence can and should lead to changes in clinical practice as new evidence becomes available. Failing to assess and integrate current evidence will likely result in deterioration of clinical performance and less than optimal patient outcomes. For these reasons, this book takes an evidence-based approach to recommending examination and intervention approaches in rehabilitation.

ARGUMENTS AGAINST EVIDENCE-BASED PRACTICE

Although EBP is widely accepted in many circles, it does have opponents. Criticisms of EBP include that everyone is already doing it, it cannot be done, it requires no clinical judgment, individual patients vary too much for it to be useful, or insurance companies will use EBP to restrict payment for patient care.

Although it may seem that EBP is widely used, the wide range of interventions and the lack of external clinical evidence for many tests, measures, and interventions demonstrate that many clinicians currently practice without evidence. For example, many clinicians treat chronic low back pain with lumbar traction, based on theoretical rationales and expert opinion that it is effective, despite the fact that systematic reviews of the literature report that there is "strong evidence that traction is not effective for the treatment of low back pain"[4] and "a lack of evidence regarding the efficacy of this intervention."[5]

It is also proposed that practicing EBP is impossible because there is too much research to read in the available time or the research is too difficult to understand. Although this argument is appealing, some clinicians do effectively practice EBP by reading selectively. For example, rather than reading all the original research in an area, the effective consumer of evidence can use condensed sources, such as databases of evidence-based analyses of common problems. These are described in detail in the next section on how to apply EBP to rehabilitation.

EBP has been described as having a "cookbook" approach that requires no clinical judgment. Some suggest that if EBP is applied, clinical decisions will be made by computers or business people rather than by clinicians. However, because EBP requires clinicians to evaluate external evidence and integrate the best external evidence with their own clinical expertise and values and the preferences of each patient, this outcome is not a logical result of EBP.

The uniqueness of each patient's problem is also proposed as a reason why EBP should not be applied. Since patients may respond differently to an intervention according to the nature and stage of their pathology, their social and psychological background and goals, and the skill of the clinician, evidence based on many other individuals is not helpful. This criticism fails to take into account that EBP is not just the application of external clinical evidence but is used to inform not replace individual clinical expertise. The individual's clinical expertise decides which, if any, available external evidence applies to a particular patient and how it can and should be integrated with patient-specific considerations to formulate, with the patient, the best clinical decision.

It has also been suggested that insurance companies may use EBP to cut costs by limiting payment for interventions until all the evidence is in. Although this is possible, this is not the intent of EBP. EBP is intended to provide the best, most effective treatment for patients whether it increases or decreases costs.

APPLYING EVIDENCE-BASED PRACTICE TO REHABILITATION

EBP requires clinical expertise and an appreciation of clinical research evidence. Clinical expertise is developed over time through interactions with patients. For an appreciation of research evidence, the clinician must take a systematic approach, frequently extending beyond the time spent directly with patients or in the clinic. Just reading a journal regularly or attending continuing education courses is not sufficient for EBP. EBP requires the critical application of research evidence to each specific patient problem. Clinicians must find and critically appraise the relevant published evidence and combine these findings with their own clinical expertise and the patient's circumstances and values to determine a course of clinical care. Having chosen this course, the clinician must execute it and follow this with evaluation of the patient's outcome. EBP should be applied to all aspects of the clinical interaction, including selection of valid and reliable tests and measures, determination of an accurate diagnosis and prognosis, and application of effective interventions.[6]

EBP requires a shift in the thought processes of many rehabilitation clinicians. Although clinical advice may rely on clinical experience, expert opinions, collegial relationships, pathophysiology, common sense, community standards, published material, and other sources, when practicing EBP the clinician must always ask, "What evidence is there to support or refute this advice?"

Applying EBP to rehabilitation is particularly challenging because trials evaluating rehabilitation interventions cannot always meet the methodological standards applied to other types of clinical trials.[7] In particular, subjects, treaters and evaluators frequently cannot be *blinded* to the application of a rehabilitation intervention because many interventions used in rehabilitation, such as manual therapy techniques, depend on the skill of the person applying them and thus necessitate at least nonblinding of the person providing the treatment. Other rehabilitation interventions, such as exercise, depend on the cooperation of the subject and thus cannot be applied without subject awareness. In addition, interventions used in rehabilitation can be difficult to describe and are frequently, by necessity, individualized. Therefore they are often not described in sufficient detail to allow a complete understanding of the intervention or replication of the study if desired. Many rehabilitation interventions also cannot be standardized because they vary with the skill, training, and experience of the provider.[8] Although these limitations may be addressed by training all providers similarly before providing an intervention, standardizing interventions, and designing similar sham interventions, complete blinding in rehabilitation studies is rare.

TYPES OF EVIDENCE

All research evidence is not equal and the evidence to be used in EBP can be classified and evaluated on a number of factors, including the study design, the types of subjects, the nature of controls, the outcome measures used, and the statistical analysis applied. One approach evaluates the quality of the question being asked by a study. All well-built questions should have four parts that can be readily remembered using the mnemonic *PICO:*

P: Patient or population. The question should apply to a specific population (e.g., adults with low back pain, children with lower extremity spasticity that is due to spinal dysraphism)

I: Intervention. The intervention should be specific (e.g., specified exercises applied for a specified period of time at a specified frequency)

C: Comparison intervention/measure. The intervention (or measure) should be compared to some current commonly used treatment (or gold standard measure) or to no intervention if no intervention is usually provided.

O: Outcome. The outcome should be defined as precisely as possible, ideally using a clinically relevant, reliable, validated measure (e.g., walking speed, level of independence with activities of daily living [ADLs])

Study Design. The simplest research design is the *case report.* A case report is a detailed description of a patient's clinical presentation, the course of treatment, and the changes in clinical presentation that occurred during and generally after that course of treatment. A case report is generally the first type of formal evaluation of a treatment approach performed. It is most valuable for describing new methods for treating a condition when little other information is available. When case reports are well written, they provide information about all aspects of the patient's presentation and care in detail, and they only require the investigator to describe an individual's course of treatment and presentation. The primary disadvantage of case reports is that they only provide information about what was done to a particular patient and what happened to that patient, without clearly indicating what caused the observed changes. Therefore one cannot be certain which,

if any, of the intervention(s) in question caused the observed changes or if these changes occurred independently of the interventions. Caution should be observed when considering applying the findings of a case report to other individuals because the changes that occurred in the subject of the report may have been unique to that individual. Case reports are therefore considered the least strong evidence for the effectiveness of an intervention for a particular problem. However, they can provide valuable information to guide controlled research studies.

A controlled research study is one in which the effects of an intervention are compared with some alternative, the control. The simplest controlled study uses only one subject whose status when an intervention is applied for a period of time is compared with the status when the intervention is not applied. This type of study provides better information about the effects of an intervention than a case report. In contrast to case reports, single-subject studies can differentiate the effects of time alone from the effects of the intervention under investigation without the time and expense of studies involving groups of subjects. Single-subject studies also eliminate the differences in initial status or individual characteristics that can confound the interpretation of studies involving groups of subjects. Studies using single subjects are particularly suitable for investigating the effects of interventions on uncommon problems where large groups of subjects may not be available and for analyzing the effects of interventions on problems whose normal progression is so variable as to obscure any effects of an intervention using a group design. Although single-subject studies have a number of advantages over case reports because they only evaluate the response of a single individual to an intervention, caution should be applied in generalizing the findings of such studies to other subjects.

In most situations, comparing the effects of providing an intervention to one group of subjects with withholding it from another group more clearly demonstrates the effects of that intervention than a single-subject study can. Group studies provide stronger evidence to support the use of a test or intervention with other individuals in clinical practice.

When well designed, studies involving groups of subjects can provide strong evidence about the effectiveness of an intervention. Studies with large homogeneous groups are preferred because they minimize the risk of failing to detect the true effects of an intervention. When small, heterogeneous groups are used, differences between groups produced by an intervention may be masked by variability within the groups. For example, if ultrasound is applied to a few patients with tendonitis of varying degrees of acuity and of varying tendons and after the treatment, no differences in pain or dysfunction are found between these patients and others who did not receive ultrasound, the failure to detect a treatment effect could be due to the fact that (1) ultrasound does not reduce the pain or dysfunction associated with tendonitis, or (2) the range of pain and dysfunction within the groups was greater than the range between the groups, or (3) ultrasound is effective for treating tendonitis only at certain depths or at certain stages of acuity. If this study was performed with a large group of subjects who all had tendonitis of the extensor carpi radialis brevis tendon in the acute inflammatory stage and if the treatment was effective, its effect will not be obscured by variations within the groups of subjects. Unfortunately, because large groups of individuals with similar characteristics are difficult to recruit, many studies in rehabilitation, particularly those involving human subjects, use small, heterogeneous samples and may thus erroneously conclude that treatments are ineffective. This is known as a type 2 error or a *false-negative* result.

Although studies using large, homogeneous groups optimize the probability of detecting small, statistically significant treatment effects, the *clinical significance* of these effects must also be taken into account when considering applying the findings to clinical practice. For example, although a study may find that applying heat before stretching the knees of patients who have had a total knee arthroplasty results in a statistically significantly greater gain in flexion range of motion than stretching without prior heating, if the difference in gains is only a few degrees, this may not be clinically significant if it does not affect patient function. A slight acceleration of recovery may also be statistically significant while not justifying the use of an intervention in general clinical care. For example, even if applying traction is found to decrease the recovery time from a low back injury from 40 days to 39 days, in most cases the cost of applying this treatment will not be justified by this small effect.

Types of Subjects. Having selected the appropriate study design based on the nature of the effect being studied and the quality and availability of prior studies, an investigator must also select suitable research subjects. Subject selection will depend on the nature of the effect being studied, the type of outcome data desired, and the availability of different types of subjects. Studies may be carried out in vitro, which means "within glass." This term describes studies that are carried out in a container or in a test tube rather than within a living organism. In vitro studies use various nonliving materials or cell cultures as subjects. In vitro studies can generally be replicated accurately and allow for very close control of subject and intervention variability; however, given how different these set ups are from patients, caution should be exercised in applying findings of these studies directly to clinical situations.

Using animals as research subjects overcomes some of the limitations of in vitro studies by allowing evaluation of the effects of rehabilitation interventions on the physical properties of tissue within a normal physiological environment. Healthy animals may be used to study the effects of rehabilitation interventions on normal processes or characteristics such as temperature or circulatory rate. Animals with pathology can be used to study the effect(s) of treatments on pathology or impairments such as muscle shortening, soft tissue injury, circulatory impairment, or pain. Studies of interventions with unknown risk may often be initiated in animals, and animal subjects allow for close control of potentially confounding variables such as activity level, age, gender, and diet. Although animal studies may support the application of clinical interventions, their evidence is limited because humans may respond differently and because these studies generally cannot provide information about the effect of an intervention on functional limitations or disabilities.

Studies using human subjects provide the best evidence for the effects on a patient's functional abilities and disabilities. Ideally, studies use patients with pathology rather than subjects without pathology because this provides information that is most readily applicable to other patients. However, because of limitations in access to subjects with problems of similar types and severity, as well as financial and ethical constraints in applying interventions with unknown effects or withholding potentially effective care from control patients, many studies are performed using human subjects without pathology. These studies may provide information about the physical and physiological effects of interventions, such as their impact on tissue length, muscle strength, or blood circulation, and may be used to investigate the effects of interventions on experimentally induced dysfunction such as pain. However, caution must be used in applying the findings of such studies to patients with pathology. For example, although electrical stimulation may not increase muscle strength more effectively than exercise in normal subjects, it has been found to augment strengthening when applied after knee surgery. Studies using groups of patients provide the best evidence about the effects of rehabilitation interventions on functional patient outcomes.

Controls. Because changes in subjects can occur whether or not an intervention has been applied, the outcome of subjects who have received an intervention must be compared with the outcome of subjects who have not received that intervention. The subjects who do not receive the intervention being evaluated are known as controls.

Controls are needed to differentiate the effects of chance, normal progression of the outcome variable, and nonspecific effects of treatment from specific effects of the intervention being evaluated. Problems addressed in rehabilitation often change or resolve over time. For example, low back pain can vary in location from one day to the next, with no clear cause, and can vary in severity among individuals; however, for most individuals, acute low back pain resolves within 6 weeks whether or not any treatment is provided. Without the use of appropriate controls it is difficult, if not impossible, to determine if the changes observed in subjects were solely due to time or were caused by the intervention being studied.

Most of the treatments provided by rehabilitation clinicians also have nonspecific effects. For example, paying attention to the patient may increase the patient's motivation, monitoring progress may improve the patient's compliance and touching the patient, either directly or with a device, may provide a sensory stimulus to block pain transmission. To control for these effects sham interventions with similar nonspecific effects to those from the intervention being studied are applied to control subjects. Such alternative interventions are known as *placebo* control interventions.

Without appropriate controls, although much time, effort, and expense may be expended, study results will not clearly show if an intervention has a specific effect and therefore will not readily improve patient care. It will not be known whether the treatments being evaluated are effective and should be used with patients or whether any observed changes in subject status were the result of chance, normal progression, or nonspecific effects of the intervention.

To most accurately determine the effects of an intervention, neither the subjects of the study nor the individuals applying the intervention should know if an active or a placebo treatment is being applied. Additionally, the choice of true or placebo intervention should be random. This is known as double-blind random application. A double-blind, *randomized controlled trial* (RCT) is the gold standard for research design. Unfortunately, it is challenging, if not impossible, to apply many rehabilitation interventions in a double-blind fashion.

Outcome Measures. In addition to evaluating a study for its design and controls, the outcome measures should also be evaluated. Outcome measures should be reliable, valid, and clinically relevant. A measure is considered to be reliable if the same or a similar result is produced when the measure is repeated. For example, goniometric measurement of active knee flexion range of motion is reliable if the same or a similar angle is reported when active knee flexion range of motion is measured repeatedly.

The *reliability* of a measure may vary for different applications or populations and with application by the same or another individual. For example, a numeric visual analog scale completed by the subject may be reliable for the assessment of pain severity in adults but be unreliable for pain assessment in infants or young children. It is important that a measure be reliable in the population being studied. Comparing the results from repeated application of a measure by one person assesses intrarater reliability. Comparing the results from repeated application of a measure by different individuals assesses interrater reliability. Studies should use measures whose reliability in the population being tested is proven, and the measures' reliability should be clearly documented in all research reports.

In contrast to reliability, which relates to the reproducibility of a measure, *validity* relates to its usefulness and the degree to which it represents the property it claims to measure. For example, for a questionnaire to be a valid measure of disability in a population, it must actually measure the reduced ability of this population to perform normal activities. Various forms of validity are assessed in different ways, such as correlation with other measures of the same characteristic, logical analysis of how the content of a measure relates to the characteristic it claims to measure, or evaluation of how accurately the measure predicts what it claims to predict. Measures may be valid by one standard but not by another. For example, although measures of abdominal strength and lumbar flexibility may have high content validity as measures of low back pain, because it appears logical that they would be related to low back pain and may be predictors of future low back pain, they are not considered to have good criterion-related or predictive validity because it has been found that abdominal strength and trunk flexibility do

not correlate with self-reports of low back pain and do not predict who will have low back pain in the future.

In addition to being reliable and valid, outcome measures should relate directly to the goal(s) of treatment and should be clinically relevant and therefore include measures of the effects of interventions on impairment, functional limitations, and disability. For example, a study on the effects of exercise for patients with knee pain should include measures of functional outcomes, such as walking speed, and disability, such as work participation, not just lower extremity strength and knee range of motion. These types of outcomes allow prediction of functional outcome in response to interventions and therefore most effectively guide practice and support reimbursement for rehabilitation.

Cost-effectiveness studies may also guide EBP. Cost-effectiveness studies evaluate the costs of achieving the benefits of an intervention. They present the costs of providing the intervention and the potential benefits and savings associated with reducing the duration and severity of a patient's disability. Potential benefits may be improved quality of life and monetary savings such as reduced loss of income to the patient, reduced employer costs associated with replacing a member of the workforce, and avoidance of costs associated with providing further care to the patient. For example, providing traction to patients with low back pain for 10 visits may cost $500; however, if it is shown that this accelerates their return to work by an average of 1 week, this treatment may be cost-effective if the costs to those patients, their employers, and their insurance carriers associated with not working for 1 week are greater than $500 and other interventions take longer or are less effective. Studies demonstrating the cost-effectiveness of interventions can provide strong support to justify reimbursement for those interventions.

Integrative Summary Reports and Studies. In some areas there are a number of original research studies with the same purpose. The findings of studies in a particular area may be summarized and evaluated in integrative summary reports. The simplest integrative summary report is a nonsystematic review or narrative report, which is a descriptive general summary of research selected by the author of the review. The methods used to collect and interpret data are often informal and subjective rather than systematic or exhaustive, with the reviewer frequently selecting studies that support their own perspective, opinion or clinical experience. The method of study selection is generally impossible to replicate and is frequently biased.

A *systematic review* is a summary of primary studies selected with a rigorous and predefined method, with precise *inclusion* and *exclusion criteria*. Published studies concerning a specific question are systematically searched for using an unbiased selection procedure. These are then abstracted, critically appraised, and synthesized, and the findings summarized. A systematic review is a comprehensive and unbiased integrative descriptive report that provides an overview of the published research on a topic. It is a scientific rather than a subjective summarization of the literature on a subject and can reveal new evidence, help to deal with the volume of literature, and produce more reliable evidence to help with decision making.

In contrast to the systematic review, which is a qualitative report, a *meta-analysis* is a quantitative review. A meta-analysis combines and analyzes the numerical data from individual primary RCTs that meet rigorous predefined standards to determine the efficacy of an intervention. Meta-analyses have a precise protocol for selection and analysis of trials.

A meta-analysis involves a sequence of systematic steps, as follows:

1. The research question is precisely defined.
2. A protocol defining the objectives of the review and the eligibility criteria for trials is established.
3. An exhaustive search of the literature to find all trials that meet the eligibility criteria is performed.
4. More than one blinded investigator tabulates the characteristics of each RCT identified and assesses its methodological quality, excluding articles not meeting the eligibility criteria.
5. The results of eligible trials are analyzed with statistical tests.
6. A critical summary of the review describing the methods of the analysis, results, potential biases, and areas for potential further study is prepared.

The quality of a meta-analysis is evaluated (as is an original study) for relevance and validity, including completeness of the search, appropriateness of the selection criteria and combination of results, and importance of the results to a specific patient.

Systematic reviews of the literature and meta-analyses regarding the efficacy of rehabilitation examination measures, prognosis, and interventions frequently report that the evidence does not support current practice. This is generally because of low subject numbers and poor descriptions of tests and interventions. Ideally, studies use large numbers of subjects and fully describe all aspects of the subjects, the test(s), and intervention(s) being evaluated. Subject descriptions should include the number of subjects, average age and age range, sex distribution, types of problem being treated, severity and acuity or duration of the problem, and any other features thought to be pertinent to the specific question. Tests and interventions should be described in sufficient detail so they can be readily replicated. This type of reporting allows clear conclusions to be drawn on the value of a test or intervention and the necessary or optimal way to examine or treat patients to produce the best clinical outcomes. When there is sufficient data available for a meta-analysis or systematic review to come to clear conclusions, these are the ideal source of evidence because they quickly provide an unbiased, systematic evaluation of the data from many high quality studies.

Statistical Analysis. With any type of study, except for the case report, if outcomes are examined with a quantifiable measure, the *statistical significance* of the results may be assessed with statistical tests. Most statistical tests evaluate the likelihood that a given result occurred as a result of chance alone rather than a true effect of the variable or intervention being evaluated. A finding is generally considered statistically significant if there is less than a 5% chance that it occurred as a result of chance alone. The probability of any difference being purely a result of chance is called the *p-value*. Some statistical tests, particularly those applied to studies of examination approaches, evaluate the degree of correlation between the test being evaluated and the current "gold standard." Other statistical tests are applied to studies of interventions and compare the outcome of the intervention being tested with that of a control.

The usefulness of tests and measures may also be evaluated by calculation of their *sensitivity* and *specificity*. Sensitivity is the probability of a positive test result in a person with the condition ($a/(a + c)$). This is also known as the true positive rate. Specificity is the probability of a negative test result in a person without the condition ($b/(b + d)$). This is also known as the true negative rate.

	Test Positive	Test Negative
Condition present	A	B
Condition absent	C	D

Ideally, a test has both high sensitivity and high specificity. If a test has high sensitivity but low specificity, it will be positive in most people with the condition but will also be positive in many people without the condition. In contrast, a test with a low sensitivity but high specificity will be negative in most patients without the condition but will also be negative in many patients who actually do have the condition.

The value of an intervention can are often be evaluated by the *number needed to treat* (NNT), which is the number of patients needed to be treated for one to benefit. The lower the NNT the more useful a treatment may be; however, this must be considered in the context of the value of the outcome.

$$\% \text{ with outcome with new intervention} -$$
$$\% \text{ with outcome with control intervention} =$$
$$\text{absolute risk reduction}$$
$$100/\text{absolute risk reduction} = \text{NNT}$$

EFFICACY AND EFFECTIVENESS

Studies examining the value of an intervention may focus on its efficacy or effectiveness. *Efficacy* is the benefit of an intervention applied under ideal and highly controlled conditions. *Effectiveness* is the benefit of an intervention applied under circumstances that more closely approximate the real world.[9] Although efficacy may be easier to evaluate with research because it involves the application of a standardized intervention, effectiveness may be more relevant to the clinical setting where patients and clinicians vary in how they carry out interventions. For example, one could evaluate the effectiveness of a set group of exercises performed in the clinic under observation or the efficacy of a prescribed home exercise program that the patient may or may not perform as instructed.

EVALUATING AND GRADING EVIDENCE

There are a variety of ways to evaluate research evidence. When evaluating the quality of a single study, one should consider the clinical relevance of the research question, the internal (avoiding bias) and external (generalizability) validity of the study, the appropriateness of data analysis and presentation and the ethical implications of the tests or interventions evaluated. Are the subjects in the study similar to the patients to whom you would want to apply the test or intervention? Are objective or reproducible diagnostic standards applied to all participants? Will the conclusions, if true, have an impact on the health of your patient? Are the outcome measures known or likely to be clinically important? To assess validity one should consider if the study is peer reviewed, whether an interested party sponsors it and if there is concealed random allocation of patients to a *comparison group*. One should evaluate if the trial is an RCT, and if so, how the groups were randomized and whether the study and *control group* are similar. Were both groups treated in exactly the same manner except for the intervention being evaluated? Were observers and subjects appropriately blinded to exposure? Are the outcomes clearly defined, objective, and clinically, as well as statistically, significant? A system may be used to collect information about the quality of a study (Table 2-2).

If a study shows no significant results, the clinician should consider whether it was adequately powered to detect an effect. If a study is inadequately powered, a type 2 error is likely. A type 2 error occurs when a study concludes that the *null hypothesis* is true (i.e., there is no effect of the intervention), when there actually is an effect. This type of error often occurs when the number of subjects is too small and is common in clinical studies with patients. To avoid a type 2 error the investigators should have performed a power analysis to determine how many subjects are needed to detect the size of effect they consider likely and relevant.

A number of grading schemes have been proposed for rating the overall quality of evidence available to support a particular intervention. The Agency for Health Care Research and Quality (AHRQ) (previously known as the AHCPR—Agency for Health Care Policy and Research) uses the following A to C rating scheme in its clinical guidelines:

A: Results of two or more RCTs in humans provide support.

B: Results of two or more controlled clinical trials in humans provide support, or when appropriate, results of two or more controlled trials in an animal model provide indirect support.
C: This rating requires one or more of the following: (1) results of one controlled trial, (2) results of at least two case series/descriptive studies on pressure ulcers in humans, or (3) expert opinion.

The Canadian Task Force Groups[10] ranks evidence according to the following three categories:

I: Evidence based on human controlled studies published in peer-reviewed journals, regardless of their level of randomization and blindness.
II: Evidence based on human noncontrolled studies published in peer-reviewed journals, regardless of their level of randomization and blindness.
III: Evidence based on human case studies published in peer-reviewed journals.

Another commonly used scheme ranks evidence between levels 1 and 3, as follows[2]:

Level 1 Evidence from at least one RCT.
Level 2a Evidence from well-controlled trials without randomization.
Level 2b Evidence from well-designed cohort of case-controlled analytic studies.
Level 2c Evidence from multiple time series with or without intervention. This also includes dramatic results from uncontrolled experiments (e.g., penicillin for treatment of infections in the 1940s).
Level 3 Opinions of experts based on clinical experience, descriptive studies, case reports, or reports of expert committees.

Although these schemes vary, they all give the highest ranking to RCTs, with more RCTs being better, and give the lowest ranking to expert opinion or case studies, with other types of trials falling in between. Any of these

TABLE 2-2	System for Evaluating the Quality of Studies			
Citation:		**Yes**	**No**	**Comments**
Question study is trying to answer				
Peer-reviewed publication?				
Type of trial (RCT, other define)?				
Appropriate control group?				
Appropriate randomization?				
Outcomes clearly defined?				
Measured outcomes relevant to the question being asked?				
Outcomes clinically significant?				
Outcomes statistically significant?				
Power analysis performed?				

RCT, Randomized control trial.

schemes or other similar schemes may be used to rank evidence to guide clinical practice.

CLINICAL PRACTICE GUIDELINES

Clinical practice guidelines are systematically developed statements that attempt to interpret current research to provide evidence-based guidelines to assist practitioner and patient decisions about appropriate health care for specific clinical circumstances.[11] Clinical practice guidelines recommend diagnostic and prognostic measures and preventive or therapeutic interventions. For any of these, the specific types of patients or problems, the nature of the intervention or test, the alternatives to the intervention being evaluated, and the outcomes of the intervention for which these guidelines apply will be stated. For example, there are guidelines for the treatment for acute low back pain and for the treatment of pressure ulcers that include evidence-based recommendations for tests and measures, interventions, prevention, and prognosis. Often, such recommendations are classified according to the strength of the evidence supporting them[12]:

Classification of recommendations

A Established as effective, ineffective, or harmful for the given condition in the specified population.

B Probably effective, ineffective, or harmful for the given condition in the specified population.

C Possibly effective, ineffective, or harmful for the given condition in the specified population.

U Data inadequate or conflicting given current knowledge; treatment is unproven.

Application of clinical practice guidelines to an individual patient depends on the similarity of the clinical circumstances of the patient to those for which the guideline was developed, the availability and feasibility of implementing the recommended intervention(s) and the value of the expected outcome(s) to the patient.[13]

FINDING REHABILITATION EVIDENCE

Clinicians may directly search the literature for individual studies related to a clinical question using a variety of databases (Table 2-3). Systematically searching for and appraising articles found in such databases is often challenging and time consuming and may yield many publi-

cations that are neither relevant nor of sufficient quality to guide clinical practice. The assistance of a librarian can be invaluable for optimizing a search strategy, but the articles will still need to be read and evaluated for their applicability and quality.

Instead of searching directly for individual studies, a search of specialized databases of systematic reviews and meta-analyses of medical and/or rehabilitation-related research can be more effective. These specialized databases offer the expertise of their authors in searching and appraising research literature and can save the clinician much time and provide a valid answer to a clinical practice question. However, many clinical questions are not addressed by these databases and must be searched for and appraised by the individual clinician. The specialized databases of systematic reviews and meta-analyses of medical and rehabilitation-related research are the Cochrane Database of Systematic Reviews, Database of Abstracts of Reviews of Effectiveness (DARE), and Patient-Oriented Evidence that Matters (POEMS). Table 2-4 gives information on the URLs and content of these databases.

From a perspective of scientific evidence, physical therapy and rehabilitation in general are still-developing fields; the scientific evidence needed to perform a review and make an evidence-based decision is frequently inadequate or unavailable. In such circumstances the clinical decision will involve more of the clinician's expertise and less evidence. In this book, every attempt has been made to provide evidence for recommendations and to clearly indicate where suggestions are made based on common practice when evidence is limited or unavailable.

EBP is a fact of professional life for all medical professionals. Although there will be modifications as the concept evolves, it is likely and reasonable that to continue doing and being reimbursed for patient care, clinicians will be asked to demonstrate with evidence the effectiveness of their clinical practice.

CHAPTER SUMMARY

This chapter describes the nature of EBP and presents arguments for and against the use of EBP in rehabilitation. This is followed by a discussion of how to apply EBP to rehabilitation and of the different types of available evidence. Evidence from individual studies can be differentiated according to the study design, the subjects, the controls, and the outcome measures. A number of studies on one

TABLE 2-3	Databases of Primary Medical and Rehabilitation Research	
Database	**URL**	**Contents**
Medline	Can be searched using a number of search engines, including www.nih.nlm.gov Medline Plus: www.medlineplus.gov PubMed: www.ncbi.nlm.nih.gov/entrez/query.fcgi?	Primary database of research published in medical journals.
Cumulative Index to Nursing and Allied Health Literature (CINAHL)	www.cinahl.com	Similar to Medline but with an allied health focus.
PEDro	www.pedro.fhs.usyd.edu.au	Australian database that critically reviews articles related to physical therapy practice but does not provide a systematic review or recommendations for practice.

TABLE 2-4	Specialized Databases of Systematic Reviews and Meta-Analyses	
Database	**URL**	**Contents**
Cochrane Database of Systematic Reviews	www.cochrane.org	Systematic reviews and meta-analyses of medically related RCTs focused on specific patient problems and interventions.
Database of Abstracts of Reviews of Effects (DARE)	http://www.ovid.com/site/products/ovidguide/daredb.htm	Structured abstracts of systematic reviews from a variety of medical journals. DARE is produced by the National Health Services' Centre for Reviews and Dissemination (NHS CRD) at the University of York, United Kingdom. DARE records cover diagnosis, prevention, rehabilitation, screening, and treatment.
Patient-Oriented Evidence that Matters (POEMS)	www.infopoems.com	Family practice database that appraises and summarizes articles related to specific medical problems.

RCTs, Randomized control trials.

topic may be presented together in integrative summary reports or studies. Methods for evaluating and grading evidence are described, and the chapter concludes with information on how to find evidence related to the clinical practice of rehabilitation.

ADDITIONAL RESOURCES

Books

Guyatt G, Drummond R. Users' guides to the medical literature: a manual for evidence-based clinical practice. Chicago, 2002, AMA Press.

Web Sites

Centre for Evidence-Based Medicine web site: www.cebm.net
APTA Hooked on Evidence web site: www.hookedonevidence.org

GLOSSARY

Bias: A systematic tendency to produce an outcome that differs from the underlying truth. There are many different types of bias.

Blinded: The participant of interest is unaware of whether patients have been assigned to the experimental or control group. Patients, clinicians, those monitoring outcomes, judicial assessors of outcomes, data analysts, and those writing the paper can all be blinded.

Case reports: Descriptions of individual patients.

Causation: The relating of causes to the effects they produce. Most clinical research is concerned with causation, and several types of causes can be distinguished.

Clinical practice guidelines: Systematically developed statements to assist practitioner and patient decisions about appropriate health care for specific clinical circumstances.

Clinical significance: The importance of a finding within a clinical context.

Comparison group: Any group to which the index group is compared. Usually synonymous with control group.

Control group: A group that does not receive the experimental intervention. In many studies, the control group receives either the standard of care currently delivered in the community or the best care that is available on the basis of the current evidence.

Correlation: The magnitude of the relationship between different variables or phenomena.

Effectiveness: How well an intervention works in real-life, non-ideal circumstances.

Efficacy: How well an intervention works in ideal circumstances.

Evidence-based practice (EBP): The conscientious, explicit, and judicious use of current best evidence in making decisions about the care of individual patients. EBP requires integration of individual clinical expertise and patient preferences with the best available external clinical evidence from systematic research.

Exclusion criteria: Conditions that preclude entrance of candidates into an investigation even if they meet the inclusion criteria.

False-negative: In a study, if a treatment is considered ineffective when it actually is effective.

Incidence: Number of new cases of a disease or condition occurring during a specified period of time.

Inclusion criteria: Criteria that define who will be eligible for a study.

Meta-analysis: An overview that incorporates a quantitative strategy for combining the results of several studies into a single pooled or summary estimate.

Null hypothesis: In the hypothesis-testing framework, the starting hypothesis, generally that an intervention has no effect, and that the statistical test is designed to consider and, possibly, reject.

Number needed to treat (NNT): The number of patients who need to be treated over a specific period of time to prevent one bad outcome or cause one good outcome.

Outcomes: Changes in health status that may be associated with exposure to an intervention.

Patient preferences: The relative value that patients place on varying health states and intervention options.

Placebo: Intervention without known or expected biological effects.

Probability: Quantitative estimate of the likelihood of a condition existing or of subsequent events.

Prognosis: The possible outcomes of a condition and the frequency with which they can be expected to occur.

P-value: A measure of how much evidence there is against the null hypothesis. The smaller the p-value the less likely the null hypothesis is true and the more likely that an intervention had an effect.

Randomized controlled trial (RCT): An experiment in which individuals are randomly allocated to receive or not receive an intervention and are then followed to determine the effect(s) of the intervention.

Reliability: Consistency or reproducibility of data.

Sensitivity: The proportion of people who truly have a designated disorder and are so identified by the test.

Specificity: The proportion of people who are truly free of a designated disorder and are so identified by a test.

Statistical significance: A result is statistically significant if the null hypothesis is rejected. That is, the probability of the observed results falls below an arbitrary predefined threshold, most often 0.05 (i.e., 5%).

Systematic review: A critical assessment and evaluation of research (not simply a summary) that attempts to address a focused clinical question using methods designed to reduce the likelihood of bias.

Validity: A study or measure is valid when its findings or results represent an unbiased estimate of the underlying truth. The extent to which an instrument measures what it is intended to measure. Internal validity of a study refers to the integrity of the experimental design. External validity of a study refers to the appropriateness by which its results can be applied to non-study patients or populations.

References

1. Sackett DL, Rosenberg WMC, Gray JAM, et al: Evidence based medicine: What it is and what it isn't, *BMJ* 312:71-72, 1996.
2. Sackett DL, Straus SE, Richardson WS, et al: *Evidence Based Medicine: How to Practice and Teach EBM,* ed 2, Edinburgh, 2000, Churchill Livingstone.
3. Isaacs D, Fitzgerald D: Seven alternatives to evidence-based practice, *BMJ* 319:1618-1618, 1999.
4. van Tulder MW, Koes BW, Assendelft WJ, et al: Chronic low back pain: exercise therapy, multidisciplinary programs, NSAIDs, back schools and behavioral therapy effective; traction not effective; results of systematic reviews, *Ned Tijdschr Geneeskd* 144(31):1489-1494, 2000.
5. Philadelphia Panel evidence-based clinical practice guidelines on selected rehabilitation interventions: Overview and methodology, *Phys Ther* 81(10):1629-1640, 2001.
6. Cormack JC: Evidence-based practice . . . what is it and how do I do it? *JOSPT* 32(10):484-487, 2002.
7. Boutron I, Tubach M, Giraudeau B, et al: Methodological differences in clinical trials evaluating nonpharmacological and pharmacological treatments of hip and knee osteoarthritis, *JAMA* 290(8):1062-1070, 2003.
8. Roberts C: The implications of variation in outcome between health professionals for the design and analysis of randomized controlled trials, *Stat Med* 18:2605-2615, 1999.
9. Fritz JM, Cleland J: Effectiveness versus efficacy: More than a debate over language, *JOSPT* 33(4):163-165, 2003.
10. Spitzer WO: The periodic health examination, *Can Med Assoc J* 121(3):1-45,1979.
11. Field MJ, Lohr KN: *Clinical Practice Guidelines: Directions of a New Program,* Washington, DC, 1990, National Academy Press.
12. Chen DK, So YT, Fisher RS: Use of serum prolactin in diagnosing epileptic seizures, *Neurology* 65:668-675, 2005.
13. Scalzitti DA: Evidence-based guidelines: Application to clinical practice, *Phys Ther* 81(10):1622-1628, 2001.

Chapter **3**

Skeletal Demineralization

Nancey A. Bookstein

OBJECTIVES

After reading this chapter, the reader will be able to:
1. Describe and differentiate among the types of skeletal demineralization.
2. Identify modifiable and nonmodifiable risk factors for skeletal demineralization throughout the lifespan.
3. Discuss tests and measures of bone density and skeletal demineralization.
4. Perform an examination to guide the selection of rehabilitation interventions for people with or at risk for skeletal demineralization.
5. Discuss evidence for and apply rehabilitation interventions to clients with or at risk for skeletal demineralization.
6. Briefly compare and contrast pharmacological interventions for the prevention and management of bone demineralization.

Skeletal demineralization refers to a loss of mass and calcium content from the bones. Skeletal demineral-

ization can vary in severity. Less severe bone loss is called *osteopenia,* and more severe bone loss is called *osteoporosis.* Skeletal demineralization may be a primary disorder or may be secondary to a variety of other diseases or disorders such as *osteomalacia* and hyperparathyroidism. Osteomalacia is a disorder in which osteoid, the new organic matrix of bone, does not mineralize correctly. Unlike other causes of bone demineralization, osteomalacia is associated with proximal muscle weakness and dull, persistent bone pain that worsens with activity. With hyperparathyroidism, the excess of parathyroid hormone causes calcium to be leached from the bones into the bloodstream, thereby causing skeletal demineralization.

Skeletal demineralization of any etiology is caused by an imbalance between bone formation and bone resorption.[1,2] When bone loss exceeds bone formation, the resultant net loss of bone mass causes skeletal fragility due to trabecular thinning and discontinuity, loss of horizontal bridges, and the occurrence of trabecular microfractures (Fig. 3-1). Although skeletal demineralization is not a disease and does not cause symptoms, individuals with less than normal bone mass are at increased risk for fractures, and these fractures can be symptomatic and impair function.

Skeletal demineralization can have many causes through the lifespan, including genetics, lack of proper nutrition, hormonal imbalances, and inadequate physical activity.[3,4] Although genetics account for much of the variance in potential *peak bone mass,* life choices, disease and health challenges, socioeconomic circumstances, and environment play important roles in both the attainment of peak bone mass and in bone loss. This chapter describes the physiological mechanisms underlying skeletal demineralization and the examination, evaluation, and interventions for patients at risk for skeletal demineralization. Postural deformities, fractures, and pain are covered in Chapters 4, 9, and 22, respectively.

In 1994 the World Health Organization (WHO) operationally defined osteoporosis as a *bone mineral density* (BMD) of 2.5 standard deviations (SD) or more below the mean for normal young white females.[5] The number of SDs from the mean for healthy young white females

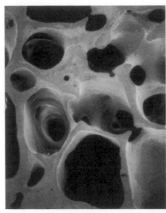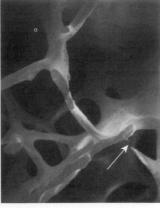

FIG. 3-1 Normal and osteoporotic bone. Arrow on osteoporotic bone shows a trabecular microfracture. *From Thibodeau GA, Patton KT:* Anatomy and Physiology, *ed 6, St. Louis, 2006, Mosby.*

is known as a *T-score*. Osteopenia, or low bone mass, in white women is defined as a T-score between −1.0 and −2.5 (i.e., 1-2.5 SD below the mean for healthy young white females). Guidelines from the National Osteoporosis Foundation (NOF) advocate considering treatment for any woman with a T-score less than or equal to −2.0.

T-scores for men based on manufacturer's normative data for young, healthy, white men from dual-energy x-ray absorptiometry (DXA), ultrasound, and quantitative computed tomography (CT) are available. However, a criterion score of −2.5 SD on DXA or ultrasound appears to underestimate the prevalence of osteoporosis in men, whereas the same criterion for quantitative CT appears to overestimate prevalence. Cut-off scores between −1.8 and −2.3 SD from the mean for DXA and ultrasound and −3.1 SD from the mean for quantitative CT are associated with a significantly increased risk of osteoporotic fractures of the spine and hip in men over 50 years of age.[6,7]

Although both diagnostic and treatment protocols have focused on white women, women from other ethnic and racial backgrounds are affected. The National Osteoporosis Risk Assessment (NORA) is an ongoing study of 200,000 postmenopausal Hispanic, Caucasian, African American, and Native American women. It has reported that all women can have osteopenia and osteoporosis and that BMD declines in all women with age, although the absolute frequency of low BMD varies by ethnic group.[8] At this time, because of limited and conflicting data, there is no consensus as to what T-score should be used to initiate pharmacological intervention in men or nonwhite women.[9] Therefore most practitioners use the cutoffs for white women in these populations.

Using the WHO definitions, the NOF estimates that there are 8 million women in the United States (US) today with osteoporosis and 22 million with osteopenia.[10] Men are also affected by BMD loss, especially with aging, although they have not received as much attention. The NOF estimates that there are 2 million men with osteoporosis and 12 million more with osteopenia in the US today and that by 2020, 3 million men will have osteoporosis and 17 million will have low bone mass.[10] Overall,

the NOF predicts that by 2020 the population prevalence of osteoporosis and low BMD will be 14 million and 48 million, respectively.[10]

The clinical significance of osteoporosis is not the condition itself but rather its association with fragility fractures that occur with minimal trauma. Such fractures are associated with significant morbidity, mortality, and economic consequences, and low bone mass is a strong, independent predictor of fracture risk.[11] White women have a 75% lifetime risk of having a clinically diagnosed fracture, with the risk of vertebral, hip, or wrist fracture in this population estimated at 14% to 15%.[11] In contrast, African American women and white men have a hip fracture risk of approximately 6%, whereas African American men have a 3% risk of hip fracture.[12] These differences are attributed largely to differences in the prevalence of osteoporosis in these populations. Low trauma hip fracture typically occurs in the older population and is associated with senile-onset osteoporosis. With no change in sex and age-specific prevalence, the worldwide incidence of fragility hip fracture is projected to increase by 310% in men and by 240% in women by 2050. Mortality within 2 years after low trauma hip fracture has been estimated to be 20% in women and up to 40% in men. Functional impairments are also common and significant after hip fracture; many patients never resume their pre-fracture functional level and approximately 50% of patients have some loss of independence and often are not able to return home after a hip fracture.[12] The National Institutes of Health (NIH) estimate that the economic burden of fragility fractures in the US is $10-15 billion annually.[13] Further information on fractures can be found in Chapter 9.

One of the major risk factors for fractures is low bone mass, identified as a T-score <−2.5, which is defined as the "fracture threshold"; fracture risk almost doubles with each SD decrease in BMD.[14] Other risk factors for fractures include an increased tendency to fall and a history of a previous fracture.[15,16]

PATHOLOGY

NORMAL BONE PHYSIOLOGY

The bones of the body form its skeleton. They provide structural support and act as a store for minerals, particularly calcium and phosphorus. The skeleton can be divided into appendicular and axial portions. The appendicular skeleton includes of the bones of the upper and lower limbs; the axial skeleton includes the bones of the cranium, vertebral column, ribs, sternum, and pelvis. All bones have cortical bone on the outside and trabecular bone on the inside, but the proportions differ between the axial and appendicular skeletons. The shafts of the long bones of the appendicular skeleton are composed primarily of cortical bone with a central marrow cavity.[17,18] The end plates of the vertebrae are also composed of cortical bone. Cortical bone is dense and solid and made up of lamellae, or compact plates. Approximately 80% of the mass of the skeleton is cortical bone.

Trabecular bone, also known as cancellous bone, has a honeycomb structure with horizontal and vertical bars filled with marrow and fat.[19] These bars of bone form struts called trabeculae, giving this type of bone its name. The axial skeleton, the pelvis, and other flat bones, as well as the ends of the long bones of the appendicular skeleton, are composed primarily of trabecular bone. Trabecular bone is responsible for about 70% of the volume of the axial skeleton, although only 35% of its weight is trabecular bone.[3] Trabecular bone is more metabolically active than cortical bone, probably because of its greater surface area, responding both more quickly and to a greater degree to changes in mineral homeostasis.[20,21]

Bone is a dynamic living tissue that undergoes constant remodeling with coupled phases of bone resorption and formation throughout the lifespan.[22] Bone remodels in response to the demands placed on it. Bone increases in length and diameter during development, responds to mechanical stresses placed on it, and repairs itself after structural damage from trauma, fatigue, or mechanical failure.[23] Approximately 3% of cortical and 7% of trabecular bone remodels each year.[24] This tissue renewal helps maintain the skeleton's structural integrity and keep blood calcium and phosphorus levels within the appropriate range. As long as there is a balance between bone resorption and bone formation, BMD stays stable. A combination of mechanical stress and metabolic and nutritional support helps the system maintain this homeostatic equilibrium. Skeletal demineralization occurs when the processes are not balanced; when bone resorption exceeds bone formation, there is a loss of bone mass.

Bone remodeling involves the balanced activity of three types of cells: osteoclasts, osteoblasts, and osteocytes.[2,25] Osteoclasts, multinucleated cells derived from macrophage precursors, resorb bone and form resorption cavities in areas of bone turnover. Osteoblasts, cells derived from fibroblast precursors, synthesize new bone matrix and osteoid to fill the cavities created by the osteoclasts. This matrix and osteoid then mineralize to form new bone. When the osteoblasts become surrounded by mineralized bone, they no longer produce matrix or osteoid. These mature osteoblasts are known as osteocytes.[2]

Bone remodeling begins with a 2-week period of bone resorption when osteoclasts erode an area of bone. Osteoblasts are attracted to the eroded area where they spend up to 3 months depositing and mineralizing new soft osteoid bone matrix.[26] Osteoblasts usually reside in the periosteum and on both sides of the epiphyseal growth plate in long bones. Calcium and phosphorus are brought to the area by the vascular system to mineralize the osteoid. Bone remodeling is controlled by levels of circulating hormones, including estrogen, testosterone, *calcitonin,* parathyroid hormone (PTH), and *1,25-dihydroxyvitamin D,* and by ongoing mechanical stresses from gravity, weight bearing, and the pull on the bones by contracting muscles.[22]

Typically, during middle adulthood, osteoblastic and osteoclastic functions are balanced and bone mass does not change significantly in men or women. During the years of skeletal growth, from birth to the late twenties, bone formation exceeds bone resorption so that absolute bone mass increases. The bones increase in both length and diameter during this period. Increases in bone length stop when the epiphyses close, which generally occurs

between the ages of 13 and 25 years.[27] Epiphyseal closure occurs earlier in girls than in boys.[28] Bone diameter continues to increase into the twenties or thirties when peak bone mass is reached.[29] Peak bone mass is then generally maintained for the next few decades until the biochemical environment of the body is affected by the hormonal changes associated with aging. Age-related bone loss begins between the ages of 45 to 50 years as the phases of bone remodeling become uncoupled and bone resorption exceeds bone formation.[12]

PATHOPHYSIOLOGY

A pattern of age-related bone loss has been identified for both cortical and trabecular bone. This type of bone loss not caused by immobilization is called involutional bone loss. Involutional bone loss is a long, slow, continuous process that occurs in both genders beginning at around age 35 to 40 years.[12] This loss accelerates in women after menopause. Osteoblast activity usually starts to decrease in midlife because of a variety of factors, including reduced mechanical loading of bone, reduced signals from impaired osteocytes, decreased calcium and vitamin D intake, and fewer hormonal signals from dropping levels of estrogen, testosterone, and growth hormones. At the same time, osteoclast function increases. Together, these changes cause bone resorption to outpace bone formation.

In 1986, Riggs and Melton defined two involutional bone loss syndromes based on clinical features and disease patterns (Table 3-1).[29] Type I, postmenopausal osteoporosis, is a high turnover state that affects women after menopause, whereas type II, senile osteoporosis, is a low turnover, or slow state, that affects both genders after the age of 70 years.[29]

During and after menopause, women produce significantly smaller amounts of the sex hormones, estrogen, progesterone, and testosterone. Because sex hormones stimulate osteoblast activity, osteoblasts become less active during menopause, and loss of bone mass accelerates partly due to unchecked osteoclast activity.[30] Estrogen or testosterone deficiency also decreases osteoclast inhibition and increases the number of osteoclasts. Estrogen and testosterone contribute to increased osteoclastic activity and the formation of deeper resorption cavities. In type I involutional bone loss, although the rate of cortical bone loss is slightly increased, the rate of trabecular bone loss is greatly increased and may be up to three times higher

TABLE 3-1	Types of Involutional Bone Loss	
	Type I	**Type II**
Population affected	Postmenopausal women	Both genders
Mechanism	Hormone-driven	Age-related after 70 years of age
Bone primarily affected	Trabecular bone	Cortical and trabecular bone
Typical fractures	Vertebral and wrist fractures	Hip fractures
Typical features	Onset ~50 years of age	Increased morbidity and mortality

than normal. This loss puts postmenopausal women at particularly increased risks for fractures of bones that are mostly trabecular. Thus vertebral compression fractures, which cause pain and spinal deformity, and Colle's fractures (fractures of the distal radius at the wrist) are associated with type I osteoporosis. Typically, over the life-span, women lose 35% to 50% of their trabecular bone mass and 25% to 30% of their cortical bone mass, while men normally lose 15% to 40% of their trabecular bone mass and 5% to 15% of their cortical bone mass.[26]

In contrast to type I involutional bone loss, which is primarily caused by increased loss of trabecular bone, type II bone loss results primarily from reduced bone formation, and the amounts of cortical and trabecular bone lost are approximately equal. With type II bone loss the osteoclasts produce normal depth resorption cavities, but the osteoblasts do not produce enough osteoid to refill them.[29] The result is a net loss of bone mass.[31,32] The cortical bone loss associated with type II involutional bone loss results in hip fractures and wedged vertebral fractures, as well as fractures of the proximal humerus, pelvis, and proximal tibia. The trabecular thinning associated with this type of bone loss causes gradual vertebral collapse, anterior wedging of thoracic vertebrae, and gradual and usually painless spinal deformities in the elderly such as the classic "dowager's hump."[25] Type II bone loss in the elderly may be due in part to a negative calcium balance caused by decreased intestinal calcium absorption, vitamin D deficiency, or secondary hyperparathyroidism.[25,33]

Primary osteoporosis occurs independent of any other disease. In contrast, secondary osteoporosis results from certain diseases or conditions or as a consequence of the treatment for a disease or condition. For example, the *glucocorticoids* used to decrease inflammation or immune response in a wide range of diseases, including rheumatoid arthritis (RA) and asthma, can cause osteopenia and osteoporosis by inhibiting osteoblast function.[34] Thus RA and asthma are associated with secondary osteoporosis. Glucocorticoids also are used to combat tissue rejection after organ transplant, so organ transplant is also associated with secondary osteoporosis. Excessive levels of glucocorticoids from adrenal disease and low estrogen or testosterone levels cause a similar degree of bone loss.[35] Other hormonal conditions associated with the development of osteoporosis include hyperthyroidism, hyperprolactinemia, and hyperparathyroidism.[33] Malignancies, including multiple myeloma, leukemia, lymphoma, and cancer of the breast and lung, are also linked with bone mineral loss, as is the use of drugs such as alcohol, marijuana, and heparin.[12] Other diseases associated with osteoporosis include renal failure, diabetes mellitus, and Down syndrome.[36]

Dietary deficiencies due to poor availability or eating disorders, such as anorexia nervosa or bulimia, and changes in the normal functioning of the gastrointestinal system that cause diseases, such as celiac sprue, can cause loss of calcium from bones. The body releases calcium from the bones in response to low calcium intake or absorption to maintain appropriate blood levels for critical activities, including nerve conduction, muscle contraction, and cardiac function.

A number of studies in animals and humans have shown that immobilization reduces BMD.[37,38,39] Donaldson found that prolonged bed rest (30 to 36 weeks) produced a 25% to 45% decrease in calcaneal bone mineral content (BMC), a mean decrease in total body calcium of 4.2%, and increased urinary and fecal calcium excretion in three healthy adult males ages 21 to 22 years.[40] With reambulation, total body calcium and BMC increased at rates similar to the rate of loss during the study so that by 30 to 36 weeks after the period of bed rest, all values for all subjects had returned to their prestudy levels. These findings are consistent with Wolff's law that states that bone morphology and density are dependent on the forces placed on the bone.[41] Bone responds by proliferating at the site of force application, or stress. When a body part is not used, as can occur after a stroke or a fracture, bone mass can be lost. Thus any disease or condition that causes disuse of a body part may also be indirectly associated with skeletal demineralization and osteoporosis.

RISK FACTORS FOR SKELETAL DEMINERALIZATION

Modifiable and nonmodifiable factors associated with the development of skeletal demineralization and osteoporosis and their sequelae are listed in Box 3-1. Female gender is associated with an increased risk of skeletal demineralization. Presently, five women are diagnosed with osteoporosis for every man.[42] This is probably due in part to increased recognition of osteoporosis in women and to the fact that, in general, females are at higher risk at an earlier age. Although women risk rapid loss of bone during and immediately after menopause as a result of estrogen deficiency, both genders lose bone mass at about the same rate after age 70. The earlier menopause begins, the longer the duration of estrogen deficiency and the greater the amount of bone loss and risk for fracture.

Race and body proportions also affect an individual's risk for skeletal demineralization; whites and Asians and those with slender, small frames are at greater risk than others.[43]

Dietary factors, primarily low calcium intake, increase the risk for skeletal demineralization. Low calcium intake

BOX 3-1	Modifiable and Nonmodifiable Risk Factors for Low Bone Mass
Modifiable Risk Factors for Low Bone Mass	**Nonmodifiable Risk Factors for Low Bone Mass**
Low calcium intake	Gender
Low vitamin D	Age
Estrogen deficiency	Race
Physical inactivity	Body size
Excessive alcohol intake	Early menopause
Excessive caffeine intake	Family history
Cigarette smoking	
Use of specific medications	
Prolonged overuse of thyroid hormone	

causes removal of calcium from its stores in the bones and teeth to meet physiological demands. Low calcium intake during childhood and adolescence results in low peak bone mass due to the continual leaching of calcium from bone. The NIH currently recommends that all men under the age of 65 and premenopausal women, as well as post-menopausal women taking hormone replacement therapy (HRT), consume 1,000 mg of calcium each day. Postmenopausal women not taking HRT, men over the age of 65, and people with osteopenia or osteoporosis should consume 1,500 mg of calcium daily.[44] Calcium intake includes calcium from all sources, including diet and supplements. Calcium intake up to a total of 2,000 mg per day appears to be safe in most individuals. However, too much supplemental calcium can increase the risk for kidney stones.[45]

Vitamin D, a fat-soluble vitamin, is essential for calcium absorption. Vitamin D is found in food and can be synthesized by the skin after exposure to ultraviolet (UV) rays from the sun.[46] Once produced in the skin or consumed in food, vitamin D must be converted in the liver and kidney into its physiological active form, 1,25-dihydroxyvitamin D. In this form, vitamin D stimulates the intestine to absorb calcium and phosphorous.[47] Adequate vitamin D levels are therefore required to avoid skeletal demineralization. An adequate intake is recommended of 200 international units (IU) for children, 400 IU for those in the 51 to 70 age bracket, and 600 IU for the healthy adult after age 70. This level can be provided by 15 minutes of sun exposure per day.[44,48] Exposure must not be compromised by sunscreen or long sleeves. In areas where there is insufficient sunlight to produce an adequate amount of vitamin D during the winter months, people should be sure to include vitamin D in their diet. Although little vitamin D occurs naturally in most foods, many countries fortify basic foods, such as milk, bread, cereals, and margarine, with vitamin D to assure adequate intake. Since the 1930s, when the federal government introduced a mild fortification program to reduce the incidence of rickets, almost all of the milk produced in the US has been is fortified with 400 IU of vitamin D per quart. Although milk, bread, and ready-to-eat cereals are usually fortified, products made from milk, such as ice cream and cheese, may not be.

Estrogen deficiency is also a risk factor for skeletal demineralization and osteoporosis. Estrogen deficiency has many causes, including delayed puberty, hypogonadism, amenorrhea, oligomenorrhea, and menopause without HRT. Therefore clinicians should include questions regarding age of menarche, activity level, menstrual regularity or irregularity, parity, age at menopause, type of menopause (i.e., natural versus surgical), and use of and type of HRT, including over-the-counter and herbal preparations, when taking a history in a patient with skeletal demineralization. Amenorrhea has many causes. Any history of eating disorders or extreme exercise training should be followed up and considered a risk factor for low bone mass or inadequate nutrition. Some studies have suggested that onset age and duration of anorexia nervosa correlate with BMD.[49] Although multiple factors appear to contribute to the low bone mass seen in such patients,[50] a history of an eating disorder should be considered a risk factor for low BMD.

A reduction in mechanical loading due to lack of physical exercise,[51] immobilization and/or long-term bed rest decreases bone density because bone requires stress for maintenance and growth.[52] Furthermore, even with activity, reduced gravitational forces cause a reduction in bone volume and density.[53-57]

Cigarette smoking and excessive alcohol intake are also risk factors for low bone mass. Smoking accelerates bone loss in both men and women and is a risk factor for hip fracture in women.[58-60] The effects of smoking on bone density begin to reverse 10 years after smoking cessation.[60] Excessive alcohol consumption predisposes individuals to hip fracture by increasing the risk of falls, as well as loss of bone density.[61] A retrospective study in 1980 found that almost 30% of a group of 200 alcoholic men had thoracic and rib fractures as compared with a less than 2% incidence of such fractures in a nonalcoholic cohort.[62]

The effects of caffeine intake on bone density are unclear. One study on over 9,500 white women ages 65 years and older found that high current caffeine intake of more than 190 mg/day was associated with an increased risk for hip fracture.[63] In contrast, a cross-sectional study of 138 healthy postmenopausal women showed no association between caffeine intake and osteoporosis,[64] and a prospective study from Taiwan with 1,037 subjects, using a multiple stepwise linear regression model, found that habitual caffeine intake from tea was associated with higher BMD.[65]

Certain disease processes are associated with low bone mass. The more common of these are included in Box 3-2. These associations may be due to direct effects of the diseases themselves or effects of medications used to treat them. For example, corticosteroids used to treat rheumatoid arthritis and anticonvulsants used to treat epilepsy cause low BMD as a side effect and primary hyperparathyroidism directly causes calcium to be leached from bone.

EXAMINATION

PATIENT HISTORY

Anyone can be at risk for developing osteopenia or osteoporosis; thus every patient should be questioned regarding family history of bone disease and risk factors for low peak bone mass. In addition, the patient history should include age and gender, past medical and surgical history, family history, functional status, present and past activity levels, history of the present condition, and the patient's goals.

The clinician should ask about current and past medication use, including prescribed, over-the-counter, and herbal preparations, because many drugs can affect bone metabolism, thereby contributing to changes in bone density. Cyclosporine, thyroid hormone, glucocorticoids, and some of the chemotherapeutic medications can cause loss of bone density.[66] High-dose methotrexate, used to treat acute lymphoblastic leukemia, has also been associated with osteoporosis and fractures.[67,68]

BOX 3-2	Risk Factors Associated with Low Bone Mass

Old age

Residence in cold geographic area

Vitamin D deficiency

Gastrectomy

Intestinal malabsorption associated with the following:

- Diseases of the small intestine
- Cholangiolitic disorders of the liver
- Biliary obstruction
- Chronic pancreatic insufficiency

Long term use of the following:

- Anticonvulsants
- Tranquilizers
- Sedatives
- Muscle relaxants
- Diuretics
- Antacids containing aluminum hydroxide
- Corticosteroids

History of the following:

- Hyperparathyroidism
- Chronic renal failure
- Renal tubular defects (decreased reabsorption of phosphate)

Data from Goodman C, Boissonnault W, Fuller K: *Pathology: Implications for the Physical Therapist,* ed 2, Philadelphia, 2003, WB Saunders.

Other preparations, such as the thiazide diuretics, may increase bone density and decrease fracture risk. A 3-year study of 320 normal men and women found that hip and spine density were higher in those taking high doses of hydrochlorothiazide than in those taking a placebo.[69] Medications specifically intended to prevent or treat skeletal demineralization should be recorded (see section on interventions).

SYSTEMS REVIEW

The systems review is used to target areas requiring further examination and define areas that may cause complications or indicate a need for precautions during the examination and intervention processes. See Chapter 1 for details of the systems review.

For patients with metabolic bone disease the cardiovascular and pulmonary systems review should include measurement of vital signs (heart rate and rhythm, respiratory rate, breathing pattern, and blood pressure as in Chapter 22). A basic review of the integumentary system should include observation of skin color, perfusion, temperature, irregularities (scratches, cuts, moles), bruising, and hair. Nails and nail beds should also be examined. For this population, the skin integrity over spinous processes, iliac crests, and ribs should be considered. Upper and lower extremity musculoskeletal screenings should include gross tests of range of motion (ROM), strength, relative flexibility, and observations of body size, symmetry, and proportion. A general assessment of posture and gait should be included. A brief review of the neuromuscular system should include gross examination of balance, coordination, reflexes, and sensation. A review of psychosocial components should include the patient's communication style, affect, cognition and language.

TESTS AND MEASURES
Musculoskeletal

Posture. Postural screening is very important in patients with osteoporosis. Because most osteoporotic fractures occur without causing symptoms, increased or increasing thoracic kyphosis may be a sign of multiple painless vertebral compression fractures. Any patient with any degree of increased dorsal kyphosis should be evaluated to identify the amount of and relationship between the thoracic and lumbar spinal curves. Although x-ray evaluation is the gold standard for measuring changes in individual vertebral height and spinal curvatures, *Debrunner's kyphometer* (Fig. 3-2, *A*) and the surveyor's *flexicurve* (Fig. 3-2, *B*) are commonly used to measure thoracic curves in patients with osteoporosis. Debrunner's kyphometer was introduced in 1972 as the first known nonradiographic method for evaluating thoracic kyphosis up to 52 degrees and was adopted for noninvasive research and routine clinical examination in 1973.[70] In 1989, after modification, the range of measurement was increased to 70 degrees. Interobserver and intraobserver reliability has been tested on 31 healthy subjects in a randomized crossover model and shown to be good for both lordosis ($0.91 < r < 0.96$) and kyphosis ($0.91 < r < 94$).[71]

The surveyor's flexicurve, a 48-cm strip of lead covered with synthetic rubber that can only be bent in one plane and that holds its shape when molded, measures kyphosis indirectly by calculating an *index of kyphosis*.[72] To use this device the patient stands as erect as possible and the flexicurve is placed with one end at the spinous process of C7 and the other end at the L5-S1 interspace. The instrument is molded to the spinous processes between these two landmarks, then removed from the patient and placed on a piece of paper so that the spinal curves may be traced with a pencil. A straight line is drawn connecting the ends of the curves. The index of kyphosis is equal to 100 times the horizontal distance of the point on the curve farthest from the straight line (I), divided by the distance from C7 to where the curve crosses the straight line (K) (Fig. 3-3). Interobserver and intraobserver reliability of this tool was described by Milne and Lauder.[73] Cross-sectional data demonstrated good correlation ($r = 0.8$) with radiographic measurement. Test/retest reliability was reported as 0.94 (I), 0.92 (K), and 0.98 (I/K) on ten subjects tested over 2 days.[73] Other reliability results have been approximately the same.[74-76]

Kyphotic posture can predispose to back pain and increase the risks of falls.[77] Thoracic flexion also increases the load on the vertebrae increasing fracture risk. Flexing the trunk by 30 degrees produces a load of 1,800 Newtons (N) on the L3 vertebral body when the arms at the chest and a load of 2,610 N when the arms are in front with a 2-kg weight in each hand.[76] Moro et al found that 500 N of force can be sufficient to produce a fracture in an elderly, cadaveric thoracic vertebra.[78] A detailed description of the examination of posture is provided in Chapter 4.

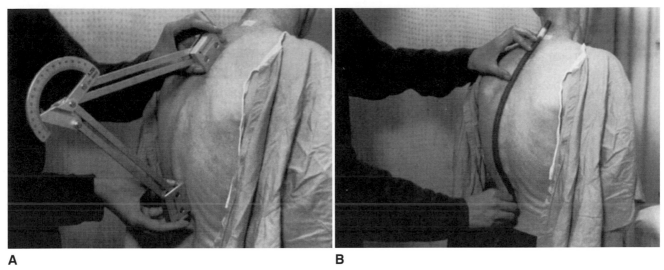

FIG. 3-2 A, Debrunner's kyphometer. **B,** Flexicurve. *From Lundon KM, Li A, Bibershtein S: Spine 23(18):1978-1985, 1998.*

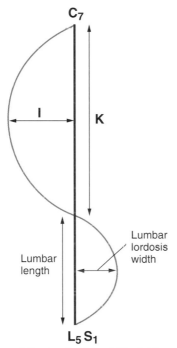

FIG. 3-3 Index of Kyphosis I/K × 100. *I,* Thoracic kyphosis width; *K,* thoracic length. Norms for I/K in women: 21-50 years of age = 7.16; 66-88 years of age = 11.12.

Anthropometric Characteristics

Height Loss. Until there is a fracture with subsequent pain, skeletal demineralization has no clinical manifestations. Vertebral compression fractures are the most common manifestation of osteoporosis, and approximately two-thirds of these fractures are asymptomatic. Almost 20% of women who have a vertebral fracture will have another vertebral fracture within the next year.[79]

Only 38% of primary care patients with vertebral fracture are diagnosed in time to be treated to decrease their fracture risk before another fracture occurs.[80] Height loss of more than 1 inch can be a herald for low bone mass, and many patients are surprised at their loss of stature when measured at an initial examination. A tape measure mounted on the wall is the easiest way to screen for such loss. A *stadiometer* is a reasonably inexpensive tool that can measure a client's height while sitting or standing and has been shown to be reliable and valid for such testing.[81] All patients at risk for or diagnosed with osteopenia or osteoporosis should have their height measured at baseline, and changes in height should be followed during the course of intervention.

Range of Motion. Changes in posture may be due to more than changes in spinal curvature from vertebral fractures. Typically, specific soft tissue changes occur as patients develop increasing kyphotic posture. Loss of flexibility and tightness in anterior soft tissue structures commonly cause decreased ROM in shoulder flexion and external rotation, hip extension, knee flexion, and ankle dorsiflexion.[82,83] ROM of the cervical spine, shoulders, hips, knees, and ankles should be examined because tightness in these areas can add to postural deformity and contribute to balance deficiencies. Standard techniques using a goniometer should be used to measure ROM.

Muscle Performance. Patients with skeletal demineralization often also have weak muscles. The muscles most commonly affected are those on constant stretch such as the shoulder depressors and retractors, hip and knee extensors, and the ankle dorsiflexors. In addition, the spinal extensors, as well as the abdominals, may be weak from disuse. Grip strength, tested by dynamometer, may correlate with overall bone density[86,87] and fracture risk.[86] Strength testing should be performed with additional caution in this population avoiding positions that increase fracture or fall risks (see Chapter 5).

Time-loaded standing (TLS) can be used to measure trunk muscle endurance in people with osteoporosis. Intraclass correlation coefficients for same day intertrial and long-term test-retest reliability were 0.89 and 0.84, respectively, in a control group and 0.81 and 0.85 in a group with osteoporosis.[87] This test measures the time that a person can stand holding a 2-lb weight in each hand. The person must stand with the shoulders flexed 90 degrees and the elbows extended. Several measures of physical function and impairment, such as the 6-minute walk test, gait velocity, and functional reach distance correlate significantly ($p \leq 0.05$) with TLS results.

Neuromuscular

Pain. When thoracic vertebral fractures cause pain in patients with skeletal demineralization, the pain usually follows a dermatomal pattern around the trunk. Anatomically, when the vertebral body collapses anteriorly, the shape of the intervertebral foramen changes and can put pressure on the dural sleeve of the exiting spinal nerve, causing pain to radiate around the anterior thoracic or abdominal wall. Patients may complain of chest pain, rib pain, shortness of breath, scapular pain, or even visceral pain, depending on the spinal nerve level affected.

Cardiovascular/Pulmonary

Aerobic Capacity and Endurance. Thoracic kyphosis, if severe, can produce a decrease in aerobic capacity due to reduced lung/chest volume. Chapter 23 includes methods of measuring and managing cardiorespiratory endurance.

Function

Gait, Locomotion, and Balance. Balance and gait should be examined in all clients with or at risk for osteoporosis because falls in this population can result in fractures. Patients with osteoporosis appear to have altered balance characteristics as a result of kyphosis, which may decrease stability during activities of daily living (ADLs), putting them at increased fracture risk.[88] The Tinetti Assessment Tool[89] measures both balance and gait. It was designed for elderly populations, is easy to administer, and has demonstrated good to excellent reliability (see Chapters 13 and 32).

Medical Tests of Bone Mineral Density. Various tests are available to assess BMD. These include screening tests readily available to the public and medical diagnostic tests. Screening tests can identify individuals whose BMD may lie significantly outside the normal range. The primary screening tests are finger densitometry and heel ultrasonography. Although these tests are inexpensive and widely available, the high incidence of false positive and false negative results of finger densitometry may give some individuals unnecessary concern and give others a false sense of security. Ultrasonography provides an indirect indication of BMC but has proved to be a good predictor of fracture risk.[90,91] Ultrasonography is typically performed at the calcaneus because this bone is superficial and mostly made of trabecular bone like the spine. All results from screening tests suggesting low bone mass should be followed up with an accurate diagnostic test

that can be used to decide if a patient should be treated and to establish a baseline from which to judge treatment results.

Until recently a fracture was required to make the diagnosis of osteoporosis because plain x-ray, the primary imaging modality available, does not detect a loss of bone mass until at least 30% to 35% of bone mineral is lost.[92] With the advent of new technology for measuring bone mass, as well as measuring levels of markers of bone turnover, earlier stages of bone loss can now be identified and osteoporosis can be diagnosed before a fracture occurs.

Presently available noninvasive diagnostic methods of assessing bone density include various types of absorptiometry, including single-photon absorptiometry (SPA), dual-photon absorptiometry (DPA), quantitative CT, and *dual-energy x-ray absorptiometry* (DXA). All forms of absorptiometry are reasonably low in cost and radiation exposure, convenient for patients, and relatively accurate. All of these techniques rely on bone absorbing or attenuating ionizing radiation. The source of the radiation for SPA and DPA are radioactive isotopes, and the source of radiation for quantitative CT and DXA is a tube that produces x-rays.

SPA, introduced in 1963, provides a one-dimensional view and is limited to peripheral sites of the distal radius and calcaneus.[93] It is of limited value for measuring bone density loss in osteoporosis because it does not differentiate between cortical and trabecular bone and cannot measure losses in deep bones such as the spine or hip.

DPA and quantitative CT are more recently developed techniques that can quantify trabecular bone mass in the spine and hip. This is important because these areas are most often affected by osteoporosis. The accuracy and precision of DPA is similar to that of CT. DPA can measure bone density in the spine, usually from L1 to L4, the femoral neck, greater trochanter, and *Ward's triangle,* as well as total body bone density.[94] Artifacts, such as compression fractures and osteophytes from degenerative joint disease, can falsely elevate DPA and quantitative CT measures in the spine but do not appear to affect hip density measurements, although errors can be caused by positioning differences during repeated studies.[95]

DXA can measure hip and spine bone density, as well as total body bone density, with high precision and accuracy. Coefficients of variation for bone densitometry have been reported to be in the range of 1% to 2%.[96] DXA also exposes the patient to less radiation and scans more quickly than other techniques. DXA provides both absolute measures of BMD and scores that can be compared with average age-matched scores and with scores expected for young women with peak bone mass.[95] Comparison with age-matched scores allows the clinician to determine an individual's relative fracture risk, while comparison with scores from young healthy women is used to determine fracture thresholds. DXA is the best method for repeated measures of BMD over time and is the gold standard for BMD measurement today (Fig. 3-4).

DXA usually provides measures of BMD in g/cm². This information can then be converted to T-scores and Z-

scores. As mentioned previously, the T-score is the number of SDs the subject's score is away from that of a normal young female. T-scores are referenced from the USA AP (anteroposterior) Spinal Referenced Population Ages 20-45 database. The Z-score is the number of SDs the subject's score is away from that of an age-, weight-, ethnicity-, and gender-matched person. Typically, the test includes examination of both hips and the lumbar spine and may also include individual and or aggregate scores for the femoral neck, Ward's triangle, and lumbar vertebrae L1 to L4.

EVALUATION, DIAGNOSIS, AND PROGNOSIS

For most individuals who fall into preferred practice pattern 4A: Primary prevention/risk reduction for skeletal demineralization, examination findings may include loss of height, thoracic kyphosis, and decreased ROM and muscle strength.[97] Individuals with a history of fracture may have chronic pain from changes in soft tissues. Complaints of acute pain will often be a result of a new frac-

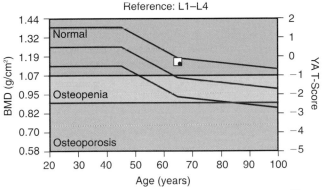

FIG. 3-4 Print out of DXA report. ▫ represents a specific patient.

ture. Individuals, especially the elderly or those with chronic medical conditions, may present with decreased balance and endurance (Table 3-2).

INTERVENTION

Interventions for patients with skeletal demineralization are intended to increase bone mass, slow bone loss, and/or reduce the risk of fractures. There are a few large, randomized controlled trials (RCTs) and a number of small clinical studies evaluating the effects of a variety of interventions in this population; however, interpretation of the findings of most of these studies is confounded by small effect sizes, questionable compliance with test or control protocol, and high drop-out rates in most studies. The following section describes rehabilitation interventions, including aerobic exercise, resistance training, and weight-bearing activities, that have been shown in some studies to improve outcomes in patients with skeletal demineralization. These interventions are followed by a brief review of medical interventions, including diet, medications, and surgery, used to improve outcomes in this population.

AEROBIC EXERCISE

Aerobic exercise can improve function and increase BMD in patients with osteoporosis. Bonaiuti and colleagues' systematic review and meta-analysis of the published studies on the effects of exercise on osteoporosis in postmenopausal women included nine studies on the effects of aerobic exercise.[98] These studies included 266 subjects who participated in aerobic exercise and 295 control subjects and demonstrated that aerobic exercise coupled with weight bearing significantly increased BMD at the spine and the wrist of postmenopausal women with osteoporosis as compared with control interventions ($p = 0.01$). Kelley reported effect size changes in bone density at the hip from a meta-analysis of the effects of aerobic exercise.[99] In this study, changes in bone density at the hip averaged an effect size of 0.43, with approximately 67%

TABLE 3-2	Evaluation and Prognosis Associated with Preferred Practice Pattern 4A: Primary Prevention/Risk Reduction for Skeletal Demineralization	
Examination Findings	**Evaluation/Likely Diagnosis**	**Prognosis Based on Outcome Research**
Height loss >1 inch	Possible asymptomatic bone loss; postural dysfunction	At potential risk for bone loss and vertebral compression fractures; improve with exercise, patient education.
Thoracic kyphosis	Potential to compromise cardiorespiratory system; decreased balance; possible single or multiple vertebral compression fractures	Can be improved or maintained with exercise, bracing, patient education; at increased risk for possible additional fractures.
Pain: Acute	Possible new fracture; decreased physical performance and function	Self-limited over 6-8 weeks; can be decreased by intermittent bed rest, modalities, positioning, bracing.
Pain: Chronic	Changes in soft tissues: tightness, weakness	Can decrease with compliance to appropriate education, exercise program, bracing.
Decreased ROM	Chronically shortened soft tissues	Can be modified with exercise.
Muscle weakness	Chronically lengthened; atrophied soft tissues	Can be modified with exercise.
Decreased balance	Increased potential for fracture from falls	Can be improved with balance training.
Decreased endurance	Compromised cardiopulmonary function; decreased mobility	Can be improved with endurance training.

Data from Itoi E, Sinaki M: *Mayo Clin Proc* 69:1054-1059, 1994; Kanis JA, Johnell O, DeLaet C, et al: *Bone* 35(2):375-382, 1994; Lui-Ambrose T, Eng JJ, Khan KM, et al: *J Gerontol A Biol Sci Med Sci* 58:M862-866, 2003.
ROM, Range of motion.

of the exercise groups demonstrating a benefit. In many of the aerobic exercise studies the type of exercise (e.g., bipedal weight bearing versus bicycling) was not defined.

Long distance running has also been found to be associated with greater BMD in men.[100] Running 15-20 miles a week is associated with higher BMD, but running farther was not associated with further increases. It is not clear if the aerobic component or the weight bearing associated with running or both are the primary cause of the increased BMD produced by this activity.

RESISTANCE TRAINING

The systematic review and meta-analysis of the effects of exercise on patients with osteoporosis included three studies on the effects of resistance exercise for specific muscle groups.[98] The exercises included back extension and flexion; hip flexion, extension, abduction, and adduction; knee flexion and extension; leg press; bench press; biceps curl; and lateral pull down. Resistance training significantly affected BMD at the spine ($p = 0.02$) but did not significantly affect BMD at the hip or the wrist ($p = 0.5$ and 0.9, respectively). Walking was also associated with significantly higher hip BMD ($p = 0.05$).

Two published meta-analyses have shown that resistance training is associated with an increase in bone mass in healthy women.[54,101] The first analysis assessed 29 studies and looked at resistance exercise in both premenopausal and postmenopausal women; exercise was defined as any external resistance added while performing exercise. Results demonstrated that there was an increase in BMD in the lumbar spine in all women who performed resistance exercise; there was also increase in BMD at the femur and radius but only in postmenopausal women. More recent studies by the same authors support the hypothesis that exercise improves and maintains BMD in the lumbar spine in postmenopausal women but finds little to support the efficacy of using resistance exercise to affect BMD at the lumbar spine or femoral neck in premenopausal women.[102,103] Although there is no absolute ratio between increase in bone mass and increase in bone strength, it appears that small gains in bone mineral can result in large improvements in bone strength[104] because new bone is usually found on bone surfaces where the greatest mechanical stress is applied.

A recent study by Sinaki and colleagues evaluated the effects of resisted back extension on lumbar extensor strength and the incidence of vertebral fractures.[105] They randomized 65 postmenopausal women to a 2-year back exercise program or a control group. The back exercise program consisted of progressive resisted back extension (Fig. 3-5) performed once a day, 5 days a week. Up to 8 years after the termination of the exercise program, the exercise group had stronger back extensor muscles and a lower incidence of vertebral fractures.

Sinaki and Mikkelson also found that not all back exercises help patients with low BMD.[106] They assigned 59 women with back pain and postmenopausal osteoporosis to 1 of 4 different exercise regimes. They found that significantly more fractures occurred in patients performing spinal flexion exercises only than in those performing spinal extension only, combined flexion and extension

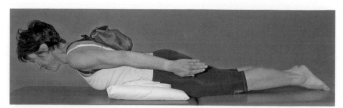

FIG. 3-5 Weighted back extension.

TABLE 3-3	Effect of Type of Spinal Exercises on the Number of New Fractures in Patients with Spinal Osteoporosis

Type of Exercise	Number of New Fractures
Spinal extension	16%
Spinal flexion	89%
Combined flexion and extension	53%
No exercise	67%

exercises, or no exercise at all (Table 3-3). Based on the findings of the two previously cited studies, resisted spinal extension exercises are recommended for patients with or at risk for skeletal demineralization and spinal flexion exercises should not be performed without combining them with spinal extension exercises.

The positive effects of resistance training on BMD have been demonstrated to occur in a range of age groups including the elderly. A group of 50- to 70-year-old sedentary postmenopausal women who participated in a resistance training program twice a week on a 5-machine circuit for 1 year had significantly increased bone density in the spine, hip, and total body after completing this program.[107]

The effect of swimming on BMD is controversial. In 1995, Taaffe et al reported that BMD among a group of swimmers and a group of controls was similar. They therefore concluded that the lack of impact loading during swimming and the low level of mechanical loading were too low to affect bone mineral acquisition.[108] However, a more recent study found that bone stiffness as measured with ultrasound was higher at the tibia, although not at the radius, in a group of young female swimmers than in a group of nonswimmers.[109] The authors of this study concluded that swimming may contribute to increasing BMD in the lower extremity but not in the upper extremity. Whether swimming does or does not increase BMD, it continues to be recommended for patients with osteoporosis because the water is a relatively safe environment in which to achieve the other benefits of exercise for those at high fracture risk.

WEIGHT-BEARING EXERCISE

Two published meta-analyses of exercise studied the effects of physical activity on bone mass in women.[54,110] One of these analyses[110] indicated that although weight-bearing exercise primarily affects BMD at the spine, there may be some effect on the hip and forearm as well. The other meta-analysis indicated that weight-bearing exercise prevents bone loss at the lumbar spine and femur.[54]

During the normal growth period, vigorous exercise can increase peak bone strength and bone mass by as much as 30%.[111] Exercise must be continued during adulthood to preserve maximum bone mass. One cross-sectional study by Ulrich and colleagues investigated the relationship between BMD and lifetime physical activity in 25 premenopausal women. Total weight-bearing physical activity was associated with total BMD ($p = 0.05$). The study suggested that physical activity in the early years (childhood through early adulthood) was more strongly associated with BMD at all sites than activity over the most recent 2-year period in those subjects.[112]

Two small RCTs examined the effects of impact exercise on BMD in children aged 9 to 12 years, one on boys[113] and the other on girls.[114] The impact exercise in these trials was a jumping program that lasted for 7 months. Both studies found that impact loading was associated with increased BMD, whereas nonimpact activities, such as swimming and resistance training, did not significantly affect bone density in children. Furthermore, girls in the study had a greater increase in BMD from impact loading, especially from gymnastics, as they approached puberty. Evidence also indicates that weight-bearing physical activity started early and continued through the period of skeletal maturation contributes to higher peak bone mass.[115] Thus it would seem prudent to recommend increasing physical activity at all ages, especially during the early years, as a form of osteoporosis prevention.

A systematic review evaluating and comparing the effects of impact and nonimpact exercise on BMD of the spine in premenopausal women ages 16 to 44 years found that both types of exercise reduced bone loss but that impact exercise may be more effective (1.6% bone loss prevented, 95% confidence interval [CI]: 1.6%-2.2%) than nonimpact exercise (1.0%, CI: 0.4%-1.6%).[116] This review included eight RCTs, and the interventions included either high impact aerobics, running and jumping (impact) or stretching, resistance training, and weight lifting (nonimpact). The duration of the exercise programs varied between 6 and 36 months. The included studies were criticized for having small sample sizes and high drop-out rates.

Epidemiological data suggest that although exercise later in life has only a small impact on BMD, being physically active reduces the incidence of hip fracture by as much as 50% in people over the age of 65.[117] This is likely due to improved balance and strength and thus a reduced incidence of falls.

In general, the evidence on the effects of resistance and impact exercise for patients with or at risk for skeletal demineralization indicates that activities should be designed to use the muscles that attach to or support the target bone(s) to stimulate those sites, while protecting potentially fragile areas, including the spine, hips, and wrists. Site-specific strengthening exercise should focus on the muscles supporting the trunk, hips, and upper extremities because these are areas at greatest risk for fracture. Strength training should be included to maintain bone density and should improve postural control and stability to decrease the risk of falls. The increase in muscle mass produced by muscle strengthening may also reduce fracture risk by providing additional protection should a fall occur.

Lower extremity weight bearing can be achieved through a variety of activities, such as walking, running, jumping rope, dancing, skiing, stair climbing, Tai Chi, and others. Walking and stair climbing activities can easily be developed into progressive programs that patients can follow. Weight-bearing activities can be done at differing speeds and varying intensities. The literature suggests that higher intensity weight-bearing activities have more impact on bone density but may put clients at increased risk for falls.[98,118,119]

BODY MECHANICS TRAINING

To avoid the increased risk of spinal compression fractures associated with spinal flexion, patients with skeletal demineralization should learn to keep the trunk in a relatively neutral position for bending and lifting activities in everyday life. Exercises or functional activities that put patients into flexed postures should be modified or avoided if possible.

Posture correction and training should address walking, standing, and sitting as tall as possible. Core stability, maintaining both a level pelvis and tension in the pelvic floor during activity, should be included. Photographs can be an effective way for patients to learn to self-adjust their posture in standing, sitting, and during activity. Patients can begin to correct posture in a supine position with knees bent and feet flat, arms flat against the supporting surface slightly away from the trunk, and palms up (Fig. 3-6). In this rest position, the patient can work on head and neck position while unloading the neck and finding the position of a neutral spine. Patients can learn to elongate the spine, as well as the extremities, while maintaining neutral positions. Maintaining good posture in sitting and standing requires constant self-monitoring. The concept of a hook attached to the top of the head and pulling the patient up from the waist may be a useful teaching tool.

While corrected posture is becoming habitual, the patient can work on gait, balance, and body mechanics with a different proprioceptive foundation. Patients should learn to use a hip hinge for all pushing, pulling, reaching, or bending activities, as well as log rolling for moving about in bed. Patients should be taught to maintain excellent body mechanics and posture while working

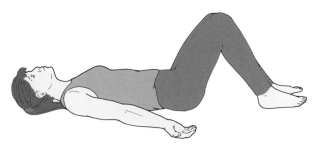

FIG. 3-6 Decompression exercise. *Redrawn from Visual Health Information, courtesy Sara Meeks Seminars.*

at a desk, doing household chores, climbing stairs, getting in and out of a car, and performing other patient-specific activities.

MEDICATIONS AND DIET

Prescribing medications, giving dietary advice, and performing invasive procedures are not generally within the practice of most rehabilitation practitioners. But since these types of interventions can be a critical components of the prevention and treatment of bone demineralization, they will be briefly discussed.

Most medications prescribed for people with skeletal demineralization are antiresorptive agents such as estrogen, *bisphosphonates, selective estrogen receptor modulators* (SERMs), calcitonin, and more recently, parathyroid hormone (PTH). Supplemental calcium is also often recommended with these medications, especially for those with poor dietary intake such as lactose-intolerant individuals and women who limit dietary intake because of concern with caloric content. Regardless of the type of compound used, the goal of any drug therapy used for this population is the prevention and reduction of fractures.

In the past, estrogen replacement was the primary therapy for the prevention of postmenopausal osteoporosis. Estrogen has the additional advantages of controlling menopausal symptoms and was thought to prevent or delay cardiovascular disease. However, data from the Women's Health Initiative (WHI) revealed that estrogen-progestin therapy does not reduce the risk of coronary heart disease and may increase the risk of breast cancer, stroke, and venous thromboembolic events.[120] Although estrogen does decrease bone loss,[121] its use is generally not recommended at this time except for short-term control of symptoms associated with menopause, Other antiresorptive agents are now preferred for the prevention and treatment of osteoporosis in postmenopausal women.

The bisphosphonates, such as *alendronate* and *risedronate*, inhibit bone resorption. They selectively bind hydroxyapatite crystals and are later released during osteoclastic bone formation. The bisphosphonate is taken up by the osteoclasts and induces a chain of intracellular events that leads to inactivation and/or apoptosis of the cell.[122] Because the actual amount of drug absorbed from each dose is minimal, strict guidelines for taking the drugs must be followed to optimize absorption. Bisphosphonates must be taken on an empty stomach with 8 to 10 ounces of water. The patient must then remain upright, without eating or drinking anything, for at least 30 minutes to allow the drug to move down into the stomach and avoid remaining in the esophagus too long and causing esophageal irritation. Bisphosphonates are contraindicated for those cannot follow these guidelines and may still cause some esophageal discomfort in susceptible patients. Both alendronate and risedronate have been shown to reduce the risk of vertebral fracture by 50% and to reduce the risk of nonvertebral fracture, including hip fractures, by 20% to 50%, according to patient characteristics.[123]

Selective estrogen receptor modulators (SERMs) have a similar mechanism of action to estrogen. They increase relative BMD by slowing bone loss. According to the Multiple Outcomes of Raloxifene Evaluation (MORE) study, which included over 7,705 women with osteoporosis, raloxifene reduced vertebral fractures in women with and without prevalent vertebral fractures by 30% and 50%, respectively.[124] Raloxifene may also reduce low density lipoprotein (LDL) and cholesterol, but because of their selective binding, SERMs do not have any adverse effects on the endometrium and do not increase the risk of breast cancer, stroke, or venous thromboembolic events.[125]

Calcitonin is a hormone secreted by the thyroid gland that decreases plasma calcium concentration by inhibiting osteoclast activity. Thus calcitonin can slow bone resorption and decrease bone loss. Exogenous calcitonin can reduce fracture risk in women 5 years or more past menopause who do not take estrogen and appears to decrease the pain associated with vertebral fractures.[126] According to the PROOF (Prevent Recurrence of Osteoporotic Fractures) study, intranasal calcitonin (200 IU/day) reduced the rate of vertebral, but not peripheral, fractures by 30% compared to placebo.[127] Calcitonin is administered either intranasally or by injection.

PTH is a hormone produced by the parathyroid gland. The primary function of PTH is to maintain blood calcium levels. PTH stimulates the release of calcium from bones when blood calcium levels fall. However, PTH also increases calcium absorption by promoting the conversion of vitamin D from its in inactive form to its active form. Intermittent administration of PTH has been found to stimulate bone formation and appears to reverse trabecular bone loss without compromising the structure or strength of cortical bone.[128] PTH has also been found to increase BMD in the spine and decrease vertebral and nonvertebral fracture risk in a wide variety of patients independent of age, baseline BMD, or number of fractures before treatment.[129,130] PTH also appears to be effective in men with low BMD and in the treatment of glucocorticoid-induced osteoporosis.[131]

Calcium consumption may be the most important modifiable factor for preventing osteoporosis.[132] Calcium intake may be increased through diet modification or oral supplements in pill, chewable, or liquid form. Diet modification should be easy, but personal taste, caloric restriction, or financial hardship makes better dietary choices difficult for some patients. Emphasizing the importance of calcium for its wide range of functions often encourages patients to be more attentive to their calcium intake. Table 3-4 provides the recommended daily calcium intake recommendations.

Sufficient vitamin D is also necessary to convert calcium into a usable form. Vitamin D intake can come from oral supplements or by sun exposure to the skin. Fifteen minutes of unfiltered sunlight daily is necessary if the patient is not taking any supplement. Sunscreens reduce vitamin D production. An SPF of only 8 filters out 97% of the UV light from the sun. The daily recommended allowance has been 400-800 IU/day but is cur-

TABLE 3-4	Calcium Requirements by Age Group
Age Group	**Daily Calcium Requirement**
Children and young adults:	
1-10 years	800 mg
11-24 years	1200 mg
Adults	1000 mg
Pregnant and lactating women	1200 mg
Postmenopausal women not on ERT	1500 mg
Men over age 65	1500 mg

ERT, Estrogen replacement therapy.

rently being revised in light of the number of children and adults that lack sufficient vitamin D.

Other dietary recommendations include avoiding excessive salt and caffeinated beverage intake. Excess salt and caffeinated beverages tend to leach calcium from bone, resulting in an increase in urinary calcium excretion.[133,134] The most common source of salt is canned or other prepared foods, and the most common source of phosphate today is soda pop.

OSTEOPOROTIC SPINAL FRACTURE INTERVENTIONS

Conservative Measures. After a painful spinal compression fracture, bed rest and narcotic analgesics are generally recommended for pain control, although this increases the risk of pneumonia, further bone loss from disuse, and deconditioning. Because of these adverse effects of bed rest, some medical practitioners have tried to used bracing to decrease pain so that patients can stay mobile during the acute recovery phase. However, patient compliance with this intervention is often poor because most spinal braces are bulky and uncomfortable. Recently, a lightweight, low-profile, adjustable brace has become available for this purpose.[135] It is designed to stimulate back extensor muscle activity, decrease pain, and improve mobility in patients with spinal compression fractures; however, its effectiveness awaits scientific testing. Others have resisted using braces for fear that patients would become dependent and stop using what muscle control they did have. Bracing continues to be used for pain relief for patients with glucocorticoid-induced osteoporosis, such as posttransplant patients. For patients dependent on antirejection drugs over a lifetime, bracing may be the only way to improve mobility.

Invasive Measures. Surgical procedures known as vertebroplasty and kyphoplasty have been developed to address the effects of skeletal demineralization on the spine. These procedures are performed percutaneously in an outpatient setting by injecting bone cement into the body of collapsed vertebrae. Vertebroplasty includes only the injection of bone cement, whereas kyphoplasty is done by inflating a collapsed area of bone and then elevating the endplates before the bone cement is injected.[136] The effectiveness of these procedures has not yet been established from RCTs, but case studies and nonrandomized trials suggest that these procedures can result in significant improvements in quality of life and functional status.[137,138]

CASE STUDY 3-1

OSTEOPOROSIS, T11 FRACTURE, AND BACK PAIN

Examination
Patient History
AB is a 79-year-old woman who presents with complaints of chronic pain and increasing weakness. She is referred to physical therapy after her last visit to the metabolic bone clinic. Her referral sheet notes that she has the medical diagnoses of osteoporosis, an old T11 fracture, and back pain. The physician's goals for her treatment are to increase her strength and decrease her pain. The patient reports that both her mother and grandmother became "humped over" with age. She states that she was active as a child and ate dairy products until she was about age 35 when she became lactose intolerant. She was a schoolteacher until she retired 15 years ago and enjoyed hiking, playing golf, and skiing. Since her husband died 5 years ago, she has developed back pain and limits her activities. She does not walk or do any other form of physical activity. AB's past medical history is significant for osteoporosis with compression fractures, pulmonary hypertension, gastroesophageal reflux disease (GERD), weight loss, depression, irritable bowel syndrome, and back pain. She had an episode of pancreatitis in 1997. Her surgical history includes a hysterectomy at age 37 and a cholecystectomy at age 41.

Her current medications include parathyroid hormone (teriparatide, Forteo), buspirone HCl (BuSpar), lansoprazole (Prevacid), oxycodone HCl (OxyContin), and conjugated estrogen (Premarin). She takes a multivitamin, a baby aspirin, and docusate sodium (Colace) daily.

AB was diagnosed with osteoporosis $4^1/_2$ years ago after a BMD test (DXA). At that time, she had a compression fracture of T11. Her most recent DXA showed that her L1-L4 T-score was −3.2 (0.548 g/cm^2); her T-score for the right femoral neck was −3.9 (0.573 g/cm^2) and for the left femoral neck was −4.37 (0.508 g/cm^2).

Tests and Measures
Musculoskeletal

Posture Kyphotic thoracic spine with a flattened lumbar curve. The Index of kyphosis = 14.2. Lower ribs are approximating the iliac crests and are lower on the right than on the left. Belly is protruded. Moderately forward head, holding cervical spine in extension. Hips and knees are slightly flexed in standing.

Anthropometric Characteristics AB is 5 feet 2 inches tall as measured in the stadiometer. AB states that she was 5 feet $4^1/_2$ inches tall when she was younger. She weighs 97 lb with clothes.

Active Range of Motion See Table 3-5.

TABLE 3-5	Range of Motion for Patient in Case Study 3-1				
	Flexion	**Extension**	**Abduction**	**External rotation**	**Dorsiflexion**
L shoulder	130°	WNL	75°	30°	NA
R shoulder	155°	WNL	115°	50°	
L hip	>100° causes low back pain	−20°	20°	30°	
R hip	WNL	−15°	20°	40°	
L knee		−15°	NA	NA	
R knee		−15°			
L ankle		NA			0°
R ankle					5°
Spine	Not tested	Unable to test			NA

Neuromuscular

Pain Patient states her pain level is 7/10 during the visit and ranges from 4 to 9/10 during a typical week. Lying down reduces low back pain for a while but then causes rib pain to increase.

Sensation Denies sensory loss.

Cardiovascular/Pulmonary

Endurance Examination had to be done over 2 nonconsecutive days because of patient fatigue. Heart rate increased to 85 bpm with strength testing of lower extremities; returned to normal after 3 minutes of rest.

Function

Gait, Locomotion, and Balance Gait is slow and deliberate. There is almost no time between heel strike and foot flat and a shortened swing phase on each side. Tinetti Assessment Score for gait is 12/16 and for balance is 9/12. AB could not complete a 6-minute walk test due to complaints of fatigue after 4 minutes.

Evaluation, Diagnosis, and Prognosis
Evaluation

AB is a 79-year-old woman with osteoporosis and vertebral compression fractures who has withdrawn from most of her normal activities. In the past 5 years, she has experienced significant back pain and has dramatically changed her lifestyle to accommodate her pain.

Impairments

- Loss of generalized flexibility in cervical spine, anterior shoulders, hip extension, knee flexion, and dorsiflexion.

- Weakness in cervical flexors, posterior scapular muscles, trunk musculature, hip, and knee extensors.

Muscle Performance

Strength Measured by MMT See Table 3-6.
- Low cardiovascular and muscular endurance
- Gait and balance abnormalities
- Low back and rib pain

Functional Limitations: By report, AB is unable to go grocery shopping or to enjoy being outside the home. She is unable to participate in housekeeping, gardening, walking, or hiking.

Diagnosis

The preferred practice pattern is 4A: Primary prevention/risk reduction for skeletal demineralization; pain from limited mobility and kyphotic posture maintaining prolonged stretch of soft tissues.

Plan of Care

Provide instruction, education, and training to the patient and her daughter regarding risk factors for fracture, impairments, functional limitations and disabilities, and a plan for intervention and wellness. Therapeutic interventions include posture awareness training, posture control training, postural stabilization, balance training, flexibility exercises, active and resistive exercises, and upright endurance training. Safety awareness in terms of body position and body mechanics during self-care and home management is coupled with injury prevention education both inside and outside the home environment.

TABLE 3-6	Strength of Patient in Case Study 3-1					
	Depression	**Retraction**	**Flexion**	**Extension**	**External rotation**	**Dorsiflexion**
L scapula	3/5	2+/5				
R scapula	3/5	2+/5				
L shoulder			4+/5	4+/5	4−/5	
R shoulder			3+/5	3/5	3−/5	
L hip			4−/5	2/5 (gluteal) 3+/5 (hamstrings)		
R hip			4−/5	2/5 (gluteal) 3/5 (hamstrings)		
L knee			4+/5	4/5		
R knee			4+/5	4−/5		
L ankle						3+/5
R ankle						3+/5
Trunk			2−/5	2+/5		

Prognosis

Patient will demonstrate adherence to an activity program that should decrease her risk factors for fracture and additional bone loss. The literature suggests that activities that include strength and balance training and graduated weight-bearing, coupled good dietary intake, will produce the best outcomes. The patient should be able to describe a diet plan and demonstrate a satisfactory activity plan within 6 visits.

Intervention

- Educate patient on how to decrease fracture risk, supplementing diet with calcium and vitamin D, and diet in general (calcium fortified foods, soda pop, caffeine).
- Plan for increasing physical activity by using a walking program 5-6 days a week, adding at least 1-3 minutes each day. AB can progress to comfortably walk 1 mile daily.
- Begin home exercise program (HEP) as follows:
  1. Supine with hands under head and elbows out; push down against surface (Fig. 3-7).

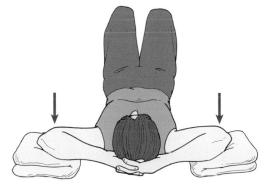

FIG. 3-7 Elbow press exercise. *Redrawn from Visual Health Information, courtesy Sara Meeks Seminars.*

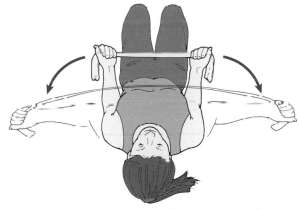

FIG. 3-8 Arm rotation. *Redrawn from Visual Health Information, courtesy Sara Meeks Seminars.*

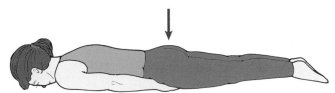

FIG. 3-9 Pelvic press. *Redrawn from Visual Health Information, courtesy Sara Meeks Seminars.*

2. Supine elastic-resisted exercise (start with low resistance and progress). External rotation (Fig. 3-8).
3. Prone lying. With arms under thighs, tighten gluteals, press pelvis into the surface (Fig. 3-9).
4. Chair rise (Fig. 3-10):
   - Sit on the edge of a strong chair with best posture.
   - Come to a standing position without using arms.
   - Sit back down slowly, maintaining best posture.
5. Wall press (Fig. 3-11):

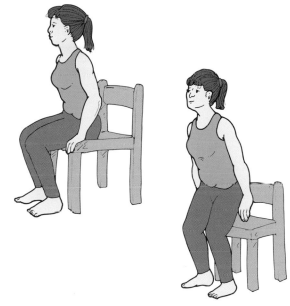

FIG. 3-10 Chair rise exercise.

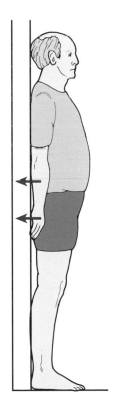

FIG. 3-11 Wall press exercise.

- Stand against wall with arms straight and palms facing wall.
- Push arms and palms against wall.

6. Walking progression:
  - Start by walking for a total of 5 minutes down the block and back.
  - Progress by adding 1-2 minutes every day until AB can walk for 30 minutes without discomfort.
  - Low level balance training using therapeutic ball and standing challenges (see Chapter 13).
  - Posture training
    1. Plumb line alignment.
    2. Tighten pelvic floor.
    3. Lift chest up, stretch neck to feel 2 inches taller.
    4. Walk as though suspended from a sky hook

Outcomes

Impairments

Pain decreased from 7/10 to 4/10 in 2 weeks
ROM increased generally by 20% in 2 weeks
Index of kyphosis decreased by 1 in 4 weeks
Strength increased by $\frac{1}{2}$-1 grade throughout in 2 weeks
Balance improved to 14/16 on Tinetti Assessment Score

Functional Limitations

In 1 week, performed light housekeeping
In 2 weeks, walked for at least 10 minutes without undue fatigue or pain
In 3 weeks, went to the grocery store for a single item
In 4 weeks, walked a mile in comfort
Please see the CD that accompanies this book for a case study describing the examination, evaluation, and intervention for a patient with osteoporosis and osteopenia.

CHAPTER SUMMARY

Skeletal demineralization affects a large and growing segment of the population. Although skeletal demineralization does not cause symptoms, it causes problems by increasing the risk of fractures. Risks for osteopenia or osteoporosis should be routinely evaluated in every client or patient. Height loss reported greater than 1 inch or any history of using glucocorticoids, eating disorders, or any nontraumatic fractures should be red flags for therapists. Patients at risk for osteopenia or osteoporosis must have appropriate education and guidance regarding diet and physical activity in order to prevent progression of bone loss.

The best treatment for skeletal demineralization is prevention through appropriate physical activity and diet during early childhood to maximize bone accretion during growth. These preventive measures including weight-bearing activities and resistive exercise regimes; cessation of smoking and limiting excess amounts of alcohol, salt, and phosphates combined with a diet rich in calcium should also continue throughout adulthood. Weight-bearing activity can include walking, running, stair climbing, dancing, tai chi, or virtually any activity that requires upright mobility against gravity. To affect bone density, resistive exercise must be site-specific, exceed normal daily loading, and be progressive. Strengthening back, hip, and knee extensor muscles and

dorsiflexors; stretching tight anterior structures; and elongating the trunk can improve posture and balance, reducing fracture risk. Specific balance training activities can also contribute significantly to reducing fall risk and thus fracture risk in those with low BMD.

The therapist may help people with or at risk for skeletal demineralization throughout the lifespan through education, exercise, pain management, and postural correction. Therapists can also provide educational and general exercise information geared to keeping exercise and activities of daily living safe for this potentially fragile population and for keeping people with skeletal demineralization safe as well as active. As illustrated by the cases, outcomes for skeletal demineralization can be positively influenced with proper guidance and compliance.

ADDITIONAL RESOURCES

Books

Nelson ME: *Strong Women, Strong Bones,* New York, 2000, GP Putnam's Sons.
Meeks S: *Walk Tall! An Exercise Program for the Prevention and Treatment of Osteoporosis,* Gainesville, Fl, 1999, Triad Publishing.

Web Sites

National Osteoporosis Foundation: www.nof.org
National Institutes of Health: Osteoporosis and Related Bone Disease—National Resource Center: www.osteo.org
International Osteoporosis Foundation: www.osteofound.org
National Osteoporosis Society (UK): www.nos.org.uk

GLOSSARY

1,25-dihydroxyvitamin D: Physiologically active form of vitamin D that stimulates absorption of calcium and phosphorus by the gut.
Alendronate: Fosamax; a bisphosphonate delivered by tablet.
Bisphosphonate: Group of antiresorptive compounds used for the prevention and treatment of osteoporosis in postmenopausal women and in men, as well as those patients with Paget's disease or steroid-induced osteoporosis.
Bone mineral density (BMD): Amount of bone mass present; typically measured in the lumbar spine and hip.
Calcitonin: Hormone (usually salmon) used for treatment of postmenopausal osteoporosis and pain from vertebral compression fracture; Miacalcin is delivered by nasal spray.
Debrunner's kyphometer: Metal device, similar to an inclinometer used to measure kyphosis
Dual-energy x-ray absorptiometry (DXA; DEXA): Gold standard measurement of BMD.
Flexicurve: A 48-cm strip of lead covered with synthetic rubber used to map the kypholordotic curve.
Glucocorticoid: Medication used to decrease inflammation in chronic conditions, such as rheumatoid arthritis, and as an antirejection drug after organ transplant.
Index of kyphosis: Mathematical equation to quantify kyphosis for repeated measures.
Osteomalacia: Lack of mineralization of the organic bone matrix.
Osteopenia: Bone mass between 1.0 and 2.5 SD below the mean for young normals.
Osteoporosis: Bone loss greater than 2.5 SD below the mean for young normals; decreased bone mass with disruption of normal architecture resulting in increased fragility and increased risk of fracture.
Peak bone mass: Greatest amount of bone accrued by the body.
Risedronate: Actonel; a bisphosphonate.

Selective estrogen receptor modulator (SERM): Compounds that act like estrogen on bone without effecting breast or uterine tissue.

Stadiometer: Measurement device to examine height; can be mounted on the wall or be free-standing.

T-score: Approximate amount of bone compared to a normal, young adult female.

Ward's triangle: Area in the femoral neck where trabeculae are typically thin and loosely arranged.

Z-score: Approximate amount of bone present compared to age- and gender-matched controls.

References

1. Junqueira LC, Carneiro J, Kelley RO: *Basic Histology,* ed 6, Norwalk, Conn, 1989, Appleton & Lange.
2. Pickles B: Biological aspects of aging. In Jackson O (ed): *Physical Therapy of the Geriatric Patient,* ed 2, New York, 1989, Churchill Livingstone.
3. Ali N, Siktberg L: Osteoporosis prevention in female adolescents: Calcium intake and exercise participation, *Pediatr Nurs* 27:132, 135-139, 2001.
4. Bemben DA, Fetters NL: The independent and additive effects of exercise training and estrogen on bone metabolism, *J Strength Condition Res* 14:114-120, 2000.
5. Kanis JA, Melton LJ III, Christiansen C, et al: The diagnosis of osteoporosis, *J Bone Miner Res* 9:1137-1141, 1994.
6. Vallarta-Ast N, Krueger D, Binkley N: Densitometric diagnosis of osteoporosis in men, *J Clin Densitom* 5:383-389, 2002.
7. Faulkner KG, Orwoll E: Implications in the use of T-scores for the diagnosis of osteoporosis in men, *J Clin Densitom* 5:87-93, 2003.
8. Faulkner K, Miller PD, Barrett-Connor E, et al: Age, ethnicity, and bone mineral density at the heel: Evidence from the National Osteoporosis Risk Assessment (NORA) program [abstract], *Bone* 23.S474, 1998.
9. Binkley NC, Schmeer P, Wasnick RD, et al: What are the criteria by which a densitometric diagnosis of osteoporosis can be made in males and non-Caucasians? *J Clin Densitom* 5 (suppl):S19-S27, 2002.
10. National Osteoporosis Foundation: *America's Bone Health: The State of Osteoporosis and Low Bone Mass in our Nation,* Washington, 2002, The Foundation.
11. National Osteoporosis Foundation: *Physician's Guide to Prevention and Treatment of Osteoporosis,* Washington, 1998, The Foundation.
12. Wehren LE: The epidemiology of osteoporosis and fractures in geriatric medicine, *Clin Geriatric Med* 19:245-258, 2003.
13. National Institutes for Health (NIH) Consensus Statement: *Osteoporosis, Prevention, Diagnosis and Therapy,* Bethesda, Md, March 27-29, 2000.
14. National Osteoporosis Foundation: Osteoporosis: Review of the evidence for prevention, diagnosis, and treatment and cost-effectiveness analysis, *Osteoporosis Int* 8:S1-88, 1998.
15. Wu F, Mason B, Horne A, et al: Fractures between the ages of 20-50 years increase women's risk of subsequent fractures, *Arch Intern Med* 162:33, 2002.
16. Cummings SR, Nevitt MC, Browner WS, et al: Risk factors for hip fracture in white women, *N Engl J Med* 332:767, 1995.
17. Steele D G, Bramblett CA: *The Anatomy and Biology of the Human Skeleton,* College Station, Tex, 1988, Texas A&M University Press.
18. Rodan GA: Introduction to bone biology, *Bone* 13:S3-S6, 1992.
19. Eriksen EF, Axelrod DW, Melsen F: *Bone Histomorphometry,* New York, 1994, Raven Press.
20. Riggs BL: Overview of osteoporosis, *West J Med* 154:63-77, 1991.
21. Riffee JM: Osteoporosis: Prevention and management, *Am Pharm* NS32(8):61-71, 1992.
22. Canalis E: Regulation of bone remodeling. In Favus M (ed): *Primer on the Metabolic Bone Mineral Diseases and Disorders of Mineral Metabolism,* ed 3, Philadelphia, 1996, Lippincott-Raven.
23. Boissonnault W, Goodman C: Pathology: Implications for the physical therapist. In Boissonnault W, ed: *Introduction to Pathology of the Musculoskeletal System,* Philadelphia, 1998, WB Saunders.
24. O'Flaherty EJ: Modeling normal aging bone loss, with consideration of bone loss in osteoporosis, *Toxicol Sci* 55:171-188, 2000.
25. Watts NB: Osteoporosis, *Am Fam Physician* 38(5):193-207, 1998.
26. Francis RM: Bone aging, osteoporosis, and osteomalacia. In Brocklehurst JC, Tallis RC, Fillit HM (eds): *Textbook of Geriatric Medicine and Gerontology,* New York, 1990, Churchill Livingstone.
27. Rosse C, Gaddum-Rosse P: *Hollinshead's Textbook of Anatomy,* ed 5, Philadelphia, 1997, Lippincott-Raven.
28. Porter RE: Normal development of movement and function: Child and adolescent. In Scully RM, Barnes MR (eds): *Physical Therapy,* Philadelphia, 1989, Lippincott.
29. Riggs BL, Melton LJ 3rd: Involutional osteoporosis, *N Engl J Med* 314:1676-1686, 1986.
30. Aloia JF: The gain and loss of bone in the human life cycle, *Adv Nutrition Res* 9:1-33, 1994.
31. Parfitt AM, Mathews CH, Villanueva AR, et al: Relationships between surface, volume, and thickness of iliac trabecular bone in aging and in osteoporosis. Implications for the microanatomic and cellular mechanisms of bone loss, *J Clin Invest* 72:1396-1409, 1983.
32. Parfitt AM: Implications of architecture for the pathogenesis and prevention of vertebral fracture, *Bone* 13(suppl 2):S41-47, 1992.
33. Parisien M, Cosman F, Mellish RW, et al: Bone structure in postmenopausal hyperparathyroid, osteoporotic, and normal women, *J Bone Miner Res* 10:1393-1399, 1995.
34. O'Brien, CA, Jia D, Plotkin LI, et al: Glucocorticoids act directly on osteoblasts and osteocytes to induce their apoptosis and reduce bone formation and strength, *Endocrinology* 145:1835-1841, 2004.
35. Hermus AR, Smals AC, Swinkels LM, et al: Bone mineral density and bone turnover before and after surgical cure of Cushing's syndrome, *J Clin Endocrinol Metab* 80:2859, 1985.
36. Goodman CC, Boissonnault WG: *Pathology: Implications for the Physical Therapist,* ed 2, Philadelphia, 2003, WB Saunders.
37. Creditor MC: Hazards of hospitalization of the elderly, *Ann Int Med* 118:219-223, 1993.
38. Maeda H, Kimmel DB, Raab DM, et al: Musculoskeletal recovery following hindlimb immobilization in adult female rats, *Bone* 14:153-159, 1993.
39. Glaser DL, Kaplan FS: Osteoporosis: Definition and clinical presentation, *Spine* 22(suppl 24), 12S-16S, 1997.
40. Donaldson CL, Hulley SB, Vogel JM, et al: Effect of prolonged bed rest on bone mineral, *Metabolism* 19:1071-1084, 1970.
41. Krolner B, Toft B, Nielsen S, et al: Physical exercise as a prophylaxis against involutional bone loss: A controlled trial, *Clin Sci* 64:541-546, 1983.
42. Lawton MT: Evaluating and managing osteoporosis in men, *Nurse Pract* 26:29-36, 2001.
43. Tobias JH, Cook DG, Chambers TJ, et al: A comparison of bone mineral density between Caucasian, Asian and Afro-Caribbean women, *Clin Sci (Lond)* 87:587-591, 1994.
44. NIH Consensus Development Panel on Optimal Calcium Intake, *JAMA* 272:1942, 1994.
45. Curhan GC, Willett WC, Knight EL, et al: Dietary factors and the risk of incident kidney stones in younger women, *Arch Intern Med* 164:885-891, 2004.
46. DeLuca HF, Zierold C: Mechanisms and functions of vitamin D, *Nutr Rev* 56:S4-S10, 1998.
47. Van den Berg H: Bioavailability of vitamin D, *Eur J Clin Nutr* 51(suppl 1):S76-S79, 1997.
48. Institute of Medicine, Food and Nutrition Board: *Dietary Reference Intakes: Calcium, Phosphorous, Magnesium, Vitamin D, and Fluoride,* Washington, 1999, National Academy Press.
49. Lloyd T, Chinchilli VM, Johnston-Rollins N, et al: Adult female hip bone density reflects teenage sports-exercise patterns but not teenage calcium intake, *Pediatrics* 106:40-44, 2000.
50. Gordon CM, Lawrence LM: Amenorrhea and bone health in adolescents and young women, *Curr Opin Obstet Gynecol* 15:377-384, 2003.
51. Siris ES, Miller PD, Barrett-Connor E, et al: Identification and fracture outcomes of undiagnosed low bone mineral in postmenopausal women: Results from the National Osteoporosis Risk Assessment, *JAMA* 286:2815-2822, 2000.
52. Wolff I, van Croonenborg JJ, Kemper HC, et al: The effect of exercise training programs on bone mass: A meta-analysis of published controlled trials in pre- and post-menopausal women, *Osteo Int* 9:1-12, 1999.
53. Caillot-Augusseau A, Lafage-Proust MH, Soler C, et al: Bone formation and resorption biological markers in cosmonauts during and after a 180-day space flight (Euromir 95), *Clin Chem* 44:578-585, 1998.
54. Greenleaf JE, Bulbulian R, Bernauer EM, et al: Exercise training protocols for astronauts in microgravity, *J Applied Physiol* 67:2191-2204, 1989.
55. Hargens AR, Whalen RT, Watenpaugh DE, et al: Lower body negative pressure to provide load bearing in space, *Aviat Space Environ Med* 62:934-937, 1991.
56. Smith EL, Raab DM: Osteoporosis and physical activity, *Acta Medica Scand* 711S:149-156, 1986.
57. Schultheis L: The mechanical control system of bone in weightless spaceflight and in aging, *Exp Gerontol* 26(2-3):203-214, 1991.
58. Cummings SR: Treatable and untreatable risk factors for hip fracture, *Bone* 18:165S, 1996.
59. Law MR, Hackshaw AK: A meta-analysis of cigarette smoking, bone mineral density, and risk of hip fracture: Recognition of a major event, *BMJ* 315(7112):841-846, 1997.
60. Krall EA, Dawson-Hughes B: Smoking increases bone loss and decreases intestinal calcium absorption, *J Bone Miner Res* 14:215, 1999.
61. Bikle DD, Genant HK, Cann C, et al: Bone disease in alcohol abuse, *Ann Intern Med* 103:42-48, 1995.
62. Israel Y, Orrego H, Holt S, et al: Identification of alcohol abuse: thoracic fractures on routine chest x-rays as indicators of alcoholism, *Alcohol Clin Exp Res* 4:420-422, 1980.
63. Cummings SR, Nevitt MC, Browner WS, et al: Risk factors for hip fracture in white women. Study of the Osteoporosis Fractures Research Group, *N Engl J Med* 332:767-773, 1995.

64. Lloyd T, Rollings N, Eggli DF, et al: Dietary caffeine intake and bone status of postmenopausal women, *Am J Clin Nutr* 65:1826-1830, 1997.

65. Wu CH, Yank YC, Tao WJ, et al: Epidemiological evidence of increased bone mineral density in habitual tea drinkers, *Arch Intern Med* 162:1001-1006, 2002.

66. Wolinsky-Friedland M: Drug-induced metabolic bone disease, *Endocrinol Metab Clin North Am* 24:395, 1995.

67. Pfeilschifter J, Diel IJ: Osteoporosis due to cancer treatment: pathogenesis and management, *J Clin Oncol* 18:1570-1593, 2000.

68. Schwartz AM, Leonidas JC: Methotrexate osteopathy, *Skeletal Radiol* 11:13-16, 1984.

69. LaCroix AZ, Ott SM, Ichikawa L, et al: Low-dose hydrochlorothiazide and preservation of bone mineral in older adults. A randomized, double-blind, placebo-controlled trial, *Ann Intern Med* 133:516, 2000.

70. Debrunner HU: Das Kyphometer, *Z Orthop* 110:389-392, 1972.

71. Ohlen G, Spangfort E, Tingvall C: Measurement of spinal sagittal configuration and mobility with Debrunner's kyphometer, *Spine* 14(6):580-583, 1989.

72. Chow RK, Harrison JE: Relationship of kyphosis to physical fitness and bone mass on post-menopausal women, *Am J Phys Med* 66:219-227, 1987.

73. Milne JS, Lauder IJ: Age effects in kyphosis and lordosis in adults, *Ann Hum Biol* 1:327-337, 1974.

74. Cutler WB, Freidmann E, Genovese-Stone E: Prevalence of kyphosis in a healthy sample of pre- and postmenopausal women, *Am J Phys Med Rehabil* 72:219-225, 1993.

75. Milne JS, Williamson J: A longitudinal study on kyphosis in older people, *Age Ageing* 12:225-233, 1983.

76. Schultz A, Andersson GB, Ortengren R, et al: Analysis and myoelectric measurements of loads on the lumbar spine when holding weights in standing postures, *Spine* 7:390-397, 1982.

77. Sinaki M: Nonpharmacologic interventions: Exercise, fall prevention, and the role of physical medicine, *Clin Geriatr Med* 19:337-359, 2003.

78. Moro M, Heckler A, Bouxsein M, et al: Failure load of thoracic vertebrae correlates with lumbar bone mineral density measured by DXA, *Calcif Tissue Int* 56:206-209, 1995.

79. Lindsay R, Silverman SL, Cooper C: Risk of new vertebral fracture in the year following a fracture, *JAMA* 285:320, 2001.

80. Neuner JM, Zimmer JK, Hamel MB: Diagnosis and treatment of osteoporosis in patients with vertebral compression fracture, *J Am Geriatr Soc* 51:483-491, 2003.

81. Watt V, Pickering M, Wales JK: A comparison of ultrasonic and mechanical stadiometry, *Arch Dis Child* 78:269-270, 1998.

82. Pearlmutter LL, Bode BY, Wilkinson WE, et al: Shoulder range of motion in patients with osteoporosis, *Arthr Care Res* 8:194-198, 1995.

83. Chow SB, Moffat M: Relationship of thoracic kyphosis to functional reach and lower-extremity joint range of motion and muscle length in women with osteoporosis or osteopenia: a pilot study, *Top Geriatr Rehabil* 20:297-306, 2004.

84. Deleted.

85. Deleted.

86. Eriksson SA, Lindgren JU: Outcome of falls in women: endogenous factors associated with fracture, *Age Ageing* 18:303-308, 1989.

87. Shipp KM, Purse JL, Gold DT, et al: Timed loaded standing: A measure of combined trunk and arm endurance suitable for people with osteoporosis, *Osteoporosis Int* 11:914-922, 2000.

88. Lynn SG, Sinaki M, Westerlind KC: Balance characteristics of persons with osteoporosis, *Arch Phys Med Rehabil* 78:273-277, 1997.

89. Tinetti ME: Performance-oriented assessment of mobility problems in elderly patients, *J Am Geriatr Soc* 34:119-126, 1986.

90. Khaw KT, Reeve J, Luben R, et al: Prediction of total and hip fracture risk in men and women by qualitative ultrasound of the calcaneus: EPIC-Norfolk prospective population study, *Lancet* 363:197-202, 2004.

91. Diez-Perez A, Marin F, Vila J, et al: Evaluation of calcaneal quantitative ultrasound in a primary care setting as a screening tool for osteoporosis in postmenopausal women, *J Clin Densitom* 6:237-245, 2003.

92. Chesnut CH 3rd: Noninvasive techniques for measuring bone mass: A comparative review, *Clin Obstet Gynecol* 30:812-819, 1987.

93. Cameron JR, Mazess RB, Sorenson JA: Precision and accuracy of bone mineral determination by direct photon absorptiometry, *Invest Radiol* 3:141-150, 1968.

94. Ostlere SJ, Gold RH: Osteoporosis and bone density measurement methods, *Clin Orthop Relat Res* 271:149-163, 1991.

95. Briney WG: Is measurement of bone density useful? *Rheum Dis Clin North Am* 19:95-106, 1993.

96. Grampp S, Genant HK, Mathur A, et al: Comparisons of noninvasive bone mineral measurements in assessing age-related loss, fracture discrimination, and diagnostic classification, *J Bone Miner Res* 12:697-711, 1997.

97. American Physical Therapy Association: *Guide to Physical Therapist Practice*, ed 2, Alexandria, Va, 1998, The Association.

98. Bonaiuti D, Shea B, Iovine R, et al: Exercise for preventing and treating osteoporosis in postmenopausal women, *The Cochrane Library*, vol 1, 2005, The Cochrane Collaboration.

99. Kelley G: Aerobic exercise and bone density at the hip in postmenopausal women: a meta-analysis, *Prev Med* 27:798-807, 1998.

100. Smith R, Rutherford OM: Spine and total body bone mineral density and serum testosterone levels in male athletes, *Eur J Appl Physiol Occup Physiol* 67:330-334, 1993.

101. Kelley GA, Kelley KS, Tran ZV: Resistance training and bone mineral density in women: a meta-analysis of controlled trials, *Am J Phys Med Rehabil* 80:65-77, 2001.

102. Kelley GA, Kelley KS, Tran ZV: Exercise and lumbar spine bone mineral density in postmenopausal women: A meta-analysis of individual patient data, *J Gerontol A Biol Sci Med Sci* 57:M599-604, 2002.

103. Kelley GA, Kelley KS: Efficacy of resistance exercise on lumbar spine and femoral neck bone mineral density in premenopausal women: a meta-analysis of individual patient data, *J Womens Health* 13:293-300, 2004.

104. Robling AG, Hinant FM, Burr DB, et al: Improved bone structure and strength after long-term mechanical loading is greatest if loading is separated into shout bouts, *J Bone Miner Res* 17:1545-1554, 2002.

105. Sinaki M, Itol H, Wollan P, et al: Stronger back muscles reduce the incidence of vertebral fractures: a prospective 10 year follow-up of postmenopausal women, *Bone* 30(6):836-841, 2002.

106. Sinaki M, Mikkelson BA: Postmenopausal spinal osteoporosis: flexion versus extension exercises, *Arch Phys Med Rehabil* 65:593-596, 2004.

107. Nelson ME, Fiaterone MA, Morganti CM, et al: Effects of high-intensity strength training on multiple risk factors for osteoporotic fractures: A randomized controlled trial, *JAMA* 272:1909-1914, 1994.

108. Taaffe DR, Snow-Harter C, Connolly DA, et al: Differential effects of swimming versus weight-bearing activity on bone mineral status of eumenorrheic athletes, *J Bone Miner Res* 10:586-593, 1995.

109. Falk B, Bronshtein Z, Zigel L, et al: Higher tibial quantitative ultrasound in young female swimmers, *Br J Sports Med* 38:461-465, 2004.

110. Berard A, Bravo G, Gauthier P: Meta-analysis of the effectiveness of physical activity for the prevention of bone loss in postmenopausal women, *Osteoporosis Int* 7:331-337, 1997.

111. Bass SL, Nowson C, Daly RM: Reducing the risk of osteoporosis: The role of exercise and diet. In Morris M, Schoo A (eds): *Optimizing Exercise and Physical Activity in Older People*, Philadelphia, 2004, Butterworth-Heinemann.

112. Ulrich CM, Georgiou CC, Gillis DE, et al: Lifetime physical activity is associated with bone mineral density in premenopausal women, *J Womens Health* 8:365-375, 1999.

113. MacKelvie KJ, McKay HA, Petit MA, et al: Bone mineral responses to a 7-month randomized controlled, school-based jumping intervention in 121 prepubertal boys: associations with ethnicity and body mass index, *J Bone Miner Res* 17:834-844, 2002.

114. Petit MA, McKay HA, MacKelvie KJ, et al: A randomized school-based jumping intervention confers site and maturity specific benefits on bone structural properties in girls: A hip structural analysis study, *J Bone Miner Res* 17:363-372, 2002.

115. MacKelvie KJ, Khan KM, Petit MA, et al: A school-based exercise intervention elicits substantial bone health benefits: A 2-year randomized controlled trial in girls, *Pediatrics* 112:e447-e452, 2003.

116. Wallace BA, Cummings RG: Systematic review of randomized trials of the effect of exercise on bone mass in pre- and postmenopausal women, *Calcif Tissue Int* 67:10-18, 2000.

117. Joakimsen RM, Magnus JH, Fonnebo V, et al: Physical activity and predisposition for hip fracture: A review, *Osteoporosis Int* 7:503-513, 1997.

118. Kohrt WM, Ehsani AA, Birge SJ Jr: Effects of exercise involving predominantly either joint-reaction or ground-reaction forces on bone mineral density in older women, *J Bone Miner Res* 12:1253-1261, 1997.

119. Heinonenn A, Kannus P, Sievanen H, et al: Randomized controlled trial of effect of high-impact exercise on selected risk factors for osteoporotic fractures, *Lancet* 348:1343-1347, 1996.

120. Rossouw JE, Anderson GL, Prentice RL, et al: Risks and benefits of estrogen plus progestin in healthy postmenopausal women: Principal results from the Women's Health Initiative randomized controlled trial, *JAMA* 288:321-333, 2002.

121. Lindsay R, Hart DM, Aitken JM, et al: Long-term prevention of postmenopausal osteoporosis by oestrogen. Evidence for an increased bone mass after delayed onset of oestrogen treatment, *Lancet* 1(7968):1038-1041, 1976.

122. Cremers S, Pillai G, Papapoulos SE: Pharmacokinetics/Pharmacodynamics of bisphosphonates: Use for optimisation of intermittent therapy for osteoporosis, *Clin Pharmacokinet* 44:551-570, 2005.

123. Delmas PD: Treatment of postmenopausal osteoporosis, *Lancet* 359:2018-2026, 2002.

124. Delmas PD, Bjarnaason NH, Mitlak BH, et al: Effects of raloxifene on bone mineral density, serum cholesterol concentrations, and uterine endometrium in postmenopausal women, *N Engl J Med* 337:1641-1647, 1997.

125. Lufkin EG, Whitaker MD, Nickelsen T, et al: Treatment of postmenopausal osteoporosis with raloxifene, *J Bone Miner Res* 13:1747-1758, 1998.

126. Lyritis GP, Tsakalakos N, Magiasis B, et al: Analgesic effect of salmon calcitonin in osteoporotic vertebral fractures: A double-blind placebo-controlled clinical study, *Calcif Tiss Int* 49:369-372, 1991.

127. Ettinger B, Black DM, Mitlak BH, et al: Reduction of vertebral fracture risk in postmenopausal women with osteoporosis treated with raloxifene: Results from a 3-year randomized clinical trial, *JAMA* 282:637-645, 1999.

128. Neer RM, Arnaud CD, Zanchettta JR, et al: Effect of parathyroid (1-34) on fractures and bone mineral density in postmenopausal women with osteoporosis, *N Engl J Med* 344:1434, 2001.

129. Crandall C: Parathyroid hormone for treatment of osteoporosis, *Arch Intern Med* 162:2297-2309, 2002.

130. Marcus R, Wang O, Satterwhite J, et al: The skeletal response to teriparatide is largely independent of age, initial bone mineral density, and prevalent vertebral fractures, *J Bone Miner Res* 18:18-23, 2003.

131. Lane NE, Sanchez S, Modin GW, et al: Parathyroid hormone treatment can reverse corticosteroid-induced osteoporosis. Results from a randomized controlled clinical trial, *J Clin Invest* 102:1627-1633, 1998.

132. Ali S, Siktberyg L: Osteoporosis prevention in female adolescents: Calcium intake and exercise participation, *Pediatr Nurs* 27:132,135-139, 2000.

133. Titze J, Rittweger J, Dietsch P, et al: Hypertension, sodium retention, calcium excretion and osteopenia in Dahl rats, *J Hypertens* 22:803-810, 2004.

134. Heaney RP, Rafferty K: Carbonated beverages and urinary calcium excretion, *Am J Clin Nutr* 74:343-347, 2001.

135. Pfeifer M, Begerow B, Minne HW: Effects of a new spinal orthosis on posture, trunk strength, and quality of life in women with postmenopausal osteoporosis: A randomized trial, *Am J Phys Med Rehabil* 3:177-186, 2004.

136. Theodorou DJ, Theodorou SJ, Duncan TD, et al: Percutaneous balloon kyphoplasty for the correction of spinal deformity in painful vertebral body compression fractures, *Clin Imaging* 26:1-5, 2002.

137. Watts NB, Harris ST, Genant HK: Treatment of painful osteoporotic vertebral fractures with percutaneous vertebroplasty or kyphoplasty, *Osteoporosis Int* 12:429-437, 2001.

138. Diamond TH, Champion B, Clark WA: Management of acute osteoporotic vertebral fractures: a nonrandomized trial comparing percutaneous vertebroplasty with conservative therapy, *Am J Med* 114-257, 2003.

Chapter 4

Posture

Amy Selinger

OBJECTIVES

After reading this chapter, the reader will be able to:
1. Describe ideal posture in sitting and standing.
2. Differentiate between anatomical position and standard (or ideal) posture.
3. Describe the position of the head, neck, shoulder, pelvis, hip, knee, and ankle in optimal erect posture.
4. Explain the difference between static and dynamic posture.
5. Provide interventions to patients with impaired posture.

*P*osture is the relative alignment of body parts, and impaired posture may be considered to be any postural abnormality that affects function. This chapter discusses normal and impaired posture in adults and the terminology used to describe posture. Information on how to examine and describe static posture, and suggestions for interventions intended to optimize posture are also provided. Although most rehabilitation clinicians assess posture and provide interventions intended to change posture and improve patient function, there is no univer-

sally agreed on definition of posture[1] and there is little research confirming a relationship between musculoskeletal pain and postural alignment.[2] Texts and articles praise the virtues of optimal alignment[3-6]; however, clinical studies have not found that alignment correlates with symptoms or function.[7] This chapter provides suggestions for postural examination, evaluation, and interventions based on the best available evidence.

Posture includes the relationship of the body parts to each other and to the body's *base of support*. The base of support is the area of the body in contact with the supporting surface.[1] In standing, the base of support is the area between the outer edges of the feet, including the posterior and lateral aspect of the heels, the lateral-most portion of the fifth toe, and the anterior-most aspect of the great toe (Fig. 4-1).[8]

Posture may be assessed statically, when the body is at rest, or dynamically with the body in motion. Static posture may be evaluated in a variety of positions, including standing, sitting, lying, or in a specific task-associated position. Dynamic posture may be assessed during a variety of activities, including walking, lifting, pushing, carrying, throwing, and cycling, or when moving from one position to another such as from sitting to standing. Because static posture is thought to be the basic posture from which other postures and movements stem, this chapter focuses on examination, evaluation, and interventions for patients with functional problems related to changes in static posture.

Although most clinicians would agree that posture and balance are crucial to the development and maintenance of independence in movements and functional activities, there is little agreement on their underlying neural mechanisms.[1] Woollacott and Shumway-Cook describe two models for understanding the neural basis for the development of posture and movement control: the reflex-hierarchical model and the systems model.[1,9] According to the reflex-hierarchical model, balance and locomotion control progress from reflexive to voluntary as a child matures. According to this model, increasing independence and control depend on inhibition of primitive reflexes and the incorporation of some reflexes into voluntary actions. Progressive maturation of sequentially higher levels of the central nervous system (CNS)

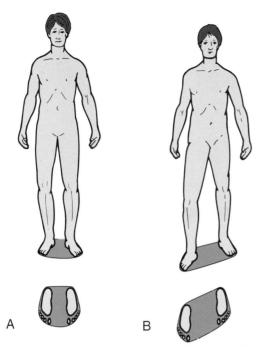

FIG. 4-1 Base of support. **A,** Feet hip width apart. **B,** Note increased base of support with one foot forward and feet further apart.

allows higher levels of behavior to replace immature behaviors.

According to the systems model of motor control, the CNS integrates information from various systems and subsystems to control balance, posture, and movement. Balance and the ability for independent stance and locomotion develop from the interactive maturation of multiple neural and mechanical components, including the visual, vestibular, and somatosensory systems' ability to detect changes in balance; muscle response synergies to control posture and balance; adaptive systems to modify sensory and motor systems in response to task or environment; body morphology (the form and structure of the individual, including such variables as height, center of mass, and size of individual segments); joint range of motion (ROM); and muscle strength (see Chapter 13 for a more detailed discussion of balance).

IDEAL ALIGNMENT

The human body can be positioned in many static postures, including standing, sitting, kneeling, quadruped, lying, and stooping. Within these basic positions there are a range of variations, such as standing on one leg or two; sitting with legs together, crossed, or apart; kneeling on one knee or two; lying on one's side; or lying supine or prone. For each of these positions the body is controlled for stability and orientation to the environment; this is *postural control. Postural orientation* is the ability to maintain the appropriate relationship between body parts and between the body and the environment during the performance of a task. The human body's unique ability to maintain an erect bipedal stance allows use of the upper extremities for fine and gross motor tasks.[6,8,10] Standing

erect has disadvantages, however, including a small base of support, a high center of gravity, and high pressures on the vertebral column, pelvis, and lower extremities.

Ideal body part alignment, also known as *good posture, ideal posture, ideal alignment,* or *neutral posture,* is the position in which the center of mass is centered over the base of support. This is a position of muscular and skeletal balance. Ideal posture is thought to minimize the risk of injury or progressive deformity to supporting structures in all functional positions. It is also thought to allow muscles, as well as the intrathoracic and abdominal organs, to function optimally.[8,11] Ideal posture requires minimal, although not the least possible, energy expenditure to maintain balanced alignment. The least amount of energy is expended in a slumped posture where ligaments rather than muscles stabilize the weight-bearing joints.[8] Ideal posture should permit efficient mechanical joint action and limit wear and tear on the joints. As such, ideal posture requires that other conditions be normal, including muscle tone, flexibility, neuromuscular control, and reflexes.[11] Poor posture, in contrast, results in increased strain on the supporting structures and inefficient balance over the base of support.[8,11]

STANDING POSTURE

Despite individual differences in body size and proportions, certain standards are proposed for ideal alignment. These standards provide general indicators of a goal for ideal alignment and a standard for comparison when examining posture, regardless of the individual's body size or proportions.[4,8] Although these standards do not necessarily describe perfect posture or alignment,[7] variations from these standards form the foundation of postural examination and evaluation. Ideal standing posture is shown in Fig. 4-2 and is described in Tables 4-1 and 4-2.

Although when standing in ideal alignment one appears to be standing completely still, one is actually constantly sway forward and back and from side to side, covering an area known as the *sway envelope.* This motion is called *postural sway.* The amplitude of postural sway can be up to 12 degrees in the sagittal plane and up to 16 degrees in the frontal plane in an adult standing with their feet 4 inches apart.[6,12] Postural sway may vary with body morphology[26,27] and gender.[27] Some have proposed that sway may act as a pump to aid venous return.[8] Studies have shown that standing postural sway increases with fatigue[13-17] and may also increase in the context of low back pain,[18] increasing age,[19] stroke,[20,21] osteoporosis,[22] and alcohol consumption[19,23,24] and during the luteal phase of the menstrual cycle.[25] Sway may be minimized by intention,[28] lightly touching a stable object,[29,30] and by visual cues.[16,31,32] Postural sway is greater in unsupported sitting than in standing, although the amount of sway depends on the individual and the particular sitting position.[33] *Scoliosis* has not been found to affect postural sway,[34] whereas changes in respiration can affect postural sway, particularly in sitting.[35] Postural sway can increase until the person reaches his or her *limit of stability.* If the limits of stability are exceeded, one must take a step, reach for support, or risk a fall.[12]

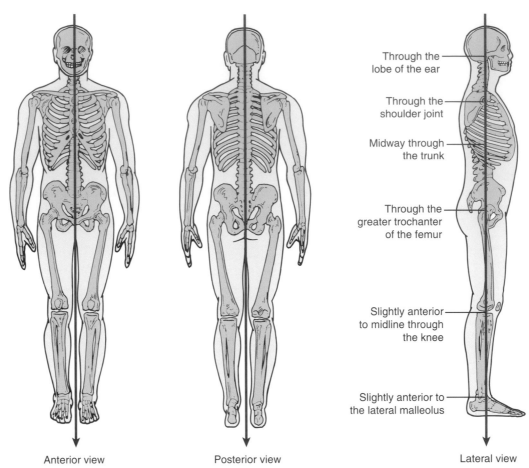

Through the lobe of the ear

Through the shoulder joint

Midway through the trunk

Through the greater trochanter of the femur

Slightly anterior to midline through the knee

Slightly anterior to the lateral malleolus

Anterior view   Posterior view   Lateral view

FIG. 4-2 Ideal standing posture. Anterior, posterior, and lateral views.

TABLE 4-1	Ideal Standing Posture from Anterior or Posterior View
Landmarks	**Ideal Alignment**
Eyes	Horizontally level.
Shoulders	Horizontally level. Superior angle slightly below the horizontal axis through T1.
Scapulae	Flat against the thorax, 30° anterior to the frontal plane, approximately 6 inches apart (or each approximately 3 inches from midline) with the medial border parallel to the spine.
Elbows	Neutral or slight *carrying angle* for males, slight to moderate carrying angle for females.
Wrists	Neutral. In neither flexion nor extension.
Hands	Face medially, toward the body.
Ribs and sternum	Ribs and the lateral contours of the rib cage symmetrical, the infrasternal angle is 90°.
Pelvis	ASISs and PSISs horizontally level.
Hips	In neutral rotation, neutral abduction and adduction.
Knees	The patellae face directly forward. Popliteal crease faces directly forward. Q angle approximately 13° in males and 18° in females.
Feet	Neither pronated nor supinated. Toes relaxed without varus or valgus. Calcaneus in mild valgus.
Spine	Vertically straight with occiput directly over sacrum.

Data from Kendall FP, McCreary EK, Provance PG: *Muscles: Testing and Function,* ed 4, Baltimore, 1993, Lippincott Williams & Wilkins; Sahrmann S: *Diagnosis and Treatment of Movement Impairment Syndromes,* St. Louis, 2002, Mosby; Winter D: *Biomechanics and Motor Control of Human Movement,* ed 3, New York, 2004, Wiley.
ASIS, Anterior superior iliac spine; *PSIS,* posterior superior iliac spine.

TABLE 4-2	Ideal Standing Posture from Side View
Landmarks	**Ideal Alignment**
Cervical spine	Slight lordosis. Supports head with minimal muscular effort without upward, downward, or sideways tilt, rotation, or retraction.
Humerus	Less than one third of humeral head anterior to anterior aspect of acromion. Proximal and distal ends are in the same (frontal) plane.
Elbow	Extension or slight flexion. Antecubital fossae face anteromedially and olecranon faces posteriorly.
Thoracic spine	Kyphosis 34° for adults and 38° for adolescents (average based on x-ray).
Ribs and sternum	Contours of ribcage symmetrical in frontal plane. No rotation of ribcage.
Lumbar spine	Lordosis 64° for adults and adolescents (average—based on x-ray).
Pelvis	ASISs in same vertical plane as pubic symphysis.
Knee	Knee is in neutral position: neither flexed nor hyperextended.
External auditory meatus, bodies of cervical vertebrae, midline of acromion, bodies of lumbar vertebrae, center of greater trochanter, point slightly anterior to midline at knee, point slightly anterior to lateral malleoli	All in vertical alignment.
Spine	Bodies of cervical vertebrae are in vertical alignment with bodies of lumbar vertebrae.

Data from Kendall FP, McCreary EK, Provance PG: *Muscles: Testing and Function,* ed 4, Baltimore, 1993, Lippincott, Williams & Wilkins; Sahrmann S: *Diagnosis and Treatment of Movement Impairment Syndromes,* St. Louis, 2002, Mosby; Winter D: *Biomechanics and Motor Control of Human Movement,* ed 3, New York, 2004, Wiley.
ASIS, Anterior superior iliac spine.

ANATOMICAL POSITION

Anatomical position is the specific alignment of the body used as the position of reference for describing the anatomical planes and axes. Although there are many possible ideal positions and postures, there is only one standard anatomical position. In anatomical position the body is erect with the head and torso upright. The arms are at the sides of the torso with the shoulders in neutral rotation, elbows extended, the cubital fossae of the elbow and the palms face forward, the fingers are extended, and the thumbs are adducted with the pad of each thumb facing forward. The lower extremities are straight and parallel, with the second toe facing straight forward (Fig. 4-3). From the anatomical position, three planes and three axes may be used to describe position, alignment, and motion of the body. In addition, the positions of the joints in anatomical position are considered the zero position for measurements of joint ROM for most joints.[4]

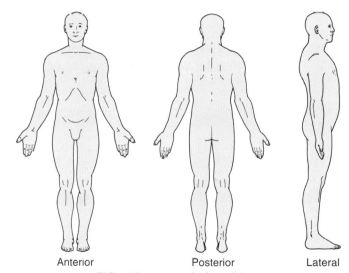

Anterior   Posterior   Lateral

FIG. 4-3 Anatomical position.

SITTING POSTURE

As with standing, there are many potential sitting postures. Sitting posture can be affected by where a person is sitting, the person's habits, and the task being performed.[37] According to Andersson, as originally described by Schoberth in 1962, there are three basic sitting postures when sitting in a chair: Anterior, middle, and posterior.[37] Anterior sitting, also known as *forward sitting,* is a posture with either anterior rotation of the pelvis or increased *kyphosis* of the spine so that more than 25% of the body's weight is transmitted through the feet to the floor and the center of gravity is anterior to the ischial tuberosities. *Middle sitting,* also known as erect sitting, is sitting with the center of gravity directly over the ischial tuberosities with approximately 25% of the body's weight transmitted through the feet to the floor. *Posterior sitting* is a posture in which the center of gravity is behind the ischial tuberosities and less than 25% of the body's weight is transmitted through the feet to the floor.[37]

Anterior sitting may be accomplished with minimal thigh support by placing the buttocks at the forward edge (front) of a chair (Fig. 4-4). This position is often used when the person is using his or her hands, such as with reaching, drafting, dentistry, and small equipment repair, as well as for eating, writing, or playing the piano. In this posture, if a desk, table, or other support surface allows, the arms can be used to take pressure off the pelvis. Within this posture, there are various ways to position the feet and the spine to balance the torso over the pelvis. *Active sitting* (described in detail later in this chapter) is an approach to anterior sitting that maintains balanced posture.[38]

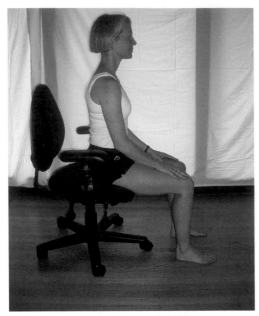

FIG. 4-4 Forward sitting.

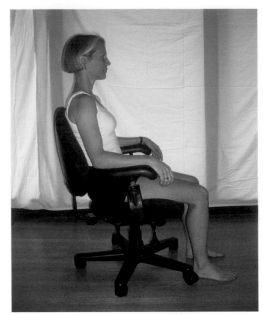

FIG. 4-6 Posterior sitting.

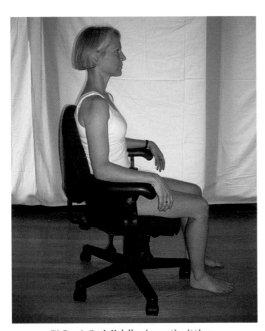

FIG. 4-5 Middle (erect) sitting.

Middle or erect sitting is generally accomplished with the thighs fully supported. The spine may be supported (with a backrest) or unsupported (without a backrest), depending on the task (Fig. 4-5). For posterior sitting, one may rotate the pelvis posteriorly and have a markedly kyphotic lumbar spine so that the spine balances above the pelvis. Alternatively, one may lean back or sit fully back in a chair with the spine supported by a slightly or markedly reclined backrest (Fig. 4-6). In posterior sitting with the spine supported by a backrest, the spine may be in neutral or kyphotic posture or any

posture in between the two that the particular backrest supports.

Intradiscal pressure may be affected by the choice of sitting posture.[37] Nachemson found that disc pressure was higher in specific postures of anterior sitting than in middle sitting and disc pressure in middle sitting, in turn, was greater than in posterior sitting.[39] Nachemson related the intradiscal pressure changes to mechanical changes within the disc itself and to back pain, suggesting that the positive relationship between the three provides a basis for the treatment of individuals with back pain.[39]

In addition to intradiscal pressure being higher in all sitting positions than in standing,[37] the primary difference between standing and any sitting posture is that sitting involves more flexion at the hips and knees. In most sitting postures, the pelvis rotates posteriorly and the lumbar *lordosis* reduces (or moves toward kyphosis).[40-43] The more acute the thigh-torso angle (also referred to as the thigh-trunk angle), the more the lumbar lordosis decreases.[44] When sitting with a thigh-torso angle of less than 90 degrees (i.e., with the hips below the knees), the lumbar lordosis typically reverses.[40] A kneeling (*Balans*) chair supports a greater thigh-torso angle (considerably greater than 90 degrees) than regular sitting chairs to more closely approximate standing and promote maintenance of the lumbar lordosis[45] (Fig. 4-7). Since the position of the rest of the torso may change in response to changes in the curvature of the lumbar spine, the position of the entire body should be considered when making adjustments to a patient's sitting posture.[46,47]

Studies have found that providing support for the lumbar spine when sitting can promote greater lordosis,[42,48] reduce intradiscal pressure,[37] and reduce low back pain.[49] Studies disagree about the effect of a forward-tilted[46,50,51] or a rearward-tilted[42,48] seat pan on sitting position and comfort[46,51,52] but agree that a reclined backrest

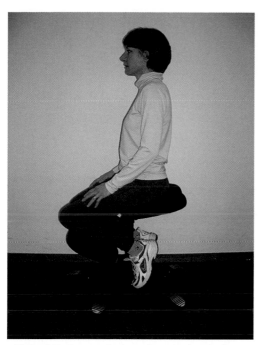

FIG. 4-7 Person in kneeling (Balans) chair.

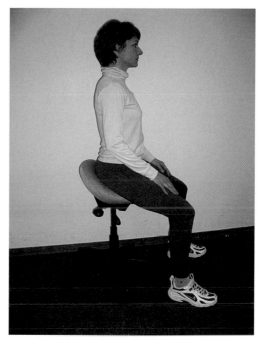

FIG. 4-8 Perching.

reduces both intradiscal pressure and pain.[49,53] Maintaining a similar lumbar lordosis in sitting as one maintains in standing is generally thought to be better than either a reduced lordosis or a kyphotic lumbar spine posture.[37,49] Changing position is thought by some to indicate discomfort[52] but is considered by others to improve comfort.[54] To decrease strain on the lumbar spine and reduce lumbar intradiscal pressure, many therapists recommend that the knees be lower than the hips and the backrest be reclined to produce an open (>90 degrees) thigh-torso angle to help maintain a lumbar lordosis when sitting. However, some individuals, particularly those with conditions such as spinal stenosis that are aggravated by lumbar extension, are more comfortable sitting with a reduced or even reversed lumbar lordosis.

For individuals who are more comfortable sitting with a lordosis (and for activities appropriate to anterior sitting), two postures have been recommended: perching and active sitting. These two postures are similar in many ways. "Perching" is sitting with an "open" thigh-torso angle by sitting at the forward edge of a seat, sitting on a seat that can tilt forward, sitting on a tall stool,[55] or sitting on a gym ball or a specialized chair (such as the Saddle Seat by Bambach or the Capisco by Hag) (Fig. 4-8). Cranz describes the ideal thigh-torso angle as being approximately 135 degrees, a position described as halfway between sitting and standing.[55] This angle corresponds to the position an individual (automatically) assumes when sidelying and the position an astronaut inherently assumes in a zero-gravity environment. Cranz notes that this angle is the same as that used to achieve stability and support in standing positions of martial arts and in the Alexander technique. The effect of sitting in this position has not been studied.

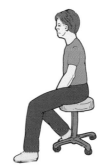

FIG. 4-9 Active sitting.

"Active" sitting is similar to perching but is described with more precise detail. Active sitting is performed with the lower extremity muscles actively supporting the sitting posture.[38] It is suggested that this posture is biomechanically better than other anterior sitting postures because it allows the spine to be in the neutral or ideal posture found in standing, uses muscles efficiently, and provides a wide base of support to stabilize the spine during static sitting, repetitive movement, and loading. Active sitting involves sitting at the front of the chair with the torso leaning forward, placing the center of gravity anterior to the ischial tuberosities[38] (Fig. 4-9). More specifically, the ischial tuberosities are positioned toward the front of the chair, the feet are anterior to the knees (or one foot is anterior to the knees and the other knee is flexed so that foot is under the torso with only the toes of that foot on the floor), the knees are lower than the hips, the pelvis is tilted slightly forward so that the torso has an apparent slight forward lean, and the lumbar lordosis is maintained in a posture similar to that in standing.

Bringing the torso forward moves weight from the ischial tuberosities to the feet, thereby reducing the activity of the lumbar erector spinae muscles. In addition, if performed with the correct balance, there is very little activity of the hip flexors. This position can easily be maintained with minimal energy expenditure and allows the torso to move in any direction through flexion, extension, abduction, or adduction of the hips and a concomitant shift in the weight-bearing emphasis of the feet and ischial tuberosities, while the spine maintains a relatively stable lordosis. The effects of this posture, as with perching, have not been reported in the peer-reviewed literature.

FORCES AFFECTING POSTURE

Both internal and external forces affect posture. Internal forces, including muscle activity and passive tension in fascia and tendons, must balance with external forces including gravity, inertia, and *ground reaction force* (GRF) for the body to maintain equilibrium.[6] All of these forces are discussed briefly in this chapter, except for inertia, which is only considered when an object is moving or accelerating. More detailed information on the forces affecting posture can be found in texts focusing on this subject.[1,4,9]

Although static posture does not involve significant active movement, active forces exert control over it. Postural control keeps the body's center of mass over its base of support and maintains stability against gravitational forces that could disrupt the upright position.[1,8,56] Postural control requires coordination between the CNS, the visual and vestibular systems, and the musculoskeletal system by using input from joint, muscle, and tendon receptors.[1,9,56] The CNS contributes to postural control by interpreting input from all sources and providing appropriate output to maintain equilibrium. To respond appropriately to this output the joints must have sufficient ROM and the muscles must have sufficient strength and coordination to respond to changes in forces acting on the body.[6] Postural adjustments may occur in response to feedback from unexpected external perturbations, as well as in a feed-forward manner in anticipation of expected self-generated perturbations.[56] Changes in either input or output may impair postural control. For example, postural control may be adversely affected by alterations in peripheral sensory input to the CNS as a result of diabetic neuropathy or by increased muscle response time (output) caused by aging.[6,56]

Gravity is a consistent and predictable force that acts on the human body. The body's *center of gravity* (COG) is the point about which gravity appears to act and the point about which all parts of the body exactly balance each other.[6,8] Although, because of differences in body size and proportions, the COG does not have exactly the same location in all individuals, it is always in the region of the pelvis when a person is standing in ideal neutral posture.[6,56] The COG for someone in neutral posture has been variously described as being located slightly anterior to the first or second sacral segment,[4] approximately at the level of the second sacral segment[6,10] anterior to the upper

part of the sacrum,[8] and in the region of the lower abdomen.[12] The closer the COG is to the center of base of support and the wider or larger the base of support the greater the stability.[8]

The *center of mass* (COM) is a theoretical point located at the exact center of the body's mass. The COM depends on the mass of each segment of the body and its location in space. The COG is the vertical projection (or the vertical component) of the body's COM.[1] In addition to gravitational forces, GRFs also affect static posture. GRFs are composed of three forces: A vertical force, a horizontal medial-lateral force, and a horizontal anteroposterior force. Because the horizontal forces during quiet standing are negligible, the GRF vector is approximately equal in magnitude but opposite in direction to the gravitational force in the erect static standing posture.[9,57] *Center of force* (COF), also known as center of pressure (COP), is the point on the supporting surface where the GRF acts and is the point from which the sway envelope is plotted (Fig. 4-10).[9,58]

Postural sway causes the *line of gravity* (LOG), a vertical line dropped from the body's COG, to move. This causes the forces acting about each joint to continually change even though a person appears to be standing still. When the LOG passes directly through a joint, no gravitational torque acts on that joint. When the LOG passes anterior to a joint, the resulting gravitational moment makes the segment proximal to the joint move anteriorly. For example, if the LOG passes anterior to the knee, the prox-

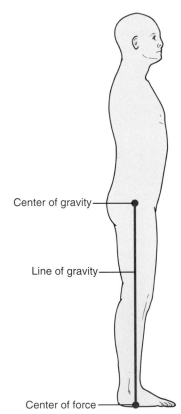

FIG. 4-10 Center of gravity (COG), line of gravity (LOG), and center of force (COF), also known as center of pressure.

Center of gravity

Line of gravity

Center of force

imal segment, the thigh, will move anteriorly, producing an extension moment at the knee. Similarly, if the LOG passes anterior to the hip, the proximal segment, the trunk, will move anteriorly, producing a flexion moment at the hip. When the LOG passes posterior to a joint, the resulting gravitational moment causes the proximal segment to move posteriorly, and when the line of gravity is lateral to the center of a joint, the segment proximal to the joint will move laterally (toward the LOG) to compensate.[59]

Changing position during activities of daily living (ADLs) or sports affects stability. If the COM moves outside the base of support, stability is reduced. This results in the individual having a greater likelihood of falling. Separating the feet increases stability by widening the base of support, lowering the COM, and making the LOG less likely to move outside the base of support. When moving through space, as with moving from sit to stand, reaching for an object or bending to wash one's hands, the COM moves in and out of the base of support, from a balanced to an unbalanced position and back again. To perform these movements the body needs postural control and dynamic stability.

When one adds a weight to the person in static standing posture, the COG is shifted toward that additional weight in proportion to its mass and its perpendicular distance from the LOG. For example, carrying a child on one's hip or carrying a suitcase in one hand shifts the COG to that side. To compensate, one may shift the hip to the ipsilateral side (the side on which the child is sitting, the arm in which the suitcase is carried) or may incline the body above the weight to the opposite side, or both, to bring the LOG closer to the center of the base of support (Fig. 4-11). Without this adjustment the additional weight could place excessive tension on certain muscle groups[8] or could cause a loss of balance as the LOG moved outside the base of support.[57]

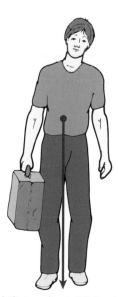

FIG. 4-11 Weight shift to adjust COG with load on one side.

PATHOLOGY

IMPAIRED POSTURE

Impaired or poor posture is posture that deviates from the ideal. Such deviations may have a variety of causes and effects. The causes of impaired posture may or may not be modifiable. Modifiable causes include changes in muscle length and strength, alterations in joint ROM, muscle spasm, and protective positioning due to pain or habit. Nonmodifiable causes of impaired posture include structural variations and damage to the basic components that maintain posture, including the bones, joints, muscles, and nervous system. Examples of structural variations include leg length discrepancy, fixed spinal scoliosis, and excessive femoral *anteversion*. Damage to the basic components that maintain posture may be caused by injury, such as a vertebral compression fracture, or diseases, such as rheumatoid arthritis or osteoarthritis. CNS disorders, such as cerebral palsy, traumatic brain injury, or stroke, may also result in impaired posture because the changes that they may cause in muscle tone, strength, and sensation may prevent attainment of ideal alignment (Table 4-3).

It is proposed, with fair support from current evidence, that modifiable postural impairments are caused by changes in muscle length and strength that result from lack of variety in movements and positions or the frequent performance of repetitive activities.[4,40] Fig. 4-12 illustrates the basic structure of skeletal muscle. Muscles are complex cells[60] (see Chapter 5 for a detailed description of skeletal muscle structure and function). Each skeletal muscle fiber is a cell with a nucleus, mitochondria, endoplasmic reticulum, ribosomes, and other organelles. Muscle fibers are cylindrical and have diameters that vary from approximately 10 to 100 µm, depending on their strength. Each muscle fiber is composed of thousands of myofibrils, and each myofibril is composed of sarcomeres. Sarcomeres are arranged end-to-end within each myofibril. The number of sarcomeres in a muscle fiber changes according to the length and diameter of the muscle fiber. The total number and arrangement of the sarcomeres within a muscle fiber are the most important determinants of the function of the muscle.

As a muscle strengthens, it gets bigger (hypertrophies) by adding more sarcomeres arranged parallel to the length of the muscle fibers. As a muscle lengthens, more sarcomeres are added in series. Immobilization of muscles in lengthened or shortened positions has been shown to cause sarcomeres to be added or lost in series, respectively. Four weeks of immobilization in a lengthened position, for example, was shown to cause the number of sarcomeres to increase by approximately 20% without any change in the length of each individual sarcomere within the lengthened muscle.[61,62]

Muscles are thought to have an ideal length and thus an ideal number of sarcomeres for optimal function and maximal force generation.[63] Shortened muscles, produced by prolonged immobilization in a shortened position, have also been shown to be stiffer (the definition of stiffness is increased tension per change in length)[63] and more

TABLE 4-3	Common Variations from Ideal Alignment
Body Area	**Variations**
Spine	Forward head, excessive kyphosis, excessive lordosis, kyphosis lordosis, swayback (hips anterior to the line of gravity, posterior pelvic tilt and reduced lordosis), flat back, scoliosis.
Rib cage and sternum	Asymmetry of the rib cage in the frontal or sagittal planes, barrel chest, *pectus excavatum* (also referred to as recurvatum), *pectus carinatum* (also referred to as *gallinatum*), increase or decrease in the infrasternal angle from 90°.
Scapulae	Elevation, depression, upward tilt, downward tilt, abduction, adduction, winging, anterior tilt
Shoulder	Forward shoulder, depressed shoulder, abduction, medial rotation, lateral rotation, flexion, extension, elevated humeral head, subluxed humeral head, humeral head more than 50% anterior to the anterior aspect of the acromion.
Elbow	Flexion, hyperextension, excessive carrying angle.
Forearm	Pronation, supination.
Wrist	Flexion, extension, ulnar deviation, *radial deviation*.
Hand/Fingers	Ulnar drift, boutonnière deformity, swan neck deformity.
Hip/Femur	Femoral anteversion (ante-torsion), femoral *retroversion* (retrotorsion), coxa vara, coxa valgum, femoral medial rotation, femoral lateral rotation.
Knee	Flexion, hyperextension, Q angle greater than 13° for males, greater than 18° for females, *patella alta, patella baja,* "squinting" *patella*.
Tibia	Tibial medial torsion, tibial lateral torsion, tibial varum.
Feet	*Pes planus, pes cavus,* calcaneal varum, excessive *calcaneal valgus*.
Toes	Hallux valgus, hammer toes, claw toe(s), mallet toe(s), overlapping toe(s), Morton's toe, bunion(s).

resistant to passive stretching than normal length muscles.[61,62,64]

After muscles are immobilized in either lengthened or shortened positions, they produce the strongest contractions at a length very close to that at which they were immobilized.[61,62] This has led investigators to conclude that a muscle adjusts its number of sarcomeres to reset ideal length to that at which it was immobilized, and that muscles adjust and optimize their number of sarcomeres in series in response to the length imposed by their most common positions.[63]

Kendall proposes that postural alignment is affected by muscle length and muscle strength and that muscles that are shorter or longer than their ideal length may cause postural deviations.[4] Muscle shortness may bring parts too close together to allow for ideal alignment, and prevent sufficient lengthening to allow for full ROM. For example, an excessively short and stiff rectus femoris could pull the anterior inferior iliac spine toward the femur, producing an anterior pelvic tilt (if *antagonist muscles* such as the hamstrings, which would prevent anterior pelvic tilt, are not similarly short and stiff) (Fig. 4-13). Similarly, a stiff or short rectus abdominis could produce a posterior pelvic tilt, a depressed ribcage, an excessively flexed thoracic spine, or any combination of these, depending on the influence of synergistic muscles and the opposing influence of antagonist muscles (Fig. 4-14).

Excessive muscle length may allow parts of the body to which the muscle(s) are attached to separate or move too far apart. For example, a lengthened serratus anterior may allow adduction and/or downward tilt of the scapula because of the unopposed pull of the shorter rhomboids (Fig. 4-15).[40]

It is commonly thought that a range of conditions may also affect posture. Muscle spasm or contracture may have similar effects to muscle shortening. For example, a functional scoliosis may develop as the result of unilateral paravertebral muscle spasm. Postural changes, including increased lumbar lordosis, anterior pelvic tilt, and posterior positioning of the head, are common during pregnancy and are thought to be related to changes in weight distribution, muscle length, and ligament laxity (Fig. 4-16).[65] Osteoporosis, aging, and ankylosing spondylitis are associated with increased thoracic kyphosis (Fig. 4-17).[66-68] Respiratory diseases are also associated with changes in posture, such as a *barrel chest*, which is associated with chronic obstructive pulmonary disease (COPD).

Although there are no published studies on postural asymmetries associated with hand dominance, in clinical practice it is often found that hand dominance correlates with a typical pattern of left-right postural asymmetry that precludes ideal alignment (Fig. 4-18). The shoulder on the dominant side is commonly slightly lower than the non-dominant shoulder and the hip on the dominant side is slightly higher than the nondominant hip (as a result of the relatively stronger dominant side muscles of the torso). It is thought that the unequal pulls caused by this dominance result in deviation of the spine away from the dominant side. The higher dominant side hip results in relative adduction of the hip on the dominant side and relative abduction of the hip on the nondominant side. This, in turn, results in an apparent leg-length discrepancy, with the dominant leg appearing to be longer than the nondominant leg, and pronation of the nondominant foot. Hand dominance is thought to begin during early childhood, long before the musculoskeletal system matures.[4]

Good posture is thought to contribute to optimal functioning of the human movement system, whereas poor or faulty posture is thought to contribute to pain or dysfunction. It has also been suggested that persistent postural faults may cause pain, dysfunction, and disability.[4] There are limited data, however, to support these assertions. One study found that posture contributes to subacromial impingement syndrome,[69] and two studies implicate posture in relation to carpal tunnel dysfunc-

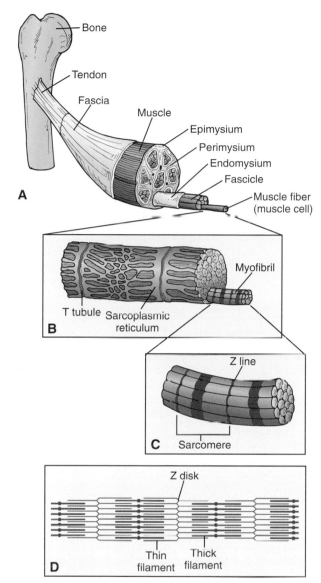

A, Skeletal muscle

FIG. 4-12 Structure of skeletal muscle. **A,** Skeletal muscle organ, composed of bundles of contractile muscle fibers held together by connective tissue. **B,** Greater magnification of single fiber showing small fibers, myofibrils in the sarcoplasm. **C,** Myofibril magnified further to show sarcomere between successive Z lines. Cross striae are visible. **D,** Molecular structure of myofibril showing thick myofilaments and thin myofilaments.

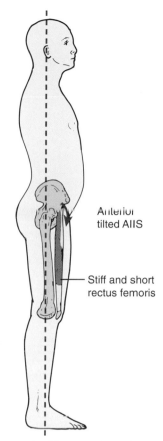

FIG. 4-13 Short and stiff rectus femoris producing an anterior pelvic tilt.

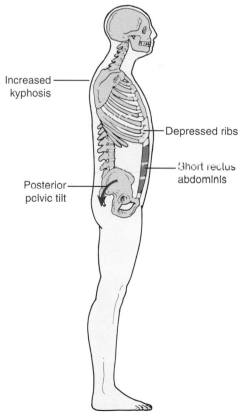

FIG. 4-14 Short rectus abdominis producing a posterior pelvic tilt.

tion.[70,71] One study identified a correlation between back pain and posture,[72] whereas two others found no correlation between acute or chronic back pain and posture.[73,74] Another study found no correlation between pain with pregnancy and posture.[65] Clearly, more research on this topic is needed.

Kendall proposed that there are three commonly observed types of impaired posture: *Kyphosis-lordosis, swayback,* and *flatback* (Fig. 4-19). These postures describe not only certain spinal postures but also an overall alignment. Hallmarks of kyphosis-lordosis posture include increased lumbar lordosis and thoracic kyphosis, anterior pelvic tilt (anterior superior iliac spines [ASIS] anterior to pubic symphysis), and forward head. Associated faulty

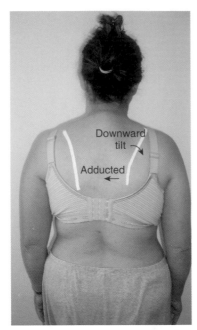

FIG. 4-15 Scapular adduction and downward tilt.

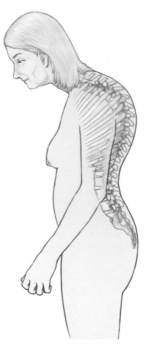

FIG. 4-17 Excessive thoracic kyphosis as a result of osteoporosis and spinal compression fractures.

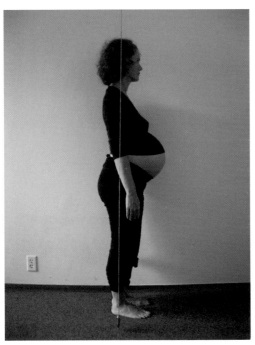

FIG. 4-16 Pregnant woman. Note increased lumbar lordosis, anterior pelvic tilt, and posterior position of the head.

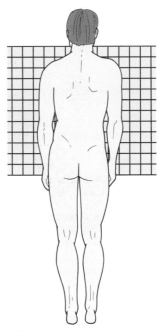

FIG. 4-18 Postural change due to handedness. Typical left hand–dominant posture.

joint postures may include abducted scapulae, forward shoulders, and either knee flexion or hyperextension (genu recurvatum). The hallmarks of flatback posture include reduced lumbar lordosis, posterior pelvic tilt (ASIS posterior to the pubic symphysis), and hip and knee hyperextension. It is common to find reductions of thoracic kyphosis, cervical lordosis, and the gluteal prominence in individuals with flatback posture. Swayback posture, like flatback posture, is characterized by a reduced lumbar lordosis and a posterior pelvic tilt, but in contrast to the flatback posture, in swayback posture the hips are anterior to the humeral heads and the lateral malleoli. It is common to find genu recurvatum, increased thoracic kyphosis, and abducted scapulae associated with swayback posture. Swayback is often mistaken for excessive lumbar lordosis because the anterior position of the lumbar-pelvic region may give the appearance of an increased lumbar lordosis, but these postures are easily

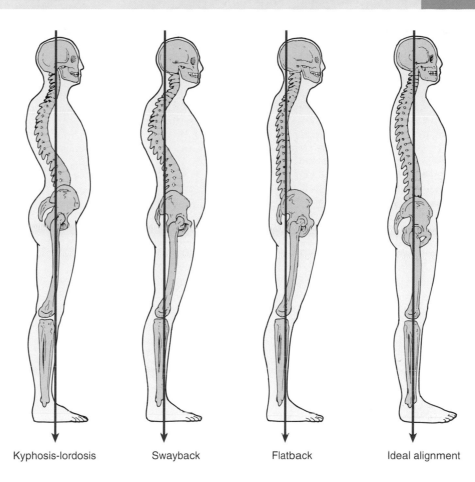

| Kyphosis-lordosis | Swayback | Flatback | Ideal alignment |

FIG. 4-19 Faulty postures: Kyphosis-lordosis, swayback, and flatback compared with ideal alignment.

differentiated by checking the alignment of the malleoli, greater trochanters, and humeral heads.[4] In all of these faulty spinal postures, kyphosis-lordosis, flatback, and swayback, forward positioning of the head, commonly known as "forward head posture," is present.[4] This is supported by a study by Christie et al, which demonstrated that at least in patients with acute low back pain, forward head posture is associated with increased thoracic kyphosis.[72]

EXAMINATION

PATIENT HISTORY

The patient history is the first component of the examination and should provide the therapist with an understanding of the patient's perception of the condition, as well as the chronology, extent, and severity of the symptoms, and the resultant physical limitations. Because impaired posture is most often addressed as a portion of a larger set of signs or symptoms, the history should address all components of the problem. From this information the therapist can begin to develop hypotheses to guide the rest of the examination, as well as the evaluation and interventions.

For the patient with impaired posture, the history should include information about the nature, location, severity, progression, and duration of symptoms, as well as information about the patient's current and past functional abilities.

SYSTEMS REVIEW

The systems review is used to target areas requiring further examination and to define areas that may cause complications or indicate a need for precautions during the examination and intervention processes. See Chapter 1 for details of the systems review.

TESTS AND MEASURES

After the patient history and systems review, specific tests and measures should be performed to rule in or rule out diagnoses suggested by these earlier components of the examination. For the experienced clinician, tests and measures related to posture begin the moment the patient presents. It is particularly helpful for the therapist to begin observation when the patient is unaware that the examination has begun. In this circumstance the patient is likely to be much more relaxed and in his or her "usual" posture. The therapist observes the patient's posture as he or she walks in and sits down to participate in the interview and during the interview itself. Although specific tests and measures are described here, the therapist can observe the patient's general appearance, height, body build, initial functional status, obvious postural deviations, and particularities of positioning while obtaining the history and performing the systems review. The therapist can also observe whether the patient uses an assistive device and whether the patient demonstrates guarding, limitation of movement, or compensatory movements.

Specific tests and measures related to posture begin with inspection or observation. Although tests and measures are described in the standard sequence used throughout this book, in the clinical setting, tests may be grouped together by patient position for the convenience of the patient and the clinician. Standing is a good position to begin the examination. After completing tests performed with the patient standing, the clinician may progress to tests performed in sitting and then lying.

Musculoskeletal

Posture. Postural assessment is typically the first component of the tests and measures for any patient with a musculoskeletal dysfunction. The therapist observes the patient from the front, the back, and the sides, ideally with the patient standing near a plumb line for vertical reference for each view and with the clinician positioned to be able to see the patient's entire body. The plumb line is used as a reference from which deviations from ideal alignment may be noted (see Fig. 4-2). It can be made from a rope or string with a weight (plumb bob) at the bottom and may be suspended from the ceiling or other fixed point. It is positioned between the examiner and the patient, in close proximity to the patient, and is aligned with a fixed point on the patient's body. If no plumb line is available, the patient may stand in front of a grid of evenly spaced horizontal and vertical lines or the clinician may imagine a vertical line against which posture may be evaluated.

In standing posture with the feet on the floor, the feet are the only fixed points. When observing from the anterior or posterior view, the plumb line should be aligned with a point midway between the feet and should divide the patient equally into left and right halves. This point represents the base of the midsagittal plane of the body.[4] Because the plumb line is aligned with the midplanes, it may aide the examiner in visualizing the LOG. Visual observation of how an individual's anatomical landmarks line up in relation to the plumb line yields information about postural alignment, including the extent to which the individual is in ideal alignment and where alignment is faulty.[4,6]

When observing the patient from the anterior view, the therapist should first scan from bottom to top to observe overall shape and alignment. Observe how far apart the feet are positioned, the alignment and positioning of the toes and for the presence of high or low arches. The tibiae should be looked at for alignment. At the knees, check patellar position, check the knee joints for *varus* or *valgus* alignment, and check the *Q angle* at the hip. Observe the hips and pelvis and step in closer to palpate the greater trochanters, ASIS, and iliac crests to determine if they are level. The torso should be observed for symmetry, and then the therapist should check the alignment of the shoulders, the neck, and the head.

When observing the patient from behind, the plumb line should divide the patient equally into left and right halves. Observe how far apart the feet are positioned, the position of the calcaneus, tibial alignment, knee varus or valgus, the relative height of the popliteal creases, and the rotation of the femurs. Observe the hips and pelvis checking that greater trochanters, PSIS, and iliac crests are level. Observe the torso for symmetry and check the alignment of the shoulders, neck, and head.

When observing the patient from the side, the plumb line should be aligned slightly anterior to the lateral malleolus. In ideal alignment the plumb line should bisect the body, with the point where the line touches the ground representing the base of the midcoronal plane. First scan from the feet to the head for an overview of the entire body and observe whether there is a forward or rearward lean. The plumb line should pass just slightly anterior to the midline of the knee, through the greater trochanter, through the bodies of the lumbar vertebrae (a line approximately bisecting the trunk), through the middle of the acromion, through the bodies of the cervical vertebrae (a line approximately bisecting the neck), through the external auditory meatus, and slightly posterior to the apex of the coronal suture. From this perspective, observe the shape of the spine. It may also be helpful to palpate the spine from the occiput to the sacrum because a tilt of the head or hypertrophied trapezii or levator scapulae may provide a misleading visual impression of the shape of the cervical spine. Likewise, a rotation of the ribcage may give one a mistaken impression of the shape or position of the thoracic spine. Hypertrophied erector spinae or a rotation as a result of scoliosis may also create a mistaken impression of the shape of the lumbar curve and again indicate a need to palpate the spine rather than relying on visual inspection alone. The clinician should consider whether the patient falls into a common category of faulty posture, kyphosis-lordosis, swayback, or flatback as previously described.

Posture is evaluated relative to ideal alignment. Postural deviations from ideal are described in terms of how the body parts have moved away from that ideal posture to achieve their current position. Anatomical position is used as the reference position from which anatomical planes and axes, as well as expressions of ROM of individual joints or parts, are described. The movements of the body, occurring in a plane about an axis, are described here in detail, using specific terminology.

The terms used to describe movements and positions of the body are based on the principle that movements occur in a plane around a given axis. For the sake of clarity, these planes and axes of reference are described briefly here. There are three types of planes and axes of reference: sagittal, frontal (or coronal), and transverse (or horizontal) planes (Fig. 4-20) and sagittal, coronal, and longitudinal axes. A sagittal plane passes from front to back (or back to front, the plane does not have a direction). The midsagittal plane passes through the midline of the body dividing it into left and right halves. A coronal plane passes from side to side, dividing the body into front and back. A horizontal plane divides the body into top and bottom portions. For each plane, there are an infinite number of possible parallel planes and only one midplane. The point at which the three midplanes intersect is the center of gravity of the body. The line of gravity is the vertical line formed by the intersection of the midsagittal and midfrontal planes.[4,8] Movements occur in a plane and around (or about) an axis that is perpendicular to

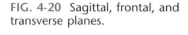

FIG. 4-20 Sagittal, frontal, and transverse planes.

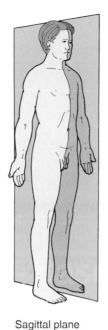
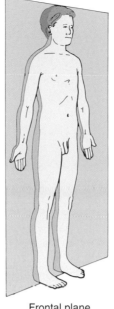
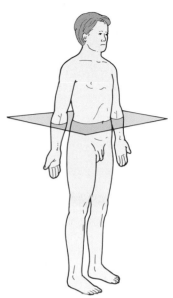
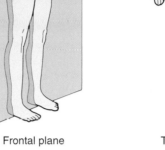

Sagittal plane   Frontal plane   Transverse plane

that plane (Fig. 4-20). Shoulder flexion, for example, occurs in a sagittal plane that passes through the shoulder joint.[8]

Axes are imaginary lines through the body at right angles to each other. A sagittal axis passes through the body from front to back. Movements of abduction and adduction occur in a coronal plane about a sagittal axis. For example, shoulder abduction occurs in a coronal plane about a sagittal axis (the coronal plane passes through the humeral head from side to side and the sagittal axis passes through the humeral head from back to front). Flexion and extension occur in a sagittal plane about a coronal axis. Shoulder flexion, for example, occurs in a sagittal plane about a coronal axis that passes from one humeral head to the other. The third axis, the longitudinal axis, passes from top to bottom when passing through the trunk and from proximal to distal when passing through an extremity. Rotation and horizontal adduction and abduction occur in a transverse plane around a longitudinal axis. Shoulder rotation occurs in a transverse plane about a longitudinal axis that extends along the center of the humerus.

Joint Positions and Motions

Flexion and Extension. As just noted, flexion and extension are movements in the sagittal plane about a coronal axis. Flexion can also be described as rotation of a bony lever around a joint to approximate the ventral surfaces (for most joints). When flexed, the distal components joined at the shoulders, elbows, wrists, fingers, and hips and the proximal components joined at the neck and torso are anterior to their anatomical or ideal position. Flexion of the knees and toes moves the distal components posteriorly. Extension is a motion of joints in the opposite direction to flexion. Anterior motion of the foot at the ankle (flexion) is called dorsiflexion. Posterior motion of the foot around the ankle (extension) is called plantarflexion. Flexion and extension of the thumb occur

in the metacarpophalangeal and interphalangeal joints and are movements in an ulnar and radial direction, respectively. Hyperextension is extension beyond the normal range or position of extension. A part may be described as being in flexion, if it is in a flexed position relative to ideal alignment, or as being in extension, if it is in an extended position relative to ideal alignment.

Abduction and Adduction. Abduction is a movement where the distal portion of a segment of the body moves away from the midline in the frontal plane about a sagittal axis. Abduction may also be used to describe a motion in which the distal portion of a segment of the body moves away from the midline in the horizontal plane about a longitudinal axis and is then referred to as horizontal abduction. Adduction is the opposite of abduction and is thus a movement of the distal component toward the midline of the body. An exception to this rule is when the torso or head moves in the frontal plane away from midline, which is referred to as lateral flexion (or sidebending) rather than abduction. Abduction of the fingers is a spreading apart of the fingers from the center of the third digit, and adduction of the fingers is a movement toward the same point. Abduction and adduction of the thumb take place at the carpometacarpal joint in a plane perpendicular to the plane of the palm. Adduction is a movement of the thumb toward the palm, and abduction is a move away from the palm. Abduction and adduction of the toes takes place around a line through the center of the second toe. Abduction may also describe the posture of a part of the body positioned farther away from midline than in ideal alignment, whereas adduction describes a part positioned closer to midline than ideal.

Rotation. Rotation describes turning about a longitudinal axis. Rotation occurs about a longitudinal axis in the transverse plane for all areas of the head and torso except the clavicles and the scapulae. The clavicles rotate about a coronal axis in the sagittal plane. The scapulae, which

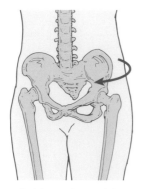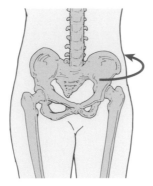

Pelvic rotation to right   Pelvic rotation to left

FIG. 4-21 Rotation of the pelvis to the right and left.

lie flush with the ribcage and as such are not in the frontal plane, rotate about a sagittal axis in a plane approximately 30 degrees anterior from the frontal plane. Rotation of the neck or pelvis is generally described as to the right or left (Fig. 4-21). Rotation of the pelvis may also be described as clockwise or counterclockwise. Rotation of the extremities occurs about an axis through the length of the long bone in that segment, with the exception of the femur. Rotation of the femur is described around an axis that connects the center of the femoral head with the center of the knee joint.[4] Extremity rotation is described as medial or internal rotation when the rotation is toward the midline, and lateral or external rotation when the rotation is away from the midline. Internal rotation may be used to describe the posture of a part of the body positioned with more rotation toward midline and external rotation may be used to describe the posture of a part of the body positioned with more rotation away from midline compared to ideal alignment.

Tilt. Tilt may describe movements of the head, pelvis, or scapulae. The head and pelvis may be tilted anteriorly, posteriorly, or laterally. The scapulae tilt anteriorly. In addition, when there is weakness, the scapulae may tilt so that the spinal border of the scapula moves away from the ribcage. This is called *scapular winging*. Anterior tilt of the head is a forward movement of the head accompanied by flexion or flattening of the cervical spine. Posterior tilt of the head is a rearward movement of the head accompanied by cervical extension or increased lordosis. Lateral tilt of the head is a sideways movement (also called lateral flexion) that is accompanied by sidebending and rotation of the cervical spine to the same side as the head. In the pelvis, anterior tilt is a downward movement of the ASISs and an accompanying upward movement of the posterior superior iliac spines (PSISs). Anterior pelvic tilt is accompanied by extension of the lumbar spine or an increase in the lumbar lordosis. Posterior pelvic tilt is an upward movement of the ASISs and an accompanying downward movement of the PSISs, which occur along with flexion, or flattening of the lumbar spine. In describing posture, the head or pelvis may be described as being in a position of anterior, posterior, or lateral tilt relative to ideal alignment, and the scapulae may be described as being in an anterior tilt or to have winging.

Protraction and Retraction. Protraction and *retraction* are terms often used to describe anterior and posterior movements at the sternoclavicular joint. These terms may also be used to describe movements of the scapulae; however, the more specific terms of abduction and adduction are recommended.[4]

Elevation and Depression. Elevation and depression are terms used to describe upward and downward gliding of the scapulae. In describing posture, a scapula may be described to be elevated or depressed if it is in a position that is elevated or depressed relative to ideal alignment.

Gliding. Gliding describes a sliding motion usually of a flat or slightly curved surface relative to another surface. This term is most often used to describe the arthrokinematic motions that occur within a joint, rather than the osteokinematic motions that are described in this chapter and as such will not be further described here.

Positions and Motions of Specific Joints. Most positions and movements of the body can be described using the previous terms; however, certain joints move or can be positioned in unique ways and are then described with unique terms. General, as well as unique, joint movements and positions are listed in Table 4-4.

Positions and Motions of the Spine. The position of the spine is critical to the examination of posture and is therefore described in additional detail here. There are a number of unique terms used to describe spinal position and posture. These include lordosis, kyphosis, and scoliosis. Lordosis is a curve that is convex anteriorly. The cervical spine and lumbar spine have a lordosis in the ideal standing position. Kyphosis is a curve that is convex posteriorly. The thoracic spine has a kyphosis in the ideal standing position. These normal curves of the spine, especially lumbar lordosis, are essential for maintaining upright posture.[75] Scoliosis is a lateral curvature of the spine. It is not normal to have any scoliosis, and therefore scoliosis is not considered a normal spinal curvature (Fig. 4-22). A scoliosis may be present in any portion of the spine. It may be confined to one portion of the spine or may extend through two or more portions of the spine. It may be a single C curve that is convex to the right or left or a "double" curve (also known as an S curve). Less frequently, scoliosis may have more than two curves.

Movements and positions of the spine as a whole include flexion, extension, side bending (lateral flexion), and rotation. Flexion of the spine is a forward movement in the sagittal plane. In the cervical and lumbar spine, flexion first flattens the normal lordotic curve and then reverses the direction of this curve. In the thoracic spine, flexion increases the normally kyphotic curve. Extension of the spine is backward movement in the sagittal plane that increases the lordosis of the cervical and lumbar spine and flattens the kyphosis of the thoracic spine. Lateral flexion is sidebending movement of the head or torso to the right or left in the coronal plane. There is less lateral flexion possible in the thoracic spine than in the cervical and lumbar spine because the ribcage restricts thoracic motion in this direction. Spinal rotation occurs in the transverse plane. In the neck, rotation is described as rota-

TABLE 4-4	Joint Positions and Movements
Joint	**Positions and Movements**
Sternoclavicular	Protraction, retraction, elevation, depression, upward rotation, downward rotation.
Glenohumeral	Flexion, extension, abduction, adduction, medial rotation, lateral rotation, horizontal abduction, horizontal adduction, *circumduction.*
Acromioclavicular	Protraction, retraction, gliding.
Scapulothoracic	Elevation, depression, abduction, adduction, anterior tilt, upward (or superior) rotation, downward (or inferior) rotation.
Elbow	Flexion, extension.
Radioulnar	Pronation (medial rotation of forearm—the palm faces posteriorly), supination (lateral rotation of the forearm—the palm faces anteriorly).
Wrist	Flexion, extension, adduction (or ulnar deviation), abduction (or radial deviation), circumduction.
Carpometacarpal	Gliding. Between trapezium and first metacarpal: Flexion, extension, abduction, adduction, slight rotation, circumduction, and opposition. Between hamate and fifth metacarpal: Flexion, extension, and slight rotation.
Metacarpophalangeal (MP)	Flexion, extension, abduction, adduction, circumduction. Thumb MP: Flexion, extension, slight abduction, adduction, and rotation.
Interphalangeal	Flexion, extension.
Pelvis	Anterior tilt, posterior tilt, lateral tilt, rotation.
Hip	Flexion, extension, abduction, adduction, medial rotation, lateral rotation, circumduction.
Knee	Flexion and extension with slight medial and lateral rotation in relation to femur during flexion and extension.
Ankle	Flexion (plantarflexion) and extension (dorsiflexion).
Subtalar and transverse tarsal joints	Supination, pronation, abduction, *inversion* (combination of adduction and supination), *eversion* (combination of abduction and pronation).
Tarso-metatarsal	Gliding.
Metatarsophalangeal	Flexion, extension, abduction, adduction.
Interphalangeal	Flexion, extension.
Spine	Flexion, extension, sidebending (lateral flexion), rotation.

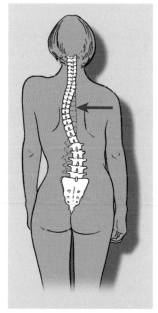

FIG. 4-22 Scoliosis. *From Thibodeau GA, Patton KT: Anatomy and Physiology, ed 6, St. Louis, 2006, Mosby.*

tion to the right or to the left and is determined by the direction that the face has turned. In the torso, rotation is described as clockwise (left side forward) or counterclockwise (right side forward). Lateral flexion and rotation of the spine occur together as coupled movements. As a result, scoliosis always has both sidebending and rotational components. In some segments of the spine, rota-

tion occurs in the same direction as the lateral flexion. In other spine segments, rotation occurs in the opposite direction from the side bend. (See Chapter 8 for a discussion of coupled movements.) The same terms used to describe spinal movements may also be used as with other parts of the body to describe the position of the spine relative to ideal alignment.

Alignment by Region. In ideal alignment (see Fig. 4-2), the lower extremities are in the optimal position for weight bearing. The pelvis is in neutral, allowing it to support the abdomen and spine in an optimal position while also assisting in the proper positioning of the lower extremities. The cervical spine is positioned vertically above the lumbar spine, with the spinal lumbar and thoracic curves supporting the ribcage in a position that permits optimal functioning of the cardiopulmonary organs. The head is balanced in the center of the torso so that minimal activity is required of the neck muscles. The following section describes ideal alignment in standing by region.

Ankle. The ankle should be in 0 degrees dorsiflexion (and 0 degrees plantarflexion), and from a lateral view. the line of reference should pass just anterior to the lateral malleolus.[4,6] Because the LOG passes anterior to the joint line, there is a dorsiflexion moment. The gastrocnemius and soleus therefore work to prevent forward motion of the tibia when standing in ideal alignment.

Knee. From a lateral view, the line of reference passes slightly anterior to the center of the knee joint. Because the LOG passes anterior to the joint line, there is an extension moment at this joint. The hamstrings therefore work to prevent hyperextension of the knee.

Hip. From a lateral view, the line of reference passes slightly posterior to the hip joint and nearly directly through the center of the greater trochanter. Because the LOG passes posterior to the joint line, there is an extension moment at this joint. The quadriceps and other hip flexors therefore work to prevent posterior rotation of the pelvis.

Pelvis. In ideal alignment, the ASISs are in the same coronal plane as the symphysis pubis. Opposing pulls of muscles on the ASISs and pubic symphysis help maintain this position. Anteriorly the rectus abdominis pulls the pelvis superiorly, while the gracilis and adductor longus pull the pelvis inferiorly. The external abdominal oblique, internal abdominal oblique, and transversus abdominis stabilize the ASISs from above, while the rectus femoris, tensor fascia lata, and sartorius stabilize from below. Posteriorly, the erector spinae and quadratus lumborum pull superiorly and the hamstrings pull inferiorly.

Shoulder. From a lateral view, the plumb line passes approximately through the center of the acromion process. According to Sahrmann, the humeral head should be positioned so that no more than 25% of its diameter is anterior to the anterior-most portion of the acromion.[40]

Peterson et al found that four techniques for measuring forward shoulder posture demonstrated clinical reliability with intraclass correlation coefficient (ICC) for intrarater reliability ranging from 0.89 to 0.91.[76] These techniques however, were unable to demonstrate validity when the measurements were compared with a radiographic measurement. Interrater reliability was not assessed nor was the ability of this measure to detect postural changes over time. The techniques included the use of a Baylor square, a double square, the "Sahrmann technique," and measurement of scapular position with a tape measure. The Baylor square, which is a carpenter's square adapted specifically for the Peterson study, measures the distance between the posterior aspect of the C7 spinous process and the anterior acromion. The double square is a modified 12-inch combination square with a second square/level mounted in an inverted position also adapted specifically for this study. It measures the distance from the wall to the anterior acromion with the subject standing with his back against the wall. The Sahrmann technique is a measure of maximum shoulder flexion achieved with full shoulder external rotation with the subject standing with his back against a wall and the arm flexed at the elbow, and the hand, elbow, and shoulder all in the same (sagittal) plane. The fourth technique, scapular position as measured with a tape measure, was the horizontal distance from the third thoracic spinous process to the medial border of the scapula. Despite the positive findings of this study, there has been no standard measurement of forward shoulder posture described in the literature. In addition it is not known whether the described measures of shoulder posture are sensitive enough to detect changes.[76]

Spine. From the posterior view, the spine should be vertically straight. The center of the occiput should be aligned with the center of the sacrum. From the lateral view, the spinal curves should be such that the bodies of the cervical vertebrae align vertically with the bodies of the lumbar spine. Those vertebral bodies should also be aligned with the external auditory meatus and the center

of the humeral head, and a vertical line continuing inferiorly should fall just posterior to the center of the hip joint, just anterior to the knee joint, and just anterior to the lateral malleolus.

Various other criteria for ideal spinal alignment have been proposed. One such criterion suggests that, in standing, the C7 vertebral body aligns with (or is just posterior to) the S1 vertebral body.[75] Pelvic alignment has been proposed to be one of the most essential elements for assuming and maintaining ideal alignment of the spine and other body parts; alignment thereof is considered to be ideal when the ASISs are in the same coronal plane as the pubic symphysis.[4,10,40] Yasukouchi found a high correlation between pelvic tilt and lumbar lordosis.[41] This is probably because pelvic alignment and the angle of inclination of the sacrum and L5 are tied together by the ligamentous tension of the sacrotuberous, sacrospinous, and iliolumbar ligaments. Soderberg asserts that the angle of inclination of the sacrum determines the position of the last lumbar vertebra, which in turn determines the position of the rest of the lumbar spine and subsequently, the entire spine, because the curves must balance with the LOG and therefore with each other.[10]

Following the examination of posture in standing, the clinician may also observe the patient's sitting posture. This examination should focus on deviations from ideal sitting posture and should include observation of where in the chair the patient sits, the tilt of the pelvis, and the alignment of the spine. The clinician should also note if and how the patient uses the backrest of the chair, as well as how and where the feet are positioned.

Range of Motion. For patients whose postural examination reveals impairment, ROM measurements of the cervical, thoracic, and lumbar spine and involved peripheral joints should be performed. ROM measurements are necessary to determine whether the patient has sufficient range available to be able to assume ideal, or at least more ideal, posture. ROM measurement technique is covered in detail in other texts.[77]

Muscle Performance. For patients with impaired posture, strength should be measured in the involved areas using manual muscle tests (see Chapter 5). Strength is measured to determine whether the patient has sufficient strength to assume an ideal posture, or at least a posture that more closely resembles ideal.

EVALUATION, DIAGNOSIS, AND PROGNOSIS

Evaluation is the organization and interpretation of the information gathered from all aspects of the examination. According to the *Guide to Physical Therapist Practice*, the purpose of the evaluation is to establish the diagnosis and prognosis.[78] The diagnosis is a classification of the signs, symptoms, syndromes, and/or categories that the evaluation discovers. The diagnostic category for impaired posture is referred to as preferred practice pattern 4B: Impaired posture.

Many factors may affect the prognosis for patients with impaired posture, which is usually one of several musculoskeletal impairments that the physical therapist will find on examination. In general, the more musculoskeletal dysfunctions that exist concurrent with the postural impairment, the longer the time required for the desired outcome. Other diagnoses will also affect the outcome and sometimes make the goals of independence or ideal posture unattainable. For example, a patient with ankylosing spondylitis may have a goal of independence in positioning for sleep, sitting, and standing without risk that the functional activity or position itself will exacerbate the progression of the disease, but ideal alignment will not be a goal because it will not be attainable. Other factors that may affect prognosis include age, length of time the patient has had the postural impairment, preexisting conditions or diseases, and the ability of the patient to adhere to the intervention.

INTERVENTION

In the management of postural impairment, each musculoskeletal dysfunction revealed in the examination is addressed with an intervention. Although individual musculoskeletal impairments may contribute to postural impairment and benefit from individual interventions, posture may also be improved through postural education, instruction, and training.

STRETCHING AND MOBILIZATION

If the evaluation reveals limitation of soft tissue ROM, interventions that assist the lengthening of these soft tissues may be employed. Soft tissue length may be limited by muscle spasm, myofascial tension, scar tissue, or lack of extensibility of soft tissue through full, normal ROM. These limitations may be managed with a variety of interventions including massage[79-81]; myofascial release[82,83]; specific stretching exercises[81,84]; and exercises that activate (contract or shorten) the muscles opposing restricted tissues.[40] Studies show that intermittent stretching programs and the proprioceptive neuromuscular rehabilitation (PNF) techniques of contract relax and hold relax can lengthen a variety of soft tissues, including muscles.[84-87] A severely shortened muscle is best lengthened gradually with a low-load stretch as can be provided by prolonged immobilization in a splint or cast.[88,85] The effectiveness of lengthening interventions may be enhanced with modalities. Modalities that increase tissue temperature, including ultrasound, diathermy, paraffin, and hot packs, have been shown to increase tissue extensibility and thus increase the lengthening obtained from a stretch.[89-95] Cryotherapy may be used before lengthening tissues in the presence of pain, muscle spasm, or inflammation and may also be used after lengthening procedures to assist in limiting the response (pain, muscle spasm, or inflammation) of the body to the tissue trauma produced by the procedures themselves. Electrical stimulation may also be used to minimize pain, inflammation, and muscle spasm before or after other interventions, as well as for neuromuscular reeducation during or after an intervention.[95]

Joint motion restrictions may be addressed with joint mobilization,[96-99] splinting,[85,100] exercises designed to use muscles that will encourage motion of the limited joint, and stretching of the joint into the direction of limited joint motion.[84,92,101] These techniques may also be assisted by therapeutic heat. Cryotherapy and electrical stimulation may be used before or after these techniques to facilitate joint motion if inflammation is present. Cryotherapy and electrical stimulation may also be used to minimize pain and inflammation after techniques used to increase joint motion.

STABILIZATION

If the evaluation reveals joint laxity, joint instability, or muscle weakness, interventions that provide stabilization to the soft tissues such as proprioceptive rehabilitation and strengthening of the surrounding muscles may be employed. Stabilization may be accomplished with splinting and education regarding proper positioning and avoidance of vulnerable positions.[4] Splinting, proprioceptive training, and strengthening exercises have been shown to improve joint stability and performance.[102-104] It is important to determine from the examination which muscles require strengthening and which do not. Posture and stability may be improved by strengthening weak muscles,[4] while avoiding further strengthening muscles that are stronger than other muscles in the same region.[40]

EXERCISE

Few studies have studied the effects of exercise on posture. Two studies with interesting outcomes provide important information to consider when determining the intervention(s) to be used. Increasing back extensor strength with back strengthening exercises was found to reduce excessive thoracic kyphosis in otherwise healthy women aged 49 to 65 years.[105] However, in a modeling study, the back extensor muscles, specifically the multifidi and erector spinae, were found to not only extend the back but also to generate compressive and shear forces. The effects of these forces should be considered when prescribing exercises for patients with poor posture and back pain. For example, exercises that activate the thoracic and lumbar erector spinae and multifidi are not recommended for individuals with intervertebral disc compression injuries because they may exert excessive compressive forces on the spinal discs. In addition, this study found that the back muscles exerted a posterior shear force on L1 through L4 and an anterior shear force on the L5 segment. Exercises that isometrically activate the back extensor muscles therefore may be deleterious to patients with translatory instability particularly at L5.[106]

CASE STUDY 4-1

CHRONIC NECK PAIN

Examination
Patient History

AD is a 31-year-old man with a past medical history that includes an umbilical hernia repair at age 4, right inguinal hernia repair at age 8, and pneumonia at age 27. He also has a history of depression. He reported long-standing neck and upper trapezius region pain for the past 10 years, which he associated with computer use. The patient is independent in ADLs. He worked 45-60 hours per week primarily at his computer. In addition, he reported spending a lot of time using his computer at home. AD bicycled 15-20 minutes to and from work 3-4 days each week and took public transportation on the other days. He also bicycled for 1-1$\frac{1}{2}$ hours once or twice each weekend for exercise. He had a regular callisthenic regime that he performed most days that included sit-ups, push-ups, standing lumbar spine rotation, standing side bending, shoulder flexion stretching, shoulder shrugs and rolls, toe touches, standing quadriceps stretch, standing calf stretch, and seated toe touches.

AD's chief complaint was of worsening neck and upper trapezius region pain. He also noted pain and a sensation of coldness in the region of the right medial palm and the tips of digits 4 and 5 with soreness over the pisiform and at the elbow at the region of the ulnar groove, the medial epicondyle of the humerus, and the olecranon process. He reported pain primarily with use of his computer input devices and some discomfort with writing and with movements involving thumb opposition.

He denies any numbness and tingling, pain with coughing or sneezing or bowel and bladder concerns. He reported an intentional 40-50 lb weight loss that he had maintained for 6 months before his initial evaluation. Medications included Effexor (venlafaxine hydrochloride), Lexapro (escitalopram oxalate), and Klonopin (clonazepam).

Tests and Measures

Musculoskeletal

Posture In standing, AD had a reduced lumbar lordosis, an excessive thoracic kyphosis that extended from C7 to L2, a low right shoulder, bilateral shoulder internal rotation, bilateral scapular depression (the superior medial angle was level with T3), bilateral scapular abduction, with more than 50% of the humeral head anterior to the acromion bilaterally, and left rotation of the cervical spine. In supine, the posterior aspect of the acromion process was more than three finger widths above the table, an indication of pectoralis minor shortness.[4] To stand with his pelvis and midthoracic spine against a wall, AD had to have his feet 4 inches from the wall, Even with his feet so far from the wall, his head was a hand's breadth (five finger widths) from the wall.

Active Range of Motion

	Movement	Result	
Cervical spine	Flexion	30°*	
	Extension	40°	
		Right	Left
	Sidebending	25°	23°
	Rotation	55°*	53°
Shoulders		Right	Left
	Flexion	145°†	150°†
	Abduction	125°	131°
	Internal rotation	48°	52°
	External rotation	78°	78°

*With pain in the right posterior cervical musculature.
†Shoulder flexion caused C6 to rotate to the left beginning at the onset of flexion.

Active shoulder flexion on the right caused C6 to rotate to the left (though more slowly than with

left shoulder flexion) and resulted in tingling in the right forearm and hand. Simultaneous flexion of the right and left shoulders caused C6 and C7 to rotate to the left.

AD's hamstrings were found to be short, both allowing only 40 degrees of passive straight leg raise.

Strength

Muscle*	Right	Left
Rhomboids	3–/5	3/5
Middle trapezius	3/5	3/5
Lower trapezius	3/5	3–/5
Shoulder external rotators	4/5	3+/5
Subscapularis	3+/5	4/5

*A complete upper extremity strength examination was performed, and all muscles tested 5/5 except for the muscles listed.

The external abdominal oblique muscles were tested for their ability to stabilize the torso against movements of the lower and upper extremities against gravity. Tested in the hooklying position, the external abdominal obliques could not prevent the lumbar spine from extending (increased lumbar lordosis) when the hip was flexed (knee brought toward the chest) or when the arms were raised (shoulder flexion) from the relaxed position of arms resting by the sides. This indicates that the lower abdominals were very weak.

Function

Ergonomics and Body Mechanics A picture of AD's workstation provided by the ergonomic consultant who referred him to physical therapy revealed that he sat in an Aeron chair (an ergonomically designed chair with a Pellicle weave surface with the following adjustable components: Arm angle, arm height, seat height, seat tilt, lumbar support height, tilt tension, and seat height) and used a keyboard, mouse, and a Wacom pen tablet while looking at two 21-inch monitors. The Wacom tablet is a pen-shaped input device used in combination with a small, flat, touch-sensitive "tablet" on which the pen writes, draws, or points and which is connected to the computer so that inputs made on the tablet are visualized on the computer monitor screen. The pen is held like a standard pen, although, in addition to standard pen components, it also has a toggle switch near the tip that may be used with the thumb or other finger. The Wacom pen and tablet are used for computer-aided drawing.

The keyboard, mouse, and Wacom tablet were positioned on the desktop. No keyboard tray was in use. AD tended to sit at the front of his chair and rest his forearms on the desk. His thoracic and lumbar spine were markedly flexed (to bring his forearms down to the desktop where they rested for support) and his cervical spine was extended (to see his monitors). His right shoulder was flexed approximately 30-40 degrees and his right wrist was slightly extended when his hand was on the mouse. His left shoulder was flexed approximately 40-45 degrees with his wrist in 20-30 degrees of extension when his hand was on the keyboard. Because of his right upper extremity discomfort, AD often reversed keyboarding and mousing arms. In fact, he reported that he generally used the mouse with his left hand and the keyboard with his right hand.

Evaluation, Diagnosis, and Prognosis

AD had swayback posture, limited cervical ROM, limited shoulder ROM, limited interscapular strength, extremely weak lower abdominals, short hamstrings, and poor habits for work. He spent a considerable amount of his day in trunk flexion. Bicycling to and from work positioned him in lumbar flexion with marked cervical extension. He tended to sit at the front of his chair seat, posteriorly tilt his pelvis, flex his lumbar spine, and lean onto the desk with his forearms to reach his mouse and keyboard with his arms. This position also contributed to his posture of excessive lumbar and thoracic spine flexion. His exercise regime of sit-ups, standing spinal flexion, and sitting spinal flexion encouraged a posture of spine flexion. Push-ups, which strengthen pectoralis major, also encouraged shoulder internal rotation and flexion, contributing to scapular abduction and therefore to excessive thoracic spine flexion.

Intervention

Because of AD's demanding work schedule and his preference, he initially attended therapy once per week. He was instructed in a home program that included exercises and postural instruction and training as the primary interventions. Although modalities could have been used as adjuncts to these interventions, they were not found to be necessary.

Treatment for AD began with instruction in home exercises and work positioning. He was instructed to discontinue those exercises of his previous home exercise program that encouraged flexion, including sit-ups, push-ups, and standing and sitting toe touches, and to start exercises to strengthen his interscapular and abdominal muscles, reduce his thoracic kyphosis, and increase his shoulder ROM. These exercises included supine scapular adduction (after prone scapular adduction was found to be too difficult) and arm slides facing a wall (Fig. 4-23). At

work, he was instructed to modify his position so that he would keep his arms at his sides with his shoulders in neutral flexion.

As AD progressed, his exercises and postural instructions were modified, and the frequency of PT sessions was reduced first to every other week and then to once per month. Posterior axial retraction and lower abdominal exercise of single hip flexion from hooklying were added. Supine scapular adduction was progressed to prone arm lifts, the first step of which involved the patient lying prone with arms overhead, adducting his scapulae without moving his trunk, holding the position for 3 seconds, and then relaxing. Foam roller exercises were added to help AD extend his thoracic spine and reduce his excessive thoracic kyphosis. All roller exercises were performed with a 6 inches × 3 feet Ethafoam roller. The roller was placed flat on the floor, and the patient was positioned face up so that the roller supported the spine from head to sacrum. The hips and knees were bent, and the feet were flat on the floor (Fig. 4-24). Roller exercises included gliding side-to-side (with the arms clasped over his abdomen, AD rolled the Ethafoam roll to the right and left by sliding his body to the left and right, respectively, as far as able with the torso remaining parallel to the floor) (Fig. 4-25); arms overhead (the arms start by the sides of the body with elbows straight and thumbs facing upward, then the shoulders were repeatedly flexed, raising the arms up and overhead as far as the shoulders could flex without any lumbar extension before the reverse action was performed) (Fig. 4-26); and snow angels (an exercise performed from the same original position with the arms at the sides of the body and the hands palms upward, and the patient then abducting and adducting the shoulder to the maximum shoulder abduction possible without any lumbar extension) (Fig. 4-27). AD was instructed to

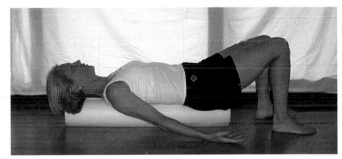

FIG. 4-24 Starting position for roller exercises.

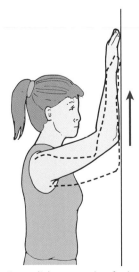

FIG. 4-23 Arm slides exercise facing a wall.

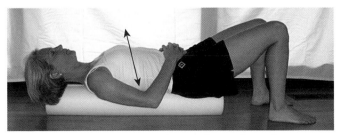

FIG. 4-25 Gliding side to side on the roller.

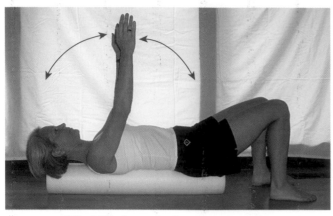

FIG. 4-26 Arms overhead on the roller.

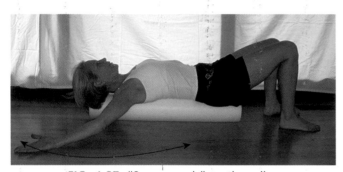

FIG. 4-27 "Snow angels" on the roller.

activate his lower abdominals to stabilize his lumbar spine for the Ethafoam roll exercises of arms overhead and snow angels.

As AD developed more abdominal and interscapular muscle strength and his torso became more stable, pectoralis minor and hamstring stretches were added. Proper posture for sitting, standing, and work was reviewed regularly.

Further progression of the exercises included progression of the prone arm lifts to include lifting the arms from the supporting surface while the scapulae were adducted. Arm slides facing the wall were progressed to back against the wall arm lifts and back against the wall arm slides. The hooklying hip flexion exercise was progressed to knee to chest leg lowering, which added further abdominal strengthening, hamstring stretching, and hip flexion ROM.

Outcomes

AD was diligent with his home exercise program and made excellent progress. He reported reduced pain soon after initiating the exercise program, and the pain steadily decreased as his exercises progressed. After 5 months, he had no pain at work or in his leisure activities. His posture improved so much that he was able to stand at the wall with his heels touching the wall with one finger width between the wall and the back of his head. The following are measurements after treatment.

Active Range of Motion

	Movement	Result	
Cervical spine	Flexion	43°	
	Extension	53°	
		Right	Left
	Sidebending	37°	37°
	Rotation	63°	64°
Shoulder		Right	Left
	Flexion	166°*	170°*
	Abduction	151°	155°
	Internal rotation	55°	60°
	External rotation	90°	90°

*Shoulder flexion did not produce any compensatory cervical motion.

Strength

Muscle	Right	Left
Rhomboids	5/5	5/5
Middle trapezius	4+/5	5/5
Lower trapezius	4–/5	4/5
Shoulder external rotators	5/5	4+/5
Subscapularis	4/5	4+/5

CHAPTER SUMMARY

Impaired posture is one of many factors that may contribute to symptoms and functional limitations.[107] The examination of posture is one component of a full patient examination, which may also include examination of other musculoskeletal, neuromuscular, integumentary, and functional aspects as appropriate to the individual patient. Evaluation may depend on examination of overall posture or of the relative alignment of one or two segments in multiple planes.[107] Regular practice of postural examination will help the clinician become familiar with ideal posture and common variations. Over time, this will improve the clinician's ability to evaluate a patient's overall posture, as well as the relative alignment of articulations and groups of articulations such as the relative alignment of the vertebrae of the cervical spine or the relative alignment of the scapula, humerus, and clavicle in their articulation at the shoulder. Interventions may help to bring posture closer to ideal and may help to alleviate symptoms related to impaired posture.

ADDITIONAL RESOURCES

Books

Sahrmann S: Diagnosis and Treatment of Movement Impairment Syndromes, St. Louis, 2002, Mosby.
Kendall FP, McCreary EK, Provance PG: Muscles Testing and Function, ed 4, Baltimore, 1993, Williams and Wilkins.

Web Sites

The Secret of Good Posture:
    www.apta.org/AM/Template.cfm?Section=Search&template=/CM/HTMLDisplay.cfm&ContentID=20457

GLOSSARY

Active sitting: Sitting with the ischial tuberosities at the forward edge of the seat, the pelvis and lumbar spine in a neutral position, the feet spread apart (either forward and back or side to side), and a slight forward lean at the hips.

Anatomical position: Erect standing posture with face forward, arms at sides of the torso, forearms supinated so that the palms face anteriorly, fingers in extension, and thumbs adducted with the pad of each thumb facing forward. Used as reference for terms relating to planes, axes, surfaces, joint motion, and directions of motion. Also the zero position for the measurement of most joint motions.

Antagonist muscles: Muscles that act in opposition to agonist muscles.

Anteversion: Anterior tipping of an organ or part. In the femur, an angle of more than the normal 15-degree anterior angulation of the femoral neck to the long axis of the shaft.

Balans chair: A kneeling chair.

Barrel chest: An increase in the anteroposterior diameter of the ribcage.

Base of support: The area of the body in contact with the supporting surface.

Calcaneal valgus: The calcaneus is angled with the inferior portion lateral to the superior portion; calcaneal eversion.

Carrying angle: A valgus angle of the elbow that may be seen clearly when the arm is positioned with the shoulder in neutral flexion/extension and full external rotation with the elbow extended.

Center of force (COF): A point on the supporting surface where the GRF acts, also known as the center of pressure (COP). Also the point from which the sway envelope is plotted.

Center of gravity (COG): A point about which gravity and the weight of a body act on one another to maintain equilibrium.

Center of mass (COM): A point that is at the center of the total body mass.

Circumduction: The movement of a limb in a circular motion.

Eversion: To turn outward, as in the foot.

Flatback: A posture of diminished lordosis of the lumbar spine.

Forward sitting: Sitting in a posture with the lumbar lordosis diminished or reversed or an increased kyphosis of the spine.

Good posture: Ideal body part alignment.

Ground reaction force (GRF): A force composed of a vertical force, a horizontal medial-lateral force, and a horizontal anteroposterior force that is approximately equal in magnitude but opposite in direction to the gravitational force in the erect static standing posture.

Ideal alignment (ideal posture, neutral posture): The position in which the center of mass is directly over the base of support.

Inversion: To turn inward, as in the foot.

Kyphosis: A posterior spinal curve or a spinal curve with a posterior convexity.

Kyphosis-lordosis: A posture with excessive thoracic kyphosis and excessive lumbar lordosis.

Limit of stability: The maximum angle that can be sustained when leaning away from the vertical, without loosing one's balance.

Line of gravity (LOG): A vertical line dropped from the body's COG.

Lordosis: An anterior spinal curve or a curve that has an anterior convexity.

Middle sitting: Sitting in a "middle position" (compared to anterior or posterior sitting) with the COM above the ischial tuberosities and the feet transmitting approximately 25% of the body weight to the floor.[37]

Patella alta: The patella is positioned more proximal than normal.

Patella baja: The patella is positioned such that the distance between the inferior pole of the patella and the tibial tubercle is less than $2/3$ of the length of the patella.

Pectus carinatum/gallinatum: Excessive prominence of the sternum.

Pectus excavatum/recurvatum: Excessive depression of the sternum.

Pes cavus: Exaggerated height of the longitudinal arch of the foot.

Pes planus: Reduced height of the longitudinal arch of the foot.

Posterior sitting: Sitting characterized by less than 25% of the body weight transmitted to the floor by the feet and the COM above or behind the ischial tuberosities.

Postural control: The ability to provide for stability and orientation to the environment regardless of position or posture.

Postural orientation: The ability to maintain the body in a position appropriate for a task, including the relationship between body segments and the relationship between the body and the environment.

Postural sway: The normal movement of a body from front to back and from side to side in standing.

Q angle: The angle formed from the intersection of a line drawn from the ASIS through the center of the patella and a line drawn from the center of the tibial tubercle through the center of the patella.

Radial deviation: A movement of the wrist in which the lateral border of the hand moves toward the radius. In anatomical position the movement occurs in the frontal plane.

Retraction: Posterior movement of the clavicle or scapula.

Retroversion: The tipping backward of an organ or part.

Scapular winging: A prominence of the vertebral border of the scapula.

Scoliosis: A lateral deviation from the normally straight vertical line of the vertebral column.

Squinting (or convergent) patellae: Patellae that appear tilted medially (toward one another).

Swayback: A posture with the pelvis in posterior tilt and the hips swayed forward in relation to the feet resulting in hip joint extension.

Valgus: The distal boney segment is aligned laterally in comparison with the proximal segment.

Varus: The distal boney segment is aligned medially in comparison with the proximal segment.

References

1. Shumway-Cook A, Woollacott M: *Motor Control: Theory and Practical Applications*, ed 2, Philadelphia, 2000, Lippincott Williams and Wilkins.
2. Raine S, Twomey LT: Attributes and qualities of human posture and their relationship to dysfunction or musculoskeletal pain, *Crit Rev Phys Rehabil Med* 6:409-437, 1994.
3. Pope MH, Bevins T, Wilder DG, et al: The relationship between anthropometric, postural, muscular and mobility characteristics of males ages 18-55, *Spine* 10:644-648, 1985.
4. Kendall FP, McCreary EK, Provance PG: *Muscles: Testing and Function*, ed 4, Baltimore, 1993, Lippincott Williams and Wilkins.
5. Kendal HO, Kendall FP, Boynton D: *Posture and Pain*, Baltimore, 1952, Williams and Wilkins.
6. Norkin CC, Levangie PK: *Joint Structure and Function: A Comprehensive Analysis*, ed 2, Philadelphia, 1992, FA Davis.
7. Danis CG, Krebs DE, Gill-Body KM, et al: Relationship between standing posture and stability, *Phys Ther* 78:502-525, 1998.
8. Luttgens K, Wells KF: *Kinesiology*, Philadelphia, 1982, Saunders CBS College Publishing.
9. Woollacott MH, Shumway-Cook M: Changes in posture control across the life span: A systems approach, *Phys Ther* 70:799-807, 1990.
10. Soderberg G: *Kinesiology*, Baltimore, 1997, Williams and Wilkins.
11. Posture and its relationship to orthopaedic disabilities: A Report of the Posture Committee of the American Academy of Orthopaedic Surgeons, 1947.
12. Nasher LM: Sensory, neuromuscular, and biomechanical contributions to human balance, Proceedings of the APTA Forum, Nashville Tenn, June 13-15, 1989.
13. Corbeil P, Blouin JS, Nougier V, et al: Perturbation of the postural control system induced by muscular fatigue, *Gait Posture* 18(2):92-100, 2003.
14. Ledin T, Fransson PA, Magnusson M: Effects of postural disturbances with fatigued triceps surae muscles or with 20% additional body weight, *Gait Posture* 19(2):184-193, 2004.
15. Vuillerme N, Forestier N, Nougier V: Attentional demands and postural sway: The effect of the calf muscles fatigue, *Med Sci Sports Exerc* 34(12):1907-1912, 2002.
16. Schieppati M, Nardone A, Schmid M; Neck muscle fatigue affects postural control in man, *Neuroscience* 121(2):277-285, 2003.
17. Nussbaum MA: Postural stability is compromised by fatiguing overhead work, *AIHA J* 64:55-61, 2003.
18. Hamaoui A, Bouisset S: Postural sway increase in low back pain subjects is not related to reduced spine range of motion, *Neurosci Lett* 357(2):135-138, 2004.

19. Rogind H, Lykkegaard JJ, Bliddal H, et al: Postural sway in normal subjects aged 20-70 years, *Clin Physiol Funct Imaging* 23(3):171-176, 2003.

20. De Haart M, Geurts AC, Huidekoper SC, et al: Recovery of standing balance in postacute stroke patients: A rehabilitation cohort study, *Arch Phys Med Rehabil* 85(6):886-895, 2004.

21. Pyoria O, Era P, Talvitie U, Relationships between standing balance and symmetry measurements in patients following recent strokes (3 weeks or less) or older strokes (6 months or more), *Phys Ther* 84(2):128-136, 2004.

22. Liu-Ambrose T, Eng JJ, Khan KM, et al: Older women with osteoporosis have increased postural sway and weaker quadriceps strength than counterparts with normal bone mass: overlooked determinants of fracture risk, *J Gerontol A Biol Sci Med Sci* 58(9):M862-M866, 2003.

23. Ahmad S, Rohrbaugh JW, Anokhin AP, et al: Effects of lifetime ethanol consumption on postural control: a computerized dynamic posturography study, *J Vestib Res* 12(1):53-64, 2002.

24. Noda M, Demura S, Yamaji S, et al: Influence of alcohol intake on the parameters evaluating the body center of foot pressure in a static upright posture, *Percept Mot Skills* 98:873-887, 2004.

25. Friden C, Hirschberg AL, Saartok T, et al: The influence of premenstrual symptoms of postural balance and kinesthesia during the menstrual cycle, *Gynecol Endocrinol* 6:433-439, 2003.

26. Allard P, Chavet P, Barbier F, et al: Effect of body morphology on standing balance in adolescent idiopathic scoliosis, *Am J Phys Med Rehabil* 83(9):689-697.

27. Farenc I, Rougier P, Berger L: The influence of gender and body characteristics on upright stance, *Ann Hum Biol* 30:279-294, 2003.

28. Mitra S, Fraizer EV: Effects of explicit sway-minimization on postural-suprapostural dual-task performance, *Hum Mov Sci* 23(1):1-20, 2004.

29. Krishnamoorthy V, Slijper H, Latash ML: Effects of different types of light touch on postural sway, *Exp Brain Res* 147(1):71-79, 2002.

30. Jeka JJ, Lackner JR: Fingertip contact influences human postural control, *Exp Brain Res* 100(3):495-502, 1994.

31. Amblard B, Cremieux J, Marchand AR, et al: Lateral orientation and stabilization of human stance: Static versus dynamic visual cues, *Exp Brain Res* 61(1):21-37, 1985.

32. Brooke-Wavell K, Perrett LK, et al: Influence of the visual environment on the postural stability in healthy older women, *Gerontology* 48(5):293-297, 2002.

33. Kantor E, Poupard L, Le Bozec S, et al: Does body stability depend on postural chair mobility or stability area? *Neurosci Lett* 308(2):128-132, 2001.

34. Bennett BC, Abel MF, Granata KP: Seated postural control in adolescents with idiopathic scoliosis, *Spine* 20:E449-E454, 2004.

35. Bouisset S, Duchene JL: Is body balance more perturbed by respiration in seating than in standing posture? *Neuroreport* 8:957-960, 1994.

36. Deleted.

37. Andersson BJ, Ortengren R, Nachemson AL, et al: The sitting posture: An electromyographic and discometric study, *Orthop Clin North Am* 6:105-120, 1975.

38. Saliba VL, Johnson GS: *Back education training*, Course Outline, San Anselmo, Calif, The Institute of Physical Art.

39. Nachemson A: Towards a better understanding of low-back pain: A review of the mechanics of the lumbar disc, *Rheumatol Rehabil* 14:129-143, 1975.

40. Sahrmann S: *Diagnosis and Treatment of Movement Impairment Syndromes*, St. Louis, 2002, Mosby.

41. Yasukouchi A, Isayama T: The relationships between lumbar curves, pelvic tilt and joint mobilities in different sitting postures in young adult males, *Appl Hum Sci* 14:15-21, 1995.

42. Andersson GB, Murphy RW, Ortengren R, et al: The influence of backrest inclination and lumbar support on lumbar lordosis, *Spine* 4:52-58, 1975.

43. Lord MJ, Small JM, Dinsay JM, et al: Lumbar lordosis: Effects of sitting and standing, *Spine* 22:2571-2574, 1997.

44. Bridger RS, Wilkinson D, van Houweninge T: Hip joint mobility and spinal angles in standing and in different sitting postures, *Hum Factors* 31:229-241, 1989.

45. Link CS, Nicholson GG, Shaddeau SA, et al: Lumbar curvature in standing and sitting in two types of chairs: relationship of hamstring and hip flexor muscle length, *Phys Ther* 70:611-618, 1990.

46. Naqvi SA: Study of forward sloping seats for VDT workstations, *J Hum Ergol (Tokyo)* 23:41-49, 1994.

47. Black K, McClure P, Polansky M: The influence of different sitting positions on cervical and lumbar posture, *Spine* 21:65-70, 1996.

48. Lengsfeld M, Frank A, van Deursen DL, et al: Lumbar spine curvature during office chair sitting, *Med Eng Phys* 22:665-669, 2000.

49. Williams MM, Hawley JA, McKenzie RA, et al: A comparison of the effects of two sitting postures on back and referred pain, *Spine* 16:1185-1191, 1991.

50. Bendix T, Biering-Sorensen F: Posture of the trunk when sitting on forward inclining seats, *Scand J Rehabil Med* 15:197-203, 1983.

51. Wu CS, Miyamoto H, Noro K: Research on pelvic angle variation when using a pelvic support, *Ergonomics* 41:317-327, 1998.

52. Vergara M, Page A: Relationship between comfort and back posture and mobility in sitting-posture, *Appl Ergon* 33:1-8, 2002.

53. Nachemson AL: Disc pressure measurements, *Spine* 6:93-97, 1981.

54. Harrison DD, Harrison SO, Croft AC, et al: Sitting biomechanics part I: Review of the literature, *J Manip Physiol Ther* 22:594-609, 1999.

55. Cranz G: *The Chair*, New York, 1998, WW Norton.

56. Horak FB: Clinical measurement of postural control in adults, *Phys Ther* 67:1881-1885, 1987.

57. Schenkman M: Interrelationship of neurological and mechanical factors in balance control, Proceedings of the APTA Forum, Nashville, Tenn, June 13-15, 1989.

58. Winter D: *Biomechanics and Motor Control of Human Movement*, ed 3, New York, 2004, Wiley.

59. Myers RS: *Saunders Manual of Physical Therapy Practice*, Philadelphia, 1995, WB Saunders.

60. Matthews GG: *Cellular Physiology of Nerve and Muscle*, ed 4, Malden, Mass, 2004. Blackwell Science.

61. Williams PE, Goldspink G: Longitudinal growth of striated muscle fibers, *J Cell Sci* 9:751-767, 1971.

62. Williams PE, Goldspink G: The effect of immobilization on the longitudinal growth of striated muscle fibers, *J Anat* 116:45-55, 1973.

63. Lieber R: *Skeletal Muscle Structure, Function, and Plasticity*, ed 2, Baltimore, 2002, Lippincott Williams and Wilkins.

64. Chleboun GS, Howell JN, Conatser RR, et al: The relationship between elbow flexor volume and angular stiffness at the elbow, *Clin Biomech* (Bristol, Avon) 12:383-392, 1997.

65. Franklin ME, Conner-Kerr T: An analysis of posture and back pain in the first and third trimesters of pregnancy, *J Orthop Sports Phys Ther* 28:133-138, 1998.

66. Milne JS, Williamson J: A Longitudinal study of kyphosis in older people, *Age Ageing* 12:225-233, 1983.

67. Ettinger B, Black DM, Palermo L, et al: Kyphosis in older women and its relation to back pain, disability and osteopenia: The study of osteoporotic fractures. *Osteoporosis Int* 4:55-60, 1994.

68. Ensrud KE, Black DM, Harris F, et al: Correlates of kyphosis in older women. The Fracture Intervention Trial Research Group. *J Am Geriatr Soc* 45:682-687, 1997.

69. Lewis JS, Wright C, Green A: Subacromial impingement syndrome: The effect of changing posture on shoulder range of motion, *J Orthop Sports Phys Ther* 35:72-87, 2005.

70. Luchetti R, Shoenhuber R, Nathan P: Correlation of segmental carpal tunnel pressures with changes in hand and wrist positions in patients with carpal tunnel syndrome and controls, *J Hand Surg* 23:598-602, 1998.

71. Liu CW, Chen TW, Wang MC, et al: Relationship between carpal tunnel syndrome and wrist angle in computer workers, *Kaohsiung J Med Sci* 19:617-623, 2003.

72. Christie HJ, Kumar S, Warren SA: Postural aberrations in low back pain, *Arch Phys Med Rehabil* 76:218-243, 1995.

73. Evcik D, Yucel A: Lumbar lordosis in acute and chronic low back pain patients, *Rheumatol Int* 23:163-165, 2003.

74. Tuzun C, Yorulmaz I, Cindas A, et al: Low back pain and posture, *Clin Rheumatol* 18:308-312, 1999.

75. Gelb DE, Lenke LG, Bridwell KH, et al: An analysis of sagittal spinal alignment in 100 asymptomatic middle and older aged volunteers, *Spine* 20:1351-1358, 1995.

76. Peterson DE, Blankenship KR, Robb JB, et al: Investigation of the validity and reliability of four objective techniques for measuring forward shoulder posture, *J Orthop Sports Phys Ther* 25:34-42, 1997.

77. Reese NB, Bandy WD: *Joint Range of Motion and Muscle Length Testing*, St. Louis, 2002, WB Saunders.

78. American Physical Therapy Association: *Guide to Physical Therapist Practice*, ed 2, Alexandria Va, 2001, The Association.

79. Hernandez-Reif M, Field T, et al: Lower back pain is reduced and range of motion increased after massage therapy, *Int J Neurosci* 106:131-145, 2001.

80. Guler-Uysal F, Kozanoglu E: Comparison of the early response to two methods of rehabilitation in adhesive capsulitis, *Swiss Med Wkly* 134:353-358, 2004.

81. Wiktorsson-Moller M, Oberg B, et al: Effects of warming up, massage, and stretching on range of motion and muscle strength in the lower extremity, *Am J Sports Med* 11:249-252, 1983.

82. Hanten WP, Chandler SD: Effects of myofascial release leg pull and sagittal plane isometric contract-relax techniques on passive straight-leg raise angle, *J Orthop Sports Phys Ther* 20:138-144, 1994.

83. Barnes JF: *Myofascial Release: The Search for Excellence*, ed 10, Paoli, Penn, 1990, Rehabilitation Services, Inc.

84. Reid DA, McNair PJ: Passive force, angle, and stiffness changes after stretching of hamstring muscles, *Med Sci Sports Exerc* 36:1944-1948, 2004.

85. Bonutti PM, Windau ME, Ables BA, et al: Static progressive stretch to reestablish elbow range of motion, *Clin Orthop* 303:128-134, 1994.

86. Decoster LC, Scanlon RL, Horn KD, et al: Standing and supine hamstring stretching are equally effective, *Athl Train* 39:330-334, 2004.

87. Voss DE, Ionta MK, Myers BJ: *Proprioceptive Neuromuscular Facilitation: Patterns and Techniques*, ed 3, Philadelphia, 1985, JB Lippincott.

88. Light KE, Nuzik S, Personius W, et al: Low-load prolonged stretch vs. high-load brief stretch in treating knee contractures, *Phys Ther* 64:330-333, 1984.

89. Lehmann JF, Masock AJ, Warren CG, et al: Effect of therapeutic temperatures on tendon extensibility, *Arch Phys Med Rehabil* 51:481-487, 1970.

90. Warren CG, Lehmann JF, Koblanski JN: Elongation of rat tail tendon: Effect of load and temperature, *Arch Phys Med Rehabil* 52:465-474, 1971.

91. Warren CG, Lehmann JF, Koblanski JN: Heat and stretch procedures: An evaluation using rat tail tendon, *Arch Phys Med Rehabil* 57:122-126, 1976.

92. Knight CA, Rutledge CR, Cox ME, et al: Effect of superficial heat, deep heat, and active exercise warm-up on the extensibility of the plantar flexors. *Phys Ther* 81:1206-1214, 2001.

93. Draper DO, Castro JL, Feland B, et al: Shortwave diathermy and prolonged stretching increase hamstring flexibility more than prolonged stretching alone, *J Orthop Sports Phys Ther* 34:12-20, 2004.

94. Safran MR, Garrett WE, Seaber AV, et al: The role of warmup in muscular injury prevention, *Am J Sports Med* 16:123-129, 1988.

95. Cameron MH: *Physical Agents in Rehabilitation: From Research to Practice,* ed 2, St. Louis, 2003, WB Saunders.

96. Shamus J, Shamus E, Gugel RN, et al: The effect of sesamoid mobilization, flexor hallucis strengthening, and gait training on reducing pain and restoring function in individuals with hallux limitus: A clinical trial, *J Orthop Sports Phys Ther* 34:368-376, 2004.

97. Nilsson N, Christensen HW, Hartvigsen J: Lasting changes in passive range motion after spinal manipulation: A randomized, blind, controlled trial, *J Manip Physiol Ther* 19:165-168, 1996.

98. Mennell JM: *Back Pain: Diagnosis and Treatment Using Manipulative Technique,* Boston, 1960, Little, Brown.

99. Twomey L: A rationale for the treatment of back pain and joint pain by manual therapy, *Phys Ther* 72:885-892, 1992.

100. Nuismer BA, Ekes AM, Holm MB: The use of low-load prolonged stretch devices in rehabilitation programs in the Pacific Northwest, *Am J Occup Ther* 51:538-543, 1997.

101. Mayer TG, Gatchel RJ, Keeley J, et al: A randomized clinical trial of treatment for lumbar segmental rigidity, *Spine* 29:2199-2205, 2004.

102. Paterno MV, Myer GD, Ford KR, et al: Neuromuscular training improves single-limb stability in young female athletes, *J Orthop Sports Phys Ther* 34:305-316, 2004.

103. Ide J, Maeda S, Yamaga M, et al: Shoulder-strengthening exercise with an orthosis for multidirectional shoulder instability: Quantitative evaluation of rotational shoulder strength before and after the exercise program, *J Shoulder Elbow Surg* 12:342-345, 2003.

104. Regis D, Montanari M, Magnan B, et al: Dynamic orthopaedic brace in the treatment of ankle sprains, *Foot Ankle Int* 16:422-426, 1995.

105. Itoi E, Sinaki M: Effect of back-strengthening exercise on posture in healthy women 49 to 65 years of age, *Mayo Clin Proc* 69:1054-1059, 1994.

106. Bogduk N, Macintosh J, Pearcy M: A universal model of the lumbar back muscles in the upright position, *Spine* 17:897-913, 1992.

107. Sahrmann SA: Does postural assessment contribute to patient care? *J Orthop Sports Phys Ther* 32:376-379, 2002.

Chapter 5

Muscle Weakness

Robert C. Manske, Michael P. Reiman

OBJECTIVES

After reading this chapter, the reader will be able to:
1. Describe the normal anatomy and physiology of skeletal muscle.
2. Differentiate between various causes of muscle weakness.
3. Apply appropriate tests and measures to examine muscle performance, including strength, power, and endurance.
4. Evaluate a patient with muscle weakness.
5. Apply interventions to safely and effectively increase muscle strength.

*M*any ailments may cause impairments in *muscular performance*, reducing *strength, power,* and *endurance,* and result in muscle weakness. Therapists often examine and provide rehabilitation to patients with muscle weakness caused by muscle strains, disuse atrophy, and muscular diseases. Impaired muscle performance may result in minor problems, such as localized muscle discomfort, or major functional problems, such as the inability to stand or ambulate. Muscles control the movement of body segments around joints and provide stability by resisting the movement of joint surfaces through joint approximation.[1] Improving muscle strength, power, and endurance are constant mainstays of physical rehabilitation. This chapter describes the anatomy and physiology of normal skeletal muscle and common pathologies that result in muscle weakness. It also discusses the examination and evaluation of patients with muscle weakness and describes principles and methods for muscle strengthening interventions.

MUSCLE STRUCTURE

The three types of muscle tissue in the body are skeletal muscle (also known as voluntary muscle or striated muscle), smooth muscle, and cardiac muscle. This chapter only discusses skeletal muscle. Skeletal muscle can be thought of as being made up of bundles within bundles. A single skeletal muscle may contain many thousands of multinucleated muscle cells known as myofibers or muscle fibers. Each myofiber is surrounded by a cell membrane known as the sarcolemma and then by a thin yet strong layer of connective tissue known as *endomysium.* Each myofiber contains hundreds or thousands of *myofibril*s, organelles, such as ribosomes and mitochondria,[1] and substances, such as glycogen, enzymes, and fat.[2] The myofibers are bundled together in groups to form fascicles. Each fascicle is covered by an outer, thicker layer of connective tissue known as *perimysium.* Groups of fascicles are held together by another strong layer of connective tissue known as *epimysium* to form the muscle itself.

The myofibrils contain overlapping parallel filaments of *actin* and *myosin* that create the appearance of alternating light and dark bands or stripes under a light microscope, giving skeletal muscle fibers a striated appearance.[3] Electron microscopy shows that the darker *A bands* contain thick myosin filaments while the lighter shaded *I bands* are composed of only the thinner actin filaments. In most of the A band there is both myosin and actin, but

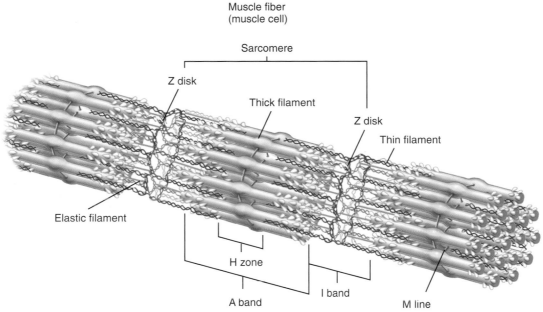

Muscle fiber
(muscle cell)

Sarcomere

Z disk

Thick filament

Z disk

Thin filament

Elastic filament

H zone

A band

I band

M line

FIG. 5-1 Basic structure of skeletal muscle. *Redrawn from Thibodeau GA, Patton KT: Anatomy and Physiology, ed 6, St. Louis, 2006, Mosby.*

in the middle of this band there are areas with only myosin filaments known as *H zones* (Fig. 5-1).[4-7]

The functional unit of the contractile system is the *sarcomere*. The sarcomere includes the actin and myosin filaments and proteins that bind them together. The thin actin filaments are made up of a long pair of polymerized molecules that form a helix.[1] A groove between this pair of molecules houses two long strands of the filamentous protein *tropomyosin*. A smaller complex polypeptide molecule, *troponin*, is attached to the tropomyosin. The troponin and tropomyosin bind the actin and myosin filaments.[4-7] A number of thick myosin filaments are usually bundled together to form long structures. Each myosin filament is composed of a globular enlargement known as a head group (the heavy meromyosin)[8] and a long tail (the light meromyosin).[9]

Muscle contraction is controlled by input from motor nerves. Each motor nerve innervates a number of muscle fibers. One motor nerve and all of the muscle fibers that it innervates are known as a *motor unit*.[2] The number of muscle fibers in a motor unit and the number of motor units in a single muscle varies. Generally, muscles used for fine motor tasks are made up of small motor units and muscles used for gross motor tasks are made up of large motor units.

PHYSIOLOGY OF MUSCLE CONTRACTION

To voluntarily activate and contract a muscle, a motor nerve impulse causes acetylcholine to be released from the axon terminal at the *motor end plate*. The acetylcholine binds to receptors on the muscle fiber and this evokes an electrical impulse, called an action potential, in the muscle fiber. This action potential spreads through the entire muscle fiber to cause a release of calcium ions. The calcium ions cause the troponin molecule to reposition the

tropomyosin molecules so that the receptor sites on the actin filament are free and the head groups of the myosin can bind with the actin molecules.[1] A cross-bridge is formed when the actin and myosin bond. This bonding of actin and myosin filaments is the basic constituent of a muscle contraction, and muscle force develops as a direct result of these cross-bridges being formed.[10] When a muscle contracts, the globular head of the myosin cross-bridge pulls on the actin filament, causing the actin and myosin filaments to slide past each other.[2] This understanding of muscle contraction is known as the sliding filament theory.[11-13] During any muscle contraction, the filaments move repeatedly so that at any given moment only about half of the cross-bridges are generating force and causing displacement.[2]

FACTORS AFFECTING MUSCLE PERFORMANCE

Many factors affect muscle performance, including the muscle fiber type and size, *force-velocity* relationships, *length-tension relationship*s, muscle architecture, neural control, fatigue, the age of the individual, cognitive strategies, and various medications, particularly corticosteroids.[14,15]

Muscle Fiber Type. Muscles are made up of two general types of fibers: type I and type II, and in most muscle, one fiber type predominates. Type I muscle fibers are slow-twitch (oxidative, red) muscle fibers. They are highly fatigue-resistant, can sustain low levels of force for long periods of time, use primarily aerobic metabolism, and have many large mitochondria. Type I muscle fibers predominate in small muscles that act across a small lever arm. They produce less force than type II muscle fibers but can sustain this force for a prolonged period of time. Postural muscles, such as those in the low back, are made up

TABLE 5-1	Muscle Fiber Type Characteristics		
	Slow-Twitch Type I	**Fast-Twitch A (FTa) Type IIa**	**Fast-Twitch B (FTb) Type IIb**
Nerve conduction velocity	Slow	Fast	Fast
Motor neuron size	Small	Large	Large
Aerobic capacity	High	Moderate	Low
Anaerobic capacity	Low	High	High
Power output	Low	Moderate-High	High
Contraction speed	Slow	Fast	Fast
Fatigue resistance	High	Reasonably resistant	Low
Recovery after exercise	Rapid	Fairly rapid	Slow
Recruitment order	First	Second	Last*

From Reiman MP: Training for strength, power, and endurance. In Manske RC (ed): *Postoperative Orthopedic Sports Medicine: The Knee and Shoulder,* Philadelphia, 2006, Elsevier Science.
*Only when very intense and rapid effort required.

of predominantly type I fibers; patients with low back pain and injuries tend to have selective wasting of type I muscle fibers.[16]

Type II muscle fibers are fast-twitch (white) fibers. Type II fibers can exert a large force for a short amount of time and then rapidly fatigue. Muscles that produce faster, explosive movements are made up predominantly of type II fibers. Type II muscle fibers can be further subdivided into type IIa and type IIb. Type IIb fibers are generally considered more true fast-twitch type fibers, whereas type IIa fibers are more similar to type I slow-twitch muscle fibers. Type IIa fibers can perform both aerobic and anaerobic metabolism, whereas type IIb fibers are optimized for anaerobic metabolism.[17,18] Table 5-1 compares the properties of the three muscle fiber types.

In general, type I fibers are recruited first, followed by type IIa fibers and finally by type IIb fibers. It has been suggested that type IIa fibers may be a pool of unused fibers that can become type IIb fibers with exercise.[19,20] Furthermore, some early studies suggested that fibers could transform from type I to type II with exercise training.[21,22] However, it is now generally accepted that this kind of change does not occur in response to training performed in rehabilitation or fitness programs.[23]

Muscle Fiber Size. The size of muscle fibers can change in response to muscle activity. If all other things are equal, the force a muscle can exert is related to its cross-sectional area rather than its volume because muscles with larger cross-sectional areas have more sarcomeres in parallel to generate force.[24]

Force-Velocity Relationships. With concentric (shortening) contractions, the amount of force generated by a muscle is inversely related to its speed of movement. Thus, when the muscle shortens more quickly, producing a faster movement, it also produces less force (Fig. 5-2). In contrast, with eccentric (lengthening) contractions, the amount of force generated initially increases when the muscle lengthens more quickly but then quickly levels off.[25,26]

Length-Tension Relationships. A muscle's capacity to produce force also depends on its length or the amount of tension in it. Muscles can produce the most force at their normal resting length, when there is the greatest number of cross-bridge sites available between the actin

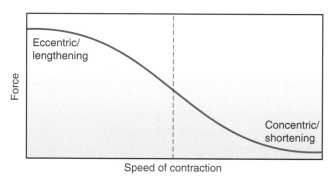

FIG. 5-2 Force–velocity curve comparison for concentric and eccentric contractions. *Redrawn from Davies G: A Compendium of Isokinetics in Clinical Usage and Rehabilitation Techniques, ed 4, Onalaska, Wis, 1992, S & S Publishers.*

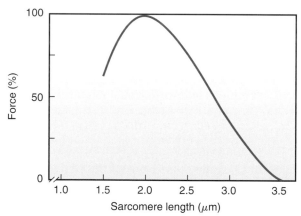

FIG. 5-3 Length-tension curve.

and myosin filaments (Fig. 5-3). Fewer sites are available when the muscle is in either a shortened or lengthened position.

Muscle Architecture. Muscles can have different shapes, or architecture (Fig. 5-4). A pennate muscle has fibers arranged in a feather-like pattern. A pennate muscle can use the length-tension relationship more effectively than a muscle in which the fibers are arranged parallel to

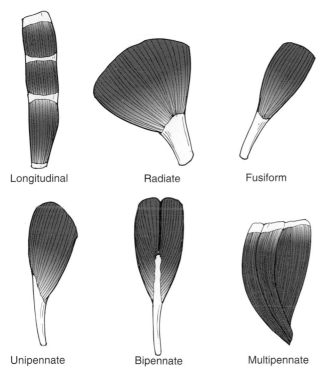

Longitudinal   Radiate   Fusiform

Unipennate   Bipennate   Multipennate

FIG. 5-4 Types of muscle fiber pennation.

the line of muscle action.[27] Pennate muscles can be unipennate, bipennate, or multipennate.[15]

Neural Control. Muscle strength generally increases as more motor units are involved in the contraction, when larger motor units contract, and when the frequency of action potentials is higher.[28] Proper coordination of movement among agonist, synergist, and antagonist muscle groups is also necessary for optimal control and function.

Fatigue. Fatigue is the reduction in force production by a muscle that occurs after repeated contractions. Fatigue can be caused by central (involving the central nervous system [CNS]) or peripheral (contractile mechanism disturbances) factors. Central fatigue involves failure of electrical excitation mechanisms. Peripherally, fatigue is influenced by adenosine triphosphate (ATP) supplies and at times by the availability or activity of acetylcholine at the motor end plate. Peripherally, limitations in oxygen transport or oxygen utilization by the muscle may also result in fatigue.[29] Fatigue of one muscle or muscle group can lead to substitution by other muscle groups or muscle injury.

Individual's Age. Muscle performance changes throughout the lifespan. Muscle strength and endurance increase linearly with chronological age in boys and girls through childhood until puberty. Muscle mass also increases in parallel with body mass at this age. The ability to increase strength rapidly accelerates during puberty, especially in boys. Strength potential is at its highest between 18 and 30 years of age.[30] Muscle mass peaks in women between the ages of 16 and 20 years and in men between the ages of 18 and 25 years. After the third decade of life strength declines by 8% to 10% per decade through

the fifth or sixth decade, with the rate of decline accelerating to 2% to 4% per year beginning in the sixth to seventh decade.[31,32]

Age-related loss of muscle strength is not uniform for all muscle groups, muscle fibers, or types of contractions. In general, lower extremity muscle strength declines more quickly than upper extremity muscle strength, and dynamic strength declines more quickly than isometric strength. According to computed tomography, after the age of 30, individual muscles in the thigh have a lower cross-sectional area and muscle density and a higher intramuscular fat content. These changes are most prominent in women.[33] The number of muscle fibers in the midsection of the vastus lateralis of autopsy specimens has also been found to be significantly lower in older men (age 70-73 years) than in younger men (age 19-37 years), with type II muscle fiber numbers declining the most.[34,35] The progressive average decline in muscle strength associated with aging may be more related to changes in patterns of use with age than to intrinsic changes in muscle produced by aging itself.[36-38]

Cognitive Strategies. Positive cognitive strategies, such as arousal, attention, imagery, and self-efficacy, are associated with enhanced muscle strength and performance,[39] whereas some types of mental preparation, such as relaxation-visualization training, have been found to have a negligible or negative impact on strength performance.[40]

Corticosteroids. Corticosteroids, used commonly as antiinflammatory and immunosuppressant agents, have potent catabolic effects. Prolonged use and high doses of corticosteroids cause protein degradation to exceed protein synthesis. This causes muscle atrophy and weakness, particularly in the limb muscles.[41]

PATHOLOGY

MUSCLE STRAIN

A muscle strain is a stretch or tear of a muscle. Muscle strains most commonly occur at the musculotendinous junction, which is the weakest area of the muscle.[42,43] Muscle strains are common and account for approximately 50% of athletic injuries.[44] A muscle strain can occur acutely, when a muscle exerts a single high load intrinsic force, or gradually, as the result of repetitive low load overuse. Additionally, a muscle strain can be caused by excessive extrinsic passive stretching of a muscle. In some instances, a strain may result from a combination of excessive intrinsic and extrinsic force. The gastrocnemius may be strained when someone lands from a jump in which the foot and ankle move into dorsiflexion, extrinsically stretching the muscle, while the gastrocnemius is also contracting eccentrically, placing an intrinsic force on the muscle. This type of movement occurs frequently during many athletic and recreational activities.

Muscle strain injuries are generally graded on a 3-point scale. In a grade I injury, a few muscle fibers are torn. With this injury, there is some minor swelling and discomfort when the muscle contracts against resistance, but the muscle can contract with normal strength. There is little if any discoloration, and little pain occurs with palpation of the area of the strain. In a grade II muscle strain injury, also known as a partial tear, there is a moderate tearing of muscle fibers without complete tearing through the muscle. Grade II muscle strains are the most common.[45,46] This injury will cause moderate pain with active contraction against resistance and the contraction will be weak. Additionally, moderate swelling, moderate pain with palpation, and pain with passive stretching will be present with a grade II muscle strain. A grade III muscle strain is a severe injury to the muscle fibers that causes complete muscle rupture. Because the muscle fibers no longer form a continuous muscle there may not be pain when contraction is attempted, but there will be profound weakness. There will also be severe swelling and discoloration and possibly a palpable gap in the muscle belly.

Factors that contribute to muscle strain injury include inadequate muscle flexibility, inadequate strength or endurance, synergistic muscle contraction, insufficient warm-up, and inadequate rehabilitation from previous injury.[47-49]

DISUSE ATROPHY

Disuse muscle atrophy refers to wasting or loss of muscle as a result of lack of use. Disuse atrophy may occur for a variety of reasons, including illness, surgery, and various disease processes (heart conditions, cancer). Most of these conditions have one thing in common—a certain amount of convalescence. With this convalescence comes muscle disuse, as well as cardiovascular deconditioning (see Chapter 23).

Loss of muscle performance after injury or surgery is often rapid and dramatic. This can be especially debilitating for patients with impaired muscle performance before their injury or surgery. Complete cessation of training will in most instances cause an immediate decline in strength.[50] If bed rest or limitations in activity are required, or if there is inflammation after trauma or surgery, this decline in strength can be compounded.

Electromyography (EMG) indicates that initial strength losses with detraining are primarily related to neural changes and that muscle atrophy occurs slightly later, with more prolonged disuse and detraining.[51] Short periods of detraining cause nonsignificant changes in fat-free mass and percentage body fat; as disuse and detraining continue, loss of strength and muscle size accelerate.[52-55] In addition, cardiovascular fitness may be lost before high force and power production, causing reduced muscle endurance.[50,56]

Muscle fibers degenerate somewhat sequentially, with *fast-twitch (type II) fibers* degenerating and losing their ability to produce force before *slow-twitch (type I) fibers*.[57-59] This sequence is thought to occur because type II fibers require a higher recruiting stimulus that is most likely not achieved during reduced use and early in rehabilitation, when contractions are weak, whereas type I fiber recruitment and activation occurs with almost all activity (Fig. 5-5).

MUSCLE DISEASES

Myopathies are nonspecific muscle weaknesses caused by an identifiable disease or condition.[60] Myopathies are gen-

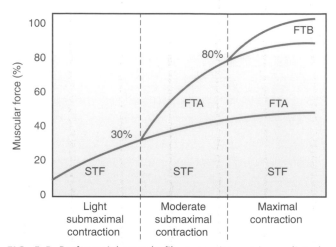

FIG. 5-5 Preferential muscle fiber recruitment is predicted by the intensity of muscle contraction. *STF,* Slow twitch fiber; *FTA,* fast twitch A; *FTB,* fast twitch B. *From Davies G: A Compendium of Isokinetics in Clinical Usage and Rehabilitation Techniques, ed 4, Onalaska, Wis, 1992, S & S Publishers.*

erally classified as hereditary or acquired. One of the more common hereditary myopathies is muscular dystrophy. In this condition, depending on the subtype of the disease, weakness can occur at any age but usually starts in childhood and progresses gradually over time. Most types of muscular dystrophy are thought to have a genetic origin and are characterized by symmetrical muscle wasting without neural or sensory deficits.[61]

NEUROLOGICAL DISEASES AFFECTING MUSCLE PERFORMANCE

Several neurological diseases can cause or be associated with muscle weakness. For example, cerebral palsy is a persistent, although not unchanging, disorder of movement and posture that appears early in life caused by a nonprogressive lesion of the developing brain (see Chapter 14).[62] Although cerebral palsy is primarily a neural condition, people with cerebral palsy may have muscle weakness.[63] Similarly, multiple sclerosis, another disease that primarily affects the CNS, is also associated with muscular weakness.[64] This weakness is associated with profound muscle fatigue[65,66] and possibly muscle fiber atrophy,[67] spasticity, sensory loss, and behavioral muscle disuse.[64]

Myasthenia gravis is an autoimmune disorder that affects the functioning of the acetylcholine receptors at the motor end plate preventing efficient neuromuscular transmission and thus causing weakness primarily characterized by fatigue.[68]

A variety of nerve root and peripheral nerve disorders can also result in muscle weakness (see Chapter 8 on spinal disorders, Chapter 18 on peripheral neuropathies, and Chapter 19 on polyneuropathies for a full discussion of the effects of peripheral nerve disorders). For example, a nerve root lesion at the C5 to T1 spinal levels, a peripheral lesion of the radial nerve at the radial tunnel, or compression of the posterior interosseous nerve as it passes between the two heads of the supinator muscle in the arcade or canal of Frohse can cause wrist extensor muscle weakness and a functional wrist drop.[69] Other neurological conditions associated with muscle weakness include post-polio syndrome, Guillain-Barré syndrome, spinal cord injury, and cerebral vascular accident.[2]

EXAMINATION

PATIENT HISTORY

As with any neuromusculoskeletal condition, a thorough patient history should be the first component of the examination. For the hospitalized patient, much of the history may be obtained through a review of the medical chart. In an outpatient setting, the therapist can generally obtain information regarding the patient's age, sex, race, employment, arm and leg dominance, general health status, past medical history including surgery, and present functional status directly from the patient. Psychosocial issues related to educational level, cultural beliefs, caregiver resources, and living environment should be discussed. Information regarding medications, laboratory or diagnostic tests, or other clinical findings should be noted.

The patient's expectations of therapy should be discussed. Patient's expectations can affect compliance with recommendations and satisfaction with treatment outcomes.

SYSTEMS REVIEW

The systems review is used to target areas requiring further examination and to define areas that may cause complications or indicate a need for precautions during the examination and intervention processes. See Chapter 1 for details of the systems review.

A musculoskeletal scanning examination should include gross tests of range of motion (ROM), strength, and relative flexibility and include observation of body size, proportion, and symmetry. The review of the neuromuscular systems may include gross examination of coordination, balance, reflexes, sensation, skin integrity, and orientation to person, place, and time.

TESTS AND MEASURES
Musculoskeletal

Anthropometric Characteristics. Limb circumference can be used to approximate muscle size. Limb circumference is generally measured with a tape measure and is often assumed to correlate with muscle power and strength, with greater circumference and muscle bulk indicating greater strength. Although limb circumference and muscle strength decrease with disuse muscle atrophy, several studies have found that the assumption that limb girth correlates with strength is misleading. Cooper et al evaluated the relationship between thigh circumference and muscle strength and power as measured by isokinetic dynamometry and found no correlation between the torques produced at the knee by the knee extensors and flexors and thigh circumference measures at three levels.[70] In addition, Hortobagyi et al also found that individual differences in muscle strength correlate poorly with segmental girth measurements.[71]

Joint swelling, generally estimated by measurement of joint circumference, can cause neuromuscularly mediated inhibition of muscle contraction. For example, knee joint effusion has been shown to inhibit quadriceps and vasti muscle contraction in a variety of patient populations.[72-74] This form of muscle weakness is thought to be a result of neurological shutdown of the quadriceps rather than true quadriceps muscle weakness. Furthermore, it takes very little joint effusion, as little as 50-60 ml of fluid in a normal knee joint, to cause reflex inhibition of the rectus femoris and vastus lateralis and a mere 20-30 ml to inhibit the vastus medialis oblique.[73]

Range of Motion. Both active ROM (AROM) and passive ROM (PROM) should be measured during the examination of a patient with suspected muscular weakness. Muscle weakness will not affect passive range of motion but may reduce AROM if strength is substantially decreased. If muscle injury or atrophy has affected strength enough to impair lifting against gravity, the patient may have decreased AROM that is readily observed during functional activities and with specific measurement of AROM. An inability to move a given segment through full AROM when PROM is full and painless generally indicates muscle strength impairment.

Muscle Performance. Patients with muscle weakness have reduced muscle performance, which is the capacity of a muscle to do work (force × distance).[75] This weakness may impair strength, power, and endurance. Strength is the ability of the muscle to exert a maximal force or torque at a specified or determined velocity. Power is the rate of work, or amount of work per unit time, and endurance refers to the ability to perform low intensity, repetitive, or sustained activities over a prolonged period of time without fatigue. Because optimal muscle performance and patient function relies on the balance and interplay among these three variables, muscle performance testing should include testing of strength, power, and endurance.

Strength can be measured in terms of force, torque, or work.[75] Functional strength relates to the ability of the neuromuscular system to produce, reduce, or control forces that are either contemplated or imposed during functional activities in a smooth, coordinated fashion.[50,72] There are various causes of decreased muscle strength, including loss of muscle mass, altered neuromuscular transmission, neuromuscular inhibition, and poor intramuscular and intermuscular coordination.[76,77]

The effect of strength on function depends on both absolute and relative strength. *Absolute strength* is the most force a muscle can generate, or the maximum amount of weight that an individual can lift once (1 RM) irrespective of their body weight. *Relative strength* is absolute strength divided by the person's body weight. Generally, women's absolute and relative upper body strength is lower than men's.[50] However, although women's absolute lower body strength is also generally less than men's, their relative lower extremity strength is generally similar to men's.[61] In most circumstances, because many functional activities involve moving external objects, absolute strength has more effect on function than relative strength. However, relative strength is more important in activities where body weight is a factor, including ambulation and sports such as wrestling and Olympic weightlifting.

Power is the amount of work produced by a muscle per unit time (force × distance/time).[1,75,78-80] Because velocity is equal to distance/time, power is equal to force × velocity. This definition emphasizes the importance of the speed component of power. The rate of force production is an essential element in the production of power. Therefore the greatest power is produced by exerting the most force in the shortest amount of time.

The ability to generate power is essential not only for sporting activity but also for many activities of daily living (ADLs). Quickly stepping forward to catch your balance and prevent falling forward is an example of an activity that requires quick application of force and thus high power. Power can be improved by either increasing strength or by reducing the amount of time required to produce force.

Endurance is often described in broad terms and refers to the ability to perform low intensity, repetitive, or sustained activities over a prolonged period of time without fatigue.[81-83] Endurance can be further broken down into local muscle endurance and general endurance. General endurance is often referred to as cardiovascular endurance. Local *muscle endurance,* however, refers to the ability of a muscle to contract repeatedly against a load (resistance), generate and sustain tension, and resist fatigue over an extended period of time.[83] Activities requiring cardiovascular endurance also require muscular endurance, although tasks requiring muscular endurance do not always require cardiovascular endurance. Muscular endurance training can also improve cardiovascular endurance.[14] The term aerobic power is sometimes used interchangeably with muscular endurance.[80]

Manual Muscle Testing. *Manual muscle testing* (MMT) is used to test the strength of individual muscles or muscle groups. MMT is performed by applying manual resistance to a limb or body part. This resistance is typically applied to the limb at a point in the limb's ROM where the muscle being tested is most efficient. Muscle strength is graded on a 0-5 numeric scale. All the grades above 1 may be scored as the number alone or with a score of the number with a + or −. Definitions of these scores are given in Table 5-2.

To test the strength of muscles with a grade higher than fair (3/5) a break test should be used.[84] This is performed by applying pressure to the tested segment, in addition to gravity, to determine the maximal effort that the subject can exert. The clinician gradually applies more pressure until the effort by the patient is overcome.[84] When a muscle can only move a body part against gravity, its strength is graded as 3/5. When testing weak muscles with less than 3/5 strength, a position that minimizes gravity and that generally involves moving the body part in the horizontal plane is used.

The MMT scale is easy to apply, but it is important to realize that these scores are relative. A score of 4 does not indicate that a muscle is twice as strong as one with a score of 2. Furthermore, validity of high scores may be limited by the strength of the clinician performing the test. MMT is the fastest and most efficient means of assessing muscle strength in the clinical setting. According to Kendall et al, muscle testing is an integral part of the patient examina-

TABLE 5-2	Muscle Testing Grading Categories	
Grade	Contraction Strength	Movement
5	Normal (100%)	Complete range of motion against gravity with maximal resistance
4	Good (75%)	Complete range of motion against gravity with some (moderate) resistance
3+	Fair +	Complete range of motion against gravity with minimal resistance
3	Fair (50%)	Complete range of motion against gravity
3−	Fair −	Some but not complete range of motion against gravity
2+	Poor +	Initiates motion against gravity
2	Poor (25%)	Complete range of motion against gravity eliminated
2−	Poor −	Initiates motion if gravity is eliminated
1	Trace	Evidence of slight contractility but no joint motion
0	None	No contraction palpated

Adapted from Magee DJ (ed): *Orthopedic Physical Assessment,* ed 3, Philadelphia, 1997, WB Saunders.

tion and provides information not obtained by other procedures.[84]

Although advantages of MMT include the speed with which it can be performed, its ready availability, and its inexpensiveness because it requires no equipment, its disadvantages include poor reliability associated with some testing procedures.[85] Frese et al[86] assessed interrater and intrarater reliability of MMT of the middle trapezius and the gluteus medius muscles performed by 11 therapists in 110 patients with various diagnoses. A small percentage of the therapists (50% to 60%) graded the muscle strength in these two muscles similarly, with the same grade (on a scale of 0-5), plus or minus one-third of a grade.[86] Rainville et al[87] evaluated the interrater reliability of two examiners grading quadriceps strength by MMT in 33 patients with L3 or L4 radiculopathy and 19 patients with L5 or S1 radiculopathy. Correlation of the two therapists' scores were moderate (kappa coefficient = 0.66) when the quadriceps strength was tested with the knee flexed, and low (kappa coefficient = 0.08) when quadriceps strength was tested with the knee extended.[87] The results of MMT may be affected by many factors other than muscle strength, including patient positioning, stabilization, effort and motivation, as well as leverage differences, sex differences, overall strength differences, age, and biomechanical and muscle length-tension relationships through the ROM, as well as various compensatory patterns.[88]

Hand-Held Dynamometers. Hand-held dynamometers may also be used to test the strength of individual muscles or muscle groups. A dynamometer is a device that can measure force. The hand-held dynamometer is a small device that fits in the examiner's hand and is placed at precise locations on a subject's limb in an effort to assess the force generated by various muscles or groups of muscles. Hand-held dynamometers are inexpensive, convenient, and lightweight; require minimal set up time and training; and can be used in a wide variety of settings.[89]

Because hand-held dynamometers overcome some of the limitations of MMT, particularly the subjectivity and nonlinearity of grading muscle force production, and because they have good to very good reliability, they are popular and well-accepted in clinical practice.[90-98] However, as with MMT, consistent locations and patient positions must be used for accurate and reliable results. These devices have been shown to quantitatively monitor strengthening regimes.[99] Recently, Leggin et al[100] found high reliability using three different hand-held dynamometers for strength testing (ICC: 0.84-0.99).

Isotonic Testing. *Isotonic* testing involves lifting a fixed mass against gravity. This testing can be performed using weight machines or free weights. There are many isotonic strength testing protocols including the 1 *repetition maximum* (RM) and the 10 RM. A 10 RM is the maximum amount of weight that can be lifted and lowered 10 times, and 1 RM is the maximum amount of weight that can be lifted once.[2] The 10 RM test was first developed by DeLorme.[101] Isotonic testing of all types has been criticized because it is limited by the "sticking point," or the weakest point, in the ROM and therefore only measures the maximum strength at this point.[88,102,103] In addition, the more recent literature calls this type of strength testing dynamic testing because it involves both a concentric (muscle shortening) and eccentric (muscle lengthening) contraction.[104]

Isokinetic Testing. *Isokinetic* strength testing measures force production during fixed velocity movement with an accommodating resistance.[88] Isokinetic strength testing is performed using an electrically powered device that maintains a chosen velocity of movement while maximizing the resistance throughout the ROM. There are many isokinetic strength testing devices available. All have components to allow testing of movement of different joints and in some instances, for testing during open and closed kinetic chain movements. Isokinetic devices can be programmed for velocities from 1 to 500 degrees per second.

Isokinetic measures can be compared with normative data for a given population or compared to the uninvolved side to determine if muscle performance is normal or abnormal. Measures can also indicate the presence of certain pathologies that produce characteristic torque curves during testing.[105] Advantages of isokinetic strength testing include its ability to measure the strength of *concentric* and *eccentric contractions* and its high reliability when applied in a standardized manner.[106] However, test-retest reliability can be poor if strength is tested with differing sequencing of angular velocities.[107] Ellenbecker therefore recommends beginning all isokinetic testing with the slowest speed in the testing sequence and progressing consistently to faster speeds to enhance reliability.[108]

Isokinetic testing can provide information about subtle changes in strength that may not be detectable by MMT.[109] Wilk et al found in 176 patients who had undergone knee arthroscopy, whose strength was graded as 5/5 bilaterally with MMT of the quadriceps and hamstrings, that isokinetic testing revealed that some patients had strength deficits of as much as 23% to 31%.[109] However, a limitation of isokinetic testing is that it does not isolate specific muscles but rather measures combined strength for moving in a single plane such as knee flexion or extension.

Isokinetic strength testing can also give a clinician copious information about a wide range of variables related to muscle strength as listed in the following:

- Peak torque
- Average peak torque
- Angle-specific peak torque
- Peak torque to body weight
- Total work
- Average power
- Peak power
- Torque acceleration energy (TAE)
- Acceleration time
- Average points variance
- Speed-specific data
- Time rate of torque development
- Time to peak torque
- Endurance ratios
- Force decay rate
- Reciprocal innervation time

Specific interpretation of these extensive test data is beyond the scope of this chapter. For further information on this complex area, readers are referred to other texts related directly to isokinetic testing,[110-112] as well as those listed in Additional Resources.

Joint Integrity. Although joint integrity does not generally limit muscle strength, limitations in joint mobility will affect joint movement and measurement of muscle strength and performance. For example, even with full strength, a patient with a severely swollen knee will probably be unable to force the knee through full AROM as a result of pain inhibition.

Neuromuscular

Arousal, Attention, and Cognition. In patients with weakness, changes in arousal, attention, or cognition are generally apparent and can be grossly assessed during the patient history. The patient's ability to maintain attention and their alertness and orientation will affect the ability to obtain a thorough and complete history and may affect cooperation both with strength testing procedures and with therapeutic interventions.

Pain. Pain may dramatically affect muscle performance and can inhibit muscle contraction, giving the impression of muscle weakness. With prolonged inhibition and the resulting prolonged disuse, pain can at times also lead to significant muscle atrophy and true weakness. Postural muscle spasm resulting from pain or injury may also affect performance on muscle strength tests.[113,114] Muscle spasms are thought to protect susceptible tissues from further damage but may also affect examination findings by limiting positioning or further muscle performance.[113,114] There are many ways to measure pain, including visual analog scales, questionnaires, and pain diagrams, as described in detail in Chapter 22.

Peripheral Nerve Integrity. Peripheral nerve integrity can be examined and evaluated clinically through a combination of strength, sensory, and reflex testing as described in detail in Chapter 18. If available, EMG may also be used to examine and evaluate peripheral nerve integrity.

Peripheral nerve compression will generally affect sensation first and will then affect motor function if it progresses. If the peripheral nerve is affected, sensory and motor loss will occur distal to the lesion in the distribution of that nerve. If the nerve is affected at the spinal nerve root, sensory loss will be in a dermatomal distribution and strength loss will be in a myotomal distribution.

Nerve injuries can be classified according to the Seddon scheme as a neurapraxia, axonotmesis, or neurotmesis.[115] Neurapraxia involves segmental demyelination, generally as a result of prolonged compression and ischemia, and usually does not affect strength. Axonotmesis, which involves axonal damage without damage to the myelin covering, may affect strength, for a period of time but full strength will generally return because the intact myelin facilitates nerve repair. Neurotmesis, the most severe type of nerve injury, involves damage to both the axon and its myelin coating, and quickly produces muscle atrophy and strength loss. In this circumstance strength will not return unless the nerves are surgically repaired. It is important to know if strength deficits are caused by nerve lesions because this type of weakness will not respond to the usual strengthening interventions unless or until nerve function recovers.

Sensory Integrity. Testing for sensory integrity is important for the examination and evaluation of peripheral nerve integrity (see Chapter 18). Furthermore, special care should be taken to protect the skin and soft tissue in patients with sensory impairment from injury during strengthening interventions.

Cardiovascular/Pulmonary

Circulation, Ventilation, and Respiration/Gas Exchange. Vital signs checked during the systems review will generally indicate if the patient with muscle weakness has cardiovascular or pulmonary problems. Vital signs of heart rate, blood pressure, and respiratory rate should be checked at the beginning of each session involving muscle exercise in patients with cardiovascular or pulmonary problems (see Chapter 22).

Aerobic Capacity and Endurance. Because aerobic capacity depends on the function of large muscle groups, aerobic capacity and endurance can be decreased in patients with muscle weakness (see Chapters 23 and 26 for information on measurement of aerobic capacity and endurance). This is especially true for sedentary individuals with large muscle group atrophy or weakness that results from chronic disuse. For example, Birk[116] and Stanghelle and Festvag[117] found that aerobic capacity was lower in patients with post-polio syndrome than in age and gender matched healthy controls.

Function

Gait, Locomotion, and Balance. Gait will often be affected by lower extremity muscle weakness. Gait assessment and intervention are discussed in detail in Chapter 32.

Assistive and Adaptive Devices. Depending on the extent of muscle weakness the patient may need to use an assistive or adaptive device (see Chapter 33). If MMT reveals the strength of lower extremity to be less than 4/5, an assistive device may be warranted to ensure safe ambulation. Crutches, a cane, or even a walker may be needed to balance and ambulate safely and efficiently.

Orthotic, Protective, and Supportive Devices. Orthotics and protective devices can improve function and safety for individuals with muscle weakness. These devices generally support a joint, or joints, to substitute for the weak muscle. The patient's current strength, functional abilities, and lifestyle will dictate which orthosis will work best for the particular situation. For example, patients with weak dorsiflexors may benefit from an ankle-foot orthosis (AFO) and those with weakness of the quadriceps and dorsiflexors may benefit from a knee-ankle-foot orthosis (KAFO)[118] (see Chapter 34).

The effects of bracing on muscle strength appear to be site specific. Studies have shown that a lumbar orthosis can increase peak muscle torque of the abdominal and back muscles in normal male volunteers[119] and that the intermittent prophylactic use of abdominal bracing does not adversely effect abdominal muscle strength and may actually reduce lost time at work.[120] Conversely, wrist extensor activity has been found to be reduced with four different wrist orthoses, but the long-term effects of extremity orthoses on strength have not been evaluated.[121]

EVALUATION, DIAGNOSIS, AND PROGNOSIS

According to the *Guide to Physical Therapist Practice,*[122] rehabilitation for patients in the preferred practice pattern 4C: Impaired Muscle Performance may take from 2-6 months with an expected range of 6-30 visits to achieve optimal performance. This range is wide because many factors may affect the frequency and duration of physical therapy visits, such as accessibility and availability of resources, age, caregiver consistency or expertise, cognitive status, comorbidities, concurrent therapeutic interventions, nutritional and overall health status, psychological and socioeconomic factors, and social support.

INTERVENTION

Interventions to reduce muscle weakness are based on the overload principle and the selective adaptation to imposed demands (SAID) principle. Training should also take into account the concepts of individuality, frequency, intensity, and duration.

OVERLOAD PRINCIPLE

The human body can continually adapt to external stimuli. If an individual encounters a load greater than usual, they will, if possible, adapt to this load by increasing strength, power, or endurance, depending on the nature of the load. This adaptive response to increased training load is called the overload principle. Once a body adapts to a given workload it will not change further unless the workload continues to increase. Therefore, to continually improve performance, the load must be progressively increased to promote progressive adaptation.[123]

Although the body initially responds to overload with fatigue, its gradual adaptation to the increased load can be used therapeutically in rehabilitation to increase strength and fitness.[124]

SAID PRINCIPLE

A systematic approach to progression of the load applied during exercise will optimize improvements in muscle performance and resultant functional ability. According to the SAID (specific adaptations to imposed demands) principle, the body adapts according to the demands placed on it. Therefore exercise for patients with muscle weakness should emphasize strength, power, and endurance according to the functional goals and needs of the individual patient.

Several factors should be considered when designing a strengthening program, including the patient's age, sex, medical history, previous training background, injury history, the body's structural integrity, functional goals, motivation, and any healing restraints related to their injury or surgery.[125] A rehabilitation training program to reduce muscle weakness also needs to consider the primary energy source used, muscle(s) actions, the mechanism of resistance, and velocity of movement required.

Energy Source. Aerobic and anaerobic energy sources may be used to produce muscle actions, depending on which component of muscle performance is mostly required. Anaerobic energy sources are used predominantly for short, intense activities and aerobic energy sources are used predominantly for longer duration, less intense activities.

Muscle Action. Muscle action refers to whether a contraction is dynamic (produces movement) or isometric (does not produce movement). Muscle action during rehabilitation exercises should match the patient's intended function, the primary function of the muscle being trained (agonist or primary mover, antagonist, stabilization), and the movement pattern of the muscle. Muscle groups are often required to perform several different types of contractions during a functional task. The muscle action requirements for each primary task should be taken into account when formulating and progressing the intervention plan, and the specific movement pattern required for functional activities should be replicated as closely as possible.

Because the CNS produces patterns of movement that are more than isolated muscle contractions, training using patterns of movement is likely to be most effective for improving functional abilities.[126,127] Patterns of movement, especially those most closely mimicking daily function, can be emphasized early in the rehabilitation process with proprioceptive neuromuscular facilitation (PNF) techniques that use mostly diagonal movement combinations.[128] However, exercises of specific, isolated muscles may also be necessary when functional activities are limited by weakness in an isolated muscle or muscle group.

Mechanism of Resistance. Muscle performance can vary, depending on the mechanism of resistance. For example, studies have shown that the quadriceps may perform poorly with open-chain activities when they are strong with closed-chain activities.[129,130] This type of residual weakness can occur after resistance training that only involves closed-chain activities.[131] Therefore strengthening programs should include activities with the same mechanism of resistance as needed for the patient's functional activity goals.

Velocity of Movement. Training has also been shown to be velocity specific, with the greatest gains in strength being made with contractions at the training velocity.[132,133] Therefore high velocity training should be used to improve performance of activities that require high velocity movement, and slower velocity training should be used to improve performance of activities that require slow velocity movement. This velocity specificity is likely based in part on fiber specificity, with type II fibers being activated more for fast movements and type I fibers being activated more for slow sustained contractions.

EXERCISE PRESCRIPTION

There are several ways to progressively overload a muscle to improve muscle performance.[134] Exercise to improve muscle performance is most readily described and prescribed according to its frequency, intensity, time, and type (the *FITT formula*).

Frequency. Frequency refers to how often exercise should be performed. The ideal frequency of exercise depends on the goals of the treatment and stage of recovery from injury or surgery. During the acute stage of healing, exercise can occur more frequently but most likely with less duration and intensity than in more advanced strengthening stages. In later advanced stages of strengthening, it is imperative to reduce the frequency of training to allow for sufficient recovery to avoid excessive fatigue, decreased performance, and overtraining.[29,134] Overtraining can be prevented by selection of the appropriate volume and frequency of exercise (periodization).[135] Periodization (Fig. 5-6) can also be used to select the optimal volume and frequency of exercise to achieve peak performance at specific times for sporting activity.

Intensity. The intensity of an exercise program should be kept inversely proportional to its volume.[130,136] The intensity is the amount of resistance used for a specific exercise and is generally set as a percentage of the individuals 1 RM (or any RM) for that particular exercise. The training volume is the total amount of work performed, whether in a particular session or in some set period of time.[134] As rehabilitation or training progresses, either the intensity or the volume of the exercise should be increased while the other is initially decreased. The relative emphasis on exercise intensity or volume depends on the individual's functional requirements and impairments. If a patient has primarily an endurance deficit, then volume should be prioritized over intensity; if a patient primarily has a strength or power deficit, then intensity should be prioritized over volume.

Duration/Time. Duration is the total number of weeks or months during which a resistance exercise program is carried out. Duration depends on multiple factors, including stage of healing, progress in rehabilitation, initial functional level, prognosis, functional goals, and presence or absence of comorbidities. In addition, duration for a maintenance program will by definition be much longer than for a recovery or rehabilitation program.

Type/Mode of Exercise. Type of exercise relates to the specific activity being performed, including the mode of resistance (e.g., free weights, elastic band, water) and type of activity being performed (e.g., isotonic, isometric, isokinetic, open chain, closed chain.). Different modes of

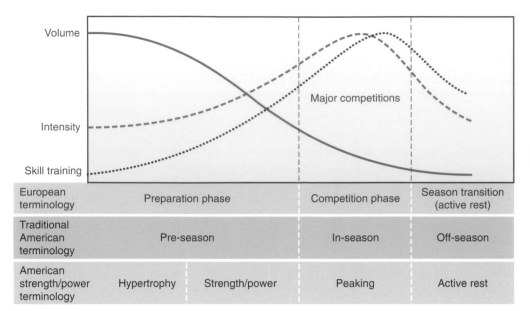

FIG. 5-6 Periodization training phases.

European terminology	Preparation phase		Competition phase	Season transition (active rest)
Traditional American terminology	Pre-season		In-season	Off-season
American strength/power terminology	Hypertrophy	Strength/power	Peaking	Active rest

resistance and types of exercise are discussed in greater detail later in this chapter.

NEUROMUSCULAR ELECTRICAL STIMULATION

Neuromuscular electrical stimulation (NMES) can be an effective component of a rehabilitation program for muscle weakness. NMES can help when the client is either unable or unwilling to volitionally elicit strong muscle contractions. NMES has been shown to accelerate functional recovery after surgery, prevent disuse atrophy, reduce ROM deficits, and improve motor control in patients with strength deficits of various etiologies.[137-139]

For NMES to increase muscle strength the electrical current must produce contractions that are at least 50% of the maximum volitional isometric contraction (MVIC) force for the targeted muscles.[140] NMES preferentially strengthens type II muscle fibers because it recruits motor units with type II fibers before those with type I fibers, which is the opposite order from voluntary contractions where type I fibers are recruited first. NMES recruits type II muscle fibers first because the axons of their motor units are larger and more superficial and offer lower resistance to electrical stimulation.[141] It is proposed that this is why NMES can accelerate strengthening and shorten rehabilitation times.[141] NMES is most effective when used in conjunction with volitional muscle contractions. This promotes strengthening of both type I and type II muscle fibers and facilitates integration of motor performance into functional use.

ADAPTATIONS TO RESISTANCE TRAINING

Strength increases because of nervous system adaptations (learning and improved coordination) and muscle *hypertrophy*.[142,143] Initially, in the first 4-6 weeks of training, strength gains are attributed to neural adaptation more than to muscle hypertrophy.[144,145] Some research also suggests that resistance training can produce muscle *hyperplasia*.[50] If hyperplasia does occur, it probably only

accounts for a small portion (5% to 10%) of the increase in muscle size produced.[50] Fig. 5-7 compares the general effects of detraining and training for strength, power, and endurance.

All activities require use of aerobic and anaerobic metabolism, although one type of metabolism generally predominates.[14,81] Strength and power training use more anaerobic metabolism and produce increases in muscle girth and muscle fiber size, as well as improvements in anaerobic capacity. In contrast, endurance training causes muscles to improve their aerobic metabolic capacity and efficiency by enhancing glycogen sparing and increasing fat utilization.[52] Endurance training also causes selective hypertrophy of type I muscle fibers,[146] which can be helpful in conditions that are associated with reductions in type I muscle fiber mass and decreases in muscle endurance such as chronic low back pain.[147-149]

Strength training is also associated with increased neuromuscular efficiency[143,150]; increased bone strength and density[151,152]; increased ligament and tendon strength and thickness[153]; improved balance and decreased the risk of falling[154]; increased gait stability and efficiency[155]; improved stair climbing and chair rising ability[155]; decreased resting blood pressure, glucose tolerance, and insulin resistance[156,157]; and decreased body fat and increased basal metabolic rate.[156]

PRECAUTIONS AND CONTRAINDICATIONS TO MUSCLE STRENGTH TRAINING

When planning and implementing a resistive exercise plan for the treatment of muscle weakness, the following precautions and contraindications should be applied:

- Additional care should be taken in very young and very old patients and in patients with comorbidities
- Limit ROM and tissue stresses as needed to respect tissue healing constraints
- Reexamine and reevaluate patients consistently to ascertain if their signs and symptoms are improving or worsening

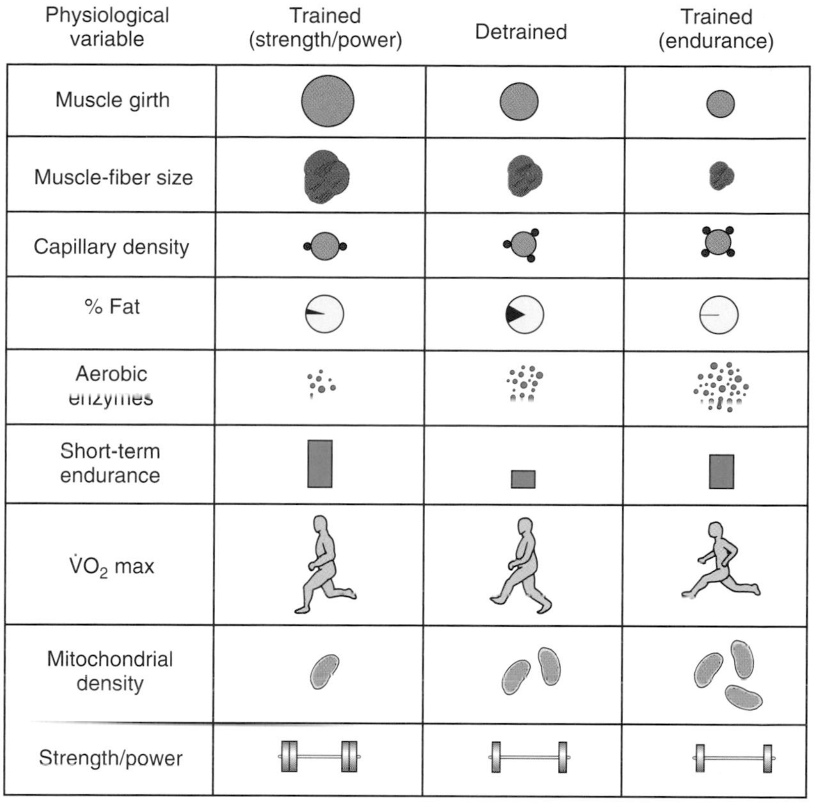

Physiological variable	Trained (strength/power)	Detrained	Trained (endurance)
Muscle girth			
Muscle-fiber size			
Capillary density			
% Fat			
Aerobic enzymes			
Short-term endurance			
$\dot{V}O_2$ max			
Mitochondrial density			
Strength/power			

FIG. 5-7 Comparison of general effects of detraining, training for strength/power, and training for endurance.

The Valsalva maneuver (an expiratory effort against a closed glottis) should be avoided during muscle contractions because this increases intrathoracic and intraabdominal pressure and leads to decreased venous return of blood to the heart. This decrease in venous return leads to a decrease in cardiac output, which then leads to a temporary drop in arterial blood pressure. The decreased arterial pressure then leads to an increase in heart rate. A heart rate increase with resistive exercise is especially contraindicated in high risk patients, such as those with a history of cardiovascular problems (cerebral vascular accident, myocardial infarction, heart failure, and hypertension) and geriatric patients.[17,50,56,61] Furthermore, the increase in intraabdominal pressure can cause damage in patients with a recent history of abdominal surgery or herniation of the abdominal wall. To prevent the Valsalva maneuver, the patient should be instructed to not hold his or her breath and to exhale when performing a contraction. The patient may be asked to count, talk, or breath rhythmically during exercise.

The clinician should try to assure that strengthening exercises activate the intended muscles. When too much resistance is applied, muscle substitution is common. For example, if trying to improve deltoid strength through resisted shoulder elevation, when too much resistance is applied the levator scapula will contract to assist. Close supervision, proper exercise instruction, and the use of a mirror for patients to monitor themselves can all help to reduce muscle substitution.

Dynamic resistance exercises are contraindicated when a muscle or joint is inflamed or swollen because exercise may provoke further inflammation or swelling and further damage the muscle or joint. However, low intensity isometric exercise can be performed if the activity does not cause pain. The patient should be carefully monitored for their immediate response to the prescribed resistance exercise and for their response over the following 24-48 hours. If severe joint or muscle pain occurs during the activity or within the 24-48 hours after exercise, the activity should be eliminated or substantially reduced and the cause of the pain should be determined.

Exercise-induced muscle soreness is muscle soreness that develops during or directly after strenuous exercise performed to the point of fatigue.[158] This response is attributed to a lack of blood flow and oxygen with a temporary buildup of metabolites, such as lactic acid and potassium, in the exercising muscle.[158] This response often subsides quickly after exercise when adequate blood flow and oxygen returns to the muscle. Implementing an appropriate cool down period of low intensity exercise (often referred to as an active recovery) can facilitate recovery from exercise-induced muscle soreness.[159]

Delayed-onset muscle soreness (DOMS) is soreness that occurs some time after vigorous or unaccustomed exercise or muscular overexertion. It often presents as a temporary stiffness and tenderness occurring approximately 12-24 hours after completion of the exercise and is clearly linked to eccentric activity.[2] Although the time course varies, the signs and symptoms can last up to 10-14 days and gradually dissipate.[81,83] The underlying mechanism of DOMS is still unclear. It has been suggested that DOMS is caused by a buildup of lactic acid in muscles or by muscle spasm after exercise,[160] but neither of these theories have been corroborated by research.[161,162] It has also been suggested that DOMS is caused by microtrauma to muscle fibers because this is common with high resistance eccentric exercise.

Acute or delayed exercise–induced muscle soreness can be avoided by gradually and systematically progressing the rehabilitation program. The American College of Sports Medicine recommends that changes in total training volume should be made in small increments of 2.5% to 5%.[134]

Strengthening exercises should also be modified for patients with osteoporosis. High resistance, explosive, or twisting type movements should be avoided, and endurance exercises or low intensity strength training should be emphasized (see Chapter 3 for further information on exercise in patients with osteoporosis).

MUSCLE STRENGTH TRAINING INTERVENTIONS

Rehabilitating muscle performance deficits is a multidimensional process. The most effective type or mode of training intervention depends on the stage of rehabilitation, the degree of muscle weakness, which muscles are primarily involved and whether they are made up primarily of slow- or fast-twitch fibers, and the primary functional task requirements of each individual client. The primary types of muscle strength training interventions are outlined in the next section with their respective advantages and disadvantages.

Isometric Muscle Strength Training. *Isometric exercises* (also known as *static exercises*) are performed by increasing tension in a muscle while keeping its length constant. To perform an isometric exercise, joint motion must be prevented. This can be achieved by pushing against an immovable object such as a wall (Fig. 5-8), immobilizing the patient with an isokinetic device or with a restraint, or when the therapist can exert sufficient force, by the patient pushing against unmoving resistance provided by the therapist. Isometric exercises against resistance provided by the therapist are often preferred early in rehabilitation because they do not involve joint movement and the intensity of muscle contraction can be more closely monitored by the clinician. However, when isometric exercises are performed against other types of resistance, high forces may be exerted making this type of exercise unsuitable early after any injury to the musculotendinous unit.

Isometric exercises can increase muscle strength but these increases are somewhat joint angle specific. Isometric exercises increase strength the most approximately 10 degrees on either side of the joint angle at which the exercise is performed.[133-135,163-165] Therefore, with isometric strengthening, exercise should be performed at multiple angles every 20 degrees to achieve strength throughout the ROM. Isometric exercises improve strength at other angles by 10% to 50% and have the most effect when performed with the muscle in a lengthened rather than a shortened position.[163-165] The advantages and disadvantages of isometric strengthening are listed in Table 5-3.

Isotonic or Dynamic Muscle Strength Training. Isotonic contractions are performed by lifting a constant weight. Isotonic contractions can be performed using free weights or weight machines and can be approximated

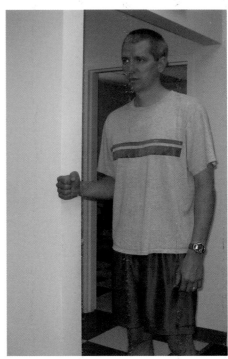

FIG. 5-8 Isometric shoulder external rotation at 0 degrees abduction.

TABLE 5-3	Advantages and Disadvantages of Isometric Strengthening
Advantages	**Disadvantages**
Can be used early in rehabilitation because there is no joint movement.	Strengthening is limited to specific joint angles.
Retards atrophy and increases "static" muscular strength.	Limited to no improvement in dynamic muscular performance.
Helps to decrease swelling.	No eccentric work.
Prevents neural dissociation.	Blood pressure concerns with Valsalva maneuver.
Joint angle-specific strengthening.	Patient motivation is likely to be less.
Can be performed anywhere.	Less proprioceptive and kinesthetic training.
No special equipment needed.	No contribution to muscular endurance.
Short periods of training time.	Can create an ischemic response in muscles.
20° strengthening overflow throughout ROM.	

Modified from Davies GJ: *A Compendium of Isokinetics in Clinical Usage*, Onalaska, Wis, 1992, S & S Publishing.
ROM, Range of motion.

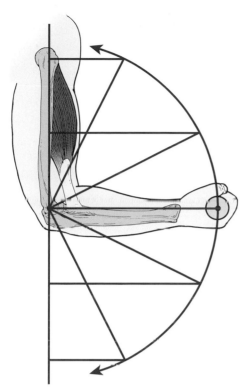

FIG. 5-9 Changing moment arm and resistive torque with elbow flexion. *Redrawn from Harmon E: The biometrics of resistance exercise. In Baechle TR (ed): Essentials of Strength Training and Conditioning. National Strength and Condition Association, ed 2, Champaign, Ill, 2000, Human Kinetics.*

with manual resistance by the therapist. Isotonic contractions have traditionally been considered to involve a constant amount of muscle tension throughout the range of motion. However, Fleck and Kraemer[50] propose calling these types of contractions "dynamic constant external resistance" (DCER) contractions because the force exerted by the muscle, whether using weight machines or free weights, is not constant but rather varies with the mechanical advantage of the joint(s) involved in the movement. DCER implies that it is the weight or external resistance that is constant and not the force developed by the muscle(s).[50] Whether the term *isotonic* or *DCER* is used, an inherent limitation with this type of exercise is that it only maximally challenges the contracting muscle at one point in the ROM where the maximum torque of the resistance matches the maximum output of the muscle. As the weight is lifted, the moment arm through which the weight acts, and therefore the resistive torque, changes as the horizontal distance from the axis of movement changes (Fig. 5-9). The mechanical advantage changes with changes in muscle length and joint angle.

Dynamic strength is the strength exhibited, or the force generated, when the length of a muscle changes while the muscle contracts. Dynamic contractions can be concentric or eccentric. *Concentric contractions* are shortening muscle contractions while eccentric contractions are lengthening muscle contractions. Eccentric contractions can produce more tension per contractile unit at a lower metabolic cost than concentric contrac-

tions.[166,167] This is because eccentric contractions use elastic elements in the muscle and metabolic processes more efficiently and require fewer motor units to be active to produce the same force than with a concentric contraction. Therefore eccentric contractions can be used early in the rehabilitation process, even if a patient cannot contract concentrically throughout the available AROM. In these situations, eccentric contractions can be introduced to allow some form of strengthening in this ROM. An example is the use of eccentric straight leg raises (SLR) in a knee rehabilitation program. Immediately after surgery, the first exercise would be quadriceps sets (an isometric contraction of the quadriceps against gravity) followed by eccentric SLRs. This exercise can be accomplished by having the rehabilitation specialist passively lift the leg and then guide the eccentric contraction as the patient lowers the leg to the starting position. In this situation the quadriceps are performing an isometric contraction and the iliopsoas is performing an eccentric contraction. Advantages and disadvantages of isotonic strengthening exercises are listed in Table 5-4.

Isokinetic Muscle Strength Training. Isokinetic training refers to muscle contractions performed at a constant angular velocity with varying resistance. The isokinetic dynamometer provides maximum resistance throughout the entire ROM. This type of resistance is referred to as accommodating resistance.

Consistent with the specificity principle, several studies have demonstrated that isokinetic strengthening produces the greatest gains in peak torque at the training velocity used but that significant gains also occur above and below this training velocity, except when the velocity is very slow (30 degrees per second or less).[168-174] Behm and Sale propose that this velocity specificity is related to neural mechanisms, including selective activation of motor units and selective activation and deactivation of co-contractions by agonist and antagonist muscles.[174] Advantages and disadvantages of isokinetic training are shown in Table 5-5.

Plyometric Muscle Strength Training. Plyometrics are high intensity, high velocity exercises, such as jumping and bounding in the lower extremities and ballistic push-ups off a wall (Fig. 5-10) in the upper extremities, intended to develop muscular power and coordination.[175,176] This type of training is based on the series elastic and stretch reflex properties of the neuromuscular unit.[175,176] *Plyometric exercise* employs high velocity eccentric and concentric muscle loading, reflexive reactions, and functional movement patterns. Because this type of training places high mechanical demands on the body, it should only be introduced when the patient has good strength and endurance.[177,178] Plyometrics should therefore be reserved for later, higher levels of rehabilitation and focus on functional activities.

It has been proposed that plyometrics should be included in all resistance training programs for both athletes and other patients because plyometric type movements are used in basic activities such as walking and running.[179] However, high velocity, low resistance (approximately 30% of maximum) dynamic weight training has been found to increase vertical jumping and

TABLE 5-4 Advantages and Disadvantages of Isotonic Strengthening

Advantages	Disadvantages
Dynamic constant external resistance that may be an advantage or disadvantage, depending on the situation.	Can maximally load the muscle at its weakest point in the ROM, especially with elastic tubing or bands.
Can improve muscular endurance.	The contracting muscle is only maximally challenged at one point in the ROM with free weights and some machines.
Concentric and eccentric muscle action.	Not safe if someone has pain during movement because patient must maintain resistance.
Use of free weights allows for multiplanar training.	At fast speeds of movement there may be an increased risk of injury.
Can use a variety of resistive devices (e.g., exercise machines, free weights, elastic tubing/bands).	Difficult to exercise at fast functional velocities.
Can use body weight for resistance.	Does not provide reciprocal concentric exercise.
Can exercise through full ROM.	Does not allow for rapid force development.
Use of functional movement patterns.	Exercise-induced muscle soreness and DOMS.
Provides motivation from achievement.	Unable to spread entire workload evenly over the entire ROM.
Inexpensive and readily available with most types of resistive devices.	
Can use manual resistance from rehabilitation specialist—allowing for specific tactile input and improved proprioceptive and kinesthetic awareness.	
More objective documentation capabilities than with isometrics.	
Various components of the program can be manipulated to maintain workload (reps, sets, weight).	
Can increase muscle strength with few repetitions.	

Modified from Davies GJ: *A Compendium of Isokinetics in Clinical Usage,* Onalaska, Wis, 1992, S & S Publishing.
ROM, Range of motion; *DOMS,* delayed-onset muscle soreness.

TABLE 5-5 Advantages and Disadvantages of Isokinetic Strengthening

Advantages	Disadvantages
Reported to cause little muscle soreness.[127]	Many physical activities far exceed the angular velocities that can be produced by isokinetic testing devices.
Concentric and eccentric strengthening of same muscle group can be performed repeatedly, or reciprocal exercise of opposing muscle groups can be performed—one muscle group always rests.	Large and expensive equipment.
Reliable measures with the equipment.	Requires assistance and time for set-up.
Helps force development (time rate of torque development).	Cannot be incorporated into a home program.
Efficiency of muscular contractions.	Most units only provide open chain movement patterns.
Can exercise at a wide range of velocities.	Most exercise performed in a single plane and at constant velocity.
Computer-based visual and/or auditory cues for feedback.	Cannot duplicate reciprocal speeds of movement used during most daily and functional activities.
Can provide maximum resistance at all points in ROM.	Eccentric loading can cause DOMS.
Can safely perform high- and low-velocity training.	Lack of personnel trained in use or interpretation of isokinetic testing and rehabilitation.
Accommodates for painful arc of motion.	Availability of equipment.
Can continue exercise as patient fatigues.	Time consuming if more than one joint is exercised/assessed.
Decreased joint compressive forces at high speed.	Some artificial parameters until the tested limb reaches the velocity of the dynamometer or decelerates.
Short duration of joint compression.	
Physiological overflow.	
Neurophysiological "pattern" for functional speeds and movements.	
Isolated muscle strengthening.	
External stabilization.	

Modified from Davies GJ: *A Compendium of Isokinetics in Clinical Usage,* Onalaska, Wis, 1992, S & S Publishing.
ROM, Range of motion; *DOMS,* delayed-onset muscle soreness.

isokinetic tested leg extension strength at high speeds more than plyometric training, suggesting that as long as the movement is fast plyometrics may not be necessary to optimize functional outcome.[180]

Plyometric drills should be preceded by a warm-up period to prepare the patient's cardiovascular and musculoskeletal system for the demands of this type of exercise. With lower extremity plyometrics, bilateral activities should precede unilateral activities, and low intensity jumps should precede higher level jumps. As with other forms of resistance training, there should be a systematic progression to more advanced drills and the patient should not be moved forward until they have mastered the previous level.

Plyometric training is proposed to reduce the risk of future injury by training muscle coactivation through neuromuscular adaptation.[181] This is particularly relevant for reducing the risk of anterior cruciate ligament (ACL) tears by training quadriceps and hamstring muscle coactivation. It has been suggested that quadriceps training and hypertrophy alone may predispose patients to ACL injuries because the hypertrophied quadriceps muscles may reduce coactivation of the hamstrings by reciprocal inhibition.[182-184] Advantages and disadvantages of plyometric strengthening are listed in Table 5-6.

Strengthening Against a Variable Load. Strengthening exercises can also be performed against forces that provide varying resistance, such as elastic bands or tubing or water. Elastic materials provide progressively more resistance as they are stretched and can provide differing amounts of resistance, depending on their composition

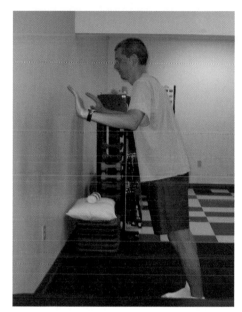

FIG. 5-10 Upper body push-up off the wall.

and thickness. Because resistance is a function of how much the elastic material is elongated, to provide consistent resistance the patient must always grasp the band or tubing in the same place.[185] Resistance will increase if a shorter section of band is used and decrease if a longer section is used. Furthermore, elastic materials provide progressively more resistance as they are lengthened, whereas the force produced by a muscle is greatest at midrange (see Fig. 5-3). Water provides resistance proportional to the relative speed of movement of the patient and the water and the cross-sectional area of the patient in contact with the water (Fig. 5-11).

INTERVENTION PROGRESSION

Several approaches have been proposed for progression of exercises to optimize muscle performance. Two of the more popular and earliest approaches are the DeLorme technique and the daily adjustable progressive resistive exercise (DAPRE) technique. The DeLorme technique was the first well-documented approach to exercise progression for muscle strengthening (Box 5-1).[101] Using this technique, exercises are performed as three sets of ten repetitions, starting with a load equal to $\frac{1}{2}$ of the 10 RM and increasing to a load equal to $\frac{3}{4}$ of the 10 RM for the second set and equal to the full 10 RM for the final set of ten repetitions.

The DeLorme technique was followed by the DAPRE technique, which was proposed to be a more adaptable progressive resistive exercise program.[186] With the DAPRE technique, a 6 RM is used to establish the initial working weight and the weight or load is increased in future sessions based on the performance during the previous training session as shown in Table 5-7. The frequency and

TABLE 5-6	Advantages and Disadvantages of Plyometric Strengthening	
Advantages	**Disadvantages**
Utilizes the series elastic and stretch reflex properties of the neuromuscular unit.	More advanced techniques requiring a high level of muscle performance capabilities prior to initiation.
Large potential influence on velocity of muscle contraction.	Higher risk of injury if not properly supervised.
Utilizes dynamic muscle co-activation for more balance between antagonistic muscle groups.	Usually reserved for more advanced stages of rehabilitation and for more advanced patients.
Can involve lower extremities, upper extremities, and trunk.	
Uses functional movements.	

FIG. 5-11 Water resistance properties.

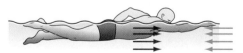
Fast-moving body results in high resistance

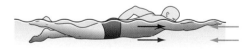
Slow-moving body results in moderate resistance

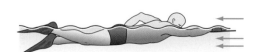
Paddles and fins increase frontal area and increase resistance

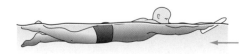
Limbs straight in front decrease frontal area and decrease resistance

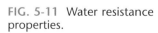

amount of weight increase are less arbitrary with this technique than with the DeLorme technique.

Because muscle performance encompasses three often very different components (strength, power, and endurance), the training for these components should reflect the needs of each component. Training that focuses on strength should involve progression of the resistance, and training that focuses on power should involve progressive changes in both resistance and speed of movement. In general, strength should be focused on before power because power requires good strength.

Endurance training should use lower loads with more repetitions than strength or power training. The speed of motion is also not a focus of endurance training. Table 5-8 highlights the recommended general training parameters for each respective component of muscle performance.

More recently, the Norwegian physiotherapist Oddvar Holten introduced the *medical exercise training* (MET) approach to muscle training.[187] This approach involves use of the Holten diagram to guide exercise progression. This diagram depicts the relationship between the maximum number of repetitions that can be performed and the percentage of maximal resistance in regard to muscle strength, strength/endurance, and endurance (Box 5-2) The diagram helps determine the muscular effort (alterations in muscular strength, endurance, or both).[156]

According to the diagram, exercise is most effective for improving endurance when 25 to 30 or more repetitions are performed at 60% to 65% of 1 RM or less and is most effective for strengthening when contractions at 90% of 1 RM are used

In summary, when selecting exercises to improve muscle performance, one should consider the following:

BOX 5-1	DeLorme Technique

Progressive Resistive Exercise
Determine 10 RM.
Patient then performs:
    10 reps at $\frac{1}{2}$ of 10 RM
    10 reps at $\frac{3}{4}$ of 10 RM
    10 reps at the full 10 RM
    Built-in warm-up
Strength progressed weekly.

TABLE 5-7	Daily Adjustable Progressive Resistive Exercise (DAPRE) Technique

Determine initial working weight (6 RM)
The patient then performs
Set 1: 10 reps of $\frac{1}{2}$ working weight.
Set 2: 6 reps of $\frac{3}{4}$ working weight.
Set 3: As many as possible with working weight.
Set 4: As many as possible with adjusted working weight according to the number of reps performed in Set 3.*
The number of reps done in Set 4 is used to determine the weight for the next day.

Reps in Set	*Adjusted Working Weight for Fourth Set	Next Exercise Session
0-2	Decrease by 5 to 10 lb	Decrease 5 to 10 lb
3-4	Same weight or decrease by 5 lb	Same weight
5-6	Same weight	Add 5 to 10 lb
7-10	Add 5 to 10 lb	Add 5 to 15 lb
>10	Add 10 to 15 lb	Add 10 to 20 lb

TABLE 5-8	Comparison of Training Characteristics for Developing Strength, Power, or Endurance

	Strength	Power	Strength and Endurance	Endurance
Load/intensity (% of 1 RM)	80%-100%	Strength/force (70%-100%) Velocity (30%-45%) or up to 10% body weight	50%-70%	Circuit training (40%-60%)
Repetitions	Very low to low 1-6	1-5 (Strength) 5-10 (Power)	12-25	Moderate to high (15-30[+])
Sets	3-5	4-6	2-3	2-5
Rest period (minutes)	3-6	2 to 4-6	30-60 seconds	45-90 seconds (1 : 1 work-rest ratio)
Speed of performance	Slow to medium (speed of effort is as fast as possible)	Fast/explosive	Slow to medium (emphasize stabilization)	Medium
Primary energy source	Phosphagen Anaerobic glycolysis	Phosphagen	Anaerobic glycolysis/aerobic	Aerobic

From Reiman MP: Training for strength, power, and endurance. In Manske RC (ed): *Postoperative Orthopedic Sports Medicine: The Knee and Shoulder,* Philadelphia, 2006, Elsevier Science.

BOX 5-2 — Holten Diagram

Dosage based off 1 RM = repetition maximum
Dosage: 100% = 1 RM
95% = 2 RM
90% = 4 RM strength
85% = 7 RM
80% = 11 RM
75% = 16 RM strength/endurance
70% = 22 RM
65% = 25 RM
60% = 30 RM endurance
Speed: >80% explosive
65%-80% breathing rhythm
<60% tissue related
Atrophy 30% 1 RM repetitions as tolerated
Mobility 10%-20% 1 RM high reps = 50
Endurance 70% 22 repetitions 3 sets
Stabilization 80% 11 repetitions 3 sets

Adapted from Fauqli HP: *Medical Exercise Therapy,* Norway, 1996, Laerergruppen for Medisinsk Treningsterapi; Torstensen TA: *Medical Exercise Therapy for Thoracic and Low Back Pain-Sciatica,* Course material, Oslo, Norway, Holten Institute.

- The requirements of the activity to which the patient is returning.
- The patient's goals for return to functional abilities.
- Advantages and disadvantages of various types of exercise.
- General and patient-specific precautions and contraindications for the type of exercise considered.
- ROM requirements for the activity and any patient restrictions in ROM.
- The ideal approach to progression for optimal functional benefit.
- The patient's motivation and social support system.
- Working weak muscles before strong muscles in situations in which fatigue of the target muscle(s) could lead to synergistic muscle compensation, especially when the focus is rehabilitation of muscle weakness.
- Developing strength and flexibility before developing power.
- Using simple exercises before initiating more complex exercises.
- Developing proximal joint and trunk stability and control before working on extremity mobility.
- Starting exercises in a more controlled environment and then progressing to a less controlled environment in regards to stationary versus dynamic surface contact and external stabilization. Initially using a stationary, externally stabilized surface to perform strengthening, and as the patient progresses, using a less stable and more dynamic surface area.
- Initiating horizontal or gravity eliminated movements before vertical or antigravity movements.
- Initiating exercises in stress-free positions before stressful positions.
- Initiating unidirectional movements before multidirectional movements.[188]

- Progressing from isometric to eccentric to concentric to plyometric types of exercises.
- Incorporating activity-specific speeds of movement in relation to the patient's functional goals.
- Ongoing reevaluation of the patient and their needs and goals, as well as the treatment plan, which is essential for rehabilitation interventions to successfully return patients with muscle weakness to optimal function.

CASE STUDY 5-1

SHOULDER PAIN AND SCAPULAR MUSCLE WEAKNESS

Examination

Patient History

HA is a 21-year-old right-handed female college volleyball player with a 2-month history of right shoulder pain with overhead movements, including serving and spiking. This pain started 2 months ago as a dull ache and has progressively worsened. She has used modalities such as ice, heat, electrical stimulation, and ultrasound in the training room, but none have helped. Radiographs and past medical history are unremarkable, except for a family history of high blood pressure.

Systems Review

Integument was normal throughout the shoulder girdle and upper trunk.

Tests and Measures

Musculoskeletal

Anthropometric Characteristics HA is a healthy, well-nourished muscular woman. She has no visible muscle atrophy around the shoulder on either side but has slightly larger muscles on the right.

Posture HA sits with a slightly forward head and bilaterally rounded shoulders. There is a positive sulcus sign with the arms at 0 degrees of abduction, indicating multidirectional laxity in both shoulders. This is consistent with later findings that suggest generalized ligamentous laxity.

Range of Motion The AROM and PROM of her cervical spine and bilateral upper extremities is slightly excessive. She also has several signs indicating generalized ligamentous laxity. These include passive fifth finger hyperextension past 90 degrees bilaterally, the ability to oppose the thumb to the forearm bilaterally, hyperextension greater than 10 degrees at the elbow bilaterally, and the ability to touch the palms flat on the floor without bending the knees. She has no discomfort with passive overpressure to the cervical spine with end ROM testing in all planes. Scapular dyskinesis (medial scapular border winging) is easily seen with AROM of the involved right shoulder.

Muscle Performance Strength testing reveals several areas of muscle weakness on the right including the shoulder external rotators, scapular upward rotators, scapular protractor muscles and scapular retractor muscles. Each of these muscles is rated at 4/5 with manual muscle testing.

Additionally, manual muscle testing of the shoulder external rotators produces some discomfort.

Reflex and Sensory Integrity Sensation is normal and symmetrical in both upper extremities in all dermatomes. Deep tendon reflexes at the biceps, triceps and brachioradialis are all normal and symmetrical.

Special Testing HA has positive impingement signs, including Neers test, Hawkins-Kennedy, and the coracoid impingement sign.

Evaluation, Diagnosis, and Prognosis

The findings from the examination indicate that HA most likely has impingement of her rotator cuff caused by rotator cuff and scapular stabilizer muscle fatigue. This fatigue is likely a result of ligamentous laxity at the shoulder in combination with the recent increased demands from playing volleyball.

Goals

Full return of muscle strength and endurance of her dominant upper extremity and a return to volleyball pain-free.

Prognosis

With rest and appropriate rehabilitation, this injury will probably resolve without the need for surgical stabilization of the shoulder.

Plan of Care

5 weeks of physical rehabilitation.

Interventions

First, HA needs to incorporate relative rest into her existing exercise program. She is therefore instructed to avoid overhead lifting, serving, setting, and spiking for several weeks while continuing with other upper extremity exercises that occur below shoulder level. Her initial interventions included moist heat followed by soft tissue mobilization to relax sore muscles and decrease muscle spasm produced by pain from overuse.

Once HA's shoulder pain subsided, she began muscular strength and endurance training exercises. First, she performed scapular and rotator cuff isometrics at a submaximal level in positions of comfort. Once HA could tolerate isometrics, she was progressed to submaximal isotonics in a limited arc with very light resistance from dumbbells and elastic tubing. As HA became able to stabilize her scapula with overhead lifting of just her arm, she gradually progressed to exercises that incorporated resisted overhead activities at different speeds.

Outcomes

After 5 weeks of physical rehabilitation, HA had full muscle strength and endurance of her dominant upper extremity and returned to volleyball pain-free. She also had no scapular winging on the right involved side. She carefully progressed her volleyball practice and playing intensity over several weeks to allow her to return to full activity safely. She has had no recurrence of symptoms.

Please see the CD that accompanies this book for a case study describing the examination, evaluation and intervention for a patient with low back pain due to muscle weakness.

CHAPTER SUMMARY

Muscle tissue is the only type of soft tissue that can generate tension enabling the skeletal system to perform functions such as maintaining posture, respiration, moving limbs, and absorbing ground reaction forces during the gait cycle. A comprehensive examination must be performed to determine the type and level of muscle performance impairment. This complex process of examination is important for many facets of rehabilitation, including evaluation, diagnosis, development of an appropriate treatment plan, and selection and implementation of interventions to improve muscle performance. Each aspect of muscle performance, including strength, power, and endurance, has its own unique characteristics and must be trained accordingly with appropriate specific interventions.

ADDITIONAL RESOURCES

Books

American College of Sports Medicine: *ACSM's Guideline for Exercise Testing and Prescription,* ed 6, Philadelphia, 2000, Lippincott Williams & Wilkins.

Baechle TR, Earle RW: *Essentials of Strength Training and Conditioning,* ed 2, Champaign, Il, 2000, Human Kinetics.

Fleck SJ, Kraemer WJ: *Designing Resistance Training Programs* ed 3, Champaign, IL., 2004, Human Kinetics.

Komi PV: *Strength and Power in Sport,* ed 2, Oxford, 2003, Blackwell Science Ltd.

Neumann DA: *Kinesiology of the Musculoskeletal System: Foundations for Physical Rehabilitation,* St. Louis, 2002, Mosby.

Web Sites

American College of Sports Medicine: www.acsm.org
National Strength and Conditioning Association: www.nsca-lift.org

GLOSSARY

A band: The densest portion of a sarcomere.
Absolute strength: A measure of the maximal amount of force generated in a movement or exercise. This is indicated by the most weight an individual can lift for 1 RM.
Actin: The thin protein of a myofibril that acts with myosin to produce muscle contraction and relaxation.
Concentric contraction: A muscle action involving shortening of the muscle length.
Delayed-onset muscle soreness (DOMS): Pain or discomfort in muscles that comes on 12-24 hours after unaccustomed exercise, particularly exercise involving eccentric muscle contractions.
Eccentric contraction: A muscle action in which tension is developed as the muscle lengthens.
Endomysium: The sheath that surrounds each muscle fiber.
Endurance: The ability to perform low intensity, repetitive, or sustained activities over a prolonged period of time without fatigue.
Epimysium: The dense outer fibrous sheath that covers an entire muscle.

Fast-twitch (type II) fibers: Muscle fibers suited to quick, explosive actions. These muscle fibers are typically larger in diameter than type I fibers.

FITT formula: A systematic method of prescribing exercise according to its frequency, intensity, time, and type to improve muscle performance.

H zone: The lighter-appearing portion in the center of an A band in a sarcomere. The H zone contains myosin but no actin.

Hyperplasia: An increase in muscle size that results from an increase in number of muscle fibers.

Hypertrophy: Increase in volume of a muscle produced by enlargement of existing cells usually as a direct result of resistance training.

I band: The portion of a sarcomere between the two A bands. The I band contains only actin filaments.

Isokinetic: A concentric or eccentric muscle action at a fixed speed with accomodating resistance.

Isometric exercise: Exercise in which muscle contraction occurs with no appreciable joint movement.

Isotonic: A concentric or eccentric muscle action moving a constant weight through a range of motion.

Length-tension relationship: A muscle's capacity to produce force depends on the length of the muscle relative to its resting length. Muscles can produce the most force near their normal resting length.

Manual muscle test (MMT): A quick and efficient way to assess and grade muscle strength by the clinician applying resistance to the subject being tested.

Medical exercise training/therapy (MET): A system of progressively graded exercise.

Motor end plate: The specialized structure at the end of the motor neuron that transmits neural impulses to the muscle fiber.

Motor unit: A motor neuron and all the muscle fibers that it innervates.

Muscle endurance (local endurance): The ability of a muscle to contract repeatedly against a load (resistance), generate and sustain tension, and resist fatigue over an extended period of time.

Muscle performance: The capacity of a muscle to do work (force × distance). The key contributing elements to muscle performance include strength, power, and endurance.

Myofibril: Rodlike structures that are contained within and run the length of the muscle fiber. The myofibril contains the contractile elements of the muscle fiber.

Myopathy: Any disease of a muscle.

Myosin: The thick protein in the myofibril that acts with actin to produce muscle contraction and relaxation.

Perimysium: A dense connective tissue sheath covering the muscle fascicles.

Plyometric exercise: Exercises involving rapid stretching of muscles by an eccentric contraction followed by a shortening of the same muscles in a concentric manner to increase muscular power and function.

Power: The work produced by a muscle per unit time (force × distance/time).

Repetition maximum (RM): The maximum amount of weight that an individual can lift a specified number of times, for example, the 10 RM is the most weight an individual can lift 10 times.

Relative strength: The maximum amount of force generated per unit of body weight. Relative strength = absolute strength/total body weight.

Sarcomere: A single contractile unit that runs from one Z band to the next Z band.

Slow-twitch (type I) fibers: Muscle fibers that are typically smaller in diameter than type II fibers and that are more suitable for long duration low force contractions.

Strength: The ability of a muscle or group of muscles to exert a maximal force or torque at a specified or determined velocity.

Tropomyosin: A muscle protein that inhibits contraction unless its position is modified by troponin so that the myosin molecules can make contact with the actin molecules.

Troponin: A complex of muscle proteins that binds to calcium to allow muscle contraction.

Velocity: Distance divided by time.

References

1. Norkin CC, Levangie PK: *Joint Structure and Function: A Comprehensive Analysis*, ed 2, Philadelphia, 1992, FA Davis.
2. Hall C, Thein-Brody L (eds): Impairment in muscle performance. In *Therapeutic Exercise. Moving Toward Function*, ed 2, Lippincott Williams and Wilkins, 2004.
3. Huxley HE: Molecular basis of contraction in cross-striated muscle. In Bourne GH (ed): *Structure and Function of Muscle*, ed 2, Academic Press, 1972, New York.
4. Huxley H: The structural basis of muscular contraction, *Proc R Soc Med* 178:131-149, 1971.
5. Lehmkuhl D: Local factors in muscle performance, *Phys Ther* 46:473-484, 1966.
6. Berne RM, Levy MN: *Physiology*, St. Louis, 1988, Mosby.
7. Garrett WE, Mumma M, Lucavecke CL: Ultrastructural differences in human skeletal muscle fiber types, *Orthop Clin North Am* 14:413-425, 1983.
8. Netter FH: *The Ciba Collection of Medical Illustrations*, vol 8, New Jersey, 1987, Ciba-Geigy.
9. Bandy WD, Dunleavy K. Adaptability of skeletal muscle: Response to increased and decreased use. In Zachazewski JE, Magee DJ, Quillen WS (eds): *Athletic Injuries and Rehabilitation*, Philadelphia, 1996, WB Saunders.
10. Williams PL, Warwick R, Dyson M, et al (eds): *Gray's Anatomy*, ed 37, London, 1989, Churchill Livingstone.
11. Huxley AF: Muscle structure and theories of contraction, *Prog Biophys Chem* 7:255-318, 1957.
12. Huxley HE, Hanson J: Changes in the cross-striation of muscle during contraction and stretch and their structural interpretation, *Nature* 173:973, 1954.
13. Huxley AF, Simmons RM: Proposed mechanism of force generation in striated muscle, *Nature* 233:533-538, 1971.
14. Thein-Brody L: Endurance impairment. In Hall CM, Thein Brody L (eds): *Therapeutic Exercise: Moving Toward Function*, Philadelphia, 1999, Lippincott Williams & Wilkins.
15. Harman E: The biomechanics of resistance exercise. In Baechle TR (ed): *Essentials of Strength Training and Conditioning*, Champaign, Il, 1994, Human Kinetics.
16. Mannion AF, Weber BR, Dvorak J, et al: Fiber type characteristics of the lumbar paraspinal muscles in normal healthy subjects and in patients with low back pain, *J Orthop Res* 15:881-887, 1997.
17. Essen B, Jansson E, Henriksson J, et al. Metabolic characteristics of fiber type in human skeletal muscle, *Acta Physiol Scand* 95:153-165, 1975.
18. Staron RS, Hagerman FC, Hikida RS, et al: Fiber type composition of the vastus lateralis muscle of young men and women, *J Histochem Cytochem* 48:623-630, 2000.
19. Adams G, Hather BM, Baldwin KM, et al: Skeletal muscle myosin heavy chain composition and resistance training, *J Appl Physiol* 74:911-915, 1993.
20. Staron RS, Karapondo DL, Kraemer WJ, et al: Skeletal muscle adaptations during the early phase of heavy-resistance training in men and women, *J Appl Physiol* 76:1247-1255, 1994.
21. Haggmark T, Jansson E, Eriksson E: Fiber type area and metabolic potential for the thigh muscle in man after knee surgery and immobilization. *Int J Sports Med* 2:12-17, 1981.
22. Howald H: Training-induced morphological and functional changes in skeletal muscle, *Int J Sports Med* 3:1-12, 1982.
23. Kraemer WJ, Patton J, Gordon SE, et al: Compatibility of high intensity strength and endurance training on hormonal and skeletal muscle adaptations, *J Appl Physiol* 78:976-989, 1995.
24. Ikai M, Fukunaga T: Calculation of muscle strength per unit cross-sectional area of human muscle by means of ultrasonic measurement. *Int Z Angew Physiol Arbeitphysiol* 26:26-32, 1968.
25. Levangie PK, Norkin CC: *Joint Structure and Function: A Comprehensive Analysis*, Baltimore, 1978, FA Davis.
26. Smith LK, Weiss EL, Lehmkuhl LD: *Brunnstrom's Clinical Kinesiology*, Philadelphia, 1996, FA Davis.
27. Josephson RK: Extensive and intensive factors determining the performance of striated muscle, *J Exp Zool* 194:135-154, 1975.
28. Enoka RM: *Neuromechanical Basis of Kinesiology*, Champaign, Il, 1988, Human Kinetics.
29. Fitts RH: Mechanisms of muscular fatigue. In *American College of Sports Medicine: Resources Manual for Guidelines for Exercise Testing and Prescription*, ed 2, Philadelphia, 1993, Lea & Febiger.

30. Hettinger TH: *Isometrisches Muskeltraining [Isometric Muscle Training],* Stuttgart, 1968, George Thieme Verlag.

31. Kisner C, Colby LA: Resistance exercise. In Kisner C, Colby LA (eds): *Therapeutic Exercise: Foundations and Techniques,* ed 4, Philadelphia, 2002, FA Davis.

32. Gajdosik RL, Vander Linden DW, Williams AK: Concentric isokinetic torque characteristics of the calf muscles of active women aged 20 to 84 years, *J Orthop Sports Phys Ther* 29:181-190, 1999.

33. Imamura K, Ashida H, Ishikawa T, et al: Human major psoas muscle and sacrospinalis muscle in relation to age: a study by computed tomography, *J Gerontol* 38:678-681, 1983.

34. Lexell J, Henriksson-Larsen K, Wimblod B: Distribution of different fiber types in human skeletal muscles: Effects of aging studied in whole muscle cross sections, *Muscle Nerve* 6:588-595, 1983.

35. Larsson L: Histochemical characteristics of human skeletal muscle during aging, *Acta Physiol Scand* 117:469-471, 1983.

36. Spirduso WW: *Physical Dimensions of Aging,* Champaign, Il, 1995, Human Kinetics.

37. Danneskoild-Samsoe B, Kofod V, Munter J, et al: Muscle strength and functional capacity in 77-81 year old men and women, *Eur J Appl Physiol* 52:123-135, 1984.

38. Mazzeo RS, Cavanagh P, Evans WJ, et al: ACSM position stand on exercise for older adults, *Med Sci Sports Exerc* 30(6):992-1008, 1998.

39. Wilkes RL, Summers JJ: Cognitions, mediating variables, and strength performance, *J Sport Psychol* 6:351-359, 1984.

40. Tenenbaum G, Bar-Eli M, Hoffman JR, et al: The effect of cognitive and somatic psyching-up techniques on isokinetic leg strength performance, *J Strength Cond Res* 9:3-7, 1995.

41. Mastaglia FL, Argov Z: Drug-induced neuromuscular disorders in man. In Walton J (ed): *Disorders of Voluntary Muscle,* ed 4, Edinburgh, 1981, Churchill Livingstone.

42. De Smet AA, Best TM: MR imaging of the distribution and location of acute hamstring injuries in athletes, *Am J Roentgenol* 174:393-399, 2000.

43. Palmer WE, Kuong SJ, Elmadbouh HM: MR imaging of myotendinous strain, *Am J Roentgenol* 173:703-709, 1999.

44. Kibler WB: Clinical aspects of muscle injury, *Med Sci Sports Exerc* 22:450-452, 1990.

45. Nguyen B, Brandser EA, Rubin DA: Pains, strains and fasciculations: Lower extremity muscle disorders, *Magn Reson Imaging Clin N Am* 8:391-408, 2000.

46. Deutsch AL, Mink JH: Magnetic resonance imaging of musculoskeletal injuries, *Radiol Clin North Am* 27:983-1002, 1989.

47. Worrell TW, Perrin DH: Hamstring muscle injury: The influence of strength, flexibility, warm-up and fatigue, *J Orthop Sports Phys Ther* 16:12-18, 1992.

48. Agre JC: Hamstring injuries: Proposed etiological factors, prevention and treatment, *Sports Med* 2:21-33, 1985.

49. Burkett LN: Causative factors in hamstring strains, *Med Sci Sports Exerc* 2:39-42, 1970.

50. Fleck SJ, Kraemer WJ: *Designing Resistance Training Programs,* ed 3, Champaign, Il, 2004, Human Kinetics.

51. Hakkinen K, Komi PV: Changes in neuromuscular performance in voluntary and reflex contraction during strength training in man, *Int J Sports Med* 4:282-288, 1983.

52. Dudley GA, Harris RT: Neuromuscular adaptations to conditioning. In Baechle TR (ed): *Essentials of Strength Training and Conditioning,* Champaign, Il, 1994, Human Kinetics.

53. Hakkinen K, Komi PV, Tesch PA: Effect of combined concentric and eccentric strength training and detraining on force-time, muscle fiber and metabolic characteristics of leg extensor muscles, *Scand J Sports Sci* 3:50-58, 1981.

54. Hakkinen K, Pakarinen A, Kyrolainen H, et al: Neuromuscular adaptations and serum hormones in females during prolonged power training, *Int J Sports Med* 11:91-98, 1990.

55. Hortobagyi T, Houmard JA, Stevenson JR, et al: The effects of detraining on power athletes, *Med Sci Sports Exerc* 25:929-935, 1993.

56. Kraemer WJ: General adaptations to resistance and endurance training programs. In Baechle TR (ed): *Essentials of Strength Training and Conditioning,* Champaign, Il, 1994, Human Kinetics.

57. Bompa TO: Periodization Training for Sports, Champaign, Il, 1999, Human Kinetics.

58. Hather BM, Tesch PA, Buchanan P, et al: Influence of eccentric actions on skeletal muscle adaptations to resistance training, *Acta Physiol Scand* 143:177-185, 1992.

59. Staron RS, Leonardi MJ, Karapondo DL, et al: Strength and skeletal muscle adaptations in heavy-resistance-trained women after detraining and retraining, *J Appl Phys* 70:631-640, 1991.

60. Boissonnault WG, Goodman CC: Bone, joint, and soft tissue disorders. In Goodman CC, Boissonnault WG, Fuller KS (eds): *Pathology: Implications for the Physical Therapist,* ed 2, Philadelphia, 2003, WB Saunders.

61. Goodman CC, Glanzman A: Genetic and developmental disorders. In Goodman CC, Boissonnault WG, Fuller KS (eds): *Pathology: Implications for the Physical Therapist,* ed 2, Philadelphia, 2003, WB Saunders.

62. Little Club: Memorandum on terminology and classification of "cerebral palsy," *Cereb Palsy Bull* 1:27-35, 1959.

63. Damiano DL, Kelly LE, Vaughn CL: Effects of quadriceps femoris muscle strengthening on crouch gait in children with spastic cerebral palsy, *Phys Ther* 75:658-671, 1995.

64. Mulcare JA, Petajan JH: Multiple Sclerosis. In *ACSM's Resources for Clinical Exercise Physiology: Musculoskeletal, Neuromuscular, Neoplastic, Immunologic, and Hematologic Conditions,* Philadelphia, 2002, Lippincott Williams & Wilkins.

65. Poser CM, Paty DW, Scheinberg L, et al: New diagnostic criteria for multiple sclerosis: Guidelines for research protocols, *Ann Neurol* 13:227-231, 1983.

66. Krupp LB, Alvarez LA, LaRocca NG, et al: Fatigue in multiple sclerosis, *Arch Neurol* 45:435-437, 1988.

67. Kent-Braun JA, Ng AV, Catro M, et al: Effects of exercise on muscle activation and metabolism in MS, *Muscle Nerve* 17:1162-1169, 1994.

68. Smith MB: The peripheral nervous system. In Goodman CC, Boissonnault WG, Fuller KS (eds): *Pathology: Implications for the Physical Therapist,* ed 2, Philadelphia, 2003, WB Saunders.

69. Magee DJ: *Orthopedic Physical Assessment,* ed 3, Philadelphia, 1987, WB Saunders.

70. Cooper H, Doods WN, Adams ID, et al: Use and misuse of the tape-measure as a means of assessing muscle strength and power, *Rheumatol Rehabil* 20(4):211-218, 1981.

71. Hortobagyi T, Katch FI, Katch VL, et al: Relationships of body size, segmental dimensions, and ponderal equivalents to muscular strength in high-strength and low-strength subjects, *Int J Sports Med* 11(5):349-356, 1990.

72. deAndrade JR, Grant C, Dixon A: Joint distention and reflex muscle inhibition in the knee, *J Bone Joint Surg Am* 47:313-322, 1965.

73. Spencer JK, Hayes KC, Alexander IJ. Knee joint effusion and quadriceps reflex inhibition in man, *Arch Phys Med Rehab* 65:171-177, 1984.

74. Stokes M, Young A: Investigations of quadriceps inhibition: Implications for clinical practice, *Physiotherapy* 70:425-428, 1984.

75. Hall C, Thein-Brody L: Functional approach to therapeutic exercise for physiologic impairments. In Hall CM, Thein-Brody L (eds): *Therapeutic Exercise: Moving Toward Function,* Philadelphia, 1999, Lippincott Williams & Wilkins.

76. Clark MA: *Integrated Training for the New Millennium,* Thousand Oaks, Calif, 2001, National Academy of Sports Medicine.

77. Clark MA: The scientific and clinical rationale for the use of closed and open chain rehabilitation. In Ellenbecker TS (ed): *Knee Ligament Rehabilitation,* New York, 2000, Churchill Livingstone.

78. McCardle WD, Katch, FI, Katch VL: *Essentials of Exercise Physiology,* ed 2, Philadelphia, 2000, Lippincott Williams & Wilkins.

79. Moffroid MT, Kusick ET: The power struggle: Definition and evaluation of power of muscular performance, *Phys Ther* 55:1098, 1975.

80. Sapega AA, Drillings G. The definition and assessment of muscular power, *J Orthop Sports Phys Ther* 5:7, 1983.

81. McCardle WD, Katch, FI, Katch VI: *Exercise Physiology: Energy, Nutrition, and Human Performance,* ed 4, Baltimore, 1996, Lippincott Williams & Wilkins.

82. Powers SK, Howley ET: *Exercise Physiology: Theory and Application,* Boston, 2001, McGraw-Hill Co.

83. Wilmore JH, Costill DL: *Physiology of Sport and Exercise,* ed 2, Champaign, Il, 1999, Human Kinetics.

84. Kendall FP, McCreary EK, Provance PG, et al: *Muscles: Testing and Function with Posture and Pain,* ed 5, Philadelphia, 2005, Lippincott Williams & Wilkins.

85. Nicholas J, Sapega A, Kraus H, et al: Factors influencing manual muscle tests in physical therapy, *J Bone Joint Surg Am* 60:186-190, 1978.

86. Frese E, Brown M, Norton BJ: Clinical reliability of manual muscle testing. Middle trapezius and gluteus medius muscles, *Phys Ther* 67(7):1072-1076, 1987.

87. Rainville J, Joube C, Finno M, et al: Comparison of four tests of quadriceps strength in L3 or L4 radiculopathies, *Spine* 28(21):2466-2471, 2003.

88. Davies GJ, Wilk K, Ellenbecker TS: Assessment of strength. In Malone TR, McPoil T, Nitz AJ (eds): *Orthopedic and Sports Physical Therapy,* ed 3, St. Louis, 1997, Mosby.

89. Wessel J, Kaup C, Fan J et al: Isometric strength measurements in children with arthritis: reliability and relation to function, *Arthritis Care Res* 12:238-246, 1999.

90. Agre JC, Magness JL et al: Strength testing with a portable dynamometer: Reliability for upper and lower extremities, *Arch Phys Med Rehabil* 68:454-458, 1987.

91. Bohannon RW: Hand-held dynamometry: Stability of muscle strength over multiple measurements, *Clin Biomech* 2:74-77, 1987.

92. Bohannon RW: The clinical measurement of strength, *Clin Rehabil* 1:5-16, 1987.

93. Bohannan RW: Make test and break test of elbow flexor muscle strength, *Phys Ther* 68:193-194, 1988.

94. Bohannon RW: Comparability of force measurements obtained with different strain gauge hand-held dynamometers, *J Orthop Sports Phys Ther* 18(4):564-567, 1993.

95. Bohannan RW, Andrews AW: Accuracy of spring and strain gauge handheld dynamometers, *J Orthop Sports Phys Ther* 10:323-325, 1989.
96. Bohannon RW: Test-retest reliability of hand-held dynamometry during a single session of strength assessment, *Phys Ther* 66:206-209, 1986.
97. Burdett RG, Whitney SL: Reliability of hand-held dynamometry in measuring muscle strength (abstract), *Phys Ther* 67:748, 1987.
98. Byl NN, Richard S, Asturias J: Intrarater and interrater reliability of the biceps and deltoids using a hand-held dynamometer, *J Orthop Sports Phys Ther* 9:399-405, 1988.
99. Wadsworth CT, Nielsen DH, Corcoran DS, et al: Interrater reliability of hand-held dynamometry: Effects of rater gender, body weight, and grip strength, *J Orthop Sports Phys Ther* 16:74-81, 1992.
100. Leggin BG, Neuman RM, Iannotti JP, et al: Intra-rater and inter-rater reliability of three isometric dynamometers in assessing shoulder strength, *J Shoulder Elbow Surg* 5(1):18-24, 1996.
101. DeLorme T, Wilkins A: *Progressive Resistance Exercises*, New York, 1951, Appleton-Century Crofts.
102. DeBries HA, Housh TJ: *Physiology of Exercise for Physical Education, Athletics and Exercise Science*, ed 5, Dubuque, Ia, 1994, Brown and Benchmark.
103. Sale DG: Testing strength and power. In MacDougall JD, Wenger HA, Green HJ (eds): *Physiological Testing of the High Performance Athlete*, ed 2, Champaign, Il, 1991, Human Kinetics.
104. Escamilla R, Wickham R: Exercise-based conditioning and rehabilitation. In Kolt GS, Snyder-Mackler L: *Physical Therapies in Sports and Exercise*, London, 2003, Churchill Livingstone.
105. Nicholas JJ: Isokinetic testing in young nonathletic able-bodied subjects, *Arch Phys Med Rehabil* 70:210-213, 1989.
106. Wilk KE, Arrigo CA, Andrews JR: Standardized Isokinetic testing protocol for the throwing shoulder: The throwers' series, *Isokinet Exerc Sci* 1:63-71, 1991.
107. Wilhite MR, Cohen ER, Wilhite SC: Reliability of concentric and eccentric measurements of quadriceps performance using the Kin Com dynamometer: The effect of testing order for three different speeds (abstract), *J Orthop Sports Phys Ther* 11:419-420, 1990.
108. Ellenbecker TS: Isokinetics in rehabilitation. In Ellenbecker TS (ed): *Knee Ligament Rehabilitation*, Philadelphia, 2000, Churchill Livingstone.
109. Wilk KE, Arrigo CA, Andrews JR: A comparison of individuals exhibiting normal grade manual muscle test and isokinetic testing of the knee extension/flexion (abstract), *Phys Ther* 72(6):71, 1992.
110. Brown LE (ed): *Isokinetics in Human Performance*, Champaign Il, 2000, Human Kinetics.
111. Dvir Z (ed): *Isokinetics. Muscle Testing, Interpretation, and Clinical Application*, ed 2, London, 2000, Churchill Livingstone.
112. Perrin DH: *Isokinetic Exercise and Assessment*, Champaign Il, 1993, Human Kinetics.
113. Korr I: The facilitated segment, *Proc IFOMT* 81-92, 1977.
114. Korr I (ed): *The Neurobiological Mechanism in Manipulative Therapy*, New York, 1978, Plenum Press.
115. Seddon H: Three types of nerve injury, *Brain* 66:237, 1943.
116. Birk TJ: Poliomyelitis and the post-polio syndrome: Exercise capacities and adaption-current research, future directions, and widespread applicability, *Med Sci Sports Exerc* 25:466-472, 1993.
117. Stanghelle JK, Festvag LV: Postpolio syndrome: A 5-year follow-up, *Spinal Cord* 35:503-508, 1997.
118. Edelstein JE: Orthotic Assessment and Management. In O'Sullivan SB, Schmitz TJ (eds): *Physical Rehabilitation: Assessment and Treatment*, ed 4, Philadelphia, 2001, FA Davis.
119. Kawaguchi Y, Gejo R, Kanamori M, Kimura T: Quantitative analysis of the effect of lumbar orthosis on trunk muscle strength and muscle activity in normal subjects, *J Orthop Sci* 7(4):483-489, 2002.
120. Walsh NE, Schwartz RK: The influence of prophylactic orthosis on abdominal strength and low back injury in the workplace, *Am J Phys Med Rehabil* 69(5):245-250, 1990.
121. Jansen CW, Olson SL, Hasson SM: The effect of use of a wrist orthosis during functional activities on surface electromyography of the wrist extensors in normal subjects, *J Hand Ther* 10(4):283-289, 1997.
122. American Physical Therapy Association: *Guide to Physical Therapist Practice*, ed 2, Alexandria, Va, 2001, The Association.
123. Wenger HA, McFadyen PF, McFadyen RA: Physiological principles of conditioning. In Zachazewski JE, Magee DJ, Quillen WS (eds): *Athletic Injuries and Rehabilitation*, Philadelphia, 1996, WB Saunders.
124. Fleck SJ, Kraemer WJ: Resistance training: physiological responses and adaptations [Part 2 of 4], *Phys Sportsmed* 16:75-107, 1988.
125. Reiman MP: Training for strength, power, and endurance. In Manske RC (ed): *Postoperative Orthopedic Sports Medicine: The Knee and Shoulder*, Philadelphia, 2006, Elsevier Science. In Press.
126. Noth J: Cortical and peripheral control. In Komi PV (ed): *Strength and Power in Sport*, London, 1992, Blackwell Scientific Publications.
127. Sherrington C: *The Integrative Action of the Nervous System*, New Haven, Conn, 1947, Yale University Press.
128. Kabat H: Studies on neuromuscular dysfunction. XIII. New concepts and techniques of neuromuscular reeducation for paralysis, *Perm Found Med Bull* 8(3):121-143, 1950.
129. Davies GJ. Descriptive study comparing open kinetic chain and closed kinetic chain isokinetic testing of the lower extremity in 200 patients with selected knee injuries (abstract). Proceedings twelfth International Congress World Confederation for Physical Therapy, Washington, DC, 1995, American Physical Therapy Association.
130. Feiring DC, Ellenbecker TS: Single versus multiple joint isokinetic testing with ACL reconstructed patients, *Isokinet Exerc Sci* 6:109-115, 1996.
131. Snyder-Mackler L, Delitto A, Bailey SL, et al: Strength of the quadriceps femoris muscle and functional recovery after reconstruction of the anterior cruciate ligament: A prospective, randomized clinical trial of electrical stimulation, *J Bone Joint Surg Am* 77:1166-1173, 1995.
132. Morrissey MC, Harman EA, Johnson MJ: Resistance training modes: Specificity and effectiveness, *Med Sci Sports Exerc* 27:648-660, 1995.
133. Kanehisa H, Miyashita M: Specificity of velocity in strength training, *Eur J Appl Physiol* 52:104-106, 1983.
134. American College of Sports Medicine: Position stand: Progression models in resistance training for healthy adults, *Med Sci Sports Exerc* 34:364-380, 2002.
135. Fry AC. The role of training intensity in resistance exercise, overtraining, and overreaching. In Kreider R, Fry A, O'Toole M (eds): *Overtraining in Sport*, Champaign, Il, 1998, Human Kinetics.
136. American College of Sports Medicine: *Principles of Exercise Prescription*, Baltimore, 1995, Williams & Wilkins.
137. Snyder-Mackler L, Delitto A, Bailey S, et al: Quadriceps femoris muscle strength and functional recovery after anterior cruciate ligament reconstruction: A prospective randomized clinical trial of electrical stimulation, *J Bone Joint Surg Am* 77:1166-1173, 1995.
138. Snyder-Mackler L, Ladin Z, Shepsis AA, et al: Electrical stimulation of thigh muscles after reconstruction of the anterior cruciate ligament, *J Bone Joint Surg Am* 73:1025-1036, 1991.
139. Carnstam B, Larsson LE, Prevec TS: Improvement of gait following functional electrical stimulation. I. Investigations on changes in voluntary strength and proprioceptive reflexes, *Scand J Rehabil Med* 9:7-13, 1977.
140. Snyder-Mackler L, Delitto A, Stralka SW, et al: Use of electrical stimulation to enhance recovery of quadriceps femoris muscle force production in patients following anterior cruciate ligament reconstruction, *Phys Ther* 74:901-907, 1994.
141. *Electrotherapy, Shortwave, and Ultrasound Update Course Material*, Wichita, Kan, 2000, International Academy of PhysioTherapeutics, Inc.
142. Moritani T, DeVries HA: Neural factors versus hypertrophy in the time course of muscle strength gain, *Am J Phys Med* 82:521-524, 1979.
143. Sale DG: Neural adaptation to resistance training, *Med Sci Sports Exerc* 20:S135-S145, 1988.
144. Siff MC, Verkhoshansky YV: *Supertraining*, ed 4, Denver, 1999, Supertraining International.
145. Morris JM, Lucas DB, Bresler B: Role of the trunk in stability of the spine, *J Bone Joint Surg Am* 43:327-351, 1961.
146. Anderson P, Henriksson J: Training induced changes in the subgroups of human Type II skeletal muscle fibers, *Acta Physiol Scand* 99:123-125, 1975.
147. Ashmen KJ, Swanik CB, Lephart SM: Strength and flexibility characteristics of athletes with chronic low back pain, *J Sports Rehab* 5:275-286, 1996.
148. Bogduk N, Twomey L: *Clinical Anatomy of the Lumbar Spine*, New York, 1987, Churchill Livingstone.
149. Bullock-Sexton JE: Local sensation changes and altered hip muscle function following severe ankle sprain, *Phys Ther* 74:17-23, 1994.
150. Haikunen K, Alen M, Kallinen M, et al: Neuromuscular adaptations during prolonged strength training, detraining, and re-training in middle aged and elderly people, *Eur J Appl Phys* 83(1):51-62, 2000.
151. Granhed H, Johnson R, Hansson T: The loads on the lumbar spine during extreme weight lifting, *Spine* 12(2):146-149, 1987.
152. Kerr D, Ackland T, Maslen B, et al: Resistance training over 2 years increases bone mass in calcium-replete postmenopausal women, *J Bone Min Res* 16:175-181, 2001.
153. Kannus P, Jozsa L, Natri A, et al: Effects of training, immobilization and remobilization on tendons, *Scand J Med Sci Sports* 7(2):67-71, 1997.
154. Gregg EW, Pereira MA, Caspersen CJ: Physical activity, falls, and fractures among older adults: a review of epidemiologic evidence, *J Am Geriatrics Soc* 48(8):883-893, 2000.
155. Benjamini Y, Rubenstein JJ, Zaichkowsky LE, et al: Effects of high-intensity strength training on quality of life parameters in cardiac rehabilitation patients, *Am J Cardiol* 80:841-846, 1997.
156. American College of Sports Medicine: *ACSM's Guidelines for Exercise Testing and Prescription*, ed 6, Philadelphia, 2000, Lippincott Williams & Wilkins.
157. Borst SE, deHoyes DV, Garzella L et al: Effects of resistance training on insulin-like growth factor-I and IGF binding proteins, *Med Sci Sports Exerc* 33:648-653, 2001.
158. Clarkson PM, Tremblay I: Exercise induced muscle damage, repair and adaptation in humans, *J Appl Physiol* 65:1-6, 1988.

159. Corder KP, Potteiger JA, Nau KL, et al: Effects of active and passive recovery conditions on blood lactate, rating of perceived exertion, and performance during resistance exercise, *J Strength Cond Res* 14(2):151-156, 2000.
160. DeVries HA: Quantitative electromyographic investigation of the spasm theory of muscle pain, *Am J Phys Med Rehabil* 45:119-134, 1966.
161. Waltrous B, Armstrong R, Schwane J: The role of lactic acid in delayed onset muscular soreness, *Med Sci Sports Exerc* 1:380, 1981.
162. Abraham WM: Factors in delayed muscle soreness, *Med Sci Sports Exerc* 9:11-20, 1977.
163. Knapik JJ, Mawdsley RH, Ramos MU: Angular specificity and test mode specificity of isometric and isokinetic strength training, *J Orthop Sports Phys Ther* 5:58-65, 1983.
164. Zatsiorsky VM: *Science and Practice of Strength Training,* Champaign, Il, 1995, Human Kinetics.
165. Thepaut-Mathieu C, Van Hoecke J, Maton B: Myoelectrical and mechanical changes linked to length specificity during isometric training, *J Appl Physiol* 64:1500-1505, 1988.
166. Abbott BC, Bigland B, Ritchie JM. The physiological cost of negative work, *J Physiol* (Lond), 117:380-390, 1952.
167. Hortobagy T, Katch FI: Eccentric and concentric torque-velocity relationships during arm flexion and extension, *Eur J Appl Physiol.* 60:395-401, 1990.
168. Moffroid MT, Whipple RH. Specificity of speed of exercise, *Phys Ther.* 50:1693-1699. 1970.
169. Seger JY, Arvidsson B, Thorstensson A. Specific effects of eccentric and concentric training on muscle strength and morphology in humans, *Eur J Appl Phys* 79:49-57, 1998.
170. Ewing JL, Wolfe DR, Rogers MA, et al: Effects of velocity of isokinetic training on strength, power, and quadriceps muscle fibre characteristics, *Eur J Appl Phys* 61:159-162, 1990.
171. Akima H, Takahashi H, Kuno S, et al: Early phase adaptations of muscle use and strength to isokinetic training, *Med Sci Sports Exer* 31:588-594, 1999.
172. Bell GJ, Syrotuik D, Martin TP, et al: Effect of concurrent strength and endurance training on skeletal muscle properties and hormone concentrations in humans, *Eur J Appl Phys* 81:418-427, 2000.
173. Lacerte M, deLateur BJ, Alquist AD, et al: Concentric versus combined concentric-eccentric isokinetic training programs: Effects on peak torque of human quadriceps femoris muscle, *Arch Phys Med Rehabil* 73:1059-1062, 1992.
174. Behm DG, Sale DG: Velocity specificity of resistance training, *Sports Med* 15:374-388, 1993.
175. Chu DA: *Jumping into Plyometrics,* Champaign, IL, 1992, Human Kinetics.
176. Radcliffe JC, Farentinos RC: *High Powered Plyometrics,* Champaign Il, 1999, Human Kinetics.
177. Verkhoshanski Y: Depth jumping in the training of jumpers, *Track Technique* 51:1618-1619, 1973.
178. Boyle M: *Functional Training for Sports,* Champaign, IL, 2004, Human Kinetics.
179. Falkel JE, Cipriani DL: Physiological principles of resistance training and rehabilitation. In Zachazewski JE, Magee DJ, Quillen WS (eds): *Athletic Injuries and Rehabilitation,* Philadelphia, 1996, WB Saunders.
180. Wilson GJ, Newton RU, Murphy AJ, et al: The optimal training load for the development of dynamic athletic performance, *Med Sci Sports Exerc* 25(11):1279-1286, 1993.
181. Anderson B: Flexibility testing, *J Strength Cond* 3(2):20-23, 1981.
182. Cowling EJ, Steel JR: Is lower limb muscle synchrony during landing affected by gender? Implications for variations in ACL injury rates, *J Electromyogr Kinesiol* 11:263-268, 2001.
183. Renstrom P, Arms SW, Stanwyck TS, et al: Strain within the anterior cruciate ligament during hamstring and quadriceps activity, *Am J Sports Med* 14:83-87, 1986.
184. Solomonow M, Baratta R, Zhou BH, et al: The synergistic action of the anterior cruciate ligament and thigh muscles in maintaining joint stability, *Am J Sports Med* 15:207-213, 1987.
185. Hughes C, Page P: Scientific basis of elastic resistance. In Page P, Ellenbecker TS (ed): *The Scientific and Clinical Application of Elastic Resistance,* Champaign, Il, 2003, Human Kinetics.
186. Knight KL: Knee rehabilitation by the daily adjustable progressive resistive exercise technique, *Am J Sports Med* 7:336-337, 1979.
187. Torstensen TA: The physical therapy approach. In Frymoyer JW, Ducker TB, Hadler NM, et al (eds): *The Adult Spine: Principles and Practice,* ed 2, vol 1, Philadelphia, 1997, Lippincott-Raven.
188. Giannakopoulos K, Beneka A, Malliou P, et al: Isolated vs. complex exercises in strengthening the rotator cuff muscle group, *J Strength Cond Res* 18(1):144-148, 2004.

Chapter 6

Connective Tissue Dysfunction

Victoria Merrell, Donna K. Everix

OBJECTIVES

After reading this chapter, the reader will be able to:
1. Describe the pathology, clinical manifestations, and prognosis of nine different types of connective tissue dysfunctions.
2. Accurately and efficiently take a history of a patient with connective tissue dysfunction.
3. Apply rheumatology specific outcome tools, tests, and measurement techniques.
4. Determine a diagnosis and prognosis for a patient with connective tissue dysfunction.
5. Apply effective rehabilitation interventions for patients with connective tissue dysfunction, including patient education, exercise, modalities, and aquatic therapy.

Connective tissue dysfunctions result from a group of diseases that generally share clinical and pathological features of widespread inflammation. These diseases are commonly known as rheumatic diseases. With the exception of osteoarthritis, the majority of the rheumatic diseases are chronic systemic inflammatory conditions with an autoimmune etiology. All of these diseases can cause joint inflammation, known as *arthritis*, as well as a range of other adverse effects.

Rheumatic diseases encompass over 100 different conditions with different clinical manifestations. All are characterized by chronic pain and progressive damage to joints and soft tissues resulting in functional impairment. Arthritis, or joint inflammation, is the most prevalent chronic condition in the United States and is the leading cause of disability.[1,2] Arthritis and the rheumatic diseases significantly limit the ability of more than 7 million Americans to participate in activities of daily living, and in vocational and leisure activities.[3] The prevalence of rheumatic disease is expected to rise so that by the year 2020, these diseases will limit an estimated 11.6 million individuals in their ability to perform daily activities.[3] This chapter focuses on a subset of rheumatic diseases that commonly cause connective tissue dysfunction, including rheumatoid arthritis and other inflammatory types of arthritis, disorders of soft tissue, and diffuse diseases of the connective tissues.

The care of individuals with rheumatic disease must be individualized and is founded on an early and accurate diagnosis. One of the challenges of working with patients with rheumatic disease is patients can have very different presentations, manifesting diverse signs and symptoms. Effective management requires an understanding of the disease process, a comprehensive examination and evaluation, and implementation of appropriate interventions to achieve realistic goals consistent with the patient's preferences. Since the rheumatic diseases involve multiple systems and have significant psychosocial ramifications, patients are best treated with a multidisciplinary approach.[4,5]

Rehabilitation plays a critical role in the management of patients with rheumatic disease and physical therapy has been identified as an integral component of care.[6,7] Rehabilitation clinicians may provide a wide range of interventions that may be beneficial adjuncts to medication and surgery. These interventions may include patient education about the disease and components of management, instruction in joint protection and energy conservation, therapeutic exercise, physical agents, and aquatic therapy. This chapter includes information on pathology; examination; evaluation, including functional outcome assessment tools; and interventions for the rheumatic diseases most commonly encountered by rehabilitation professionals. These include systemic lupus erythematosus, rheumatoid arthritis, spondyloarthropathies, polymyalgia rheumatica, polymyositis and dermatomyositis, scleroderma, Sjögren's syndrome, crystal-induced arthropathies, and juvenile rheumatoid arthritis.

PATHOLOGY

SYSTEMIC LUPUS ERYTHEMATOSUS

Etiology. *Systemic lupus erythematosus* (SLE) is an autoimmune disease that results from the body producing antibodies directed against its own tissue. In SLE, autoantibodies react with antigens to produce circulating immune complexes that deposit in tissues causing a range of biochemical, pharmacological, and morphological changes. The clinical spectrum of SLE is broad, ranging from fatigue and mild *arthralgias* to severe and unremitting kidney inflammation *(nephritis)* that may ultimately cause renal failure (see Box 6-1). SLE may impact any or all organ systems and is most damaging if there is renal, myocardial, or neurological involvement. Although no single cause of SLE has been identified, numerous influential factors, including viral, genetic, environmental, and hormonal, are proposed.

Genetics. There is evidence that genetic factors predispose individuals to SLE. SLE occurs more often in relatives than in the general population. The prevalence of *lupus* in first-degree relatives is between 0.4% and 5%, which is a several hundred-fold increase over the prevalence in the general population.[8] The prevalence of SLE is also three times higher in African Americans than would be expected given their representation in the general population, and SLE is more common in certain Native American tribes and particularly in females within that population.[9]

Environmental Factors. Environmental factors, including chemical exposure, ultraviolet radiation, diet, and viral infections, may trigger the expression of SLE in some individuals.[10] Drug-induced lupus comes on in response to a drug and resolves when the drug is no longer present and is almost always associated with exposure to one of three medications: hydralazine, procainamide, or methyldopa.[11] Aromatic amines (used in certain hair dyes) have also been associated with drug-induced lupus. The mechanism of this effect remains unclear and only a small proportion of people exposed to these drugs or chemicals develop lupus.[12,13] Exposure to ultraviolet (UV) radiation, particularly UVA and UVB, may exacerbate lupus symptoms, possibly by promoting the formation of anti–DNA antibodies.[12] The effects of diet on SLE are poorly substantiated and are based only on expert opinion or observational studies.

Hormonal Influences. Ninety percent of patients with lupus are women, and 90% of these patients develop lupus in their childbearing years.[14] It is thought that this is because of the profound differences between the impact of female sex hormones (estrogens) and male sex hor-

| BOX 6-1 | Diagnostic Criteria for Systemic Lupus Erythematosus |

1. Malar rash: Fixed erythema, flat or raised, over the malar eminences, tending to spare the nasolabial folds.
2. Discoid rash: Erythematous raised patches with adherent keratotic scaling and follicular plugging; atrophic scarring may occur in older lesions.
3. Photosensitivity: Skin rash as a result of unusual reaction to sunlight, by patient history or physician observation.
4. Oral ulcers: Oral or nasopharyngeal ulceration, usually painless, observed by a physician.
5. Arthritis: Nonerosive arthritis involving two or more peripheral joints, characterized by tenderness, swelling, or effusion.
6. Serositis
   A. Pleuritis: Convincing history of pleuritic pain or rub heard by a physician or evidence of pleural effusion OR
   B. Pericarditis: Documented by electrocardiogram (ECG) or rub or evidence of pericardial effusion.
7. Renal disorder
   A. Persistent proteinuria >0.5 gm per day or >3+ if quantitation not performed OR
   B. Cellular casts may be in red cell, hemoglobin, granular, tubular, or mixed.
8. Neurological disorder
   A. Seizures: In the absence of offending drugs or known metabolic derangements OR
   B. Psychosis: In the absence of offending drugs or known metabolic derangements.
9. Hematologic disorder
   A. Hemolytic anemia
   B. Leukopenia
   C. Thrombocytopenia.
10. Immunologic disorder
    A. Positive LE cell preparation OR
    B. Anti-DNA: Antibody to native DNA in abnormal titer OR
    C. Anti-Sm: Presence of antibody to Sm nuclear antigen OR
    D. False positive test for syphilis.
11. ANA: An abnormal titer of ANA by immunofluorescence or an equivalent assay at any point in time and in the absence of drugs known to be associated with drug-induced lupus syndrome.

A person has SLE if any 4 or more of the 11 criteria are present, serially or simultaneously, during any interval of observation.

From Tan EM, Cohen AS, Fries JF, et al: *Arthritis Rheum* 25:1271-1277, 1982.
LE, Lupus erythematosus; *ANA*, antinuclear antibody; *SLE*, systemic lupus erythematosus.

mones (androgens) on the immune system. Estrogens promote immune responses and increase the production of autoantibodies while androgens are more immunosuppressive. Thus female sex hormones appear to promote both disease activity and etiology.[15]

Diagnosis. The diagnosis of SLE is based on the criteria devised by the American College of Rheumatology. The presence of 4 of the 11 criteria listed in Box 6-1 confirm the diagnosis of SLE.

Clinical Features. Although SLE can involve all organ systems, its most common symptoms are fatigue and

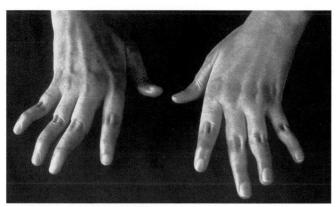

FIG. 6-1 Jaccoud's arthritis. A nonerosive deforming arthropathy of the hands that occurs in patients with SLE. *Reprinted from the Clinical Slide Collection on the Rheumatic Diseases, copyright 1997. Used by permission of the American College of Rheumatology.*

arthralgia (joint pain). Arthralgias occur in 80% to 90% of patients with SLE; however, arthritis (joint inflammation) occurs in fewer than half of these cases. The joint pain and inflammation, when present, tends to be symmetrical with a predilection for the knees, wrists, and interphalangeal joints. The shoulders, hips, ankles, and elbows are less commonly involved.[14] When arthritis is present in patients with SLE it is generally not deforming; however, 10% of patients with SLE develop a nonerosive deforming arthropathy of the hands, referred to as Jaccoud's arthritis (Fig. 6-1), which mostly affects the joint capsule and surrounding ligaments, causing joint instability and subluxation rather than the joint contractures and bony ankylosis associated with erosive arthritides.

Avascular necrosis occurs in 3% to 52% of patients with SLE, and involvement is frequently bilateral and asymptomatic. Avascular necrosis is thought to be caused by the corticosteroids used to treat SLE rather than by the disease itself because patients who have been treated with higher doses of steroids for prolonged periods are at greatest risk for developing this problem. Prolonged corticosteroid use may also cause or accelerate osteoporosis in this population.[14]

Systemic manifestations of SLE include fever, malaise, weight loss, anorexia, and weakness. Fatigue occurs in 80% to 100% of patients and is often the most debilitating symptom, affecting quality of life and interfering with family and social relationships.[14] Myalgias, muscle tenderness, and muscle weakness may be present in up to 69% of patients with SLE.[16]

SLE commonly causes skin rashes, including malar, discoid, or subacute lesions. The term *lupus* was derived from the Latin word for "wolf" and is used to describe the butterfly-shaped rash (Fig. 6-2) reported by 35% of patients with lupus.[17] Acute inflammatory rashes may occur on the malar regions of the face, on the trunk, and upper extremities, or between the interphalangeal joints. *Discoid lupus* is manifested by a chronic, scaly, and scarring rash with a predilection for the sun exposed areas of the body. Subacute nonscarring symmetrical rashes resembling psoriatic skin lesions are seen in 9% of patients with

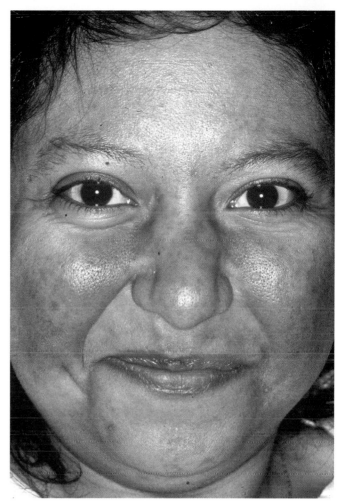

FIG. 6-2 Lupus rash. Erythematous rash (butterfly rash) extending across the malar regions of the face and across the bridge of the nose. *Reprinted from the Clinical Slide Collection on the Rheumatic Diseases, copyright 1997. Used by permission of the American College of Rheumatology.*

lupus, and patients may also have mouth or nose sores, alopecia, urticaria, *purpura, Raynaud's phenomenon, livedo reticularis,* vasculitis, and *panniculitis.*[12]

Approximately 50% of patients with lupus develop kidney disease (lupus nephritis), and 78% of patients develop *proteinuria* (protein in the urine), the most common renal abnormality caused by lupus, at some period during the disease.[14] Lupus also has hematological manifestations, including anemia, *leukopenia* or lymphopenia, thrombocytopenia, and a false positive syphilis test. In addition, lupus may affect the cardiopulmonary system by causing *pleurisy* or *pericarditis,* or more rarely, endocarditis, pneumonitis, thrombophlebitis, and coronary artery disease.

Neuropsychiatric symptoms occur in 25% to 80% of patients with SLE at some time during the course of the illness. SLE can also cause seizures, stroke, headaches, psychosis, and organic brain syndromes, but depression is the most common psychiatric disorder in patients with lupus and may be caused by the disease itself or be a reaction to the stresses associated with chronic illness.

RHEUMATOID ARTHRITIS

Rheumatoid arthritis (RA) is a chronic, systemic inflammatory disease of unknown etiology. It is characterized by symmetrical polyarthritis of the peripheral joints, morning stiffness, malaise, and fatigue. The disease course is variable, although there are often exacerbations and remissions, and the disease may completely remit or progress aggressively to result in profound disability.

The cause of RA has not been identified; however, research suggests that there are genetic influences.[18] The concordance rate for RA in monozygotic twins is 15% which is four times higher than in dizygotic twins.[19] Disease transmission in RA is complicated and may involve numerous genetic loci.

The inflammation and tissue destruction in RA are caused by complex interactions between antigen-presenting cells and T cells. Clonal expansion of T cells stimulates synovial secretion of proinflammatory *cytokines,* including *interleukin-1* (IL-1) and tumor necrosis factor-alpha (TNF-α).[20] RA also causes synovial proliferation, with the synovium changing from a single cell layer to a multicellular composition containing growth factors, lymphocytes, and inflammatory cytokines. The overgrown synovium, referred to as *pannus,* invades and destroys articular cartilage and bone.[21]

Diagnosis. There is no diagnostic test for RA that is 100% sensitive or specific. The diagnostic criteria for RA drafted by the American College of Rheumatology (ACR) are listed in Box 6-2. Disease presentation may vary among individuals and over time, delaying the initial diagnosis. Although *rheumatoid factor* is detectable in the serum of most patients with rheumatoid arthritis, it can also be found in patients with other diseases including SLE, Sjögren's syndrome, and liver or chronic lung disease. Furthermore, 20% to 30% of patients with RA do not have a positive rheumatoid factor test.

Clinical Features

Articular Manifestations. Articular manifestations of RA include morning stiffness, synovial inflammation, and structural damage. Morning stiffness correlates with the degree of inflammation and usually lasts more than 2 hours as opposed to the brief morning stiffness that occurs with osteoarthritis. Pain and swelling are key features of joints affected by RA. Acute *synovitis* may cause redness, warmth, and swelling in superficial joints; however, synovitis that affects deeper joints, such as the hips and shoulders, may be difficult to appreciate on physical examination. Persistent synovitis may lead to loss of cartilage, bony erosion, and ultimately, irreversible structural damage.[22]

Joint Specific Manifestations

Hands. The wrists and the metacarpophalangeal (MCP) and proximal interphalangeal (PIP) joints of the hands are commonly involved in RA.[22] Radial deviation at the wrist is often associated with ulnar deviation at the fingers (zigzag deformity)[23] (Fig. 6-3). This deformity is caused by chronic synovitis at the wrists and MCP joints, weakening of the extensor carpi ulnaris muscle, the ulnar bias of the power grasp,[24] and inappropriate action of the intrinsic muscles.[25]

Swan-neck deformities, which involve flexion of the MCP and distal IP (DIP) joints and hyperextension of the PIP joint, may develop due to persistent MCP synovitis with concomitant intrinsic muscle tightness (Fig. 6-4). Chronic inflammation at the PIP joint with avulsion of the extensor hood may lead to a *boutonnière deformity* (flexion at the PIP joint and hyperextension at the DIP joint) (Fig. 6-5).

Dorsal swelling within the synovial sheaths of extensor tendons at the wrist is also a common early manifestation

---

BOX 6-2	**Diagnostic Criteria for Rheumatoid Arthritis**

1. Morning stiffness: Morning stiffness in and around the joints, lasting at least 1 hour before maximal improvement.
2. Arthritis of 3 or more joint areas: At least 3 joint areas simultaneously have had soft tissue swelling or fluid observed by a physician. The 14 possible areas are right or left PIP, MCP, wrist, elbow, knee, ankle, and MTP joints.
3. Arthritis of hand joints: At least one area swollen in a wrist, MCP, or PIP joint.
4. Symmetrical arthritis: Simultaneous involvement of the same joint areas on both sides of the body.
5. Rheumatoid nodules: Subcutaneous nodules, over bony prominences, or extensor surfaces, or in juxtaarticular regions, observed by a physician.
6. Serum rheumatoid factor: Demonstration of abnormal amounts or serum rheumatoid factor by any method for which the result has been positive in <5% of normal control subjects.
7. Radiographic changes: Radiographic changes typical of rheumatoid arthritis on posteroanterior hand and wrist radiographs, which must include erosions or unequivocal bony decalcification localized in or most marked adjacent to the involved joints.

A patient has RA if 4 of the 7 criteria have been satisfied.

From Arnett FC, Edworthy SM, Bloch DA, et al: *Arthritis Rheum* 31:315-324, 1988.
PIP, Proximal interphalangeal; *MCP,* metacarpophalangeal; *MTP,* metatarsophalangeal; *RA,* rheumatoid arthritis.

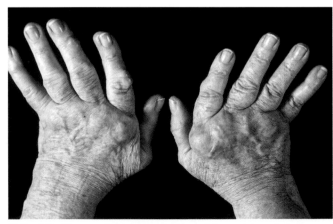

FIG. 6-3 Zigzag deformity at the wrists and hands in patient with RA. *Reprinted from the Clinical Slide Collection on the Rheumatic Diseases, copyright 1997. Used by permission of the American College of Rheumatology.*

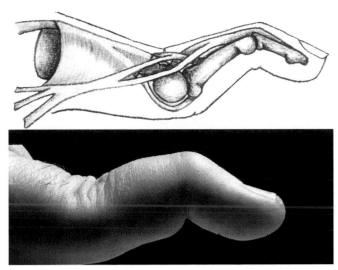

FIG. 6-4 Swan-neck deformity in patient with RA. *From Ruby LK, Cassidy C: Hand Clinics: Rheumatoarthritis of the Hand and Wrist, Vol. 12, No. 3, Philadelphia, 1996, WB Saunders.*

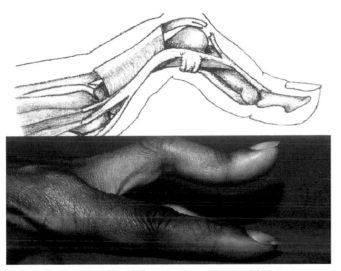

FIG. 6-5 Boutonnière deformity in patient with RA. *Reprinted from the Clinical Slide Collection on the Rheumatic Diseases, copyright 1997. Used by permission of the American College of Rheumatology.*

of RA. Synovial proliferation may also compromise the integrity of the radioulnar joint leading to stretching or rupture of the ulnar collateral ligament and subluxation of the ulnar head.

Flexor *tenosynovitis* and nodule formation may compromise finger flexion, and tendons may rupture due to persistent inflammation and resulting attenuation. Tendons may also become inflamed or rupture if they rub on the jagged edges of eroded carpal bones or the ulnar styloid.

Foot and Ankle. RA can cause synovitis at the metatarsophalangeal (MTP), talonavicular, and ankle joints. Synovitis at the MTP joint weakens the joint capsules and ligaments, leading to plantar subluxation of the metatarsal heads and cock-up deformities at the toes.[22] Inflammation

at the talonavicular joint results in pronation and eversion of the foot and flattening of the longitudinal arch. The tarsal tunnel may be subjected to increased stress that results from structural changes, and synovitis within the tarsal tunnel may cause compression of the posterior tibial nerve, which is manifested by paresthesias at the plantar aspect of the foot.

Hips. The hips are rarely involved in RA, and early manifestations of synovitis at the hips are difficult to detect on physical examination due to their deep location. Hip synovitis may produce pain at the groin, anteromedial knee, low back, or thigh that is reduced by positioning the hip in flexion and external rotation.[22]

Knees. Synovitis at the knee is not uncommon in RA and is easily detected on physical examination. Synovitis produces *effusions* that distend and stretch the joint capsule and contribute to ligamentous attenuation. A palpable synovial or *Baker's cyst* may also occur posteriorly in the popliteal fossa if some synovium becomes trapped and separated from the rest of the joint.

Elbows. The elbows are affected in 20% to 65% of individuals with RA. Patients may attempt to minimize pain from elbow synovitis by holding the joint in flexion and pronation. This commonly causes flexion contractures that impair function because a loss of as little as 30 degrees of extension may interfere with performance of activities of daily living (ADLs), such as dressing, feeding, grooming, hygiene, and sit-to-stand transfers.

Shoulders. RA of the shoulder may involve synovitis at the glenohumeral joint and inflammation within the surrounding bursae and rotator cuff tendons. Standard radiographic tests of the shoulders in RA commonly reveal erosions (69%) and superior subluxation (31%).[26] Patients may not be aware of the resulting loss of motion until significant restrictions occur since most daily activities do not require extremes of shoulder range. A person may lose as much as 50% of shoulder range of motion (ROM) before this interferes with functional activities.

Cervical Spine. RA of the cervical spine generally first presents with neck pain and stiffness. Neck pain may be caused by joint inflammation or by chronic tension in the posterior cervical muscles that results from postural strain, emotional stress, deconditioning, and altered biomechanics. Synovitis of the transverse ligament at C1, which stabilizes the odontoid process, may cause the ligament to become lax. Such ligamentous laxity or ligament rupture can cause C1-C2 instability or subluxation, which can result in cervical myelopathy (spinal cord compression).[27] Atlantoaxial (C1-C2) subluxation may initially cause pain and tenderness in the suboccipital region, as well as headaches, and progress to upper extremity paresthesias, lower extremity weakness, and instability. If not stabilized, paralysis or death will eventually occur. Patients can sometimes feel the bones sublux and report that it feels as though their head may "slip off." Atlantoaxial subluxation may also compress the vertebral arteries (the vertebral arteries pass through the foramina in the processes of C1 and C2) and induce visual disturbances (blurred vision or diplopia), loss of equilibrium, lightheadedness, dizziness, or other signs of posterior circulation stroke.[28] Inflammation at the apophyseal joints may also lead to pain and instability at multiple levels throughout the cervical spine.[22] Since C1-C2 subluxation has the potential for such bad sequelae, any examination findings suggestive of this pathology should be discussed immediately with the physician for consideration of further evaluation and management.

Systemic and Other Nonarticular Manifestations of Rheumatoid Arthritis. Systemic manifestations of RA include fatigue, malaise, subjective weakness, depression, and low-grade fever. These symptoms may precede the typical joint findings and may correlate with the degree of inflammation.

Common cutaneous manifestations of RA are rheumatoid nodules and Sjögren's syndrome. Rheumatoid nodules are subcutaneous masses, which may be soft and amorphous or firm and rubberlike, that tend to develop the extensor surfaces of the forearm and may form within tendons or ligaments. Sjögren's syndrome, which is characterized by dry eyes and dry mouth, occurs in 10% to 15% of patients with RA. RA can also cause photosensitivity, Raynaud's phenomenon, and *vasculitis*.

A small percentage of people with RA may have cardiac or pulmonary involvement, including pleurisy, interstitial lung disease, pericarditis, and myocarditis. It is important that therapists know if a patient has cardiopulmonary involvement and any restrictions this may cause before implementing an intervention program.

SPONDYLOARTHROPATHIES

The spondyloarthropathies are a group of inflammatory diseases involving the synovium, entheses, spine, and peripheral joints.[29] These diagnoses are strongly associated with the *HLA-B27* antigen. Ankylosing spondylitis, reactive arthritis (Reiter's syndrome), psoriatic arthritis, and a spondylitis related to inflammatory bowel disease are categorized in this group.[30] This discussion focuses on ankylosing spondylitis with lists highlighting features of the other spondyloarthropathies.

Ankylosing Spondylitis. *Ankylosing spondylitis* (AS) is a chronic systemic inflammatory disorder, primarily causing *enthesitis* and synovitis of the axial skeleton that almost always involves the sacroiliac joints. The predominant symptoms are low back pain (LBP) and stiffness that worsen with inactivity. Fatigue, malaise, weight loss, low-grade fever, and anorexia are also common.[30]

The onset of AS is between late adolescence and early adulthood, with an average of 26 years of age. Symptoms are reported to commence earlier in persons with lower socioeconomic status.[31] Juvenile onset is more common in North American natives (Amerindians).[32] Involvement of one or a few peripheral joints (known as oligoarthritis), usually a knee or MTP joint, without spinal involvement, is a typical presentation of AS in children.[30]

In AS, chronic inflammation at the enthesis (the site of ligament insertion into bone) causes fibrosis and then ossification of the ligaments and joint capsule, ultimately causing ankylosis (fusion) of the affected joints.[32] Enthesitis occurs in many areas of the spine including around the diskovertebral, costovertebral and costotransverse joints and at the attachments of the interspinous and paravertebral ligaments.[30] "Squaring" of vertebrae occurs

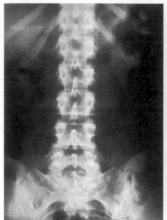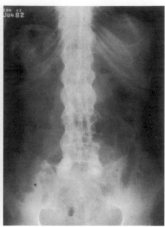

FIG. 6-6 Bamboo spine in ankylosing spondylitis. *Reprinted from the Clinical Slide Collection on the Rheumatic Diseases, copyright 1997. Used by permission of the American College of Rheumatology.*

because of bony erosion at the ligamentous insertions at the corners of the vertebral bodies.[32] The term bamboo spine describes the typical appearance of the spine on x-ray when AS has caused complete fusion of the vertebral column, with syndesmophytes and ossification extending to the posterior longitudinal and interspinous ligaments (Fig. 6-6).[33] The inflammation usually progresses upward from the sacroiliac joints toward the cervical spine. Without intervention, this can result in a fixed, extremely forward flexed spine.

Factors affecting prognosis in AS include severity of disease at onset, development of extraarticular complications, stage of disease when diagnosis was confirmed and treatment was initiated, flexion deformity of the spine, and patient compliance.[32] During pregnancy, sacroiliitis may produce pain and hinder delivery.

Etiology

Genetics. AS is much more common in men than in women, with a male : female ratio of 3-5 : 1.[32,33] The role of the HLA-B27 antigen in the pathogenesis of AS is undefined, although it is present in 90% to 95% of cases.[30] The presence of the HLA-B60 antigen has been shown to be associated with a threefold increase in the risk of developing AS.[34]

Diagnosis. The New York criteria from 1968 are used to make a diagnosis of AS.[35,36] Radiographic evidence of sacroiliitis is required. Other criteria include history of pain at the thoracolumbar junction or lumbar spine; limitation of motion in the lumbar spine, including flexion, lateral flexion and extension; and limitation of chest expansion to 2.5 cm (1 inch) or less at the fourth intercostal space.[34]

Clinical Features

Axial Spine. LBP is the first complaint in 75% of people with AS.[32] It can be unilateral and intermittent, but over time it becomes more persistent and bilateral. Tenderness or pain on palpation of the sacroiliac joints or LBP with hyperextension of the hip is common.[37] The back becomes stiff, and the lumbar lordosis fails to reverse with forward bending. Posture typically includes a forward head, protracted and internally rotated shoulders, increased thoracic kyphosis, and flattened lumbar spine.

Back pain combined with inactivity and stiffness can cause difficulties with sleeping, getting in and out of bed, and with dressing and grooming. As the thoracic spine and rib cage become stiff, chest expansion may be limited requiring the diaphragm to work harder during breathing.[33] Progression to cervical spine fusion may occur, limiting cervical rotation and extension and causing difficulties with driving.[32]

Initially, the pain and stiffness associated with AS improves with exercise or a hot shower or bath, but as the joints fuse, although pain may be less, the stiffness no longer resolves.[33] Spinal fractures and spinal cord compression may occur with increased disease severity.[30]

Peripheral Joints. AS can cause arthritis in the hips, knees, ankles, and MTP joints. Hip disease is typically bilateral, and pain combined with decreased ROM may lead to contractures in the hips and knees. The upper extremity joints are rarely involved, but with increased thoracic kyphosis, the shoulders may be affected.[30]

Other. Acute anterior *uveitis* (acute iritis) occurs in 25% to 30% of patients with AS and usually subsides in 2-3 months. Symptoms include eye pain, increased tearing, photophobia, and blurred vision and tend to be unilateral.[32]

Reactive Arthritis (Reiter's Syndrome). *Reactive arthritis,* also known as *Reiter's syndrome* (RS), is a systemic disease that typically begins suddenly (within days or weeks) after a venereal infection or gastroenteritis.[38,39] Joint and eye inflammation, enthesopathy, cutaneous lesions, malaise, fever, and fatigue are common manifestations. The prognosis for reactive arthritis is good with symptoms generally fully resolving in 3-12 months.

Diagnosis
Clinical Features
Musculoskeletal. Joint pain and inflammation are the principal musculoskeletal symptoms of RS. These range from mild arthralgias to severe, disabling polyarthritis.[40] Involvement is asymmetrical and usually affects the hips, knees, and ankles, but it is also common to see shoulder, elbow, wrist, and small joints in the hands and feet involved as in RA. Generalized stiffness often also occurs as a result of inactivity. Enthesopathy and tenosynovitis most often arise in the plantar fascia and Achilles tendon and can impair ambulation. Enthesitis may also occur at the symphysis pubis, iliac crest, greater trochanter, and anterolateral ribs.[33]

Skin and Mucous Membranes. A skin rash known as keratoderma blenorrhagicum (or pustulosis palmoplantaris) is the most frequent skin lesion in RS. This rash usually occurs on the sole of the foot or the palm of the hand and initially has flaky plaques like psoriasis, but later, these lesions develop pustules and become scaly.

Psoriatic Arthritis. *Psoriatic arthritis* (PA) is an autoimmune inflammatory disorder involving chronic activation of T helper-1 (TH-1) cells. PA usually affects the skin and joints, but one third of patients also develop some type of eye inflammation.[41,42]

Psoriasis that primarily affects the skin generally starts between the ages of 5 and 15 years. Although psoriatic skin lesions precede joint manifestations in 75% of cases, the joints are affected first 10% of the time and 15% of patients have simultaneous onset of skin and joint symptoms.

When psoriasis starts in childhood, symptoms frequently resolve. In adults, the prognosis for prolonged symptoms or progression is worse if there is a family history, disease onset before age 20, presence of HLA-DR3 or HLA-DR4 antigens, erosive or polyarticular disease, or extensive skin involvement.

Diagnosis
Clinical Features
Musculoskeletal. In PA, enthesitis frequently occurs where the Achilles tendon and the plantar fascia attach to the calcaneus. Spondylitis may occur and result in fusion similar to AS. Usually the arthritis associated with PA affects large joints like the knees and one or two DIP or PIP joints in an asymmetrical pattern. In women, symmetrical polyarthritis, mainly affecting the small joints of the hands, feet, wrists, ankles, knees, and elbows (similar to RA), is more common; in men, involvement of the DIP joints with associated changes in the nail bed or asymptomatic and asymmetrical spinal arthritis (sacroiliitis) is more common. When there is severe involvement of the skin of the scalp, there is also often cervical spine arthritis.

PA is also associated with soft tissue swelling that creates "sausage-like" digits. *Dactylitis,* (inflammation of a finger or toe) as a result of to tenosynovitis and arthritis of the DIP or PIP joints, can also occur. If bony ankylosis occurs in these joints it will cause a "claw" or "paddle" deformity.

Skin. The typical psoriatic lesion is a well-demarcated, erythematous plaque with a scaly appearance (Fig. 6-7). The nails are also often involved, with pitting as the most frequent characteristic. The nails can crack, turn brownish yellow (oil-drop sign), and separate from the underlying nail bed (onycholysis).

POLYMYALGIA RHEUMATICA

Polymyalgia rheumatica (PMR) is a systemic inflammatory disorder that primarily causes pain and stiffness in the

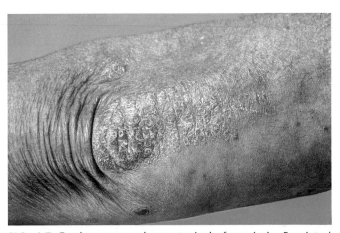

FIG. 6-7 Erythematous plaque typical of psoriasis. *Reprinted from the Clinical Slide Collection on the Rheumatic Diseases, copyright 1997. Used by permission of the American College of Rheumatology.*

neck, shoulder, and pelvic girdle muscles and rarely involves the distal extremities.[43,44] Low-grade fever, fatigue, anorexia, anemia, weight loss, depression and an elevated erythrocyte sedimentation rate (ESR) are common in PMR. Muscle biopsy reveals type II muscle fiber atrophy.[43] The incidence of PMR is estimated to be 10-53 cases per 100,000 with a peak age of onset of 60 to 80 years old. The etiology of this disease is unknown, although an immunological component is suspected.[43]

Giant cell arteritis (GCA), also known as temporal *arteritis,* cranial arteritis, or granulomatous arteritis, is a vasculitis of the medium and large arteries that commonly occurs together with PMR. About 50% of individuals with GCA have PMR-type complaints with muscular aches and pains. However, although only 10% of patients with PMR have GCA,[44] because GCA can cause sudden irreversible loss of vision, patients with PMR are generally evaluated for GCA. GCA commonly causes fatigue, tenderness around the temporal and occipital arteries and the scalp, jaw pain, visual disturbances, and headaches, often with severe pain in the temple area. Up to $^2/_3$ of patients with GCA experience claudication of the jaw muscles causing pain with chewing, and many have tingling of the tongue, loss of taste, and pain in the mouth and throat.[43]

Etiology

Genetics. PMR is more common in women than men with a ratio of 2-3 : 1, and PMR almost exclusively affects whites, especially Scandinavians and people of northern European descent.[44,45] There appears to be a familial predisposition to PMR and GCA.[43]

Diagnosis. The diagnosis of PMR is based on the clinical findings of proximal muscle weakness, aching, and stiffness for at least 4 weeks.[45] An ESR, in the range of 50-100 mm/hour, supports the diagnosis of PMR.[43,44]

Clinical Features

Musculoskeletal. The symptoms of PMR are usually bilateral and symmetrical tenderness of periarticular structures including bursae, joint capsules, and tendons. Synovitis of the hands, wrists, and knees may be present, and flexor tenosynovitis can lead to carpal tunnel syndrome.[44] Stiffness occurs after prolonged sitting and after getting out of bed in the morning. Pain is common at night and is then aggravated by movement.[43]

Vascular. PMR does not cause vascular changes; however, GCA, which is associated with PMR, is primarily a vascular disease. GCA causes the vessels to initially become filled with inflammatory infiltrates. They may then become thickened, tender, and nodular, causing a diminished or absent pulse, and blood clots can develop at the sites of inflammation.[43] Frequently, the vessels in the neck and head are affected by GCA but rarely the ones in the brain are also affected. Without intervention, GCA causes irreversible blindness in 25% to 50% of cases as a result of occlusion of the orbital or ocular arteries. Rapid initiation of treatment with corticosteroids can prevent this visual loss.[43]

POLYMYOSITIS AND DERMATOMYOSITIS

Polymyositis (PM) and *dermatomyositis* (DM) are rare autoimmune diseases that cause chronic inflammation in striated muscle. DM also has a dermatological component. The most prominent feature of both of these diseases is proximal weakness, affecting the muscles of the hips and shoulders with ocular and facial muscle weakness being very rare. The joints, lungs, heart, and GI systems can also be affected. There are two age peaks, between 10 and 15 years of age for children and between 45 and 60 years of age for adults.

Etiology. The etiology of these diseases is unknown, but viruses, infectious agents, genetic components, immune system dysfunction, and presence of autoantibodies are proposed influences.[46] In PM there is a cell-mediated immune response against myofibrils that causes infiltration of the muscles by T-lymphocytes and macrophages and atrophy of type II fibers.[46-48] In DM the B cells proliferate, and there is antibody-mediated injury to the capillaries and small arterioles in muscle.[46]

Symptoms of muscle pain, morning stiffness, weakness, fatigue, malaise, chills, fever, or weight loss generally come on rapidly. In DM, symptoms may appear briefly and then remit spontaneously without treatment. This form of *myositis* has the best functional outcome.

Before corticosteroids were used to treat DM, up to 50% of patients died from its complications. Now, the 5-year survival rate is 90%.[49] Risk factors for poor outcome include older age of onset, malignancy, delayed initiation of corticosteroids, pharyngeal dysphagia with aspiration pneumonia, interstitial lung disease (ILD), myocardial involvement, and complications from corticosteroids and other *immunosuppressive drugs.* Children with DM have a poor prognosis if GI vasculitis and sepsis occur.[49]

Genetics. PM and DM occur more often in women than in men, with a higher incidence in African Americans than in whites, with ratios of 2.5 : 1 and 3-4 : 1, respectively. There is an increased prevalence of PM and DM in monozygotic twins and first-degree relatives.[49] There is an increased risk of developing inflammatory muscle disease if HLA-DR3 is present.[46]

Environmental Factors. PM and DM onset is more frequent in winter and spring months, especially in children, after exposure to viral and bacteria infections.[49]

Diagnosis. Standards are still being developed for the diagnosis of PM and DM, but the most commonly used classification criteria are those developed by Bohan and Peter.[50] These criteria include symmetrical proximal muscle weakness, elevated serum skeletal muscle enzymes, muscle biopsy evidence of myositis, and electromyographic pattern characteristic of myositis. DM also requires the presence of a typical rash.[48-51]

Clinical Features

Musculoskeletal. Muscle weakness is the most prevalent clinical feature of PM and DM, with the shoulder and pelvic girdle muscles being affected most significantly. In about 50% of cases the neck flexor muscles are weak, and rarely, the ocular and facial muscles are affected.[47,49] About 50% of patients with PM and DM complain of muscle pain, but it is the muscle weakness that most impacts function, affecting tasks such as reaching overhead, dressing, toilet transfers, and stair climbing. Decreased neck flexor strength also impairs the ability to lift the head off of a pillow, and pharyngeal muscle weakness may cause swallowing difficulty.[46] Muscle shortening as a result of atrophy and fibrosis can also reduce joint ROM and cause contractures that impair function.[49] EMG studies are abnormal in 85% to 90% of patients with PM or DM.[46]

Skin. The rash associated with DM has a typical erythematous or heliotrope (purple) color and presents on the upper eyelids, malar areas (cheeks), bridge of the nose, nasolabial folds, and the "V" areas of the anterior neck and upper chest, "shawl sign" of posterior shoulder and neck, extensor surface of the elbows and knees, on the MCP and PIP joints, and around the nails. The skin also has a scaly characteristic. "Mechanic" or "machinist" hands, with rough skin with cracks or fissures over the distal digital pad, are also typical of DM.[49] As the disease progresses, the skin becomes shiny, atrophic, and hypopigmented.[49]

Cardiac. Although cardiac muscle involvement is common in PM and DM, it is generally asymptomatic until the disease is advanced. Rhythm abnormalities are the most frequent cardiac manifestations and infrequently, congestive heart failure may occur as the result of myocardial inflammation or fibrosis.[46,49]

Pulmonary. There are four common pulmonary effects of PM and DM. Initially, persons may be asymptomatic with only radiographic evidence of bibasilar fibrosis or measurable decreased vital capacity. Later, aspiration pneumonia may occur as a result of pharyngeal dysphagia. More commonly, patients have slowly progressive interstitial lung disease that is symptomatically masked by the myopathy. A few patients develop aggressive pulmonary involvement with diffuse alveolitis, a nonproductive cough and rapidly progressive dyspnea leading to respiratory distress syndrome.[49]

Gastrointestinal. Pharyngeal dysphagia may cause nasal regurgitation and dysphonia, as well as swallowing difficulties that can lead to aspiration pneumonia. Patients report that food "sticks" (especially bread and meat) because of dysmotility of the lower esophagus.[49] Weakness of the lower esophageal sphincter causes gastric reflux and heartburn. Constipation is common and is caused by colonic hypomotility.[49] The vasculitis and ischemia that occurs in children can also cause life-threatening GI hemorrhage or perforation.[49]

Malignancy. The link between myositis and malignancy is controversial. The prevalence of malignancy in patients with myositis has a wide estimated range of 4% to 42%.[51,52] The highest risk for neoplasm appears to be in the first 3 years after the diagnosis of myositis, although in some cases the malignancy is diagnosed before the myositis. The incidence of malignancy is higher in DM than in PM. Some sources recommend that all patients with myositis be screened for malignancy.[51]

Other. The peripheral vascular system is often affected by Raynaud's phenomenon especially in DM.[49]

SCLERODERMA

Scleroderma (Sc) is an autoimmune connective tissue disease characterized by fibrosis of the skin and internal organs. "Scleroderma" means hardening of the skin, and taut, hidebound skin is the most characteristic feature of Sc.[53] How the immune system is activated in Sc is not fully understood, but it is thought that viruses, including par-

vovirus B19 and cytomegalovirus, may play a role in susceptibility to the disease.[53]

The two types of Sc are limited and diffuse.[54] "Limited cutaneous" or "localized" scleroderma primarily affects the skin distal to the elbows and knees and affects the lungs, although there may be some involvement of the skin of the face or neck. Fatigue and Raynaud's phenomenon are also common in this form of the disease.

"Diffuse" Sc or *systemic sclerosis* (SSc) is the more aggressive form of the disease. In this form of the disease there is fibrosis of the internal organs, musculoskeletal structures (tendons, muscle, joints, synovium), blood vessels, the gastrointestinal (GI) tract, lungs, heart, and kidneys, as well as much of the skin over the trunk and proximal extremities. Raynaud's phenomenon can appear shortly before the skin fibrosis.[55] Thickening of the skin occurs within months of disease onset and progresses rapidly over 2 to 3 years. The extent of skin involvement is a predictor of the progression of the clinical course of SSc.[53] Later the skin may begin to soften, but contractures may have already developed.[55]

Approximately 50% of patients with SSc have GI and pulmonary disease, and most have cardiopulmonary involvement that can become life threatening. The 10-year survival rate in SSc is about 40% to 60%.[55] Poor prognosis is linked with late age of onset, African American or Native American descent, diffuse skin involvement, presence of tendon rubs, pulmonary function with diffusing capacity less than 40% of predicted values, presence of large pericardial effusion, proteinuria, hematuria, renal failure, low hemoglobin, elevated erythrocyte sedimentation rate, and an abnormal electrocardiogram.[55]

Etiology

Genetics. Sc is rare in children and seldom runs in families, but there is a tendency for other autoimmune and connective tissue diseases to occur in relatives.[53] More women have the disease with an average ratio of 3 : 1 women to men. The average age of onset is between 35 and 65 years of age.[53]

Environmental Factors. The equal concordance rates for Sc in monozygotic and dizygotic twins and the occurrence of disease in conjugal pairs indicate that the environment may impact the occurrence of Sc.[53] There is an increased risk for diffuse Sc with occupational exposure to silica dust,[54,55] and although cases of scleroderma have been reported after exposure to a wide range of other substances, no correlation between these exposures and this disease has been proved.[53,55-62]

Diagnosis. The diagnosis of Sc is based on the criteria devised by the Subcommittee for Scleroderma Criteria of the American Rheumatism Association.[63] The major required criterion is skin thickening proximal to the MCP joints. Minor criteria include *sclerodactyly,* digital ischemia, abnormal skin pigmentation, pulmonary fibrosis, Raynaud's phenomenon, and lower esophageal dysphagia and dysmotility. A diagnosis requires one major and two or more minor criteria.

Clinical Features

Musculoskeletal. The earliest symptoms of Sc are often joint and muscle pain and stiffness without signs of inflammation.[55] Pain with joint motion accompanied by a tendon friction rub may indicate inflammation or fibrosis of the tendon sheaths or adjacent tissues.

Swelling and fibrosis can also limit motion, particularly in the fingers and face, and fibrosis around the carpal tunnel may result in carpal tunnel syndrome. Vascular involvement can further reduce hand function by causing pain and skin ulceration. A progressive loss of hand function may occur as pain and decreased flexibility lead to inactivity, which cause muscle weakness and atrophy that then cause further loss of flexibility and more pain. Patients with Sc often cannot perform simple functional fine motor tasks such as fastening buttons or snaps, opening jars, or tying shoes.

Skin. Skin changes in Sc occur in three phases of varying duration. The first phase begins with puffiness and edema in the distal phalanges, sometimes together with mild inflammation, erythema, and itching. The second phase is characterized by progressive tightening of the skin leading to fibrosis, decreased flexibility, and severe drying. The fibrotic tissue binds to the deeper tissues as the skins thins out, creating a tethering effect. The third phase is characterized by skin atrophy without inflammation or fibrosis.[55]

Sclerodactyly (scaring together of the fingers) and the neck sign (thick horizontal folds of skin on the anterior neck) are also associated with Sc. Decreased elasticity of the facial skin can make the person appear expressionless with pursed lips, decreased oral aperture, a pinched nose, and smooth facial creases creating a mouselike appearance *(mauskopf)* (Fig. 6-8). In SSc, there may also be mixed hypopigmentation and hyperpigmentation of the skin that creates a tanned or "salt and pepper" discoloration. Subcutaneous calcium deposits can also form in the fingers, forearms, or other areas of pressure in patients with limited SSc.[55]

Vascular. Raynaud's phenomenon occurs in about 90% to 95% of patients with Sc.[64] Sc can also adversely affect circulation by causing proliferation of smooth muscle cells around blood vessels narrowing the vessel which can cause blood clots to form in the vessels. These vascular effects can cause arterial insufficiency and digital ischemia, leading to ulceration that can occasionally necessitate digital amputation (Fig. 6-9).[53,54,65]

Cardiac. Fibrosis of the heart and its vessels usually occurs late in the course of SSc and is associated with a poor prognosis. The most common symptoms of cardiac involvement are dyspnea with exertion, palpitations, and chest discomfort.[55]

Pulmonary. Impaired lung function resulting from pulmonary fibrosis is almost universal in Sc. The most common symptom is dyspnea with exertion. Pulmonary function tests may help detect reduction in lung volumes or diffusing capacity before symptoms begin (see Chapter 26). Pulmonary fibrosis can also lead to pulmonary hypertension, which is the primary cause of death in limited Sc. Less frequent pulmonary problems include aspiration caused by esophageal dysfunction, chronic cough, respiratory distress, pulmonary hemorrhage, and pneumothorax. There is also an increased prevalence of lung cancer in patients with Sc.[55]

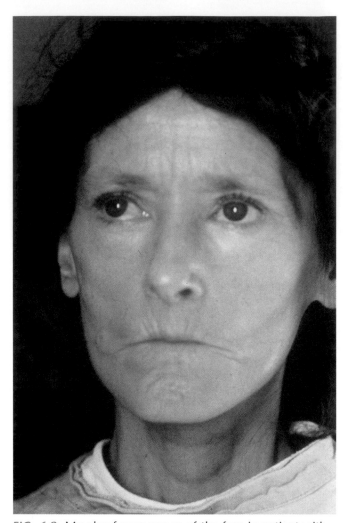

FIG. 6-8 Mauskopf appearance of the face in patient with scleroderma. *Reprinted from the Clinical Slide Collection on the Rheumatic Diseases, copyright 1997. Used by permission of the American College of Rheumatology.*

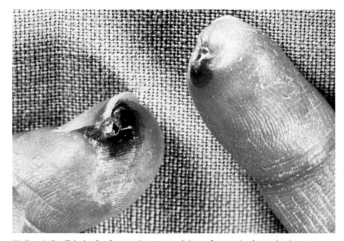

FIG. 6-9 Digital ulceration resulting from ischemia in a patient with scleroderma. *Reprinted from the Clinical Slide Collection on the Rheumatic Diseases, copyright 1997. Used by permission of the American College of Rheumatology.*

Gastrointestinal. Sc can cause difficulty chewing food, loss of teeth, and malnutrition because of the decreased perioral aperture, dry mucosal membranes, and periodontal disease. Heartburn, dysphagia, and dyspepsia are also common, and patients frequently have a sensation of food "sticking" because of lower esophageal dysmotility. Esophageal involvement can also lead to reflux of acid from the stomach into the esophagus, which can result in esophageal erosions, bleeding, stricture, and possibly adenocarcinoma, and to aspiration, unexplained cough, hoarseness, and chest pain.

Other Clinical Signs and Symptoms. Sc is a chronic disease and depression occurs in 50% of cases.[55] There can also be sexual dysfunction in males as a result of neurovascular involvement, causing impotence. SS often accompanies Sc so there is a need for fastidious dental care, as well as artificial tears for corneal lubrication. Trigeminal neuralgia may also occur, and thyroid fibrosis can lead to hypothyroidism.[55]

SJÖGREN'S SYNDROME

Sjögren's syndrome (SS) is an autoimmune disorder primarily characterized by inflammation of the exocrine glands.[66] Involvement of the salivary and lacrimal glands results in decreased production of saliva and tears causing dry mouth *(xerostomia)* and dry eyes *(xerophthalmia)*, respectively. Additional features of SS include synovitis, neuropathy, and vasculitis. Patients with SS may present to rehabilitation because of the effects of the synovitis on their functional abilities or when they have secondary SS caused by another rheumatic disease such as RA.

The pathogenesis of SS is unknown; however, it is thought that a virus triggers the autoimmune process in genetically predisposed individuals. Because women are more often affected by SS than men it is also proposed that hormones play a role in the development of SS.[67]

Diagnosis. Diagnostic criteria for SS are shown in Box 6-3.

Clinical Features. The cardinal features of SS are dry eyes and dry mouth. Additional manifestations include dry skin, hypothyroidism, nonproductive cough, peripheral neuropathy, lymphoid malignancy, and increased urinary frequency. Patients may also develop musculoskeletal manifestations, including myalgias, arthralgias, and arthritis.

CRYSTAL-INDUCED ARTHROPATHIES

Gout. *Gout* is caused by deposition of uric acid crystals in the joints and connective tissue. Although gout is related to high uric acid levels in the blood *(hyperuricemia)*, many people with hyperuricemia do not develop gout. Uric acid levels are influenced by genetic and environmental factors.

Clinical Features. Gout is characterized by three stages: hyperuricemia, acute intermittent gout, and chronic tophaceous gout. The rate and degree of progression varies among patients.[68] Hyperuricemia is common, and in most people, never results in clinical symptoms of gout.[68] Clinical gout initially presents with warmth, swelling, pain, and erythema at a single joint. The pain progresses from mild twinges to intense and severe pain. The initial attack is most often at the first MTP joint.[69] Other joints commonly involved in the initial stages of gout include the ankles, heels, midfoot, and knees. The joint symptoms may be accompanied by systemic symptoms, including fever, chills, and malaise. Such acute episodes may last for hours to weeks and can recur at varying intervals.[68]

Chronic tophaceous gout may develop in individuals who have had acute intermittent gout for over 10 years. The involved joints become chronically swollen and painful. *Tophi*, which are deposits of uric acid crystals around the joints, then develop, correlating with the severity and duration of hyperuricemia (Fig. 6-10). Tophi occur most often at the fingers, wrists, ears, knees, olecranon bursae, and Achilles tendons.[68]

Pseudogout. *Pseudogout* is similar to gout but is caused by deposition of calcium pyrophosphate dehydrate (CPPD) crystals, rather than urate crystals, in joints and periarticular tissues. The crystals are mostly deposited in the cartilage. Acute joint inflammation (arthritis) results from the release of CPPD crystals from the cartilage or

---

BOX 6-3	**Diagnostic Criteria for Primary Sjögren's Syndrome**

Symptoms and Objective Signs of Ocular Dryness
Schirmer's test less than 8 mm wetting per 5 minutes.
Positive rose bengal or fluorescein staining of cornea and conjunctiva to demonstrate keratoconjunctivitis sicca.

Symptoms and Objective Signs of Dry Mouth
Decreased parotid flow rate using Lashley cups or other methods.
Abnormal biopsy of minor salivary gland.

Evidence of a Systemic Autoimmune Disorder
Elevated rheumatoid factor >1 : 160
Elevated ANA >1 : 160
Presence of anti-SS-A/Ro or anti-SS-B/La antibodies

Data from Fox RI, Robinson C, Curd J, et al: *Scand J Rheumatol* Supplement 61:28-30, 1986.
ANA, Antinuclear antibody.

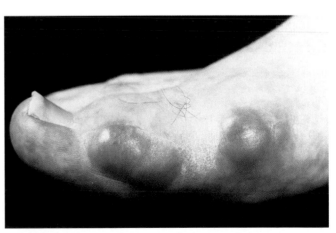

FIG. 6-10 Gouty tophi around the joints of the great toe. *Reprinted from the Clinical Slide Collection on the Rheumatic Diseases, copyright 1997. Used by permission of the American College of Rheumatology.*

other tissues into the joint space. Phagocytosis of the CPPD by synovial lining cells leads to cellular proliferation and release of inflammatory mediators that cause the acute inflammation.[70]

Clinical Features. Acute pseudogout is characterized by inflammation at one or two joints that lasts for days or weeks. Fifty percent or more of the attacks affect the knees, but any joint may be involved. Acute attacks may be induced by acute illness, surgery, or trauma. Patients are generally symptom-free between bouts.

JUVENILE RHEUMATOID ARTHRITIS

Juvenile RA (JRA) is the most common connective tissue disease in children. It is a chronic inflammatory disease that starts before the age of 16 and causes joint symptoms for more than 6 weeks. Although the etiology of JRA is unknown, environmental triggers in genetically predisposed individuals have been hypothesized.[71] Research has linked specific HLA genotypes to the type and course of JRA,[72] and viral diseases, such as rubella and parvovirus, have been implicated as triggers for disease expression.[73]

The pathology of JRA resembles that of adults with RA. There is hyperplasia of the synovial lining with clusters of lymphocytes, plasma cells, and other immunologically active cells. Synovial proliferation with pannus formation may result in cartilaginous degradation, bony erosion, and subsequent joint destruction.

Diagnosis

Clinical Features. JRA is divided into three different subtypes based on clinical manifestations and course within the first six months of illness. The subtypes are pauciarticular, polyarticular, and systemic JRA.[74]

Pauciarticular Juvenile Rheumatoid Arthritis. *Pauciarticular* JRA involves four or fewer joints and is the most common form of JRA. The joint inflammation tends to be milder than in the other subtypes and extraarticular manifestations are rare. Children with pauciarticular JRA respond well to medical treatment, and joint symptoms often remit within several years. Pauciarticular JRA may have an early or late onset. Early onset is considered to be before the age of 5 years and is most common in girls. JRA commonly affects the knees, ankles, wrists, and elbows, with the knees being involved in 75% of the cases. The hips are generally spared. Chronic uveitis occurs in 20% of patients.[75] Late-onset pauciarticular arthritis presents after 9 years of age and generally occurs in boys. The lower extremity joints are affected asymmetrically, and enthesitis is common. The presence of HLA-B27 and the absence of rheumatoid factor are common in late-onset pauciarticular JRA, and 40% of patients go on to develop disease manifestations consistent with the spondyloarthropathies.

Polyarticular Juvenile Rheumatoid Arthritis. Polyarticular JRA is the second most common form of JRA and involves five or more joints in a symmetrical presentation, including both large and small joints. As many as 20 joints may be involved at one time, including joints of the cervical spine, the costovertebral joints, and the temporomandibular joints (TMJs). This type of JRA is more common in girls. The prognosis for patients with poly-

articular disease is not as favorable as in pauciarticular JRA, especially in individuals who are rheumatoid-factor positive.

Systemic-Onset Juvenile Rheumatoid Arthritis. Systemic-onset JRA (SOJRA) is the least common subtype of JRA, occurring in only 10% of patients. It may present at any age during childhood and has no gender predominance. High spiking fevers twice daily and the presence of a rash on the trunk and proximal extremities are characteristic. The arthritis may coincide with systemic features or manifest weeks to months later. Children with SOJRA often feel ill, fatigued, and lose their appetite, resulting in weight loss, with constitutional symptoms and rash being most notable during febrile episodes.

EXAMINATION

The first component of the examination of the patient with connective tissue dysfunctions is a thorough patient history. This is followed by a systems review and specific tests and measures. Patient observation should occur throughout the examination. The competencies for working with patients with rheumatological diseases, as developed by the Association of Rheumatology Health Professionals, require that a patient examination and evaluation be performed to identify an individual's abilities and functional limitations before treatment is initiated. The findings of the examination may be documented on a rheumatology-specific examination form (see Additional Resources on the CD that accompanies this book) and supplemented by an initial intake questionnaire (multisystem medical history form, also on the CD that accompanies this book).

PATIENT HISTORY

Most of the key information needed for diagnosis, evaluation, and selection of interventions for patients with connective tissue dysfunctions can be identified from the patient history. Physical and psychological needs and concerns should be considered to understand how the patient's condition affects their functional abilities. Medical aspects of the disease also need to be considered since connective tissue dysfunctions are associated with chronic, systemic processes.

The initial phase of the history should cover the patient's experience with the disease, including their expectations and goals for treatment. Involving the patient in goal setting develops rapport, helps to gain trust and confidence and, improves adherence to treatment.

Demographic information, including the patient's age, sex, occupation, and diagnosis, is usually collected when the patient initially registers for care. This information can be helpful in making a diagnosis as certain rheumatological diseases have specific gender and racial distributions.

After getting a general impression of the patient's condition and experience of their disease, the interviewer should try to determine the chronology of the patient's symptoms, including how and when the symptoms began and how they evolved. Sometimes symptoms are still evolving when the patient is referred for rehabilitation. If a definitive diagnosis has not been made or an "overlap" syndrome exists that does not specifically fit into one diagnostic category, the therapist's observation and feedback may help the physician make a medical diagnosis. People with rheumatological diseases usually have a range of symptoms that began at a certain point, with varying periods of time elapsing until they are "officially diagnosed."

After obtaining information about the development of symptoms, the current presenting symptoms, including pain, stiffness, swelling, weakness, fatigue, and anxiety, should be explored. Certain details of the patient's pain may help to differentiate the patient's pathology and stage of involvement and thus suggest which types of interventions are most likely to be effective.

Stiffness is related to how much force it takes or how difficult it is to move or bend a joint. Subjectively, the term stiffness may be used to describe pain with movement, an ache, or decreased ROM, as well as passive resistance to motion. With connective tissue dysfunction resulting from inflammation, morning stiffness may be prolonged, lasting for several hours. Stiffness associated with inflammation can also be severe, present in the morning and evening, and cause difficulty with moving joints and performing functional tasks. Degenerative or mechanical pathologies cause stiffness after inactivity, making it difficult to initiate movement.[76,77] This is referred to as the "gel" or "gelling" phase. Swelling can also be a sign or symptom of active joint disease.

Although weakness is generally caused by loss of muscle strength, complaints of generalized weakness are often related to fatigue, whereas localized weakness is more likely a result of true muscle weakness. Fatigue is a common manifestation of systemic rheumatic diseases. Belza describes this as an enduring, subjective sensation of debilitating and generalized tiredness or exhaustion.[78] The fatigue from rheumatic diseases can be so overwhelming that it limits the ability to perform any task and robs patients of their independence. It is often a marker of the amount of disease activity and can be used to monitor the effectiveness of treatment.

The patient's past medical history with regards to this and other conditions and prior interventions (medical, surgical, rehabilitative, and alternative/complementary) and their effectiveness may also provide information relevant to the plan of care.[79-81] In addition, the patient's social history may play a part in how they experience their symptoms and which interventions will be most appropriate and effective. It has been shown that people with rheumatic diseases have a better quality of life and less pain if they have a stronger support structure, including family, friends, and neighbors.[82]

Rheumatic diseases can cause fear and anxiety because they are chronic, progressive diseases. Fear may be related to a sense of loss of control and independence, anger, abandonment, or isolation.[83] The patient may worry about becoming "crippled" or feel that pain is a sign of more damage. Denial and depression are common in patients with a variety of chronic medical conditions.[84,85] Psychological interventions can be important adjuncts to the treatment plan and should be included in the interview process.[86]

SYSTEMS REVIEW

The systems review is used to target areas requiring further examination and to define areas that may cause complications or indicate a need for precautions during the examination and intervention processes. See Chapter 1 for details of the systems review.

TESTS AND MEASURES
Musculoskeletal

Posture. Postural assessment may initially be performed with the patient standing, with attention to deviations from normal spinal curves (see Chapter 4). As previously discussed, patients with *spondyloarthropathy* may develop forward-head positioning with increased thoracic kyphosis and loss of lumbar lordosis. Forward-head positioning may be quantified by measuring either the tragus-to-wall or occiput-to-wall distance as the patient stands with the back to the wall.

Anthropometric Characteristics. All joints should be inspected for deformities, malalignment, and swelling. Increased girth may be caused by intraarticular effusion, synovial thickening, periarticular soft tissue inflammation, or extraarticular fat pads. Warmth, a sign of inflammation, may be detected by palpation.

The hands and wrists are examined for alignment, intrinsic wasting, swelling, nail changes, and joint deformities. This examination may reveal disease-specific patterns that may clarify the diagnosis. The MCP and PIP joints are generally involved in RA; osteoarthritis more often affects the PIP and DIP joints. Synovial swelling produces symmetrical enlargement of the joint, while extraarticular swelling may be diffuse and asymmetrical. The MCP joints are palpated for swelling with the examiner's thumbs at the dorsal aspect of the joint, while the index fingers palpate the volar aspect of the MCP head. The PIP joints are best palpated by compressing anteroposteriorly with the thumb and index finger, while palpating medially and laterally with the other thumb and index finger. The wrists may be inspected for signs of synovitis, including warmth, tendon thickening, and nodules. Ulnar subluxation may occur with chronic *inflammatory arthritis* and is often referred to as the piano key sign. The subluxed ulna appears as a prominence at the dorsolateral aspect of the wrist and may lead to attrition and eventual rupture of the extensor digitorum communis tendons. Swelling of the wrist may be associated with tenosynovitis or intraarticular swelling of the wrist joint itself. Tenosynovitis tends to manifest more locally, whereas wrist synovitis is more diffuse, protruding anteriorly or posteriorly from beneath the tendons.

Synovitis can cause elbow flexion contractures. Synovitis at the elbow is most readily detected in the triangular recess between the olecranon process, the lateral epicondyle of the humerus, and the radial head when the elbow is in 70 degrees of extension, or the open packed position. The elbow should also be inspected for nodules, tophi, and olecranon *bursitis.*

At the shoulder, rheumatic diseases can affect the glenohumeral joint, rotator cuff, subacromial bursae, or bicipital region. The shoulder girdle should be observed from the front and the back, and the two shoulders should be compared. The shoulder should also be palpated for muscle atrophy, warmth, and tenderness. Effusions are best observed anteriorly, medial to the bicipital groove, and laterally, below the acromion.

The knee joint is inspected for swelling, muscle atrophy, varus or valgus deformities, flexion contractures, and Baker's cysts. A large synovial effusion can cause a flexion contracture. Knee joint effusion or synovitis may be identified by a suprapatellar swelling with fullness of the distal anterior thigh. An effusion as small as 4-8 ml may be detected by the presence of a bulge sign. The bulge sign is detected by the examiner stroking the medial aspect of the knee proximally and laterally with the palm of one hand to move the fluid from the area and then tapping the lateral aspect of the knee. A positive bulge sign is when a fluid wave or bulge appears medially.

The ankle and foot should be examined in weight-bearing and non–weight-bearing positions and dynamically during gait. Visual inspection may reveal nodules, calluses, swelling, nail changes, and foot deformities. The feet and toes are often affected in gout, osteoarthritis, and RA. Deformities may include hallux valgus (lateral deviation of the great toe), hammer toes (hyperextension of the MTP joint), subluxation of the metatarsal heads, and severe forefoot pronation with medial arch collapse.

Range of Motion. Active ROM (AROM) and passive ROM (PROM) should be measured and recorded at all peripheral joints. Causes of limitations may include pain, weakness, muscle shortening, or swelling. Joint *crepitus* may be noted as a grinding or grating sensation that is either palpable or audible with movement of joints or supportive structures. The goniometer is the instrument of choice for measuring peripheral joint motion, and the tape measure is the most convenient instrument for measuring spinal motion.[6]

Spine ROM should initially be examined with the patient in standing with attention to deviations from the normal spinal curves. Mobility testing for the cervical and lumbar spine should be performed actively in all planes of motion. *Schober's test* may be employed to quantify motion at the lumbar spine. This test is performed by placing marks at the lumbosacral junction and 10 cm up along the spine, with the patient standing (Fig. 6-11). The patient then bends forward as far as possible, and the increase in distance between the two marks is measured with a flexible tape measure. This distance should increase by at least 5 cm if lumbar spine mobility is normal. Thoracic mobility may be assessed by measuring chest circumference at the level of the nipples (T4) during exhalation and inhalation. It is normal for the chest circumference to increase by at least 5 cm from maximum exhalation to maximum inhalation.

Muscle Performance. Connective tissue dysfunction may be associated with generalized or localized weakness. There may be weakness in more than one area that may be distributed asymmetrically or symmetrically or be more pronounced centrally or peripherally. Approximately 1% to 5% of strength can be lost just as a result of inactivity rather than as a direct consequence of a particular disease process.[87,88]

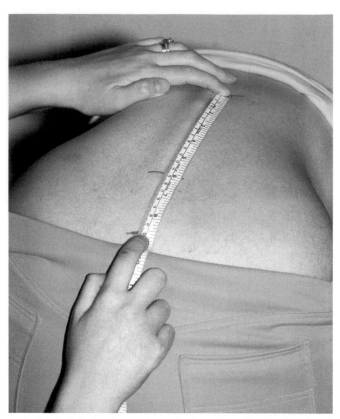

FIG. 6-11 Schober's test for spinal mobility in AS. *Reprinted from the Clinical Slide Collection on the Rheumatic Diseases, copyright 1997. Used by permission of the American College of Rheumatology.*

Muscle performance and strength deficits may be tested with functional strength assessment tools and other standardized measures (see Chapter 5). For patients with connective tissue dysfunction, it is recommended that strength be tested functionally rather than graded by manual muscle testing (MMT) because MMT may be unreliable in this population of patients who are often unable to assume standardized testing positions and in whom joint pain often limits test performance.[6]

Neuromuscular

Pain. Pain should be quantified using a visual analog scale (VAS) or other descriptive scale (see Chapter 22). Additionally, the location of painful and tender areas should be determined and documented.

Peripheral Nerve Integrity. Inflammation associated with connective tissue dysfunction may indirectly affect peripheral nerve function. For example, entrapment neuropathies are commonly seen in the rheumatic diseases, and synovitis may result in nerve compression at the carpal tunnel (median nerve), medial epicondyle (ulnar nerve), and tarsal tunnel (posterior tibial nerve). See Chapter 18 for a complete discussion of tests and measures to examine and evaluate peripheral nerve integrity.

Integumentary

Integumentary Integrity. Cutaneous manifestations of connective tissue dysfunction may be a primary manifestation of the underlying disease process or a secondary manifestations of vascular insufficiency or medications. In particular, corticosteroid medications may cause skin thinning and fragility that may impact selection of rehabilitation interventions, adaptive equipment, and assistive devices. Common cutaneous manifestations of diseases that cause connective tissue dysfunction include: nail changes, rashes, reduced skin elasticity, cutaneous plaques, subcutaneous nodules, ulcerations, Raynaud's phenomenon or trophic changes.[6]

Sc primarily affects the skin. The extent of skin thickening in Sc can be measured by pinching the skinfold between the fingertips and grading the thickening as mild, moderate, or extreme, or by measuring the skin thickness. Serial measurements of skin involvement may be used to define the stage and follow the course of the disease.[89]

Function. Functional status and the ability to perform activities in the home, community, and at work may be assessed with a variety of validated instruments. These include the Button test, Grip Strength test, Jepson Hand Function test, Timed-Stands test, and the Keitel Index. All of these tests involve direct observation of the patient performing a task and rely on patient cooperation and motivation to be valid. All of these tools have been validated in patients with chronic rheumatic diseases and are sensitive to change. The Button, Grip Strength, and Timed-Stands tests are easy to use in the clinical environment because they are quick and the standardized equipment is inexpensive. As with other tests and measures, these functional tests can be used to indicate the patient's baseline condition and to measure progress over the course of treatment or time. Table 6-1 contains tools to measure function in this population.

Gait, Locomotion, and Balance. Gait examination is an integral part of the examination of patients with connective tissue dysfunction. All phases of gait should be analyzed with specific attention to joint position, alignment, and compensatory patterns. Patients should be examined with and without assistive devices and from all angles. The 6-minute walk test has been demonstrated to be valid and sensitive change in patients with chronic rheumatic diseases.[90-92]

Self-Care and Home Management/Work, Community, and Leisure Integration. Most tests of self-care and home management for this population are based on self-administered questionnaires. Three self-report measures specifically designed to assess function in patients with arthritis are the Functional Status Index (FSI),[93,94] the Arthritis Impact Measurement Scale (AIMS),[96] and the Health Assessment Questionnaire (HAQ).[95] The FSI evaluates 18 items that encompass gross mobility skills, personal care, hand activities, home chores, and social activities. It scores the amount of help required to perform the task, ranging from 0 (independent) to 4 (unable to execute). It also asks the patient to report the level of difficulty and pain when performing these activities. The FSI was developed specifically for examination of patients with arthritis and has been validated in this population.[97]

The two questionnaires most often used to assess functional outcome in patients with connective tissue dys-

functions are the AIMS and the HAQ. Both have been extensively validated and have been translated into multiple languages. The most comprehensive health status tool is the AIMS2, which is a 1992 revision of the original AIMS developed in 1980.[98] The AIMS2 assesses the impact of chronic arthritis diagnoses on physical and psychosocial health, functional status, patient satisfaction, priorities for health status improvement, and recognition of problems related to arthritis. The AIMS2 enhanced the original instrument by adding new subscales for patient satisfaction and patient priorities for improving health status and new domains for mobility skills, self-care, household tasks, social activities, support structure, work, and levels of tension and mood.[99] Meenan et al[98] found that the internal consistency coefficients for the 12 scales were 0.72-0.91 for patients with RA and 0.74-0.96 for individuals with osteoarthritis. They also demonstrated validity of this scale with the finding that patient designation of an area as a problem or as a priority for improvement was significantly associated with AIMS2 scale scores in that area. This tool is most suitable for clinical research because it is lengthy, requiring a minimum of 20 minutes to complete, and has a complex scoring method. A shortened version called the AIMS-SF reduces the items surveyed by half but needs further study to assess its validity, reliability, and sensitivity.[100]

There are several versions of the HAQ.[101] The original version was developed in 1980, is 20 pages in length, and includes information about medications, use of health care services, co-morbidities, pain, function, global disease severity, and economic costs. The second revision, which is used most often, includes 24 questions regarding activities of daily living, a VAS for pain in the last week, and global disease severity.[102] The 24 questions are scored from 0 (no problem) to 3 (unable to perform with help). The modified HAQ (MHAQ)[103] includes 8 functional items and additional items regarding patient satisfaction with their function and ability to perform routine activities, stress, and learned helplessness.[104] The more recent revised version of the HAQ, the HAQ II, is a 10-item questionnaire that has been demonstrated to be more reliable than the HAQ (reliability of 0.88 versus 0.83 for the HAQ).[105] The HAQ II correlated as well or better with clinical and outcome variables than the HAQ and the MHAQ. The Multi-Dimensional Modified HAQ (MDHAQ) combines the MHAQ with information on activity level, pain, fatigue, psychological distress, global status, and medications and is best suited for the clinical environment. The Clinical HAQ (CLINHAQ) is a compilation of instruments, including the HAQ functional disability scale, a VAS (of pain, global disease severity, sleep disturbance, gastrointestinal distress, and fatigue), a pain diagram, and the anxiety and depression scales from AIMS.[106] The HAQ functional disability scale, HAQ II, MHAQ, and CLINHAQ each take about 5 minutes to complete and are most useful in the clinical setting. The HAQ has also been modified for use in patients with specific diseases, including Sc,[107] PA,[108] and AS (HAQ-S),[109] and also for children (CHAQ).[110]

Some other instruments have been designed for measuring functional ability in patients with particular

TABLE 6-1	Standardized Measures for Evaluating Physical Functioning in Patients with Chronic Rheumatic Disorders Using Direct Observation		
Measurement Tool	**Purpose**	**Measurement Method**	**Comments**
Grip strength test	Measurement of hand, wrist, and forearm strength.	Patient squeezes the cuff of a sphygmomanometer inflated to 30 mm Hg as hard as possible. The highest level on the mercury column of 3 attempts is recorded. May also be measured with a Martin Vigorimeter.	Motivation, handedness, pain threshold, and muscle weakness will affect scores, as will involvement of any joint from the elbow to the hand. Grip strength measures have been shown in clinical trials to be sensitive to change in disease activity.
Thumb to index strength test	Hand and finger function.	Measured with a Martin Vigorimeter.	Same as grip strength measurement.
Time to walk 50 feet	Measurement of LE function.	Individual walks 50 feet on a flat surface using any aides or assistive devices. Time is recorded to the nearest 0.1 second.	Motivation can affect performance. Low reliability, insensitive to changes in disease activity.
6-minute walk test	Field test of fitness.	Measures the distance the patient can walk in 6 minutes.	Motivation can affect performance. Low correlation with standard laboratory tests of physical fitness. Sensitive to change in exercise clinical trial in fibromyalgia. Little information available for other disorders.
Jepson Hand Function test, Grip Ability test, Grip Function test, Arthritis Hand Function test	Various measurements of hand function tested in persons with arthritis. Activities tests are based on ADLs.	Specific tasks (e.g., picking up cards, pouring water from a jug, writing) are performed in presence of evaluator.	May be used in clinical trials of specific hand treatments, following hand surgery, and in long-term outcome studies. Some tests require special equipment.
Button test	Measurement of hand function that can be used in clinical practice.	Standard board with 5 buttons. Patients are timed while they unbutton and button using right and left hands separately, with scores from both hands averaged.	Motivation is an important factor. Useful in disorders that affect hand function (e.g., RA).
Timed-Stand test	Measurement of LE function.	Measures number of seconds it takes the patient to stand up and sit down 10 times from a chair using only the LEs.	Motivation, age, and nonmusculoskeletal comorbid conditions may affect scores. Sensitivity to change has not been determined.
Keitel Index	UE and LE extremity function with emphasis on ROM.	Measures performance of 24 standard tasks requiring peripheral and axial joint motion. Performance is evaluated by a trained observer. Takes 10-15 minutes to complete.	Motivation may be a factor. Time and personnel to observe and score tasks are a factor in its use. Scale is sensitive to short-term change.

Adapted from Robbins L, Burckhardt CS, Hannan MT, et al (eds): *Clinical Care in the Rheumatic Diseases*, ed 2, Atlanta, 2001, Association of Rheumatology Health Professionals.
Data from Pincus T, Callahan LF: *J Rheumatol* 19:1051-1057, 1992; Anderson JJ, Felson DT, Meenan RF, et al: *Arthritis Rheum* 32:1093-1099, 1989; Newcomer KL, Krug HE, Mahowald ML: *J Rheumatol* 20:21-27, 1993; Kalla AA, Smith PR, Brown GMM, et al: *Br J Rheumatol* 34:141-149, 1995; Sullivan M, Ahlmen M, Bjelle A, et al: *J Rheumatol* 20:1500-1507, 1993; Walker JM, Helewa A: *Physical Therapy in Arthritis*, Philadelphia, 1996, WB Saunders.
LE, Lower extremity; *ADLs,* activities of daily living; *RA,* rheumatoid arthritis; *UE,* upper extremity; *ROM,* range of motion.

rheumatological diagnoses. The McMaster Toronto Arthritis Patient Preference Disability Questionnaire (MACTAR)[111] is designed to measure limitations in activities, including physical function, self-care, household tasks, work, leisure activity, social roles, and sexuality and ranks the importance of performing these tasks without pain, in patients with arthritis. It is a valid and highly responsive tool but is time consuming and therefore costly to administer because the interviewer has to elicit patient responses and preferences by asking them to describe these limitations.[112] The Western Ontario and McMaster Universities Osteoarthritis Index (WOMAC)[113] is a tool specifically developed for use in patients with osteoarthritis. It has been validated and translated into several languages, focuses on lower extremity mobility and function, and takes about 10 minutes to administer. It correlates strongly with other measures of pain, fatigue, and psychological distress and is appropriate for use in the clinic. With its focus on lower extremity function, this tool is most useful with patients with hip and knee involvement, although it has been used in patients with RA and fibromyalgia.[114]

Indices specifically valid and reliable in patients with spondyloarthropathies include the HAQ-S,[109] the Bath Ankylosing Spondylitis Functional Index (BASFI),[115] and the Dougados Functional Index (DFI). The BASFI has been found to be more responsive than the HAQ-S or the DFI, especially in physical therapy trials since it is more responsive to changes in function.[116,117] One measure designed to specifically to measure hand function in patients with Sc is the Hand Mobility in Scleroderma (HAMIS) test. This measure has been found to be reliable in this population.[118]

A few instruments were specifically developed for assessing the outcome of pediatric patients with connective tissue dysfunctions. These measures are limited by the complexities involved working with children, including variability in developmental roles and tasks and changes in growth and behavior from infants to toddlers to adolescents.[119] The CHAQ is used most often and includes age-appropriate activities.[110] More comprehensive indices include the Juvenile Arthritis Quality of Life Questionnaire[120] and the Childhood Arthritis Health Profile (CAHP),[121] which address not only function but also health quality of life issues such as pain, psychosocial functioning, and areas concerning family, friends and school. The Juvenile Arthritis Functional Assessment Scale (JAFAS) includes 10 activities of daily living that are assessed by a health professional.[122] In children over 7 years of age, this instrument has been useful in differentiating children with JRA from healthy children. The Juvenile Arthritis Functional Assessment Report (JAFAR) is a longer modified version of the JAFAS designed as a self-report instrument with separate versions for proxy reports by parents or self-administration by the child.[123]

EVALUATION, DIAGNOSIS, AND PROGNOSIS

Information from all aspects of the examination, including the patient history, systems review, and tests and measures, are interpreted together by the clinician to derive a treatment diagnosis. Patients falling into the preferred practice pattern 4D: Impaired joint mobility, motor function, muscle performance, and range of motion associated with connective tissue dysfunction, as described in the *Guide to Physical Therapist Practice*,[124] typically have decreased ROM, muscle guarding, or weakness, pain, swelling or effusions, joint instability and some limitation in their ability to perform functional tasks that may require adaptive equipment or assistance from others. According to the *Guide*, 80% of patients in this preferred practice pattern can be expected to demonstrate optimal joint mobility, muscle performance, and ROM and the highest level of functioning in home, work, community, and leisure environments over the course of 2 weeks to 6 months of physical therapy interventions, with 3 to 36 visits. A number of factors, including accessibility and availability of resources, adherence to interventions, age, chronicity and severity of the condition, co-morbidities, level of impairment, decline in functional independence, living environment, overall health status, psychological and socioeconomic factors, and the amount of social support, may require a new episode of care or may modify the frequency of visits or the duration of an episode of care.

INTERVENTION

Interventions for connective tissue dysfunctions are most effective when a multidisciplinary approach that includes patient education for self-management and cognitive behavioral interventions is used in addition to medical and physical interventions. A partnership between the clinician and the patient is also critical, since success depends on ongoing participation and compliance with home exercise programs and an appreciation of the principles of pain management, rest, joint protection, use of adaptive equipment for ambulation and ADLs, energy conservation, and splinting.

This section first discusses the general approach to management of functional limitations related to connective tissue dysfunctions and inflammatory arthritis, including RA, PA, RS, SLE, crystal-induced arthropathies, and Sc, with reference to disease-specific variations. Physical therapy management of the spondyloarthropathies, polymyositis/dermatomyositis, polymyalgia rheumatica, and JRA are discussed subsequently because of differences in the treatment approach for these conditions.

RHEUMATOID ARTHRITIS AND OTHER INFLAMMATORY CONDITIONS

The examination and evaluation provide the foundation for individualizing interventions and therapeutic goals in patients with inflammatory connective tissue dysfunctions. Rehabilitation interventions to reduce pain; increase and maintain joint mobility, muscle strength, and cardiovascular fitness; conserve energy and reduce fatigue; and optimize function should be started early before irreversible joint deformities occur. The interventions employed to accomplish these objectives include patient education, rest (joint protection, energy conservation, and splinting), physical agents, and therapeutic exercise.

Patient Education. Patient education is integral to promoting self-management in inflammatory arthritis. The ACR guidelines for the treatment of rheumatoid arthritis include patient education as a first line of treatment.[125] Quality education for patients with arthritis should foster self-management behaviors to help patients achieve or maintain optimal health status or quality of life.[126] Patient education is most effective when it helps patients incorporate behavioral change into their lifestyles. This can be done through interactive methods that build confidence and improve skills such as decision-making, problem-solving, self-monitoring, and communication with health care providers. This may be done in groups or individually. A meta-analysis of clinical trials on the effects of patient education in patients with arthritis found that educational interventions that included behavioral techniques produced greater changes in pain, functional disability, and tender joints than interventions that relied exclusively on transmitting information.[127] Cognitive behavioral interventions may also decrease health care utilization by promoting patient independence.[128]

Informational educational may also improve outcomes in arthritis. The arthritis education program with the most substantial evidence supporting its effectiveness is the Arthritis Self-Management Program (ASMP) developed at

Stanford University. This arthritis self-help course is taught through the Arthritis Foundation in the United States. A 4-year study demonstrated that participation in this program resulted in a persistent 20% decrease in pain, a 43% reduction in physician visits and an estimated savings of $648 per year per patient with RA.[129] In addition, Scholten et al found in a study with 68 patients with RA that participation in a multidisciplinary patient education program covering disease pathogenesis, drug therapy, exercise, use of joint protection devices, orthopedic perspectives, psychological counseling, dietetics, and information about unproved remedies resulted in sustained better clinical outcomes.[130]

Patient education programs have also been demonstrated to enhance perceived ability to control various aspects of arthritis and to promote self-management techniques.[131] Patients participating in a self-management course on SLE experienced reduced fatigue and depression and improved coping skills and self-efficacy.[132] In a patient education program for children with JRA and their parents, the parents' self-reported competencies on medical, exercise, pain, and social support issues improved significantly, whereas the children showed minimal improvement.[133]

Rest and Joint Protection. Rest is a key component in the management of arthritis and includes both general and joint-specific rest. The management of inflammatory arthritis requires a fine balance between activity and rest. Recommendations for rest may be included as part of the patient education program and specific techniques may be reviewed by an appropriate health professional and practiced by patients to enhance adherence.

Recommendations for general rest during the active phases of inflammatory arthritis are for 8-10 hours of sleep per night with 30-60 minutes of rest during the day. Instruction in energy conservation techniques may help patients with pacing and planning of scheduled rest periods to avoid undue fatigue and joint flares.

Joint-specific rest is recommended for joints with active inflammation to avoid activity-related injuries, provide periods of unloading, and promote function and activity in spite of joint swelling and pain. Joint-specific rest may include activity modification, use of assistive devices or adaptive equipment, and protective or supportive splinting. Some pieces of adaptive equipment can help maintain and promote independence in people with connective tissue dysfunctions. Fig. 6-12 shows practice application of a dressing stick, a reacher, and a long

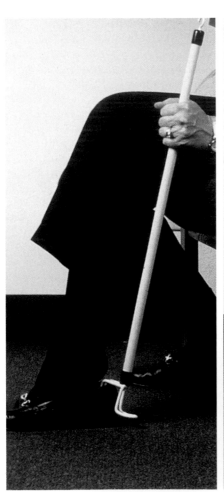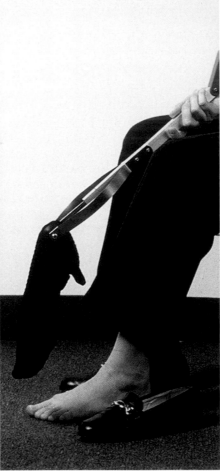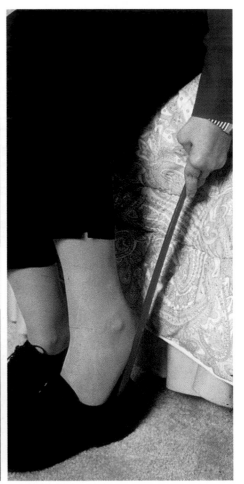

FIG. 6-12 Examples of assistive equipment used in daily activities for individuals with arthritis. *Reprinted from the Clinical Slide Collection on the Rheumatic Diseases, copyright 1997. Used by permission of the American College of Rheumatology.*

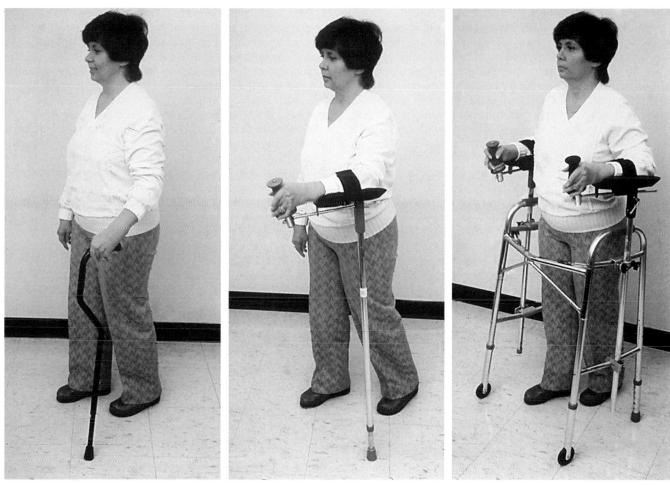

FIG. 6-13 Assistive devices used to aid ambulation in patients with arthritis. *Reprinted from the Clinical Slide Collection on the Rheumatic Diseases, copyright 1997. Used by permission of the American College of Rheumatology.*

handled shoe horn. This type of equipment can make the difference between independence and relying on another person for ADLs.

Various assistive devices (Fig. 6-13), as described in Chapter 33, can be used to aid ambulation. Device selection may be difficult in this population because of systemic disease and involvement of multiple areas including the hands. A platform crutch or walker may be helpful to reduce lower extremity weight bearing and distribute the weight-bearing forces to a large area of the upper extremity. If a platform walker is used, it should have wheels because it will generally be too heavy and awkward to lift.

A systematic review of the literature confirms the effectiveness of instruction in joint protection and energy conservation techniques, introduction to the use of adaptive equipment, and provision of splints for improving functional outcomes in patients with RA.[134] Specifically, 95% of subjects demonstrated increased ADL ability after participating in a 3-week joint protection course for women with RA.[135] Sometimes a simple change in the physical environment, like replacing the tap head of the faucet with a lever tap, can increase independence with household tasks.[136]

Although some studies have found that splinting reduces pain in patients with rheumatoid arthritis,[137] a Cochrane Database review of the literature found insufficient evidence to draw firm conclusions about the effectiveness of wrist splints in decreasing pain or increasing function for persons with RA.[138] Evidence suggests that resting hand and wrist splints do not impact ROM or pain, although patients preferred wearing a resting splint to not wearing one.[138] There is sufficient evidence, however, that extra depth shoes and molded insoles decrease pain in weight-bearing activities such as standing, walking, and stair climbing.[138]

Physical Agents. Electrotherapy modalities and thermotherapy agents are used in patients with arthritis to decrease pain and inflammation, reduce stiffness, and increase mobility. Some studies support the use of thermotherapy, low level laser therapy and transcutaneous electrical nerve stimulation (TENS) in patients with arthritis.[139] In an overview of arthritis-related literature on physical interventions for pain management in arthritis, Minor and Sanford[140] found that physical agents were most effective when combined with exercise.

Heat. Heat has been demonstrated to provide analgesia, promote relaxation, reduce muscle spasm, and enhance flexibility of muscles and periarticular structures. Heat is the most commonly used physical agent in arthritis care by health professionals and patients. Methods of delivering superficial heat include hot packs, warm water, and paraffin baths. There are few published studies on the impact of superficial heat on arthritis management. The majority of the studies have been reported on the use of paraffin alone or paraffin and exercise with RA patients. Studies have revealed short-term pain relief with the use of paraffin alone. However, functional benefits have only been demonstrated when paraffin was combined with exercise.[141] Ultrasound, a form of deep heat, has not been shown to relieve pain or improve motion in patients with arthritis.[142] Only one systematic review exists on the efficacy of therapeutic ultrasound in the management of RA. The review found a significant difference between experimental and control groups on reduced number of painful and swollen joints; however, a combined program of ultrasound and exercise did not have this effect.[143]

The stage of the disease process must be taken into account when selecting thermal modalities for the treatment of inflammatory arthritis. When there is acute inflammation, heat may cause symptom exacerbation.[144] Heat may also increase joint damage by promoting the activity of collagenase and thereby accelerating collagen breakdown.

Cold. Cold has been used to reduce pain, inflammation, and muscle spasm in patients with arthritis. Cold may be applied with cold packs, ice massage, and cold water immersion. In a study on patients with RA of the knee, cold packs applied 3 times daily for 1 month resulted in decreased pain, increased mobility, improved sleep, and decreased use of analgesic medications.[145]

Heat and Cold. There is no evidence that heat or cold alter the immunological processes in inflammatory arthritis; however, both appear to help reduce the pain associated with muscle spasm, fibrosis, and tissue trauma associated with biomechanical stress. In a review of the literature, there was no effect of heat or ice versus control on objective measures of disease activity (joint counts, medication intake, mobility) in RA.[146] A systematic review on the use of ice packs or hot packs in RA also revealed no effect on measures of disease activity, pain, medication intake, ROM, grip force, or hand function when compared with the control group.[147] However, both heat and cold have been shown to improve function and decrease pain when used in conjunction with an exercise program.[148]

Topical Applications. Although iontophoresis and phonophoresis are commonly used in clinical practice to deliver antiinflammatory agents to patients with inflammatory conditions, this practice has not been shown by research to reduce symptoms or improve function in patients with chronic inflammatory arthritis.[140]

Electrotherapy. The research on the use of TENS for inflammatory arthritis primarily focuses on RA affecting the wrist. A systematic review of the literature found that well-designed studies did demonstrate that TENS can reduce pain and improve hand function without adverse effect in patients with RA.[149]

Low Level Laser Therapy. Meta-analyses of trials on low level laser therapy (LLLT) found that LLLT reduced pain and morning stiffness and increased ROM more than placebo interventions in patients with RA.[150,151]

Exercise. Connective tissue dysfunctions result in pain, stiffness, and fatigue, with a concomitant decline in function, because of decreased ROM, muscle strength, and aerobic capacity. Joint immobilization may also lead to weakening of cartilage and periarticular structures, whereas the regular joint motion and intermittent weight bearing that occurs with many forms of exercise may enhance joint health.[152] Despite previous beliefs that exercise may harm individuals with arthritis, current research has found that various forms of exercise can safely help patients with rheumatic disease.[153] People with arthritis can generally follow recommendations for health and fitness applied in the healthy population as depicted in Box 6-4, while adhering to general and joint specific recommendations for pacing and rest. A meta-analysis found that aquatic therapy, stationary cycling, and weight-bearing exercise are safe for patients with RA and improve their flexibility, strength, endurance, function, cardiovascular fitness, and general health without increasing joint symptoms.[154]

BOX 6-4   Recommendations for Health and Fitness in the Apparently Healthy Population

Physical Activity for General Health
Mode: Whole body, repetitive activities
Frequency: On most days of the week
Intensity: Moderate; 55%-70% age-predicted maximal heart rate; RPE 12-13/2-4
Duration: 30 minutes accumulation (3 10-minute bouts)

Exercise Training for Cardiovascular Fitness
Mode: Rhythmic, aerobic exercise
Frequency: 3-5 days/week
Intensity: 70%-85% age-predicted maximal heart rate; RPE 14-16/4-7
Duration: 20-30 minutes continuous

Exercise Training for Muscular Fitness (Strength and Endurance)
Mode: Dynamic, resistance exercise for major muscle groups
Frequency: 2-3 days/week on alternate days
Volume: 8-10 exercises; resistance adequate to induce fatigue after 8-12 repetitions, or 10-15 reps if over 50-60 years of age or frail

Exercise for Musculoskeletal Flexibility
Mode: Gentle stretching; static or PNF technique
Frequency: 2-3 days/week minimum
Duration: Hold position for 10-30 seconds for static; 6-second contraction followed by 10-30 second assisted stretch for PNF
Repetitions: 3-4 repetitions for each stretch

Data from ACSM Guidelines for Exercise Testing and Prescription, ed 6, Philadelphia, 2000, Lippincott Williams & Wilkins.
RPE, Rate of perceived exertion; *PNF,* Proprioceptive neuromuscular facilitation.
RPE scale 6-20 scale/0-10 scale.

Range of Motion Exercise. ROM exercises can alleviate stiffness, increase or maintain joint mobility, and increase the flexibility and elasticity of periarticular structures. Active and active-assisted exercise is recommended in patients with inflammatory arthritis, avoiding over-stretching inflamed tissues. During periods of acute inflammation, joint ROM may be maintained by performing at least one to two repetitions through the full ROM daily.[155] The number of repetitions may be gradually increased as the acute joint symptoms subside and become subacute or chronic. Active ROM exercise in combination with relaxation has also been shown to produce functional gains and pain reduction in patients with RA.[156]

Strengthening Exercise. Loss of muscle strength, endurance, and power in patients with arthritis may be caused by the inflammatory disease process, disuse atrophy, side effects of medications, inhibition due to joint pain and inflammation, and loss of mechanical joint integrity. Studies show that muscle conditioning programs can improve strength, endurance, proprioception, and function without increasing pain or disease activity in patients with RA.[157]

Table 6-2 outlines the purpose and recommendations for isometric and dynamic muscle conditioning exercise for individuals with arthritis. Based on a review of the evidence, Stenström and Minor[158] derived specific strengthening recommendations for patients with RA:

strengthening exercises may be static or dynamic at a load level of 50% to 80% of maximal voluntary contraction, 2-3 times per week. The exercise may be performed against body weight or using resistance training equipment such as weights or elastic bands (Fig. 6-14), with gradual progression in either a supervised clinical environment or at home with professional guidance.

Aerobic Exercise. Many studies suggest that people with arthritis can exercise regularly and vigorously enough to improve cardiovascular fitness and endurance without increasing joint symptoms.[154,159] Evidence-based recommendations for aerobic exercise in RA are as follows: the goal for the intensity level of aerobic exercise should be moderate to hard (60% to 85% of maximum heart rate) and exercise should be performed 3 times weekly for 30-60 minutes.[158] Exercise may be either land-based or performed in an aquatic environment with progressive adjustment in intensity. A summary of the results from the review of the evidence on aerobic and strengthening exercise in RA is shown in Table 6-3.

Aquatic Therapy. Aquatic therapy is physical therapy performed in the water environment and may incorporate mobility exercises, strengthening activities, aerobic conditioning, and functional tasks. Exercise performed in water can reduce pain, probably because of the sensory input from hydrostatic pressure and temperature, muscle relaxation, and reduced joint compression.[178] Aquatic fitness programs have resulted in improved activity level, functional status, mobility, strength, exercise tolerance, and mood in patients with RA (Fig. 6-15).[179,180] Community-based exercise programs like the Arthritis Foundation's Aquatic Program have been found to not only increase ROM and strength but also provide social support and camaraderie.[181]

Exercise and Juvenile Arthritis. Children with JRA have joint pain, swelling, and mobility limitations that lead to reduced physical activity, fitness, and function.[182] Various types of exercise have been shown to result in decreased disease severity and activity,[183] increased mobility,[183] strength,[184] and aerobic fitness,[183] and improved function in children with arthritis. In a review of the literature on exercise and physical activity in children with arthritis, Klepper[185] made the following observations:

1. Children with JRA may participate in either aquatic or land-based exercise programs without disease exacerbation.

TABLE 6-2	Purposes, Recommendations, and Precautions for Isometric and Dynamic Muscle Conditioning Exercise in Patients with Connective Tissue Dysfunction
Isometric	**Dynamic**
PURPOSE	
Minimize atrophy.	Maintain and increase dynamic strength and endurance.
Improve tone.	
Maintain and increase static strength and endurance.	Increase muscle power.
Prepare for dynamic and weight-bearing activity.	Improve function.
	Enhance synovial blood flow.
	Promote strength of bone and cartilage.
RECOMMENDATIONS	
Perform at functional joint angles.	Able to perform 8-10 reps against gravity before increasing resistance.
Breathe normally; do not hold breath.	
Intensity: ≤70% MVC.	Use functional movements.
Duration: 6 seconds.	Modify ACSM guidelines as appropriate.
Frequency: 5-10 reps daily.	
PRECAUTIONS	
Decreased muscle blood flow.	May increase biomechanical stress on unstable or malaligned joint.
May increase intraarticular pressure.	Need for power grip.
May increase blood pressure.	

From Robbins L, Burckhardt CS, Hannan MT, et al (eds): *Clinical Care in the Rheumatic Diseases,* ed 2, Atlanta, 2001, Association of Rheumatology Health Professionals.
reps, Repetitions; *ACSM,* American College of Sports Medicine.

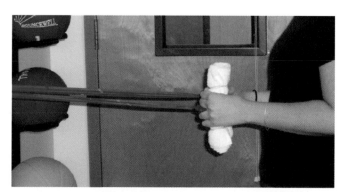

FIG. 6-14 Strengthening exercise with elastic band.

TABLE 6-3   Summary of the Results from 15 Randomized Controlled Studies on Aerobic and Strengthening Exercise in Patients with Connective Tissue Dysfunction

Author, Year	Aerobic Capacity	Muscle Strength	ROM	Performance Tests	Pain	ADL	HRQoL	Disease Activity
Minor et al, 1989[160]	+	0	0	+	0	NR	+	0
Ekdahl et al, 1990[161]	+	+	0	+	0	0	NR	+
Baslund et al, 1993[162]	+	NR	NR	NR	NR	NR	NR	0
Hansen et al, 1993[163]	0	0	NR	0	0	0	NR	0
Hoenig et al, 1993[164]	NR	+	0	+	NR	NR	NR	+
Häkkinen et al, 1994[165]	NR	+	NR	NR	NR	0	NR	0
Lyngberg et al, 1994[166]	0	+	NR	0	0	0	NR	0
Stenström et al, 1996, 1997[167,168]	NR	–	0	0	NR	NR	0	0
van den Ende et al, 1996[169]	+	+	+	0	0	0	0	+
Komatireddy et al, 1997[170]	0	0	NR	+	+	0	0	+
Boström et al, 1998[171]	NR	0	0	NR	0	0	0	0
Häkkinen et al, 1999, 2001[172,173]	NR	+	NR	0	0	+	NR	+
McMeeken J et al, 1999[174]	NR	+	NR	+	+	+	NR	NR
van den Ende et al, 2000[175]	NR	+	0	0	–/0*	0	NR	+
Westby et al, 2000[176]	+	NR	NR	NR	NR	0	NR	0

From Stenström CH, Minor MA: *Arthritis Rheum* 49(3):428-434, 2003.
ROM, Range of motion; *ADL,* activities of daily living; *HRQoL,* health-related quality of life; +, improvement; 0, no change; *NR,* not reported; –, deterioration compared with control/comparison groups.
*Pain increased temporarily during the first phase but did not differ from controls at later assessments.

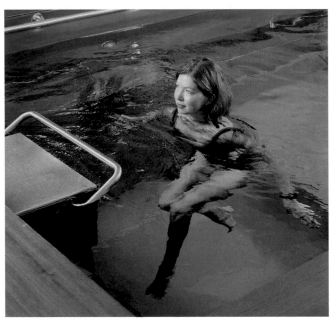

FIG. 6-15 Aquatic exercise.

2. Participation in an aquatic or land-based exercise program twice a week for 6 weeks may reduce disease activity and improve exercise endurance.
3. Studies suggest that exercise on land may promote greater gains in strength and function than aquatic exercise programs.
4. Weight-bearing exercise is necessary for developing adequate bone growth and bone density in children.
5. Individualized and supervised strengthening exercise appears to be safe and effective in children as young as 8 years of age.

6. Individualized exercise may be more appropriate for children with severe disease, whereas children with mild to moderate disease may benefit from group exercise programs.
7. Children with mild disease should be able to participate in most sport with proper screening and physical conditioning. However, highly competitive contact sports should be avoided during active disease.

SPONDYLOARTHROPATHIES

Dagfinrud[186] and van der Linden[187] report positive results from physical therapy interventions for patients with AS, although there is insufficient evidence to indicate that specific interventions are beneficial. More research is needed to determine the effectiveness of particular exercises and physical therapy techniques. A few studies on AS document statistically significant improvements in physical parameters, including cervical and thoracolumbar ROM, vital capacity, straight leg raise, and fitness levels with a reduction in pain and stiffness, but these were completed in an inpatient setting where intensive daily treatment was applied for 3-4 weeks.[188] For example, van Tubergen[189] evaluated the effects of a combined spa and exercise regime, including lying supine, group physical exercise, hydrotherapy, walking, sports, and a visit to a spa in Austria or the Netherlands. This comprehensive approach is rare and almost impossible to replicate in the typical outpatient setting today where treatment is given a few times per week.[190]

The few published studies on interventions for patients with AS do, however, give some direction for intervention. They note that exercise needs to be ongoing to maintain improvements and that more disabled patients are generally more motivated to exercise.[191] Interventions that promote self-management significantly improve self-efficacy and self-reported levels of exercise and function.[192] Group exercise also more effectively improves pain, stiffness, thoracolumbar mobility, fitness, and global health scores than individual treatment sessions.[193] Hydrotherapy may also be used safely, although patients with AS may feel a sensation of chest pressure when immersed in chest-deep water.[194]

In the clinical setting, based on the limited available evidence and typical findings in the patient examination, the following interventions are recommended for patients with spondyloarthropathies. The focus of treatment is postural reeducation because these diagnoses primarily affect the spine. In AS, the inflammatory process progresses from the sacroiliac joint superiorly throughout the spine producing a fused spine, so it is critical to keep the spine erect to minimize fusion in flexion. Flexibility exercises for the spine, hips, and shoulders should be emphasized to prevent a forward flexed posture and maintain the ability to reach overhead. With thoracic spine involvement the rib cage is also affected, so breathing exercises are recommended to optimize expansion with inhalation and exhalation movements. To maintain upright posture, the anterior axial structures, especially the pectoral and hip flexor muscles should be stretched and the posterior spinal extensors, specifically the scapular and hip extensor muscles, should be strengthened. Abdominal muscle strengthening may also help support the spine and improve posture.

POLYMYALGIA RHEUMATICA

Currently there is no published research evaluating the effects of physical therapy interventions on patients with PMR. The interventions recommended are those thought to lessen the impairments and functional limitations typically found during the examination. Since proximal weakness is the most significant clinical finding in PMR, the focus of treatment is strengthening exercises for the hip and shoulder girdle muscles. Depending on the duration of symptoms and flexibility limitations, ROM activities for the hips and shoulders may also be indicated. When shoulder ROM is limited, patients often complain of shoulder pain and difficulty in functional tasks that require reaching overhead or behind, such as washing and dressing. Systemic corticosteroids, which are frequently given to treat symptoms of PMR, do not always resolve joint restrictions even though they generally relieve pain and stiffness. Soft tissue and joint mobilization may improve ROM and function in such circumstances.

Postural reeducation is usually also recommended for patients with PMR. These patients are often older women with a forward flexed posture at baseline before their diagnosis. Stretching anterior structures, especially the pectoral muscles, and strengthening the hip, spinal extensors, and abdominal muscles can reduce trunk weakness and provide a more effective base of support and foundation for extremity motion. This can improve independence with functional activities. Proprioceptive neuromuscular facilitation (PNF) techniques may also be used to improve trunk stability and extremity strength. Aquatic therapy can safely be used to increase endurance, reduce fatigue and strengthen the trunk and extremities.

POLYMYOSITIS AND DERMATOMYOSITIS

Historically, exercise was considered contraindicated for patients with myositis, especially in the acute stages, because it was thought that this would cause more muscle damage and increase muscle enzyme levels, potentially damaging the kidneys. However, it has been shown that although creatinine phosphokinase (CPK), the primary product of skeletal muscle breakdown, levels do rise in patients with PM during isometric exercise, the CPK levels fall rapidly after the exercise ceases.[195] Furthermore, a number of studies demonstrate that exercise is safe in patients with myositis and results in increased strength, respiratory function, and aerobic capacity, as well as improved well-being and function, without significantly elevating muscle enzyme levels.[196-199] Most studies demonstrating a benefit of exercise only lasted for 2-12 weeks[195,196,198,200]; however, one long-term study over 6 months demonstrated significant improvements in ADLs, peak isometric torque of lower extremity muscle groups, and a statistically significant increase in VO_2 max without changing CPK levels.[199] A case study of a single individual who participated in a year-long exercise program had similar findings, suggesting that the benefits of exercise in this population can persist over time. Given this evidence, it is recommended that patients with myositis participate in vigorous strengthening and conditioning programs to address their functional deficits. Exercise programs based on PNF techniques, weight lifting, and other land-based conditioning activities, as well as aquatic exercises, have been shown to help individuals with myositis regain independence with functional tasks.[197,199]

SCLERODERMA

Because Sc tends to tighten the soft tissues and thus reduce joint ROM and soft tissue flexibility, interventions intended to maintain joint ROM and soft tissue flexibility are often used. Two areas to focus on are the face, especially around the mouth for activities like eating and brushing teeth, and the fingers to maintain the ability to perform fine motor skills and ADLs. There are few published studies in this area and no randomized controlled trials; however, a recent study in 10 subjects with Sc found that mouth opening significantly improved and that eating, speaking, and oral hygiene measures became easier after an 18-week exercise program of mouth stretching and oral augmentation exercises.[201] A much earlier study in 9 patients with Sc demonstrated increased mouth opening after 6 months of mouth stretching and oral augmentation exercises.[202] Most recently, Sandqvist and colleagues[203] found that the use of paraffin significantly improved finger, thumb, and wrist flexibility and perceived stiffness and skin elasticity in patients with Sc. These studies suggest that stretching activities and the use of paraffin can improve ROM and function in patients with Sc, although it is probable that this benefit will be short-lived since this is a progressive disease.

CASE STUDY 6-1

RHEUMATOID ARTHRITIS

Examination

Patient History

CH is a 52-year-old woman who presents with pain and mobility limitations at the shoulders, wrists, MCPs/PIPs, knees, ankles, and feet. She was diagnosed with RA 3 years earlier after experiencing peripheral joint symptoms for 10 years. She was quite active before diagnosis but now reports a significant loss of function. She finds dressing and grooming activities, meal preparation, and housework difficult. Her walking is limited to one block by pain at her ankles and feet, and she climbs stairs nonreciprocally. CH's sleep is disturbed by shoulder and foot pain, and she reports feeling stiff for $1\frac{1}{2}$ hours in the morning. She also suffers from fatigue and a general feeling of being unwell. Her medications for arthritis are methotrexate and acetaminophen, which she has been taking for 1 month. Her goals are to decrease pain, improve function, and prevent the progression of arthritis.

Systems Review

Skin has no apparent abnormalities or compromise of skin integrity.

Tests and Measures

Musculoskeletal

Anthropometric Characteristics CH has swan-neck deformities at the left ring and small fingers and a Boutonnière deformity at the right small finger. Her MCP joints and ankles are swollen bilaterally. CH has bilateral calcaneal valgus positioning and bilateral forefoot pronation.

Range of Motion CH has mobility limitations at the shoulders, elbows, wrists, right knee, and ankles as shown in Table 6-4.

Strength CH's grip strength measured with a sphygmomanometer was 100 mm Hg on the left and 110 mm Hg on the right.

Neuromuscular

Arousal, attention, cognition	Alert
Pain	7/10
Peripheral nerve integrity	Reflexes and sensation are intact.

Function

Gait, Locomotion, and Balance CH has an antalgic gait pattern with decreased step length, decreased cadence, limited push off at terminal stance, and accentuated pronation at midstance. Walk time for 50 feet was 35 seconds. In 1 minute she walked 105 feet, compared with an age-adjusted average of approximately 194 feet.

Self-Care and Home Management CH has difficulty with dressing (buttons, shoes, socks), sit to stand transfers, and negotiating stairs. She can button 5 buttons in 1 minute.

Evaluation, Diagnosis, and Prognosis

CH presents with aggressive RA that was not medically managed over the first 7 years of symptom presentation. She now has deformities and decreased ROM in multiple joints bilaterally. These impairments have resulted in profound functional limitations.

Goals

1. Decrease morning stiffness to less than 1 hour.
2. Increase number of buttons on timed test by 2.
3. Increase shoulder ROM by 10 degrees in all planes.
4. Decrease flexion contractures at elbows by 10 degrees or greater.
5. Decrease time on the 50-foot walk test to 30 seconds.
6. Increase walking tolerance to $\frac{1}{2}$ mile.
7. Patient to sleep through the night without being awakened by joint pain.
8. Increase grip strength force by 5 mm Hg.
9. Patient to be independent with a home exercise program (HEP).

Diagnosis

CH falls into the preferred practice pattern 4D: Impaired joint mobility, motor function, muscle performance, and ROM associated with connective tissue dysfunction.

Prognosis

It is expected that CH's symptoms may improve over the next few months because she started taking methotrexate 1 month ago. She has already noted a reduction in joint pain and fatigue. Her prognosis for achieving the set goals is fair to good.

Plan of Care

CH is to be seen 2 times per week for 6-8 weeks, including a comprehensive approach to management focused on patient education, joint protection, and exercise.

Interventions

CH is to be educated about the disease, the role of medications, and the components of self-management. She should have instruction in joint protection and energy conservation techniques with introduction to adaptive

TABLE 6-4	Range of Motion for Patient in Case Study 6-1		
Joint	**AROM**	**Left**	**Right**
Shoulder	Flexion	100°	124°
	Abduction	65°	70°
	Internal rotation	60°	63°
	External rotation	58°	62°
Elbows	Flexion	138°	138°
	Extension	−30°	−18°
Wrists	Flexion	40°	26°
	Extension	38°	24°
Knees	Flexion	125°	118°
	Extension	0°	3°
Ankles	Dorsiflexion	0°	5°
	Plantarflexion	40°	40°

equipment and practice within relevant contexts. She will be fitted with daytime functional splints for swan-neck deformities and boutonnière deformities and resting splints fabricated for night time use.

Exercise

CH was instructed in a HEP, including ROM, strengthening, and aerobic conditioning exercise. ROM exercises were to be performed daily (1-10 repetitions [reps]) for all joints. Strengthening exercises were progressed from isometrics to elastic band–resisted exercises for upper and lower extremities (2-3 times per week, 2 sets of 10 reps per exercise). Aerobic conditioning was progressed to 30 minutes of cumulative exercise to be performed 4-5 times per week, including a combination of stationary cycling, walking, and suspended exercise in the water, as well as instruction in an aquatic therapy program to be performed in a community setting. The aquatic program could be done independently or through the Arthritis Foundation at the YMCA.

Orthotics

Custom foot orthotics to accommodate existing foot deformities and provide enhanced arch support were fabricated. Foot wear recommendations were made for supportive shoes with good arch support, good heel cushion, and a wide toe box.

Outcomes

CH responded well to the interventions. She was compliant with all aspects of her home program, and she achieved all of the set goals over the course of 6 weeks. She was able to perform her dressing activities, meal preparation, and work activities (engraving) with decreased difficulty. She was able to take short walks (15 minutes) and had enough energy to participate in social activities such as going out to dinner and movies.

   Please see the CD that accompanies this book for case studies describing the examination, evaluation and interventions for patients with SLE and AS.

CHAPTER SUMMARY

Connective tissue dysfunctions primarily result from rheumatic diseases with various pathologies and generally autoimmune or unknown etiologies. A thorough understanding of these conditions and the effectiveness of different interventions assists the clinician in selecting appropriate, individualized interventions specific to patient needs. Since these diseases are generally chronic and progressive, patients may need frequent reexamination and modification of their home program and other interventions. Visits may need to be scheduled judiciously to accommodate restrictions in the patient's health care coverage.

   Patients should be educated about their disease and instructed in activity modification, the use and benefits of adaptive equipment, joint protection, pacing, and the importance of learning to manage their disease. Interventions should emphasize enhancing function to promote independence while also managing pain. Exercise is one of the most effective interventions for people with connective tissue disorders, since increasing muscular strength to support the joints improves biomechanical efficiency and reduces pain and fatigue. Exercise can be performed at home, in a community-based setting, or in the aquatic environment. Outcome measures will help determine which interventions are most effective and enable health care providers to achieve the goal of improving the quality of life for patients with connective tissue disorders.

ADDITIONAL RESOURCES

Useful Forms

Health Assessment Questionnaire: www.aramis.stanford.edu/ HAQ.html
Evaluation Form

Books

Banwell BF, Gall V (eds): *Clinics in Physical Therapy: Physical Therapy Management of Arthritis,* New York, 1988, Churchill Livingstone.
Kelley W, Harris ED, Ruddy S, Sledge CB (eds): *Textbook of Rheumatology,* ed 4, 1993, Philadelphia, WB Saunders.
Klippel JH, Crofford LJ, Stone JH, et al (eds): *Primer on the Rheumatic Diseases,* ed 12, Atlanta, 2001, Arthritis Foundation.
Klippel JH, Dieppe PA (eds): *Rheumatology,* ed 2, Philadelphia, 1998, Mosby.
Melvin JL: *Rheumatic Disease in the Adult and Child: Occupational Therapy and Rehabilitation,* ed 3, Philadelphia, 1989, FA Davis.
Melvin JL, Jensen GM (eds): *Rheumatologic Rehabilitation Series, vol 1. Assessment and Management,* Bethesda, Md, 1998, The American Occupational Therapy Association.
Robbins L, Burckhardt CS, Hannan MT, et al (eds): *Clinical Care in the Rheumatic Diseases,* ed 2, Atlanta, 2001, Association of Rheumatology Health Professionals.
Walker JM, Helewa A: *Physical Therapy in Arthritis,* Philadelphia, 1996, WB Saunders.

Web Sites

American College of Rheumatology (ACR) and Association of Rheumatology Health Professionals (ARHP): www.rheumatology.org
American Juvenile Arthritis Organization (Council of the Arthritis Foundation): www.arthritis.org/communities/about_ajao.asp
Arthritis Foundation: www.arthritis.org
The Arthritis Society (Canada): www.arthritis.ca
Lupus Foundation of America, Inc.: www.fmpartnership.org
National Institute of Arthritis and Musculoskeletal and Skin Diseases: www.nih.gov/niams
National Psoriasis Foundation: www.psoriasis.org
Scleroderma Foundation: www.scleroderma.org
Sjögren's Syndrome Foundation: www.sjogren's.org
Spondylitis Association of America: www.spondylitis.org

Videos

PACE—People with Arthritis Can Exercise Level I and II: Available through the Arthritis Foundation: www.arthritis.org/afstore/storehome.asp
Yoga for Arthritis: Pathways to Better Living with Arthritis and Related Conditions
Videos for students and practitioners: www.mobilityltd.com
Water Workout: www.spondylitis.org/materials/video.aspx
Back In Action: Available through the Spondylitis Association: www.spondylitis.org/materials/video.aspx
Tai Chi for Arthritis: www.taichiproductions.com/shop/product.php?product=8

Good Moves For Every Body and Good Moves 2: www.muhealth.org/
~shrp/goodmove/video.html
ROM Dance videotapes: www.taichihealth.com/catalog/
default.php?cPath=22
Pool Exercise Program (PEP): Available through the Arthritis
Foundation

GLOSSARY

Ankylosing spondylitis (AS): A form of inflammatory arthritis that has a predilection for the sacroiliac joints, axial spine, and ligamentous/tendinous insertions.

Arteritis: Inflammation of the arteries.

Arthralgias: Joint pain.

Arthritis: Encompasses over 100 types of rheumatic diseases but literal translation means inflammation of the joint.

Avascular necrosis: Necrosis of bone due to ischemia.

Baker's cyst: A cystic swelling within the popliteal space posterior to the knee as a result of mechanical irritation or synovial inflammation.

Boutonnière deformity: A finger deformity with flexion at the PIP joint and hyperextension at the DIP joint.

Bursitis: Inflammation at the bursa, which may be due to trauma, frictional forces, or rheumatic disease.

Crepitus: Grating, grinding, or popping sensations/sounds that occurs with movement of a joint.

Cytokines: Proteins secreted by a variety of cells to help regulate immunological responses (e.g., interleukin, tumor necrosis factor, lymphokines, and interferon).

Dactylitis: Inflammation of a finger or toe.

Dermatomyositis (DM): Diffuse inflammatory disease of striated muscle that leads to symmetric proximal muscle weakness with a dermatological component.

Discoid lupus: A form of lupus that involves skin disease with distinctive erythematous scaly plaques.

Effusion: Excess fluid in the joint resulting from joint irritation or inflammation of the synovium.

Enthesitis: Inflammation where ligaments and tendons attach to bone.

Gout: A disease characterized by acute episode of arthritis resulting from the deposition of uric acid crystals at the joint or in surrounding tissues.

HLA-B27: A genetically determined antigen associated with ankylosing spondylitis.

Hyperuricemia: Abnormal amount of uric acid in the blood.

Immunosuppressive drugs: Substances that suppress or interfere with the normal immune response.

Inflammatory arthritis: Systemic arthritis that involves inflammation of the synovium of the joint.

Interleukin-1 (IL-1): Substance from monocytes and macrophages important in the acute phase response.

Leukopenia: Abnormal decrease in white blood cells.

Livedo reticularis: A semipermanent bluish mottling of the skin of the legs and hands.

Lupus: A chronic inflammatory autoimmune disease that may affect the skin, joints, and internal organs.

Mauskopf: Loss of facial expression due to tightening/tautness of the skin resulting from scleroderma.

Myositis: Inflammatory disease of striated muscle.

Nephritis: Inflammation of the kidney.

Pannus: Excessive proliferation of synovial and granulation tissue that invades joint surfaces.

Panniculitis: Inflamed condition of a layer of fatty connective tissue in the anterior wall of the abdomen.

Pauciarticular: Involvement of few joints.

Pericarditis: Inflammation of the pericardium.

Pleurisy: Inflammation of the pleura.

Polymyalgia rheumatica (PMR): Condition characterized by stiffness and pain at the shoulder girdle without weakness; usually seen in women over 50 years of age in conjunction with an elevated ESR.

Polymyositis (PM): Diffuse inflammatory disease of striated muscle that leads to symmetric proximal muscle weakness.

Proteinuria: Protein in the urine.

Pseudogout: Synovitis due to the deposition of calcium pyrophosphate dehydrate crystals resulting in arthritis; articular chondrocalcinosis.

Psoriatic arthritis (PA): A spondyloarthropathy with concomitant psoriasis.

Purpura: Condition characterized by hemorrhage into the skin.

Raynaud's phenomenon: An intermittent vasoconstriction of the distal small arteries, arterioles and capillaries that results in blanching, erythema, and cyanosis of the hands.

Reactive arthritis: Spondyloarthropathy with enteric or venereal infectious trigger.

Reiter's syndrome (RS): Triad of arthritis, conjunctivitis and urethritis.

Rheumatoid arthritis (RA): Systemic disease characterized by inflammation of the joint synovium.

Rheumatoid factor: An immunoglobulin found in the serum of 50% to 95% of adults with rheumatoid arthritis.

Schober's test: A measurement of spinal mobility in patients with spondyloarthropathy.

Sclerodactyly: Sclerosis and tapering of the fingers in progressive systemic sclerosis.

Scleroderma (Sc): A chronic disease of unknown etiology that causes sclerosis of the skin and organs (GI tract, heart, lungs, and kidneys) and arthritis.

Sjögren's syndrome (SS): Disease of the lacrimal and parotid glands resulting in dry eyes and mouth; frequently occurs with RA, SLE, and SS.

Spondyloarthropathy: Inflammation of the spine and sacroiliac joints. Describes a category of diseases including ankylosing spondylitis, reactive arthritis/Reiter's syndrome, psoriatic arthritis and all may include an inflammatory bowel disease as well.

Synovitis: Inflammation of the synovium.

Systemic lupus erythematosus (SLE): Systemic inflammatory disease characterized by small vessel vasculitis and a diverse clinical presentation.

Systemic sclerosis (SSc): A chronic disease of unknown etiology that causes sclerosis of the skin and organs (GI tract, heart, lungs, and kidneys) and arthritis.

Tenosynovitis: Inflammation of the synovial lining of the tendon sheaths.

Tophi: Deposits of uric acid crystals around the joints.

Uveitis: Inflammation of the iris, ciliary body and choroids, or the entire uvea.

Vasculitis: Inflammation of the blood or lymph vessels.

Xerostomia: Dry mouth.

Xerophthalmia: Dry eyes.

References

1. Yelin E, Callahan LF: The economic cost and social and psychological impact of musculoskeletal conditions, *Arthritis Rheum* 38:1351-1362, 1995.
2. Lawrence RC, Helmick CG, Arnett FC, et al: Estimates of the prevalence of arthritis and selected musculoskeletal disorders in the United States, *Arthritis Rheum* 41:778-799, 1998.
3. Centers for Disease Control and Prevention: Arthritis prevalence and activity limitations—United States, *MMWR* 43:433-438, 1990.
4. Vliet Vlieland TP: Multidisciplinary team care and outcomes in RA, *Curr Opin Rheumatol* 16(2):153-156, 2004.
5. Maravic M, Bozonnat MC, Sevezan A, et al: Preliminary evaluation of medical outcomes (including quality of life) and costs in incident RA cases receiving hospital-based multidisciplinary management, *Joint Bone Spine* 67(5):425-33, 2000.
6. Gall V: Patient evaluation. In Banwell BF, Gall V (eds): *Clinics in Physical Therapy: Physical Therapy Management of Arthritis*, New York, 1988, Churchill Livingstone.
7. Clark BM: Physical therapy and occupational therapy in the management of arthritis, *CMAJ* 163 (8):999-1005, 2000.
8. Winchester RJ, Nunoz-Roldon A: Some genetic aspects of systemic lupus erythematosus. *Arthritis Rheum* 25:833, 1982.
9. Ballou SP, Kahn M, Kusher A: Clinical features of systemic lupus erythematosus. Differences related to race and age of onset, *Arthritis Rheum* 25:55,1982.
10. Manson JJ, Isenberg DA: The pathogenesis of systemic lupus erythematosus, *Neth J Med* 61(11):343-346, 2003.

11. Atzeni F, Marrazza M, Sarzi-Puttini P, et al: Drug-induced lupus erythematosus, *Reumatismo* 147-154, 2003.
12. Wallace D: *The Lupus Book*, Oxford, 2000, Oxford University Press.
13. Jimenez AJ, Sabio JM, Perez AF, et al: Hair dye treatment use and clinical causes in patients with systemic lupus erythematosus and cutaneous lupus, *Lupus* 11(7):430-434, 2002.
14. Schur P: Clinical features of SLE. In Kelley WN, Sledge CB, Harris ED, et al (eds): *Textbook of Rheumatology*, ed 4, Philadelphia, 1993, WB Saunders.
15. Merrill JR, Dinu AT, Lahita RG: Autoimmunity: The female connection, *Med Gen Med* 1(1), 1999.
16. Stevens MB: Musculoskeletal manifestations. In Schur PH (ed): *The Clinical Management of Systemic Lupus Erythematosus*, Orlando, Fl, 1983, Grune and Stratton.
17. Buyon J: Systemic lupus erythematosus: Clinical and laboratory features. In Klippel JH, Crofford LJ, Stone JH (eds): *Primer on the Rheumatic Diseases*, ed 12, Atlanta, 2001, Arthritis Foundation.
18. Stastny P: Association of the B-cell alloantigen DRw4 with rheumatoid arthritis, *N Engl J Med* 298:869-871, 1978.
19. Silman AJ, MacGregor AJ, Thomson W, et al: Twin concordance rates for rheumatoid arthritis: results from a nationwide study, *Br J Rheumatol* 32:903-907, 1993.
20. Arend WP, Dayer JM: Inhibition of the production and effects of interleukin–I and tumor necrosis factor alpha in rheumatoid arthritis, *Arthritis Rheum* 38:151-160, 1995.
21. Goronzy JJ, Weyand CM: Rheumatoid arthritis: Epidemiology, pathology, and pathogenesis. In Klippel JH, Crofford LJ, Stone JH, et al (eds): *Primer on the Rheumatic Diseases*, ed 12, Atlanta, 2001, Arthritis Foundation.
22. Anderson RJ: Rheumatoid arthritis: Clinical and laboratory features. In Klippel JH, Crofford LJ, Stone JH, et al (eds): *Primer on the Rheumatic Diseases*, ed 12, Atlanta, 2001, Arthritis Foundation.
23. Hastings DE, Evans JA: Rheumatoid wrist deformities and their relation to ulnar drift, *J Bone Joint Surg Am* 57:930, 1975.
24. Inglis AE: Rheumatoid arthritis in the hand, *Am J Surg* 109:368,1965.
25. Sweazey RL, Fiegenberg, DS: Inappropriate intrinsic muscle action in the rheumatoid hand, *Ann Rheum Dis* 30:619, 1972.
26. DeSmet A, Ting YM, Weiss JJ: Shoulder arthrography in rheumatoid arthritis, *Diagn Radiol* 116:601, 1975.
27. Thomas WH: Surgical management of the rheumatoid cervical spine, *Orthop Clin North Am* 6(3):793, 1975.
28. Lipson SJ: Rheumatoid arthritis of the cervical spine, *Clin Orthop Rel Res* 182:143 149, 1984.
29. Dougados M, van der Linden S, Juhlin R, et al: The European Spondyloarthropathy Study Group preliminary criteria for the classification of spondyloarthropathy, *Arthritis Rheum* 34:1218 1227, 1991.
30. Keat ACS, Arnett FC: Spondyloarthropathies: Introduction. In Klippel JH, Dieppe PA (eds): *Rheumatology*, ed 2, vol 2, Philadelphia, 1998, Mosby.
31. Russell AS: Spondyloarthropathy: Ankylosing spondylitis. In Klippel JH, Dieppe PA (eds): *Rheumatology*, ed 2, vol 2, Philadelphia, 1998, Mosby.
32. Khan MA: Spondyloarthropathies: Ankylosing spondylitis. In Klippel JH, Dieppe PA (eds): *Rheumatology*, ed 2, vol 2, Philadelphia, 1998, Mosby.
33. Helewa A, Stokes B: Spondyloarthropathies. In Robbins L, Burckhardt CS, Hannan MT, et al (eds): *Clinical Care in the Rheumatic Diseases*, ed 2, Atlanta, 2001, Association of Rheumatology Health Professionals.
34. Reveille JD: Seronegative spondyloarthropathies: Epidemiology, pathology, and pathogenesis. In Klippel JH, Crofford LJ, Stone JH (eds): *Primer on the Rheumatic Diseases*, ed 12, Atlanta, 2001, Arthritis Foundation.
35. van der Linden S, Valkenburg HA, Cats A: Evaluation of diagnostic criteria for ankylosing spondylitis. A proposal for modification of the New York criteria, *Arthritis Rheum* 27:361-368, 1984.
36. Goei The HS, Steven MM, van der Linden SM, et al. Evaluation of diagnostic criteria for ankylosing spondylitis: A comparison of the Rome, New York and modified New York criteria in patients with a positive clinical history screening test for ankylosing spondylitis, *Br J Rheumatol* 24:242-249, 1985.
37. Blackburn WD Jr, Alarcon JS, Ball JV: Evaluation of patients with back pain of suspected inflammatory nature, *Am J Med* 85:766-770, 1998.
38. Willkens RF, Arnett FC, Bitter T, et al: Reiter's syndrome: Evaluation of preliminary criteria for definite disease, *Arthritis Rheum* 24:844-849, 1981.
39. Simon DG, Kaslow RA, Rosenbaum J, et al: Reiter's syndrome following epidemic shigellosis, *J Rheumatol* 8:969-973, 1981.
40. Leirisalo M, Skylv G, Kousa M, et al: Follow-up study on patients with reactive arthritis with special reference to HLA-B27, *Arthritis Rheum* 25:249-289, 1982.
41. Veale D, Rogers S, Fitzgerald O: Classification of clinical subsets in psoriatic arthritis, *Br J Rheumatol* 33:133-138, 1994.
42. Breathnach SM: Spondyloarthropathies: Psoriatic arthritis: Etiology and pathogenesis. In Klippel JH, Dieppe PA (eds): *Rheumatology*, ed 2, vol 2, Philadelphia, 1998, Mosby.
43. Hazleman BL: The vasculitides: Polymyalgia rheumatica and giant cell arteritis. In Klippel JH, Dieppe PA (eds): *Rheumatology*, ed 2, vol 2, Philadelphia, 1998, Mosby.
44. Paget SA: Polymyalgia rheumatica. In Robbins L, Burckhardt CS, Hannan MT, et al (eds): *Clinical Care in the Rheumatic Diseases*, ed 2, Atlanta, 2001, Association of Rheumatology Health Professionals.
45. Weyand CM, Goronzy, JJ: Vasculitides: Giant cell arteritis, polymyalgia rheumatica and Takayasu's arteritis. In Klippel JH, Crofford LJ, Stone JH (eds): *Primer on the Rheumatic Diseases*, ed 12, Atlanta, 2001, Arthritis Foundation.
46. Wortmann RL: Inflammatory and metabolic diseases of muscle. In Klippel JH, Crofford LJ, Stone JH (eds): *Primer on the Rheumatic Diseases*, ed 12, Atlanta, 2001, Arthritis Foundation.
47. Tanimoto K, Nakano K, Kano S, et al: Classification criteria for polymyositis and dermatomyositis, *J Rheumatol* 22:668-674, 1995.
48. Targoff IN, Miller FW, Medsger TA Jr, et al: Classification criteria for idiopathic inflammatory myopathies, *Curr Opin Rheumatol* 9:527-535, 1997.
49. Medsger TA, Oddis CV: Inflammatory muscle disease: Clinical features. In Klippel JH, Dieppe PA (eds): *Rheumatology*, ed 2, vol 2, Philadelphia, 1998, Mosby.
50. Bohan A, Peter JB: Polymyositis and dermatomyositis, *N Engl J Med* 292:344-347, 1975.
51. Buchbinder R, Forbes A, Hall S, et al: Incidence of malignant disease in biopsy proven inflammatory myopathy, *Ann Intern Med* 134(12):1087-1095, 2001.
52. Leandro MJ, Isenberg DA: Rheumatic diseases and malignancy—is there an association? *Scand J Rheumatol* 30(4):185-188, 2001.
53. White B: Systemic sclerosis and related syndromes: A. Epidemiology, pathology, and pathogenesis. In Klippel JH, Crofford LJ, Stone JH, et al (eds): *Primer on the Rheumatic Diseases*, ed 12, Atlanta, 2001, Arthritis Foundation.
54. LeRoy EC, Black C, Fleischmajer R, et al: Scleroderma (systemic sclerosis): Classification, subsets and pathogenesis, *J Rheumatol* 15:202-205, 1988.
55. Wigley FM: Systemic sclerosis: Clinical features. In Klippel JH, Crofford LJ, Stone JH, et al (eds): *Primer on the Rheumatic Diseases*, ed 12, Atlanta, 2001, Arthritis Foundation.
56. Laing TJ, Schottenfeld D, Lacey JV Jr, et al: Potential risk factors for undifferentiated connective tissue disease among women: Implanted medical devices, *Am J Epidemiol* 154(7):610-617, 2001.
57. Nietert PJ, Silver RM: Systemic sclerosis: Environmental and occupational risk factors, *Curr Opin Rheumatol* 12(6):520-526, 2000.
58. Garabrant DH, Lacey JV Jr, Laing TJ, et al: Scleroderma and solvent exposure among women, *Am J Epidemiol* 157(6):493-500, 2003.
59. Povey A, Guppy MJ, Wood M, et al: Cytochrome P2 polymorphisms and susceptibility to scleroderma following exposure to organic solvents, *Arthritis Rheum* 44(3):662-665, 2001 Mar.
60. Czirjak L: Exposure to solvents in female patients with scleroderma, *Clin Rheum* 21(2):114-118, 2002.
61. Kono T, Ishii M, Negoror N, et al: Scleroderma-like reaction induced by uracil-tegafur (UFT), a second generation anticancer agent, *J Am Acad Dermatol* 42(3):519-520, 2000.
62. Yamamoto T, Nishioka K: Analysis of the effect of halofuginone on bleomycin-induced scleroderma, *Rheumatology* (Oxford) 41(5):594-596, 2002.
63. Subcommittee for Scleroderma Criteria of the American Rheumatism Association Diagnostic and Therapeutic Criteria Committee: Preliminary criteria for classification of system sclerosis (scleroderma), *Arthritis Rheum* 23:581-590, 1980.
64. Prescott RJ, Freemont AJ, Jones CJP, et al: Sequential dermal microvascular and perivascular changes in the development of scleroderma, *J Pathol* 166:255-263, 1992.
65. Wigley FM, Wise RA, Miller R, et al: Anticentromere antibody as a predictor of digital ischemic loss in patients with systemic sclerosis, *Arthritis Rheum* 35:688-693, 1992.
66. Fox RI, Saito I: Criteria for diagnosis of Sjögren's syndrome, *Rheum Dis Clin North Am* 20:391-407, 1994.
67. Fox RI, Maruyama T: Pathogenesis and treatment of Sjögren's syndrome, *Curr Opin Rheumatol* 9:393-399, 1997.
68. Edwards NL: Gout: Clinical and laboratory features. In Klippel JH, Crofford LJ, Stone JH, et al (eds): *Primer on the Rheumatic Diseases*, ed 12, Atlanta, 2001, Arthritis Foundation.
69. Kelley W, Schumacher HR: Gout. In Klippel JH, Crofford LJ, Stone JH, et al (eds): *Primer on the Rheumatic Diseases*, ed 12, Atlanta, 2001, Arthritis Foundation.
70. Schumacher HR: Acute inflammatory arthritis. In Robbins L, Burckhardt CS, Hannan MT, et al (eds): *Clinical Care in the Rheumatic Diseases*, ed 2, Atlanta, 2001, Association of Rheumatology Health Professionals.
71. Taylor J, Erlandson DM: Pediatric rheumatic diseases. In Robbins L, Burckhardt CS, Hannan MT, et al (eds): *Clinical Care in the Rheumatic Diseases*, ed 2, Atlanta, 2001, Association of Rheumatology Health Professionals.
72. Glass D, Giannini E: Juvenile rheumatoid arthritis as a complex genetic trait, *Arthritis Rheum* 42:2261-2268, 1999.
73. Cassidy J: Juvenile rheumatoid arthritis. In Kelley WN, Sledge CB, Harris ED, et al (eds): *Textbook of Rheumatology*, ed 4, Philadelphia, 1993, WB Saunders.

74. Cassidy JT, Levinson JE, Bass JC, et al: A study of classification criteria for a diagnosis of juvenile rheumatoid arthritis, *Arthritis Rheum* 29:274, 1986.

75. Cassidy JT, Petty RE (eds): *Textbook of Pediatric Rheumatology,* ed 4, Philadelphia, 2001, WB Saunders.

76. Verzijl N, Degroot J, Thorpe SR, et al: Effect of collagen turnover on the accumulation of advanced glycation end products, *J Biol Chem* 275:39027-39031, 2000.

77. Kjaer M: Role of extracellular matrix in adaptation of tendon and skeletal muscle to mechanical loading, *Physiol Rev* 84(2):649-698, 2004.

78. Belza B: The impact of fatigue on exercise performance, *Arthritis Care* 7:176-180, 1994.

79. Casimiro L, Barnsley L, Broseau L, et al: Acupuncture and electroacupuncture for the treatment of RA, *Cochrane Database Syst Rev* 4:CD003788, 2005.

80. Feldman DE: Factors associated with the use of complementary and alternative medicine in juvenile idiopathic arthritis, *Arthritis Rheum* 51(4):527-532, 2004.

81. Soeken KL: Selected CAM therapies for arthritis-related pain: The evidence from systematic reviews, *Clin J Pain* 20(1):13-18, 2004.

82. Badley EM: The effect of osteoarthritis on disability and health care use in Canada, *J Rheumatol* 22(suppl 43):19-22, 1995.

83. Parker JC, McRae C, Smarr K, et al: Coping strategies in rheumatoid arthritis, *J Rheumatol* 15:1376-1383, 1988.

84. Blalock S, DeVellis R, Brown GK, et al: Validity of the center for epidemiological studies depression scale in arthritis populations, *Arthritis Rheum* 32:991-997, 1989.

85. Katz P, Yelin E: Prevalence and correlates of depressive symptoms among persons with rheumatoid arthritis, *J Rheumatol* 20:790-796, 1993.

86. Astin JA: Psychological interventions for rheumatoid arthritis: A meta-analysis of randomized controlled trials, *Arthritis Rheum* 47(3):291-302, 2002.

87. Smith E, Gilligan C: Physical activity prescription for the older adult, *Physician Sports Med* 11:8, 1983.

88. Hicks J: Exercise for patients with inflammatory arthritis, *J Musculoskeletal Med* 6:10, 1989.

89. Rodnan GP, Lipinski E, Luksick J: Skin thickness and collagen content in progressive systemic sclerosis and localized scleroderma, *Arthritis Rheum* 22:130, 1979.

90. Guyatt GH, Sullivan MJ, Thompson PJ, et al: The 6-minute walk: A new measure of exercise capacity in patients with chronic heart failure, *Can Med Assoc J* 132(8):919-923, 1985.

91. Lipkin DP, Scriven AJ, Crake T, et al: Six minute walking test for assessing exercise capacity in chronic heart failure, *Br Med J* 292:653-655, 1986.

92. Bittner V, Weiner Dh, Yusuf F, et al: Prediction of mortality and morbidity with a 6-minute walk test in patients with left ventricular dysfunction, *JAMA* 270:1702-1707, 1993.

93. Jette AM: The functional status index: Reliability and validity of a self-report functional disability measure, *J Rheumatol* 14(suppl 15):15-19, 1987.

94. Jette AM: Using health-related quality of life measures in physical therapy outcomes research, *Phys Ther* 73:528-537, 1993.

95. Fries JF, Spitz P, Kraines RG, et al: Measurement of patient outcomes in arthritis, *Arthritis Rheum* 23:137-145, 1980.

96. Meenan RF, Gertman PM, Mason JH: Measuring health status in arthritis. The arthritis impact measurement scales, *Arthritis Rheum* 23:146-152, 1980.

97. Jette AM: Physical disablement concepts for physical therapy research and practice, *Phys Ther* 74:380-386, 1994.

98. Meenan RF, Mason JH, Anderson JJ, et al: AIMS2: The content and properties of a revised and expanded Arthritis Impact Measurement Scales Health Status Questionnaire, *Arthritis Rheum* 35(1):1-10, 1992.

99. Hawley DJ: Clinical outcomes: Issues and measurement. In Melvin JL, Jensen GM (eds): *Rheumatologic Rehabilitation Series, vol 1: Assessment and Management,* Bethesda, Md, 1998, The American Occupational Therapy Association.

100. Haavardsholm EA, Kvien TK, Uhlig T, Smedstad LM, Guillemin F: Comparison of agreement and sensitivity to change between AIMS 2 and a short form of AIMS2 (AIMS2-SF) in more than 1000 rheumatoid arthritis patients, *J Rheumatol* 27:2810-2816, 2000.

101. Wolfe F: Which HAQ is best? A comparison of the HAQ, MHAQ and RA-HAQ, a difficult 8-item HAQ (DHAQ) and a rescored 20-item HAQ (HAQ20): Analyses on 2,491 rheumatoid arthritis patients following leflunomide initiation, *J Rheumatol* 28:982-989, 2001.

102. Ramey DR, Raynauld J, Fries JF: The health assessment questionnaire, *Arth Care Res* 5:119-129, 1992.

103. Pincus T, Wolfe F: An infrastructure of patient questionnaires at each rheumatology visit: improving efficiency and documenting care, *J Rheumatol* 27:2727-2730, 2000.

104. Wolfe F, Pincus T: Data collection in the clinic, *Rheum Dis Clin North Am* 21:321-358, 1995.

105. Wolfe F, Michaud K, Pincus T: Development and validation of the health assessment questionnaire II: A revised version of the health assessment questionnaire, *Arthritis Rheum* 50(10):3296-3305, 2004.

106. Hawley DJ, Wolfe F: Depression is not more common in rheumatoid arthritis: A 10 year longitudinal study of 6,608 rheumatic disease patients, *J Rheumatol* 20:2025-2031, 1993.

107. Poole JL: Concurrent validity of the HAQ disability index in scleroderma, *Arth Care Res* 8(3):189-193, 1995.

108. Husted JA, Gladman DD, Long JA, et al: A modified version of the health assessment questionnaire (HAQ) for psoriatic arthritis, *Clin Exp Rheumatol* 13:439-443, 1995.

109. Daltroy LH, Larson MG, Roberts NW, et al: A modification of the Health Assessment Questionnaire for the spondyloarthropathies, *J Rheumatol* 17(7):946-950, 1990.

110. Singh G, Athreya BH, Fries JF, et al: Measurement of health status in children with juvenile rheumatoid arthritis. *Arthritis Rheum* 37:1761-1769, 1994.

111. Tugwell P, Bombardier C, Buchanan WW, et al: The MACTAR patient preference disability questionnaire—an individualized functional priority approach for assessing improvement in physical disability in clinical trials in rheumatoid arthritis, *J Rheumatol* 14:446-451, 1987.

112. Verhoeven AC, Boers M, van der Linden S: Validity of the MACTAR questionnaire as a functional index in a rheumatoid arthritis clinical trial, *J Rheumatol* 27:2801-2809, 2000.

113. Bellamy N, Buchanan WW, Goldsmith CH, et al: Validation study of WOMAC: A health status instrument for measuring clinically important patient relevant outcomes to antirheumatic drug therapy in patients with osteoarthritis of the hip or knee, *J Rheumatol* 15:1833-1840, 1988.

114. Wolfe F: Determinants of WOMAC function, pain and stiffness scores: Evidence for the role of low back pain, symptoms counts, fatigue and depression in osteoarthritis, rheumatoid arthritis and fibromyalgia, *Rheumatology* (Oxford) 38:355-361, 1999.

115. Calin A: Ankylosing spondylitis: Defining disease status and the relationship between radiology, metrology, disease activity, function and outcome, *J Rheumatol* 22:740-744, 1995.

116. Ruof G, Stucki G: Comparison of the Dougados Functional Index and the Bath Ankylosing Spondylitis Functional Index. A literature review, *J Rheumatol* 26:955-960, 1999.

117. Heikkla S, Viitanen J, Kautiainen H, Kauppi M: Sensitivity to change of mobility tests; effects of shot term intensive physiotherapy and exercise on spinal, hip and shoulder measurements in spondyloarthropathy, *J Rheumatol* 27:1251-1256, 2000.

118. Sandqvist G: Hand mobility in scleroderma (HAMIS) test: the reliability of a novel hand function test, *Arth Care Res* 13(6):369-374, 2000.

119. Feldman BM, Grundland B, McCullough L, et al: Distinction of quality of life, health related quality of life, and health status in children referred for rheumatologic care, *J Rheumatol* 27:226-233, 2000.

120. Duffy CM, Arsenault L, Duffy KNW, et al: The juvenile arthritis quality of life questionnaire development of a new responsive index for juvenile rheumatoid arthritis and juvenile spondyloarthritides, *J Rheumatol* 24:738-746, 1997.

121. Tucker LB, DeNardo BA, Abetz LN, et al: The Childhood Arthritis Health Profile (CAHP): Validity and reliability of the condition-specific scales (abstract), *Arthritis Rheum* 38(suppl 9):S183, 1995.

122. Lovell DJ, Howe S, Shear E, et al: Development of a disability measurement tool for juvenile rheumatoid arthritis: The Juvenile Arthritis Functional Assessment Scale, *Arthritis Rheum* 32:1390-1395, 1989.

123. Howe S, Levinson J, Shear E, et al: Development of a disability measurement tool for juvenile rheumatoid arthritis: The Juvenile Arthritis Functional Assessment Report for children and their parents, *Arthritis Rheum* 34:873-880, 1991.

124. American Physical Therapy Association: *Guide to Physical Therapist Practice,* ed 2, Alexandria, Va, 2001, The Association.

125. Guidelines for the management of rheumatoid arthritis. American College of Rheumatology Ad Hoc Committee on Clinical Guidelines, *Arthritis Rheum* 39:713-722, 1996.

126. Brady TJ, Sniezek JE, Conn DL: Enhancing patient self-management in clinical practice, *Bull Rheum Dis* 49:1-4, 2001.

127. Superio-Cabuslay E, Ward MM, Lorig KR: Patient education interventions in osteoarthritis and rheumatoid arthritis: A meta-analytic comparison with nonsteroidal anti-inflammatory drug treatment, *Arth Care Res* 9:292-301, 1996.

128. Young LD, Bradley LA, Turner RA: Decreases in health care resource utilization in patients with rheumatoid arthritis following a cognitive behavioral intervention, *Biofeedback Self Regul* 20:259-268, 1995.

129. Lorig KR, Mazonson PD, Holman HR: Evidence suggesting that health education for self-management in patients with chronic arthritis has sustained health benefits while reducing health care costs, *Arthritis Rheum* 36:439-446, 1993.

130. Scholten C et al: Persistent functional and social benefits 5 years after a multidisciplinary arthritis training program, *Arch Phys Med Rehabil* 80(10):1282-1287, 1999.

131. Barlow JH, Williams B, Wright CC: Instilling the strength to fight the pain and get on with life: Learning to become an arthritis self-manager through an adult education programme, *Health Educ Res* 14(4):533-544, 1999.

132. Sohng K: Effects of a self-management course for patients with systemic lupus erythematosus, *J Adv Nurs* 42(5):479-486, 2003.

133. Andre M, Hagelberg S, Stenstrom CH: Education in the management of juvenile chronic arthritis. Changes in self-reported competencies among adolescents and parents of young children, *Scand J Rheumatol* 30(6):323-7, 2001.

134. Steultjens EM, Dekker J, Bouter LM, et al: Occupational therapy for rheumatoid arthritis, *Cochrane Database Syst Rev* 1:CD003114, 2004.

135. Nordenskiob U, Grimby G, Hedberg M, et al: The structure of an instrument for assessing the effects of assistive devices and altered working methods in women with rheumatoid arthritis, *Arth Care Res* 9:358-367, 1996.

136. Sweeney GM, Catchpole N, Clarke AK: Choosing lever taps for people with rheumatoid arthritis, *Br J Occup Ther* 57:263-265, 1994.

137. Philips CA: Management of the patient with rheumatoid arthritis. The role of the hand therapist, *Hand Clin* 5:291-309, 1989.

138. Egan M, Brosseau L, Farmer M, et al: Splints/orthoses in the treatment of rheumatoid arthritis, *Cochrane Database Syst Rev* 1:CD004018, 2003.

139. Ottawa panel evidence-based clinical practice guidelines for electrotherapy and thermotherapy interventions in the management of rheumatoid arthritis in adults, *Phys Ther* 84(11):1016-1043, 2004.

140. Minor M, Sanford M: Physical interventions in the management of pain in arthritis, *Arth Care Res* 6:197-206, 1993.

141. Dellhag B, Wollersjo I, Bjelle A: The effect of active hand exercise and wax bath treatment in rheumatoid arthritis patients, *Arth Care Res* 5:87-92, 1992.

142. Falconer J, Hayes KW, Chang RW: Therapeutic ultrasound in the treatment of musculoskeletal conditions, *Arth Care Res* 3:85-91, 1990.

143. Casimiro L, Brosseau L, Robinson VA, et al: Therapeutic ultrasound for the treatment of rheumatoid arthritis (Cochrane review), *Cochrane Database Syst Rev* 3:CD003787, 2002.

144. Feibel A, Fast A: Deep heating of joints: A reconsideration, *Arch Phys Med Rehabil* 57:513, 1976.

145. Kangilaski J: "Baggietherapy:" Simple pain relief for arthritic knees, *JAMA* 246:317-318, 1981.

146. Welch V, Brosseau L, Shea B, et al: Thermotherapy for treating rheumatoid arthritis, *Cochrane Database Syst Rev* 2:CD002826, 2001.

147. Brosseau L, Robinson V, Pelland L, et al: Thermotherapy for treating rheumatoid arthritis: A meta-analysis, *Phys Ther Rev* 7:203-208, 2002.

148. Williams J, Harvey J, Tannenbaum H: Use of superficial heat versus ice in the rheumatoid arthritic shoulder, *Physiother Canada* 38:6-13, 1986.

149. Brosseau L, Yonge K, Marchand S, et al: Efficacy of transcutaneous electric nerve stimulation for rheumatoid arthritis: A systematic review, *Phys Ther Rev* 7:199-208, 2002.

150. Brosseau L, Welch V, Wells GA, et al: Low level laser therapy for osteoarthritis and rheumatoid arthritis: A meta-analysis, *J Rheumatol* 27:1961-1969, 2000.

151. Brosseau L, Robinson V, Wells GA, et al: Low level laser therapy for treating rheumatoid arthritis (Cochrane review), *Cochrane Database Syst Rev* 4:CD002049, 2005.

152. Houlbrooke K, Vause K, Merrilees MJ: Effects of movement and weightbearing on the glycosaminoglycan content of sheep articular cartilage, *Aust J Physiother* 36:88-91, 1990.

153. Minor M: Arthritis and exercise. "The times they are a-changin," *Arth Care Res* 9:79-81, 1996.

154. Van den Ende CHM, Vliet TPM, Munneke M, et al: Dynamic exercise therapy for rheumatoid arthritis (Cochrane review), *Cochrane Database Syst Rev* 4:CD000322, 1999.

155. Melvin J: *Rheumatic Disease in the Adult and Child: Occupational Therapy and Rehabilitation*, ed 3, Philadelphia, 1989, FA Davis.

156. Van Deusen J, Harlowe D: The efficacy of the ROM dance program for adults with rheumatoid arthritis, *Am J Occup Ther* 41:90-95, 1987.

157. Rall LC, Meydani SN, Kehayias JJ, et al: The effect of progressive resistance training in rheumatoid arthritis: increased strength without changes in energy balance or body composition, *Arthritis Rheum* 39:415-426, 1996.

158. Stenström C, Minor M: Evidence for the benefit of aerobic and strengthening exercise in rheumatoid arthritis, *Arthritis Rheum* (Arth Care Res) 49:428-434, 2003.

159. Westby MD, Wade JP, Rangno KK, et al: A randomized controlled trial to evaluate the effectiveness of an exercise program in women with rheumatoid arthritis taking low dose prednisone, *J Rheumatol* 27:1674-1680, 2000.

160. Minor MA, Hewett JE, Webel RR, et al: Efficacy of physical conditioning exercises in patients with rheumatoid arthritis and osteoarthritis, *Arthritis Rheum* 32:1396-1405, 1989.

161. Ekdahl C, Andersson SI, Moritz U, et al: Dynamic versus static training in patients with rheumatoid arthritis, *Scan J Rheumatol* 19:17-26, 1990.

162. Baslund B, Lyngberg K, Andersen V, et al: Effect of 8 wk of bicycle training on the immune system of patients with rheumatoid arthritis, *J Appl Physiol* 75:1691-1705, 1993.

163. Hansen TM, Hansen G, Langgaard AM, et al: Long term physical training in rheumatoid arthritis: a randomized trial with different training programs and blinded observers, *Scan J Rheumatol* 22:107-112, 1993.

164. Hoenig H, Groff G, Pratt K, et al: A randomized controlled trial of home exercise on the rheumatoid hand, *J Rheumatol* 20:785-789, 1993.

165. Häkkinen A, Häkkinen K, Hannonen P: Effects of strength training on neuromuscular function and disease activity in patients with recent-onset inflammatory arthritis, *Scand J Rheumatol* 23:237-242, 1994.

166. Lynberg K, Harreby M, Bentzen H, et al: Elderly rheumatoid arthritis patients on steroid treatment tolerate physical training without an increase in disease activity, *Arch Phys Med Rehabil* 75:1189-1195, 1994.

167. Stenström CH, Arge B, Sundbom A: Dynamic training versus relaxation training as home exercise for patients with inflammatory rheumatic diseases: A randomized controlled study, *Scand J Rheumatol* 25:28-33, 1996.

168. Stenström CH, Arge B, Sundbom A: Home exercise and compliance in inflammatory rheumatic diseases: A prospective clinical trial, *J Rheumatol* 24:470-476, 1997.

169. Van den Ende CHM, Hazes JMW, le Cessie S, et al: Comparison of high and low intensity training in well controlled rheumatoid arthritis: Results of a randomized clinical trial. *Ann Rheum Dis* 55:798-805, 1996.

170. Komatireddy GR, Leitch RW, Cella K, et al: Efficacy of load resistive muscle training in patients with rheumatoid arthritis functional class II and III, *J Rheumatol* 24:1531-1539, 1997.

171. Boström C, Harms-Ringdahl K, Nordemar R: Effect of static and dynamic shoulder rotator exercises in woman with rheumatoid arthritis, *Scand J Rheumatol* 27:281-290, 1998.

172. Häkkinen A, Sokka T, Kotaniemi A, et al: Dynamic strength training in patients with early rheumatoid arthritis increases muscle strength but not bone mineral density, *J Rheumatol* 26:1257-1263, 1999.

173. Häkkinen A, Sokka T, Kotaniemi A, et al: A randomized two-year study of the effects of dynamic strength training on muscle strength, disease activity, functional capacity, and bone mineral density in early rheumatoid arthritis, *Arthritis Rheum* 44:515-522, 2001.

174. McMeeken J, Stillman B, Story I, et al: The effects of knee extensor and flexor muscle training on the timed-up-and-go test in individuals with rheumatoid arthritis, *Physiother Res Int* 4:55-67, 1999.

175. Van den Ende CHM, Breedveld FC, le Cessie S, et al: Effect of intensive exercise on patients with active rheumatoid arthritis: A randomized clinical trial, *Ann Rheum Dis* 59:615-621, 2000.

176. Westby MD, Wade JP, Rangno KK, et al: A randomized controlled trial to evaluate the effectiveness of an exercise program in women with rheumatoid arthritis taking low dose prednisone, *J Rheumatol* 27:1674-1680, 2000.

177. Verhagen AP, de Vet HCW, de Bie RA, et al: Balneotherapy for rheumatoid and osteoarthritis, *Cochrane Database Syst Rev* 4:CD000518, 2003.

178. McNeal RL: Aquatic therapy for patients with rheumatic disease, *Rheum Dis Clin North Am* 16:915-929, 1990.

179. Sanford-Smith M, MacKay-Lyons M, et al: Therapeutic benefit of aquaerobics for individuals with rheumatoid arthritis, *Physiother Can* 50:40-46, 1998.

180. Hall J, Skevington SM, Maddison PJ, et al: A randomized controlled trial of hydrotherapy in rheumatoid arthritis, *Arth Care Res* 9:206-215, 1996.

181. Suomi R: Effects of arthritis exercise programs on functional fitness and perceived ADL measures in older adults with arthritis, *Arch Phys Med Rehabil* 84(11):1589-1594, 2003.

182. Wallace CA, Levinson JE: Juvenile rheumatoid arthritis: Outcome and treatment for the 1990s. In Athreya B (ed). *Rheumatic Disease Clinics of North America*, Philadelphia, 1991, WB Saunders.

183. Klepper S: Effects of an eight week physical conditioning program on disease signs and symptoms in children with chronic arthritis, *Arth Care Res* 12:52-60, 1999.

184. Fisher NM, Venkatraman JT, O'Neil K: The effects of resistance exercise on muscle function in juvenile arthritis, *Arthritis Rheum* 44(suppl 9):S276, 1999.

185. Klepper S: Exercise and fitness in children with arthritis: Evidence of benefits for exercise and physical activity, *Arthritis Rheum* 49:435-443, 2003.

186. Dagfinrud H, Kvien TK, Hagen KB: Physiotherapy interventions for ankylosing spondylitis, *Cochrane Database Syst Rev* 18(4):CD002822, 2004.

187. van der Linden S, van Tubergen A, Hidding A: Physiotherapy in ankylosing spondylitis: what is the evidence? *Clin Exp Rheumatol* 20(6 suppl 28):S60-S64, 2002.

188. Viitanen JV, Heikkila S: Functional changes in patients with spondyloarthropathy. A controlled trial of the effects of short-term rehabilitation and a 3-year follow-up, *Rheumatol Int* 20(5):211-214, 2001.

189. van Tubergen A, Land ewe R, van der Heijde D, et al: Combined spa-exercise therapy is effective in patients with ankylosing spondylitis: a randomized controlled trial. *Arthritis Rheum* 45(5):430-438, 2001.

190. Kraal G, Stokes B, Groh J, et al: The effects of comprehensive home physiotherapy and supervision on patients with ankylosing spondylitis—an 8-month follow-up, *J Rheumatol* 21:261-263, 1994.

191. Falkenbach A: Disability motivates patients with ankylosing spondylitis for more frequent physical exercise, *Arch Phys Med Rehabil* 84(3):382-383, 2002.

192. Sweeney S: The effect of a home based exercise intervention package on outcomes in ankylosing spondylitis: a randomized controlled trial, *J Rheumatol* 29(4):763-766, 2002.
193. Analay Y: The effectiveness of intensive group exercise on patient with ankylosing spondylitis, *Clin Rehabil* 17(6):631-636, 2003.
194. Helliwell PS: A randomized trial of 3 different physiotherapy regimes in ankylosing spondylitis, *Physiotherapy* 82(2):85-90, 1996.
195. Hicks JE: Isometric exercise increases strength and does not produce sustained creatinine phosphokinase increases in a patient with polymyositis, *J Rheumatol* 20(8):1399-1401, 1993.
196. Varju C, Petho E, Kutas R, et al: The effect of physical exercise following acute disease exacerbation in patients with dermato/polymyositis, *Clin Rehabil* 17:83-87, 2003.
197. Lawson Mahowald M: The benefits and limitation of a physical training program in patients with inflammatory myositis, *Curr Rheumatol Rep* 3(4):317-324, 2001.
198. Alexanderson H: The safety of a resistive home exercise program in patients with recent onset active polymyositis or dermatomyositis, *Scand J Rheumatol* 29(5):295-301, 2000.
199. Wiesinger GF: Benefit of 6 months long-term physical training in polymyositis/dermatomyositis patients, *Br J Rheumatol* 37(12):1338-1342, 1998.
200. Alexanderson H: Safety of a home exercise programme in patients with polymyositis and dermatomyositis: a pilot study, *Rheumatology* (Oxford) 38(7):608-611, 1999.
201. Pizzo G, Scardina GA, Messina P: Effects of a nonsurgical exercise program on the decreased mouth opening in patients with systemic scleroderma, *Clin Oral Invest* 7(3):175-178, 2003.
202. Naylor WP, Douglass CW, Mix E. The nonsurgical treatment of microstomia in scleroderma: A pilot study, *Oral Surg Oral Med Oral Pathol* 57(5):508-511, 1984.
203. Sandqvist G, Akesson A, Eklund M: Evaluation of paraffin bath treatments in patients with systemic sclerosis, *Disabil Rehabil* 26(16):981-987, 2004.

Localized Inflammation

L. Vince Lepak III

OBJECTIVES

After reading this chapter, the reader will be able to:
1. Explain the phases of the inflammatory process.
2. Describe how various pathologies contribute to and are affected by localized inflammation.
3. Identify the signs and symptoms of localized inflammation.
4. Plan an appropriate examination that recognizes and measures signs and symptoms associated with localized inflammation.
5. Develop an evidence-based intervention plan for an individual with localized inflammation.

Inflammation is the body's first response to tissue damage or injury. As the first line of defense, it is critical to the survival of the human organism. Inflammation is defined as a localized protective response elicited by injury or destruction of tissues that destroys, dilutes, or walls-off the injurious agent, as well as the injured tissue. However, the acute or chronic response of inflammation to various stimuli makes a strict definition difficult to fit all situations.[1] It is not one process but rather an overlapping sequence of interactions between stimuli and the body's cellular and biochemical defenses designed to destroy offending pathogens and initiate tissue healing. The extent of the response depends both on the body's reactivity and the mode and extent of cellular injury.[1]

PATHOLOGY

According to the *Guide To Physical Therapist Practice*, localized inflammation is a pathology that has a multifactorial impact on an individual.[2] The diagnostic classification associated with localized inflammation is preferred practice pattern 4E: Impaired joint mobility, motor function, muscle performance, and range of motion associated with localized inflammation. The *Guide* lists a wide range of risk factors for this preferred practice pattern, including abnormal response to provocation, ankylosing spondylitis, bursitis, capsulitis, epicondylitis, fasciitis, gout, osteoarthritis, prenatal and postnatal soft tissue inflammation, synovitis, and tendinitis. A number of these are also risk factors for other preferred practice patterns, particularly pattern 4D: Impaired joint mobility, motor function, muscle performance, and range of motion associated with connective tissue dysfunction (see Chapter 6). To separate these, this chapter focuses on inflammation that is primarily due to local insult or degeneration, whereas Chapter 6 focuses on the systemic inflammatory and autoimmune disorders. In addition, Chapter 28 provides a more detailed discussion of tissue healing particularly as it relates to wounds.

The earliest descriptions of inflammation were derived from clinical observation, including what continues to be described as the five classical (cardinal) signs of inflammation: rubor (redness), calor (heat), dolor (pain), tumor (swelling), and functiona laesa (loss of function).[3] These classical signs and symptoms are readily observed by the rehabilitation professional and direct the examination, evaluation, and interventions related to inflammatory conditions. Physicians are aided in their diagnostic process by the tools of the modern laboratory[1] and are able to intervene at the biochemical level with medications to control inflammation, whereas other rehabilitation clinicians, including physical therapists and occupational therapists, primarily use physical interventions and patient education to influence and modify inflammation.

A wide range of stimuli can provoke localized inflammation in the musculoskeletal system. These include trauma from crush, contusion, avulsion, rupture, sprain, or strain, as well as infection, physical or chemical agents (thermal injury or chemical irritation), derangement of joint components, degeneration, crystal deposition, foreign bodies, immune reactions, and overuse. In response to any of these stimuli, a cascade of events, known collectively as the inflammatory response, occurs. This response should be balanced, first initiating inflammation and then limiting its extent and duration to avoid harm.[4] When inflammation is prolonged, it is known as chronic inflammation. Since the classical signs of inflammation are often absent with chronic inflammation, it may not be recognized until enough tissue damage has occurred to create impairments and limit function. Chronic inflammation often persists because the body cannot resolve the initial damage or because the initial stimulus did not initiate a sufficient acute inflammatory response to trigger completion of the cascade of events needed to resolve the condition. In addition, the ongoing presence of infectious agents, foreign bodies, metabolic byproducts, exogenous irritants (mechanical or chemical), and persistent immune responses can all contribute to maintaining a chronic inflammatory state.[5]

This chapter outlines the major events of the inflammatory process in the musculoskeletal system and describes factors that can cause pathological or chronic inflammation. Inflammatory conditions commonly encountered and treated by rehabilitation professionals are described, including a summary of the pathophysiology of each. This is followed by discussion of evidence-based examination, evaluation, and interventions for successfully managing localized inflammatory conditions.

STAGES OF TISSUE HEALING

The first stage of tissue healing is the inflammatory stage (phase I). This stage is designed to initiate healing; prevent further damage; rid the body of pathogens, foreign material, and nonviable tissue; and thus prepare the way for tissue repair through collagen proliferation (phase II or proliferation). Phase III, remodeling or maturation, occurs when the initial weak collagen produced during the proliferation phase is gradually replaced by stronger collagen. This phase can last 2 years or longer. Fig. 7-1 illustrates the stages of tissue healing.

Phase I—Inflammatory Phase. Inflammation usually resolves 24-72 hours after the initial trauma, but repeated agitation and associated risk factors can delay its completion and lead to secondary injuries.[6] Inflammation is designed to protect the body and promote repair by destroying, diluting, or sequestering the injurious agent and the injured tissue. Initially, for the first 5-10 minutes, a vasoconstrictive vascular response is initiated to help contain the insult. This response is triggered by the release of norepinephrine from blood vessels and serotonin from mast cells and platelets.[7] At the same time, *neutrophils* begin to migrate and release proinflammatory *cytokines* that attract and stimulate additional inflammatory cells.[8]

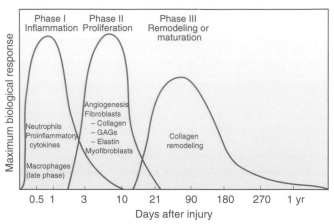

FIG. 7-1 Stages of tissue healing: Inflammation, proliferation, and remodeling. *GAGs,* Glycosaminoglycans.

The initial vasoconstriction is quickly followed by prolonged vasodilation and increased capillary permeability triggered by the release of *histamines* and *prostaglandins.* The increased capillary permeability allows more fluid, plasma proteins, white blood cells, and fibrin to enter the area.[7,9] Fibrin plugs form in the blood vessels and wall off the injured area. At this point, the clinical signs of inflammation, redness, heat, swelling, and often pain, appear. The rise in tissue temperature creates a favorable environment for cellular multiplication and metabolic reactions. Eventually, other leukocytes are attracted to the area by chemotaxis and they assist with phagocytosis.[7]

During the inflammatory phase, *macrophages* are the predominant cells. They rid the area of debris, microorganisms, and residual neutrophils, through phagocytosis. A vast array of growth factors (*angiogenesis* growth factor, platelet-derived growth factor, *fibroblast* growth factor, and others) and cytokines (interleukin-1 and tumor necrosis factor) are also released during the inflammatory response. These facilitate tissue repair, stimulate specific immune responses, promote the release of chemotactic factors that attract fibroblasts, and help regulate the production of collagen through the release of matrix metalloproteinases (MMPs), which are primarily produced by fibroblasts. The environment becomes hypoxic and acidic, allowing the macrophages and fibroblasts to flourish.[9,10]

The end of the inflammatory phase is signaled by the release of fibrinolysin, an enzyme that helps open the lymphatic channels. Pain and loss of function now occur as a result of increased sensitivity of the pain receptors, activation of neurologically mediated reflexes, and increased pressure on surrounding structures from edema.[11]

Phase II—Proliferation Phase. The proliferation phase begins as the number of fibroblasts increases and the number of macrophages decreases. Fibroblasts are the dominant cell type of the proliferation phase. They synthesize MMPs, collagen and other proteins, fibronectin, glycosaminoglycans, and elastin. Some fibroblasts differentiate into *myofibroblasts,* which are responsible for wound contraction.[6,10] Granulation and angiogenesis are also associated with this phase.

Proliferation starts a few days after the initial insult and is usually complete within 3 weeks, although it can last for as long as 6-12 weeks. In the early portion of this phase, type III collagen, which is fairly weak, is produced and loosely arranged in a disorganized fashion in the damage area. During this phase, this collagen gradually aligns itself to some degree with the stress imposed on it and starts to be replaced by stronger type I collagen.[6]

Phase III—Remodeling or Maturation Phase. Phase III, the remodeling or maturation phase, begins by day 21 after the initial injury and may continue for months or years. This phase is characterized by a continual restructuring of the collagen from weak unorganized fibers to stronger fibers (type I) that are continually being reorganized to meet the demands of imposed mechanical forces.

COMPONENTS OF THE FUNCTIONAL JOINT COMPLEX

A quick review of the functional joint complex can help the reader understand the specific inflammatory conditions of the musculoskeletal system. These generally involve synovial or diarthrodial joints because these joints' capacity for movement makes them vulnerable to injury and thus local inflammation. The typical synovial joint (Fig. 7-2) includes hyaline cartilage at the articulating ends of the bone, menisci, ligaments, a joint capsule, bursae, tendons, and muscles. In some places, particularly in areas close to bones, tendons are surrounded by tendon sheaths that form tunnels to protect the tendons and bathe them in synovial fluid. There may also be fascia that extends beyond the tendons or ligaments to provide greater strength and stability.

Lining the joint capsule of all synovial joints is a well-vascularized, well-innervated tissue known as synovium. Within the joint, synovial fluid facilitates movement through lubrication and nutrient exchange to adjacent relatively avascular tissues such as tendons and cartilage. Synovial fluid is an ultrafiltrate of plasma that is cleared by the lymphatics.[12] The constituents of synovial fluid change in the presence of inflammation, and physicians may remove some of this fluid with a needle and analyze it to help with diagnosis. In addition, synovial fluid pressure may rise in response to inflammation. This rise can

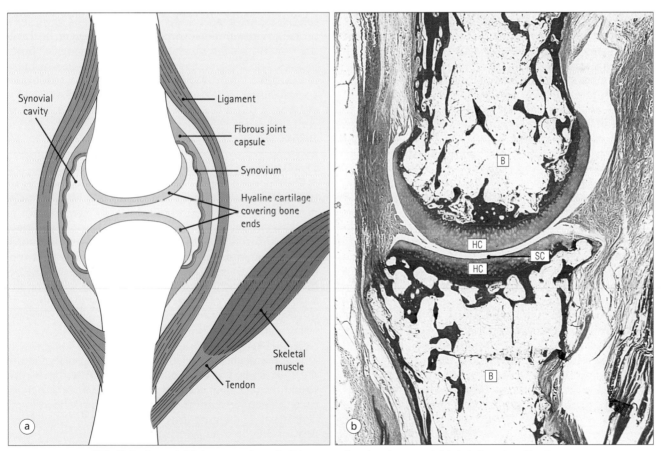

FIG. 7-2 Synovial joint complex. **A,** Diagram of a simple synovial joint showing the two articulating bone ends separated from each other by synovial fluid and enclosed within a fibrocollagenous capsule. Surrounding ligaments and tendinous muscle attachments prevent excess movement. **B,** Low power micrograph of an interphalangeal joint of the finger. Note the ends of the articulating bone *(B),* the hyaline cartilage *(HC)* and the joint capsule enclosing the synovial cavity *(SC),* which contains synovial fluid. The synovial cavity is lined internally by synovium. ©Fleshandbones.com.

decrease capillary perfusion[12] and inhibit muscle activation around the joint.[13]

Cartilage. Normal adult articular cartilage is composed primarily of an extracellular matrix of collagen, proteoglycans, and a few chondrocytes. Chondrocytes make up 1% to 2% of the articular cartilage and are responsible for maintaining a balance between the synthesis and breakdown of the cartilage matrix.[12] The chondrocytes synthesize the collagens and proteoglycans that build up cartilage and the proteinases that degrade collagens. Unfortunately, cartilage has a limited capacity for repair.[14]

The structural characteristic of articular cartilage is determined primarily by its hyaline extracellular matrix, which is 65% to 80% water (water content progressively decreases from superficial to deeper zones).[12] Water passes freely between cartilage and synovial fluid. Articular cartilage generally has no blood supply or lymphatics and receives its nutrition primarily from the synovial fluid within the joint. The biochemical composition of cartilage and the structure of the matrix give it special properties, including elasticity, compressibility, and self-lubrication.

Normally, cartilage is protected from wear by a form of self-lubrication that occurs as weight bearing gradually deforms the cartilage, pushing water out of the interior onto hydrophilic surface tissues. This "squeeze-film" of lubrication is re-imbibed by the cartilage when the pressure is removed.[12] Movement through physiological range of motion helps nourish the articular cartilage by providing intermittent hydrostatic pressure changes that increase the diffusion of fluid and maintain or increase proteoglycan and collagen synthesis. However, joint motion without loading or compression does not provide enough nutrition to maintain cartilage integrity over time.[15] Immobilization and weightlessness, as well as excessive loading (obesity), developmental abnormalities (e.g., Perthes' disease), and joint incongruities, can lead to articular cartilage degradation.[16] Furthermore, damage to any of the structures that protect cartilage by absorbing excessive weight-bearing forces, including muscles, tendons, and ligaments around a joint as well as the subchondral bone, can cause wear on the cartilage to be increased.[15]

SPECIFIC INFLAMMATORY CONDITIONS

Osteoarthritis. Osteoarthritis (OA) or degenerative joint disease is the most common type of arthritis in the United States and the world.[17] OA is responsible for 59 million physician visits each year, is the primary reason for total hip and knee replacements (see Chapter 10), is the leading cause of lower extremity (LE) disability among the elderly, and is a leading cause of disability in persons 15 years or older.[18,19] OA can interfere with a wide range of activities of daily living (ADLs), including ambulation, bathing, dressing, eating, drinking, home maintenance, taking medication, toileting, sleeping, using a telephone, and writing.[17] The knees are affected by OA more commonly than any other joint, and this is the primary reason that individuals have difficulty climbing stairs and walking.[19]

OA is characterized by the breakdown of the joint's cartilage and periarticular bone changes (osteophyte forma-

tion and subchondral sclerosis).[20,21] The structural changes that occur in OA appear first in cartilage, with the development of edema in the extracellular matrix, or microcracks, and increasing variability in chondrocyte quality and quantity. As destruction of the cartilage progresses, fissuring and pitting occur parallel and perpendicular to the collagen fibrils down to the subchondral bone. The subchondral bone can then be eroded, and subchondral microcysts may develop. Fragments of cartilage may also fall into the joint. These are phagocytosed in the synovial fluid and cause mild synovial inflammation. In OA, the synovial cells also produce a range of inflammatory mediators and cytokines that can alter the cartilage matrix and stimulate chondrocytes to synthesize destructive enzymes, particularly stromelysin and collagenase, to further degrade the cartilage.[12,22,23] *Osteoblasts* from exposed subchondral bone may also synthesize proteolytic enzymes that further contribute to the degenerative process.[24]

Eburnated bone (bone that appears polished and shiny, indicating a full thickness loss of articular cartilage)[25] attempts to regenerate, causing subchondral bone sclerosis and a buildup of bony outgrowths at the joint margins called osteophytes. Osteophytes are covered with poor quality cartilage. As OA progresses the chondrocytes produce more type I and type III collagens with shorter proteoglycans and also more type VI collagen instead of the type II collagen produced by chondrocytes in healthy joints.[26] The collagen fibers are also arranged more loosely, diminishing their ability to hold water and self-lubricate and making them more brittle and more vulnerable to enzymatic degradation. Vascular changes also affect subchondral bone synthesis and degradation. Increased vascularity of the damaged bone may play a role in bone hyperplasia[27], whereas avascular necrosis can cause subchondral bone breakdown.

Prolonged synovitis associated with the joint damage from OA can also cause capsular fibrosis and limitations in joint range of motion (ROM).[16] Reflexive inhibition of muscle contraction that results from pain and swelling can further contribute to functional losses by causing muscle atrophy and imbalanced forces around the joint. Joint narrowing that is a result of the erosive changes in the bone may also lead to ligament instability. Together, these structural changes may lead to biomechanical instabilities that create a cycle of joint degeneration and local synovial inflammation (Fig. 7-3).

Pain-free joint motion requires an intact joint with relatively few degenerative changes. Damage or degeneration of the articular cartilage, synovium, capsule, ligamentous structure, or other components of the functional joint complex can decrease ROM, cause pain, and lead to joint instability, malalignment, or mechanical disturbances.[28] Any loss of congruency or stability in the normal complex may initiate or accelerate degenerative changes (OA), leading to loss of mobility and joint deformities.[29]

The exact causes of OA are not known, but a variety of systemic or local risk factors are known to be associated with OA. Systemic factors include age, gender, ethnicity, hormonal status and bone density, nutritional factors, and genetics. Local factors include obesity, joint injury, joint

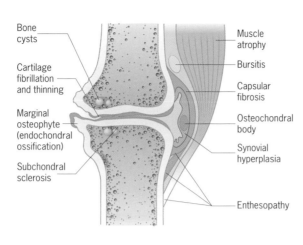
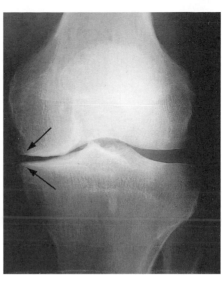

Bone cysts

Cartilage fibrillation and thinning

Marginal osteophyte (endochondral ossification)

Subchondral sclerosis

Muscle atrophy

Bursitis

Capsular fibrosis

Osteochondral body

Synovial hyperplasia

Enthesopathy

FIG. 7-3 Diagram and x-ray of a knee showing early OA. There is medial compartment narrowing owing to cartilage thinning with subarticular sclerosis and marginal osteophyte formation *(arrows)*. ©*Fleshandbones.com.*

deformity (congenital or developmental), occupational factors, sports participation, and muscle weakness.[19,30] The primary risk factors for the development of OA appear to be increased age, obesity, hip injury, congenital or developmental hip disorders, and a genetic predisposition to the disorder.[21]

The prevalence of OA increases with age.[31] Approximately 50% of people over the age of 65 have radiographic signs of OA. This increases to 80% for persons 75 years old and older.[21]

Obesity may contribute to OA by increasing compressive and shearing forces applied through the weight-bearing joints of the body. However, factors associated with obesity other than weight bearing clearly also affect the development of OA because although the presence of obesity correlates most with the development of OA in weight-bearing joints, it also correlates with OA at other joints, including those of the hands. Individuals with a *body mass index* (BMI) of 35 kg/m^2 have been found to be twice as likely to develop OA at the first carpometacarpal joint as people of similar age, gender, and associated risk factors with a BMI between 20 and 24.9 kg/m^2.[32]

Twin and sibling studies of the prevalence of OA and joint replacement suggest that there is a strong genetic component and inherited susceptibility to primary OA.[33,34] Inherited traits that have been linked to the development of OA include alterations in the structure and mechanical properties of cartilage, genetic joint dysplasias, joint instability and ligamentous laxity, obesity, and issues related to bone mechanics such as an increased valgus or varus joint angle.

Trauma, particularly if it results in intraarticular damage, is also associated with the development of OA. A study found that 40% of men and 20% of women who are 55 to 64 years of age with OA of the knee had a history of trauma affecting the stability of the knee, including articular surface fracture and ligament or meniscal tear or dislocation.[19] Women with a history of severe trauma to the knee have three times the risk of developing knee OA, and prior trauma in men results in a fivefold to sixfold increase in risk.[19,35] It has been reported that the risk of

developing knee OA increases tenfold after an anterior cruciate ligament or meniscal repair.[36] Joint injuries may increase the risk of OA because weakened tissues are less able to withstand compressive and shear forces and may increase forces on the joint by altering its alignment and biomechanics.

Occupational or nonoccupational repetitive stress has also been identified as a risk factor for the development of OA.[22] Studies have shown that OA occurs more often in dominant than nondominant hands and has a lower occurrence in paralyzed hands.[37,38] Prolonged or repetitive standing, bending, walking long distances over rough ground, lifting and moving heavy objects, and previous major trauma to the hip are also associated with an increased risk of hip OA.[19] Studies have also shown an increased occurrence of OA in the weight-bearing joints of elite athletes.[39] High-impact sports have the greatest effect, while low-impact recreational exercise does not appear to increase the risk for developing OA.[36]

Developmental factors affecting the congruity of the joints, such as joint deformities, dysplasia, and structural deformities, may also influence the development of OA in affected or neighboring joints.[19] Examples of such disorders include multiple epiphyseal dysplasia, developmental displacement of the hip, Legg-Calvé-Perthes disease, acetabular dysplasia, genu varum, and genu valgum.[19,30]

There is a positive relationship between high subchondral bone density and the occurrence of OA and an inverse relationship between the occurrence of OA and osteoporosis.[40,41] The mechanism for these correlations is not clear. Although high bone mineral density may increase the likelihood of OA, it may also slow progression of the disease.[30]

Bursitis. Bursae are fluid-filled sacs located at numerous points throughout the body (Fig. 7-4). They are designed to provide a smooth gliding surface between bones, tendons, ligaments, muscles, and skin.[42] Bursae may become inflamed by trauma, overuse, or as part of a more systemic inflammatory process (e.g., rheumatoid arthritis, crystal arthropathies, or infection). Detecting the

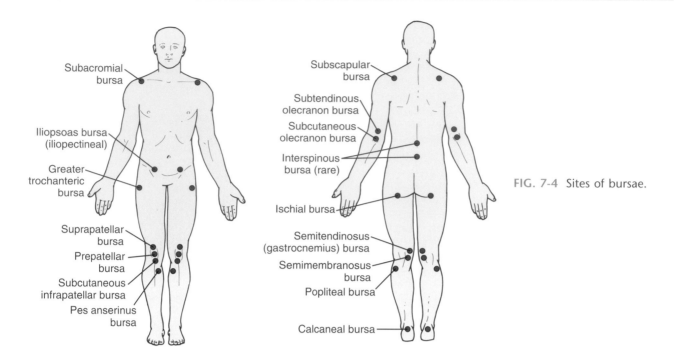

FIG. 7-4 Sites of bursae.

classical signs of inflammation with bursitis can be difficult if the bursa is deep or the response is mild. Unrecognized, chronic bursitis will lead to effusion, thickening of the bursal wall, deposits of fibrin, and the development of a cartilage-like material around the bursa that may need to be surgically excised to relieve symptoms. Bursitis can cause pain that limits a person's ability to engage in normal daily activities (e.g., reaching overhead, ambulation, and participating in work or recreational activities). Bursae are widely distributed, and bursitis may occur at any bursa.

In the pelvic and hip region, the greater trochanteric bursa, which is located beneath the site where the gluteus maximus inserts into the greater trochanter, is one of the more commonly affected.[43,44] Initial onset is usually insidious and thought to be secondary to repetitive strains and stresses. Females who are 40 to 69 years of age are disproportionately affected, although trochanteric bursitis can affect anyone at any age.[43] Trochanteric bursitis typically causes aching pain at the lateral thigh. Occasionally, patients describe their symptoms as sharp or a numbness that extends into the low back or the knee. Lying on the affected side and prolonged standing or walking (running for younger athletes) often aggravates symptoms and there is usually tenderness with palpation over the bursa and pain with resisted muscle testing of the hip abductors.[43]

Bursae around the knee that are commonly affected by bursitis are the pes anserinus bursa and the infrapatellar bursa. The pes anserinus is the common insertion for the sartorius, gracilis, and semitendinosus muscles, and its bursa is located just proximal to the insertion. This bursa may become inflamed by overtraining, tight hamstrings, or trauma. When inflamed, the pain can be severe enough to limit running and stair climbing and can even cause difficulty with rising from a chair.[45] Signs and symptoms of inflammation should be detectable approximately 2

inches below the medial joint line of the knee. There are two infrapatellar bursae (superficial and deep). The superficial infrapatellar bursa (clergyman knee) is located between the patellar tendon and the skin, and the deep infrapatellar bursa is located just proximal to where the patellar tendon inserts into the tibial tuberosity, inferior to the infrapatellar fat pad. The superficial bursa should be readily palpable under the skin, and if it is inflamed, the deep bursa can be palpated on both sides of the patellar tendon.[46-48]

In the upper extremity (UE), the subacromial bursa is a common cause of shoulder pain.[49] In the acute condition, active shoulder elevation may be limited and a painful arc may be present. This bursa is readily accessible by extending the humerus and palpating inferior to the anterior aspect of the acromion.[50] Olecranon bursitis is another common bursitis of the UE. It is usually caused by trauma however, overuse (typing, weightlifting), infection, and arthritis can also cause this bursa to become inflamed. It is critical that the therapist differentiate between septic and nonseptic olecranon bursitis. Septic bursitis will generally develop more quickly and become more severe, making the patient seek treatment sooner. With septic bursitis there are also commonly accompanying integumentary changes (cellulitis, overlying skin lesions), and the patient is likely to be febrile. If septic olecranon bursitis is suspected, the patient should be immediately referred to their physician for further testing (aspiration).[42]

Bursitis can be difficult to diagnosis in some cases and may require an MRI to confirm the diagnosis. Several uncommon areas for bursitis include interspinous,[51] intermetatarsophalangeal,[52] and lesser trochanteric bursitis.[53]

Capsulitis. Capsulitis is an inflammation of the joint capsule. Although any synovial joint capsule may be affected, glenohumeral joint capsulitis is the most common.[54] Glenohumeral joint capsulitis is often referred to as adhesive capsulitis of the shoulder or frozen shoul-

TABLE 7-1	Stages of Adhesive Capsulitis in the Shoulder			
Findings	Stage 1	Stage 2 "Freezing Stage"	Stage 3 "Frozen Stage"	Stage 4 "Thawing Phase"
Duration of symptoms	0 to 3 months	3 to 9 months	9 to 5 months	15 to 24 months
Pain	Pain with active and passive ROM	Chronic pain with active and passive ROM	Minimal pain except at end ROM	Minimal pain
ROM	Limitation of forward flexion, abduction, internal rotation, external rotation	Significant limitation of forward flexion, abduction, internal rotation, external rotation	Significant limitation of ROM with rigid "end-feel"	Progressive improvement in ROM
Examination under anesthesia	Normal or minimal loss of ROM	ROM essentially identical to ROM when the patient is awake	ROM identical to ROM when patient awake	Data not available
Arthroscopy	Diffuse glenohumeral synovitis, often most pronounced in the anterosuperior capsule	Diffuse, pedunculated synovitis (tight capsule with rubbery or dense feel on insertion of arthroscope)	No hypervascularity seen, remnants of fibrotic synovium seen, capsule feels thick on insertion of arthroscope, diminished capsular volume	
Pathological changes	Hypertrophic, hypervascular synovitis, rare inflammatory cell infiltrates, normal underlying capsule	Hypertrophic, hypervascular synovitis with perivascular and subsynovial scar, fibroplasias, and scar formation in the underlying capsule	"Burned out" synovitis without significant hypertrophy or hypervascularity, underlying capsule shows dense scar formation	

Data from Hannafin JA, Chiaia TA: *Clin Orthop* 372:95-109, 2000.
ROM, Range of motion.

der. Risk factors for adhesive capsulitis include female gender, diabetes mellitus, recent trauma to the shoulder, and immobility of the shoulder. Adhesive capsulitis occurs most commonly after the age of 40, and approximately 25% of those who develop adhesive capsulitis in one shoulder will subsequently develop it in the other shoulder. The four stages of adhesive capsulitis with different pathological changes, signs, and symptoms are listed in Table 7-1.

Ligament Sprain. A ligament sprain is a stretch or tear of a ligament. Ligament sprains are graded according to severity. A first-degree sprain is one where there is minimal loss of structural integrity. There is no loss of motion, little or no swelling, and little to no functional loss, although there is usually some localized tenderness and slight bruising. Patients can generally return to activity immediately with some protection and can resume full unprotected activity within 10 days to 2 weeks. A second-degree sprain is one where the ligament is weakened. Initially there is loss of motion, bruising, and swelling with pain at the limits of motion. Immobilization and/or protection are necessary to prevent further injury and it may take 2 to 3 months for the patient to return to full activity. A third-degree sprain is when the ligament is completely torn; this causes excessive motion and potential joint instability, significant bruising, and often bleeding within the joint.[55]

LE sprains are more common than UE or axial sprains because of the forces placed on the LE. Ankle sprains and knee sprains are both common, particularly in sports participants. The history should help clarify the exact mechanism of injury, which, in conjunction with a careful physical examination with attention to palpation and provocative tests of ligaments, should allow isolation of the specific structure(s) involved. Fractures can often occur in conjunction with ligament sprains. Therefore if the patient cannot bear weight after an injury consistent with a ligament sprain, they should be referred to the physician immediately for x-rays.[56]

Muscle Strain. A muscle strain is a stretch or a tear of a muscle and is the most common injury in sports. Muscle strains typically occur near the myotendinous junction of muscles crossing two or more joints.[57] When muscle damage occurs, force production is initially reduced due to muscle fiber disruption and inflammation. It has also been found that muscle function is reduced further approximately 24 hours after the initial injury. Although the mechanism for this delayed effect is poorly understood, it is thought to be caused by a neutrophil-mediated response that results in further muscle injury.[58] As with ligaments sprains, muscle strains are categorized into three degrees according to severity. These degrees reflect similar types of tissue damage and physical findings as in ligaments sprains and cause similar functional limitations for similar periods of time.[55] One notable physical finding with a third-degree muscle strain (i.e., a complete tear) is that the muscle will not be able to generate any force and will be seen to "ball up" when contraction is attempted (Fig. 7-5).

Tendinitis. Tendinitis is an acute inflammatory condition of the tendon and its surrounding structure that may lead to degeneration (tendinosis or angiofibroblastic dysplasia), if not treated appropriately (Fig. 7-6). Often, persistent low-grade inflammation and gradual weakening

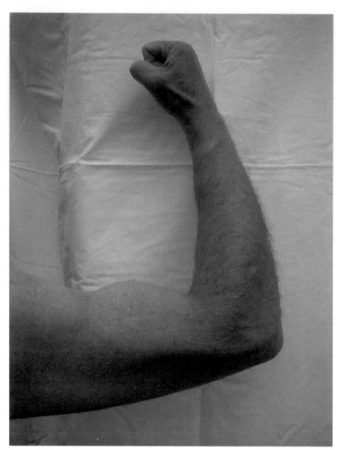

FIG. 7-5 Third-degree muscle strain (complete tear) of the biceps. Note that the muscle belly has balled up during contraction.

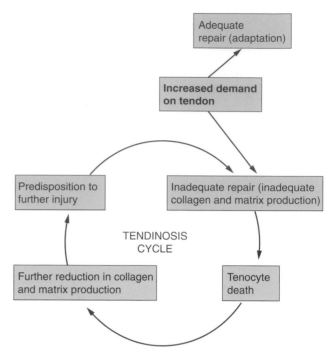

FIG. 7-6 Tendinosis cycle. *Redrawn from Leadbetter WB:* Clin Sports Med *11:533-578, 1992.*

of the tissues goes unrecognized until macrotrauma occurs (partial tear). Overuse and abnormal biomechanics are primarily responsible for eventual tendon failure.[59] Associated risk factors include but are not limited to a sudden increase in physical activity, age (peak incidence 30-50 years of age), decreased vascularity, abnormal joint alignment or altered ROM, and strength deficits or imbalances.[60]

Current and recent studies indicate that the chronic tendon disorders that commonly occur at the shoulder, elbow, knee, or ankle involve a degenerative process (called tendinosis), as well as or more than an inflammatory process (appropriately called tendonitis).[59,60] Since both degeneration and inflammation may occur together, some authors prefer to use the term tendinopathy.[60] Tendinitis (tendinosis, tendinopathy) can be divided into the following 5 stages, which range from less to more severe:[55]

Grade I: Least severe pain, only occurs with activity, does not interfere with performance, generalized tenderness, and disappears before the next exercise session.

Grade II: Minimal pain with activity, localized tenderness, does not interfere with activity intensity or duration.

Grade III: Interferes with activity but usually disappears between sessions, localized tenderness.

Grade IV: Interferes with intensity of training and does not disappear between activity sessions, significant localized pain, tenderness, crepitus, and swelling.

Grade V: Most severe form, interferes with sports and ADLs, symptoms are chronic or recurrent, signs of tissue changes and altered muscle function.

Tenosynovitis. Tenosynovitis, or paratendinitis, refers to an inflammation of the synovial sheath. Like tendinitis, the term tenosynovitis is used to describe both inflammatory and noninflammatory conditions.[61] The tendons at the wrist and ankle have synovial sheaths that encompass them to help the tendons glide freely as they pass between bone and the retinaculum (Fig. 7-7). The synovial sheath produces synovial fluid to help reduce friction and protect the tendon.[61] Synovial sheaths may become damaged or inflamed as the result of systemic disease (rheumatic conditions), trauma, overuse, or retinacular thickening. This may result in the tendon sheath thickening that can cause nodular swelling or narrowing of the tendon.[61,62]

De Quervain's tenosynovitis is stenosing tenosynovitis of the synovial sheaths surrounding the abductor pollicis longus and the extensor pollicis brevis tendons just proximal to the wrist. It is one of the more common examples of tenosynovitis in the UE. In trigger finger and trigger thumb, stenosis of the tendon sheath and hypertrophy or swelling of the flexor tendon lead to a snapping or locking of the digit.[62,63]

The diagnosis of tenosynovitis is based on signs and symptoms.[64] Finkelstein's test is the discriminative test for de Quervain's tenosynovitis[61]; unfortunately there are no discriminative clinical tests for trigger finger.

Fasciitis. In the extremities there are two functional types of fascia, the superficial fascia and the deep fascia. The superficial layer acts as the basal layer of the skin. It

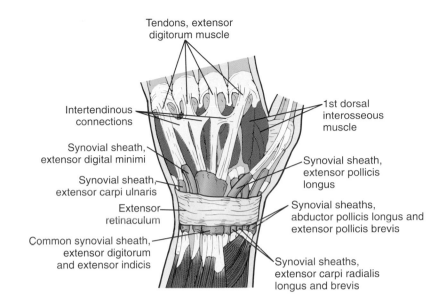

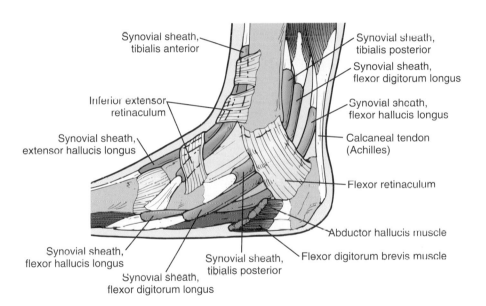

FIG. 7-7 Synovial sheaths of the wrist and ankle.

is designed to allow movement of the skin, to provide support and give shape, and to protect deeper structures from excessive pressures. The deeper fascia is much thicker, and the fibers are more organized and have major muscular and bony attachments. It serves a similar function to its more superficial counterpart. The plantar aponeurosis is the one of the thickest fascia in the body and is composed of superficial and deep fascia.[64]

Plantar Fasciitis. Plantar fasciitis is a localized inflammatory condition of the plantar aponeurosis. It is frequently cited as the most common cause of unilateral localized heel pain in sedentary or athletic adults.[65-67] The condition generally develops over 6 weeks (in patients who seek immediate care) to 12 months.[68,69]

Plantar fasciitis is thought to be caused by overuse although the exact mechanism is unclear. A recent matched case-control study (n = 50) linked three risk factors to plantar fasciitis: limited dorsiflexion, obesity

(BMI $>30 \, kg/m^2$), and a workday that involved self-reported weight bearing for most of the day. The authors acknowledge that it is impossible to know if these risk factors, particularly the limited dorsiflexion and obesity, were the cause or the result of plantar fasciitis and that their findings could not be generalized to an athletic population.[66] Others suggest that shoes with poor cushioning, pes cavus or planus, increase in running/walking distance or intensity, or a hard running/walking surface may increase the risk for plantar fasciitis.[68,69]

Currently there is no gold standard for the diagnosis of plantar fasciitis except clinical symptoms (pain with weight bearing especially during the initial steps in the morning or after sitting for prolonged periods) and signs (reproduction of symptoms with palpation at the medial tubercle of the calcaneus).[66,69] Important differential diagnoses include rupture of the plantar fascia, enthesopathies, stress fracture, infection, cancer, *Paget's disease,* fat pad atrophy, tarsal tunnel syndrome, injury to the medial calcaneal branch of tibial nerve, and S1 radiculopathy.[68]

Tensor Fascia Lata Fasciitis. Tensor fascia lata fasciitis, also known as iliotibial band friction syndrome (ITBFS), is an overuse injury with a population specific incidence. This syndrome is caused by repetitive rubbing of the iliotibial band over the lateral femoral condyle during knee flexion and extension. Most friction is reported to occur with movement through 30 degrees of knee flexion, although this was not substantiated in a study using magnetic resonance imaging (MRI) (16 subjects with ITBFS) and MR arthrography (6 cadaver knees).[70] Perceived causes for ITBFS include certain anthropometric and biomechanical characteristics (e.g., genu varum), inadequate flexibility of the iliotibial band, weak hip abductor (gluteus medius), inappropriate foot wear, and training surface conditions (hilly or crowned).[71]

Prenatal and Postnatal Soft Tissue Inflammation. The physiological changes that occur during pregnancy predispose women to a range of soft tissue inflammation conditions. During pregnancy, hormonal changes, ligament laxity, weight gain and redistribution, and soft tissue swelling place the woman at risk for musculoskeletal strains that may cause injury or exacerbate prior injuries. Common musculoskeletal impairments prenatally and postnatally include low back pain, pubic pain, hip and knee pain, carpal tunnel syndrome, and de Quervain's tenosynovitis.[72]

Low back pain is the most common musculoskeletal disorder among pregnant women. Predisposing factors include previous injury, prior pregnancies, and increasing age. Although the incidences of herniated discs are relatively low with pregnancy, there is a higher incidence of spondylolisthesis in *multiparous* women (see Chapter 8).

Pelvic pain during pregnancy generally occurs if the pubic symphysis widening causes inflammation. This usually begins during the tenth to twelfth weeks of pregnancy. Walking and bending exacerbate pain, and gait analysis may reveal an increased waddling gait.

Hip pain can be the result of pubic symphysis pain, sacroiliac pain, bursitis, or hip joint pathology *(osteonecrosis or osteitis pubis)*. Knee pain is usually the result of tracking difficulties. Carpal tunnel syndrome (the second most common musculoskeletal disorder during pregnancy after low back pain) and de Quervain's tenosynovitis are the result of swelling and inflammation.

EXAMINATION

PATIENT HISTORY

The patient history should include the patient's description of their current condition and its evolution. This will help the clinician determine the stage and severity of the disorders and, the likely structures involved.[73] A description of the activity when the symptoms started may also indicate the mechanism of injury and the likely affected tissues.

The nature of a patient's symptoms may also clarify their diagnosis. Stiffness after inactivity that eases with movement is generally thought to indicate inflamma-

tion.[73,74] Stiffness that lasts more than an hour and occurs primarily in the morning is commonly associated with arthritic inflammation, although these symptoms are not always present and cannot be considered diagnostic.[73,74]

A visual analog scale (VAS; see Chapter 22) can be used to establish a baseline for symptom severity before or during an activity and at rest. The responsiveness of symptoms to activity also gives an indication of severity, with pain that occurs at rest indicating a more severe problem than pain that only occurs during or after activity.[75]

General demographics should include information, such as age, gender, race/ethnicity, education, and language, because these can affect the probability of certain pathologies as previously noted. Social history can elicit cultural beliefs and behaviors, resources, and support that affect the client's condition. Growth and development, living environment, general health status, prior level of fitness, family history, and past medical and surgical history are all factors that contribute to the client's reason for seeking care.[2]

An employment or work history should focus on information about repetitive movements, exposure time, environmental risk factors (temperature, humidity, equipment), posture-related risk factors (excessive or sustained postures), and psychological stresses. All of these factors can contribute to localized inflammation.[76]

SYSTEMS REVIEW

The systems review is used to target areas requiring further examination and to define areas that may cause complications or indicate a need for precautions during the examination and intervention processes. See Chapter 1 for details of the systems review.

The systems review can help differentiate between constitutional (systemic) signs and symptoms that masquerade as a musculoskeletal injury. Fever and chills, diaphoresis (unexplained perspiration), night sweats (can occur during the day), nausea, vomiting, diarrhea, pallor, dizziness or syncope (fainting), fatigue, and rapid weight loss are all manifestations of nonmusculoskeletal pathology. The therapist's role is not to differentiate among the various causes of systemic signs and symptoms but to identify when a client's history and physical examination are inconsistent with the presence of a musculoskeletal injury.[77]

TESTS AND MEASURES
Musculoskeletal

Posture. Posture should always be examined because an individual may develop or assume an unwanted position as a result of pain arising from localized inflammation. When a part is injured, the body naturally splints the area to prevent further injury. This immobilization can lead to faulty biomechanics, which can perpetuate stress and strains on bones, joints, ligaments, capsules, and muscles.[78] Postural asymmetry or altered alignment may correlate with gait abnormalities and altered ROM.[79]

Anthropometric Characteristics. Anthropometric characteristics (palpation, girth, volume measurements) are primarily used to measure soft tissue edema or joint effusion. These may take several days to develop or become apparent. Effusion can be difficult to detect and even harder to quantify. Changes are more easily appreciated in small superficial joints like the interphalangeal joints than in larger or deeper joints like the hip and the lumbar zygapophyseal joints. Effusion may be detected by placing fingers or thumbs on either side of a joint, then exerting pressure on the joint effusion with one hand, while the other examining hand attempts to detect an impulse wave.[80]

Girth[81] and volumetric measurements can be used to detect joint effusion, edema, or muscle atrophy. Volumetric measurements have been considered the gold standard. However, both methods have consistently shown good to high interrater and intrarater reliability (intraclass correlates [ICCs]: .82-1.0) on both the UE and LE.[82,83] They cannot be used interchangeably, and they may not be sensitive to small changes in interstitial edema.[84,85] Pretreatment and posttreatment measurements should be taken because differences between limbs can exist without pathology.[82,83] However, some authors suggest that more than 1.5 cm difference in the girth of the lower extremities indicates the presence of edema if there is no prior pathology.[86] Even if girth measurements are not different and there are no clinical signs, complaints of increased pressure within or around a joint may indicate edema or effusion.[84] There are other ways of detecting and quantifying localized inflammation (computed tomography, bioelectric impedance), but they are expensive and require special training and equipment.

Palpation is also used to detect temperature changes and joint line tenderness. Localized temperature changes are difficult to reliably detect through palpation[87] because of variations between individuals (age, gender, BMI, diurnal variations) and environmental factors (ambient temperatures, clothing). When palpation is used to detect joint line tenderness, if the examiner can reproduce the client's pain with a pressure that does not blanch the examiner's nail (approximately 4 kg/cm^2), the presence of localized pathology may be indicated.[80]

Range of Motion. Measures of ROM can help identify inflamed structures and provide important information about impairments and functional limitations. If inflammation and effusion are present, there will usually be a loss of active and passive ROM and a "boggy" or sluggish end-feel.[80] A goniometer is commonly used to measure ROM and has been found to be reliable and valid in a wide range of populations.[88,89]

Muscle Performance. Assessment of motor performance is necessary to characterize limitations of functional joint use, identify muscle or tendon injuries, track patient progress, and to help design an appropriate intervention program to facilitate recovery. However, results of strength testing should be interpreted with caution in this population because motor performance may be impaired by pain.

Although there are multiple methods to assess muscle strength, manual muscle testing (MMT) is appropriate for testing muscle performance in most patients with localized inflammation (see Chapter 5). MMT results are often graded on 5 point nonlinear scale. The reliability and sen-

sitivity of this scale becomes more questionable in the against gravity grades. It is recommended that the same therapist perform the MMT in a standardized position, since the intrarater reliability is better than the interrater reliability.[90]

Hand-held dynamometers may also be used to measure strength in this population. They provide a quantitative linear measure of strength, and as with MMT, have better intrarater reliability than interrater reliability.[91] To improve reliability with handheld dynamometers, an "isometric make test" should be used rather than an "isometric break test."[92] The therapist should place the hand-held dynamometer consistently in the same place for repeated testing.[93]

Joint Integrity and Mobility. When examining the integrity of the joint and its accessory (joint play/component) motions, it is important to note if there is laxity or hypomobility and in what direction. This should be compared to the uninvolved limb to determine what is normal and abnormal (pathological) for the individual.[94]

Neuromuscular

Pain. Pain can impact an individual's ability to function, their emotional state, and their quality of life. Common measurement scales, including the horizontal or vertical VAS, the verbal rating scale (VRS), verbal descriptor scales (VDS), and faces pain scales (FPS), can be used to assess pain in patients with localized inflammation (see Chapter 22). Although pain is a hallmark sign of localized inflammation, the absence of pain does not necessarily indicate that patient does not have pathology or functional deficits.[95]

Cardiovascular/Pulmonary

Aerobic Capacity and Endurance. Several standardized walking tests (2-minute, 6-minute, 12-minute, Shuttle, and Self-Paced) can be used to assess exercise tolerance and cardiovascular fitness in individuals with or without cardiopulmonary pathologies, including those with localized inflammation (see Chapter 23). These measures may also give the examiner insight into the individuals' ability to perform ADLs.[96]

Integumentary

Integumentary Integrity. The examination of patients with localized inflammation should include assessment for local warmth, swelling and redness (edema or effusion), temperature changes, tenderness, and muscle atrophy or hypertrophy.

Function

Gait, Locomotion, and Balance. In a patient with localized inflammation, impairments of ROM, edema, strength, sensation, pain, or other concomitant factors can affect gait, locomotion, and balance. A person's ability to ambulate depends on their ability to develop acceleration while maintaining relative stability. Impairments may cause noticeable compensations, deviations, or substitutions in the gait pattern. In general, patients with localized inflammation involving the lower extremities (e.g., trochanteric bursitis) may have reduced gait speed or a noticeable limp as a result of pain (known as an antalgic gait).[96] An antalgic gait may also indicate a long-term hip pathology (e.g., OA of the hip joint), resulting in weak hip abductors and a characteristic *Trendelenburg gait* (see Chapter 32).[74,97] Balance may also be impaired in patients with localized inflammation. This is largely due to changes in gait caused by pain or weakness (see Chapter 13).

Assistive and Adaptive Devices/Orthotic, Protective, and Supportive Devices. Patients with localized inflammation commonly use assistive and adaptive devices, as well as orthotic, protective, and supportive devices, to compensate for decreased muscle performance, ROM impairments, and loss of balance and to protect an inflamed area from further injury, inflammation, and damage. These devices should be examined for fit, function, and effectiveness.

Ergonomics and Body Mechanics. Ergonomics and body mechanics should always be examined in patients with localized inflammation because this may identify tasks or activities that contribute to the client's condition. The demands, frequency, duration of exposure, or position of the joints during activity can over time cause microtrauma that then causes localized inflammation. Therefore a thorough evaluation of the patient's ergonomics and body mechanics at work, home, and in the leisure environment may help to establish, reduce, or prevent the cause(s) of their condition.

EVALUATION, DIAGNOSIS, AND PROGNOSIS

No one examination finding is more important than any other single finding in detecting localized inflammation. Rather, it is the combination of examination findings from the patient history, systems review, and tests and measures that allow for diagnosis and intervention planning. This is particularly true in patients with localized inflammation in whom the sensitivity and specificity of many tests and measures for specific pathologies are not known.[73,80]

According to the *Guide to Physical Therapist Practice,* patients who fall into the preferred practice pattern 4E: Impaired joint mobility, motor function, muscle performance, and ROM associated with localized inflammation often have the following abnormal examination findings: Temperature changes, joint swelling, loss of ROM, altered function, joint line tenderness, *fluctuance,* and localized pain when the inflamed tissues are stressed.[80] These patients should demonstrate steady improvement and optimal return to function within 6 to 24 physical therapy visits over 2 to 4 months.[2] The optimal number of visits and time frames for each client is determined in part by the pathology, the duration of the event, and any associated concomitant factors that could influence management (e.g., age, cognitive status, overall health status, smoking, social support).

Currently, there is evidence to suggest that involvement in a rehabilitation program can improve the outcomes of individuals with inflammatory conditions of the joint and surrounding soft tissues such as OA[98] and rheumatoid arthritis.[99] Rehabilitation can limit the formation of edema,[100] help control pain,[101] and allow the person to return to function earlier.[102] The rehabilitation

specialist can use physical agents, manual therapy, bracing (splinting and orthotics), strengthening and stretching exercise, work site modification (ergonomics and tool modification), and patient education to promote recovery and protect the client from further injury.

Outcomes for patients with localized inflammation may be measured in various ways. In addition to changes in impairment findings on the examination, various self-administered health status instruments are available to assess the status of patients at a higher level. The Western Ontario and McMaster Universities Arthritis Index (WOMAC) is an instrument specifically designed to examine pain, stiffness, and physical function in clients with primary OA of the knee and/or hip.[103] The SF-36v2, a generic self-administered measure of health-related quality of life, has been used to measure the impact of variety of diseases and conditions on the general population and may also be used to measure outcome in patients with localized inflammation. This tool measures physical functioning, role limitations that result from physical and emotional health, pain, general health perceptions, vitality, social functioning, mental health, and perceived change in health and takes 5-10 minutes to complete.[103]

INTERVENTION

The rehabilitation professional should consider the management of inflammatory conditions in two stages, the acute stage and the restorative stage.[11] During the acute stage, interventions should focus on controlling the inflammatory process, minimizing further injury, promoting healing, and minimizing or eliminating any associated signs and symptoms. Often, clinicians use physical agents, bracing, or wraps to help protect and limit swelling. Prolonged immobilization should be avoided because this can cause weakness and loss of ROM.[104] Patient education should include joint protection, rest, and edema management principles. Other principles of treatment at this stage include promoting healing, reducing or eliminating pain, and maintaining current cardiovascular fitness. This stage usually lasts a few days to a week, depending on the severity of the injury and the tissues involved.[11]

The second stage or the restorative stage begins as the acute stage or inflammatory phase subsides. The timing of this will vary depending on the injury and the extent of the damage. This stage coincides with the proliferative phase of tissue healing. The goals of this stage are to establish full pain-free ROM, increase or restore flexibility, improve or restore cardiovascular and muscular fitness and performance (strength, power, and endurance), and address any other neuromuscular deficits (proprioception, coordination, agility, and balance). The ultimate outcome of this stage should be to return the individual to their prior or desired level of function.[11]

PROTECT, REST, ICE, COMPRESSION, AND ELEVATION

PRICE is an acronym for protect, rest, ice, compression, and elevation. This acronym is used to describe the interventions recommended during the acute stage of localized inflammation. These interventions are intended to limit swelling and speed the client's return to activity.

Protection can be accomplished through the use of tape, bracing, an orthosis, or, in severe cases, casting. With acute soft-tissue musculoskeletal injuries a flexible or semi rigid orthosis is preferred to a rigid cast because experimental and clinical trails have shown that controlled motion results in greater patient satisfaction, early ROM and less strength loss, and a quicker return to activity than does complete immobilization.[102,105] The ideal device (taping, brace, inflatable cast) should limit the amount of torque applied to the injured area while avoiding disuse associated with prolonged immobilization. This "relative" rest is designed to limit damage to the injured structure while stimulating collagen alignment, preventing adhesions, improving circulation and proprioception, and maintaining muscle strength.[105]

Ice, compression, and elevation limit the formation of edema by reducing local tissue blood flow to the affected area. Ice limits hemorrhaging and edema formation by causing vasoconstriction of small vessels. Ice is also helps to control pain. Compression can reduce blood flow to an area. Moderate compression (40 mm Hg) is recommended because it sufficiently reduces local intramuscular blood flow by about 50%.[106] Elevation of the limb is the final component of PRICE. Elevation limits hemorrhage and reduces edema by reducing the arterial pressure in the elevated limb.

PHYSICAL AGENTS

Cryotherapy. Cryotherapy is the therapeutic application of cold or ice to a patient. Cryotherapy is often used to treat patients with acute localized inflammation because it reduces the formation of edema and hematoma associated with acute trauma and inflammation. Ice produces these effects by causing vasoconstriction, decreasing microvascular permeability, and reducing the rate of local tissue metabolism.[100,107] These effects may also protect the surrounding tissues from secondary trauma that result from pressure and enzymatic reactions.[108] Ice has been shown to reduce the formation of edema associated with injury in controlled clinical trials with animals. For example, a recent study found that ice significantly reduced edema, as compared with a control intervention, in rats after a contusion injury to muscle (n = 50, $p <$ 0.001).[100] Systematic reviews of the literature have found that there is good evidence that cryotherapy can reduce pain associated with soft tissue injuries.[108,109]

Cryotherapy may also be used during the restorative stage of rehabilitation in patients with localized inflammation. In particular, cryotherapy has been shown to help maintain improved ROM after the application of heat with stretching.[110] It is hypothesized that decreasing the viscoelasticity of the tissues in the stretched position helps maintain the new length and/or that nociceptive input is decreased, allowing tissues that were otherwise too sensitive to stretch to be engaged.[110]

Cryotherapy can be applied for localized inflammation using ice or cold gel packs, ice baths, cold compression pumps, or with ice massage. Differences in the thermodynamic properties of these agents may affect their rates of cooling, particularly of the superficial tissues. Ice packs have been shown to provide more rapid cooling of superficial tissues than gel packs at the same temperature.[108] This is probably because when ice changes from a solid to a liquid it has a greater capacity to absorb heat from the tissues. This difference in effect is less pronounced in deeper tissues because the effect is distributed over a larger volume of tissue.

Body fat may also insulate the deeper tissues from cooling as was demonstrated by Myrer et al's study that compared cooling rates of the calf soft tissue in 30 healthy college students with varying amounts of overlying fat, as measured by skinfold.[111] Ice was applied to all subjects for 20 minutes, and tissue temperature at 1- and 3-cm depth was measured every 10 seconds. Subjects with the least amount of subcutaneous fat (≤8 mm) cooled the most and the fastest, by 14.43° C at 0.72° C/min and by 6.22° C at 0.31° C/min at 1 cm and 3 cm depths, respectively. Those with the most subcutaneous fat (≥20 mm) cooled the least and the slowest, by 5° C at 0.25° C/min and by 2.42° C at 0.12° C/min at 1 cm and 3 cm depths, respectively.[111] This evidence suggests that patients with localized inflammation that lies deep to large amounts of adipose, or probably any other tissue, may benefit less from local application of cryotherapy than those with less overlying subcutaneous fat (Fig. 7-8).

Cryotherapy has been shown to improve clinical parameters in patients with localized inflammation. It has been shown to improve ROM, strength, and function in clients with radiographically confirmed OA at the knee when compared to standard treatment or a placebo.[112] A recent systematic review of randomized controlled clinical (RCT) trials using cryotherapy found marginal evidence (Physiotherapy Evidence Database [PEDro] Scale score of 3.4 out of 10) for the treatment of impairments (pain, ROM, edema) associated with acute soft-tissue injuries. Ice with exercise appeared to be the most effective combination. The most effective duration, mode, and frequency of cryotherapy application after an acute injury is unknown.[109] The Association of Chartered Physiotherapists in Sports Medicine recommend a 20-30 minute period of application, an interface (soft towel) between the subject and cooling agent, and that cold applied to an area

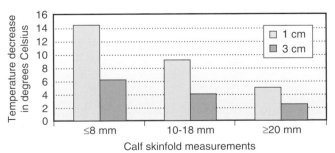

INTRAMUSCULAR TEMPERATURE CHANGES AFTER 20 MINUTES OF ICE PACKS

FIG. 7-8 Effect of adipose tissue on muscle cooling with ice packs.[111] *Data from Myrer WJ, Myrer KA, Measom GJ, et al: J Athl Train 36:32-36, 2001.*

of little muscle or adipose near superficial nerves be limited to 10 minutes.[113] These recommendations are made to reduce the risk of frostbite because full-thickness skin damage may occur with prolonged application of ice and/or when there is no interface between the cold modality and patient.[114]

Thermotherapy. Thermotherapy (heat) is used to decrease pain, promote relaxation, decrease muscle spasm, lower skin impedance, decrease the stiffness of joints, promote collagen extensibility, increase local tissue metabolism, promote vasodilatation, and accelerate healing.[115,116] However, it should not be used in the acute stage of an injury because it may worsen edema and inflammation. There are many modalities that produce heat: hot packs, ultrasound, diathermy, paraffin baths, fluidotherapy, whirlpools, and infrared lamps. These modalities can be divided into two broad categories of superficial (<1 cm) and deep (>1 cm) heat. Ultrasound and diathermy are the only heating modalities listed that are considered deep heaters. The rest are superficial heating agents that can be categorized as moist or dry and as having a constant or declining source of energy.[115]

When heating modalities are properly applied, metabolic, vascular, neuromuscular, and soft tissue extensibility are affected. Heat increases the rate of metabolic activity, which increases oxygen consumption and phagocytosis. Increases in tissue temperature are also usually associated with vasodilatation and an increase in blood flow to the area that helps provide nutrients and leukocytes to that area, thereby increasing the rate of clearing metabolites, decreasing pain or muscle spasm, and increasing capillary permeability and fluid exchange. Neuromuscular effects of heat include decreased pain, general relaxation, decreased skin impedance, decreased muscle spasm and spasticity, and increases in nerve conduction velocity and neuronal firing.[115] Thermotherapy is often used to promote flexibility and soft tissue extensibility,[117] which should decrease joint stiffness in patients with chronic localized inflammation. Superficial heat can be used to promote muscle relaxation and flexibility,[118] but it will probably not increase the blood flow to the underlying muscles.[115] It is recommended that the targeted tissues be heated between 104° F (40° C) to 113° F (45° C) for 5-10 minutes to increase their extensibility.[115]

Ultrasound. Therapeutic ultrasound (US) has been studied and used to manage a variety of conditions from soft tissue injuries to malignant tumors for over 70 years.[119] Current indications for rehabilitation specialists include contractures (joint capsule, scar tissue, or other soft tissue shortening), facilitating stretching,[120] pain control,[121] noninfected dermal ulcers,[122] surgical skin incisions, tendon injuries and repairs,[123] bone fractures,[124-126] calcium deposits,[127] acceleration of inflammation,[128] drug delivery (phonophoresis),[129-132] and conservative management of grade I or II tears of the meniscus.[133]

Therapeutic US produces thermal and nonthermal effects. Thermal effects include increased collagen extensibility, alterations in blood flow, changes in nerve conduction velocity, increased cell membrane permeability, increased tissue metabolism, and increased pain threshold.[115,119,134,135] Thermal US is recommended for use only

in the later stages of localized inflammation because, as with other forms of heat, thermal US may exacerbate edema and inflammation in the early stages.

Nonthermal effects of US include increased cell membrane permeability, increased intracellular calcium, increased rate of protein synthesis by fibroblasts, production of stronger collagen fibers, altered enzymatic activity, accelerated angiogenesis, increased macrophage responsiveness, accelerated bone healing, increased release of inflammatory mediators (prostaglandin E_2 and leukotriene B_4), and decreased length of the inflammatory stage of tissue healing.[119,132,134,136,137] Pulsed US is recommended in the acute stage of rehabilitation for patients with localized inflammation because its mechanical nonthermal effects may help stimulate and accelerate the inflammatory phase, leading to earlier resolution, and help relieve pain.[119,137,138] Even in degenerative conditions that lack clinical signs or symptom of inflammation, such as tendinosis, US may facilitate recovery.[119]

Phonophoresis, the use of US to facilitate transdermal drug delivery, is also a recommended intervention during the acute stage of rehabilitation for patients with localized inflammation.[132]

Selection of the optimal US treatment parameters, is based on the goals of the treatment (thermal or nonthermal), the depth of the tissue involved, and the area of the tissue involved (Fig. 7-9). Specific information on the application, precautions, and contraindications related to the application of US can be found in a text on physical agents.[132]

Electrical Stimulation. Electrical stimulation (ES) can be used to address the impairments (edema, pain, ROM, and force deficits) associated with localized inflammation. There is some evidence that ES may retard the formation of edema associated with acute localized inflammation. A number of studies using animal models found that negative polarity (i.e., cathode) reduces the formation of edema for up to 8 hours after tissue injury.[139-142] However, not all studies have shown such an effect,[143,144] and a recent study demonstrated that although cathodal ES retarded the formation of edema in the hind paws of rats after trauma, it was no more effective than immersion in cool water at 12.8° C (55° F) for a similar period of time. Similarly, Michlovitz and colleagues found that ice and ES were no more effective than ice alone in improving pain, edema, or ROM in patients with acute lateral ankle sprains.[145]

The studies that did find reduction of edema formation in response to ES applied within the first 24 hours after injury, using a monophasic pulsed current with a pulse rate of around 120 pulses per second, a current amplitude sufficient to produce a strong sensation, and a treatment duration of 20-90 minutes, with the cathode at the site of inflammation.

Transcutaneous electrical nerve stimulation (TENS) has been used effectively to treat acute and chronic conditions.[101,146,147] Reducing the pain allows increased activity levels, which lead to a quicker return to function and fewer visits.[101] Two prominent theories for this effect are the gate control theory and the release of endogenous opioids. The gate control theory of pain was originally

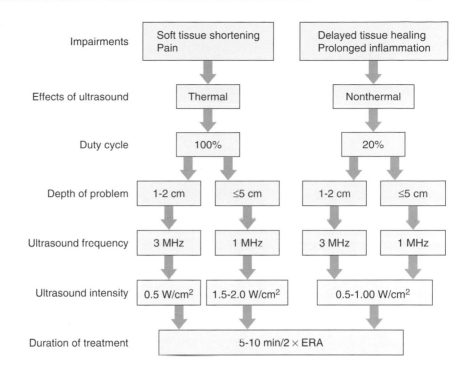

FIG. 7-9 US treatment parameters. *ERA,* Effective radiating area. *Redrawn from Cameron MH: Physical Agents in Rehabilitation: From Research to Practice, ed 2, St. Louis, 2002, WB Saunders.*

proposed by Melzack and Wall.[148] It is based on the theory that stimulation of larger diameter myelinated neurons (type I and II fibers) temporarily blocks the transmission from smaller diameter neurons (type III and IV fibers). Stimulating the larger diameter neurons decreases or inhibits the transmission of the smaller (nociceptive) neurons, reducing pain.[101,146,148] Descending inhibitory pathways may also be activated, reducing the amount of nociceptive input.[101,146]

There is also evidence that TENS may control pain by promoting the release of endogenous opioids. Opioids activate pathways from the periaqueductal gray and rostral ventral medulla, which inhibits transmission of nociceptive stimuli from spinothalamic tract cells.[101] Increased concentrations of endorphins and *enkephalins* have been measured in the bloodstream and cerebrospinal fluid of animals and humans after the use of high-frequency and low-frequency TENS, with the frequency of the stimulation affecting the type of opioid released.[101,149]

ES can also be used to promote ROM, increase muscular strength or endurance, and facilitate motor recruitment through stimulation of motor nerves sufficiently to produce muscle contractions. When used in this context, ES is referred to as neuromuscular ES (NMES). NMES and voluntary exercise with similar regimens both produce significant increases in strength (see Chapter 5). Adding NMES to exercise enhances strengthening, although this may not be true in individuals without pathology or strength deficits.[150-152] The optimal parameters, precautions, and contraindications for applying ES to improve muscle performance are discussed in chapter 5 of this book.

Iontophoresis. Iontophoresis is the application of an electrical current to promote transdermal drug delivery. The principle of iontophoresis is that low–amperage, direct monophasic electrical current will repel drug ions

with the same charge into and through the skin to the inflamed structure. Iontophoresis has been used successfully to delivery antiinflammatory drugs, such as dexamethasone, in sufficient concentrations to provide a therapeutic effect, although in lower concentrations than typical with localized injection.[153] Human studies have demonstrated that the delivery of dexamethasone by iontophoresis can produce immediate improvements in impairments associated with localized inflammation, including improved ROM and decreased pain.[154-156]

MANUAL THERAPY

Early mobilization has been suggested to promote early ROM and prevent joint contracture in patients with localized inflammation. However, there is limited evidence to support the use of manual therapy in acute and chronic inflammatory conditions.

One randomized controlled trial (RCT) reported that adding early passive joint accessory mobilization (anteroposterior) of the talocrural joint to the standard treatment of RICE (rest, ice, compression, elevation) in 17 patients with acute ankle sprains resulted in significantly quicker gains in pain-free dorsiflexion ROM and stride speed than in the control group (n = 18) who used RICE alone ($p < .01$ and $p < .05$, respectively), but there was no difference in how long it took for the subjects to return to normal activity.[157]

Another RCT examined the effectiveness of manual therapy and exercise in patients with OA of the knee and found this combination was more effective than placebo US (0.1 W/cm^2) or exercise alone at producing functional gains (6-minute walk test and WOMAC scale scores) and reducing the need for surgical intervention at 4-week, 8-week, and 1-year follow-up.[98] Placzek et al also reported successfully using an inferior and posterior mobilization at the shoulder to increase ROM, decrease pain, and improve functional scores in 31 patients with adhesive capsulitis (7.8 ± 2 months average duration of symptoms).[158] There was no control group, but all of the patients had failed to make substantial gains in physical therapy for 3 weeks before the intervention.[158]

THERAPEUTIC EXERCISE

Therapeutic exercise does not necessarily change the course of localized inflammation but may lessen the pain and disability associated with inflammatory conditions such as OA.[159] Exercise and physical activity can increase muscle strength and endurance, retard bone loss, control joint swelling and pain, improve joint lubrication, reduce joint stiffness, maintain or improve flexibility, increase aerobic fitness and reduce fatigue, reduce postural sway, prevent exacerbations and risk factors associated with a sedentary lifestyle, and promote weight management in patients with localized inflammation.[159-165] Exercise should address muscle performance, cardiovascular conditioning, flexibility, and proprioception.

The American College of Sports Medicine (ACSM) recommends that people with arthritis begin exercise slowly and progress gradually, avoiding rapid or repetitive movements of affected joints.[161] Since no one type of exercise has been proved to be more beneficial than another, it is recommended that exercises be well tolerated by the patient, focus on areas of deficits, and address the functional needs of the patient[166,167] (see Chapters 5 and 23). Exercises should be adapted to patients with localized inflammation to avoid overuse of and exacerbation of symptoms in areas with localized inflammation. For strengthening, exercise intensity may be progressed according to standard protocols.[168]

During an exacerbation of an inflammatory condition, repetitive movement involved in most strengthening exercises should be avoided. However, it is important to maintain ROM during such periods. Each joint should be moved through its full available ROM at least several times each day to prevent contractures. Static isometric exercises may also be performed to maintain strength. As inflammation resolves, isotonic or dynamic exercise may be started, initially emphasizing low resistance and high repetitions (reps).[169]

Cardiovascular fitness programs for patients with localized inflammation should use low-impact exercises that use large muscle groups in a smooth and continuous manner. Examples include walking, bicycling, swimming, and even dancing.[166,170,171] Exercise intensity is most readily guided by the patient's perceived level of exertion. A level between 11 and 16 on the Borg scale of perceived exertion is appropriate for most patients with localized inflammation.[172] (Chapter 23 includes a discussion of perceived exertion scales including the Borg scale.)

Patients with localized inflammation benefit from exercises to enhance flexibility because poor flexibility increases the risk of injury and interferes with function. Stretching of major muscle groups should be emphasized. Static stretching should be performed slowly to the point of mild discomfort and held for 10-30 seconds. Longer durations do not appear to significantly enhance flexibility. If proprioceptive neuromuscular facilitation (PNF) techniques are used, a 6 second contraction should be held, followed by static stretching for 10-30 seconds. For either method, each muscle group should be stretched at least 3 times 2-3 days each week.[171,173]

Proprioception may decline with age and joint disorders such as OA at the knee.[30] Inadequate proprioception can lead to repetitive trauma at the joint. In particular, patients with a history of recurrent injuries to the same area and those reporting a feeling of instability or giving way at a joint may benefit from proprioceptive exercises.[57,174] Support sleeves have also been recommended to increase proprioceptive input to enhance a feeling of stability.[175]

Aquatic exercises can be used as an exercise regime when a client has impaired ROM, strength, muscle power, endurance, or balance. As with any other tool, it may not be appropriate for all individuals within a specified practice pattern. The physical properties of water can unload a joint if the water depth is sufficient, while providing varying amounts of resistance, depending on the speed of the movement, depth of the part, the direction of movement, viscosity of the water, and the surface area of the part being moved. The effects of the hydrostatic forces can result in a physiological changes (e.g., increased cardiac output by 32%, decreased vital capacity by 8%) when the client is immersed up to their neck.[176] Therefore appropriate screening must be performed before its implementation.

ORTHOTICS

Orthotics, including braces, taping, and splints, are recommended for patients with localized inflammation to limit the load imposed on the affected structures. This can help the individual return to activity sooner and limit exacerbation of inflammation and local tissue damage. Shoe orthoses, or even shoes with good support, can limit excessive pronation or decrease the demand placed on the Achilles' tendon. A brace, strap, or taping placed over the patellar tendon can assist in the recovery of jumper's knee (patellar tendinitis/tendinosis), although it does little to reduce the load to the tendon.[177] Other devices include straps for lateral epicondylitis, neoprene sleeves for knee OA[175] or an unloading brace for unilateral medial compartment OA,[178] compression boots[179] or stabilizing braces for lateral ankle sprains,[180] hand splints for patients with arthritis affecting the hands, orthoses for the spine, and others depending on the patient's condition and needs (see Chapter 34).

PATIENT EDUCATION

Patient education is aimed at empowering individuals to manage their pathology and its effect on their daily life.[181] Effective education allows the patient to become their own diagnostician about what activities are harmful or helpful and allows them to recognize an exacerbation and implement an appropriate plan to manage it.

Patient education should include information about pathology, methods to reduce inflammation and pain, joint protection strategies, methods to increase function (exercise and ADL training), modification of the home and work environment, and coping strategies. Therapists

BOX 7-1	Common Joint Protection Principles

1. Respect pain.
2. Avoid improper postures or positions.
3. Avoid staying in one position for a long time.
4. Use the strongest and largest joints and muscles for the job.
5. Avoid sustained joint activities.
6. Maintain muscle strength, joint ROM and conditioning.
7. Use assistive devices and/or splints.

From Schwarz SP: *250 Tips for Making Life with Arthritis Easier,* Atlanta, 1997, Longstreet Press.

may use handouts, videotapes, or other educational methods to augment education through direct verbal communication.

JOINT PROTECTION AND TOOL MODIFICATION

Box 7-1 lists common joint protection techniques.[99] Assistive devices can also be used to reduce joint impact during ambulation. Recommendation for joint protection may range from elevating toilets and seats for those with LE or spinal impairments to changing or enlarging the grips of commonly used kitchen or work appliances to providing assistive devices for getting dressed (e.g., buttonhook device). There is evidence from randomized controlled trails to support that joint protection reduces pain and improves function in patients with localized inflammation[182] and may even slow the progression of inflammatory diseases.[99]

To optimize recommendations for joint protection to prevent or reduce functional deficits associated with localized inflammation, an assessment of environmental barriers in the home, community and/or work, is recommended (see Chapter 35 of this book). Vibration, mechanical shock, high palmar and gripping loads, external loads, hard and sharp edges, poor postures, and repetitive movements, as well as extremes of temperature, humidity, and psychological stress, may all impact the occurrence of and functional limitations associated with localized inflammation.[183,184]

PACING STRATEGIES (CONSERVATION OF ENERGY)

Pacing strategies involve breaking down daily activities into manageable tasks and devising a strategy for accomplishing those tasks. Pacing requires finding a balance between rest and activity. If a client's symptoms are exacerbated by their current level of activity, they may still be able to complete those activities if they do small amounts at a time. For example, neither mowing the whole yard nor vacuuming the whole house has to be done all at one time or all in 1 day. If the yard takes 3 hours to mow, the person could incorporate an hour of rest for every hour of mowing or they could mow the front yard 1 day and the back yard the next. This takes more time overall, but this strategy may allow the person to achieve their own goals without further injury.

PSYCHOSOCIAL MANAGEMENT OF CHRONIC INFLAMMATORY DISEASES

Many chronic diseases like arthritis have no cure and will likely have periods of exacerbation with an unpredictable course. These may necessitate day-to-day adjustments in activity, as well as long-term adaptations to a gradual decline in functional capacity, with gradually increasing economic burden over several years.[181] These factors and others can result in stress, depression, and learned helplessness.

Learned helplessness occurs when the client stops trying because they feel helpless. They loose motivation because they do not feel that their efforts will affect the outcome. To combat these issues, it has been recommended that interventions for patients with chronic conditions involving localized inflammation include stress management, coping skills, cognitive restructuring, problem solving, behavior modification, altering a patient's perception and responses to pain, teaching the difference between harm and hurt, and educating family members about the patient's condition.[185]

CASE STUDY 7-1

OSTEOARTHRITIS

Examination
Patient History
JJ is a 53-year-old man who presents with complaints of right knee pain, which was diagnosed as being caused by OA. JJ had a right meniscectomy 30 years ago for a torn meniscus. He complains of morning stiffness and difficulty standing for more than 1 hour, walking for long periods (>20-30 minutes), and getting up and down from the floor. An x-ray of his right knee taken 3 weeks ago revealed unilateral medial compartment OA at the right knee with eburnated bone per the radiologist's report.

Systems Review

System	Results
Cardiovascular/ Pulmonary:	BP 140/90 mm Hg. No peripheral edema. HR 80 bpm, RR 14.
Integumentary:	Presence of well-healed surgical scar right knee. No trunk, head, or UE skin color changes. Decreased hair growth on both legs.
Musculoskeletal:	ROM: Limited right knee. JJ appears to have some atrophy of the right thigh. He is overweight and has a slight limp on the right and anterior trunk lean with initial contact on right during ambulation.
Neuromuscular:	Height is 5 foot 9 inches, JJ weighs 200 lb. Bilateral genu varus. Gross coordination, balance, and locomotion appear intact.

During communications with the therapist, JJ had no apparent deficits and appeared to be an informational type of learner.

Tests and Measures
Musculoskeletal

Posture JJ has a kyphotic-lordotic posture while standing and the lordosis reduces when sitting. Bilateral genu varus, 9 cm between medial femoral epicondyles with medial malleoli touching.

Anthropometric Characteristics Palpation of the right knee did not reveal temperature changes. Effusion of the right knee was detectable by palpating along the medial and lateral joint lines. There was no effusion of the left knee.

Circumferential Measurements

Area	Right	Left
10 cm above medial knee joint line	50 cm	53 cm
Knee joint line	43 cm	42.5 cm
10 cm below medial joint line	41.5 cm	42 cm

Range of Motion Bilaterally UE active ROM (AROM) without deficits, able to reach behind head and back with both UE without difficulty. Bilaterally LE within normal limits except at the knee which were as follows:

Flexion/extension	Right	Left
AROM (sitting)	115-15°	135-0°
Passive ROM (supine)	120-8°	140-0°

Muscle Performance MMT: Both UE 5/5, both LE 5/5 except both hip flexors 4/5, right quadriceps 4/5 (within available AROM), left 5/5. Extensor lag noted on right.

Joint Integrity and Mobility Right knee accessory (joint play/component) movements in all directions were decreased when compared to left.

Neuromuscular

Pain VAS:

What is pain currently? 2/10

When your pain is at its worst? 6/10

When your pain is at its best? 1/10

Reflex Integrity 2+ deep tendon reflexes (DTR) all extremities.

Sensory Integrity Circumferential dermatome testing at midthighs, knees, and midcalves revealed no deficits to light touch.

Cardiovascular/Pulmonary

Aerobic Capacity and Endurance Using a pedometer, JJ was able to ambulate 402 m (1318.9 feet) in 6 minutes with some shortness of breath, but he was able to converse (respiratory rate increased to 22). He was able to ascend 10 steps in 24.45 seconds.

Integumentary

Integumentary Integrity JJ has a well-healed 10 cm scar along anteromedial aspect of right knee.

Function

Gait, Locomotion, and Balance JJ has an anterior trunk lean at initial contact and decreased stance time on right. When going up and down stairs, he is not able to use a step-over gait because of knee pain and instability. No apparent balance deficits.

WOMAC LK3.1 (self-administered health status instrument) three subscales: Pain = 11/20, stiffness = 6/8, and physical function = 40/68.

Evaluation, Diagnosis, and Prognosis

The diagnosis for this patient is local inflammation of his knee joint caused by OA that limits his ability to engage in work, leisure, and household maintenance. The preferred practice pattern is 4E: Impaired joint mobility, motor function, muscle performance, and ROM associated with localized inflammation.[2] History and physical examination are consistent with OA. He describes a unilateral stiffness in the morning that diminishes quickly. Weight-bearing activities increase his pain. History of trauma,[19,29,35] prior meniscectomy,[36] genu varum,[36] participation in high impact sports,[36] and borderline obesity (BMI 29.5)[19] are all consistent with his given medical diagnosis of OA.

Goals

1. JJ will perform his job duties while standing for more than 2 hours in 1 month.
2. JJ will get up and down from the floor without difficulty in 1 month.
3. JJ will carry 24 lb (grandson's projected weight) up and down the steps without fear of falling in 2 months.
4. JJ will mow his yard in 1½ hours without exacerbating his knee pain in 3 months.

Prognosis

Prognosis for JJ's condition is good. He should demonstrate steady improvement and optimal return to function within 2-4 months.

Plan of Care

JJ will be seen initially 3 times a week for 2 weeks, then 2 times a week for 2 weeks, then 2 weeks later, and then for a final time 1 month later for final program adjustment. Interventions will initially concentrate on restoring ROM and improving strength. Pain should subside as ROM and strength improve. Patient will also be enrolled in the Arthritis Foundation aquatics program and given UE strengthening exercises to promote weight loss and cardiovascular endurance. Patient will progress to land-based exercises as tolerated. Patient will be referred back to his physician for possible pharmacological management, management of hypertension, and possible referral to nutritionist for weight loss.

Intervention
Weeks 1-2

Flexibility: Bicycle ergometer for 5 minutes. Followed by grade III and IV joint mobilization (distraction, anteroposterior glide, and medial/lateral tilt), followed by supervised stretching (hamstrings, quadriceps, and calves) 20-30 seconds, 4 reps on both legs.

Strengthening: NMES (30 pps, 10 seconds on: 50 seconds off, 15 reps, intensity to maximal tolerance) to the right quadriceps in an open chain, attempting to reach terminal knee extension. Using a 3-inch step, with patient practicing controlled concentric and eccentric step-ups, 15 reps and 3 sets with right LE.

Home exercise program (HEP)

1. Flexibility: 2-3 times a day, 20-30 second static stretch, 3-4 reps of hamstrings and knee flexion.
2. Ambulating: 10 minutes 3 times a day (with attention to strong quadriceps contraction at heel strike), 5 days a week

3. Strengthening: 3 days a week, 15 reps, and 3 bouts of heel/toe raises, wall slides, standing leg curls (2 lb ankle cuff weight), seated leg extensions (2 lb ankle cuff weight).
4. Aerobic: UE ergometer 10 minutes, progressing to 15 minutes over 2 weeks at a light to moderate pace (11-12 on the Borg scale). Patient enrolled and participated in an aquatic aerobic conditioning program for 30 minutes 2 times a week.

Bracing: JJ was fitted with a brace designed to unload the medial compartment in patients with arthritis.

Weeks 3-4

Examination: JJ states his knee still feels unsteady when he becomes fatigued. He is still experiencing morning stiffness but can stand for longer periods of time before resting. He feels more in control when going up and down stairs. Gait: No anterior trunk lean at initial contact on right. Knee active ROM (sitting): Right 125-5 degrees, left 138-0 degrees. Passive ROM (supine): Right 130-3 degrees, left 143-0 degrees. Firm end-feel on right for flexion and extension. Effusion still present in right knee.

Exercise: Recumbent bicycling for 20-30 minutes at 50%-75% heart rate reserve maintaining a conversational pace. Followed by joint mobilization (described in week 1).

Strengthening: Machine leg press and curls. Progressed to a 5-inch step with patient practicing controlled concentric and eccentric step-ups, 15 reps, and 3 sets with right LE. Initiated upper body dumbbell training (military press, upright row, chest press, and biceps curls).

HEP Adjustments: JJ will continue with flexibility training. Ambulation modified by increasing duration to 20 minutes, 2 bouts, 5 days per week. Patient to continue with strengthening and increase ankle cuff weights to 3 lb. Add 5-inch stair training to HEP.

Patient to continue with Arthritis Foundation aquatics program, perform UE dumbbell training and leg extension press and curls on gym machines, and perform UE ergometry on gym machines for 15 progressing to 20 minutes at a moderate progressing to a hard pace (12-15 on the Borg scale) or follow-up with therapist in 2 weeks.

Week 6

Examination: 6-minute walk test: 453.3 meters (1487.2 feet) without shortness of breath (SOB) or anterior trunk lean on initial contact, able to ascend 10 stairs using step-over gait in 16.46 seconds. JJ can stand and work for more than 2 hours without discomfort. AROM (sitting): Right 130-2 degrees, left 135-0 degrees. PROM (supine): Right 135-0 degrees, left 140-0 degrees. Hard end-feel on both knees extension and firm for flexion extension. Effusion not detectable. MMT: Knee extension bilaterally 5/5, no extensors lag. JJ states morning stiffness is decreased, and he has lost approximately 8 lb in the last 6 weeks. He states he is only doing his flexibility training once a day but has continued with aquatics and gym training.

WOMAC LK3.1: Pain = 7/20, stiffness = 3/8, and physical function = 20/68.

HEP Adjustments: Continue with flexibility training daily, home strengthening program (progress to a 7-inch step), ambulate 30 minutes 5-7 days a week, and continue with aquatics/gym training at current perceived exertion levels. Follow-up and plan to discharge in 1 month.

Week 10

Examination: 6-Minute walk test: 460.4 meters (1510.4 feet) without SOB. Able to ascend 10 stairs using step over gait in 11.15 seconds. AROM (sitting): Right 135-3 degrees, left 138-0 degrees. PROM (supine): Right 140-1 degrees, left 145-0 degrees. There was no detectable joint effusion of either knee. Patient is able to mow yard in 1½ hours, although his knee feels stiff the next day. He is able to get up and down from the ground without difficulty. He has carried his grandson up and down the stairs, using a step-to-step gait but does not feel comfortable doing this with a step-over-step gait. Patient has continued faithfully with his HEP. Patient did follow-up with his physician and was referred to a nutritionist for assistance with meal planning and weight loss. Antihypertensive medication was considered but was not started because JJ's blood pressure measured 130/80 mm Hg at this time and was thought to be lower because of his weight loss and exercise. BP 130/80 mm Hg, HR 70 bpm, RR 12.

VAS pain scores: What is pain currently? 1/10 When your pain is at its worst? 3/10 When your pain is at its best? 1/10.

WOMAC LK3.1: Pain = 3/20, stiffness = 2/8, and physical function = 13/68.

HEP Adjustments: Patient to continue with flexibility training and walking program 5-7 days a week. He should continue with the aquatics and gym program indefinitely. He can stop the home strengthening program except for the step up/down exercise. He will need to continue this for another month or two and can now perform while holding 10 lb for the first month, progressing to 20 lb the second month (progressive exercise to simulate carrying grandchild). JJ has met all his goals, reports significant gains in his health status (WOMAC), and is independent in his HEP. He is ready to be discharged from physical therapy.

Please see the CD that accompanies this book for a case study describing the examination, evaluation, and intervention for a patient with lateral epicondylitis (tendinosis).

CHAPTER SUMMARY

This chapter describes the inflammatory process and how various pathologies associated with localized inflammation present. An organized and detailed review of the examination, evaluation, diagnosis, prognosis, and management of individuals in preferred practice pattern 4E is provided. Evidence for the use of interventions, including physical agents and therapeutic exercises, to reduce or minimize the impact the physiology or impairments associated with localized inflammation is presented. Case studies are used to provide an example of how this information is applied to practice. This chapter is to be used in conjunction with other chapters in this text to provide the most effective approach to management of clients with localized inflammation in your practice.

ADDITIONAL RESOURCES

Web Sites

Arthritis Foundation: www.arthritis.org/
The American College of Rheumatology: www.rheumatology.org/
The Bone and Joint Decade: www.boneandjointdecade.org/
National Institutes for Arthritis, Musculoskeletal, and Skin Diseases: www.niams.nih.gov/

GLOSSARY

Angiogenesis: Development and formation of blood vessels.

Body mass index (BMI): Relative measure of body fat calculated by dividing body weight (kilograms) by height squared (meters). It is sometimes referred to as the Quetelet index.

Cytokines: Proteins secreted by a variety of cells to help regulate immunological responses (e.g., interleukin, tumor necrosis factor, lymphokines, and interferon).

Enkephalins: Endogenous pentapeptide opiates (Leucine or Methionine) with analgesic activity and a short half-life.

Fibroblast: Connective tissue cell that secretes proteins (collagen, glycosaminoglycans, elastin, and glycoproteins) to help form the extracellular matrix. Fibroblasts have the ability to differentiate into other cells (e.g., osteoblasts, chondrocytes, and myofibroblasts).

Fluctuance: Abnormal condition in which the area under the skin being palpated feels "boggy" or viscous. It is an indication of pus accumulating, especially if the surrounding area is indurated.

Histamine: Chemical substance produced by mast cells with a wide range of effects, including capillary dilatation, vessel wall permeability, contraction of bronchial smooth muscle, increased gastric secretions, and decreased blood pressure.

Macrophage: Large cell whose primary role is phagocytosis and removal of pathogens. Macrophages produce a variety of substances (e.g., H_2O_2, ascorbic acid, fibronectin, lactic acid, and angiogenesis growth factor) to promote angiogenesis and wound debridement.

Multiparous: Having borne more than one child.

Myofibroblasts: Fibroblasts that differentiated to resemble smooth muscle (contains myofilaments) for the specialized function of approximating (contracting) the borders of an injury.

Neutrophils (granulocytes): Phagocytic white blood cells.

Osteoblasts: Bone forming cell.

Osteonecrosis: Necrosis of the bone (also avascular necrosis and ischemic necrosis of the bone).

Osteitis pubis: Noninfectious inflammation of the pubis.

Paget's disease: Chronic skeletal disorder characterized by inflammation of bones, resulting in thickening and softening of bones.

Prostaglandins: Originally recognized near the prostate, these hormone-like chemicals are found in almost all tissues in the body. They are potent biological mediators that have proinflammatory and antiinflammatory effects and that influence a variety of other physiological functions (e.g., metabolism, temperature regulation, and nerve conduction).

Trendelenburg gait: Disorder of the hip abductors caused by weakness or an inhibition. During the stance phase, the body weight is transferred to the affected side and the hip abductors on the affected side are unable to support the pelvis, resulting in a pelvic drop or tilt toward the swing limb. Although typically seen in adults, this gait pattern may be seen in children with a slipped capital femoral epiphysis.

References

1. Ballou SP, Kushner I: Laboratory evaluation of inflammation. In Harris Ed, Budd RC, Firestein GS, et al (eds): *Kelley's Textbook of Rheumatology*, ed 7, Philadelphia, 2005, WB Saunders.

2. American Physical Therapy Association: *Guide to Physical Therapist Practice*, ed 2, Alexandria, Va, 2001, The Association.

3. Klippel JH: Mediators of inflammation, tissue destruction, and repair. In Klippel JH, Crofford LJ, Stone JH, et al (eds): *Primer on the Rheumatic Diseases*, ed 12, Atlanta, 2001, Arthritis Foundation.

4. Mohammed FF, Smookler DS, Khokha R: Metalloproteinases, inflammation, and rheumatoid arthritis, *Ann Rheum Dis* 62(suppl II):ii43-ii47, 2003.

5. Trowbridge HO, Emling RC: Chronic inflammatory processes. In Trowbridge HO, Emling RC (eds): *Inflammation: A review of the process*, ed 5, Carol Stream, Ill, 1997, Quintessence Publishing.

6. Kannus P, Parkkari J, Jarvinen TL, et al: Basic science and clinical studies coincide: active treatment approach is needed after a sports injury, *Scand J Med Sci Sports* 13:150-154, 2003.

7. Gogia P: *Clinical Wound Management*, Thorofare, NJ, 1995, Slack.

8. Tidball JG: Inflammatory cell response to acute muscle injury, *Med Sci Sports Exerc* 27:1022-1032, 1995.

9. Kirsner RS, Bogensberger G: The normal process of healing. In Kloth LC, McCulloch JM, (eds): *Wound Healing: Alternatives in Management*, ed 3, Philadelphia, 2002, FA Davis.

10. Williams DT, Harding K: Healing responses of skin and muscle in critical illness, *Crit Care Med* 31(S8):S547-S557, 2003.

11. Houglum PA: Soft tissue healing and its impact on rehabilitation, *J Sport Rehabil* 1:19-39, 1992.

12. Goldring SR, Goldring MB: Biology of the normal joint. In Harris Ed, Budd RC, Firestein GS, et al (eds): *Kelley's Textbook of Rheumatology*, ed 7, Philadelphia, 2005, WB Saunders.

13. Geborek PU, Moritz, Wollheim FA: Joint capsular stiffness in knee arthritis: Relationship to intraarticular volume, hydrostatic pressures, and extensor muscle function, *Rheumatology* 16:1351-1358, 1989.

14. Klippel JH: The musculoskeletal system. In Klippel JH, Crofford LJ, Stone JH, et al (eds): *Primer on the Rheumatic Diseases*, ed 12, Atlanta, 2001, Arthritis Foundation.

15. Mow VC, Hung CT. Biomechanics of articular cartilage. In Nordin M, Frankel VH (eds): *Basic Biomechanics of the Musculoskeletal System*, ed 3, Philadelphia, 2001, Lea & Febiger.

16. Walker JM: Pathophysiology of inflammation, repair, and immobility. In Walker JM, Helewa A (eds): *Physical Rehabilitation in Arthritis*, ed 2, St. Louis, 2004, WB Saunders.

17. Zhang Y, Niu J, Kelley-Hayes M, et al: Prevalence of symptomatic hand osteoarthritis on functional status among the elderly: The Framingham study, *Am J Epidemiol* 156:1021-1027, 2002.

18. Jackson DW, Simon TM, Aberman HA: The articular cartilage repair dilemma. Symptomatic articular cartilage degeneration: The impact in the new millennium, *Clin Ortho Rel Res* 391S:S14-S25, 2001.

19. Felson DT, Zhang Y: An update on the epidemiology of knee and hip osteoarthritis with a view to prevention, *Arthritis Rheum* 41:1343-1355, 1998.

20. Brooks P: Inflammation as an important feature of osteoarthritis, *Bull World Health Organ* 81:689-690, 2003.

21. Cooper C, Campbell L, Byng P, et al: The epidemiology of osteoarthritis in the peripheral joints: Occupational activity and the risk of hip osteoarthritis, *Ann Rheum Dis* 55:680-682, 1996.

22. Martel-Pelletier J, Alaaeddine N, Pelletier JP: Cytokines and their role in the pathophysiology of osteoarthritis, *Front Biosci* 4:D694-D703, 1999.

23. Goldring MB: The role of cytokines as inflammatory mediators in osteoarthritis: lessons from animal models, *Connect Tissue Res* 40:1-11, 1999.

24. Klippel JH: Osteoarthritis. In Klippel JH, Crofford LJ, Stone JH, et al (eds): *Primer on the Rheumatic Diseases*, ed 12, Atlanta, 2001, Arthritis Foundation.

25. Shepstone L, Rogers J, Kirwan J, et al: The shape of the distal femur: A palaeopathological comparison of eburnated and non-eburnated femora, *Ann Rheum Dis* 58:72-78, 1999.

26. Goldring MB: The role of the chondrocytes in osteoarthritis, *Arthritis Rheum* 43:1916-1926, 2000.

27. Trueta J: *Studies of the Development and Decay of the Human Frame*, Philadelphia, 1968, WB Saunders.

28. Buckwalter JA: Articular cartilage injuries, *Clin Orthop* 402:21-37, 2002.

29. Buckwalter JA, Martin JA: Sports and osteoarthritis, *Curr Opin Rheumatol* 16:634-639, 2004.

30. Felson DT (conference chair): Osteoarthritis: New insights. Part 1: The disease and its risk factors, *Ann Intern Med* 133:635-646, 2000.

31. Oliveria SA, Felson DT, Reed JL, et al: Incidence of symptomatic hand, hip, and knee osteoarthritis among patients in a health maintenance organization, *Arthritis Rheum* 38:1134-1141, 1995.

32. Haara MM, Heliövaara M, Kröger H, et al: Osteoarthritis in the carpometacarpal joint of the thumb: Prevalence and associations with disability and mortality, *J Bone Joint Surg Am* 86(7):1452-1457, 2004.

33. Loughlin J: Genetic epidemiology of primary osteoarthritis, *Curr Opin Rheumatol* 13:111-116, 2001.

34. Holderbaum D, Haqqi TM, Moskowitz RW: Genetics and osteoarthritis: Exposing the iceberg, *Arthritis Rheum* 42:397-405, 1999.

35. Zhang Y, Glynn RJ, Felson DT: Musculoskeletal disease research: Should we analyze the joint or the person? *J Rheumatol* 23:1130-1134, 1996.
36. Conaghan PG: Update on osteoarthritis, Part 1: Current concepts and the relation to exercise, *Br J Sports Med* 36:330-333, 2002.
37. Acheson R, Chan Y, Clemmett AR: New Haven survey of joint diseases. XII. Distribution and symptoms in the hands with reference to handedness, *Ann Rheum Dis* 29:275, 1970.
38. Needs CJ, Webb J, Tyndall A: Paralysis and unilateral arthritis: is the association established? *Clin Rheumatol* 4:176, 1985.
39. Kujala UM, Kettunen J, Paananen H, et al: Knee osteoarthritis in former runners, soccer players, weight lifters, and shooters, *Arthritis Rheum* 38:539-546, 1995.
40. Foss MVI, Byers PD: Bone density, osteoarthritis of the hip and fracture of the upper end of the femur, *Ann Rheum Dis* 31:259, 1972.
41. Dequeker J: The relationship between osteoporosis and osteoarthritis, *Clin Rheum Dis* 11:271, 1985.
42. Shell D, Perkins R, Cosgarea A: Septic olecranon bursitis: Recognition and treatment, *J Am Board Fam Pract* 8:217-220, 1995.
43. Shbeeb MI, Matteson EL: Trochanteric bursitis (greater trochanter pain syndrome), *Mayo Clin Proc* 71:565-569, 1996.
44. Akisue T, Yamamoto T, Marui T, et al: Ischiogluteal bursitis: Multimodality imaging findings, *Clin Orthop* 406:214-217, 2003.
45. Gnanadesigan N, Smith RL: Knee pain: Osteoarthritis or anserine bursitis? *J Am Med Dir Assoc* 4:164-166, 2003.
46. Aydingoz U, Oguz B, Aydingoz O, et al: The deep infrapatellar bursa: Prevalence and morphology on routine magnetic resonance imaging of the knee, *J Comput Assist Tomogr* 28:557-561, 2004.
47. Dutton M (ed): The knee joint complex. In *Orthopaedic Examination, Evaluation, & Intervention*, New York, 2004, McGraw-Hill.
48. Talbot-Stern J: Bursitis, Emedicine December 28, 2004. Available at http://www.emedicine.com/emerg/topic74.htm
49. van der Windt DA, Koes BW, de Jong BA, et al: Shoulder disorders in general practice: incidence, patient characteristics, and management. *Ann Rheum Dis* 54:959-964, 1995.
50. Dutton M (ed): The shoulder complex. In *Orthopaedic Examination, Evaluation, & Intervention*, New York, 2004, McGraw-Hill.
51. DePalma MJ, Slipman CW, Siegleman E, et al: Interspinous bursitis in an athlete, *J Bone Joint Surg Br* 86:1062-1064, 2004.
52. Matsumoto K, Okabe H, Ishizawa M, et al: Intermetatarsophalangeal bursitis induced by a plantar epidermal cyst, *Clin Orthop* 385:151-156, 2001.
53. Webner D, Drezner JA: Lesser trochanteric bursitis: A rare cause of anterior hip pain, *Clin J Sport Med* 14:242-244, 2004.
54. Lee MH, Ahn JM, Muhle C, et al: Adhesive capsulitis of the shoulder: Diagnosis using magnetic resonance arthrography, with arthroscopic findings as the standard, *J Comput Assist Tomogr* 27:901-906, 2003.
55. Reid DC: Connective tissue healing and classification of ligament and tendon pathology. In Reid DC: *Sports Injury Assessment and Rehabilitation*, New York, 1992, Churchill Livingstone.
56. DiGiovanni BF, Partal G, Baumhauer JF. Acute ankle injury and chronic lateral instability in the athlete, *Clin Sports Med* 23:1-19, 2004.
57. Järvinen TA, Kääriäinen M, Järvinen M, et al: Muscle strain injuries, *Curr Opin Rheumatol* 12:155-161, 2000.
58. Tidball JG: Interactions between muscle and the immune system during modified musculoskeletal loading, *Clin Orthop* 403S:100-109, 2002.
59. Dutton M (ed): The response of biological tissue to stress. In *Orthopaedic Examination, Evaluation, & Intervention*, New York, 2004, McGraw-Hill.
60. Almekinders SC, Temple JD: Etiology, diagnosis, and treatment of tendinitis: an analysis of the literature, *Med Sci Sports Exerc* 30:1183-1190, 1998.
61. Moore JS: De Quervain's tenosynovitis: Stenosing tenosynovitis of the first dorsal compartment, *J Occup Environ Med* 39:990-1002, 1997.
62. Moore JS: Flexor tendon entrapment of the digits (trigger finger and trigger thumb), *J Occup Environ Med* 42:526-545, 2000.
63. Gorsche R, Wiley JP, Preston J, et al: Prevalence and incidence of stenosing flexor tenosynovitis (trigger finger) in meat-packing plant, *J Occup Environ Med* 40:556-560, 1998.
64. Palastanga N, Field D, Soames R (eds): *Anatomy and Human Movement: Structure and Function*, Oxford, 1989, Heinemann Medical Books.
65. DiGiovanni BF, Nawoczenski DA, Lintal ME, et al: Tissue-Specific plantar fascia-stretching exercise enhances outcomes in patients with chronic heel pain: A prospective, randomized study, *J Bone Joint Surg Am* 85:1270-1277, 2003.
66. Riddle DL, Pulisic M, Pidcoe P, et al: Risk factors for plantar fasciitis: A matched case-control study, *J Bone Joint Surg Am* 85:872-877, 2003.
67. Wearing SC, Smeathers JE, Urry SR: The effect of plantar fasciitis on vertical foot-ground reaction force, *Clin Orthop* 409:175-185, 2003.
68. Buchbinder R: Plantar fasciitis, *N Engl J Med* 350:2159-2166, 2004.
69. Singh D, Angel J, Bentley G, et al: Fortnightly review: Plantar fasciitis, *BMJ* 315:172-175, 1997.
70. Muhle C, Ahn JM, Yeh L, et al: Iliotibial band friction syndrome: MR imaging findings in 16 patients and MR arthrographic study of six cadaver knees, *Radiology* 212:103-110, 1999.
71. Austermuehle PD: Common knee injuries in primary care, *Nurse Pract* 26:32-38, 41-45, 2001.
72. Ritchie JR: Orthopedic considerations during pregnancy, *Clin Obstet Gyn* 46:456-466, 2003.
73. Yazici Y, Gibofsky A: A diagnostic approach to musculoskeletal pain, *Clin Cornerstone* 2:1-10, 1999.
74. Hooper MM, Holderbaum D, Moskowitz RW: Clinical and laboratory findings in osteoarthritis. In Koopman WJ, Moreland LW (eds): *Arthritis and Allied Conditions: A Textbook of Rheumatology*, ed 15, Philadelphia, 2005, Lippincott Williams & Wilkins.
75. Chumbley EM, O'Connor FG, Nirschl RP: Evaluation of elbow injuries, *Am Fam Physician* 61:691-700, 2000.
76. Muggleton JM, Allen R, Chappell PH: Hand and arm injuries associated with repetitive manual work in industry: A review of disorders, risk factors and preventive measures, *Ergonomics* 42:714-739, 1999.
77. Goodman CC, Snyder TE: *Differential Diagnosis in Physical Therapy*, ed 3, Philadelphia, 2000, WB Saunders.
78. Kendall FP, McCreary EK, Provance PG, et al: Posture. In Kendall FP, McCreary EK, Provance PG, et al (eds): *Muscles Testing and Function with Posture and Pain*, ed 5, Philadelphia, 2005, Lippincott Williams & Wilkins.
79. Hertling D, Kessler RM: Assessment of musculoskeletal disorders and concepts of management. In Hertling D, Kessler RM (eds): *Management of Common Musculoskeletal Disorders*, ed 3, Philadelphia, 1996, Lippincott.
80. Cibulka MT, Threlkeld J: The early clinical diagnosis of osteoarthritis of the hip, *JOSPT* 34:461-467, 2004.
81. Ross M, Worrell TW: Thigh and calf girth following knee injury and surgery, *JOSPT* 27:9-15, 1998.
82. Soderberg GL, Ballantyne BT, Kestel LL: Reliability of lower girth measurements after anterior cruciate ligament reconstruction, *Physiother Res Int* 1:7-16, 1996.
83. Sander AP, Hajer NW, Hemenway K, et al: Upper-extremity volume measurements in women with lymphedema: A comparison of measurements obtained via water displacement with geometrically determined volume, *Phys Ther* 82:1201-1212, 2002.
84. Amber J, Fu M, Wainstock J, et al: Lymphedema following breast cancer treatment, including sentinel lymph node biopsy, *Lymphology* 37:73-91, 2004.
85. Cornish BH, Thomas BJ, Ward LC, et al: A new technique for the quantification of peripheral edema with application in both unilateral and bilateral cases, *Angiology* 53:41-47, 2002.
86. Whitney SL, Mattocks L, Irrgang JJ, et al: Reliability of lower extremity girth measurements, *J Sports Rehab* 4:108-115, 1995.
87. Murff RT, Armstrong DG, Lanctot D, et al: How effective is manual palpation in detecting subtle temperature differences? *Clin Podiatr Med Surg* 15:151-154, 1998.
88. Brosseau L, Balmer S, Tousignant M, et al: Intra- and intertester reliability and criterion validity of the parallelogram and universal goniometers for measuring maximum active knee flexion and extension of patients with knee restrictions, *Arch Phys Med Rehabil* 82:396-402, 2001.
89. Norkin CC, White DJ: *Measurement of Joint Motion: A Guide to Goniometry*, ed 3, Philadelphia, 2003, FA Davis.
90. Hislop HJ, Montgomery J: *Muscle Testing: Techniques of Manual Examination*, ed 6, Philadelphia, 1995, WB Saunders.
91. Wadsworth C, Neilsen D, Corcoran C, et al: Interrater reliability of hand-held dynamometry: Effects of gender, body weight, and grip strength, *JOSPT* 16:74-81, 1992.
92. Stratford P, Balsor B: A comparison of make and break tests using a hand-held dynamometer and the Kin com, *JOSPT* 19:28-32, 1994.
93. McMahon L, Brudett R, Whitney S: Effects of muscle group and placement site on reliability of hand held dynamometry strength measurements, *JOSPT* 15:236-242, 1992.
94. Irrgang JJ, Safran MR, Fu FH: The knee: Ligamentous and meniscal injuries. In Zachazewski JE, Magee DJ, Quillen WS (eds): *Athletic Injuries and Rehabilitation*, Philadelphia, 1996, WB Saunders.
95. McGhee JL, Burks FN, Sheckels JL, et al: Identifying children with chronic arthritis based on chief complaints: Absence of predictive value for musculoskeletal pain as an indicator of rheumatic disease in children, *Pediatrics* 110:354-359, 2002.
96. Johnson DL, Bealle DP, Brand JC, et al: The effect of a geographic lateral bone bruise on knee inflammation after acute anterior cruciate ligament rupture, *Am J Sports Med* 28:152-155, 2000.
97. Feletar M, Littlejohn G: The value of clinical signs in rheumatology, *Aust Fam Physician* 28:1223-1227, 1999.
98. Deyle GD, Henderson NE, Matekel RL, et al: Effectiveness of manual physical therapy and exercise in osteoarthritis of the knee, *Ann Intern Med* 132:173-181, 2000.
99. Hammond A, Freeman K: One-year outcomes of a randomized controlled trial of an educational-behavioral joint protection program for people with rheumatoid arthritis, *Rheumatology* 40:1044-1051, 2001.
100. Deal DN, Tipton J, Rosencrance E, et al: Ice reduces edema, *J Bone Joint Surg Am* 84-A:1571-1578, 2002.
101. Sluka KA, Walsh D: Transcutaneous electrical nerve stimulation: basic science mechanisms and clinical effectiveness, *J Pain* 4(3):109-121, 2003.

102. Hockenbruy RT, Sammarco GJ. Evaluation and treatment of ankle sprains; Clinical recommendations for a positive outcome, *Physician Sportsmed* 29:57-64, 69-70, 2001.

103. Finch E, Brooks D, Stratford PW, et al: SF-36 (Medical Outcomes Study 36-Item Short-Form Health Survey). In *Physical Rehabilitation Outcome Measures: A Guide to Enhanced Clinical Decision Making*, ed 2, Baltimore, 2002, Lippincott Williams & Wilkins.

104. Buckwalter JA: Activity vs. rest in the treatment of bone, soft tissue and joint injuries, *Iowa Orthop J* 15:29-42, 1995.

105. Kannus P. Immobilization or early mobilization after an acute soft-tissue injury? *Physician Sportsmed* 28:55-56, 59-60, 62-63, 2000.

106. Thorsson O, Hemdal B, Lilja B, et al: The effect of external pressure on intra-muscular blood flow at rest and after running, *Med Sci Sports Exerc* 19:469-473, 1987.

107. Bleakley C, McDonough S, MacAuley D: The use of ice in the treatment of acute soft-tissue injury: A systematic review of randomized controlled trails, *Am J Sports Med* 31:251-261, 2004.

108. Ogilvie-Harris DJ, Gilbart M: Treatment modalities for soft tissue injuries of the ankle: A critical review, *Clin J Sport Med* 5:175-186, 1995.

109. Bleakley S, McDonough S, MacAuley D: The use of ice in the treatment of acute soft-tissue injury: A systematic review of randomized controlled trials, *Am J Sports Med* 32:251-261, 2004.

110. Lin Y: Effects of thermal therapy in improving the passive range of knee motion: Comparison of cold and superficial heat applications, *Clin Rehabil* 17:618-623, 2003.

111. Myrer WJ, Myrer KA, Measom GJ, et al: Muscle temperature is affected by overlying adipose when cryotherapy is administered, *J Athl Train* 36:32-36, 2001.

112. Brosseau L, Yonge KA, Robinson V, et al: Thermotherapy for treatment of osteoarthritis, *Cochrane Database Syst Rev* 4:CD004522, 2003.

113. Kerr KM: Commentary, *Br J Sports Med* 34:383, 2000.

114. Graham CA, Stevenson J: Frozen chips: An unusual case of severe frostbite injury, *Br J Sports Med* 34:382-384, 2000.

115. Cameron MH: Thermal agents: Cold and heat. In Cameron MH (ed): *Physical Agents in Rehabilitation: From Research to Practice*, ed 2, Philadelphia, 2003, WB Saunders.

116. Taylor BF, Waring CA, Brashear TA: The effects of therapeutic application of heat or cold followed by static stretch on hamstring muscle length, *JOSPT* 21:283-286, 1995.

117. Draper DO, Castro JL, Feland B, et al: Shortwave diathermy and prolonged stretching increase hamstring flexibility more than prolonged stretching alone, *JOPST* 34:13-20, 2004.

118. Funk D, Swank A, Adams K, et al: Efficacy of moist heat pack application over static stretching on hamstring flexibility, *J Strength Cond Res* 15:123-126, 2001.

119. Speed CA: Therapeutic ultrasound in soft tissue lesions, *Rheumatology* 40:1331-1336, 2001.

120. Draper DO, Ricard MD: Rate of temperature decay in human muscle following 3 MHz ultrasound: The stretching window revealed, *J Athl Train* 30:304-307, 1995.

121. Esenyel M, Caglar N, Aldemir T: Treatment of myofascial pain, *Am J Phys Med* 79:48-52, 2000.

122. Uhlemann C, Heinig B, Wollina U: Therapeutic ultrasound in lower extremity wound management, *Int J Low Extrem Wounds* 2:152-157, 2003.

123. Ng CO, Ng GY, See EK, et al: Therapeutic ultrasound improves strength of Achilles tendon repair in rats, *Ultrasound Med Biol* 29:1501-1506, 2003.

124. Busse JW, Bhandari M, Kulkarni AV, et al: The effect of low-intensity pulsed ultrasound therapy on time to fracture healing: A meta-analysis, *CMAJ* 166:437-441, 2002.

125. Giannini S, Giombini A, Moneta MR, et al: Low-intensity pulsed ultrasound in the treatment of traumatic hand fracture in an elite athlete, *Am J Phys Med Rehabil* 83:921-925, 2004.

126. Heckman JD, Pyaby JP, McCabe J, et al: Acceleration of tibial fracture-healing by non-invasive, low-intensity pulsed ultrasound, *J Bone Joint Surg Am* 76-A:26-34, 1994.

127. Ebenbichler GR, Erdogmus CB, Resch KL, et al: Ultrasound therapy for calcific tendinitis of the shoulder, *N Engl J Med* 340:1533-1538, 1999.

128. Dyson M: Mechanisms involved in therapeutic ultrasound, *Physiotherapy* 73:116, 1987.

129. Bare AC, Christie DS, McAnaw MB, et al: Phonophoretic delivery of 10% hydrocortisone through the epidermis of humans as determined by serum cortisol concentrations, *Phys Ther* 76:738-749, 1996.

130. Cagnie B, Vinck E, Rimbaut S, et al: Phonophoresis versus topical application of ketoprofen: Comparison between tissue and plasma levels, *Phys Ther* 83:707-712, 2003.

131. Baskurt F, Ozcan A, Algun C: Comparison of effects of phonophoresis and iontophoresis of naproxen in the treatment of lateral epicondylitis, *Clin Rehabil* 17:96-100, 2003.

132. Cameron MH: Ultrasound. In Cameron MH (ed): *Physical Agents in Rehabilitation: From Research to Practice*, ed 2, Philadelphia, 2003, WB Saunders.

133. Muche JA: Efficacy of therapeutic ultrasound treatment of a meniscus tear in a severely disabled patient: A case report, *Arch Phys Med Rehabil* 84:1558-1559, 2003.

134. Baker KG, Robertson VJ, Duck FA: A review of therapeutic ultrasound: Biophysical effects, *Phys Ther* 81:1351-1358, 2001.

135. Dyson M: Mechanisms involved in therapeutic ultrasound, *Physiotherapy* 76:116-120, 1990.

136. Johns LD: Nonthermal effects of therapeutic ultrasound: The frequency resonance hypothesis, *J Athl Train* 37:293-299, 2002.

137. Leung MC, NG GY, Yip YY: Effect of ultrasound on acute inflammation of transected medial collateral ligaments, *Arch Phys Med Rehabil* 85:963-966, 2004.

138. Hay-Smith EJ: Therapeutic ultrasound for postpartum perineal pain and dyspareunia (review), *Cochrane Database Syst Rev* 2:CD000495, 2000.

139. Mohr T, Akers TK, Landry RG: Effect of high voltage stimulation on edema reduction in the rat hind limb, *Phys Ther* 67:1703-1707, 1987.

140. Reed BV: Effect of high voltage pulsed electrical stimulation on microvascular permeability to plasma proteins, *Phys Ther* 68:491-495, 1988.

141. Bettany JA, Fish DR, Mendel FC: Influence of high voltage pulsed direct current on edema formation following impact injury, *Phys Ther* 70:219-224, 1990.

142. Dolan MG, Mychaskiw AM, Mattacola CG, et al: Effects of cool-water immersion and high-voltage electrical stimulation for 3 continuous hours on acute edema in rats, *J Athl Train* 38:325-329, 2003.

143. Cosgrove KA, Alon G, Bell SF, et al: The electrical effect of two commonly used clinical stimulators on traumatic edema in rats, *Phys Ther* 72:227-233, 1992.

144. Griffin JW, Newsome LS, Stralka SW, et al: Reduction of chronic posttraumatic hand edema: a comparison of high voltage pulsed current, intermittent pneumatic compression, and placebo treatments, *Phys Ther* 70:279-286, 1990.

145. Michlovitz S, Smith W, Wattkins M: Ice and high voltage pulsed stimulation in treatment of acute lateral ankle sprains, *JOSPT* 9:301-304, 1998.

146. Garrison DW, Foreman RD: Effects of transcutaneous electrical nerve stimulation (TENS) electrode placement on spontaneous and noxiously evoked dorsal horn cell activity in the cat, *Neuromodulation* 5:231-237, 2002.

147. Osiri M, Welch V, Brosseau L, et al: Transcutaneous electrical nerve stimulation for knee osteoarthritis (review), *Cochrane Database Syst Rev* 4;CD002823, 2000.

148. Melzack R, Wall PD: Pain mechanisms: A new theory, *Science* 333:325-326, 1965.

149. Hughes GS, Lichstein PR, Whitlock D, et al: Response of plasma beta-endorphins to transcutaneous electrical nerve stimulation in health subjects, *Phys Ther* 64:1062-1066, 1984.

150. Lewek M, Stevens J, Snyder-Mackler L: The use of electrical stimulation to increase quadriceps femoris muscle force in an elderly patient following total knee arthroplasty, *Phys Ther* 81:1565-1571, 2001.

151. Stevens JE, Mizner RL, Snyder-Mackler L: Neuromuscular electrical stimulation for quadriceps muscle strengthening after bilateral total knee arthroplasty: A case series, *JOSPT* 34:21-29, 2004.

152. Alon G, McCombe SA, Koutsantonis S, et al: Comparison of the effects of electrical stimulation and exercise on abdominal musculature, *JOSPT* 567-573, 1987.

153. Glass JM, Stephen RL, Jacobsen SC: The quantity and distribution of radiolabeled dexamethasone delivered to tissue by iontophoresis, *Int J Dermatol* 19:519-525, 1980.

154. Bertolucci LE: Introduction of anti-inflammatory drugs by iontophoresis: Double blind study, *JOSPT* 4:103-108, 1982.

155. Harris PR: Iontophoresis: Clinical research in musculoskeletal inflammatory conditions, *JOSPT* 4:109-112, 1982.

156. Gudeman SD, Eisele SA, Heidt RS, et al: Treatment of plantar fasciitis by iontophoresis of 0.4% dexamethasone: A randomized, double-blind, placebo-controlled study, *Am J Sports Med* 25:312-316, 1997.

157. Green T, Refshauge K, Crosbie J, et al: A randomized controlled trial of passive accessory joint mobilization of acute ankle inversion sprains, *Phys Ther* 81:984-994, 2001.

158. Placzek JD, Roubal PJ, Freeman DC, et al: Long term effectiveness of translational manipulation for adhesive capsulitis, *Clin Orthop* 356:181-191, 1998.

159. Sevick MA, Bradham DD, Muender M, et al: Cost-effectiveness of aerobic and resistance exercise in seniors with knee osteoarthritis, *Med Sci Sports Exerc* 32:1534-1540, 2000.

160. Iversen MD, Liang MH, Bae SC: Selected arthritides: Rheumatoid arthritis, osteoarthritis, spondyloarthropathies, systemic lupus erythematosus, polymyositis/dermatomyositis, and systemic sclerosis. In Frontera WR, Dawson DM, Slovik DM (eds): *Exercise in Rehabilitation Medicine*, Champaign, Ill, 1999, Human Kinetics.

161. Minor MA, Kay DR: Arthritis. In Durstine JL, Moore GE (eds): *ACSM's Exercise Management for Persons with Chronic Diseases and Disabilities*, Champaign, Ill, 1997, Human Kinetics.

162. Andersen RE, Blair SN, Cheskin LJ, et al: Encouraging patients to become more physically active: The physician's role, *Ann Int Med* 127:395-400, 1997.

163. Bloomfield SA, Smith SA: Osteoporosis. In Durstine JL, Moore GE (eds): *ACSM's Exercise Management for Persons with Chronic Diseases and Disabilities*, Champaign, Ill, 1997, Human Kinetics.

164. Messier SP, Royer TD, Craven TE, et al: Long-term exercise and its effect on balance in older, osteoarthritis adults: Results from the fitness, arthritis, and seniors trial (FAST), *J Am Geriatr Soc* 48:131-138, 2000.

165. Messier SP, Loeser RF, Mitchell MN, et al: Exercise and weight loss in obese older adults with knee osteoarthritis: A preliminary study, *J Am Geriatr Soc* 48:1062-1072, 2000.

166. American College of Sports Medicine position stand: The recommended quantity and quality of exercise for developing and maintaining cardiorespiratory and muscular fitness and flexibility in healthy adults, *Med Sci Sports Exerc* 30:975-991, 1998.

167. Buljina AI, Taljanovic MS, Avdic DM, Hunter TB. Physical and exercise therapy for treatment of the rheumatoid hand, *Arthritis Care Res* 45:392-397, 2001.

168. American College of Sports Medicine position stand: Progression models in resistance training for healthy adults, *Med Sci Sports Exerc* 34:364-380, 2002.

169. Bennett K: Therapeutic exercise for arthritis. In Hall CM, Brody LT (eds): *Therapeutic Exercise: Moving Toward Function*, Philadelphia, 1999, Lippincott Williams & Wilkins.

170. Kudlacek S, Pietschmann F, Bernecker P, et al: The impact of a senior dancing program on spinal and peripheral bone mass, *Am J Phys Med Rehabil* 76:447-481, 1997.

171. Noreau L, Moffet H, Droler M, et al: Dance-based exercise in rheumatoid arthritis: Feasibility in individuals with American college or rheumatology functional class III disease, *Am J Phys Med* 76:109 113, 1997.

172. Borg GAV: Psychophysical bases of perceived exertion, *Med Sci Sports Exerc* 14.377-381, 1982.

173. Krivickas LS. Training flexibility. In Frontera WR, Dawson DM, Slovick DM (eds): *Exercise in Rehabilitation Medicine*, Champaign, Ill, 1999, Human Kinetics.

174. van Os AG, Bierma-Zeinstra SMA, Verhagen AP, et al: Comparison of conventional treatment and supervised rehabilitation for treatment of acute lateral ankle sprains: A systematic review of the literature, *JOSPT* 35:95-105, 2005.

175. Felson DT (conference chair): Osteoarthritis: New insights. Part 2: Treatment approaches, *Ann Intern Med* 133:726-737, 2000.

176. Brody LT. Aquatic physical therapy. In Hall CM, Brody LT (eds): *Therapeutic Exercise: Moving Toward Function*, ed 2, Baltimore, Md, 2005, Lippincott Williams & Wilkins.

177. Khan KM, Maffulli N, Coleman BD, et al: Patellar tendinopathy: some aspects of basic science and clinical management, *Br J Sports Med* 32:346-355, 1998.

178. Antich TJ: Orthoses for the knee: The tibiofemoral joint. In Nawoczenski DA, Epler ME (eds): *Orthotics in Functional Rehabilitation of the Lower Limb*, Philadelphia, 1997, WB Saunders.

179. Owens A, Menasche R, Kenney J, et al: Effectiveness of the auto edema reduction (AER) boot for treatment of edema in acute ankle sprains: A single case study, *J Man Manip Ther* 8:115-126, 2000.

180. Epler ME: Orthoses for the ankle. In Nawoczenski DA, Epler ME (eds): *Orthotics in Functional Rehabilitation of the Lower Limb*, Philadelphia, 1997, WB Saunders.

181. Riemsma RP, Kirwan J, Taal E, et al: Patient education for adults with rheumatoid arthritis (review), *Cochrane Database Syst Rev* 2:CD003688, 2003.

182. Steultjens EM, Dekker J, Bouter LM, et al: Occupational therapy for rheumatoid arthritis (review), *Cochrane Database Syst Rev* 1:CD003114, 2004.

183. Muggleton JM, Allen R, Chappell PH: Hand and arm injuries associated with repetitive manual work in industry: A review of disorders, risk factors and preventive measures, *Ergonomics* 42:714-739, 1999.

184. Melhorn MJ: Cumulative trauma disorders and repetitive strain injuries, *Clin Orthop* 351:107-126, 1998.

185. Cameron MH: Pain. In Cameron MH (ed): *Physical Agents In Rehabilitation: From Research To Practice*, ed 2, Philadelphia, 2003, WB Saunders

Spinal Disorders

Cynthia Chiarello

OBJECTIVES

After reading this chapter, the reader will be able to:
1. Identify the pathophysiological and mechanical basis of selected common pathological conditions of the spine.
2. Discuss the importance of classification systems in relation to the diagnosis and management of spinal dysfunction.
3. Explain the components of a scanning and detailed spinal examination.
4. Describe the evidence to support the use of various examination and intervention procedures used in the management of spinal disorders.

*M*usculoskeletal spinal disorders are an immense problem in industrialized societies resulting in tremendous personal and economic costs. Low back pain (LBP) is usually defined as pain extending from the twelfth rib inferiorly to the gluteal fold, whereas neck pain is pain between the occiput and the third thoracic vertebra.[1] It is estimated that 70% to 85% of the population will experience back or neck pain at some time in their life and between 14% and 50% of adults have LBP at some time during any single year.[2-7] The prevalence of chronic neck pain or uninterrupted neck pain of more than 6 months' duration has been reported to be 18%,[8] and the point prevalence, or the number of individuals with LBP at a given point in time, has been reported to be between 13.7 and 28.7 per hundred.[3] Additionally, 56% of American adults had back pain for at least 1 day in the previous year, 34% had pain for 6 days or more, and 14% had pain for more than 30 days.[9] In the United States (US), LBP is the most common reason for activity limitation in individuals under the age of 45, and approximately 2% of the workforce receives compensation for LBP annually.[2] Although variations in epidemiological methods may account for differences in the estimates of LBP, pregnant and postpartum women comprise a segment of society frequently excluded from these statistics. LBP during a normal pregnancy is common, with prevalence rates varying from 48% to 90%.[10-14] Furthermore, back pain during pregnancy cannot be explained by biomechanical factors alone[15] and is two to three times more common during pregnancy than in the general population.[10,14,16]

It is a commonly held belief that LBP almost always resolves within 4-6 weeks. However, there is evidence to suggest that this is not the case. For example, one study found that only 30% of patients with back pain in primary care practices were pain-free within 4 weeks, whereas 70% to 80% still had symptoms.[17] In addition, it may appear that back pain has resolved in many patients because they do not return to their health care provider with this complaint, but this may reflect a disillusionment or dissatisfaction with the medical establishment rather than a resolution of symptoms.[17] It is reported that although up to 75% of individuals with new episodes of back pain return to work within 4 to 6 weeks, many remain symptomatic.[17] Furthermore, even if an episode of back pain passes, this does not imply a resolution of the problem since the hallmark of LBP is recurrence, with as many as 85% of individuals experiencing multiple episodes. In fact, the strongest predictor for back pain is a previous episode of back pain.[2,18] Thus it appears that many individuals with spinal disorders and their inherent functional sequelae may never experience a complete resolution of their problem.

According to the National Health Interview Survey, musculoskeletal impairment was the most common impairment for those under the age of 65, with spine impairments being the most frequent subcategory of musculoskeletal impairment at 51.7%.[2] It is reported that LBP is the most frequent reason for referral to outpatient physical therapy, representing over 25% of outpatient discharges from both hospital-based and private physical therapy practices.[19] Because spine-related pain is such a large-scale problem, affecting much of the population, it is imperative that physical therapists (PTs) are well equipped to manage spinal problems.

PTs play a critical role in the management of patients with spinal disorders. PTs are required to have an in-depth knowledge of musculoskeletal examination and evaluation in order to determine the most appropriate interventions, assess outcomes, recognize serious pathology, and make referrals to other health professionals when indicated. This chapter provides the reader with an understanding of techniques of examination and intervention for patients with spinal disorders, assuming that the reader is already familiar with the basics of anatomy and spinal biomechanics.[20,21]

PATHOLOGY

PHASES OF SPINAL DEGENERATION

Structural changes seen on plain x-rays, computed tomography (CT), or magnetic resonance imaging (MRI) do not usually relate to symptoms that localize to the back or neck.[22] However, progressive degenerative changes in the facet joints and the intervertebral discs of the spine are often associated with symptoms.[22] This degeneration can

be considered to occur in three phases, progressing from a clinical picture of restricted movement during phase I (dysfunction), followed by hypermobility in phase II (unstable), and then again by stability in the final phase, phase III (stabilization) (Fig. 8-1).[22,23]

RADICULOPATHY

In general, a *radiculopathy* occurs when nerve conduction in the axons of a spinal nerve or its roots is impeded by compression or ischemia.[21] Numbness results when conduction is blocked in sensory nerves, and weakness occurs when motor nerves are obstructed. Signs of radiculopathy include muscle wasting, motor weakness, depressed deep tendon reflexes, and sensory changes in the distribution of the involved nerve root.[9] Symptoms commonly include central spinal pain, with or without associated pain radiating from the neck or back to the limb. When a single nerve root is affected, the signs and symptoms are limited to the specific distribution of that nerve root, simplifying the diagnostic process. The typical sensory, motor, and reflex changes caused by disturbances at individual nerve roots are shown in Table 8-1. This chart may not correlate exactly with an individual's symptoms because more than one nerve root may be involved and because innervation patterns vary between individuals. In addition, muscles may receive motor innervation from multiple or unexpected nerve roots, and the area of skin with sensory innervation from one root may also be innervated by other nerves at the borders.[23]

Encroachment on the central spinal canal or neural foramina can cause radicular symptoms (Fig. 8-2). A space-occupying lesion, such as a bony spur, soft tissue fibrosis and hypertrophy, tumor, or a protruding disc narrowing the intervertebral foramen, may cause encroachment. Osteoarthrosis of the uncovertebral joints in the cervical spine or other arthritic changes in facet joints, as well as

FIG. 8-1 The phases of spinal degeneration as described by Kirkaldy-Willis. *Adapted from Kirkaldy-Willis W, Gernard T: Managing Low Back Pain, ed 4, New York, 1991, Churchill Livingstone.*

	FACET JOINTS	CLINICAL PRESENTATION	INTERVERTEBRAL DISC
PHASE I DYSFUNCTION	Synovitis	Restricted movement	Circumferential and radial annular tears
	Minimal cartilage degeneration	Unilateral radicular symptoms	
PHASE II UNSTABLE	Joint capsule laxity	Increased movement	• Tears all the way through the annulus
	Facet joint subluxation	Unilateral radicular symptoms	• Complete internal disc disruption • Circumferential annular bulging
	Subperiosteal osteophytes		• Loss of disc height
PHASE III STABILIZATION	Periarticular fibrosis	Restricted movement	Ossification
	Osteophytes	Multilevel bilateral radicular symptoms	

TABLE 8-1	Sensory, Motor, and Reflex Nerve Root Innervation		
Nerve Root	**Sensory Distribution**	**Motor Distribution**	**Reflexes**
C4	Top of the shoulder	Trapezius, rhomboid	None
C5	Lateral arm	Deltoid, biceps, brachioradialis	Biceps
C6	Lateral forearm, thumb, and index finger	Biceps, extensor carpi radialis longus and brevis	Brachioradialis
C7	Middle finger	Triceps, pronator teres	Triceps
C8	Medial forearm, little and ring finger	Interossei, flexor digitorum profundus	None
T1	Medial arm	Interossei	None
L2	Proximal anteromedial thigh	Iliopsoas, adductors	None
L3	Distal anteromedial thigh, knee, and upper leg	Adductors, quadriceps	None
L4	Medial leg and foot	Tibialis anterior, quadriceps	Patellar
L5	Lateral leg and dorsum of the foot	Extensor hallucis longus	Hamstring, Achilles
S1	Lateral foot, posteromedial thigh and leg	Peroneus longus and brevis, gluteus maximus,	Achilles
S2	Posterolateral thigh	Gastrocnemius, soleus, gluteus maximus	Achilles

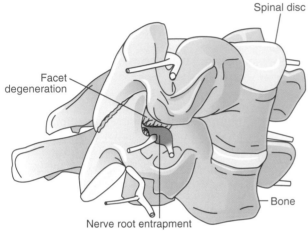

FIG. 8-2 Neural foraminal stenosis causing nerve root entrapment and radiculopathy.

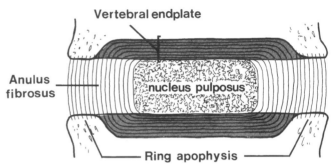

FIG. 8-3 Cross-section through the intervertebral disc and vertebral body showing the components of the disc: The vertebral end plate, annulus fibrosus, and nucleus pulposus. *Adapted from Bogduk N:* Clinical Anatomy of the Lumbar Spine and Sacrum, *ed 3, New York, 1997, Churchill Livingstone.*

degenerative changes of the ligamentum flavum or facet joint capsule, may also cause intervertebral foraminal encroachment.[23] Nerve root sleeve fibrosis or hyperplasia can also cause foraminal impingement or fibrous adhesions to the pedicle, resulting in nerve root compression. Spinal nerve roots are particularly susceptible to injury because they do not have dense connective tissue between their fibers and because the connective tissue covering the nerve, the perineurium, may be missing or not well developed.[23,24]

Encroachment on the nerve roots may cause injury by mechanical and chemical means. Mechanical nerve compression can directly damage the nerve, and indirectly, compression may cause damage by impairing blood flow to the nerve or by tethering it to surrounding structures, thus reducing its mobility and making it vulnerable to irritation from stretch.[24] A nerve that is compressed but not swollen will not cause pain, but compression of a swollen or stretched nerve root generally does cause pain.[24]

Chemical irritation may be produced by direct contact of *nucleus pulposus* material with the spinal nerves. This can reduce nerve conduction and cause biochemically mediated inflammatory, microvascular, and structural injury to the nerve.[24] Synovial cytokines, which come

from facet joint leaking, and T cells, which are present during inflammation, have also been found to impair nerve function.[24]

INTERVERTEBRAL DISC DISEASE

Intervertebral disc (IVD) disease is responsible for a large proportion of spinal disorders. It is estimated that 5.7 million new cases of IVD disease will be diagnosed each year.[25] The IVD has a unique structure that allows for mobility at the interbody joint while maintaining weight-bearing capabilities and withstanding mechanical stress. The IVD is made up of three components (Fig. 8-3): An outer cartilaginous ring, the *annulus fibrosus* (AF) (Fig. 8-4); an inner gelatinous core, the nucleus pulposus (NP); and vertebral end plates (VEP) that cover the disc from above and below. Details of each of these components are described in Table 8-2.

In a healthy, normal IVD the interaction of these components accounts for the disc's mechanical weight-bearing properties. When the disc is loaded in compression, as occurs in standing, the weight of the head, arms, and trunk are transmitted through the VEP to the viscoelastic NP. Since the NP cannot be compressed, it exerts the force centrifugally in all directions, producing distraction of the annular fibers. This annular tension prevents further

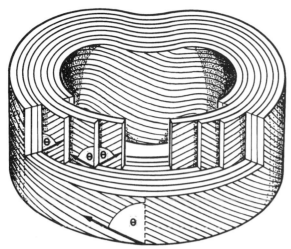

FIG. 8-4 Annulus fibrosus structure showing fiber orientation. *θ,* Angle of fibers from verticle. *Adapted from Bogduk N: Clinical Anatomy of the Lumbar Spine and Sacrum, ed 3, New York, 1997, Churchill Livingstone.*

expansion of the NP, and thus the weight is borne on both the NP and AF (Fig. 8-5). The radial force exerted by the NP supports the AF and places pressure on the VEP, allowing for the load to be transmitted from one vertebra to the next.[20]

The unique structure of the IVD also allows for complex spinal movements. All spinal movements affect the IVD, the interbody and zygapophyseal (facet) joints, the posterior ligaments, and the muscles around the spine. During bending, including flexion, extension, and lateral flexion to either side, the IVD is compressed on the concave side of the curve and stretched on the convex side of the curve. The NP tries to escape the compressive force by moving to the convexity.[20] For example, in spinal flexion, the anterior annular fibers buckle, the posterior annular fibers are under tension, and the NP moves posteriorly to escape the anterior compression. The load on the disc causes the pressure within the nucleus to rise. If there are degenerative changes, such as clefts or fissures within the disc, the additional pressure may lead to rupture of annular lamellae and herniation of the NP.[20] Torsion or twisting movements occur when all points on one vertebra move circumferentially in a direction opposite to the adjacent vertebra.[20]

TABLE 8-2	Characteristics and Function of the Components of the Intervertebral Disc		
	Annulus Fibrosus (AF)	**Nucleus Pulposus (NP)**	**Vertebral End Plates (VEP)**
Structure and location	Fibers arranged in 10-12 layers, or lamellae, forming concentric rings encircling the NP. The lamellae are thicker anteriorly and laterally and thinner posteriorly. The fibers lie parallel within each lamella but are oriented at 65-70° from vertical, successively in opposite directions between layers (see Fig. 8-4).	Oval-shaped mass in central or posterior-central disc. Enclosed by collagen fibers from inner layers of AF.	Boundary between the cancellous core of the vertebral body and the IVD. VEPs extend centrally from an apophyseal ring and completely enclose the NP from above and below.
Composition	The AF is 60%-70% water. Dry components are 50%-60% collagen (predominantly type I) and 20% proteoglycans to bind water. Chondrocytes near the nucleus and fibroblasts near the annular periphery synthesize collagen and proteoglycans.	The NP is a hydrated, gelatinous, semifluid mass, 70%-90% water. Dry components are 65% proteoglycans and 15%-20% collagen (predominantly type II). Chondrocytes near the VEP synthesize proteoglycans and collagen.	VEPs are composed primarily of hyaline cartilage in the area closest to vertebral body and of fibrocartilage near the NP. VEPs also contain proteoglycans, collagen fibers, and chondrocytes, with more water and proteoglycans and less collagen centrally.
Properties	Resists tensile loads. Half the lamellae resist torsional loads in each direction.	Deforms under pressure but cannot be compressed.	Strongest and stiffest posterolaterally and weakest centrally.
Function	Principal load-bearing component of the IVD.	Reallocates applied loads in all directions to the AF and the VEPs.	Anchor the IVD to the vertebral bodies. Prevent extrusion of the NP into the vertebral body. Distribute and transfer load to the vertebral body. Site for diffusion of nutrients to the IVD.
Degenerative changes	The border between the NP and the AF becomes difficult to differentiate. Three types of tears occur: 1. Peripheral: Isolated to outer layers, parallel and adjacent to the VEPs. 2. Circumferential: Rupture between lamellae. 3. Radial: Continuous with clefts that radiate from the NP.	Water and proteoglycan content decreases, causing the NP to become dryer, more fibrotic, and less distinct from the AF. The disc becomes weaker as the NP becomes less able to distribute loads. Horizontal clefts develop between the VEPs and the center of the disc.	Thinning, fissures, horizontal cleft formation, and fractures increase with age. Ossification and local calcification result in diminished disc nutrition.

During a twisting movement, the attachments of fibers from the AF oriented in the direction of the twist will separate and resist the motion. Farfan originally determined that torsion could cause tears primarily in the posterolateral annulus.[26] When stress exceeds the mechanical capabilities of the disc or when the disc degenerates, lesions may develop.[26]

Bogduk proposed a mechanism relating mechanical stresses to the initiation of disc disruption, herniation, and degeneration.[20] A healthy disc, without any previous injury, can withstand compression without NP herniation. Under continued or excessive loading in compression, in compression with flexion, as occurs with heavy lifting in untrained individuals, or with an unanticipated fall, the VEP develops fractures. These VEP fractures may damage the NP, leading to proteolysis and de-aggregation of proteoglycans and reduced water-binding capability. This will cause a decrease in disc height and make the annulus bulge radially. Diminished hydrostatic pressure in the NP alters its mechanical properties, so it will herniate through clefts or fissures in the AF under the normal minor compression that occurs with daily flexion or flexion together with rotation. Various types of IVD herniations are listed in Table 8-3 and shown in Fig. 8-6.

There is ample evidence that with conservative management, IVD herniations diminish in size or completely resolve with a concomitant resolution of symptoms.[27-30] Some individuals' symptoms resolve before morphological changes are observed on MRI, and some people become asymptomatic without regression of the hernia-

tion. The exact mechanism of disc resorption has not been fully elucidated, and yet, it is hypothesized that nuclear extrusion triggers an immune response to the disc fragments. Neovascularization follows, with the release of macrophages that produce inflammatory cytokines and proteinases that degrade the disc fragments.[27]

It is difficult to distinguish normal age-related changes in the IVD from pathological degenerative changes. Although the incidence of degenerative changes increases with age, evidence suggests that degenerative changes in the IVD are not always entirely age-related. Once disc structure changes, usually as a result of injury, degeneration starts and then progresses over time.[31] Many spinal degenerative changes are asymptomatic,[32,33] yet some studies show an association between degenerative changes and pain.[34-36] A systematic review of the literature by van

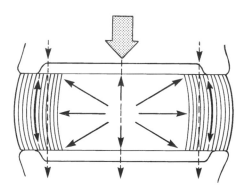

FIG. 8-5 Force distribution in the nucleus pulposus and annulus fibrosus in response to compression. *Adapted from Bogduk N: Clinical Anatomy of the Lumbar Spine and Sacrum, ed 3, New York, 1997, Churchill Livingstone.*

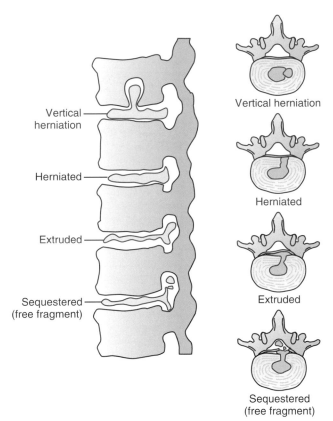

FIG. 8-6 Types of disc herniation: Vertical herniation, herniated, extruded, and sequestered.

TABLE 8-3	Types of Intervertebral Disc Herniations
Herniation	**Characteristics**
Intraspongy	Nuclear material travels from its central location posterolaterally into the annular fibers. No change in the arrangement of the outermost annular fibers.
Protrusion	Bulging of outer annular fibers as a result of migration of nuclear material through annular tears. Outer annular fibers remain intact to contain nuclear material.
Extruded	Nuclear material extrudes through ruptured annular fibers but remains attached to the disc.
Sequestrated	Nuclear material, extruded through ruptured annular fibers, forming a free fragment within spinal canal.
Schmorl's node	Vertical extrusion of nuclear material through the VEP into the substance of the vertebral body.

VEP, Vertebral end plate.

Tudler and colleagues[37] concluded that degenerative changes in the spine seen on radiological studies are associated with nonspecific LBP. More recently, using MRI to examine the lumbar spines of men with LBP and sciatica, Luoma and associates[38] reported that degenerative changes, including decreased water and proteoglycan content of the NP and anterior and posterior disc bulging, were significantly related to LBP during the preceding 12 months. They conclude that although degenerative changes are not diagnostic of LBP, the presence of these changes makes LBP more likely and that a greater number of degenerated discs has a greater association with the presence of pain. Therefore the appearances of degenerative changes on diagnostic imaging studies should be correlated with salient features of the examination to determine if a patient's pain is caused by the observed changes.

The most frequently cited age-related change in the IVD is dehydration of the NP. Over time the NP changes from a translucent, mucoid, gelatinous structure that behaves hydrostatically under load to an opaque, white fibrocartilaginous structure, which is barely distinguishable from the AF.[20,31,39-41] The IVD is avascular and receives nutrients by diffusion through the VEP. NP dehydration may be caused by decreased VEP permeability with aging.[40] As cellular nutrition and oxygenation diminishes, the number of viable cells and the amount of hydrophilic proteoglycan aggregates decrease.[42] The disc's fluid content determines its mechanical response to loading, and it loses fluid as its load bearing changes from fluid pressurization of the NP to elastic deformation of the annulus, increasing the risk for annular injury.[41] When degenerated, dehydration and reduced hydrostatic pressure also make the disc stiffer, lowering the failure stress of the annulus and further increasing the risk of annular tears and fissures.[42]

Disc dehydration also makes the disc get thinner and lose height, increasing compression of the facet joints and reducing the size of the intervertebral foramen. This increases the risk for nerve root impingement. If the IVD herniates, it may become even thinner. Loss of disc height appears to be related to degenerative changes and not age alone, since average lumbar disc height has been found to increase up to the fifth to seventh decade[43,44]; the decline in overall body height with age is due to decreased height of the vertebral bodies.[45]

The AF also dehydrates and degenerates to some degree with age. After the age of 50, the AF commonly has peripheral tears or rim lesions in the outer layer, circumferential tears or a split between the AF layers, and radial tears extending from the NP to the outer annulus.[46] Annular tears are have been observed to occur together with mechanical changes in the vertebral bone and intervertebral joint complex,[47] suggesting that these degenerative changes may not necessarily be a function of age but rather reflect progression over time after an injury has occured.[31]

SPINAL STENOSIS

Spinal stenosis is a narrowing of the spinal canal, intervertebral foramina, or radicular canals, resulting from the bony or soft tissue encroachment that reduces the space between the spinal cord and the vertebral elements.[48-51] Spinal stenosis occurs most often in the elderly, may occur at one or several spinal levels, and can have a variety of causes.[48] Spinal stenosis does not always cause symptoms, and the amount of narrowing is not necessarily proportional to the intensity of symptoms. Because asymptomatic stenosis is common, as with other degenerative spinal changes, diagnosis is established by agreement between signs, symptoms, and imaging studies.[48]

Cervical spinal stenosis may be classified into clinically relevant syndromes according to the portion of the spinal cord producing the symptoms[52] (Table 8-4). Classification of lumbar spinal stenosis is based on either etiology or anatomical location. Arnoldi[53] subdivided the etiology of spinal stenosis into congenital, which includes developmental, or degenerative. Congenital stenosis usually becomes symptomatic in the fourth to fifth decade, whereas degenerative spinal stenosis usually becomes symptomatic in the sixth to seventh decade in patients with a history of pain and disability. Although rare, congenital or developmental stenosis is due to either idiopathic or developmental narrowing of the spinal canal and by itself does not necessarily cause compression of nerves but rather makes the patient more vulnerable to other sources of narrowing. Acquired stenosis is more common and is usually due to degenerative changes such as bone or ligamentous hypertrophy and IVD protrusion[48] (Table 8-5).

Classification of lumbar spinal stenosis based on the anatomical location of the narrowing relates clinically relevant presenting symptoms and is used to guide surgical intervention. Central stenosis (Fig. 8-7) at the level of the disc is mainly caused by facet joint hypertrophy, buckling of the ligamentum flavum, disc protrusion, degenerative spondylolisthesis, or a combination.[48,49] The nerve root canal, or lateral recess, and the intervertebral foramen, which together make up the canal through which the nerve root exits the spinal canal, are involved in lateral

TABLE 8-4	Classification of Cervical Spinal Stenosis Syndromes	
Clinical Syndrome	**Parts of Spinal Cord Affected**
Transverse lesion syndrome	Corticospinal, spinothalamic, and posterior cord tracts
Motor system syndrome	Corticospinal tracts and anterior horn cells
Central cord syndrome	More pronounced motor and sensory deficits in the upper extremities than in the lower extremities
Brown-Séquard syndrome	Ipsilateral motor deficits with contralateral sensory deficits
Brachialgia and cord syndrome	Radicular upper extremity pain together with motor or sensory long-tract signs

TABLE 8-5	Etiological Classification of Lumbar Spinal Stenosis
Type of Stenosis	Origin/Characteristics
DEVELOPMENTAL OR CONGENITAL SPINAL STENOSIS	
Idiopathic	Anomalous unusually small size and shape of vertebral canal.
Achondroplastic	Bone dysplasia seen in congenital dwarfism.
ACQUIRED SPINAL STENOSIS	
Degenerative	Bulging of annulus into canal secondary to disc collapse.
	Buckling of ligamentum flavum. Osteophyte formation with sclerosis and hypertropic changes in laminae and facets.
Combined congenital and degenerative	Degenerative changes in individuals with congenital or developmental vertebral canal narrowing.
Spondylotic or spondylolisthetic	Compromise to vertebral canal because of anterior vertebral slippage with or without fracture.
Iatrogenic	Accelerated degenerative changes after spinal fusion or laminectomy.
Posttraumatic	Complication of fracture with bone fragments in the canal.
Pathological	Metabolic bone diseases such as Paget's disease, tumor, or infection.

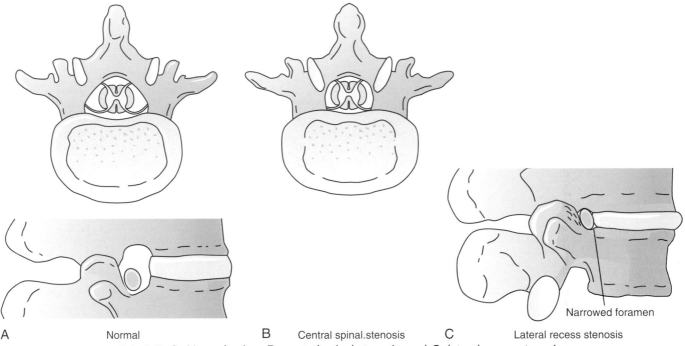

A   Normal   B   Central spinal.stenosis   C   Lateral recess stenosis

FIG. 8-7 **A,** Normal spine; **B,** central spinal stenosis; and **C,** lateral recess stenosis.

stenosis. The degenerative changes seen in lateral stenosis, including facet joint hypertrophy and osteophytes, decreased disc height, and protrusion of the disc posterolaterally into the intervertebral foramen, are common causes of radiculopathy.[48,49,54] The degenerative changes seen in central stenosis can cause lateral stenosis, but lateral stenosis can occur alone.

There is considerable individual variation in spinal cord volume and size, and in the shape of the vertebral canal, which results in variation in the amount of space available for the cord within the bony canal.[20,21,50] In the cervical spine, where stenosis can cause cord compression and myelopathy (pathology of the spinal cord), the size of the canal has been shown to affect the risk for symptomatic stenosis. The normal anterior to posterior (AP) cervical spinal canal diameter is 17-18 mm and a diameter less than 13 mm is diagnostic of congenital stenosis.[52] The ratio of the AP diameter of the spinal cord to its transverse diameter is used as a measure of cord flattening and the severity of cervical stenosis. A ratio of less than 0.40 indicates substantial spinal cord flattening and is associated with neurological impairment from myelopathy.[52] In the lumbar spine, the normal AP diameter of the spinal canal ranges from 14-25 mm.[54] A diameter of less than 10 mm indicates stenosis.[55] However, in the lumbar spine the size of the vertebral canal does not appear to be associated with the degree of stenosis or the severity of clinical symptoms.[54]

Spinal stenosis also has a dynamic component because the dimensions of the spinal canal and intervertebral foramina, as well as the volume of the spinal cord, change with flexion and extension of the spine. The spinal canal narrows with extension and widens with flexion in both normal and degenerated spines.[55-59] In the lumbar spine, Inufusa[55] demonstrated an 11% increase in the size of the central canal and a 12% increase in the size of the intervertebral foramina with flexion and 11% and 15% decreases, respectively, with extension. For degenerated spines, the effects of movement are even greater, with the spinal canal area decreasing by up to 67% in extension. According to the "rule of progressive narrowing," the greater the degenerative narrowing the greater the decrease in spinal canal area during extension.[59] The spinal cord stretches with flexion, decreasing its cross-sectional area, and thickens with extension, increasing its cross-sectional area.[60] Thus spinal flexion, which increases spinal and intervertebral canal area and decreases spinal cord area, optimizes the space for neurovascular structures and tends to minimize symptoms in patients with spinal stenosis, whereas spinal extension tends to aggravate symptoms.

Patients with cervical spinal stenosis frequently present with signs and symptoms of nerve root and spinal cord involvement with or without neck pain.[50,60] Patients with primarily cervical nerve root involvement have pain, sensory, reflex, and motor disturbances in the distribution of the nerves involved.[50,60] With cervical spinal cord involvement the clinical presentation depends on the area of the cord compressed, but most patients report an insidious onset of clumsiness in the hands and lower limbs, worsening handwriting, difficulty with grasping or holding objects, or diffuse hand numbness, with possible balance difficulties and an awkward gait.[50]

Lumbar spinal stenosis is clinically characterized by disabling chronic and progressive LBP, unilateral or bilateral leg pain, and lower extremity weakness. Since the L3-4 and L4-5 segments are most often affected, cauda equina compression can produce radicular symptoms with motor, sensory, and reflex changes in the affected nerve root distributions.[48,49,51] Neurological symptoms are present in only about 50% of patients during examination but may become evident in many more with symptom-provoking activities such as walking.[48]

The hallmark of lumbar spinal stenosis is *neurogenic claudication,* which is activity-dependent pain radiating into the thigh, leg, or both that increases with prolonged standing or lumbar extension and that is relieved by sitting, lying down, or lumbar flexion. Patients with lumbar spinal stenosis generally walk with a forward-stooped posture with lumbar flexion.[61] Neurogenic claudication can be distinguished clinically from vascular claudication because although both are characterized by aggravation of symptoms and signs with ambulation, neurogenic claudication is increased by increasing lumbar lordosis of the spine even without activity and improves with increased spinal flexion. Vascular claudication, however, is aggravated by lower extremity activity performed in any position, including cycling in a sitting flexed position, and is reduced by rest in any position.[48] In addition, patients with neurogenic claudication tend to have worse symptoms walking down hill because this puts the spine in extension and less pain with walking up hill as this puts the spine in flexion.[54] In contrast, patients with vascular claudication tend to have more pain with walking up hill because this requires stronger muscle contractions and thus greater blood supply.

SPONDYLOLYSIS AND SPONDYLOLISTHESIS

Spondylolysis is a bilateral defect in the pars interarticularis of a vertebra that decreases the ability of the posterior elements to stabilize the motion segment.[62] *Spondylolisthesis* is when a vertebra translates forward in the sagittal plane with respect to an adjacent vertebra. The intact facet joint or the pedicles usually resist this forward slippage. Spondylolysis can progress to or occur with spondylolisthesis or may occur alone. MRI studies have shown that spondylolysis is associated with hypermobility whereas spondylolisthesis is associated with normal spinal mobility.[63] Spondylolysis and spondylolisthesis are usually diagnosed radiologically. As with other radiological findings, caution must be exercised when attributing symptoms to these abnormalities since both spondylolysis and spondylolisthesis can be asymptomatic.

Spondylolisthesis is common in the lumbar spine and rare in the cervical spine. When spondylolisthesis does occur in the cervical spine, it is usually due to defects in the pars lateralis of the pedicles of C2, C4, or C6.[60] In the lumbar spine, spondylolisthesis can be classified by etiology as described in Table 8-6 and illustrated in Fig. 8-8.[64]

Age appears to play a role in the development of spondylolisthesis. There have been no reported cases of spondylolysis or spondylolisthesis in utero or at birth.[62,65] Spondylolysis and spondylolisthesis begin to occur during adolescence, possibly as a result of rapid growth and

TABLE 8-6	Classification of Spondylolisthesis
Type	**Description**
Congenital	Congenital abnormality with inadequacy of the upper sacrum or dysplasia of the posterior arch of L5. Allows for forward slippage of L5 on S1.*
Isthmic	Defect in pars interarticularis may be due to recurrent microfracture elongating the pars,* acute fracture of the pars, or flexion, extension, or rotational trauma.† Is graded by the amount of forward slippage.
Degenerative	The upper vertebral body moves forward on the lower vertebral body as a result of spondylotic degenerative changes in the disc and zygapophyseal joints. Degenerative facet arthrosis allows the disc to give way and the inferior articular process to move forward as the superior process becomes more eroded.*†
Traumatic	Rare, acute fracture in a vertebra not in the pars interarticularis.*
Pathological	Weakening of the pars interarticularis, pedicle, or facet joint because of metabolic bone diseases or tumors that allow forward slippage of superior vertebrae.*

*From Esses S: *Textbook of Spinal Disorders,* Philadelphia, 1995, JB Lippincott.
†From Kirkaldy-Willis W, Gernard T: *Managing Low Back Pain,* ed 4, New York, 1991, Churchill Livingstone.

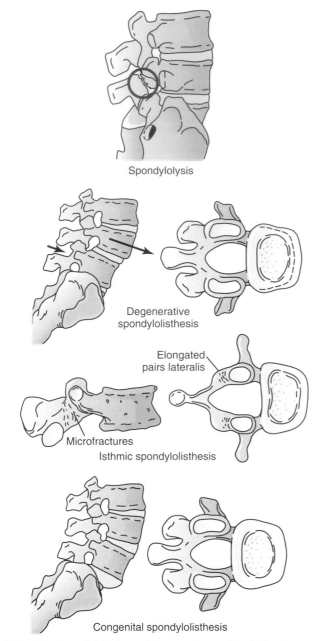

Spondylolysis

Degenerative
spondylolisthesis

Elongated
pairs lateralis

Microfractures
Isthmic spondylolisthesis

Congenital spondylolisthesis

FIG. 8-8 Spondylolysis and types of spondylolisthesis: Degenerative, isthmic, and congenital.

increased athletic participation. A landmark study evaluated the natural history of spondylolisthesis by following a group of children for 45 years from the age of 6.[65] The incidence of spondylolisthesis was initially 4.4% and rose to 6% by adulthood. The subjects with spondylolisthesis did not report pain in childhood or adolescence, even though most forward slippage occurred before skeletal maturity. No slippage ever occurred in subjects with only a unilateral pars defect. In subjects with slippage, the progression of slippage diminished with age, and while some subjects experienced LBP, this was not related to progression of the slippage, although the degree of slippage was associated with the amount of decrease in disc height and severity of foraminal stenosis.

In adults, patients who present with pain and are found to have spondylolisthesis have similar symptoms to those with spine-related pain without spondylolisthesis. A cross-sectional clinical study of patients with spondylolisthesis and symptoms found that 62% of the patients had LBP and sciatica, 31% had only LBP, and 7% had only sciatica.[66] The most common signs were a positive straight leg raise, which was present in 12% of the patients, and sensory disturbance in the L5 distribution, which was present in 13% of the patients.

WHIPLASH-ASSOCIATED DISORDERS

The Québec Task Force on Whiplash-Associated Disorders describes *whiplash-associated disorders* (WAD) as the bony or soft tissue injuries of the neck and related areas that occur following a rear or side collision in which the neck is subjected to acceleration–deceleration energy transfer.[67] The annual incidence of whiplash ranges from 30 to 188 per 100,000.[68-71] Most WADs are caused by motor vehicle accidents, but WAD may also be caused by sports-related injuries and falls. WAD most commonly causes neck pain, headache, and decreased cervical spine mobility but can also cause neck stiffness and low back and shoulder pain, as well as visual disturbances and dizziness.[72,73]

The Québec Task Force developed the following three category *classification system* for WAD:[67]

Grade I: The patient has no physical signs but feels neck pain, stiffness, and tenderness.

Grade II: The patient has neck symptoms and signs of musculoskeletal dysfunction.

Grade III: The patient has neck signs and symptoms and also neurological signs.

Imaging studies are recommended for WAD if serious pathology, such as fracture, is suspected.[73]

Although the IVDs, facet joints, and vascular and neurological systems may sometimes be involved in WAD, the ligaments and muscles generally sustain most damage as a result of direct stretching or neuromuscular reflex contractions.[73] In studying the effect of low velocity collisions on muscles, using electromyography (EMG), Kumar found that the position of the head relative to the direction of impact may determine which muscles are injured.[74] During the collision impact, muscles contralateral to the side of impact are stretched and injured. The contralateral splenius capitis was injured during side impact, and the sternocleidomastoid muscles were at greatest risk for injury in rear end impacts.[74] Furthermore, occupants aware of imminent impact had a lower maximal EMG activity, suggesting that this reduces the potential for injury.[74] With acute WAD, there is typically a decreased active cervical range of motion (AROM), more EMG activity in the superficial neck flexors, and generalized hypersensitivity to a many stimuli independent of psychological distress, suggesting central nervous system (CNS) sensitization.[75] Individuals with moderate and severe WAD also had lower pain thresholds, altered kinesthetic awareness, more psychological distress, and more fear of movement or re-injury. Generalized hyperexcitability and CNS sensitization are also common in patients with chronic WAD.[75]

Many individuals with WAD improve rapidly but some continue to experience significant pain and disability. Patients with symptoms at 3 months tend to continue to have symptoms for 2 years or more.[73] Several factors have been linked to delayed recovery and poor outcome, including sociodemographic status, crash-related features, litigation, and various other physical and psychosocial factors. There are conflicts in the literature as to which factors are the most prognostic of a delayed or difficult recovery. There is strong evidence and agreement that a high initial pain intensity immediately after the injury predicts a difficult and extended recovery.[68-71] A population-based cohort study found that neck pain on palpation; pain or numbness from neck to shoulders, arms, or hands; or headache and muscle pain at presentation predict a longer recovery.[69] It has been suggested that high initial pain intensity and disability produce poorer outcomes because of increased CNS sensitization.[75] Although some report that older age, female gender, and an insurance system that compensates for pain and suffering are associated with slower progress and greater chronicity and disability,[69-71,74] a systematic review of the literature found that older age, female gender, high acute psychological response, angular deformity of the neck, rear-end collision, or compensation system were not prognostic of delayed recovery.[72]

BACK PAIN DURING PREGNANCY AND POSTPARTUM

Back pain during pregnancy is common. Large-scale population-based studies have found that 35% to 90% of women have back pain during pregnancy.[10-12,14,76,77] Epidemiological studies also report that back pain during pregnancy is 2-3 times more common than at other times in life.[10,12] Although many factors may be associated with an increased risk of back pain during pregnancy, a history of back pain before pregnancy is the most consistent and well-substantiated risk factor.[13,15,78-80] Having back pain during pregnancy does not affect the pregnancy outcome[77] and does not appear to be associated with weight gain before or during pregnancy.[79] Back pain during pregnancy may severely limit activities of daily living (ADLs) beyond the typical limitations experienced during pregnancy and more than a third of women who have back pain during pregnancy find that this pain limits their activities.[12,14] Women who experience back pain during pregnancy also require significantly more sick leave time, with at least 20% of pregnant women not attending work as a result of back pain alone.[80-82] The increase in back pain during pregnancy does not appear to be caused by the biomechanical changes of pregnancy, with only a large sagittal and transverse diameter of the abdomen and a large lumbar lordosis being very weakly correlated with back pain.[15]

Back pain during pregnancy and postpartum may originate from the lumbar spine (above the sacrum) or from the sacroiliac (SI) joint structures (also called posterior pelvic pain, [PPP]).[15,83-85] Pain from the lumbar spine generally increases with forward flexion, causes decreased lumbar ROM, is elicited with palpation of the lumbar spine muscles, has negative SI joint provocations tests, has occurred previously, and improves with exercise and education.[15,83,85] In contrast, with PPP, which is four times more common than lumbar spine pain during pregnancy, lumbar ROM is normal; pain is located in the buttocks and posterior pelvis; is worse with walking, standing, or turning in bed; may decrease with an SI belt; is elicited with palpation of the gluteal and hip muscles; has positive SI *provocation tests;* and usually begins during pregnancy.[83,84] Women with PPP do not appear to benefit from back exercises and education addressing the lumbar spine.[85] There is some evidence that PPP is associated with increasing levels of the hormone relaxin[15,86] and poor function of the pelvic musculature.[87] Lumbar pain and PPP can coexist during pregnancy.[10,14,16,78]

Current evidence indicates that back pain during pregnancy is not a normal consequence of pregnancy that can be predicted to resolve with delivery. Approximately 15% to 65% of women report substantial persistent back and pelvic pain postpartum,[12] and if a woman has back pain during pregnancy, she is at increased risk of pain postpartum[16,83] and has a poor prognosis for improvement immediately after delivery.[81,83,85,88] One study found that immediately after delivery about two-thirds of women report they have back pain, with most recovering from this within 4-5 months, but with over one-third still having pain 1 year later and 7% reporting the pain as severe.[89] Another study found that 68% of women who had back pain during pregnancy of at least moderate intensity continued to have recurrences of back pain throughout life with a concurrent diminution in their health.[76,90] Given the high frequency of recurrent back pain in the general population, it is not clear if this represents a greater incidence than would be expected in a control population. Postpartum pain does not appear to be related to the use of epidural anesthesia or to the type of delivery.[77] Some risk factors for pain persisting 2 years or more after delivery are onset of severe pain early in gestation and inability to decrease weight to prepregnancy levels.[77]

SYSTEMS FOR CLASSIFICATION OF SPINAL DISORDERS

Back and neck disorders are not caused by only one specific pathological entity.[91-97] Similar signs and symptoms may have a variety of causes, and very often the precise cause is not known.[98] Even when degenerative changes are seen on imaging, the presence and degree of degenerative change is known to not correlate well with symptom intensity or degree of disability[32,37,99] Therefore classification systems have been developed to categorize these disorders into syndromes based on a combination of pathology, clustering of signs and symptoms, and duration of symptoms. Such classification systems can help with clinical decision making, determining prognosis, evaluating the quality of care, conducting research, and selecting interventions for patients with spinal disorders.[100] Currently, several classification systems are being investigated for clinical usefulness, reliability, and validity.

The Québec Task Force on Spinal Disorders classification system is most frequently referred to by physicians and the medical literature. The three classification systems most often used by PTs are the McKenzie Classification System,[101] the Movement System Impairment-Based Classification,[94-97,102] and the Treatment-Based Classification System.[93]

The Québec Task Force on Spinal Disorders Diagnostic Classification System for Spinal Disorders. In 1987 the Québec Task Force (QTFC) on Spinal Disorders presented a diagnostic classification system for spinal disorders that could be used to assist in making clinical decisions, determining a prognosis, assessing quality of care, and carrying out scientific research.[103] Patients are classified using simple clinical criteria determined through history, physical examination, radiological tests, and reaction to treatment. This system classifies activity-related spinal disorders into 11 categories and further divides these categories by duration of symptoms and work status (Table 8-7). The first four categories are divided by symptom duration into acute (<7 days), subacute (7 days to 7 weeks), or chronic (>7 weeks) stages and by whether the patient is or is not working. The first category, believed to be the largest, includes spinal pain in the lumbar, thoracic, or cervical areas without neurological signs or distal radiation. Subsequent QTFC categories reflect increasing severity with the addition of radiating pain patterns and/or neurological signs. QTFC categories 5 through 7 rely on additional imaging studies and diagnostic testing, and categories 8 and 9 are based on the patient's status after surgical intervention. Individuals with chronic pain syndrome are placed in QTFC category 10 because of the complex interaction with psychosocial factors and work status, and category 11 is reserved for all other syndromes.[103]

The validity but not the reliability of the QTFC system has been examined. A prospective cohort study of patients with lumbar spinal stenosis and 2 months of sciatica found that symptom severity was worse in patients in higher categories but that the categories did not correlate with functional abilities. QTFC category was predictive of surgery, with 7% of patients in QTFC category 1 receiving surgery and 84% in QTFC category 6 receiving surgery.[104] Surprisingly, those who did not have surgery had a better outcome 1 year later if they were initially placed in a higher QTFC category.

Another prospective cohort study of workers with subacute pain found that the first four QTFC categories had poor discriminative validity, demonstrated by the low correlation between category and scores on functional status measures, but that the system did have good predictive validity.[105] Patients in QTFC categories 3 and 4 (with distal radiation of symptoms) had higher pain levels and lower functional status and fewer had returned to work at a 1-year follow-up than patients in categories 1 and 2 (without distal radiation of symptoms). One study found that the QTFC category correlated with pain and disability at the time of examination in patients with acute work-related LBP but that it did not predict pain or disability at discharge from rehabilitation or 1 year later.[106]

The McKenzie Diagnostic Classification System for Spinal Disorders. The McKenzie approach to classifying patients with back pain is the system most commonly used by PTs.[107] This system was developed by analyzing patients' responses to movements in several planes, integrating Cyriax's manual therapy principles, and relating these clinical findings to existing literature on IVD disease.[107] Initially, a patient's symptoms are classified as mechanical if the pain changes with movements or positions or as nonmechanical, indicating inflammatory or other medical conditions, if symptoms do not change with movement or positions.[108] Patients with mechanical symptoms without serious medical pathology, neurological deficits, or constant, severe sciatica are then put into treatment categories based on their history, posture, and specific movement testing performed in standing, sitting, supine, and prone positions. Examination findings of particular interest include loss of ROM and rapid changes in the intensity or location of pain and symptoms with repeated or sustained movements.

Movement testing first tests whether repeated and sustained movements centralizes or peripheralizes the patient's symptoms (Fig. 8-9). *Centralization* refers to pain or other symptoms that originate from the spine, that are felt lateral to the midline or distally, and that rapidly move proximally or centrally in response to specific movements.[101,109] Movements that cause centralization are believed to be therapeutic. Peripheralization refers to pain or other symptoms moving laterally or distally in response to specific movements. Movements that cause peripheralization should be avoided or minimized.

Back pain is then also classified into one of the following three syndromes: postural, dysfunction, or derangement. The examination findings and suggested interventions for each of these syndromes are summarized in Table 8-8. *Postural syndrome* is thought to be caused by prolonged abnormal stresses that produce mechanical deformation or vascular insufficiency and then pain in

TABLE 8-7	The Québec Task Force Classification of Spinal Disorders
QTFC Category	**Definition**
1	Pain without radiation
2	Pain with proximal radiation (above the knee)
	Acute: Duration of symptoms: <7 days; working or not working
3	Pain with distal radiation (below the knee)
	Subacute: Duration of symptoms: 7 days to 7 weeks; working or not working
4	Pain with distal radiation and neurological signs
	Chronic: Duration of symptoms: >7 weeks; working or not working
5	Presumptive compression of a spinal nerve root on a simple x-ray
6	Compression of a spinal nerve root confirmed by specific imaging techniques
7	Spinal stenosis
8	Postsurgical 1-6 months after the intervention
9	Postsurgical >6 months after the intervention
10	Chronic pain syndrome
11	Other diagnoses

From Spitzer W: *Spine* 12(7):S1-S53, 1987.

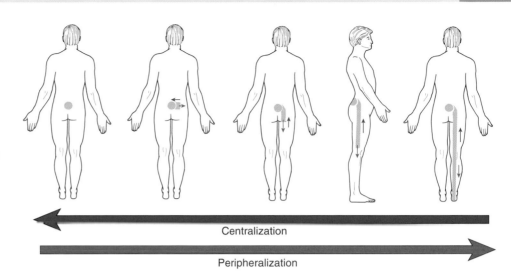

FIG. 8-9 Centralization occurs when symptoms move toward the midline or site of origin. Peripheralization occurs when symptoms move away from the midline or site of origin. *Adapted from Magee DJ:* Orthopedic Physical Assessment, *ed 4, Philadelphia, 2002, WB Saunders.*

Centralization

Peripheralization

TABLE 8-8   The McKenzie Classification System for Spinal Disorders

Category	Examination Findings	Suggested Interventions
Postural syndrome	Lumbar posture is poor in sitting and standing but without deformity. Pain occurs only with sustained postures and is not reproduced by repeated movements.	Promote postural correction. Avoid sustained end-range positions.
DYSFUNCTION SYNDROMES		
Flexion	Poor posture with loss of movement or function. No pain or radiation with movement. Pain at end-range of flexion that does not worsen with repetition. Loss of flexion ROM. Symptoms appear stable without rapid changes.	End-range flexion exercises.
Extension	Poor posture with loss of movement or function. Pain at end-range of extension. Loss of extension ROM. Symptoms appear stable without rapid changes.	End-range extension exercises.
Adherent root	Intermittent sciatic pain. Loss of flexion ROM with deviation during range. Flexion reproduces lower extremity pain that ceases on standing.	Stretching exercises for adherent nerve root.
Side-gliding	Poor posture occurs with loss of movement or function. Loss of side-gliding ROM with intermittent central LBP at end-range of side-glide, which does not worsen with repetition.	End-range gliding exercises.
DERANGEMENT SYNDROMES		
One	Central or symmetrical LBP without postural deformity of lumbar spine. Repeated flexion may peripheralize or worsen pain. Repeated extension centralizes, diminishes, or eliminates pain.	Initially repeated extension exercises.
Two	Central or symmetrical LBP, with or without buttock or thigh pain. Lumbar kyphosis.	Initially prone lying or sustained extension position followed by repeated extension exercises.
Three	Unilateral LBP, with or without buttock or thigh pain. No postural deformity of lumbar spine. Repeated flexion may peripheralize or worsen pain. Repeated extension centralizes, diminishes, or eliminates pain.	Usually repeated extension exercises centralize pain. If not, side-glide with extension.
Four	Unilateral or asymmetrical LBP with or without buttock or thigh pain. Lateral shift postural deformity. Flexion and extension increase pain.	Correction of lateral shift followed by extension exercises.
Five	Unilateral or asymmetrical LBP with or without buttock or thigh pain. Constant or intermittent leg pain extends below the knee. Repeated flexion peripheralizes or worsens pain. Repeated extension centralizes, diminishes, or eliminates pain.	Usually repeated extension exercises centralize pain. If not, side-glide or rotation followed by extension exercises.
Six	Unilateral or asymmetrical LBP with or without buttock or thigh pain. Constant leg pain extends below the knee. Lateral shift postural deformity. Flexion and extension increase pain.	Correction of lateral shift followed by extension exercises.
Seven	Unilateral or bilateral LBP with or without buttock or thigh pain. Deformity of accentuated lordosis. Repeated flexion centralizes, diminishes, or eliminates pain.	Flexion exercises.

From McKenzie R: *The Lumbar Spine: Mechanical Diagnosis and Therapy,* Waikane, New Zealand, 1981, Spinal Publications; Razmjou H, Kramer JF, Yamada R: *J Orthop Sports Phys Ther* 30(7):368-383, 2000; Riddle DL, Rothstein JM: *Spine* 18(10):1333-1344, 1993.
ROM, Range of motion; *LBP,* low back pain.

normal articular or contractile structures.[101,110,111] The *dysfunction syndrome* is characterized by pain that results from mechanical deformation of abnormal adaptively-shortened soft tissue following maintenance of poor positioning after degeneration, trauma, or a derangement. This pain is intermittent and occurs with a loss of ROM in a specific direction. The *derangement syndrome* is characterized by anatomical disruption of the structures of the intervertebral joints. McKenzie originally attributed a derangement to internal disruption of the IVD or herniation of the NP but later stated that pain from derangement can also be caused by displacement of articular structures. In a derangement, spinal movement is painful and limited in the direction of displacement.[101,110,111]

The reliability of the McKenzie classification system has been investigated in a number of studies, with some indicating it has good reliability, particularly when used by therapists with training in the system, and others suggesting that it has questionable reliability.[99,108,110-113] One study found only 39% agreement in categorization among 49 randomly paired PTs performing repeated independent examinations of 363 patients with LBP.[111] However, this study was criticized because the patients were examined repeatedly, which may have altered the location and intensity of pain and symptoms.[108] Since detection of the presence and direction of a lateral shift are thought to be the most difficult components of the McKenzie examination, one study specifically evaluated this component and found only 47% agreement between 10 PTs for the presence of a clinically relevant lateral shift.[113]

Studies evaluating the reliability of the McKenzie classification system when used by therapists with additional training have yielded more positive results. One study found 90% or greater interexaminer agreement in assessing pain behavior and the response of pain to repeated movements, 80% agreement for finding lumbar deformity, 70% agreement for finding end-range pain, and 55% agreement for finding a lateral shift, between 2 PTs with some additional McKenzie training.[112] A similar study with 45 patients and 2 PTs with McKenzie certification found 93% agreement between examiners for placing patients into the three major syndromes, 97% agreement for placing patients into derangement subsyndromes, 78%

agreement for the presence of lateral shift, 98% agreement for the relevance of the lateral component to the classification, and 100% agreement for the presence of a sagittal plane deformity.[108] Kilpikoski[110] reported a 95% agreement between 2 therapists with specific McKenzie training for classifying patients into the main syndromes, 95% agreement of the centralization of pain, 77% agreement for the presence of a lateral shift and 79% agreement for the direction of the shift. In one study comparing physical therapy students' abilities to classify patients using the McKenzie system to experienced PTs, an 88% agreement overall was reported in classifying patients, with 86% agreement among the students and 90% among the experienced therapists.[99]

Overall, despite conflicting reports, most of the evidence indicates that therapists can reliably categorize low back patients according to the McKenzie classification system, particularly if they have some additional training in the use of this system.

The Delitto Treatment-Based Diagnostic Classification System for Spinal Disorders. Delitto, Erhard, and Bowling[93] developed a system for classifying patients with LBP into categories to direct management. The patients are categorized based on the history of their condition, history suggesting possible nonmusculoskeletal causes for back pain, the responses of signs and symptoms to movement tests, and alignment of body structures.[94,114] This treatment-based system has two to three levels reflecting the clinical decisions needed for patient classification (Fig. 8-10).

The first level is based on whether the patient can be managed primarily and independently by the PT or by the PT in consultation with another health care practitioner or if referral to another health care practitioner is required. Information for classification at this level is obtained from patient self-reports, a medical screening questionnaire, a modified *Oswestry Low Back Pain Disability Questionnaire*, pain diagrams, pain scale, and Waddell's screening for abnormal illness behavior.[93,100,114]

The second level of classification is based on stages and severity of disability. In stage I, also referred to as acute,[114,115] patients cannot sit for more than 30 minutes, stand for more than 15 minutes, and walk more than ¼

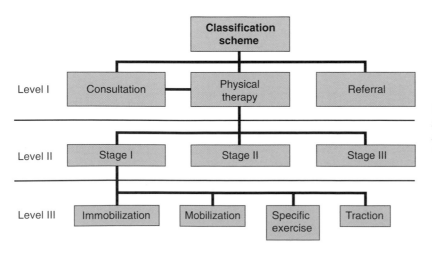

FIG. 8-10 The treatment-based classification system for low back pain. *Adapted from Delitto A, Erhard RE, Bowling RW:* Phys Ther *75(6):470-485; discussion 485-479, 1995.*

mile and have an Oswestry score of greater than 30.[93] In stage II, which reflects a less severe problem, patients have an Oswestry score between 15 and 30, but their back pain still prevents them from performing instrumental ADLs (IADLs).[93] In stage III, patients can perform IADLs and score less than 15 on the Oswestry, but they cannot perform sustained activities requiring high physical demands.[93]

The third level of classification only applies to patients in stage I and consists of four categories: immobilization, *mobilization,* specific exercise, and traction.[115] Patients are placed into these categories based on key examination findings, and each category designates specific recommended treatments.[114] Patients in the immobilization category have findings indicating lumbar segmental instability. Patients in the mobilization category have findings indicating that they need lumbar or SI mobilization or *manipulation.* Patients in the specific exercise category have centralization during the examination, and patients who appear to have nerve root compression without centralization are placed into the traction category (Table 8-9).

Patient classification may change during an episode of back pain. Thus patients receive interventions specific to their individual presentation, and these interventions are modified as the patient's presentation changes.[115]

Patient classification according to the treatment-based approach has moderate interrater reliability.[114] This system has also demonstrated validity in directing effective treatment. In a randomized controlled trial (RCT), the outcome of patients with LBP treated for 4 weeks directed by this classification system had greater improvement in disability, were more likely to return to work, and were more satisfied with treatment and there was a trend toward lower costs than for patients treated according to clinical practice guidelines for patients with acute work-related LBP.[115]

Movement System Impairment-Based Classification. Van Dillen, Sahrmann, and associates[94-97] proposed

an alternative classification system for LBP that focuses on movement system impairments and is unrelated to symptom acuity. The fundamental principle of this system is that the habitual movements and postures individuals adopt in reaction to the stresses of functional activities differ from a kinesiological ideal to eventually cause LBP.

In this system, patients are categorized according to the direction of spinal alignment or motion that produces or exacerbates symptoms.[94-97] During the examination the patient performs trunk and limb movements and holds various trunk positions to determine which lumbar movement dysfunction or movement or alignment pattern is most consistently associated with an increase in symptoms.[94,115] Active limb movements are part of this examination because patients tend to habitually use limb movement strategies that overemphasize spinal movement and thus affect their LBP and ability to perform ADLs. Patients are then classified into one of five mutually exclusive categories: lumbar flexion, lumbar extension, lumbar rotation, lumbar rotation with extension, or lumbar rotation with flexion.[96,102] Treatment strategies focus on limiting direction-specific motions or alignments that increase symptoms and on ameliorating impairments in muscle force and joint flexibility thought to effect the lumbar movement dysfunction.[94]

The interrater reliability of this approach for interpreting responses of symptom behavior was found to be good (98% to 100%) and for judgment of alignment and movement acceptable (65% to 100%).[95] The face validity of this approach is also supported by a study in which 83% of 185 patients with LBP were found to have symptoms with one of seven primary tests, and of these, 95% had decreased symptoms with the corresponding movement correction.[97]

The pertinent features of this system (symptoms, key tests and signs, associated signs, differential movement diagnosis and associated diagnoses, and screening for

TABLE 8-9 The Delitto Treatment-Based Diagnostic Classification System for Spinal Disorders

Classification	Examination Findings	Treatment
MOBILIZATION		
SI pattern	Unilateral symptoms without signs of nerve root compression, positive findings for SI region dysfunction (pelvic asymmetry, standing, and seated flexion tests)	Joint mobilization or manipulation techniques and spinal AROM exercises
Lumbar pattern	Unilateral symptoms without signs of nerve root compression, asymmetrical restrictions of lumbar side-bending motion, lumbar segmental hypomobility	Joint mobilization or manipulation techniques and spinal AROM exercises
SPECIFIC EXERCISE		
Flexion pattern	Patient preference for sitting versus standing, centralization with lumbar flexion motions	Lumbar flexion exercises, avoidance of extension activities
Extension pattern	Patient preference for standing versus sitting, centralization with lumbar extension motions	Lumbar extension exercises, avoidance of flexion activities
Immobilization	Frequent previous episodes, positive response to prior manipulation or bracing as treatment, presence of "instability catch" or lumbar segmental hypermobility	Trunk strengthening and stabilization exercises
Traction	Radicular signs present, unable to centralize with movements, may have lateral shift deformity	Mechanical or auto-traction

Adapted from Delitto A, Erhard RE, Bowling RW: *Phys Ther* 75(6):470-485; discussion 485-479, 1995.
SI, Sacroiliac; *AROM,* active range of motion.

potential medical diagnosis) are described in detail in Sahrmann's text.[116]

EXAMINATION

The clinician follows a series of hierarchical steps to develop a diagnosis and plan of care for patients with spinal dysfunction (Fig. 8-11). An extensive interview incorporating self-reported pain and disability is needed to establish not only the history of this episode and the patient's medical, social, and occupational status but also to establish if the patient should be referred to other specialists. The history and systems review allows the clinician to develop a preliminary diagnosis or working hypothesis. After completing the patient history and

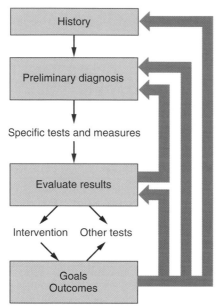

FIG. 8-11 Relationships between examination, evaluation, and patient management.

systems review, the clinician performs a scanning examination to determine which structures are involved and to establish a musculoskeletal diagnosis. The scanning examination establishes which impairments and limitations require intervention and may indicate a need for more in-depth testing of specific movement impairments. The scanning examination may also point to the need for further detailed investigation to establish a diagnosis and an effective intervention program. The clinician combines findings from the patient history, systems review, and the scanning and specific examination to evaluate the patient, determine their diagnosis and prognosis, and plan interventions.

PATIENT HISTORY

In patients with spinal dysfunction, taking a thorough, carefully directed history is the first and one of the most important steps in determining a physical therapy diagnosis. A preliminary diagnosis is developed by comparing the patient's reported signs and symptoms to established patterns. The clinician can determine if the patient's condition is probably mechanical or nonmechanical and whether it is acute, subacute, or chronic. The patient's responses to specific questions will then direct selection of specific tests and measures. The patient history includes information about the patient's psychosocial and occupational status and relevant medical history, as well as information about the location and severity of pain, sensory changes and weakness, the effects of movement or postural and position changes on symptoms, and whether symptoms centralize or peripheralize with position changes (Table 8-10).

Certain specific questions should also be asked when there are problems in specific spinal regions. For patients with neck disorders, the clinician should ask if the patient experiences dizziness, tinnitus, vertigo, nausea, or blurred vision to determine if the vertebral arteries may be involved.[117] For patients with upper cervical spine and

TABLE 8-10	Questions to Address Specific Areas of the History in Patients with Spinal Disorders
Area of History	**Questions**
Chief complaint	What brings you to physical therapy today?
Duration	How long have you had these symptoms?
Nature of disorder	What do the symptoms feel like?
Location	Where are your symptoms?
Behavior	Are the symptoms constant or intermittent?
	What activities/postures/movements make the symptoms better? Worse?
	How does rest affect your pain?
	Are there positions or movements that seem to make your symptoms better? Worse?
	What is the effect of coughing, sneezing, or straining on your symptoms?
	Are you getting better or worse?
	How disabling/painful are your symptoms?
	How easily provoked are your symptoms?
	How long after symptoms occur does it take for them to subside?
	What are your symptoms like first thing in the morning? During the day? Evening? Night?
Etiology	Do you know what caused it to start?
	Is it a result of an injury? If so, can you describe how the injury occurred (e.g., motor vehicle collision, LOC, type of impact)?
	Have you had previous episodes? How did they respond to treatment?

LOC, Loss of consciousness.

temporomandibular joint (TMJ) disorders, the therapist should also ask about headaches and try to determine if the headaches are related to the musculoskeletal disorder. For patients with thoracic spine involvement, one should ask if the symptoms are affected by deep breathing as this may indicate involvement of the ribs. For patients with lumbar spine involvement, the clinician should ask about the effects of sitting, standing, and walking to differentiate symptoms caused by spinal stenosis from those caused by IVD dysfunction and about genitourinary symptoms because these may indicate sacral nerve root involvement. When SI joint dysfunction is suspected, the therapist should ask if symptoms increase with prolonged or unilateral weight bearing and with changing positions.[118]

During the history, the therapist also screens the patient for indicators of serious medical pathology or red flags (Box 8-1). The presence of any red flags (also referred to as Waddell signs) increases the likelihood that the patient's problem is not of musculoskeletal origin and therefore the patient should be referred to a physician for medical diagnosis and possible intervention.

Certain psychosocial, cognitive, and behavioral factors, such as believing that back pain is harmful or potentially severely disabling, can increase the risk of an individual with acute LBP developing protracted pain and disability[8,118] (Table 8-11). Patients with these risk factors may benefit from referral to psychosocial health professionals to develop strategies to prevent pain behavior, adoption of a sick role, inactivity, re-injury, and recurrences.[119]

Signs and symptoms of organic problems or findings from the physical examination that indicate the presence of pathology or disease should be distinguished from signs of nonorganic problems that deviate from the usual presentation of the disease (Table 8-12).[19,120]

Several reliable self-report questionnaires used as outcome measures for patients with spinal disorders can also be useful components of the examination. Patients can complete these questionnaires before the initial examination and at intervals during a period of treatment. This can save valuable clinician time and be used to evaluate progress. Generic health status indices, such as the SF-36 Health Survey, can be used to gauge the general health and well-being of the patient.[121] Several condition-specific questionnaires, such as the Oswestry Low Back Pain Disability Questionnaire,[122] the Roland-Morris Questionnaire,[123] and the *Neck Disability Index* (NDI),[124] are also available. The Oswestry Low Back Pain Disability Questionnaire is a valid and reliable 10-section self-report measure that is responsive to change in patients with LBP.[124-128] A reduction by 6 points or more in the Oswestry score indicates improvement in patients with LBP.[129] The Roland-Morris Questionnaire is another valid and reliable condition-specific outcome measure for patients with LBP.[125,127,130] A change of 5 points on this scale reflects a clinically relevant improvement.[131] The NDI is a 10-item self-administered questionnaire similar to the Oswestry that measures neck pain and disability. It has a test-retest reliability of 0.89.[132] It is the most commonly used and most extensively validated outcome measure among several diverse patient populations.[133] Although these questionnaires are widely used for most patients, their results may be questionable when reading and comprehension skills are limited or when English is not the patient's preferred language.

SYSTEMS REVIEW

The systems review is used to target areas requiring further examination and to define areas that may cause complications or indicate a need for precautions during the examination and intervention processes. See Chapter 1 for details of the systems review.

TESTS AND MEASURES

Many clinical tests are available for examining patients with spinal disorders. The usefulness of these tests depends on their clinical relevance, as well as their reliability, validity, sensitivity, and specificity. The following section describes clinical tests for the spine, including indications for the test, basic procedures for performing the test, interpretation of findings, and when available, the evidence regarding the test.

Scanning Tests and Measures. A scanning examination of the spine is used to rule in or out involvement of various structures and to determine if symptoms are of musculoskeletal origin. Findings may indicate need for more specialized tests or a higher level of skill and experience in interpretation. The scanning examination determines whether muscles, nerves, joints, or joint structures are causing symptoms and determines if predisposing factors contributed to symptom onset. During this part of the examination, the therapist tries to implicate specific structures by placing them under mechanical stress and checking if this reproduces the patient's symptoms.

BOX 8-1	Red Flags or Waddell Signs: Indicators of Possible Serious Medical Pathology

Presentation age <20 years or onset >55 years
Violent trauma (e.g., fall from a height, traffic accident)
Constant, progressive pain that does not change with
   movement or position
Thoracic pain
History of:
   Carcinoma
   Systemic steroid use
   Drug abuse
Human immunodeficiency virus (HIV)
Systemically unwell
Unexplained weight loss
Persistent severe restriction of lumbar flexion
Widespread neurological symptoms (numbness,
   weakness)
Structural deformity
Test results:
   Erythrocyte sedimentation rate (ESR) >25 mm
   Plain x-ray showing vertebral collapse or bone destruction

Adapted from Waddell G: The Back Pain Revolution, Churchill Livingstone, 2004, New York.

TABLE 8-11	Psychosocial Risk Factors for Developing Chronic Back Pain
Risk Factors	**Examples**
Attitudes and beliefs about back pain	Belief that pain is harmful or disabling resulting in fear-avoidance behaviors (e.g., guarding and fear of movement)
	Belief that all pain must be abolished before attempting to return to work or normal activity
	Expectation of increased pain with activity or work, lack of ability to predict capability
	Catastrophizing, thinking the worst, misinterpreting bodily symptoms
	Belief that pain is uncontrollable
Behaviors	Use of extended rest, disproportionate "downtime"
	Reduced activity level with significant withdrawal form activities of daily living
	Irregular participation or poor compliance with physical exercise, tendency for activities to be in a "boom-bust" cycle
	Avoidance of normal activity and progressive substitution of lifestyle away from productive activity
Compensation issues	Lack of financial incentive to return to work
	Delay in accessing income support and treatment cost, disputes over eligibility
	History of claim(s) due to other injuries or pain problems
	History of extended time off work due to injury or other pain problem
	History of previous back pain, with a previous claim(s) and time off work
	Previous experience of ineffective case management (e.g., absence of interest, perception of being treated punitively)
Diagnosis and treatment	Health professional sanctioning disability, not providing interventions that will improve function
	Experience of conflicting diagnoses or explanations for back pain, resulting in confusion
	Diagnostic language leading to catastrophizing and fear (e.g., fear of ending up in wheelchair)
	Dramatization of back pain by health professional producing dependency on treatments and continuation of passive treatment
	Number of times visited health professional in last year (excluding present episode of back pain)
	Expectation of a "techno-fix" (e.g., requests to treat as if body were a machine)
	Lack of satisfaction with previous treatment for back pain
	Advice to withdraw from job
Emotions	Fear of increased pain with activity or work
	Depression (especially long-term low mood), loss of sense of enjoyment
	More irritable than usual
	Anxiety about and heightened awareness of body sensations (includes sympathetic nervous system arousal)
	Feeling under stress and unable to maintain sense of control
	Presence of social anxiety or disinterest in social activity
	Feeling useless and not needed
Family	Overprotective partner/spouse, emphasizing fear of harm or encouraging catastrophizing (usually well-intentioned)
	Solicitous behavior from spouse (e.g., taking over tasks)
	Socially punitive responses form spouse (e.g., ignoring, expressing frustration)
	Extent to which family members support any attempt to return to work
	Lack of support person to talk to about problems
Work	History of manual work, notably from the following occupational groups: fishing, forestry, and farming workers; construction, including carpenters and builders; nurses; truck drivers; laborers
	Work history, including patterns of frequent job changes, experiencing stress at work, job dissatisfaction, poor relationships with peers or supervisors, lack of vocational direction
	Belief that work is "harmful" and that it will do damage or be dangerous
	Unsupportive or unhappy current work environment
	Low educational background, low socioeconomic status
	Job involves significant biomechanical demands, such as lifting, manual handling of heavy items, extended sitting, extended standing, driving, vibration, maintenance of constrained or sustained postures, inflexible work schedule preventing appropriate breaks
	Job involves shift work or working unsociable hours
	Minimal availability of selected duties and graduated return to work pathways, with unsatisfactory implementation of these
	Negative experience of workplace management of back pain (e.g., absence of a reporting system, discouragement to report, punitive response from supervisors and managers)
	Absence of interest from employer

Musculoskeletal

Posture. Deviations from normal postural alignment are frequently seen in many types of spinal disorders. A forward head, rounded or protracted shoulders, and exaggerated thoracic kyphosis frequently accompanies neck and shoulder dysfunctions. Areas of flatness or diminished spinal curves can indicate mobility restrictions. McKenzie believes that diminished lumbar lordosis is both a precursor and indicator of posterior displacement of the nucleus in IVD disease.[101] An exaggerated lordosis often accompanies spondylolisthesis. With increasing age, both thoracic kyphosis and lumbar lordosis have been shown to increase.[134] Taken alone, postural abnormalities are not pathognomonic for any specific dysfunction[135,136] and

TABLE 8-12	Signs and Symptoms Differentiating Physical Causes of Spinal Pain from Illness Behavior	
	Physical Disease	**Illness Behavior**
PAIN		
Distribution	Localized, anatomical	Nonanatomical, regional, magnified
Description	Sensory	Emotional
SYMPTOMS		
Pain	Musculoskeletal or neurological distribution	Whole leg pain
		Pain at the tip of the tailbone
Numbness	Dermatomal distribution	Whole limb numbness
Weakness	Myotomal distribution	Whole extremity giving way
Time pattern	Varies with time and activity	Never free of pain
Response to treatment	Variable benefit	Intolerance of treatments
		Emergency hospitalization
SIGNS		
Tenderness	Musculoskeletal distribution	Superficial, nonanatomical
Axial loading	Neck pain	LBP
Simulated rotation	Nerve root pain	LBP
SLR	Limited on formal examination	Marked improvement with distraction
	No improvement on distraction	
Strength	Consistent myotomal distribution of weakness	Regional, jerky, giving way
Sensory changes	Dermatomal distribution	Regional

Adapted from Waddell G: *The Back Pain Revolution,* New York, 2004, Churchill Livingstone.
LBP, Low back pain; *SLR,* straight leg raises.

have not been shown to be good predictors for the severity of back pain.[135] However, in conjunction with other signs and symptoms, postural analysis can be a useful adjunct in diagnosis of spinal dysfunction and intervention planning. To examine posture, the therapist observes the patient in standing from the front, side, and rear view. Bony landmarks are palpated and assessed for symmetry, depth, and alignment. Verbal and tactile cues may be given to determine whether the patient can volitionally correct deviations (see Chapter 4).

Range of Motion. ROM is examined to evaluate the quantity and quality of movement and the effect of movement on symptoms. Spinal ROM is the most commonly assessed impairment in patients with spinal disorders and is an integral component of diagnosing back pain, predicting outcome, and assessing responses to interventions.[102,137] Spinal ROM normally decreases with age.[134,138-140] AROM is usually estimated by comparison with the expected norm or measured with an inclinometer and is documented on a movement diagram indicating the plane(s) in which movement is limited and any symptoms produced at the end of range (Fig. 8-12).

The quality of movement can also be very revealing. Any hesitancy or reluctance to complete a motion or slight deviations in movement direction, hitching, or catching may occur to accommodate a hypomobile or painful segment. Momentary reflexive muscle contraction may also occur when trying to stabilize a hypermobile segment. Portions of the spine that appear to move as a block or flattening of an expected curvature can also point to hypomobility, whereas excessive bending at a single segment implies hypermobility. Any alterations in the smooth quality of movement require specific mobility examination of the involved segments. It is important to differentiate between movements that provoke discomfort as a result of muscle tightness or novelty of the movement

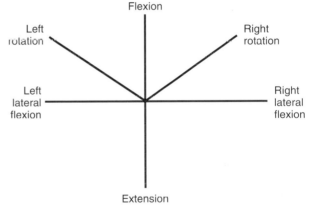

FIG. 8-12 A short-hand method of recording spinal range of motion. The therapist marks the locations of diminished range and any symptoms that occur during or at the end of motion.

and true symptom reproduction. Symptoms caused by any movement that produces the same pain for which the patient sought medical intervention is important diagnostically as it can reveal the nature of the disorder or provide insight into the mechanism of injury.

AROM in the cervical spine is measured with the patient seated (proper lumbosacral support is necessary for examining the cervical spine). The therapist asks the patient to sequentially flex, extend, rotate, and sidebend to each side. After completing each movement, the therapist applies overpressure to the movement by applying gentle graded pressure in the direction of the movement and noting the effect on range and symptoms. Fig. 8-13 shows positions of the therapist and the patient and the therapist's hands for applying overpressure to end-range cervical ROM. Passive ROM (PROM) of the cervical spine

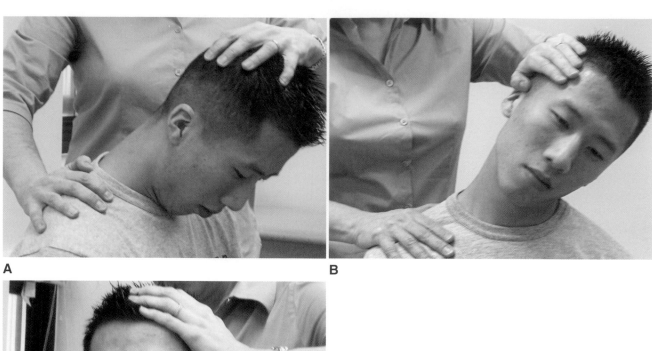

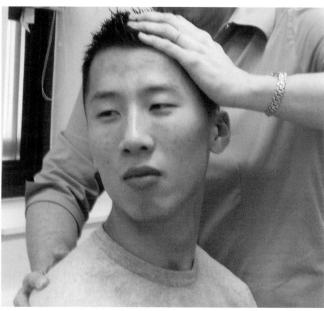

FIG. 8-13 Cervical spine range of motion with overpressure. Note hand placement. **A,** Flexion with overpressure. **B,** Sidebending with overpressure. **C,** Rotation with overpressure.

is examined with the patient supine on an examining table and the therapist standing while cradling the patient's head.

AROM of the thoracic and lumbar spine are assessed similarly to the cervical spine but with the patient standing. The therapist observes cardinal plane movements but before adding overpressure, and movements are repeated 5-10 times in each plane, while the therapist notes changes in symptoms. Any movements that cause pain or symptoms to peripheralize are stopped. Centralization of symptoms are carefully observed and repeated since these movements are incorporated into the intervention plan. The proper therapist and patient position and hand placement for applying overpressure to the thoracolumbar spine are shown in Fig. 8-14.

Most human activity involves multidimensional rather than simple cardinal plane movement. Therefore the clinician should also examine the range and effects of combined spinal movements. Selection of combined

movement testing should be guided by information in the patient history, indicating motions or positions associated with symptoms or that replicate the position of injury. To perform combined movements the patient should move to end-range in one plane and then superimpose movement in the other plane. Any sequence of movements can be combined as long as the full limit of one motion is reached before adding any additional movement.

Most studies indicate that spinal ROM can be examined reliably when measurement devices, such as inclinometers, are employed.[141-144] Fewer studies have investigated the reliability of observational assessment of spinal ROM. Interexaminer reliability has been reported as good (kappa = 0.43-0.76) for PTs examining spinal AROM and ROM that provokes symptoms in lateral bending, extension, and flexion,[145] whereas it is moderate (kappa = 0.6) for measuring sidebending and poor (kappa = 0.17-0.39) for measuring combined spinal movements in patients with LBP.[146]

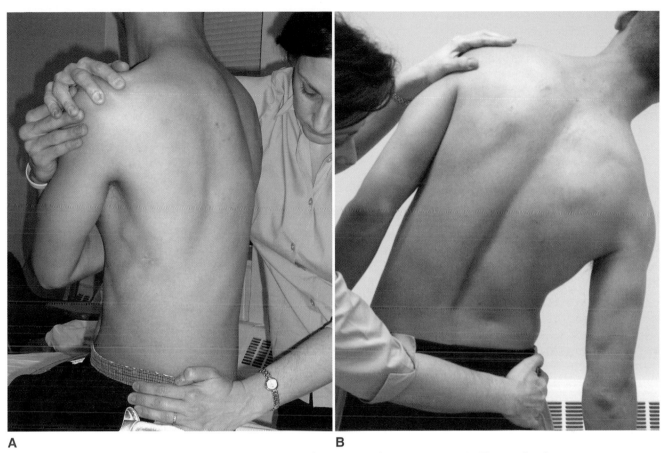

A   **B**

FIG. 8-14 Thoracolumbar spine range of motion with overpressure. **A,** Thoracolumbar rotation. **B,** Thoracolumbar lateral flexion.

The sensitivity and specificity of ROM measurements for diagnosing spinal disorders have also been studied. One study reported that cervical rotation to the involved side of less than 60 degrees and cervical flexion of less than 55 degrees has high sensitivity (0.89) for diagnosing cervical radiculopathy, whereas specificity was poor (0.49 for rotation and 0.41 for flexion).[147] Reduced lumbar motion has also been found to correlate moderately to weakly (r – 0.25 to 0.47) with disability[148-150] and chronic LBP.[151,152] A population-based epidemiological study found that lumbar rotation and lateral flexion and total trunk flexion were moderately associated with severity of back pain (kappa = 0.47),[135] and measures of spinal motion have been shown to correlate strongly ($r = 0.60$, $p = 0.005$) with measures of physical performance such as functional reach, moving from supine to sitting, and turning in place while standing.[134]

Passive Range of Motion of Single Intervertebral Joints. *Passive physiological intervertebral mobility* (PPIVM) testing is a routine part of the spinal examination. PPIVM testing assesses motion at each segmental level during passive motion into flexion, extension, side flexion, and rotation. To test PPIVM, the therapist palpates each segment as it is passively moved through its normal ROM. PPIVM testing techniques for various areas of the spine are illustrated in Fig. 8-15.

To evaluate the outcome of PPIVM testing, the therapist notes whether the movements provoke symptoms, judges end-feel, and decides whether the amount of available movement is normal, reduced (hypomobile), or excessive (hypermobile). This information, along with the results from the rest of the examination, is used to determine appropriate interventions. Painful hypomobile segments may benefit from mobilization or manipulation followed by stretching and strengthening of related muscles, whereas hypermobile segments may benefit from stabilization. During this testing, irritable hypermobile segments may be found in which a reflex muscle spasm is elicited during the passive testing, which prevents movement into the excessive painful range. Precise palpation skills are required for accurate determination of PPIVM.

The reliability and validity of manual palpation skills have been extensively studied, although many studies have statistical and methodological flaws.[153,154] Content validity is difficult to determine because there is no agreement on a reference gold standard, and reliability studies are often limited because they included only asymptomatic patients. Furthermore, variability in palpation techniques and terminology make comparisons between studies problematic. Despite these limitations, the evidence regarding the reliability and validity of these tests

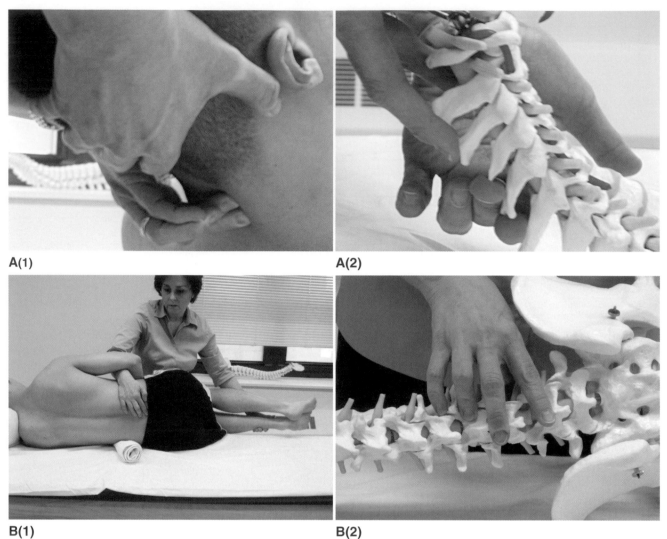

A(1)   A(2)

B(1)   B(2)

FIG. 8-15 **A(1),** Cervical spine flexion passive physiological intervertebral mobility. One hand cradles the occiput while the other palpates movement between the spinous processes; **A(2),** cervical spine passive physiological intervertebral mobility showing hand placement on skeletal model. Note the location of the therapist's index and middle finger palpating motion between adjacent spinous processes. **B(1),** Lumbar spine flexion passive physiological intervertebral mobility. One hand palpates spinal movements while the other produces lumbar spine flexion by moving the legs cranially; **B(2),** lumbar spine flexion passive physiological intervertebral mobility showing hand placement on skeletal model. Note the location of the therapist's index and middle finger palpating motion between adjacent spinous processes.

does provide some useful information. In the cervical spine, studies have found excellent (kappa = 0.81) intrarater and fair-to-moderate (kappa = 0.38 to 0.52) interrater agreement for PPIVM testing in patients with and without neck pain.[155-157] In the thoracolumbar spine, intrarater agreement for PPIVM has been found to be excellent ($r = 0.81$ to 0.91),[158] whereas interrater reliability has ranged from poor for stiffness (21% to 29% agreement; $ICC_{(1,1)} = 0.03$ to 0.37),[159] to moderate to excellent for mobility (51% to 98% agreement).[160] When examining spinal motion in a mechanical model, sensitivity for the detection of abnormalities was found to be poor (0.510 to 0.636), whereas specificity was found to be good (0.868 to 0.902), indicating that although abnormalities that are

present are often not detected on examination, when the examination does detect a problem, there probably really is one.[153]

Muscle Length. Examination for muscle tightness or loss of extensibility should precede evaluation for weakness since tight muscles influence movement patterns and inhibit their antagonists. When testing for tightness, when muscle attachments are passively moved apart, they should move easily with a soft or springy pain-free end-feel. Tight muscles will limit range with a firm and painful end-feel. In patients with cervical and thoracic spinal dysfunction, the length of the upper trapezius, levator scapulae, and pectoralis major muscles should be examined. In lumbosacral dysfunction, the length of the lumbar erector spinae, hip flexors, hamstrings, piriformis, quadratus lumborum, and hip adductors should be examined.

Muscle Performance. Specific manual muscle testing (MMT) is completed to determine if there is nerve root involvement. Additionally, muscle strength must be examined in the trunk and extremities to further evaluate for weakness, pain with contraction, or abnormal patterns of muscle activity (see Chapter 5).

Janda[161-163] proposes that trunk and extremity muscles can interact with the spinal joints to produce pain in patients with spinal dysfunction.[164-166] In response to pain from a specific spinal segment, muscle tone increases to hold or immobilize the involved spinal segment in as painless a position as possible and to reduce stresses on the motion segment. The decreased segmental motion alters proprioceptive input from the joint, perpetuating muscle spasm and promoting development of trigger points. The decreased mobility of the spinal segment itself can also produce pain and the ongoing increase in muscle tone also results in muscle imbalance, which can further contribute to pain and altered movement patterns. Certain muscles react in typical ways, either with overreaction and tightness or with inhibition and weakness (Table 8-13). The predisposition of muscles to react by over activity or inhibition is exemplified by the shoulder crossed syndrome[165] and pelvic crossed syndrome.[166] In the shoulder crossed syndrome, the levator scapulae, upper trapezius, sternocleidomastoid, and pectoral muscles become overactive and tight, whereas the lower

scapular stabilizers and deep neck flexors are inhibited and weakened. This can produce a protracted head and rotated scapulae, stressing the cervicocranial and cervicothoracic junctions and the C4 and C5 spinal segments and decreasing the stability of the glenohumeral joint. A similar imbalance is created between shortened and tight hip flexors and lumbar erector spinae and weakened abdominal and gluteal muscles in the pelvic crossed syndrome.[166] Janda[165,166] recommends providing resistance to weak and inhibited muscles and stretching tight muscle to improve muscle balance and posture and reduce symptoms.

To examine muscles for normal patterns of movement, the therapist asks the patient to actively perform a specific movement while observing the pattern of coordination and sequencing of muscle activity. Deviations from the expected pattern of muscle recruitment signify impairment of muscle function and suggest the need for muscle reeducation and control as an intervention. Test movements, procedures, and altered movement patterns for examining trunk movement patterns are listed in Table 8-14.

Janda's work is widely accepted as a valuable contribution to manual medicine, and his concepts have been integrated into today's orthopedic physical therapy practice. His work has served as a foundation for other clinicians and researchers and is often discussed and cited.[167-170] Despite this secondary substantiation of scholarship, there is little primary evidence in the English literature in support of Janda's principles. Knowledge in this country comes mainly from Janda's writing in books and from discussions of his principles by other authors.[167-170]

Mechanical Provocation Tests. Mechanical provocation tests involve application of a series of maneuvers that may aggravate or diminish a patient's presenting symptoms. A change in symptom severity indicates that the disorder is mechanical in nature and should be responsive to physical intervention. These maneuvers apply compressive or distractive forces to pain producing structures.[171] In the spine a series of specific provocation tests, called foraminal closure or *quadrant tests*, which stress spinal neurovascular structures and facet joints are used to rule in or rule out nerve root irritation by closing down (placing the facet joint into a closed packed position) or opening up the intervertebral foramen. These tests are not intended to identify the specific cause of nerve root irritation. A positive test can indicate the presence of a space-occupying lesion, such as a herniated disc, edema, or local capsular restrictions.

Quadrant/Foraminal Closure Tests. There are many different variations of foraminal closure tests for the cervical spine. Spurling's test involves cervical sidebending and extension together with axial compression or overpressure.[170,172] Reproduction of symptoms in the neck or arm corresponding to the side of bending constitutes a positive test. When symptoms occur with sidebending away from the side of pain, an intervertebral disc dysfunction is implicated. If pain is reproduced with lateral flexion toward the side of pain, foraminal encroachment is thought to be the cause.[170,172] Maitland describes separate upper and lower cervical spine quadrant tests.[173] To test foraminal closure in the upper cervical spine, with the

TABLE 8-13	Muscles That Commonly Become Tight or Weak in Response to Spinal Disorders

Tight Muscles	Weak Muscles
CERVICOTHORACIC AREA	
Pectoralis major and minor	Serratus anterior
Upper trapezius	Rhomboids
Levator scapulae	Middle and lower trapezius
Sternocleidomastoid	Deep neck flexors
Suboccipitals	Suprahyoid
Erector spinae	Mylohyoid
LUMBOSACRAL AREA	
Erector spinae	Gluteus maximus, medius, and
Iliopsoas	minimus
Rectus femoris	Rectus abdominis
Tensor fascia lata	Transversus abdominis
Hamstrings	Vastus medialis and lateralis
Quadratus lumborum	
Piriformis	
Short hip adductors	
Gastrocnemius, soleus	

Adapted from Janda V: *Movement patterns in pelvic and hip region in pathogenesis of vertebrogenic disease,* Prague, 1964, Charles University; Janda V: *Procedings Kongressmand Manulle Medizin* 127-130, 1968; Janda V: *Storungen Archive fur Physikalische Therapit* 20:113-116, 1968; Janda V: Muscles and motor control in cervicogenic disorders: Assessment and management. In Grant R (ed): *Physical Therapy of the Cervical and Thoracic Spine,* New York, 1988, Churchill Livingstone; Janda V: Evaluation of muscular imbalance. In Liebenson C (ed): *Rehabilitation of the Spine: A Practitioner's Manual,* Philadelphia, 1996, Williams & Wilkins.

TABLE 8-14   Examination of Movement Patterns

Test Movement	Procedure	Aberrant Patterns
CERVICOTHORACIC REGION		
Head and neck flexion	Supine patient actively raises head.	The cervicocranial junction hyperextends, the jaw projects forward at the beginning of the movement when SCM is strong and deep neck flexors are weak.
Push-up	Slowly perform full push-up and return to prone. Prime mover: Serratus anterior.	Weakened serratus anterior cannot stabilize scapula against rib cage.
Shoulder abduction	In sitting with elbow flexed, shoulder is abducted. If shoulder begins to elevate, movement is stopped.	Glenohumeral abduction, scapular rotation, and shoulder girdle elevation are examined for abnormal muscle activity and diminished contributions of specific joints to movement.
LUMBOSACRAL REGION		
Hip extension	Prone patient actively extends one hip. Prime mover: Gluteus maximus.	If weak, gluteus maximus contracts later than hamstrings and erector spinae and erector spinae may initiate the movement.
Hip abduction	Leg is actively abducted from sidelying. Prime movers: Gluteus medius, minimus, and tensor fascia lata.	Lateral rotation with hip abduction occurs with strong tensor fascia lata and weak gluteus medius. Lateral rotation indicates iliopsoas is active to substitute hip flexion for abduction.
Curl-up	Full sit-up progressively flexing cervical thoracic and lumbar spine from hooklying position.	Iliopsoas can be palpated to determine its contribution to movement or ask patient to actively plantar flex ankles, minimizing its use.

Adapted from Janda V: *Movement patterns in pelvic and hip region in pathogenesis of vertebrogenic disease,* Prague, 1964, Charles University; Janda V: *Procedings Kongressmand Manulle Medizin* 127-130, 1968; Janda V: *Storungen Archive fur Physikalische Therapit* 20:113-116, 1968; Janda V: Muscles and motor control in cervicogenic disorders: Assessment and management. In Grant R (ed): *Physical Therapy of the Cervical and Thoracic Spine,* New York, 1988, Churchill Livingstone; Janda V: Evaluation of muscular imbalance. In Liebenson C (ed): *Rehabilitation of the Spine: A Practitioner's Manual,* Philadelphia, 1996, Williams & Wilkins.
SCM, Sternocleidomastoid.

patient sitting, the therapist stands at the side, grasps the patient under the chin with one hand and the forehead with the other, extends the upper cervical spine (chin forward), rotates upper cervical spine (small oscillation) to one side, and then laterally flexes (tilt the crown of patient's head).[173] To test foraminal closure in the lower cervical spine, with the patient sitting with normal cervical lordosis, the therapist stands at the side and places a hand on the patient's right temple, rotates the patient's head to one side, sidebends to the same side, and extends. Gentle overpressure is applied by the therapist's hand on the patient's temple (Fig. 8-16). In a blinded prospective study, Spurling's test was found to have good interrater reliability in the classical form (with only sidebending and overpressure) and the modified form (with sidebending, rotation, and extension with overpressure).[147] Spurling's test has been found to be very specific for diagnosing cervical radiculopathy, but its sensitivity is only moderate to fair.[147,174] This suggests that a patient with a positive Spurling's test is very likely to have cervical radiculopathy, but a negative Spurling's test does not rule out the presence of cervical radiculopathy.

To perform a quadrant test for the thoracolumbar spine, the patient stands with feet slightly apart with the therapist guarding posterolaterally. The therapist places a hand across the patient's chest on the anterolateral shoulder on the side opposite the lateral flexion and places the other hand on an upper lumbar vertebra. The patient is moved into sidebending, rotation to the same side, and backward bending. Each movement is taken to the end of the available range before superimposing the next movement. If these movements are asymptomatic, overpressure

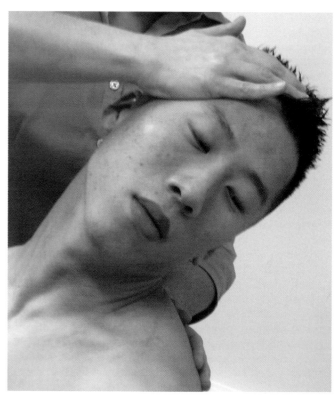

FIG. 8-16 Spurling's test. A foraminal closure in which the therapist rotates the head to one side, side bends to the same side and extends. Gentle overpressure is applied by the therapist's hand on the patient's temple.

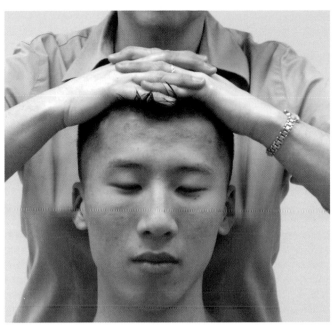

FIG. 8-17 Cervical spine compression test.

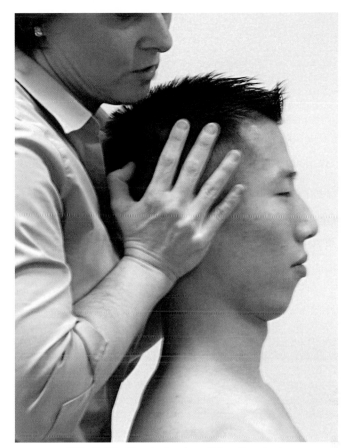

FIG. 8-18 Cervical spine distraction test.

is added. If the patient is still asymptomatic, the patient is moved into rotation and sidebending to the opposite side.

Cervical Compression. Cervical compression is a provocation test used to assess for nerve root impingement that results from encroachment on structures within the intervertebral foramen. To perform the test, with the patient sitting, the therapist clasps both hands across the top of patient's head and applies a downward force on the head (Fig. 8-17). A positive test reproduces the patients presenting symptoms because compression mechanically constricts the intervertebral foramen. Very good interexaminer reliability (kappa = 0.70) has been reported for the cervical compression test in patients with neck dysfunction.[175] However, this test is not diagnostically specific because increased symptoms can be due to a disc herniation or fragment or acute inflammation of the soft tissue structures such as the facet joint capsule.

Cervical Distraction. The cervical distraction test is a provocation test in which relief of symptoms constitutes a positive finding. With the patient sitting, the therapist grasps the patient's head with palms under the mastoid process and fingers pointing to the crown of the head. To impart a distraction force, the therapist leans back lifting the patient's head (Fig. 8-18). This test is also frequently performed with the patient in supine with a traction force imparted to the head and neck. The distraction force mechanically alleviates compression on the nerve root or intervertebral structures. In a blinded prospective study of patients with neck dysfunctions, Wainner et al[147] found very good interexaminer reliability (kappa = 0.69) for the cervical distraction test and that this test was highly specific (0.90) for cervical radiculopathy.

Joint Integrity and Mobility. Before palpating spinal joints for accessory mobility, the therapist should palpate the regions' bony and soft tissue structures. This assists in

determining the nature of the dysfunction and pain response and may help detect structural abnormalities. Palpation of soft tissue structures, which was discussed under pain assessment, is usually performed in conjunction with palpation for bony positional changes. In the cervical spine, the bony structures palpated include the spinous processes, articular pillars or the row of zygapophyseal joints, mastoid process, and base of the skull. In the thoracic spine, the structures of the scapula and shoulder are palpated in addition to the spinous processes, transverse processes, vertebral lamina, and ribs. In the lumbar spine, in addition to spinous and transverse processes and vertebral lamina, palpation of the structures of the hip and pelvis, such as the iliac crests, posterior superior iliac spines (PSISs), ischial tuberosities, greater trochanters, and the sacrum, is included. While palpating, the therapist notes symptom provocation, condition irritability, and any obvious positional abnormalities. Palpation between spinous processes can reveal a step or a large difference in the depth of adjacent segments, suggesting the possibility of a spondylolisthesis that may be further evaluated by diagnostic imaging.

To palpate the spinal structures, the patient is positioned prone on a firm surface with the thoracic and lumbar spine supported in neutral and the cervical spine positioned in neutral to 30 degrees of flexion to disengage the facet joints. Using the pads of the index and middle fingers, the therapist carefully traces the bony structures.

The therapist begins palpating the lumbosacral spine by finding the PSISs, then moves medially to the midline of the sacrum at approximately the S2 level. The clinician palpates all parts of the sacrum and then move superiorly. The first space felt is the interspinous space between the sacrum and L5. Thus the next spinous process is that of L5. The spinous processes and interspinous spaces moving superiorly are palpated. The transverse processes of L4-L2 are palpable through the paraspinal muscles 2-3 cm lateral to the spinous processes. In the cervical spine, the therapist begins at the base of the skull and proceeds palpating inferiorly. The largest spinous process, C2, is easily palpable. As the cervical spinous processes are bifid, it is important not to make judgments on vertebral position based on spinous process location. In the cervical spine, the articular pillars can be found approximately at the level of the corresponding spinous process just lateral and deep to the paravertebral musculature. The thoracic spine can be palpated beginning either from the cervical or lumbar spine.

To determine the accessory mobility of the intervertebral joints, the therapist imparts a posterior to anterior (PA) mobilization force to the spinous processes, transverse processes, articular pillars, and the sacrum. To ensure reproducibility and comparability to subsequent examinations, the therapist should apply a grade III mobilizing force, which is one that moves the bony prominence through all of its available accessory range. During this procedure, end-feel, the depth and smoothness of movement, symptom provocation, and amount of movement are assessed. To execute a mobilizing force, it is important for the therapist's hand to apply force to the bony prominence. To ensure adequate contact and force, the therapist's thumbs are usually used for contact with the cervical spine, the hypothenar space medial to the pisiform for contact with the thoracic and lumbar spine, and the heel of the hand for contact with the sacrum (Fig. 8-19).

The reliability and validity of procedures for testing accessory mobility of the intervertebral joints varies, depending on the measure used.[153,154,176] There is good agreement between therapists for symptom provocation[136,177] and pain with percussion of the spinous processes that correlates with functional limitations and disability.[135] Although grading of movement depth is less consistent,[176] clinically it is most important that clinicians judge segments similarly to be hypermobile or hypomobile to make the same treatment decisions.[154]

Neuromuscular. Neurological screening is an important component of the scanning examination to determine if spinal nerve function is affected in patients with spinal or radicular symptoms. Results of neurological screening tests should be documented in all patients with spinal disorders and should routinely be rechecked.

Pain. The severity, nature, and location of pain should be examined (see Chapter 22). To determine if specific structures are causing pain, the musculoskeletal soft tissues should be palpated in the areas overlying the spinal region being evaluated. The patient should be placed in a comfortable, supported position that allows easy access to the area being examined, while maintaining the spinal

segments in a neutral to slightly open-packed (flexed) position. The therapist should gently place his or her finger pads on the structure being examined and apply gradually more pressure over each section of muscle, noting symptoms. Temperature, the presence and degree of sweating and swelling, and ease of skin mobility while examining the skin and subcutaneous tissue should be noted. Abnormally warm tissues may indicate an inflammatory process, whereas cool or immobile tissues may indicate a long-standing problem. The muscles should be palpated more deeply to detect generalized tenderness, tender or trigger points, and spasm.

Peripheral Nerve Integrity. Sensory modalities are screened using light touch, pin prick, and vibration in various dermatomal distributions (see Table 8-1). In a blinded prospective trial, good interrater reliability was found between physical therapists examining pin prick sensation for C5 and T1 spinal levels and moderate interrater reliability for the other cervical spinal levels.[147] This test was diagnostically accurate for cervical radiculopathy at C5 and has high specificity for ruling in cervical radiculopathy at any level.[147] A high level of agreement (96% to 98%) has also been reported between two PTs examining sensation in patients with low back symptoms.[136]

Motor function is assessed by testing the strength of the limb muscles that are representative of each nerve root distribution using manual muscle testing (MMT) and by comparing the strength of one side with the strength of the other side (see Table 8-1). Many extremity muscles are innervated by more than one nerve root so care must be exercised in extrapolating from findings of motor weakness to the presence of nerve root involvement. Upper extremity MMT has been found to be highly specific for ruling in cervical radiculopathy,[147] and excellent agreement has been reported (96% to 98%) between two PTs examining lower extremity strength in patients with low back symptoms.[136]

Reflex Integrity. Deep tendon reflexes are diminished with some types of spinal nerve root impingement. To assess reflexes, the muscle tendon in tapped with a reflex hammer and the response is compared to the other side. Good reliability between PTs has been reported for upper extremity reflex testing in patients with cervical spine disorders, and this test was also found to be highly specific for cervical radiculopathy.[147]

Neurodynamic Tests. *Neurodynamic tests* mechanically stress nervous tissue in an attempt to determine if spinal nerve roots and peripheral nerves are causing pain. Nervous tissue may become inflamed in response to injury, resulting in the production of fibrous adhesions within the connective tissue in the nerves and surrounding structures and pain when the tissue is stressed.[24,50] If mechanical stress on a nerve evokes pain, this suggests that the nerve has impaired mobility.[170] In all of the neurodynamic tests, the examiner carefully positions the patient and applies a tensile force to the nerve, noting symptoms. A series of *sensitizing maneuvers* are then applied in a sequential manner to successively apply additional mechanical stress to the tissues. When using extremity tests, the uninvolved extremity is assessed first and responses are compared to the affected side. The

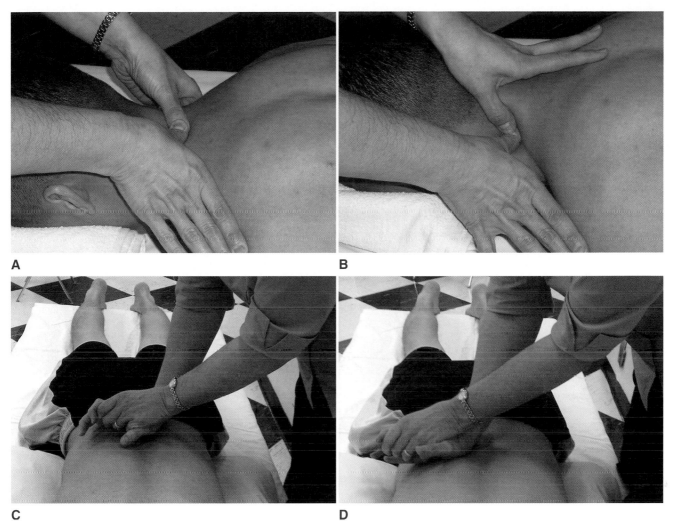

FIG. 8-19 **A,** PA pressure on a cervical spinous process; **B,** PA pressure on a cervical articular pillar; **C,** PA pressure on a lumbar spinous process; **D,** PA pressure on a lumbar articular pillar.

examiner is advised to carefully differentiate between discomfort as a result of stretching overlying tight muscles, increased resistance that results from a protective muscle spasm, and true reproduction of distal symptoms in the distribution of the stressed nerve(s).

Straight Leg Raise Test. The most common neurodynamic test is the straight leg raise (SLR) test, which is used to evaluate for involvement of lumbosacral nerve roots and the sciatic nerve. To perform the SLR test, the patient lies supine and the opposite hip and knee are extended to stabilize the pelvis. The therapist passively lifts the test leg keeping the leg in neutral rotation and the knee in extension. It is important to document whether pain occurs unilaterally or bilaterally, if there is resistance to movement, the hip range when symptoms occur and the type of symptoms elicited. The amount of hip flexion at which symptoms occur can be measured with a goniometer. Sensitizing maneuvers, such as reducing the hip flexion slightly when symptoms occur and then sequentially adding ankle dorsiflexion, medial hip rotation, and neck flexion, can be used to localize symptom etiology to the

sciatic nerve[178] (Fig. 8-20). The SLR test is considered positive if symptoms are reproduced by any of these maneuvers.

With straight leg raising the sciatic nerve starts to move within the first 30 degrees of straight leg elevation, with the greatest movement occurring in the lumbosacral nerve roots at the L5 to S2 level with 60-80 degrees of hip flexion.[179] Further leg elevation produces greater stretch on structures other than the sciatic nerve such as muscles and joints.[170] When SLR testing on the unaffected side reproduces symptoms on the affected side, it is called a crossed SLR or *crossover sign* and is highly correlated with large central disc protrusions.[180]

A systematic review of the literature on SLR testing found intrarater and interrater reliability to be good in most studies.[179] Interrater reliability between physical therapists for measuring SLR testing in patients with low back was found to be high (kappa = 0.83 for a 96% agreement).[136] In a population-based epidemiological study of over 4,000 patients with LBP, a passive SLR test that produced pain in the thigh or lumbosacral area was found to

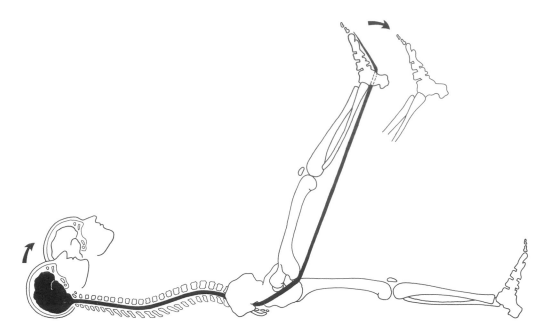

FIG. 8-20 Diagram of the excursion of the sciatic nerve during a straight leg raise and with the addition of the sensitizing maneuver of cervical flexion. *From Butler DS:* Mobilisation of the Nervous System, *New York, 1991, Churchill Livingstone.*

be a good predictor of back pain severity.[135] The sensitivity of the SLR test for a nerve root adhesion or space-occupying lesion has been reported to be between 72% and 97% but with poor specificity of 11% to 66%.[181,182] This implies that patients with lumbosacral nerve root involvement are very likely to have a positive SLR test and that those with a negative SLR test probably do not have lumbosacral nerve root involvement; however, many patients with a positive SLR test may not have lumbosacral nerve root involvement.

Prone Knee Bend Test. The prone knee bend test is intended to mechanically stress the femoral nerve and the L2 and L3 nerve roots. Like the SLR test, symptom reproduction is thought to indicate a nerve root lesion due to impingement or a space occupying lesion. This test may also stress the anterior hip joint, and an increase in symptoms in the SI region may result from anterior rotation of the ilium produced by tension through the rectus femoris. To perform the test, the patient lies prone and the therapist stabilizes the patient's pelvis and passively flexes the knee, maintaining neutral hip rotation (Fig. 8-21). The test is considered positive when the maneuver reproduces the patient's symptoms. Although this test has not been as extensively studied as the SLR test, PTs have demonstrated 99% interrater reliability when applying this test in patients with LBP.[136]

Slump Test. To further tension the lumbar or sacral nerve roots, it may be necessary to completely flex the spine. The slump test, devised by Maitland,[173] combines the extremes of the SLR test with ankle dorsiflexion and neck flexion in a sitting position with thoracolumbar spinal flexion. Hall demonstrated the need to maximally flex the lumbar spine when performing the SLR test in sidelying to increase the stress placed on the sciatic nerve roots.[183] However, not all patients require this degree of symptom provocation. It is recommended that the slump test only be performed if a dural lesion is strongly suspected in a patient with a negative SLR test, although this

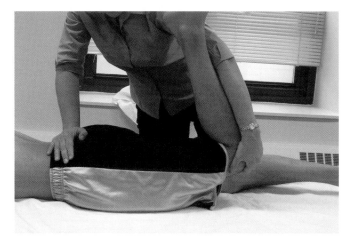

FIG. 8-21 Prone knee bend. Note that the therapist stabilizes the pelvis as she is lifting the femur into hip extension while maintaining knee flexion.

should rarely be needed given the high sensitivity of the SLR test alone.

Although there are variations to the procedure, to perform the slump test as described by Maitland,[173] the patient sits with thighs fully supported on a plinth. The patient is then asked to "slump," fully flexing the thoracic and lumbar spine without flexing the neck. The therapist exerts an overpressure through the thoracolumbar spine to add further flexion. If asymptomatic, the patient fully flexes their neck and the therapist adds overpressure. The patient then sequentially extends the knee on the symptomatic side and if possible, dorsiflexes the ankle on the same side (Fig. 8-22). This is a difficult position to maintain and usually the sensitizing maneuvers are added and released before progressing to a position that places the spinal cord and nerve roots on this much tension. If symptoms are provoked, the sensitizing maneuver is reversed and the effect on symptoms is noted. For example, if full

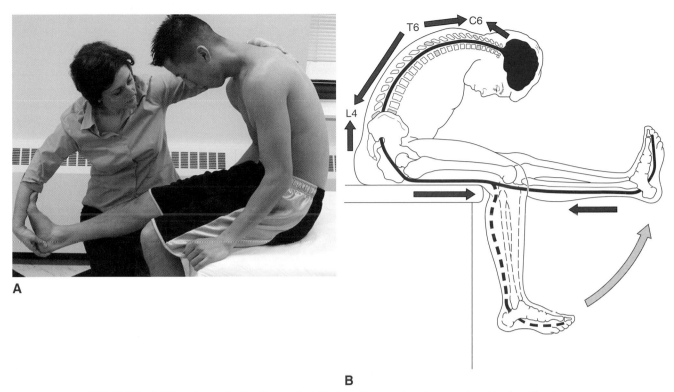

FIG. 8-22 **A,** The slump test with cervical flexion, knee extension, and ankle dorsiflexion added as sensitizing maneuvers. **B,** Excursion of the spinal cord and sciatic nerve in a maximal slump position with cervical flexion, knee extension, and ankle dorsiflexion. *B, Adapted from Magee DJ:* Orthopedic Physical Assessment, *ed 4, Philadelphia, 2002, Saunders.*

neck flexion provokes symptoms, the patient extends their neck, which is expected to diminish symptoms. The slump test should be interpreted with caution because many subjects without pathology will become symptomatic with this maneuver, giving it low specificity for nerve involvement.[184]

Upper Limb Tension Tests. The upper limb tension tests (ULTTs), primarily developed by Butler, are based on the brachial plexus tension test originally developed by Elvy.[173,185] As with the SLR and prone knee bend tests that place the lower extremity nerves under stress, the ULTTs place the upper extremity nerves and the cervical spine nerve roots under mechanical stress and sequentially add sensitizing maneuvers to provoke symptoms. There are four ULTTs that combine movements of upper extremity and cervical spine to bias, stressing the median, ulnar, and radial nerves (see Chapter 18 for detailed descriptions and illustrations of ULTTs).

Special Tests

Vertebral Artery Test. In the cervical spine, the vertebral arteries pass through the foramen transversarium, which is a hole in the transverse processes, en route to the cerebral circulation. The arteries turn sharply at the C1 and C2 vertebrae before entering the foramen magnum (Fig. 8-23). In patients with vascular disease or significant osseous and soft tissue encroachment, there is a potential for arterial occlusion with extremes of cervical rotation and extension. This can cause dizziness, vertigo, tinnitus,

nausea, speech deficits, dysphagia, diplopia or blurred vision, and if maintained, cerebral ischemia and stroke. The vertebral artery test is used to determine whether extremes of movement of the cervical spine will compromise the vertebral artery and thus the cerebral circulation. If any symptoms occur, the test is positive and high-velocity or maintained end-range techniques of the cervical spine are contraindicated.[173,186]

There are several variations of the vertebral artery test, all of which use combinations cervical extension and rotation with some adding traction or compression. In one method, the patient extends the head and neck, with assistance from the therapist to hold the position at the limit of their range, and holds for 30 seconds. The patient then rotates their head completely to one side, and the therapist maintains pressure to hold the position for 30 seconds. If this is asymptomatic, the patient returns to the neutral position for a 10-second rest and then the therapist assists the patient to fully rotate to the other side and then extend followed by a 30-second hold (Fig. 8-24). Throughout the procedure the therapist carefully watches and questions the patient for any occurrence of symptoms. If symptoms occur during any component of the test, the therapist concludes the procedure and does not add more compromising maneuvers. If neurological signs, such as nystagmus and dysphagia, result, the patient's physician should be contacted immediately.[187]

After analyzing ipsilateral and contralateral blood flow in several cervical positions, Arnold found that only full

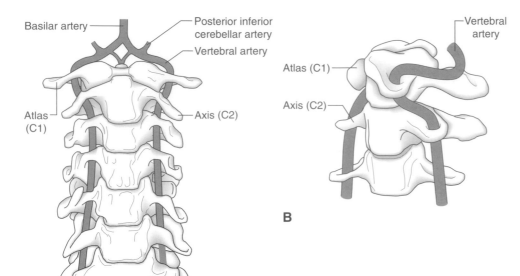

FIG. 8-23 **A,** Location of the vertebral artery within the foramen transversarium of the cervical spine. **B,** Twisting of the vertebral artery in the upper cervical spine with rotation. *Adapted from Gibbons P, Tehan P:* Manipulation of the Spine Thorax and Pelvis: An Osteopathic Perspective, *New York, 2004, Churchill Livingstone.*

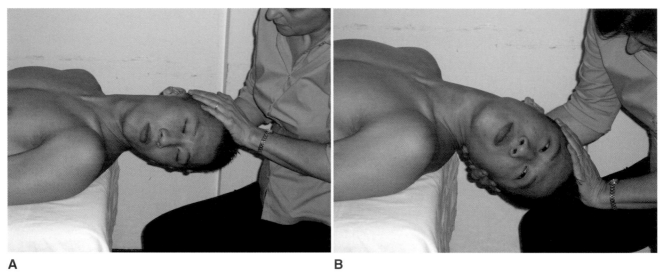

FIG. 8-24 Supine vertebral artery test. **A,** Phase I with cervical spine rotation. **B,** Phase II with cervical spine rotation and extension.

range of cervical rotation and a maneuver in which the atlantoaxial joint was placed in lateral flexion and contralateral rotation produced sufficient stress to reduce vertebral basilar blood flow. The vertebral artery test can be performed in sitting or supine; however, it is suggested that the test may be more accurate when performed while sitting because blood must be pumped against gravity against any vascular restrictions. However, in supine, more range may be obtained, which potentially causes greater occlusion. When the patient presents with symptoms, such as positional dizziness, a static test can first be performed in which the patient remains stationary and the head and neck are moved, followed by a dynamic test in which the head is held stationary and the body is

rotated.[173] If the patient is symptomatic with the static test and not with the dynamic test this suggests the patient has a vestibular disorder rather than a vascular disorder.[173] Despite the absence of data on the sensitivity and specificity of these screening tests for identifying patients who should not be treated vigorously, experts still suggest that these tests be used to screen patients who may be at risk for vascular occlusion.[186-188]

Sacroiliac Joint Tests. The prevalence of SI dysfunction among patients with LBP has been reported to be between 13% and 30%.[189] SI dysfunction is defined as an alteration in joint mobility occurring with changed positional relations between the sacrum and the ilium.[190,191] Mobility dysfunction of the SI joint is considered to be either sacroiliac (abnormal postioning of the sacrum on a normally positioned ilium) or iliosacral (abnormal positioning of the ilium on a normally positioned sacrum).[167,190] SI dysfunction may be identified by palpation of lumbosacral and lower extremity landmarks and special tests for pain provocation, movement, and pelvic position in conjunction with a history of buttock and leg pain made worse with unilateral weight bearing.

Landmark Palpation. During the postural and structural examination, the therapist should examine for asymmetry in the paired anatomical landmarks of the sacrum, pelvis, and lower extremity. Although there is considerable anatomical variability and asymmetry in the level of the iliac crests, anterior superior iliac spines (ASISs), the PSISs in all planes, and lower extremity landmarks, the absence of a leg length discrepancy suggests the need for specific evaluation of the SI joint (Fig. 8-25). Intrarater reliability for landmark palpation of the ASIS and PSIS in standing and asymmetry of the ASIS and PSIS have been reported to be high (ICC = 0.99 for landmark palpation, 0.75 and 0.70 for ASIS and PSIS asymmetry, respectively).[191]

Standing Flexion Test. The standing flexion test is used to determine the side of an iliosacral lesion. To perform the standing flexion test the patient stands with feet hip distance apart, bearing weight symmetrically. The therapist is positioned with eyes level to the PSISs and the thumbs are placed on or just under the PSISs. The patient bends forward keeping their knees straight (Fig. 8-26). The amount of cranial movement of the PSISs is observed. The

test is considered positive for restricted mobility if the PSIS on one side moves more cephalad, or moves before, the one on the other side. As the spine and sacrum flex the innominate should remain upright on the stable lower extremity and the ilium should move up on the sacrum. If movement of the ilium on the sacrum is restricted they will remain linked and the PSIS will move forward and upward during spinal flexion.

Sacral Fixation Test. Like the standing flexion test, the sacral fixation test (also known as Gillet's test, the marching test, or the stork test) is used to test for the presence and side of an iliosacral lesion. The patient and therapist are positioned as described for the standing flexion test. The therapist places one thumb on a PSIS and the other on the adjacent part of the sacrum. The patient stands on one leg while flexing the opposite hip and knee to at least 90 degrees. The therapist palpates the PSIS on the side of the flexing leg (Fig. 8-27). The procedure is repeated on both sides. With normal iliosacral mobility, the innomi-

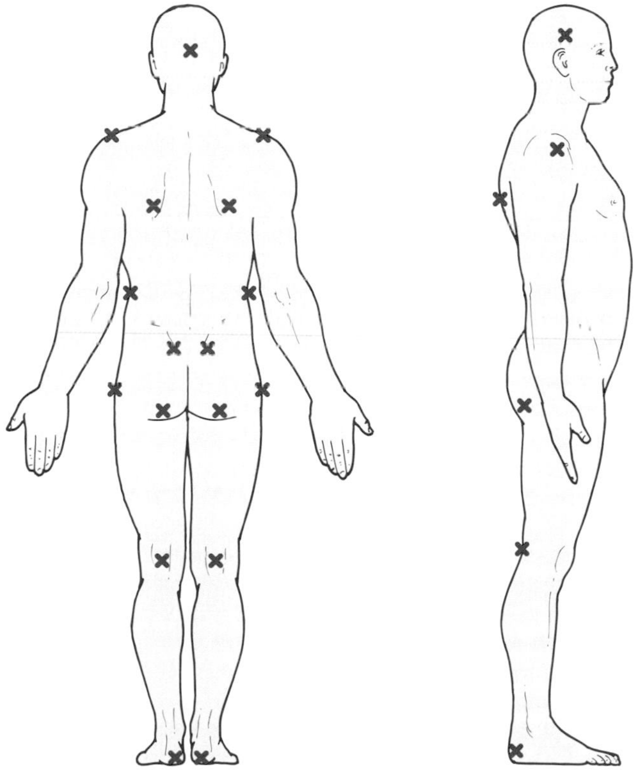

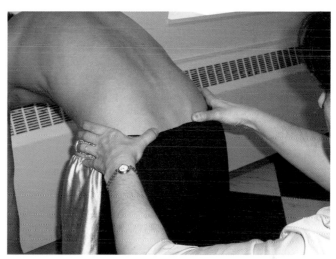

FIG. 8-26 Standing flexion test. Note that therapist's eyes are level with the posterior superior iliac spines.

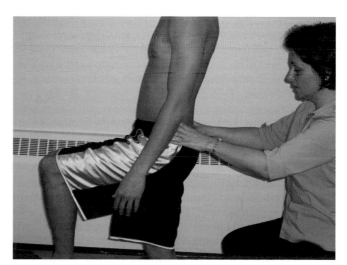

FIG. 8-27 Sacral fixation test (also called Gillet's test, marching test, or stork test).

FIG. 8-25 Landmarks palpated for symmetry as part of the sacroiliac examination.

nate rotates backward and caudally on the side of the flexing leg, thus the PSIS should move posteriorly and down. A test is considered positive for restricted mobility if little or no PSIS movement occurs.

Sitting Flexion Test. The sitting flexion test is also used to test for the presence and side of a iliosacral lesion. The subject sits on a level surface with feet supported on a stool. The therapist is positioned with eyes level with the PSISs and the thumbs are placed on or just under the PSISs bilaterally. The patient flexes the trunk fully forward until their elbows are between their knees while the therapist palpates for cranial movement of either PSIS. A test is considered positive for restricted mobility if either PSIS moves cranially because in sitting the ischial tuberosities and thus the ilia cannot move, so with SI joint hypomobility the sacrum will pull the PSIS cranially.

Long Sitting Test (Supine to Sit Test). The long sitting test is used to examine for abnormal movement of the innominate on the sacrum and to determining the direction of innominate rotation. This test is performed with the patient starting supine and the therapist standing at the patient's feet with their thumbs just distal to the apex of the malleoli. The patient then moves into a long sitting position with knees extended, and the therapist observes for changes in the position of the malleoli. In a patient with a posteriorly rotated innominate, the limb will appear short when the patient is supine because the acetabulum is more cranial. This leg will then appear to lengthen in long sitting as the acetabulum moves forward. In a patient with an anteriorly rotated innominate, the lower extremity appears long in supine and shorter in long sitting (Fig. 8-28).

Compression Tests. There are various tests that apply shearing and compressive forces through the SI joints in order to provoke symptoms and determine the side of involvement. A common compression test has the patient lie supine, the examiner crosses their arms, places the palm of each hand against the medial aspect of the ASISs, and then gradually pushes the ASISs apart. This test applies compressive forces through the SI joints and has been shown to exhibit good reliability (kappa = 0.77),[192] but many patients find this maneuver uncomfortable. A more comfortable method of applying compression to the SI joints is to have the patient lie supine while the examiner cups one ASIS in the palm of their hand and imparts a force at a 45-degree angle, approximately perpendicular to the angle of the SI joint. This test examines mobility and the response to provocation, much like a PA test. This test is considered positive if symptoms on the side tested increase or the joint has reduced mobility.

Other tests use the patient's thigh as a lever arm to impart a force through the SI joint. Porterfield and DeRosa[193] recommend testing SI mobility by placing the patient supine with the hip flexed to 90 degrees and imparting a downward force at varying angles of abduction and adduction. With the hip in 90 degrees of flexion and in neutral rotation, this test is known as the posterior pelvic pain provocation (PPPP) test.[84] This test is recommended for differentiating pelvic dysfunction from other sources of back pain in pregnant women and has been found to have a 71% positive predicative value and a negative predictive value of 88% for diagnosing pelvic dysfunction in this population.[84]

A systematic review of studies on SI mobility and provocation tests revealed that the studies had adequate methodological quality but that the reliability of individual SI joint tests were mixed, with only some studies demonstrating adequate reliability for some tests.[194,195] The incidence of false positive tests has been reported to be as high as 20% for provocation tests,[190] and no single provocation test has shown a statistically significant association with response to sacroiliac joint nerve blocks.[196] It is recommended that the clinician use a number of SI joint tests together since consistent results from a cluster of tests has been found to be sensitive (82%) and specific (88%) for identifying SI joint dysfunction in patients with LBP.[118]

Limb Length Inequality. *Limb length inequality* (LLI) is a difference in length between the two lower extremities. Anatomical or true LLI occurs when one of the bones in the lower extremity, from the head of the femur to the ankle mortise, is shorter than the one on the other side.[197] Functional or apparent LLI is when one lower extremity is shorter than the other while the bones are of equal length. In functional LLI, the length discrepancy is caused by adaptive soft tissue shortening, joint contractures, ligamentous laxity, or axial malalignment.[197] There is no agreement on the amount of LLI that is clinically significant or requires correction. LLI has been linked to back pain, but this relationship is controversial and is not completely supported.[197-201] Practically speaking, when LLI is observed in patients with LBP, correction should be attempted and implemented if it helps alleviate symptoms.

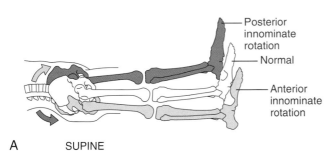

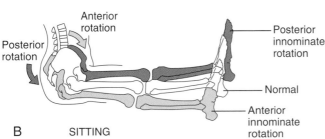

FIG. 8-28 Relationship between leg length in supine and long sitting and an anteroposterior innominate rotation. *Redrawn from Wadsworth CT (ed): Manual Examination and Treatment of the Spine and Extremities, Baltimore, 1998, Williams & Wilkins. In Magee D: Orthopedic Physical Assessment, ed 4, Philadelphia, 2002, Saunders.*

The standard method of assessing anatomical LLI is radiography. Clinically, physical therapists assess LLI directly by measuring between two fixed points, such as the umbilicus and the medial malleolus, with a tape measure and indirectly by having the patient stand and palpating the ASISs or iliac crests bilaterally and adding shims or blocks of various heights under the shorter leg until the landmarks become level. Direct clinical measurements using a tape measure have been found to have high to questionable reliability.[198,202,203] Hoyle and associates recorded ICC $_{(3,1)}$ for tape measurements for two examiners measuring from ASIS to medial malleolus of 0.98-0.99, whereas the discrepancy between examiners' measurements ranged between 0-28.5 mm.[202] Errors in direct clinical measurements are subject to error because of inaccurate palpation of landmarks, differences in limb girth, iliac asymmetries that may obscure actual limb differences, and joint contractures.[197] For clinical LLI correction, the indirect method of placing blocks or shims under the shorter limb until the pelvic landmarks, including the greater trochanters, ASISs, PSISs, iliac crests, and ischial tuberosities, become level is recommended because it has the greatest direct impact on selection of interventions.[197]

Examination of Neighboring Joints. When examining a patient with a spinal disorder, it is important to screen neighboring joints to determine if the spine is the primary site of origin of the patient's symptoms.[170,172] Upper cervical spine symptoms frequently occur in patients with TMJ dysfunctions. Neck pain can be referred from the shoulder or the shoulder may develop problems secondary to neck dysfunction. In primary long-standing shoulder dysfunctions, the thoracic spine may become hypermobile or hypomobile. Pain from the lumbar spine is frequently referred to the hip, and lumbosacral dysfunctions can be caused by hip pathologies, especially when gait is affected, causing abnormal forces to be transmitted through the SI joints to the spine.

Detailed Tests and Measures. The results of the scanning examination can be used to develop initial diagnostic hypotheses, prioritize the patient problem list, and develop a plan of care for most patients with spinal pain. However, some patients require more in-depth examination. These patients are usually not in the acute phase of the condition and can withstand the more vigorous examination procedures that may be needed to make an accurate physical therapy diagnosis. The techniques involved in the detailed examination require advanced palpation and observation skills. It is recommended that students or clinicians unfamiliar with these procedures work under the direct mentorship of an experienced manual therapist to master these techniques. The following sections provide the reader with a brief overview some of the more frequently used advanced examination techniques for patients with spinal disorders.

Detailed Mobility Examination

Position Testing of the Spine. Position testing of the spine is a technique in which spinal facet joints, lamina, or transverse processes are palpated dynamically and statically to determine the position and movement behavior of one vertebra relative to the vertebra directly below it. In examining the cervical spine, the articular pillars or facets are palpated; in the thoracic and lumbar spine the transverse processes or lamina are palpated. In dynamic testing the examiner palpates the spinal landmarks as the patient actively moves through flexion and extension. This is usually performed with the patient sitting. In static position testing the patient is positioned in a neutral prone position and in a flexed and an extended position and the spinal landmarks are palpated in each position (Fig. 8-29).

Position testing is performed to determine the precise location, position, and direction of movement limitations. Knowledge of normal spinal mechanics is essential for correct diagnosis of a specific movement restriction. In flexion the facet joints separate or open, and in extension they compress or close. In sidebending the facets close on the concavity of the curve and open on the convexity. In rotation, the facets compress or close on the side toward which the rotation occurs. In flexion from the head down,

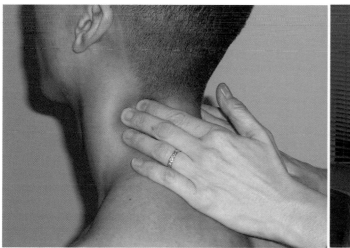
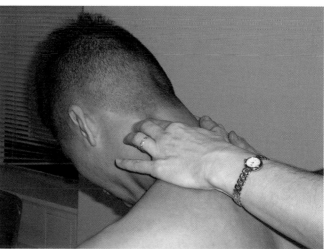

A   **B**

FIG. 8-29 Position testing of the cervical spine. **A,** Neutral. **B,** Flexion.

the superior vertebra rotates and translates anteriorly and the facets, lamina, or transverse processes will be felt more prominently. In extension the superior vertebra rotates and translates posteriorly causing the facets, lamina, and transverse processes to be less prominent.[20,167] If a vertebra has a movement restriction, it will not move in this predicted manor. When the clinician feels an asymmetry in the depth of the landmarks, they can determine the nature of the motion restriction from the position of the patient when the asymmetry was noted (e.g., flexion or sidebending) and the position of the landmarks. The position of the spinal joint found in the examination is described in the past tense[167] and noted with capital letters. For example, in *FRSrt* the upper vertebra is flexed, rotated, and sidebent to the right in relation to the lower vertebra. The vertebra is restricted in the movements of extension, rotation, and sidebending to the left.[167] In the cervical spine and when the thoracic and lumbar spine are flexed or extended, rotation and sidebending occur to the same side. However, when the thoracic and lumbar spines are in neutral, rotation and sidebending occur to opposite sides. Once the movement restriction is determined, the clinician can determine the specific intervention necessary. For example, if a vertebra is positioned in flexion, rotation, and sidebending to the right (FRSrt), specific manual therapy techniques can be used to promote extension and rotation and sidebending to the left to correct this abnormality.[167]

Position Testing of the Sacrum. SI dysfunctions are suspected when the sitting flexion test and tests of sacral mobility are positive. Position testing can be used to further diagnose the exact nature of the sacral dysfunction. For this type of testing the sacral sulci and inferior lateral angles of the sacrum are palpated for depth and symmetry. The sacral sulci are the indentations filled with soft tissue immediately medial to the PSISs. The inferior lateral angles are the lateral prominence as the sacrum bends inward toward the coccyx (Fig. 8-30).

As in position testing of the spine, knowledge of sacral mechanics is critical to an accurate diagnosis. When the

lumbar spine moves into extension, the sacrum moves into *nutation* (i.e., anterior rotation, forward flexion), the sacral base moves anteriorly and inferiorly and the sacral apex moves posteriorly and superiorly.[20] Thus the depth of the sacral sulci should symmetrically become deeper, and the inferior lateral angles should become more prominent as they move more posteriorly and inferiorly. When the spine flexes, the sacrum counter-nutates or rotates posteriorly, the sacral base moves posteriorly and superiorly, and the sacral apex moves anteriorly and inferiorly. Thus the sacral sulci become more superficial (less deep) and the inferior lateral angles become deeper during *counter-nutation*.[167]

To perform this test the sacral sulci and inferior lateral angles are first palpated with the patient prone with the spine in neutral. The patient then moves into a prone prop or a "sphinx" position (spinal extension and sacral nutation), and the landmarks are again palpated. To test for sacral position in spinal flexion, the patient is seated, the landmarks are palpated, and the patient then slumps forward, flexing the lumbar spine. Any deviations from the expected movement patterns during these tests indicate a specific SI dysfunction. Asymmetrical positions of the sacral sulci and inferior lateral angles indicate a sacral torsion or unilaterally flexed or extended sacrum.[167] Bilateral changes indicate a sacrum that is unable to flex or extend. Specific muscle energy and mobilization techniques are recommended to correct each of these sacral dysfunctions.[170]

Tests for Spinal Instability. Certain findings from the patient history and scanning examination may indicate the need for specific testing for spinal instability. These findings include a history of spinal trauma, multiple previous episodes of LBP brought on by minimal provocation, short-term relief from spinal manipulation, self-manipulation, and a decrease in symptoms with the use of a spinal orthotic or brace.[93] Findings from the scanning examination consistent with instability include abnormal movements during active ROM, hypermobility, and symptom provocation during passive intervertebral motion testing. A quick speeding up or slowing down of motion combined with lateral bending or rotation during flexion and extension ROM assessment, known as an "instability catch," can also suggest that the patient cannot control motion of a vertebral segment.[22,170] A medical diagnosis of spinal instability is made by comparing the sagittal plane rotation and translation exhibited by a motion segment during flexion and extension lateral x-rays to normal values. However, this procedure only evaluates for stability at end-range and does not capture functional instability during midrange movements.[204]

Clinical segmental spinal instability is the condition in which a force produces more displacement in a spinal motion segment than is expected in a normal spine.[204] Panjabi[205,206] describes spinal stability as depending on three stabilizing subsystems. The passive subsystem, composed of the facet joints and joint capsules, the spinal ligaments, and the musculotendinous passive elastic system, stabilizes the spine at end-range. The active subsystem is composed of the small, intersegmental spinal muscles,

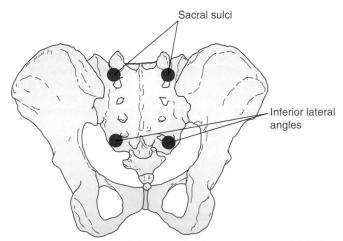

FIG. 8-30 Location of the sacral sulci (superior) and inferior lateral angles (inferior) of the sacrum.

Sacral sulci

Inferior lateral angles

which provide proprioceptive feedback on spinal positions, and the larger multisegmental muscles that produce and control spinal movements. The third subsystem, neural control, receives input for the active and passive subsystems and controls stability through muscular activity. Segmental instability occurs when the capacity of the spine's stabilizing is exceeded. Injury to any of the components of any of the subsystems increases demand on the other subsystems.[204] For example, IVD injuries, degenerative changes in the disc and facet joints, and spondylolisthesis reduce the passive subsystem's contribution to spinal stability. Muscle atrophy, disuse, imbalance, and inhibition that result from injury affect the active subsystem's ability to provide spinal stability. Spinal injury can also impair neuromuscular control and improved neuromuscular control can improve function in patients with structural spinal injuries or abnormalities.[204]

To confirm a diagnosis of clinical lumbar instability, Hicks et al recommend completing the prone instability test, the Beighton ligamentous laxity scale, and an AROM examination for aberrant movement because these examination procedures demonstrated high interrater reliability among PTs in patients with segmental instability.[207] To perform the prone instability test, the patient stands facing the end of a plinth, leans over at the hips, grasps the plinth, and supports his or her upper body on the plinth. The PT applies PA pressure on each lumbar spinous process to assess for mobility and symptom provocation. The patient then raises both feet off the floor, actively contracting the lumbosacral musculature, and the therapist repeats the PAs. The test is considered positive for instability at that level if symptoms are provoked only during active muscle contraction (Fig. 8-31).

The Beighton scale is a test for generalized ligamentous laxity test in which one point is given for each of the following indicators of laxity: Passive extension of the fifth metacarpophalangeal (MCP) joint past 90 degrees, passive apposition of the thumb to the forearm, hyperextension of the elbow past 10 degrees, hyperextension of the knee past 10 degrees, and trunk flexion allowing the palms to be placed flat on the floor. A score of $\geq^5/_9$ indicates the presence of generalized ligamentous laxity.

Other tests for instability, such as the AP shear test, are often recommended, however, the literature indicates instability can be diagnosed based on the previously mentioned examination procedures alone. Patients with segmental instability are likely to benefit from spinal stabilization exercises.

Craniovertebral Joint Examination. The upper cervical spine, which consists of the joints between the occiput and atlas and the joints between the atlas and axis, is mechanically and functionally distinct from the lower cervical spine. The first cervical vertebra, the atlas, has a larger transverse than AP diameter, a large transverse processes containing the foramen transversarium for the vertebral artery, and an articular facet for the odontoid process but does not have a vertebral body, pedicles, lamina, or a spinous process. The concave paired superior articular processes of the atlas articulate with the convex occipital condyles. There is a synovial joint between the odontoid process, or dens, located on C2, the axis, and the anterior aspect of the anterior tubercle. The dens acts as a pivot around which C1 rotates and the joint between C1 and C2 accounts for almost half of the rotation seen in the cervical spine. The specialized structures of the upper cervical spine allow the head to move independently of the neck and allow the individual to orient the visual field and sense organs of the head in multiple planes. Because of these anatomical, mechanical, and functional distinctions of the upper cervical spine, the upper cervical spine requires special consideration during examination.

In addition to a careful assessment of the vertebral artery (as described earlier), the joints of the upper cervi-

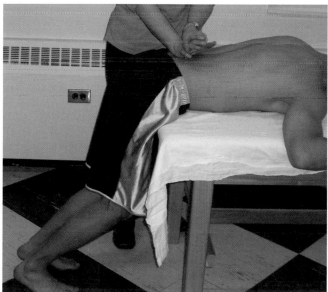

B

A

FIG. 8-31 Tests for instability. **A,** The therapist performs a PA while the patient's feet remain on the ground. **B,** The PA is performed with the patient's feet elevated.

cal spine are examined for ROM, PPIVM, and passive accessory intervertebral mobility, as well as pain provocation. Tests for stability of the joints of the upper cervical spine are extremely important because of the proximity of vital neurovascular structures. The Sharp-Purser test is used to determine the integrity of the transverse portion of the cruciate ligament that prevents forward translation of C1 on C2. Additional ligamentous tests include tests for rotational and lateral flexion stresses on the alar ligament as well as tests to examine the integrity of the tentorial membrane and other upper cervical spine supporting structures.[170,172] Use and interpretation of these tests requires skills that are beyond the scope of this entry-level text. It is not recommended that the novice implement upper cervical spine examination procedures without adequate training and supervision. However, it is important to recognize when these structures should be examined by an appropriately qualified clinician.

EVALUATION, DIAGNOSIS, AND PROGNOSIS

After completing the examination, the PT has much information to synthesize in performing the evaluation component of patient management. From the history, the therapist obtains information about the severity and chronicity of the current condition. Acute, subacute, and chronic conditions may require different intervention approaches. Information about the behavior of symptoms informs the therapist about how vigorous testing and interventions can be. The history also provides important prognostic information. For patients with psychosocial factors that increase the risk for developing chronic disability (see Table 8-11), the clinician should select interventions that avoid dependency and focus goals and outcomes on functional improvements rather than on pain relief.[119]

Most patients with back pain do not have a specific medical diagnosis.[208] The literature is unclear as to the typical course of back pain and who requires or would benefit from physical therapy interventions. It is often reported that as many as 90% of patients with mechanical LBP recover within 6 weeks and another 5% recover in 12 weeks with or without any intervention.[208] However, systematic literature reviews have found that back pain abates for substantially less than 50% of patients in 1 month and that at 3 months, more than 40% are still experiencing symptoms.[208,209] Furthermore, 25% to 50% of patients will have a recurrence within the first year,[207] and the lifetime recurrence rate is 85%.[2] How is the PT to use this information when evaluating a specific patient at a specific point in time? Back pain is a symptom not a medical or physical therapy diagnosis. Both the high percentage of patients with continuing symptoms and the high recurrence rate suggest that the cause for the initial episode was never identified and addressed and supports the need to conduct a thorough biomechanical examination to identify the mechanical origin of the patient's symptoms. Information from the history and from specific tests and measures is used to determine the mechanical or musculoskeletal source of the presenting symptoms and to place the patient into a diagnostic category to direct the type of intervention. Although up to 98% of all back pain is mechanical,[210] patients who present with symptoms suggesting a nonmechanical spine or visceral source of symptoms should be referred to the appropriate health care practitioner.

Although patients with spinal disorders fall into the *Guide to Physical Therapy Practice*[211] preferred practice pattern 4F: Impaired joint mobility, motor function, muscle performance, range of motion, and reflex integrity associated with spinal disorders, a more specific diagnosis is necessary to direct optimal intervention. The classification systems and the evidence in support of their use discussed in this chapter provide the PT with specific examination criteria to place a patient into a diagnostic category to direct interventions. The plan of care is directed toward techniques that target the mechanical dysfunctions identified during the examination. Active involvement of the patient in the intervention and in setting goals will help ensure patient participation and provide the patient with information need to reduce the risk of recurrence.

INTERVENTION

Spinal pain is a symptom with many different causes. However, much of the literature on the effectiveness of interventions for spinal pain treats spinal pain as though it were a single diagnosis requiring one approach to treatment. This may dilute the over-all treatment effect and lead to erroneous conclusions. There is abundant literature on the effectiveness of various types of treatment in the management of spinal disorders. Systematic reviews[212-214] and meta-analyses[215] have tried to integrate the available research to provide clinicians with evidence for making treatment decisions. Unfortunately, the patient and treatment selection process is seldom factored into the assessment of research used to determine the level of evidence in support of a specific approach. Therefore the clinician should exercise caution in interpreting whether a treatment has merit for a specific patient.

MOBILIZATION AND MANIPULATION

Mobilization and manipulation are manual therapy techniques in which skilled passive movements are applied to joints and related soft tissues at a variety of speeds and amplitudes.[211] Manual therapy is not the sole purview of a single profession and is and always has been practiced by many different practitioners. Manipulative treatment for the spine was used in ancient times by Hippocrates, Galen, and others in Greece, Rome, Asia, the Middle East, and South America.[167] The modern practice of manual therapy, previously known as bone setting, was first documented in the US in the late 1800s with the introduction of osteopathy by Dr. Andrew Still and of chiropractic by DD Palmer, both in the 1890s.[167] Manual therapy has since been further developed by various PTs and physicians, as well as osteopaths and chiropractors.

James Mennell, a British physician who wrote *The Art and Science of Joint Manipulation* in 1949, believed that facet joint dysfunction was the primary pathology responsible for back pain. He advocated manipulating the

TABLE 8-15	Maitland's Grades of Mobilization
Mobilization Grade	**Description**
Grade I	A small amplitude movement near starting position of the range.
Grade II	A large amplitude movement that carries well into the range. It can occupy any part of the range that is free of any stiffness or muscle spasm.
Grade III	A large amplitude movement that does move into stiffness or muscle spasm. Usually the movement is from midrange to the end of the range.
Grade IV	A small amplitude movement stretching into stiffness or muscle spasm at the limit of range.

From Maitland G, Banks K, English K, et al (eds): *Maitland's Vertebral Manipulation,* ed 6, Boston, 2001, Butterworth-Heinemann.

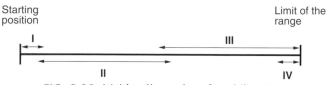

FIG. 8-32 Maitland's grades of mobilization.

facets by stabilizing one articular surface and moving the other articular surface to the point of pain and then applying a spring thrust through the pain. His son, John Mennell, explained "joint play" in his book *Joint Pain,*[216] as accessory movement that must be restored for normal joint mobility. John recommended that trained PTs work with medical professionals to provide joint manipulation.

James Cyriax, a British orthopedist who first published his *Textbook of Orthopaedic Medicine* in 1954, was an enthusiastic proponent of the use of manipulation by PTs because of their training and expertise in understanding the musculoskeletal system. Cyriax believed that spinal dysfunction was caused by disc displacement irritating and impinging on the dura and inhibiting nerve root mobility. He recommended the application of a high-velocity thrust to the spine after carefully positioning the patient, while assistants applied spinal traction by pulling on the patient's trunk and feet.

Geoffrey Maitland, an Australian PT, distinguished between mobilization and manipulation in his book *Vertebral Manipulation,* which was published in 1964.[173] He described mobilization as a gentler coaxing movement performed within or at the limit of the available range. He recommends that a series of graded passive oscillatory movements or mobilizations be applied to the spine at a level below the pain threshold. Maitland's system for grading mobilization is widely used today (Table 8-15; Fig. 8-32).

Freddy Kaltenborn, a Norwegian PT who later also trained as a chiropractor and an osteopath, developed the Nordic system of spinal mobilization in the 1960s, based on the work of Mennell and Cyriax. Kaltenborn treated loss of mobility by localizing the level of lesion, locking the joints above and below, and then delivering a thrust with minimum force in the direction of the limitation to normalize joint movement. He applied arthrokinematic principles to joint mobilization, developing the convex-concave rule for determining the direction of mobilizing force. Kaltenborn added traction to mobilizations performed parallel or perpendicular to the plane of the joint to reduce pain and restore mobility to hypomobile joints.

The effect of manual therapy for reducing pain and improving mobility in patients with spinal disorders is thought to be mediated by mechanical and neurophysiological mechanisms. Mechanically, joint mobilization and manipulation directly impart external forces to the joints of the spine and the overlying muscles, ligaments, and soft tissue structures. These forces may restore more normal joint play and articular relationships,[167] separate facet joint surfaces, release trapped synovial folds, break intraarticular adhesions and scar tissue, and stretch specific joint capsules and muscles.[217] There is evidence that these mechanical effects can decrease pain caused by IVD disease.[218] IVD pressure is also reduced during maneuvers with a longitudinal traction or rotational component. Neurophysiologically, manual therapy alters central sensory processing and thereby increases the pain threshold.[218] During mobilization and manipulation, reflex changes and altered motor neuron excitability can reduce muscle spasm by interfering with the pain-spasm cycle and may thereby improve posture and movement.[217,218]

There is has been more research investigating the effectiveness of spinal manipulative therapy (SMT) than almost any other intervention for spinal disorders. In many RCTs, SMT has been found to be more effective than placebo or no intervention for acute, subacute, and chronic spinal disorders.[211,219,220] However, when the literature is systematically examined through critical reviews and meta-analyses in which methodological quality of the research are considered, SMT, either alone or in combination with other interventions, has not been found to be any better than other approaches for treating patients with spinal disorders.[211,219,220]

Clinical guidelines for the treatment of spinal pain, based on expert review of RCTs and qualitative assessments by panel members, make various recommendations.[220] For example, although guidelines from the US, New Zealand, and Finland state that spinal manipulation may be useful in the first 4-6 weeks after the onset of symptoms, Israeli guidelines do not recommend manipulation at all, guidelines from the Netherlands recommend using SMT with an active approach only after 6 weeks, guidelines from the United Kingdom, Germany, and Australia do not consider SMT any more effective than other interventions, and Switzerland considers SMT only optional.

When spinal mobilization has been used selectively and based on examination findings and a clinical patient classification system, rather than applied to all patients with spinal disorders, it has been shown to allow patients to return to work sooner and to produce a predictable clinical outcome.[221-223] For example, in one study, patients with 4 of the following 5 variables: symptoms of less than 16 days' duration, lumbar hypomobility, at least one hip with more than 35 degrees of internal rotation, no symptoms distal to the knee, and a fear-avoidance belief questionnaire score of less 19 were found to have a 95% chance of a successful outcome from a lumbosacral manipulation.[223] Future research that takes into account the inherent heterogeneity of patient subgroups may further clarify the utility of spinal mobilization and manipulation in patients with spinal disorders.

Patients with musculoskeletal disorders characterized by intermittent pain, diminished ROM, and hypomobility are most likely to respond to mobilization or manipulation. Specific indications for mobilization or manipulation are listed in Table 8-16. Precautions to the use of spinal mobilization and manipulation are relative contraindications or situations when great care should be exercised before implementing the techniques. Because the development of skill and clinical judgment are a vital part of the decision to use manual therapy, precautions should be considered as contraindicated for the novice clinician. Contraindications are absolute circumstances and patient presentations in which it is unsafe to use these techniques. Precautions and contraindications for mobilization and manipulation are listed in Table 8-17.

There are many types of mobilization procedures. Descriptions of characteristics of various types of manual therapy procedures appear in Table 8-18. Joint mobilization is a gentle type of manual therapy as the sustained rhythmic passive accessory movements are performed to patient tolerance, with the patient always able to stop the movement. As such, mobilization is a safe and effective intervention that can more readily be used by novice clinicians. In general, gentle oscillatory mobilizations (grades I and II) are used to diminish acute and subacute pain. More forceful mobilizations (grades III, III+, and IV) are used for immobility and stiffness. Table 8-19 summarizes which techniques should be used, depending on the findings of the examination.

Guidelines as to when a therapist should use a gentler or more vigorous approach are listed in Table 8-20. Irritable conditions require a gentle approach to prevent exacerbation of symptoms, while more vigorous techniques, including spinal joint manipulation, which is performed at the limit of range and is not under the control of the patient and cannot be stopped once initiated, may be used for nonirritable conditions. Manipulation should only be performed after adequate training under the tutelage of qualified, experienced clinicians (Fig. 8-33).

MUSCLE ENERGY TECHNIQUE

The muscle energy technique (MET) was developed by integrating the resistive duction principles of Ruddy with the principles of proprioceptive neuromuscular facilitation (PNF).[224] MET is a form of manual therapy in which the patient voluntarily contracts a specific muscle from a controlled position in an exact direction, at varying levels of intensity, against a force applied by the therapist.[225] MET can be used to relax hypertonic muscles, mobilize restricted joints, strengthen weak muscles, stretch muscles and related connective tissue, reduce local edema, and improve local circulation.[167,224,225] MET is an active technique that requires the patient to participate with the therapist to improve function.

The mechanism of METs has yet to be substantiated. Based on principles of neurophysiology and motor control, it is believed that in the presence of dysfunction, the muscles at a spinal segment are facilitated to become hypertonic in response to nociceptive input.[226] This hypertonicity restricts movement of structures innervated by that segment, leading to local circulatory congestion, changes in connective tissue mobility, and pain. Once a segment becomes facilitated, it is both hypersensitive and hyperactive so that a small, normally tolerated stimulus will cause an overactive response without selectivity for a specific muscle or organ.[224,226] MET uses postisometric relaxation and reciprocal inhibition to decrease the tone in the hypertonic muscles to reestablishing their normal resting length and block nociceptive input.[226]

The system of muscle energy treatment depends on accurate localization and classification of the dysfunction. The dysfunction is classified according to findings from a series of specific palpatory, movement, and provocation tests. There is a specific MET for each diagnostic classification.

To perform an isometric MET the patient is positioned comfortably, permitting the operator to control all patient positions and movements. The operator moves the patient

TABLE 8-16	**Indications for Joint Mobilization**
Symptom Characteristics	**Examination Findings**
Mechanical origin	Symptoms are aggravated by certain movements or postures and are relieved by rest or other positions.
Diminished ROM	Loss of active or passive osteokinematic movement found on examination of ROM, PPIVM, and position testing.
Joint hypomobility	Diminished arthrokinematic movement determined by diminished passive mobility (PA) and position testing.
Joint asymmetry	Asymmetrical movement at individual joints as determined by PPIVM and position testing.
Tissue texture abnormality	Abnormal resistances to movement as a result of pain, spasm, trigger points, or thickened and stiff soft tissues overlying the joint.
Pain	Neuromusculoskeletal pain on movement, palpation, and elicited by provocation tests.

ROM, Range of motion; *PPIVM,* passive physiological intervertebral mobility; *PA,* posterior to anterior.

TABLE 8-17	Precautions and Contraindications to Mobilization and Manipulation*

Precautions	Contraindications
MOBILIZATION	
Neurological signs	Malignancy involving the spinal column
Rheumatoid arthritis	Cauda equina lesions affecting bowel or bladder function
Osteoporosis	Spinal cord involvement
Spondylolisthesis	Active inflammatory (e.g., RA) or infective arthritis
Hypermobility	Rheumatoid collagen necrosis of vertebral ligaments
Pregnancy	Bone disease and severe osteoporosis
Previous malignancy	Instability
Dizziness	Vertebral artery disease
Steroid use	Fracture or dislocation
Cervical trauma	
Internal derangement	
Psychological issues	
MANIPULATION*	
Disc lesions	Frank spinal deformity caused by old pathology
Ankylosing spondylitis after acute stage	Generalized congenital hypermobility (Ehlers-Danlos syndrome)
Congenital anomalies	Osteoporosis
Neurological dysfunction	Lower limb neurological symptoms caused by cervical or thoracic dysfunction
Irritable conditions	Undiagnosed pain
	Protective joint spasm
	Evidence of involvement of more than two adjacent nerve roots of the lumbar spine

RA, Rheumatoid arthritis.
*Precautions and contraindications listed under manipulation are in addition to those listed for mobilization.

TABLE 8-18	Characteristics of Manual Therapy Procedures

Characteristics	Procedural Techniques of Manual Therapy
Types of mobilizations	**Active:** Patient exerts mobilizing force by muscular contraction. **Passive:** Clinician exerts mobilizing force. **Combined:** Clinician and patient work together to exert mobilizing force through active movement and passive force application.
Type of movement	**Physiological:** Mobilizing force is directed to restore normal physiological motions: Flexion, extension, rotation, or lateral flexion. **Nonphysiological:** Mobilizing force is directed to restore arthrokinematic and accessory motions. Such movements include joint compression and distraction, gliding and gliding varying the direction of force such as cranially or caudally. These techniques include central or unilateral PAs and transverse vertebral pressures.
Direction of mobilizing force	**Into the pain:** The mobilization maneuver is in the direction of a motion restriction that produces pain. This may reproduce pain and is used to restore movement in subacute or chronic conditions. **Away from the pain:** The maneuver is performed in the direction opposite to the motion restriction.
Types of levers	**Indirect techniques:** The clinician uses limbs, pelvis or shoulder girdle as natural levers to impart a mobilizing force indirectly to the spinal column or sacroiliac joint. **Direct techniques:** The mobilizing force is exerted by application of manual pressure on the vertebral processes to influence the intervertebral joints. These are sometimes referred to as "pressure techniques" because the therapist uses the heel of the hand, thumb, hypothenar eminence or pisiform to apply pressure to the spinous or transverse processes.
Spinal location	**Regional:** Repetitive, rhythmic, passive movement is applied to the vertebral region in two or more segments. Useful for mobilizing larger sections of spine when specific techniques cannot be used. **Specific:** Therapist uses various techniques to localize the mobilizing force (such as locking) to restrict movement to a single segment.
Locking	Spinal motion segments are positioned so that no (or minimal) movement is possible. All spinal segments, except the one to be mobilized are locked. Segments not to be moved are placed in an extreme position. **Ligamentous locking:** Spinal joints, which are not to receive the mobilizing force, are positioned at the limit of possible range so that capsular and ligamentous tension to holds these segments, localizing the mobilization to the desired joint. **Facet locking:** Patient is placed in various combinations of movement patterns to constrain facet movement.

PAs, Posterior to anteriors.

TABLE 8-19	Manual Therapy Technique Selection According to Patient Symptoms
Patient Symptom	**Techniques**
Pain	Grade I and II mobilization.
	For acute pain or pain throughout the range, the technique should be gentle, pain-free, and comfortable to avoid exacerbation.
	Slow, smooth, rhythmic physiological and nonphysiological movements with as large an amplitude as can be comfortably tolerated for short duration.
Stiffness	Firm techniques, mobilizations using grade III, grade III stretch mobilizations, and grade IV and V manipulation at the end of the range to stretch tissues in the direction of restriction.
	With subacute and chronic stiffness the techniques are applied for longer mobilizing into the painful movement limitation while still respecting discomfort.
Spasm	Grades I and II mobilization to decrease pain.
	Gentle techniques to avoid provoking a protective muscle reaction.
	Active techniques to inhibit overactive muscles.

TABLE 8-20	Guidelines for Selecting Gentle or Vigorous Manual Therapy Techniques	
Gentle Technique	**Vigorous Technique**	
Severe pain	Moderate or mild pain	
Widespread radiation	Nonirritable condition	
Severe joint irritability	Intermittent pain	
Range limitation because of pain	Pain relieved by rest	
Motion produces distal pain	Minimal radiation	
Postural or reactive spasm	Not static or reactive spasm	
Recent neurological deficit	Range limited by soft tissue	
Pain caused by cough or sneeze	No neurological deficit	

through a series of precise movements to locate the barrier to motion by palpation of movement in three planes; sagittal (flexion and extension), frontal (lateral flexion), and horizontal (rotation). After finding the barrier, the patient is moved slightly into a position just before the barrier is engaged, which is known as the interbarrier zone. The patient is then performs a low force isometric contraction of the muscle opposing the motion for approximately 10 seconds and then relaxes for 3-5 seconds. The operator then repositions the patient to the new barrier and repeats the procedure.[167,224] After completion of the MET, the patient is reexamined to determine if the procedure has corrected the dysfunction.

A sample of MET procedures is found in Fig. 8-34. Contraindications to MET procedures include unstable joints, fractures, severe rheumatoid arthritis, severe osteoporosis, malignancy, cauda equina syndrome, and open wounds. Because the patient must actively participate with the operator throughout the procedure, this intervention is also not recommended for patients who cannot cooperate because of a language barrier, personality factors, or other reasons that preclude cooperation.

There is a paucity of literature on the effectiveness of MET. Most published trials that used MET included it as a component of an osteopathic treatment program.[227-231] In these trials, comparing standard treatment (medication, active physical therapy, and modalities),[229] sham osteopathic interventions, or no interventions[230] with osteopathic interventions that included MET in patients with LBP, no significant differences in a variety of outcomes persisted for more than 2 months after treatment.[231]

Three RCTs specifically examined the effect of MET on patients with spine-related symptoms or dysfunction. One study with asymptomatic subjects with limited spinal ROM found a statistically significant increase in cervical spine[232] and lumbar spine[233] ROM after eight sessions of MET. In another study, patients with acute LBP treated with MET in addition to neuromuscular reeducation and resistance exercises had statistically significant greater improvements in Oswestry Low Back Pain Disability Index scores than patients treated with neuromuscular reeducation and resistance exercises alone.[234] These studies suggest that MET may provide some benefit to appropriately selected patients but that further research into the effectiveness of this approach is needed.

EXERCISE

Exercise is one of the most commonly used interventions for the management of spinal disorders, yet the literature on its efficacy is contradictory.[213,220,235,236] PTs prescribe exercises by integrating the results of the examination with their knowledge of pertinent literature and disease processes and an individual patient's functional needs. Exercises can include activities to improve impaired muscle performance, deconditioning, disuse and atrophy, endurance, hypomobility or hypermobility, neuromuscular control, balance and coordination, and posture and alignment. Exercises are not confined to the trunk and consist of programs that also train the pelvic, hip, and shoulder muscles. An individualized program is the hallmark of a physical therapy exercise prescription.

Numerous studies in the literature purport to examine the application and efficacy of exercise in nonspecific back pain.[237-244] In much of the literature, exercise is characterized as a program with a focus on a certain direction of movement (flexion or extension), as a general conditioning program, or as some other specific program of exercises. Systematic reviews[213,236,244,245] and meta-analyses[246,247] have been conducted to evaluate the literature in its totality.

One systematic review analyzed the literature to evaluate the effectiveness of exercise therapy, including specific

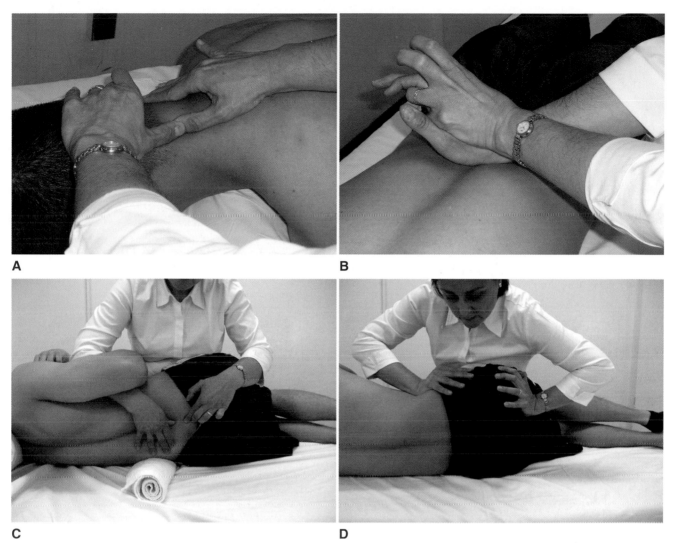

FIG. 8-33 Selected rotatory mobilization techniques. **A,** Transverse vertebral pressure in the cervical spine. **B,** Transverse vertebral pressure in the lumbar spine. **C,** The "lumbar roll." **D,** Iliosacral rotation.

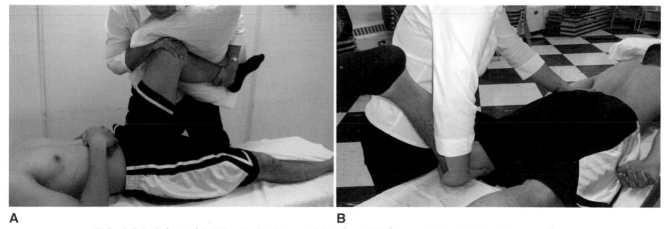

FIG. 8-34 Selected METs. **A,** Supine position for MET for an anterior innominate with barriers in flexion, adduction, and internal rotation. **B,** Prone position for MET for a posterior innominate with barriers in extension, abduction, and external rotation.

exercises, such as abdominal, flexion, extension, static, dynamic, strengthening, stretching, or aerobic, for the treatment of nonspecific LBP.[213] Only 39 RCTs were of adequate methodological quality, with pain and either generic or specific back pain self-report questionnaires used as the outcome measures. The authors concluded that there was strong evidence that exercise therapy and specific flexion and extension exercises were no more effective for the treatment of back pain than other treatments.[213] Although the evidence for chronic LBP was less clear, exercise was shown to be more effective than a general practitioner's care in this group but no more effective than conventional physiotherapy (defined as hot packs, massage traction, mobilization, short-wave diathermy, ultrasound, stretching, flexibility and coordination exercises, and electrotherapy).

Mior[248] believes that the lack of support for any form of exercise is due to a failure to recognize that although exercise provides psychological and physical benefits, inappropriate movement can cause loading that leads to further injury. Van Tulder's[213] review did not evaluate whether the exercise prescribed was specifically selected as appropriate for the patients treated. Research on all interventions for spinal disorders, including that on exercise, is limited by the fact that usually all patients with LBP are given the same treatment. It is recommended that patients in future studies are appropriately classified before being assigned to an intervention.

In addition, self-reports of pain and function provide a limited view of the outcome of exercise programs. A meta-analysis of RCTs on the impact of exercise alone or as part of a multidisciplinary intervention in patients with nonspecific, nonacute LBP found strong evidence that exercise decreases sick days for up to 1 year after the intervention.[247]

A review of the literature examining the safety and efficacy of exercise in treating back pain found that exercise for patients with acute, subacute or chronic LBP is safe and does not add to the risk of future back injuries or absences from work.[235] In addition to improvements in pain after exercise, Rainville found that there is substantial evidence that exercise improves flexibility and strength. Furthermore, exercises were found to improve the behavioral, cognitive, affect, and disability aspects of back pain.[235]

To address the impact of exercise on the structures producing impaired muscle performance implicated in nonspecific LBP, Hubley-Kozey et al[249] reviewed the literature using strength, endurance, neuromuscular control, flexibility, or posture as outcomes. They found moderately strong evidence that trunk extensor exercises significantly improve trunk extensor strength and endurance, that trunk flexor strength training improves trunk flexor strength and endurance, and that both types of exercise decrease pain and disability. Only minimal evidence could be found for the effectiveness of exercises to improve spinal mobility, posture, and neuromuscular performance. These authors noted that the current confusion about the usefulness of exercise in spinal disorders is likely due to failure to categorize both the exercises and the nature of the spinal disorder in most studies.

The following specific exercise intervention programs for patients with spinal disorders are most frequently employed and investigated by physical therapists.

MCKENZIE APPROACH TO INTERVENTION

The McKenzie approach to intervention, which emphasizes patient self-management through exercise and education, is one of the most popular methods of intervention among PTs for patients with spinal dysfunction and for treating patients with LBP.[107] In examining physical therapy practices in Britain and Ireland, Foster found that 47% of the therapists ranked the McKenzie approach to management of LBP as most frequently used.[250]

McKenzie's approach to intervention and management of spinal pain is integrated with the examination process in which patients are classified into subgroups for the purpose of directing treatment. During the examination the patient undergoes a series of repeated end-range test movements to determine whether a mechanical maneuver centralizes (draws toward the spinal midline) or peripheralizes (spreads distally or laterally) their symptoms. For most patients, movements toward extension will centralize symptoms; in other patients, symptoms will centralize with lateral movement in the frontal plane (called side gliding); and in a very few, symptoms will centralize with other directions of movement.[101,251] The direction of the movement that centralizes or abolishes symptoms forms the basis for beginning the intervention program. Patients are advised to perform a series of 10-15 repetitions of each movement noted in the examination to centralize their symptoms. These exercises are repeated as frequently as every 2 hours for a patient in acute pain. Once the symptoms stay centralized, a patient in the acute stage is advised to maintain a lordotic posture for 24-48 hours to promote tissue healing. As soon as a patient can tolerate additional movement without symptoms peripheralizing, exercises in other movement planes are introduced.[101]

As noted in Table 8-8, exercise prescription is linked to the classification according to the patient's syndrome. For example, a patient with a derangement four syndrome would present with a lateral shift or a posture in which the shoulders are typically shifted away from the side of pain (Fig. 8-35, *A*). To produce a centralization of symptoms the therapist would instruct the patient in self-correction of the lateral shift (Fig. 8-35, *B*), and if this did not produce centralization the therapist would assist the patient with manual correction (Fig. 8-35, *C*). With repeated lateral shift correction, the symptoms would be expected to move from the leg to the lumbosacral midline at which time extension exercises are added. This may begin with simple prone lying, followed by the patient assuming a prone on elbows position (Fig. 8-35, *D*) and continued with press-up exercises (Fig. 8-35, *E*). These movements are to be done as passive mobility exercises and with minimal contraction of the paraspinal muscles. The repetitive nature of McKenzie exercises have been shown to elicit hemodynamic stress, which increases as the number of exercise repetitions increases.[252] Patients with cardiopulmonary co-morbidities or those at risk for

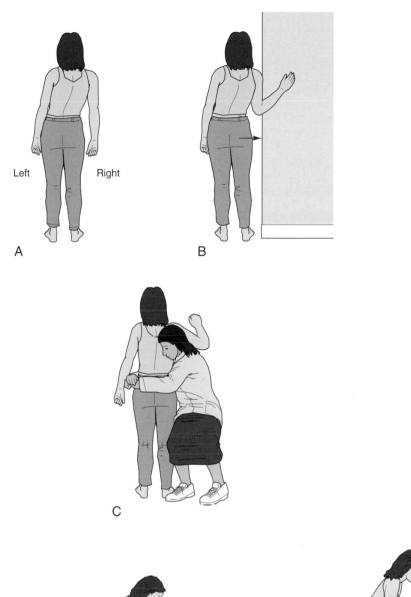

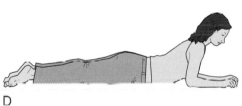

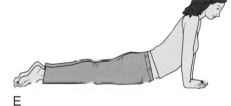

FIG. 8-35 **A,** Lateral shift with shoulders shifted to the right. **B,** Self-correction of lateral shift. **C,** Manual correction of lateral shift. **D,** Prone on elbows. **E,** Press-up.

such disease should therefore be carefully monitored while performing repetitions of McKenzie exercises.[252]

In the McKenzie approach, passive treatment modalities such as hot packs or ultrasound are frowned upon with the therapist guiding the patient into an active role for symptom management. Patients gain confidence in their ability to manage pain, should symptoms recur, by gaining an understanding of the relationship between their pain and movement. Prevention of future episodes of pain is facilitated by postural education and prophylactic exercises. It is a common misconception that the McKenzie approach is synonymous with extension exercises. Using McKenzie examination procedures for patients with nonspecific LBP in a prospective randomized

study, Donelson[251] found that 40% of the subjects experienced centralization and symptom reduction with a repeated end range extension, whereas 7% experienced centralization and symptom reduction with repeated end-range flexion.

In some studies investigating the McKenzie approach to intervention, all patients receive the same treatment rather than an individualized program[241,253-255] or receive additional interventions not considered to be part of the McKenzie method, such as joint manipulation,[240,256] active spinal extension,[253] or hip extension.[257]

To assess the effectiveness and cost of treatment, Cherkin et al[237] randomly assigned patients with nonspecific LBP of 7 days' duration to the McKenzie method, chiropractic manipulation, or an educational booklet. Although the authors reported that the mean number of chiropractic visits was 50% greater than the mean number of physical therapy visits, they report that outcomes including symptoms, function, patient satisfaction, disability, pain recurrences, and additional provider visits were similar for the McKenzie physical therapy and chiropractic manipulation.[237] A limitation of this study is that patients were not examined and then selected as suitable for the McKenzie approach before being assigned to the treatment.

In a similar RCT, Petersen et al[258] compared the effectiveness of the McKenzie method to intensive dynamic strength training for patients with chronic LBP. The McKenzie group showed a faster initial decrease in pain at 2 months, whereas long-term groups had similar outcomes. Only Schenk et al[233] examined patients with LBP and categorized them as having a lumbar posterior derangement before randomly assigning them to either a McKenzie extension (or extension with lateral shift correction) exercise or to a mobilization treatment group. The McKenzie exercise group demonstrated a clinically and statistically significant greater decrease in both pain and Oswestry scores than did the mobilization group.[233]

Clare and associates[239] conducted a systematic review of studies with sufficient methodological quality, where treatment was individualized and selected according to McKenzie principles and provided by therapists specifically trained in this approach, and appropriate outcomes were measured. The McKenzie approach was found to be statistically and clinically more effective than other treatments in decreasing pain and disability at 3 months, although long-term effects were not reported.[239]

SPINAL STABILIZATION EXERCISES

Spinal stabilization exercises are specifically designed to target the muscles that control segmental stability. The theoretical rationale for spinal stabilization exercises comes from the work of Panjabi,[205,206] who defines spinal instability as a loss of control or excessive motion in the spinal segment's neutral zone that is related to injury, spinal degenerative changes, and muscle weakness. The neutral zone is the portion of movement within the ROM that is not resisted by the passive structures such as the bones and ligaments.[205,206] Stabilization exercises are specifically designed to target the multifidus (MF) and transverses abdominis (TrA) muscles, which work together, contracting before the initiation of arm and leg movement, to stiffen the spine.[169,259-261] Spinal stiffness protects the spine from reactive forces to reduce the risk of spinal injury.[262]

In normal trunk function, co-contraction of the TrA and MF muscles stabilizes the spine when the limbs are moved and occurs independently of contraction of the larger, multisegmental, superficial muscles of the trunk, such as the erector spinae and rectus abdominis, which move the trunk. In patients with chronic LBP, as well as those with experimentally chemically induced back pain, motor control of the TrA has been found to be impaired, with delayed onset of contraction with limb movement.[262,263] The MF is also reflexively inhibited in pa-

tients with LBP, exhibiting weakness, loss of control, and a decreased cross-sectional area.[264-266] Poor outcome after disc surgery has been attributed to loss of MF function.[267,268]

Exercises focusing on training the TrA and MF have also been shown to help patients with LBP. A RCT compared the effects of 4 weeks of isometric exercises for the TrA together with the MF with the effect of gradually returning to normal activities as tolerated in a group of patients with LBP and found that although both groups' symptoms significantly decreased,[266] the group that did not perform the exercises was 12.4 times more likely to experience a recurrence of back pain at 1 year and 9 times more likely to experience recurrences 2 and 3 years after the initial episode.[269]

The hallmark of stabilization exercises is drawing in of the abdominal wall, also called abdominal bracing, which generates a co-contraction of Tra and MF (Fig. 8-36). As the emphasis of stabilization exercise is motor control of the deep spinal muscles, a low level continuous contraction, less than 30% to 40% of a maximum voluntary contraction is used. Accurate replication of the correct holding co-activates only the TrA and MF without activating other trunk muscles.[169] Control is developed through repeated practice, which allows patients with back pain to learn or relearn how to isolate TrA and MF contraction to maintain spinal stability.

Therapists can teach patients techniques to master abdominal bracing with co-contraction. These include focusing on contracting the TrA or MF one at a time, verbal and visual cues, different postures and positions, facilitation and feedback techniques, and techniques to decrease activity of overactive global muscles.[169] Verbal cues that can help to elicit TrA contraction are "draw in your abdomen" and "pull your navel up and in toward your spine." The therapist can check by palpation for a contraction of the TrA and can teach the patient to self-check by palpating between the lateral border of the rectus abdominis and the ASIS. Contraction of the TrA has been found to occur with contraction of the diaphragm[270] and the pelvic floor musculature.[271] Therefore to facilitate contraction of TrA in patients who have lost the perception of muscle contraction, patients can be asked to contract their pelvic floor muscles or to deeply sigh with expiration.[169] When overactivity of global muscles interferes with local muscle contraction, EMG biofeedback from the external oblique and rectus abdominis muscles can help teach the patient to isolate muscle contraction. To promote an isolated contraction of the MF, the therapist palpates just lateral to the spinous process at the location of the MF and asks the patient to "bulge your muscle up into my fingers."

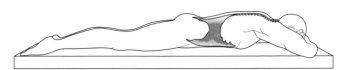

FIG. 8-36 Co-activation of transversus abdominis and multifidus.

Stabilization exercises are initiated in a non–weight-bearing position to diminish the use of global muscles. Once the patient masters the technique of drawing in or abdominal hollowing in supine and prone, the activity is progressed to sitting, sidelying, standing, and ultimately walking. With progression to more challenging positions, the patient must maintain a neutral spinal position and hold the co-contraction of the TrA and MF with a normal breathing pattern. At this point, stabilization exercises can be integrated into light functional activities in which the local muscles support the spine while the global muscles move the trunk. This can be accomplished by moving the extremities during reaching, turning, and leaning. A fre-quently used exercise is to ask the patient to contract the TrA and MF from a crooklying position (supine with hips and knees flexed, feet flat), while raising an arm, leg, and both (Fig. 8-37). Pressure biofeedback from the small of the back can be used to ensure that the proper position is maintained throughout the exercise. For greater challenges the trunk can be inclined while the patient holds an upright posture. Finally, actively controlling the spine in neutral with abdominal bracing can be performed while walking increasing distances.

Incorporation of abdominal stabilization exercises with greater loads in functional tasks can also be tailored to the demands of the patient's work, leisure and other usual

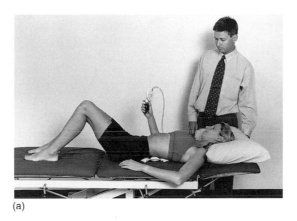
(a)

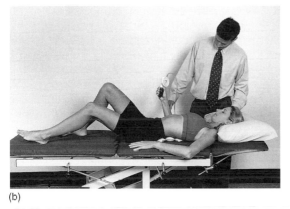
(b)

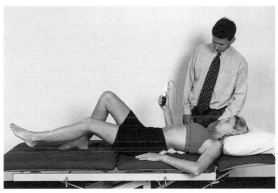

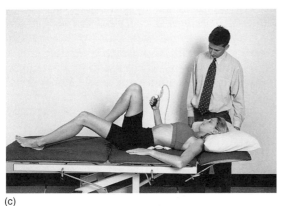
(c)

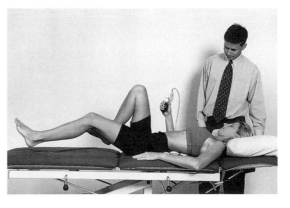

FIG. 8-37 Patient in supine position with biofeedback unit under spine. Instructed in co-contraction with leg movement. *From Richardson C:* Therapeutic Exercise for Lumbopelvic Stabilization, *ed 2, Philadelphia, 2005, Churchill Livingstone.*

activities. External load can be increased with several types of exercises, body positioning, decreasing stability of the body position, and equipment. Therapists are urged to be creative in developing an individualized program. In a commonly used exercise, the patient extends an arm, leg, and both to increase spinal load from a quadruped position. This can be made more difficult by placing a small ball or balance board under the hand. Bridging from a hooklying position is performed, and stability is challenged by using a single leg for support, a ball under the foot, or by increasing speed. Many exercises incorporate the use of a large gym ball to challenge stability. Exercises that train the global muscles, such as the erector spinae, quadratus lumborum, and abdominal obliques, can be added by using a variety of exercise equipment and functional movements as long as the patient maintains control of an abdominal brace throughout the activity.

INTERVENTIONS FOR COMMON PATHOLOGICAL CONDITIONS

Spinal Stenosis. Traditionally, patients with spinal stenosis have undergone surgical intervention as the disorder was believed to be progressive. Therefore much of the literature on the management of spinal stenosis addresses the effectiveness of surgical management.[272,273] However, in the absence of progressive neurological deficits, the condition may be relatively stable, and conservative management, including medication, epidural injections, bracing, and physical therapy, can have favorable outcomes.[51,104,274-276] The studies of conservative interventions all have methodological flaws, such as lack of patient randomization or generally grouped patients (i.e., surgery versus nonsurgery), not specifying the type of intervention, and to date there are no published RCTs specifically examining the effectiveness of conservative interventions in spinal stenosis.[51,274,275] There are ongoing RCTs comparing different conservative management strategies and comparing conservative management with surgery, and case studies have reported positive results for physical therapy interventions in patients with spinal stenosis.[277,278]

Symptoms of spinal stenosis are exacerbated by positions and movements that cause compressive loading and spinal extension and are diminished with flexion or unloading. Therefore physical therapy interventions are directed towards encouraging flexion or unloading of the spine.[279]

Manual therapy may initially be used to improve intervertebral flexion and restore segmental mobility to assist in postural restoration. Whitman specifically recommends PA and rotation mobilizations or manipulations to the thoracolumbar spine and PA mobilizations to the hip to restore hip extension mobility.[278] A therapeutic exercise program of stretching and strengthening exercises to decrease extension forces on the lumbar spine is recommended.[280] This typically includes active and passive stretching of the iliopsoas and rectus femoris (hip flexors) and the lumbar paraspinals and strengthening of the abdominals and gluteals. The hip flexors may be stretched in supine, sidelying, half-kneeling, or in unilateral stand-

ing. Lumbar paraspinal stretching may be performed in supine, quadruped, or sitting. Postural awareness exercises and stabilization exercises to strengthen the abdominals and unload the spine are also recommended.[51] A flexion-biased stabilization program for abdominal strengthening has also been shown to reduce symptoms in patients with spinal stenosis,[281,282] as have pelvic tilts and bridging exercises.[280]

Bicycle exercise is recommended for general conditioning in patients with spinal stenosis because the seated position keeps the spine in flexion. Inclined treadmill walking, which also flexes the spine, may also be well tolerated by patients with spinal stenosis. Body weight support with a harness during treadmill ambulation has also been shown to increase ambulation duration and distance before the onset of symptoms in patients with spinal stenosis.[51,278] Aquatic therapy may be useful for both strengthening and conditioning as the support of the water reduces spinal compression forces. Physical therapy treatment programs in which manual therapy was reinforced with therapeutic exercise and a graded walking program have been shown to significantly improve patients' impairments, functional limitations, and disability for up to 18 months.[277,278]

Spondylolisthesis. Surgical stabilization to prevent the progression of slippage is generally recommended for management of patients with severe spondylolisthesis with radicular signs or significant pain and for those who fail to improve with conservative intervention.[204,283] However, most patients with spondylolysis and spondylolisthesis respond well to nonoperative treatment consisting of modalities for pain relief, bracing, exercise, electrical stimulation, and activity modification.[284] Patients are referred to physical therapy to reduce pain, restore mobility and function, and to strengthen and stabilize the spine.[284] There is some disagreement in the literature as to the relative effectiveness of physical therapy and surgery in the management of spondylolisthesis. For example, in a prospective randomized study of exercise in 111 patients with spondylolisthesis, Moller and Hedlund[285] reported a significantly lower disability rating index and pain index at a 2-year follow-up for patients who received a posterolateral fusion than for those who received exercises. Specific exercises were not delineated but were reported to include back and abdominal muscle strengthening and postural training. In contrast, good results were reported in patients with mild to moderate spondylolisthesis treated with a spinal orthotic that prevented excessive lumbar lordosis in conjunction with physical therapy that emphasized hamstring and lumbodorsal stretching and abdominal strengthening.[286,287]

The type of exercises that provide the greatest benefit to these patients remains unclear; however, most recommend that extension exercises be avoided in patients with spondylolisthesis because these can increase anterior shearing force on the vertebrae, which could result in additional slippage.[288] In addition, some common abdominal strengthening exercises, such as supine straight leg raises, bent leg raises, and static cross-knee curl-ups, also exert high mechanical loads on the lumbar spine and are therefore not recommended for patients at risk for bone slippage.[289] In a comparison of the effects of flexion, extension, or combined flexion-extension exercises in nonsurgical candidates with pain secondary to spondylolisthesis, Gramse et al found that the flexion exercises were the most effective, resulting in less need for back supports or job modification and less limitation of activities by pain.[290] Sinaki and Lutness[291] also compared flexion exercises to extension exercises in patients with spondylolisthesis and found that after 3 months, 58% of those who performed flexion exercises were asymptomatic as compared to 6% who performed extension exercises. After 3 years, 62% of those who performed flexion exercises remained symptom-free, whereas none of the extension group remained asymptomatic. The authors concluded that when conservative treatment is indicated, back flexion or isometric back strengthening exercises should be implemented.[291] Conversely, in a RCT in patients with retrodisplacement and spondylolisthesis, Spratt and Weinstein[292] found extension exercises to significantly decrease pain and hypothesized that radiographic instability could indicate advanced discogenic disease. Finally, O'Sullivan and associates,[293] in a RCT, examined the effect of a 10-week exercise program for the deep stabilizing muscles, including the internal oblique, TrA, and lumbar MF in patients with spondylolysis or spondylolisthesis and chronic LBP. The patients who performed the stabilization exercises had statistically significant reductions in pain and functional disability scores as compared to a control group. These findings persisted at 3, 6, and 30 months' follow-up. The authors conclude that training the spinal stabilizing muscles provide dynamic spinal stability while keeping the spinal motion segment in a neutral zone during functional activities.[293] With this approach, the risks of increasing spinal compression with dynamic flexion exercises or anterior shearing with spinal extension exercises are eliminated, providing the clinician with a safe and effective exercise approach for patients with spondylosis or spondylolisthesis.

Whiplash. The Québec Task Force on WAD reviewed published RCTs for evidence regarding interventions typically used for treatment of whiplash.[67] No research was found to support the use of traction, rest, or soft cervical collars. Soft cervical collars and extended periods of rest encouraged inactivity and delayed recovery. Activity, on the other hand, was found to be helpful, with active exercise producing both short- and long-term benefits and joint mobilization producing short-term results. No acceptable research was found regarding passive modalities, such as acupuncture, transcutaneous electrical nerve stimulation, ultrasound, electrical stimulation, laser, or short-wave diathermy. Despite the recommendations of the Québec Task Force on WAD, passive modalities, soft cervical collar, and rest are still frequently used to treat whiplash.

In 2002, seven experts, using study selection recommendations from the Dutch Royal Physical Therapy Association, developed evidence-based clinical practice guidelines for the physical therapy management of WAD from published RCTs, systematic reviews, and prospective studies.[68] These clinical guidelines recommend that the patient history include information about impairments, disabilities, problems that might preclude participation in normal activities, prognostic factors, Waddell signs, and the patient's work history. The Visual Analog Scale (VAS), the NDI, and the Coping Strategies Questionnaire are recommended assessment tools. Based on case series and expert consensus, in the absence of higher quality evidence, the guidelines advise the therapist to perform the following examination procedures for patients with WAD:

- Observe posture and overt pain behavior
- Measure cervical ROM, including movement quality and symptom provocation
- Test for muscular stability, cervical proprioception, muscle strength, regional sensory changes, and neurological screening

In the development of a treatment plan for WAD, the primary goal of physical therapy is a rapid return to usual activities and prevention of chronicity. Prognostic factors, which may indicate a predisposition for the WAD to become chronic, are decreased cervical spine mobility, previous trauma to the neck, and the presence of three Waddell signs. The therapist is advised to consult the physician if the patient has vertigo, memory problems, passive coping strategies, or difficult pain behavior.

The guidelines for the treatment for a normal recovery from WAD are divided into five phases as delineated in Table 8-21.

CASE STUDY 8-1

LOW BACK PAIN AND INTERVERTEBRAL DISC HERNIATION

Examination
Patient History

MJ is a 39-year-old woman who presents with a 3-month history of LBP and radiating symptoms to her right posterior thigh and lateral calf. The symptoms started when MJ was bending and lifting a food service tray from a low tray holder to a raised cleaning bin. At that time, she experienced centralized LBP progressing to her right posterior thigh and lateral calf and noticed some foot slap during ambulation. She has experienced similar episodes before and 1-year ago received physical therapy for an episode of these symptoms that resulted in a full recovery. MJ had a transforaminal epidural corticosteroid injection 4 days ago, which relieved her lateral calf pain. Her past medical history includes mitral valve prolapse repair 5 years ago. Plain x-rays showed no bony abnormalities, and MRI reveals the right L4/L5 IVD to have a lateral herniation with nerve root compression.

Tests and Measures
Musculoskeletal

Posture The patient has a slightly increased lumbar lordosis and thoracic kyphosis. There is no apparent lateral shift. The patient demonstrates a decreased tolerance to

TABLE 8-21	Goals and Interventions for Patients with Whiplash-Associated Disorder	
Recovery Phase	Goals of Treatment	Interventions
Phase 1 (<4 days)	Decrease pain. Provide information. Explain the consequences of whiplash.	**Education:** Nature of injury, natural course of whiplash, avoid factors that lead to chronicity. **Exercise therapy:** Frequent cervical AROM within limits of pain. NSAIDs in consultation with physician.
Phase 2 (4 days-3 weeks)	Provide information. Improve function. Return patient to normal activities.	**Education:** Reassure about benign nature of symptoms. **Exercise therapy:** Graded activities such as muscle stabilization exercises and ROM to prevent fear of movement. **Functional activities:** Reaching, walking, postural control.
Phase 3 (3-6 weeks)	Provide information Explain consequences of whiplash. Improve function. Increase activities.	**Education:** To prevent chronicity correct pessimistic beliefs and passive coping strategies. **Exercise therapy:** Muscle strengthening and stabilization. Postural correction and awareness. **Functional activities:** Increase graded activities required for prior usual activities.
Phase 4 (6 weeks-3 months)	Provide information. Explain consequences of whiplash. Improve activity levels. Improve participation.	**Education:** Restore patient's confidence that symptoms do not indicate chronicity. **Exercise therapy:** Provide a personalized graded exercise program. Give alternative ways of performing tasks by changing frequency and speed. **Functional activities:** Increase activities on time-dependent basis.
Phase 5 (>3 months)	Provide information. Explain consequences of whiplash. Improve activity levels. Improve participation.	**Education:** Recovery may be delayed. Promote healthy behaviors. Encourage feelings of self-control and optimistic attitudes about pain. Consider the need for psychological referral if symptoms persist for this long. **Functional activities:** Continue graded activities.

AROM, Active range of motion; *NSAIDs,* nonsteroidal antiinflammatory drugs.

weight bearing on the right lower extremity with the right hip held in slight external rotation and knee flexion for comfort.

Active Range of Motion

Flexion	50% of normal with pain
Extension	10% of normal with pain
Right sidebending	50% of normal with pain
Left sidebending	100% with pain on return
Right rotation	100% without pain
Left rotation	100% without pain

Muscle Length Thomas test 5 degrees above neutral hip flexion bilaterally.

Muscle Performance Abdominal muscles are weak, grossly 3+/5 and producing lumbosacral pain at their limit.

Joint Integrity and Mobility Pain with grade II PA on all lumbar spinous processes; hypomobile thoracolumbar junction; PROM of single intervertebral joints—PPIVM: Not tested secondary to pain.

Neuromuscular

Pain Pain is worsened by walking and sitting for more than 5-10 minutes and with rising from sitting. Pain improves with lying supine and prone. Pain scale: 7/10 currently. Minimal pain is elicited on palpating bilateral paraspinal muscle (right > left). There is pain to palpation throughout the right buttock with a trigger point in the right piriformis.

Peripheral Nerve Integrity Sensation is intact to light touch throughout the L5-S2 dermatomes. Strength by MMT is 5/5 throughout both lower extremities except right extensor hallucis longus 4-/5 and right gluteus medius 4-/5. The patient cannot heel walk on the right.

Reflex Integrity Knee and ankle jerk are WNL bilaterally.

Neurodynamic Tests

SLR Test + at 45 degrees on the right with symptom provocation to the right thigh.

Prone Knee Bend Test WNL bilaterally, slight stretching pain in the anterior thigh.

Slump Test + with symptom provocation in the right lower extremity.

Cardiovascular/Pulmonary: MJ's cardiopulmonary status is stable and periodically evaluated by a cardiologist.

Special Tests

SI Joint Tests Compression test and sitting and standing flexion tests are negative bilaterally.

Evaluation, Diagnosis, and Prognosis

Abnormal findings include the following:

Impairments	Functional Limitations
Postural malalignment	Unable to sit for more than 5-10 minutes
Pain with movement	Limited prolonged weight bearing.
Diminished active ROM with pain	Limited ambulation
Impaired lumbar joint arthrokinematics (↓PAs)	Unable to perform employment duties
Diminished lower extremity and abdominal strength	
Decreased neural mobility (+SLR and +slump)	

Diagnosis

The patient's symptoms of increased pain with sitting and standing from sitting suggest that disc herniation and increased intradiscal pressure in sitting and standing from sitting may be contributing to her symptoms. Clinical signs that support the hypothesis that a space-occupying lesion is impairing nerve transmission of L5/S1 are a positive SLR and slump test, the loss of strength in the right extensor hallucis longus, and gluteus medius, and the trigger point in the piriformis muscle. Diminished right sidebending and extension produce pain resulting from closing of facet or adding additional compression through the intervertebral foramen.

Prognosis

Factors that suggest a more prolonged recovery include the fact that the patient has not been able to work for 2 weeks because of this condition and that she has had other episodes of LBP. However, the fact that the patient is very motivated, willing to actively participate in her care, and expresses a strong desire to return to work since she is the sole financial support for her family are all positive prognostic factors.

Goals

Reduced pain, normal trunk ROM, normal lower extremity and abdominal strength, pain-free sitting, standing, and walking for greater than 1 hour. Ability to perform duties as a nurse's aid.

Intervention

MJ was seen initially for physical therapy twice a week for 4 weeks. The initial interventions emphasized pain modulation, restoration of spinal mobility and personal responsibility, thus giving the patient the tools to exert some control over her symptoms. Pain modulation was achieved by applying ice to the lumbosacral spine and right buttock and performing grade I and II PAs to the lumbar spinous processes. Restoration of spinal mobility was initiated with prone press-ups throughout the day and instructions to engage the transverses abdominis in supine. The patient was also educated in positioning, body mechanics, and the use of a lumbar roll and was instructed to begin short bouts of walking within her apartment. Interventions progressed to include grade III and IV unilateral PAs and transverse vertebral rotations to mobilize the facet joints restricting active mobility. A more vigorous stabilization program was initiated, which began in supine and was progressed to quadruped and then to using a therapeutic gym ball. Stretching of the right piriformis and bilateral hip flexor muscles was begun. Later interventions included training in postural awareness and proper lifting techniques.

After completing 8 sessions over 4 weeks, the patient was seen 3 more times in physical therapy over the following 3 weeks. Her trunk strengthening was advanced, and she was educated in proper body mechanics and ergonomics for her work duties and prevention of future episodes.

Outcomes

At 4 weeks, MJ's pain and mobility improved, enabling a return to work at her prior job as a nurse's aide, although with light duty restrictions.

Please see the CD that accompanies this book for case studies describing the examination, evaluation and interventions for a patient with low back pain and spinal stenosis and for a patient with whiplash-associated disorder.

CHAPTER SUMMARY

Patients with spinal disorders may have back or neck pain with or without radiation of symptoms to the extremities. Spinal disorders for which a pathoanatomical diagnosis can be made and for which physical therapy may be helpful include radiculopathy, intervertebral disc disease, spinal stenosis, spondylolisthesis, and whiplash-associated disorders. However, despite the abundance of research on the diagnosis of spinal disorders, for the overwhelming majority of patients a definitive pathoanatomical diagnosis cannot be made and therefore classification systems that are independent of pathology have been developed to direct treatment. Three of these classification systems, the McKenzie approach, the treatment-based approach, and the impairment-based approach are described in this chapter. Evaluation of the findings of a thorough systematic examination which includes a patient history and tests of general and specific spinal joint mobility, muscle length and strength and neuromuscular function, can guide the clinician in selection of interventions. Interventions which have been shown to help patients with spinal disorders described in this chapter include joint mobilization and specific kinds of exercise.

ADDITIONAL RESOURCES

Useful Forms

Neck Disability Index Form
Oswestry Low Back Pain Disability Questionnaire
Roland-Morris Disability Questionnaire

Books

Dutton M: *Manual Therapy of the Spine: An Integrated Approach,* New York, 2002, McGraw-Hill.
Lee D: *The Pelvic Girdle: An Approach to the Examination and Treatment of the Lumbopelvic-Hip Region,* ed 3, New York, 2004, Churchill Livingstone.
Richardson C, Hodge P, Hides J: *Therapeutic Exercise for Lumbopelvic Stabilization: A Motor Control Approach for the Treatment and Prevention of Low Back Pain,* ed 2, New York, 2004, Churchill Livingstone.
Saunders HD, Saunders R: Evaluation, *Treatment and Prevention of Musculoskeletal Disorders,* ed 4, vol I, Bloomington, Minn, 2004, Educational Opportunities.
Vleeming A, Mooney V, Dorman T, et al: *Movement, Stability, and Low Back Pain: The Essential Role of the Pelvis,* New York, 1997, Churchill Livingstone.

Web Sites

North American Spine Society: www.spine.org
American Academy of Orthopedic Surgeons: www.aaos.org

Journal of Orthopedic and Sports Physical Therapy: www.jospt.org
Spine Society of Australia: www.spinesociety.org.au/
British Cervical Spine Society: www.boa.ac.uk/BCSS/

GLOSSARY

Annulus fibrosus: Outer component of the intervertebral disc.

Centralization: Proximal or central movement of distal pain or symptoms that originate from the spine in response to specific movements.

Classification system: A method used to categorize spinal pain disorders that are independent of pathology on diagnostic imaging. Frequently depends on the patient's presenting signs and symptoms and is related to intervention.

Counter-nutation: The movement in which the anterior aspect of the base (top) of the sacrum moves backward and upward relative to the ilium.

Crossover sign (crossed SLR sign): Reproduction of presenting symptoms with a SLR on the side contralateral to the pain.

Derangement syndrome: One of the major categories of the McKenzie classification system characterized by anatomical disruption of the structures of the intervertebral joints.

Dysfunction syndrome: One of the major categories of the McKenzie classification system characterized by pain that results from mechanical deformation of adaptively-shortened soft tissue after maintenance of poor positioning after degeneration, trauma, or a derangement.

Limb length inequality (LLI): A difference in length between the two lower extremities. In anatomical LLI, one of the bones of the lower extremity is short. In functional LLI, shortening of one of the lower extremities occurs without shortening of the bones.

Manipulation: A manual therapy technique in which a high-velocity thrust is applied at the limits of range.

Mobilization: A manual therapy technique in which graded passive movements are imparted within the anatomical limits of joint range.

Neck Disability Index (NDI): A self-report questionnaire that assesses limitations in ADLS as a result of neck pain.

Neurodynamic tests: Manual provocation tests that mechanically stress nervous tissue to determine if spinal nerve roots and peripheral nerves are causing pain.

Neurogenic claudication: A condition characterized by aggravation of neurological signs and symptoms, such as pain, paresthesias, and lower extremity cramping with ambulation, or by increasing lumbar lordosis of the spine. Symptoms improve with a change in posture.

Nucleus pulposus: Gelatinous inner core of the IVD.

Nutation: The movement in which the anterior aspect of the base (top) of the sacrum moves forward and downward relative to the ilium.

Oswestry Low Back Pain Disability Questionnaire: A disease-specific self-report questionnaire that assesses pain and disability in LBP.

Passive physiological intervertebral mobility (PPIVM): A spinal examination technique in which the passive motion at each segmental level is palpated in flexion, extension, side flexion, or rotation.

Postural syndrome: One of the major categories of the McKenzie classification system characterized by pain that results from maintenance of poor posture.

Provocation tests: Tests in which a series of maneuvers are applied that may aggravate or diminish a patient's presenting symptoms. A change in symptom severity indicates that the disorder is mechanical in nature.

Quadrant tests: A series of provocation tests that compress the contents of the intervertebral foramen and neighboring facet joints.

Radiculopathy: Irritation of a nerve root at any level of the spine.

Sensitizing maneuvers: Movements sequentially added to the distal extremity during a neurodynamic test to provoke symptoms that further stretch the nerves under examination.

Spinal stenosis: Narrowing of the spinal canal or intervertebral foramina because of bony or soft tissue encroachment so that the space between the spinal cord or nerve roots and the vertebral elements is compromised.

Spondylosis: A bilateral defect in the pars interarticularis of a vertebra that decreases the ability of the posterior elements to stabilize the motion segment.

Spondylolisthesis: Translation of vertebra forward in the sagittal plane with respect to an adjacent vertebra.

Whiplash-associated disorders (WAD): Bony or soft tissue injuries of the neck and related areas that occur after a rear or side motor vehicle collision in which the neck is subjected to acceleration-deceleration energy transfer.

References

1. Cote P, Cassidy JD, Carroll L: The treatment of neck and low back pain: Who seeks care? Who goes where? *Med Care* 39(9):956-967 2001.
2. Andersson G: Epidemiological features of chronic low-back pain, *Lancet* 354(9178):581-585, 1999.
3. Loney PL, Stratford PW: The prevalence of low back pain in adults: a methodological review of the literature, *Phys Ther* 79(4):384-396, 1999.
4. Cassidy JD, Carroll LJ, Cote P: The Saskatchewan health and back pain survey. The prevalence of low back pain and related disability in Saskatchewan adults, *Spine* 23(17):1860-1866; discussion 1867, 1998.
5. Cote P, Cassidy JD, Carroll L: The Saskatchewan Health and Back Pain Survey. The prevalence of neck pain and related disability in Saskatchewan adults, *Spine* 23(15):1689-1698, 1998.
6. Bovim G, Schrader H, Sand T: Neck pain in the general population (see comment), *Spine* 19(12):1307-1309, 1994.
7. Croft PR, Lewis M, Papageorgiou AC, et al: Risk factors for neck pain: A longitudinal study in the general population, *Pain* 93(3):317-325, 2001.
8. Guez M, Hildingsson C, Stegmayr B, et al: Chronic neck pain of traumatic and non-traumatic origin: a population-based study, *Acta Orthop Scand* 74(5):576-579, 2003.
9. Waddell G: *The Back Pain Revolution*, ed 2, New York, 2004, Churchill Livingstone.
10. Endresen E: Pelvic pain and low back pain in pregnant women: An epidemiological study, *Scand J Rheumatol* 24:135-141, 1995.
11. Fast A, Shapiro D, Ducommun EJ, et al: Low back pain in pregnancy, *Spine* 12(4):368-371, 1987.
12. Kristiansson P, Svardsudd K, Schoultz B: Serum relaxin, symphyseal pain, and back pain during pregnancy, *Am J Obstet Gynecol* 175(5):1342-1347, 1996.
13. Orvieto R, Achiron A, Ben-Rafael Z, et al: Low back pain of pregnancy, *Acta Obset Gynecol Scand* 73:209-214, 1994.
14. Ostgaard H, Andersson GBJ, Karlsson K: Prevalence of back pain in pregnancy, *Spine* 1991;16(5):549-552, 1991.
15. Ostgaard HC, Andersson GB, Schultz AB, et al: Influence of some biomechanical factors on low-back pain in pregnancy, *Spine* 18(1):61-65, 1993.
16. Kristiansson P, Svardsudd K, Schoultz B: Back pain during pregnancy, *Spine* 21(6):702-709, 1996.
17. Hestbaek L, Leboeuf-Yde C, Manniche C: Low back pain: What is the long-term course? A review of studies of general patient populations, *Eur Spine J* 12(2):149-165, 2003.
18. Waddell G, Bircher M, Finlayson D, et al: Symptoms and signs: Physical disease or illness behaviour? *Br Med J* (Clin Res Ed) 289(6447):739-741, 1984.
19. Jette AM, Smith K, Haley SM, et al: Physical therapy episodes of care for patients with low back pain (see comment), *Phys Ther* 74(2):101-110; discussion 110-115, 1994.
20. Bogduk N: *Clinical Anatomy of the Lumbar Spine and Sacrum*, ed 3, New York, 1997, Churchill Livingstone.
21. Bogduk N: The anatomy and pathophysiology of neck pain, *Phys Med Rehabil Clin N Am* 14(3):455-472, 2003.
22. Kirkaldy-Willis W, Gernard T: *Managing Low Back Pain*, ed 4, New York, 1991, Churchill Livingstone.
23. Goldstein B: Anatomic issues related to cervical and lumbosacral radiculopathy. *Phys Med Rehabil Clin N Am* 13(3):423-437, 2002.
24. Lipetz JS: Pathophysiology of inflammatory, degenerative, and compressive radiculopathies, *Phys Med Rehabil Clin N Am* 13(3):439-449, 2002.
25. An HS, Thonar EJ, Masuda K: Biological repair of intervertebral disc, *Spine* 28(15 suppl):S86-92, 2003.
26. Farfan HF, Cossette JW, Robertson GH, et al: The effects of torsion on the lumbar intervertebral joints: the role of torsion in the production of disc degeneration, *J Bone Joint Surg Am* 52(3):468-497, 1970.
27. Benoist M: The natural history of lumbar disc herniation and radiculopathy, *Joint Bone Spine* 69(2):155-160, 2002.
28. Saal JA, Saal JS, Herzog RJ: The natural history of lumbar intervertebral disc extrusions treated nonoperatively, *Spine* 15(7):683-686, 1990.

29. Maigne JY, Rime B, Deligne B: Computed tomographic follow-up study of forty-eight cases of nonoperatively treated lumbar intervertebral disc herniation, *Spine* 17(9):1071-1074, 1992.

30. Komori H, Shinomiya K, Nakai O, et al: The natural history of herniated nucleus pulposus with radiculopathy, *Spine* 21(2):225-229, 1996.

31. Vernon-Roberts B, Fazzalari NL, et al: Pathogenesis of tears of the anulus investigated by multiple-level transaxial analysis of the T12-L1 disc, *Spine* 22(2):2641-2646, 1997.

32. Boden SD, Davis DO, Dina TS, et al: Abnormal magnetic-resonance scans of the lumbar spine in asymptomatic subjects: A prospective investigation, *J Bone Joint Surg Am* 72(3):403-408, 1990.

33. Jensen MC, Brant-Zawadzki MN, et al: Magnetic resonance imaging of the lumbar spine in people without back pain (see comment), *N Engl J Med* 331(2):69-73, 1994.

34. Erkintalo MO, Salminen JJ, Alanen AM, et al: Development of degenerative changes in the lumbar intervertebral disk: Results of a prospective MR imaging study in adolescents with and without low-back pain, *Radiology* 196(2):529-533, 1995.

35. Paajanen H, Erkintalo M, Kuusela T, et al: Magnetic resonance study of disc degeneration in young low-back pain patients, *Spine* 14(9):982-985, 1989.

36. Tertti MO, Salminen JJ, Paajanen HE, et al: Low-back pain and disk degeneration in children: a case-control MR imaging study, *Radiology* 180(2):503-507, 1991.

37. van Tulder MW, Assendelft WJ, Koes BW, et al: Spinal radiographic findings and nonspecific low back pain. A systematic review of observational studies, *Spine* 22(4):427-434, 1997.

38. Luoma K, Riihimaki H, Luukkonen R, et al: Low back pain in relation to lumbar disc degeneration, *Spine* 25(4):487-492, 2000.

39. Rannou F, Corvol M, Revel M, et al: Disk degeneration and disk herniation: the contribution of mechanical stress, *Joint Bone Spine* 68(6):543-546, 2001.

40. Bibby SR, Jones DA, Lee RB, et al: The pathophysiology of the intervertebral disc, *Joint, Bone, Spine* 68(6):537-542, 2001.

41. Ferguson SJ, Steffen T: Biomechanics of the aging spine, *Eur Spine J* 12(suppl 2):S97-S103, 2003.

42. Gordon SL, Weinstein JN: A review of basic science issues in low back pain, *Phys Med Rehabil Clin N Am* 9(2):323-342, 1998.

43. Lundon K, Bolton K: Structure and function of the lumbar intervertebral disk in health, aging, and pathologic conditions, *JOSPT* 31(6):291-303; discussion 304-306, 2001.

44. Thompson RE, Pearcy MJ, Downing KJ, et al: Disc lesions and the mechanics of the intervertebral joint complex, *Spine* 25(23):3026-3035, 2000.

45. Twomey L, Taylor J: Age changes in lumbar intervertebral discs, *Acta Orthop Scand* 56:496-499, 1985.

46. Amonoo-Kuofi HS: Morphometric changes in the heights and anteroposterior diameters of the lumbar intervertebral discs with age, *J Anat* 175:159-168, 1991.

47. Shao Z, Rompe G, Schiltenwolf M: Radiographic changes in the lumbar intervertebral discs and lumbar vertebrae with age (see comment), *Spine* 27(3):263-268, 2002.

48. Arbit E, Pannullo S: Lumbar stenosis: A clinical review, *Clin Orthop Rel Res* 384:137-143, 2001.

49. Spivak JM: Degenerative lumbar spinal stenosis, *J Bone Joint Surg Am* 80(7):1053-1066, 1998.

50. Rao R: Neck pain, cervical radiculopathy, and cervical myelopathy: Pathophysiology, natural history, and clinical evaluation, *J Bone Joint Surg Am* 84-A(10):1872-1881, 2002.

51. Fritz JM, Delitto A, Welch WC, et al: Lumbar spinal stenosis: A review of current concepts in evaluation, management, and outcome measurements, *Arch Phys Med Rehabil* 79(6):700-708, 1998.

52. Rao R: Neck pain, cervical radiculopathy, and cervical myelopathy: pathophysiology, natural history, and clinical evaluation, *Instr Course Lect* 52:479-488, 2003.

53. Arnoldi CC, Brodsky AE, Cauchoix J, et al: Lumbar spinal stenosis and nerve root entrapment syndromes: Definition and classification, *Clin Orthop Rel Res* 115:4-5, 1976.

54. Nagler W, Hausen HS: Conservative management of lumbar spinal stenosis. Identifying patients likely to do well without surgery, *Postgrad Med* 103(4):69-71, 76, 81-83, 1998.

55. Inufusa A, An HS, Lim TH, et al: Anatomic changes of the spinal canal and intervertebral foramen associated with flexion-extension movement, *Spine* 21(21):2412-2420, 1996.

56. Wilmink JT, Penning L: Influence of spinal posture on abnormalities demonstrated by lumbar myelography, *AJNR Am J Neuroradiol* 4(3):656-658, 1983.

57. Wilmink JT, Penning L, van den Burg W: Role of stenosis of spinal canal in L4-L5 nerve root compression assessed by flexion-extension myelography, *Neuroradiology* 26(3):173-181, 1984.

58. Schonstrom N, Lindahl S, Willen J, et al: Dynamic changes in the dimensions of the lumbar spinal canal: an experimental study in vitro, *J Orthop Res* 7(1):115-121, 1989.

59. Penning L, Wilmink JT: Posture-dependent bilateral compression of L4 or L5 nerve roots in facet hypertrophy. A dynamic CT-myelographic study, *Spine* 12(5):488-500, 1987.

60. Esses S: *Textbook of Spinal Disorders*, Philadelphia, 1995, JB Lippincott.

61. Thomas SA: Spinal stenosis: History and physical examination, *Phys Med Rehabil Clin N Am* 14:29-39, 2003.

62. Stone AT, Tribus CB: Acute progression of spondylolysis to isthmic spondylolisthesis in an adult, *Spine* 27(16):E370-372, 2002.

63. McGregor AH, Anderton L, Gedroyc WM, et al: The use of interventional open MRI to assess the kinematics of the lumbar spine in patients with spondylolisthesis, *Spine* 27(14):1582-1586, 2002.

64. Wiltse LL, Newman PH, Macnab I: Classification of spondylolysis and spondylolisthesis, *Clin Orthop Rel Res* 117:23-29, 1976.

65. Beutler WJ, Fredrickson BE, Murtland A, et al: The natural history of spondylolysis and spondylolisthesis: 45-year follow-up evaluation, *Spine* 28(10):1027-1035; discussion 1035, 2003.

66. Moller H, Sundin A, Hedlund R: Symptoms, signs, and functional disability in adult spondylolisthesis, *Spine* 25(6):683-689; discussion 690, 2000.

67. Spitzer WO, Skovron ML, Salmi LR, et al: Scientific monograph of the Quebec Task Force on Whiplash-Associated Disorders: Redefining "whiplash" and its management (see comment)(erratum appears in *Spine* 20(21):2372, 1995), *Spine* 20(8 suppl):1S-73S, 1995.

68. Scholten-Peeters GG, Verhagen AP, Bekkering GE, et al: Prognostic factors of whiplash-associated disorders: A systematic review of prospective cohort studies, *Pain* 104(1-2):303-322, 2003.

69. Suissa S, Harder S, Veilleux M: The relation between initial symptoms and signs and the prognosis of whiplash, *Eur Spine J* 10(1):44-49, 2001.

70. Cote P, Cassidy JD, Carroll L, et al: A systematic review of the prognosis of acute whiplash and a new conceptual framework to synthesize the literature (see comment), *Spine* 26(19):E445-458, 2001.

71. Sterner Y, Toolanen G, Gerdle B, et al: The incidence of whiplash trauma and the effects of different factors on recovery, *J Spin Disord Tech* 16(2):195-199, 2003.

72. Scholten-Peeters GG, Bekkering GE, Verhagen AP, et al: Clinical practice guideline for the physiotherapy of patients with whiplash-associated disorders (see comment), *Spine* 27(4):412-422, 2002.

73. McClune T, Burton AK, Waddell G: Whiplash associated disorders: a review of the literature to guide patient information and advice, *Emerg Med J* 19(6):499-506, 2002.

74. Kumar S, Ferrari R, Narayan Y: Electromyographic and kinematic exploration of whiplash-type neck perturbations in left lateral collisions, *Spine* 29(6):650-659, 2004.

75. Sterling M, Jull G, Vicenzino B, et al: Characterization of acute whiplash-associated disorders, *Spine* 29(2):182-188, 2004.

76. Stapleton DB, MacLennan AH, Kristiansson P: The prevalence of recalled low back pain during and after pregnancy: A South Australian population survey, *Aust N Z J Obstet Gynaecol* 42(5):482-485, 2002.

77. To WW, Wong MW: Factors associated with back pain symptoms in pregnancy and the persistence of pain 2 years after pregnancy, *Acta Obstet Gynecol Scand* 82(12):1086-1091, 2003.

78. Ostgaard H, Andersson GBJ: Previous back pain and risk of developing back pain in a future pregnancy, *Spine* 16(4):432-436, 1991.

79. Padua L, Padua R, Bondi R, et al: Patient-oriented assessment of back pain in pregnancy, *Eur Spine J* 11(3):272-275, 2002.

80. Ostgaard HC: Assessment and treatment of low back pain in working pregnant women, *Semin Perinatol* 20(1):61-69, 1996.

81. Ostgaard HC, Zetherstrom G, Roos-Hansson E: Back pain in relation to pregnancy: A 6-year follow-up, *Spine* 22(24):2945-2950, 1997.

82. Goldman L, Ishigami S, Raynovich K, et al: A comparison of back pain characteristics of pregnant, postpartum, and not pregnant women, *J Sect Wom Health* 24(3):14-21, 2000.

83. Mens JMA, Vleeming A, Stoeckart R, et al: Understanding peripartum pelvic pain, *Spine* 21(11):1363-1370, 1996.

84. Ostgaard H, Zetherstrom G, Roos-Hansson E: The posterior pelvic pain provocation test in pregnant women, *Eur Spine J* 3:258-260, 1994.

85. Ostgaard HC, Zetherstrom G, Roos-Hansson E, et al: Reduction of back and posterior pelvic pain in pregnancy, *Spine* 19(8):894-900, 1994.

86. Sturesson B, Uden G: Pain pattern in pregnancy and "catching" of the leg in pregnant women with posterior pelvic pain, *Spine* 22(16):1880-1883, 1997.

87. Noren L, Ostgaard S, Johansson G, et al: Lumbar back and posterior pelvic pain during pregnancy: A 3-year follow-up, *Eur Spine J* 11(3):267-271, 2002.

88. Ostgaard HC, Andersson GB: Postpartum low-back pain, *Spine* 17(1):53-55, 1992.

89. Svensson H, Andersson GBJ, Hagstad A, et al: The relationship of low-back pain to pregnancy and gynecologic factors, *Spine* 15(5):371-375, 1990.

90. Borkan JM, Koes B, Reis S, et al: A report from the Second International Forum for Primary Care Research on Low Back Pain. Reexamining priorities, *Spine* 23(18):1992-1996, 1998.

91. Powell MC, Wilson M, Szypryt P, et al: Prevalence of lumbar disc degeneration observed by magnetic resonance in symptomless women, *Lancet* 2(8520):1366-1367, 1986.

92. Childs JD, Fritz JM, Piva SR, et al: Clinical decision making in the identification of patients likely to benefit from spinal manipulation: A traditional versus an evidence-based approach, *JOSPT* 33(5):259-272, 2003.

93. Delitto A, Erhard RE, Bowling RW: A treatment-based classification approach to low back syndrome: identifying and staging patients for conservative treatment (see comment), *Phys Ther* 75(6):470-485; discussion 485-489, 1995.

94. Van Dillen LR, Sahrmann SA, Norton BJ, et al: Reliability of physical examination items used for classification of patients with low back pain, *Phys Ther* 78(9):979-988, 1998.

95. Van Dillen LR, Sahrmann SA, Norton BJ, et al: Effect of active limb movements on symptoms in patients with low back pain, *JOSPT* 31(8):402-413; discussion 414-408, 2001.

96. Van Dillen LR, Sahrmann SA, Norton BJ, et al: Movement system impairment-based categories for low back pain: Stage 1 validation, *JOSPT* 33(3):126-142, 2003.

97. Van Dillen LR, Sahrmann SA, Norton BJ, et al: The effect of modifying patient-preferred spinal movement and alignment during symptom testing in patients with low back pain: A preliminary report, *Arch Phys Med Rehabil* 84(3):313-322, 2003.

98. Borkan JM, Cherkin DC: An agenda for primary care research on low back pain, *Spine* 21(24):2880-2884, 1996.

99. Fritz JM, Delitto A, Vignovic M, et al: Interrater reliability of judgments of the centralization phenomenon and status change during movement testing in patients with low back pain (see comment), *Arch Phys Med Rehabil* 81(1):57-61, 2000.

100. Fritz JM: Use of a classification approach to the treatment of 3 patients with low back syndrome, *Phys Ther* 78(7):766-777, 1998.

101. McKenzie R: *The Lumbar Spine: Mechanical Diagnosis and Therapy,* Waikane, New Zealand, 1981, Spinal Publications.

102. Maluf KS, Sahrmann SA, Van Dillen LR: Use of a classification system to guide nonsurgical management of a patient with chronic low back pain (see comment), *Phys Ther* 80(11):1097-1111, 2000.

103. Spitzer W: Scientific approach to the assessment and management of activity-related spinal disorders: A monograph for clinicians: Report of the Quebec Task Force on Spinal Disorders, *Spine* 12(7):S1-S53, 1987.

104. Atlas SJ, Deyo RA, Keller RB, et al: The Maine Lumbar Spine Study, Part III: 1-year outcomes of surgical and nonsurgical management of lumbar spinal stenosis (see comment), *Spine* 21(15):1787-1794; discussion 1794-1785, 1996.

105. Loisel P, Vachon B, Lemaire J, et al: Discriminative and predictive validity assessment of the Quebec Task Force classification, *Spine* 27(8):851-857, 2002.

106. Werneke M, Hart DL: Discriminant validity and relative precision for classifying patients with nonspecific neck and back pain by anatomic pain patterns, *Spine* 28(2):161-166, 2003.

107. Battie MC, Cherkin DC, Dunn R, et al: Managing low back pain: attitudes and treatment preferences of physical therapists, *Phys Ther* 74(3):219-226, 1994.

108. Razmjou H, Kramer JF, Yamada R: Intertester reliability of the McKenzie evaluation in assessing patients with mechanical low-back pain (see comment), *JOSPT* 30(7):368-383; discussion 384-369, 2000.

109. Donelson R: The McKenzie approach to evaluating and treating low back pain, *Orthop Rev* 19(8):681-686, 1990.

110. Kilpikoski S, Airaksinen O, Kankaanpaa M, et al: Interexaminer reliability of low back pain assessment using the McKenzie method, *Spine* 27(8):E207-214, 2002.

111. Riddle DL, Rothstein JM: Intertester reliability of McKenzie's classifications of the syndrome types present in patients with low back pain (see comment), *Spine* 18(10):1333-1344, 1993.

112. Kilby J, Stigant M, Roberts A: The reliability of back pain assessment by physiotherapists, using a "McKenzie algorithm," *Physiotherapy* 76(9):579-583, 1990.

113. Donahue MS, Riddle DL, Sullivan MS: Intertester reliability of a modified version of McKenzie's lateral shift assessments obtained on patients with low back pain (see comment), *Phys Ther* 76(7):706-716; discussion 717-726, 1996.

114. Fritz JM, George S: The use of a classification approach to identify subgroups of patients with acute low back pain. Interrater reliability and short-term treatment outcomes, *Spine* 25(1):106-114, 2000.

115. Fritz JM, Delitto A, Erhard RE: Comparison of classification-based physical therapy with therapy based on clinical practice guidelines for patients with acute low back pain: A randomized clinical trial, *Spine* 28(13):1363-1371; discussion 1372, 2003.

116. Sahrmann SA: *Diagnosis and Treatment of Movement Impairment Syndromes,* St. Louis, 2002, Mosby.

117. Grant R: Vertebral artery concerns: premanipulative testing of the cervical spine. In Grant R (ed): *Physical Therapy of the Cervical and Thoracic Spine,* New York, 1884, Churchill Livingstone.

118. Cibulka MT: Understanding sacroiliac joint movement as a guide to the management of a patient with unilateral low back pain, *Man Ther* 7(4):215-221, 2002.

119. New Zealand Acute Low Back Pain Guide: Guide to Assessing Yellow Flags in Acute Low Back Pain. Available at: http://www.acc.co.nz/injury-prevention/back-injury-prevention/treatment-provider-guides/.

120. Waddell G, McCulloch JA, Kummel E, et al: Nonorganic physical signs in low-back pain, *Spine* 5(2):117-125, 1980.

121. Ware JE: SF-36 health survey update, *Spine* 25(24):3130-3139, 2000.

122. Fairbanks JCT, Couper J, Davies JB, et al: The Oswestry Low Back Pain Disability questionnaire, *Physiotherapy* 66:271-273, 1980.

123. Roland M, Morris R: A study of the natural history of back pain. Part I. Development of a reliable and sensitive measure of disability in low-back pain, *Spine* 8:141-144, 1983.

124. Vernon H: The neck disability index: patient assessment and outcome monitoring in whiplash, *J Musculoskeletal Pain* 4:95-104, 1996.

125. Resnik L, Dobrzykowski E; Guide to outcomes measurement for patients with low back pain syndromes, *JOSPT* 33(6):307-318, 2003.

126. Leclaire R, Blier F, Fortin L, et al: A cross-sectional study comparing the Oswestry and Roland-Morris Functional Disability scales in two populations of patients with low back pain of different levels of severity, *Spine* 22(1):68-71, 1997.

127. Beurskens AJ, de Vet HC, Koke AJ, et al: Measuring the functional status of patients with low back pain. Assessment of the quality of four disease-specific questionnaires, *Spine* 20(9):1017-1028, 1995.

128. Triano JJ, McGregor M, Cramer GD, et al: A comparison of outcome measures for use with back pain patients: Results of a feasibility study (see comment), *J Manipulative Physiol Ther* 16(2):67-73, 1993.

129. Fritz JM, Irrgang JJ: A comparison of a modified Oswestry Low Back Pain Disability Questionnaire and the Quebec Back Pain Disability Scale, *Phys Ther* 81(2):776-788, 2001.

130. Stratford PW, Binkley JM: Measurement properties of the RM-18. A modified version of the Roland-Morris Disability Scale, *Spine* 22(20):2416-2421, 1997.

131. Riddle DL, Stratford PW, Binkley J: Sensitivity to change of the Roland-Morris Back Pain Questionnaire: Part 2, *Phys Ther* 79(10):939-948, 1998.

132. Vernon H, Mior S: The Neck Disability Index: A study of reliability and validity (erratum appears in *J Manipulative Physiol Ther* 15(1):1992), *J Manipulative Physiol Ther* 14(7):409-415, 1991.

133. Pietrobon R, Coeytaux RR, Carey TS, et al: Standard scales for measurement of functional outcome for cervical pain or dysfunction: a systematic review (see comment), *Spine* 27(5):515-522, 2002.

134. Schenkman M, Shipp KM, Chandler J, et al: Relationships between mobility of axial structures and physical performance, *Phys Ther* 76(3):276-285, 1996.

135. Michel A, Kohlmann T, Raspe H: The association between clinical findings on physical examination and self-reported severity in back pain. Results of a population-based study. *Spine* 22(3):296-303; discussion 303-304, 1997.

136. Strender LE, Sjoblom A, Sundell K, et al: Interexaminer reliability in physical examination of patients with low back pain, *Spine* 22(7):814-820, 1997.

137. Deyo RA, Andersson G, Bombardier C, et al: Outcome measures for studying patients with low back pain, *Spine* 19(18 suppl):2032S-2036S, 1994.

138. Fitzgerald GK, Wynveen KJ, Rheault W, et al: Objective assessment with establishment of normal values for lumbar spinal range of motion, *Phys Ther* 63(11):1776-1781, 1983.

139. Gracovetsky S, Newman N, Pawlowsky M, et al: A database for estimating normal spinal motion derived from noninvasive measurements, *Spine* 20(9):1036-1046, 1995.

140. McGill SM, Yingling VR, Peach JP: Three-dimensional kinematics and trunk muscle myoelectric activity in the elderly spine: A database compared to young people, *Clin Biomechan* 14(6):389-395, 1999.

141. Keeley J, Mayer TG, Cox R, et al: Quantification of lumbar function. Part 5. Reliability of range-of-motion measures in the sagittal plane and an in vivo torso rotation measurement technique, *Spine* 11(1):31-35, 1986.

142. Mayer TG, Kondraske G, Beals SB, et al: Spinal range of motion. Accuracy and sources of error with inclinometric measurement, *Spine* 22(17):1976-1984, 1997.

143. Chiarello CM, Savidge R: Interrater reliability of the Cybex EDI-320 and fluid goniometer in normals and patients with low back pain, *Arch Phys Med Rehabil* 74(1):32-37, 1993.

144. Batti'e MC, Bigos SJ, Sheehy A, et al: Spinal flexibility and individual factors that influence it, *Phys Ther* 67(5):653-658, 1987.

145. Strender LE, Lundin M, Nell K: Interexaminer reliability in physical examination of the neck, *J Manipulative Physiol Ther* 20(8):516-520, 1997.

146. Haswell K, Williams M, Hing W: Interexaminer reliability of symptom-provoking active sidebend, rotation and combined movement assessments of patients with low back pain, *J Manipulative Physiol Ther* 12(1):11-20, 2004.

147. Wainner RS, Fritz JM, Irrgang JJ, et al: Reliability and diagnostic accuracy of the clinical examination and patient self-report measures for cervical radiculopathy, *Spine* 28(1):52-62, 2003.

148. Deyo RA, Diehl AK: Measuring physical and psychosocial function in patients with low-back pain, *Spine* 8(6):635-642, 1983.

149. Sullivan MS, Dickinson CE, Troup JD: The influence of age and gender on lumbar spine sagittal plane range of motion. A study of 1126 healthy subjects, *Spine* 19(6):682-686, 1994.

150. Waddell G, Somerville D, Henderson I, et al: Objective clinical evaluation of physical impairment in chronic low back pain (see comment), *Spine* 17(6):617-628, 1992.

151. Mellin G: Measurement of thoracolumbar posture and mobility with a Myrin inclinometer, *Spine* 11(7):759-762, 1986.

152. Mellin G: Correlations of spinal mobility with degree of chronic low back pain after correction for age and anthropometric factors, *Spine* 12(5):464-468, 1987.

153. Najm W, Seffinger M, Mishra S, et al: Content validity of manual spinal palpatory exams. A systematic review, *BMC Complement Altern Med* 9(3):50-57, 2003.

154. Huijbregts PA: Spinal motion palpation: a review of reliability studies, *J Manipulative Physiol Ther* 10(1):24-39, 2002.

155. Deboer KF, Harmon R Jr, Tuttle CD, et al: Reliability study of detection of somatic dysfunctions in the cervical spine, *J Manipulative Physiol Ther* 8(1):9-16, 1985.

156. Schoensee SK, Jensen G, Nicholson G, et al: The effect of mobilization on cervical headaches, *JOSPT* 21(4):184-196, 1995.

157. Jull G, Zito G, Trott P, et al: Inter-examiner reliability to detect painful upper cervical joint dysfunction, *Aust J Physiother* 43(2):125-129, 1997.

158. Jull G, Bullock M: A motion profile of the lumbar spine in an ageing population assessed by manual examination, *Physiother Pract* 3(2):70-81, 1987.

159. Maher C, Adams R: Reliability of pain and stiffness assessments in clinical manual lumbar spine examination, including commentary by Shields RK with author response, *Phys Ther* 74(9):801-811, 1994.

160. Phillips DR, Twomey LT: A comparison of manual diagnosis with a diagnosis established by a uni-level lumbar spinal block procedure, *Man Ther* 1(2):82-87, 1996.

161. Janda V: *Movement patterns in pelvic and hip region in pathogenesis of vertebrogenic disease*, Prague, 1964, Charles University.

162. Janda V: Muskelfunktion in Beziehung zur Entwicklung Vertebragener Storungen, *Procedings Kongressmand Manulle Medizin* 127-130, 1968.

163. Janda V: Die Beduntung Muskularer Filhaltung als Pathogeneticher Faktor Vertebragner, *Storungen Archive fur Physikalische Therapit* 20:113-116, 1968.

164. Jull GA, Janda V: Muscles and motor control in low back pain: Assessment and management. In Twomey LT, Taylor JR (eds): *Physical Therapy of the Low Back*, vol 1, New York, 1987, Churchill Livingstone.

165. Janda V: Muscles and motor control in cervicogenic disorders: Assessment and management. In Grant R (ed): *Physical Therapy of the Cervical and Thoracic Spine*, New York, 1988, Churchill Livingstone.

166. Janda V: Evaluation of muscular imbalance. In Liebenson C (ed): *Rehabilitation of the Spine: A Practitioner's Manual*, Philadelphia, 1996, Williams & Wilkins.

167. Isaacs E, Bookhout M: *Bourdillion's Spinal Manipulation*, vol 6, Boston, 2002, Butterworth Heinemann.

168. Richardson C, Hodges PW, Hides JA: *Therapeutic Exercise for Lumbopelvic Stabilization: A Motor Control Approach for the Treatment and Prevention of Low Back Pain*, New York, 2004, Churchill Livingstone.

169. Richardson C, Jull G, Hodges PW, et al: *Therapeutic Exercise for Spinal Stabilization in Low Back Pain*, New York, 1999, Churchill Livingstone.

170. Dutton M: *Orthopaedic Examination, Evaluation and Intervention*, New York, 2004, McGraw-Hill.

171. Wainner RS, Gill H: Diagnosis and nonoperative management of cervical radiculopathy, *JOSPT* 30(12):728-744, 2000.

172. Magee DJ: *Orthopedic Physical Assessment*, Philadelphia, 2002, WB Saunders.

173. Maitland G, Banks K, English K, et al (eds): *Maitland's Vertebral Manipulation*, ed 6, Boston, 2001, Butterworth-Heinemann.

174. Tong HC, Haig AJ, Yamakawa K: The Spurling test and cervical radiculopathy. *Spine* 27(2):156-159, 2002.

175. Viikari-Juntura E, Martikainen R, Luukkonen R, et al: Longitudinal study on work related and individual risk factors affecting radiating neck pain, *Occup Environ Med* 58(5):345-352, 2001.

176. Binkley J, Stratford PW, Gill C: Interrater reliability of lumbar accessory motion mobility testing, *Phys Ther* 75(9):786-792; discussion 793-795, 1995.

177. Maher CG, Latimer J, Adams R: An investigation of the reliability and validity of posteroanterior spinal stiffness judgments made using a reference-based protocol, *Phys Ther* 78(8):829-837, 1998.

178. Breig A, Troup JD. Biomechanical considerations in the straight-leg-raising test. Cadaveric and clinical studies of the effects of medial hip rotation, *Spine* 4(3):242-250, 1979.

179. Rebain R, Baxter GD, McDonough S: A systematic review of the passive straight leg raising test as a diagnostic aid for low back pain (1989 to 2000), *Spine* 27(17):E388-395, 2002.

180. Supik LF, Broom MJ: Sciatic tension signs and lumbar disc herniation, *Spine* 19(9):1066-1069, 1994.

181. Deyo RA, Rainville J, Kent DL: What can the history and physical examination tell us about low back pain? (see comment), *JAMA* 268(6):760-765, 1992.

182. Andersson GB, Deyo RA: History and physical examination in patients with herniated lumbar discs, *Spine* 21(24 suppl):10S-18S, 1996.

183. Hall T, Hepburn M, Elvey RL: The effect of lumbosacral posture on a modification of the straight leg raise test, *Physiotherapy* 79(8):566-570, 1993.

184. Johnson EK, Chiarello CM: The slump test: the effects of head and lower extremity position on knee extension, *JOSPT* 26(6):310-317, 1997.

185. Kenneally M: The upper limb tension test: The straight leg raise test of the arm. In Grant R (ed): *Physical Therapy of the Cervical and Thoracic Spine*, New York, 1989, Churchill Livingstone.

186. Di Fabio RP: Manipulation of the cervical spine: risks and benefits (see comment), *Phys Ther* 79(1):50-65, 1999.

187. Terrett A: Contraindications to cervical spine manipulation. In Giles L, Singer K (eds): *Clinical Anatomy and Management of Cervical Spine Pain*, Boston, 1998, Butterworth-Heinemann.

188. Arnold C, Bourassa R, Langer T, et al: Doppler studies evaluating the effect of a physical therapy screening protocol on vertebral artery blood flow, *Man Ther* 9(1):13-21, 2004.

189. Schwarzer AC, Aprill CN, Bogduk N: The sacroiliac joint in chronic low back pain, *Spine* 20:31-37, 1995.

190. Dreyfuss P, Dryer S, Griffin J, et al: Positive sacroiliac screening tests in asymptomatic adults, *Spine* 19:1138-1143, 1994.

191. Levangie P: Four clinical tests of sacroiliac joint dysfunction: The association of test results with innominate torsion among patients with and without low back pain, *Phys Ther* 79(11):1043-1057, 1999.

192. Laslett M, Williams M: The reliability of selected pain provocation tests for sacroiliac joint pathology, *Spine* 1243-1249, 1994.

193. Porterfield J, DeRosa C: *Mechanical Low Back Pain: Perspectives In Functional Anatomy*, Philadelphia, 1998, WB Saunders.

194. van der Wurff P, Hagmeijer RHM, Meyne W: Clinical tests of the sacroiliac joint. Part 1: A systematic methodological review. Part 1: Reliability, *Man Ther* 5(1):30-36, 2000.

195. Cibulka MT, Koldehoff R: Clinical usefulness of a cluster of sacroiliac joint tests in patients with and without low back pain (see comment), *JOSPT* 29:83-89; discussion 90-82, 1999.

196. Maigne JY, Aivaliklis A, Pfefer F: Results of sacroiliac joint double block and value of sacroiliac pain provocation tests in 54 patients with low back pain, *Spine* 21(16):1889-1892, 1996.

197. Brady RJ, Dean JB, Skinner TM, et al: Limb length inequality: clinical implications for assessment and intervention, *JOSPT* 33(5):221-234, 2003.

198. Friberg O: Clinical symptoms and biomechanics of lumbar spine and hip joint in leg length inequality, *Spine* 8(6):643-651, 1983.

199. Grundy PF, Roberts CJ: Does unequal leg length cause back pain? A case-control study, *Lancet* 2(8397):256-258, 1984.

200. Soukka A, Alaranta H, Tallroth K, et al: Leg-length inequality in people of working age. The association between mild inequality and low-back pain is questionable (see comment), *Spine* 16(4):429-431, 1991.

201. ten Brinke A, van der Aa HE, van der Palen J, et al: Is leg length discrepancy associated with the side of radiating pain in patients with a lumbar herniated disc? *Spine* 24(7):684-686, 1999.

202. Hoyle D, Latour M, Bohannon R: Intraexaminer, interexaminer and inter-device comparability of leg length measurements obtained with measuring tape and metrecom, *JOSPT* 14:263-268, 1991.

203. Woerman AL, Binder-Macleod SA: Leg length discrepancy assessment: accuracy and precision in five clinical methods of evaluation, *JOSPT* 5(5):230-239, 1984.

204. Fritz JM, Erhard RE, Hagen BF: Segmental instability of the lumbar spine, *Phys Ther* 78(8):889-896, 1998.

205. Panjabi MM: The stabilizing system of the spine. Part I. Function, dysfunction, adaptation, and enhancement, *J Spinal Disord* 5:383-389, discussion 397, 1992.

206. Panjabi MM. The stabilizing system of the spine. Part II. Neutral zone and instability hypothesis, *J Spinal Disord* 5:390-396; discussion 397, 1992 Dec.

207. Hicks GE, Fritz JM, Delitto A, et al: Interrater reliability of clinical examination measures for identification of lumbar segmental instability, *Arch Phys Med Rehabil* 84(12):1858-1864, 2003.

208. Wheeler AH: Diagnosis and management of low back pain and sciatica, *Am Fam Phys* 52:1333-1341, 1995.

209. Von Korff M, Saunders K: The course of back pain in primary care, *Spine* 21(24):2833-2837; discussion 2838-2839, 1996.

210. Hicks GS, Duddleston DN, Russell LD, et al: Low back pain, *Am J Med Sci* 324(4):207-211, 2002.

211. American Physical Therapy Association: *Guide to Physical Therapist Practice*, ed 2, Alexandria, Va, 2001, The Association.

212. Assendelft WJ, Morton SC, Yu EI, et al: Spinal manipulative therapy for low back pain, *Cochrane Database System Rev* 1:CD000447, 2004.

213. van Tulder MW, Malmivaara A, Esmail R, et al: Exercise therapy for low back pain, *Cochrane Database System Rev* 2:CD000335, 2000.

214. van Tulder MW, Esmail R, Bombardier C, et al: Back schools for non-specific low back pain, *Cochrane Database System Rev* 2:CD000261, 2000.

215. Ottenbacher K, DiFabio R: Efficacy of spinal manipulation/mobilization: A meta-analysis, *Spine* 10(9):833-837, 1985.
216. Mannell J: *Joint Pain: Diagnosis and Treatment Using Manipulative Techniques*, Boston, 1964, Little, Brown.
217. Mior S: Manipulation and mobilization in the treatment of chronic pain, *Clin J Pain* 17(suppl 4):S70-76, 2001.
218. Pickar JG: Neurophysiological effects of spinal manipulation, *Spine* 2(5):357-371, 2002.
219. Koes BW, Bouter LM, van Mameren H, et al: The effectiveness of manual therapy, physiotherapy, and treatment by the general practitioner for nonspecific back and neck complaints. A randomized clinical trial (see comment), *Spine* 17(1):28-35, 1992.
220. Koes BW, van Tulder MW, Ostelo R, et al: Clinical guidelines for the management of low back pain in primary care: An international comparison (see comment), *Spine* 26(22):2504-2513; discussion 2513-2514, 2001.
221. Swenson R, Haldeman S: Spinal manipulative therapy for low back pain, *J Am Acad Orthop Surg* 11(4):228-237, 2003.
222. Hurwitz EL, Morgenstern H, Harber P, et al: A randomized trial of medical care with and without physical therapy and chiropractic care with and without physical modalities for patients with low back pain: 6-month follow-up outcomes from the UCLA low back pain study (see comment), *Spine* 27(20):2193-2204, 2002.
223. Childs JD, Fritz JM, Flynn TW, et al: A clinical prediction rule to identify patients with low back pain most likely to benefit from spinal manipulation: A validation study (see comment), *Ann Intern Med* 141(12):920-928, 2004.
224. Greenman PE: *Principles of Manual Medicine*, ed 2, Baltimore, 1996, Williams & Wilkins.
225. Goodridge JP: Muscle energy technique: Definition, explanation, methods of procedure, *J Am Osteopath Assoc* 81(4):249-254, 1981.
226. Mitchell FL, Mitchell PKG: *The Muscle Energy Manual: Concepts and Mechanisms—The Musculoskeletal Screen, Cervical Region Evaluation and Treatment*, vol 1, East Lansing, Mich, 1995, MET Press.
227. Gibson T, Grahame R, Harkness J, et al: Controlled comparison of short-wave diathermy treatment with osteopathic treatment in non-specific low back pain, *Lancet* 1(8440):1258-1261, 1985.
228. MacDonald RS, Bell CM: An open controlled assessment of osteopathic manipulation in nonspecific low-back pain (erratum appears in *Spine* 16(1):104, 1991), *Spine* 15(5):364-370, 1990.
229. Andersson GB, Lucente T, Davis AM, et al: A comparison of osteopathic spinal manipulation with standard care for patients with low back pain (see comment), *N Engl J Med* 341(19):1426-1431, 1999.
230. Licciardone JC, Stoll ST, Fulda KG, et al: Osteopathic manipulative treatment for chronic low back pain: a randomized controlled trial, *Spine* 28(13):1355-1362, 2003.
231. Williams NH, Wilkinson C, Russell I, et al: Randomized osteopathic manipulation study (ROMANS): Pragmatic trial for spinal pain in primary care, *Fam Pract* 20(6):662-669, 2003.
232. Schenk RJ, Adelman K, Rouselle J: The effects of muscle energy technique on cervical range of motion, *J Manipulative Physiol Ther* 2:179-183, 1994.
233. Schenk RJ, Jozefczyk C, Kopf A: A randomized trial comparing interventions in patients with lumbar posterior derangement, *J Manipulative Physiol Ther* 11(2):95-102, 2003.
234. Wilson E, Payton O, Donegan-Shoaf L, et al: Muscle energy technique in patients with acute low back pain: a pilot clinical trial, *JOSPT* Sep 2003;33(9):502-512.
235. Rainville J, Hartigan C, Martinez E, et al: Exercise as a treatment for chronic low back pain, *Spine* 4(1):106-115, 2004.
236. Schonstein E, Kenny D, Keating J, et al: Physical conditioning programs for workers with back and neck pain: A cochrane systematic review, *Spine* 28(19):E391-395, 2003.
237. Cherkin DC, Deyo RA, Battie M, et al: A comparison of physical therapy, chiropractic manipulation, and provision of an educational booklet for the treatment of patients with low back pain (see comment), *N Engl J Med* 339(15):1021-1029, 1998.
238. Bronfort G, Evans R, Nelson B, et al: A randomized clinical trial of exercise and spinal manipulation for patients with chronic neck pain, *Spine* 26(7):788-797, discussion 798-789, 2001.
239. Clare HA, Adams R, Maher CG: A systematic review of efficacy of McKenzie therapy for spinal pain, *Aust J Physiother* 50(4):209-216, 2004.
240. Delitto A, Cibulka MT, Erhard RE, et al: Evidence for use of an extension-mobilization category in acute low back syndrome: a prescriptive validation pilot study (see comment), *Phys Ther* 73(4):216-222; discussion 223-218, 1993.
241. Dettori JR, Bullock SH, Sutlive TG, et al: The effects of spinal flexion and extension exercises and their associated postures in patients with acute low back pain (see comment), *Spine* 20(21):2303-2312, 1995.
242. Koes BW, Bouter LM, van Mameren H, et al: Randomised clinical trial of manipulative therapy and physiotherapy for persistent back and neck complaints: results of one year follow up (see comment), *BMJ* 304(6827):601-605, 1992.
243. Maher CG: Effective physical treatment for chronic low back pain, *Orthop Clin North Am* 35(1):57-64, 2004.
244. Tveito TH, Hysing M, Eriksen HR: Low back pain interventions at the workplace: A systematic literature review, *Occup Med* (Lond) 54(1):3-13, 2004.
245. Pengel HM, Maher CG, Refshauge KM: Systematic review of conservative interventions for subacute low back pain, *Clin Rehabil* 16(8):811-820, 2002.
246. Koes BW, Bouter LM, van der Heijden GJ: Methodological quality of randomized clinical trials on treatment efficacy in low back pain, *Spine* 20(2):228-235, 1995.
247. Kool J, de Bie R, Oesch P, et al: Exercise reduces sick leave in patients with non-acute non-specific low back pain: A meta-analysis, *J Rehabil Med* 36(2):49-62, 2004.
248. Mior S: Exercise in the treatment of chronic pain, *Clin J Pain* 17(4 suppl):S77-85, 2001.
249. Hubley-Kozey CL, McCulloch TA, McFarland DA: Chronic low back pain: A critical review of specific therapeutic exercise protocols on musculoskeletal and neuromuscular parameters, *J Manipulative Physiol Ther* 11(2):78-87, 2003.
250. Foster NE, Thompson KA, Baxter GD, et al: Management of nonspecific low back pain by physiotherapists in Britain and Ireland. A descriptive questionnaire of current clinical practice, *Spine* 24(13):1332-1342, 1999.
251. Donelson R, Grant W, Kamps C, et al: Pain response to sagittal end-range spinal motion. A prospective, randomized, multicentered trial (see comment), *Spine* 16(6 suppl):S206-212, 1991.
252. Al-Obaidi S, Anthony J, Dean E, et al: Cardiovascular responses to repetitive McKenzie lumbar spine exercises, *Phys Ther* 81(9):1524-1533, 2001.
253. Stankovic R, Johnell O: Conservative treatment of acute low-back pain. A prospective randomized trial: McKenzie method of treatment versus patient education in "mini back school" (see comment), *Spine* 15(2):120-123, 1990.
254. Nwuga G, Nwuga V: Relative therapeutic efficacy of the Williams and McKenzie protocols in pack pain management, *Physiother Pract* 1:99-105, 1985.
255. Underwood MR, Morgan J: The use of a back class teaching extension exercises in the treatment of acute low back pain in primary care, *Fam Pract* 15:9-15, 1998.
256. Erhard RE, Delitto A, Cibulka MT. Relative effectiveness of an extension program and a combined program of manipulation and flexion and extension exercises in patients with acute low back syndrome (see comment), *Phys Ther* 74(12):1093-1100, 1994.
257. Bushwell J: Low back pain: A comparison of two treatment programs, *NZ J Physiother* August:13-17, 1982.
258. Petersen T, Kryger P, Ekdahl C, et al: The effect of McKenzie therapy as compared with that of intensive strengthening training for the treatment of patients with subacute or chronic low back pain: A randomized controlled trial (see comment), *Spine* 27(16):1702-1709, 2002.
259. Hodges PW, Richardson CA: Feedforward contraction of transversus abdominis is not influenced by the direction of arm movement, *Exp Brain Res* 114(2):362-370, 1997.
260. Hodges PW, Richardson CA: Contraction of the abdominal muscles associated with movement of the lower limb, *Phys Ther* 77(2):132-142; discussion 142-134, 1997.
261. Moseley GL, Hodges PW, Gandevia SC: Deep and superficial fibers of the lumbar multifidus muscle are differentially active during voluntary arm movements, *Spine* 27(2):E29-36, 2002.
262. Hodges PW, Richardson CA: Inefficient muscular stabilization of the lumbar spine associated with low back pain. A motor control evaluation of transversus abdominis, *Spine* 21(22):2640-2650, 1996.
263. Hodges PW, Moseley GL, Gabrielsson A, et al: Experimental muscle pain changes feedforward postural responses of the trunk muscles, *Exp Brain Res* 151(2):262-271, 2003.
264. Hides JA, Stokes MJ, Saide M, et al: Evidence of lumbar multifidus muscle wasting ipsilateral to symptoms in patients with acute/subacute low back pain, *Spine* 19(2):165-172, 1994.
265. Hides JA, Richardson CA, Jull GA: Magnetic resonance imaging and ultrasonography of the lumbar multifidus muscle. Comparison of two different modalities, *Spine* 20(1):54-58, 1995.
266. Hides JA, Richardson CA, Jull GA: Multifidus muscle recovery is not automatic after resolution of acute, first-episode low back pain, *Spine* 21(23):2763-2769, 1996.
267. Sihvonen T, Herno A, Paljarvi L, et al: Local denervation atrophy of paraspinal muscles in postoperative failed back syndrome, *Spine* 18(5):575-581, 1993.
268. Rantanen J, Hurme M, Falck B, et al: The lumbar multifidus muscle five years after surgery for a lumbar intervertebral disc herniation. *Spine* 18(5):568-574, 1993.
269. Hides JA, Jull GA, Richardson CA: Long-term effects of specific stabilizing exercises for first-episode low back pain, *Spine* 26(11):E243-248, 2001.
270. Hodges PW, Cresswell AG, Daggfeldt K, et al: In vivo measurement of the effect of intra-abdominal pressure on the human spine, *J Biomech* 34(3):347-353, 2001.

271. Sapsford RR, Hodges PW, Richardson CA, et al: Co-activation of the abdominal and pelvic floor muscles during voluntary exercises, *Neurourol Urodyn* 20(1):31-42, 2001.
272. Ciol MA, Deyo RA, Howell E, et al: An assessment of surgery for spinal stenosis: time trends, geographic variations, complications, and reoperations, *J Am Geriatr Soc* 44(3):285-290, 1996.
273. Katz JN: Lumbar spinal fusion. Surgical rates, costs, and complications, *Spine* 20(24 suppl):78S-83S, 1995.
274. Atlas SJ, Keller RB, Robson D, et al: Surgical and nonsurgical management of lumbar spinal stenosis: Four-year outcomes from the maine lumbar spine study, *Spine* 25(5):556-562, 2000.
275. Simotas AC, Dorey FJ, Hansraj KK, et al: Nonoperative treatment for lumbar spinal stenosis. Clinical and outcome results and a 3-year survivorship analysis, *Spine* 25(2):197-203; discussions 203-194, 2000.
276. Simotas AC: Nonoperative treatment for lumbar spinal stenosis, *Clin Orthop Rel Res* 384:153-161, 2001.
277. Fritz JM, Erhard RE, Delitto A, et al: Preliminary results of the use of a two-stage treadmill test as a clinical diagnostic tool in the differential diagnosis of lumbar spinal stenosis, *J Spinal Disord* 10(5):410-416, 1997.
278. Whitman JM, Flynn TW, Fritz JM: Nonsurgical management of patients with lumbar spinal stenosis: A literature review and a case series of three patients managed with physical therapy, *Phys Med Rehabil Clin N Am* 14(1):77-101, 2003.
279. Rademeyer I: Manual therapy for lumbar spinal stenosis: a comprehensive physical therapy approach, *Phys Med Rehabil Clin N Am* 14(1):103-110, 2003.
280. Bodack MP, Monteiro M: Therapeutic exercise in the treatment of patients with lumbar spinal stenosis, *Clin Orthop Rel Res* 384:144-152, 2001.
281. Hilibrand AS, Rand N: Degenerative lumbar stenosis: Diagnosis and management, *J Am Acad Orthop Surg* 7(4):239-249, 1999.
282. Rittenberg JD, Ross AE: Functional rehabilitation for degenerative lumbar spinal stenosis, *Phys Med Rehabil Clin N Am* 14(1):111-120, 2003.
283. Lonstein JE: Spondylolisthesis in children: Cause, natural history, and management. *Spine* 24:2640-2648, 1999.
284. McNeely ML, Torrance G, Magee DJ: A systematic review of physiotherapy for spondylolysis and spondylolisthesis, *Man Ther* 8(2):80-91, 2003.
285. Moller H, Hedlund R: Surgery versus conservative management in adult isthmic spondylolisthesis—a prospective randomized study: Part 1 (see comment), *Spine* 25(13):1711-1715, 2000.
286. Bell DF, Ehrlich MG, Zaleske DJ. Brace treatment for symptomatic spondylolisthesis. *Clin Orthop* 236:192-198, 1988.
287. Steiner ME, Micheli LJ. Treatment of symptomatic spondylolysis and spondylolisthesis with the modified Boston brace, *Spine* 10:937-943, 1985.
288. Neumann DA: Kinesiology of the musculoskeletal system: Foundations for physical rehabilitation, Philadelphia, 2002, Mosby.
289. Axler CT, McGill SM: Low back loads over a variety of abdominal exercises: searching for the safest abdominal challenge, *Med Sci Sports Exerc* 29(6):804-811, 1997.
290. Gramse RR, Sinaki M, Ilstrup DM: Lumbar spondylolisthesis: A rational approach to conservative treatment, *Mayo Clin Proc* 55(11):681-686, 1980.
291. Sinaki M, Lutness MP, Ilstrup DM, et al: Lumbar spondylolisthesis: Retrospective comparison and three-year follow-up of two conservative treatment programs, *Arch Phys Med Rehabil* 70(8):594-598, 1989.
292. Spratt KF, Weinstein JN, Lehmann TR, et al: Efficacy of flexion and extension treatments incorporating braces for low-back pain patients with retrodisplacement, spondylolisthesis, or normal sagittal translation, *Spine* 18(13):1839-1849, 1993.
293. O'Sullivan PB, Phyty GD, Twomey LT, et al: Evaluation of specific stabilizing exercise in the treatment of chronic low back pain with radiologic diagnosis of spondylolysis or spondylolisthesis, *Spine* 22(24):2959-2967, 1997.

Chapter 9

Fractures

Julie A. Pryde, Debra H. Iwasaki

OBJECTIVES

After reading this chapter, the reader will be able to:
1. Describe fractures and their subtypes using the proper terminology.
2. Identify local and systemic factors affecting fracture healing.
3. Recognize fractures commonly seen in adults and children.
4. Discuss mechanisms of injury of fractures and how these relate to fracture patterns and soft tissue injury.
5. Differentiate between primary and secondary fracture healing.
6. Outline the components of a comprehensive examination of a patient with a fracture.
7. Select and apply evidence-based interventions for patients with fractures.

The treatment and prevention of fractures is an important aspect of musculoskeletal medicine. Fracture treatment and rehabilitation is a challenge requiring a cooperative effort from all members of the health care team, including the physician or other health provider and the rehabilitation specialist. With the significant cost of this treatment and high potential for disability, it is imperative that the rehabilitation specialist understands the principles of fracture healing and the biomechanical principles of fixation to optimize the patients' functional outcome. Fracture patterns, orthopedic intervention and treatment timing, and medical and psychosocial issues, as well as the patient's age and functional needs, must all be considered when designing a rehabilitation program.

It is important for the rehabilitation specialist to understand the depth and complexity of fracture management and its implications in health care today. In 2002 in the United States, over 9 million patients were seen in physician offices for fracture management. The treatment of fractures is the third most common surgical procedure for men of all ages, after cardiac catheterization and prostatectomy.[1] The cost of fracture care in the United States is substantial; nearly one-third of patients with fractures require admission to the hospital. According to the American Academy of Orthopedic Surgeons (AAOS), in 2002, 152,000 people underwent surgical fixation of the femur due to a fracture[2] and half of all inpatient hospital days were due to fractures of the proximal femur.[3] Certain populations have typical fracture patterns. For example, fractures of the forearm, rib, and hip are most common in the elderly. The occurrence of hip fractures is highest in white women and lowest in African American men.[4] After the age of 50, the incidence of fractures increases considerably, doubling for every 5-year increase in age.[5]

NORMAL BONE

Through their relationship with each other and with muscles, bones give form to the body, support tissue, protect organs, and permit movement. Mature bone is a rigid connective tissue consisting of cells, fibers, ground substance, and minerals containing elements such as calcium. Minerals give bones their inherent rigidity, and the bone cells, osteoblasts and osteoclasts, are the living part of the bone that give it the ability to grow, repair, and change shape. Osteoblasts synthesize bone, and osteoclasts reabsorb bone, primarily during the process of growth and repair.

In addition to their structural function, bones have a crucial role in chemical homeostasis since they store many minerals, including calcium and phosphate. Bones also play a major role in blood cell formation in adults because blood cells are first formed in the bone marrow.

Bone can be described as *cortical* (also known as compact) or *cancellous* (also know as spongy). These types of bone differ in their amount of solid matter and number and size of spaces. All bones have a thin outer layer of periosteum that covers the dense outer layer of cortical bone, which surrounds a central mass of cancellous bone (Fig. 9-1). Cortical bone provides strength for weight bearing and rigidity for muscular attachments. Some bones have a medullary (also known as marrow) canal centrally within the cancellous bone. Blood cells are formed in the medullary canal.

There are 206 bones in the human body. Bones may be classified according to their location. The 80 bones of the axial skeleton include the bones of the skull, pelvis, ribs, sternum, vertebrae, and scapulae. The other 126 bones are part of the appendicular skeleton. Bones can also be classified according to their shape. *Long bones,* such as the femur and humerus, are longer than they are wide. They have a tubular midportion, the *diaphysis,* which widens into a broader neck portion, the *metaphysis.* The end of the bone, the *epiphysis,* is widest in order to distribute the force of weight bearing over a wide area. In children, the epiphysis and metaphysis are separated from each other by a cartilaginous growth plate, which is the *epiphyseal growth plate* (Fig. 9-2). This plate is where the bone grows in length. After puberty, the epiphyseal plate calcifies and the epiphysis and metaphysis merge so that by adulthood this demarcation is undetectable.

Short bones, such as the carpals and tarsals, are cuboidal in shape and are found exclusively in the ankle and wrist. They have a thin layer of cortical bone covering cancellous bone with no central medullary canal. Flat bones, such as those of the skull and pelvis, serve a protective function. These bones are made up of cortical

plates that lie roughly parallel to one another and sandwich a cancellous central core. *Irregularly-shaped bones* are found throughout the body and include the mandible and the vertebrae. *Sesamoid bones* develop in certain tendons in areas where those tendons cross the ends of long bones. They protect the tendon from excessive wear and increase the mechanical advantage of the muscle by changing its angle of attachment. The patella is an example of a sesamoid bone. *Accessory bones* are the supernumerary bones that develop when additional ossification centers appear and form extra bones. Many bones develop from this process but normally fuse together to form one. If one of these parts fail to fuse to the main bone, an "extra" bone appears. An accessory navicular is a common example of such a bone in the foot. *Heterotopic bone* may develop within soft tissue or around joints in areas where it is not normally present. Such bone often develops after blunt trauma or closed head injury.

PATHOLOGY

FRACTURES AND THEIR CAUSES

A *fracture* is commonly defined as a break in the continuity of a bone. This term applies to all bony disruptions, ranging from small hairline fractures to multifragmentary or *comminuted fractures.* Bones fracture when the stress applied to them exceeds their strength. The most common cause of fractures in normal bone is trauma. This trauma may be direct or indirect, depending on whether a force is applied directly to the bone or at a distance from it. For example, with direct trauma, a bone may be fractured by an object falling on it or striking it. With direct trauma there is often soft tissue injury around the fracture, and the fracture is often comminuted (in more than two pieces). This is the most common mechanism of injury for a fracture of the distal end of the fourth or fifth metacarpal (known as a *boxer's fracture*) and for a transverse fracture of the distal end of the radius just above the wrist with displacement of the hand backward and outward, known

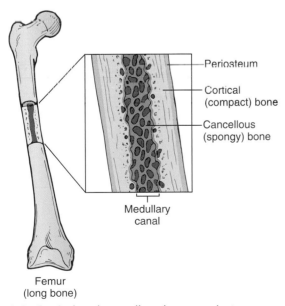

FIG. 9-1 Cortical and cancellous bone, periosteum, medullary canal.

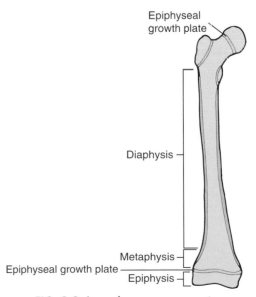

FIG. 9-2 Long bone components.

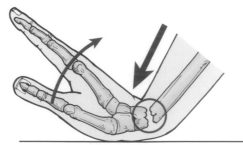

FIG. 9-3 A Colles' fracture caused by a direct force.

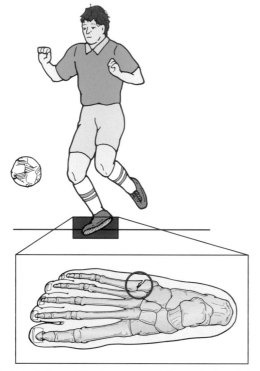

FIG. 9-4 A Jones' fracture caused by an indirect force.

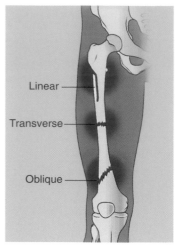

FIG. 9-5 Fracture classification by direction: Linear, transverse, or oblique. *From Thibodeau GA, Patton KT:* Anatomy and Physiology, *ed 6, St. Louis, 2006, Mosby.*

portion of the joint is fixed. This is often seen in patellar and olecranon fractures.

Regardless of where a force is applied, the stress generated may be compressive, tensile, or shear in nature or a combination. In long bones in particular, the type of force will affect whether, how, where, and along which path a fracture will occur. This is because bones are anisotropic, meaning that they respond differently to forces applied in different directions. With normal use, most of the forces applied to bone are compressive so most of the mineral in the bone aligns to resist such forces. It will therefore take more compressive force than tensile or shear force to fracture a bone. In addition, if the load is applied rapidly, the bone must absorb more energy at one time than if a load is applied slowly. This also increases the likelihood of fracture. This is why injuries with rapid loading, such as those sustained in a motor vehicle accident or from a gunshot wound, cause more damage to the bone, with more comminution and displacement.

CLASSIFICATION OF FRACTURES

Fractures may be classified according to direction, mechanism, whether the skin is broken or not, and location. A fracture that runs parallel to the bone is known as a *linear fracture*. A *transverse fracture* is one that runs approximately perpendicular to the long axis of a bone. Transverse fractures are caused by tensile or bending forces. With application of an uneven force, an *oblique fracture* that runs at approximately a 30-degree angle to the long axis of the bone may occur (Fig. 9-5).

A *compression fracture* occurs when the bone is compressed beyond its limits of tolerance (Fig. 9-6). These fractures are often seen in the vertebral bodies as a result of a flexion injury or without trauma in patients with osteoporosis. Compression fractures of the calcaneus are also common when patients fall from a height and land on their feet. *Avulsion fractures* are caused by a sudden muscular contraction or pulling by a ligament in which the area of bone where the tendon or ligament attaches is pulled away from the rest of the bone. These fractures are common in the fifth metatarsal as a result of pulling by

as a *Colles' fracture* (Fig. 9-3). With indirect trauma, a fracture may be caused when a bending or twisting stress is applied at a distance from the resultant fracture. For example, a fall on an outstretched hand may result in a radial head fracture, whereas an inversion stress at the ankle may result in a fifth metatarsal fracture (Fig. 9-4).

The risk for a fracture and the pattern of the fracture depends largely on the nature of the applied force and the properties of the bone. A fracture may arise when a force is applied repetitively over time or from a single application of force. The degree of damage depends on the amount of energy applied to the bone and the volume and brittleness of the bone. A fracture is more likely to occur if the force is great or the bone is small or brittle. People with osteoporosis have more brittle bones and therefore sustain fractures more easily, whereas children have more elastic bones, allowing their bones to bend rather than break. When a bone bends, it may sustain a "greenstick" fracture, which is a partial fracture of the bone only on one side. When the force is applied at a distance from the fracture site, strong muscle contractions across the joint may produce a separated or distracted fracture if the distal

Compression

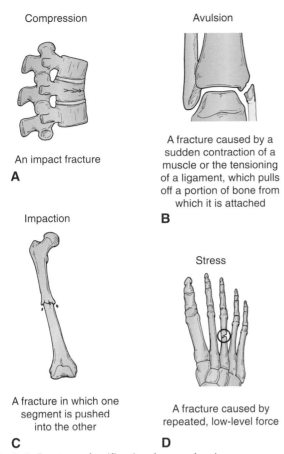

An impact fracture

A

Avulsion

A fracture caused by a sudden contraction of a muscle or the tensioning of a ligament, which pulls off a portion of bone from which it is attached

B

Impaction

A fracture in which one segment is pushed into the other

C

Stress

A fracture caused by repeated, low-level force

D

FIG. 9-6 Fracture classification by mechanism. **A,** Compression fracture; **B,** avulsion fracture; **C,** impaction fracture; **D,** stress fracture.

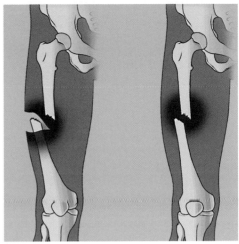

FIG. 9-7 Open fracture and closed fracture. *From Thibodeau GA, Patton KT:* Anatomy and Physiology, *ed 6, St. Louis, 2006, Mosby.*

the peroneus brevis and at the distal fibula with inversion sprains. An *impaction fracture* occurs when one fragment is driven into another. This type of fracture is common in tibial plateau fractures in adults. A *stress fracture* is caused by repeated low force trauma that eventually causes the bone to break. Stress fractures may extend through all or only part of the way through the bone. These types of fractures are common in soldiers or runners[6-9] and are far more common in women.[10] They often occur in the lower extremity (LE), most often in the fibula, tibia, or metatarsals.[11,12] Stress fractures are most commonly seen in women who participate in track and field, followed by crew, basketball, lacrosse and soccer.[13] Stress fractures of the calcaneus are also seen in military personnel and pubic rami fractures are seen in swimmers and runners.[14-16] Stress fractures of the pars interarticularis are seen in adolescent girls participating in sports that require repetitive hyperextension of the lumbosacral region such as gymnastics, cheerleading, and dance.[17,18] Stress fractures may be caused by compression, as occurs with repetitive striking of the heel during marching or running, or by distraction when a muscle pulls on the bone.

A fracture that does not communicate with the external environment, where the skin barrier is intact, is referred to as a *closed fracture*. Most closed fractures are accompanied by soft tissue injuries. *Open fractures* are exposed to the external environment as a result of skin

and soft tissue damage (Fig. 9-7). This includes cases with a grossly exposed bone, as well as fractures accompanied by a small puncture wound that communicates to the fracture. The soft tissue damage may be caused by an external force or by the fragments of exposed bone. An open fracture is far more prone to complications than closed fractures because of the potential for contamination.[19,20] (Closed and open fractures were previously referred to as simple and compound fractures, respectively, but these terms have fallen out of favor because they are not descriptive.)

A fracture may be located in the proximal, middle, or distal third of the bone. The location of a fracture is generally described by the bone affected and with the long bones, whether it is in the diaphysis, metaphysis, or epiphysis of the bone. Diaphyseal fractures may also be described as being in the proximal, middle, or distal third. A fracture may also be described by anatomical landmarks such as a fracture of the femoral neck or intertrochanteric fracture of the femur. Finally, an eponym may also be used to describe a specific type of fracture such as a Monteggia fracture or a Jones fracture. A Monteggia fracture is a fracture of the proximal third of the ulna with a dislocation of the radial head; a Jones fracture is a fracture of the base of the fifth metatarsal.

RISK FACTORS FOR FRACTURES

The most common cause of fractures is trauma. The incidence of fractures and the types of fractures sustained vary with age, race, and co-morbidities. In the geriatric population, especially those with osteoporosis, the most common fractures are hip fractures; in children, forearm and leg fractures are more common.

Osteoporosis accounts for the largest number of fractures among the elderly. A woman's risk of developing a hip fracture is equal to her combined risk of developing breast, uterine, and ovarian cancer.[21] It is estimated that 8 million American women and 2 million American men have osteoporosis, putting them at risk for the pain and disability associated with fracture.[22] Approximately 50% of postmenopausal white women and 25% of men will incur an osteoporotic fracture in their lifetime.[23] Women have a higher risk of fracture than men of the same race, and whites generally have a higher risk of fracture than African-Americans of the same gender.[24] Over 90% of hip fractures are associated with osteoporosis, and most are associated with a fall.[25] Nationally, it is estimated that the direct costs for osteoporotic hip fractures was $18 billion in 2002.[22] National statistics show that 10% to 20% of people with hip fractures die within 6 months, 50% cannot walk without an assistive device, and 25% require long-term aid.[26] The most common sites of osteoporotic fractures are the vertebrae, hip, wrist, and proximal humerus.[27] Chapter 3 contains more information on the pathology, examination, evaluation, and management of patients with osteoporosis.

Fractures in the elderly are also frequently associated with a history of poor balance and falls, especially falls to the side in which the patient lands on the greater trochanter[28] (see Chapter 13). Certain anthropometric characteristics, including tallness, long femurs, and low body weight, are also associated with increased hip fracture risk.[29] Some risk factors for fractures, such as advanced age, low body mass index, and low levels of physical activity, probably affect fracture incidence through the linked characteristics of osteoporosis, propensity toward falling, and the inability to absorb impact.[29]

Some fracture patterns occur most commonly or only in children. These include *greenstick fractures* and *torus fractures*. Greenstick fractures, as previously described, only occur in children and adolescents because these fractures only happen in somewhat elastic bones. A torus fracture is buckling of the bone that occurs most commonly in the forearm bones of children. With this type of fracture the bone becomes compressed at the point of impact, producing only a change in angulation of the cortex. Epiphyseal fractures also only occur in skeletally immature patients. When an epiphyseal fracture occurs at the end of a long bone near the joint, the disruption may halt or impair bone growth.

Certain diseases can weaken bone to such an extent that minor trauma results in a fracture. Fractures that occur under such circumstances may be called pathological fractures. Pathological fractures are associated with benign and malignant tumors, osteogenesis imperfecta, Paget's disease, osteomalacia, osteoporosis, and bone cysts. Approximately 75% of malignant tumors in bone are metastatic from a primary cancer elsewhere, most commonly the breast, thyroid, kidney, lung, or prostate[30]; 50% of bony metastases occur in the spine, usually in the thoracic or lumbar regions. A high index of suspicion for pathological fracture is necessary in patients with a history of cancer. Vertebral compression fractures are frequently seen in patients with advanced osteoporosis and are one of the most common pathological fractures. Because these fractures are not associated with significant trauma, they may go undetected unless there is a high level of suspicion on the part of the clinician.

FRACTURE HEALING

A fracture initiates a sequence of events that may ultimately restore the injured bone to its original state. Frac-

tures in bone heal with like tissue without scar formation. This allows them to regain their prior mechanical and structural integrity. To understand the different processes that contribute to bone healing, it is helpful to view these events as distinct processes occurring in the bone itself and in the adjacent soft tissues. Depending on the type of fracture, its location, and the method by which it is treated, these responses may occur simultaneously or sequentially.

Primary and Secondary Fracture Healing. The type of fracture healing, primary or secondary, depends on the method of treatment or fixation. Primary healing, which is also known as direct union or contact healing, will occur if the intramedullary vasculature is intact, there is cortical contact, and fracture fixation provides compression across the fracture, reduces the interfragmentary gap to less than 1 mm, and eliminates motion at the fracture site. This type of fracture healing is usually achieved by the surgical insertion of implants, such as plates and screws, but can occur without surgical fixation with certain types of fractures, including impacted epiphyseal, metaphyseal fractures, and vertebral compression fractures.

During primary healing, new bone grows directly across the compressed fracture site to unite the fracture without *callus* formation.[31] First, osteoclasts in the intact portion of the bone form cutting cones that move across the fracture site, forming new haversian canals. These cutting cones contain blood vessels that revascularize the bone fragments, restoring microcirculation. Osteoblasts then follow to fill in the canals with osteons that bridge the fracture site. This is followed by generation of new bone that unites the fracture.

It takes approximately 5-6 weeks for a fracture to close by primary healing.[32] Although the healed bone is initially weak, with time and repeated static and cyclic loading, extensive remodeling occurs and the new bone regains the full strength of intact undamaged bone. Initially, when the bone is weak, the fracture site is stabilized and strengthened by the fixation device. When a rigid or stable fixation device is used, the site can be strong immediately after fixation, allowing for early initiation of weight bearing, functional activity, and rehabilitation. Early activity can shorten recovery time by reducing loss of range of motion (ROM), strength, and function. However, surgical implantation of a fixation device, as opposed to using an external cast and avoiding surgery, subjects the tissues to a surgical procedure with its own inherent trauma and risks.

If motion across a fracture site is minimized but not eliminated, a fracture will close by secondary healing. Secondary healing, also known as callus healing or indirect healing, is an ordered process initiated by a cascade of signaling factors. This cascade of events starts with formation of a fibrous callus around the fracture site and ends with its conversion to bone. The callus initially stabilizes the fracture. The callus must be big enough to compensate for its relatively poor strength. Some motion at the fracture site is required to induce callus formation. However, there is fine line between enough motion to induce the callus and too much motion that can prevent healing. Secondary healing occurs in fractures treated with stress sharing devices such as casts, Kirschner wires (K wires), intramedullary rods, and external fixation devices. These devices align the bone fragments but do not compress the fracture gap, therefore allowing for some degree of motion. Secondary healing is the most common type of bone healing.

Secondary healing involves not only the response of the bone itself but also of the periosteum and the soft tissue around the fracture site. The response from the periosteum is thought to be critical to callus formation and is enhanced by slight motion and inhibited by rigid fixation.[33] Secondary healing is rapid and can bridge a gap as large as half of the diameter of the fractured bone.

Fractures are considered clinically healed when the bone is stable and pain-free. Roentgenographic/radiological healing has occurred when trabecular or cortical bone crosses the fracture site as evidenced by x-ray.[34] Panjabi et al found by comparing radiographic evaluation of fracture healing to failure strength of healing osteotomies that the best radiological indicator of clinical healing was cortical continuity and the poorest indicator was the callus area. In general, radiographic information alone is not sufficient to accurately assess the biomechanical strength of a healing fracture.[35]

Stages of Fracture Healing. Fracture healing generally occurs in three stages:[36] Inflammatory, repair, and remodeling, although some authors break these into six stages. These stages may overlap and events that begin in one stage may continue into the following stage. The length of each stage varies with the location and severity of the fracture and associated injuries and other local and systemic factors.

The inflammatory stage of fracture healing typically lasts 1-2 weeks. When a bone is injured, both the bone and its blood supply are disrupted. Disruption of the blood vessels in and around the bone leads to formation of a hematoma at the injury site. The organization of this hematoma is the first step of fracture repair. The hematoma causes various molecules and cells to initiate the healing process.[37,38] Such molecules, including cytokines, interleukins, and various growth factors, regulate the early stages of healing, including cell proliferation and differentiation. Open fractures or those treated surgically may not have a hematoma at the fracture site and may therefore heal more slowly.

Soon after the hematoma forms, inflammatory cells, including neutrophils, macrophages, and phagocytes, invade the area. Along with osteoclasts, these cells remove the damaged and necrotic tissue near the distal edges of the fracture and lay the groundwork for the repair stage to begin. Radiographically, the fracture line becomes more visible as the necrotic material is removed, which is why some hairline fractures are not evident on x-ray until days after the initial injury.

The repair stage usually begins within 2 weeks of the fracture and lasts several months. It is characterized by the differentiation of mesenchymal stem cells into cell types necessary for tissue restoration, including osteoblasts, osteoclasts, chondroblasts, fibroblasts, and angioblasts. The fracture site is invaded by chondrocytes and fibroblasts, which lay down a matrix for the callus composed of collagen, glycosaminoglycan (GAG), and proteoglycans. Initially, a soft callus composed mainly of fibrous tissue and cartilage with small amount of bone is formed. Osteoblasts then mineralize this soft callus, converting it to a hard callus and increasing the stability of the fracture. However, this immature bone is still weaker than normal bone, particularly in response to torque, and therefore must be protected. Delayed union or nonunion, as described later in this chapter, generally result from errors in this phase of healing. The repair stage ends when the fracture is clinically stable. Radiographically, the fracture line begins to disappear during this stage.

During the remodeling stage, which can take months or years to complete, osteoblasts and osteoclasts replace the immature, poorly organized bone with mature, organized laminar bone, making the fracture site more stable. The ultimate goal of this stage is to restore the bone to its original strength and structure, giving it the ability to withstand the usual stresses placed on it. During this stage, areas of bone that sustain little stress are reabsorbed by osteoclasts, while more bone is laid down by osteoblasts in areas with high stress. Mechanical loading of the fracture site is needed to facilitate strong callus formation, fracture alignment, and ultimately lamellar remodeling.[39] Over time, the medullary canal inside the bone reforms and angular, although not rotational, deformities may correct. By the end of remodeling, the fracture line is no longer visible radiographically and the bone at the fracture site should have the same stiffness as normal bone and the same or greater strength than normal bone. Because a fully healed fracture is often stronger than the surrounding bone, subsequent application of an excessive load to the whole bone generally does not cause a fracture at the original fracture site but rather above or below the fracture site.[40] Additionally, despite successful fracture healing, the overall density of the bones in the involved limb may be decreased for years.[41]

Prognosis for Fracture Healing. Although the length of time for fracture healing varies, there is a typical rate at which fractures heal and some predictable variability based on the location and nature of the fracture and the type of fixation. For example, a distal radial fracture is expected to heal within 6-8 weeks, whereas a midshaft femur fracture may require 6 months.

The location and stability of the fracture can also affect how much callus forms. For example, metaphyseal fractures tend to heal with little callus formation because there is little surrounding periosteum and because the interdigitation and impaction of the fracture keeps the site stable and limits the fracture gap. In contrast, diaphyseal fractures tend to form a large callus because they are not impacted and have a larger fracture gap and more periosteum.

Fractures caused by high-speed or high-force impacts often heal slowly because there is more soft tissue and vascular damage in the area of the fracture and more fracture comminution. Open fractures also tend to heal more slowly than closed fractures because of the amount of soft tissue damage and bone loss, as well as fracture displacement and increased infection risk. Infection around a fracture not only compromises healing but may also lead to chronic infection of the bone known as *osteomyelitis.* Intraarticular fractures may also heal slowly because they can require extensive surgical intervention to assure good joint alignment.

Some fractures heal more slowly than expected or fail to heal at all. Slow healing is known as *delayed union* and failure to heal is known as *nonunion.* Nonunion is generally defined as failing to heal after 6-8 months.[42] When a fracture fails to heal, cartilage or fibrocartilage forms over the fracture surfaces and the cavity between the fracture surfaces fills with fluid that resembles normal joint or bursal fluid. This false joint or *pseudoarthrosis* may or may not be painful but will always be unstable. A fibrous union formed by dense cartilage or fibrocartilage band may also be an end result and although it will stabilize the fracture site and may be painless, this union does not restore normal strength.

Common risk factors for delayed fracture healing include diabetes mellitus, smoking, long-term steroid use, nonsteroidal antiinflammatory drugs (NSAIDs) and other medications, and poor nutrition.[43] Diabetes is thought to impair fracture healing by causing a defect in collagen or collagen cross-linking.[43] Cigarette smoking interferes with osteoblast activity.[44] Nicotine can also impair healing by causing vasoconstriction and inhibiting angiogenesis, both of which can reduce blood flow to the fracture site.[45,46] Humans who smoke have been found to have more complications with fracture healing, including infections, amputations and nonunions or *malunions,* and slower healing rates than their nonsmoking counterparts.[47,48] In animal studies, those exposed to nicotine also healed more slowly and had a higher percentage of nonunions.[49] Nicotine has also been shown to inhibit vascularization of bone grafts in rabbits, although the exact mechanism remains unclear.[50,51] Castillo and colleagues evaluated healing in patients with traumatic unilateral open tibial fractures and found that current and previous smokers were 37% and 32%, respectively, less likely than nonsmokers to achieve union. Current smokers were twice as likely to develop an infection and 3.7 times as likely to develop osteomyelitis. Previous smokers were 2.8 times more likely to develop osteomyelitis but were at no greater risk for developing other types of infection.[52] Clinical observations parallel these studies. With over 50 million smokers in the United States, it is important that the clinician and the patient take into consideration that smoking may delay fracture healing and increase the risk of complications and thus contribute to a poorer functional outcome.

Corticosteroids can delay fracture healing and increase the risk for fractures.[53,54] Delayed healing is thought to be due to decreased synthesis of organic bone matrix components and slowed differentiation of osteoblasts from mesenchymal cells. NSAIDs are also thought to slow fracture healing. The evidence for this is from a variety of animal studies and one retrospective series using high doses of intramuscular ketorolac after spinal fusion in human subjects. A dose-dependent relationship was found between that particular NSAID and nonunion rates.[55] Certain antibiotics, specifically fluoroquinolones such as ciprofloxacin and levofloxacin, have also been shown to delay fracture healing, especially early in the course of fracture repair. Randomized controlled trials (RCTs) have shown that animals given these drugs after a fracture have fractures with less mature callus formation and decreased torsional strength and stiffness, suggesting that administration of fluoroquinolones during the early stages of fracture repair may also compromise fracture healing in humans.[56,57]

Nutrition also influences fracture repair as the energy required for the body to heal a fracture is substantial. To synthesize large volumes of collagen, proteoglycans, and other matrix constituents, cells need a steady supply of the components of these molecules—specifically proteins and carbohydrates. Fractures that would heal rapidly in well-nourished patients may fail to heal in patients with severe malnutrition. Jensen et al found a 42% incidence of clinical or subclinical malnutrition in patients undergoing orthopedic procedures.[58] It has been reported that a single long bone fracture can temporarily increase metabolic requirements by 20% to 25% and that multiple injuries or infections can increase this requirement by as much as 50%.[59] Specifically, it has been shown that fracture callus strength is reduced in patients with protein deficiencies.[60] Therefore it is important that patients eat a balanced diet to optimize their healing potential.

A patient's age can also influence the rate of fracture healing. Infants have the most rapid rate of fracture healing and the rate of fracture healing declines with age.[61] Fracture healing in adults and the elderly follows the same sequence, but in the elderly it is often slower and less effective. For some fractures, age-related changes are significant enough to alter the treatment patterns. For example, a nondisplaced closed femoral fracture in a 3-year-old child may be effectively managed with a cast with restoration of tissue structure and function in 6 weeks, whereas a 70-year-old patient may require surgery and may take up to 6 months for an outcome that is much less predictable.

The amount of soft tissue damage also affects the rate of fracture healing. The time for a bone to heal is greatly prolonged in fractures that have more soft tissue stripping or damage. Studies have shown that muscle damage slows bone healing.[62] If the fracture site loses its intrinsic vascularity as a result of periosteal stripping from surgery or injury, comminution, or a large initial displacement, the extrinsic blood supply becomes imperative for fracture healing. The extrinsic blood supply of bone comes mainly from the muscles, as well as the soft tissues, that surround it. Experimentally, ischemic bone will not revascularize until the surrounding soft tissue envelope does so. Therefore if the soft tissue envelope is damaged, bone healing will be delayed.[63] Most studies show that the incidence of nonunion is higher with open fractures than with closed fractures. Godina also found that delayed closure time increased total healing time. The average healing time is 6 months for primary closure and 12.8 months for delayed closure.[64]

The presence of infection can also slow or prevent fracture healing. Infection may cause necrosis of normal tissue, as well as edema and thrombosis of blood vessels.[65]

If bone necrosis is present, healing depends entirely on ingrowth of vessels from the living side of the fracture and surrounding soft tissues. This type of healing occurs more slowly, and healing is less predictable.[66] Necrosis can be caused by irradiation, infection, surgical trauma, prolonged use of corticosteroids, and sickle cell anemia. Bone that has been irradiated often heals at a much slower rate than normal bone. This is especially important for pathological fractures treated with radiation.[67] Pathological fractures caused by malignancies also often fail to heal if the neoplasm is left untreated. This is also true of infected bone, which requires removal of the underlying infection and debridement.

The presence of osteoporosis does not impair fracture healing but may increase the time it takes to restore the mechanical strength of the bone. The decreased bone mass may also reduce the strength of the interface between a hardware implant used for internal fixation, which may lead to failure and subsequent delayed union or nonunion of the fracture site.[68]

Types of Fracture Fixation. If a fracture is inherently stable, as with a torus fracture of the radius as described previously, then a cast or a brace will exert sufficient force to limit interfragmentary motion. A cast is an externally applied circumferential plaster or fiberglass device that allows for secondary healing. Usually the joints above and below the fracture site are immobilized to prevent rotation or translation at the fracture site. Splints and braces, which are removable, can also be used for fracture stabilization. They offer the advantage of being removable for ROM and hygiene but also the disadvantage of possibly allowing for excessive motion with the noncompliant patient.

Many fractures require surgical placement of additional internal or external fixation to maintain stability while they are healing (Fig. 9-8). The surgical procedure required for placement of these fixation devices may alter normal healing by injuring soft tissues, blood vessels, or periosteum around the fracture site.

A variety of techniques are currently used to surgically fix fractures. Many factors influence the selection of fixation method, but the most crucial is the need for sufficient stability to achieve fracture healing. The biomechanics of fracture fixation is based on the principles of stress

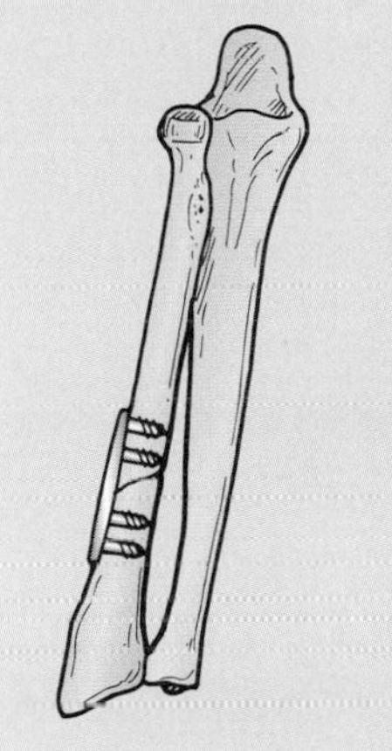

Type of Fixation: Compression Plate and Screws	
Biomechanics	Stress shielding
Type of bone healing	Primary
Speed of recovery	Slow
Advantages	Allows perfect alignment of the fracture Holds bone in compression allowing for primary healing
Disadvantanges	Stress shielding at the site of the plate Some periosteal stripping inevitable
Other information	May initially need secondary support such as a splint or cast
Applications	Tibial plateau fracture Displaced distal radial fracture

A

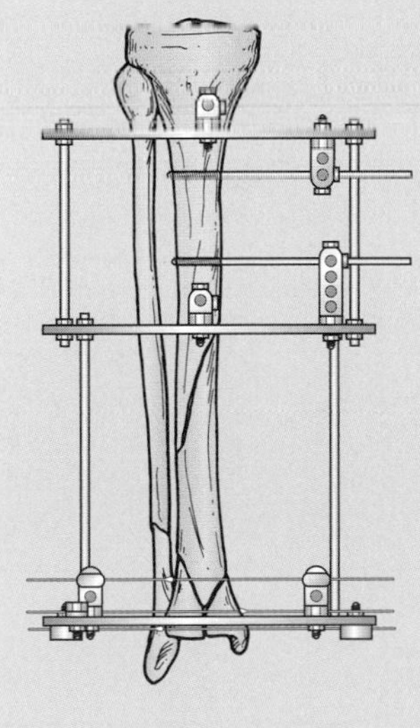

FIG. 9-8 Fracture fixation methods. **A**, Compression plate and screws, **B**, external fixator devices.

Type of Fixation: External Fixator Devices	
Biomechanics	Stress sharing
Type of bone healing	Secondary
Speed of recovery	Fast
Advantages	Allows access to soft tissue if wounds are open
Disadvantanges	Pin tract infections Cumbersome
Other information	Mainly used if patients have associated soft tissue injuries that prevent ORIF or if patient is too sick to undergo lengthy surgery
Applications	Open tibial fractures Severely comminuted distal radial fractures

B

Continued

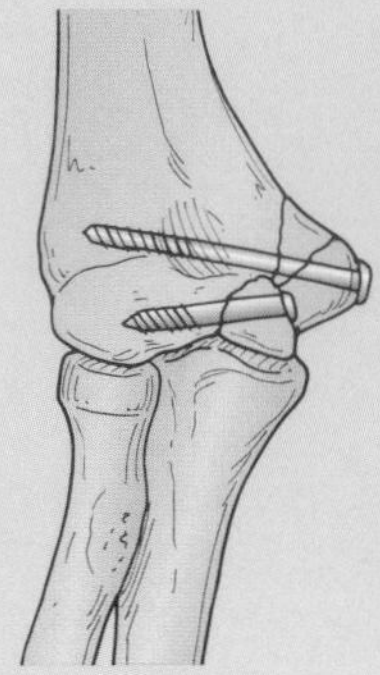

C

Type of Fixation: Screws, Pins, or Wires	
Biomechanics	Stress sharing
Type of bone healing	Secondary
Speed of recovery	Fast
Advantages	Minimal incision size often needed Less chance of growth plate damage with the use of smooth wires (Kirschner wires/K-wires)
Disadvantanges	Difficult to get perfect alignment Hardware may need to be removed after healing is achieved
Other information	Often needs secondary support such as a splint or cast
Applications	Displaced patellar fractures Pediatric displaced supracondylar humeral fractures

D

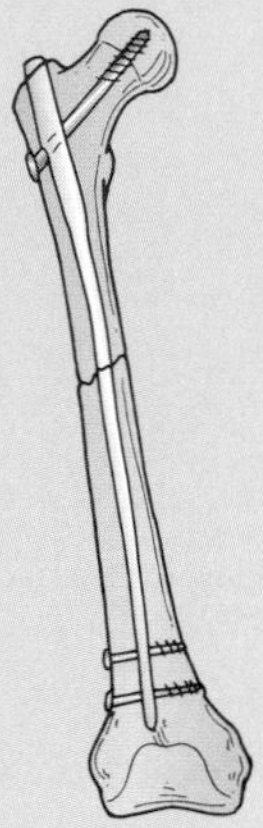

Type of Fixation: Rods/Nails	
Biomechanics	Stress sharing
Type of bone healing	Secondary
Speed of recovery	Fast
Advantages	Smaller incision than plates so often less soft tissue damage caused by surgery Early weight bearing possible
Disadvantanges	Disruption of endosteal blood supply Reaming may cause fat emboli
Other information	Reamed rods are most commonly used
Applications	Midshaft tibial and femoral fractures

E

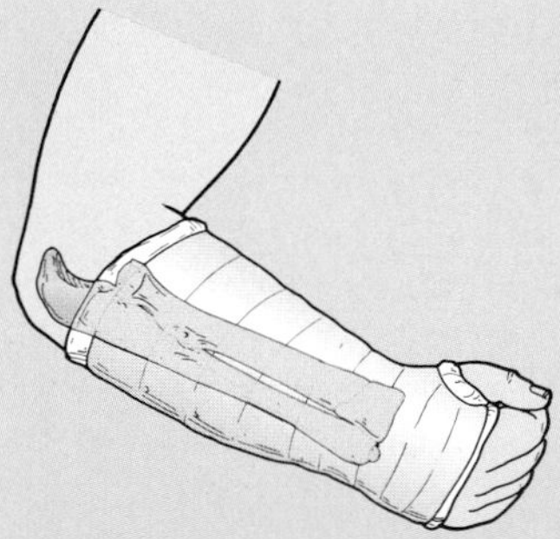

Type of Fixation: Short or Long Cast of Plaster or Fiberglass; Brace	
Biomechanics	Stress sharing
Type of bone healing	Secondary
Speed of recovery	Fast
Advantages	Noninvasive Easy to apply Inexpensive
Disadvantanges	Skin breakdown or maceration Reduction of fracture may be lost if cast becomes loose Potential for harmful pressure on nerve/blood vessels
Other information	Most commonly used means of fracture support
Applications	Torus fracture of the wrist Nondisplaced lateral malleolar fracture

FIG. 9-8—cont'd **C,** Screws, pins, or wires; **D,** rods/nails; **E,** short or long cast of plaster or fiberglass; brace.

shielding or stress sharing. A stress-shielding device transfers stress to the implanted device and holds the fractured ends of bones together under compression so that no callus forms. The fracture heals by primary healing with no motion across the fracture, and all stresses in the area are absorbed by the plate. A compression plate is an example of a stress-shielding device. A stress-sharing device, such as a cast, intramedullary rod, or external fixator, absorbs only part of the forces at the fracture site. This allows for "micromotion" of the fracture site, which induces callus formation through secondary healing.

Most implanted fracture fixation devices are made of stainless steel, titanium, or occasionally a cobalt-chromium alloy. These devices can have a wide range of forms. A common device is the intramedullary rod. This is a long straight piece of metal placed in the bone. These are commonly used for fixation of fractures of long bones, most frequently the shaft of the femur, tibia, or humerus. They restore bone alignment and allow early weight bearing and mobilization of the joints above and below the fracture site. Intramedullary rods are load sharing and allow for secondary fracture healing through callus formation.

K wires hold fragments of bone together before rigid fixation. They lack sufficient mechanical stability to be used as primary support for weight-bearing bones but can be used in conjunction with other stronger wires or with other forms of external fixation such as casts or splints.

Plates are stress-shielding devices that take the load of the bone to allow for primary healing without callus formation. They are used most frequently in the upper extremity (UE) and the fibula where early load bearing is not as important. Plates are also used for periarticular and periprosthetic fractures where good alignment and lack of callus are most important. Because primary healing is slow, compression plating often requires a non–weight-bearing period, as well as secondary support, such as a cast or splint, to prevent hardware failure that results from cyclic loading.

EXAMINATION

The examination of a patient who has sustained a fracture should follow a format that will allow the clinician to "paint" a picture of the patient and develop an intervention program that will optimize the patient's functional outcome. The examination should include a patient history, a systems review, and tests and measures.

PATIENT HISTORY

A thorough history of a patient with a fracture should include information about the patient's current presenting concerns, their prior level of function, and their goals for therapy. Direct communication with patients about their goals is important because their goals may differ from those of the physical therapist (PT) or physician. Additionally, information from family members and other caregivers, especially when the patient is a child, is elderly, or has impaired cognitive abilities or other special needs, may allow the therapist to develop a realistic and appropriate plan of care for the patient. The patient's goals should be considered when selecting and prioritizing interventions. For example, if the patient's primary functional goal is independent toileting, then the therapist should focus on dynamic balance, safe transfers, and increasing strength or ROM to enable to patient to remove and replace clothing, as well as to achieve being able to rise from sitting to get on and off of the commode. Alternatively, if the patient's goal is to be able to sleep in his or her bed on the second floor, the therapist may need to address endurance, as well as managing stairs.

The patient history for patients with a fracture should also include demographic information and a social history, as well as information about their living environment. Attention should be paid to the presence of stairs or other environmental barriers, as well as bathroom access, especially for patients with LE fractures with a limited weight-bearing status. The PT may wish to examine the patient's home to ascertain if the patient will be able to safely negotiate his or her environment and to determine if environmental adaptations, such as hand rails, may need to be installed or if assistive devices, such as shower chairs, raised commodes, or reachers, are necessary or helpful for the patient during recovery. The availability of caregivers or family members to assist in the rehabilitation and recovery of the patient should also be noted.

The patient history should include information about when and where the fracture occurred, how it has been managed thus far, and what limitations or precautions have been recommended. The date of injury will help the clinician know the stage of healing. If the fracture involved a joint, current mobility and long-term functional outcome will more likely be affected than with an extraarticular fracture. The method and duration of fracture immobilization will influence the rate of recovery and the nature and duration of activity and weight-bearing precautions. Information about the surgery and the fixation devices used can be found in the operative report and information about the surgical restrictions should be noted by the surgeon on the referral or in the standard protocol.

A general medical history may also alert the clinician to any factors that may delay fracture healing, such as diabetes, osteoporosis or smoking, or that may delay or impair functional recovery such as a stroke. The patient's current medications may give insight into their ongoing medical problems, their pain level, and the possible risk for side effects that could delay fracture healing or functional recovery. The use and quantity of analgesic medications may give an indication of the patient's pain level. Antiinflammatory medications may impact pain and swelling, as well as the rate of tissue healing, and anticoagulants may limit the vigor of therapy. The use of other medications, alcohol, or tobacco can also be noted at this time.

SYSTEMS REVIEW

The systems review is used to target areas requiring further examination and to define areas that may cause complications or indicate a need for precautions during the examination and intervention processes. See Chapter 1 for details of the systems review.

TESTS AND MEASURES

When performing tests and measures on a patient with a fracture it is important to respect ROM, resistance, and weight-bearing restrictions. Tests and measures should start with an overall observation of the patient, their posture, and their willingness to move. This is important not only for the area in question but also for the rest of the involved upper or lower quarter. It is optimal to check the joints above and below the involved area to ensure that nothing is overlooked that may jeopardize an optimal outcome. For example, it is important to examine the wrist and shoulder in a patient that has sustained a fracture at the elbow.

Musculoskeletal

Anthropometric Characteristics. The girth around a joint and/or volume measurements, as well as observation and palpation, may be used to assess for the presence of edema. Girth and volume measurements of the involved side should be compared with those of the uninvolved side to determine if a change has occurred. Edema is an indicator of inflammation and soft tissue injury. Loss of skin landmarks and wrinkles suggests moderate swelling, and a delay in capillary refill indicates severe swelling.[69]

Girth measurements around the middle of a limb segment may also be used to assess for muscle atrophy. Muscle atrophy is common after prolonged immobilization but may also occur if a peripheral nerve was injured at the time of the fracture. For example, axillary and radial nerve injuries commonly occur in conjunction with proximal humeral fractures. Atrophy that results from disuse can be differentiated from atrophy that results from nerve injury by peripheral nerve examination as described later.

Swelling in the limb may also indicate a more sinister pathology such as a deep venous thrombosis (DVT). Trauma, surgery and prolonged immobilization are risk factors for local DVT formation.[70] In the LE, a DVT can occur proximal or distal to the popliteal artery. Proximal DVTs (PDVTs) are considered more dangerous as they are often larger and more likely to lead to pulmonary embolus. A prospective study by Geerts et al found that PDVTs occur in up to 66% of patients with isolated LE fractures seen in a trauma unit.[71] With hospitalizations getting shorter, it is more likely that rehabilitation professionals in both the inpatient and outpatient setting will see patients with DVTs. Although the Homan sign, the presence of pain in the calf when the toes are passively dorsiflexed, is often used clinically to screen for the presence of DVT, the poor sensitivity and specificity of this test make it inappropriate for clinical use.[72] It is recommended that clinicians use a clinical decision rule (CDR) (Box 9-1) that includes the presence of swelling and pain, as well as various other aspects of the patient history and physical examination, to more accurately estimate DVT risk.[73-75]

Range of Motion. Passive ROM (PROM) and active ROM (AROM) of the joint above and below the fracture, as well as muscle length, should be examined. If the fracture involves the hand, wrist, or foot, measure the ROM of the individual joints, as well as the functional range of combined movements. In addition to measuring the

---

BOX 9-1   Clinical Decision Rule for Proximal Deep Venous Thrombosis

- Active cancer within 6 months or diagnosis or palliative care
- Paralysis, paresis, or recent plaster immobilization of the LE
- Recently bedridden >3 days or major surgery within 4 weeks of application of the clinical decision rule
- Localized tenderness along the distribution of the deep venous system—firm palpation in the center of the posterior calf, popliteal space, and along the femoral vein along the anterior thigh
- Entire LE swelling
- Calf swelling >3 cm compared to the asymptomatic LE measured 10 cm below the tibial tuberosity
- Collateral superficial veins (nonvaricose)
- Alternative diagnosis as likely or greater than that of DVT such as cellulitis, calf strain or postoperative swelling

Score each as 1 point if positive except for the final bullet, which is scored as (−2). Interpret scores as follows:
<0: Probability of PDVT is 3% (confidence level 95%)
1-2: Probability of PDVT is 17% (confidence level 17%)
>3: Probability of PDVT is 75% (confidence level 75%)

Data from Wells PS, Anderson DR, Bormanis J, et al: *Lancet* 350:1795-1817, 1997 and Wells PS, Hirsh J, Anderson DR, et al: *J Intern Med* 243:15-23, 1998.
LE, Lower extremity; *DVT,* deep vein thrombosis; *PDVT,* proximal DVT.

---

quantity of the motion, also examine for the quality of movement, including the presence of stiffness, muscle spasm, or guarding during the movement. Loss of ROM and joint stiffness are particularly common after an intra-articular fracture and prolonged joint immobilization.

Muscle Performance Strength testing of the primary muscle groups around the fracture site, as well as a general screening for the strength of the involved upper or lower quarter, should be performed. The quality of the movement and any compensatory or accessory movements should be noted. For example, when testing forward flexion of the shoulder after a humeral fracture, trapezius activity instead of deltoid recruitment should be noted. Strength may be tested by manual muscle testing (MMT), hand-held dynamometry, or isokinetic means (see Chapter 5). Loss of strength because of disuse atrophy and inefficient motor recruitment is common after prolonged immobilization.

Joint Integrity and Mobility. The integrity of the joints above and below the fracture should be examined through testing accessory joint motions and ligament stability (see Chapter 11).

Neuromuscular

Pain. It is important for the clinician to determine if the patient has pain, and if so, its location, severity, quality, frequency, and how these symptoms change in relation to both rest and activity (see Chapter 22 for details of pain measures). Symptoms may occur not only at the fracture site but also in other areas affected by changes in biomechanics, sleeping positions, or gait changes. For example, immobilization of the UE with a sling may result in cervical pain, and gait deviations caused by a LE fracture may cause back pain. The response of symptoms to activity will give the clinician an appreciation of the severity and irritability of this patient's presentation.

Peripheral Nerve Integrity. Peripheral nerve integrity is generally determined through a combination of strength testing, sensory testing, and reflex testing (see Chapter 18). Electromyography may also be used in select cases. Peripheral nerve integrity should be examined in patients with fractures commonly associated with peripheral nerve injury, such as humeral shaft fractures, and in patients who report sensory changes or pain that is electrical in quality.

Integumentary

Integumentary Integrity. Evaluate the area of the fracture for any signs of inflammation such as swelling, redness, and temperature changes. These findings are normal early in fractures treated with both immobilization and surgical fixation. These findings should be differentiated from signs of infection, which often include fever and constitutional symptoms. The healing of any incision and the mobility of the scar should also be examined. Soft tissue mobility testing may be limited by tissue healing constraints, especially if the fracture was open and required skin grafts.

Function

Gait, Locomotion, and Balance. For the patient with a LE fracture, examine gait (see Chapter 32) and balance (see Chapter 13). These tests may be limited at the initial examination by weight-bearing restrictions but should be repeated as weight-bearing restrictions are lifted.

After a LE fracture, it is common for patients to have gait deviations secondary to weight-bearing restrictions, pain, decreased strength, decreased proprioception and balance, and use of assistive devices or braces. Weight-bearing restrictions and pain with weight bearing will often cause the patient to use a "limb shortening strategy," with increased hip flexion, knee flexion, and ankle dorsiflexion, in an attempt to keep the extremity from full contact with the floor. Decreased strength or balance often results in the patient shortening his or her step length and may decrease the length of time in stance phase of the affected extremity. Additionally, the patient may tend to shuffle his or her feet to decrease the amount of time in single limb support. A patient using assistive devices or braces may tend to ambulate with a "jerky" motion to advance his or her limb following the assistive device.

Assistive and Adaptive Devices/Orthotic, Protective, and Supportive Devices. Patients with weight-bearing restrictions should be provided with an assistive device, and the device should be checked for correct fit and appropriate use (see Chapter 33). The therapist should note if the patient is safe to use the specific device alone or with a trained individual or family member. If a brace or other protective device is used, note if the fit is appropriate, the alignment is appropriate, and it is functional.

EVALUATION, DIAGNOSIS, AND PROGNOSIS

Most patients who fall into preferred practice pattern 4G: Impaired joint mobility, muscle performance, and range of motion associated with fracture have a history of trauma leading to fracture followed by some type of immobilization.[76] Tests and measures generally reveal decreased strength, decreased ROM, and reduced joint mobility, as well as pain and edema. For those with LE fractures there are also often impairments in gait and balance, and the patient often requires an assistive device for ambulation.

According to the *Guide to Physical Therapist Practice*,[76] the expected range of number of visits per episode of care for a patient with a fracture is between 6 and 18. Where a patient will fall within this range may depend on the type of fracture and how it is managed. Fractures that are immobilized for a long period of time, involve a joint or need surgical correction, and those associated with significant soft tissue injury tend to need more physical therapy. Patient motivation may also affect the required duration of treatment.

The factors that influence prognosis for functional recovery after a fracture may be broadly placed into two categories: (1) extrinsic factors and (2) intrinsic factors. Extrinsic factors are those not under the control of the patient that may lead to delayed healing of the bone or soft tissue, thereby delaying functional return. The following is a list of such extrinsic factors:

Extrinsic factors

Type of fracture
Degree of comminution
Size of the fracture gaps
Accuracy of the reduction
Stability of the fixation
Whether or not the fracture was grafted
Involvement of the articular surface of the joint
Wound healing
Presence of infection
Degree of devitalization/presence of osteoporosis
Patient's age
Events during postoperative care
Amount of surrounding soft tissue damage
Nerve damage
Vascular compromise
Presence of heterotopic ossification
Development of reflex sympathetic dystrophy (RSD)
Medications that interfere with healing
Co-morbidities

Intrinsic factors are factors under the patient's control that may lead to delayed functional recovery. These include the following:

Intrinsic factors

Noncompliance with physician's restrictions
Noncompliance with home exercise program

Noncompliance with wound care management
Poor effort and lack of motivation
Smoking or use of other nicotine products
Poor nutrition[77]

INTERVENTION

There are many intervention strategies and tools that can help a patient achieve optimal return of function following a fracture. In the following section, specific interventions are identified and the reader is provided with evidence-based rationales and a clear explanation of how and when to apply each intervention. It is important to note that all interventions should be directly related to specific functional outcome goals and that these goals should be based on the limitations found during the initial examination and work in conjunction with the specific restrictions set forth by the referring physician (e.g., weight-bearing and ROM limitations).

COMMUNICATION AND DOCUMENTATION

One of the most important aspects of managing the patient with a fracture is communication between the members of the management team: the physician, the PT, the patient, and the caregiver. It is imperative that orders for rehabilitation, especially limitations and/or restrictions be clearly delineated. It is the responsibility of the clinician to request a clarification of orders or any additional material deemed necessary (e.g., radiology report, operative report) before commencing treatment. The therapist should send a copy of the initial evaluation, goals, management plan, and periodic progress reports, including any problems that may have arisen, to the referring physician so that all members of the team have current information about the patient's status.

EXERCISE

Aerobic Conditioning. Most fractures are caused by trauma, and many are associated with co-morbidities, multiple surgical procedures, lengthy hospital stays, and significant decreases in functional mobility. All of these factors contribute to a more sedentary lifestyle. There is little literature evaluating the specific benefits of aerobic exercise for patients with fractures, but one can extrapolate from the benefits for a sedentary population. These include lowering blood pressure, building stronger bones, improving muscle strength, improving flexibility, decreasing anxiety and depression, controlling weight, and improving functional abilities.[78-83]

The American College of Sports Medicine (ACSM) defines aerobic exercise as "any activity that uses large muscle groups, can be maintained continuously, and is rhythmic in nature." Aerobic exercise stresses the cardiovascular system above that which it is taxed at rest and makes it more efficient at delivering oxygenated blood to the working muscles and removing metabolic waste from the body (see Chapter 32). ACSM guidelines for healthy aerobic activity include the following:

Exercise 3-5 days each week
Warm up for 5-10 minutes before aerobic activity
Maintain the exercise intensity for 30-45 minutes
Gradually decrease the intensity of the workout
Stretch to cool down for 5-10 minutes

When designing the aerobic component of an exercise program for a patient recovering from a fracture, one must keep in mind the restrictions placed on the patient by the physician. Given these restrictions, the therapist can be creative in implementing an aerobic conditioning program that matches the patient's current ability and can progress the program in intensity, length, and variety to most closely match the patient's desired functional outcome. Choices of aerobic training may include but are not limited to walking, treadmill jogging or running, stair climbing, elliptical training, stationary biking, dancing, swimming, and using a cross country skiing machine, an upper body ergometer, or a rowing machine.

An example of adapting these activities for a patient with a fracture would be stationary bicycling with only the uninvolved leg (and both arms) for the patient who sustained a LE fracture and may not bear weight on that limb (Fig. 9-9). Additionally, an athlete who sustained a LE stress fracture and is training for a specific competition but has not been cleared for full weight bearing may benefit from body weight–supported treadmill jogging (Fig. 9-10) or by jogging in water, with or without the use of a vest flotation device (Fig. 9-11). If the patient has pain with impact but does not have a weight-bearing restriction, he or she may benefit from cross training on an elliptical trainer. As with all aerobic conditioning programs, it is ideal to alternate the mode of exercise, when possible, to recruit additional muscle groups, overcome plateaus in aerobic capacity, and avoid monotony of endurance training.

Balance, Coordination, and Agility Training. After a period of prolonged immobilization or altered weight-bearing after a fracture, patients may have an abnormal or altered sense of balance. The patient's body must adapt to changes in center of gravity (COG) and must modify pos-

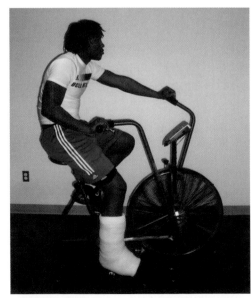

FIG. 9-9 Patient with a lower extremity fracture performing aerobic conditioning on a stationary bike.

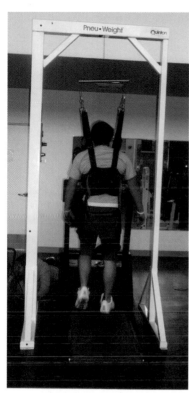

FIG. 9-10 Patient with a lower extremity stress fracture performing aerobic conditioning while partially unweighted using harness and treadmill.

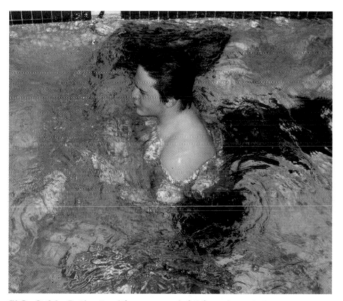

FIG. 9-11 Patient with non–weight-bearing status performing aerobic conditioning in pool with current for resistance and wearing a flotation device.

tural reflex reactions to accommodate these changes. COG may be changed slightly by simple alterations in position such as when the UE is kept in a sling in front of the patient with a clavicle fracture. Conversely, the COG may be altered significantly when an external fixator is applied for a complex tibial fracture, and the patient is required to not bear weight on that lower extremity and must use bilateral axillary crutches.

Additionally, a joint effusion, which is often associated with acute trauma, may contribute to an *arthrogenic muscle inhibition,* whereby swelling in the joint produces an alteration of the afferent somatosensory feedback leading to an abnormal efferent response.[84] This has been well documented in reference to inhibition of the quadriceps muscle after acute effusion of the knee and inhibition of the peroneus longus muscle after acute effusion of the ankle.[85-87] A recent study by Palmieri et al, however, found that injecting 60 cc of sterile saline into healthy knees improved the subject's ability to maintain a one-legged stance.[88] They proposed two possible explanations for their findings. First, their subjects' artificially imposed knee joint effusions did not accompany any structural damage, which would normally be seen with a clinical population presenting with a knee joint effusion. Second, tension within the otherwise healthy knee joint capsule may have enhanced proprioceptive feedback, thereby promoting improved postural control.[88]

Others factor that may contribute to impaired coordination and balance, especially when the task demands significant force output, include disuse atrophy and altered neuromuscular control. If the task is too demanding for the patient to perform, he or she may attempt to recruit compensatory muscles to complete the task, thereby modifying his or her stabilizing posture and counterbalance force.

Most of the research on the effects of balance, coordination, and agility training on functional recovery from fractures has been conducted on elderly patients with hip fractures. In a RCT with 42 subjects from 64 to 94 years of age who were 7 months status-post a fall-related hip fracture, authors found that patients assigned to a daily home exercise program (HEP) consisting of "step-ups" onto a 5- or 10-cm block had a reduced subjective fall risk, stronger quadriceps ($p < 0.01$), and faster walking speed ($p < 0.05$) than a control group who were not assigned a HEP.[89] A more recent study by the same authors found that 4 months of weight-bearing exercises (sit to stand, lateral step-ups, forward step-up and -over, foot tapping, and a stepping grid) improved balance ($p < 0.001$) and functional performance ($p < 0.001$) more than a similar duration of non–weight-bearing exercise (supine hip abduction, hip flexion, heel slides, terminal knee extensions, and ankle dorsiflexion and plantarflexion) or no intervention (control) in a group of 120 subjects (79 ± 9 years) who had completed the usual care after a fall-related hip fracture.[90]

Another RCT was carried out with 57 female geriatric patients (mean age = 82 ± 4.8 years) who were recently admitted to acute care or inpatient rehabilitation with a history of recurrent or injurious falls, including some patients with acute fall-related fractures. The investigators found that patients who participated in a 3-month ambulatory training program that included balance training and progressive resistive exercises performed significantly better on the Tinnetti Performance-Oriented Mobility Assessment (see Chapters 13 and 32) ($p < 0.001$) and the Timed Up-and-Go test (see Chapters 13 and 32) ($p < 0.001$), walked faster ($p < 0.001$), and had stronger quadriceps muscles ($p < 0.001$) than a control group of patients who performed flexibility exercises, calisthenics, ball games, and memory tasks while seated. Additionally, the incidence of falls during the 6 months after the initiation of the program was lower in the ambulatory training group than in the control group (45% versus 60%).[91]

In summary, there is strong evidence to support ongoing functional, weight-bearing group exercise or HEPs for elderly patients with or without cognitive impairments who have sustained fall-related hip fractures. These programs also appear to be cost-effective when weighed against the substantial cost of hospitalizations for injuries sustained from subsequent falls.

Stretching. After immobilization following a fracture, patients often have decreased ROM, joint stiffness, and decreased flexibility of the musculotendinous unit and surrounding fascial layers. There is no literature that specifically addresses flexibility or loss of flexibility in patients with fractures. However, a number of animal studies show that immobilization causes microscopic changes in connective tissue structure. For example, muscle immobilized in a shortened position leads to a decrease in the number of sarcomeres in series, thereby decreasing the muscle's overall length and subsequent flexibility.[92,93] Other animal studies have shown that collagen fibril arrangement in the endomysium changes from a longitudinal arrangement to a more circumferential arrangement after approximately 2-3 weeks of immobilization.[94,95] Since long-term functional limitations are more often complicated by soft tissue dysfunction rather than the actual damage to bone, interventions should address soft tissue restrictions and lack of flexibility in the muscle groups surrounding the fracture site as early as it is safe to do so.

A number of different stretching techniques may be used to increase ROM and flexibility and reduce joint stiffness. These include ballistic, static, and passive stretching as well as techniques based on proprioceptive neuromuscular facilitation (PNF). These techniques are described in Table 9-1.

The evidence evaluating which stretching method to use, the ideal duration of stretching, and the timing of stretching in relationship to a workout to elicit maximal gains in muscle length is contradictory. Possible explanations for these discrepancies may include inadequate controls, lack of baseline measurements, varied training programs, different instruments for measuring flexibility, and utilization of different muscle groups.[96] In regard to

the length of time needed to produce detectable significant changes in muscle length, Bandy and Irion found that a 30-second or 60-second static passive stretch increased hamstring flexibility more than a 15-second stretch or no stretching ($p < 0.05$) in a group of 57 subjects ranging in age from 21 to 37 years, with limited hamstring muscle flexibility (defined as a loss of 30 or more degrees of knee extension with hip flexed 90 degrees).[97] A more recent study of 93 subjects, ranging in age from 21 to 39 years with tight hamstrings (as defined above), by the same group found that hamstring stretching for 30 seconds or 1 minute, 1 or 3 times, 5 days each week for 6 weeks increased hamstring flexibility significantly more than not stretching at all. However, 30-second and 1-minute stretches were equally effective and 3 stretches in a session were no more effective than only 1 stretch in a session.[98] These findings suggest that at least 30 seconds of static stretching per day, 5 times per week for 6 weeks is sufficient to increase hamstring flexibility.

In regard to timing of stretching, the ACSM's guidelines state that muscles, tendons, ligaments, and joints may be "more responsive to stretching after the endurance phase," but data to support this are lacking.[99] A study by Funk et al found that hamstring flexibility was significantly increased if PNF stretching was performed after 60 minutes of exercise ($p < 0.05$) when compared to baseline and without exercise. In this study, there were no differences in hamstring flexibility observed with static stretching across time.[100]

There are no clinical trials to date that demonstrate a correlation between stretching method and functional gains; however, many medical professionals recommend static stretching because it is relatively simple to learn, does not require a partner, and is less likely to exceed the limits of tissue extensibility than a resistive or ballistic style stretch. Additionally, static stretching may facilitate the inhibition of muscle contraction by the Golgi tendon organs (GTO), thereby allowing greater increases in hamstring length.[101]

Proponents of PNF-style stretching argue that it may produce greater gains in flexibility than other types of stretching because autogenic inhibition and reciprocal inhibition allow the muscle to relax more effectively.[102] Others propose that this approach is effective because the tactile cues involved provide a neurologically-enhanced training stimulus.[96] Still others advocate a viscoelastic theory, where increases in flexibility are caused by repeated repositioning of the collagenous and elastin fibers within the connective and contractile tissue.[102] Recent studies have shown that submaximal contractions (with contract-relax PNF programs) are sufficient to produce gains in muscle length.[103] A limitation of PNF-style stretching, however, is that it usually requires a partner to provide resistance and a subsequent stretching force.

Ballistic stretching rapidly stretches the muscle fibers activating the intrafusal muscle spindles and leading to a reflexive and protective muscle contraction of the stretched muscle.[104] This may increase the chance of injury to the muscle or tendon and may cause muscle soreness, especially in sedentary individuals who are not

TABLE 9-1	Stretching Techniques
Technique	**Description**
Ballistic	Quick, repetitive bouncing movements
Static	Slow, sustained stretching
Passive	Slow, sustained stretching by an external force
PNF	Contraction of a lengthened muscle, followed by stretching, either actively or passively; may need the assistance of a partner

PNF, Proprioceptive neuromuscular facilitation.

accustomed to the rapid stretch.[105] In highly trained individuals, however, ballistic stretching rarely causes injury and this type of stretching may actually help prepare the musculotendinous unit for highly explosive activity.

Strengthening. One of the primary complications of fractures is weakness secondary to immobilization, disuse, swelling, pain, or direct muscle trauma. The PT must keep in mind that strengthening exercises may be limited by restrictions in ROM, use of splints or braces, and weight-bearing status. Although the therapist may want to use the most functional approaches for strengthening, he or she should communicate with the surgeon to ensure that sufficient fracture healing has occurred to progress through the stages of strengthening.

Chapter 5 contains general recommendations for interventions to address weakness and impaired muscle performance. However, strengthening interventions may need to be adapted from the standard application because of activity restrictions placed on the patient. For example, for a patient with a tibial fracture and weak quadriceps, during resisted straight leg raises, resistance should be applied at the proximal leg or distal thigh rather than distal to the fracture. Similarly, a patient with a fracture of the distal radius may not be able to use hand-held weights in the initial stages of rehabilitation to strengthen their shoulder girdle but may be able to use an elastic band or tubing applied to the distal humerus to provide appropriate resistance.

Presently, there is no specific evidence in the literature to support the use of any particular mode of exercise, such as isometric, concentric, eccentric, open kinetic chain, or closed kinetic chain, with patients who have sustained fractures. However, a recent study did compare the effects of 6 months of extended physical therapy, consisting of progressive resistance training, with a low-intensity HEP in 90 community dwelling men and women over the age of 65, who had had surgical repair of a proximal femur fracture within the past 4 months. The results indicated that after completion of the program the patients who participated in the intensive exercise had significantly higher levels of physical function, quality of life, and reduced disability as determined by their Physical Performance Score (PPT) ($p < 0.003$) and their Functional Status Questionnaire (FSQ) ($p < 0.01$) as compared to the low-intensity exercise group.[106] These findings suggest that higher intensity strengthening exercises and more hours of therapy may be more effective than low-intensity exercise and less therapy in achieving functional goals for patients with fractures. It is imperative that PTs continue performing research that evaluates the need for aggressive rehabilitation at a time when reimbursement for therapies is limited.

FUNCTIONAL TRAINING

Gait Training. Many patients with LE fractures have gait deviations and may benefit from gait training (see Chapter 32). In patients with fractures, the PT must ensure that the patient has sufficient ROM, strength, balance, and pain control before advancing gait, or they may cause the patient to adopt additional compensatory strategies that may further affect their ability to ambulate. When patients

are recovering from LE fractures, it is common for a physician to advance the patient's weight-bearing status as their healing status progresses. They may start with non-weight bearing (NWB), and advance through toe-touch weight bearing (TTWB), to partial weight bearing (PWB), to full weight bearing as tolerated (WBAT). These restrictions may be based on a number of factors such as the severity of the injury, whether or not the fracture was stabilized, the length of time from the initial injury, and whether or not the bone shares weight-bearing responsibilities (i.e., fibula versus tibia). When a patient is PWB, the surgeon may give specific restrictions regarding percentage of body weight that the patient may apply through his or her affected limb. Many patients have difficulty determining the amount of pressure that is equal to a portion of their body weight, for example, 25% of their body weight. One solution that has been suggested to help remedy this problem is to determine what 25% of their total weight is and have them use a bathroom scale to apply the 25% weight on their affected limb as they gait train (i.e., a 200 lb patient will be allowed to apply 50 lb on the affected limb). This may enable the patient to get a more accurate feeling of what 25% PWB is and provides the patient with direct feedback while practicing within their limitations.

Youdas et al trained 10 healthy subjects in 50% PWB with a variety of assistive devices (axillary crutches, forearm crutches, a wheeled walker, and a single-point cane) utilizing the bathroom scale method. They found that subjects were able to effectively reproduce the 50% reduction in body weight on the tested limb while using axillary crutches or forearm crutches while walking across a forceplate, but they were not able to do so with a wheeled walker or single-point cane.[107] This study has limited applications since it was conducted on a small number of subjects (n = 10) and all of the subjects were healthy.

A study by Dabke et al assessed the ability of 6 healthy volunteers (mean age = 30 yrs) and 23 patients (mean age = 41 yrs) who had sustained a LE fracture or had surgery to their LE to reproduce a specified weight-bearing force while walking across a force plate. These individuals had been trained to apply the designated amount of force on their affected limb on a bathroom scale a few days earlier. The authors found that 4 of 6 volunteers and 21 of 23 patients exerted significantly more force ($p < 0.001$) than they had been trained to do (on average 27% and 35% of body weight more than prescribed, respectively). They concluded that the subjects were unreliable in their ability to reproduce the "allowable" forces, thus they were unable to comply with the physician's guidelines.[108] One difficulty with this type of study is that subjects were trained statically by standing and pushing their affected limb down onto the scale for training, but they were tested dynamically as they ambulated across the force plate. Another criticism of the method is that it is difficult for patients to gait train while they are looking down at a moving dial on a bathroom-type scale.

A study by Li et al found that modifying the percentage of body weight practiced during the training period affected the outcome in 12 healthy subjects who were trained with the bathroom scale method in 3-point gait utilizing 10%, 50%, and 90% of their body weight. The authors found that subjects were more consistent with placing 50% of their body weight during level walking than either the 10% or 90%.[109] In a true clinical setting, however, it is rare that a physician will give either 10% or 90% weight-bearing restrictions. Despite the number of limitations of the bathroom scale method in providing feedback for PWB training, it is presently the best readily available tool to assist patients in complying with weight-bearing restrictions.

Assistive Devices. Following a fracture, a patient is usually immobilized or has other restrictions placed on him or her by the surgeon to allow proper healing. These restrictions, combined with pain, swelling, and weakness will often prevent the patient from independently performing activities of daily living (ADLs) or from participating in independent ADLs (IADLs). With an UE fracture involving the wrist or hand, the patient loses the ability to perform even simple tasks that require two hands. Similarly, if a patient has a LE fracture and cannot bear full weight on his or her extremity, the patient will need to use an assistive device for mobility, which may further encumber the use of the upper extremities. This patient may now need to use a backpack or other type of carrier to carry his or her belongings. There are numerous assistive devices to aide patients who are recovering from fractures with resuming ADLs and IADLs. These range from wheelchairs, walkers, and crutches to assist with mobility to reachers that enable a person to grasp something is placed beyond their reach (see Chapter 33 for more information on assistive devices).

Injury Prevention. Throughout the rehabilitation process, the therapist should reevaluate the patient's ability to safely negotiate his or her environment. If a patient does not have the strength, balance, or cognitive ability to safely move in his or her environment before discharge from the hospital, the therapist should contact social services to ensure that services are brought into the home and that a plan for follow-up is in place.

Since fractures occur when external forces exceed the inherent strength of the bone, the focus of fracture prevention has been on improving bone density (with osteoporotic patients) and with reducing the incidence of falls (via balance, agility, strength training, and education programs) (see Chapters 3 and 13).

MANUAL THERAPY

Passive Range of Motion. Physical therapy should focus on the restoration of ROM once sufficient healing or stable fixation has occurred. Early motion will help to decrease the incidence of adhesions, decrease atrophy of articular cartilage, and help prevent capsular or ligamentous contractures.[110,111] If the patient does not have sufficient strength to perform active ROM exercises, the therapist may want to begin with PROM activities.

PROM is the amount of motion that is produced solely by an external force, without any active muscle contraction. The external force may be applied by the clinician, gravity, or an external device. If the patient is hesitant to move the extremity, the therapist may want to begin by manually moving the patient's joint into the allowed ROM while the patient lies in a relaxed position. The therapist can maintain the joint in the end-range position briefly and then slowly return the joint back to its resting position. When performing manual PROM on a patient, it is important for the therapist to provide gentle but firm contact with the patient's extremity at all times. In order to relax, the patient must trust that the therapist will not make any sudden moves or push into a region of pain. If the patient is fearful, he or she will tend to muscle guard and block motion from occurring.

The therapist can also teach patients how to use gravity and their opposing limb to independently perform PROM as a part of their HEP. For example, while performing supine wall slides to increase knee flexion ROM, patients can be instructed to use gravity to allow their heel to slide down the wall, thereby flexing the knee. After a brief holding period in the flexed position, patients can use the opposite LE to push the heel up the wall and assist the knee back into extension. Similarly, to obtain terminal knee extension, patients can be taught to lie prone with their knee hanging off the edge of a bed. Gravity will produce a force on the lower leg to help achieve terminal knee extension.

A more technical device that has been developed to assist with PROM is the continuous passive motion (CPM) machine. CPM machines are electrically powered devices that provide a slow and controlled passive mechanical force to move a joint through a prescribed or preset ROM. The clinician is able to control the ROM, as well as the speed of motion (Fig. 9-12) Although many physicians continue to prescribe CPM machines after LE surgical procedures, the literature shows mixed results in terms of both short- and long-term benefits.[112,113] A meta-analysis on the efficacy of CPM after total knee arthroplasty (TKA) was conducted in 2004. The authors reviewed 178 articles, 14 of which met their inclusion criteria, and results were pooled whenever possible. Their goal was to compare the benefits of CPM and physical therapy with the benefits of physical therapy alone after TKA. They found that those patients who received physical therapy and CPM had greater knee flexion ROM and used less analgesic medication 2 weeks after surgery, and they had significantly shorter lengths of stay in the hospital. However, they also found that the use of CPM did not significantly improve

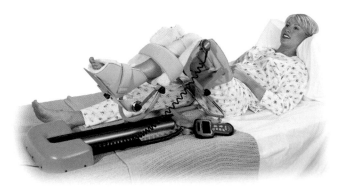

FIG. 9-12 Continuous passive motion. *Photo courtesy Chattanooga Group.*

passive knee flexion at the end of treatment or at 6-week, 3-month, and 6-month follow-up.[114] This study did not evaluate other long-term effects or functional outcomes. Future studies should address long-term functional benefits and should weigh the benefits against the cost of using this form of PROM.

Joint Mobilization and Manipulation. After prolonged immobilization, it is not uncommon for the joints surrounding a fracture site to become stiff. A number of animal studies have shown that a variety of factors contribute to joint stiffness after immobilization. These include proliferation of intraarticular connective tissue and its adhesion to cartilage,[115-118] increased cross-linking between the collagen fibrils and ground substance or decreased lubrication between collagen fibrils;[110,119-121] and adaptive shortening of the capsule.[122,123] If joint hypomobility after immobilization is not addressed, the joint may remain dysfunctional and may alter the biomechanics and integrity of other joints above or below the injured site. For example, patients who sustain a LE fracture may develop back pain because reduced LE joint motion places abnormal biomechanical forces on the spine.

To combat the detrimental effects of immobilization, therapists will often perform joint mobilizations. Joint mobilizations are manual therapy techniques that involve passively moving one articular surface across another. A search of the Medline and CINAHL databases between the years 1950 and 2006 using the key words joint mobilization, benefits, fracture, and function revealed no peer-reviewed articles that assessed the use of joint mobilization to improve ROM or functional outcome after immobilization or fracture. Clinically, however, joint mobilizations have been found to help restore arthrokinematics, improve osteokinematics, decrease muscle spasms, and relieve pain.

Maitland[124] identified the following five grades of mobilization, which vary in the amplitude of oscillation, from the beginning point in the ROM through the point of limitation of motion:

Grade I: Small amplitude oscillation at the beginning of the ROM.

Grade II: Large amplitude oscillation within the midrange of available motion.

Grade III: Large amplitude oscillation up to the point of limitation of joint motion.

Grade IV: Small amplitude oscillation at the end of the point of limitation of joint motion.

Grade V: Small amplitude quick-thrust manipulation initiated at the point of limitation of joint motion.

The grade of the mobilization depends on the specific goal of the treatment. In general, grades I and II are used to reduce pain and muscle spasm, and grades III and IV reduce stiffness. Rhythmic oscillations may be used to stimulate joint mechanoreceptors in an attempt to decrease the transmission of pain to the brain.[124]

Even though performing mobilizations in grades I to IV is not aggressive or invasive, the therapist should clear the patient of any contraindications before commencing treatment. These include inflammatory arthritis, malignancy, bone disease, joint instability, congenital bone deformities, and vascular disorders that may be compromised with joint mobilization. Additionally, one must be certain that the fracture has healed sufficiently to allow for forces to be applied across the fracture site. If there is any uncertainty or if the patient has any pain during or after mobilization, the technique should be delayed.

ELECTROTHERAPEUTIC MODALITIES

Electrotherapeutic modalities may be used to control pain or edema associated with a fracture, facilitate specific muscle strengthening, and perhaps most importantly with fracture patients, improve tissue healing. It is important to note that the successful use of modalities to produce the desired outcome depends on the appropriate selection and application of modality variables. Continued research is needed in this field to further define which treatment variables produce the best results.

Electrical Stimulation to Control Pain. Pain is the most common symptom associated with fractures. Clinicians debate which method most effectively controls pain with the fewest side effects. Transcutaneous electrical nerve stimulation (TENS) is one of the primary electrotherapeutic modalities that can relieve pain. A few benefits of the use of TENS over other methods of pain management are that it is noninvasive and well tolerated by most patients. TENS is thought to decrease pain, according to the gate theory of pain control, by selectively stimulating A-beta nerve fibers, thereby interfering with the transmission of noxious stimuli from the periphery to the brain via small myelinated A-delta nerve fibers and small unmyelinated C nerve fibers.

Conventional TENS (with a pulse frequency of 100 to 150 pps, a pulse duration of 50-80 µsec, and an intensity above sensory but below motor threshold) has been found to be comfortable and effective in decreasing pain.[125-127] TENS has also been found to cause a release of endorphins in the spinal cord.[128] Motor level electrical stimulation with a low pulse frequency of less than 10 pps has been found to stimulate the production of endogenous opiates, which have also been found to decrease one's perception of pain.[129,130]

Most of the research studying the use of TENS on patients with fractures has been performed on patients with rib fractures secondary to blunt chest trauma. These patients experience a considerable amount of pain, which if not adequately controlled, may lead to atelectasis, alveolar collapse, ventilation-perfusion mismatch, and respiratory distress.[131] All of these conditions will contribute to more extensive injury and a longer hospital stay.

An early study on the effectiveness of TENS for pain relief after rib fracture in 24 consecutive patients (mean age = 55.3 years, range = 18 to 85 years) who were randomly allocated to either a TENS group or a NSAID group (Naproxen sodium 250 mg 3 times a day) found that patients in the TENS group had less of a drop in their arterial oxygen level ($p < 0.01$), a greater increase in the peak expiratory flow rates (PEFR; $p = 0.025$; indicating better breathing), and more effective and continuous pain relief as measured on a visual analog scale (VAS; $p < 0.01$ for both scores).[132]

A larger, more recent study involved 100 consecutive patients admitted to an emergency service with minor rib fractures (defined as less than four fractured ribs, without flail chest or fractures to the first or second ribs) randomly allocated to one of four groups. Group 1 received 275 mg oral Naproxen sodium 4 times a day for 3 days. Group 2 received TENS (80 Hz, 12 mA, 50 µs) for 30 minutes, 2 times a day. Group 3 received 275 mg oral Naproxen sodium 4 times a day for 3 days, as well as inactive TENS unit applied for 30 minutes, 2 times a day. Group 4 received placebo tablets 4 times a day for 3 days. All patients were asked to rate their pain on a 0-10 VAS on admission ("Day 0"), as well as the day after admission, just before discharge ("Day 1") and on the third day after treatment had been completed ("Day 3"). Results indicated that on the third day, the active TENS group had less pain than the other three groups ($p < 0.05$), who did not differ significantly from each other.[133]

This study suggests that TENS can be an effective means of managing pain after minor rib fractures. TENS also avoids the complications of sedation, nausea and vomiting, constipation, and respiratory depression, as well as platelet and renal dysfunction associated with the use of narcotics and NSAIDs.[131] More clinical trials are needed to evaluate the effect of TENS on pain associated with other types of fractures.

Electrical Stimulation. Monophasic pulsed electrical current, particularly high voltage pulsed current (HVPC), has been studied for its effects on edema formation after trauma. A number of animal studies have shown stimulation with the negative pole at a submotor level to reduce the formation of edema.[134-136] Proposed mechanisms for this effect include repelling negatively charged ions and cells from the area of inflammation and decreasing the permeability of the microvascular membrane.[137] Additionally, when electrical stimulation produces muscle contractions, these contractions may reduce edema by improving lymphatic and venous return. One human subjects study compared the effects of HVPC, intermittent pneumatic compression (IPC), and a placebo treatment on the reduction of posttraumatic hand edema but found no significant difference between the HVPC group and the placebo group.[138] There is no specific evidence to date that supports the use of electrical stimulation to decrease edema or inflammation in patients with fractures.

Electrical Stimulation to Improve Strength. Neuromuscular electrical stimulation (NMES) is often used clinically as an adjunct to strengthening exercises and to retard the effects of disuse atrophy. Most studies in this area involve postoperative LE injuries, including anterior cruciate ligament (ACL) reconstructions, meniscectomies, lateral releases, and TKA.[139-146] The effect of this intervention is based on the fact that electrical stimulation can produce strong muscle contractions and that strong muscle contractions can increase strength, according to the overload principle. It is assumed that this increased strength will then translate to an increase in function. There are no high quality studies on the use of NMES for increasing muscle strength in patients with fractures. One recent RCT with 12 women over 75 years of age with a hip fracture did attempt to evaluate the effect of electrical stimulation on function and strength by stimulating the quadriceps muscle but found little effect.[147] However, since

they set the current intensity at the minimum level that produced a visible muscle contraction, a strengthening effect would not be expected. See Chapter 5 for information on optimal use of electrical stimulation for muscle strengthening.

Electrical Stimulation to Promote Fracture Healing. Since the 1950s researchers have been interested in finding biological applications for electricity, especially as it pertains to the healing of fractures. Of particular interest is the potential benefit for improved fracture healing with nonunions, which account for approximately 5% to 10% of all fractures in the United States annually.[148,149] In the laboratory, electromagnetic fields have been found to stimulate the biological processes involved in osteogenesis via stimulation of extracellular matrix synthesis, increases in proteoglycan and collagen synthesis, and inhibition of osteoclastic bone resorption.[150-152]

Currently, there are three clinical methods to deliver electrical stimulation to bone. The first method involves the application of direct current (DC) directly to the fracture site using percutaneous or surgically implanted electrodes. Since this invasive procedure is beyond the scope of physical therapy practice, this section will focus on two noninvasive techniques, capacitive coupling and pulsed electromagnetic fields. Capacitive coupling (CC) uses external electrodes applied to the skin with conductive gel to produce an electrical field at the fracture site. Pulsed electromagnetic fields (PEMF), or inductive coupling (IC), uses electromagnetic coils placed over the fracture site without contact with the skin. These can be secured to the outside of a cast.

Simonis et al performed a prospective, randomized, double-blind clinical trial examining the effects of PEMF versus "dummy" treatment on 34 tibial fractures that were "un-united" at least 1 year after the initial fracture and had no metal implant bridging the fracture gap and no radiological progression of healing within the 3 months before initiation of the study. Each patient received an oblique fibular osteotomy followed by the application of an external fixator. The patients were randomly assigned to receive PEMF with 3-ms pulses and a 40-ms interval between pulses, peak current of 6 A at 150 V passed through the active coils. An identical electrical device was applied to the "dummy group," but the electrical current passed through a small secondary coil, which was not in contact with the patient's body so that no current was passed around the fracture and no electromagnetic field was produced. Each group wore the device for 14 hours a day for 6 months. The fractures were considered to be healed if there was a loss of distinction at the fracture gap, evidence of cortical bridging, or evidence of trabecular bridging on radiographs. The authors found that there was a statistically significant correlation between tibial union and PEMF use ($p = 0.02$). In the active group, 16 of 18 fractures healed, whereas in the dummy group only 8 of 16 fractures healed. A flaw of this study was that there were more smokers in the dummy group than in the PEMF group. After adjusting for smoking status, the effect was weaker and no longer statistically significant ($p = 0.07$).[153]

Linovitz et al conducted a similar prospective, randomized, double-blind, placebo-controlled trial to study the effects of magnetic fields on the healing of primary noninstrumented posterolateral lumbar spine fusions.[154] Patients with one- or two-level fusions between L3 and S1 with either autograft or a combination of autograft and allograft were randomized into a treatment group (a single posterior coil centered over the fusion site providing a magnetic field 30 minutes a day for 9 months) or a placebo group. 201/243 patients were evaluated at 3, 6, and 9 months postoperatively, and 3 months after completing the study. There was a statistically significant increase in rate of fusion ($p = 0.003$ by Fisher's exact test) in the treated group with 64% of the patients in this group demonstrating radiographic fusion at 9 months compared to 43% of the patients in the placebo group. Interestingly, when the investigators stratified the results by gender, women in the treatment group demonstrated a statistically significant improvement in fusion rate over women in the placebo group but there was no significant difference in healing between groups in the male patients. The investigators did not report whether there was an interaction between age and gender or multiple levels of fusion and gender, which may help to explain the difference found between genders.

PEMF has also been found to improve healing after other bone procedures including femoral intertrochanteric osteotomies[155] and tibial osteotomies.[156,157] A meta-analysis to examine the role of electrical and electromagnetic stimulation on bone healing was conducted in 2002.[158] The authors found 20 studies that assessed the effect of electrical stimulation (primarily PEMF) on healing. Patients with a wide range of diagnoses were included in this study. They included Perthes disease, aseptic necrosis of the femoral head, nonunion or delayed union in long bones, spinal fusion, leg lengthening procedures, Charcot joints, and fresh fractures. Of the 20 RCTs, 15 trials supported the effectiveness of electrical stimulation and five failed to show clinical significance. The authors acknowledged that many of the studies that failed to show significance had methodological limitations and concluded that overall, one could not overlook the positive findings associating electrical stimulation with tissue repair. Again, more RCTs need to be performed with specific fracture populations.

PHYSICAL AND MECHANICAL AGENTS

Ultrasound. Ultrasound (US) is a form of mechanical energy that can be transmitted through biological tissues, via a piezoelectric crystal, as high frequency acoustical pressure waves. PTs have used US for its thermal, as well as nonthermal, effects on soft tissues (muscles, tendons, ligaments, joint capsules, and so on) for many years. Use of US as a modality in patients with fractures, however, has been negligible in the physical therapy community because it was previously thought to be contraindicated in the area of a healing fracture.[159] However, recent evidence shows that low-intensity pulsed US (LIPUS) can promote fracture healing. The FDA cleared the use of LIPUS for accelerating fresh fracture healing in October 1994 and for the treatment of established nonunions in February 2000. The FDA-approved device used in clinical trials is the EXOGEN 2000+. The

TABLE 9-2	Exogen 2000+ LIPUS Parameters
Parameters	**Exogen 2000+**
Time	20 minutes
SATA intensity	30 mW/cm²
SATP intensity	0.16 W/cm²
Frequency	1.5 MHz
Duty cycle	20% pulsed

SATA, Space average temporal average; *SATP,* space average temporal peak.

parameters are preset within this unit and are listed in Table 9-2.

There are a number of proposed mechanisms for the effectiveness of LIPUS on delayed union or nonunion fractures. These include influences on gene expression at all stages of healing, increasing blood vessel formation at the site of the clot, increasing growth factor release, increasing synthesis of cartilage matrix proteins by chondrocytes, increasing cartilage formation at the fracture callus, increasing the progression of bridging at the bone gap, and increasing blood flow at the fracture site during and shortly after the US stimulus has been removed.[160-165]

Nolte et al conducted a study to determine the effects of LIPUS on 29 nonunion fractures in various parts of the body. All patients had no evidence of healing by x-ray within the 3 months before enrolling in the study. They were treated for 20 minutes per day until the surgeon determined that the fracture was healed (3 of 4 cortices were bridged). The results indicated that 25 of 29 nonunions went on to heal ($p < 0.0001$) with average healing time of 152 days.[166]

Another clinical trial randomly assigned 67 subjects with open or closed fresh tibial fractures to either the treatment group (LIPUS) or the control group (sham). There was a significant decrease in time to clinical healing 86 ± 5.8 days for the treatment group as compared to 114 ± 10.4 days for the sham group ($p = 0.01$). Similarly, x-rays showed a significant decrease in radiologic healing time 96 ± 4.9 days for the treatment group as compared to 154 ± 13.7 days for the control group ($p = 0.0001$).[167]

Kristiansen et al also looked at the healing rate of 60 fresh dorsally angulated distal radius fractures. Patients were randomly assigned to the treatment group (LIPUS plus cast and splint) or the control group (sham plus cast and splint). All subjects received the intervention daily for 10 weeks starting within 7 days of the fracture. Healing, as determined by x-ray, was statistically faster in the treatment group (61 ± 3.4 days) than in the control group (98 ± 5.2 days) ($p < 0.0001$).[165]

Mayr et al assessed the effects of LIPUS on the healing rate of 30 acute nondisplaced scaphoid fractures. They found that healing, as determined by computed tomography (CT) scan, averaged 43 days in the treatment group, compared with 62 days in the control group.[168] These studies show that LIPUS may improve the healing of fresh fractures, as well as delayed union or nonunion fractures, at a variety of sites throughout the body. More research is needed to assess the effects of LIPUS on stress fractures.

CASE STUDY 9-1

COLLES' FRACTURE

Examination
Patient History
JT is a 35-year-old right-hand dominant cafeteria worker who sustained a Colles' fracture to her right UE (RUE) 6 weeks ago after tripping and falling onto an outstretched arm. She was treated conservatively with a cast, which was removed yesterday, and she is now being referred to physical therapy for initial evaluation and rehabilitation. JT enjoys cooking, playing the piano, and doing arts and crafts with her children. She reports no pain at rest but has a dull ache, rated as 4/10 pain, with attempts to move her wrist. She reports that her wrist gets sore and tired after attempting to eat a few bites with her fork in her right hand. She would like to return to work and hobbies as soon as possible. JT's past medical history is significant for a 4-year history of cigarette smoking, but JT reports that she stopped smoking before having her children.

Tests and Measures
Musculoskeletal
Anthropometric Characteristics Significant atrophy of right forearm musculature (both flexors and extensors). No swelling. Visible callous formation on the dorsal aspect of the radius, 2 inches proximal to the joint line.

Range of Motion AROM of right wrist: Flexion = 45 degrees, extension = 30 degrees, radial deviation = 5 degrees, ulnar deviation = 8 degrees. JT has difficulty opposing her thumb to her fifth finger.

Muscle Performance Grip strength with hand-held dynamometer on 3 trials is 14 psi, 16 psi, 17 psi at position 3. MMT to right wrist is grossly 3+/5 within her available range.

Joint Integrity and Mobility Decreased joint mobility to anterior to posterior and posterior to anterior glides at the radiocarpal and intercarpal joints.

Neuromuscular
Sensory Integrity Sensation is intact to light touch on the entire RUE

Motor Function—Control and Learning Mildly decreased coordination and dexterity with quick finger opposition.

Function: JT reports that she cannot dry her hair, tie her child's shoe laces, write down telephone messages, or prepare dinner for her family. In addition, to return to work she needs to be able to use a large chef's knife, twist a can opener, and lift and carry 15-20 lb trays of cafeteria food.

Evaluation, Diagnosis, and Prognosis
JT has decreased ROM and significant muscle atrophy and associated loss of strength and endurance. The impairments have resulted in a decreased ability to care for herself and her children. In addition, she is unable to work because she must rely heavily on her dominant hand for chopping, mixing, and carrying large trays of food to return to work. JT's diagnosis is preferred practice pattern 4G: Impaired joint mobility, muscle performance, and ROM associated with fracture.

Goals
At the end of her physical therapy sessions (likely 10-12 visits), JT will have full ROM in her wrist and hand. She will have no residual swelling. She will have 4+/5 strength throughout her RUE as compared to her left. Although she may continue to have a callus formation around her fracture site, her radius will be well-healed. She will be independent with all ADLs and will be able to care for her husband and children. She will be able to return to work in limited capacity at first and will wean into full capacity.

Plan of Care
JT will begin outpatient physical therapy 3 times per week for 2 weeks, then 2 times per week for an additional 2 weeks. At that time she will be assessed for discharge to a HEP.

Intervention
1. JT will receive joint mobilizations to the radiocarpal and intercarpal joints to improve joint mobility.
2. JT will apply static stretches to increase ROM.
3. JT will begin strengthening exercises for her entire RUE, including her shoulder girdle, elbow, wrist, and hand intrinsics to increase both static and dynamic strength.
4. JT will do manual dexterity exercises with her right hand to improve her coordination.
5. JT will also do functional training to mimic the activities that she will have to do for 6-8 hours per day to prepare her for her return to work. These activities may include knife skills, stirring a pot and carrying trays with gradually increasing weight back and forth from a makeshift countertop to a makeshift oven or refrigerator.
6. JT will apply ice after therapy to decrease the risk of pain or swelling following exercise and mobilization.

Please see the CD that accompanies this book for a case study describing the examination, evaluation and interventions for a patient with a delayed union fracture.

CHAPTER SUMMARY

A fracture is a break in a bone. The many different types of fractures are categorized based primarily on their location and the mechanism of injury. Fractures may initially be treated with immobilization and in many cases, surgical fixation, to promote healing. After a thorough examination of a patient with a fracture, the PT should carefully consider all of the findings to develop an appropriate comprehensive plan to address the deficits found. Interventions, including exercise, PROM, joint mobilization, and various physical agent modalities, may accelerate and enhance the functional recovery from fractures and in some cases, accelerate fracture healing.

ADDITIONAL RESOURCES

Journal

The Journal of Bone and Joint Surgery

Books

Bucholz RW, Heckman JD (eds): *Rockwood and Green's Fractures in Adults*, ed 5, Philadelphia, 2001, Lippincott.

Buckwalter JA, Einhorn TA, Simon SR (eds): *Orthopaedic Basic Science: Biology and Biomechanics of the Musculoskeletal System*, ed 2, Chicago, 2000, American Academy of Orthopedic Surgeons.

Schatzker J, Tile M: *The Rationale of Operative Fracture Care*, ed 2, New York, 1996, Springer.

Web Site

American Academy of Orthopedic Surgeons: www.aaos.org

GLOSSARY

Accessory bone: Supernumerary bones that develop when secondary ossification centers appear and form extra bones. Such bones are commonly seen in the foot and are often mistaken for fractures.

Arthrogenic muscle inhibition: Reflex inhibition of a muscle secondary to an acute joint effusion.

Avulsion fractures: Fractures caused by a tendon or ligament pulling off a small piece of bone to which it is attached.

Boxer's fracture: A fracture of fourth and/or fifth metacarpal often seen after the patient strikes an object or person.

Callus: A combination of cartilage, bone and fibrous tissue that fills and surrounds the fracture site during the process of fracture healing.

Cancellous bone: Spongy bone.

Closed fracture: A fracture without a break in the overlying skin.

Colles' fracture: A metaphyseal fracture of the distal radius that is dorsally angulated.

Comminuted fracture: A fracture that forms more than two pieces of bone.

Compression fracture: A fracture in which cancellous bone collapses and compresses on itself. Typically this occurs in the vertebral bodies.

Cortical bone: The dense outer layer of bone.

Delayed union: Progression of healing of a fracture that is slower than average.

Diaphysis: The central tubular portion of a long bone.

Epiphysis: The end of a long bone.

Epiphyseal growth plate: A horizontal growth plate located at the ends of immature long bones.

Fracture: A break in a bone.

Greenstick fracture: A fracture through only one side of a bone. These fractures are common in children.

Heterotopic bone: Abnormal bone formation within a tendon, muscle, or joint.

Impaction fracture: A fracture in which a bony fragment, generally cortical, is forced or impacted into cancellous bone. Typically this occurs at the ends of long bones.

Irregularly-shaped bones: Bones such as those in the jaw or the spinal column that are of various shapes—examples of which are the mandible and the vertebrae.

Linear fracture: A fracture that runs parallel to the long axis of a bone.

Long bones: Tubular shaped bones.

Malunions: Fractures that have united with angulation or rotation to a degree that gives a displeasing appearance or adversely affects function.

Metaphysis: The part of a long bone between the diaphysis and the epiphysis where the bone starts to widen.

Nonunion: The failure of a fracture to heal.

Oblique fracture: A fracture at approximately 30 degrees to the long axis of the bone.

Open fracture: A fracture in which the skin is broken exposing the fracture site to the external environment.

Osteomyelitis: Inflammation of the bone caused by a pathological organism.

Pseudoarthrosis: A false joint that develops at the site of a fracture

Sesamoid bone: A bone within a tendon.

Stress fracture: A fracture caused by repeated, prolonged, or abnormal stress.

Torus fracture: A fracture that warps but does not completely break one side of the cortex of the bone, also known as a buckle fracture. This fracture is most commonly seen in children.

Transverse fracture: A fracture perpendicular to the long axis of the bone.

References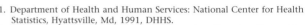

1. Department of Health and Human Services: National Center for Health Statistics, Hyattsville, Md, 1991, DHHS.
2. http://www.aaos.org/wordhtml/research/stats/top5hosp.htm#hospvis1
3. Mehta AJ: An introduction. In Mehta AJ (ed): Rehabilitation of Fractures. Physical medicine and rehabilitation state of the art reviews, *Phys Med Rehabil* 9:1-11, 1995.
4. Kellie SE, Brody JA: Sex specific and race-specific hip fracture rates, *Am J Public Health* 80:326-328, 1990.
5. Jette AM, Harris BA, Cleary PD, et al: Functional recovery after hip fracture. *Arch Phys Med Rehabil* 68:735-740, 1987.
6. Daffner RH: Stress fractures: Current concepts, *Am J Radiology* 159:245-252, 1992.
7. Greaney RB, Gerber FH, Laughlan RL: Distribution and natural history of stress fractures in US marine recruits, *Radiology* 146:339-346, 1983.
8. Milgrom C, Giladi M, Chisin R, et al: The long term followup of soldiers with stress fractures, *Am J Sports Med* 13:398-400, 1985.
9. Pester S, Smith PC: Stress fractures in the lower extremity of soldiers in basic training, *Orthop Rev* 21:297-303, 1992.
10. Lappe JM, Stegman MR, Recker RR: The impact of lifestyle factors on stress fractures in female army recruits, *Osteoporos Int* 12:35-42, 2001.
11. Beals RK, Cook RD: Stress fractures of the anterior tibial diaphysis, *Orthopedics* 14:869-875, 1991.
12. Childers RL, Meyers DH, Turner PR: Lesser metatarsal stress fractures: A study of 37 cases, *Clin Podiatr Med Surg* 7:633-644, 1990.
13. Bennell, KL, Brukner PD: Epidemiology and site specificity of stress fractures, *Clin Sport Med* 16:179-196, 1997.
14. Kim SM, Park CH, Gartland JJ: Stress fracture of the pubic ramus in a swimmer, *Clin Nuc Med* 12:118-119, 1987.
15. Thorne DA, Deltz FL: Pelvic stress fracture in female runners, *Clin Nuc Med* 11:828-829, 1986.
16. Wilson ES, Katz FN: Stress fractures: An analysis of 250 consecutive cases. *Radiology* 92:481-486, 1969.
17. Bellah RD, Summerville DA, Treves ST, et al: Low back pain in adolescent athletes: Detection of stress injury to the pars interarticularis with SPECT, *Radiology* 180:509-512, 1991.
18. Letts M, Smallman T, Afanasiev R, et al: Fracture of the pars interarticularis in adolescent athletes: a clinical—biomechanical analysis, *J Pediatr Orhtop* 6:40-46, 1986.
19. Gustillo RB, Anderson JT: Prevention of infection in the treatment of one thousand and twenty five open fractures of long bones: Retrospective and prospective analyses, *J Bone Joint Surg* 58A:453-458, 1976.
20. Gustillo RB, Gruninger RP, Davis T: Classification of Type III (severe) Open Fractures relative to treatment and results, *Orthopedics* 10:1781-1788, 1987.
21. National Osteoporosis Foundation: Important disease facts (web site), http://www.nof.org/osteoporosis/index.htm
22. National Osteoporosis Foundation: Fast facts: Disease statistics (web site), http://www.nof.org/osteoporosis/diseasefacts.htm
23. Griffin LY, Garrick JG (eds): Women's musculoskeletal health: Update for the new millennium, *Clin Orthop Relat Res* 372:3-22, 2000.
24. Baron JA, Karagas M, Barrett J, et al: Basic epidemiology of fractures of the upper and lower limbs among Americans over 65 years of age, *Epidemiology* 7:612-618, 1996.
25. Riggs B, Melton L (eds): *Osteoporosis: Etiology, Diagnosis and Management*, ed 2, New York, 1995, Press.
26. Riggs BL, Melton LJ: The world wide problem of osteoporosis: insights afforded by epidemiology. *Bone* 15:505-511S, 1995.
27. Lenchik L, Sartoris DJ: Current concepts in osteoporosis, *AJR Am J Roentgenol* 168:905-911, 1997.
28. Parkkari J, Kannus P, Palvenen M, et al: Majority of hip fractures occur as a result of a fall and impact on the greater trochanter of the femur: A prospective controlled study with 206 consecutive patients, *Calcif Tissue Int* 65(3):183-187, 1999.
29. National Institutes of Health (NIH) Consensus Statement: *Osteoporosis, Prevention, Diagnosis, and Therapy*, Bethesda, Md, 2000, The Institutes.
30. Goodman CC, Randall T: Musculoskeletal neoplasms. In Goodman CC, Fuller KS, Boissonnault WG (eds): *Pathology: Implications for the Physical Therapist*, ed 2, Philadelphia, 2003, WB Saunders.

31. Schenk R, Willenegger H: Zum histolgischen Bild der sogenannten Primarheilung der Knockenkompaakta nach experimentellen Osteotomien am Hund, *Experimenta* 19:593, 1963.
32. Heppenstell RB: Fracture healing. In Heppenstall RB (ed): *Fracture Treatment and Healing,* Philadelphia, 1980, WB Saunders.
33. Day SM, Ostrum RF, Chao EYS: Bone injury, regeneration and repair. In Buckwalter JA, Einhorn TA, Simons SR (eds): *Orthopedic Basic Science: Biology and Biomechanics of the Musculoskeletal System,* Chicago, 2000, American Academy of Orthopedic Surgeons.
34. Wood GW: General principles of fracture treatment. In Calane ST (eds): *Campbells Operative Orthopaedics,* ed 10, St. Louis, 2004, Mosby.
35. Panjabi MM, Walter SD, Karuda M, et al: Correlations of radiographic analysis of healing fractures with strength: A statistical analysis of experimental osteotomies, *J Orthop Res* 3:212-218, 1985.
36. Mckibbin B: The biology of fracture healing in long bones, *J Bone Joint Surg Br* 60:150-162, 1978.
37. Grundnes O, Reikerras O: The importance of the hematoma for fracture healing in rats, *Acta Orthop Scand* 64:340-342, 1993.
38. Grundnes O, Reikeras O: The role of the hematoma and periosteal sealing for fracture healing in rats, *Acta Orthop Scand* 64:47-49, 1993.
39. Einhorn TA, Bennarens F, Burstein AH: The contributions of dietary protein and mineral to the healing of experimental fractures. A biomechanical study, *J Bone Joint Surg Am* 68:1389-1395, 1996.
40. White AA, Panjabi MM, Southwick WO: The four biomechanical stages of fracture repair, *J Bone Joint Surg* 59:188-189, 1977.
41. Wiel HE, Lips P, Nauta J, et al: Loss of bone in the proximal part of the femur following unstable fractures of the leg, *J Bone Joint Surg Am* 76A:230-236, 1994.
42. Day SM, Ostrum RE, Chao EYS, et al: Bone injury regeneration and repair. In Buckwalter JA, Einhorn TA, Simon SR (eds): *Orthopedic Basic Science: Biology and biomechanics of the Musculoskeletal System,* Chicago, 2000, American Academy of Orthopaedic Surgeons.
43. Herbsman H, Powers JC, Hirschman A, et al: Retardation of fracture healing in experimental diabetes, *J Surg Res* 8:424-431, 1968.
44. De Vernejoul MC, Bielakoff J, Herve M, et al: Evidence for defective osteoblastic function. A role for alcohol and tobacco consumption in osteoporosis in middle-aged men, *Clin Orthop Relat Res* 179:107-115, 1983.
45. Daftari TK, Whitesides TE, Hellen JG, et al: Nicotine on the revascularization of bone graft: An experimental study in rabbits, *Spine* 19:904-911, 1994.
46. Ueng SWN, Lin SS, Wang CR, et al: Bone healing of tibial lengthening is delayed by cigarette moking: study of bone mineral density and torsional strength of rabbits, *J Trauma* 46:110-115, 1999.
47. McKee MD, DiPasqualle DJ, Wild LM, et al: The effect of smoking on clinical outcome and complication rates following Ilizarov reconstruction, *J Ortho Trauma* 17:663-667, 2003.
48. Harvey EJ, Agel J, Selznick HS, et al: Deleterious effect of smoking on healing open tibial-shaft fractures, *Am J Orthop* 31:518-521, 2002.
49. Raikin SM, Landsman JC, Alexander VA, et al: Effect of nicotine on the rate and strength of healing of long bones fracture healing, *Clin Orthop Relat Res* 353:231-237, 1998.
50. Riebel GD, Boden SD, Whitesides TE, et al: The effect of nicotine on incorporation of cancellous bone graft in an animal model, *Spine* 20:2198-2202, 1995.
51. Ueng SW, Lee SS, Lin SS, et al: Hyperbaric oxygen therapy mitigates the adverse affects of cigarette smoking on bone healing of tibial lengthening: an experimental study on rabbits, *J Trauma* 47:752-759, 1999.
52. Castillo RC, Bosse MJ, MacKenzie EJ, et al: Impact of smoking on fracture healing and risk of complications in limb threatening open tibia fractures, *J Orthop Trauma* 19:151-157, 2005.
53. Hogevold HE, Grogaard B, Reikeras O: Effects of short term treatment with corticosteroids and indomethacin on bone healing: a mechanical study of osteotomies in rats, *Acta Orthop Scand* 63:607-611, 1992.
54. Adinoff AD, Hollister JR: Steroid induced fractures and bone loss in patients with asthma, *N Engl J Med* 309:265-268, 1983.
55. Glassman SD: The effect of postoperative nonsteroidal anti-inflammatory drug administration on spinal fusion, *Spine* 23:834-838, 1998.
56. Huddleston PM, Steckelberg JM, Hanssen AD, et al: Ciprofloxacin inhibition of experimental fracture-healing, *J Bone Joint Surg Am* 82:161-173, 2000.
57. Perry AC, Pirpa B, Rouse MS, et al: Levofloxacin and trovafloxacin inhibition of experimental fracture-healing, *Clin Orthop Relat Res* 414:95-100, 2003.
58. Jensen JG, Jensen TG, Smith TK, et al: Nutrition in orthopedic surgery. *J Bone Joint Surg Am* 64A:1263-1272, 1983.
59. Jensen JE, Jensen TG, Smith TK, et al: Nutrition in orthopedic surgery, *J Bone Joint Surg Am* 64A:1263-1272, 1982.
60. Einhorn TA, Bonnarens F, Burstein AH: The contributions of dietary protein and mineral to the healing of experimental fractures: A biomechanical study, *J Bone Joint Surg Am* 68A:1389-1395, 1986.
61. Buckwalter JA, Woo SL-Y, Goldberg VM, et al: Soft tissue aging and musculoskeletal function, *J Bone Joint Surg Am* 75A:1533-1548, 1993.
62. Rhinelander FW, Phillips RS, Steel WM, et al: Microangiography and bone healing. II. Displaced closed fractures, *J Bone Joint Surg Am* 50A:643-662, 1986.
63. Holden HE: The role of blood supply to the soft tissue in the healing of diaphyseal fractures, *J Bone Joint Surg Am* 54A:993-1000, 1972.
64. Godina M: Early microsurgical reconstruction of complex trauma of the extremities, *Plast Reconstr Surg* 78:285-292, 1986.
65. Andriole VT, Nagel DA, Southwick WO: A paradigm for chronic human osteomyelitis, *J Bone Joint Surg Am* 55A:1511-1515, 1973.
66. Boyd HB, Salvatore JE: Acute fracture of the femoral neck: Internal fixation or prosthesis? *J Bone Joint Surg Am* 46A:1066-1068, 1964.
67. Widmann RF, Pelker RR, Friedlander GE, et al: Effects of prefracture irradiation on the biomechanical parameters of fracture healing, *J Orthop Res* 11:422-428, 1993.
68. Buckwalter JA, Einhorn TA, Bolander ME, et al: Healing of the musculoskeletal tissues. In Rockwood CA, Bucholz RW, Heckman JD, et al (eds): *Rockwood and Green's Fractures in Adults,* Philadelphia, 1996, Lippincott Williams and Wilkins.
69. Tull F, Borrelli J: Soft tissue injury associated with closed fractures: evaluation and management, *J Am Acad Orthop Surg* 11:431-438, 2003.
70. Kahn SR: The clinical diagnosis of deep vein thrombosis integrating incidence, risk factors and symptoms and signs, *Arch Phys Med* 158:2315-2323, 1998.
71. Geerts WH, Code KL, Jay RM, et al: A prospective study of venous thromboembolism after major trauma, *N Engl J Med* 331:1601-1606, 1991.
72. O'Donnell TF, Abbott WM, Athanasoulis CA, et al: Diagnosis of deep vein thrombosis in the outpatient by venography, *Surg Gynecol Obstet* 150:69-74, 1980.
73. Wells PS, Hirsh J, Anderson DR, et al: Accuracy of clinical assessment of deep vein thrombosis, *Lancet* 345:1326-1330, 1995.
74. Wells PS, Anderson DR, Bormanis J, et al: Value of assessment of pretest probability of deep-vein thrombosis in clinical management, *Lancet* 350:1795-1798, 1997.
75. Wells PS, Hirsh J, Anderson DR, et al: A simple clinical model for the diagnosis of deep vein thrombosis combined with impedance plethysmography: Potential for the improvement in the diagnostic process, *J Intern Med* 243:15-23, 1998.
76. American Physical Therapy Association: *Guide to Physical Therapist Practice,* ed 2, Alexandria, Va, 2001, The Association.
77. Koval KJ, Maurer SG, Su ET, et al: The effects of nutritional status on outcome after hip fracture. *J Ortho Trauma* 13:164-169, 1999.
78. Ketelhut RG, Franz IW, Scholze J: Regular exercise as an effective approach in anti-hypertensive therapy, *Med Sci Sport Exerc* 36(1):4-8, 2004.
79. Turner CH, Robling AG. Designing exercise regimens to increase bone strength, *Exer Sport Sci Rev* 31(1):45-50.
80. Tsutsumi T, Don BM, Zaichkowsky LD: Physical fitness and psychological benefits of strength training in community dwelling older adults, *Appl Human Sci* 16(6):257-266, 1997.
81. Fox KR: The influence of physical activity on mental well-being, *Public Health Nutri* 2(3a):411-418, 1999.
82. DiLorenzo TM, Bargman EP, Stucky-Ropp R: Long-term effects of aerobic exercise on psychological outcome, *Prev Med* 28:75-85, 1999.
83. Cramer SR, Nieman DC, Lee JW: The effects of moderate exercise training on psychological well-being and mood state in women, *J Psychosom Res* 35:537-449, 1991.
84. Hopkins JT, Ingersoll CD, Krasue BA, et al: Effect of knee joint effusion on quadriceps and soleus motoneuron excitability, *Med Sci Sport Exerc* 33:123-126, 2001.
85. Palmieri RM, Ingersoll CD, Hoffman MA, et al: Arthrogenic muscle response following artificial ankle joint effusion, *J Athl Train* 37:S-25, 2002.
86. Spencer JD, Hayes KC, Alexander IJ: Knee joint effusion and quadriceps reflex inhibition in man, *Arch Phys Med Rehabil* 65:171-177, 1884.
87. Hopkins JT, Palmieri RM: Effects of ankle joint effusion on lower leg function, *Clin J Sport Med* 14(1):1-7, 2004.
88. Palmieri RM, Ingersoll CD, Cordova ML, et al: The effect of simulated knee joint effusion on postural control in healthy subjects, *Arch Phys Med Rehabil* 84:1076-1079, 2003.
89. Sherrington C, Lord SR: Home exercise to improve strength and walking velocity after hip fracture: A randomized controlled trial, *Arch Phys Med Rehabil* 78:208-212, 1997.
90. Sherrington C, Lord SR, Herbert RD: A randomized controlled trial of weight-bearing versus non-weight-bearing exercise for improving physical ability after usual care for hip fracture, *Arch Phys Med Rehabil* 85:710-716, 2004.
91. Hauer K, Rost B, Rutschle K, et al: Exercise training for rehabilitation and secondary prevention of falls in geriatric patients with history of injurious falls, *J Am Geriatr Soc* 49:10-20, 2001.
92. Coutinho EL, Gomes ARS, Franca CN, et al: Effect of passive stretching on the immobilized soleus muscle fiber morphology, *Braz J Med Biol Res* 37(12):1853-1861, 2004.
93. Williams PE: Use of intermittent stretch in the prevention of serial sarcomere loss in immobilized muscle, *Ann Rheum Dis.* 49:316-317, 1990.

94. Okita M, Yoshimura T, Nakano J, et al: Effects of reduced joint mobility on sarcomere length, collagen fibril arrangement in the endomysium, and hyaluronan in rat soleus muscle. *J Muscle Res Cell Motil* 25(2):159-166, 2004.

95. Jarvinen TAH, Joza L, Kannus P, et al: Organization and distribution of intramuscular connective tissue in normal and immobilized skeletal muscles. An immuno-histochemical, polarization and scanning electron microscopic study, *J Muscle Res Cell Motil* 23:245-254, 2002.

96. Sady SP, Wortman M, Blanke D: Flexibility training: Ballistic, static, or proprioceptive neuromuscular facilitation? *Arch Phys Med Rehabil* 63:261-263, 1982.

97. Bandy WD, Irion JM: The effect of time on static stretch on flexibility of the hamstring muscle, *Phys Ther* 74(9):845-852, 1994.

98. Bandy WD, Irion JM, Briggler M: The effect of time and frequency of static stretching on flexibility of the hamstring muscle. *Phys Ther* 77:1090-1096, 1997.

99. American College of Sports Medicine: *ACSM Guidelines for Exercise Testing and Prescription,* ed 6 Philadelphia, 2000, Lippincott Williams and Wilkins.

100. Funk DC, Swank AM, Milka BM: Impact of prior exercise on hamstring flexibility: A comparison of proprioceptive neuromuscular facilitation and static stretching, *J Strength Cond Res* 17(3):489-492, 2003.

101. Davis DS, Ashby PE, McCale KL, et al: The effectiveness of 3 stretching techniques on hamstring flexibility using consistent stretching parameters, *J Strength Cond Res* 19(1):27-32, 2005.

102. Burke DG, Culligan CJ, Holt LE: The theoretical basis of proprioceptive neuromuscular facilitation, *J Strength Cond Res* 14(4):496-500, 2000.

103. Feland JB, Marin HN: Effect of submaximal contraction intensity in contract-relax proprioceptive neuromuscular facilitation stretching, *Br J Sports Med* 38:e18, 2004.

104. Wallin D, Ekblom B, Grahn R, et al: Improvement of muscle flexibility: A comparison between two techniques. *Am J Sports Med* 13(4):263-268, 1985.

105. Etnyre BR, Abraham LD: Gains in range of ankle dorsiflexion using three popular stretching techniques, *Am J Phys Med* 65(4):189-196, 1986.

106. Binder EF, Brown M, Sinacore DR, et al: Effects of extended outpatient rehabilitation after hip fracture: A randomized controlled trial, *JAMA* 292:837-846, 2004.

107. Youdas JW, Kotajarvi BJ, Padjett DJ, et al: Partial weight bearing gait using conventional assistive devices, *Arch Phys Med Rehabil* 86:394-398, 2005.

108. Dabke HV, Gupta SK, Holt CA, et al: How accurate is partial weightbearing? *Clin Orthop Relat Res* 421:282-286, 2004.

109. Li S, Armstrong CW, Cipriani D: Three-point gait crutch walking: Variability in ground reaction force during weight-bearing, *Arch Phys Med Rehabil* 82:86-92, 2001.

110. Behrens F, Kraft EL, Oegema TR: Biochemical changes in articular cartilage after joint immobilization by casting or external fixation, *J Orthop Res* 7(3):335-343, 1989.

111. Videman T: Connective tissue and immobilization. Key factors in musculoskeletal degeneration, *Clin Orthop Rel Res* 221:26-32, 1986.

112. Pope RO, Corcoran S, McCaul K, et al: Continuous passive motion after primary total knee arthroplasty. Does it offer any benefits? *J Bone Joint Surg B,* 79B:914-917, 1997.

113. Chen B, Zimmerman JR, Soulen L, et al: Continuous passive motion after total knee arthroplasty, *Am J Phys Med Rehabil* 79:421-426, 2000.

114. Brosseau L, Milne S, Wells G, et al: Efficacy of continuous passive motion following total knee arthroplasty: A metaanalysis, *J Rheumatol* 31:2251-2264, 2004.

115. Finsterbush A, Friedman B: Early changes in immobilized rabbits knee joints: A light and electron microscopic study, *Clin Orthop Relat Res* 92:305-319, 1973.

116. Schollmeier G, Uhthoff HK, Sarkar K, et al: Effects of immobilization on the capsule of the canine glenohumeral joint. A structural functional study, *Clin Orthop Relat Res* 304:37-42, 1994.

117. Hall MC: Articular changes in the knees of adult rat after prolonged immobilization in extension, *Clin Orthop Relat Res* 34:184-195, 1964.

118. Thaxter TH, Mann RA, Anderson CE: Degeneration of immobilized knee joints in rats; histological and autoradiographic study, *J Bone Joint Surg Am* 47:567-585, 1965.

119. Peacock EE: Comparison of collagenous tissue surrounding normal and immobilized joints, *Surg Forum* 14:440-441, 1963.

120. Akeson WH, Amiel D, Mechanic GL, et al: Collagen cross-linking alterations in joint contractures: Changes in the reducible cross-links in periarticular connective tissue collagen after nine weeks of immobilization, *Connect Tissue Res* 5(1):15-19, 1977.

121. Akeson WH: An experimental study of joint stiffness, *J Bone Joint Surg Am* 43:1022-1034, 1961.

122. Trudel G, Uhthoff HK: Contractures secondary to immobility: Is the restriction articular or muscular? An experimental longitudinal study in the rat knee, *Arch Phys Med Rehabil* 81(1):6-13, 2000.

123. Trudel G, Jabi M, Uhthoff HK: Localized and adaptive synoviocyte proliferation characteristics in rat knee joint contractures secondary to immobility, *Arch Phys Med Rehabil* 84(9):1350-1356, 2003.

124. Maitland GD: *Peripheral Manipulation,* ed 3, Oxford, 1991, Butterworth-Heinemann.

125. Cameron MH: *Physical Agents In Rehabilitation: From Research to Practice,* ed 2 St. Louis, 2003, WB Saunders.

126. Levin MF, Hui-Chan CW: Conventional and acupuncture-like transcutaneous electrical nerve stimulation excite similar afferent nerve fibers, *Arch Phys Med Rehabil* 74(1):54-60, 1993.

127. Starkey C: *Therapeutic Modalities,* ed 2, Philadelphia, 1999, FA Davis.

128. Solar G, Job I, Mingano J, et al: Effective transcutaneous electrotherapy in CSF B-endorphin content in patients without pain problems, *Pain* 10:169-172, 1981.

129. Mannheimer JS, Lampe GN: *Clinical Transcutaneous Electrical Nerve Stimulation,* Philadelphia, 1984, FA Davis.

130. Hughes GS Jr, Lichstein PR, Whitlock D, et al: Response of beta-endorphins to transcutaneous electrical nerve stimulation in healthy subjects, *Phys Ther* 64(7):1062-1066, 1984.

131. Karmarker MK, Ho AMH: Acute pain management of patients with multiple fractured ribs, *J Trauma* 54:615-625, 2003.

132. Sloan JP, Muwanga CL, Waters EA, et al: Multiple rib fractures: Transcutaneous nerve stimulation versus conventional analgesia, *J Trauma* 26(12):1120-1122, 1986.

133. Oncel M, Sencan S, Yildiz H, et al: Transcutaneous electrical nerve stimulation for pain management in patients with uncomplicated minor rib fractures, *J Card Thor Surg* 22:13-17, 2002.

134. Taylor K, Fish DR, Mendel FC, et al: Effect of a single 30-minute treatment of high voltage pulsed current on edema formation in frog hind limbs, *Phys Ther* 72(1):63-68, 1992.

135. Bettany JA, Fish DR, Mendel FC: High-voltage pulsed direct current: effect on edema formation after hyperflexion injury, *Arch Phys Med Rehabil* 71(9):677-681, 1990.

136. Mendel FC, Wylegala JA, Fish DR: Influence of high voltage pulsed current on edema formation following impact injury in rats, *Phys Ther* 72(9):668-673, 1992.

137. Reed BV: Effect of high voltage pulsed electrical stimulation on microvascular permeability to plasma proteins: A possible mechanism in minimizing edema, *Phys Ther* 68:491-495, 1988.

138. Griffin JW, Newsome LS, Stralka SW, et al: Reduction of chronic posttraumatic hand edema: A comparison of high voltage pulsed current, intermittent pneumatic compression, and placebo treatments, *Phys Ther* 70(5):279-286, 1990.

139. Gould N, Donnermeyer D, Pope M, et al: Transcutaneous muscle stimulation as a method to retard disuse atrophy, *Clin Orthop Rel Res* 164:215-220, 1982.

140. Laughman RK, Youdas JW, Garrett TR, et al: Strength changes in the normal quadriceps femoris muscle as a result of electrical stimulation, *Phys Ther* 63(4):494-499, 1983.

141. Snyder-Mackler L, Delitto A, Stralka SW, et al: Use of electrical stimulation to enhance recovery of quadriceps femoris muscle force production in patients following anterior cruciate ligament reconstruction, *Phys Ther* 74(10):901-907, 1994.

142. Delitto A, Rose SJ, McKowen JM, et al: Electrical stimulation versus voluntary exercise in strengthening thigh musculature after anterior cruciate ligament surgery, *Phys Ther* 68(5):660-663, 1988.

143. Fitzgerald GK, Piva SR, Irrgang JJ: A modified neuromuscular electrical stimulation protocol for quadriceps strength training following anterior cruciate ligament reconstruction, *J Orthop Sports Phys Ther* 33(9):492-501, 2003.

144. Lewek M, Stevens J, Snyder-Mackler L: The use of electrical stimulation to increase quadriceps femoris muscle force in an elderly patient following total knee arthroplasty, *Phys Ther* 81(9):1565-1571, 2001.

145. Avramidis K, Strike PW, Taylor PN, et al: Effectiveness of electrical stimulation of the vastus medialis muscle in the rehabilitation of patients after total knee arthroplasty, *Arch Phys Med Rehabil* 84:1850-1853, 2003.

146. Stevens JE, Mizner RL, Snyder-Mackler L: Neuromuscular electrical stimulation for quadriceps muscle strengthening after bilateral total knee arthroplasty: a case series, *J Orthop Sports Phys Ther* 34:21-29, 2004.

147. Lamb SE, Oldham JA, Morse RE, et al: Neuromuscular stimulation of the quadriceps muscle after hip fracture: A randomized clinical trial, *Arch Phys Med Rehabil* 83:1087-1092, 2002.

148. Einhorn TA: Enhancement of fracture healing, *J Bone Joint Surg Am* 77A:940-956, 1995.

149. Alpert SW, Ben-Yishay A, Koval KJ: *Fractures and Dislocations: A Manual of Orthopedic Trauma,* New York, 1994, Lippincott-Raven.

150. Skerry TM, Pead MJ, Lanyon LE: Modulation of bone loss during disuse by pulsed electromagnetic fields, *J Orthop Res* 9(4):600-608, 1991.

151. Nagai M, Ota M: Pulsating electromagnetic field stimulates mRNA expression in bone morphogenetic protein -2 and -4, *J Dental Res* 73:1601-1605, 1994.

152. Aaron RK, Ciombor D, Simon BJ: Treatment of nonunions with electric and electromagnetic fields, *Clin Orthop Relat Res* 419:21-29, 2004.

153. Simonis RB, Parnell EJ, Ray PS, et al: Electrical treatment of non-union: a prospective, randomized, double-blind trial, *Injury* 34:357-362, 2003.

154. Linovitz RJ, Pathria M, Bernhardt M, et al: Combined magnetic fields accelerate and increase spine fusion: A double blind, randomized, placebo controlled study. *Spine* 27(13):1383-1388, 2002.

155. Borsalino G, Bagnacani M, Bettati E, et al: Electrical stimulation of human femoral intertrochanteric osteotomies: Double-blind study. *Clin Orthop Relat Res* 237:256-263, 1988.

156. Mammi GI, Rocchi R, Cadossi R, et al: The electrical stimulation of tibial osteotomies: A double-blind study, *Clin Orthop* 288:246-253, 1993.

157. Traina G, Sollazzo V, Massari L: Electrical stimulation of tibial osteotomies: A double-blind study. In Bersani F (ed): *Electricity and Magnetism in Biology and Medicine*, New York, 1999, Kluwer Academic/Plenum.

158. Akai M, Hayashi K: Effects of electrical stimulation on musculoskeletal systems; a meta-analysis of controlled clinical trials, *Bioelectromagnetics* 23:132-143, 2002.

159. Busse JW, Bhandari M: Therapeutic ultrasound and fracture healing: A survey of beliefs and practices, *Arch Phys Med Rehabil* 85:1653-1656, 2004.

160. Duarte LR: The stimulation of bone growth by ultrasound, *Arch Orthop Trauma Surg* 101:153-159, 1983.

161. Ryaby JT, Bachner EJ, Bendo J, et al: Low-intensity pulsed ultrasound increases calcium incorporation in both differentiating cartilage and bone cell cultures, *Trans Orthop Res Soc* 14:15, 1989.

162. Wu CC, Lewallen DG, Bolander MF, et al: Exposure to low-intensity pulsed ultrasound stimulates aggrecan gene expression by cultured chondrocytes, *Trans Orthop Res Soc* 21:622, 1996.

163. Rawool D, Goldberg B, Forsberg F, et al: Power Doppler assessment of vascular changes during fracture treatment with low-intensity ultrasound, *Trans Radiol Soc North Am* 83:1185, 1998.

164. Rubin C, Bolander M, Ryaby JP, et al: The use of low-intensity ultrasound to accelerate the healing of fractures, *J Bone Joint Surg Am* 83A(2):259-270, 2001.

165. Kristiansen TK, Ryaby JP, McCabe J, et al: Accelerated healing of distal radius fractures with the use of specific, low-intensity ultrasound. A multicenter, prospective, randomized, double-blind, placebo-controlled study, *J Bone Joint Surg Am* 79A: 961-973, 1997.

166. Nolte PA, van der Krans A, Patka P, et al: Low-intensity pulsed ultrasound in the treatment of nonunions, *J Trauma* 51:693-703, 2001.

167. Heckman JD, Ryaby JP, McCabe J, et al: Acceleration of tibial fracture-healing by non-invasive, low-intensity pulsed ultrasound, *J Bone Joint Surg Am* 76A(1):26-34, 1994.

168. Mayr E, Rudzki MM, Rudzki M, et al: Acceleration by pulsed, low-intensity ultrasound of scaphoid fracture healing, *Handchir Mikrochir Plast Chir* 32:115-122, 2000.

Chapter 10

Joint Arthroplasty

Julie A. Pryde

CHAPTER OUTLINE

OBJECTIVES

After reading this chapter, the reader will be able to:
1. List the surgical considerations and options available for joint arthroplasty and arthrodesis.
2. Understand the postoperative precautions and restrictions following specific joint arthroplasty procedures.
3. Discuss the current research on joint arthroplasty and its limitations.
4. Understand the goals of total joint replacement surgery.
5. Design safe and effective, evidence-based rehabilitation programs for patients after joint arthroplasty.

Joint arthroplasty is any reconstructive joint procedure, with or without an implant, designed to relieve pain and/or restore joint motion.[1] Most joint arthroplasty involves a joint implant and is known as joint replacement surgery. Over the past four decades, joint replacement surgery has become the most successful surgery for patients with severe debilitating arthritis.[2] These procedures have also been used successfully in the management of joints affected by *avascular necrosis*, fractures, and tumors.[3-5]

Joint replacement procedures, such as total hip and total knee replacements, are types of joint arthroplasty.

Hip or knee joint replacements have become some of the most common procedures in orthopedic surgical practice in the United States, with an estimated 152,000 total hip arthroplasties (THA) and 360,000 total knee arthroplasties (TKA) performed in the United States in 2000.[6] The number of these procedures is steadily increasing as the population ages and the age of patients having these surgeries decreases.[7] Although the average age of a patient undergoing THA is 69 years, this procedure is increasingly being performed on patients less than 50 and more than 75 years old.[8]

Total joint replacement has emerged as one of the most successful and common procedures for the treatment of joint degeneration as a result of arthritis, and arthritis accounts for the majority of elective joint replacement surgeries.[9] Over 21 million people in the United States have arthritis, and as the population ages, this number will undoubtedly increase.[10] Arthritis is the leading cause of long-term disability in the United States and the second leading cause of decreased physical activity.[11] As health care–related expenditures increase, joint replacement surgeries have emerged as an accepted cost-effective and efficacious treatment for the management of arthritis.[12,13] For example, the cost-effectiveness of a THA has been found to be similar to or better than that of a coronary artery bypass graft (CABG) or renal dialysis.[14]

The knee is the joint most frequently affected by osteoarthritis (OA)[15,16] and therefore is the most common joint replaced. Although many conservative measures may initially reduce the pain and disability associated with OA of the knee, with severe arthritis, TKA is necessary to optimize functional outcome.

PATHOLOGY

The term *arthroplasty* refers to any reconstructive joint procedure, with or without joint implant, designed to relieve pain and/or restore joint motion.[1] There are a number of different types of arthroplasty. Total joint replacements involve removing both the proximal and distal joint surfaces and replacing them with an artificial joint implant. The primary components of these implants are made of an inert metal, such chromium cobalt, titanium, or stainless steel, or of ceramic. Some components of specific joint implants are made of high-density polymer plastics such as polyethylene. These include the glenoid component of the shoulder, the patella resurfacing "button" and spacer of the knee, and in some hips, the liner of the acetabulum. Implants can be attached to the bone with cement *(methylmethacrylate),* screws, or other hardware or without cement, using either biological fixation by ingrowth of bone into a porous-coated implant or by being tightly press-fit.

Hemiarthroplasty involves removing and replacing only one side of the joint, or one compartment in the case of the knee. This procedure is gaining favor[17] and is often used when one side of a joint is damaged and the other side is intact. This often occurs with trauma that damages the long bones, causing, for example, a displaced femoral neck fracture or a 4-part humeral head fracture (Fig. 10-1). Hemiarthroplasty may also be indicated for unicompartmental arthritis, avascular necrosis, or when a tumor needs to be excised. Hemiarthroplasty of the knee, shoulder, and hip is generally successful, reducing pain and improving function.

A bipolar or unipolar hemiarthroplasty can be used to treat fractures on or around the femoral neck that can not be treated by open reduction internal fixation. In a unipolar hip arthroplasty the femoral head and neck are replaced with a prosthetic implant with a stationary head that articulates with a single bearing. This type of device is often used in elderly patients who place lower demands on the prosthesis as a result of their ambulatory and medical status. This is also the least expensive type of implant used. The more complex bipolar hip prosthesis has a fixed femoral head component capped with a plastic acetabular bearing attached to the femoral ball and a mobile metal cup attached to the plastic bearing. The metal cup can move freely along the cartilaginous acetabular surface, which is thought to lessen the potential for pain and destructive wear.

Under special circumstances, such as when there is joint infection, joint ankylosis, or failure of a prior arthroplastic procedure, a number of alternative arthroplastic procedures that do not involve replacement of the joint with an implant may be performed. These include *resec-*

tion arthroplasty, also known as excisional arthroplasty, which involves removal of one or both articular surfaces of a joint, allowing a fibrotic scar to form in the space that remains, and *fascial arthroplasty,* which involves debriding the joint and placing a foreign material, such as fascia, between the two joint surfaces. These procedures, although used less commonly, are still appropriate in selected cases.

In the hip, one type of resection arthroplasty, Girdlestone pseudarthrosis, which dates back to 1923, can be used as a temporary intervention or permanent treatment of joint infection or when ankylosis of the hip has placed it in an unsuitable position for function. This may be seen in some patients with spinal cord injury, severe Parkinsonism, multiple sclerosis, or head injury. In this procedure the femoral neck and head are resected at the level of the intertrochanteric line and the remaining end of the femur is left free to articulate with the acetabulum. Although this procedure improves perineal care and allows for a pain free joint with relatively good motion, the hip generally has poor stability, and the involved lower extremity is shortened. These result in gait deviations and the need for an assistive device during ambulation. A similar procedure, the resection arthroplasty, can be performed in the knee after an infected prosthesis is removed. This also generally produces an unstable joint.

When a total joint replacement fails as a result of fracture or loosening, or in other patient-specific circumstances, *arthrodesis,* also known as joint fusion, may be performed. Arthrodesis is the creation of a bony union across a joint. This procedure can alleviate the pain associated with arthritis by eliminating motion across the joint. It is also used to treat fractures across a joint that can not otherwise be managed. Arthrodesis may occur spontaneously, for example, as the result of infection, or be surgically produced. Unfortunately, since arthrodesis eliminates motion, it generally also impairs function, and with spontaneous arthrodesis, functional outcomes are worse because the joint fuses in the position that produces the least pain rather than in the position that optimizes function.

Surgical arthrodesis can be performed in almost any joint, including those of the spine. The most commonly fused joints are the ankle, wrist, spine, and thumb. The technique used to produce fusion is similar in all joints. The articular cartilage is removed from the joint surfaces, and the joint is positioned at an optimal angle for function and to maximize the contact area between bony surfaces for optimal stabilization and fusion. The joint is filled with autologous or cadaveric bone chips or pieces to produce a graft, and the joint position is maintained with internal fixation hardware, such as rods, plates, or screws, or by an external fixation, such as a cast or external fixator (Fig. 10-2). Over time, the bone graft solidifies to permanently immobilize the joint.

There are many indications for arthrodesis (Box 10-1). However, because of the poor functional results for most joints, this procedure is avoided if possible. For example, in the elbow, the loss of motion produced by a fusion prevents most functional uses of the extremity, including feeding and personal hygiene. However, in some joints,

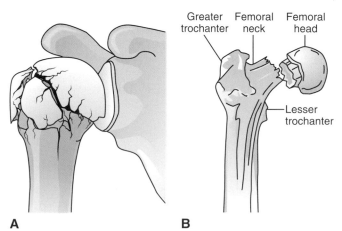

A   **B**

FIG. 10-1 Traumatic causes for joint replacement. **A,** Four-part humeral head fracture. **B,** Displaced femoral neck fracture. *A From www.orthogastonia.com; B from www.painanddisability.com.*

Greater trochanter   Femoral neck   Femoral head

Lesser trochanter

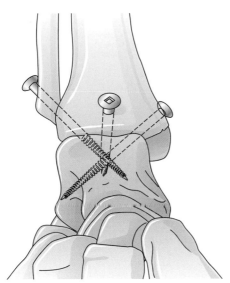

FIG. 10-2 Surgically fused ankle.

BOX 10-1   Indications for Arthrodesis

- Painful, degenerative, posttraumatic arthritis or RA that can not be helped by arthroplasty
- Avascular necrosis or osteonecrosis that can not be treated by arthroplasty
- Neurological disease that resulted in an unstable joint
- Neuropathic joints
- Infection such as chronic osteomyelitis
- Failed total joint arthroplasty caused by infection, resulting in severe bone loss, and precluding a revision arthroplasty
- Deltoid or quadriceps femoris paralysis

RA, Rheumatoid arthritis.

---

such as the tibiotalar joint in the ankle, where the functional limitations produced by arthrodesis are much less severe and the alternative procedures have limited success, this procedure is often used.

EXAMINATION

Examination of a patient after joint arthroplasty is similar to the examination of a patient in any of the other musculoskeletal preferred practice patterns. The examination should follow the standard format and include all information needed for the clinician to create a picture of the patient's problem. During the examination, it is important to respect range of motion (ROM), resistance, and weight-bearing restrictions. Examination and evaluation are part of each patient encounter and should guide the intervention plan.

PATIENT HISTORY

The patient history should begin with demographic information, a social history, and information about the patient's living environment. Information about physical barriers, such as stairs, and areas with limited access, such as bathrooms, may be important to consider for someone with a lower extremity arthroplasty, especially if their weight-bearing status is limited. This information will help determine the need for assistive devices, such as raised commodes, reachers, and shower chairs, during the recovery period. The availability of caregivers' or family members' assistance should also be ascertained.

It is important to determine patients' perceptions of their overall health and the prescribed and over-the-counter medications they are taking. It is particularly important to determine if the patient is currently using an antiinflammatory medication or anticoagulant because this may limit the vigor of therapy. For example, Coumadin makes patients more prone to bleeding and bruising and therefore aggressive soft tissue mobilization should be avoided. It is also important to note any prior surgeries, injuries, or other musculoskeletal problems that may limit or impact the rehabilitation process.

Next, it is important to establish the nature, location, and severity of a patient's current symptoms. Whatever the symptom, the therapist should also note whether it is constant (all the time) or intermittent (comes and goes) or if it is varying (changes in intensity) or nonvarying (does not change in intensity). The therapist should find out what their symptom level is at rest, what brings on the symptoms, and at what level of intensity that specific activity causes their symptoms. In addition, the therapist should find out how long it takes for symptoms to settle back to their baseline.

One should also ask about the patient's level of function before the arthroplasty and the expectations for recovery. For example, was this patient a limited household ambulator who wants to increase his or her walking in the community or does this patient plan on returning to golfing or dancing? This information will help set appropriate patient-specific goals.

SYSTEMS REVIEW

The systems review is used to target areas requiring further examination and to define areas that may cause complications or indicate a need for precautions during the examination and intervention processes. See Chapter 1 for details of the systems review.

TESTS AND MEASURES
Musculoskeletal

Posture. The position of the joint and how the patient holds the joint in relationship to his or her body may give the clinician important clues as to the function of that area of the body (see Chapter 4). It is important to look at the entire upper or lower quarter of the affected side of the body to determine how this area may function. For example, a patient who holds the total shoulder adducted, internally rotated, and elevated may have an upper quarter dysfunction. This is due to having prolonged limitations in glenohumeral ROM and using compensatory motions such as hiking the shoulder to achieve arm elevation. This may lead to trapezius and levator scapulae muscle overuse and spasm, which may also lead to cervical symptoms. After a total knee replacement, knee pain and effusion may result in an antalgic gait and limitations in knee extension may cause lumbar and hip symptoms such as pain.

Anthropometric Characteristics. The clinician should evaluate the patient's joint overall, looking for signs of inflammation such as swelling, redness, and temperature changes. All of these findings should be expected directly after a surgery of this nature. Swelling, which is the last of these signs to dissipate, may often take as long as 6 months to resolve. These findings should be differentiated from signs of infection that often include systemic fever and constitutional symptoms.

Girth should also be measured. Increased joint girth may indicate a joint effusion, whereas reduced limb girth above or below the joint may be due to muscle atrophy. Girth measurements should be noted by consistent landmarks, such as the medial joint line or medial malleolus, to improve the reliability of measurements between sessions and clinicians and to optimize sensitivity to changes over time. Measures should also be compared to the uninvolved side.

Swelling in the lower extremities may also be a sign of thromboembolic disease. Joint replacement surgery places patients at high risk for deep vein thrombosis (DVT) and pulmonary emboli (PE). Furthermore, as hospital stays become shorter, these patients may present in the inpatient or outpatient setting. Warwick et al reported that 64% of the venous thromboembolism complications among 1,162 patients after hip arthroplasty occurred after discharge from the hospital.[18]

Many clinicians rely on the Homan's test to help in the diagnosis of a DVT. A positive Homan's test is pain in the calf when the ankle is passively dorsiflexed. This test, however, has been proven to have almost no diagnostic value because of its poor specificity and sensitivity.[19] A clinical decision rule (CDR) has been developed to assist clinicians in determining the likelihood of a DVT based on nine clinical and medical history findings.[20,21] Patients could be categorized in high-, moderate-, and low-risk groups based on their CDR scores.[22] A random sample of 1,500 physical therapists (PTs) found that years of clinical experience, board certification status, practice setting, or geographical location did not improve recognition rates of high DVT risk.[23] Risk factors for DVT are shown in Box 10-2.

Range of Motion/Joint Mobility. Passive ROM (PROM) and active ROM (AROM) at the involved joint and joints above and below should be measured. The clinician should look for the quality and quantity of motion, as well as end-feel. ROM should be noted for both the affected and unaffected side. Joint precautions, as well as ROM restrictions, should be respected, as noted by the physician. For the knee, close attention should be paid to the mobility of the patella because restrictions in its mobility may result in restrictions of knee ROM and function.

Muscle Performance. Strength testing of the muscle groups crossing the involved joint, as well as a general screening of the involved limb, should be performed. Manual muscle tests are generally appropriate for this purpose (see Chapter 5). The restrictions and precautions from the prescribing clinician should be noted, particularly after upper extremity arthroplasty.

BOX 10-2	Risk Factors for Deep Vein Thrombosis

Strong Risk Factors
Fracture (pelvis, femur, tibia)
THA or TKA
Major general surgery
Major trauma
Spinal cord injury

Moderate Risk Factors
Arthroscopic knee surgery
Central venous lines
Chemotherapy
CHF or respiratory failure
Hormone replacement therapy
Malignancy
Oral contraception therapy
CVA
Pregnancy: Postpartum
Previous venous thromboembolism
Thrombophilia

Weak Risk Factors
Bed rest >3 days
Immobility due to sitting (e.g., prolonged air travel)
Increasing age
Laparoscopic surgery
Obesity
Pregnancy: Antepartum
Varicose veins

From Anderson FA, Spencer FA: *Circulation* 107(S):19-116, 2003. *THA,* Total hip arthroplasty; *TKA,* total knee arthroplasty; *CHF,* congestive heart failure; *CVA,* cerebrovascular accident.

Neuromuscular

Pain. The pain quality, intensity, duration, and frequency should be noted, as well as these levels in relationship to rest and activity. The location of pain should also be noted since there may be pain not only in the operative area but also in areas affected by changes in biomechanics or alterations in gait or sleeping positions. For example, an antalgic gait may cause back pain, and shoulder immobilization may cause neck pain. The types and doses of analgesic medication used may also give the clinician an indication of how the patient's pain is responding to current interventions (see Chapter 22).

Integumentary. The healing status and mobility of the incision should also be noted. Soft tissue mobility testing may be limited because of tissue healing constraints. Obesity, diabetes, peripheral vascular disease, steroid and tobacco use, prior infection, and malnutrition all increase the risk for poor wound healing. Morbid obesity has been shown to increase the risk of poor wound healing and infection more than tenfold (22% versus 2% for poor healing and 10% versus 0.6% for infection) after a total knee replacement.[24] Poor nutritional status, which may impair immune function, has also been associated with a threefold increased rate of wound complications.[25]

Function

Gait, Locomotion, and Balance. If the patient has undergone a lower extremity joint replacement, balance and proprioception should be examined and addressed throughout the treatment. These may be difficult to examine fully during the initial examination because of pain and ROM and strength deficits (see Chapter 13). Gait and transfers should also be examined and assessed (see Chapter 32).

EVALUATION, DIAGNOSIS, AND PROGNOSIS

According to the *Guide to Physical Therapy Practice,*[26] the preferred practice pattern for most patients with joint replacement is 4H: Impaired joint mobility, motor function, muscle performance, and ROM associated with joint arthroplasty.

The results of total joint arthroplasty have improved over time; hip, knee, and shoulder procedures currently have the best outcomes. Extensive evidence shows that 85% to 90% of patients report pain reduction after TKA.[2,27,28] Patients who have had a THA have significantly increased maximum walking speed, stride length, and cadence and oxygen consumption with walking.[29] Patients who have undergone a total shoulder arthroplasty (TSA) feel that the impact of the procedure on their health is comparable to that of THA or CABG.[30] Replacement of other joints, such as the ankle, wrist, elbow, and first metatarsophalangeal (MTP), are less successful because of limited advances in technology and limited use.[31]

Outcome studies after total joint replacement reveal that although pain and mobility are almost always improved, improved functional ability does not necessarily follow. Studies have shown that 1 year after knee and hip replacement surgeries, impairments and functional limitations often persist, even in the absence of pain.[32-34] These impairments include decreased muscle strength and limitations in the ability to climb stairs. It is therefore imperative that rehabilitation professionals follow the findings of ongoing research so these approaches produce better functional outcomes.

INTERVENTION

Preoperative patient education has been advocated for many years as important to the overall rehabilitation of patients undergoing joint arthroplasty. Many medical centers offer a multidisciplinary, team-taught, preoperative group class for patients planning to have an arthroplastic procedure and their families. These classes cover information about the procedure, the rehabilitation process, and the early postoperative period. Hough, Crosat, and Nye described an educational program for clients undergoing THA.[35] Although no formal evaluation was undertaken, it was noted that surgeons and staff reported fewer dislocations, fewer phone calls to surgeons, less medication use, and an ability to walk sooner in those patients that attended the preoperative class.[35] In a pilot study, patient satisfaction, length of hospital stay, and physical therapy input on patients undergoing THA were all positively impacted in the group of patients receiving the preoperative class and informational booklet.[36] Another study of patients with complex needs (co-morbid conditions or limited social support) undergoing TKA or THA found that patients who underwent a preoperative, multidisciplinary educational session regarding the in-hospital phase of their treatment, early discharge planning, and how to optimize functional capacity were discharged from the hospital more quickly and achieved discharge criteria earlier than those that did not receive this visit.[37]

Education, exercise, and functional mobility training, including gait training if appropriate, are the three main components of rehabilitation after arthroplasty. Postoperative rehabilitation aims to optimize function, while ensuring adherence to ROM and weight-bearing precautions and preventing complications such as DVTs and pneumonia. There are few prospective, randomized trials showing one protocol to be better than another. Therefore most rehabilitation procedures are based on expert opinion, local customs, and anecdotal evidence rather than on high-quality research studies.

TOTAL HIP ARTHROPLASTY

The first recorded total hip replacement was performed more than 150 years ago by Sir Anthony White, a surgeon at London's Westminster hospital. However, it was not until the early 1960s that Sir John Charnley, also in England, popularized what is known today as the total hip arthroplasty. Since then, advancements in biologically compatible implants and fixation and surgical techniques have continued to produce ever better results in THA. Recent refinements include "mini" open, one-, and two-incision techniques that result in less soft tissue damage, particularly of the muscles. The two main surgical approaches to THA are the anterior and the posterolateral; the posterolateral approach is the most common. The joint may also be cemented or uncemented, depending on the patient's life expectancy, bone quality, and activity level. An uncemented acetabular component is used for most patients because it lasts longer. A cemented acetabular component is only used for the patient with a life expectancy of less than 10 years. Indications for uncemented femoral components vary with surgeon preference but are usually reserved for younger patients. Implants are modular so they can be customized to the specific anatomy of each patient. The components are usually made of metal alloy such as titanium or cobalt chrome. Highly polished ceramic femoral head components are also used in limited patient populations. In most patients, the alloy or ceramic femoral head component articulates with a polyethylene plastic acetabular insert. Metal or ceramic heads that articulate with metal liners are also available for active, younger patients (Fig. 10-3).

Pathology. The THA procedure exposes the acetabulum and proximal femur and then removes the femoral head and neck. The proximal femoral medullary canal is reamed to prepare it to accept the femoral component. The acetabulum is prepared by rasping and articular cartilage debridement. Most acetabular components just press-fit into place, but some are held in with screws.

These components are rarely cemented. If the femoral component is cemented, the methylmethacrylate cement is first put into the proximal femur under pressure, and then the femoral component is inserted. If there is no cement, the proximal femur is underreamed so that the femoral component can be impacted into the femur (Fig. 10-4). Reduction and stability testing is performed before the soft tissue is closed. In some patients, the joint capsule is resected before soft tissue closure.

THA revision may be needed for a variety of reasons, including infection, component failure, or mechanical loosening. According to data from United States hospital databases, approximately 18% of all THA procedures are revisions.[38] For a revision, bone grafting, whether autologous or allograft, is often necessary to fill architectural defects caused by the primary arthroplasty, to fill defects made when the initial implant was removed, or if there was a fracture or poor bone stock that results from severe osteoporosis. Postoperative care must consider the unique demands of these patients and the specific limitations imposed by their surgery.

Prognosis. The primary indications for THA are pain and disability. Although some authors have attempted to define specific criteria for the appropriateness of THA, the subjective nature of patients' symptoms will always require patients to weigh the risks and benefits of such procedures according to their own values.[39] Studies have not found a direct and predictable correlation between preoperative status and THA outcome.[40-42] One study examining the relationship between baseline pain and functional status with the outcomes of THA in an elderly population found that the worse a patient's preoperative status, the greater the gains they made in level of activity, presence and severity of pain with walking, the need for an assistive device with walking, the distance the patient was able to walk and the ability to perform specific ADLs. Yet, patients with a better preoperative status had better overall outcomes.[43]

Common physical impairments after THA include decreased muscle strength, limited hip ROM and flexibility, and abnormalities of gait. Persistent, although improved, muscle strength deficits after THA have been documented in several studies. One study showed that strength on the operative side was 84% to 89% of the nonoperative side in men and 79% to 81% of the nonoperative side in women 1 year after surgery.[44] A prospective found that hip flexion, extension, and abduction strength in 40 patients with uncemented THA was increased by an average of 150% and 250% from preoperative levels at 6 months and 1 year, respectively; however, none of the subjects achieved the same strength on the operative side as

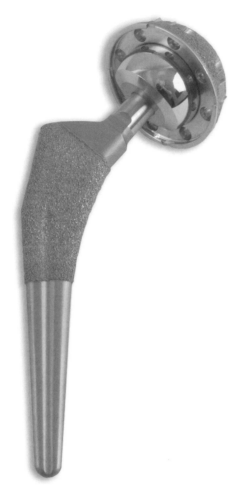

FIG. 10-3 Typical hip replacement components: Metal head with metal acetabular liner. *Image courtesy Biomet.*

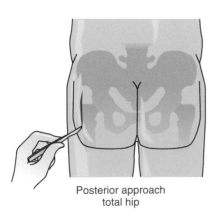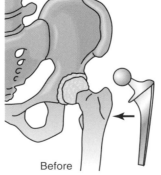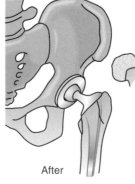

Posterior approach total hip

A

Before

B

After

C

FIG. 10-4 Total hip arthroplasty procedure.

on the nonoperative side.[45] Neither the length of hospitalization nor the type or number of inpatient physical therapy visits was listed nor did any of the patients receive outpatient physical therapy after hospital discharge.

Leg length discrepancy can affect patient satisfaction and prognosis for overall function after THA. Many patients report a sensation that their operated leg is longer than the nonoperated leg. This may be due to a true leg length discrepancy caused by a limited amount of bone being resected from the femoral neck, the implant being longer than the patient's original anatomy, or because the acetabulum's center of rotation has changed. The perception of a leg length discrepancy, without an actual discrepancy, may also result from temporary periarticular soft tissue imbalances because of use of an abduction pillow or from years of compensation resulting from long-standing arthritis. A true leg length discrepancy of more than 1 cm will often cause patient dissatisfaction.[45]

Driving. An important activity of daily life that most patients are anxious to resume is driving. After THA, the decision to allow a patient to resume driving is based on a combination of factors including discontinuation of postsurgical precautions, side of the surgery, reaction times, and use of narcotic pain medication. Note that the physician, not the therapist, has to decide when a patient can resume driving. Patients in the United States return to their preoperative driving reaction times with their right leg (for braking) in 4-6 weeks postoperatively with a right THA and as early as 1 week postoperatively with a left THA. Reaction times of patients with OA of the hip are slower than age-matched subjects with normal hips.[46]

Athletic Participation. Athletic activity after total joint replacement depends in part on preoperative activity. Patients who have not participated in a specific sport or activity before surgery are less likely to achieve a high level of skill and may have an increased risk of injury. The technical aspects of joint reconstruction are also important predictors of functional outcome and athletic activity after joint replacement.[47] Another important consideration is implant fixation. Athletic activity increases the stress on fixation, and several studies have shown that increased activity level contributes to the loosening and ultimately the failure of implants.[48-50] Kilgus et al demonstrated that active patients with cemented implants had a revision rate that was twice that of their less active counterparts, but this difference was not seen until 10 years after replacement.[51]

Wear of the polyethylene liner, which depends on how much it is used, influences the survival of total joint replacements. A prosthetic joint should wear like a car tire, in that wear is a function of use or the number of cycles that the joint goes through not how old it is. It is thought that walking is the most important physical activity affecting the wear of hip and knee replacements.[52] One study notes that patients who have undergone total knee or hip replacements walk on average 1 million steps per year,[53] which is less than their healthy age-matched counterparts.[54] It was also noted that men walk on average 28% more than women and those under 60 walked 30% more than those over 60. This may be why younger patients tend to wear out their total joint replacements faster than

older patients. Polyethylene wear not only causes prosthetic failure but also produces polyethylene debris that can stimulate *osteolysis* and weakening of the bone.[55-57]

Fixation of the prosthesis also affects implant success or failure. In this case, activity may improve prognosis because exercise can increase bone density and thus improve implant fixation. Some studies have shown that there is a lower rate of prosthetic loosening in active patients.[58,59] This may be because of improved bony ingrowth in noncemented implants and protection of the implant by greater hip abductor strength.[60]

Overall, the evidence suggests that there should be a balance between too little and too much activity, with too little activity leading to decreased bone density and early prosthetic loosening (before 10 years), whereas too much activity may lead to prosthetic wear and late loosening (after 10 years).

There is limited research on the prevalence or effects of athletic activity after total hip replacement. Mallon and Callaghan[61] surveyed physician members of the Hip Society and patients who had undergone total hip replacement and previously played golf. Of the 47 Hip Society members, 96% permitted or did not discourage their patients from participating in golf. Of the surgeons, 65% recommended that their patients use a golf cart. One hundred and fifteen active golfers were surveyed at least 3 years after having a primary unilateral THA. These patients played golf an average of 3.7 times per week and noticed a 1.1-stroke increase in handicap and 3.3-yard increase in drive length after their hip replacement. It was also noted that hybrid and uncemented hips loosened less often than cemented implants. The relationship between tennis and THA was evaluated in 58 tennis players who underwent 75 THAs.[62] Only 14% of the patients stated that their surgeons approved of their return to playing tennis. These players had an average rating of 4.25 before surgery and 4.12 after surgery. On average, they played 3 times per week, returned to tennis 6.7 months after surgery, and 4% required revision surgery a mean of 8 years after their initial THA.

In a survey of 54 members of the Hip Society regarding their recommendations for athletic and sports participation for their patients who had hip replacement surgery, 42 athletic events were evaluated. Each surgeon was asked to rate the activity as recommended/allowed, allowed with experience, no opinion, or not recommended (Box 10-3).[63] McGrory et al surveyed 28 orthopedic surgeons to ascertain their guidelines for athletic participation after THA and concluded that most agreed that high-impact activities, such as baseball and running, should be avoided but that low-impact activities, such as golf and scuba diving, were recommended. The only sport that they did not uniformly agree on was cross-country skiing.[64]

Intervention

Preoperative Rehabilitation. Preoperative rehabilitation of arthritic joints has been suggested to improve postoperative rehabilitation and the effectiveness of joint replacement operations. Yet, the benefit of preoperative PT for THA has not been supported by research. In a study by Wijgman et al, patients who underwent preoperative

BOX 10-3	Activity After Total Hip Arthroplasty—1999 Hip Society Recommendations		
Recommended/Allowed	**Allowed with Experience**	**Not Recommended**	**No Conclusion**
Stationary biking	Low-impact aerobics	High-impact aerobics	Jazz dancing
Croquet	Road biking	Baseball/softball	Square dancing
Ballroom dancing	Bowling	Basketball	Fencing
Golf	Canoeing	Football	Ice skating
Horseshoes	Hiking	Gymnastics	Roller or inline skating
Shooting	Horseback riding	Handball	Rowing
Shuffleboard	Cross-country skiing	Hockey	Speed walking
Swimming		Jogging	Downhill skiing
Doubles tennis		Lacrosse	Stationary skiing machine
Walking		Racquetball	Weight lifting
		Squash	Weight machines
		Rock climbing	
		Soccer	
		Singles tennis	
		Volleyball	

physical therapy before a THA did show improvements in some measurement instruments over control groups at discharge and day 14, but there were no differences between the two groups in the time it took patients to begin standing, ambulating, negotiating stairs, or the duration of hospital stay.[65] These authors concluded that preoperative physical therapy was not useful for patients undergoing THA.

Postoperative Rehabilitation. After THA, inpatient rehabilitation generally follows a preset protocol, depending on the nature of the surgery, the patient, and the preferences of the surgeon. In general, the following goals should be attained before hospital discharge:

- Adhere to hip precautions and weight-bearing status restrictions
- Ambulate on flat surfaces for 100 feet with the use of an assistive device
- Attain functional transfers (toilet, bed) and activities of daily living (ADLs)
- Adhere to interventions to reduce the risk of bed rest hazards such as DVTs, pneumonia, pressure ulcers, and PE
- Obtain ROM within precaution limits and initiate strengthening of knee and hip musculature
- Attain independence in initial home exercise program (HEP)

Zavadak and colleagues have shown a progression in the attainment of functional milestones necessary for safe discharge to a home environment after arthroplasty.[66] They found that it took an average of 5.5 therapy sessions for a patient to transfer from sit to stand independently, 8.1 sessions to ambulate 100 feet and transfer from supine to sit, and 9.5 sessions to independently climb stairs. Discharge may be delayed if the patient lives alone or has no resources for help, and may be facilitated if a strong family support system is available. It was also noted that only 40% of all patients undergoing joint replacement surgery could perform these tasks independently, whereas 80% were considered proficient when standby assistance or

verbal cueing was available. After elective THA and TKA, patients needing continued inpatient rehabilitation after hospitalization tended to live alone (51% versus 17%), were significantly older (71.4 versus 65.1 years of age), had more comorbid conditions, and had significantly greater pain levels.[67] With improvements in surgical technique, pain control, and rehabilitation, anecdotally patients seem to be recovering more quickly and achieving independence sooner after undergoing THA with most hospitalized for 3-5 days.

Precautions, Restrictions, and Complications. One of the most important aspects of inpatient PT is to educate the patient about weight-bearing restrictions imposed by the surgeon and other precautions that must be followed after a total hip replacement. Weight-bearing restrictions after arthroplasty are not standardized and are generally based on individual surgeon preference. Few published studies are available to guide the prescription of the weight-bearing status, and there are no outcome studies supporting empirical weight-bearing restrictions used in common clinical practice.[68] Many factors not easily characterized in prospective studies can affect weight-bearing status, including the type of implant, the quality and type of fixation, the degree of bony integrity, the integrity and strength of the soft tissue envelope, and the presence of any periprosthetic fractures. Growing evidence does support the safety of allowing patients with cemented, noncemented, and hybrid primary total hip replacements to weight bear as tolerated on the operated extremity immediately after surgery.[69]

Definitions of weight-bearing status are also not standardized and therefore can lead to confusion among practitioners. Full weight-bearing implies that the patient may put all of his or her weight on the involved limb, whereas non–weight-bearing means that they must keep all of their weight off of the limb. The confusion begins with terms such as touch-down weight-bearing (TDWB) and partial weight-bearing (PWB). PWB is best described by percentage of total body weight the patient may place on the affected limb. Some authors state that PWB is 30% to 50% of body weight.[70,71] TDWB generally means that the patient may touch the affected foot to the floor for help with balance only and has been described as 10% to 15% of body weight.[72]

Studies show that most patients have difficulty estimating the percentage of body weight they actually place on their lower extremity and that most place between 69% and 85% of their total body weight on an extremity with the use of an assistive device.[73] In a study using both healthy volunteers and patients who had had lower extremity surgery or fracture, most of the patients put 35% more weight on the affected extremity than allowed. These subjects were trained on the amount of allowable body weight using a conventional bathroom scale and were tested using force plates in a gait laboratory setting.[74] On comparing methods to train patients to weight bear partially, Gray et al found that weight-bearing on the therapist's hand or a bathroom scale were ineffective (23% and 26% accuracy, respectively), whereas force platforms were effective (66% accuracy).[75] In contrast, Youdas et al found that 10 healthy subjects were trained to offload approximately 50% of their body weight with axillary and forearm crutches using a bathroom scale for feedback during a 3-point PWB gait pattern at a self-selected pace.[76] These results were confirmed through the use of force plates. However, pain, decreased upper extremity strength, or balance may alter this in patients who have undergone total joint replacements.

Reduced weight-bearing is achieved by use of assistive devices such as walkers, crutches, and canes. Determination of the appropriate assistive device depends not only on the weight-bearing status but also on the individual patient. Walkers are usually the first choice for most patients after a THA because these provide the greatest stability and the largest base of support. They reduce the contact forces at the hip to 1 times body weight during ambulation and 0.5 times body weight during double leg stance[77,78] (see Chapters 32 and 33).

ROM restrictions are prescribed postoperatively to prevent dislocation of the prosthetic joint. Patients with weak periarticular structures, such as those with collagen disease, revision surgeries, or previous dislocations, are at the greatest risk for dislocation. Other causes of dislocation include malpositioned prosthesis, trauma, and falls. The risk of dislocation appears to be the greatest during the first week after surgery when patients are least familiar with the ROM restrictions and when the periarticular soft tissues are the weakest. The rate of prosthetic hip dislocation in the postoperative phase has been reported to be between 2.1% and 3.1% for an initial replacement and 8.3% for those undergoing revision surgery.[79,80] The rate of dislocation decreases over time and levels off between 10-13 weeks postsurgery.[81] How long ROM restrictions should be adhered to is not standardized. Most surgeons require that precautions be maintained for 12 weeks after the surgery, although others recommend adherence to these restrictions for the life of the prosthesis (Fig. 10-5). A

No! **Yes**

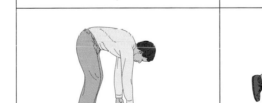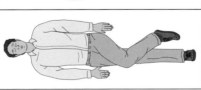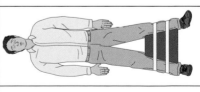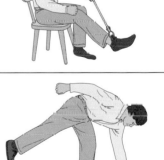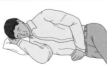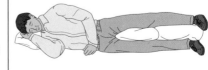

FIG. 10-5 Total hip arthroplasty: Positions to be avoided and recommended alternatives.

prospective randomized trial of 265 patients with 303 primary anterolateral-approach total hip replacements, comparing dislocation rates within 6 months after THA with and without ROM restrictions, found that only one patient dislocated and this patient was in the "restricted" group.[81] Furthermore, patients without restrictions returned to side sleeping, riding in and driving cars, and work sooner and had a higher rate of satisfaction with their recovery.[81] This suggests that ROM restrictions may not reduce dislocation rates.

To avoid overstressing healing tissues and risking injury or dislocation, the rehabilitation professional should know the anatomical approach used in the surgical procedure. This will give an appreciation of which structures were structurally compromised and which motions are least stable. The movements the surgeon used to dislocate the hip during the surgical procedure will have the greatest instability and risk of dislocation after the procedure. For example, after a THA with a posterior approach, hip flexion greater than 90 degrees, hip adduction and internal rotation should be avoided to prevent femoral head dislocation in a posterior direction. Similarly, after THA with an anterolateral approach, the hip should be protected from extremes of extension and external rotation. With the minimally invasive anterior approach, ROM precautions are often not necessary because of the limited soft tissue damage, minimal soft tissue release, and the high degree of stability achieved intraoperatively.

Although there is sparse evidence to support specific guidelines for total joint precautions, given the risk for dislocation with excessive forces postoperatively and frequent reference to such precautions in the literature and in common practice, it is prudent for the clinician to adhere to and instruct patients in total joint precautions. These precautions should be presented to the patient in functional terms. For example, a patient who underwent a THA with a posterior approach who is told not to exceed 90 degrees of hip flexion may not realize that bending over to put on stockings or pull on pants is exceeding this limitation. Patients should be instructed to avoid low seats and toilets without risers because this will increase hip flexion and probably exceed the limitation imposed by the surgeon. It is also important to tell the patient to avoid reaching their hand past their knees. For example, patients will be unable to pick objects off the floor without the help of a "reacher." Patients should also be told that when rising up from a chair, they should slide the hips forward and then stand. Patients should be reminded to not stand with feet turned in (internal rotation) or sit cross-legged.

It is also important to obtain the appropriate assistive devices and equipment to allow the patient to be discharged from inpatient care safely after a THA. Adaptive equipment and assistive devices, such as toilet seat risers (Fig. 10-6) and long-handled reachers, are often used to assist patients in adhering to the ROM restrictions while performing ADLs. Hip abduction pillows and splints and knee immobilizers (these prevent excessive hip flexion by limiting knee flexion) are also commonly prescribed to prevent restricted movements when the patient is in bed. Although these devices are commonly used, their effectiveness has not been studied.

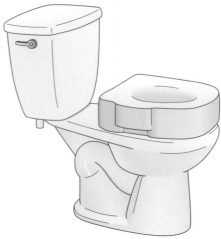

FIG. 10-6 Raised toilet seat to be used after total hip arthroplasty.

Prevention of Thromboses. One of the most common causes of severe complications after joint arthroplasty is the formation of intravascular blood clots (thrombi), which generally form in the deep veins of the legs and can cause severe complications if they embolize (move) to the lungs, resulting in a PE, which is one of the most common causes of death after lower extremity arthroplasty. Kakkar et al reported that 29% of thrombi occur before postoperative day 12 and 23% occur between postoperative days 13 and 24.[82] Thus the risk is greatest during the first 3 weeks after surgery.

Prophylaxis for thromboemboli can be broadly divided into 2 categories—nonpharmacological and pharmacological. Nonpharmacological thromboprophylaxis interventions include elastic compression stockings, early ambulation, and intermittent pneumatic compression (IPC). Elastic compression stockings are traditionally used as an adjunct to other methods because other treatment methods have been found to be more effective.[83] Early ambulation is also associated with a lower incidence of symptomatic thromboembolic disease.[84] IPC devices can be helpful but are only effective if used at all times when the patient is not walking. How long each day such devices must be used is unknown, although it is presumed that the longer the better.[85]

The optimal method of thromboprophylaxis after total joint arthroplasty is controversial. A combination of pharmacological and nonpharmacological methods seems most beneficial. A protocol that used aspirin, elastic stockings, exercise, and intermittent compression devices yielded good clinical results.[86] The principle pharmacological prophylactic agents used by most surgeons are Coumadin or low molecular weight heparin (LMWH). The optimal duration of this prophylaxis is unknown, but there is evidence to suggest that prophylaxis for THA should extend for 4-6 weeks as the chance for a DVT in this patient population lasts longer than for a patient with a TKA.[87] The therapist should know if these drugs have been used since they may predispose patients to bruising or bleeding with vigorous activity or mobilization.

Therapists should also recognize signs and symptoms of DVT, which include increased pain and swelling in the lower extremities (see Box 10-2). It is important to communicate any such findings to the surgeon.

Exercise. As with other aspects of rehabilitation after THA, exercise protocols are based mainly on clinical experience and preferences rather than on research-derived evidence. A THA exercise program reported as a consensus of several practitioners included ankle pumps, quadriceps and gluteal sets, and active hip flexion.[88] Patients are encouraged to sit on the side of the bed, stand with the walker, and begin supine knee and hip flexion exercises postoperatively on day 1. In another protocol, active assist ROM (AAROM) and strengthening were initiated on day 2.[89] Some facilities only used walking programs, whereas other postoperative protocols included instruction in specific exercises and functional training.[90]

The surgical disruption of muscles, ligaments, and capsules during hip joint replacement surgery can affect muscle strength, stability, and joint proprioception. Hip abductor strengthening has been described as the single most important exercise for the patient to return to a nonantalgic gait.[91] Hip abductor strengthening after THA has been shown to prevent a Trendelenburg gait (see Chapter 32) and improve hip stability,[92,93] and patients with greater hip abduction strength demonstrate quicker early postoperative functional progress.[94] Vaz et al also found a correlation between distance walked during a 6-minute walk test and hip abductor torque in patients after THA.[95]

Muscle strengthening programs after THA must respect surgeon-imposed restrictions, as well as tissue healing and pain. This is achieved by starting with exercises that place the least amount of stress on the joint and soft tissue envelope, progressing to functional activities. A progression of isometrics followed by isotonic antigravity activities, such as knee extension exercises, then progressing to pulleys, weights, and elastic resistance bands is recommended. Closed kinetic-chain activities, such as step-ups and mini-squats, allow for a progression to functional ADLs and recreational activities. These activities most often involve some degree of weight bearing and muscle co-contraction, which often adds to joint stability.

Another intervention that has shown promise after THA is partial body weight–supported treadmill walking. A randomized controlled trial (RCT) showed that this activity resulted in faster return to symmetrical unassisted ambulation, greater gluteus medius activity, and more hip extension ROM than conventional physical therapy alone.[96]

When considering exercise prescription and patient education regarding activity level, it is important to consider the amount of stress placed on the joint components during specific activities. Some limited single-subject studies have questioned assumptions made by clinicians as to specific exercises used in the early stages of rehabilitation after THA. These studies found that some exercises that are traditionally considered low level, such as maximal contraction gluteal sets, unassisted heel slides, and manually resisted isometric hip abduction, may actually generate greater acetabular contact forces than are generated by weight-bearing activities.[97-99] The clinician may therefore find that these exercises may not be appropriate for patients with weight-bearing restrictions. However, if weight-bearing is not an issue, these exercises may be well tolerated.

The most recent in-vivo instrumented hip studies, although limited by number of participants and difficulty with instrumentation, yield further valuable information to guide exercise prescription.[100,101] Data obtained through a triaxial telemeterized total hip replacement implanted in patients as part of a THA procedure demonstrated that single leg stance transmits a force of approximately two times body weight (BW) to the hip joint, straight leg raises impart a force of 1.5-1.8 BW and stair climbing imparts a force of 2.6 BW and a significant torsional stress on the femoral stem component. Torsional stresses may cause femoral loosening.[102] Bergmann et al described hip joint forces that varied with walking speed ranging from 3.0-4.5 BW on the stance leg and usually below 1.0 BW during swing phase.[103] During jogging, hip forces reached 5.0 BW. In a subsequent publication, Bergmann et al, reported peak hip forces of 2.7 BW during level walking, 1.5 BW with straight leg raises, and 2.5 BW with a bilateral pelvic bridge. Stair climbing caused hip forces to rise to 2.0-3.5 BW, which increased with stair descent causing high torsional moments. Rising from a low chair also imposes a high load across the hip joint, which approaches 8 times BW.[104] Both the direction and the magnitude of this force places the hip at a high risk for posterior dislocation with this activity, especially during early healing when the soft tissue envelope is weak. The use of armrests when rising from a chair decreased forces markedly.[105] Abduction exercises against resistance created forces of 1.3 BW, whereas cycling caused only a small increase in forces, except when accelerating quickly, which caused a force of 2.7 BW. The lowest hip forces were recorded when the patient was bare footed or wearing soft soled shoes.

The effectiveness of exercise after initial hospitalization for THA was prospectively evaluated by Sashika.[106] A non–RCT of a HEP in 23 patients 6-48 months after surgery compared 3 different interventions: (1) ROM and isometric strengthening exercises; (2) ROM, isometric, and eccentric strengthening exercises; and (3) no exercise program. Hip ROM, isometric strength, gait speed, and cadence were evaluated after 6 weeks. Hip abduction strength improved in all groups, with the greatest gains in the group performing eccentric exercise, and gait speed and cadence improved in both exercise groups. Similarly, a randomized controlled study found that THA patients who adhered to a HEP of 30 minutes of walking and bilateral isotonic strengthening of the hip muscles had better hip muscle strength, walking speed, and function than a matched control group who did not exercise.[107] The evidence indicates that most of the benefits of rehabilitation are achieved by 3-6 months after surgery[108]; however, patients may continue to make gains for up to 2 years.[109]

Postural stability after THA has not been investigated thoroughly, although it stands to reason that after an incision of the joint capsule and muscular structures, with subsequent disarticulation and joint replacement, that a patient's proprioception may change. Wykman found that double limb stance sway was decreased 12 months after surgery in 21 patients who underwent THA for hip OA.[110] Exercises to improve balance are also recommended after THA because poor balance has been shown to be highly predictive of falls and subsequent disability in the elderly.[111] The evidence regarding the effects of THA on balance is conflicting. One study found that patients who undergo a THA have significantly better postural stability in bilateral stance 12 months after surgery than preoperatively.[112] However, THA patients tested in single leg stance had significantly decreased postural stability on the surgical side.[113] The authors speculated that this may be due to muscular weakness, especially in the hip abductors and hip flexors. It therefore appears important to work on strength and balance control to limit falls in this patient population. Activities, such as single leg balancing and weight shifts, are recommended (see Chapter 13 for other interventions to improve balance).

Modalities. Research on the use of modalities in the treatment of total hip replacement is very limited. For example, only one study was found that examined the use of cryotherapy after THA.[114] This study demonstrated that local cooling reduces surgery-related pain after THA. Cryotherapy is also thought to limit bleeding and swelling by constricting blood vessels and may reduce tissue metabolism and inflammation, preventing secondary soft tissue damage. Ice also has a local anesthetic effect and reduces muscle spasms. Although this local treatment does not penetrate to the depth of the hip joint and capsule, it may modulate pain by gating at the spinal cord level and by producing anesthesia of the skin in the area.

The use of ultrasound (US) over a cemented joint replacement or one with polyethylene plastic components is contraindicated since these materials may be rapidly heated by US.[115] US may, however, be used on noncemented and all metal component joints because US does not rapidly heat metal or loosen screws or plates.[116] The effect of US on cemented joints with or without plastic components is in all likelihood minimal since little US will penetrate to the depth of most prosthetic joints; however, it is recommended that the clinician err on the side of caution and not use this modality over such materials.[117] Diathermy is contraindicated in patients with metal implants, including total hip replacements, because the metal can become very hot and damage adjacent tissues.

TOTAL KNEE ARTHROPLASTY

According to the National Institutes of Health (NIH) Consensus Study on total knee replacement, the use of rehabilitation services is the most understudied aspect of perioperative management of total knee replacement patients.[118] Postoperative physical therapy and rehabilitation "greatly influence the outcome of total knee arthroplasty."[119]

The three main types of component design used for uncomplicated primary knee replacements are the *cruciate retaining* knee, the *posterior stabilized* knee, and the *mobile bearing* knee. There are negligible functional differences between these prostheses, thus selection usually depends on the preference of the surgeon. In the posterior cruciate retention design, the posterior cruciate ligament supplements the anteroposterior (AP) stability of the prosthesis. In the posterior stabilized implant, the cruciate ligaments are resected and AP stability is provided by the conformity of the components and by a central tibial spine. Huang et al assessed muscle strength ratios of 50 knees after TKA and found no difference in hamstring to quadriceps ratio among posterior stabilized and cruciate retaining prosthetic designs. However, even after 6-13 years, the ratios were not the same as in controls who had not had TKAs.[120] A mobile bearing knee has a polyethylene insert that articulates with the femoral component and with the metallic tibial tray, thus creating a dual surface articulation. This feature is intended to reduce the stress and fatigue wear on the polyethylene insert and possibly the osteolysis caused by polyethylene particles that may contribute to joint replacement failure (Fig. 10-7).

TKAs also vary in their method of fixation. The prosthesis can be cemented or uncemented, or a combination of the two, known as a hybrid. The hybrid fixation, where the tibial component is cemented and the femoral component is uncemented, is gaining popularity; however, cemented TKAs are still the most common.

A more recent trend in knee replacement is a minimally invasive surgical approach, in which the quadriceps muscle is either not cut or only a small 1-2 cm "snip" in the vastus medialis oblique muscle is made. This avoids damage to the extensor mechanism and thereby allows better quadriceps contraction than with the traditional approaches where the quadriceps tendon is cut. The skin incision is also much shorter (3-5 inches versus 8-12 inches in the traditional TKA), which limits soft tissue trauma. The same clinically proven implants as used in the traditional total knee replacement are utilized (Fig. 10-8). This modified procedure is gaining popularity because it appears to cause less pain and blood loss and results in

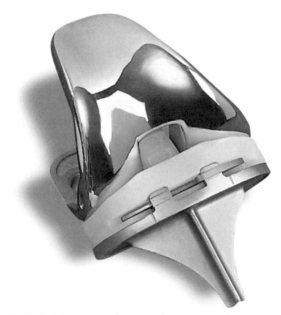

FIG. 10-7 Total knee replacement components for a mobile bearing knee. *Image courtesy Biomet.*

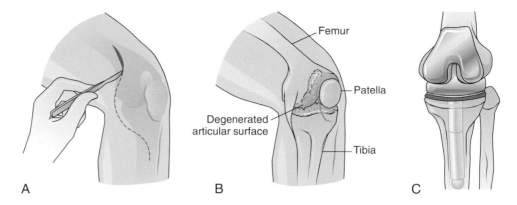

FIG. 10-8 Total knee arthroplasty procedure.

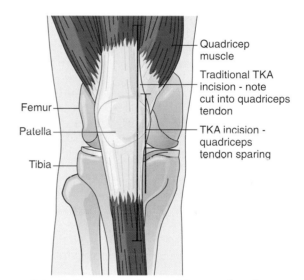

FIG. 10-9 Incisions for total knee arthroplasty.

a shortened hospital stay, improved ROM and strength, and less time on crutches or a walker. However, there is still limited research on outcomes for minimally invasive TKAs.

Another advancement in TKA is computer-assisted surgery. Although this technique is not widely used, some centers report excellent results because of improved alignment of the lower extremity when compared to the conventional technique. The potential benefits in long-term outcome and functional improvement require further clinical investigation.[121]

Pathology. For the TKA procedure, a longitudinal incision of the skin is made along the anterior aspect of the knee from just proximal to the patella to just distal to the tibial tubercle (Fig. 10-9). The quadriceps are then either split or moved aside to expose the joint. The knee is then flexed and the entire knee joint, including the ends of the tibia and femur, as well as the menisci and anterior cruciate ligament (and possibly the posterior cruciate ligament depending on the implant), are excised and the prosthesis is placed. If there are knee deformities, soft tissue and ligament balancing are performed to achieve optimal alignment. The wounds are then thoroughly irrigated, a drain placed, and the incision is closed with sutures.

Examination. The examination of the patient with a TKA is similar to that presented in the general arthroplasty examination section with a few added components specific to the knee in general such as assessing patellar mobility. It is also important to assess the extensor mechanism's extensibility, as well as its ability to generate a contraction and ultimately adequate force. This should be done through passive ROM and manual muscle testing, respectively.

Prognosis. Studies comparing preoperative and postoperative knee total ROM after TKA report a mean increase of 8 degrees.[122] After TKA, quadriceps strength is commonly less than it was preoperatively for up to 2 months after the surgery,[123] and generally remains below that of the uninvolved side,[124,125] and that of age-matched people without OA,[126-128] even after strength training. Weakness directly after surgery is most likely caused by pain, effusion, and soft tissue injury, as well as by muscle atrophy and limited volitional control. Quadriceps weakness impairs function and has been correlated with an increased risk of falling,[129] as well as decreased ambulation

speed,[130] decreased performance in sit to stand transfers,[131] and decreased ability to negotiate stairs.[132]

According to one prospective study, early quadriceps weakness after TKA is due to impaired volitional control of the muscle and to a lesser extent, atrophy. Pain had surprisingly little effect on muscle activation. Thus pain control alone will not be sufficient to improve strength, and efforts must be made to directly address voluntary muscle activation early in the postoperative period, using modalities, such as biofeedback and electrical stimulation, if needed to offset these deficiencies.[133]

A survey assessed activities considered important and limiting to patients that had undergone TKA.[134] Of those surveyed, 40% felt that squatting was an important task and 75% reported some limitation in this activity. It was not noted whether this limitation was due to lack of ROM or strength, but many patients noted that it was difficult to descend stairs and participate in heavy domestic chores that are affected by lower extremity strength.[135] These finding were also corroborated in a study using the WOMAC (Western Ontario and McMaster Universities Osteoarthritis Index), which found that patients who were 3 months' post-TKA reported that descending stairs, doing heavy domestic duties, and getting in and out of a car or bath were among their most difficult tasks.[136] In a study of 397 knee patients, the Activities of Daily Living Scale (ADLS) proved to be a reliable, valid, and responsive patient-reported instrument for assessing functional limitations in patients with knee pathology. This scale is part of the knee outcome survey (KOS) developed at the University of Pittsburgh. The functional limitations in this survey include difficulty walking on level surfaces and stairs and standing, kneeling, sitting, and rising from a chair.[137] Approximately 1-year after TKA, patients have been found to be 51% slower in ascending and descending stairs than age- and gender-matched controls.[138] Stair climbing has also been found to be much more demanding for patients after TKA than for healthy controls.[139] Therefore rehabilitation efforts should focus on activities that help patients improve performance of these ADLs.

Athletic Participation. Indications for total knee replacement have expanded over the last decade to include improvement in athletic participation. Recommendations regarding which athletic activities patients may participate in after TKA must take into account biomechanics, joint stability, strength, prior experience, and level of participation. Tibiofemoral and patellofemoral biomechanics in the TKA have shown peak loads of 2 times BW with level walking and 3.1 times BW while descending stairs.[140] Bradbury et al[141] evaluated sports participation after TKA in 160 patients who underwent 208 TKAs. Forty-nine percent of the patients participated in sports at least 1 time per week before surgery, and 65% participated in sports at least 1 time a week after surgery. Twenty percent of patients returned to high-impact sports, such as tennis, whereas 91% returned to low-impact activities.

A biomechanical study tested the compressive forces generated on three different TKA implant designs during four recreational activities: Cycling, power walking, downhill skiing, and mountain hiking. The authors measured the amount of implant surface area that was loaded to the polyethylene yield point and found that cycling and power walking were the safest activities, whereas downhill skiing and mountain hiking were associated with significant overloaded areas.[142] Some activities, such as mountain hiking, may be modified to reduce the joint loads. For example, avoiding steep descents, walking slowly when going downhill, and using ski poles or hiking poles when hiking can reduce the load on the knee joint by as much as 20%.[143]

Mallon and Callaghan and Mallon et al surveyed 72 surgeon members of the Knee Society regarding knee replacement surgery in active golfers.[61,144] Ninety-two percent recommended or did not discourage their patients with a TKA from playing golf, 66% recommended that their patients use a golf cart, and 96% noted no increase in complications in patients who played golf. The authors also surveyed 83 amateur golfers with a unilateral TKA at an average minimum of 3-years after their TKA. Patients returned to golf on average 18 weeks after surgery, noting a 4.6-stroke rise in their handicap and a 12.2-yard decrease in their drive length. Of these golfers, 87% reported using a cart and 84% reported no pain during play, but 35% reported a mild ache after the round of golf. LaPorte et al[145] reported on 11 male tennis players with a total of 18 TKAs with an average age at time of surgery of 72 years. All patients were satisfied with their results at their annual follow-up of 3 years. Their average National Tennis Player ranking was 3.94 before and 3.72 after arthroplasty. Fifty-two percent of surgeons did not recommend that their patients play tennis after TKA. The results of a survey of 58 members of the Knee Society regarding recommendations for participation in 42 different athletics and sports activities after TKA are shown in Box 10-4.[146]

Driving. Another important aspect in returning to normal life and independence after TKA is returning to driving. Brake response time after TKA returns to preoperative level as early as 3-weeks' postoperatively, and at 9-weeks' postoperatively, there is a significant improvement over baseline measurements.[147] Based on these findings, it is recommended that patients undergoing TKA be allowed to return to driving 6 weeks after surgery.

BOX 10-4   Activity After Total Knee Arthroplasty—1999 Knee Society Recommendations

Recommended/Allowed	Allowed with Experience	Not Recommended	No Conclusion
Low-impact aerobics	Road biking	Racquetball	Fencing
Stationary biking	Canoeing	Squash	Roller or inline skating
Bowling	Hiking	Rock climbing	Downhill skiing
Golf	Rowing	Soccer	Weight lifting
Dancing	Cross-country skiing	Singles tennis	
Horseback riding	Stationary skiing machine	Volleyball	
Croquet	Speed walking	Football	
Walking	Doubles tennis	Gymnastics	
Swimming	Weight machines	Lacrosse	
Shooting	Ice skating	Hockey	
Shuffleboard		Basketball	
Horseshoes		Jogging	
		Handball	

Intervention

Preoperative Exercise. There are few controlled studies evaluating the benefit of preoperative PT for patients undergoing TKA. Studies by Weidenheilm et al[148] and Mattsson et al,[149] both done on patients scheduled to undergo *unicompartmental knee replacement,* reported similar findings. In both studies the patients who underwent preoperative physical therapy showed a slight improvement in pain, subjective stability of the knee during walking, and an improvement in gait speeds over the control group. However, 3 months after surgery, there were no significant differences between groups. One study comparing a preoperative physical therapy exercise group, a cardiovascular conditioning group, and a control group of patients undergoing total knee replacement found that neither exercise group showed a statistically significant difference in their postoperative course compared with the controls.[150] This could be because the chronicity of the preoperative symptoms made them resistant to a limited amount of physical therapy or because the preoperative pain prevented patients from performing sufficient exercise to improve outcomes. Alternatively, the total knee replacement surgery could be so effective that it overshadows the relatively smaller benefit of preoperative exercise, or the initial response to the trauma of the surgery may negate any benefits of preoperative exercise. Thus preoperative physical therapy is not generally thought to improve long-term outcomes or significantly shorten hospital stays in patients undergoing total knee replacement.

Postoperative Rehabilitation. The following guidelines for rehabilitation progression should be tailored to the individual patient. The rehabilitation professional should evaluate the findings from the examination to determine when milestones are met and when rehabilitation can proceed and not rely on a "cookbook" approach or "protocol." The therapist must, however, respect tissue healing parameters and the postsurgical precautions.

Immediate postoperative recovery of the patient with a TKA centers on achieving functional milestones. Inpatient rehabilitation programs and functional milestones are similar to those of THA, including ambulation with an assistive device, independent transfers, achievement of ROM, initiation of strengthening, and understanding and performance of an appropriate HEP. Since postoperative hospital stays have become shorter, the clinician must educate the patient, family members, and other caregivers as to the importance of these milestones.

Most surgeons advocate the same rehabilitation parameters after total knee replacement for implants with cemented or biological fixation, although some advocate limited weight bearing for up to 6 weeks for uncemented implants. It is customary for full weight bearing to be allowed with all primary TKAs unless certain other conditions, such as severe osteoporosis, fracture, concomitant osteotomies, or bone grafts, are present. This may not be the case with revision TKAs, especially if bone grafting or tibial tuberosity osteotomies were performed. It is always prudent to contact the surgeon if there is any doubt as to the weight-bearing status of the patient.

During the initial phase of outpatient rehabilitation, the focus should be on tissue healing and reducing pain and inflammation. It is during this period that modalities, such as cold and compression, are used to decrease pain and swelling. A study by Ivey et al found that cryotherapy reduced pain and swelling after TKA.[151] A prospective study using continuous flow cold therapy on 30 patients undergoing bilateral staged primary TKA showed that the patients had less pain when the cooling device was used, used less analgesic medication for this procedure, and had improved wound healing and less blood loss.[152] Anecdotally, combination pneumatic compression/cryotherapy devices have also shown promise (Fig. 10-10).

The use of *continuous passive motion* (CPM) machines (see Fig. 9-12) after TKA remains controversial. No study to date has offered conclusive evidence of the long-term benefits of the use of CPM. CPM is considered a cost-effective intervention that facilitates early knee flexion after TKA. Studies suggest that CPM promotes greater earlier knee flexion ROM, decreased postoperative knee pain, fewer days of inpatient rehabilitation, decreased DVT incidence, and a decreased need for surgical manipulation.[153,154] McInnes reported on a RCT that compared immediate and 6-week outcomes of subjects treated with CPM and physical therapy versus physical therapy alone.[155] They found that adding CPM to physical therapy resulted in increased initial active knee flexion ROM, decreased swelling, and reduced the number of manipulations but did not affect initial active or passive knee extension ROM or quadriceps strength. At 6 weeks, there were no differences noted. A meta-analysis of the effectiveness of CPM after TKA reported that CPM in conjunction with physical therapy had favorable results when compared with physical therapy alone but did not significantly improve passive or active knee extension.[156] Use of a CPM machine can be started immediately postoperatively, although some surgeons advocate waiting until postoperative day 2 to avoid disruption of the incision.

Achieving knee flexion early in rehabilitation allows patients more independence in ADLs since 65 degrees of

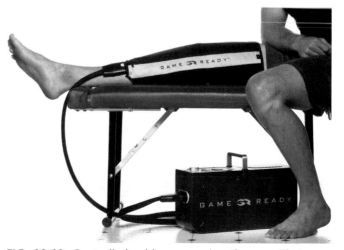

FIG. 10-10 Controlled cold compression therapy. *Photo courtesy GameReady.*

flexion is required for a normal swing phase during gait, and 105 degrees is needed to rise comfortably from sitting. Final postoperative knee flexion ROM depends on the type of implant used, the preoperative ROM,[157] and the mobility of the patient's soft tissues. Aggressive rehabilitation and adequate pain control are also paramount to prevent postoperative contractures and optimize flexion ROM. It has been suggested that a lack of physical therapy can contribute to decreased functional ROM after TKA.[158]

To achieve optimal results, ROM activities for the patient with a TKA should be initiated soon after surgery. Patients often have a flexion contracture immediately after surgery because of irritation of the joint and hemarthrosis. This will resolve with time and appropriate rehabilitation. ROM activities can include passive knee flexion and extension, as well as active heel slides and supine wall slides. Forward and backward pedaling on a stationary bicycle can also increase flexion ROM. With the saddle of the bicycle high, a patient with limited flexion can often "rock" back and forth and ultimately complete a backward revolution. This is an excellent way for a patient to improve ROM in a safe and self-controlled manner.

Full extension ROM is also essential for a normal gait pattern and for efficient function of the lower extremity. A limitation of as little as 5 degrees of extension may require a quadriceps force of 30% of a person's BW to stabilize the knee, with more force being needed as the amount of knee flexion limitation increases.[159] Therefore a patient who cannot achieve full extension during gait will expend more energy walking. They may also have limited knee stability as a result of compromised strength of the quadriceps muscles after TKA. Full extension can be achieved in a variety of ways (Fig. 10-11). First, the patient should not sleep with a pillow under the knee, although this will be a position of comfort. To achieve full extension, the patient may lie prone with the knee on the edge of the bed, allowing gravity to extend the knee. Another option is to lie supine and place a pillow under the heel, allowing the knee to extend. To further intensify this stretch the patient may use a slow-sustained pressure manually or from a small weight such as a phone book or weighted bag to achieve full extension. Backward walking may also help the patient who has difficulty achieving full extension. This may be done in a pool or on land.

Prevention and early recognition of ROM limitations are essential to prevent *arthrofibrosis,* a potential complication of any knee surgery. Arthrofibrosis is a process that occurs when diffuse scar tissue or fibrous adhesions form within or around a joint. This periarticular scarring can restrict flexion, extension, or patellar mobility. Manual patellar mobilization, as well as mobilization of the soft tissues of the quadriceps and patellar tendon, is critical to restoring normal extensor mobility and ultimately a functional knee. The patella should be mobilized in all planes, mediolateral and superoinferior, and the tendons should be manually mobilized medially and laterally (Fig. 10-12). Gentle patellar and scar mobilization initiated after the incision site is stable may also help prevent contractures and promote functional ROM. Patellar mobilization is very important because the suprapatellar pouch is often

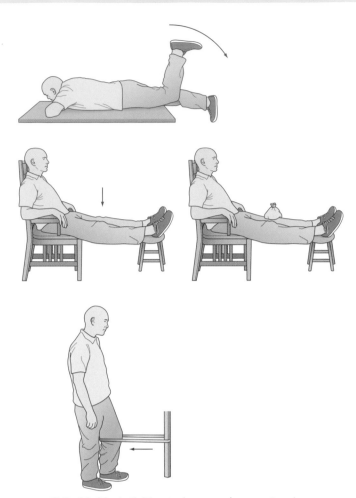

FIG. 10-11 Activities to increase knee extension.

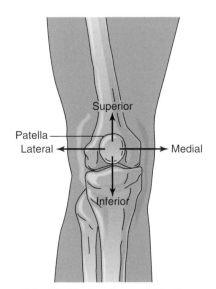

FIG. 10-12 Patellar mobilization.

where adhesions that limit ROM develop. These mobilizations should also be taught to patients so that they can be performed at home. Decreased superior mobility of the patella interferes with the ability of the quadriceps muscles to straighten the knee and may also result in an *extensor lag.* An extensor lag occurs when the range of

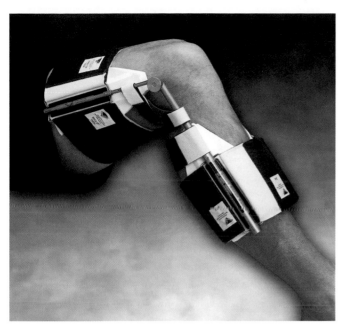

FIG. 10-13 Dynamic splinting of the knee for increased ROM. Low load prolonged stretching device that can be used to improve knee flexion or extension ROM. *Courtesy Dynasplint Systems, Inc.*

active extension is less than the passive extension of the joint. In the case of the knee, this may also be known as a quadriceps lag because it is caused by the quadriceps muscles not being able to straighten the knee fully even though the patient may have full passive extension. Full inferior glide of the patella is essential to maximize flexion ROM.

If rehabilitation techniques are not effective in achieving functional ROM, it may be necessary to add bracing, such as dynamic splinting (Fig. 10-13), or have surgical intervention through arthroscopic release or manipulation under anesthesia to maximize ROM. Early motion is the key for the successful rehabilitation of the postoperative knee.[160]

Pool therapy is an excellent adjunct for gait training, ROM, strengthening, and ultimately recreation in patients after TKA. One study in Germany with 25 patients reported that hydrotherapy was superior to the "standard rehabilitation program" in the rehabilitation of patients with TKA.[161] Another activity that often helps patients achieve full knee extension ROM is standing closed-chain knee extensions using a resistance band (or towel) placed at the distal thigh and held by the therapist (see Fig. 10-11) for feedback. This activity will also improve extension by increasing active extension force and gently stretching the posterior capsule.

Electrical Stimulation. Neuromuscular electrical stimulation (NMES) is an alternative and potentially more effective means than exercise alone of decreasing persistent quadriceps weakness in the appropriate patient. It adds to active exercise alone by recruiting a greater proportion of type II fibers. These fibers have a higher incidence of atrophy in patients with a history of severe OA.[162] It has been shown that NMES used alone or in combination with

volitional exercise is helpful in regaining functional quadriceps strength in this patient population.[163] In a case study of an elderly patient with disuse atrophy after TKA, NMES was used to supplement volitional exercise of the quadriceps femoris and resulted in an increase of force production from 50% (involved/uninvolved) at 3-weeks postsurgery to 86% at 8-weeks postsurgery.[164] NMES has also been shown to increase walking speed in a prospective randomized controlled study of 30 TKA patients treated for 4 hours a day for a period of 6 weeks.[165] NMES has also been reported to improve the functional capacity of the quadriceps and to attenuate disuse atrophy associated with TKA.[166]

Exercise. Rehabilitation after TKA must restore the function of muscles that cross the knee joint as well as those muscles that influence the proximal and distal motion segments. During the initial stages, regaining motor control of the quadriceps muscles should be emphasized. In patients with an acute knee effusion as a result of acute or surgical trauma, reflex inhibition of the quadriceps is common.[167-169] Strengthening exercise after TKA should start with quadriceps isometrics and straight legs raises. Open-chain lower extremity strengthening activities can be progressed as tolerated to promote voluntary quadriceps control. Repetitive open-chain exercises, especially in the range of 40 degrees to full extension, may increase soft tissue irritation that can occur in the early postoperative period.[140] Electrical stimulation, biofeedback, and tactile stimulation can be used for quadriceps facilitation. In addition, hip adduction and abduction strengthening exercises, as well as hamstring curls, may be added to strengthen all muscle groups around the knee joint. As strength improves and pain decreases, closed-chain strengthening should be added to improve function. Most patients with chronic knee joint arthritis have altered quadriceps function especially for performing closed kinetic-chain activities such as stair stepping.[170-172] Closed-chain exercises may include mini-squats, front and lateral step-ups, stool pulls, and lunges as tolerated (Fig. 10-14). These activities improve quadriceps, hamstring, and overall lower extremity strength.[173,174] The patient should avoid activities that increase load on the joint because this may damage the replaced surfaces. Such activities include squats and leg press performed at more than 90 degrees of flexion. Some rehabilitation professionals feel that TKA patients should be treated similarly to patients with patellofemoral pain syndrome since many of these patients have very limited quadriceps strength and dysfunction of their extensor mechanism. Gym equipment may also be used for a variety of closed-chain strengthening activities. Stationary cycling, pool therapy, and a walking program may be added to achieve optimal function and allow patients to ultimately return to participation in selected recreational sports activities. However, activities that involve high impact should be avoided because these increase wear on the components and can hasten the need for revision.

Sensorimotor functions, such as proprioception, joint position sense, and balance, are all important for function of the lower extremities. Proprioception is the conscious and unconscious perception of limb position in

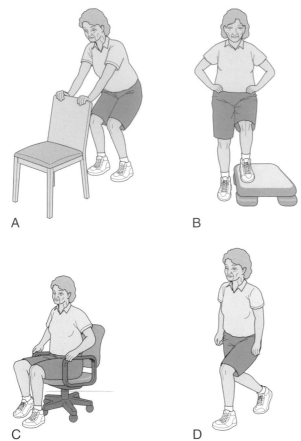

FIG. 10-14 Sample of closed kinetic chain exercises for the lower extremity. **A,** Mini-squat; **B,** step-up; **C,** stool pull/push; **D,** lunges.

space, including the awareness of joint position and movement.[175] Balance is the ability to maintain a posture or postural control during movement.[176] Elderly people and patients with arthritis and with TKAs have been shown to have a poorer joint position sense than young people without OA, and reestablishing joint position sense and balance are important for optimizing patient outcomes.[177-180] Some studies have shown that proprioception and balance improve after a total knee replacement, although not consistently for all types of implants and not to levels equal to age-matched subjects without joint disease.[181-185] Some studies have postulated that improvement in joint position sense and balance after TKA is due to reestablishment of soft tissue tension and joint space, reduction of pain and chronic inflammation, and the resumption of ADLs.[185] Since balance and proprioception can impact the frequency of falls and subsequent injury, rehabilitation programs for TKA should include activities that will improve these functions (see Chapter 13).

SHOULDER ARTHROPLASTIES

Shoulder arthroplasty is not as common as THA or TKA and most general orthopedic surgeons have limited experience with it. However, the number of TSAs has increased substantially over the past decade from approximately

10,000 in 1990 to 20,000 in 2000.[6] TSAs involve replacement of both the glenoid and the humeral head, whereas hemiarthroplasties involve the replacement of only the humeral component. Because of the need for careful soft tissue balancing and implant insertion, this procedure is considered by many to be mainly for pain relief, although Jensen et al found that many patients were able to return to prior recreational activities such as golf.[186]

Pathology. Both constrained and nonconstrained TSA prostheses are currently used. A constrained TSA has a ball and socket design that reduces humeral motion. A nonconstrained TSA more closely resembles the normal anatomical motion of the shoulder joint, allowing for more humeral motion, and is the type of prosthesis most commonly used. A semiconstrained prosthesis with a hood on the superior aspect of the glenoid that helps with stability is sometimes used for patients with irreparable rotator cuff tears. The humeral component of total shoulder replacements can be either press-fit or cemented, whereas the glenoid portion is always cemented. Symptomatic loosening of the glenoid component is usually associated with pain, whereas loosening of the humeral component is often asymptomatic. The implant may loosen if an eccentric load is placed on the glenoid by the humeral component, especially if the humeral head migrates superiorly as a result of poor deltoid or rotator cuff function from weakness or a tear. Postoperatively, 1% to 13% of patients with TSAs develop rotator cuff tears.[187]

Another less common form of shoulder arthroplasty is the Copeland surface replacement of the humeral head, which replaces only the damaged joint surface and restores the anatomy with minimal bone resection. This procedure is indicated for patients with rheumatoid arthritis (RA) and OA if the bone is strong and the joint is not severely damaged.[188]

Shoulder arthroplasty involves an incision from a point superomedial to the coracoid process down toward the anterior insertion of the deltoid on the upper arm. If the surgery is undertaken because of a humeral fracture, the soft tissue attachments of the tuberosities are preserved and reattached to the humeral shaft and stem before the wound is closed so that the rotator cuff can function. If the surgery is undertaken because of arthritis, the subscapularis muscle and the joint capsule are taken down. The humeral head is then removed and the glenoid is inspected. If it is significantly worn, it is replaced. The humeral canal is then reamed, and the humeral component is inserted, with or without cement, depending on the shoulder's condition and the surgeon's preference. The final components are then placed and the subscapularis is repaired. The deltopectoral interval and the skin are then closed (Fig. 10-15).

Prognosis. Over the past 2 decades, TSA and hemiarthroplasty of the shoulder have been successfully used to treat a wide variety of shoulder conditions. Most total shoulder replacements are performed on patients with OA, RA, avascular necrosis, or posttraumatic fractures.[189] A retrospective study indicates that patients of surgeons with a higher annual caseload of shoulder arthroplasties have fewer complications and shorter hospital lengths of stay than patients of surgeons who perform fewer of these pro-

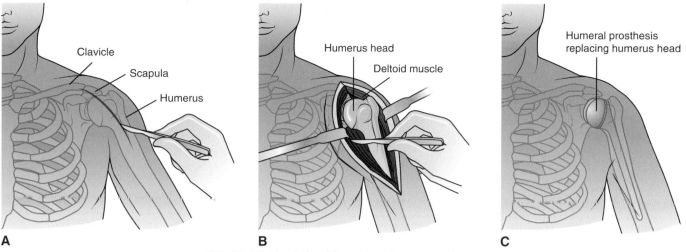

A   B   C

FIG. 10-15 Total shoulder arthroplasty procedure.

cedures.[190] It has also been shown that centers where more of these procedures are performed have better outcomes and lower complication rates.[191]

The outcome depends on factors common to all total joint replacements as well as those specific to the shoulder, most importantly, the status of the rotator cuff muscles. In patients with minimally retracted or non-retracted rotator cuff tears that are limited to the supraspinatus tendon, a multicenter study has shown that the outcome of shoulder arthroplasty done for OA is similar to that for patients without rotator cuff tears. However, if the infraspinatus or, less importantly, the subscapularis is involved, the outcome is poorer.[192] Although patients often have limited ROM, strength, and function before surgery, TSA can primarily be expected to relieve pain rather than improve other symptoms. Meta-analyses have found that more than 90% of patients with shoulder OA, RA,[193] or osteonecrosis[194,195] and over 70% of patients with shoulder fractures do have complete or near-complete relief of pain after TSA.[196,197]

Functional results after TSA vary, depending largely on the underlying cause. Patients with OA or osteonecrosis tend to get the best ROM, reaching 75% to 80% of normal and being able to achieve an average forward flexion ROM of greater than 140 degrees and external rotation ROM of 45 degrees, as well as reaching their hand behind their back to approximately 2-3 levels above their presurgical ROM. Flexion after hemiarthroplasty performed in patients with humeral fractures can range from 90-120 degrees.[198] Outcome is best with a well-reduced fracture, a motivated patient, and an appropriate rehabilitation program with a maximum recovery of function usually occurring within 6-12 months of the surgery.[199-201] Patients with RA or dislocation *arthropathy* have poorer functional outcomes than other patients, regaining on average 50% to 60% of normal motion because they often have poor soft tissue and bone quality. Patients with arthropathy a result of a rotator cuff tear also fare poorly, generally achieving only 33% to 50% of normal motion.[202] Some patients who have a TSA for recurrent instability have pain and arthrosis after surgery, at times because of continued multidirectional instability, overtightening of the soft tissues, or progressive cartilage wear.[203,204]

Strength after TSA is generally sufficient to allow ADLs, as well as light recreational fitness activities such as golf, light fitness training, gardening, and swimming. Goldberg et al documented a self-reported increase in the performance of functional tasks in patients who underwent TSA for the treatment of OA.[205] Patients rated their ability to perform a total of 12 tasks, including lifting, tucking in their shirt, underhand toss, and sleeping on the affected side, at specific intervals before and up to 5 years after surgery. Before surgery, patients reported that they could perform 3.8 of the tasks, 1 year after surgery they could perform 9.5 of the tasks, and 5 years after surgery they could perform 10 of the tasks.

The surgeon and rehabilitation professional need to communicate and characterize the anticipated functional improvement after TSA in a way the patient can understand. Shoulder-specific functional gains in relation to pre-operative shoulder function are the most effective way to present this information. TSA for the treatment of primary OA significantly increases shoulder function from 4 out of 12 to 9 out of 12 tasks.[206] Patients with better preoperative function tend to have better postoperative function, although patients with the poorest preoperative function may have the greatest improvement overall. On average, patients reported that they gained two-thirds of the functions that had been absent preoperatively. Thus TSA can provide substantial improvement in shoulder function.

TSA also significantly improves quality of life for patients with OA. Self-assessed health status improved significantly after TSA and to a similar degree as for hip arthroplasty and CABG surgery, although for none of these procedures did health status reach the level of healthy subjects without indications for these procedures.[207] A retrospective study of 138 patients who underwent hemiarthroplasty as a result of a fracture found that the variables most predictive of a decrease in functional outcome included advanced age, presence of a preoperative persistent neurological deficits, the use of alcohol or tobacco, and the need for an early reoperation.[208]

In patients undergoing Copeland surface replacement for the treatment of RA, a case series of 75 shoulders between 1986 and 1998 noted improvements of 50 degrees in flexion, to 100 degrees of total flexion motion, with 96% of patients reporting improved satisfaction compared to their preoperative status.[209]

The major complications of TSA are loosening of the glenoid component, instability, and late rotator cuff tears, although sepsis and nerve injury have also been reported. TSA failure is primarily due to loosening of the glenoid component, which has a risk of 1% per year.[210,211] A meta-analysis of 838 cases of TSA found a reported incidence of postoperative dislocation of 1.2% over a follow-up period of 20-54 months.[199] The incidence of instability was higher after hemiarthroplasty alone, with a reported rate of 6.7% in a meta-analysis of 4 series with a total of 152 cases.[197] Activities that involve repetitive impact, vibration, heavy lifting, pulling, pushing, or jerking maneuvers may jeopardize implant stability; thus realistic expectations must be set to foster compliance for long-term implant survival.[212] Results for TSA survivorship are generally good with 93% survivorship at 10 years and 87% at 15 years, according to a retrospective analysis of patients between 1975-1981.[213]

Interventions. The rehabilitation clinician must consider a number of unique anatomical and biomechanical features of the shoulder when designing a rehabilitation program for patients after TSA. First, the shoulder is not a weight-bearing joint but still achieves joint compressive loads equal to the weight of the arm when it is abducted. Lifting a weight, tossing a ball, or swinging a racquet or golf club significantly increase this load. Second, the glenohumeral joint is quite unstable because there is little contact between the bones and because it is subjected to shear forces in many directions. Stability in a TSA is achieved through the prosthetic components and appropriate tension in the soft tissues. Patients with OA and those with generalized joint laxity may have persistent glenoid retroversion despite attempts at surgical correction and can therefore be prone to posterior instability especially with shoulder elevation and horizontal adduction.[214] The risks of anterior instability may be increased by anteversion of the glenoid or by anterior capsule insufficiency.[215] Patients with RA are more likely to have multidirectional instability as a result of rotator cuff or capsuloligamentous instabilities. An optimal functional outcome requires restoration of an optimal scapulohumeral rhythm and upper quarter length-tension relationships, as well as functional strength.

Rehabilitation begins with PROM on the day of or the day after the surgery. Early mobilization promotes appropriate collagen formation, decreases pain, and minimizes the adverse effects of immobility.[216,217] The amount of external rotation and forward flexion PROM achieved by the surgeon at the time of wound closure should guide rehabilitation.[218] Ideally, the shoulder should externally rotate 40 degrees without excessive tension on the subscapularis.[219] The extent and amount of activity allowed depends on the extent of soft tissue damage and the quality of the repair. During surgery, the subscapularis muscle is cut and then repaired. Therefore passive

external rotation and active internal rotation are limited for the first 4-6 weeks after surgery. Elements of the surgery that may limit or alter the rehabilitation process include rotator cuff repairs and subscapularis z-plasty lengthening.

Patient-conducted flexibility programs performed several times a day after TSA to improve shoulder ROM and flexibility have been reported.[220] A home-based program that started with PROM and progressed through AAROM at week 5 and eventually to elastic-band strengthening at week 10 has also been described.[221] This program was coordinated and instructed by a PT but was completed by the patient at home. Some patients with RA, traumatic arthritis, and osteonecrosis did not maintain flexion ROM postoperatively, which may be due to weakened, thinned rotator cuff muscles or an excessive inflammatory response. Muscle weakness has been implicated as a risk factor for not regaining flexion ROM after humeral fracture and TSA.[222] Self-motivated patients with OA and no other shoulder pathology who undergo TSA may benefit from an independent home-based program coordinated and supervised by a rehabilitation professional, but patients with additional shoulder pathology may need a clinic-based program.

Neer described limited goal rehabilitation (LGR) for patients with deficient rotator cuff or deltoid strength or patients with significant bony deficiency, such as severe osteoporosis, who could not tolerate a typical rehabilitation program. Patients with rotator cuff arthropathy, those with long-standing RA, or those with certain revision arthroplasty may also fall into this category. The goal of LGR is only pain relief and joint stability but not necessarily functional ROM or strength.

Current programs for TSA rehabilitation are based on experience, without research into their effectiveness or superiority. Typically there is a progression from PROM to AROM, followed by progressive strengthening and stretching. The patient is usually in a sling for 2 weeks for an uncomplicated TSA with a longer period of protection of 4-6 weeks if the surgery involved a rotator cuff repair or fracture. It is important to instruct the patient to take his or her arm out of the sling frequently to perform ROM exercise for the joints distal to the shoulder for a few minutes to avoid problems with stiffness in these areas. PROM, and possibly AAROM, are initiated on postoperative day 1. These activities include pendulum exercises in the standing position, as well as supine PROM flexion and PROM/AAROM into external rotation to a limit of usually 40 degrees. Pendulum or Codman's exercises facilitate relaxation and initiate early glenohumeral joint motion and scapulohumeral mobility.[223,224] This exercise is also useful as a "warmup" activity and often helps modulate pain and spasm of the shoulder girdle musculature. It is important to teach the patient the correct way to do this activity because vigorous motions done actively can avulse the anterior capsule and subscapularis repair, or in the case of fractures, tuberosity displacement, which can have devastating complications. This exercise may be too painful for patients with generalized soft tissue laxity because of the distractive force of the hanging upper limb, which is equal to approximately 14% of total BW.[225]

The goal of inpatient therapy is to teach patients ROM activities that they can do at home. Initially, supine PROM in the scapular plane will allow for the greatest impingement free arc of motion with the least soft tissue stress.[226] This position allows the humeral head to be centered in the glenoid and the capsule to be relaxed with the appropriate tension on the ligaments and the muscles. An electromyography (EMG) study of shoulder rehabilitation exercises found that the passive exercise of forward elevation and external rotation generated the least amount of electrical activity in the deltoid and rotator cuff musculature.[227] Less activity was noted in the supraspinatus and middle deltoid with elevation in the scapular plane if the elbow was bent rather than extended. These exercises should be initiated in the supine position and progressed to sitting because the supine position allows the patient to be more relaxed and is helpful in isolating glenohumeral motion and discouraging scapulothoracic substitution patterns. This should progress to AAROM as soon as possible if there are no contraindications, such as a fracture or soft tissue injury, to allow for activation of shoulder girdle muscles. In patients with rotator cuff repairs, assisting external rotation with a cane may be preferable to having the therapist assist because the latter has been found to be associated with higher levels of EMG activity in the rotator cuff muscles.[228] External rotation is one of the hardest and most painful motions to regain, but it is important to achieve good ROM in this direction because external rotation ROM of less than 40-45 degrees is associated with significant functional limitations. Patients are typically discharged from the hospital 48-72 hours after TSA surgery and are given instructions to continue with their ROM program at home.

Outpatient therapy can be started, and AROM activities can be initiated 10-14 days postoperatively. As pain decreases and the patient can demonstrate adequate shoulder girdle control during supine exercise, more functional upright ROM activities should be started. Upright ROM activities, such as wall walking, cane or wand activities, and pulleys, help improve functional ROM and strengthen the rotator cuff muscles.[224] The first 6 weeks should focus on regaining ROM, and once the subscapularis has had time to heal, strengthening can be initiated as tolerated. The strengthening program should start with isometric contractions in various directions and at a variety of angles and gentle scapular stabilization. Scapulothoracic strengthening can be initiated with rowing motions, serratus anterior strengthening, scapular clocks, and table-top activities such as weight shifts. To avoid straining the anterior soft tissues of the shoulder, rowing motion should only go as far back as the midcoronal line of the body (Fig. 10-16).

Shear stresses on the glenoid component of shoulder implants are thought to be the primary cause for loosening and ultimately failure of shoulder arthroplasty. Therefore it is important that the rotator cuff minimize glenohumeral joint shear. It has been shown that the glenohumeral joint reaction forces gradually increase to 90% BW at 90 degrees of flexion,[229] and the humeral head migrates superiorly if the rotator cuff is weak or fatigued, loading and ultimately causing failure of the glenoid.[230-232]

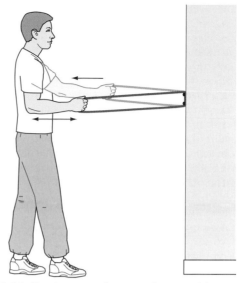

FIG. 10-16 Rowing exercise stopping at mid-coronal line.

It is important to strengthen but not overstress the rotator cuff during rehabilitation. Supine AROM exercises are a good way to start to strengthen the rotator cuff and deltoid muscles. In this position, the sheer forces on the glenohumeral joint are minimized.[233] This activity can be initiated 2 weeks after an uncomplicated TSA or hemiarthroplasty in patients with an intact rotator cuff and no fracture and can be progressed to standing when the patient has control of the extremity in supine. The patient should be reminded that pain-free motion below 90 degrees with NO weight can be performed throughout the day but that lifting, pulling, or pushing with the extremity should be avoided until instructed by the surgeon or rehabilitation professional.

Isometric strengthening can be initiated 1 week after TSA if done in a submaximal progression. However, because of the subscapularis repair performed as part of the TSA, internal rotation should not be performed for 6 weeks after a TSA. In patients with rotator cuff repairs, isometrics of the involved muscles should not be initiated for 4-8 weeks after the surgery, depending on the nature of the tear and its repair. With fractures, isometrics should not be performed for 3-4 weeks after the surgery to allow for a callus to form at the fracture site. Multiple angle isometrics can also improve strength in very weak patients, especially with external rotation.[234]

Isotonic rotator cuff strengthening should be initiated 6-12 weeks postoperatively in patients with intact rotator cuffs and 3-6 months postoperatively in those with rotator cuff repairs. Initially, all shoulder flexion movements should be done with the elbow flexed to reduce the upper limb moment arm. The patient may use manual resistance, hand weights, elastic bands, or aquatic therapy to provide resistance for strengthening the upper quarter. Elastic resistance training should be used primarily for midrange strengthening where it is safest and easiest to control. Aquatic activities have the advantage of providing resistance that varies with the speed of motion, buoyancy to support the arm, and potentially the comfort of warmth if the pool is heated to a therapeutic level.

By 3-6 months after TSA the patient should be encouraged to continue with a HEP of stretching and strengthening because gains in strength and function may be seen for up to 18-24 months after the procedure.

Athletic Participation. Although there is limited published research on shoulder replacement and athletic activity restrictions, 11 published reports were evaluated to compare loosening with different approaches to humeral head component fixation.[235] This evaluation found that both cemented and press-fit humeral components were associated with loosening rates of less than 1% but suggested that young, active patients who wish to return to recreational activities should have a cementless humeral component. A retrospective study of 24 golfers who underwent TSA found that 23 (96%) of the subjects were able to return to playing golf in an average of 4.5 months.[186] Patients with handicaps noted a 5-stroke improvement. Thirty-five members of the Shoulder and Elbow Society were surveyed regarding their recommendations for return of their TSA patients to athletic and recreational activity.[236] Surgeons were asked to rate 42 activities as recommended or allowed, allowed with experience, not recommended, and no conclusion; their recommendations are listed in Box 10-5.

TOTAL ELBOW ARTHROPLASTY

Pathology. Total elbow arthroplasty (TEA) (Fig. 10-17) is useful when conservative management of a painful or unstable elbow, caused by OA or RA, is unsuccessful. Elbow involvement occurs in 20% to 40% of patients with RA, may be bilateral, and may significantly impair a patient's ability to work or perform ADLs. TEA may also be used for primary management of a distal humeral fracture in certain patients.

Four main designs of elbow prostheses have been developed: Constrained, semiconstrained, unconstrained, and resurfacing. Currently, a semiconstrained hinge type and an unconstrained surface replacement are used most often. The semiconstrained hinge prosthesis allows 5-10 degrees of valgus and varus tilt and axial rotation. The unconstrained prosthesis still has some inherent stability by virtue of the interlocking shape of the components.[237]

Prognosis. Relief of pain is the primary goal of TEA.[238] Improved motion after TEA is the next most important goal. Improved motion is especially important if there is concomitant disease of the shoulder as limitations in ROM of both joints will severely restrict function.

Early results of TEA were compromised by design flaws in the prostheses that led to an unacceptable number of complications. Through subsequent improvements in implant design, cement, interfaces, and high-density polyethylene bearings, the average lifespan and functional performance of these implants have improved significantly. After a TEA the patient is usually permanently restricted from lifting more than 5 lb (2.25 kg) repetitively or more than 10 lb (4.5 kg) for a single episode.

TEAs generally last from 8-15 years.[239] In patients with RA who have undergone TEA with a semiconstrained prosthesis, these implants last about as long as a THA.[240] In 21 patients who underwent this procedure because of trauma, Cobb and Morrey found that 4 years after the procedure all were satisfied with the results, 15 reporting excellent and 5 reporting good scores on the Mayo Elbow Performance Score.[241] Seventeen patients reported no pain, and 3 reported mild pain. The average arc of motion for these patients was 25-130 degrees of flexion-extension.[241]

Some patients experience a loss of elbow extension strength after TEA, which may be because of scarring and adhesions of the triceps as a result of the approach used in the surgery. This can limit many ADLs, including rising from a chair using armrests. Surgical techniques that spare the triceps may result in fewer difficulties with ADLs by improving the strength and function of the elbow.

The infection rate of TEA is high when compared to other joint replacement surgeries. Postoperative infection rates of the elbow are 8% to 12% as compared to 0.8% for total shoulder replacements.[242] This may be due to the rel-

BOX 10-5	Activity After Total Shoulder Arthroplasty—1999 American Shoulder and Elbow Society		
Recommended/Allowed	**Allowed with Experience**	**Not Recommended**	**No Conclusion**
Cross-country skiing	Golf	Football	High-impact aerobics
Stationary skiing machine	Ice skating	Gymnastics	Baseball/softball
Speed walking and jogging	Shooting	Hockey	Fencing
Swimming	Downhill skiing	Rock climbing	Handball
Doubles tennis			Horseback riding
Low impact aerobics			Lacrosse
Road or stationary biking			Racquetball or squash
Bowling			Inline or roller skating
Canoeing			Rowing
Croquet			Soccer
Shuffleboard			Singles tennis
Horse shoes			Volleyball
Ballroom dancing			Weight training

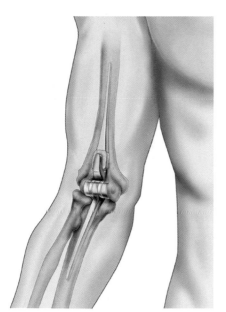

FIG. 10-17 Elbow prosthesis (Zimmer® Coonrad-Morrey Total Elbow System). *Image courtesy Zimmer, Inc.*

ative subcutaneous exposure, the potential for olecranon bursa infection, and the extent of the reflection of the muscles over the distal humerus and proximal ulna.

Intervention. Limited information is available on therapeutic interventions after TEA. Some protocols have been published in textbooks from centers where many of these procedures are performed; however, there is little published research in this area. The following suggestions are based primarily on expert recommendations.

Use of compressive cryotherapy has been shown to decrease postoperative swelling in patients undergoing elbow surgery.[243] Since such swelling may lead to soft tissue problems that may restrict ROM, early icing and compression are recommended. Active rehabilitation should begin 5-7 days after the semiconstrained TEA, when the elbow may be removed from its postsurgical extension splint. This thermoplastic extension splint should be placed anteriorly and worn at night and between exercise sessions for 6 weeks after the surgery and then be discontinued. This splint promotes elbow extension, which is often the hardest motion to maintain after surgery and the most critical for functional weight bearing on the upper extremity. Full extension may not be achieved if there were long-standing soft tissue contractures before surgery. However, many functional activities, such as reading a newspaper, drinking from a glass, pouring liquid from a pitcher, and using silverware, may be performed with limited elbow movement in midrange from 130 degrees of flexion to 30 degrees of extension and from 50 degrees of supination to 50 degrees of pronation.[244]

With the semiconstrained TEA, AAROM exercises are begun on day 7. These can include flexion-extension, as well as pronation and supination at 90 degrees of elbow flexion. Pronation and supination are performed at 90 degrees of flexion because in this position the bones, rather than the ligaments, provide the most joint stabil-

ity.[245] The elbow should also be kept close to the body during all exercises to avoid stretching the newly reconstructed collateral ligaments. If patients have difficulty avoiding varus stress on the joint, a hinged elbow brace with no ROM restrictions may be used to provide lateral stability. For 6 weeks after TEA patients should also avoid ADLs that require motions in the scapular or frontal plane.

AROM and NMES for the biceps and triceps can usually be started 2 weeks after a semiconstrained TEA, unless a triceps splitting or reflecting surgical approach was used. In this circumstance, the triceps should not perform forceful extension for 3-6 weeks (depending on the physician) to ensure proper healing of the extensor mechanism. For patients who use an assistive mobility device, such as a cane, walker, or crutches, a platform should be added to allow upper extremity weight bearing without active elbow extension (see Chapter 33).

At week 6 (or 12, depending on the surgeon) after a semiconstrained TEA, if the joint is stable and extension ROM is good, extension splint use may be discontinued and ROM exercises may be performed away from the body. At this time, light resistance exercises for the elbow can be started, within the patient's comfort level. Some authors recommend not performing concentric or eccentric strengthening exercises but instead rely on only gentle isometrics and ADLs to increase strength.[246]

With an unconstrained TEA, splinting the elbow at between 30-90 degrees of flexion is recommended to prevent posterior dislocation and to promote implant stability.[247,248] The length of time and position of immobilization for optimal outcome has not been adequately studied and is therefore primarily determined by surgeon preference. When the degree of flexion immobilization exceeds 30 degrees the residual flexion contracture worsens.[249] Therefore a 30-degree extension splint should be worn full time for 2 weeks and thereafter only at night and during high-risk activities. The goal of this splint is to encourage a flexion contracture of 30 degrees to promote stability of the implant and prevent it subluxing or dislocating posteriorly. The ROM goal for flexion is at least 130 degrees to allow for performance of most ADLs.

With an unconstrained TEA, PROM and AAROM limited to between 30 and 150 degrees of flexion should begin within 7 days after the surgery. The joint should only be moved to the point of tissue tension and aggressive PROM should be avoided. Sagittal plane precautions are also applied, and the patient should be encouraged to perform home exercises many times each day. For the first 2-3 months, lifting is limited to 1-2 lb and thereafter a lifelong limit of 5 lb is imposed. Most strength and function will return with the routine performance of ADLs. Therefore strengthening programs are generally not needed unless the patient is so severely limited that weakness prevents the performance of ADLs. In this case, only midrange isometric strengthening activities should be used because concentric and eccentric strengthening activities may adversely affect implant stability. Patients are also cautioned not to participate in any upper extremity impact sport, such as golf or tennis, after undergoing any TEA.

TOTAL WRIST ARTHROPLASTY

Although the wrist was one of the first joints to be treated with prosthetic replacement, total wrist arthroplasty (TWA) is rare in mainstream orthopedic practice.[250] This may be because symptomatic wrist arthritis is rare, because prostheses are limited, and because of the availability of other acceptable forms of treatments such as limited or complete joint fusion or other surgical procedures that relieve pain while retaining some wrist ROM.[251] Wrist implants have had trouble with component loosening, rapid wear, and breakage, especially at the distal component of the prosthesis. Meuli reported that of 40 implants, 6 failed within the first year but overall most patients were satisfied with the outcome after 5 years and 33 of the patients reported significant improvements in their ADLs.[252]

TWA is generally used to treat patients with RA that affects the wrist and low functional demands. In these patients, who often have many upper extremity joints involved, TWA can preserve motion at the wrist to help compensate for loss of motion in other joints. Patients with traumatic or degenerative arthritis of the wrist usually do not have other joints of the upper extremity involved and are generally candidates for more conservative approaches. In addition, if a patient, such as a musician, needs increased motion a TWA may be warranted. If a patient wished to return to an impact sport, such as golf, he or she should anticipate the need for a revision because of the high risk of implant loosening. Patients with an arthrodesis (fusion) of one wrist and an arthroplasty on the other generally prefer the arthroplasty to the fusion because of the associated reduction in pain and deformity despite high complication rates.[253,254] Studies have shown that 75% to 90% of patients report pain relief with TWA with an average ROM of 36 degrees of extension, 29-41 degrees of flexion, 7-10 degrees of radial deviation, and 13-20 degrees of ulnar deviation.[255,256] It has been reported that at the wrist, 60 degrees of extension, 54 degrees of flexion, 17 degrees of radial deviation, and 40 degrees of ulnar deviation are sufficient to perform all routine ADLs; however, most activities (with the notable exceptions of perineal care and pushing off armrests to rise from a chair) can be completed with 40 degrees of flexion and extension, 10 degrees of radial deviation, and 30 degrees of ulnar deviation.[257] Appropriate candidates for TWA are those with severe pain from RA and elderly patients with severe OA.

Pathology. The TWA procedure starts with a dorsal incision over the wrist. In many cases, a dorsal tenosynovectomy of the extensor tendons is also necessary. For a rigid implant, the distal portions of the radius and ulna, some of the carpals, and a small portion of the proximal aspect of the third metacarpal are removed. A rigid stemmed prosthesis is then press fit into the third metacarpal intramedullary canal and the distal radius. In most cases, this implant is cemented in place (Fig. 10-18).

Intervention. Since very limited information on interventions after TWA was found in the literature, the following information is based on expert opinion from texts, journals, and protocols from medical centers that routinely perform these procedures.

For a TWA to be successful, the patient must have intact and functioning wrist extensor tendons, as well as a stable radiocarpal joint. If this is not the case, ligament reconstruction is often necessary.[258] Rehabilitation after wrist arthroplasty requires balancing ROM and stability needs. The duration of postoperative immobilization depends on the stability of the prosthesis intraoperatively and is usually about 2-4 weeks. If there is any tendency toward instability, the period of immobilization should be extended. In patients with RA, who are those most com-

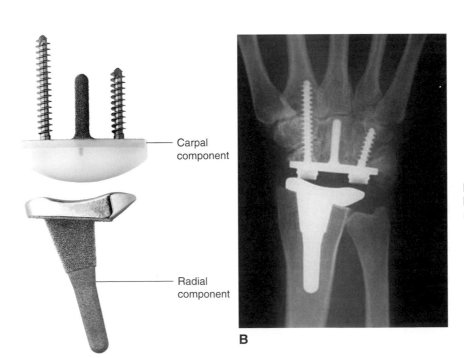

Carpal
component

Radial
component

A

B

FIG. 10-18 **A,** Wrist prosthesis (implant). **B**, X-ray of wrist implant. *A Image courtesy KMI.*

monly having wrist arthroplasty, longer immobilization does not necessarily lead to long-term stiffness. Immobilization should be in a position of neutral flexion and extension to allow the volar and dorsal portions of the capsule to heal with equal lengths for more optimal balance of the joint. Initial placement of the forearm in supination may reduce the risk of early volar dislocation of the prosthesis.[250] Because TWA is associated with substantial postoperative swelling, the hand should be elevated and finger motion should be started early.

After the cast and sutures are removed at 2 weeks, the patient should be fitted with a molded wrist splint to be used for the following 2-4 weeks, during which time an active ROM program for the wrist should be initiated. This program should include active flexion, extension, pronation, and supination of the wrist. Passive ROM is discouraged for the first 8 weeks postoperatively at which time light strengthening through isometrics may also be initiated. Unrestricted use of the hand and wrist is not allowed for the first 3 months. Long-term activity restrictions, although not well defined, should include avoidance of repetitive forceful motion and impact loading.

FINGER ARTHROPLASTY

Arthroplasty of the fingers and thumb are used to treat a wide variety of painful conditions that limit hand function. Whether the etiology is OA, RA, or posttraumatic arthritis, a wide variety of both implant and nonimplant arthroplasties can successfully improve function. Implant arthroplasty has been successful in the metacarpophalangeal (MCP) and proximal interphalangeal (PIP) joints, whereas ligament reconstruction tendon interposition (LRTI) has become a mainstay in the treatment of basal or carpometacarpal (CMC) arthritis, although implant arthroplasty is also used for CMC arthritis.

Metacarpophalangeal Arthroplasty. MCP arthroplasty has been performed since the 1950s.[259] Since that time, advances in technology have led to the development of a variety of techniques and implants. Implants may have a single or two-piece hinge design, be constrained or nonconstrained, and be fixed with or without cement. Implants may be silicone, metallic, or ceramic coated, however, a hinged silastic spacer is used most commonly for MCP and PIP joint reconstruction in patients with RA.[260] This design is referred to as a "load distributing flexible hinge." It acts like an internal splint to maintain alignment. It does not simulate normal joint mechanics but does provide pain relief and a useful arc of motion.[261]

Contraindications to MCP arthroplasty include infection, inadequate bone stock or soft tissue covering, and an irreparable musculotendinous system. Patients with juvenile RA may not have large enough intramedullary canals to accept implants, so a simple resection arthroplasty may be performed on these patients.[262,263] It is also important to consider what other joints are involved in patients with complex RA deformities. For example, a fixed radial deviation of the wrist will lead to recurrent ulnar deviation of the fingers even after successful MCP arthroplasty.[264]

Many surgical approaches are used for placement of MCP arthroplasties. For example, for a single-digit arthroplasty of the MCP joint, the extensor mechanism of the

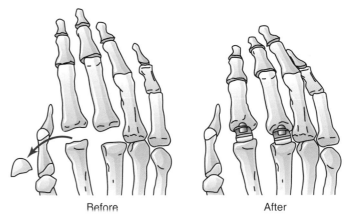

FIG. 10-19 Metacarpophalangeal arthroplasty: Before and after. *Copyright of Medical Multimedia Group, LLC.*

finger is exposed through a longitudinal incision, whereas, if multiple joints are to be replaced, a transverse incision is more common. The extensor mechanism is dissected so that it can be relocated at the time of wound closure. If the patient has RA with ulnar drift, the drift is then corrected. If possible, the sagittal bands of the MCP capsule are preserved. The capsule is incised to expose the MCP joint. The proximal phalanx is cut to remove the articular surface and an awl is then inserted into the intramedullary canal of both the proximal phalanx and metacarpal until the appropriate fit is obtained. Trial implants are inserted, and the joint is tested for stability and ROM. The final implant can be press-fit or cemented, depending on the prosthesis chosen. Then the extensor mechanism is relocated, and the wound is closed (Fig. 10-19).

Prognosis. The goal of MCP arthroplasty is to decrease pain, enhance joint stability, and ultimately improve hand function. By restoring skeletal alignment and improving tendon mechanics, the patient should regain more effective and efficient finger function.

The final result of a finger implant arthroplasty in patients with RA is not a normally functioning joint, but a painless arthroplasty with a functional ROM.[265] The largest meta-analysis to date reviewed all the published series of MCP joint arthroplasty used for the treatment of RA and found that this procedure effectively corrected the ulnar drift deformity and improved the aesthetic appearance of the hand.[266] Nalebuff states that the 40 degrees of MCP joint motion typical after uncomplicated MCP arthroplasty (as opposed to normal flexion ROM of 85 degrees for the MCP) provides good overall hand function if PIP motion is normal.[267] A goal of 70 degrees of MCP flexion is recommended. Grip strength does not increase after MCP arthroplasty, possibly because usually other joints are also invoved.[268,269] However, two studies found that hand function does improve, particularly functions requiring pinch, span, and hook grip.[270,271] Patient satisfaction with this procedure may be more affected by pain relief and aesthetic appearance than by more readily measurable outcomes such as strength and ROM.[272]

Intervention. Therapy regimens after MCP arthroplasty should protect the joint, improve ROM, and safely progress the patient back to activity. Although many articles describe surgical technique and outcomes for MCP arthroplasty, few describe their postoperative regimen with any specificity, making comparisons of therapy intervention protocols difficult.[261,273,274] For example, in a review of 64 studies that described results of MCP arthroplasty, only 5 described their postoperative regimen.[275] The main differences between rehabilitation protocols were the use of passive or active MCP extension and the splinting of the MCPs in extension[276] versus flexion.[277] One of the difficulties with performing studies of the rehabilitation for this procedure is its relative infrequency compared with other arthroplasties such as hips and knees. For example, one group took 3 years to find 43 hands to include in their research.[274]

Postoperative rehabilitation is recognized as an important factor in the successful outcome of joint arthroplasty of the hand.[278] In general, therapy regimens after MCP arthroplasty are based on the principles of tissue healing and scar formation; however, there are wide differences in splinting, exercise protocols, and time frames.[279] All of the regimens started therapy within 2-5 days after surgery. CPM machines are rarely used as they have not been shown to increase the ROM after this procedure.[280] Initially the goals of therapy are to monitor wound healing, decrease edema, and prevent scar adherence. Tissue healing after this procedure is often impaired because many of the patients are on long-term corticosteroid treatment for RA. Additionally, as ulnar drift is common in this population, the postoperative splint is usually fashioned in slight radial deviation to align the digits with the corresponding metacarpal. In addition, to optimize finger ROM, the PIP may be splinted in extension with the MCP in flexion. Some authors advocate using dynamic splints, whereas others recommend passive or resting splints.[280-282] Most allow patients to begin retraining the hand and begin active ROM at the MCP within 7-10 days after surgery. Patient may begin to use their hands for ADLs and light activities at about 1 month, although night splints are often continued for 4 months to help reduce extensor lags. It is important to obtain motion early because capsular tightness that persists beyond 3-4 weeks after surgery may limit final functional outcome.

Interphalangeal Joint Arthroplasty. The normal PIP joint has the greatest arc of motion of any joint of the hand and therefore plays a critical role in hand function.[283] Arthroplasty of the PIP and distal interphalangeal (DIP) joints may be indicated for the treatment of pain, stiffness, deformity, instability, and loss of cartilage in the joint. Typically, these finding are sequelae of OA, RA, or trauma. An acceptable alternative treatment to arthroplasty may be arthrodesis, depending on the patient's functional needs and limitations. For example, a patient who needs a powerful grip and joint stability, such as a laborer, may be better served by an arthrodesis than an arthroplasty, which may be prone to loosening and failure. PIP function, especially of the fourth and fifth fingers, generally will significantly impact the overall function of the hand, whereas DIP function will have less functional impact. Therefore, in the fourth and fifth digits, a PIP arthroplasty may be preferred to arthrodesis.[284]

Prognosis. The primary goals of interphalangeal joint arthroplasty are to relieve pain and to improve hand function. The ROM goals for the PIP joint of the fourth and fifth fingers are 60-70 degrees of flexion and neutral extension. In a retrospective review of a series of 70 PIP arthroplasties in 48 patients, there were no significant changes in flexion ROM after PIP arthroplasty but extension ROM did increase, improving the functional motion of the joint.[285] Pinch and grip strength did not change significantly, but overall pain relief was good in 70% of patients. Patients who had these implants placed because of RA had poorer outcomes than those who had the procedure performed because of degenerative or posttraumatic arthritis.

Less flexion of the interphalangeal joints is needed for functional use of the index and middle finger than for the fourth and fifth fingers.[286] With DIP arthroplasty of these fingers, 30 degrees of flexion and neutral extension are acceptable. When assessing the functional outcomes from these procedures, the function of the hand as a whole should be considered. If the arthroplasty of the PIP joint is on the same finger as an MCP arthroplasty, the overall function of that finger will be more severely impacted than if the PIP was fused and the MCP was treated with an arthroplasty.[283] Patients with PIP arthroplasty with simple joint contractures or joint surface incongruity on the same digit tend to fare better than those with tendon imbalances such as swan-neck deformities.[287,288]

CASE STUDY 10-1

TOTAL KNEE ARTHROPLASTY

Examination
Patient History
MV is a 66-year-old woman with a long-standing history of OA affecting her right knee. She underwent a cemented primary TKA 2 weeks ago. She spent 4 days as an inpatient and received physical therapy and CPM. She was discharged home 10 days ago. She lives with her husband in a 2-story home with 12 stairs up to the second story. She has been referred to outpatient physical therapy with a prescription for evaluation and treatment for "s/p R TKA." Her goal for therapy is to be able to "stroll through the streets of Venice" on her upcoming trip to Europe in the fall (6 months from now). Currently, her pain is a constant 4/10 but increases to 6/10 with activity. This is controlled with ice and hydrocodone and acetaminophen. MV's past medical history includes hypertension and hypercholesteremia. Both are controlled with medication.

Tests and Measures
Musculoskeletal

Anthropometric Characteristics Effusion of the right knee. Girth is 55 cm on the right and 45 cm on the left measured at the level of the medial joint line.

Range of Motion AROM and PROM of the right knee: 10-95 degrees.

Muscle Performance Strength 3+/5 hamstrings and quadriceps with poor control of the quadriceps with straight leg raise.

Integumentary: Well-healed 15 cm incision on the anterior right knee. No signs of infection.

Function

Gait, Locomotion, and Balance MV ambulates with a front wheeled walker with an antalgic gait and weight bearing as tolerated. She has a decreased ability to go from sit to stand and requires minimal assistance if the chair does not have arms.

Evaluation, Diagnosis, and Prognosis

MV presents with increased pain and swelling, impaired ROM, strength, motor control and balance. The impairments have resulted in decreased ability to walk, move from sitting to standing and perform ADLs such as household chores.

Diagnosis

MV's diagnosis is preferred practice pattern 4H: Impaired joint mobility, motor function, muscle performance, and ROM associated with joint arthroplasty.

Goals

Decrease pain and swelling of the right knee, increase ROM and strength, and improve ambulation so that the patient can return to a normal level of function.

Plan of Care

The plan is for outpatient treatment to include therapeutic modalities, joint mobilization, therapeutic exercise, aerobic conditioning, ROM, and gait training, 3 times a week for 4 weeks, then 2 times a week for 2 weeks. The patient will be reevaluated at the end of the treatment time to determine the need for continued treatment or discharge to a home exercise program at the end of the sessions.

Interventions

- PROM and AROM exercises in supine, prone and seated to facilitate increased flexion and extension. Exercises to include activities on a stationary bicycle, as well as clinician- and patient-directed ROM.
- Soft tissue mobilization of the scar and peripatellar area, and patellar mobilizations, to improve ROM and soft tissue extensibility.
- Open and closed kinetic chain strengthening activities to improve strength and ultimately function. If quadriceps strength is not responding to active strengthening techniques, NMES will be utilized.
- Balance and proprioception will be improved through single leg balance activities.
- Aerobic capacity and endurance will be improved through cycling and treadmill walking.
- Ice and electrical stimulation or a cryotherapy/pneumatic compression device will be used at the end of the treatment session to control pain and swelling.

Please see the CD that accompanies this book for a case study describing the examination, evaluation and interventions for a patient after a shoulder hemiarthroplasty.

CHAPTER SUMMARY

Joint arthroplasty can effectively treat painful and disabling joint pathologies. It is one of the most widely performed orthopedic surgical procedures in the United States that will doubtless increase in frequency with the increasing longevity of the population. Understanding and implementing appropriate rehabilitation interventions for patients who have undergone joint arthroplasty and arthrodesis is essential. Studies of patient outcomes, although not extensive, have demonstrated that patients who undergo these procedures have limitations in ROM, strength, proprioception, and ultimately function. These limitations are decreased by appropriate rehabilitation. Through thoughtful evaluation and appropriate patient-specific, goal-oriented, evidence-based interventions, the quality of life of patients who have undergone joint arthroplasty can be improved by physical rehabilitation.

ADDITIONAL RESOURCES

Web Sites

FDA article on joint replacement surgery: www.fda.gov/fdac/features/2004/204_joints.html

National Institute of Arthritis and Musculoskeletal and Skin Diseases (NIAMS): www.niams.nih.gov

American Academy of Orthopaedic Surgeons (AAOS): www.aaos.org

American College of Rheumatology (ACR): www.rheumatology.org

GLOSSARY

Arthrodesis: The surgical fusion of the bony surfaces of a joint with internal fixation such as pins, plates, nails and/or bone graft.

Arthrofibrosis: Increased fibrous tissue in a joint that limits ROM.

Arthropathy: Any disease or abnormal condition affecting a joint.

Arthroplasty: Any reconstructive joint procedure with or without an implant that is designed to relieve pain and restore motion

Avascular necrosis: Death of bone cells as a result of loss of a blood supply.

Continuous passive motion (CPM): A machine that that passively moves a joint at a prescribed speed and through a prescribed ROM.

Cruciate retaining (or sparing) TKA: A total knee replacement in which the posterior cruciate is retained for stability.

Extensor lag: When the knee's PROM into extension exceeds the AROM into extension. This term is synonymous with quadriceps lag.

Fascial arthroplasty: Removal of the bone from one or both of the articular surfaces of a joint and allowing a fibrotic scar to form in the space that remains.

Hemiarthroplasty: Replacement of one side of a compartment of a joint. For example, in the shoulder, replacement of the humeral component only.

Methylmethacrylate: Epoxy cement used in cemented total joint surgery to attach the implant to the bone surface.

Mobile bearing TKA: A total knee replacement in which a polyethylene insert articulates with the femoral component and the metallic tibial tray.

Osteolysis: Softening or destruction of bone.

Posterior stabilized TKA: A total knee replacement in which both cruciate ligaments are excised and the stability of the knee depends on the implant.

Resection arthroplasty: Removal of one or both articular surfaces of a joint (also known as excisional arthroplasty).

Unicompartmental knee replacement: Replacement of one compartment, medial or lateral tibiofemoral compartment, of the knee.

References

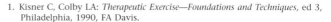

1. Kisner C, Colby LA: *Therapeutic Exercise—Foundations and Techniques,* ed 3, Philadelphia, 1990, FA Davis.

2. Callahan CM, Drake BG, Heck HA, et al: Patient outcomes following tricompartmental total knee replacement. A meta-analysis, *JAMA* 271:1329-1357, 1994.

3. Mont MA, Rifal A, Baumgarten KM, et al: Total knee arthroplasty for osteonecrosis, *J Bone Joint Surg Am* 84:599-603, 2002.

4. Neer CS: Displaced proximal humerus fractures. II. Treatment of three and four-part displacement, *J Bone Joint Surg Am* 52:1090-1103, 1970.

5. Schneiderbauer MM, Von Knoch M, Schleck CD, et al: Patient survival after hip arthroplasty for metastatic disease of the hip, *J Bone Joint Surg Am* 86:1684-1689, 2004.

6. www.aaos.org/wordhtml/research/stats/arthropl.htm

7. Quaim JP, Michet CJ Jr, Wilson MG, et al: Total knee arthroplasty: a population based study, *Mayo Clin Proc* 66:589-595, 1991.

8. Total hip replacement, *NIH Consens Statement* 12(5):1-31, 1994.

9. Ethgen O, Bruyere O, Richy F, et al: Health related quality of life in total hip and total knee arthroplasty: A qualitative and systematic review of the literature, *J Bone Joint Surg Am* 86:963-974, 2004.

10. Lawrence RC, Helmick CG, Arnett FC, et al: Estimates of the prevalence of arthritis and selected musculoskeletal disorders in the United States, *Arthritis Rheum* 41(5):778-779, 1998.

11. Badley EM: The effect of osteoarthritis on disability and health care use in Canada, *J Rheumatol Suppl* 43(suppl):19-22, 1995.

12. Hawker G, Wright J, Coyte P, et al: Health-related quality of life after knee replacement, *J Bone Joint Surg Am* 80:163-173, 1998.

13. Liang MH, Cullen KE, Larson MG, et al: Cost effectiveness of total joint arthroplasty for osteoarthritis, *Arthritis Rheum* 29:937-943, 1986.

14. Chang RW, Pellsier JM, Hazen GB: A cost effective analysis of the total hip arthroplasty for osteoarthritis of the hip, *JAMA* 275:858-865, 1996.

15. Felson DT, Anderson JJ, Naimark A, et al: Obesity and knee osteoarthritis: The Framington study, *Ann Intern Med* 109:18-24, 1988.

16. Felson DT: Epidemiology of hip and knee arthritis, *Epidemiol Rev* 10:1-28, 1988.

17. Callahan CM, Drake BG, Heck DA, et al: Patient outcomes following unicompartmental or bicompartmental knee arthroplasty: A meta-analysis, *J Arthroplasty* 10:141-150, 1995.

18. Warwick D, Williams MH, Bannister GC: Death and thromboembolic disease after total hip replacement: a case series of 1162 patients with no routine chemo prophylaxis, *J Bone Joint Surg Br* 77B:6-10, 1995.

19. O'Donnell TF, Abott WM, Athanasoulis CA, et al: Diagnosis of deep vein thrombosis in the outpatient by venography, *Surg Gynecol Obstet* 150:69-74, 1980.

20. Wells PS, Hirsh J, Anderson DR, et al: Accuracy of clinical assessment of deep vein thrombosis, *Lancet* 345:1326-1330, 1995.

21. Wells PS, Anderson DR, Bormanis J, et al: Value of assessment of pretest probability of deep vein thrombosis in clinical management, *Lancet* 350:1795-1798, 1997.

22. Wells PS, Hirsh J, Anderson DR, et al: A simple clinical model for the diagnosis of deep vein thrombosis combined with impedance plethysmography: Potential for an improvement in the diagnostic process, *J Intern Med* 243:15-23, 1998.

23. Riddle DL, Hillner BE, Wells PS, et al: Diagnosis of lower-extremity deep vein thrombosis in out patients with musculoskeletal disorders: A national survey study of physical therapists, *Phys Ther* 84(8):717-728, 2004.

24. Winiarsky R, Barth P, Lotke P: Total knee replacement in morbidly obese patients, *J Bone Joint Surg Am* 80:1770-1774, 1998.

25. Marin LA, Salido JA, Lopez A, et al: Preoperative nutritional evaluation as a prognostic toll for wound healing, *Acta Orthop Scand* 73:2-5, 2002.

26. American Physical Therapy Association: *Guide to Physical Therapist Practice*, ed 2, Alexandria, Va, 2001, The Association.

27. Harris WH, Sledge CB: Total hip and total knee arthroplasty (2), *N Engl J Med* 323:801-807, 1990.

28. Hawker G, Wright J, Coyte P, et al: Health related quality of life after knee replacement, *J Bone Joint Surg Am* 80:163-173, 1998.

29. Macnicol MF, McHardy R, Chalmers J: Exercise testing before and after total hip arthroplasty, *J Bone Joint Surg Br* 62B:326-331, 1980.

30. Boorman RS, Kopjar B, Fehringer E, et al: The effect of total shoulder arthroplasty on self assessed health status is comparable to that of total hip arthroplasty and coronary artery bypass grafting, *J Shoulder Elbow Surg* 12:158-163, 2003.

31. Namba RS, Skinner HB: Adult reconstructive surgery. In Skinner HB (ed): *Current Diagnosis and Treatment in Orthopedics*, New York, 2000, McGraw-Hill.

32. Finch E, Walsh M, Thomas SG, et al: Functional ability perceived by individuals following total knee arthroplasty compared to age matched individuals without knee disability, *JOSPT* 23:3-11, 1998.

33. Long WT, Dorr LD, Healy B, et al: Functional recovery after noncemented total hip retrieved hip arthroplasty, *Clin Orthop* 288:73-77, 1993.

34. Walsh M, Woodhouse LJ, Thomas SG, et al: Physical impairments and functional limitations: A comparison of individuals 1 year after total knee arthroplasty with control subjects, *Phys Ther* 78:248-258, 1998.

35. Hough D, Crosat S, Nye P: Client education for total hip replacement, *Nurs Manage* 22:80I-80J, 80N, 80P, 1991.

36. McGregor AH, Rylands H, Owen A, et al: Does preoperative hip rehabilitation advice improve recovery and patient satisfaction? *J Arthroplasty* 19:464-468, 2004.

37. Crowe J, Henderson J: Pre-arthroplasty rehabilitation is effective in reducing hospital stay, *Can J Occup Ther* 70(2):88-96, 2003.

38. National Hospital Discharge Survey Summary 1997-2001, Hyattsville, Md, 2002, National Center for Health Statistics.

39. Quintana JM, Arostegul I, Azkarate J, et al: Evaluation of explicit criteria for total joint replacement, *J Clin Epidemiol* 53:1200-1208, 2000.

40. Braeken AM, Lochhaas-Gerlach JA, Gollish JD: Determinants of 6-12 month post-operative functional status and pain after elective total hip replacement, *Int J Qual Health Care* 9:413-418, 1997.

41. Fortin PR, Clarke AE, Joseph L, et al: Outcomes of total hip and knee replacement; preoperative functional status predicts outcomes at six months after surgery, *Arthritis Rheum* 42:1722-1728, 1999.

42. MacWilliam CH, Yood MU, Verner JJ: Patient related risk factors that predict poor outcome after total hip replacement, *Health Serv Res* 31:623-638, 1996.

43. Holtzman J, Saleh K, Kane R: Effect of baseline functional status and pain on outcomes of total hip arthroplasty, *J Bone Joint Surg Am* 84:1942-1948, 2002.

44. Shih CH, DuYK, Lin Yh, et al: Muscular recovery around the hip joint following total hip arthroplasty, *Clin Orthop* 302:115-120, 1994.

45. Bitar AA, Kaplan RJ, Stitik TP, et al: Rehabilitation of orthopedic and rheumatologic disorders. 3. Total hip arthroplasty rehabilitation, *Arch Phys Med Rehabil* 6:S56-S60, 2005.

46. Ganz SB, Levin AZ, Peterson MG: Improvement in driving reaction time after total hip arthroplasty, *Clin Orthop Relat Res* 413:192-200, 2003.

47. Healy WL, Iorio R, Lemos MJ: Athletic activity after joint replacement, *Am J Sports Med* 29:377-388, 2001.

48. Dubs L, Gschwend N, Munzinger U: Sports after total hip arthroplasty, *Arch Orthop Trauma Surg* 101:161-169, 1983.

49. Perrin T, Door LD, Perry J, et al: Functional evaluation of total hip arthroplasty with five to ten year followup evaluation, *Clin Orthop* 195:252-260, 1985.

50. Schmalzried TP, Shepherd EF, Dorey FJ, et al: Wear is a function of use, not time, *Clin Orthop* 381:36-46, 2000.

51. Kilgus DJ, Dorey FJ, Finerman GA, et al: Patient activity, sports participation and impact loading on the durability of cemented hip replacements, *Clin Orthop* 269:25-31, 1991.

52. Seehom BB, Walbridge NC: Walking activities and the wear of prostheses, *Ann Rheum Dis* 44:838-843, 1985.

53. Schmalzried TP, Szuszczwicz ES, Northfield MR, et al: Quantitative assessment of walking after total hip or knee replacement, *J Bone Joint Surg Am* 80:54-59, 1998.

54. Wallbridge N, Dowson D: The walking activity of patients with artificial hip joints, *Eng Med* 11:95-96, 1982.

55. Jasty M, Goetz DD, Bragdon CR, et al: Wear of the polyethylene acetabular components in total hip arthroplasty: An analysis of one hundred and twenty eight components retrieved at autopsy or revision operations, *J Bone Joint Surg Am* 79:349-358, 1997.

56. Sieber HP, Rieker CB, Kottig P: Analysis of 118 second generation metal on metal retrieved hip implants, *J Bone Joint Surg Br* 81:46-50, 1999.

57. Cuckler JM, Bearcroft J, Asgian CM: Femoral head technologies to reduce polyethylene wear in total hip arthroplasty, *Clin Orthop* 317:57-63, 1995.

58. Dubs L, Gschwend N, Munzinger U: Sport after total hip arthroplasty, *Arch Orthop Trauma Surg* 101:161-169, 1983.

59. Gschwend N, Frei T, Morscher E, et al: Alpine and cross country skiing after total hip replacements: 2 cohorts of 50 patients each, one active, the other inactive in skiing, followed for 5-10 years, *Acta Orthop Scand* 71:243-249, 2000.

60. Long WT, Dorr LD, Healy B, et al: Functional recovery of noncemented total hip arthroplasty, *Clin Orthop* 288:73-77, 1993.

61. Mallon WJ, Callaghan JJ: Total hip arthroplasty in active golfers, *J Arthroplasty* 7(supp):339-346, 1992.

62. Mont MA, LaPorte DM, Mullick T, et al: Tennis after total hip arthroplasty, *Am J Sports Med* 24:60-64, 1999.

63. Healy WL, Iorio R, Lemos M: Athletic activity after total joint replacement, *Am J Sports Med* 29:377-388, 2001.

64. McGrory BJ, Stuart MJ, Sim FH: Participation in sports after hip and knee arthroplasty: review of literature and survey of surgeon preferences, *Mayo Clin Proc* 70:342-348, 1995.

65. Wijgman AJ, Deekers GH, Waltje E, et al: No positive effect of preoperative exercise therapy and teaching in patients to be subjected to total hip arthroplasty, *Ned Tijdschr Geneeskd* 138:949-952, 1994.

66. Zavadak KH, Gibson KR, Whitley DM, et al: Variability in the obtainment of functional milestones during the acute care admission after total joint replacement, *J Rheumatol* 22:482-487, 1995.

67. Munin MC, Kwoh CK, Glenn NW, et al: Predicting discharge outcomes after elective hip and knee arthroplasty, *Am J Phys Med Rehabil* 74:294-301, 1995.

68. Huo MH, Carbone JJ: Conversion total hip replacement. In Callagan JJ, Rosenberg AG, Rubash HJ (eds): *The Adult Hip*, Philadelphia, 1998, Lippincott.

69. Kishida Y, Sugano N, Sakai T, et al: Full weight bearing after cementless total hip arthroplasty, *Int Orthop* 25:25-28, 2001.

70. Goodman CC, Boissonault WG, Fuller KS: Bone, joint, and soft tissue disorders. In Goodman CC, Boissonault WG, Fuller KS: *Pathology: Implications for the Physical Therapist,* Philadelphia, 2003, Saunders.

71. Munin MC, Hockenberry PS, Flynn PG, et al: Rehabilitation. In Callagan JJ, Rosenberg AG, Rubash HJ (eds): *The Adult Hip,* Philadelphia, 1998, Lippincott.

72. Brandler VA, Mullarkey CF, Stulberg SD: Rehabilitation after total joint replacement for osteoarthritis: An evidence based approach, *Physical Medicine and Rehabilitation: State of the Art Reviews* 15:175-197, 2001.

73. Baxter MI, Allington BA, Koepke GH: Weight distribution variables in the use of crutches and canes, *Phys Ther* 49:360-365, 1969.

74. Dabke HV, Gupta SK, Holt CA, et al: How accurate is partial weightbearing? *Clin Orthop Relat Res* 421:282-286, 2004.

75. Gray FB, Gray C, McClanahan JW: Assessing the accuracy of partial weightbearing instruction, *Am J Orthop* 27:558-560, 1998.

76. Youdas, JW, Kotajarvi BJ, Padgett DJ, et al: Partial weight bearing gait using conventional assistive devices, *Arch Phys Med Rehabil* 86:394-398, 2005.

77. Davy DT, Kotzar GM, Brown RH, et al: Telemetric force measurements across the hip and after total arthroplasty, *J Bone Joint Surg Am* 70:40-45, 1988.

78. Strickland EM, Fares M, Krebs De, et al: In vivo acetabular contact pressures during rehabilitation. I. Acute phase, *Phys Ther* 72:691-699, 1992.

79. Krotenberg R, Stitik T, Johnson MV: Incidence of dislocation following hip arthroplasty for patients in the rehabilitation setting, *Am J Phys Med Rehabil* 74:444-447, 1995.

80. Phillips CB, Barrett JA, Losina E, et al: Incidence rates of dislocation, pulmonary embolism, and deep infection during the first six months after elective total hip replacement, *J Bone Joint Surg Am* 85:20-26, 2003.

81. Peak EL, Parvizi J, Ciminiello M, et al: The role of patient restrictions in reducing the prevalence of early dislocation following total hip arthroplasty. A randomized prospective study, *J Bone Joint Surg Am* 87:247-253, 2005.

82. Kakkar VV, Fok PJ, Murray WJ: Heparin and dihydroergotatamine prophylaxis against thrombo-embolism of the hip arthroplasty, *J Bone Joint Surg Br* 67:538-542, 1985.

83. Hui AC, Heras-Palou C, Dunn I, et al: Graded compression stockings for prevention of deep vein thrombosis after hip and knee replacement, *J Bone Joint Surg Br* 78:550-554, 1996.

84. Haas S: Prevention of venous thromboembolism: Recommendations based on the International Consensus and the American College of Chest Physicians Sixth Consensus Conference on Antiembolic Therapy, *Clin App Thromb Hemost* 7:171-177, 2001.

85. Bitar AA, Kaplan RJ, Stitil TP, et al: Rehabilitation of orthopedic and rheumatologic disorders. 3. Total hip arthroplasty rehabilitation, *Arch Phys Med Rehabil* 86:S56-S60, 2005.

86. Sarmiento, A, Goswami ADK: Thromboembolic prophylaxis with the use of aspirin, exercise, graded elastic stockings or intermittent compression devices in patients managed with total hip arthroplasty, *J Bone Joint Surg* 81:339-346, 1999.

87. Geerts WH, Pineo GF, Heit JA, et al: Prevention of venous thromboembolism: The Seventh ACCP Conference on antithrombolytic therapy, *Chest* 126:338S-400S, 2004.

88. Enloe, LJ, Shields RK, Smith K, et al: Total hip and knee replacement treatment programs: A report using consensus, *JOSPT* 23:3-11, 1996.

89. Brander VA, Stulberg, SD, Chang RW: Rehabilitation following hip and knee arthroplasty, *Phys Med Rehabil Clin North Am* 5.815-836, 1994.

90. Enloe LJ, Shields RK, Smith K, et al: Total hip and total knee replacement treatment programs: A report using consensus, *JOSPT* 23:3-11, 1996.

91. Cameron HU: The Cameron anterior osteotomy. In Bono JV et al (ed): *Total hip arthroplasty,* New York, 1999, Springer Verlag.

92. Beber CA, Coventry FR: Management of patients with total hip replacement, *Phys Ther* 52:823-828, 1972.

93. Burton DS, Imrie SH: Total hip arthroplasty and postoperative rehabilitation, *Phys Ther* 53:132-140, 1973.

94. Munin MC, Kwoh CK, Glynn NW, et al: Predicting discharge outcome after elective hip and knee arthroplasty, *Am J Phys Med Rehabil* 74:294-301, 1995.

95. Vaz MD, Kramer JF, Rorabeck CH, et al: Isometric hip abductor strength following total hip replacement and its relationship to functional assessments, *JOSPT* 18:526-531, 1993.

96. Hesse S, Werner C, Seibel H, et al: Treadmill training with partial body weight support after total hip arthroplasty: A randomized controlled study, *Arch Phys Med Rehabil* 84:1767-1773, 2003.

97. Givens-Heiss DL, Krebs DE, Riley PO, et al: In-vivo acetabular contact pressures during rehabilitation. Part II. Post acute phase, *Phys Ther* 72:700-705, 1992.

98. Krebs DE, Elbaum L, Riley PO, et al: Exercise and gait effects on in vivo hip contact pressures, *Phys Ther* 71:301-309, 1991.

99. Krebs DE, Robbins CE, Lavine L, et al: Hip biomechanics during gait, *JOSPT* 28:51-59, 1998.

100. Bergmann G, Graichen F, Rohlmann A, et al: Hip joint forces during load carrying, *Clin Orthop* 335:190-201, 1997.

101. Davy DT, Kotzar GM, Brown RH, et al: Telemetric force measurements across the hip and after total arthroplasty, *J Bone Joint Surg Am* 70:45-50, 1988.

102. Lim LA, Carmichael SW, Cabanela ME: Biomechanics of total joint arthroplasty, *Anat Rec* 257:110-116, 1999.

103. Bergmann G, Graichen F, Rohlmann A, et al: Hip joint loading during walking and running, measured in two patients, *J Biomechanics* 16:969-999, 1993.

104. Nordin M, Frankel VH: Biomechanics of the hip. In Nordin M and Frankel VH: *Basic Biomechanics of the Musculoskeletal System,* ed 3, Philadelphia, 2001, Lippincott Williams & Wilkins.

105. Bergmann G: Loads acting at the hip joint. In Sedel L, Cabanela ME (eds): *Hip Surgery: Materials and Developments,* London, 1998, Martin Dunitz.

106. Sashika H, Matsuba Y, Watanabe Y: Home program of physical therapy: Effect on disabilities of patients with total hip arthroplasty, *Arch Phys Med Rehabil* 77:273-277, 1996.

107. Jan HW, Hung JY, Liu JC, et al: Effects of a home program of strength, walking speed, and function after total hip replacement, *Arch Phys Med Rehabil* 85:1943-1951, 2004.

108. Gogia PP, Christiansen CM, Schmidt C: Total hip replacement in patients with osteoarthritis of the hip: Improvements in pain and functional status, *Orthopedics* 17:145-150, 1994.

109. Munin MC, Hockenbury PS, Flynn PG: Rehabilitation. In Callagan JJ, Rosenberg AG, Rubash HJ (eds): *The Adult Hip,* Philadelphia, 1998, Lippincott.

110. Wykman A, Goldie J: Postural stability after total hip replacement, *Int Orthop* 13:235-238, 1989.

111. Gehlsen GM, Whaley MS: Falls in the elderly. Part II. Balance, strength and flexibility, *Arch Phys Med Rehabil* 71:739-741, 1990.

112. Guralnik JM, Ferrucci L, Simonsick EM, et al: Lower extremity function in persons over the age of 70 as a predictor of subsequent disability, *N Engl J Med* 332:556-561, 1995.

113. Trudelle-Jackson E, Emerson R, Smith S: Outcomes of total hip arthroplasty: A study of patients one year postsurgery, *JOSPT* 32:260-267, 2002.

114. Saito N, Horiuchi H, Kobayashi S, et al: Continuous local cooling for pain relief following total hip arthroplasty, *J Arthroplasty* 19:334-337, 2004.

115. Normand H, Darlas Y, Solassol A, et al: Etude experimente de l'effet thermique des ultra sons sur le materiel prosthetique, *Ann Readaptation Med Phys* 32:193-201, 1989.

116. Skoubo-Kristensen E, Sommer J: Ultrasound influence on internal fixation with rigid plates in dogs, *Arch Phys Med Rehabil* 63:371-373, 1982.

117. Cameron MH: Ultrasound. In Cameron MH (ed): *Physical Agents in Rehabilitation: From Research to Practice,* ed 2, St. Louis, 2003, WB Saunders.

118. Rankins EA, Alarcon GS, Chang RW: NIH Consensus statement on total knee replacement, Dec 8-10, 2003, *J Bone Joint Surg Am* 86:1328-1335, 2004.

119. Arthroplasty of the ankle and knee. In Canale ST (ed): *Campbell's Operative Orthopaedics,* ed 10, St. Louis, 2003, Mosby.

120. Huang CH, Cheng CK, Lee YT, et al: Muscle strength after successful total knee replacement, *Clin Ortho Relat Res* 328:147-154, 1996.

121. Bathis H, Perlick L, Tingart M, et al: CT-free computer assisted total knee arthroplasty versus conventional technique: Radiographic results of 100 cases, *Orthopedics* 27:476-480, 2004.

122. Callahan CM, Drake BG, Heck DA, et al: Patient outcomes following tricompartmental total knee replacement: A meta-analysis, *JAMA* 271:1349-1357, 1994.

123. Rossi MD, Brown LE, Whitehurst M, et al: Comparison of knee extensor strength between limbs in individuals with bilateral total knee replacement, *Arch Phys Med Rehabil* 83:523-526, 2002.

124. Berman AT, Bosacco SJ, Israelite C: Evaluation of total knee arthroplasty using isokinetic testing, *Clin Orthop* 271:106-113, 1991.

125. Rossi MD, Hasson S: Lower limb force production in individuals after unilateral total knee arthroplasty, *Arch Phys Med Rehabil* 85:1279-1284, 2004.

126. Gill GS, Joshi AB, Mills DM: Total condylar knee arthroplasty: 16-21 year results, *Clin Orthop* 367:210-215, 1999.

127. Konig A, Walther M, Kirschner S, et al: Balance sheets of knee and functional scores 5 years after total knee arthroplasty for osteoarthritis: A source of patient information, *J Arthroplasty* 15:289-294, 2000.

128. Finch E, Walsh M, Thomas SG, et al: Functional ability perceived by individuals following total knee arthroplasty compared to age matched individuals without knee disability, *JOSPT* 27:255-263, 1998.

129. Lord SR, Rogers MW, Howland A, et al: Lateral stability, sensorimotor function and falls in older people, *J Am Geriatr Soc* 47:1077-1081, 1999.

130. Connelly DM, Vandervoot AA: Effects of detraining on knee extensor strength and functional mobility in a group of elderly women, *JOSPT* 26:340-346, 1997.

131. Moxley Scarborough D, Krebs DE Harris BA: Quadriceps muscle strength and dynamic stability in elderly persons, *Gait Posture* 10:10-20, 1999.
132. Walsh M, Woodhouse LJ, Thomas SG, et al: Physical impairments and functional limitations; a comparison of individuals 1 year after total knee arthroplasty with control subjects, *Phys Ther* 78:248-258, 1998.
133. Mizner RL, Pettersen SC, Stevens JE, et al: Early quadriceps strength loss after total knee arthroplasty. The contributions of muscle atrophy and failure of voluntary muscle activation, *J Bone Joint Surg Am* 87:1047-1053, 2005.
134. Weiss JM, Noble PC, Conditt MA, et al: What functional activities are important to patients with knee replacements? *Clin Orthop* 404:172-188, 2002.
135. Jones CA, Voaklander DC, Suarez-Almazor ME: Determinants of function after total knee arthroplasty, *Phys Ther* 83:696-706, 2003.
136. Whitehouse SL, Lingard EA, Katz JN, et al: Development and testing of a reduced WOMAC function scale, *J Bone Joint Surg Br* 85:706-711, 2003.
137. Irrgang JJ, Synder-Macker L, Wainner RS, et al: Development of a patient-reported measure of function of the knee, *J Bone Joint Surg Am* 80:1132-1145, 1998.
138. Walsh M, Woodhouse LJ, Thomas SG, et al: Physical impairments and functional limitations: A comparison of individuals 1 year after total knee arthroplasty with control subjects, *Phys Ther* 78:248-258, 1998.
139. Jevsevar DS, Riley PO, Hodge WA, et al: Knee kinematics and kinetics during locomotor activities of daily living in subjects with knee arthroplasty and healthy control subjects, *Phys Ther* 73:229-242, 1993.
140. Bizzini M, Boldt JG: Rehabilitation before and after total knee arthroplasty. In Munzinger U, Boldt J, Keblish P (eds): *Primary Knee Arthroplasty*, Berlin, 2004, Springer.
141. Bradbury N, Borton D, Spoo G, et al: Participation in sports after total knee replacement, *Am J Sports Med* 26:530-535, 1998.
142. Kluster MS, et al: Endurance sports after total knee replacement. A biomechanical investigation, *Med Sci Sport Exerc* 32:721-724, 2000.
143. Schwameder H, Roithner R, Muller E, et al: Knee joint forces during downhill walking with hiking poles, *J Sport Sci* 17:969-978, 1999.
144. Mallon WJ, Liebelt RA, Mason JB: Total joint replacement and golf, *Clin Sport Med* 15:179-190, 1996.
145. LaPorte DM, Mont MA, Hungerford DS, et al: Characterization of tennis players after total knee arthroplasty. Proceedings of the sixty-sixth annual meeting of the AAOS, Anaheim, Calif, 1999.
146. Healy WL, Iorio R, Lemos MJ: Athletic activity after joint replacement, *Am J Sports Med* 29:377-388, 2001.
147. Pierson JL, Earles DR, Wood K: Brake response time after total knee arthroplasty: When is it safe for patients to drive? *J Arthroplasty* 18:840-843, 2003.
148. Weidenheilm L, Mattsson E, Brostrom LA, et al: Effect of preoperative physical therapy in unicompartmental prosthetic knee replacement, *Scand J Rehabil Med* 25:33-39, 1993.
149. Mattsson E: Energy costs of level walking, *Scand J Rehabil Med* 23(suppl):1-48, 1989.
150. D'Lima DD, Colwell CW, Morris BA, et al: The effect of preoperative exercises on total knee replacement outcomes, *Clin Orthop Relat Res* 326:174-182, 1996.
151. Ivey M, Johnston RV, Uchida T: Cryotherapy for postoperative pain relief following knee arthroplasty, *J Arthroplasty* 9:285-290, 1994.
152. Morsi E: Continuous-flow cold therapy after total knee replacement, *J Arthroplasty* 17(6):718-722, 2002.
153. Walker RH, Morris BA, Argulo DL, et al: Postoperative use of continuous passive motion, transcutaneous electrical nerve stimulation and continuous cooling pad flowing total knee arthroplasty, *J Arthroplasty* 6:151-156, 1991.
154. Brosseau L, Milne S, Wells G, et al: Efficacy of continuous passive motion following total knee arthroplasty: A meta-analysis, *J Rheumatol* 31:2251-2264, 2004.
155. McInnes J, Larson MG, Daltroy LH, et al: A controlled evaluation of continuous passive motion in patients undergoing total knee arthroplasty, *JAMA* 268:1423-1428, 1992.
156. Milne S, Brosseau L, Robinson V, et al: Continuous passive motion following total knee arthroplasty, *Cochrane Database Syst Rev* (2):CD004260, 2003.
157. Ritter MA, Harty LD, Davis KE, et al: Predicting range of motion after total knee arthroplasty, *J Bone Joint Surg Am* 85:1278-1285, 2003.
158. Mauerhan DR, Mokris JG, Ly A, et al: Relationship between the length of stay and manipulation rate after total knee arthroplasty, *J Arthroplasty* 13:896, 1998.
159. Perry J, Antonelli D, Ford W: Analysis of knee-joint forces during flexed knee stance, *J Bone Joint Surg Am* 57(A):961-967, 1975.
160. Millett PJ, Johnson B, Carlson J, et al: Rehabilitation of the arthrofibrotic knee, *Am J Orthop* 32(11):531-538, 2003.
161. Erler K, Anders C, Fehlberg G, et al: Objective assessment of results of special hydrotherapy in inpatient rehabilitation following knee prosthesis implantation, *Zorthop Ihre Grenzgeb* 139(3):352-358, 2001.
162. Glasberg MR, Glasberg JR, Jones RE: Muscle pathology in total knee replacement for severe osteoarthritis: A histochemical and morphometric study, *Henry Ford Hosp Med J* 34:37-40, 1986.
163. Avramidis K, Strike PW, Taylor PN: Effectiveness of electrical stimulation of the vastus medialis muscle in the rehabilitation of patients after total knee arthroplasty, *Arch Phy Med Rehab* 84:1850-1853, 2003.
164. Lewek M, Stevens J, Synder-Mackler L: The use of electrical stimulation to increase the quadriceps femoris muscle force in an elderly patient following a total knee arthroplasty, *Phys Ther* 81:1565-1571, 2001.
165. Avramidis K, Strike PW, Taylor PN: Effectiveness of electrical stimulation of the vastus medialis muscle in the rehabilitation of patients after total knee arthroplasty, *Arch Phys Med Rehabil* 84:1850-1853, 2003.
166. Martin TP, Gunderson LA, Blevins FT, et al: The influence of functional electrical stimulation on the properties of the vastus lateralis fibres following total knee arthroplasty, *Scand J Rehabil Med* 23:207-210, 1991.
167. Hopkins JT, Ingersoll CD, Krause BA, et al: Effect of knee effusion on quadriceps and soleus motoneuron pool excitability, *Med Sci Sports Exer* 33:123-126, 2001.
168. Spencer JD, Hayes KC, Alexander IJ, et al: Knee joint effusion and quadriceps reflex inhibition in man, *Arch Phys Med Rehabil* 65:171-177, 1984.
169. Hopkins JT, Ingersoll CD, Edwards JE, et al: Cryotherapy and transcutaneous electrical neuromuscular stimulation decrease arthrogenic muscle inhibition of the vastus medialis after knee joint effusion, *J Athl Train* 37:25-31, 2002.
170. Hinman RS, Bennell KL, Metcalf BR, et al: Delayed onset quadriceps activity and altered knee joint kinematics during stair stepping in individuals with knee osteoarthritis, *Arch Phys Med Rehabil* 83:1080-1086, 2002.
171. Fisher NM, Pendergast DR: Reduced muscle function in patients with osteoarthritis, *Scan J Rehabil Med* 57:588-594, 1998.
172. O'Reilly SC, Jones A, Muir KR, et al: Quadriceps weakness in knee osteoarthritis: the effect of pain and disability, *Ann Rheum Dis* 57:588-594, 1998.
173. Worrell TW, Borchert B, Erner K, et al: Effect of lateral step up exercise protocol on quadriceps and lower extremity performance, *JOSPT* 18:646-653, 1993.
174. Blackburn JR, Morrissey MC: The relationship between open and closed kinetic chain strength of lower limb and jumping performance, *JOSPT* 27:430-435, 1998.
175. Lephart SM, Pinciviero DM, Rozzi SL: Proprioception of the ankle and knee, *Sports Med* 25:149-155, 1998.
176. Wescott SL, Lowes LP, Richardson PK: Evaluations of postural stability in children: Current theories and assessment tools, *Phys Ther* 77:629-645, 1997.
177. Simmons S, Lephart S, Rubash H, et al: Proprioception after unicondylar knee arthroplasty versus total knee arthroplasty, *Clin Orthop* 331:179-184, 1996.
178. Andriacchi TP, Galante JO, Fermier RW: The influence of total knee replacement design on walking and stair climbing, *J Bone Joint Surg Am* 64:1328-1335, 1992.
179. Kaplan FS, Nixon JE, Reitz M, et al: Age related changes in proprioception and sensation of joint position, *Acta Orthop Scand* 56:72-74, 1985.
180. Skinner HB, Barrack RL, Cook SD: Age related decline in proprioception, *Clin Orthop* 184:208-211, 1984.
181. Warren PJ, Olanlokum TK, Cobb AG, et al: Proprioception after knee arthroplasty. The influence of prosthetic design, *Clin Orthop* 297:182-187, 1993.
182. Cash RM, Gonzalez MH, Garst J, et al: Proprioception after arthroplasty: role of the posterior cruciate ligament, *Clin Orthop* 331:172-178, 1996.
183. Barrett DS, Cobb AG, Bentley G: Joint proprioception in normal, osteoarthritic and replaced knee, *J Bone Joint Surg Br* 73:53-56, 1991.
184. Pagnano MW, Cushner FD, Scott WN: Whether to preserve the posterior cruciate ligament in total knee arthroplasty, *J Am Acad Orthop Surg* 6:176-187, 1998.
185. Swanik CB, Lephart SM, Rubash HE: Proprioception, kinesthesia and balance after total knee arthroplasty with cruciate retaining and posterior stabilized prosthesis, *J Bone Joint Surg Am* 86:328-334, 2004.
186. Jensen KL, Rockwood CA: Shoulder arthroplasty in recreational golfers, *J Shoulder Elbow Surg* 7:362-367, 1998.
187. Cuomo F, Checroun A: Avoiding pitfalls and complications in total shoulder arthroplasty, *Orthop Clin North Am* 29:507-518, 1998.
188. Rydholm U: Surface replacement of the humeral head in rheumatoid shoulder, *J Shoulder Elbow Surg* 2:286-295, 1993.
189. Smith KL, Matsen FA: Total shoulder arthroplasty vs hemiarthroplasty. Current trends, *Orthop Clin North Am* 29:491-506, 1998.
190. Hammond JW, Queale WS, Kim TK, et al: Surgeon experience and clinical and economic outcomes for shoulder arthroplasty, *J Bone Joint Surg Am* 85:2318-2324, 2003.
191. Jain N, Pietrobin R, Hocker S, et al: The relationship between surgeon and hospital volume and outcomes for shoulder arthroplasty, *J Bone Joint Surg Am* 86:496-505, 2004.
192. Edwards TB, Boulahia A, Kempf JF, et al: The influence of rotator cuff disease on the results of shoulder arthroplasty for primary osteoarthritis, *J Bone Joint Surg Am* 84:2240-2248, 2002.

193. Matsen FA III, Lippitt SB, Sidles JA, et al: *Practical Evaluation and Management of the Shoulder,* Philadelphia, 1994, WB Saunders.
194. Tanner MW, Cofield RH: Prosthetic arthroplasty for fractures and fracture dislocations of the proximal humerus, *Clin Orthop* 179:116-128, 1983.
195. Hattrup SJ: Indications, techniques and results of shoulder arthroplasty in osteonecrosis, *Orthop Clin North Am* 29:445-451, 1998.
196. Goldman RT, Koval KJ, Cuomo F, et al: Functional outcome after humeral head replacement for acute three and four part proximal humeral fractures, *J Shoulder Elbow Surg* 4:81-86, 1995.
197. Zyto K, Wallace WA, Frostick SP, et al: Outcome after hemiarthroplasty for three- and four-part fractures of the proximal humerus, *J Should Elbow Surg* 7:85-89, 1998.
198. Bigliani LU: Proximal humeral fractures. In Post, M, Flatow EL, Bigliani LU, et al (eds): *The Shoulder: Operative Techniques,* Baltimore, 1998, Lippincott Williams & Wilkins.
199. Mighell MA, Kiom GP, Collinge CA, et al: Outcomes of hemiarthroplasty for fractures of the proximal humerus, *J Shoulder Elbow Surg* 12:6, 2003.
200. Bioleau P, Trogani C, Walsh G, et al: Shoulder arthroplasty for the sequela of fractures of the proximal humerus, *J Shoulder Elbow Surg* 10:4, 2001.
201. Prekash U, McCurty DW, Dent JA: Hemiarthroplasty for severe fractures of the proximal humerus, *J Shoulder Elbow Surg* 11:428-430, 2002.
202. Namba RS, Skinner HB: Adult reconstructive surgery. In Skinner HB (ed): *Current Diagnosis and Treatment in Orthopedics,* ed 2, New York, 2000, McGraw-Hill.
203. Van der Zwaag HM, Brand R, Obermann WR, et al: Glenohumeral osteoarthrosis after Putti-Platt repair, *J Shoulder Elbow Surg* 8:252-258, 1999.
204. Bigliani LU, Weinstein DM, Glasgow MT, et al: Glenohumeral arthroplasty for arthritis after instability surgery, *J Shoulder Elbow Surg* 4:87-94, 1995.
205. Goldberg BA, Smith K, Jackins S, et al: The magnitude and durability of functional improvement after total shoulder arthroplasty for degenerative joint disease, *J Shoulder Elbow Surg* 10:464-469, 2001.
206. Fehringer EV, Kopjar B, Boorman RS, et al: Characterizing the functional improvement after total shoulder arthroplasty for osteoarthritis, *J Bone Joint Surg Am* 84:1349-1353, 2002.
207. Boorman RS, Kopjar B, Fehringer E, et al: The effect of total shoulder arthroplasty on self assessed health status is comparable to that of total hip arthroplasty and coronary artery bypass grafting, *J Shoulder Elbow Surg* 12:158-163, 2003.
208. Robinson CM, Page RS, Hill RM, et al: Primary hemiarthroplasty for the treatment of proximal humeral fractures, *J Bone Joint Surg Am* 85:1215-1223, 2003.
209. Levy O, Funk L, Sforza G, et al: Copeland surface replacement arthroplasty of the shoulder in rheumatoid arthritis, *J Bone Joint Surg Am* 86:512-518, 2004.
210. Sperling JW, Cofield RH, Rowland CM: Neer hemiarthroplasty and Neer total shoulder arthroplasty in patients 50 years old or less: Long term results, *J Bone Joint Surg Am* 80:464-473, 1998.
211. Rodosky MW, Bigliani LU: Indications for glenoid resurfacing in shoulder arthroplasty, *J Shoulder Elbow Surg* 5:231-248, 1996.
212. Parsons IM, Weldon EJ, Titelman RM, et al: Glenohumeral arthritis and its management, *Phys Med Rehabil Clin N Am* 15:447-474, 2004.
213. Torchia ME, Cofield RH, Settergren CR, et al: Total shoulder arthroplasty with the Neer prosthesis: Long term results, *J Shoulder Elbow Surg* 6:495-505, 1997.
214. Wirth M, Rockwood CJ: Complications of shoulder arthroplasty, *Clin Orthop* 307:37-46, 1994.
215. Noble J, Bell R: Failure of total shoulder arthroplasty: Why does it occur? *Semin Arthroplasty* 6:280-288, 1995.
216. Melzak R, Wall P: Pain mechanisms: A new theory, *Science* 150:971-979, 1960.
217. Arem AJ, Madden JW: Effects of stress on healing wounds, *J Surg Res* 20:93-97, 1976.
218. Kelley M, Leggin B: Shoulder rehabilitation. In Iannotti JP, Williams GR Jr (eds): *Disorders of the Shoulder: Diagnosis and Management,* Philadelphia, 1999, Lippincott Williams & Wilkins.
219. Hayes PR, Flatow EL: Total shoulder arthroplasty in the young patient, *Instr Course Lect* 50:73-83, 2001.
220. O'Kane JW, Jackins S, Sidles JA, et al: Simple home program for frozen shoulder to improve patient's assessment of shoulder function and health status, *J Am Board Fam Pract* 12:270-277, 1999.
221. Boardman ND, Cofield RH, Bengtson KA: Rehabilitation after total shoulder arthroplasty, *J Arthroplasty* 16:483-486, 2001.
222. Boileau P, Caligaris-Cordero B, Payeur F, et al: Prognostic factors during rehabilitation after shoulder prostheses for fracture, *Rev Chir Orthop Reparatrice Appar Mot* 85:106-116, 1999.
223. McCann P, Wotten M, Kadaba M: A kinematic and electromyographic study of shoulder rehabilitation exercises, *Clin Orthop* 288:179-188, 1993.
224. Dockery M, Wright T, LeStayo P: Electromyography of the shoulder: An analysis of passive modes of exercise. *Orthopedics* 21:1181-1184, 1998.
225. Dahm DL, Smith J: Rehabilitation and activities after shoulder arthroplasty. In Morrey BF (ed): *Joint Replacement Arthroplasty,* ed 3, Philadelphia, 2003, Churchill Livingstone.
226. Saha A: Mechanism of shoulder movements and a plea for recognition of the zero position of the glenohumeral joint, *Clin Orthop* 173:3-10, 1983.
227. McCann PD, Wooten MS, Kadaba MP, et al: A kinematic and electromyographic study of shoulder rehabilitation exercises, *Clin Orthop Relat Res* 288:179-188, 1993.
228. Dockery M, Wright T, LeStayo P: Electromyography of the shoulder: An analysis of passive modes of exercise, *Orthopedics* 21:1181-1184, 1998.
229. Poppen N, Walker P: Forces at the glenohumeral joint in abduction, *Clin Orthop* 135:165-172, 1978.
230. Flatow EL: Prosthetic design considerations in total shoulder arthroplasty, *Semin Arthroplasty* 6:233-244, 1995.
231. Anglin C, Wyss UP, Pichora DR: Mechanical testing of shoulder prostheses and recommendations for glenoid design, *J Shoulder Elbow Surg* 9:323-331, 2000.
232. Stone KD, Grabowski JJ, Cofield RH, et al: Stress analysis of glenoid components in total shoulder arthroplasty, *J Shoulder Elbow Surg* 8:151-158, 1999.
233. Poppen NK, Walker PS: Forces at the glenohumeral joint in abduction. *Clin Orthop* 135:165-170, 1978.
234. Basti J: Rehabilitation of shoulder arthroplasty. In Bigliani LU, Flatow EL (eds): *Shoulder Arthroplasty,* New York, 2005, Springer.
235. Cofield RH: Revision procedures for shoulder arthroplasty. In Morrey BF, An KN, Cabanells ME (eds): *Reconstructive Surgery for Joints,* ed 2, New York, 1996, Churchill Livingstone.
236. Healy WL, Iorio R, Lemos MJ: Athletic activity after joint replacement, *Am J Sports Med* 29:377-388, 2001.
237. King GJ, Glauser SJ, Westreich A, et al: In vitro stability of an unconstrained total elbow prosthesis: Influence of axial load and joint flexion angle, *J Arthroplasty* 8:291-298, 1993.
238. Connor PM, Morrey BF: Total elbow arthroplasty in patients who have juvenile rheumatoid arthritis, *J Bone Joint Surg Am* 80:678-688, 1998.
239. Ewald FC, Simmons ED, Sullivan JA, et al: Capitellocondylar total elbow replacement in rheumatoid arthritis: Long term results, *J Bone Joint Surg Am* 75:498-507, 1993.
240. Gill DR, Morrey BE: The Conrad-Morrey Total elbow arthroplasty in patients that have rheumatoid arthritis: A 10- to 15-year follow-up study, *J Bone Joint Surg Am* 80:1327-1335, 1995.
241. Cobb TK, Morrey BF: Total elbow replacement as primary treatment for distal humeral fractures in elderly patients, *J Bone Joint Surg Am* 82:826-832, 1997.
242. Sjoder SO, Lundberg A, Blomgren CA: Late results of Souter-Strathclyde total elbow prosthesis in RA: 6/19 implants loose after 5 years, *Acta Orthop Scand* 66:391-394, 1995.
243. Adams RA, Morrey BF: The effectiveness of a compressive Cryo cuff after elbow surgery: A prospective randomized study. Proceedings of the sixty-sixth annual meeting of the AAOS, Anaheim, Calif, 1999.
244. Morrey BF, Askew LJ, An KN, et al: A biomechanical study of normal functional elbow motion, *J Bone Joint Surg Am* 63:872-877, 1981.
245. Morrey BF, An KN: Articular and ligamentous contributions to the stability of the elbow joint, *Am J Sports Med* 11:315-318, 1983.
246. Amis AA, Dowson D, Wright V, et al: Elbow force predictions for some strenuous isometric actions, *J Biomechanics* 13:765-775, 1980.
247. Kudo H, Iwano K, Nishino J: Total elbow arthroplasty with the use of a non-constrained humeral component inserted with out cement in patients who have rheumatoid arthritis, *J Bone Joint Surg Am* 81:1268-1280, 1999.
248. Maloney WJ, Schurman DJ: Cast immobilization after total elbow arthroplasty: a safe cost-effective method of initial post-operative care, *Clin Orthop* 245:117-122, 1989.
249. Allen DM, Nunley JA, Bonzani PJ: Surgical and postoperative management of the rheumatoid elbow. In Mackin EJ, Callahan AD, Osterman AL, et al (eds): *Hunter, Mackin, and Callahan's Rehabilitation of the Hand and Upper Extremity,* ed 5, St. Louis, 2002, Mosby.
250. Adams BD, Khoury JG: Total wrist arthroplasty. In Weiss APC, Hastings H (eds): *Surgery of the Arthritic Hand and Wrist,* Philadelphia, 2002, Lippincott Williams & Wilkins.
251. Adams BD: Total wrist arthroplasty, *Semin Arthroplasty* 11(2):72-81, 2000.
252. Meuli HC: Total wrist arthroplasty, *Clin Orthop* 342:77-83, 1997.
253. Goodman MJ, Millender LH, Nalebuff ED, et al: Arthroplasty of the rheumatoid wrist with silicone rubber: An early evaluation, *J Hand Surg* 5A:114-121, 1980.
254. Vicar AJ, Burton RJ: Surgical management of rheumatoid wrist fusion or arthroplasty, *J Hand Surg* 11A:790-797, 1986.
255. Cobb TK, Beckenbaugh RD: Biaxial total wrist arthroplasty, *J Hand Surg* 21A:1101-1121, 1996.
256. Menon J: Universal total wrist implant: Experience with a carpal component fixed with three screws, *J Arthroplasty* 13:515-523, 1998.
257. Ryu J, Cooney WP, Askew LJ, et al: Functional ranges of motion at the wrist, *J Hand Surg* 16A:409-419, 1991.
258. Bednar JM, Von Lersner-Benson C: Wrist reconstruction: Salvage procedures. In Mackin EJ, Callahan AD, Osterman AL, et al (eds): *Hunter,*

Mackin, and Callahan's Rehabilitation of the Hand and Upper Extremity, ed 5, St. Louis, 2002, Mosby.

259. Brannon EW, Klein G: Experiences with finger a finger joint prosthesis, *J Bone Joint Surg Am* 41:87-102, 1959.

260. Murray PM: New generation implant arthroplasties of the finger joints, *J Am Acad Orthop Surg* 11:295-301, 2003.

261. Wilson TG, Sykes PJ, Niranjan NS: Long-term follow-up of Swanson's silastic arthroplasty of the metacarpal phalangeal joints in rheumatoid arthritis, *J Hand Surg* 18B:81-91, 1993.

262. Tupper JW: The metacarpophalangeal volar plate arthroplasty, *J Hand Surg Am* 14:371-375, 1989.

263. Vainio K: Vainio arthroplasty of the metacarpophalangeal joints in rheumatoid arthritis, *J Hand Surg Am* 14:367-368, 1989.

264. Shapiro JS: The wrist in the rheumatoid arthritis, *Hand Clin* 12:477-498, 1996.

265. Gellman H, Stetson W, Brumfield R, et al: Silastic metacarpophalangeal joint arthroplasty in patients with rheumatoid arthritis, *Clin Orthop Relat Res* 342:16-21, 1997.

266. Chung KC, Kowalski CP, Myra KH, et al: Patient outcomes following Swanson silastic metacarpophalangeal joint arthroplasty in the rheumatoid hand: A systematic review, *J Rheumatol* 27:1395-1402, 2000.

267. Nalebuff EA: The rheumatoid hand: Reflections on metacarpophalangeal arthroplasty. *Clin Orthop Relat* Res 182:150-159, 1994.

268. Bieber EJ, Weiland AJ, Volenc-Dowling S: Silicone rubber implant arthroplasty for metacarpophalangeal joints for rheumatoid arthritis, *J Bone Joint Surg Am* 68:206-209, 1986.

269. Blair WF, Shurr DG, Buckwalter JA: Metacarpophalangeal joint arthroplasty with a silastic spacer, *J Bone Joint Surg Am* 66:365-370, 1984.

270. Rothwell AG, Cragg KJ, O'Neill LB, et al: Hand function following Silastic arthroplasty of the metacarpophalangeal joint in the rheumatoid hand, *J Hand Surg* 22B:90-93, 1997.

271. Chung KC, Kotsis SV, Kim HM: A prospective outcome of Swanson metacarpophalangeal joint arthroplasty for the rheumatoid hand, *J Hand Surg* 29A:646-652, 2004.

272. Synnott K, Mullett H, Faull H, et al: Outcome measures following metacarpophalangeal joint replacement, *J Hand Surg* 25B:601-603, 2000.

273. Cook SD, Beckenbaugh RD, Redondo J, et al: Long term follow up of pyrolytic carbon metacarpophalangeal implants, *J Bone Joint Surg Am* 81:635-648, 1999.

274. Pereira JA, Belcher HJCR: A comparison of metacarpophalangeal joint silastic arthroplasty with or without crossed intrinsic transfer, *J Hand Surg* 26B:229-234, 2001.

275. Massey-Westropp N, Krishnan J: Post-operative therapy after metacarpophalangeal arthroplasty, *J Hand Ther* 16:311-314, 2003.

276. Ring D, Simmons BP, Hayes M: Continuous passive motion following metacarpophalangeal joint arthroplasty, *J Hand Surg* 23A:505-511, 1998.

277. Groth G, Watkins M, Paytner P: Effect of an alternative flexion splinting protocol on midjoint ROM (letter), *J Hand Ther* 9:68-69, 1996.

278. Mannerfelt L, Anderson K: Silastic arthroplasty of the metacarpophalangeal joints in rheumatoid arthritis, *J Bone Joint Surg Am* 57:484-489, 1975.

279. Madden JW, De Vore G, Arem AJ: A rational post-operative program for metacarpophalangeal joint implant arthroplasty, *J Hand Surg* 2A:358-366, 1997.

280. Ring D, Simmons BP, Hayes M: Continuous passive motion following metacarpophalangeal joint arthroplasty, *J Hand Surg* 23A:505-511, 1998.

281. Burr N, Pratt AL: MCP joint arthroplasty case study: The Mount Vernon static regime. *Br J Hand Ther* 4:137-140, 1999.

282. Burr N, Pratt AL, Smith PJ: An alternative splinting and rehabilitation protocol for metacarpophalangeal joint replacements in patients with rheumatoid arthritis, *J Hand Ther* 15:41-47, 2002.

283. Amadio PC, Murray PM, Linscheid RL: Arthroplasty of the proximal interphalangeal joint. In Morrey B (ed): *Joint Replacement Arthroplasty*, Philadelphia, 2003, Churchill Livingstone.

284. Feldon PG, Nalebuff EA, Terrano AL, et al: Rheumatoid arthritis and other connective tissue diseases. In Green DP, Hotchkiss RN, Pederson WC (eds): *Green's Operative Hand Surgery*, vol 2 and 4, New York, 1999, Churchill Livingston.

285. Takigawa S, Meletiou S, Sauerbier M, et al: Long-term assessment of Swanson implant arthroplasty in the proximal interphalangeal joint of the hand, *J Hand Surg* 29A:785-795, 2004.

286. Theisen L: Proximal interphalangeal and distal interphalangeal joint arthroplasty. In Aiell B, Clark GL, Wilgis EFS (eds): *Hand Rehabilitation: A Practical Guide*, ed 2, New York, 1997, Churchill Livingstone.

287. Swanson AB: Flexible implant arthroplasty of the proximal interphalangeal joints of the fingers, *Ann Plastic Surg* 3:346-354, 1979.

288. Swanson AB, Maupin BK, Gajjar NV, et al: Flexible implant arthroplasty in the proximal interphalangeal joint of the hand, *Hand Surg* 10A:796-805, 1985.

Chapter 11

Soft Tissue Surgery

Christopher J. Durall, Robert C. Manske

CHAPTER OUTLINE

OBJECTIVES

After reading this chapter, the reader will be able to:

1. Differentiate different types of nonmineralized connective tissue, including bursa, synovium, cartilage, fascia, ligament, capsule, and tendon.
2. Compare and contrast the mechanical properties of the different types of nonmineralized connective tissue.
3. Discuss the effects of immobilization and remobilization on connective tissue.
4. Describe in general terms the rehabilitation process after soft tissue surgery.
5. Discuss the different types of surgeries performed on bursae, synovium, cartilage, fascia, ligaments, capsules, and tendons.
6. Explain unique elements of the rehabilitation process after surgery on bursae, synovium, cartilage, fascia, ligaments, capsules, and tendons.
7. Provide safe and effective rehabilitation to a patient after a soft tissue surgery.

*M*any musculoskeletal pathologies and injuries require surgical intervention and a period of postoperative rehabilitation to maximize functional recovery. Tissues that undergo surgery are subjected to trauma, albeit controlled trauma. As with other forms of trauma, the affected tissues undergo a healing process. After surgery there is often a period of immobilization. Thus, to most effectively manage postoperative rehabilitation, the physical therapist (PT) must understand the healing process and how immobilization affects musculoskeletal tissues. Tissue healing is reviewed in detail in Chapter 28.

This chapter discusses the rehabilitation of individuals with impairments and functional limitations after soft tissue surgery. The effects of immobilization are described as well as remobilization parameters and interventions for rehabilitation. The chapter includes a discussion of the unique properties of nonmineralized (or soft) *connective tissue,* an overview of soft tissue postoperative rehabilitation, tissue-specific rehabilitation recommendations, and case studies. Skeletal muscle, although an integral soft tissue in the musculoskeletal system, is not often surgically repaired and thus will not be covered in this chapter.

PATHOLOGY

NONMINERALIZED CONNECTIVE TISSUES OF THE MUSCULOSKELETAL SYSTEM

All body structures are comprised of various combinations of four types of tissue: Connective, epithelial, nerve, and muscular. Aside from muscle, the structures of the musculoskeletal system are all composed of connective tissues. Connective tissues perform many highly specialized metabolic and biomechanical functions in the body, including providing structural support and facilitating movement. Although there are many forms of connective tissue with disparate functions, all connective tissues have an abundant *extracellular matrix* but are relatively devoid of cells. The extracellular matrix, produced by the cells, consists of ground substance and fibers, which give the tissues their unique characteristics (Fig. 11-1). *Cartilage,* for example, has a firm, yet flexible extracellular matrix, whereas bone has a rigid extracellular matrix.

The ground substance of connective tissue contains interstitial fluid, *proteoglycan molecules,* and proteins that "glue" the cells to the matrix (e.g., fibronectin).[1] The proteoglycan molecules are hydrophilic and combine readily with water to form a fluid or semisolid gel (depending on the type and abundance of proteoglycan in the matrix)

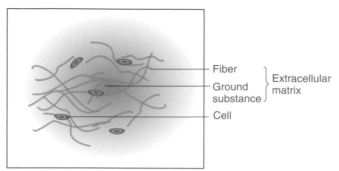

FIG. 11-1 Constituents of connective tissue.

that lubricates and creates space between adjacent fibers in the extracellular matrix. Space between fibers is needed to prevent the fibers adhering to one another.[1] The ground substance reduces friction between fibers and prevents the formation of fibrous adhesions.

There are three types of connective tissue fibers: *Collagen,* reticular, and elastic. All are formed from varying proportions of collagen and elastin proteins. Collagen proteins undergo little elongation in response to tensile loading, whereas elastin proteins are more extensible or rubber-like.[2] Tissues with a high collagen content, such as *tendon*s and *ligament*s, resist or transmit tensile forces well, whereas tissues with a relatively high elastin content, such as skin, are more pliable.[1]

There are many different types of collagen fibers, but our discussion is limited to types I, II, and III, which are most prevalent. Type I collagen, which is the most abundant, has the greatest tensile strength and is found in many connective tissues, including tendon, bone, and ligaments. The function of type I collagen is resisting tension. In contrast, type II collagen is most effective at resisting pressure and appropriately is abundant in the hyaline cartilage lining weight-bearing joints. Type III collagen, the second most abundant type of collagen, is found in skin, blood vessels, and the granulation tissue of healing wounds. Type III collagen fibers are more delicate than type I and are gradually replaced by type I collagen fibers during tissue healing.[3]

Connective tissue can be classified as dense, or loose, and as regular, or irregular, according to the density and orientation, respectively, of its fibers. Dense regular connective tissue has a high concentration of fibers arranged in a regular or unidirectional manner. Dense regular connective tissue has a relatively poor vascular supply and therefore heals less well than other more well-vascularized tissues.[4] This is in part why tendons and ligaments, which are comprised of dense regular connective tissue, often heal slowly or incompletely.

Dense irregular connective tissue, as is found in joint *capsule*s, has densely packed fibers with multidirectional orientation. This tissue also has relatively low vascularity and therefore heals slowly.[4]

Unlike dense connective tissue, loose connective tissue has relatively few fibers and therefore relatively low tensile strength. Loose connective tissue is found in the superfi-

cial *fascia* throughout the musculoskeletal system. In contrast to dense connective tissue, loose connective tissue is relatively well vascularized and thus heals more readily.[4]

Synovium is a specialized connective tissue on the innermost portion of the capsule of synovial joints. Synovial cells secrete fluid that is thought to serve two main purposes: Joint lubrication and nourishment of the avascular articular cartilage.[5] Synovial cavities may be contiguous with pouches containing synovial fluid known as *bursae,* which are located at frictional interfaces in the musculoskeletal system.

Bone and cartilage are also specialized connective tissues. As with other connective tissues, bone and cartilage have cells (osteoblasts and chondrocytes, respectively) that secrete an extracellular matrix. The firm, slightly yielding yet resilient matrix of cartilage is ideal for damping compressive loads and reducing friction at joints, and the rigid, calcified matrix of bone provides structural support and protection.

Although there are several forms of cartilage, articular cartilage and fibrocartilage are the forms most commonly affected by orthopedic surgery. Articular cartilage is a specialized form of hyaline cartilage that covers the ends of bones in diarthrodial joints. This type of cartilage has a high proteoglycan and water content to allow it to distribute compressive loads.[5] Fibrocartilage has properties of dense connective tissue and properties of hyaline cartilage.[2,4] It has more type I collagen and thus greater tensile strength than articular cartilage but more proteoglycan and water than dense connective tissue, so it can also tolerate pressure loading.[4,5] Fibrocartilage often forms temporarily at fracture sites and is a permanent component of the intervertebral disks of the spine, the menisci at the knee and wrist, the labrum at the shoulder, and the acetabulum at the hip.

Unlike other connective tissues, cartilage is avascular and alymphatic. It is nourished by the diffusion of nutrients from the synovial fluid and by capillaries in adjacent connective tissue. The lack of a direct vascular supply precludes an inflammatory response to injury and gives cartilage a poor healing potential. Articular cartilage far from the bony surface, which relies entirely on diffusion of nutrients and oxygen through the cartilage matrix, has almost no ability to heal.[4,5] If articular cartilage close to subchondral bone is injured, it may heal with a mixture of hyaline cartilage and fibrocartilage.[5]

Biomechanics of Nonmineralized Connective Tissue. Connective tissues have many different functions that can often be surmised by examining the tissues' components. For instance, tissues with a high collagen fiber content and a relatively low proteoglycan content, such as ligament and tendon, are well suited to attenuating tensile loads, whereas connective tissues with a relatively high proteoglycan content, such as articular cartilage, are better suited to attenuating compressive loads.[1,4]

Tissues with high tensile strength have an abundance of collagen fibers that are oriented to most effectively withstand imposed forces. Collagen fibers in tendons, for example, are aligned parallel to the tensile forces developed within their associated muscles. This allows the large tensile forces developed by muscles to be transmitted to their bony attachments without damaging the tendons. While most of the collagen fibers in ligaments are also aligned parallel to each other to withstand longitudinal forces, some fibers course diagonally to withstand oblique forces that may be placed on a ligament.

Articular cartilage, which covers the articulating ends of bones, provides a low-friction, wear-resistant surface and is also slightly compressible to dampen forces on the bone.[4] Fibrocartilage, which has mechanical properties of both articular cartilage and dense regular connective tissue, dampens compressive loads and also assists ligaments and joint capsules in constraining joint movement.

Connective tissue undergoes deformation when loaded, yet it has a remarkable ability to return to its original length and shape when the load is removed, as long as the load is not excessive in magnitude or duration.[1,4] This characteristic deformability and resilience of connective tissue allows it to attenuate shock and transmit forces.[4] When connective tissue is stressed, it deforms in a predictable manner, which is demonstrated graphically by the "stress-strain" curve (Fig. 11-2). The first part of this curve, the "toe" region, corresponds to low forces of a magnitude similar to those applied during clinical stress testing. The second part of this curve, the "linear" region, corresponds to a moderate amount of force. Collagen fibers lose their wavy appearance and straighten, and the tissue's structural stiffness increases in response to this range of force. If the tissue is deformed with brief, low, or

moderate magnitude loads, it will exhibit elasticity by quickly returning to its prior length and shape after the load is removed.[6] If the load is increased further, the tissue will eventually deform beyond its elastic limit and change permanently, demonstrating plastic deformation.[6] The permanent increase in tissue length as a result of plastic deformation is often the goal of stretching exercises or mobilization techniques. If even greater loads are applied, individual fibers and eventually the entire tissue will tear and fail.[6]

The rate of loading (stress) also influences connective tissue deformation (strain). In general, low magnitude loads applied for longer durations will cause greater tissue deformation than transient, high magnitude loads.[6] This behavior, known as *viscoelasticity,* explains why low magnitude, long duration stretching is more effective than high magnitude, short duration stretching for increasing connective tissue mobility or length.

Effects of Immobilization and Remobilization on Nonmineralized Connective Tissue. After surgery, immobilization may be needed to prevent disruption of the surgical repair. However, prolonged immobilization results in the loss of ground substance and subsequent dehydration and approximation of the embedded fibers in the extracellular matrix.[7-9] These microstructural changes contribute to the formation of fibrous adhesions and increased friction between fibers, leading to reduced tissue length and strength.[1,9-12]

Numerous experimental studies have shown that controlled remobilization after injury or surgery can reverse many of the adverse effects of immobilization.[13-15] Mechanical stress of the appropriate magnitude and direction can stimulate collagen synthesis and optimize its alignment,[13,16-18] whereas too much or too little stress can impair collagen synthesis.[19-22] For example, controlled muscle contraction can make collagen fibers in tendons orient in the direction of force transmission from the muscle to the skeletal attachment. This optimizes the structural integrity and functionality of the tissue.[13,18]

During tissue healing, much of the initial collagen formed is type III, which is weaker than type I collagen.[19,23] As the connective tissue matures, which may take up to a full year after a period of immobilization,[9] most of the type III collagen is replaced by type I collagen.[19] Thus healing connective tissue may be weaker than fully mature tissue for many months after an injury or a period of immobilization.[3,24] Clinically, it is important to remember that mechanical forces that may be safe for mature, healthy tissue may injure healing tissue for up to a year after the injury.

In his seminal study, Noyes demonstrated that 8 weeks of lower limb immobilization caused a substantial loss of ligament tensile strength.[9] He immobilized the knees of 92 rhesus monkeys for 8 weeks and found that at the end of this period the maximum failure load of the ligaments was 39% less than in nonimmobilized control monkeys and energy absorbed to failure was 32% less than in nonimmobilized control monkeys. Even after 5 months of reconditioning after immobilization, there was only partial recovery of the ligament strength. Immobilization

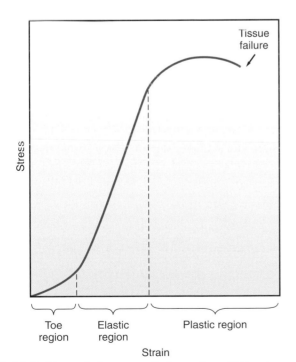

FIG. 11-2 Stress-strain curve. *Redrawn from Birkkey J: Physiother Canada 41(1):24-30, 1980.*

was thought to weaken the ligaments by a number of mechanisms, including changing the ligament force–elongation relationship, causing histological changes at the bone-ligament junction, altering mechanisms of failure, and changing the glycosaminoglycan collagen fiber relationship.

Vailas et al examined histological changes and the ultimate separation force in the knee medial collateral ligaments (MCLs) of rats after surgical repair; 2 or 8 weeks of immobilization was followed in some by a period of exercise.[8] The exercise was 65 minutes of continuous treadmill running at approximately 70% of maximum aerobic capacity. The ligaments from the rats immobilized for 8 weeks were smaller and weaker and contained significantly less total collagen than ligaments from rats immobilized for 2 weeks, and the ligaments from the rats who exercised were significantly heavier and stronger and contained more collagen than the ligaments from the rats who did not exercise.

Tipton and colleagues examined the influence of exercise on MCL strength in seven groups of dogs exposed to different amounts of exercise.[13] The most inactive dogs had the weakest ligaments, whereas the most active animals had the strongest ligaments. Likewise, physical activity was shown to positively influence fiber bundle diameter—trained dogs had the largest fiber bundles, whereas the immobilized group had the smallest bundles.

The studies described clearly demonstrate that non-mineralized connective tissue in animals weakens with immobilization and becomes stronger in response to the stress of physical activity. Several investigators have hypothesized that human connective tissue responds similarly, but this has not been tested experimentally.[8-10,16,17] Thus, although the clinical practice of prescribing therapeutic exercise to increase the tensile strength of non-mineralized connective tissues in patients is logical and supported by studies in animals, it has not been definitively proved to be effective in humans.

OVERVIEW OF REHABILITATION AFTER SOFT TISSUE SURGERY

Although rehabilitation after soft tissue surgery varies slightly according to the type of tissue operated on, there is considerable overlap for all tissue types, with most focusing on remobilization, increasing range of motion (ROM), decreasing edema, and returning to an optimal level of functional activity. This section describes general, non–tissue-specific postoperative rehabilitation. Unique considerations for each type of nonmineralized connective tissue are discussed in the following sections.

EXAMINATION

PATIENT HISTORY

When feasible, the therapist should review the medical chart before meeting the patient to gather pertinent information such as the patient's age, sex, race, language, education, cultural beliefs, family/caregiver resources, social interactions/support, employment, hand/leg dominance, living environment (architectural barriers, projected

discharge destination), general health status (including physical activity and if the patient is a smoker), medical/surgical history, chief complaint(s), functional status and activity level, medications, laboratory or diagnostic test results, and other clinical findings (e.g., nutrition, hydration). Salient information in the chart should be briefly discussed with the patient (e.g., job description/requirements). Likewise, important information relevant to the patient's rehabilitation that is not included in the chart (e.g., living environment) should be discussed. The therapist should also be cognizant of any relative or absolute contraindications to movement or activity and communicate these clearly to the patient.

The patient's present functional status and their anticipated long-term functional goals should be discussed. Plans and expectations regarding return to activity should be brought up early so that the clinician and patient can reach agreement and fully understand each other's concerns. For instance, the patient may have unrealistic expectations regarding how quickly they can return to full activity. The therapist should also briefly explain the generic intervention process, as well as the specific patient's unique rehabilitation considerations based on the type of connective tissue affected.

SYSTEMS REVIEW

The systems review is used to target areas requiring further examination and to define areas that may cause complications or indicate a need for precautions during the examination and intervention processes. See Chapter 1 for details of the systems review.

TESTS AND MEASURES
Musculoskeletal

Posture. The affected limb position should be observed. Patients tend to assume a position that is comfortable, but in some instances the most comfortable position, if maintained for prolonged periods, may lead to undesirable adaptive tissue shortening.

Anthropometric Characteristics. Limb circumference should be measured bilaterally at several locations around and over affected joints to assess for swelling or soft tissue atrophy.[25] At the knee, for instance, circumferential measurements can be taken at four locations as described by Manske and Davies (Table 11-1). Soderberg et al[26] found

TABLE 11-1	Circumferential Location and Clinical Rationale
Location of Measurement	**Clinical Rationale**
20 cm proximal to joint line	Quadriceps atrophy (generalized)
10 cm proximal to joint line	Quadriceps atrophy (more specific to vastus medialis oblique) or suprapatellar pouch for effusion
Joint line	General joint effusion
15 cm distal to joint line	Gastrocnemius/soleus atrophy or lower leg edema

From Manske RC, Davies GJ: *Crit Rev Phys Rehabil Med* 15(2):141-166, 2003.

that these measurements showed high interrater reliability (ICC 0.82-1.0) using a similar protocol.

Range of Motion. ROM should be assessed both actively and passively in joints affected by the surgery. Surgical restrictions, as well as the patient's symptom response, should guide the passive motion assessment.

Muscle Performance. High-intensity strength testing is often contraindicated in the initial postoperative period since high levels of muscle tension may damage surgically repaired tissue.[27] Bearing in mind that postoperative joint effusion and/or pain can impair muscle performance,[28] it may be appropriate though to ascertain if the patient can move the affected body segment through their available ROM against gravity (criteria for a "fair" (3/5) muscle grade). More strenuous strength testing can be performed in the later phases of rehabilitation. Muscles important to the function of the affected joints but not directly affected by the repair may be strenuously strength tested initially.

Joint Integrity and Mobility. The indications and appropriate vigor for clinical stress and mobility testing varies considerably with joint structure and is typically not well tolerated after orthopedic operative procedures and may be contraindicated, depending on the type of procedure performed.

Neuromuscular

Arousal, Attention, and Cognition. The astute therapist will form an opinion about a patient's arousal, attention, and cognition while obtaining the patient history and performing the systems review as described. In essence, the patient should be able to interact meaningfully with the therapist and ideally should not be easily distracted or have difficulty following through with directions.

Pain. Pain or other symptoms can be recorded and tracked using a visual analog scale (VAS). Commonly, this scale ranges from 0 (pain-free) to 10 (severe pain). Qualifiers (e.g., boring, stabbing, achy) may also be used to help identify the specific nociceptors affected.

Peripheral Nerve Integrity. Peripheral nerve integrity is assessed through testing of reflex integrity, sensory integrity, and muscle performance.

Reflex Integrity. Deep tendon reflexes may be assessed if there are no contraindications to movement or muscle contraction.

Sensory Integrity. Superficial skin sensation may often be reduced or compromised in a patient after soft tissue surgery because of severing of superficial nerves or compression by local swelling.[29] Sensation testing should be conducted regularly to assess for nerve regeneration.

Motor Function—Control and Learning. Motor function is generally quickly assessed during the systems review by observing the patient's coordination and movement in response to simple requests (e.g., "try to straighten your knee").

Cardiovascular/Pulmonary

Circulation, Ventilation, and Respiration/Gas Exchange. Vital signs should be assessed in the inpatient setting at the beginning of each rehabilitation session (see Chapter 22). In addition, in the outpatient setting, vital signs should be recorded during the initial evaluation and again if the patient experiences marked or inexplicable symptom changes. Vital signs should be monitored regularly in all patients with cardiopulmonary compromise. Circulation can be quickly assessed by palpating for skin temperature, pulses, and by viewing skin color and capillary refill.

Integumentary

Integumentary Integrity. During the initial examination and at each subsequent meeting, the surgical site should be carefully inspected for any indicators of an adverse reaction (e.g., erythema, swelling, wound drainage, heat). The skin color and presence of scar formation should also be noted. Wound healing, as well as scar formation and compliance, should be monitored throughout the rehabilitation process. The integument in any areas subjected to prolonged pressure or shear should also be monitored regularly for the development of pressure ulcers (see Chapter 28). Because of decreased oxygen perfusion, ischemia, and low oxygen tension, soft tissue healing may be delayed in individuals with systemic diseases, such as diabetes or peripheral vascular disease, and in individuals who smoke.[30] A list of postoperative "red flags" or signs and symptoms that merit further investigation and/or physician notification can be found in Box 11-1. These warning signs and symptoms may indicate the presence of infection or disruption of the surgical repair and should be carefully documented and quickly communicated to the surgeon.

Function

Gait, Locomotion, and Balance. For surgeries involving the lumbar spine, pelvis, or lower extremities, gait should be assessed since postoperative pain, swelling, and weakness can affect stride length, stride width, and stance time[31] (see Chapter 32). Weight-bearing restrictions imposed by the surgeon should be clearly communicated to the patient. For surgeries involving one or both upper extremities, functional ability can be assessed with instruments like the Melbourne Assessment of Unilateral Upper Limb Function.[32]

Orthotic, Protective, and Supportive Devices. The therapist should determine if the patient's functional ability would improve by the use of orthotic, protective, or

BOX 11-1	Postoperative Red Flags: Signs and Symptoms That Merit Further Investigation or Physician Notification

- Erythema
- Increased edema
- Colored or purulent drainage
- Increased local tissue temperature
- Fever or other systemic manifestations (e.g., hyperhidrosis)
- Unexplainable marked increase in pain
- Excessive mobility after a stabilizing procedure
- Significant loss of mobility after a releasing procedure

support devices. Previously dispensed devices should be inspected on and off the patient to determine if the fit and usage of the device is appropriate. The patient should also be observed using any devices to ensure that the devices are used safely.

Ergonomics and Body Mechanics. Ergonomics and body mechanics are not typically assessed formally during the initial examination but may be appropriate to examine later in the rehabilitation process.

Environmental Barriers, Self-Care, and Home Management. Environmental barriers and self-care and home management should have been discussed during the patient history.

Work, Community, and Leisure Integration. Work, community, and leisure integration are not typically assessed formally during the initial examination but should be examined and evaluated later in the rehabilitation process.

EVALUATION, DIAGNOSIS, AND PROGNOSIS

After the physical therapy examination, a physical therapy diagnosis and prognosis should be established. According to the *Guide to Physical Therapist Practice,*[33] rehabilitation for patients in the preferred practice pattern 4I: Impaired joint mobility, motor function, muscle performance, and ROM associated with bony or soft tissue surgery may take from 1-8 months (roughly 6-70 visits), although there are many factors, such as adherence to the intervention program; age; caregiver consistency and expertise; chronicity or severity of condition; concurrent medical, surgical, and therapeutic interventions; and overall health status, including nutritional status, that may require modification of the frequency and duration of physical therapy visits.[34] At present, specific evidence-based data on the prognosis or outcome of patients in this practice pattern are not available.

INTERVENTION

The process of tissue healing (see Chapters 7 and 28) consists of an inflammatory phase, a fibroplastic proliferation phase, and a maturation phase. The intervention process after soft tissue surgery is divided into three phases that roughly correspond with the three phases of healing: Immediate postoperative phase (also known as the maximum protection phase), the intermediate phase (also known as the moderate protection phase), and the advanced strengthening/return to activity phase (also known as the minimum protection phase). Unfortunately, the phases of healing are not punctuated with obvious beginning or end points. Likewise, the signs and symptoms indicating that a patient is ready to advance from one phase of rehabilitation to the next are often subtle. Nonetheless, some criteria can be used to guide rehabilitation progression decisions.

Although this chapter primarily addresses postoperative rehabilitation, preoperative interventions are valuable as well. Restoring or maximizing joint motion and strength before orthopedic surgery has been shown to reduce postoperative recovery time.[35,36] Additionally, obtaining preoperative data of the patient's performance

and functional ability can assist with postoperative goal setting.

IMMEDIATE POSTOPERATIVE PHASE

During the immediate postoperative period, the surgically affected connective tissues undergo an inflammatory response. While the inflammatory response is necessary for healing, the associated pain and edema can impede the rehabilitation process.[37-39] Goals of the immediate postoperative period include protection of the soft tissues from harmful stress, minimizing the adverse effects of immobilization, and controlling pain and inflammation. Bracing and assistive devices (e.g., crutches, splints) can be used to protect the tissues from excessive stress after spine, pelvic, or upper or lower extremity surgery. A scale can be used to help the patient quantify their weight bearing. Aquatic therapy and unloading devices may be appropriate for patients with weight-bearing restrictions. After upper extremity surgery, slings, splints, or immobilizers can be used to protect the soft tissues.

Several interventions have been shown to be effective for pain modulation, including cryotherapy,[40] manual therapy,[41] exercise,[42,43] and electrical stimulation.[44] Cryotherapy, which causes local vasoconstriction and increases blood viscosity, or monophasic pulsed electrical current may be used to limit edema formation during the inflammatory response.[45-47]

To minimize the adverse effects of immobilization and to stimulate collagen synthesis and proper collagen alignment, movement should begin as soon after surgery as the surgeon deems safe. As discussed earlier, connective tissue must be stressed appropriately if it is to become sufficiently robust. Early motion can be achieved through either passive ROM (PROM) or active assisted ROM (AAROM).[42,43] If the surgeon has not imposed joint motion limits, the therapist may want to consider imposing motion limits based on the patient's pain and swelling response to movement. Patients who take analgesic medications may have greater pain tolerance to movement or exercise, but they also may be at greater risk of iatrogenic injury and therefore should be advised to exercise below their pain threshold.

INTERMEDIATE POSTOPERATIVE PHASE

The intermediate phase begins when the acute inflammatory reaction has subsided, typically 1 week after surgery.[48,49] Goals of the immediate postoperative period include pain and edema reduction; restoration of normal functional movement patterns; increased joint motion and muscle strength; and improved neuromuscular coordination, timing, strength, and endurance, and *proprioception*. During this phase, it is important to continue protecting the soft tissues with bracing, splinting, assistive devices, and gradual, symptom-limited exercise progression.

Edema remaining after the acute inflammatory response can cause pain[50] and impair muscle performance.[37-39] Interventions that have been found to be effective in reducing edema during this phase include elevation,[51] compression,[52] motor-level electrical stimulation,[53] and exercise.[54] Elevation of the edematous segment above heart level promotes venous and lymphatic return via the effects of gravity.[51] Compressive wraps or garments can reduce edema by driving extracellular fluid into the venules and lymphatic vessels.[54] Exercise can also promote proximal movement of venous and lymphatic fluid since contracting and relaxing muscles compresses and decompresses venous and lymphatic vessels, pumping the fluid proximally.[54] If necessary, motor-level electrical stimulation can be used to induce the muscle contractions and thus enhance circulation.[53]

Because dense, regular connective tissue is poorly vascularized, interventions that increase local circulation and metabolism may facilitate tissue healing.[55] Local circulation may be increased with thermotherapy[56,57] (e.g., hot packs, paraffin baths, fluidotherapy, continuous ultrasound), massage,[58] exercise,[56,59] and electrical stimulation.[53,60]

Strengthening exercises should be initiated during this phase, when the muscle-tendon unit can safely tolerate tensile loading. After tendon repairs, resistance exercise may be delayed for several weeks or months, depending on surgeon preference.[61-64] The intensity of strengthening exercises (see Chapter 5) should be progressed, based on the patient's symptom response. If joint movement is contraindicated, isometric exercises should be considered. Concentric and eccentric muscle actions should be predicated on the appropriateness of joint movement. Adjacent or synergistic motion segments should also be exercised to reduce atrophic changes from reduced activity.

Remaining functional limitations, such as gait impairments (see Chapter 32) and reduced hand function, should be addressed during this phase. Activities intended to enhance position-sense (proprioception), balance (see Chapter 13), neuromuscular control, and cardiovascular fitness (see Chapter 23) should be instituted as early in the process as possible.[65] Any lingering motion deficits should be addressed with stretching and/or mobilization.

Objective and subjective criteria should be used to determine when a patient is ready to progress to the advanced strengthening and return to activity phase. Criteria recommended by other authors include pain, swelling, surgical repair stability, joint motion, muscle strength, and functional test results, but there are no published studies on the validity of these criteria.[66,67] Based on clinical experience, it is recommend that the following criteria be satisfied (at a minimum) before advancing a patient to the advanced strengthening and return to activity phase: A stable surgical repair; no pain during activity; minimal, transient postexercise pain; no swelling; joint AROM and PROM within normal limits (or comparable to the contralateral side); and bilateral deficits less than 25% with manual muscle testing (MMT), isokinetic testing, and functional testing. The reader is referred to works by Brotzman and Wilk,[67] Maxey and Magnusson,[66] and Manske[68] as excellent examples of criterion-based postoperative rehabilitation programs.

ADVANCED STRENGTHENING AND RETURN TO ACTIVITY PHASE

During the last phase of rehabilitation, the patient should be advanced to their maximum functional potential.

Goals during the advanced strengthening and return to activity phase include restoration of full ROM, strength, endurance, and proprioception and maximization of functional ability. During this phase, more strenuous and stressful exercises are introduced. Jumping, hopping, and running may be introduced for patients recovering from lower extremity surgery, and diagonal patterns that mimic overhand sports may be initiated for patients recovering from upper extremity surgery. High-intensity sport- or work-specific activities should be introduced to prepare the patient for return to activity. To reduce the risk of reinjury, resistance exercise intensity should ultimately be consistent with the intensity of the patient's work, sport, or activities of daily living (ADLs).

Ideally, at the end of this phase, the patient will return to work, sports activities, and ADLs without functional limitations. Some patients, however, do not regain full functional ability after soft tissue surgery and rehabilitation. Despite this, every attempt must be made to maximize their functional ability.

The next section includes common surgical procedures performed on soft tissue and unique rehabilitation considerations for each. Table 11-2 provides information about unique signs and symptoms for each surgical procedure.

TABLE 11-2	Considerations After Surgery to Different Types of Soft Tissue
Tissue	**Considerations**
Bursal	Infection
	Symptom limited
	Complex regional pain syndrome
Cartilage	Immobilization time frames
	Joint hypomobility following immobilization
	ROM limitations
	Excessive swelling
	Inability to bear weight secondary to pain
	Painful "grinding," "catching," or "popping"
	Complex regional pain syndrome
Fascial	Immobilization time frames
	Complex regional pain syndrome
Ligament	Immobilization time frames
	Joint hypomobility following immobilizations
	Active ROM limitations
	Passive ROM limitations
	Muscle flexibility limitations
	Feeling or sensation of "instability"
	Contracture
	Inadequate soft tissue mobility
	Complex regional pain syndrome
Tendon	Immobilization time frames
	Joint hypomobility following immobilizations
	Active ROM limitations
	Passive ROM limitations
	Muscle flexibility limitations
	Inadequate tendon resiliency
	Contractures
	Inadequate soft tissue mobility
	Complex regional pain syndrome

ROM, Range of motion.

SOFT TISSUE–SPECIFIC POSTOPERATIVE REHABILITATION

Bursae or Synovium. Surgery to bursae and synovium is generally performed when these structures are pathologically inflamed or hypertrophied. Surgical procedures include incision and drainage of inflamed bursae (also known as decompression), and excision of chronically infected and thickened bursae or synovium (also known as bursectomy and synovectomy, respectively).

Examination. Assessment of joint mobility and strength should be limited by symptoms in the surgical region. Bursae are compressed against bone by tendons, so activities that increase pressure of the tendon against the bone, such as MMTs, may still provoke pain after a bursal decompression (see Table 11-2).

Prognosis. Several studies report that outcomes after bursal decompression or bursectomy are favorable,[69-72] which is probably a result of these procedures directly addressing the symptomatic tissues. Fox reported that 85% of patients had increased functional ability and less pain 1 year after arthroscopic trochanteric bursectomy.[70] Ogilvie-Harris and Gilbart reported that 86% of patients were pain-free after olecranon bursectomy.[71] In the same study, the authors reported that 66% of patients were pain-free after prepatellar bursectomy, whereas 24% had some residual tenderness and 10% had pain on kneeling.

Intervention. Postoperatively, the affected region is generally immobilized with a splint for comfort. Typically no muscles are cut for bursal procedures so the rehabilitation can progress on a symptom-limited basis.

Cartilage Surgery. Cartilage may be treated surgically to promote repair of damage and to stimulate new cartilage growth. The procedures performed on articular cartilage include lavage (washing out of the joint to remove loose cartilage fragments and degradative enzymes), autologous osteochondral cylinder transplantation, autologous chondrocyte implantation, and various chondro-stimulating techniques.[73] Autologous osteochondral cylinder transplantation involves harvesting one or more osteochondral "plugs" from a healthy donor site and transplanting them into the region of articular cartilage degeneration. Autologous chondrocyte implantation involves obtaining a few healthy chondrocytes from the patient and then growing the cells on a culture medium to increase their number. These cells are then implanted into a region of cartilage damage in the same patient.[74] Chondro-stimulating techniques include drilling, abrasion, and microfracture. All of these are intended to stimulate mesenchymal cells in the subchondral bone to produce new cartilage.[73] Unfortunately, the mesenchymal cells synthesize primarily fibrocartilage rather than hyaline cartilage, and fibrocartilage does not distribute forces as well as the hyaline cartilage it is replacing.[75,76] It is also prone to fibrillation and breakdown over time.[77] Although not yet used clinically, some studies suggest that placing growth factors in an area of cartilage damage may also help promote repair.[78,79]

The procedures performed to repair fibrocartilage damage include debridement (removal of damaged portion of fibrocartilage), removal of the entire fibrocarti-

lage (e.g., knee meniscectomy), repair with sutures or bioabsorbable tacks, and fibrocartilage replacement or transplant (e.g., knee meniscal allograft transplantation).

Examination. After cartilage surgery, weight-bearing restrictions are commonly imposed. The therapist should ensure that the patient adheres to these restrictions. A standard floor scale can be used to determine the amount of weight being borne on the surgical leg (see Table 11-2).

Prognosis. Favorable long-term outcomes have been reported after autologous osteochondral cylinder transplantation for the treatment of small- and medium-sized focal chondral and osteochondral defects at the knee[80] and talus,[81,82] as well as after osteochondral allograft implantations to repair articular defects in the distal femur.[83] Two prospective, randomized clinical trials (RCTs) showed better clinical outcomes with autologous osteochondral cylinder transplantation than with autologous chondrocyte implantation for the repair of articular defects in the distal femur.[84,85]

Outcomes after arthroscopic repair of traumatic triangular fibrocartilage complex injury at the wrist have been reported to be favorable, with good or excellent results in most cases.[86,87] Outcomes after labral injuries at the hip depend on the stage and extent of the labral and chondral lesion[88] but appear to be favorable in many cases.[89] Glenoid labral injuries at the shoulder also appear to respond favorably to surgical fixation[90] or debridement in most cases.[91]

Regarding knee meniscal surgeries, short-term recovery and overall functional outcome are better after a partial meniscectomy than after a total meniscectomy.[92,93] However, long-term outcomes appear to be determined largely by the type of meniscal tear.[94] Outcomes after posterior horn tears appear less favorable than bucket-handle or anterior horn tears[95] (Fig. 11-3). When meniscal allografts are used, patients who receive deep-frozen meniscal transplants have less pain and swelling and can squat and climb stairs more easily than those who receive lyophilized (i.e., freeze-dried) transplants.[96]

Intervention. Aquatic therapy and/or unloading devices may be used to allow walking with reduced weight bearing. The transition from full weight bearing to impact loading should be made gradually. For instance, an elliptical exerciser can be employed for weight-bearing exercise without impact loading before transitioning to treadmill walking or jogging. Deficits in muscle performance should be addressed, but the impact of joint compression or shear must be considered when prescribing specific exercises.

Fascial Surgery. Surgery to fascial tissue is generally performed to relieve tension or pressure, to increase joint movement or to reduce fascial compartment pressure. Orthopedic surgeries involving fascia consist primarily of fasciotomies, also known as fascial releases. *Retinaculum*—essentially thick fascia—can also be released if necessary (e.g., lateral patellar retinacular release, carpal tunnel retinacular release). After a fascial or retinacular release, new fascia develops in the space formed by the incision, resulting in physiological lengthening of the fascia.[97]

Examination. When a fascial or retinacular release is performed to increase joint ROM, joint mobility must be

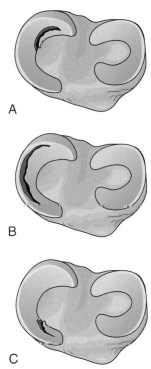

FIG. 11-3 Common meniscal tear patterns. **A,** Posterior horn tear. **B,** Bucket-handle tear. **C,** Anterior horn tear.

assessed regularly. Otherwise the examination may proceed as described in the general examination section.

Prognosis. Outcomes after fasciotomies for chronic exertional compartment syndrome of the lower leg(s) appear to be favorable in most cases. Howard and colleagues reported that 81% of patients with anterior/lateral compartment fasciotomy and 50% of patients with deep posterior compartment fasciotomy had clinically significant improvement.[98] In this same study, 79% of patients were satisfied with the outcome of the operation, but 22% of patients reported lower activity levels than before the operation. Additionally, 6% of patients continued to have exercise-induced pain and required revision surgery. In a similar investigation, Verleisdonk et al found that 87% of patients with chronic exercise-induced compartment syndrome in the anterior compartment of the leg experienced marked symptom reduction.[99]

In a study of outcomes after a lateral retinacular release for patellofemoral pain, Aderinto and Cobb found that 80% of patients experienced pain reduction, 16% were unchanged, and 4% were worse.[100] At follow-up (mean 31 months; range 12-65 months), 33% of patients were very satisfied, 26% satisfied, and 41% dissatisfied with their knee. Dzioba found that 85% of the patients with good-to-excellent outcome ratings at a 2-year follow-up also had good-to-excellent outcome ratings at 4 years.[101] In a similar investigation by Jackson et al, 56% of patients experienced good or excellent outcomes at 6 years, whereas 20% of patients did not receive any benefit from the procedure.[102]

Intervention. When a fascial or retinacular release is performed to increase joint ROM, interventions that pre-serve or improve mobility, such as joint-specific mobilizations and AAROM or PROM exercises, should be used. When a fascial release is performed to relieve tissue tension or pressure, the therapist should avoid untoward tissue tension or pressure throughout the rehabilitation process.

Ligament and Capsular Surgery. Orthopedic surgeries on ligamentous tissues are generally performed to repair ligament ruptures or partial ruptures and include primary repairs and reconstructions using autogenous (the patient's own) or allogenous (from a donor) tissue. Capsular surgeries are generally performed to repair torn or attenuated capsular restraints and include capsular reconstructions and capsular shortening procedures. Several synonyms have been used to describe capsular shortening procedures, including imbrication,[103] capsulorrhaphy,[104] and reefing.[105]

Intracapsular ligamentous reconstructions (i.e., grafts) undergo a process of remodeling commonly known as *ligamentization*.[106-108] The newly transplanted ligament goes through four distinct phases: (1) avascularity and necrosis, (2) revascularization, (3) cellular repopulation, and (4) structural remodeling.[108] Immediately after transplantation the graft undergoes necrosis because of its loss of blood supply. During this phase the collagen becomes disorganized and ultimately breaks down. The tensile strength of the reconstructed tissue quickly drops well below that of the original graft.[107] Extraarticular ligaments and capsular tissue heal more readily than intraarticular structures and typically do not lose much strength initially because they have more vascular perfusion. Thus the extraarticular MCL heals more quickly and readily than the intraarticular anterior cruciate ligament (ACL), but in both cases, the stresses applied during rehabilitation must be systematically controlled to avoid damaging the repair.

Examination. Because surgically repaired ligament and capsule can be easily overstressed early in the postoperative period, forceful testing of ROM should be avoided during this period, particularly in the direction that would stretch the repaired tissue.

After intraarticular ACL reconstruction, a ligament arthrometer can be used to assess the integrity of the repair. The KT-1000 (MEDmetric Corporation, San Diego, Calif), a ligament arthrometer (see Fig. 11-6), has been shown to objectively and quantitatively measure the amount of anterior translation of the tibia on the femur.[109-111]

Prognosis. Outcomes after capsular and ligamentous repairs are usually good. Because of the extensive use of ligament repairs and reconstructions throughout the body, the number of studies describing outcomes is extensive. Furthermore, many different procedures are used at each of the various locations of ligament repair. For example, numerous studies have found that patients have good functional outcomes when measured shortly after or even up to 10 years after ACL repair or reconstruction.[115-121] In general, with modern surgical and rehabilitation techniques, most patients can return to full participation in sports or other strenuous activities, after ligament reconstruction.[122]

Intervention. During the immediate postoperative period, soft tissue healing restrictions will also limit interventions. In most cases, protected ROM rather than complete immobilization is recommended to minimize capsular or ligamentous tissue stress. The exact restrictions vary, depending on the specific requirements of the repair, the stresses expected on full return to activity, the tissue quality, the type of tissue used for the repair (autograft, allograft, or synthetic), and the referring physician's beliefs regarding soft tissue healing time frames. For example, immediately after thermal capsulorrhaphy of the shoulder performed to treat shoulder instability, patients should not fully abduct or externally rotate their arm to avoid overstretching the healing tissue and making the shoulder unstable again. Similarly, after the classic Bankart repair of the anterior glenoid labrum and capsule of the shoulder, forceful full ROM should be avoided as this would jeopardize the surgical repair and fixation. In some instances however, obtaining full ROM is an early goal, most notably for knee extension after ACL reconstruction or repair.

Because ligaments and joint capsules not only constrain and guide joint movement but also provide proprioceptive or joint position sense via mechanoreceptors embedded within the ligament or capsule,[112] surgical repair or reconstruction may quickly restore joint integrity, but joint proprioception may remain impaired unless specifically addressed in the rehabilitation program.[113,114]

Tendon Surgery. Tendon surgeries are generally performed when there are partial tears or ruptures of tendons. Tendon surgeries include tenodesis, tendon transplants, tendon primary repair, tenotomy, and tendon debridement. Although the terms tendon transplant, primary repair, and debridement are self-explanatory, the terms tenodesis and tenotomy are less clear. Tenodesis is any surgical fixation of a tendon. Tenodesis is commonly performed with the tendon of the long head of the biceps, and during this procedure the long head may be moved to a new location to help restore its functional use. Tenotomy means surgical removal of a portion of a tendon.

Examination. After surgery to a tendon, stress on the tissue should be limited during both the examination and interventions. As with ligaments and capsules, forceful examination of PROM should be avoided. In addition, strength testing of the muscle(s) attached to the involved tendon should not be performed initially as contraction of the muscle will stress the tendon and may cause it to rupture. For example, performing full active finger flexion immediately after repair of the flexor tendons may cause the tendon to rupture.

The duration and degree of force restriction depends on the specific requirements of the repaired tendon, the stresses it is expected to tolerate for full return to activity, the tissue quality, the repair tissue type (autograft, allograft or synthetic), and the physician's beliefs regarding soft tissue healing time frames. During the immediate postoperative period, the patient should strictly adhere to soft tissue healing restrictions to optimize soft tissue healing and functional outcomes.

Prognosis. There is extensive literature concerning patient outcomes after tendon repair. A thorough review of this literature is beyond the scope of this chapter; however, a few examples follow. Many authors report that surgical reconstruction of tendons, such as the Achilles tendon, have favorable outcomes, including increased strength and function and decreased risk of rerupture.[61,63,64,123] The flexor tendons of the hands are also frequently surgically repaired or reconstructed and the outcome of these procedures varies, depending on numerous factors, including the patient's age, health, lifestyle, as well as associated damage to skin, vascular system, nerves, and skeletal structures.[124-127]

Intervention. As with the other soft tissue injuries previously described, surgical procedures to tendons generally require a brief period of immobilization to allow for tissue to form in and around the area of the repair. The duration of immobilization depends on a range of factors, including the health and age of the patient, the type of repair, which tendon was repaired, the quality of repaired tissue, and the surgeon's beliefs regarding healing times for the various tissues. For example, after flexor tendon repairs, recommendations regarding early activity vary. Some favor immobilization,[128] others favor early passive mobilization,[129,130] and yet others favor early active mobilization.[131-134]

After a lower extremity tendon rupture and repair, a brace or immobilizer is generally recommended to limit forces from weight bearing and to limit ROM during ambulation. After an upper extremity tendon rupture and repair, a splint or sling may also be needed to limit or prevent active contraction of the ruptured tendon. The duration of immobilization a surgeon recommends is likely to vary among patients and is generally influenced not only by which tendon is repaired but also by the size of repair, the quality of the tendon, the location of the tear (muscle, tendon, or muscle-tendon junction), the type of fixation (suture, staple, anchor), the presence of other concomitant injuries, and the age and general health of the patient.

A wide variety of immobilization protocols after Achilles tendon repair are described in the literature.[135-140] These include casting for 4 to 9 weeks, possibly using a heel lift after the cast is removed and restricting weight bearing from weight bearing as tolerated to no weight bearing during the period of cast immobilization. Since there is a risk of poor outcome when restrictions are not followed, the clinician involved in patient rehabilitation should obtain patient-specific guidelines from the referring physician regarding the nature and duration of restrictions after any tendon repair.

CASE STUDY 11-1

REHABILITATION AFTER ANTERIOR CRUCIATE LIGAMENT REPAIR (SEMITENDINOSUS-GRACILIS)

Examination
Patient History
CM is a 28-year-old man working full time in the United States Armed Forces. He ruptured the ACL of his right knee

while playing football 4 months before surgery. CM is a muscular man and previously won several bodybuilding contests. CM underwent an arthroscopically assisted semi-tendinosus-gracilis hamstring ACL reconstruction (ACLR) and a partial medial meniscectomy and was seen by the therapist 3 days after this surgery. He was then placed in a motion–controlled, double-hinged knee brace locked in full extension for ambulation. He was ambulating weight bearing as tolerated, per the physician's orders.

Systems Review

There was visible edema and erythema at the right knee.

Tests and Measures

Musculoskeletal

Anthropometric Characteristics Girth measurements were as follows:

Knee	Right	Left
20 cm proximal to the knee joint line	56 cm	54 cm
10 cm proximal to the knee joint line	45 cm	43 cm
Knee joint line	39 cm	37 cm
15 cm distal to the knee joint line	41 cm	40 cm

Passive Range of Motion Right knee: 3-50 degrees of knee flexion. Left knee: 5-0-135 degrees.

Muscle Performance CM had 5/5 strength by MMT of all tested lower extremity muscles on the right. Knee flexion and extension strength were not tested to their limits initially to avoid excessive stress on the reconstructed ligament and on the gracilis and semitendinosus tendons. CM was noted to have an extensor lag (he was not able to actively extend his knee to its full passive range of motion) during active straight leg raising.

Neuromuscular

Sensory Integrity Light touch sensation was slightly diminished in the area around the tibial incision but was normal on the remainder of the right lower extremity. Proprioception at the knee, as reflected by balance, was not tested during the initial examination because at this time balance would likely be impaired by many other factors, including reduced weight bearing and altered muscle firing patterns that result from intraarticular effusion.

Integumentary

Integumentary Integrity The incision at the medial tibia was clean without signs of infection, although the skin was slightly warmer in and around the right knee than in other areas.

Function

Gait CM was able to ambulate with bilateral axillary crutches on a level surface with a step-to gait. Following instructions to weight bear as tolerated, he was measured to place approximately 50% of his body weight on his right lower extremity without increasing his symptoms.

Evaluation, Diagnosis, and Prognosis

CM's impairments included pain, swelling, decreased ROM, and decreased muscular strength. These impairments were the likely cause of his inability to ambulate on level surfaces with a normal gait pattern, his inability to ambulate up and down stairs or steps with a normal gait

pattern, and his inability to return to normal leisure and recreational activities. CM falls into the preferred practice pattern 4I: Impaired joint mobility, motor function, muscle performance, and ROM associated with bony or soft tissue surgery.

Goals

1. Return of a normal gait pattern within 2 weeks
2. Full knee ROM in 4 weeks
3. Return to straight line jogging in 12 weeks

Prognosis

Excellent; achievement of goals is expected.

Plan of Care

Directed at alleviating impairments and allowing full return of normal ADLs and recreational activities without symptoms of knee instability. See Box 11-2 for a thorough review of postoperative goals for ACL reconstruction.

Intervention

CM was initially seen in therapy 3 times a week for 3 weeks, followed by 2 times a week until the ninth week, at which time he was decreased to 1 visit per week. Immediate therapy consisted of modalities for pain relief and edema control. Electrical stimulation with elevation and cold therapy were used, and CM was instructed to use compressive hose or a compressive wrap at all times when not in therapy. Additionally, attainment of full passive extension was stressed since he was not able to get his knee fully extended at this time. Prone hangs and sitting with foot and ankle over a bolster were initial components of his home exercise program. This was to be performed hourly to obtain full knee extension as soon as possible (Figs. 11-4 and 11-5). Weight bearing as tolerated was allowed until a normal heel-toe gait cycle could be performed without compensations.

Initial exercises consisted of quadriceps sets, straight leg raises, and heel slides to increase motor activation of the quadriceps and hamstring muscles and to disperse synovial fluid within the joint, allowing soft tissue movement and motion and decreasing the risk of problematic scar tissue and adhesions. Because the hamstrings were used as an autograft reconstruction source, hamstring stretching was delayed for 4 weeks, and hamstring resistance exercises were delayed for 6 weeks to reduce the risk of developing tendinopathy of the remaining hamstring tendons.

By the end of the first week of therapy, CM's knee extension had returned to 3 degrees, but his passive knee flexion was still limited to 70 degrees. To address the restriction of knee flexion ROM, manually-assisted quadriceps muscle-stretching, aggressive patellar inferior glide mobilization, and posterior tibial glide mobilization were added. Within 1-2 weeks of initiating this more aggressive approach, CM's knee flexion increased to 115 degrees.

By 4 weeks after surgery, CM's quadriceps strength had improved so that he could perform a straight leg raise without an extensor lag. His knee flexion ROM was 125 degrees passively. At this time, exercises were advanced to stationary cycling for a warm-up period of up to 10

BOX 11-2   Anterior Cruciate Ligament Repair Rehabilitation Protocol

General Guidelines
- Assume 8 weeks for complete graft revascularization
- Rarely use CPM
- Isolated hamstring strengthening began 6 weeks postoperatively
- Supervised physical therapy takes 3-9 months

Activities of Daily Living Progression
- Bathing/showering without brace after suture removal
- Sleep with brace locked in extension for 1 week
- Driving: Wait 1 week for automatic vehicles with left leg repair
- Wait 4-6 weeks for standard vehicles or right leg repair
- Brace locked in extension for 1 week for ambulation
- Crutches and brace for ambulation as needed for 6 weeks
- Weight bearing as tolerated immediately postoperative

Phase I: Immediate Postoperative Phase (Postoperative through 6 Weeks)
Goals
- Protect graft fixation (8 weeks)
- Minimize the effects of immobilization
- Control inflammation and swelling
- Immediate full knee passive extension
- Quadriceps activation
- Patient education

Restrictions
- Weight bearing as tolerated with axillary crutches as needed for 6 weeks
- Hamstring mobilization and stretching in 4 weeks

Brace
0-1 week: Locked in full extension for weight bearing and sleeping

1-6 weeks: Unlocked for ambulation, remove for sleeping

Therapeutic Exercises
- Gentle heel slides
- Quadriceps setting
- Patellar mobilization
- Non–weight-bearing gastrocnemius and soleus stretching
- SLR in all planes (SLR times 4) with brace locked in full extension until quadriceps prevent extensor lag
- Quadriceps isometrics at 60 and 90 degrees
- Gluteal setting
- Weight shifting
- Static balance exercises
- Heel raises—bilateral progressing to unilateral

Clinical Milestones
- Full knee extension
- SLR without extensor lag
- No limp or pain during gait
- 90 degrees of knee flexion
- No signs of active inflammation
- No increased effusion or edema
- No increased pain

Phase II: Intermediate Phase (6-8 Weeks)
Goals
- Restore normal gait
- Maintain full knee extension
- Progress flexion ROM

- Protect graft
- Initiate *open kinetic-chain* hamstring exercises

Comments
Discontinue use of the brace and crutches, as allowed by the physician, when the patient has full extension and can perform SLR without extensor lag.

Therapeutic Exercise
- Wall slides 0-45 degrees, progressing to mini-squat
- Multi-Hip (4-way) machine)
- Stationary bicycling (high seat, low tension promoting ROM)
- Closed-chain terminal extension with resistive tubing or weight machine
- Heel raises
- Balance exercises (e.g., single leg balance)
- Hamstring curls
- Aquatic therapy with emphasis on normalization of gait
- Continue hamstring stretches, progress to weight-bearing gastrocnemius and soleus stretches

Clinical Milestones
- Maximize ROM
- Good quadriceps recruitment
- Maintenance of full passive knee extension

Advanced Strengthening Phase III (8 Weeks-6 Months)
Goals
- Full ROM
- Improve strength, endurance, and proprioception of lower extremity to prepare for full functional activities
- Avoid overstressing graft or graft fixation
- Protect patellofemoral joint

Therapeutic Exercise
- Continue flexibility exercises as appropriate
- StairMaster: Begin short steps, avoid knee hyperextension
- NordicTrack knee extension: 90-45 degrees of knee flexion
- Advanced closed kinetic-chain strengthening (single leg squats, leg press 0-45 degrees, step-ups begin at 2 inches progressing to 8 inches)
- Progress proprioceptive activities (slide board, use of ball, racquet with balance activities, and so on)
- Progress aquatic program to include pool running, swimming (no breast stroke)

Criteria for Advancement
- Full pain-free ROM
- No evidence of patellofemoral joint irritation
- Strength and proprioception approximately 70% of uninvolved leg
- Physician clearance to initiate advanced *closed kinetic-chain* exercises and functional progression

Return to Activity: Phase IV (9 Months+)
Goals
- Safe return to athletics
- Maintenance program for strength and endurance

Comments
Physician may recommend a functional brace for use during sports for the first 1-2 years after surgery.

Modified from Manske RC, Prohaska D, Livermore R: Anterior cruciate ligament reconstruction using the hamstring/gracilis tendon autograft. In Manske RC (ed): *Postsurgical Orthopedic Sports Medicine: Knee and Shoulder,* Philadelphia, 2005, Elsevier Science.
CPM, continuous passive motion; *SLR,* straight leg raises; *ROM,* range of motion.

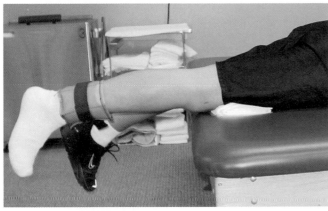

FIG. 11-4 Prone hang exercise used to increase passive knee extension. Patient lies prone with their leg off the mat. A cuff weight can be placed at the ankle to apply additional force.

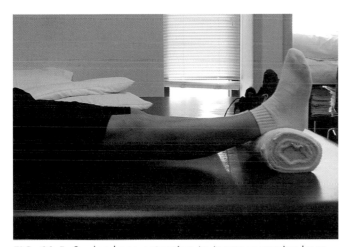

FIG. 11-5 Supine knee extension to increase passive knee extension.

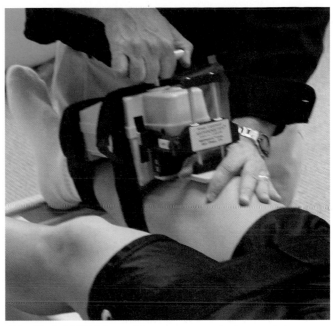

FIG. 11-6 KT-1000 used to measure anterior cruciate ligament tightness/laxity.

minutes, leg press motions with just the right leg and with both legs, bilateral heel raises, closed-kinetic chain terminal knee extensions, and static balance exercises. Gentle hamstring stretching exercises were also begun.

At 8 weeks after the surgery, gentle hamstring strengthening was started, using light weights to perform isotonic contractions on a hamstring curl machine.

At 12 weeks, knee extension ROM has maintained at 3 degrees of hyperextension, and knee flexion has increased to normal at 135 degrees. KT-1000 measurements of ligament laxity (Fig. 11-6) revealed a side-to-side difference of 0.5 mm at 15 lb, 0.75 mm at 20 lb, 1.5 mm at 30 lb, and 1.5 mm with application of the maximum manual force. Isokinetic strength testing showed that the peak torque of the right quadriceps was 78% of that on the left and the peak torque of the hamstrings on the right was 70% of that on the left.

Because CM performed so well on his 3-month re-examination, he is now allowed to begin straight line jogging on level ground. In addition, functional activities will begin with gentle jumps followed by hops, large zigzag type motions, and figure-of-eights. This will progress to more aggressive sports-specific agility drills and plyometric exercises if indicated, but contact sports and full athletic activity will not be allowed until at least 6 months after surgery. ACL repair rehabilitation protocols can be found in Box 11-2.

Please see the CD that accompanies this book for case studies describing the examination, evaluation, and interventions for a patient undergoing rehabilitation after knee meniscal repair, and for a patient undergoing rehabilitation after Achilles tendon repair.

CHAPTER SUMMARY

This chapter provided a framework for rehabilitation following soft tissue surgery based on available scientific evidence and clinical empiricism. Several factors should be considered when designing postoperative rehabilitation programs including the biomechanics of healing and mature connective tissue, the effects of immobilization and remobilization on connective tissue, and the prognosis for a successful outcome after different orthopedic procedures. The case studies provide examples of how the concepts and evidence presented may be applied to specific patients.

ADDITIONAL RESOURCES

Books

Brotzman SB, Wilk K: *Clinical Orthopaedic Rehabilitation,* ed 2, Philadelphia, 2003, Mosby.
Lundon K: *Orthopedic Rehabilitation Science: Principles for Clinical Management of Nonmineralized Connective Tissue,* St. Louis, 2003, Butterworth-Heinemann.
Manske RC: *Postsurgical Orthopedic Sports Rehabilitation: Knee and Shoulder,* St. Louis, 2006, Mosby.
Maxey L, Magnusson J: *Rehabilitation for the Postsurgical Orthopedic Patient,* St. Louis, 2001, Mosby.

Web Sites

www.aaos.org: American Academy of Orthopedic Surgeons
www.aossm.org: American Orthopaedic Society for Sports Medicine
www.orthoteers.com: Largest Orthopaedic e-textbook on the Web
www.physsportsmed.com: *The Physician and Sportsmedicine* online
www.wheelessonline.com: *Wheeless Textbook of Orthopaedics*

GLOSSARY

Bursae: Type of nonmineralized connective tissues consisting of small pouches of synovial fluid; usually located at areas of high friction in the musculoskeletal system.

Capsules: Type of dense, irregular nonmineralized connective tissue that surrounds and supports joints.

Cartilage: Type of specialized nonmineralized connective tissue that supports and cushions the skeleton (e.g., articular cartilage and fibrocartilage).

Closed kinetic-chain exercises: Exercises in which the distal limb or body part is fixed. During this form of exercise, muscles and joints act in a predictable pattern or sequential order.

Collagen: The most abundant structural protein in the body and an integral component of connective tissue.

Connective tissue: One of the four types of tissue in the body from which all structures are derived; connective tissue supports, binds, or separates more specialized tissues and organs of the body.

Extracellular matrix: A component of connective tissue, consisting of ground substance and fibers produced by the connective tissue cells.

Fascia: Type of loose nonmineralized connective tissue that divides and binds muscles and organs in the body.

Ligaments: Type of dense, regular nonmineralized connective tissue that connects bone to bone or bone to cartilage and helps stabilize joints.

Ligamentization: The process of remodeling that an intraarticular graft undergoes. This process is broken into four distinct phases: (1) Avascularity and necrosis, (2) revascularization, (3) cellular repopulation, and (4) structural remodeling.

Open kinetic-chain exercises: Exercises in which the distal limb or body part is free to move without causing any appreciable motion at another joint. During this form of exercise, muscles and joints do not act in a predictable pattern or sequential order because the distal end is free to move on its own.

Proprioception: Position sense coming from skin, ligaments, tendons, muscles, and joint capsule, integrated to maintain joint stability.

Proteoglycan molecules: Biological molecules that consist of a protein core with glycosaminoglycan side chains; a major component of cartilage.

Retinaculum: Thickened fascia (see *Fascia*).

Synovium: Type of specialized nonmineralized connective tissue on the innermost portion of the capsule of synovial joints. Synovial cells secrete fluid that lubricates joint surfaces and nourishes articular cartilage.

Tendons: Type of dense, regular nonmineralized connective tissue that connects muscle to bone or other tissue.

Viscoelasticity: Behavior of structures in which the relationship between stress and strain depends on time. In connective tissues, low magnitude loads (stress) applied for longer durations will cause greater tissue deformation (strain) than transient, high magnitude loads.

References

1. Culav EM, Clark CH, Merrilees MJ: Connective tissues: matrix composition and its relevance to physical therapy, *Phys Ther* 79:308-319, 1999.
2. Akeson WH, Amiel D, Lee J, et al: Cartilage and Ligament: Physiology and Repair Processes. In Nicholas JA, Hershman EB (eds): *The Lower Extremity and Spine in Sports Medicine*, ed 2, St. Louis, 1995, Mosby.
3. Liu SH, Yang R-S, al-Shaikh R, et al: Collagen in tendon, ligament, and bone healing: a current review. *Clin Orthop* 318:265-278, 1995.
4. Ker RF: The design of soft collagenous load-bearing tissues, *J Exper Biol* 202:3315-3324, 1999.
5. Newman AP: Articular cartilage repair, *Am J Sports Med* 26(2):309-324, 1998.
6. Bader DL, Bouten C: Biomechanics of soft tissue. In Dvir Z (ed): *Clinical Biomechanics*, Philadelphia, 2000, Churchill Livingstone.
7. Houlbrooke K, Vause K, Merrilles MJ: Effects of movement and weightbearing on glycosaminoglycan content of sheep articular cartilage, *Aus J Physiotherapy* 36:88-91, 1990.
8. Vailas AC, Tipton CM, Matthes RD, et al: Physical activity and its influence on the repair process of medial collateral ligaments, *Connect Tissue Res* 9(1):25-31, 1981.
9. Noyes FR: Functional properties of knee ligaments and alterations induced by immobilization: A correlative biomechanical and histological study in primates, *Clin Orthop* 123:210-242, 1977.
10. Vailas AC, Zernicke RF, Grindeland RE, et al: Suspension effects on rat femur-medial collateral ligament-tibia unit, *Am J Physiol* 258(3 Pt 2):R724-728, 1990.
11. Woo SL, Gomez MA, Sites TJ, et al: The biomechanical and morphological changes in the medial collateral ligament of the rabbit after immobilization and remobilization, *J Bone Joint Surg Am* 69(8):1200-1211, 1987.
12. Amiel D, Woo SL, Harwood FL, et al: The effect of immobilization on collagen turnover in connective tissue: A biochemical-biomechanical correlation, *Acta Orthop Scand* 53(3):325-332, 1982.
13. Tipton CM, James SL, Mergner W, et al: Influence of exercise on strength of medial collateral ligaments of dogs, *Am J Physiol* 218(3):894-902, 1970.
14. Fronek J, Frank C, Amiel D, et al: The effects of intermittent passive movement (IPM) in the healing of medical collateral ligament (abst), *Proc Orthop Res Soc* 8:31, 1983.
15. Noyes FR, Torvik PJ, Hyde WB, et al: Biomechanics of ligament failure. II. An analysis of immobilization, exercise, and reconditioning effects in primates, *J Bone Joint Surg Am* 56(7):1406-1418, 1974.
16. Tipton CM, Vailas AC, Mathers RD: Experimental studies on the influences of physical activity on ligaments, tendons, and joints: A brief review, *Acta Med Scand Suppl* 771:157-168, 1986.
17. Buckwalter JA, Grodzinsky AJ: The effects of loading on healing bone, fibrous tissue and muscle: Clinical Implications, *J Am Acad Orthop Surg* 7:291-299, 1999.
18. Hildebrand KA, Frank CB: Scar formation and ligament healing, *Can J Surg* 41(6):425-430, 1998.
19. Forrest L: Current concepts in soft connective tissue wound healing, *Br J Surgery* 70:133-140, 1983.
20. Hayashi K: Biomechanical studies of the remodeling of knee joint tendons and ligaments, *J Biomech* 29(6):707-716, 1996.
21. Provenzano PP, Martinez DA, Grindeland RE, et al: Hindlimb unloading alters ligament healing, *J Appl Physiol* 94(1):314-324, 2003.
22. Shiiba M, Arnaud SB, Tanzawa H, et al: Regional alterations of type I collagen in rat tibia induced by skeletal unloading, *J Bone Miner Res* 17(9):1639-1645, 2002.
23. Williams IF, McCullagh KG, Silver IA: The distribution of types I and III collagen and fibronectin in the healing equine tendon, *Connect Tissue Res* 12(3-4):211-227, 1984.
24. Mason ML, Allen HS: The rate of healing of tendons: An experimental study of tensile strength, *Ann Surg* 113:424-459, 1941.
25. Burks RT, Friederichs MG, Fink B, et al: Treatment of postoperative anterior cruciate ligament infections with graft removal and early reimplantation, *Am J Sports Med* 31(3):414-418, 2003.
26. Soderberg GL, Ballantyne BT, Kestel LL: Reliability of lower extremity girth measurements after anterior cruciate ligament reconstruction, *Physiother Res Int* 1(1):7-16, 1996.
27. Beynnon BD, Fleming BC: Anterior cruciate ligament strain in-vivo: a review of previous work, *J Biomech* 31(6):519-525, 1998.
28. Lewek M, Rudolph K, Axe M, et al: The effect of insufficient quadriceps strength on gait after anterior cruciate ligament reconstruction, *Clin Biomech* 17(1):56-63, 2002.
29. Grossman MG, Ducey SA, Nadler SS, et al: Meralgia paresthetica: diagnosis and treatment, *J Am Acad Orthop Surg* 9(5):336-344, 2001.
30. Hunt TK, Hoph H, Hussain Z: Physiology of wound healing, *Adv Skin Wound Care* 13(2):6-11, 2000.
31. Torry MR, Decker MJ, Viola RW, et al: Intra-articular knee joint effusion induces quadriceps avoidance gait patterns, *Clin Biomech* 15(3):147-159, 2000.
32. Johnson LM, Randall MJ, Reddihough DS, et al: Development of a clinical assessment of quality of movement for unilateral upper-limb function, *Dev Med Child Neurol* 36(11):965-973, 1994.
33. American Physical Therapy Association: *Guide to Physical Therapist Practice*, Alexandria, Va, 1998, American Physical Therapy Association.
34. American Physical Therapy Association: Guide to physical therapist practice, *Phys Ther* 81:277-294, 2001.
35. McHugh MP, Tyler TF, Gleim GW, et al: Preoperative indicators of motion loss and weakness following anterior cruciate ligament reconstruction, *JOSPT* 27(6):407-411, 1998.

36. Shelbourne KD, Patel DV, Martini DJ: Classification and management of arthrofibrosis of the knee following anterior cruciate ligament reconstruction, *Am J Sports Med* 24(6):857-862, 1996.

37. De Andrade JR, Grant C, Dixon A: Joint distention and reflex muscle inhibition in the knee, *J Bone Joint Surg Am* 47A:312-322, 1965.

38. Spencer JD, Hayes KC, Alexander IJ: Knee joint effusion and quadriceps reflex inhibition in man, *Arch Phys Med Rehab* 65:279-283, 1981.

39. Stokes M, Young A: The contribution of reflex inhibition to arthrogenous muscle weakness, *Clin Sci* 67:7-14, 1984.

40. Benson TB, Copp EP: The effects of therapeutic forms of heat and cold on the pain threshold of the normal shoulder, *Rheumatol Rehabil* 13:101-104, 1974.

41. Hoving JL, Koes BW, de Vet HC, et al: Manual therapy, physical therapy, or continued care by a general practitioner for patients with neck pain. A randomized, controlled trial, *Ann Intern Med* 136(10):713-722, 2002.

42. O'Reilly SC, Muir KR, Doherty M. Effectiveness of home exercise on pain and disability from osteoarthritis of the knee: a randomised controlled trial, *Ann Rheum Dis* 58:15-19, 1999.

43. Van Baar ME, Assendelft WJ, Dekker J, et al: Effectiveness of exercise therapy in patients with osteoarthritis of the hip or knee. A systematic review of randomized clinical trials, *Arthritis Rheum* 42(7):1361-1369, 1999.

44. Chabal C, Fishbain A, Weaver M et al: Long term transcutaneous electrical nerve stimulation (TENS) use: Impact on medication utilization and physical therapy costs, *Clin J Pain* 14(1):66-73, 1988.

45. Clarke R, Hellon R, Lind A: Vascular reactions of the human forearm to cold, *Clin Sci* 17:165-179, 1958.

46. Bettany JA, Fish DR, Mendel FC: High-voltage pulsed direct current: effect on edema formation after hyperflexion injury, *Arch Phys Med Rehabil* 71(9):677-681, 1990.

47. Bettany JA, Fish DR, Mendel FC. Influence of high voltage pulsed direct current on edema formation following impact injury, *Phys Ther* 70(4):219-224, 1990.

48. Esclamado RM, Damiano GA, Cummings CW. Effect of local hypothermia on early wound repair, *Arch Otolaryngol Head Neck Surg* 116(7):803-808, 1990.

49. Kirsner RS, Eaglstein WH. The wound healing process, *Dermatol Clin* 11(4):629-640, 1993.

50. Chleboun GS, Howell JN, Baker HL, et al: Intermittent pneumatic compression effect on eccentric exercise-induced swelling, stiffness, and strength loss, *Arch Phys Med Rehabil* 76(8):744-749, 1995.

51. Xia ZD, Hu D, Wilson JM, et al: How echographic image analysis of venous oedema reveals the benefits of leg elevation, *J Wound Care* 13(4):125-128, 2004.

52. Partsch H, Winiger J, Lun B: Compression stockings reduce occupational leg swelling, *Dermatol Surg* 30(5):737-743, 2004.

53. Cook HA, Morales M, La Rosa EM, et al: Effects of electrical stimulation on lymphatic flow and limb volume in the rat, *Phys Ther* 74:1040-1046, 1994.

54. Hiatt WR: Contemporary treatment of venous lower limb ulcers, *Angiology* 43(10):852-855, 1992.

55. Nanbu PN, Wakabayashi T, Yamashita R, et al: Heat treatment enhances healing process of experimental pseudomonas corneal ulcer, *Ophthalmic Res* 36(4):218-225, 2004.

56. Greenberg RS: The effects of hot packs and exercise on local blood flow, *Phys Ther* 52(3):273-278, 1972.

57. Baker KG, Robertson VJ, Duck FA: A review of therapeutic ultrasound: biophysical effects, *Phys Ther* 81(7):1351-1358, 2001.

58. Ek AC, Gustavsson G, Lewis DH: The local skin blood flow in areas at risk for pressure sores treated with massage, *Scand J Rehabil Med* 17(2):81-86, 1985.

59. Rendell MS, Green SS, Catania A, et al: Post-exercise cutaneous hyperaemia resulting from local exercise of an extremity, *Clin Physiol* 17(3):213-224, 1997.

60. Currier DP, Petrilli CR, Threlkeld AJ: Effect of graded electrical stimulation on blood flow to healthy muscle, *Phys Ther* 66(6):937-943, 1986.

61. Assal M, Jung M, Stern R, et al: Limited open repair of Achilles tendon ruptures. A technique with a new instrument and findings of a prospective multicenter study, *J Bone Joint Surg Am* 84A(2):161-170, 2002.

62. Carter TR, Fowler PJ, Blokker C: Functional postoperative treatment of Achilles tendon repair, *Am J Sports Med* 20:459-462, 1992.

63. Cetti R, Christensen SE, Ejsted R, et al: Operative versus nonoperative treatment of Achilles tendon rupture. A prospective randomized study and review of the literature, *Am J Sports Med* 21(6):71-79, 1993.

64. Mandelbaum BR, Myerson MS, Foster R: Achilles tendon ruptures. A new method of repair, early range of motion, and functional rehabilitation, *Am J Sports Med* 23:392-395, 1995.

65. Liu-Ambrose T, Taunton JE, MacIntyre D, et al: The effects of proprioceptive or strength training on the neuromuscular function of the ACL reconstructed knee: A randomized clinical trial, *Scand J Med Sci Sports* 13(2):115-123, 2003.

66. Maxey L, Magnusson J: *Rehabilitation for the Postsurgical Orthopedic Patient*, St. Louis, 2001, Mosby.

67. Brotzman SB, Wilk K: *Clinical Orthopaedic Rehabilitation*, ed 2, Philadelphia, 2003, Mosby.

68. Manske RC: *Postsurgical Orthopedic Sports Rehabilitation: Knee and Shoulder*, St. Louis, 2006, Mosby.

69. Chen WS, Wang CJ: Recalcitrant bicipital radial bursitis, *Arch Orthop Trauma Surg* 119(1-2):105-108, 1999.

70. Fox JL: The role of arthroscopic bursectomy in the treatment of trochanteric bursitis, *Arthroscopy* 18(7):E34, 2002.

71. Ogilvie-Harris DJ, Gilbart M: Endoscopic bursal resection: the olecranon bursa and prepatellar bursa, *Arthroscopy* 16(3):249-253, 2000.

72. Wilson-MacDonald J: Management and outcome of infective prepatellar bursitis, *Postgrad Med J* 63(744):851-853, 1987.

73. Minas T, Nehrer S: Current concepts in the treatment of articular cartilage defects, *Orthopedics* 20(6):525-538, 1997.

74. Ronga M, Grassi FA, Bulgheroni P: Arthroscopic autologous chondrocyte implantation for the treatment of a chondral defect in the tibial plateau of the knee, *Arthroscopy* 20(1):79-84, 2004.

75. Chen FS, Frenkel SR, Di Cesare PE: Repair of articular cartilage defects: Part 2: Treatment options, *Am J Orthop* 28(2):88-96, 1999.

76. O'Driscoll SW: The healing and regeneration of articular cartilage, *J Bone Joint Surg Am* 80(12):1795-1812, 1998.

77. Newman AP: Articular cartilage repair, *Am J Sports Med* 26(2):309-324, 1998.

78. Tanaka H, Mizokami H, Shiigi E, et al: Effects of basic fibroblast growth factor on the repair of large osteochondral defects of articular cartilage in rabbits: dose-response effects and long-term outcomes, *Tissue Eng* 10(3-4):633-641, 2004.

79. Wakitani S, Imoto K, Kimura T, et al: Hepatocyte growth factor facilitates cartilage repair. Full thickness articular cartilage defect studied in rabbit knees, *Acta Orthop Scand* 68(5):474-480, 1997.

80. Hangody L, Fules P: Autologous osteochondral mosaicplasty for the treatment of full-thickness defects of weight-bearing joints: Ten years of experimental and clinical experience, *J Bone Joint Surg Am* 85A(suppl)2:25-32, 2003.

81. Assenmacher JA, Kelikian AS, Gottlob C, et al: Arthroscopically assisted autologous osteochondral transplantation for osteochondral lesions of the talar dome: An MRI and clinical follow-up study, *Foot Ankle Int* 22(7):544-551, 2001.

82. Hangody L, Kish G, Modis L, et al: Mosaicplasty for the treatment of osteochondritis dissecans of the talus: Two to seven year results in 36 patients, *Foot Ankle Int* 22(7):552-528, 2001.

83. Aubin PP, Cheah HK, Davis AM, et al: Long-term followup of fresh femoral osteochondral allografts for posttraumatic knee defects, *Clin Orthop* 391(suppl):S318-327, 2001.

84. Bentley G, Biant LC, Carrington RW, et al: A prospective, randomised comparison of autologous chondrocyte implantation versus mosaicplasty for osteochondral defects in the knee, *J Bone Joint Surg Br* 85(2):223-230, 2003.

85. Horas U, Pelinkovic D, Herr G, et al: Autologous chondrocyte implantation and osteochondral cylinder transplantation in cartilage repair of the knee joint. A prospective, comparative trial, *J Bone Joint Surg Am* 85A(2):185-192, 2003.

86. Miwa H, Hashizume H, Fujiwara K, et al: Arthroscopic surgery for traumatic triangular fibrocartilage complex injury, *J Orthop Sci* 9(4):354-359, 2004.

87. Shih JT, Lee HM, Tan CM: Early isolated triangular fibrocartilage complex tears: management by arthroscopic repair, *J Trauma* 53(5):922-927, 2002.

88. McCarthy JC: The diagnosis and treatment of labral and chondral injuries, *Instr Course Lect* 53:573-577, 2004.

89. O'Leary JA, Berend K, Vail TP: The relationship between diagnosis and outcome in arthroscopy of the hip, *Arthroscopy* 17(2):181-188, 2001.

90. O'Neill DB: Arthroscopic Bankart repair of anterior detachments of the glenoid labrum. A prospective study, *J Bone Joint Surg Am* 81(10):1357-1366, 1999.

91. Martin DR, Garth WP Jr: Results of arthroscopic debridement of glenoid labral tears, *Am J Sports Med* 23(4):447-451, 1995.

92. Andersson-Molina H, Karlsson H, et al: Arthroscopic partial and total meniscectomy: A long-term follow-up study with matched controls, *Arthroscopy* 18(2):183-189, 2002.

93. Howell JR, Handoll HH: Surgical treatment for meniscal injuries of the knee in adults, *Cochrane Database Syst Rev* 2:CD001353, 2000.

94. Englund M, Roos EM, Roos HP, et al: Patient-relevant outcomes fourteen years after meniscectomy: Influence of type of meniscal tear and size of resection, *Rheumatology* (Oxford) 40(6):631-639, 2001.

95. Hede A, Larsen E, Sandberg H: The long-term outcome of open total and partial meniscectomy related to the quantity and site of the meniscus removed, *Int Orthop* 16(2):122-125, 1992.

96. Wirth CJ, Peters G, Milachowski KA, et al: Long-term results of meniscal allograft transplantation, *Am J Sports Med* 30(2):174-181, 2002.

97. Larson RL, Cabaud HE, Slocum DB, et al: The patellar compression syndrome: surgical treatment by lateral retinacular release, *Clin Orthop* (134):158-167, 1978.

98. Howard JL, Mohtadi NG, Wiley JP: Evaluation of outcomes in patients following surgical treatment of chronic exertional compartment syndrome in the leg, *Clin J Sport Med* 10(3):176-184, 2000.

99. Verleisdonk EJ, Schmitz RF, van der Werken C: Long-term results of fasciotomy of the anterior compartment in patients with exercise-induced pain in the lower leg, *Int J Sports Med* 25(3):224-229, 2004.

100. Aderinto J, Cobb AG: Lateral release for patellofemoral arthritis, *Arthroscopy* 18(4):399-403, 2002.

101. Dzioba RB: Diagnostic arthroscopy and longitudinal open lateral release. A four year follow-up study to determine predictors of surgical outcome, *Am J Sports Med* 18(4):343-348, 1990.

102. Jackson RW, Kunkel SS, Taylor GJ: Lateral retinacular release for patellofemoral pain in the older patient, *Arthroscopy* 7(3):283-286, 1991.

103. Cole BJ, Mazzocca AD, Meneghini RM: Indirect arthroscopic rotator interval repair, *Arthroscopy* 19(6):E28-31, 2003.

104. Khan AM, Fanton GS: Electrothermal assisted shoulder capsulorraphy—monopolar, *Clin Sports Med* 21(4):599-618, 2002.

105. Ghanem I, Wattincourt L, Seringe R: Congenital dislocation of the patella. Part II: Orthopaedic management, *J Pediatr Orthop* 20(6):817-822, 2000.

106. Amiel D, Kleinert JB, Roux RD, et al: The phenomenon of "ligamentization:" Anterior cruciate ligament reconstruction with autogenous patellar tendon, *Orthop Res Soc* 4(2):162-172, 1986.

107. Arnoczky SP, Tarvin GB, Marshall JL: ACL replacement using patellar tendons. *J Bone Joint Surg Am* 64A:217-224, 1982.

108. Lane JG, McFadden K, Bowden K, et al: The ligamentization process: A 4 year case study following ACL reconstruction with a semitendinosus graft, *Arthroscopy* 9(2):149-153, 1993.

109. Anderson A, Lipscomb A: Preoperative instrumented testing of anterior and posterior knee laxity, *Am J Sports Med* 17:387-392, 1989.

110. Daniel DM: Assessing the limits of knee motion. *Am J Sports Med* 19:139-147, 1991.

111. Kowalk DL, Wojtys EM, Disher J, et al: Quantitative analysis of the measuring capabilities of the KT-1000 knee ligament arthrometer, *Am J Sports Med* 21:744-747, 1993.

112. Barrack RL, Skinner HB: The sensory function of knee ligaments. In Daniel D, Akeson WH, O'Connor DD, eds: *Knee Ligaments: Structure, Function, Injury, and Repair*, New York, 1990, Raven Press.

113. Fremerey R, Lobenhoffer P, Skutek M, et al: Proprioception in anterior cruciate ligament reconstruction. Endoscopic versus open two-tunnel technique. A prospective study, *Int J Sports Med* 22(2):144-148, 2001.

114. Reider B, Arcand MA, Diehl LH, et al: Proprioception of the knee before and after anterior cruciate ligament reconstruction, *Arthroscopy* 19(1):2-12, 2003.

115. Harter RA, Osternig LR, Singer KM, et al: Long-term evaluation of knee stability and function following surgical reconstruction for anterior cruciate ligament insufficiency, *Am J Sports Med* 16:434-443, 1988.

116. Johnson RJ, Eriksson E, Haggmark T, et al: Five- to ten-year follow-up evaluation after reconstruction of the anterior cruciate ligament, *Clin Orthop* 183:122-140, 1984.

117. Natri A, Jarvinen M, Latvala K, et al: Isokinetic muscle performance after anterior cruciate ligament surgery: Long-term results and outcome predicting factors after primary surgery and late-phase reconstruction, *Int J Sports Med* 17(3):223-228, 1996.

118. Otto D, Pinczewski LA, Clingeleffer A, et al: Five-year results of single-incision arthroscopic anterior cruciate ligament reconstruction with patellar tendon autograft, *Am J Sports Med* 26:181-188, 1998.

119. Shelbourne KD, Gray T: Anterior cruciate ligament reconstruction with autogenous patellar tendon graft followed by accelerated rehabilitation: A two- to nine-year follow-up, *Am J Sports Med* 25:786-795, 1997.

120. Williams RJ, Hyman J, Petrigliano F, et al: Anterior cruciate ligament reconstruction with a four-strand hamstring tendon autograft, *J Bone Joint Surg Am* 86A(2):225-232, 2004.

121. Risberg MA, Holm I, Tjomsland O, et al: Prospective study of changes in impairments and disabilities after anterior cruciate ligament reconstruction, *JOSPT* 29(7):400-412, 1999.

122. D'Amato MJ, Bach BR: Anterior cruciate ligament reconstruction in the adult. In DeLee JC, Drez D, Miller MD, eds: *DeLee and Drez's Orthopedic Sports Medicine: Principles and Practice,* ed 2, Philadelphia, 2003, WB Saunders.

123. Sodatis JJ, Goodfellow DB, Wilber JH: End-to-end operative repair of Achilles tendon rupture, *Am J Sports Med* 25:90-95, 1997.

124. Culp RW, Taras JS: Primary care of flexor tendon injuries. In Hunter JM, Mackin EJ, Callahan AD (eds): *Rehabilitation of the Hand: Surgery and Therapy,* vol 1, ed 4, St. Louis, 1995, Mosby.

125. Falkenstein N, Weiss-Lessard S: *Hand Rehabilitation: A Quick Reference Guide and Review,* St. Louis, 1999, Mosby.

126. Schneider LH: Flexor tendons: Late reconstruction. In Green DP, Hotchkiss RN, Pederson WC (eds): *Green's Operative Hand Surgery,* vol 2, ed 4, New York, 1999, Churchill Livingstone.

127. Stewart KM, van Strien G: Postoperative management of flexor tendon injuries. In Hunter JM, Mackin EJ, Callahan AD (eds): *Rehabilitation of the Hand: Surgery and Therapy,* vol 1, ed 4, St. Louis, 1995, Mosby.

128. Cifaldi D, Collins D, Swhwarze L: Early progressive resistance following immobilization of flexor tendon repairs, *J Hand Ther* 4:11-15, 1991.

129. Duran R, Houser R: Controlled passive motion following flexor tendon repair in zones 2 and 3. In *AAOS Symposium on Tendon Surgery in the Hand,* St. Louis, 1975, Mosby.

130. Kleinert HE, Kutz JE, Cohen MJ: Primary repair of zone 2 flexor tendon lacerations. In *AAOS Symposium on Tendon Surgery in the Hand,* St. Louis, 1975, Mosby.

131. Cullen K, Tolhurst P, Lang D, et al: Flexor tendon repair in zone 2 followed by controlled active mobilization, *J Hand Surg* 14B:392-395, 1989.

132. Allen BN, Frykman GK, Unsell RS, et al: Ruptured flexor tendon tenorrhaphies in zone II: repair and rehabilitation. *J Hand Surg* 12A:18-21, 1987.

133. Gratton P: Early active mobilization after flexor tendon repairs. J Hand Ther 6:285-289, 1993.

134. Small J, Brennan M, Colville J: Early active mobilization following flexor tendon repair in zone 2, *J Hand Surg* 14B:383-391, 1989.

135. Beskin JL, Sanders RA, Hunter SC, et al: Surgical repair of Achilles tendon ruptures, *Am J Sports Med* 15:1-8, 1987.

136. Crolla RM, Leeuwwn DM, Ramshortst B, et al: Acute rupture of the tendo calcaneus. Surgical repair with functional after treatment, *Acta Orthop Belg* 53:492-494, 1987.

137. Inglis AE, Scott WN, Sculco TP, et al: Ruptures of the tendo Achillis. An objective assessment of surgical and non-surgical treatment, *J Bone Joint Surg Am* 58A:990-993, 1976.

138. Kellam JF, Hunter GA, McElwain JP: Review of the operative treatment of Achilles tendon rupture, *Clin Orthop* 201:80-83, 1985.

139. Quigley TB, Scheller AD: Surgical repair of the ruptured Achilles tendon, *Am J Sports Med* 8:244-250, 1980.

140. Wills CA, Washburn S, Caiozzo V, et al: Achilles tendon rupture: A review of the literature comparing surgical versus nonsurgical treatment, *Clin Orthop* 207:156-163, 1986.

Chapter 12

Amputations and Prostheses

Joan E. Edelstein

CHAPTER OUTLINE

OBJECTIVES

After reading this chapter, the reader will be able to:
1. Identify the incidence, etiologies, and levels of upper and lower extremity amputation.
2. Perform a rehabilitation examination and evaluation of patients with amputation.
3. Develop preoperative and postsurgical interventions for the residual limb and the entire patient with an amputation.
4. Describe prosthetic options for patients with all levels of upper and lower extremity amputations.
5. Design a basic prosthetic training program for patients fitted with upper and lower extremity prostheses.
6. Compare the functional outcomes of patients according to etiology, amputation level, and prosthetic components.

Amputation is a specialty area in rehabilitation. In 1996, the rate of amputation in the United States was 52.4 per 100,000, with most being lower extremity amputations.[1] Most lower extremity amputations become necessary because of underlying vascular disease or diabetes, whereas most upper extremity amputations are needed because of trauma. A minority of amputations are needed because of malignancy or congenital limb anomalies. Many people with amputation are fitted with a prosthesis (a replacement for a body part). Regardless of site or design, a prosthesis does not substitute fully for the appearance or function of the anatomic extremity.

PATHOLOGY

Acquired amputation results from peripheral vascular disease, trauma, and more rarely, diseases such as osteogenic sarcoma, meningitis, and *Hansen's disease* (leprosy). Occasionally, a patient may elect amputation to eliminate a nonfunctional extremity. Another etiology is congenital extremity absence or malformation, evident at birth; sometimes the malformed extremity is revised surgically to facilitate prosthetic fitting and improve function.

Amputation surgery is classified as closed when the skin is sutured, or open when the skin is not sutured. *Open amputation* is much less common in civilian practice and is indicated when the operative site is contaminated. This procedure usually involves severing the muscle without suturing *(guillotine amputation)*. Traction is then applied to the open edges of the skin to retain its length so that, upon secondary closure, there will be enough skin for coverage. With a *closed amputation* the skin edges are stapled or sutured together and the underlying muscles may be sutured to one another *(myoplasty)* or sutured through holes drilled in the bone *(myodesis)*. The cut ends of bones are beveled to reduce the likelihood of sharp osteophytes which can be painful. Nerves are severed under tension so that they retract within muscle bellies rather than terminating near the skin. This reduces the risk of local pain.[2]

The most common etiology of amputation in the United States is peripheral vascular disease (PVD), particularly arteriosclerosis.[3] The typical patient with PVD is a man in his mid-sixties with a history of diabetes, coronary artery disease, hypertension, and smoking.[4,5] Diabetes increases the risk for amputation by causing both PVD and neuropathy. Thromboangiitis obliterans, a disease characterized by inflammation and occlusion of the small- and medium-sized arteries, and thrombophlebitis, inflammation of veins, often with clotting, are primary PVDs that increase the risk of amputation. In patients with PVD, amputation is generally the last resort, after the patient has endured years of treatment for intermittent claudication (cramping in the calf after a brief period of walking), recurrent skin ulcers, and edema. The precipitating event for amputation in patients with PVD is usually skin ulceration that fails to heal followed by osteomyelitis (infection of bone) and/or gangrene (see Chapter 29).

Trauma is also a common cause of amputation, particularly upper extremity amputation. Patients who sustain trauma requiring amputation usually also sustain injury to many other systems and areas, complicating their recovery, but are generally younger than other patients who undergo amputation.[6]

Very occasionally (less than 1/1,000 live births), an infant is born with one or more absent or abnormal extremities. This may be caused by intrauterine exposure to teratogens, such as thalidomide and x-rays, or by amniotic bands that constrict the distal portion of the developing extremity. Congenital limb deficiencies are more common in the lower than the upper extremity.[7] Limb anomalies are classified as transverse—where the distal portion is absent—or longitudinal—where the proximal portion is absent but the distal portion is present.[8] A transverse anomaly may be further subcategorized as partial or complete, with termination being through the diaphysis or through the joint (resembling a disarticulation), respectively. Since congenital anomalies occur in children, the family should be involved in all stages of habilitation, and habilitation should be structured to help the child reach developmental milestones.

Some malignancies that affect bone, such as Ewing's osteogenic sarcoma, are treated with amputation. Osteogenic sarcoma most commonly occurs at the distal end of the humerus or femur in adolescence or young adulthood. The patient may undergo shoulder or hip disarticulation, or *transpelvic* (hemipelvectomy), *transhumeral,* or *transfemoral amputation* as part of the treatment of this disease. These patients may also receive radiation or chemotherapy, or both. Radiation can effect rehabilitation because radiation can make the skin more fragile, whereas chemotherapy can reduce the patient's energy level. Radiation and chemotherapy may also reduce the patient's appetite, resulting in weight loss that can disturb socket fit.

Hansen's disease (leprosy) is caused by infection with *Mycobacterium leprae. M. leprae* infects sensory nerves, causing sensory loss. Sensory loss leads to ulceration from repeated trauma that is complicated by bony and soft tissue resorption. This resorption, known as autoamputation, may cause loss of the ends of the digits, portions of the nose, and other body parts.

Rarely, a viable body part is amputated when patients decide that their overall function would be better without it than with it. For example, a patient contracted poliomyelitis in infancy, which markedly interfered with the growth of his left leg. In adolescence he chose to have the leg amputated above the knee and wear a prosthesis rather than wearing a shoe with an 8- to 12-inch lift for the rest of his life. Similarly, there is a published report of several men with spinal cord injury who underwent bilateral hip disarticulation, after developing deep pressure ulcers, to allow them to transfer much more easily from bed to wheelchair.[9]

TYPES OF AMPUTATION

Amputations can be classified as minor, referring to amputations distal to the wrist or ankle, or major, referring to more proximal amputations.

Lower Extremity Amputations

Minor Lower Extremity Amputations. Partial foot amputation is removal of any portion of the foot (Fig. 12-1). The most common levels for this type of amputation are phalangeal, *transmetatarsal,* and midtarsal disarticulation (also known as Chopart's disarticulation). Ray resection refers to removal of a metatarsal and its phalanges.

The main concern with phalangeal amputation in patients with PVD is the possibility of further amputation. Transmetatarsal amputation shortens the foot considerably and with the loss of the metatarsal heads, compels the patient to bear substantial weight on the calcaneus. During gait, late stance is altered by the loss of metatarsophalangeal hyperextension, and during swing phase, the shortened foot can slip from the shoe.

Ray resection creates a foot that is abnormally narrow. This reduces the base of support in standing, and the absence of one or more metatarsal heads and their muscular attachments reduces the strength of plantar flexion during terminal stance. Loss of the first ray is particularly disabling because this part of the foot usually takes much of the load when walking on level and irregular surfaces.

The Chopart's disarticulation involves amputation between the talus and navicular on the medial side of the foot and between the calcaneus and the cuboid on the lateral side of the foot. With this procedure, the triceps surae are kept intact and the dorsiflexors are transected, causing the foot to assume a plantarflexed position, unless the Achilles tendon is sectioned or otherwise attenuated. Standing on a plantarflexed foot places stress on the amputation scar, produces a very small weight-bearing area, and severely compromises terminal stance.

Major Lower Extremity Amputations. A *Syme's amputation* involves transsection of the distal tibia and fibula through broad cancellous bone with preservation of the calcaneal fat pad (Fig. 12-2). All the foot bones are removed, and the skin overlying the calcaneal fat pad is sutured to the anterior portion of the distal shank. The

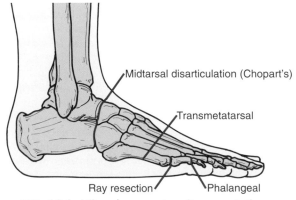

FIG. 12-1 Minor lower extremity amputations.

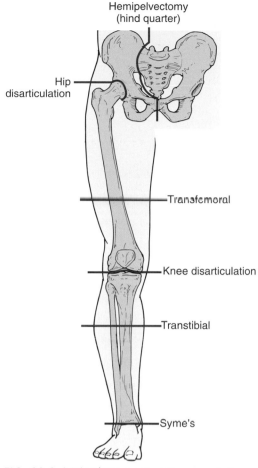

FIG. 12-2 Major lower extremity amputations.

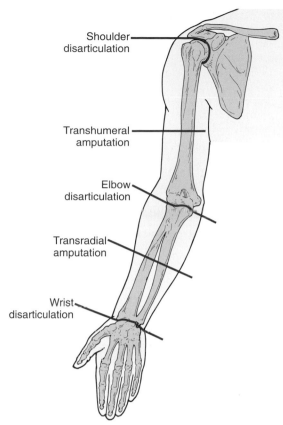

FIG. 12-3 Major upper extremity amputations.

residual limb tends to be bulbous distally. Although the amputated leg is slightly shorter than the sound extremity, the patient can move short distances without a prosthesis. Walking long distances requires a prosthesis to equalize leg length and provide foot function, thereby lessening the risk of back pain.

Other major lower extremity amputations are the following:

- Ankle disarticulation (separation of the foot at the ankle).
- Transtibial (amputation through the tibia and fibula), previously known as below-knee knee amputation (any of a group of amputations and separations in the vicinity of the anatomic knee joint).
- Transfemoral (amputation through the femur), previously known as above-knee amputation.
- Hip disarticulation (separation of the femur from the acetabulum).
- Transpelvic amputation (removal of any portion of the pelvis and all distal parts), previously known as hemipelvectomy.

Unlike distal amputations, which are usually necessary because of PVD, hip disarticulation and transpelvic amputation are most often required because of a malignancy in the bone or less commonly because of trauma or soft-tissue infection.[10]

- *Translumbar amputation* (removal of the entire pelvis and all distal), previously known as hemicorporectomy, requires creation of a urinary diversion, as well as a colostomy.

Upper Extremity Amputations

Minor Upper Extremity Amputations. Partial hand amputation or removal of any portion of the hand is a minor upper extremity amputation.

Major Upper Extremity Amputations. Major upper extremity amputations are classified as follows (Fig. 12-3):

- Wrist disarticulation (separation of the radius from the proximal carpals or separation between the proximal and distal row of carpals).
- *Transradial amputation* (through the radius and ulna), previously known as below-elbow.
- Elbow disarticulation (separation of the humerus from the ulna or amputation through the most distal portion of the humerus).
- Transhumeral amputation (through the humerus), previously known as above-elbow.
- Shoulder disarticulation (separation of the humerus from the scapula).
- Forequarter (removal of any portion of the thorax, together with any portion of the shoulder girdle and all distal parts).

Transradial and Transhumeral Amputations. Transradial and transhumeral amputations are classified according to the relative lengths of the residual limb and the sound extremity (Fig. 12-4).

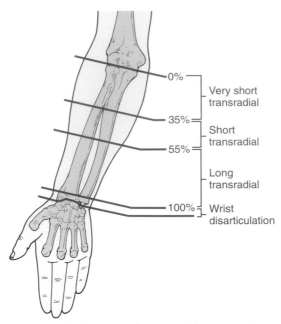

FIG. 12-4 Classification of transradial amputations.

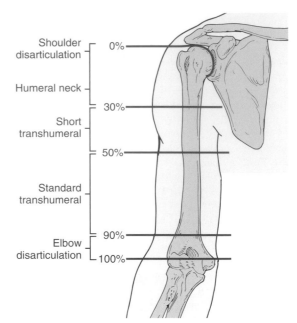

FIG. 12-5 Classification of transhumeral amputations.

For transradial amputations, the length of the sound side is measured from the medial humeral epicondyle to the ulnar styloid. On the amputated side the length is measured from the medial humeral epicondyle to the bony end of the residual limb. Classification is as follows:

Length of Amputated/ Length of Sound	Classification
100%	Wrist disarticulation
55%-100%	Long transradial
35%-55%	Short transradial
0%-35%	Very short transradial

For transhumeral amputations the length of the sound side is measured from the scapular acromion to the lateral humeral epicondyle (Fig. 12-5). On the amputated side the length is measured from the acromion to the bony end of the residual limb. Classification is as follows:

Length of Amputated/ Length of Sound	Classification
90%-100%	Elbow disarticulation
50%-90%	Standard transhumeral
30%-50%	Short transhumeral
0%-30%	Humeral neck
0%	Shoulder disarticulation

To classify an amputation in an adult with bilateral upper extremity amputation, expected sound extremity length can be estimated from the person's height, with the forearm being 14% of height and the upper arm being 19% of height. For example, on a 6-foot tall man, bilat-eral transradial amputations that are 5 inches long from the medial humeral epicondyle are approximately 50% of usual sound extremity length and would therefore be classified as short transradial amputations.

EXAMINATION

PATIENT HISTORY

A thorough patient history should be the first component of the examination. For the hospitalized patient, much of the history may be obtained through a review of the medical chart. In an outpatient setting the therapist can generally obtain information regarding the patient's age, sex, race, employment, arm and leg dominance, general health status, past medical history including surgery, and present functional status directly from the patient. Psychosocial issues related to educational level, cultural beliefs, caregiver resources, and living environment should also be discussed. Information regarding medications, laboratory or diagnostic tests, or other clinical findings should also be noted.

The patient's expectations of therapy should also be discussed. Patients' expectations can affect compliance with recommendations and satisfaction with treatment outcomes.

SYSTEMS REVIEW

The systems review is used to target areas requiring further examination and to define areas that may cause complications or indicate a need for precautions during the examination and intervention processes. See Chapter 1 for details of the systems review.

TESTS AND MEASURES
Musculoskeletal

Posture. All patients should have a postural assessment, with particular reference to pelvic alignment, scoliosis, and kyphosis (see Chapter 4). Severe postural abnormality compromises prosthetic fitting and the patient's function.

Anthropometric Characteristics. The length and the girth of the residual limb should be measured because these will affect the type of prosthesis and the snugness or looseness of the socket, respectively.

For the upper extremity, limb length should be measured relative to the landmarks described in the section on classification. For the lower extremity, there is no well-established system of classification, therefore limb length should be measured relative to bony anatomical landmarks such as the tibial tuberosity, head of the fibula, medial tibial plateau, greater trochanter, and the ischial tuberosity. When there is a unilateral residual limb, its length should also be compared to that of the intact, contralateral body segment. In the lower extremity the residual limb is usually described as being short (upper third), moderate (middle third), or long (lower third).

The girth of the residual limb should be measured at various distances from stable bony landmarks. Although there is no standard for landmark selection, convenient sites are the acromion and medial humeral epicondyle for transhumeral and transradial residual limbs, respectively, and the greater trochanter and medial tibial plateau for transfemoral and transtibial residual limbs. Girth should also be measured over time, and final prosthetic fitting should be delayed until edema has resolved and atrophy has peaked, so that limb volume is stable and fit will remain good.

Range of Motion. For the individual with a lower extremity amputation, range of motion (ROM) of all joints on both lower extremities and the hips should be measured. For those with upper extremity amputation, ROM should be measured at all joints of both upper extremities, as well as the shoulder. Joint ROM restrictions should be addressed early to avoid contractures from inactivity, faulty positioning, and muscle imbalance. For example, after a transtibial amputation, knee and hip flexion contractures, which can compromise dressing, transfers, and prosthetic use, are common. After a transfemoral amputation, hip flexion, abduction, and external rotation contractures are common because of muscle imbalances and persistent sitting. In patients with transradial amputations, forearm pronation and supination are often limited because of fibrosis of the interosseous membrane, and without the hand there is much less need to rotate the forearm. With a very short transradial amputation, elbow motion may be limited. Transhumeral amputation predisposes patients to reduced glenohumeral and scapular motion, whereas shoulder disarticulation and *forequarter amputation* predisposes to thoracic scoliosis.

Muscle Performance. Strength of the entire affected extremity should be tested using manual muscle tests to determine if muscle strengthening interventions are needed to optimize function and prosthetic use.

Neuromuscular

Arousal, Attention, and Cognition. Depression is common among people with amputations. Nearly 30% of 914 subjects with amputation who responded to the Center for Epidemiologic Study Depression Scale (a 10-point questionnaire) reported significant depressive symptoms.[11] Phantom limb pain, residual limb pain, and back pain were major contributors to depression in this group.

Pain and Sensory Integrity. Phantom sensation and pain are among the most vexing symptoms after amputation.[9] Most patients remain aware of the missing part *(phantom sensation)* for the rest of their lives. For some individuals, anxiety and depression are associated with this phantom sensation.[12] The patient should be reassured that phantom sensation is a normal concomitant of amputation. There may also be pain in a portion of the residual limb (local pain) or pain may be felt in the missing body part *(phantom pain)*. Because the hand has a relatively large cerebral representation, phantom sensation or phantom pain are often quite prominent after amputation of the hand. The phantom limb may feel foreshortened or otherwise distorted, and pain sensations may vary and include burning, electric shocks, or other abnormal unpleasant feelings. For most patients, phantom pain subsides within the first year after amputation.

Cardiovascular/Pulmonary

Circulation. Regardless of the etiology of amputation, the remaining extremity and the residual limb must have an adequate blood supply to maintain viability. Poor circulation increases the risk of ulceration and gangrene. Routine examination for circulatory status should include visual inspection looking for color changes, palpation of all portions of the residual limb, and after a lower extremity amputation, palpation of the contralateral foot and assessment of peripheral pulses throughout the legs. One should also palpate skin temperature because abnormal warmth suggests infection, whereas cold skin indicates circulatory insufficiency. Circulation may be further examined with Doppler ultrasound and transcutaneous oxygen assessments (see Chapter 30).

Integumentary

Integumentary Integrity. The skin should be examined to check for healing and mobility of the amputation scar, for early signs of dermatitis in reaction to materials contacting the skin, and after a prosthesis has been provided, for signs of excessive or persistent pressure, particularly at the margins of the prosthetic brim or on the torso beneath the suspension apparatus. Soap, lotion, or other topical preparations, as well as the sock or liner used with the prosthesis or the material of the prosthesis itself, can cause skin irritation. The skin in contact with the prosthesis may not initially be accustomed to so much wear and pressure and may also be unusually fragile if the area has been grafted or irradiated. Redness that does not quickly resolve with removal of pressure is the first stage of a pressure ulcer (see Chapter 28).

For the person with lower extremity amputation, the skin should be inspected on the sound leg, as well as on the residual limb. After an amputation, the sound foot is vulnerable to breakdown because it has to support more weight. The risk for breakdown of the contralateral leg is greatest in patients with an amputation caused by a systemic disease, particularly PVD and diabetes, because the risk factors for amputation affect the entire body.

In addition to skin inspection and palpation, in people with diabetes, tactile sensation of the sound foot should be tested regularly with a 10-gm monofilament to evaluate for loss of protective sensation that results from neuropathy (see Chapter 31).

EVALUATION, DIAGNOSIS, AND PROGNOSIS

According to the *Guide to Physical Therapist Practice*,[13] rehabilitation for patients with amputation is in the preferred practice pattern 4J: Impaired motor function, muscle performance, ROM, gait, locomotion, and balance associated with amputation.

Medicare and Medicaid categorize patients with unilateral transfemoral and transtibial amputations according to the following functional levels:[14]

Level 0: Patient does not have ability or potential to transfer safely with or without assistance and a prosthesis does not enhance quality of life or mobility. Not a prosthetic candidate, no prosthesis allowed, no components can be used.

Level 1: Has ability or potential to use a prosthesis for transfer or ambulation on a level surface at a fixed cadence. Typical of limited and unlimited household ambulator.

Level 2: Has ability or potential for ambulation with the ability to traverse low level environmental barriers such as curbs, stairs, or uneven surfaces. Typical of the limited community ambulator.

Level 3: Has ability or potential for ambulation with variable cadence. Typical of the community ambulator who has the ability to traverse most environmental barriers and may have vocational, therapeutic or exercise activity that demands prosthetic utilization beyond simple locomotion.

Level 4: Has ability or potential for prosthetic utilization that exceeds basic ambulation skills exhibiting high impact, stress, or energy levels. Typical of the prosthetic demands of the child, active adult or athlete.

An individual patient's functional level is determined by their prescribing physician, and this level is used by most insurance companies, as well as Medicare and Medicaid, as the basis for reimbursement for prosthetics.

The prognosis for patients with an amputation caused by PVD, particularly those with concurrent diabetes, is for future amputations.[15-17] For patients with diabetes, the interval between amputations averages less than 20 years.[18] Future amputation surgeries may include surgical revision of the initial amputation because of poor wound healing and/or amputation of the contralateral extremity because of systemic disease effects and increased use. Using an appropriate well-fitting prosthetic may delay further amputation by distributing body weight and reducing the load on the sound side.

Walking with a lower extremity amputation and a prosthesis increases energy consumption and reduces walking speed as compared with walking with intact extremities.[19-23] Adults with Syme's amputation caused by

vascular disease walk 33% slower and consume 30% more energy per unit distance than nondisabled subjects.[19] Subjects with longer residual limb lengths used significantly less energy than those with shorter limbs while walking at a comparable pace. Adults with transtibial amputation caused by vascular disease walked 44% slower than adults of similar age who had amputations at similar levels as a result of trauma, but the subjects with traumatic amputation still walked 12% slower than normal with 12% higher energy cost per unit distance. The rate of oxygen consumption per unit distance was increased by 58% for the dysvascular group and by 33% for those who sustained trauma.[19]

After transfemoral amputation, energy cost per unit time has been found to be within normal range but is increased by up to 116% per unit distance while comfortable walking speed is slower, most likely because of the increased energy demand.[21] Eight people with hip disarticulation were found to walk 41% more slowly than those without amputations, while 10 adults with transpelvic amputation walked 51% slower. The energy cost per unit distance was 43% and 75% greater than normal for these groups, respectively.[22]

A meta-analysis of several studies with small sample sizes of individuals with bilateral amputations found that their walking speed was decreased and varied according to level of amputation, from 15% for those with bilateral transtibial amputation to 48% for those with bilateral transfemoral amputation, with as much as a 260% rise in energy cost per unit distance.[23]

Although residual limb length and etiology of amputation affect energy consumption, the data are inconclusive with regard to the effect of various prosthetic components. Published research consists largely of studies on small, heterogeneous samples, with subjects not blinded to the component being evaluated, and components seldom applied in a random manner.[24] Comparison of the energy cost and gait efficiency in seven young adults with traumatic transtibial amputation using the solid ankle, cushioned heel (SACH) foot and the Flex-Foot showed a minimal difference in oxygen consumption per unit distance at slower walking speed. Subjects wearing the Flex-Foot demonstrated a 10% lower oxygen consumption while walking at an average 9% higher self-selected walking velocity.[25] Physically active young men used slightly less energy with a foot with a shock-absorbing spring, as compared with walking and running with a SACH foot or Flex-Foot.[26] Other studies comparing the energy cost of the SACH and various dynamic elastic response feet have failed to show a significant difference in energy consumption between these devices.[27,28]

No statistically significant difference in energy consumption has been reported between walking with transfemoral prostheses equipped with a locked or an unlocked knee unit; however, energy consumption may increase significantly when subjects walk with the knee at a setting to which they were unaccustomed. Older subjects walked faster with the locked knee, whereas younger subjects walked better with the unlocked knee.[29] Young adults with transfemoral amputations have been shown to walk faster with less energy expenditure with prostheses with computerized knee units than with other types of knee units.[30-32] Computer-controlled knee units also decreased energy expenditure of three adults wearing hip disarticulation prostheses.[33] Lower energy cost and faster speed was exhibited by subjects wearing an ischial containment transfemoral socket when compared with the quadrilateral design.[34]

Unsurprisingly, given the high energy cost of ambulating with bilateral prostheses, studies have demonstrated that it is more energy efficient for people with bilateral transtibial[35] or bilateral transfemoral amputations[36] to use a wheelchair than ambulate with protheses. Six adults with bilateral transtibial amputations caused by PVD averaged a 12% reduction in velocity at a 157% greater energy cost when walking as compared with wheeling.[35] A 41-year-old woman with traumatic transfemoral amputations walked 69% slower than she moved in her wheelchair with a 707% increase in energy consumption.[36]

Unilateral lower extremity amputation is associated with an overall lower activity level.[37] This is not thought to be the result of deconditioning as resting heart rate is not different.[37] A prospective study of 46 elderly adults with unilateral amputation caused by PVD found that poor balance on the sound leg and cognitive impairment were most predictive of diminished future function and activity level.[38]

Several recent reports have evaluated the effects of different prosthetic components on objective measures of function. Thirteen subjects with unilateral traumatic transtibial amputation averaged 83% more steps per day when wearing a polyethylene foam liner than with an elastomeric gel liner.[39] Ten adults with transfemoral amputation caused by vascular disease walked at similar velocity regardless of the weight of the prosthesis, with as much as 1625 gm added to the basic prosthesis.[40]

Various instruments have been used to evaluate the overall function of individuals with lower extremity amputations, although no single instrument measures all aspects of mobility.[41] A meta-analysis of studies published between 1978 and 1998 found that the Stanmore Harold Wood Mobility Scale was used in most studies.[41,42] A 1-year follow-up of all individuals with unilateral amputation at a regional amputee rehabilitation center found that almost all those younger than 50 years achieved functional community mobility. Half of the older adults with transtibial amputation were also community ambulators, whereas fewer than a quarter of those with transfemoral amputation were able to walk in the community.[43] Quality of life after amputation appears to be more affected by body image, as indicated on the Amputee Image Body Scale, than by age, level of amputation, or number of co-morbidities.[44] Scores on the Amputee Mobility Predictor[45] are correlated with the Medicare 5-level coding scale described earlier.[46] Another useful instrument is the Sickness Impact Profile-68, which predicted functional outcome in 69% of 46 patients older than 60 years with unilateral amputation caused by vascular disease.[38] The Houghton Scale is also responsive to functional change among adults with amputations caused by trauma or vascular disease.[47] Scores on the Prosthetic Evaluation Questionnaire,[48] which includes a 4-item function scale,

2 mobility scales, and 4 psychosocial questions, are inversely correlated with walking distance among adults with unilateral transtibial amputation.[49] Balance confidence accounted for most of the mobility performance as measured by the Prosthetic Evaluation Questionnaire and the Houghton Scale.[50] The Locomotor Capabilities Index,[51] a 14-item self-report, with demonstrated internal consistency and test-retest reliability, confirmed that those with transtibial amputation were more independent than individuals with transfemoral amputation. The Trinity Amputation and Prosthesis Experience Scales[52] has been used to assess consumer satisfaction after amputation; troublesome areas include delay in fitting the first prosthesis and negative perceptions regarding prosthetists' interpersonal manner.[49] The Orthotics and Prosthetics Users' Survey[53] is a self-report of functional status, general health, employment, and satisfaction with clinic services that demonstrates internal consistency and construct validity. Physiological measures, such as electrocardiography and peak heart rate, have shown that although the average physical and cardiac condition is poor in adults with vascular amputation, most succeeded in prosthetic training with or without a walker.[54]

Interviews of 32 adults who averaged a year between amputation and return to work indicated that reintegration into the work force was delayed by problems with the residual limb, particularly wound healing; many subjects were employed in less physically demanding jobs after rehabilitation.[55] Socket discomfort, phantom pain and skin disorders are common among those with traumatic amputations.[56]

Because most upper extremity amputations involve only one hand, and one can do most daily and vocational activities without a prosthesis, many individuals eventually opt to discard the prosthesis.[57] Factors contributing to ongoing prosthetic use among adults include graduation from high school, employment, emotional acceptance of the amputation, and the perception that the prosthesis is expensive. Those with transradial amputation are more likely to persist with prosthetic use compared with those having other levels of amputation. Early fitting for people with traumatic amputation, as well as posttraumatic counseling, contribute to continued prosthetic usage in this group.[50]

INTERVENTION

PREOPERATIVE AND POSTSURGICAL MANAGEMENT

The goal of preoperative care is to prepare the patient for life after amputation surgery and to begin rehabilitation. Postoperatively, regardless of whether the patient is eventually fitted with a prosthesis, the individual should engage in a structured program aimed at hastening wound healing and fostering maximum function. The level of amputation, the surgical procedure, and the patient's health all influence the early management program.

Rehabilitation should begin preoperatively, except in cases of congenital anomaly or trauma involving immediate severance of the extremity. The optimum preoperative program involves psychological counseling, joint mobility, general conditioning, and functional activities.

Every effort should be made to prevent the formation of contractures. Active ROM exercises are helpful, and for those with lower extremity amputation, bed and wheelchair positioning should also be part of the early rehabilitation program. While in bed, the patient should lie prone as much as tolerated; for those who experience difficulty breathing when prone, side-lying is preferable to the supine position. When the person is supine, some well-intentioned caregivers place pillows under the lumbar spine, beneath the residual limb, or between the thighs to increase comfort; such pillow placement, however, fosters the development of contractures.

General conditioning exercises aimed at improving strength and endurance can help reverse deconditioning, which is common among older adults with PVD.[54] Gentle strengthening exercises for the trunk and all extremities are recommended. Functional activities provide constructive activity and foster self-care. Candidates for lower extremity amputation should be taught bed-to-wheelchair and chair-to-chair transfers before their surgery, and those who are candidates for immediate postoperative ambulation should learn three-point transfers with the aid of a walker or a pair of crutches.

The individual who is scheduled for upper extremity amputation should be encouraged to gain proficiency in one-handed activities. Most patients, while initially clumsy, achieve reasonable proficiency in one-handed dressing, grooming, and dining. Even if a prosthesis is to be prescribed, the patient will rely more on the remaining hand because it is sensate and more agile than any mechanical device. If the amputation will occur on the dominant side, early care should also address change of dominance. The patient may eventually write with the prosthesis on the preamputation dominant side; however, other activities, such as managing buttons, using a knife when cutting meat, and tying shoe laces, are generally easier with the dexterous, sensate sound hand whether or not it is dominant.

EARLY POSTOPERATIVE MANAGEMENT

The goals of early postoperative management are to foster wound healing and promote maximum function. Early rehabilitation begins as soon as the patient is medically stable after surgery and ends when a prosthesis is fitted. For the person who is not a candidate for a prosthesis, early rehabilitation ends when the residual limb is no longer painful and the individual achieves maximum function. In either instance, care focuses on the residual limb, as well as the patient as a whole. Residual limb care should focus on wound healing, pain reduction, edema control, joint mobility, and strengthening. Holistic care at this time includes psychosocial counseling, general conditioning, care of the remaining foot (in the case of lower extremity amputation), and functional activities.

Wound Healing. Wound healing is fundamental to recovery from amputation surgery (see Chapters 28 and 31). An open wound is vulnerable to infection, which may have serious consequences, including gangrene with subsequent reamputation, and sepsis, which can be fatal. Interventions aim to create a clean, stable wound environment to facilitate healing. Modalities that may hasten healing include electrical stimulation, ultraviolet, US, intermittent pneumatic compression, hydrotherapy, and negative pressure,[59] although not all modalities are appropriate for those with PVD. Chapters 28 through 31 provide additional information about wound care and healing.

Edema Control. Edema control promotes wound healing, reduces pain, and facilitates prosthetic fitting. The larger the extremity circumference, the more postoperative edema is likely to be present. Thus there will be more edema, followed by more volume loss, after a transfemoral amputation than after a transtibial, transradial, or transhumeral amputation. Ideally, edema control measures are introduced at the time of surgery; however, if the patient is medically unstable, edema control is sometimes delayed. Edema control measures should be used until the patient is wearing a prosthesis for most of the day, or until the wound has healed and the residual limb is no longer painful. Limb volume changes continue to occur for an average of 120 days after surgery.[60] Interventions intended to stabilize limb volume after amputation of the upper or lower extremity include soft dressings (elastic bandage and elastic shrinker socks), semirigid dressings (Unna bandage and air splints), and rigid (plaster or plastic) dressings. A thin dressing should be placed directly on the amputation wound, particularly if sutures or staples are in place. Although abundant anecdotal reports support the effectiveness of various dressings, relatively little evidence confirms the effectiveness of any specific alternative.[61]

Soft dressings are used most commonly,[62] possibly because the materials are relatively inexpensive and dressing application and removal are simple. Elastic bandages should be applied in a figure-of-eight pattern, avoiding circular turns.[63] Elastic bandages have several disadvantages. They must be reapplied several times a day because they tend to loosen as the patient moves about. Although individuals with transtibial amputation generally can bandage themselves, it is very difficult for those with transfemoral amputation to wrap the residual limb and torso effectively. If the transfemoral bandage rolls distally, the patient is apt to develop an adductor roll, a mass of tissue in the medial thigh; the roll is subject to chafing and subsequent breakdown. Furthermore, pressure beneath the dressing varies with each application making volume stabilization relatively ineffective.[64-67]

Shrinker socks are closed-ended tubes made of fabric knitted with elastic threads. They are relatively easy to roll onto the amputation limb, and when properly applied, compress the limb uniformly.[66] The transtibial sock usually remains snugly on the distal thigh; however, the transfemoral sock requires a belt with garters for suspension. Newer versions of shrinker socks include elasticized shorts[68] and gel socks.[69]

Semirigid dressings, especially the *Unna dressing*, overcome most of the problems with soft dressing.[70-72] The Unna dressing is made of gauze permeated with zinc oxide and calamine, with glycerin and gelatin added as moisture-retention agents. The bandage is applied over a thin sterile wound dressing and is placed obliquely on the residual limb, with turns requiring cutting the bandage, rather than twisting it. This nonextensible bandage adheres to the skin, assuring suspension and constant compression and, is relatively thin, making it especially suitable for transfemoral amputations. It can be placed high in the groin to prevent an adductor roll.

Usually the Unna bandage is left in place until sutures are removed unless there are signs of infection, in which case the bandage is removed immediately. With transtibial, transradial, and transhumeral amputations, sutures are generally removed 7-10 days after surgery; with transfemoral amputations, sutures are usually removed slightly later, at around 14 to 18 days after surgery. The bandage can be removed by cutting it with bandage scissors.

Rehabilitation, especially for those with transfemoral amputation, is significantly accelerated by the Unna dressing.[72] Survival curves comparing patients fitted with Unna dressings with those using elastic bandaging showed that the time from surgery to prosthetic fitting in 30% of each group was 34 days for the Unna group and 64 days for the elastic bandage group. Of those who received prostheses, time from admission to the rehabilitation unit to readiness for fitting averaged 21 days for the Unna group and 29 days for the elastic bandaging group.

An alternative to the Unna semirigid dressing is an air splint. This is an inflatable plastic limb encasement. It is easy to apply and remove and is self-suspending. Inflation ensures uniform pressure within the splint because a gas in a closed container distributes pressure uniformly.[73] The splint may be augmented with an aluminum frame, permitting limited weight bearing.[74,75] The drawbacks of air splints include bulkiness and susceptibility to punctures.

Rigid dressings can also be used to assist with edema reduction after amputation. These dressings are made of a series of layers. The first layer, next to the skin, is an elasticized cotton sock. Elastic plaster and then a reinforcing layer of regular plaster are wrapped over the sock. Cotton or Dacron webbing straps are plastered in place to provide suspension.[76,77] The rigid dressing remains on the residual limb until suture removal, although it may be removed if the wound becomes infected or pain is intolerable. The rigid dressing may be the foundation for an immediate postoperative prosthesis (IPOP) if a *pylon* with foot is plastered into the dressing. Compared with soft dressings, some investigators report that rigid dressings foster faster wound healing and volume stabilization with fewer surgical revisions, while also accelerating rehabilitation.[78,79] Others, however, found no difference in infection rate or time to prosthetic fitting with this type of dressing.[80] Sometimes a rectangular window is cut near the suture line to permit wound inspection. After inspection, the window is plastered in place. Alternatively, the plaster may be bivalved, so that it can be removed for wound examination.[81] Polyethylene may be substituted for plaster.[82,83] Application of rigid dressings requires considerable skill.[84] The cast is also relatively heavy, so the suspension straps must be kept taut. Suspension for a transfemoral rigid dressing requires a shoulder harness, making sitting awkward. The cast is removed with a cast cutter.

Pain Management. One of the benefits of compressive amputation limb dressings is reduction in pain.[78] However, the cause of pain or other unpleasant sensations should be removed whenever possible.[85] Local pain may respond to removal of an irritant, if one can be identified. Occasionally, a neuroma near fascia can cause either local or phantom pain. In this circumstance, excision of the neuroma may help. Directly after surgery, or trauma resulting in amputation, a patient-controlled anesthesia pump may be effective for pain control.[6] Conservative approaches to phantom pain control include massage, whether effleurage, tapotement, or friction.[86-90] Massage provides sensory input and may serve as a counterirritant. Other interventions are resistive exercise of the contralateral extremity; relaxation,[91] acupuncture,[92] and various modalities such as ultrasound, transcutaneous electrical nerve stimulation,[93,94] and biofeedback.

Joint Mobility. Joint mobility should be preserved with active exercise,[95] positioning, and/or splinting. To prevent flexion contractures after transtibial or transradial amputation, the nearest proximal joint should be kept extended with a splint or a rigid or semirigid dressing. When in bed, the patient should spend as much time as tolerated in a prone position. Regardless of position, the individual should not have pillows placed under the lumbar spine, between the thighs, or under the thigh or transtibial residual limb. When in the wheelchair, the patient should sit in good posture without a pillow between the thighs; the transtibial residual limb should rest on an extension support projecting from the wheelchair seat so that the knee can be extended.

Strengthening. Strengthening the muscles of the residual limb facilitates eventual prosthetic use. The patient with an upper extremity amputation is usually a young, healthy man who can readily preserve or increase strength of the proximal musculature, including the shoulder girdle, to allow use of prostheses that are controlled with shoulder motions. Those with lower extremity amputation are often older and have more co-morbidities and are therefore less able to increase strength. Nonetheless, they should try to strengthen the hip extensors and abductors[96,97] because these muscles are important during stance phase when walking with any prosthesis at or below the transfemoral level. Individuals with transtibial amputation should also work on knee extensor strength because strong knee extension is essential for transferring from one seat to another and for best use of a prosthesis. Without active exercise, isokinetic and isometric quadriceps strength will decrease significantly.[98] Various types of resistance, including manual, active, elastic, pulley, and isokinetic resistance, can be used to increase strength of patients with amputation and to reduce energy consumption when the patient walks with a prosthesis[99] (see Chapter 5). Exercises suitable for younger and older adults with lower extremity amputation are listed in Table 12-1.

Holistic Care. Holistic care of the patient should occur along with treatment focused on the residual limb. Peer counseling for the patient and family helps put their experiences in a larger context. For example, knowing that others are coping with phantom sensation, anxiety, and a vigorous exercise program can be reassuring.

The physical therapist (PT) should design a general conditioning program that challenges the individual. In addition, the person with lower extremity amputation,

TABLE 12-1	Exercises for Adults with Lower Extremity Amputation
Exercise	**Technique**
Bridging	Lie on back with head on pillow and arms folded across chest.
	Towel roll under residual limb.
	Bend sound leg.
	Push residual limb into towel while lifting buttock on amputated side.
	Hold 5 seconds.
Hip extension	Lie on chest with arms folded under head.
	Keep thighs close together.
	Lift residual limb to clear the other thigh while keeping abdomen on mat.
Hip abduction: Sidelying	Lie on sound side, with bottom knee bent.
	Lift residual limb.
Quadriceps sets	Lie on back, with sound knee bent.
	Slowly tighten thigh muscles in residual limb while counting to 5.
Knee extension	Sit on chair.
	Straighten knee, holding position for 3 seconds.
Straight leg raise	Recline on back, propping yourself on your elbows.
	Bend sound knee.
	Raise residual limb 4 inches, holding position for 5 seconds.
	Slowly return to starting position.
Hip adduction	Sit on mat with hands bent for support.
	Place towel roll between thighs.
	Squeeze roll for 5 seconds.

particularly the adult with arteriosclerosis, should be instructed in meticulous care of the remaining extremity and avoidance of activities that increase the risk of poor healing and further amputation. Activities that are especially deleterious and that aggravate the effects of PVD include smoking, bathing in hot water, using a heating pad, exposing the feet to a radiator or fire, and wearing circular garters. In addition, using chemical corn or callus removers; walking barefoot; wearing a shoe without hose; wearing hose with mends, holes, or an elastic top; and wearing flip-flop sandals increase the risk of trauma and infection.

Foot care should occur on a daily basis and include inspecting the foot using a mirror and looking for redness, blisters, cuts, toenail discoloration, and edema. The feet should be washed in lukewarm water and dried well, especially between the toes. The feet should be lubricated with moisturizing lotion after drying, but lotion should not be used between the toes. Toenails should be trimmed straight across, and if they are thick or the patient has sensory loss, they should be trimmed by a podiatrist. Shoes should be checked for wrinkled linings, protruding tacks, and debris.

The person with lower extremity amputation should practice standing on the intact foot with the aid of a walker or a pair of crutches. Some therapists begin standing practice in parallel bars. If this is done, it is important to discourage the patient from pulling on the bars because this is not an effective approach for using a cane.

During the early postoperative period, before the patient has a prosthesis, they may have a rigid dressing with a pylon. The pylon is fixed into the rigid dressing at one end and into a prosthetic foot at the other end to make an IPOP. The pylon should be detached whenever the patient leaves the physical therapy department to prevent unsupervised weight bearing. Until sutures are removed, the person should bear a maximum of 25 lb on this temporary prosthesis. Loading can be monitored with the aid of a bathroom scale. The individual can progress to three-point gait and transfers during this phase.[76]

Adjustable sockets that can be attached to a pylon and foot are also commercially available for people using semirigid or soft dressings. The socket circumference and depth can be adjusted to fit over the dressing using straps and padding. As with the IPOP, this prosthesis can be used for practicing three-point transfers and gait with assistive devices.

Most people with lower extremity amputation use a wheelchair on a temporary or permanent basis. The wheelchair should have its rear wheels displaced posteriorly, so that the rearward transposition of the seated person's center of gravity will not cause the wheelchair to tip backward. The person with a unilateral amputation and no expectation for a prosthesis should have one swing-out footrest to support the sound lower extremity, and individuals who can be expected to wear a prosthesis should have a pair of swing-out footrests to support the prosthetic foot and the sound foot. To facilitate transfers, wheelchairs for patients with bilateral amputations who are not candidates for prostheses should have no footrests.

Someone with an upper extremity amputation should practice one-handed activities to foster resumption of self-care. A temporary prosthesis facilitates edema control and aids with accomplishing bimanual activities. If the dominant hand was amputated, the patient should be guided to change hand dominance to accomplish manipulative tasks. With the possible exception of handwriting, the sound hand will become the dominant extremity whether or not a prosthesis is provided. As soon as possible, the patient should be encouraged to bathe, groom, dress, feed, and toilet independently, using the sound upper extremity. Occasionally, the patient may rely on adaptive equipment, such as a combination fork and spoon, or on trunk motion to perform a particular task.

LOWER EXTREMITY PROSTHETIC OPTIONS

A prosthesis does not always benefit the person with an amputation. It is contraindicated for those with severe cardiovascular or pulmonary disease that would make the exertion needed to use the prosthesis functionally unsafe or if the prosthesis allows the individual to perform activities that place excessive strain on the heart.[100] Few patients with dementia are candidates for a prosthesis, especially if the person cannot comprehend instructions for donning the prosthesis and using it safely. Very occasionally, the individual with cognitive deficits can use a prosthesis if the caregiver is extraordinarily supportive. If the patient is not motivated, prosthetic prescription should be delayed until the person appears interested in rehabilitation.

Medical factors that influence but do not preclude prosthetic prescription include neuropathy, arthritis, lack of skin integrity, contracture, and weakness.

For the patient who is a candidate for a prosthesis, the only absolute limitations to specific prescriptions are size and cost. Nearly all components are manufactured in adult size, but the options for children are much more limited. Medicare regulations or other insurance guidelines regarding reimbursement may proscribe expensive components. Because of the dearth of objective research, selection must be guided by expert opinion and experience.[24]

Partial Foot Amputations. No prosthesis is necessary after a phalangeal amputation because the absence of one or more phalanges has minimal effect on standing and walking, although amputation of the first or fifth phalanges compromises late stance. However, the patient will walk more comfortably and the shoe will look better with a filler in the toe box, the distal portion of the shoe. Ideally, a custom-made filler that fits the residual foot precisely should be used to minimize the risk of abrasion that can compromise the amputation scar and cause calluses or ulceration. If the entire toe is removed, the plantar aponeurosis supports the longitudinal arch less effectively, making a longitudinal arch support helpful. With any ray resection the patient should be provided with a custom-made foot prosthesis to restore the width of the foot and increase the weight-bearing area.

Transmetatarsal amputation shortens the foot considerably. A custom-made, total-contact resilient socket attached to a shoe-filler is recommended to protect the residual limb from abrasion. The shoe should have the fastening on the proximal dorsal surface, as well as a padded tongue, longitudinal arch support, and a cushioned- or beveled-heel rocker sole. These can restore normal function in the late stance phase of gait and avoid an unsightly transverse crease in the upper portion of the shoe. The plantar surface of the insert should also be curved to facilitate late stance.[101]

Since Chopart and similar intertarsal amputations produce a short foot, which can easily slip from the shoe

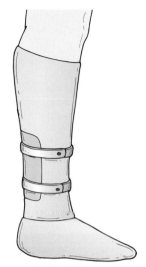

FIG. 12-6 Syme's prosthesis with opening in socket wall to permit entry of bulbous limb.

during swing phase, the patient should wear a shoe that fastens high on the dorsum of the foot. Ideally, a partial foot prosthesis that replaces the forefoot and midfoot is used. Sometimes the prosthesis is attached to a posterior upright that fastens around the proximal portion of the leg.

Syme's Amputation and Ankle Disarticulation. After a Syme's amputation or an ankle disarticulation, gait is optimized with use of a prosthesis with a foot specifically manufactured for this type of amputation and a custom-made plastic socket that encases the leg up to the level of the tibial tuberosity. The socket may have no opening on the side walls, particularly if the amputation limb is relatively streamlined. An elastic liner inside the socket facilitates donning. Alternatively, the socket may have an opening in the medial wall, especially if the amputation limb is bulbous (Fig. 12-6). The opening makes donning easier but will need to be closed after donning; a piece of plastic on the medial wall allows uniform weight bearing.

Lower Extremity Prosthetic Options

Amputation	Prosthesis	Balance	Gait
Toe	Toe filler Longitudinal arch support	Minimal effect, may have pes planus	Late stance: Propulsion
Ray	Sole wedge	Minimal effect, tend to load the unaffected border	Minimal effect
Transmetatarsal and midtarsal	Total-contact resilient socket + toe filler Shoe with fastening on proximal dorsal surface Firm shoe counter Padded tongue Longitudinal arch support Cushion or beveled heel Rocker sole	Tend to shift posteriorly and onto contralateral foot	Late stance: Decreased propulsion during swing phase Prosthesis should remain on foot
Syme's	Syme's foot: Keel accommodates long socket Socket: Expandable, no medial opening, or medial opening	Minimal effect, if end-bearing	Comparable to transtibial

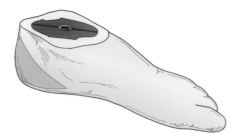

FIG. 12-7 Solid ankle cushion heel (SACH) foot.

Transtibial Amputation. The transtibial prosthesis consists of a foot, shank, socket, and suspension. Prosthetic feet are mass-produced in sizes to fit 6-month-old infants to adults with very large feet. All feet support weight when the wearer stands or is in the stance phase of gait, and all absorb shock at heel contact. They respond passively to the amount and direction of the load applied by the wearer. Feet are designed to simulate metatarsophalangeal hyperextension during late stance and remain in neutral position during swing phase. No prosthetic foot provides sensory feedback, and none plantarflexes when the knee is flexed nor plantarflexes to permit tip-toe walking. Prosthetic feet, with or without a shoe, may fail to attenuate impact force after initial contact during the stance phase of gait.[102]

Foot. Feet may be classified as nonarticulated and articulated. Nonarticulated feet have no separation between the foot and the prosthetic shank but do permit some passive motion in all planes. They may be further classified according to the amount of energy stored during stance phase and released at late stance and early swing phase. Because they have no moving parts, nonarticulated feet are relatively lightweight and durable.

The SACH foot is the basic nonarticulated foot (Fig. 12-7). It consists of a rubberlike compressible heel, a rigid longitudinal support known as the *keel,* and a rubber-like toe section and overall covering. At heel contact, the wearer compresses the heel cushion. At late stance, as the person transfers weight forward, the foot hyperextends at the junction between the distal end of the keel and the toe section. The SACH foot is inexpensive and is available in the largest range of sizes and includes designs to accommodate high-heeled shoes. Other relatively simple feet have a flexible keel that yields slightly when the wearer steps on an uneven surface.

Feet that store more energy are sometimes known as dynamic or energy response feet. They are also nonarticulated but incorporate an elastic element that the wearer stresses during early or mid-stance and that recoils during late stance, simulating the propulsive action of the triceps surae.[103] Flex-Foot is one example of a dynamic energy response foot (Fig. 12-8). It has a carbon-fiber leaf spring extending from the toe to the proximal shank and a carbon-fiber heel section. The long leaf spring stores considerable energy as the wearer moves forward on the foot.[104] The Flex-Foot is appreciably more expensive than a SACH foot.

Articulated feet have a separation between the foot and the shank, allowing motion to occur around one or more

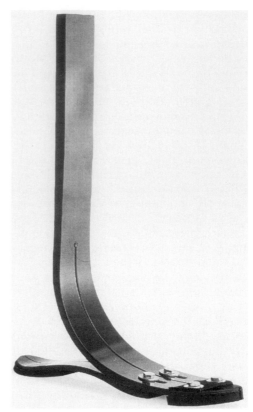

FIG. 12-8 Flex-Foot. *Photo courtesy Ossur North America, Aliso Viejo, Calif.*

axial bolts. Plantarflexion in early stance is somewhat faster than with a nonarticulated foot because once the patient applies minimal load to the rear foot, the foot moves downward. Compressible bumpers control this motion. Some articulated feet allow only sagittal plane motion (single-axis) (Fig. 12-9), whereas others allow triplanar motion (multiple-axis). Comparison of gait with the SACH foot and a multiple axis foot, the Greissinger Plus, worn by nine men indicated that the spatial and temporal parameters of gait were significantly improved when subjects wore the multiaxial foot.[105]

Shank. The shank is the portion of the prosthesis between the foot and the socket. It must be rigid enough to support the wearer's weight. Most shanks are shaped to match the contour of the contralateral leg. They may be exoskeletal (crustacean) with a rigid weight-bearing plastic or wood shell, or endoskeletal, consisting of a central weight-bearing metal or plastic pylon and a cosmetic cover. The pylon allows slight adjustment of alignment and some newer models of pylon have a shock-absorbing mechanism.[106] A torque absorber may also be installed in the shank to absorb transverse stress that would otherwise be transmitted to the skin of the residual limb. This is particularly helpful for people who play golf or walk on uneven terrain.

Socket. The socket is considered the most important part of the prosthesis because this component contacts the wearer's skin. Sockets for permanent, definitive prostheses are custom-made of plastic that is either entirely rigid or flexible on the inside with a rigid frame. The flexible

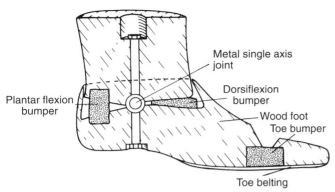

FIG. 12-9 Single-axis foot. *From Ferqason J: Prosthetic feet. In Lusardi MM, Nielsen CC (eds):* Orthotics and Prosthetics in Rehabilitation, *St. Louis, 2000, Butterworth-Heinemann.*

plastic is thought to dissipate heat more effectively than the rigid socket; however, construction of a flexible socket and rigid frame takes more time than making an entirely rigid socket. All sockets are designed to contact portions of the residual limb. Areas of the residual lower limb that tolerate pressure best are the patellar ligament, triceps surae belly, and pes anserinus, also known as the medial tibial flare. Areas that do not tolerate pressure well are the tibial tuberosity, crest, and condyles, as well as the fibular head, hamstring tendons, and distal ends of the tibia and fibula.

The basic transtibial socket is known as patellar tendon bearing (PTB), although there is also some loading throughout the residual limb. The PTB socket has a prominent indentation at the patellar ligament. Tests with an indenter connected to a force transducer confirm that subjects tolerated the highest pressure over the midpatellar ligament and that pressure tolerance decreases with age.[107] Newer socket designs include total surface-bearing[108-110] and hydrostatic[111] models. Total surface-bearing sockets have the basic contours of the PTB socket but are designed to be worn with a compressible liner and are especially suited for suspension by a distal attachment. The hydrostatic design has smoother contours and is most appropriate for short, fleshy residual limbs. With this type of socket, distal tissue cushions the bottom of the socket.

Most transtibial sockets are worn with one or more interfaces or liners.[112,113] The oldest type of interface is a thermoplastic foam concentric replica of the socket. In addition to cushioning impact, the liner makes it easier to alter the size of the socket. As the residual limb atrophies, the prosthetist can add material to the inside of the socket; the flexible liner also creates a smooth surface against the wearer's skin. In addition to the liner, or in place of it, the patient wears one or more socks made of wool, cotton, or Orlon acrylic. Sock thickness is described by ply, referring to the number of threads woven together. The individual should not wear more than 15 ply of socks because thicker padding obscures the concavities and convexities within the socket. A nylon sock worn next to the skin provides a smooth surface to reduce the risk of abrasion. In addition to or instead of socks and the resilient socket liner, the patient may wear a liner made of sili-

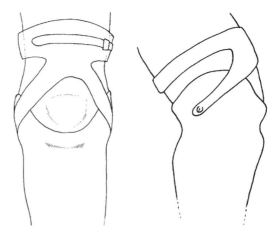

FIG. 12-10 Supracondylar cuff. *From Berke G: Transtibial prostheses. In Lusardi MM, Nielsen CC (eds):* Orthotics and Prosthetics in Rehabilitation, *St. Louis, 2000, Butterworth-Heinemann.*

cone[114,115,39] or polyurethane,[116] sometimes with gel-filled or mineral oil-filled channels to equalize pressure within the socket.

Suspension. The fourth component of the transtibial prosthesis is provision for suspension during swing phase and whenever the prosthesis is hanging such as during climbing stairs and ladders. The simplest, least expensive, and most adjustable suspension is the supracondylar cuff (Fig. 12-10). This is attached to the proximal portion of the socket and buckled or strapped around the distal thigh. Some people augment the supracondylar cuff with a waist belt and fork strap. The fork strap extends anteriorly from the waist belt to the socket and incorporates an elastic segment. Alternatively, the person may wear a rubberized sleeve from the distal thigh to the proximal portion of the prosthesis. The sleeve creates a smooth contour about the knee that makes it more attractive when the wearer sits. However, the sleeve requires two strong hands to don and will not fit a very large thigh.

A transtibial prosthesis can also be suspended using a silicone liner and a metal pin that lodges in a receptacle in the proximal portion of the shank (Fig. 12-11). Testing with force sensors reveals that during swing phase the liner squeezes proximally while creating a large suction distally.[117] This distal suction may compromise skin health. Other modes of suspension include a webbing strap or lanyard extending from the distal portion of the liner through a hole in the socket to a proximal attachment. Alternatively, the contour of the socket brim may be designed to provide suspension. *Supracondylar suspension* features a brim extending over the medial and lateral femoral epicondyles and the socket covers the patella to accommodate a very short residual limb (Fig. 12-12). Donning is easy because the patient does not have to fasten any straps or buckles; however, prosthetic fit is not readily adjustable.

The oldest mode of suspension is the thigh corset, consisting of a leather or flexible plastic corset around the thigh secured with straps or lacing. The corset is attached

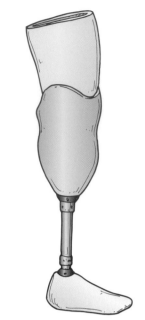

FIG. 12-11 Distal pin suspension.

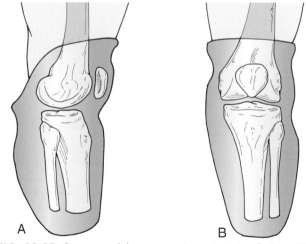

FIG. 12-12 Supracondylar suspension. **A,** Lateral view; **B,** anterior view.

to the socket by a pair of metal side bars with single-axis hinges. This type of suspension provides mediolateral stability, is readily adjustable, and supports some weight on the thigh. However, the corset is more difficult to don than other types of suspension, can cause pressure atrophy of the thigh, retains heat, is heavy, and is bulky at the knee.

Prosthesis Alignment. Prosthesis alignment is adjusted to optimize the wearer's stability and ease of movement. In the sagittal plane, the socket is flexed slightly to enhance quadriceps function, reduce the tendency of the residual limb to slide downward in the socket, and increase loading on the patellar tendon. The farther anterior the prosthetic foot is placed relative to the socket, the more stable the prosthesis. For a frail patient, the foot

is located forward, so that the weight line passes well in front of the knee. For an athletic person, the foot is located slightly behind the socket, so that the knee is easy to flex.

In the frontal plane, the socket is adducted slightly to enhance loading on the proximal medial aspect of the residual limb. The foot is slightly medial to the socket to augment proximomedial loading and to maintain a relatively narrow walking base. Regardless of socket and foot alignment, the prosthesis should be shaped to present an attractive appearance.

Knee Disarticulation. The prosthesis for a knee disarticulation consists of a foot, shank, knee unit, socket, and suspension. Any foot and shank can be used. The knee unit should have a relatively small vertical dimension, so that when the wearer sits the prosthetic knee does not protrude noticeably. The socket covers the residual limb to the proximal thigh. Two socket designs are generally used. The older design has an anterior opening and fastens with straps or laces. It is best suited to the person with an amputation limb with a bulbous end, as is characteristic of a true disarticulation. The newer socket does not have an anterior opening; instead, it has a flexible liner, similar to that of the Syme's prosthesis. It is appropriate for the individual with a streamlined residual limb, without protruding femoral epicondyles. This latter type of prosthesis usually does not require an additional suspension unit as the socket is usually effective at keeping the prosthesis on.

Transfemoral Amputation. The transfemoral prosthesis consists of a foot, shank, knee unit, socket, and suspension. Any foot can be included in the transfemoral prosthesis; however, the basic SACH foot and the single-axis foot are more likely to be used than more sophisticated designs. The patient who is hesitant about applying weight to the prosthesis may do better with a single-axis foot because this will plantarflex with less force than needed for a SACH or other nonarticulated foot. The prosthesis can have an endoskeletal or an exoskeletal shank. An endoskeletal shank, in addition to being adjustable and with its cover, more cosmetic, is lighter in weight than an exoskeletal shank. The thigh portion, between the socket and knee unit, may have a torque absorber or a unit that enables manually locked thigh rotation, or both. However, the transfemoral endoskeletal cover is subject to considerable erosion at the knee when the wearer sits or kneels.

Many designs of knee units are available. These have different axes, friction mechanisms, extension aids, and stabilizer mechanisms (Table 12-2), although a given unit may not have all these features. All knees are designed to flex when the wearer sits.

Knee Units

Axis. The axis connects the proximal and distal parts of the unit. The single axis with a transverse bolt is most common (Fig. 12-13). It is simple in design and works well for most patients. The polycentric axis has two or more pairs of pivoting side bars arranged so that when the knee is flexed the instant center of rotation is the intersection of the longitudinal axes of the bars. Usually the

TABLE 12-2	Knee Unit Component Options
Components	**Options**
Axis	• Single • Polycentric

Friction mechanism	• Constant/sliding
	• Variable/fluid
	  ○ Hydraulic
	  ○ Pneumatic

Extension aid	• External • Internal
Stabilizer mechanism	• Manual lock • Brake

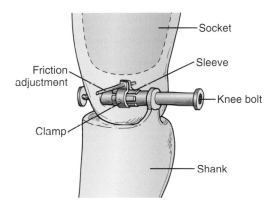

FIG. 12-13 Single-axis knee unit.

intersection is posterior to the weight line, making the prosthesis stable through a longer portion of stance phase.[118] However, because it has more moving parts, the polycentric axis unit is not as durable as the single-axis version.

Friction Mechanism. A friction mechanism resists shank movement during the swing phase of gait to prevent excessive knee flexion during early swing (known as high-heel rise) and abrupt extension at late swing (known as terminal impact). Most knee units have some way to adjust the amount of friction. Either the single-axis or the polycentric axis can be combined with any type of friction mechanism. A constant, or sliding, friction knee unit is simplest. It has one or two adjustable clamps around the knee axis that keep friction constant throughout stance phase. In contrast, a variable, or fluid, friction unit provides different amounts of friction throughout swing phase, typically more at early and late swing and less at midswing. Sliding friction units use solid parts, such as a clamp rubbing on another solid structure such as the knee bolt, to generally provide constant friction. Fluid friction units have a cylinder containing either oil (hydraulic) or air (pneumatic) to generally provide variable friction. All fluid units vary friction with the speed of knee motion. When the wearer walks slowly, the friction is low, providing little restriction to shank movement. When the wearer walks quickly or runs, the unit provides more friction to resist excessive shank motion. Consequently, the motion of the prosthetic leg more closely resembles that of the

contralateral sound leg at all walking speeds. There are also new computer-controlled fluid friction control mechanisms available that use information from ankle and knee motion sensors to adjust resistance according to gait velocity and alterations in terrain.[31] Hydraulic and pneumatic units are more complex, heavier, and more expensive than sliding friction units. Hydraulic units offer a greater range of cadence response and they tend to cost and weigh slightly more than pneumatic units.

Extension Aid. An extension aid is a mechanism for extending the shank at the end of swing phase so that the wearer can be assured of a straight knee at the time of heel contact. An external elastic webbing over the knee unit, known as a kick strap, is the simplest type of extension aid. An internal extension aid has elastic webbing or a coil spring that recoils at late swing to extend the shank. The internal unit is more cosmetic and when the user sits, keeps the knee flexed. All fluid units have an internal extension aid.

Stabilizer Mechanism. The final feature of a few knee units is a stabilizer mechanism. The simplest stabilizer is a manual lock, consisting of a spring-loaded pin designed to lodge in a receptacle in the proximal shank. The locking unit provides maximum stability, not only during early stance phase, when control is needed but throughout the entire gait cycle.[119] With this type of device the wearer walks with a stiff knee and must unlock the unit when sitting. A braking stabilizer is one that provides considerable friction to resist knee motion only during early stance. Braking stabilizers are available with a sliding friction unit, known as weight-activated units, as well as with several hydraulic units. The sliding friction braking unit stabilizes the knee during early stance if the wearer initiates stance phase with the knee extended or flexed less than 25 degrees. The unit is designed to protect against inadvertent knee collapse if the person should happen to catch the foot on an object or irregularity in the walking surface; however, if the wearer begins stance phase with the knee flexed more than 25 degrees, the knee will flex and may cause a fall. Hydraulic swing and stance phase control knee units (Fig. 12-14) give the patient the closest approximation of normal gait kinematics. Microprocessor-controlled stance flexion units (Fig. 12-15) increase friction at heel contact, regardless of the angle of the prosthetic knee, to absorb shock and enable the wearer to walk more normally with controlled knee flexion in early stance.

The thigh section, between the socket and the knee unit, may be equipped with a manually locked rotator unit to allow the person to sit tailor fashion. A torque absorber can also be installed in the thigh section to accommodate stress in the transverse plane.[120]

Socket. Increasingly, people with transfemoral amputation are being fitted with a flexible socket seated in a rigid frame. As compared with an entirely rigid socket, the flexible socket/frame combination is more comfortable when the person sits because the flexible plastic conforms to the contour of the chair. It is also cooler because the thin plastic transmits body heat, and it is easier to modify the flexible thermoplastic by applying heat or removing

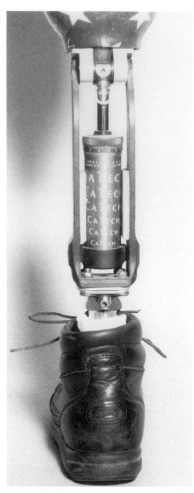

FIG. 12-14 Hydraulic knee unit. *From Psonak R: Transfemoral prostheses. In Lusardi MM, Nielsen CC (eds): Orthotics and Prosthetics in Rehabilitation, ed 2, St. Louis, 2006, Butterworth-Heinemann.*

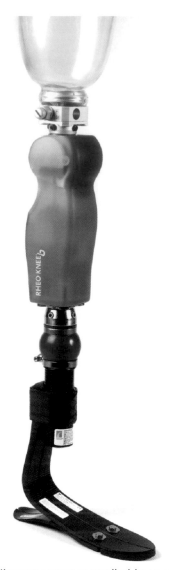

FIG. 12-15 Microprocessor-controlled knee unit. *Photo of Rheo Knee courtesy Ossur.*

material.[121] The flexible socket, however, is somewhat more difficult to fabricate.

Although sockets for people with transfemoral amputations are custom made and thus have a unique shape, there are two principal designs, the quadrilateral and ischial containment. Unlike the transtibial residual limb, which is rather bony, the transfemoral residual limb is fleshy with few bony prominences. The socket must accommodate the greater trochanter, and the proximal brim of the socket must not press excessively on the ischiopubic ramus. Although the ischial tuberosity tolerates loading, some sockets encase the tuberosity and try to minimize applying force to it. Sockets can be made of either flexible or rigid plastic. With the quadrilateral socket, the ischial tuberosity rests on the posterior brim of the socket and supports considerable weight. The anterior wall of the socket has a sizable convexity over the femoral (Scarpa's) triangle to disperse the contact force over the sensitive structures in this area and to provide posteriorly directed force to maintain ischial seating. The medial brim is level with the posterior brim, while the lateral and anterior brims are approximately 2.5 inches higher. The ischial containment socket (Fig. 12-16) extends above the ischial

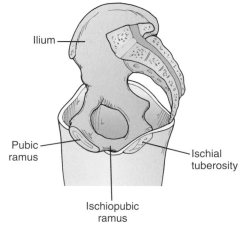

FIG. 12-16 Medial view of an ischial containment socket.

Ilium

Pubic ramus

Ischial tuberosity

Ischiopubic ramus

tuberosity with the medial brim covering part of the ischiopubic ramus. The anterior wall is somewhat lower than the posterior wall. Because the mediolateral width of the ischial containment socket is relatively narrow, this socket is intended to provide greater stability to the femur than the broader quadrilateral socket.

Suspension. Suspension of the transfemoral prosthesis usually involves suction that is controlled with an air expulsion valve in the distal portion of the socket. Total suction suspension eliminates the need for a sock or liner. The socket must fit snugly at the brim, and the patient's limb volume must not fluctuate. Total suction optimizes control of the prosthesis and is the lightest mode of suspension. Some people wear an elasticized fabric belt over the proximal prosthesis and lower torso to enhance suspension. Partial suction involves use of the suction valve and creates a difference in pressure between the socket interior and exterior. However, this pressure differential is not sufficient to suspend the prosthesis so auxiliary suspension is essential. This is usually provided with a Dacron polyester webbing belt wrapped around the lower torso, known as a Silesian belt (Fig. 12-17). The person can wear socks or a gel-filled liner with partial suction to accommodate day-to-day changes in thigh volume. The Silesian belt also controls the tendency of the prosthesis to be internally rotated when the wearer dons it and resists abduction of the prosthesis. Some people prefer a roll-on silicone or polyurethane liner with or without a distal pin,

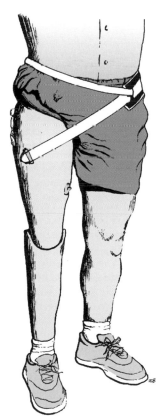

FIG. 12-17 Silesian belt. *From Psonak R: Transfemoral prostheses. In Lusardi MM, Nielsen CC (eds):* Orthotics and Prosthetics in Rehabilitation, *ed 2, St. Louis, 2006, Butterworth-Heinemann.*

or a webbing lanyard suspension, similar to that used with some transtibial prostheses. An alternative to the Silesian belt is the pelvic band that consists of a single-axis hip hinge attached superiorly to a leather belt around the torso and distally to the socket. The pelvic band provides better control of hip abduction, adduction, and rotation but is bulkier and apt to irritate the low back when the wearer sits. Very few people cannot tolerate any suction in the socket. In such instances, a hole can be made in the distal section to provide some ventilation for the residual limb and a pelvic band can be used for suspension.

A new concept in prosthetic suspension is osseointegration, in which hardware is secured proximally to the skeleton. The hardware has provisions for attaching and detaching the distal portion of the socket. Limited experience in Sweden and the United Kingdom have demonstrated that patients achieve greater comfort, function, and quality of life with this type of suspension; however, meticulous surgery and prosthetic fitting are essential.[122,123]

Reimbursement. Medicare allows reimbursement for the following types of prostheses for people with transfemoral amputations:

Level 1: SACH or single-axis foot, manually locked, single-axis, polycentric, or weight-activated knee, any suspension or liner, all socket designs.

Level 2: All L1 components, also flexible keel or multi-axial feet, rotator, and torque absorber.

Level 3: All L1 and L2 components, dynamic response feet, hydraulic/pneumatic knees, dynamic or shock-absorbing pylons. All components allowed.

Level 4: All L1, L2, and L3 components. All existing components.

Alignment. A transfemoral prosthesis is aligned with the socket in slight flexion and adduction. Socket flexion facilitates hip extensor contraction that helps the wearer control the prosthetic knee during early stance phase. Socket adduction helps to stabilize the hip abductors and thus minimize lateral trunk bending during stance phase. The placement of the knee axis relative to the greater trochanter and ankle depends on the patient and the type of knee unit. For the weaker patient, the prosthesis should be aligned with the axis posterior to the line between the trochanter and the ankle to provide maximum stability. For the stronger athletic patient, the axis should be on the line between trochanter and ankle to allow for greater mobility. If the knee unit has a hydraulic friction mechanism, the knee axis must be placed slightly anterior to the line between trochanter and ankle.

Hip Disarticulation and Transpelvic Amputation. The prosthesis for a person with hip disarticulation or transpelvic amputation consists of a socket for weight bearing and suspension, a hip joint, thigh section, knee unit, shank, and foot. The socket encompasses the entire lower trunk. The hip disarticulation socket is designed to support weight on the ipsilateral ischial tuberosity and both iliac crests. The hemipelvectomy socket relies on abdominal compression, the contralateral iliac crest, and sometimes, the lower thorax for weight bearing. The hip joint is either a single-axis joint that allows movement only in the sagittal plane or a ball and socket joint adjusted to limit motion to flexion and extension only. Regardless of design, the hip joint has an extension aid to limit flexion when the wearer walks. The knee unit must have an extension aid and can have any type of axis, friction mechanism, and stabilizer. Endoskeletal shank and thigh sections are preferable because they are considerably lighter than exoskeletal alternatives and any type of foot can be used.

Translumbar Amputation. After translumbar amputation the patient is fitted with a socket to allow sitting in a wheelchair. The socket may have apertures to enable the patient to urinate and defecate while wearing it; otherwise, the individual must transfer out of the socket for toileting. Some patients may have cosmetic non–weight-bearing legs attached to the socket to present a normal appearance when wearing shoes and trousers or a skirt.

Bilateral Amputations. Patients may sustain bilateral amputation either simultaneously, usually as a result of trauma or a congenital deformity, or more commonly, sequentially, with amputation of one leg followed by amputation of the other, as the result of PVD and/or diabetes. If one leg is amputated first, it can be fitted with a prosthesis to reduce the load on the intact lower extremity that is usually also at high risk for amputation because of the patient's underlying medical condition. Additionally, a unilateral prosthetic will allow the person to learn to use a prosthetic.

In general, selection of prosthesis components for the individual with bilateral amputations should apply the same principles as selection for someone needing a unilateral prosthesis. The individual with bilateral transtibial and transfemoral amputations should have prostheses with feet that are identical in design and manufacture because patients can detect subtle differences between the actions of dissimilar feet. However, the feet should be shorter than preamputation size to ease transition during stance phase, and they should be wider to increase stability.

Bilateral transfemoral prostheses may be short, nonarticulated "stubbies" (Fig. 12-18). These prostheses provide greater stability than longer, articulated prostheses. Typically, the shortest length of stubbies equals the length of the longer residual limb. This type of prosthesis has a posteriorly directed, curved base to protect the individual from falling backward. When walking, the person uses short crutches or canes and has a waddling gait. Transfers from adult-sized chairs and climbing 8-inch stairs are very difficult with stubbies. If prostheses with articulating feet and knees are used after bilateral transfemoral amputation, shanks several inches shorter than the wearer's preamputation height are recommended to improve balance. Any knee unit can be used, and the units need not be identical; however, a pair of knees with bilateral manual locks should be avoided because their stiffness hinders walking. A weight-activated friction brake makes stair climbing more difficult, although climbing is very arduous under any circumstance. A pair of hydraulic swing and stance control knee units is generally ideal because they provide needed stance phase stability and do not interfere with swing phase. Identical short, wide, single-axis feet are also recommended.

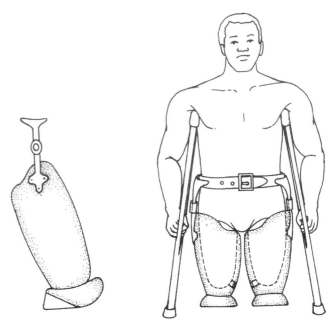

FIG. 12-18 Bilateral transfemoral, short, nonarticulated prostheses (stubbies). *From May BJ: Assessment and treatment of individuals following lower extremity amputation. In O'Sullivan SB, Schmitz TJ (eds):* Physical Rehabilitation: Assessment and Treatment, *ed 3, Philadelphia, 1994, FA Davis.*

Basic Lower Extremity Prosthetic Training. Before starting training, the clinician should ascertain that the prosthesis fits properly and provides the appropriate stability for the patient. At a minimum the patient should be taught how to don the prosthesis (Table 12-3) and transfer from one seat to another. Without these skills, it is unlikely that the person will persist with prosthetic use.

Dressing. The easiest sequence for dressing is the following:

1. Don undergarments.
2. Place the trouser leg or panty hose on the prosthesis.
3. Put a sock (if worn) and shoe on the prosthesis.
4. Don the prosthesis.

Transfers. Moving from bed to chair requires the person to place the sound, or stronger, leg closer to the chair, lean forward at the waist, and rise. The sitting technique also requires the stronger leg to be closer to the chair so that the person can feel the chair with the back of the sound leg and can benefit from hip and, in the case of transtibial amputation, knee extensor strength. Starting with a sturdy armchair or wheelchair makes transfers easier. Eventually, the patient should be able to transfer to and from a toilet, automobile, and other seating surfaces.

Balance and Gait Training. The goal of balance and gait training is to enable the patient to place equal weight on the prosthesis and sound leg, or in the case of someone with bilateral amputations, on both prostheses. Fear of falling often limits gait training.[124] The person must be able to shift weight to advance each leg. Training aims to help the patient walk with steps of equal length and to

TABLE 12-3	Donning a Lower Extremity Prosthesis
Prosthesis	**Technique**

Syme's or transtibial prosthesis	1. Don the sock or other interface on the residual limb.
	2. Lodge the residual limb in the socket.
	3. Fasten the suspension device.
	  a. Distal pin suspension: Enter the socket taking care to position the pin into its receptacle at the base of the socket. The pin will lock into place.
	  b. Lanyard suspension: Feed the end of the lanyard through the slot at the base of the socket, then pull the strap proximally to fasten it.
	  c. Thigh corset: Fasten the corset loosely while the person sits, then fasten the corset snugly after the wearer stands, so that the amputation limb is properly seated in the socket.

Knee disarticulation	1. Don the sock or other interface on the residual limb.
	2. If the socket has an anterior opening:
	  a. Lodge the amputation limb in the socket.
	  b. Fasten the straps to close the socket.
	3. If the socket has a suction valve:
	  a. Remove the valve.
	  b. Place the thigh in the socket.
	  c. Draw the distal end of the sock through the valve hole.
	  d. Stand near a stable piece of furniture.
	  e. Flex and extend the contralateral hip and knee while tugging down on the sock.
	  f. Withdraw the entire sock.
	  g. Install the valve.

Transfemoral prosthesis	1. Remove the suction valve.
	2. To pull the thigh into the socket:
	  a. Don a knitted fabric tube to the level of the groin.
	  b. Place the thigh in the socket.
	  c. Draw the distal end of the fabric through the valve hole.
	  d. Stand near a stable piece of furniture.
	  e. Flex and extend the contralateral hip and knee while tugging down on the fabric.
	  f. With total suction, withdraw the entire fabric, then install the valve.
	  g. With partial suction, tug on the fabric enough to draw the skin of the proximal thigh into the socket, then tuck the end of the fabric back into the socket; then install the valve and fasten the Silesian belt or pelvic band.
	3. To push the thigh into the socket:
	  a. Lubricate the thigh with a nongreasy lotion.
	  b. Push the thigh into the socket.
	  c. Install the valve is installed.
	  d. Fastens any auxiliary suspension if present.

control the knee unit if a transfemoral prosthesis is worn. Proprioceptive neuromuscular facilitation (PNF) techniques and emphasis on body awareness have been found to be more effective than traditional gait training.[125,126] A study with 50 adults fitted with their first unilateral transfemoral prosthesis found that those who received PNF bore significantly more weight on the prosthesis and took more symmetrical steps than those who had traditional training, including weight-shifting, balancing, stool-stepping, and gait exercises.[125] A study comparing training parts of the gait sequence with training of gait as a whole found both increased walking velocity equally.[127] Since adults with unilateral transtibial amputation often have sensory and proprioceptive deficits on the intact leg,[128] it is suggested that gait training also include mechanisms to compensate for these deficits.

Devices that provide partial weight support, including parallel bars or harness and frame units,[129,130] can accustom the patient to safe standing and walking and reduce the energy demand of walking with a prosthesis. Frail patients may also benefit from use of a tilt table to acclimate to upright posture before gait training. The type of walker used has also been shown to influence the final gait selected by a patient. All subjects with unilateral or bilateral transtibial prostheses, or with unilateral transfemoral prostheses, halted with each step when they used a four-footed walker without wheels, whereas only 55% of the subjects halted when using a two-wheeled walker.[131]

Exercises for patients with unilateral or bilateral transtibial or transfemoral prostheses have been developed empirically (Table 12-4). These are intended to promote practice of the elements of walking, including weight shifting in various directions, single-limb stance, narrow-based gait, and forceful hip and knee extension.

Wearing Schedule. Although the PT should encourage the patient to persist with the rehabilitation program, the therapist should also carefully monitor the residual limb for skin irritation and assess the patient for fatigue during development of a prosthetic wear schedule. Initially, the patient should wear the prosthesis for 5-15 minutes, then remove it so that the skin may be assessed. The period of wear can then gradually be increased to tolerance. Fre-

TABLE 12-4	Exercises for Unilateral or Bilateral Transtibial or Transfemoral Prosthetic Wearers
Method	**Technique**
Side-to-side shifting	• Stand between 2 chairs or in parallel bars, feet 2-4 inches apart. Hold the chair backs. • Shift weight from the pelvis to right and left. • Do not bend at the waist.
Forward-backward shifting	• Stand between 2 chairs or in parallel bars, feet 2-4 inches apart. Hold the chair backs. • Shift weight from the pelvis forward and backward. • Do not bend at the waist.
Single-limb stance	• Stand between 2 chairs or in parallel bars, with step stool in front of the sound leg. Hold the chair backs. • Step slowly onto stool with the sound foot. Eventually remove hands from the chairs or parallel bars. • Stepping quickly on the stool reduces the effectiveness of the exercise because less time is spent bearing weight on the prosthesis.
Side-stepping	• Stand facing a sturdy table. Place hands on table for balance. • Side-step to sound side, moving from the pelvis. • Keep the torso erect without bending at the waist.
Braiding	• Stand with the feet 2-4 inches apart. • Cross the prosthesis in front of the sound leg. • Bring sound leg on line with prosthesis. • Cross prosthesis behind sound leg. • Bring the sound leg on line with the prosthesis. • Rotate the trunk while moving the legs. • Keep the torso erect.
Ball rolling	• Stand with the prosthesis next to a sturdy table. • Place a tennis ball in front of the sound foot. • Place sound foot on ball and roll it in all directions. • Keep the torso erect.
Elastic band	• Secure one end of the elastic band to a sturdy table leg. • Place the other end of rubber around the sound ankle. • Hold onto a chair while kicking sound leg backward and forward, and side to side. • Keep the torso erect and the knee on the amputated side extended.
Knee flexion/extension	• Stand with the sound leg next to a sturdy table. • Place the sound foot 6 inches in front of the prosthetic foot. • Flex the hip on the amputated side to flex the knee on the same side. • Extend the hip on the amputated side to extend the knee on the same side. • Repeat knee flexion/extension on the sound side. • Repeat with the prosthetic foot in front of the sound foot. • Keep the torso erect.
Leg swing	• Swing the prosthesis forward and backward rhythmically. • Keep the torso erect.

Heel strikes	• Start with the prosthesis behind the trunk.
	• Balance on the prosthetic toe.
	• Push on front socket wall, swing through, and then quickly push on back socket wall.
	• Performing this exercise slowly may allow the knee to flex inadvertently.
	1. Coin toss
	  ◦ Toss coins on floor.
	  ◦ Hit the prosthetic heel on coins called at random.
	  ◦ Keep the knee on the prosthetic side extended.
	2. Tiny steps
	  ◦ Walk with short steps, emphasizing rapid hip flexion, then extension.
	  ◦ Performing this exercise slowly may allow the knee to flex inadvertently.
	3. Step-ups
	  ◦ Place stool in front of prosthesis.
	  ◦ Lead with prosthesis to step up on stool.
	  ◦ Push on back socket wall.
	  ◦ Performing this exercise slowly may allow the knee to flex inadvertently.

quent removal and reapplication of the prosthesis is also important to allow the patient to practice donning and doffing.

Gait Compensations. Even under the best of circumstances, gait with a prosthesis differs from the walking pattern of a nondisabled person. Gait with a transtibial prosthesis is characterized by a longer step length, step time, and swing time, as well as higher activity of the biceps femoris on the amputated side. Increasing walking speed does, however, reduce some gait asymmetry.[132] Gait with a transfemoral prosthesis is also asymmetrical.[133,134] Gait asymmetries are caused by a combination of anatomical and prosthetic limitations. Anatomical limitations include lack of distal sensation, muscle severance, and skeletal discontinuity that prevents closed-chain action during stance phase. Pain from stress on the intact contralateral knee may also contribute to gait asymmetry.[135] In addition, pain, contracture, weakness, instability, incoordination, and slow gait velocity may be correctable causes of gait changes. Slow walking with a unilateral transtibial or transfemoral prosthesis produces an inefficient pendulum mechanism of gait during swing phase, which correlates with increased energy cost.[136] A transfemoral prosthesis also alters the spatiotemporal distribution of the center of pressure in both feet.[137]

Prosthetic limitations that interfere with gait include weight asymmetry, with the prosthesis always being lighter than the missing body part, and limited excursion of prosthetic feet. Other prosthetic limitations that may be eliminated include improper donning, use of an inappropriate shoe, socket misfit or malalignment, malfunctioning components, and improper prosthesis height (Tables 12-5 and 12-6).

Caring for the Residual Limb and the Prosthesis. An essential part of rehabilitation is instruction in the care of the residual limb and prosthesis. The skin should be protected against abrasions that if untended can make wearing the prosthesis uncomfortable.[138-140] The patient who has accommodated to daily wear of the prosthesis should check the skin each evening. Reddened or discolored areas should resolve within 10 minutes. If not, the wearer should return to the prosthetist for socket or harness adjustment. Flexibility and strength should be maintained so that the person can control the prosthesis and perform the full range of activities effectively. Hip or knee flexion contractures compromise stability in standing and walking, and hip and knee extensor strength are needed to be able to rise from a chair easily and for maximum ambulatory function.

Prosthetic care involves keeping the socket clean by wiping it with a damp cloth nightly, brushing the knee unit and articulated foot to remove debris, and inspecting the appliance for signs of wear or malfunction. When any abnormality becomes evident, the prosthesis should be returned promptly to the prosthetist for repair.

UPPER EXTREMITY PROSTHETIC OPTIONS

Partial Hand. Those who lose fingers or other parts of the hand may choose to wear cosmetic replacements. If the thumb is absent, the patient may elect surgery to create a thumb-like opposition post either by rotating an adjacent metacarpal or by transplanting the great toe. While the appearance is abnormal, most patients obtain useful function with the sensate segment. Partial hand prostheses are rarely satisfactory because they block the wearer from using sensation on the portion of the hand covered by the prosthesis.

Transradial Prosthesis. The transradial prosthesis consists of a terminal device (TD), wrist unit, socket, suspension, and control mechanism.

TABLE 12-5	Causes of Common Gait Deviations with a Transtibial Prosthesis	
Deviations/Compensations	**Prosthetic Causes**	**Anatomical Causes**
EARLY STANCE		
Excessive knee flexion: Buckling	High shoe heel	Flexion contracture
	Insufficient plantarflexion	Weak quadriceps
	Stiff heel cushion	
	Socket too far anterior	
	Socket excessively flexed	
	Cuff tabs too posterior	
Insufficient knee flexion	Low shoe heel	Extensor hyperflexion
	Excessive plantarflexion	Weak quadriceps
	Soft heel cushion	Anterodistal pain
	Socket too far posterior	Arthritis
	Socket insufficiently flexed	
MIDSTANCE		
Excessive lateral thrust	Excessive foot inset	
Medial thrust	Foot outset	
LATE STANCE		
Early knee flexion: Drop off	High shoe heel	Flexion contracture
	Insufficient plantar flexion	
	Heel too short	
	Dorsiflexion stop too short	
	Socket excessively flexed	
	Cuff tabs too posterior	
Delayed knee flexion: Walking uphill	Low shoe heel	Extensor hyperreflexia
	Excessive plantarflexion	
	Heel too long	
	Dorsiflexion stop too stiff	
	Socket too far posterior	
	Socket insufficiently flexed	

TABLE 12-6   Causes of Common Gait Deviations with a Transfemoral Prosthesis

Deviations/Compensations	Prosthetic Causes	Anatomical Causes
LATERAL DISPLACEMENTS		
Abduction stance	Long prosthesis	Abduction contracture
	Abducted hip joint	Weak abductors
	Inadequate lateral wall adduction	Lateral distal pain
	Sharp or high medial wall	Adductor redundancy
		Instability
Circumduction swing	Long prosthesis	Abduction contracture
	Locked knee unit	Poor knee control
	Loose friction	
	Inadequate suspension	
	Small socket	
	Loose socket	
	Foot plantarflexed	
TRUNK SHIFTS		
Lateral bend stance	Short prosthesis	Abduction contracture
	Inadequate lateral wall adduction	Weak abductors
	Sharp or high medial wall	Hip pain
		Instability
		Short amputation limb
Forward flexion: Stance	Unstable knee unit	Instability
	Inadequate socket flexion	
Lordosis: Stance	Short walker or crutches	Hip flexion contracture
		Weak extensors
Medial (lateral) whip: Heel off	Faulty socket contour	With sliding friction unit: Fast pace
	Knee bolt externally (internally) rotated	
	Foot malrotated	
	Prosthesis donned in malrotation	
Foot rotation at heel contact	Stiff heel cushion	
	Malrotated foot	
EXCESSIVE KNEE MOTION		
High heel rise: Early swing	Inadequate friction	
	Slack extension aid	
Terminal impact late swing	Inadequate friction	Forceful hip flexion
	Taut extension aid	
REDUCED KNEE MOTION		
Vault: Swing	Same as circumduction	With sliding friction unit: Fast pace
Hip hike: Swing	Same as circumduction	
Uneven step length	Uncomfortable socket	Hip flexion contracture
	Insufficient	Instability

Terminal Device. The TD is a mass-produced substitute for the anatomical hand and may be in the form of a prosthetic hand or a hook. Prosthetic hands and hooks are made in sizes ranging from those small enough for a 6-month-old infant to those large enough for a large adult hand.

In comparison with an anatomical hand, the TD has the following limitations:

- Appearance: The shape of the human hand changes with the activity being performed, whereas prosthetic hands have a stylized shape and are covered by a glove to resemble the wearer's skin color. Some people increase the lifelike effect by adding nail polish, rings, bracelets, and even adhesive bandages to the glove. The glove is susceptible to discoloration and damage from abrasion.
- Prehension pattern: The human hand can move in a near-infinite number of positions. Although most TDs can be opened and closed, their fingers only move in one plane. The prosthetic hand has a basic posture of a three-jaw chuck, in which the thumb opposes the index and long fingers. The ring and little fingers of the prosthetic hand do not move. Hooks provide finger-tip prehension.
- Grasp size: The anatomical adult hand can grasp a basketball and span an octave on the piano. TDs have a maximum grasp size of approximately 4 inches, adequate for most basic tools.
- Grasp force: Healthy young men achieve prehension forces in excess of 120 lb. Most daily activities, however, require 7 lb or less of grasp force, although vocational and avocational tasks may need more forceful prehension. Depending on TD design, grasp force ranges from 1-50 lb.[141]
- Sensation: The human hand has receptors that detect movement, heat, cold, light touch, and deep pressure. TDs provide no sensory feedback, other than visual cues.

TDs may be passive or active. A passive TD has a wire armature in each finger to allow the wearer to bend or straighten the digit with the other hand, or with pressure against a firm surface. This type of hands is lightweight, inexpensive, and durable and can be used to hold packages, stabilize paper while the wearer is writing, and improves overall appearance.

Active hands have a wearer-controlled mechanism to allow prehension. A myoelectrically controlled hand is one with a battery-powered motor that is activated by contraction of the remnants of forearm muscles. In the usual transradial arrangement, the person has skin electrodes embedded in the socket of the prosthesis (Fig. 12-19). One electrode lies over the forearm flexors and another electrode lies over the extensors. Isometric flexor muscle contraction generates an action potential, which is detected by the electrode that in turn transmits the signal to the motor that triggers the closing mechanism. With some versions, the longer the patient maintains the contraction, the greater the force of closure and more closely the three radial prosthetic fingers approach one another. Most myoelectric hands are designed to provide grasp forces ranging from less than 1 lb to approximately 35 lb. Relaxation of the forearm muscles causes the fingers to remain in the position they were in just before relaxation, and the hand is opened by the wearer contracting the extensor muscles.

Myoelectric hands are popular because they have a good appearance and provide useful grasp force and because most transradial prostheses with myoelectric terminal devices do not require a harness over the torso. A multicenter comparison of 120 children fitted with both myoelectric and cable-controlled hands revealed that although 78% preferred the myoelectric hands, at a 2-year follow-up only 44% continued to wear the myoelectric TD.[142] More recently developed hands include force sensors that automatically adjust grip force to maintain grasp of a heavy object without additional muscular contraction.

Electric switch-controlled hands are also available. These have a battery-powered motor that is operated by the wearer using a pull switch or similar mechanism attached to a harness. These switch-controlled hands are less expensive than myoelectric ones but do require the patient to wear a harness.

Limitations of motorized hands are that they require occasional recharging of the battery and the relative delicacy of the mechanism requiring that the patient refrain from immersing the hand in fluids. Also, the prosthesis, whether myoelectric or switch-controlled, is relatively heavy, and finger action rather slow.

Another option for hand prostheses are cable-controlled hands. Depending on the mechanism, the wearer can either close (*voluntary closing* [VC]) or open (*voluntary opening* [VO]) the three radial fingers by applying tension to a cable attached to a harness. These hands are less expensive and lighter than electric hands, but the mechanism is still relatively fragile and must be protected

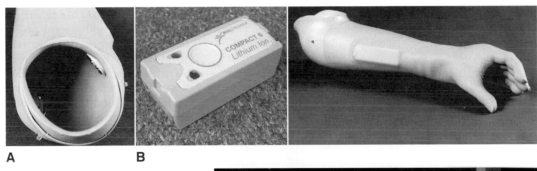

A   B

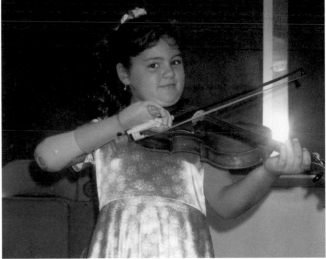

FIG. 12-19 Myoelectric transradial prosthesis. **A,** Electrode placement within the socket. **B,** The battery pack is positioned in the forearm. **C,** Playing the violin with a myoelectric prosthesis. *A and B From Zenie J: Prosthetic options for persons with upper extremity amputation. In Lusardi MM, Nielsen CC (eds):* Orthotics and Prosthetics in Rehabilitation, *ed 2, St. Louis, 2006, Butterworth-Heinemann. C Courtesy MH Mandelbaum Orthotic & Prosthetic Services.*

C

against immersion, debris, and rough use. Also, the grasp force with VO hands is approximately 4 lb, which is insufficient for many functional tasks.

Hooks are the primary alternative to prosthetic hands. Although a hook does not resemble the natural hand, it does provide the wearer with a versatile tool to assist in performance of many activities. Hooks are manufactured in sizes to fit 6-month-old infants to adults with moderately large hands. Cable-controlled hooks are the lightest, least expensive, and most durable TDs. Cable-controlled hooks consist of a moving tine, known as a finger, which pivots toward a fixed finger, providing pinch. A cable is attached distally to a projection on the moving finger and proximally to the harness. Hooks are made of aluminum, steel, or titanium and have neoprene-lined fingers. Most VO hooks (Fig. 12-20) have one or more rubber bands proximally that determine grasp force. An experienced wearer usually has enough bands to provide 5-8 lb of grasp force. The patient exerts force through the harness to open the hook and tension of the rubber bands causes closure. VC hooks (Fig. 12-21) have a mechanism that responds to the tension the wearer applies to the cable. As the wearer increases the cable tension the grip force increases up to about 60 lb. Relaxation of cable tension allows the hook to open.

The relatively slender fingers of a hook TD allow the wearer to see the object being manipulated better than with a prosthetic hand. This is important because all prostheses lack tactile sensation. One can also operate a cable-controlled hook with greater accuracy and speed than

other devices, and the small contact area of the hook allows manipulation of very small objects. Hooks with myoelectric mechanism are also occasionally prescribed. These provide substantial grasp force but weigh more and are more expensive than cable-controlled hooks.

Wrist Unit. With any type of upper extremity amputation the TD is generally attached to a wrist unit that provides rotation to enable pronation and supination of the TD. With a friction wrist unit, the TD is turned by the wearer who twists it with the sound hand, or nudges it against a firm surface. A rubber washer or a clamp within the unit maintains the desired position, although there are devices with locking mechanisms to provide greater stability. With a locking wrist unit, the patient must unlock the unit, turn it, and then lock it manually. A few wrist units have a mechanism to allow the wearer to select 0, 25, or 50 degrees of palmar flexion. This feature is important to those who cannot position the TD at the midline by internally rotating the shoulder. The typical candidate for a wrist flexion unit is someone with bilateral transhumeral amputations.

Socket. The prosthesis for a patient with a transradial amputation has a plastic forearm proximal to the wrist unit that attaches to a custom-made plastic socket. The amputation limb fits into the socket. The length of the socket-forearm combination should equal the length of the sound forearm.

Suspension. An upper extremity prosthesis is secured to the patient's body either by a snugly fitted socket or by a harness. Socket suspension requires that the proximal brim of the socket encase the humeral epicondyles; this design is known as supracondylar suspension. Myoelectric

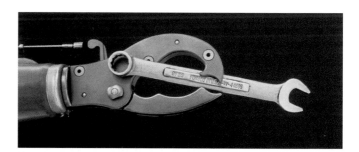

A

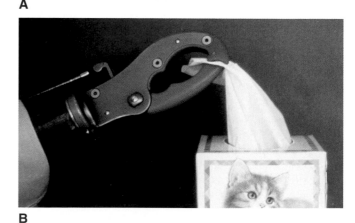

B

FIG. 12-20 Voluntary-opening hook. *Courtesy Hosmer Dorrance Corporation, Campbell, Calif.*

FIG. 12-21 Voluntary-closing hooks. *Courtesy T.R.S., Inc., Boulder, Colo.*

transradial prostheses usually have supracondylar suspension. The Muenster socket, developed in Muenster, Germany, is a type of socket that encases the epicondyles and the olecranon. This is indicated for short and very short residual limbs. An alternative to supracondylar or Muenster suspension is a roll-on flexible plastic suspension sleeve, with electrodes embedded in it if myoelectric control is to be used.

A harness can also be used to both suspend an upper extremity prosthesis and transmit shoulder motion to a cable-controlled TD. This harness is usually made of Dacron tape and has a transradial figure-of-eight design. The harness is made with two strips of tape riveted to the medial and lateral sides of the socket and then joined in an inverted Y strap over the anterior aspect of the upper arm. The strap then passes through the deltopectoral triangle to the back of the torso, crossing the spine to pass under the contralateral axilla and then around the contralateral shoulder, to form an axillary loop. From there, the strap passes back over the spine to the distal portion of the scapula, where it is known as the control attachment strap because it is buckled to the control cable. The figure-of-eight harness is easy to don and is relatively inconspicuous because it does not cross the front of the chest. The figure-of-nine harness is similar, having an axillary loop and a control attachment strap, but it lacks the inverted Y portion because the figure-of-nine harness is worn with a supracondylar or Muenster socket. Patients who cannot tolerate an axillary loop can wear a transradial chest strap harness. This type of harness includes a strap that encircles the chest and a broad shoulder saddle that lies over the ipsilateral shoulder and is attached to the chest strap. The control attachment strap extends from the posterior portion of the chest strap to the control cable. The patient must unbuckle the strap when doffing the harness. Some people complain that this type of harness is uncomfortable or unsightly.

Control Systems. Upper extremity prostheses, except passive hands, require a control system to control the TD and wrist unit. For a myoelectric prosthesis the wearer uses muscles within the socket to activate electrodes to achieve finger opening and closing. Cable controlled prostheses use a single steel cable attached distally to the TD and proximally to the control attachment strap (Fig. 12-22). This cable is encased in a steel tubular housing secured distally to the socket and proximally to the proximal portion of the socket or to a flexible plastic or leather pad placed over the triceps muscle. The housing prevents the cable from bowstringing when the wearer bends the elbow. Flexing the glenohumeral joint or abducting the scapula applies tension to the cable, and this tension opens or closes the TD, depending on its mechanism.

Transhumeral Prostheses. The transhumeral prosthesis includes all the components used in a transradial prosthesis with the addition of a forearm section and an elbow unit (Fig. 12-23).

Terminal Device and Wrist Unit. Any type of TD and wrist unit can be included in a transhumeral prosthesis. Some patients with a short transhumeral or *humeral neck amputation* or a shoulder disarticulation or forequarter amputation may require a wrist flexion unit to position

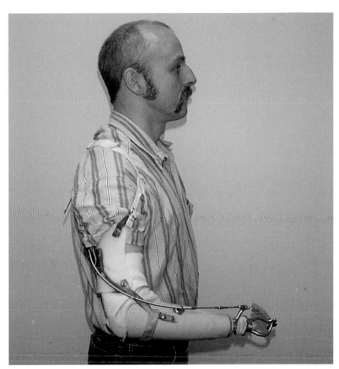

FIG. 12-22 Transradial prosthesis. *Courtesy Hosmer Dorrance Corporation, Campbell, Calif.*

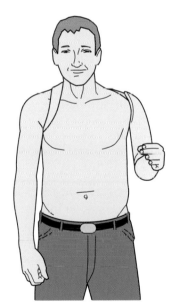

FIG. 12-23 Transhumeral prosthesis.

the TD close to the mouth, chest, and perineum. In all instances, the wrist unit is bonded to the distal end of the forearm arm section that is a plastic truncated cone the same length as the missing anatomical forearm.

Elbow Unit. Prostheses for amputations at the standard transhumeral level and higher require an elbow unit that enables elbow flexion and extension, locking, and rotation. The elbow unit has a turntable to provide transverse rotation. The patient can position the forearm manually by pushing it away from or toward the chest. The turntable is needed even if the glenohumeral joint is unimpaired because the cylindrical residual limb encased in a cylindrical socket would rotate inside the socket, rather than transmitting anatomical shoulder rotation to the distal portion of the prosthesis.

The elbow unit is embedded in the proximal portion of the forearm section. Elbow units provide a hinge for elbow flexion and extension; most also have a lock to secure the desired elbow angle and a turntable to allow the wearer to rotate the forearm horizontally. Young children are usually fitted with a passive elbow unit with a hinge with a friction clamp that maintains the desired elbow angle.

Older children and adults are generally fitted with a cable-controlled locking elbow unit that can be locked in seven, eleven, or more positions, depending on the design. Tension on the locking cable locks and then unlocks the unit, triggering an alternator mechanism within the unit. Tension on a separate cable flexes and extends the elbow. Myoelectrically controlled elbow units enable elbow flexion and extension, as well as locking. The elbow motor is activated by different skin electrodes than those that operate the TD. Some people are fitted with a hybrid prosthesis that combines a myoelectrically controlled hand with a cable-controlled elbow unit.

Socket. The transhumeral socket is custom made of plastic. The patient with an elbow disarticulation can be fitted with a socket that terminates at the proximal portion of the upper arm. Those with higher amputations need a socket that extends superiorly to maintain stable fit, although such higher trim lines do somewhat restrict shoulder motion.

Suspension. Transhumeral prostheses usually require harness suspension because there are no bony prominences available for their suspension. The usual harness is the transhumeral figure-of-eight harness. This is similar to the transradial figure-of-eight harness with the addition of an elbow lock control strap and more suspension straps. A few patients are fitted with a transhumeral chest strap harness.

Control Systems. Cable control of the transhumeral prosthesis is usually achieved with two cables, each encased in steel housing. One cable extends from the control attachment strap on the back of the harness to the TD. This cable has proximal and distal housing sections. If the elbow unit is unlocked, tension on the cable causes elbow flexion; controlled relaxation of the cable allows the elbow to extend. If the elbow unit is locked, tension on the same cable activates the TD. The second cable extends from the elbow unit locking mechanism to the anterior support strap of the harness. Tension on this cable locks and unlocks the elbow unit alternatively.

Electrically powered elbow units are less commonly prescribed. These are activated by switches in the harness or elsewhere in the prosthesis, or by skin electrodes placed over the remnants of the anterior and posterior deltoid muscles.

Controls Training. Once the prosthesis is custom made for the patient, it should be assessed carefully. Often the therapist performs the examination and reports the findings to others on the clinical team. Controls training should not proceed until the clinical team is certain that the prosthesis fits and operates properly; otherwise, the wearer is apt to exert unnecessary effort to achieve adequate function. Controls training involves instructing the patient to operate all components of the prosthesis, as well to don the appliance.

Transradial Prosthesis. Donning is an essential skill. The patient first dons a T-shirt to protect the skin from irritation by the harness straps. Then the amputation limb is placed in a cotton, wool, nylon, or silicone sock. The patient then inserts the residual limb into the socket and then places the sound hand through the axillary loop. If a chest strap is used for suspension, the person should place the residual limb in the socket, wrap the chest strap around the torso, and then fasten the strap in the front.

A supracondylar or Muenster socket fits very snugly. To don this, the residual limb is first put in tubular stockinet with the distal end of the stockinet extending beyond the end of the residual limb. The patient then inserts the residual limb in the socket, taking care to place the end of the stockinet through a hole drilled through the end of the socket. The stockinet continues through another hole in the plastic forearm. The person tugs on the stockinet to draw the skin and subcutaneous soft tissue into the socket. If the socket is part of a myoelectrically controlled prosthesis, the patient continues pulling on the stockinet until it is pulled completely out of the prosthesis, so that the skin is in direct contact with the socket and its electrodes. If the socket is part of a cable-controlled prosthesis, the patient pulls on the stockinet until the socket is well positioned, then tucks the end of the stockinet into the forearm cavity.

TD operation with a myoelectrically controlled prosthesis begins before construction of the prosthesis. The therapist uses an electrode to determine where on the forearm the greatest voltage can be measured when the patient forcefully contracts the flexor or extensor muscles. The patient then practices isolated contraction of the flexors while maintaining relaxation of the extensors, and vice versa. Once optimal electrode positions are found, the electrodes are embedded in the socket so that they overlie these chosen sites. With the finished prosthesis on, the patient then practices opening the TD to different distances, as well as closing the TD with various amounts of force. The rehabilitation program emphasizes endurance exercises for the forearm musculature to reduce fatigue when the patient is engaging in a prolonged task.

Cable-controlled TD training begins with the prosthesis on the patient. The best position for early training is with the elbow flexed approximately 90 degrees because the wearer can see the TD easily and the harness and cable are in the easiest position for TD operation. The therapist resists glenohumeral flexion until the patient observes the TD open or close. If the TD is voluntary opening, it will open; if it is voluntary closing, it will close. The patient practices glenohumeral flexion until the motion can be done without external resistance and the TD operates reliably. Control motion should be confined to the amputated side because tensing the contralateral musculature can interfere with performance of bimanual activities. The next step in training involves having the patient keep the elbow flexed while attempting to operate the TD by abducting the scapula. This maneuver achieves TD operation close to the body.

With a VC TD the wearer practices closing it gently, then forcefully, and then with intermediate amounts of force. Control of a VO TD includes drills in opening the hand or hook at various distances. The patient also practices relaxing cable tension to allow the device to snap closed. The most difficult control procedure requires the wearer to close the TD partially by maintaining tension on the control attachment strap.

Regardless of TD design, after mastering the basic opening and closing maneuvers, the patient then practices operating the TD with the elbow extended, fully flexed, and at intermediate angles and with the shoulder in all positions.

Positioning the TD involves using the wrist unit. An array of soft and firm balls, cubes, disks, and prisms of various sizes, known as a form board, can be used to practice grasping, holding, and releasing commonly shaped objects. Most pieces on the form board can be grasped with the TD pronated. Some items, such as disks, are easier to manage if the TD is placed halfway between pronation and supination. A large, rigid ball is most readily secured in a hook turned to the supinated position; with a prosthetic hand, the ball is easier to grasp with the TD pronated. The therapist teaches the patient to rotate the wrist unit to position the TD appropriately. If the wrist unit has a locking mechanism, the wearer must unlock it, rotate the TD, and then relock the wrist unit.

Transhumeral Prosthesis. Donning a transhumeral prosthesis with a figure-of-eight harness is easiest with the prosthesis placed on a table with the harness untangled. The patient wears a T-shirt and a residual limb sock, inserts the sound extremity into the axillary loop, and then places the residual limb in the socket. If the prosthesis has a chest strap, the individual dons the socket, encircles the chest with the chest strap, and then secures it.

TD operation and positioning is taught first with the elbow lock engaged. TD and wrist unit operation are performed in the same way as for a transradial prosthesis. The therapist also teaches the patient to rotate the forearm in the horizontal plane by pulling or pushing the forearm so that the elbow unit pivots at the turntable.

Elbow unit control begins with the elbow unlocked. The therapist shows the patient that the same glenohumeral flexion or scapular abduction that operates the TD also flexes the elbow because the cable connected to the TD also passes in front of the elbow hinge. To extend the elbow, the patient gradually relaxes the shoulder or scapular musculature.

The second step in elbow unit control is elbow locking and unlocking. Training should start with the prosthesis off the patient. The therapist shows the patient that the elbow lock is an alternator mechanism, that is, the first pull on the elbow lock cable locks the unit. The next pull unlocks it; a soft clicking sound occurs when the alternator engages. The patient pulls on the elbow lock cable with the sound hand until smooth, reliable action is achieved. Then with the prosthesis on the patient, the therapist

unlocks the elbow and supports the forearm with one hand while using the other hand to resist an oblique movement composed of humeral hyperextension and shoulder girdle depression until the elbow locks. Repeating the movement unlocks the unit. The patient then practices rapid elbow locking and unlocking while the therapist continues to support the forearm. The final step in elbow unit controls training requires coordination of elbow flexion and locking. The patient flexes the elbow to the desired angle, then locks it quickly. If the locking motion is done slowly, the forearm would extend. Flexion of the elbow hinge requires shoulder flexion, and elbow locking needs shoulder hyperextension.

Use Training. Use training emphasizes employing the prosthesis as an assistive device, complementing maneuvers of the sound hand. Most daily activities, such as drinking from a cup, are naturally performed with one hand. The individual who wears a prosthesis would do the same and generally hold the cup in the intact hand. A few tasks, however, are ordinarily done bimanually. These activities form the basis of use training. In general, the prosthesis performs the more stationary portion of the task. The therapist should allow the patient to experiment with various techniques, offering cues only when the individual is stymied. Techniques used by people with hemiplegia often work well for those with an amputation. Some adaptive aids, such as a cutting board with protruding nails to stabilize objects on the board, can be useful. Use training is beneficial whether the patient has an active or passive TD.

Washing the face can be done entirely with one hand. Nevertheless, it is usually easier to stabilize the wash cloth with the prosthesis while soaping it with the soap held in the sound hand. To wash the sound hand, one can hold the bar of soap in the TD while moving the hand over the soap. One does not wear a prosthesis while showering or tub bathing. Grooming may challenge the ingenuity of the patient. Most appliances, however, can be managed with one hand. A toothbrush, for example, is used with one hand. Extracting toothpaste from a pump dispenser can be done by pressing on the nozzle control with the forearm on the amputated side while the sound hand holds the brush. With a toothpaste tube, one can press on the tube with the forearm. An electric or manual shaver suits one-handed use, as do simpler hair styles and makeup.

Dressing involves practice with buttoning, using a zipper, and managing other garment fasteners. The prosthesis can be used to stabilize the fabric while the sound hand manipulates the closure. Some people use a button hook to facilitate buttoning. Shirts, jackets, and coats are most readily donned by slipping the prosthesis into the sleeve and then maneuvering the intact arm in the other sleeve. Pullover shirts and sweaters are most manageable if the garment is laid on a bed or table. The prosthesis enters its sleeve first, following by introducing the head through the neck opening and the sound arm into its sleeve. Trousers and skirts are easy to don if the sound hand holds one side of the waistband and the prosthesis holds the other side. The prosthesis stabilizes the distal end of the zipper while the sound hand pulls the slider.

Dining can be entirely one-handed, depending on the menu. The activity that is most often accomplished with the aid of a prosthesis is cutting meat. The prosthesis holds the fork, while the sound hand grasps the knife. After one or more morsels are cut, the wearer switches utensils to spear food and bring it to the mouth with the fork held in the intact hand.

Writing can be done either with the sound hand or terminal device. If the nondominant hand is absent, then the person generally holds the pen in the sound hand. The TD stabilizes the paper, especially when the writing surface is firm such as a glass counter at a bank. If the dominant hand was amputated, the patient may have learned to change dominance in the preprosthetic phase of rehabilitation. Alternatively, the individual with a transradial amputation can hold a pen in the TD, relying on shoulder and elbow motion to shape the letters. Because they lack natural elbow motion, those with a transhumeral amputation generally find it easier to learn to write with the sound hand.

Vocations. The prosthesis serves as a useful tool to aid in the performance of the clerical aspects of most school and professional endeavors. Machinery may also be adapted, often with little cost or effort, to suit the capabilities of most people who wear a prosthesis. Unlike those with more distal amputations, people with transhumeral amputations will have difficulty reaching overhead with the prosthesis. Keyboard control can be aided by use of a keyboard designed for one-handed use. Alternatively, one can press the key with the tip of the hook or with the eraser end of a pencil held in the TD using a one-finger, "hunt and peck" technique. Driving is aided by a spinner knob bolted to the steering wheel.

Care of the Residual Limb and Prosthesis. The residual limb must be kept clean and dry. Nightly use of a moisturizing lotion should keep the skin supple. The patient should inspect the torso and both arms for signs of reddening at the margins of the prosthesis and along the path of the harness, with particular attention to the contralateral axilla.

TD care is simplest with the cable-controlled hook. The device should be kept clean and wiped dry if unintentionally immersed. One should check the neoprene lining for deep cracks, which indicate that the lining needs replacement. Rubber bands on a hook should be changed when they become brittle.

With a prosthetic hand, care of the glove includes avoiding sharp or rough textured objects. The glove can be cleaned with a slightly moistened soapy cloth. One should never place the hand on a varnished surface. The wearer should avoid exposing the glove to solvents, such as gasoline, kerosene, or turpentine, or staining agents like ballpoint pen ink, newsprint, tobacco, mustard, grape juice, and beet juice. Nail polish can be worn but must be removed by scraping rather than with acetone.

The socket should be wiped each evening with a moistened soapy cloth. Unless the prosthesis is myoelectrically controlled, one should wear a fresh sock daily. Most harnesses can be unbuckled from the rest of the prosthesis. The Dacron strap can then be laundered. If the housing on the control cable becomes unwound, it would snag clothing and possibly cause the control cable to break and then the housing would require replacement. A clean T-shirt worn under the harness protects the skin and the harness.

ADVANCED ACTIVITIES

Depending on the individual's stamina and motivation, the rehabilitation program may go considerably beyond basic training. For the person with lower extremity amputation, advanced activities may include climbing stairs and curbs, kneeling, stepping over obstacles, running, and jumping.

Sometimes the side of amputation is pertinent. For example, transferring into the passenger side of a car is easier for someone wearing a right lower extremity prosthesis than a left one. The person would simply swing the intact left leg into the car, then lift or otherwise move the prosthesis into place. Driving, however, is easier for the person with a left prosthesis because the individual can use the intact, sensate right foot to operate the accelerator and brake pedals of a vehicle with automatic transmission. The adult who wears a right prosthesis can cross the left leg over the right to use the sound foot for pedaling. Alternatively, the person can attach a pedal extension to enable right foot operation. People with unilateral or bilateral transtibial amputation can also operate the car with the prosthetic feet, relying on proprioception from the knee and hip for safe operation; however, it is prudent to check the state motor vehicle regulations to determine whether such operation is permissible. Hand controls are indicated for the individual with bilateral transfemoral amputations, with or without prostheses.

Bicycling is easier if a toe clip is added to the pedal on the amputated side. A prosthesis is more effective at pulling the pedal than pushing it. Some individuals with lower extremity amputations bicycle without a prosthesis. Skiing can be performed with short rudders attached to the ski poles whether or not the person wears a leg prosthesis. Those with bilateral leg amputation often use a sled for winter fun.

Sports that require running or jumping can be enjoyed by people with leg amputation. Even with an energy-storing prosthetic foot, the athlete gets more propulsive force from the sound leg; consequently, the individual usually runs with a hop-skip progression. Runners with bilateral amputations generally wear a pair of Flex-Feet or other energy-storing feet designed for running. Jumping also relies on the power generated by the sound leg. Regular participation in vigorous activity has been shown to be associated with positive body image.[142]

Some people with upper extremity amputation may develop considerable manipulative skill for vocational and avocational pursuits. Many musical instruments can be played by children and adults with upper extremity amputation. The most accessible are brass wind instruments because the valves are ordinarily operated with one hand while the prosthesis stabilizes the instrument. One may have to switch hands; for example, a trumpet is designed to be played with the right hand controlling the valves. It can, however, be played with the left hand. Conversely, the French horn, normally played with the left hand, can be operated in reverse. The trombone is well suited to people with amputations because most models have no valves. Guitars and other stringed instruments, ordinarily fingered with the left hand, can have the strings reversed. This may also require changing the position of the bridge, depending on the instrument. A pick or bow can be adapted so it is secured in the TD or in an elastic cuff worn on the forearm. Piano compositions for one-handed performance exist in the beginner, intermediate, and advanced repertory.

Sports are well within the reach of individuals with upper or lower extremity amputation, whether or not they wear regular or modified prostheses or use modified equipment. Special TDs can be exchanged for the usual one to hold a bowling ball or golf club, manage a baseball catcher's mitt, and perform gymnastic stunts. Professional football, basketball, and baseball players with limb deficiencies are role models for their skilled one-handed prowess. Accounts of athletes who overcame major impairments may inspire some patients.[143-145] Many sports organizations are open to people with disabilities. Participation is an excellent way of integrating into the community, as well as garnering the physiological benefits of exercise

CASE STUDY 12-1

CLOSED AMPUTATION LEFT TIBIA

Examination
Patient History
AB is a 72-year-old retired machinist. He is a widower who was diagnosed with type 2 diabetes 7 years ago. He tests his blood glucose daily and relies on diet to control his glucose levels. Four years ago, he began to experience intermittent claudication in his left leg. Angiography revealed blockage of the left peroneal artery, for which he underwent successful angioplasty. After the surgery, the claudication resolved but started to return a year ago when he cut his left hallux on a shard of glass. A week later, the wound still had not healed, and the toe was now discolored. His physician repeated the angiogram and found that the angioplasty had occluded. Within 2 weeks the entire forefoot became gangrenous. Two vascular surgeons recommended immediate amputation at the musculotendinous junction of the left leg. AB presents 3 weeks after a closed amputation through the proximal tibia with myodesis. Postoperatively, the limb was dressed with elastic bandage compressive dressing.

Systems Review
BP was 165/92 mm Hg. Pulse rate was 84 bpm. Well-healed amputation scar on left lower limb.

Tests and Measures
Musculoskeletal
Anthropometric Characteristics The amputation limb is 7 inches long from the medial tibial plateau to the bony end of the tibia. The circumference has smooth contours with no proximal constriction or distal tissue redun-

dancy. The right ankle has normal alignment, and the second and third toes show mild claw deformity.

Range of Motion Knee flexion 0 to 125 degrees bilaterally; hip flexion, extension, adduction, abduction, external rotation, and internal rotation within normal limits bilaterally. No restriction of trunk or upper extremity motion.

Muscle Performance Left: Quadriceps 3/5; hamstrings 4/5; hip musculature within normal limits. Right: Ankle, knee, and hip strength within normal limits.

Joint Integrity and Mobility Both knees have mild crepitus and no mediolateral or anteroposterior laxity. Both hips have full passive motion without pain.
Neuromuscular
Sensory Integrity Sensation is intact on the residual left limb and the entire right lower extremity
Cardiovascular
Circulation Skin temperature normal to touch on right foot and left amputation limb.
Integumentary
Integumentary Integrity Left: The amputation scar is well healed, nonadherent, and with minimal invagination. Color and temperature are normal. Ample granulation tissue is evident, with no exudate.

Right: There is interdigital dermatitis and dorsal calluses on the second and third toes.

Evaluation, Diagnosis, and Prognosis
AB has had a left transtibial amputation likely as the result of diabetic arteriosclerosis.

Goals
1. Community ambulation with a prosthesis and cane within 6 months.
2. Indoors: Walk 50 yards in 3 minutes without a cane.
3. Resume independent homemaking in his apartment.

Prognosis
AB's prognosis is good.

Intervention
Postoperative Management
AB was instructed in a ROM and general conditioning exercise program by his therapist. He quickly progressed to doing this program independently. He was instructed to wear his temporary prosthesis 8-10 hours daily. Transfer and mobility training included 3 point transfer (weight bearing on sound foot and both hands on parallel bars or walker), ambulation, relying on bimanual support standing within parallel bars, and progression to ambulation with a walker. He wore his elastic shrinker sock at night. AB was reexamined at 4 weeks postoperatively.

Prosthetic Management
A definitive prosthesis was successfully fitted for AB at 6 weeks postoperatively. Therapy intervention included donning and doffing his prosthesis, balance facilitation, and gait training. Emphasis for AB's therapy was on left knee control, safe ADL performance, and increasing his endurance. He successfully transferred to chairs with and

without armrests, including automobile transfers. AB was instructed in and was able to independently climb curbs and stairs with a handrail. AB resumed driving after training.

Please see the CD that accompanies this book for case studies describing the examination, evaluation, and interventions for a patient undergoing rehabilitation after a left transfemoral amputation and for a patient undergoing rehabilitation after a right long transradial amputation

CHAPTER SUMMARY

Amputation is a relatively infrequent occurrence in the civilian world. Lower extremity amputation is much more common than upper extremity amputation, with PVD being the principal cause. People with transtibial, transfemoral, transradial, and transhumeral amputations are most frequently seen in rehabilitation. The functional outcome of adults with unilateral lower extremity amputation depends on amputation level, as well as the individual's general health. Ambulation with a prosthesis is slower and consumes more energy per distance than able-bodied gait. People fitted with a unilateral upper extremity prosthesis can accomplish activities of daily living, although many tasks can also be done one-handed. Advanced activities for all patients involve maneuvering over all types of terrain and engaging in recreational activities. In all instances, the goal of rehabilitation is to enable the patient to engage in the broadest range of endeavors.

ADDITIONAL RESOURCES

Useful Forms

Transfemoral Examination Questions
Transtibial Examination Questions

Books

Burgess EM, Rappoport A: *Physical Fitness: A Guide for Individuals with Lower Limb Loss,* Washington, DC, 1990, Department of Veterans Affairs.

Carroll K, Edelstein JE: *Prosthetics and Patient Management: A Comprehensive Clinical Approach,* Thorofare, NJ, 2006, Slack.

Engstrom B, Van De Ven C: *Therapy for Amputees,* ed 3, New York, 1999, Churchill Livingstone.

Ham R, Cotton L: *Limb Amputation: From Aetiology to Rehabilitation,* London, 1991, Chapman & Hall.

Harmarville Rehabilitation Center: *Learning and Living after Your Leg Amputation.* Pittsburgh, 1983, The Center.

Karacoloff LA, Hammersley CS, Schneider FJ (eds): *Lower Extremity Amputation,* ed 2, Gaithersburg, Md, 1992, Aspen Publishers.

Lusardi MM, Nielsen CC (eds): *Orthotics and Prosthetics in Rehabilitation,* Boston, 2005, Elsevier.

May BJ: *Amputations and Prosthetics: A Case Study Approach,* ed 2, Philadelphia, 2002, FA Davis.

Meier RH, Atkins DJ: *Functional Restoration of Adults and Children with Upper Extremity Amputations,* New York, 2004, Demos Medical Publishing.

Mensch G, Ellis PM: *Physical Therapy Management of Lower Extremity Amputations,* Gaithersburg, Md, 1986, Aspen.

Murdoch G, Wilson AB (eds): *Amputation: Surgical Practice and Patient Management,* Oxford, 1996, Butterworth Heinemann.

Seymour R: *Prosthetics and Orthotics: Lower Limb and Spinal,* Philadelphia, 2002, Lippincott Williams & Wilkins.

Shurr DG, Michael JW: *Prosthetics and Orthotics,* ed 2, Upper Saddle River, NJ, 2002, Prentice Hall.

Smith D, Bowker JH, Michael JW (eds): *Atlas of Limb Prosthetics: Surgical, Prosthetic, and Rehabilitation Principles,* ed 3, Chicago, 2004, American Academy of Orthopaedic Surgeons.

Winchell E: *Coping with Limb Loss,* Garden City Park, NY, 1995, Avery Publishing Group.

Journals

Journal of Prosthetics and Orthotics: www.oandp.org/jpo
Journal of Rehabilitation Research and Development: www.vard.org/jour/jourindx.html
O&P (Orthotics and Prosthetics) Business News: www.oandpbiznews.com/

Web Sites

American Academy of Orthotists and Prosthetists: www.oandp.org
American Amputee Soccer Association: www.ampsoccer.org
American Association of Adapted Sports Programs: www.aaasp.org
American Board for Certification in Orthotics & Prosthetics, Inc.: www.abcop.org
American Orthotic and Prosthetic Association: www.aopnet.org
Amputee Coalition of America: www.amputee-coalition.org
Amputees in Motion: www.usinter.net
Association of Birth Defect Children, Inc.: www.birthdefects.org
Association of Children's Prosthetic-Orthotic Clinics: www.acpoc.org
Barr Foundation: www.oandp.com/barr
Association of Brånemark Osseointegration Centers: www.branemark.se
Disabled Sports USA: www.dsusa.org
Eastern Amputee Golf Association: www.eaga.org
Family Center on Technology and Disability: www.fctd.info
Helping Hands Group: www.helpinghandsgroup.org
Rehabilitation Engineering and Assistive Technology Society of North America (RESNA): www.resna.org/
International Center for Disability Resources on the Internet: www.icdri.org
International Child Amputee Network: www.child-amputee.net
International Society for Prosthetics and Orthotics: www.ispo.ws/
Limb Differences: www.limbdifferences.org
National Amputee Golfers Association: www.nagagolf.org
National Center on Physical Activity and Disability: www.ncpad.org
National Disability Sports Alliance: ndsaonline.org
Pedorthic Footwear Association: www.pedorthics.org
United Amputee Services Association: www.oandp.com/resources/organizations/uasa/
Wheelchair Sports USA: www.wsusa.org

GLOSSARY

Closed amputation: Amputation surgery in which the skin is sutured.

Forequarter amputation: Amputation through any portions of the scapula, clavicle, and thorax.

Guillotine amputation: Amputation surgery in which all portions of the limb are severed at the same level.

Hansen's disease: Leprosy, a communicable disease caused by mycobacterium leprae which may result in autoamputation of the digits, nose, and ears.

Humeral neck amputation: Amputation through the proximal portion of the humerus.

Keel: Longitudinal supporting structure of a prosthetic foot.

Myodesis: Amputation surgical procedure in which one muscle group is sutured to another group.

Myoplasty: Amputation surgical procedure in which muscles are sutured to bone through holes drilled in the bone.

Open amputation: Amputation surgery in which the skin is not sutured, because of infection. Secondary closed amputation is usually planned.

Phantom pain: Discomfort experienced in the missing limb segment.

Phantom sensation: Awareness of the missing limb segment.

Pylon: Endoprosthetic vertical support substituting for the shank.

Supracondylar suspension: Mode of suspension of a transtibial prosthesis in which the brim terminates immediately above the femoral epicondyles, or a transradial prosthesis in which the brim terminates immediately above the humeral epicondyles.

Syme's amputation: Amputation through the distal portion of the tibia and fibula, with the calcaneal fat pad sutured to the distal end of the amputation limb; all tarsals and distal structures are removed.

Transfemoral amputation: Amputation through the femur, previously known as above-knee.

Transhumeral amputation: Amputation through the humerus, previously known as above-elbow.

Translumbar amputation: Amputation through the lumbar spine, previously known as hemicorporectomy.

Transmetatarsal amputation: Amputation through the metatarsals.

Transpelvic amputation: Amputation through the pelvis, previously known as hemipelvectomy.

Transradial amputation: Amputation through the radius and ulna, previously known as below-elbow.

Unna dressing: Postoperative limb dressing composed of gauze permeated with zinc oxide, calamine, glycerin, and gelatin.

Voluntary closing: Mode of terminal device operation in which the patient volitionally closes the fingers and springs cause opening.

Voluntary opening: Mode of terminal device operation in which the patient volitionally opens the fingers and rubber bands or springs cause closing.

References

1. Dillingham TR, Pezzin LE, MacKenzie EJ: Limb amputation and limb deficiency: Epidemiology and recent trends in the United States, *South Med J* 95:875-883, 2002.
2. Bowker JH: The choice between amputation and limb salvage. In Bowker JH, Michael JW, (eds): *Atlas of Limb Prosthetics: Surgical, Prosthetic, and Rehabilitation Principles*, ed 2, St. Louis, 1992, Mosby–Year Book.
3. Mayfield JA, Reiber GE, Maynard C, et al: Trends in lower limb amputation in the Veterans Health Administration, 1989-1998, *J Rehabil Res Dev* 37:23-30, 2000.
4. Armstrong DG, Lavery LA, van Houtun WH, et al: The impact of gender on amputation, *J Foot Ankle Surg* 36:66-69, 1997.
5. Group TG: Epidemiology of lower extremity amputation in centres in Europe, North America and East Asia: The global lower extremity amputation study group, *Br J Surg* 87:328-337, 2000.
6. Pasquina PF: Optimizing care for combat amputees: Experiences at Walter Reed Army Medical Center, *J Rehabil Res Dev* 41:vii-xv, 2004.
7. Rijnders LJ, Boonstra AM, Groothoff JW, et al: Lower limb deficient children in The Netherlands: Epidemiological aspects, *Prosthet Orthot Int* 24:13-18, 2000.
8. Fisk JR: Terminology in pediatric limb deficiency. In Smith DG, Michael JW, Bowker JH, (eds): *Atlas of Amputations and Limb Deficiencies*, ed 3, Rosemont, Ill, 2004, American Academy of Orthopaedic Surgeons.
9. Lawton RL, DePinto V: Bilateral hip disarticulation in paraplegics with decubitus ulcers, *Arch Surg* 122:1040-1043, 1987.
10. Chansky HA: Hip disarticulation and transpelvic amputation: surgical management. In Smith DG, Michael JW, Bowker JH, (eds): *Atlas of Amputations and Limb Deficiencies*, ed 3, Rosemont, Ill, 2004, American Academy of Orthopaedic Surgeons.
11. Darnall BD, Ephraim P, Wegener ST: Depressive symptoms and mental health service utilization among persons with limb loss: Results of a national survey, *Arch Phys Med Rehabil* 86:650-658, 2005.
12. Ehde DM, Smith DG: Chronic pain management. In Smith DG, Michael JW, Bowker JH, (eds): *Atlas of Amputations and Limb Deficiencies*, ed 3, Rosemont, Ill, 2004, American Academy of Orthopaedic Surgeons.
13. American Physical Therapy Association: *Guide to Physical Therapist Practice*, ed 2, Alexandria, Va, 2001, The Association.
14. HCFA Common Procedure Coding System: Washington, DC, 2001, US Government Printing Office.
15. Robinson-Whelen S, Bodenheimer C: Health practices of veterans with unilateral lower-limb loss: Identifying correlates, *J Rehabil Res Dev* 41:453-460, 2004.
16. Johannesson A, Larsson GU, Oberg T: From major amputation to prosthetic outcome: A prospective study of 190 patients in a defined population, *Prosthet Orthot Int* 28:9-21, 2004.
17. Dillingham TR, Pezzin LE, Shore AD: Reamputation, mortality, and health care costs among persons with dysvascular lower-limb amputations, *Arch Phys Med Rehabil* 86:480-485, 2005.
18. Thornhill HL, Jones GD, Brodzka W, et al: Bilateral below-knee amputations: Experience with 80 patients, *Arch Phys Med Rehabil* 67:159-163, 1986.
19. Gonzalez EG, Edelstein JE: Energy expenditure during ambulation. In Gonzalez EG, Myers SJ, Edelstein JE, et al (eds): *Downey & Darling's Physiological Basis of Rehabilitation Medicine*, ed 3, Boston, 2001, Butterworth Heinemann.
20. Gailey RS, Wenger MA, Raya M, et al: Energy expenditure of trans-tibial amputees during ambulation at self-selected pace, *Prosthet Orthot Int* 18:84-91, 1994.
21. Jaegers SMHJ, Vos LD, Rispens P, et al: The relationship between comfortable and most metabolically efficient walking speed in persons with unilateral above-knee amputation, *Arch Phys Med Rehabil* 74:521-525, 1993.
22. Nowroozi F, Saronelli ML, Gerber LH: Energy expenditure in hip disarticulation and hemipelvectomy, *Arch Phys Med Rehabil* 64:300-303, 1983.
23. Waters RL, Mulroy SJ: Energy expenditure of walking in individuals with lower limb amputations. In Smith DG, Michael JW, Bowker JH, (eds): *Atlas of Amputations and Limb Deficiencies*, ed 3, Rosemont, Ill, 2004, American Academy of Orthopaedic Surgeons.
24. van der Linde H, Hofstad CJ, Geurts ACH, et al: A systematic literature review of the effect of different prosthetic components on human functioning with a lower limb prosthesis, *J Rehabil Res Dev* 41:555-570, 2004.
25. Nielsen PH, Schurr DG, Golden JC, et al: Comparison of energy cost and gait efficiency during ambulation in below-knee amputees using different prosthetic feet, *J Prosthet Orthot* 1:24-31, 1989.
26. Hsu MJ, Nielsen DH, Yack HJ, Shurr DG. Physiological measurements of walking and running in people with transtibial amputations with 3 different prostheses, *JOSPT* 29:526-533, 1999.
27. Torburn L, Powers CM, Gutierrez R, et al: Energy expenditure during ambulation in dysvascular and traumatic below-knee amputees: A comparison of five prosthetic feet, *J Rehabil Res Dev* 32:111-119, 1995.
28. Casillas JM, Dulieu V, Cohen M, et al: Bioenergetic comparison of a new energy-storing foot and SACH foot in traumatic and vascular below-knee amputations, *Arch Phys Med Rehabil* 76:39-44, 1995.
29. Isakov E, Susak Z, Becker E: Energy expenditure and cardiac response in above-knee amputees while using prosthesis with open and locked knee mechanisms, *Scand J Rehab Med* 12(suppl):108-111, 1985.
30. Schmalz T, Blumentritt S, Jarasch R: Energy expenditure and biomechanical characteristics of lower limb amputee gait: The influence of prosthetic alignment and different prosthetic components, *Gait Posture* 16:255-263, 2002.
31. Chin T, Sawamura S, Shiba R, et al: Effect of an Intelligent Prosthesis (IP) on the walking ability of young transfemoral amputees: Comparison of IP users with above bodied people, *Am J Phys Med Rehabil* 82:447-451, 2003.
32. Perry J, Burnfield JM, Newsam CJ, et al: Energy expenditure and gait characteristics of a bilateral amputee walking with C-Leg prostheses compared with stubby and conventional articulating prostheses, *Arch Phys Med Rehabil* 85:1711-1717, 2004.
33. Chin T, Sawamura S, Shiba R, et al: Energy expenditure during walking in amputees after disarticulation of the hip: A microprocessor-controlled swing-phase control knee versus a mechanical-controlled stance-phase control knee, *J Bone Joint Surg Br* 87:117-119, 2005.
34. Gailey RS, Lawrence D, Barditt C: The CAT-CAM socket and quadrilateral socket: A comparison of energy cost during ambulation, *Prosthet Orthot Int* 17:95-100, 1993.
35. DuBow LL, Witt PL, Kadaba MP, et al: Oxygen consumption of elderly persons with bilateral below knee amputations: Ambulation vs. wheelchair propulsion, *Arch Phys Med Rehabil* 64:255-259, 1983.
36. Wu Y-J, Chen S-Y, Lin M-C, Lan C, et al: Energy expenditure of wheeling and walking during prosthetic rehabilitation in a woman with bilateral transfemoral amputations, *Arch Phys Med Rehabil* 82:265-269, 2001.
37. Bussman JB, Grootscholten EA, Stam HJ: Daily physical activity and heart rate response in people with a unilateral transtibial amputation for vascular disease, *Arch Phys Med Rehabil* 85:240-244, 2004.
38. Schoppen T, Boonstra A, Groothoff JW, et al: Physical, mental, and social predictors of functional outcome in unilateral lower-limb amputees, *Arch Phys Med Rehabil* 84:803-811, 2003.
39. Coleman KL, Boone DA, Laing LS, et al: Quantification of prosthetic outcomes: Elastomeric gel liner with locking pin suspension versus polyethylene foam liner with neoprene sleeve suspension, *J Rehabil Res Dev* 41:591-602, 2004.

40. Meikle B, Boulias C, Pauley T, et al: Does increased prosthetic weight affect gait speed and patient preference in dysvascular transfemoral amputees? *Arch Phys Med Rehabil* 84:1657-1661, 2003.
41. Rommers GM, Vos LD, Groothoff JW, et al: Mobility of people with lower limb amputations: Scales and questionnaires, *Clin Rehabil* 15:92-102, 2001.
42. Hanspal RS, Fisher K: Prediction of achieved mobility in prosthetic rehabilitation of the elderly using cognitive and psychomotor assessment, *Int J Rehabil Res* 20:315-318, 1997.
43. Davies B, Datta D: Mobility outcome following unilateral lower limb amputation, *Prosthet Orthot Int* 27:186-190, 2003.
44. Miller CA: Factors related to quality of life in elderly persons following lower limb amputation, *J Geriatr Phys Ther* 27:115, 2004.
45. Gailey RS, Roach KE, Applegate EG, et al: The Amputee Mobility Predictor: An instrument to assess determinants of the lower-limb amputee's ability to ambulate, *Arch Phys Med Rehabil* 83:613-627, 2002.
46. Levin AZ: Functional outcome following amputation, *Topics Geriatr Rehabil* 4:253-261, 2004.
47. Devlin M, Pauley T, Head K, et al: Houghton Scale of Prosthetic Use in people with lower-extremity amputations: Reliability, validity, and responsiveness to change, *Arch Phys Med Rehabil* 85:1339-1344, 2004.
48. Legro M, Reiber GD, Smith DG, et al: Prosthesis Evaluation Questionnaire for persons with lower limb amputations: Assessing prosthesis-related quality of life, *Arch Phys Med Rehabil* 79:931-938, 1998.
49. Trantowski-Farrell R, Pinzur MS: A preliminary comparison of function and outcome in patients with diabetic dysvascular disease, *J Prosthet Orthot* 15:127-132, 2003.
50. Miller WC, Deathe AB, Speechley M: Psychometric properties of the Activities-specific Balance Confidence Scale among individuals with a lower-limb amputation, *Arch Phys Med Rehabil* 84:656-661, 2003.
51. Franchignoni F, Orlandini D, Gerriero G, et al: Reliability, validity, and responsiveness of the Locomotor Capabilities Index in adults with lower-limb amputation undergoing prosthetic training, *Arch Phys Med Rehabil* 85:743-748, 2004.
52. Gallagher PM, MacLachlan M: The Trinity Amputation and Prosthesis Experience Scales and quality of life in people with lower-limb amputation, *Arch Phys Med Rehabil* 85:730-736, 2004.
53. Heinemann AW, Bode RK, O'Reilly C: Development and measurement properties of the Orthotics and Prosthetics Users' Survey (OPUS): A comprehensive set of clinical outcome instruments, *Prosthet Orthot Int* 27:191-206, 2003.
54. Cruts HE, de Vries J, Zilvold G, et al: Lower extremity amputees with peripheral vascular disease: Graded exercise testing and results of prosthetic training, *Arch Phys Med Rehabil* 68:14-19, 1987.
55. Bruins M, Geertzen JH, Groothoff JW, et al: Vocational reintegration after a lower limb amputation: A qualitative study, *Prosthet Orthot Int* 27:4-10, 2003.
56. Pezzin LE, Dillingham TR, MacKenzie EJ, et al: Use and satisfaction with prosthetic limb devices and related services, *Arch Phys Med Rehabil* 85:723-729, 2004.
57. Datta D, Selvarajah K, Davey N: Functional outcome of patients with proximal upper limb deficiency—acquired and congenital, *Clin Rehabil* 18:172-177, 2004.
58. Weed R, Atkins DJ: Return to work issues for the upper extremity amputee. In Meier RH, Atkins DJ (eds): *Functional Restoration of Adults and Children with Upper Extremity Amputation*, New York, 2004, Demos Medical Publishing.
59. Knight CA: Peripheral vascular disease and wound care. In O'Sullivan SB, Schmitz TJ (eds): *Physical Rehabilitation: Assessment and Treatment*, ed 4, Philadelphia, 2001, FA Davis.
60. Lilja M, Oberg T: International forum: Proper time for permanent prosthetic fitting, *J Prosthet Orthot* 9:90-98, 1997.
61. Smith DG, McFarland LV, Sangeorzan BJ, et al: Postoperative dressing and management strategies for transtibial amputations: A critical review, *J Rehabil Res Dev* 40:213-224, 2003.
62. Choudhury SR, Reiber GE, Pecoraro JA, et al: Postoperative management of transtibial amputations in VA hospitals, *J Rehabil Res Dev* 38:293-298, 2001.
63. May BJ: *Amputations and Prosthetics: A Case Study Approach*, ed 2, Philadelphia, 2002, FA Davis.
64. Isherwood PA, Robertson JC, Ross A: Pressure measurements beneath below-knee amputation stump bandages: Elastic bandaging, the Puddifoot dressing and a pneumatic bandaging technique compared, *Br J Surg* 62:982-986, 1975.
65. Kane TJ, Pollack EW: The rigid versus soft postoperative dressing controversy: A controlled study in vascular below-knee amputees, *Am J Surg* 189:244-247, 1980.
66. Manella KJ: Comparing the effectiveness of elastic bandages and shrinker socks for lower extremity amputees, *Phys Ther* 61:334-337, 1981.
67. Mueller MJ: Comparison of removable rigid dressings and elastic bandages in prosthetic management of patients with below-knee amputations, *Phys Ther* 62:1438-1441, 1982.
68. Little CE, Kirby RL, Conner M: Spandex shorts to assist stump shrinkage in lower-limb amputees: A pilot study, *Physiother Canada* 49:126-128, 1997.
69. Graf M, Freijah N: Early trans-tibial oedema control using polymer gel socks, *Prosthet Orthot Int* 27:221-226, 2003.
70. Menzies H, Newham J: Semirigid dressings: The best for lower extremity amputees, *Physiother Canada* 30:225-228, 1978.
71. MacLean N, Fick GH: The effect of semirigid dressings on below-knee amputations, *Phys Ther* 74:668-673, 1994.
72. Wong CK, Edelstein JE: Unna and elastic postoperative dressings: Comparison of their effects on function of adults with amputation and vascular disease, *Arch Phys Med Rehabil* 81:1191-1198, 2000.
73. Bonner FJ, Green RF: Pneumatic air leg prosthesis: Report of 200 cases, *Arch Phys Med Rehabil* 63:383-385, 1982.
74. Ham R, Richardson P, Sweet A: A new look at the Vessa PPAM aid, *Physiotherapy* 75:494-495, 1989.
75. Lein S: How are physiotherapists using the Vessa pneumatic post-amputation mobility aid? *Physiotherapy* 78:318-322, 1992.
76. Burgess EM, Romano RL: The management of lower extremity amputees using immediate postsurgical prostheses, *Clin Orthop* 57:137-146, 1968.
77. Sarmiento A, May BJ, Sinclair WF: Immediate post-operative fitting of below-knee amputations, *Phys Ther* 50:10-18, 1970.
78. Mooney V, Harvey JP, McBride E, et al: Comparison of post-operative stump management: Plaster vs. soft dressings, *J Bone Joint Surg Am* 53A:241-249, 1971.
79. Baker WH, Barnes RW, Shurr DG: The healing of below knee amputations: a comparison of soft and plaster dressings, *Am J Surg* 133:716-718, 1977.
80. Woodburn KR, Sockalingham S, Gilmore H, et al: A randomised trial of rigid stump dressing following trans-tibial amputation for peripheral arterial insufficiency, *Prosthet Orthot Int* 28:22-27, 2004.
81. Wu Y, Keagy RD, Krick HJ, et al: An innovative removable rigid dressing technique to below-the-knee amputation, *J Bone Joint Surg Am* 61A:724-729, 1979.
82. Swanson VM: Below-knee polyethylene semi-rigid dressing, *J Prosthet Orthot* 5:10-15, 1993.
83. Schon LC, Short KW, Soupiou O, et al: Benefits of early prosthetic management of transtibial amputees: A prospective clinical study of a prefabricated prosthesis, *Foot Ankle Int* 23:509-514, 2002.
84. Cohen SI, Goldman LD, Salzman EW, et al: The deleterious effect of immediate postoperative prosthesis in below-knee amputation for ischemic disease, *Surgery* 76:992-1001, 1974.
85. Finnoff J: Differentiation and treatment of phantom sensation, phantom pain, and residual-limb pain, *J Am Podiatric Med Assoc* 91:23-33, 2001.
86. Houghton AD, Saadah E, Nicholls G, et al: Phantom pain: Natural history and association with rehabilitation, *Ann Royal Coll Surg Engl* 76:22-25, 1994.
87. Arena JG, Sherman RA, Bruno GM, et al: The relationship between situational stress and phantom limb pain: Cross-lagged correlational data from six month pain logs, *J Psychosomatic Res* 34:71-77, 1990.
88. Hanley MA, Jensen MP, Ehde DM, et al: Psychosocial predictors of long-term adjustment to lower-limb amputation and phantom limb pain, *Disability Rehabil* 26:882-893, 2004.
89. Wainapel S, Thomas A, Kahan B: The use of alternative therapies by rehabilitation outpatients, *Arch Phys Med Rehabil* 79:1003-1005, 1998.
90. Leskowitz ED: Phantom limb pain treated with therapeutic touch: A case report, *Arch Phys Med Rehabil* 81:522-524, 2000.
91. Oakley DA, Whitman LG, Halligan PW: Hypnotic imagery as a treatment for phantom limb pain: Two case reports and a review, *Clin Rehabil* 2002; 16:368-377.
92. Xing G: Acupuncture treatment of phantom limb pain: A report of 9 cases, *J Traditional Chinese Med* 18:199-201, 1998.
93. Wartan SW, Hamann W, Wedley JR, et al: Phantom pain and sensation among British veteran amputees, *Br J Anaesthesia* 78:652-659, 1997.
94. Carabelli RA, Kellerman WC: Phantom limb pain: Relief by application of TENS to contralateral extremity, *Arch Phys Med Rehabil* 66:466-467, 1985.
95. Meier RH, Atkins DJ: Postoperative and preprosthetic preparation. In Meier RH, Atkins DJ (eds): *Functional Restoration of Adults and Children with Upper Extremity Amputation*, New York, 2004, Demos Medical Publishing.
96. Nadolleek H, Brauer S, Ilses R: Outcomes after trans-tibial amputation: The relationship between quiet stance ability, strength of the hip abductor muscles and gait, *Physiother Res Int* 7:203-214, 2002.
97. Powers CM, Boyd LA, Fontaine CA, et al: The influence of lower extremity muscle force on gait characteristics in individuals with below knee amputations secondary to vascular disease, *Phys Ther* 76:369-377, 1996.
98. Isakov E, Burger H, Gregoric M, et al: Isokinetic and isometric strength of the thigh muscles in below-knee amputees, *Clin Biomech* 11:233-235, 1996.
99. Pitetti K, Snell PG, Stray-Gundersen J, et al: Aerobic training exercises for individuals who had amputation of the lower limb, *J Bone Joint Surg Am* 66A:914-920, 1987.
100. Fletcher DD, Andrews KL, Butters MA, et al: Rehabilitation of the geriatric vascular amputee patient: A population-based study, *Arch Phys Med Rehabil* 82:776-779, 2001.

101. Mueller MJ, Strube MJ: Therapeutic footwear: Enhanced function in people with diabetes and transmetatarsal amputation, *Arch Phys Med Rehabil* 78:952-956, 1997.

102. Klute GK, Berge JS: Modelling the effect of prosthetic feet and shoes on the heel-ground contact force in amputee gait, *Proc Inst Mech Eng* 218:173-182, 2004.

103. Hafner BJ, Sanders JE, Czerniecki JM, et al: Transtibial energy-storage-and-return prosthetic devices: A review of energy concepts and a proposed nomenclature, *J Rehabil Res Dev* 39:1-11, 2002.

104. Perry J, Boyd LA, Rao SS, et al: Prosthetic weight acceptance mechanics in transtibial amputees wearing the Single Axis, Seattle Lite, and Flex Foot, *IEEE Trans Rehabil Eng* 5:283-289, 1997.

105. Marianakis GNS: Interlimb symmetry of traumatic unilateral transtibial amputees wearing two different prosthetic feet in the early rehabilitation stage, *J Rehabil Res Dev* 41:581-590, 2004.

106. Gard SA, Konz RJ: The effect of a shock-absorbing pylon on the gait of persons with unilateral transtibial amputation, *J Rehabil Res Dev* 40:109-124, 2003.

107. Lee WC, Zhang M, Mak AF: Regional differences in pain threshold and tolerance of the transtibial residual limb: including the effects of age and interface material, *Arch Phys Med Rehabil* 86:641-649, 2005.

108. Narita H, Yokogushi K, Skii S, et al: Suspension effect and dynamic evaluation of the total surface bearing transtibial prosthesis: A comparison with the patellar tendon bearing transtibial prosthesis, *Prosthet Orthot Int* 21:175-178, 1997.

109. Yigiter K, Sener G, Bayar K: Comparison of the effects of patellar tendon bearing and total surface bearing sockets on prosthetic fitting and rehabilitation, *Prosthet Orthot Int* 26:206-212, 2002.

110. Selles RW, Janssens PJ, Jongenengel CD, et al: A randomized controlled trial comparing functional outcome and cost efficiency of a total surface-bearing socket versus a conventional patellar tendon-bearing socket in transtibial amputees, *Arch Phys Med Rehabil* 86:154-161, 2005.

111. Goh JCH, Lee PVS, Chong SY: Comparative study between patellar-tendon-bearing and pressure cast prosthetic sockets, *J Rehabil Res Dev* 41:491-502, 2004.

112. Mak AFT, Zhang M, Boone DA: State of the art research in lower-limb prosthetic biomechanics-socket interface, *J Rehabil Res Dev* 38:161-174, 2001.

113. Sanders JE, Nicholson BS, Zachariah SG, et al: Testing of elastomeric liners used in limb prosthetics: Classification of 15 products by mechanical performance, *J Rehabil Res Dev* 41:175-186, 2004.

114. Datta D, Vaidya SK, Howitt J, et al: Outcome of fitting an ICEROSS prosthesis: Views of transtibial amputees, *Prosthet Orthot Int* 20:111-115, 1996.

115. Boonstra AM, Van Duin W, Eisma W: International forum: silicone suction socket versus supracondylar PTB prosthesis with Pelite liner: Transtibial amputees' preference, *J Prosthet Orthot* 8:96-99, 1996.

116. Astrom I, Stenstrom A: Effect on gait and socket comfort in unilateral trans-tibial amputees after exchange to a polyurethane concept, *Prosthet Orthot Int* 28:28-36, 2004.

117. Beil TL, Street GM: Comparison of interface pressures with pin and suction suspension systems, *J Rehabil Res Dev* 41:821-828, 2004.

118. Blumentritt S, Scherer HW, Wellershaus U, et al: Design principles, biomechanical data and clinical experience with a polycentric knee offering controlled stance phase knee flexion, *J Prosthet Orthot* 9:18-24, 1997.

119. Devlin M, Sinclair LB, Colman D, et al: Patient preference and gait efficiency in a geriatric population with transfemoral amputation using a free-swinging versus a locked prosthetic knee joint, *Arch Phys Med Rehabil* 83:246-249, 2002.

120. Van der Linden ML, Twiste N, Rithalia SV: The biomechanical effects of the inclusion of a torque absorber on trans-femoral amputee gait, *Prosthet Orthot Int* 26:35-43, 2002.

121. Fishman S, Edelstein JE, Krebs DE: Icelandic-Swedish-New York above-knee prosthetic sockets: Pediatric experience, *J Pediatr Orthop* 7:557-562, 1987.

122. Branemark R, Branemark PI, Rydevik B, et al: Osseointegration in skeletal reconstruction and rehabilitation, *J Rehabil Res Dev* 38:175-181, 2001.

123. Sullivan J, Uden M, Robinson KP, et al: Rehabilitation of the trans-femoral amputee with an osseointegrated prosthesis: The United Kingdom experience, *Prosthet Orthot Int* 27:114-120, 2003.

124. Miller WC, Deathe AB, Speechley M, et al: The influence of falling, fear of falling, and balance confidence on prosthetic mobility and social activity among individuals with lower extremity amputation, *Arch Phys Med Rehabil* 82:1238-1244, 2001.

125. Yigiter K, Sener G, Erbahceci F, et al: A comparison of traditional prosthetic training versus proprioceptive neuromuscular facilitation resistive gait training with transfemoral amputees, *Prosthet Orthot Int* 26:213-217, 2002.

126. Sjodahl C, Harnlo GB, Persson BM: Gait improvement in unilateral transfemoral amputees by a combined psychological and physiotherapeutic treatment, *J Rehabil Med* 33:114-118, 2001.

127. Hyland N, Ketki P, Magistrado J: Comparison of gait training strategies for individuals with transtibial amputation, *J Geriatr Phys Ther* 27:106-107, 2004.

128. Kavounoudias A, Tremblay C, Gravel D, et al: Bilateral changes in somatosensory sensibility after unilateral below-knee amputation, *Arch Phys Med Rehabil* 86:633-640, 2005.

129. Matjacic Z, Burger H: Dynamic balance training during standing in people with trans-tibial amputation: A pilot study, *Prosthet Orthot Int* 27:214-220, 2003.

130. Hunter D, Smith Cole E: Energy expenditure of below knee amputees during harness supported treadmill ambulation, *JOSPT* 21:268-276, 1995.

131. Tsai HA, Kirby RL, MacLeod DA, et al: Aided gait of people with lower-limb amputations: Comparison of 4-footed and 2-wheeled walkers, *Arch Phys Med Rehabil* 84:584-591, 2003.

132. Nolan L, Wit A, Dudzinski K, et al: Adjustments in gait symmetry with walking speed in transfemoral and transtibial amputees, *Gait Posture* 17:142-151, 2003.

133. Jaeger SM, Arendzen JH, de Jongh JH: Prosthetic gait of unilateral transfemoral amputees: A kinematic study, *Arch Phys Med Rehabil* 76:736:743, 1995.

134. Hoffman MD, Sheldahl LM, Buley KJ, et al: Physiological comparison of walking among bilateral above-knee amputee and able-bodied subjects, and a model to account for the differences in metabolic cost, *Arch Phys Med Rehabil* 78:385-392, 1997.

135. Norvell DC, Czerniecki JM, Reiber GE, et al: The prevalence of knee pain and symptomatic knee osteoarthritis among veteran traumatic amputees and nonamputees, *Arch Phys Med Rehabil* 86:487-493, 2005.

136. Detrembleur C, Vanmarsenille J-M, De Cuyper F, et al: Relationship between energy cost, gait speed, vertical displacement of centre of body mass and efficiency of pendulum-like mechanism in unilateral amputee gait, *Gait Posture* 21:333-340, 2005.

137. Schmid M, Beltrami G, Zambarbieri D, et al: Centre of pressure displacements in trans-femoral amputees during gait, *Gait Posture* 21:255-262, 2005.

138. Lyon CC, Kulkarni J, Zimerson E, et al: Skin disorders in amputees, *J Am Acad Dermatol* 44:/223-/234, 2001.

139. Hachisuka K, Nakamura T, Ohmine S, et al: Hygiene problems of residual limb and silicone liners in transtibial amputees wearing the total surface bearing socket, *Arch Phys Med Rehabil* 82:1286-1290, 2001.

140. Dudek NL, Marks MB, Marshall SC, et al: Dermatologic conditions associated with use of a lower-extremity prosthesis, *Arch Phys Med Rehabil* 86:659-663, 2005.

141. Smaby N, Johanson ME, Baker B, et al: Identification of key pinch forces required to complete functional tasks, *J Rehabil Res Dev* 41:215-224, 2004.

142. Kruger LM, Fishman S: Myoelectric and body-powered prostheses, *J Pediatr Orthop* 13:68-75, 1993.

143. Legro MW, Reiber GE, Czerniecki JM, et al: Recreational activities of lower-limb amputees with prostheses, *J Rehabil Res Dev* 38:319-325, 2001.

144. Ralston A: *Between a Rock and a Hard Place*, New York, 2004, Atria Books.

145. Plitt T: Wresting with an exceptional life, *USA Today* November 18, 2004, 11A.

Chapter 13

Balance and Fall Risk

Toni Tyner, Diane D. Allen

OBJECTIVES

After reading this chapter, the reader will be able to:
1. Identify the relationship between balance disorders and fall risk.
2. Define terminology used in the physical therapy management of balance disorders.
3. Specify the central and peripheral components of postural control mechanisms.
4. Compare and contrast the roles of the visual, vestibular, and somatosensory systems in postural control.
5. Identify and differentiate between pathologies that can result in impaired balance.
6. Relate common age-related changes in postural control mechanisms to fall risk in the elderly.
7. Identify and describe examination procedures used in the management of patients with balance disorders or who are at increased risk for falls.
8. For a patient with a balance disorder, use the results of the examination to evaluate impairments, develop a physical therapy diagnosis and prognosis, and design a plan of care.
9. Select and apply appropriate interventions to improve balance and reduce fall risk in patients with loss of balance or increased fall risk.

*P*oor balance and falls adversely affect the lives of thousands. More than one-third of adults aged 65 years and older fall each year.[1] When people fall, 20% to 30% sustain moderate to severe injuries such as hip fractures or head trauma that reduce their mobility and independence and increase their risk for premature death.[2] The risk of sustaining severe injury from a fall is higher for older adults and those with co-morbidities such as stroke, Parkinson's disease, vestibular dysfunction, amputation, arthritis, and head trauma. Falls may result in pain, injury, and disability, and, after falling, individuals may lose confidence in their ability to perform routine activities. A heightened fear of falling can also lead to restriction of activities.[3] Although not all falls can be prevented, the poor balance that precipitates some of them can be improved to reduce the risk for falls and their consequences.

Balance is the ability to locate and maintain one's center of gravity (COG) within or over one's *base of support* (BOS).[4,5] Sensory and motor systems are used to maintain an upright position during static and dynamic tasks in multiple and changing environments. Balance is sometimes referred to as *postural control* because it involves controlling the position or posture of the body at rest or when moving. The term posture implies holding a particular static position (see Chapter 4). The terms postural control and balance, as used in this chapter, refer to the ability to move efficiently and effectively in a variety of environments and situations without falling. Postural control involves the use of many systems to obtain information about the environment and produce appropriate movements and responses. The visual, somatosensory, and vestibular systems relay information about the position and movement of the body, particularly the head, in relation to the environment and the position and movement of the environment in relation to the body.[3,6-9] The neuromuscular and musculoskeletal systems allow for voluntarily or reactive motions in response to the sensory input. The cognitive system interprets sensory input to select and coordinate motor output in terms of posture and movement. Cognition is particularly important for functional balance because it "provides us with the collective ability to anticipate or adapt our actions in response to changing task demands and the environment."[3] Redundancy among the systems allows for compensation if a system is compromised.[2]

Postural control may need to change in response to changing task demands, such as differences in lighting, stability, or evenness of the supporting surface, or mechanical *perturbations*. To live and move freely in the environment, people need to have effective static balance, *automatic and reactive postural responses*, anticipatory control, and volitional postural movements[4,10] (Box 13-1). A lack or dysfunction of any type or component of postural control can hinder a person's ability to meet particular task demands and increase the risk of falling.

Evaluation of a person's postural control and fall risk requires examination of his or her usual tasks, the types of postural control required to perform these tasks, and the person's ability to use the needed types of postural control. Fall risk is affected by intrinsic factors such as age, gender, low body mass index, cognitive impairments, previous falls, presence of chronic diseases, and medication use.[3,11-19] In addition, extrinsic factors related to the task and environmental conditions, such as clothing, particularly footwear in older adults,[20] living situation, and social situation, may also increase or decrease the risk of falls.

The *Guide to Physical Therapist Practice* defines preferred practice pattern 5A as: Primary prevention/risk reduction for loss of balance and falling.[21] This practice pattern refers specifically to primary prevention, which is prevention before a fall occurs, although secondary prevention, which is risk reduction for further falls after a fall has occurred, and tertiary prevention, reduction of the functional sequelae of poor balance, may also help reduce the

frequency and functional sequelae of falls (Table 13-1). Fall prevention or risk reduction requires examination, evaluation, and interventions for patients thought to be at increased risk for falling. Early determination of fall risk can be used to select patients most likely to benefit from interventions shown to reduce the risk of falls.[13,22,23] Although improving balance can reduce fall risk, falls may still occur, particularly if environmental challenges or intrinsic risk factors change.

Many pathologies and impairments can affect postural control. Therefore patients with various diagnoses in different practice settings, including acute care, long-term care, inpatient rehabilitation, outpatient practice, and community sites, may benefit from interventions to reduce their risk of loss of balance and falls. Fig. 13-1 gives an overview of the circumstances under which patients

---

BOX 13-1 Postural Control

Static Postural Control
- Normal sway
- Reflex reactions
  - Righting reactions
  - VOR
  - VSR

Automatic or Reactive Postural Responses
- Occur in response to a stimulus.
- Occur rapidly, less than 250 msec.
- Four common automatic postural strategies:
  - Ankle strategy
  - Hip strategy
  - Suspensory strategy
  - Stepping strategy

Anticipatory Postural Responses
- Similar to automatic but occur before an actual stimulus.
- Involve a "postural set" to offset forces.
- Functioning anticipatory reactions limit need for rapid reactive responses.

Volitional Postural Movements
- Under conscious control.
- Weight shifts.
- Trained responses, like those in gymnastics or advanced sport activities.

VOR, Vestibulo-ocular reflex; *VSR,* vestibulospinal reflex.

TABLE 13-1 Fall Prevention for Individuals with Increased Fall Risk

Type of Patient	Type of Prevention	Examples of Intervention
Individual of advanced age	Primary	Muscle strengthening and endurance program focused on lower extremities. Patient education in reducing environmental hazards that represent fall risk.
Individual with a history of falls	Secondary	Exercise program and gait training focused on components and types of postural control that show deficits. Assessment and modification of patient's environment as appropriate.
Individual with CNS pathology with chronic or progressive balance deficits	Tertiary	Exercise program, instruction in ADLs, and gait training with assistive devices as needed. Patient and caregiver instruction on fall prevention and safety.

Adapted from American Physical Therapy Association: *Phys Ther* 81:9-744, 2001.
CNS, Central nervous system; *ADL,* activities of daily living.

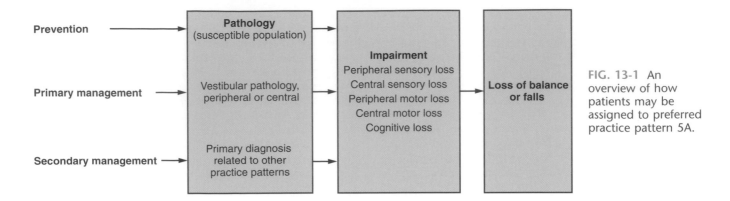

FIG. 13-1 An overview of how patients may be assigned to preferred practice pattern 5A.

may be assigned to preferred practice pattern 5A and the impairments that typically result in loss of balance or falls.

PATHOLOGY

CAUSES OF BALANCE DYSFUNCTION

Balance dysfunction during normal tasks in an ordinary environment occurs when postural control systems function inadequately. Current theories of balance are based on a systems approach that assumes that balance is controlled by many interacting systems. When one or more of these systems has a problem, the other systems adapt as much as possible to prevent falling while still accomplishing the task.

According to the dynamic equilibrium theory of balance control (Fig. 13-2),[10] sensory and motor systems interact to dynamically control equilibrium and allow adjustment to displacement of a person's COG through appropriate changes in the BOS.[24] The sensory system receives information about the environment, and the neuromuscular and musculoskeletal systems allow for motor planning and motor output in response to this information. This interaction can provide the static, adaptive, anticipatory, and reactive control required for people to move and respond in a changing environment.[24] Since changes in any of these contributing systems may result in loss of balance or a fall, the examination of the patient assigned to preferred practice pattern 5A should include tests of the musculoskeletal, neuromuscular and sensory systems, as well as their controlled interactions (Fig. 13-3).

Various pathologies or impairments can cause problems with balance (Table 13-2). The intrinsic causes of balance problems can be grouped into the following five categories: (1) Peripheral sensory, (2) central sensory, (3) peripheral motor, (4) central motor, and (5) cognitive.[25] The next section of this chapter reviews these causes of balance problems and provides examples of each.

Peripheral Sensory Impairments. Vision, vestibular sensation, and *somatosensation* all contribute to postural control, and if impaired, can result in balance dysfunction. The visual system includes the eyes with the visual receptors; the optic nerves that project, via connections, to the occipital region of the brain; and the nerves and muscles of the oculomotor system. Visual receptors detect light and differences in light patterns to

allow us to identify objects and obstacles. Vision also detects relative motion of the environment and thus provides orientation to help maintain balance. The central visual field is used most for environmental orientation to tell us where we are in space. Peripheral vision, also known as ambient vision, provides information about movement relative to the environment; including head movements and postural sway.[9] Vision contributes to anticipatory and responsive postural control. Any pathology that impairs vision, such as glaucoma, macular degeneration, cataracts, diplopia, or visual field cuts, can impair balance (Fig. 13-4).[26]

The visual and vestibular systems work together to generate eye movements that allow observation of moving or stationary objects when the head is moving or stationary. This helps maintain upright posture and allows a person to keep track of their position in space.[26]

Although eye movements are a form of motor output, because of their intimate link with vision and the vestibular system, problems with eye movements are generally considered with peripheral sensory impairments. Important occulomotor functions relating to balance include conjugation, saccades, smooth pursuit, *vestibulo-ocular reflex* (VOR), and nystagmus. Problems with any of these can interfere with orientation to the environment. Eye

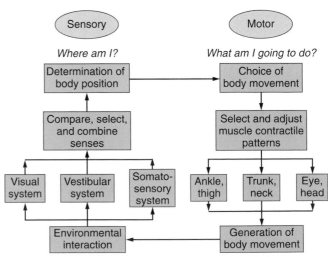

FIG. 13-2 The dynamic equilibrium model of balance control. *Courtesy NeuroCom.*

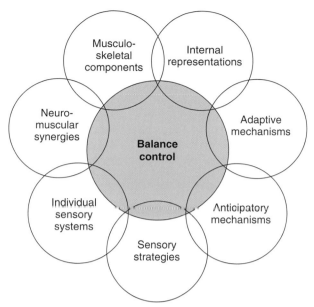

FIG. 13-3 Interaction of the systems that contribute to balance control. *Redrawn from Shumway-Cook A, Woollacott MH: Motor Control: Theory and Practical Applications, ed 2, Philadelphia, 2001, Lippincott Williams & Wilkins.*

movements should be conjugate, with the two eyes moving together, so that an image always falls on corresponding points of the two retinas. Diplopia (double vision) will occur if the eyes do not move together. Saccades ensure that the gaze can move quickly from one point of fixation to another so that sensory information can be rapidly gathered and responded to. Smooth pursuit allows a moving object to be visually followed while keeping the image on the center of the retina. The VOR, which maintains eye fixation as the head turns, is a combination of smooth-pursuit movements and saccades elicited by movement of the head. The VOR is normally suppressed when one follows a moving object while moving one's head, as when watching a moving car or a

running pet. Nystagmus is involuntary back-and-forth, up-and-down, or rotating movement of the eyes that occurs in response to the environment or the body "spinning." Nystagmus that lasts for only a few beats after spinning can be normal, but spontaneous, position-induced or persistent nystagmus is usually pathological. Table 13-3 summarizes normal eye movements and impairments.

The *vestibular system* includes the labyrinths and their mechanoreceptors (peripheral components of the system), the vestibulocochlear nerve (cranial nerve VIII), the vestibular nuclei in the brainstem, central projections to the cerebellum and vestibular cortex (central components), and the long tracts of nerves arising from the vestibular nuclei that influence motor neuron pools in the spinal cord.

The peripheral components of the vestibular system are located in the inner ear, also known as the labyrinth (Fig. 13-5). These components include the cochlea, the vestibule (which contains the otolithic organs, the saccule and the utricle), and the semicircular canals. The cochlea provides the structure for hearing receptors. The otolithic organs and semicircular canals contain hairlike receptors that respond to head positions and movements.

The receptors in the otolithic organs, which are embedded in gelatinous acellular membranes beneath masses of many calcium carbonate crystals, respond to changes in head velocity (acceleration) but not to movement at a constant velocity. Utricle receptors respond to linear acceleration and deceleration in a horizontal plane as occurs, for example, when first stepping onto a moving walkway at the airport. Saccule receptors respond to linear acceleration and deceleration in a vertical plane, as occurs when jumping. Since the right and left otoliths work together to give information about acceleration, a problem on either side can cause balance problems. Generally, the body responds to otolithic stimulation by contracting the postural extensor muscles, and dysfunction of the otoliths usually causes difficulty with maintaining a static posture against gravity.[24]

There are three connected semicircular canals in each inner ear, the anterior, posterior, and horizontal. Each semicircular canal has an endolymph-filled swelling called

TABLE 13-2		Causes of Balance Problems	
System	Area	Areas of Impairment	Consequences
Sensory	Peripheral	Visual system, receptors. Vestibular system, receptors. Somatosensory system, receptors: primarily lower extremities.	Decreased ability to sense the position or movement of the head or body in relation to a static or dynamic environment.
	Central	Cortical areas responsible for interpreting and integrating sensory information.	Decreased ability to combine information from relevant sensory input; perception of space, true vertical or horizontal may be distorted.
Motor	Peripheral	Muscles, joints, motor units.	Decreased ability to execute balance strategies or reactions to postural sway.
	Central	CNS areas responsible for planning, coordinating, and affecting motor control.	Decreased ability to plan and coordinate postural control under static and dynamic conditions.
Cognitive	Central	Cortical and limbic areas responsible for attention, arousal, and judgment.	Decreased ability to remember previously successful strategies, or judge and attend to potential dangers.

CNS, Central nervous system.

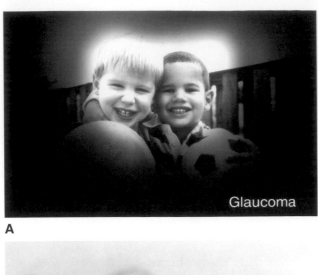

A

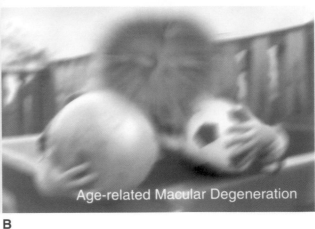

B

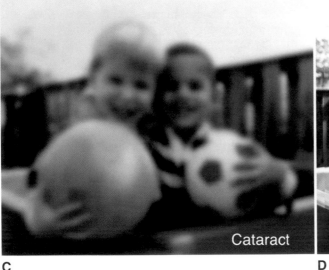

C

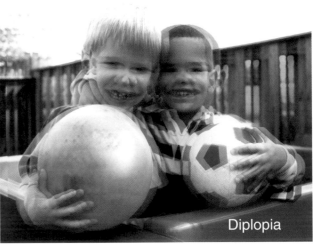

D

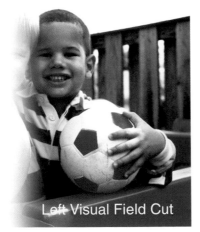

E

FIG. 13-4 Consequences of various visual impairments.
A, Glaucoma; **B,** macular degeneration; **C,** cataracts;
D, diplopia; **E,** left visual field cut. *Courtesy National Eye Institute, National Institutes of Health.*

the ampulla, which contains calcium carbonate crystals and hair cells that project into the cupula, a structure like the acellular membrane in the otolithic organs, which spans the opening of the ampulla. Receptors in the semi-circular canals detect movements of the head, particularly angular or rotational acceleration. The anterior and pos-terior canals are positioned vertically and respond to up and down motions of the head (nodding) and rolling (sidebending); the horizontal canal (positioned in the middle) responds to head rotation to the right and left.

TABLE 13-3	Normal Eye Movements	
Type	**Description**	**Impairments that Increase Risk of Loss of Balance or Falls**
Conjugate	Eyes move at the same time to follow object moving across visual field.	Paresis/paralysis of extraocular eye muscles of one eye, diplopia.
Convergence	Eyes move toward each other to follow object approaching face head-on.	Paresis/paralysis of extraocular eye muscles, diplopia.
Smooth pursuit	Eyes move to follow image whether head or image is moving, or both.	Impaired tracking resulting from acute vestibular lesions, coordination deficits resulting from cerebellar lesions.
Saccades	Quick recovery phase to resume smooth pursuit after eyes slip off an image during head or image movement, or both; function of the VOR.	Slowed movement resulting from CNS disorders, such as MS or PD, or deficits, either peripheral or central.
Nystagmus	Multiple slow movements of eyes interspersed rhythmically by quick recovery phases; normal if noted at ends of ranges of eye movements and after spinning (for a few seconds).	Inability to fix gaze normally, resulting from uncompensated peripheral or central vestibular deficits; vertical or oblique nystagmus may result from CNS disorders.

VOR, Vestibulo-ocular reflex; *CNS,* central nervous system; *MS,* multiple sclerosis; *PD,* Parkinson's disease.

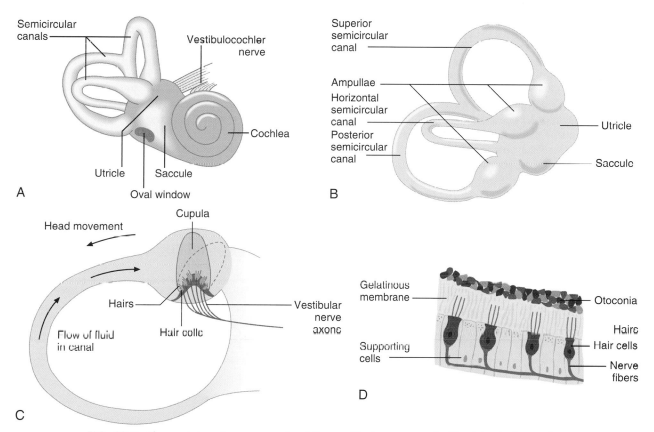

FIG. 13-5 The peripheral components of the vestibular system. **A,** The labyrinth; **B,** the vestibule; **C,** semicircular canal; **D,** movement receptor. *From Lundy-Ekman L: Neuroscience: Fundamentals for Rehabilitation, ed 2, St. Louis, 2002, Saunders.*

Together, the semicircular canals provide information about dynamic movement, help to align the head and body in space, and are critical for controlling visual gaze and ocular movements.

Vestibular disorders[24,25] vary but can be grouped into two primary categories: (1) deficiencies, which occur with vestibular neuronitis, labyrinthitis, or acoustic neuromas, and (2) distortions, which occur in benign paroxysmal positional vertigo (BPPV). BPPV is generally caused by semicircular canal dysfunction, such as canalithiasis, when crystals become dislodged and float in the canal, or cupulolithiasis, when crystals adhere to the cupula. Symptoms common to both categories are *vertigo* or reduced balance when the person moves his or her head.[27]

The positions of the vestibular receptors in the otolithic organs and semicircular canals make them most responsive when the individual is upright or supine. Sidelying causes the least stimulation because the otolithic cilia register no gravitational force. Bending the neck or turning the head increases firing on the side of the direction of the movement and decreases firing on the opposite side. Dysfunction of either side will cause vertigo, a sensation of the person or the room spinning (Fig. 13-6). Fortunately, with time, most patients adjust to such altered sensory input, and the sensation of vertigo resolves.

The central components of the vestibular system receive information from the peripheral components. Input arriving via cranial nerve VIII to the vestibular nuclei in the brainstem is combined with information from the cerebellum to coordinate head and eye movements and control equilibrium. The central components of the vestibular system also send information to the reticular formation, which facilitates arousal and motor responses. These connections result in increased extensor tone and postural responses, activation of cervical musculature for head position, and eye reflex reactions.

The vestibular system is one of the nervous system's most important tools for controlling posture. It has four primary roles: (1) sensing and perceiving self-motion, (2) orienting to vertical, (3) controlling the *center of mass*, and (4) stabilizing the head.[28] In perceiving self-motion, the vestibular system can help differentiate self-motion from environmental motion[24] and thus compensate for misinformation from another sense. For example, if the eyes see movement in the environment, but the labyrinths register no concurrent head movement, the brain can abort any postural adjustments triggered by visual information initially intended to react to body movement (Fig. 13-7). By sensing, integrating, and producing motor responses the vestibular system can orient the head and body to vertical and activate antigravity muscles and *automatic postural responses* to control the stability of the head and the body's center of mass (COM).

Information about muscle length, stretch, tension, and contraction and about pain, temperature, pressure, and joint position is provided by somatosensory receptors located in joints, ligaments, muscles, and the skin. This information allows individuals to know where they are in space and to glean information from their environment needed for postural control.[29] Receptors, particularly in the feet, ankles, knees, hips, back, and neck, provide information needed for static and dynamic balance control. Simply anesthetizing the soles of the feet will prevent an otherwise normal individual from being able to balance on one leg.[30] Disease or trauma can impair peripheral sensory receptor and sensory nerve function and limit or

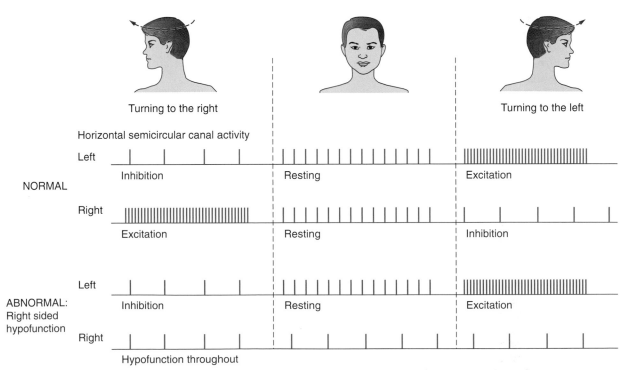

FIG. 13-6 Responses of the horizontal semicircular canals to head turning to the right and left, with normal functioning *(top)* and with right-sided hypofunction *(bottom)*.

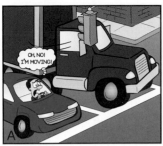
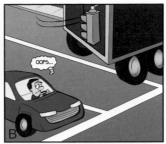

FIG. 13-7 As you sit in your car at a stop sign, the truck next to you starts to move forward. Visual information suggests you are moving backward and you slam on your brakes and brace **(A)**. An instant later, information from the labyrinths lets you know you really are not moving and you relax **(B)**.

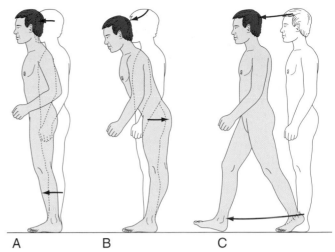

FIG. 13-8 Strategies used to maintain balance. **A,** Ankle strategy; **B,** hip strategy; **C,** change-in-support strategy.

impair their information-gathering capabilities, causing data to be inaccurate or absent. Patients with altered sensory integrity diagnosed in any preferred practice patterns may therefore also have impairments or disability associated with loss of balance and falling.

Using information from the vestibular system, neck proprioceptors, vision, and somatosensation, the brain maps the position and movement of the entire body and its immediate environment.[31] We perceive our position and motion in space by using information from the visual system regarding our surroundings, information from the vestibular system about head movement, and information from the somatosensory system regarding the support surface and position and motion of body segments with respect to each other. Although the close relationship of all this information can make it difficult to separate the impacts and roles of each system, particularly when one is dysfunctional, knowledge of the different systems and careful selective examination and evaluation is needed to guide selection of interventions likely to reduce loss of balance and falls.

Central Sensory Impairments. Sensory information from the periphery, including vision, vestibular sense, and somatosensation from both sides of the body, is integrated in the central nervous system (CNS).[5] This is needed because information from a single system does not distinguish specific movements and positions. For example, information from the somatosensory system alone cannot discriminate between a tilting body and a tilting support surface, and input from the visual or vestibular system alone cannot distinguish movement of the body from movement in the surrounding environment.[4] If this central processing is impaired, a person will have difficulty with certain balance tasks. For example, if one cannot integrate information from the right and left sides of the body, one may have difficulty maintaining balance when turning or performing other asymmetrical movements.

Central processing is particularly important when there are sensory conflicts within or between sensory systems. Conflict can occur within a system if there is disproportional information from the two sides. For example, if there is damage to the vestibular system on one side (see Fig. 13-6), then symmetrical head movements may be interpreted as turning, triggering inappropriate postural adjustments that could cause a loss of balance. In this case, in order to compensate, the central processing system must relearn what sensory input to expect with various head movements.[32] When there is conflict between systems, the central processing system must select which input(s) to use to drive motor responses or reactions. If one system provides inaccurate or conflicting information while the other two systems concur, then the concurrent systems will be relied on. However, if more than one sensory system provides inadequate or inaccurate information, or if sensory conflict is not resolved quickly, selection of an appropriate motor response will be difficult and decreased or poorly controlled movement, unsteadiness, *dizziness*, or falls may result.

Certain common environments or activities, such as descending stairs, walking in busy traffic or on escalators, walking on uneven ground, moving in dimly lit or overly bright areas, and making quick movements or turns, can also create sensory conflict. These environments are particularly challenging for individuals with limited or inaccurate sensory input from one or more systems.

CNS disease, such as stroke, multiple sclerosis, cerebral palsy or brain tumors, as well as trauma, can adversely affect central sensory processing, particularly if there is parietal lobe involvement.[24,28] This is because the parietal lobes process complex sensory and perceptual information, especially information related to somatosensation, spatial relations, body schema, and motor learning.

Peripheral Motor Impairments. The peripheral motor system executes all of the movements required for postural control. Strategies utilized for postural control are specific to the demands of the task. Although most people also have upper extremity reactions when balance is disturbed,[30] the most studied of the postural strategies for responding to balance perturbations include variations of three basic lower extremity strategies: The ankle, hip, and stepping (change-in-support) strategies (Fig. 13-8).[30] These basic strategies may be used to prevent falls during a wide range of tasks.[33]

The *ankle strategy* primarily controls body sway during stance. It starts with early activation of the ankle dorsiflexor or plantarflexor muscles followed by recruitment of hip and then trunk musculature to create small shifts in the alignment of the COM over the BOS. When someone uses an ankle strategy in quiet standing, the upper and lower body sway together in the same direction, with the body moving as a single entity over the ankle joints. The ankle musculature can generate relatively small forces to control sway through a small range of motion (ROM) at a slow speed.

When the COG moves more quickly over the BOS, moves unexpectedly laterally, or sways more than a very small amount, a *hip strategy* is used to control balance. Hip strategy involves activation of large hip and trunk muscles first, including the hip abductors, followed by ankle muscle activation. When a patient uses hip strategy in standing, the upper and lower body move in opposite directions to maintain balance. If the COG suddenly shifts forward, the upper trunk will move rapidly backward and the pelvis will move forward; the arms may also flail before balance is regained.

The *stepping strategy* initiates establishment of a new BOS when the boundaries of stability are exceeded or even approached.[30] Boundaries of stability vary among individuals: A person with reduced boundaries will use a stepping strategy in response to smaller movement of the COG than a person with normal boundaries. When using a stepping strategy, the individual takes a step to avoid a fall.

The various strategies have several requirements to function well. The ankle strategy requires good ankle ROM in midrange, adequate plantar and dorsiflexor strength, intact sensation in the feet and ankles, and a broad, firm surface of support. Hip strategies require adequate hip strength and ROM along with somatosensation about the hips and trunk. Lateral hip strategies specifically require hip abductor and adductor muscles. Stepping strategies require adequate lower body strength for weight bearing on the stepping leg and adequate ROM at the ankles, knees, and hips. Central processing speed and the ability to initiate and coordinate the timing of movements are also critical.

Musculoskeletal problems, such as weakness, reduced ROM, and skeletal asymmetry, can diminish balance.[34] Decreased ankle ROM has been specifically correlated with decreased balance in community-dwelling elderly women.[34] In elderly nursing home residents, those who had experienced two or more falls in the past year had weaker knee flexors and extensors and ankle muscles than those who had not fallen; the peak torque in the ankle dorsiflexors of fallers was only 9.5% of that of nonfallers.[35] Fig. 13-9 shows the muscles used for stabilization during normal forward and backward sway, using ankle or hips strategies for maintaining balance.[10] Although weakness or diminished power in the lower extremity muscles can affect balance,[35,36] good functioning of other muscles, such as the scapulothoracic stabilizers that normally control forward movement of the COM when the arms are raised, can also be important to prevent falls during functional activities.[37] Joint problems, particularly those

	Ankle strategy	Hip strategy
Forward sway	Paraspinals Hamstrings Gastrocnemius	Abdominals Quadriceps
Backward sway	Abdominals Quadriceps Tibialis anterior	Paraspinals Hamstrings

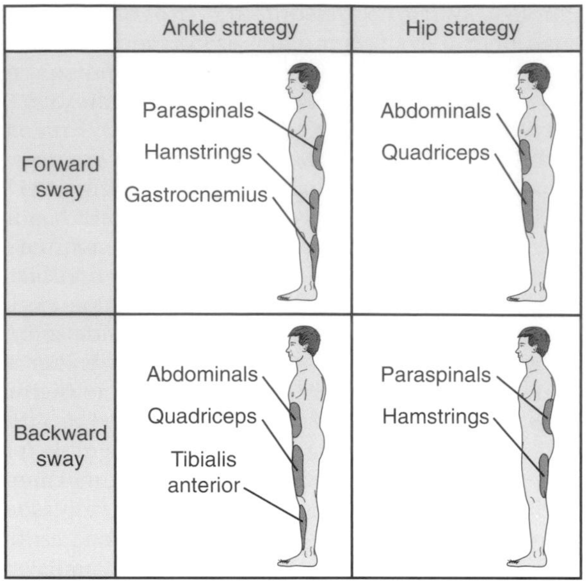

FIG. 13-9 Muscles used for stabilization during forward and backward sway, using ankle or hip strategies to maintain balance.

that cause pain or instability like arthritis,[38] as well as lower extremity amputations, can also cause abnormal weight shifting and asymmetrical weight bearing that can reduce balance options.

Central Motor Impairments. The CNS directs the execution of postural control and movement through the peripheral motor system. The central motor systems refine reflexive movements and initiate and coordinate voluntary movement needed for balance. They determine reaction time and movement speed and also coordinate and inhibit movement patterns. Motor planning provides timing, sequencing, and force modulation, as well as limb, joint, and muscle selection, for an activity.[4] Problems in areas of the CNS that control motor output, primarily the motor cortex, the basal ganglia, and the cerebellum, can cause difficulties with motor control that affect static, anticipatory, adaptive, and reactive postural control.[4,39] People who have had a stroke, head injury, or multiple sclerosis affecting these areas of the brain and people with diseases affecting these areas of the brain, such as Parkinson's disease,[40] cerebellar ataxia,[41] and Huntington's disease[42] generally have problems with balance.

Cognitive Impairments. Once learned, postural control functions automatically, without much conscious thought. However, cognition, attention, and memory still play important roles in balance. In a trial with 60 subjects, Hauer and colleagues found that performing dual tasks impaired postural control in older patients with cognitive impairments and a history of falls more than in those without cognitive impairments or in healthy adults.[43] The investigators concluded that the additional cognitive demands decreased postural stability because they reduced attention in the cognitively impaired subjects and that this may explain the increased incidence of falls in individuals with cognitive impairments.[43] Attention is important for balance because it is needed for the individual to collect information about the immediate environment. Attention deficits may limit anticipatory control by decreasing awareness of hazards. Cognitive problems, including poor judgment, distractibility, and limited multi-tasking skills, also increase fall risk.

Not only do cognitive problems affect balance, they also limit an individual's ability to learn or relearn balance skills. Jensen et al found that after a balance training intervention, those who fell less often were those who had a higher level of cognition as indicated by higher scores on the Mini-Mental State Examination (MMSE).[44] The study was a nonblinded, cluster-randomized controlled trial (RCT) comparing the effects of a multifactorial fall and injury prevention program with usual care in 378 older subjects. Individuals who have had a stroke, head injury, multifocal cerebral infarcts, tumors, or dementia may have significant changes in cognition that can increase their risk of falling.

IMPACT OF POOR BALANCE AND LIMITED POSTURAL CONTROL ON GAIT

Although much of the research on balance has been evaluated standing, the same principles apply to gait. Walking involves moving toward the boundaries of stability with each step and then catching oneself with a stepping strategy. Individuals with a history of falls have more and faster sway during the stance phase of gait than those who have not fallen[10]; they also have slower motor responses and altered motor organization during gait. Several changes that coincide with advanced aging, including multisystem degeneration and musculoskeletal and neuromuscular changes, can result in responses to postural perturbations like those seen in individuals who fall. Individuals with balance disorders and the elderly often walk slower to improve accuracy during gait and use hip rather than ankle strategies when stance is perturbed. Without a functioning ankle strategy, the amount and direction of sway during standing can also affect progression through the stance phase of gait. Central sensory, central motor, and cognitive impairments can slow planning and execution of postural control during gait and impair problem solving when gait is challenged. With poor balance, gait speed is reduced, time in unilateral stance is decreased, initiation of swing phase of gait is delayed, step length is shortened, and toe clearance is reduced during the swing phase of gait.[3]

NEUROLOGICAL DISORDERS THAT AFFECT BALANCE

Many neurological disorders adversely affect balance. The problems can be compounded in older adults in whom the remaining systems typically available to compensate for singular deficits may also have problems. Fig. 13-10 summarizes the effects of common neuromuscular

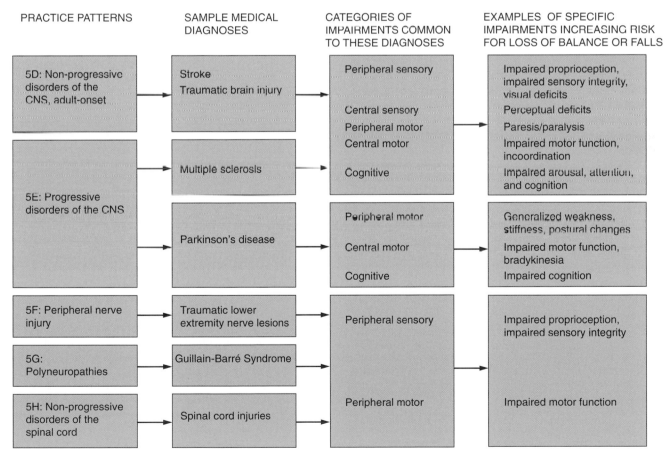

FIG. 13-10 Effects of common neuromuscular disorders on balance and falling. *CNS,* Central nervous system.

disorders on balance and falling. This section addresses some of the specific effects on balance of Parkinson's disease, cerebellar degeneration, stroke, multiple sclerosis, vestibular disorders and multisensory disequilibrium resulting from peripheral neuropathy, diabetes, or other systemic illness.

Parkinson's disease (PD) is a progressive disease of gradual onset caused by disruption of the dopamine pathways in the substantia nigra (see Chapter 17). Tremor, rigidity, flexed or forward posture, slowing of movements, or bradykinesia, all seen with PD, prolong reaction times and diminish balance strategies and fall prevention options. PD often causes unsteadiness and increased postural sway because of slowed response times when turning, negotiating stairs, experiencing perturbations, or completing transitional movements. Loss of balance and falling are common in patients with PD, especially falling backward.[45-47]

Cerebellar degeneration may occur in chronic alcoholics and in patients with certain metabolic, degenerative, or inherited disorders.[41] Ataxia, a muscular incoordination seen especially with voluntary movement, and dysmetria are frequently seen in patients with cerebellar lesions or degeneration. Ataxia and dysmetria decrease the effectiveness of balance strategies and impair occulomotor control, increasing the risk of falls. Symptoms of cerebellar dysfunction include delayed or exaggerated postural reactions, progression of gait instability and *disequilibrium,* incoordination of eye and limb movements, nystagmus, tilting to one side, and a wide-based stance and gait pattern.[41]

After a stroke or head trauma (see Chapter 16), people often have problems with balance and falls.[48-50] This can be due to paresis, sensory loss, visual field defects, or impaired spatial perception. Additionally, brainstem lesions that affect the vestibular nuclei can cause vertigo, disequilibrium, and incoordination; basal ganglia lesions can cause slowed or involuntary movement; and cerebellar lesions can cause ataxia.

Multiple sclerosis (MS), a CNS demyelinating disorder (see Chapter 17), affects balance by impairing function in multiple locations of the brain and spinal cord.[51] Symptoms depend on the locations of the lesions and may include vertigo, nystagmus, and imbalance with disruption of central vestibular pathways or interruption of vestibular integration. Optic neuritis may result in blurred vision and inaccurate visual input. Motor and cerebellar pathway disruption lead to weakness, incoordination, and poor motor control. If MS affects the posterior columns, the resulting changes in somatosensory input will also alter postural control.

Multisensory disequilibrium refers to combined dysfunction of the vestibular, visual, and somatosensory systems. Diabetes can cause vestibulopathy, retinopathy, and peripheral neuropathy resulting in changes in all three sensory systems. Aging may also result in impairment of all three sensory systems along with the motor systems critical to postural control.[52] Common symptoms of multisensory disequilibrium include imbalance when walking, especially in dim lighting or on uneven surfaces, sensory complaints such as numbness and tingling in the lower extremities and feet, poor proprioception, poor use of the vestibular system, and poor vision.

EXAMINATION

The examination of patients at risk for loss of balance and falling includes global and specific components. Global components help the clinician confirm that the patient's problems are both appropriate for physical therapy and within the realm of preferred practice pattern 5A, relevant to loss of balance and falling. Specific components pinpoint the impairments or functional limitations that lead to loss of balance or falling. The examination provides information for evaluation of the cause(s) of loss of balance and/or falls and for selection of appropriate and effective interventions. This chapter focuses on the components of the examination relevant to patients who have problems with loss of balance and fall risk.

PATIENT HISTORY

The history, obtained through interview or from review of records or other sources, should include standard demographic information such as the patient's age, as well as background information about his or her living situation, prior level of function, and current functional status. Social and medical histories should also be covered, including previous diagnostic tests and current diagnoses and medications. The clinician is looking for possible sources of fall risk or causes for loss of balance. Anything potentially impairing the peripheral or central sensory or motor systems or the cognitive abilities of the patient should be noted.

The type and overall number of medications should be noted. Medications that lower blood pressure may increase fall risk if they cause excessively low blood pressure or orthostatic (postural) hypotension. Sedative hypnotic medications are also thought to affect balance. However, a study of elderly community dwellers found no difference in sedative hypnotic use between fallers and non-fallers, although fallers more often took more than four medications.[13] A study of the effect of number of medications taken by 885 community-dwelling older adults (mean age 81), controlling for number of chronic diseases, age, and hospitalizations in the past year, found that those with better balance took fewer medications than those with impaired balance.[53] It should be noted, however, that another study specifically evaluating the effect of number of medications on fall risk found no difference in the number of medications used by older community dwellers with or without a history of falls.[54]

It is also important to ascertain the fall history for patients in this preferred practice pattern, including the number, time, and circumstances of any falls or loss of balance, even when these do not result in injury or actually falling to the ground. The number of previous falls is directly related to the risk of falling again.[38] In addition, the circumstances surrounding a fall can tell the clinician which type of postural control may have malfunctioned, indicating impairments that may require intervention. For example, someone who tripped while ascending well-lighted, evenly rising stairs may have weakness in the hip or ankle dorsiflexors that hindered voluntary postural control. In contrast, tripping on the last of a long line of steps rather than the first few is most likely a result of reduced muscular endurance rather than weakness. Someone who fell when a shopping cart bumped a hip may have slowed initiation of movement that hindered reactive postural control. Patient goals for the prevention of falls or loss of balance should also be clarified.

A number of targeted standardized self-report instruments, including the Balance Efficacy Scale (BES), the Activities-Specific Balance Confidence (ABC) scale, and the Dizziness Handicap Inventory (DHI), have been developed to collect information about a patient's history of loss of balance or falls.[3]

The BES consists of 18 questions asking clients about their level of confidence (0% to 100%) performing daily life tasks. A higher level of confidence is thought to reflect greater perception of "self-efficacy," a proposed mediator of performance. The BES has been shown to improve in older adult fallers after an 8-week balance training program that also improved other balance measures.[55]

The ABC also records respondents' confidence in their ability to maintain balance in various situations.[56-58] Its 16 items range from mobility inside the home to walking in a crowded mall or on an icy sidewalk. Test-retest reliability of this measure in older adults over a 2-week period was 0.92.[56] Lower confidence as recorded on the ABC correlates with slower self-selected gait velocity and lower balance scores after hip fracture[59] and with slower walking speed and greater postural sway in community-dwelling elders.[57] ABC scores were also lower in community-dwelling elderly subjects who reported having fallen in the past year, and the difference between scores in fallers and non-fallers was statistically significant ($p = 0.03$) in one study[60] but not in another ($p = 0.06$).[57] The borderline differentiation between fallers and non-fallers is reflected in the moderate sensitivity (51.9% of fallers correctly identified) and higher specificity (81.5% of non-fallers correctly identified) of the ABC in older adults.[60] ABC scores reflected overall mobility with lower confidence levels (<50%) associated with significant mobility limitations (gait speed <0.5 msec), and high confidence levels (>90%) associated with lack of chronic health conditions in a retirement-age population.[58]

The DHI records self-perceived physical, functional, and emotional effects imposed by vestibular system disease.[61] The DHI has 25 questions scored 0, 2, or 4 with a higher score indicating greater perceived handicap. The average score of one group of 106 consecutive patients with vestibular complaints was 32.7 ± 21.9, out of the total 100 points possible with patients who experienced more episodes of dizziness in the previous year scoring higher.[61] Test-retest reliability (0.97) and internal consistency (0.89) are high. Some authors suggest that a change in score of at least 18 points reflects a significant change in the subject's perceived handicap.[61] Attempts to correlate this patient self-report measure with clinical measures have found no correlation with caloric testing,[61] weak correlation with slow and fast speeds of rotary chair testing,[62] moderate correlation with the Sensory Organization Test (SOT),[62] good correlation with postural sway,[63] and equivocal correlation with posturography.[64,65]

Complaints or data gathered from the patient history that should alert the therapist to a fall risk include imbalance, dizziness, vertigo, *oscillopsia*, nausea and/or vomiting, diminished strength, sensation changes (diminished or paresthesia), hearing loss, tinnitus, or vision changes. Such complaints must be followed by questions asked to determine their different qualities, temporal features, functional conditions, and anatomical extent of the particular problem.[66] For example, allowing the patient or client to describe dizziness further, as *lightheadedness* or a sense of spinning, can help to differentiate between postural hypotension and a vestibular problem.[24] Vertigo, which is the sensation of motion of either self or surroundings, usually has vestibular origins, whereas lightheadedness is usually due to cerebral hypoperfusion. Oscillopsia, which is the illusion of visual motion, can be spontaneous, but words that bounce with reading usually indicate a cerebellar problem, and visual motion induced by head movements might indicate loss of the VOR bilaterally.

Temporal features of the complaint should include precipitating events, rate of onset, duration, termination, and easing or aggravating conditions (Table 13-4). Sporadic or short-term complaints characterize conditions like BPPV, postural hypotension, transient ischemic attacks (TIAs), migraine, panic attacks, or Ménière's disease.[66] Longer-term conditions that cause intense acute complaints include peripheral vestibular disorders like labyrinthitis or vestibular neuritis. More chronic symptoms, whether progressive or stable, generally arise from chronic neurological conditions such as multiple sclerosis, Parkinson's disease, or stroke.

Information should also be obtained about the tasks and environments in which problems occur, including whether imbalance or disequilibrium occurs at rest, during movement, or both. The effects of low light conditions, walking on uneven or unstable terrain, movement, spinning images, flashing lights, and coincidental balance challenges should also be evaluated.

Obtaining accurate information about different features of a patient's complaints takes skilled questioning since patients generally alter their activities to avoid dizziness, loss of balance, and falls. They may avoid situations that require use of a poorly developed motor strategy, keep the head still and the eyes closed when conflicts arise between vision and vestibular sense, or stop performing an activity altogether. Patients may also not be aware of their compensations until specific questioning elicits this information.

SYSTEMS REVIEW

The systems review is used to target areas requiring further examination and to define areas that may cause complications or indicate a need for precautions during the examination and intervention processes. See Chapter 1 for details of the systems review.

TESTS AND MEASURES

In the next component of the examination, the clinician selects specific tests and measures to confirm or reject hypotheses about causes of the patient's loss of balance or

TABLE 13-4	Features of Balance Complaints in Patients with Different Disorders		
Patient Complaint	**Duration**	**Functional Conditions**	**Possible Disorder**
Vertigo, lightheaded, nausea	Seconds	Dynamic; lying down, sitting up or turning over in bed, bending forward	BPPV
Lightheaded	Seconds	Positional; standing up from a sitting or supine position	Orthostatic hypotension
Vertigo, lightheaded, disequilibrium	Minutes	Spontaneous	TIAs
Vertigo, dizziness, motion sickness	During movement	Usually movement induced	Migraine
Dizzy, nausea, diaphoresis, fear, palpitations, paresthesias	Minutes	Spontaneous or situational	Panic attack
Vertigo, disequilibrium, ear fullness from hearing loss and tinnitus	Hours	Spontaneous, exacerbated by head movements	Ménière's disease
Intense disequilibrium, vertigo, nausea	Continuous for 2-3 days	At rest and during movement	Acute unilateral peripheral vestibular hypofunction
Dizzy, disequilibrium	Continuous	Head movements, walking; worse in dark or uneven surface	Bilateral, or chronic unilateral, peripheral vestibular pathology
Disequilibrium	Stable or progressive	Turning, negotiating stairs, experiencing perturbations, or completing transitional movements	MS, PD, cortical stroke
Disequilibrium, may have oscillopsia from nystagmus	Stable, or progressive if degenerative disorder	Disequilibrium while on feet; oscillopsia while reading	Cerebellar disorders
Vertigo, disequilibrium, lateropulsion, oscillopsia, sensory loss	Stable/improves in days	Spontaneous, exacerbated by head movements	Brainstem stroke

BPPV, Benign paroxysmal positional vertigo; *TIA,* transient ischemic attacks; *MS,* multiple sclerosis; *PD,* Parkinson's disease.

fall risk suggested by the history and systems review. The accumulated examination findings will then allow the clinician to complete the evaluation, make a diagnosis and prognosis, and intervene effectively.

Musculoskeletal

Posture. The relative location of the COG over the BOS (centered or too close to one edge) in a patient's typical sitting and standing positions should be examined[10] (see Chapter 4). For patients using an assistive device, standing posture with and without the device should be noted, along with the size of the BOS (wide or narrow), and the height of the COG (stooping versus upright posture). Although poor standing posture does not correlate with force-plate measured instability in people with vestibular hypofunction,[67] postural disturbances can be a sign of CNS lesions or deficiencies in ROM at various joints. Postural asymmetries and abnormalities can also be a clue to pain, fatigue, or other dysfunction. Head tilt, particularly combined with skew deviation and torsion of the eyes, may indicate vestibular involvement and disorders of perception of vertical.[27]

Range of Motion and Muscle Performance. ROM and muscle performance (see Chapter 5) should be examined when the systems review or history suggests these could be impaired. In patients with poor standing balance, ROM and muscle performance at the ankles should be tested; in those with poor sitting balance, hip ROM and trunk strength should be tested. Ankle ROM has been shown to have moderately high correlation with the ability to accomplish gait and reaching balance tasks in standing and moderate, although significant, correlation with standing up and turning balance tasks in older women.[34] Loss of strength in one or both lower limbs is a significant fall risk factor for hospitalized older adults.[36] Neck ROM

must also be checked before performing any of the head-moving vestibular tests.

Neuromuscular

Arousal, Attention, and Cognition. Cognition and attention affect balance because movement choices are based on perception and memory of consequences. Although there are many tests of cognition,[68] a commonly used standardized measure is the MMSE.[69] The MMSE is a quick test of orientation, memory, reading, verbalization, copying a drawn figure, and writing and is scored from 0 to 30, with a higher score indicating better cognitive function. This test has been found to be reliable, with a test-retest reliability or 0.89 to 0.99,[69] and valid, correlating highly with verbal and performance aspects of the Wechsler Adult Intelligence Scale (WAIS) (0.78 and 0.66, respectively).[69] Patients admitted to a geriatric rehabilitation facility who had scores less than 18 on the MMSE were almost twice as likely to fall as those with higher scores.[70] In addition to cognition, MMSE scores have been linked to attention deficits, or an inability to concentrate on physical performance while a computational task is attempted at the same time. Older adults with MMSE scores of 24 or above show no dual-task performance deficits during balance activities, compared to those with lower scores.[43]

Therapists can also test attention directly by presenting clients with multiple tasks or multitasking skills. One reported method notes the ability to walk and talk at the same time.[71,72] If, while walking with the clinician, the subject must stop walking to take part in conversation, then the test is recorded as positive; if the subject can continue walking while talking, then the test is recorded as negative. For elderly subjects who cannot divide attention sufficiently to talk while walking, this fact alone positively predicted falls in 83%. For those who did not stop walking when talking, 76% did not have falls in the subsequent 6 months.[71]

Cranial Nerve Integrity. Testing of cranial nerve integrity is a particularly important component of the examination of patients with decreased balance and increased fall risk because of the critical contributions of vision and the vestibular system to maintenance of balance.[66] If the patient complains of diplopia (double vision) or blurred vision or balance problems in low light conditions, a vision screen should be performed, including simple tests of visual acuity, visual fields, light reflex (direct and consensual), accommodation, and convergent and conjugate eye movements. Any problems should be referred appropriately, but compensatory methods can be taught to patients if visual problems affect balance. Testing of conjugate eye movements should specifically note smooth pursuit and whether nystagmus is evoked other than at the ends of the range of eye motion. If nystagmus is noted at the change of direction within about 30 degrees of center, this may indicate central vestibular problems if there is no other confounding eye pathology.[63]

If a patient reports hearing loss or tinnitus, an auditory screen should be performed, recognizing that any lesion affecting hearing might similarly affect the vestibular system, which shares cranial nerve VIII.

If a patient reports vertigo or oscillopsia or if nystagmus is noted during vision testing, vestibular testing should be performed. The goal of vestibular testing is to localize the lesion to the right and/or left side and to the central or peripheral components of the vestibular system. The severity of symptoms during symptom-inducing tests may also be used as a baseline for comparison following intervention. Vestibular testing is intended to provoke the patient's symptoms through movements similar to those used for functional activities. Because these tests provoke unpleasant sensation, patients generally do not like them repeated. This may explain the paucity of reliability data for some tests and differences in results obtained by well-trained and inexperienced clinicians. The clinician should select among available tests according to the history regarding times and functional conditions where symptoms occur and by the availability of specialized testing equipment. Referral to a setting where specialized equipment is available may be necessary in some cases to make an accurate physical therapy diagnosis.

Vestibular testing may begin with observation of the eyes for alignment and any spontaneous nystagmus in room light.[63] Skew deviations and nystagmus can occur during the most acute stage of peripheral vestibular lesions, even when objects can be seen for optical fixation. When a skew deviation makes one eye appear higher than the other (Fig. 13-11), the skew is named by the eye that appears elevated even though the skew is caused by the other eye dropping because of loss of tonic vestibular input.[63]

The head thrust test is performed by the patient keeping gaze stationary (fixed on the therapist's nose, for example) while the therapist turns the patient's head passively slowly and then quickly to one side or the other and

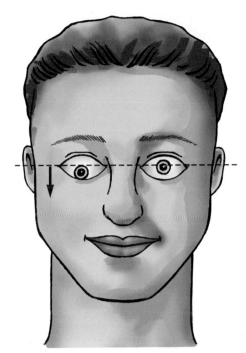

FIG. 13-11 Eye position with a left skew deviation.

then slowly and quickly in a vertical direction.[27] The slow motion is performed to check that the patient can comfortably move through the necessary range, and the fast motion is the actual test. With normal vestibular function, patients should be able to maintain gaze on the stationary object without difficulty at all speeds (Fig. 13-12, *A*). Failure to maintain gaze on the stationary object in response to fast motion to one side, followed by corrective saccades, suggests a unilateral lesion (Fig. 13-12, *B* and *C*), whereas saccades in response to motion to both sides suggest bilateral lesions. Although the specificity of this test is fairly high at 95%, its sensitivity for identifying people with vestibular hypofunction is low at 35%, possibly because of inconsistencies in speed of head movement.[72] Having the patient tilt the head forward 30 degrees and ensuring that the rapid head thrusts are unpredictable in timing and direction may improve the sensitivity of this test.[73]

Frenzel glasses are +20 or +30 (magnifying) lenses mounted on a frame that prevents the subject from fixating on objects while allowing the observing clinician, with the help of a light, to examine the subject's magnified eyes. Either these glasses, or a darkened room to limit fixation, along with an infrared camera for the clinician to watch eye movement, may be required for the careful observation of nystagmus needed for some tests.[74] A couple of beats of nystagmus in response to rapid rotation of the head or at extreme end-ranges of motion of the eyes is considered normal, but nystagmus with other characteristics generally indicates some abnormality. Nystagmus may be evaluated using the head-shaking test, the Hallpike-Dix maneuver, or the rotary chair test. The direction of nystagmus is considered to be the direction of the rapid saccades. Table 13-5 reviews the interpretation of directions of nystagmus with these tests.

TABLE 13-5	Nystagmus Related to Particular Vestibular Lesions Under Various Conditions			
	Vestibular Lesion			
Condition	Peripheral	Central	Unilateral	Bilateral
Spontaneous	Acute only: Mostly horizontal, quick toward normal side in the absence of fixation	Remains visible in room light ≥2 weeks after onset, may be purely vertical, may be pendular	Acute: Quick toward normal side	None
Head shaking test	Horizontal: Quick toward normal side	Vertical, may be pendular	Horizontal: Quick toward normal side	None
Hallpike-Dix test	Up- or down-beating and torsional or horizontal, depending on canal involved; latency of 1-40 seconds; symptoms resolve in 30-60 seconds	Persistent even if test is repeated several times in a short period, vertical, no latency, lasts longer than 30-60 seconds	Only noted when performed to one side	Noted when performed to each side
Rotary chair test	Longer duration than normal	Diverse patterns, pendular, dysrhythmic movement		

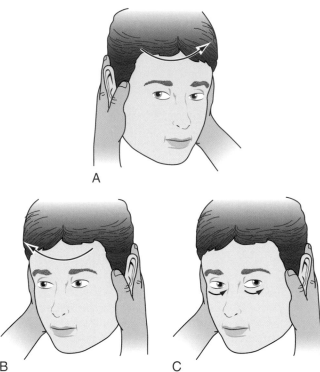

FIG. 13-12 The head thrust test. The test is started with the eyes fixated on a target, and the head in slight cervical flexion to improve test sensitivity. **A,** Normal response to rapid head thrust to the left: the eyes smoothly move to the right maintaining fixation on the target. **B,** Abnormal response to rapid head thrust to the right. The eyes initially lose the target and move with the head. **C,** Then make small saccades to the left to regain fixation on the target.

In the head-shaking test, the patient sits, with eyes closed, Frenzel glasses on, and head tilted forward 30 degrees (so that the horizontal semi-circular canal is parallel to the ground). The therapist passively moves the patient's head from side to side horizontally 20 times over 40 seconds, then stops and asks the patient to open their eyes. People with a unilateral peripheral vestibular problem will have horizontal nystagmus toward the normal side.[27]

The Hallpike-Dix test can be performed in two different ways.[27] In the first, the patient long-sits on the plinth, the therapist rotates the patient's head horizontally 45 degrees, then, while holding the rotation, supports the patient in moving quickly to a supine position with the head off the edge of the plinth and the neck extended 30 degrees (Fig. 13-13, *A*). In the second method, the patient short-sits on the side of the plinth, the therapist rotates the head away from the coming direction of movement by 45 degrees, then, while holding the rotation, supports the patient in moving quickly to a sidelying position opposite to the rotation of the head (Fig. 13-13, *B*). The ear closest to the ground indicates the side being tested in both ways of performing the Hallpike-Dix maneuver. If nystagmus occurs, it will be up-beating and torsional if the posterior semicircular canal is involved (incidence = 63% to 87%), down-beating and torsional if the anterior semicircular canal is involved (incidence = 12% to 36%), and horizontal only if the horizontal semicircular canal is involved (incidence = 1%). In theory, if the nystagmus starts a few seconds after the position change and resolves within 60 seconds, then the cause is likely canalithiasis: Calcium carbonate debris is free-floating in the canal. If the nystagmus lasts as long as the position is maintained, then cupulolithiasis is more likely: Debris is weighing down the cupula in the direction of gravity.[27]

The rotary chair test involves rotating a seated patient 10 times in 20 seconds, with the patient's head tilted forward 30 degrees, and then observing for the duration of the nystagmus when tested both clockwise and counterclockwise. Postrotatory nystagmus lasting more than a few beats is considered abnormal in lighted environments where the eyes should easily fixate on an object. More recent advances in technology have converted the simple manual rotation of a chair, used for nearly a century, to a motorized version in a darkened room controlled by computer. The parameters of significance are the duration of the slow and fast phases of the nystagmus, measured with specialized equipment.[74]

Other vestibular tests include the clinical dynamic visual acuity (DVA) test and the Fukuda step test. Static

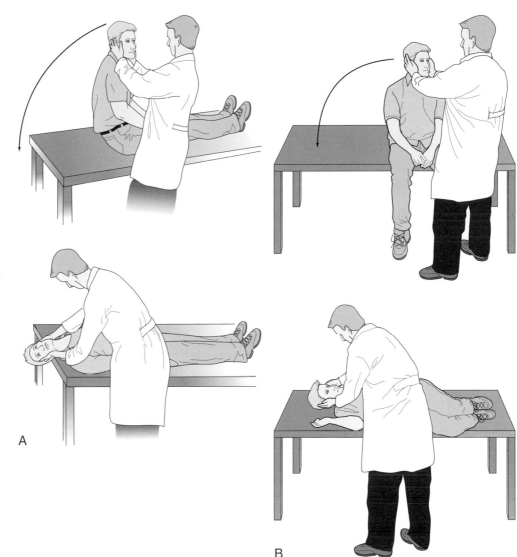

FIG. 13-13 The Hallpike-Dix test. **A,** Starting in long-sitting position. **B,** Starting in short-sitting position. *Adapted from Herdman SJ: Phys Ther 70(6):381-388, 1990.*

A

B

visual acuity is generally assessed with the head in a static position, recorded by the line number on an eye chart that the patient can still read accurately. For the dynamic visual acuity test, the patient reads the chart while the therapist rotates the patient's head left and then right within 1 second. If the line the patient can read decreases by only one, the test is considered normal. If it decreases by 3 or more lines, the patient may have vestibular hypofunction. A computerized version of the dynamic visual acuity test was found to have a sensitivity and specificity of 94.5% and 95.2%, respectively, for the detection of vestibular dysfunction. Statistics for the manual version have yet to be obtained.[72]

For the Fukuda step test,[63] the patient is instructed to march in place for 50 steps with arms raised to shoulder height in front, first with eyes open and then with eyes closed. Moving forward by up to 50 cm and rotating by up to 30 degrees is considered a normal result. Patients with unilateral vestibular deficits affecting the long vestibulospinal tracts may rotate more than 30 degrees when their eyes are closed. Since patients with bilateral vestibular hypofunction may fall during this test,[72] appro-priate guarding is essential. However, the high numbers of false positives and false negatives for the Fukuda step test limit its utility.[63]

Peripheral Nerve Integrity. If the patient history or systems review suggest the presence of motor or sensory losses, particularly in the distal lower extremities, periph-eral nerve integrity should be tested (see Chapter 18).

Motor Function—Control and Learning. In addition to testing for muscle performance or weakness during the musculoskeletal component of the tests and measures, the clinician may also need to test motor control, tone, and coordination that relate to CNS functions. The patient's ability to isolate muscle activity should be observed; dependence on synergistic movements as in poststroke hemiparesis can limit a patient's options for postural control, particularly when encountering unexpected envi-ronmental obstacles. Use of a measure of motor recovery after stroke, such as the Fugl-Meyer Assessment, can doc-ument the extent of synergy dependence in patients after a stroke.[75,76] The Fugl-Meyer Assessment also includes a specific balance component that has been shown to be valid and reliable.[77,78]

Cerebellar screening is critical for the examination of a patient at risk for loss of balance or falls. All coordinated movement is processed in the cerebellum, including movements that require upright control and those that can be performed with the trunk and head fully supported. Nonequilibrium tests, those that require no upright control, might include the finger-to-nose or heel-to-shin movements to test for dysmetria, or the pronation-supination or toe-tapping movements to test for dysdiadochokinesia, the term for uncoordinated rapid alternating movements.

Equilibrium tests require that the patient assumes and maintains the upright position, coordinating motor output with the sensory input of the upright position. In this sense, equilibrium is synonymous with balance. Disequilibrium is when performance on these tests is poor or people report the sense of being off-balance. Common tests of equilibrium include the Romberg, Sharpened Romberg, one-legged stance, and tandem-walking. The first three of these tests also are considered tests of quiet standing balance and may be categorized as such by some authors.[4] The Romberg test is essentially the same as the first two conditions of the Clinical Test of Sensory Balance (CTSIB): Standing for 30 seconds with feet together, first with eyes open and then with eyes closed. A positive Romberg test is one in which, when the eyes are closed, the patient starts to fall and makes no attempt to correct this. The Sharpened Romberg repeats the Romberg test but with the feet lined up in tandem, heel to toe. Patients who rely on a wide BOS to maintain upright stance will have trouble with the Sharpened Romberg, particularly with the weaker (less capable) leg behind the stronger one. The one-legged stance test documents how long the patient can stand on each leg alone, up to 30 seconds, and is difficult for patients who have pathologies that restrict the ability to maintain control over a small BOS.[55] Likewise, patients with an ataxic or wide-based gait will have trouble walking on a line, or heel-to-toe as in the tandem walk. Difficulty with tandem walking correlates significantly with fall risk in older hospitalized patients.[36]

Standing with successively smaller bases of support is a balance test that was standardized for the Frailty and Injuries Cooperative Studies of Intervention Techniques (FICSIT) trials.[79] The FICSIT-3 includes 3 conditions of timed static standing (for up to 10 seconds) with eyes open: (1) feet together, (2) stride stance, and (3) tandem stance. The FICSIT-4 test adds a fourth condition, single-legged stance, to raise the ceiling for very able subjects (Fig. 13-14).[23] The conditions were thought to be sequential in difficulty, so if a person could not complete 10 seconds of an easier condition, the clinician would not have the person attempt the next harder condition.

In the FICSIT trials, common data were collected across 8 sites, from 2,559 older subjects, ranging from quite fit to frail.[23] The FICSIT-3 is scored as follows:

0 = Subject refuses or fails first condition (so no other conditions attempted).

0.5 = Subject achieves first condition (feet together) but holds it for less than 10 seconds.

1.0 = Subject holds first condition for 10 seconds but refuses or fails second condition.

1.5 = Subject holds first condition for 10 seconds and achieves second condition (stride stance) but cannot hold second condition for full 10 seconds.

2.0 = Subject holds (first and) second condition for 10 seconds but refuses or fails third condition (tandem stance).

3.0 = Subject holds (first and) second condition for 10 seconds and achieves third condition but cannot hold third condition for full 10 seconds.

4.0 = Subject holds (first and second and) third condition for full 10 seconds.

The FICSIT-4 test revises the definition for a score of 4.0, requiring that the subject also achieves but cannot hold the fourth condition and adds a level:

5.0 = Subject holds (first and second and third and fourth condition [single-legged stance]) for full 10 seconds.

For example, a person who could stand for 10 seconds with feet parallel but for less than 10 seconds with feet in stride stance would score 1.5 on the FICSIT test.[23] The reliability of this test averaged 0.66 across multiple sites. This test has also been shown to correlate with other balance and gait measures but has not been evaluated for its validity in predicting falls.

Neuromotor Development and Sensory Integration. Central integration of vestibular, visual and somatosensory systems for balance control can be examined with the CTSIB, also known as the "foam and dome" test for its characteristic equipment[8] (Fig. 13-15). The "foam" can be a cushion or cut piece of foam that provides a compliant surface on which the patient can stand. The "dome" can be devised from a large Japanese lantern, cut out at the back so that it can be positioned over the head of the patient. The dome creates a condition in which the visible environment (the inside of the lantern) moves with the body and head, thereby eliminating any horizontal and vertical visual cues. With the dome on, the patient receives false visual information about the body's movement because the environment moves at the same rate as sway. The integrated brain should be able to compare vestibular input to that false visual input and determine that the body is actually swaying. When, in addition to faulty visual input, the patient stands on a compliant surface that interferes with the somatosensory system's evaluation of sway, the vestibular system must reconcile differences between faulty sensation and movement of the head.

Postural sway is noted qualitatively during each condition. Passing the test requires that a patient maintain the position for the full 30 seconds for each trial of each tested condition. Moving the arms or feet, opening the eyes during eyes closed conditions, or swaying to the extent of a near fall under any condition stops the clock for that trial, decreasing the overall points. A modified CTSIB deletes conditions 3 and 6, the ones requiring a dome for sway-referenced vision.[63] The CTSIB has been found to be a reliable test. Agreement between two raters using this test was 68% to 100% for patients after stroke,[28] and inter-rater and intrarater reliability was 99% in a study with

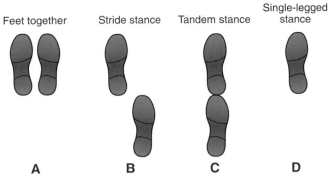

Feet together   Stride stance   Tandem stance   Single-legged stance

A   B   C   D

FIG. 13-14 **A** to **C**, Stance positions for FICSIT-3 test. **A** to **D**, Stance positions for FICSIT-4 test. *Redrawn from Hasson S: Clinical Exercise Physiology, St. Louis, Mosby, 1994.*

young and old healthy subjects and patients with vestibular disorders.[6]

The SOT (also known as the EquiTest) is a version of the CTSIB that uses computerized force-plate technology and dynamic posturography to gather similar information (Fig. 13-16). Scores on the SOT correlate well (90%) with scores on the CTSIB in people with vestibular disorders,[80] and the validity of this test was supported by a study with 47 community-dwelling elders, in which it was found that people who had fallen 2 or more times in the previous 6 months had significantly shorter stance duration than non-fallers in conditions 4-6 (those on the unstable surface) of the SOT.[29]

Cardiovascular. Cardiovascular tests may be indicated if the vital signs examined in the systems review reveal deficits. Postural hypotension, a source of light-headedness and loss of balance, will not be detected if blood pressure is only measured with the patient in one position. Therefore blood pressure and heart rate should be measured before and after transition from lying to

FIG. 13-15 Conditions for the Clinical Test of Sensory Integration in Balance (CTSIB). The patient stands with feet together and arms crossed for 30 seconds 3 times each under 6 different conditions: *1,* Normal vision, fixed surface; *2,* Absent vision (eyes closed), fixed surface; *3,* Sway referenced vision (with the dome on), fixed surface; *4,* Normal vision, compliant surface (standing on the foam); *5,* Absent vision, compliant surface; *6,* Sway-referenced vision, compliant surface. *Redrawn from Hasson S: Clinical Exercise Physiology, St. Louis, 1994, Mosby.*

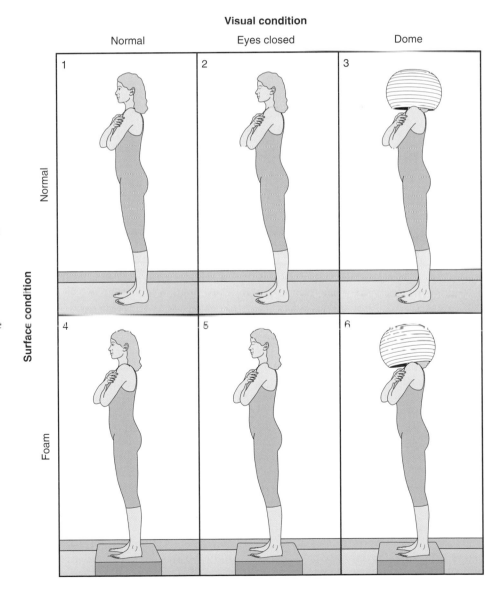

Visual condition

Normal   Eyes closed   Dome

Surface condition

Normal

Foam

1   2   3

4   5   6

Visual condition

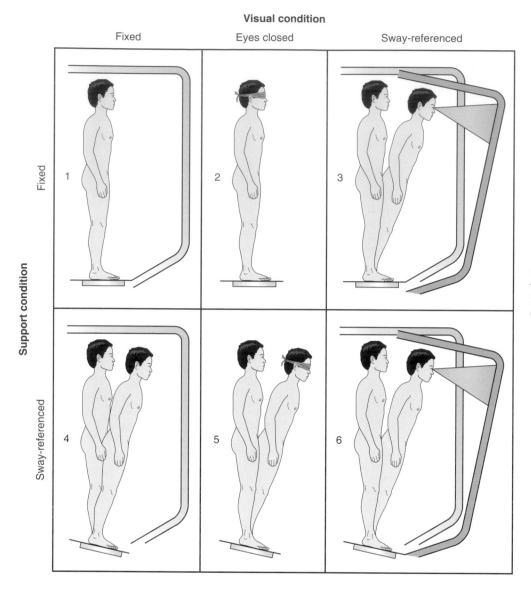

FIG. 13-16 Support and visual conditions for the Sensory Organization Test (SOT).

standing. A fall in systolic blood pressure of more than 20 mm Hg or an increase in heart rate of more than 10 beats per minute indicates the presence of postural hypotension (see Chapter 22).

The vertebral artery compression test should also be performed in people complaining of dizziness. For this test the patient is supine and the neck is extended and then rotated to one and then the other side (Fig. 13-17, *A*). Reproduction of symptoms suggests vertebral artery compression on the side of the direction of rotation. BPPV and vertebral artery compression can be differentiated by repeating the vertebral artery test in sitting, with the patient forward flexed at the hips before extending and rotating the neck (Fig. 13-17, *B*). If symptoms occur in this position, they can more clearly be attributed to vertebral artery compression than to BPPV because in this position head rotation should not affect the semicircular canals.[81]

Integumentary. Integumentary integrity should be observed on the plantar aspects of the feet because

avoidance of painful areas may decrease the patient's BOS and decrease balance.

Function

Locomotion and Balance. Functional testing is especially important in people with increased fall risk, since most falls do not occur in static, but rather in dynamic and functional situations. Many tests may be needed to cover the basic functional tasks of balance: Static balance, *anticipatory postural control* (client initiated movement requiring balance adjustment), and reactive postural control (client responds to unexpected need for balance adjustment).[10,82]

Tinetti's Performance-Oriented Mobility Assessment (POMA)[83] is a balance test developed specifically for older adults that has since been used with a limited number of other populations.[84,85] The instrument has a 7-item gait subscale and a 9-item balance subscale. Each item can receive 1-2 criterion-referenced points. Balance activities assessed include sitting, rising from sitting, standing with

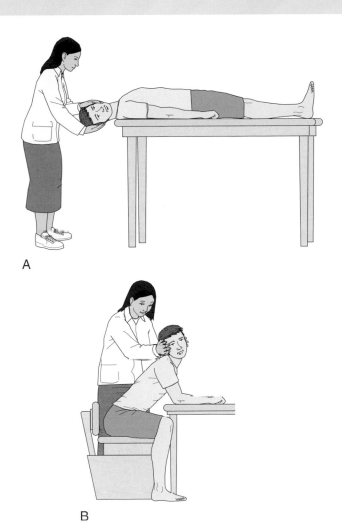

FIG. 13-17 A, Supine vertebral artery compression test.
B, Sitting vertebral artery compression test.

eyes open or closed, nudge test, tandem stance, single limb stance, reaching, bending, and turning 360 degrees. Scores from the balance and gait subscales total 28 in normally functioning adults. A score of 19 or less indicates a high risk for falling; 19-24 points indicate a moderate risk.[83] This instrument has high interrater (85% agreement) and intrarater[86] reliability, and low scores on the POMA have been shown to correlate with fall risk in elderly adults.[87-89] Two modifications to the POMA have focused it more for community-dwelling elderly (POMA IA, with a possible score of 40), or for people who are frail and at risk for injury (POMA II, with a possible score of 54).[12,90]

The Dynamic Gait Index (DGI)[10] was developed to assess walking under various dynamic conditions. It consists of eight walking tasks that patients would likely perform on a daily basis. The tool examines (1) walking on a level surface, (2) capacity for changing gait speed, (3 and 4) ability to walk and turn the head in horizontal and vertical directions, (5) balance for rapid directional changes, (6 and 7) capacity for stepping over and around an obstacle, and (8) stair performance. Each item is scored 0-3, lower scores indicating greater impairment. A score of 19 or less correlates with a history of more falls.[22,54] Interrater reliability (0.96) and test-retest reliability (0.98) are both high.[22] In a sample of 54 community-dwelling older adults, using a cut-off score of 19, this test was found to have a 66.7% sensitivity and a 61.5% specificity for identifying individuals who had fallen once or more in the previous 6 months.[60] In another study using the same cut-off score, the DGI was found to have 59% sensitivity and 64% specificity for identifying individuals who had fallen twice or more in the previous 6 months.[54]

While initially developed for determining fall risk in an elderly adult population, the DGI has also been used to evaluate fall risk in people with vestibular problems. A study of adults with vestibular dysfunction found that a score of 19 or less on the DGI was associated with a $2\frac{1}{2}$ times greater chance of falling in the past 6 months than a score of more than 19.[91] The authors concluded that the DGI can identify fallers with vestibular dysfunction regardless of age. However, this tool has only moderate interrater reliability (overall kappa = 0.64) when used in people with vestibular disorders.[92]

The Timed Up and Go (TUG) test,[93-94] combines several common functions that patients are likely to encounter many times each day. It requires the subject to rise from a standard chair, walk 3.0 m (10 feet) at a comfortable pace to a mark placed on the floor, turn around, walk back to the starting point, and return to sitting in the chair. The score is the number of seconds the subject takes to complete the test. The developers of this test report inter- and intra-rater reliability of 0.99 for the TUG in 60 patients at a day hospital.[94] Using a cut-off score of 20 seconds, this test was found to be 87% sensitive and specific for distinguishing community-dwelling individuals who had not fallen from those who reported 2 or more falls in the previous 6 months.[95] Although most healthy individuals without neurological impairments can complete the TUG in less than 10 seconds, the range for people with impairments and disabilities is quite wide. People who take up to 20 seconds to complete the test remain quite functionally independent, whereas people who take more than 30 seconds will need assistance with activities of daily living (ADLs). People who take longer than 20 seconds to complete the test are considered at high risk for falling.[94] When additional cognitive (counting backwards by threes) or manual tasks (carrying a cup of water) are added to the TUG, subjects take longer to complete the test but the test does not identify fallers any more accurately.[96] Since the TUG was developed, it has been used quite widely to examine and document mobility function in patients with various diagnoses.[86,96-99]

The Berg Balance Scale (BBS) was developed for elderly adults, with 14 items testing various sitting and standing balance activities using a 0-4 scale.[100] Based on the criterion assigned to each item, a score of 4 is given if the client is fully able to perform the activity. A score of 0 indicates inability to perform any aspect of the item. Scores below 45 out of the maximum 56 indicate impaired balance and greater risk for falls. Interrater reliability is 0.99, intrarater reliability is 0.98.[101] Evidence for validity includes a relatively high correlation with a global balance rating by a physical therapist ($r = 0.81$), and moderate correlation with postural sway as measured using a computerized balance platform that records changes in force.[101]

When used as a predictive tool, a score of 45 or less on the BBS is only 53% sensitive but 92% specific for falls in the 6 months *after* the test.[102] The low sensitivity may be because those with greater physical impairment and thus lower BBS scores may have environmental and behavioral adaptations in place to compensate for fall risk, thus lowering their number of falls.

The BBS has been used as an indicator of fall risk in many studies assessing the effectiveness of interventions intended to improve balance and reduce fall risk.[103] Subjects in a residential care facility had higher BBS scores, by an average of 5.6 points, after a 4- to 5-week physical therapy program, and retained that improvement when tested a month later.[104] Subjects after stroke had higher BBS scores by an average of 14 points after a 4-week course of rehabilitation.[49] Subjects who had central balance dysfunction had significantly higher BBS scores after outpatient vestibular and balance therapy.[105]

The BBS takes about 20 minutes to complete; Kornetti et al suggest, after a Rasch analysis of the BBS, that it may be unnecessary to administer all of the items if the criterion scoring is weighted appropriately for difficulty.[103] In their sample of 100 veterans, if a person was able to pass the item tandem stance (with a score of 4), while receiving a passing score also on 2 out of 3 of the following—alternating foot on stool (score of 3), standing on one leg (score of 2), and look behind while standing (score of 2)—then the person had a score above the cut-off of 45 for the entire test, indicating low risk for falling without considering the other items.[103]

The Functional Reach test provides a quick clinical assessment of anticipatory postural control in the anterior direction.[16] A yardstick is taped to the wall at shoulder height. The patient stands with the tested shoulder next to the wall, then, without touching the wall or using any other support, reaches forward as far as possible along the wall without moving the feet or losing balance (Fig. 13-18). Most people can reach more than 10 inches. A reach of 6 inches or less indicates limited functional balance. In a sample of 128 people ranging in age from 21 to 87 years, the test-retest reliability of this test was 0.81; in persons with PD, it was 0.84.[106] Test-retest reliability is this low because twisting of the trunk or other angulation of the body can alter functional reach. Therefore, a lateral reach test has been suggested and this has been found to have high test-retest reliability (>0.94). For the lateral reach test, standing still for 10 seconds with both arms stretched to the sides at shoulder height helps standardize the starting position.[107]

The Physical Performance Test (PPT) is a simple clinical test that takes about 10-15 minutes to complete.[108] In the 7-item version, patients write a sentence, simulate eating, put a jacket on and take it off, lift a book, turn 360 degrees in standing, pick up a penny from the floor, and walk 50 feet. The 9-item version also scores the time it takes to

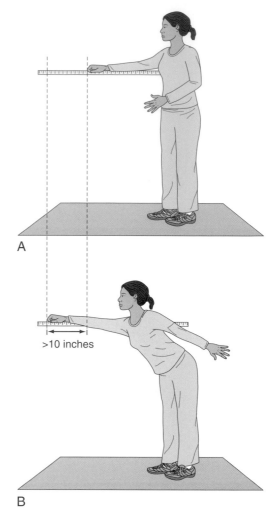

FIG. 13-18 The Functional Reach test. **A,** Starting position. **B,** Normal functional reach of more than 10 inches.

climb a flight of stairs and the number of flights (up to 4) the patient is able to climb. Each item has 5 levels of performance, scored 0-4, based on completion of the task and the time taken. Higher scores equal higher level of performance. The interrater reliability of this test has been reported to be good, but the statistical result was reported as a Pearson correlation coefficient when it should probably have been assessed as a kappa value.[87] The 7-item PPT has been found to predict recurrent falls in 84 community-dwelling frail veterans with a sensitivity of 78% and specificity of 71%, using a cut-off score of 15 out of the total possible of 28.[109] Using a cut-off score of 14/28, patients admitted to a geriatric rehabilitation unit were more than 3 times as likely to fall during hospitalization if they had lower PPT scores instead of higher scores.[70]

EVALUATION, DIAGNOSIS, AND PROGNOSIS

After completing the examination of a patient with poor balance, the therapist evaluates the data and makes clinical judgments to determine a diagnosis, prognosis, and plan of care. According to the *Guide to Physical Therapist Practice,*[21] the conditions that might result in a higher risk for loss of balance and falling include advanced age, alteration in auditory, visual or somatosensation, dementia, depression, dizziness, fear of falling, history of falls, medications, musculoskeletal diseases, neuromuscular diseases, prolonged inactivity, and vestibular pathology. The condition alone, however, does not tell the clinician much about the movement dysfunction or appropriate management of the patient. The clinician needs additional data from the examination to determine the specific problems at the level of impairments, functional limitations, and disabilities. Prognosis for patients with poor balance and increased fall risk depends on many variables, including severity of the condition, concurrent medical conditions, overall health status, and cognitive status, to name a few. If underlying pathology can be corrected or alleviated, then return to normal function may be achievable. However, in many patients, falls cannot be completely prevented, but balance can be improved and the risk of falling reduced through therapeutic exercise, balance training, and lifestyle modification.

In establishing the plan of care for patients with poor balance at risk for falls, the overall or primary goal is to minimize impairments and maximize function. According to the *Guide to Physical Therapist Practice,*[21] more specific goals and outcomes of intervention for patients or clients with balance problems could include (1) resolve or prevent impairment; (2) improve functional balance, particularly during gait; (3) decrease the risk of falls; (4) improve the ability to see clearly and focus during head movement or when in a moving environment; (5) improve overall general physical condition and activity level; (6) reduce social isolation caused by fear of falling; and (7) decrease the patient's disequilibrium and oscillopsia.

INTERVENTION

Current theories underlying interventions for balance and fall prevention focus on the individual, the task, the environment, and their interactions.[10] In general, improving individual capabilities, manipulating the task and/or the environment, and progressing tasks from lower to higher demands can improve balance and reduce fall risk. However, the same interventions are not indicated for all patients with balance deficits.[13,22,110]

FLEXIBILITY EXERCISES

Flexibility exercises can increase ROM in patients with limited ROM and consequent poor balance.[34,111] Patients with balance problems and increased fall risk often have tight trunk flexors, hip flexors, and ankle plantarflexors that may be lengthened by spinal extension, hip extension in a prone position, and heel cord stretching, respectively. Decreased tightness in these muscle groups should improve balance, although few studies have specifically evaluated the effects of flexibility exercises on balance. In one study of 46 men and women with Parkinson's disease, however, the group receiving 10 weeks of progressive exercise to improve spinal flexibility had a significant improvement in both axial rotation and the functional reach test compared to the control group.[111] Stretching is also frequently added to a strengthening program[112] or included in multi-factorial interventions that have been reported to improve balance and reduce fall risk.[13,105,113,114]

STRENGTH TRAINING

Studies have found that strength affects balance and that strengthening exercises, even when they do not produce measurable changes in strength, can improve balance or reduce fall risk, particularly in older adults.[37,114,115] Strengthening functional groups of muscles together may more effectively improve balance than strengthening specific muscles in isolation. Brown et al found in a group 16 frail healthy older adults (75-88 years of age) no correlation between the strength of individual muscles and balance but a fair correlation between the strength of functional muscle groups combined (e.g., hip extensors, knee extensors, and plantarflexors together) and balance.[37]

Although many studies report strength changes as a result of strength training (see Chapter 5), some specifically relate changes to improved balance or reduced fall risk. Douris et al found that lower body exercise like walking activities and active leg movements, whether performed in a therapy pool or on land, improved balance in 11 older adults as indicated by significantly higher scores on the BBS.[116] Aquatic exercise provides an added degree of safety since a loss of balance in the water is less likely to result in an injurious fall.

Buchner et al studied the effects of strength and endurance training programs on balance and prospectively reported falls, as well as a number of other outcomes, in 105 adults ages 68 to 85 with poor balance and reduced strength.[115] Subjects were initially unable to perform 8 steps of a tandem gait pattern without problems and had knee extensor strength below the 50th percentile for their height and weight, without other diagnoses or known problems. All exercise was performed in a supervised setting for 1 hour three times per week, for 24-26 weeks, and thereafter independently by the subjects without supervision. The exercises consisted of strength training using weight machines (n = 25), endurance training using bicycles (n = 25), combined strength and endurance training (n = 25), or no intervention for a control group (n = 30). Follow-up continued up to 25 months after intervention.[115] No differences in balance measures were found between the four groups, using the FICSIT-3 test, as well as a wide and narrow balance beam walk, and a 30-second standing test in which subjects attempted to maintain a level position on a tilt board. However, when they combined the exercise groups together, those who exercised had a significantly reduced fall incidence compared to those in the control group. The percentage of persons who fell and the number of falls were lower in the exercise groups: 42% of the exercisers reported falling in the first year compared to 60% of those not in any exercise group, and the average rate of falls per year was 0.49 in the exercise groups and 0.81 in the control groups. Participating in some kind of exercise was also associated with fewer outpatient clinic visits ($p < 0.06$) and a lower probability of hospital costs over $5,000 in the following year ($p < 0.05$).[116]

Strengthening exercises for patients with poor balance and increased fall risk usually focus on the lower extremities, particularly the ankle and hip muscles, and include task specific activities such as weight shifting, step-up or step-over-objects exercises, and single-leg or tandem standing activities. Standing activities on uneven surfaces can also be used to activate and strengthen the ankle muscles (dorsiflexors and plantarflexors). Continuing exercises to increase endurance, as well as strength, should include monitoring the vital signs and perceived exertion of the patient or client. (See Chapter 5 for other types of exercise and Chapters 22 and 23 for approaches to patient monitoring.)

SENSORY TRAINING OR RETRAINING

Sensory training is intended to optimize the function of the visual, vestibular, and proprioceptive sensory systems to enhance delivery of information to the CNS where it can be integrated and processed, and then used to control balance. Although sensory training and retraining typically augment other types of balance training included in multidimensional or multifactorial training,[3,13,22,117] sensory training can prove effective when combined with limited numbers of other interventions. In a small study (n = 29) of the effects of combined sensory and muscular training on balance, the experimental group showed improvements in one-leg balance with eyes closed, as well as several dynamic measures of postural sway, whereas the "usual activity" group showed no significant changes.[118] The intervention consisted of two 60-minute sessions each week for 12 weeks and focused on balance exercises challenging the visual system (opened/closed eyes), vestibular system (utilizing head movements), somatosensory system (standing on compliant surfaces), and muscular training (one-leg stance and COG activities).

Training differs depending on whether the sensory systems are functioning poorly or not at all. Poorly functioning sensory systems can be trained to assist with balance by "forcing" them to be more active. To force any one system to function better, one should minimize or provide confounding input from the other systems. Thus, to improve visual system balance functions, such as VOR and gaze stabilization, somatosensory and vestibular input should be confounded. This can be achieved by having the patient stand on a soft or moving surface and also move the head. To force use of an underused proprioceptive or vestibular system, the patient could close the eyes. To specifically force use of proprioceptive systems, the patient could stand on a firm surface while both visual information and vestibular information are removed by having the patient close the eyes or read while moving the head. To force use of the vestibular system, visual and proprioceptive information can be minimized or confounded by having the patient close the eyes or read while standing on a compliant surface.

Another common method of sensory training or retraining is to *enhance* the feedback provided via one sensory system until the patient learns to associate the sensation from the other systems with balance in a particular activity. For example, to enhance visual feedback, patients could watch a computer screen that indicates how much sway is occurring as measured by the change in pressure of the patients' feet on a force platform. After sufficient training, patients are expected to be able to perform the newly learned tasks without the external feedback. Sihvonen et al found that a 4-week visual feedback-based program improved balance functions in frail elderly women living in residential care homes compared to those who were randomly selected to receive no training.[119] Improvements were noted in dynamic control of weight shift and postural sway and in BBS scores.

Visual feedback has not been shown to be more effective than other types of feedback. Walker et al compared the effects of visual feedback on balance with the effects of verbal and tactile cues given to patients during weight shifting activities in 46 inpatients after an acute stroke.[120] All subjects received 2 hours of physical and occupational therapy per day, 5 days a week, individualized for tolerance and ability, and two thirds of the subjects received an additional 30 minutes per day of balance training with visual feedback. All subjects had significant improvements in gait speed, TUG test, and BBS scores over approximately 4 weeks, but the additional 30 minutes of visual feedback training provided no additional benefit. Geiger et al obtained similar results in a group of 13 outpatients in the acute to chronic stages of stroke.[48]

Compensatory strategies can be used when a system does not and cannot be trained to function. Simoneau et al suggest reducing the height of shelving when patients cannot control their increased postural sway when their heads are tilted back.[9] Adding high contrast and vertical visual cues can optimize a patient's ability to maintain stability in a particular environment.[9] Compensatory strategies may also involve using environmental assistance such as lights, reflective tape at the edge of surface changes, timing of activities, shopping carts, or canes. Visually fixating on an object 20 to 30 feet ahead can improve balance in persons with vestibular problems or poor functioning of the VOR. When walking, as the person passes the object, he or she should pick a new point for visual fixation. This strategy helps to stabilize the head and reduce dizziness.

PERCEPTUAL TRAINING

Perceptual training for patients with balance problems focuses on integrating all sensory information relevant to certain environmental conditions, particularly vertical orientation relative to gravity and surface orientation relative to the BOS. Patients who lack perception of the vertical or of the surface generally need to retrain their automatic postural responses to use all available sensory information.

Individuals at risk for falls often have lost their internal sense of true vertical and may have additional trouble controlling movement at or around the midline of the body. Activities in midline that require movement in vertical directions, or activities that move in, out of, and back into a full upright position can promote greater facility with these functions. Progressive use of developmental postures can grade the BOS and height of the COG for the patient as activities progress through more challenging tasks. Exercises could include moving the body's COG in various directions and then returning to midline. Further progression could incorporate factors such as having the body on a firm surface with the eyes open and then closed, the body on a compliant surface with the eyes open and then closed, stationary and then dynamic movements, and movements with and without manipulation of something in the hands while performing a balance task [121] The goal is to develop an accurate internal representation of true vertical and midline that is not dependent on vision or verbal cues.

Tips for Finding Vertical

- Complete a postural assessment using a plumb line or computerized equipment to determine the COG.
- Increase sensory awareness utilizing verbal cues:
  - Sit or stand tall.
  - Are your ears directly above your shoulders?
  - Is your nose in line with your belly button?
  - Is there equal weight on your feet? (Two side-by-side bathroom scales can confirm this.)
- Increase sensory awareness utilizing visual cues:
  - Utilizing a door jam for a vertical reference.
  - Using a mirror and looking for a vertical stripe or button placket on a shirt.
  - Utilizing visual feedback on computerized equipment.
- Hold center and move limbs; start with arms, progress to one leg at a time.
- Hold steady with perturbation.
- Move away from vertical, then back with eyes closed. Open eyes to see if vertical was attained.

Similar progressions can help improve perception of the surface upon which the BOS rests. Surface orientation exercises focus on activities performed on several gradations of firm to compliant and dynamic surfaces. The use of mats, wobble boards, Swiss balls, and variations can progress activities so that patients must use available sensory information to attain and retain balance on the progressively more challenging surfaces. Visual information can be minimized by closing the eyes or distracting vision, while vestibular information can be confounded by patients moving their head or by the clinician creating movement of the environment. For advanced activities, challenges may be combined.

POSTURAL AWARENESS TRAINING

Training a patient to be aware of posture could incorporate some of the sensory or perceptual training suggestions discussed previously but could also include COG training

and postural strategy training, which focus on attaining and regaining an upright posture.

COG training requires a progressively smaller BOS for succeeding trials of activities that shift the COG progressively closer to the edge and then outside of the BOS. One study that used this approach with subjects 60 years or older who scored less than 45 on the BBS and received treatment for 45 minutes twice a week for 6 weeks, found that both the experimental and the "current practice" group, who received transfer, bed mobility, and gait training, improved in BBS scores, number of falls, and a Falls Handicap Inventory (FHI). However, only COG training produced significant improvements in walking speed and quality-of-life scores.[122]

Tips for COG Training

- Shift weight over the BOS, circumscribing the *cone of stability*. Sequence weight shifts from easier-to-harder directions:
  - Forward-backward
  - Lateral
  - Forward diagonal
  - Backward diagonal
- Progress weight-shifting activities from head movements only, to trunk and limb movements that have a greater effect on the COG.
- Progress weight-shifting activities to performing them over a smaller BOS:
  - Normal stance
  - Tandem stance
  - Single-leg stance
- Progress weight-shifting activities to performing them on more compliant surfaces.

Postural strategy training involves selecting postural tasks that require each type of strategy (ankle, hip, or stepping strategies; Fig. 13-19) and then practicing the task first in a protected environment and then in progressively more challenging environments or at faster speeds.[10] Postural strategy training is designed to help clients select and implement, efficiently and effectively, the most appropriate strategy to prevent falls. By varying the task, support surface, BOS, and the intensity of a perturbation one can promote selection of certain strategies. For example, standing quietly on a firm, broad surface promotes the use of ankle strategies to control postural sway. A narrow or unsteady surface will tend to trigger hip strategies while large perturbations that move the COG outside the BOS or cause fear of falling will trigger a stepping strategy. Careful guarding during practice sessions is particularly critical for individuals with a higher fall risk or limited mobility. Because older adults tend to require multiple steps to recover from loss of balance and have particular difficulty with lateral instability even with anterior-posterior displacement,[30] practice of lateral weight transfer, rapid foot movement, and cross-over steps may be particularly helpful in this population.

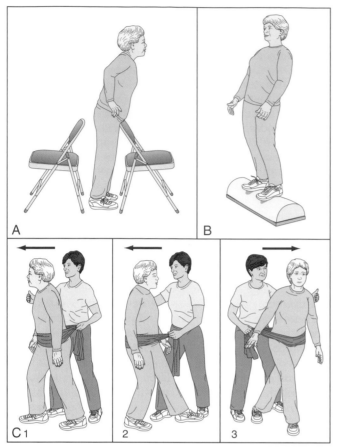

FIG. 13-19 Postural strategy training. **A,** Using ankle strategy. **B,** Using hip strategy. **C,** Using stepping strategies: *(1)* Forward, *(2)* backward, and *(3)* sideways.

Tips for Postural Strategy Training
- Closely guard patients.
- Determine that joint ROM allows the requested movement.
- Start with voluntarily-controlled strategies, then request a specific action within the patient's ability.
- Progress to involuntary strategies, and then to rapid automatic responses. Stay within the patient's ability.
- Start with easier directions (usually forward), progress to more difficult ones. The easier-to-harder sequence is usually anterior, posterior, side to side, then diagonal.

TASK-SPECIFIC TRAINING: LOCOMOTION

Locomotion, particularly gait, generally requires an advanced level of postural control. Balance during gait can be made more challenging by increasing its speed, number of stops and starts, variation of surfaces, and closing the eyes. A treadmill can be used to alter gait velocity and adding head and eye movements can increase the challenge of this controlled activity. Further challenges include walking around stationary and then moving

obstacles; being in quiet or more distracting environments, such as grocery stores or malls; carrying objects; and performing dual tasks, such as walking and talking. In a study of 32 residents of a long-term care facility and outpatients age 66-98 years old, 6 months of perturbed gait exercise on a split treadmill (one with separate right and left belts) resulted in significantly greater improvement in balance and reaction time than in untreated controls.[123] Those in the experimental group also had 21% fewer falls, which was not statistically significant.

Assistive devices (see Chapter 33) are prescribed for use during gait to compensate for certain types of balance problems. Although assistive devices may improve balance by increasing the BOS, they can increase fall risk in some circumstances because they can inhibit stepping strategies, particularly laterally.[124] Research has evaluated the effects of ambulation aids on balance and weight-bearing patterns on several populations of patients, including those with stroke, PD, and lower extremity amputation. Laufer examined the effects of standard and quad canes on postural sway and weight-bearing patterns in 30 patients with hemiparesis and 20 age-matched controls[125] and found that the quad cane reduced postural sway in both groups whichever foot was forward in stride stance, whereas the standard cane only reduced sway when the affected foot was forward and neither type of cane changed asymmetrical weight-bearing patterns in those with hemiparesis. This study provides support for the clinical belief that quad canes provide greater stability in static positions than standard canes.

VESTIBULAR REHABILITATION

Vestibular rehabilitation is widely used in the management of patients with disequilibrium, dizziness, a history of loss of balance or falls, and gait instability caused by peripheral or central vestibular dysfunction.[73] Vestibular rehabilitation has been shown by a number of studies to help patients with peripheral and central vestibular disorders, although outcomes are better for patients with peripheral disorders.[73,126-128]

In a RCT with 42 patients 50 years or older with dizziness of central or age-related origin, patients who participated in balance training and vestibular rehabilitation twice a week for 6 weeks had significantly greater improvement in their ability to stand on one leg with eyes closed (SOLEC) than a control group who received no intervention.[129] However, several other outcome measures, including dizziness, were no different between these groups.

Dysfunction resulting from vestibular loss may resolve through spontaneous cellular recovery, vestibular adaptation, compensation, habituation, or canalith repositioning. Vestibular rehabilitation may incorporate all of these except spontaneous cellular recovery.

Adaptation exercises are designed to help the nervous system adapt to a change in or loss of vestibular input. In essence, the brain must relearn which vestibular signal patterns from the two sides indicate movement of the head in which directions. This learning requires practice of moving the head that is often avoided because moving the head and eye movements initially provokes dizziness. To improve patient adherence, adaptation exercises should start with minimal stimuli and gradually be made more challenging. An adaptation response can be triggered by as small a stimulus as a retinal slip, the movement of a visual image across the retina.[24] This can be progressed by varying visual input and/or head and body movement and continually reorienting to one's head position in space. Adaptation exercises can incorporate movements called X 1 (times one) and X 2 (times two) viewing. X 1 viewing involves keeping the eyes fixed on a stationary visual target while the subject moves the head back and forth, and up and down (Fig. 13-20, *A*). X 2 viewing involves maintaining visual fixation on a visual target when the head and target move in the same or opposite directions (Fig. 13-20, *B*). These exercises can be performed sitting, standing, or walking and may involve horizontal or vertical movements progressing from small to large and from slower to faster.[24]

Tips for Adaptation Exercises
- Exercise 1-2 minutes to patient tolerance but provoke symptoms.
- Change the frequency of the movement and the range of head movement.
- Exercise can be completed in the dark using mental imagery—gains will occur, but not to the same extent as with actual head and eye movement.
- Exercise should stress the patient's ability and be guided by the patient's ability to manage symptoms and keep the target in focus.

When the vestibular system is not working well, balance can require compensation with increased use of the other sensory systems, either vision or somatosensation or both, as discussed in the section on sensory training. Compensation specifically directed toward dysfunction of the VOR includes use of a number of possible strategies (Table 13-6).

Gaze stabilization exercises can be used to help patients learn to keep an image on the fovea during head movements. These exercises are designed to decrease eye saccades *during* head movement and to compensate by moving the eyes either before or after the head moves. Different patients will prefer different strategies so it is best to provide situations and gaze stabilization exercises and let patients choose their own strategy.[24,130] Gaze stabilization strategies are appropriate for both training and compensation. They can be used if the VOR is unlikely to return, as with bilateral vestibular loss, as well as in the initial stages of an acute unilateral lesion when a patient is too symptomatic to tolerate adaptation exercises. Exercises may start with X 1 viewing (see Fig. 13-20), as in

X 1 Viewing

Eyes fixed on target, head moves and target stays stationary. Head may move side to side or up and down.

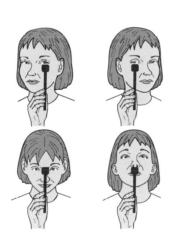

A

X 2 Viewing

Eyes fixed on target, head moves same direction as moving target.

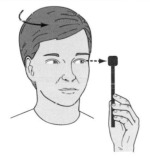

Eyes fixed on target, head moves opposite direction as moving target.

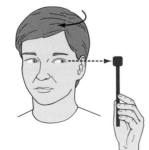

B

FIG. 13-20 **A,** X 1 viewing. **B,** X 2 viewing.

TABLE 13-6	Compensatory Strategies for Vestibulo-Ocular Reflex Dysfunction
Alternative Strategy	**Technique**
Cervico-ocular reflex	Very slow head movements, may allow eyes to compensate.
Saccade modification	Using saccades as a compensatory strategy, move eyes then head between 2 targets.
Create predictable tasks	Central preprogramming is possible if it is a predictable task.
Visual tracking	Use visual tracking to maintain gaze stability during head movement.
Visual fixation	While walking, patient fixates on object 20-30 feet away. Once past the object, the patient picks another object and continues to maintain visual fixation.
Move eyes first	When turning, teach patient to move eyes first, focus on object, then turn the head, and then the body, all in the target direction.
Stop	When dizziness starts or imbalance begins, stop and focus on an object. Let symptoms pass before moving.

adaptation exercises, for less than a minute with the client sitting, and the visual target placed on a plain background. Exercises can be progressed by increasing the distance between targets or the complexity of targets. Only a few patients with bilateral vestibular loss may eventually tolerate X 2 viewing.

Progression of Gaze Stabilization Exercises

- Start with a simple target, single letter, or plain business card taped on the wall. While sitting, have the patient move the head in the direction that it is easiest to focus (side to side OR up and down) progress to include both motions. If you note corrective saccades with the exercise, slow the movement.
- Using two targets have the patient focus on one with eyes and head aligned, and then move eyes to the other target without moving the head, focus, then move the head, keeping the target in focus. Keep targets close enough together that when focusing on one the other can be seen using peripheral vision.
- Use an imaginary target. Have the patient focus on a real target then close the eyes. Tell the patient to keep the eyes on that target as visualized, have the patient move the head slightly, still looking at the target. Then have the patient open the eyes and check to see if he or she has stayed with the target.

Habituation exercises involve repeated exposure to a symptom-causing stimulus or movement to reduce the pathological response to that movement. These exercises can help with balance in patients with vestibular hypofunction or BPPV. In contrast to adaptation exercises that use mostly head and eye movements to learn what altered signals mean, habituation generally focuses on whole body movements and repeats these until the patient no longer reacts adversely to the stimuli. The patient is provided with a list of functional motions to rate according to which motions trigger symptoms: none, some, or a lot.[7,24] The clinician picks a few of the motions that trigger moderate symptoms. The patient then repeats these motions with the goal of eventually generalizing the lack of symptoms to all functional motions.

Tips for Habituation Exercises

- No more than four motions should be selected.
- Motions should be completed 2-3 times, twice per day.
- Movements should be quick enough and through enough range to produce mild to moderate but not severe symptoms. Progress speed and range as symptoms resolve.
- Rest between each motion for symptoms to stop or calm. Symptoms should diminish after a minute or at least within 5-10 minutes of the routine; if not, regress speed and range.

- Habituation exercises typically show results within 4 weeks, but are generally continued for 2 months.
- Orthostatic hypotension should be checked before starting exercises incorporating rapid changes in height of the head in relation to the heart.

CANALITH REPOSITIONING TREATMENTS OR MANEUVERS

If examination reveals a unilateral vestibular problem consistent with BPPV, the most effective intervention may be a canalith repositioning treatment or maneuver. Examination should reveal which canal requires intervention. Correct canal identification and determination of the stability of the debris, whether it is free-floating, as in canalithiasis, or adhering to the cupula, as in cupulolithiasis, can affect the success of treatment as different directions and speeds of movement should be used for these different situations. Three basic bedside interventions are used: Canalith repositioning treatments, liberatory maneuvers, and Brandt-Daroff habituation exercises.

Canalith repositioning treatment (CRT; also known as the Epley maneuver) is used for canalithiasis of the anterior or posterior canals. The Hallpike-Dix is first performed in the direction that provokes symptoms, ending in a supine position with the head turned toward the affected side. This position is maintained for 1-2 minutes, and then the clinician slowly rotates the patient's head through moderate neck extension toward the unaffected side and keeps it there briefly. Finally, the clinician rolls the patient into sidelying with the head turned 45 degrees (nose down) and then helps the patient slowly sit up. The patient is then fit with a soft neck collar and told not to bend over, lie back, move their head up or down, or tilt the head for the rest of the day.[24] Patients are encouraged to sleep on an extra pillow that evening to keep the head elevated and prevent the debris from moving back into the canal.[131] A modification of CRT designed for the horizontal canal keeps the patient's head in the plane of the horizontal canal, level with the table; this maneuver is sometimes referred to as the barbecue roll.

The liberatory maneuver developed by Semont et al can be used to treat posterior or anterior canalithiasis or cupulolithiasis.[132] After the provoking position is determined, the patient is moved to the provoking sidelying position with head turned up and kept in the position for 2-3 minutes. The patient is then turned to the opposite eardown position with the therapist maintaining the alignment of the neck on the body; the speed of the movement depends on whether the initial nystagmus indicated canalithiasis or cupulolithiasis, determined by the length of the initial nystagmus. If the examination suggests the presence of cupulolithiasis, the movement should be rapid to jar the debris from the cupula. If canalithiasis is suspected, the movement may be slow. To treat the posterior canal the head is turned toward the uninvolved side and the patient is laid on the involved side (nose up); to treat anterior canal the head is turned toward the involved side and the patient laid on the involved side (nose down). Following the maneuver, patients should remain vertical for the rest of the day and sleep with multiple pillows that night. Initially, individuals were to remain vertical for 48 hours, including while they slept, and avoid the provoking position for a week after treatment; such rigid restrictions are now thought to be unnecessary. The liberatory maneuver is typically preferred over Brandt-Daroff exercises, since it often requires only a single treatment. It is believed this maneuver will float the debris through the canal system to the common crus.[24]

Brandt-Daroff exercises were developed as a particular type of habituation exercises, but now are thought to help dislodge or refloat debris out of the semicircular canals.[133,134] They have the advantage that patients can perform them on their own as a home program, perhaps after a liberatory maneuver is performed in the office. For these exercises the patient moves rapidly from sitting into the semi-sidelying position that causes their vertigo and holds that position until the vertigo stops or diminishes. The patient then sits up again rapidly and stays sitting for 30 seconds (Fig. 13-21). Patients are generally instructed to perform these movements ten times every 3 hours until patients have no episodes of vertigo for 2 consecutive days.[24]

Tips for Canalith Repositioning Treatment
- Identify involved canal.
- Determine if the patient has canalithiasis or cupulolithiasis.
- Consider any precautions for neck movement or joint protection.
- Instruct the patient on what to expect during and after treatment.

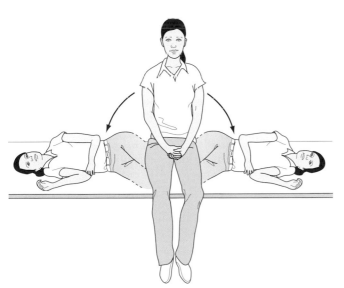

FIG. 13-21 Brandt-Daroff exercises. Note that the patient moves only to the side that reproduces their vertigo. *Redrawn from Brandt T, Daroff RB: Arch Otolaryngol 106:484-485, 1980.*

MULTIDIMENSIONAL OR MULTIFACTORIAL TRAINING

Multiple risk factors and multiple problems contribute to most individuals' falls. Therefore it can be important to target interventions toward multiple factors simultaneously. Multifactorial interventions normally include gait training, strengthening programs, balance training, training in appropriate assistive device use, review of health management (monitoring blood pressure, numbers and types of medications, vision correction, and assessment of dementia) and environmental assessment or modification, including a home safety evaluation and patient and/or caregiver education regarding fall risk.[135] Programs are targeted to the specific areas identified in the examination. Several studies have shown that falls can be prevented through appropriately targeted examination and implementation of multidimensional interventions.[13,22,111,118] These interventions have been tested in individual and group settings, with community-dwelling elderly, homebound elderly, and nursing home residents and in acute care settings. Most of the studies report similar components to their interventions (Table 13-7).

To assess the effects of a multidimensional exercise program on balance and mobility, Shumway-Cook and colleagues conducted a prospective clinical investigation with 105 community-dwelling older adult fallers.[22] Subjects were divided into 3 groups: Control group, fully adherent exercise group, and a partially adherent exercise group.[22] Although both exercise groups showed a reduction in fall risk; the fully adherent exercise group decreased their fall risk by 33% compared to the partially adherent exercise group, which reduced their fall risk by 11%. The control group showed an 8% increase in fall risk.

TABLE 13-7	Components of Multidimensional Balance Training
Exercise and Progression	**Activities**
Balance exercises	• Balance recovery
• Sitting	• Using sensory information for postural orientation (center alignment)
• Standing	
• Walking	• Anticipatory postural adjustment activities
	• Integration of sensory and motor strategies for posture and balance control
	• Functional activities
Mobility retraining	• Various light conditions
• Unperturbed gait	• No distractions—distractions
• Perturbed gait	• Variety of surfaces
• Transfers	• With and without head movements
• Stair climbing	• With and without cognitive tasks

SPECIFIC EXERCISES AS DETERMINED BY THE THERAPIST BASED ON IMPAIRMENT

Weakness	Strengthening
Fatigue	Endurance training
Limited ROM	Stretching

Interestingly, these researches found that age, gender, number of medications, number of co-morbidities, living situation, performance of clinical measures of balance and mobility (other than Tinetti's POMA), frequency of imbalance, and fall history did not limit their subjects' positive responses to exercise. A multidimensional intervention can thus reduce falls and improve balance for a variety of patients. The only variable that emerged as a predictor for exercise adherence was the type of assistive device used for gait: Patients who used a walker as the primary assistive device for gait were less likely to follow through with exercises than those who used a cane or no assistive device.[22]

Rose noted the importance of fostering problem-solving skills to achieve balance and function versus training specific transfer and gait skills to improve balance and reduce falls.[111] Her program focused on manipulating task goals and performance environments to develop a repertoire of postural strategies that could be adapted to various demands. Three core ingredients were (1) COG control training, (2) strategy training, and (3) multisensory training. This intervention primarily focused on a technology-based activities utilizing a support surface that could be computer programmed, but similar situations can be set-up in a standard clinic as evidenced in other studies.[22,13,118]

Hart-Hughes et al conducted a study in which a "Fall Clinical Team" provided an interdisciplinary, specialized, and individualized care plan to 571 veterans at-risk for falls and fall-related injuries.[118] At the time of discharge and at 3-month follow-up a statistically significant reduction in the number of falls was reported. In regard to fall prevention, at the start of the study, 19% reported no falls in the 3 months prior; at the end of the study 64% reported no falls in the 3 months prior.[118] It is important to note that in this study, grab bars, shower chairs, and other devices were recommended to provide a safe home environment. These may have contributed to a reduced fall rate but are common in multifactorial interventions.

Tinetti et al conducted a study with 301 community dwelling individuals over 70 years of age with risk factors for falling in which the control group received usual health care plus social visits.[13] The experimental group received a combination of adjustment in their medications, behavioral instructions, and exercise programs targeted to their specific risk factors. At a 1-year follow-up, 35% of the intervention group had fallen compared to 47% of the control group ($p = 0.04$). The exercise programs in this intervention consisted of gait or transfer training, as needed, and a progressive, competency-based balance and strengthening exercise program. Subjects were instructed to perform the exercises twice a day for 15-20 minutes per session. Intervention lasted 3 months.[13]

Chang et al completed a systematic review and meta-analysis of 61 RCTs on interventions for the prevention of falls in older adults and concluded that the most effective intervention was a multifactorial falls risk assessment and management program.[114] They also concluded that strengthening and balance specific exercise programs were effective in reducing the risk of falling. The goals of a multidimensional program are (1) to resolve, prevent, or reduce underlying impairments; (2) to utilize effective and efficient task-specific sensory and motor strategies; and (3) to adapt and train task-specific strategies to allow functional tasks to be performed in changing environmental situations.[22] Challenging multiple systems at the same time by challenging the individual (taking them to their outer *limit of stability*), changing the environment (darker, uneven surface, movement around the individual), adding complexity to the task (reading while walking, doing multiplication tables while balancing on a Dyna-disc) simulates "lifelike" situations and provides opportunity for the therapist to train the patient in integration of postural control.

PATIENT- OR CLIENT-RELATED INSTRUCTION: EDUCATION AND SAFETY

Even if patients have the potential for improving their postural control over time, the risk for falls may be so great that compensatory strategies will be required. Teach patients to stop, hold onto a stable surface, and refocus if they feel dizzy or unbalanced. When turning, they should move their eyes first, focus, and then turn their head and body to help minimize dizziness.

All individuals should be taught to identify safety hazards at home and in the community; for people with poor balance, hazards might include poor lighting, uneven surfaces, and visually conflicting environments. Compensation for such hazards might include using night lights, carrying pocket flashlights, securing throw rugs, and safely using extension cords. A home safety checklist should be used to assess environmental hazards and help educate the patient, client, care-provider, and/or family. Safety checklists typically include external factors that impact fall risk but should review internal factors to heighten awareness of risks.

INJURY PREVENTION OR REDUCTION

A primary focus of fall prevention and balance intervention is to reduce or prevent injury from falls. The previously mentioned interventions—strengthening, ROM, general conditioning, use of assistive devices, sensory and multisensory training, vestibular rehabilitation, and patient education, as well as environmental modification—can all be used to reduce or prevent injury from falls. Research regarding the effect of external hip protectors on reducing injuries from falls is equivocal, with some studies suggesting that these are helpful and others reporting no benefit. A RCT with 561 subjects in the Netherlands, including individuals residing in nursing homes as well as those residing in the community, found that hip protectors did not prevent hip fracture: 4 out of 18 fractures in the intervention group occurred while hip protectors were being worn.[136]

The most important considerations in making home modifications to reduce falls are modifications of surfaces, lighting, obstacles, and activity in the home (see Chapter 35). Adding grab bars and other safety devices to bathrooms may help reduce the risk of falls.[118] However, some evidence suggests that changing a familiar environment may increase the risk of falls for the elderly, particularly if they are used to using furniture in its current location for maintaining balance.

CASE STUDY 13-1

BALANCE

Examination
Patient History
FA is an 84-year-old woman who was independent in all ADLs, including driving, until 3 days ago when she fell and fractured her left humerus and broke her glasses. She underwent open reduction internal fixation (ORIF) of the left humerus, and the fracture is stable. Her past medical history includes an arrhythmia controlled by flecainide (Tambocor). She has a hearing aid for her right ear and states she needs one for the left. She had cataract surgery last year and wears glasses for all ADLs. She admits that her confidence in balance has been decreasing. She has problems on uneven surfaces, such as her brick patio or grass, and in dark areas, such as movie theaters, outside at night, or her interior hallway. She notes problems with balance in the shower when she tips her head back and closes her eyes to wash her hair. She generally ambulates without an assistive device but uses a walking stick for her walks around the block. Until this most recent fall, she has stayed active walking once a day for 30 minutes, going out with friends, and gardening. Her score on the ABC scale was 70%.

Tests and Measures
Musculoskeletal
Posture Slight forward head and kyphosis. COG was relatively forward. ROM (excluding left upper extremity) was WNL with the exception of bilateral ankle dorsiflexion to 10 degrees.

Muscle Performance Lower extremities: 4+/5, with the following exceptions: 4-/5 peroneals, dorsiflexors, hip abductors, and hip flexors.

Neuromuscular
Arousal, Attention, and Cognition MMSE: 28/30
Cranial Nerve Integrity
Vision: Smooth pursuits and saccades: Normal.
Vestibular: Horizontal/vertical VOR intact. No nystagmus or report of dizziness.
Head thrust test: – for nystagmus or dizziness.
DVA test: + with a 4 line change.
Sensory Integrity Light touch was impaired bilaterally in a stocking distribution; proprioception was absent in the left great toe; and vibration was diminished bilaterally.

Motor Function—Control and Learning Shin-to-heel and finger-to-nose tests were normal, and smooth and sharpened Romberg was positive.
Neuromotor Development and Sensory Integration
Modified CTSIB:

Condition	Time
Eyes open firm surface	30 seconds
Eyes closed firm surface	5 seconds, 8 seconds, 8 seconds = 7 seconds
Eyes open foam	20 seconds, 23 seconds, 26 seconds = 23 seconds
Eyes closed foam	Unable

Function Unable to stand on one leg; requires moderate assist to get up from floor.
Tinetti's POMA: 18/28 = high risk of falls.
DGI: 18/24, <19 correlates with increased fall risk.
TUG: 12 seconds.
Gait Cautious, unsteady, short steps, and forward lean. Ambulates 60 feet before losing balance and/or needing a rest. Cannot turn head and maintain path. Functional reach 4 inches forward, 2 inches backward.

Evaluation, Diagnosis, and Prognosis
Abnormal Findings
1. Lower extremity weakness bilaterally in hip abductors and flexors, ankle dorsiflexors, and evertor
2. Poor use of the somatosensory system for maintaining balance, diminished sensation.
3. Poor use of the vestibular system for maintaining balance.
4. Diminished limits or cone of stability noted when reaching; increased risk of falls.
5. High risk of falls, indicated by Tinetti's POMA, DGI, and Functional Reach tests and inability to stand on one leg.
6. Limited functional gait; velocity drops with head turns; path deviates; loss of balance noted.

Diagnosis
Fall risks are decreased strength, decreased somatosensation, limited vision without glasses, and decreased visual acuity with head movement (+DVA). This patient falls into the following preferred practice patterns: 4G: Impaired joint mobility, muscle performance, and ROM associated with fracture and 5A: Primary prevention/risk reduction for loss of balance and falling.

Plan of Care
FA will be seen in the acute care setting until she is medically stable. She may need to transfer to another level of care (skilled nursing) to work on balance and mobility issues before she returns home alone. Plan of care for the acute setting includes education to effect safe ambulation, improve strength, promote vestibular system use for balance, and increase limits of stability.

Goals
1. Patient will demonstrate safe and appropriate use of an assistive device for all ambulation within 1 week.
2. Patient will be able to get up from the floor with minimal assistance in 1 week.
3. Patient will stand unsupported with eyes closed, minimal sway, for an average of 10 seconds in 3 trials within 1 week.
4. Patient will demonstrate functional reach to 6 inches forward and 4 inches backward within 1 week.

Intervention
1. Therapeutic exercises: Lower extremity strengthening, plantarflexor stretching.
2. COG activities: Limit of stability exercises; weight shifting exercises; ankle, hip and stepping strategy practice.

3. Dynamic gait activities: Obstacles, gait training with head turns, curb training
4. Vestibular activities: Uneven surfaces, dark environment, gaze stability exercises

Outcome

After 3 days, patient was transferred to a skilled nursing facility for 3 weeks and then was able to return home where she modified the lighting and marked curbs with tape.

Please see the CD that accompanies this book for case studies describing the examination, evaluation and interventions for a patient with a history of multiple falls and for a patient with vertigo caused by canalithiasis.

CHAPTER SUMMARY

This chapter discusses the pathology, examination, evaluation, and intervention for patients with impaired balance and increased fall risk. Poor balance can result in reduced activity and falls. Reduced activity has many secondary sequelae, including reduced participation and reduced fitness. Falls can result in fractures, particularly for those with fragile bones. Impaired balance may have many causes, including cognitive, vision, vestibular, sensory, or motor dysfunction. This chapter describes components of the examination needed to differentiate among these causes and guide the selection of interventions. Interventions can help improve balance and decrease fall risk. Procedural interventions that can improve balance include exercises that address musculoskeletal impairments found in the examination and specific balance exercises and mobility retraining. Education in safety and injury prevention can also be helpful for patients in this practice pattern. Evidence demonstrates that rehabilitation intervention can reduce the risk of loss of balance and falls, particularly in the elderly, and thus reduce injury risk and increase participation in activities.

ADDITIONAL RESOURCES

Useful Forms

Activities-Specific Balance Confidence (ABC) scale
Balance Efficacy Scale (BES)
Berg Balance Scales (BES)
Dizziness Handicap Inventory (DHI)
Dynamic Gait Index (DGI)
Fugl-Meyer Assessment
Mini-Mental Status Examination (MMSE)
Performance-Oriented Mobility Assessment (POMA)
Physical Performance Test (PPT)

GLOSSARY

Ankle strategy: A coordinated small amplitude motor sequence used to maintain balance particularly when standing with feet about hip width apart.
Anticipatory postural control: Motor activity that occurs before a planned movement to maintain balance when a shift in the center of mass is anticipated.
Automatic postural responses: Motor responses that maintain or restore balance when unexpected events or environmental demands occur; also known as reactive postural responses.
Balance: Process by which one controls the body's center of mass with respect to the BOS, whether the body is stationary or moving.

Base of support (BOS): The area defined by the outer boundaries of one's contact with external supportive surfaces; the foundation over which the center of mass moves during balance activities.
Center of mass (COM): Sometimes known as center of gravity (COG), this is the central point of the object or body given the current location and mass of all parts of the object or body.
Cone of stability: Approximate shape of the area around a standing body, with the small end of the cone around the BOS, within which stability may be maintained without changing the BOS.
Disequilibrium: Unsteadiness, clumsiness in upright movement, increased postural sway.
Dizziness: A lay term that may include giddiness, swimming sensation, sensation of whirling or reeling, faintness, lightheadedness, or vertigo.
Hip strategy: A moderate amplitude coordinated motor sequence used to maintain balance particularly when the standing BOS is small or sway is perceived to be too far for an ankle strategy to correct.
Lightheaded: Faintness, typically resulting from inadequate cerebral perfusion.
Limit of stability: Maximum distance an individual is able or willing to lean in any direction without changing the BOS.
Oscillopsia: The illusion of visual motion.
Perturbations: Disturbances, either internal or external, to a system, as in disturbances to balance.
Postural control: Effective and efficient management of the body while holding still or moving in a particular environment.
Reactive postural responses: Also known as automatic postural responses, this is motor activity used to maintain or restore balance when unexpected events or environmental demands occur.
Somatosensation: Sensory input from the body from cutaneous and internal exteroceptive and proprioceptive receptors.
Stepping strategy: Coordinated motor sequence that may be large in amplitude used to restore balance when the center of mass is displaced beyond stability limits over the current BOS.
Vertigo: The illusion of movement of self or the environment.
Vestibular system: The anatomical components and physiological functions that allow sensation of head movement and head position relative to gravity, and that initiate some of the body's response to head movement and position.
Vestibulo-ocular reflex (VOR): A sensorimotor connection that links the sensation of head movement (or stability) to eye movement so that functional vision is less interrupted by head position or movement.

References

1. National Center for Injury Prevention and Control: Falls and hip fractures among older adults, August 5, 2004. Available at: http://www.cdc.gov/ncipc/factsheets/falls.htm.
2. Clark S, Rose DJ, Fujimoto K: Generalizability of the limits of stability test in the evaluation of dynamic balance among older adults, *Arch Phys Med Rehabil* 78:1078-1084, 1997.
3. Rose DJ: *Fallproof: A Comprehensive Balance and Mobility Training Program,* Champaign, Ill, 2003, Human Kinetics.
4. Allison L, Fuller K: Balance and vestibular disorders. In Umphred D (ed): *Neurological Rehabilitation,* ed 4, St. Louis, 2001, Mosby.
5. Nashner L: Sensory, neuromuscular, and biomechanical contributions to human balance. In Duncan PW (ed): *Balance: Proceedings of the APTA Forum,* Alexandria, Va, 1990, American Physical Therapy Association.
6. Cohen H, Blatchly CA, Gombash LL: A study of the clinical test of sensory interaction on balance, *Phys Ther* 73:346-354, 1993.
7. Shepard NT, Solomon D: Functional operation of the balance system in daily activities, *Otolaryngol Clin North Am* 33(3):455-469, 2000.
8. Shumway-Cook A, Horak FB: Assessing the influence of sensory interaction on balance, *Phys Ther* 66:1548-1550, 1986.
9. Simoneau GG, Leibowitz HW, Ulbrecht JS, et al: The effects of visual factors and head orientation on postural steadiness in women 55-70 years of age, *J Gerontol* 47(5):M151-158, 1992.
10. Shumway-Cook A, Woollacott MH: *Motor Control: Theory and Practical Applications,* ed 2, Philadelphia, 2001, Lippincott Williams & Wilkins.

11. Tinetti ME, Doucette JT, Claus EB: The contribution of predisposing and situational risk factors to serious fall injuries, *J Am Geriatr Soc* 43(11):1207-1213, 1995.

12. Tinetti ME, Speechley M, Ginter SF: Risk factors for falls among elderly persons living in the community, *N Engl J Med* 319(26):1701-1707, 1988.

13. Tinetti ME, Baker DI, McAvay G, et al: A multifactorial intervention to reduce the risk of falling among elderly people living in the community, *N Engl J Med* 331(13):821-827, 1994.

14. Tinetti ME, Doucette JT, Claus EB, et al: Risk factors for serious injury during falls by older persons in the community, *J Am Geriatr Soc* 43(11):1207-1213, 1995.

15. Tromp AM, Pluijm SF, Deeg DH, et al: Fall-risk screen test: a prospective study on predictors for falls in community-dwelling elderly, *J Clin Epidemiol* 54(8):837-844, 2001.

16. Duncan PW, Weiner DK, Chandler J, et al: Functional reach: a new clinical measure of balance, *J Gerontol* 45(6):M192-197, 1990.

17. Urton MM: A community home inspection approach to preventing falls among elderly, *Public Health Rep* 106(2):197-195, 1991.

18. Boulgarides LK, McGinty SM, Willett JA, et al: Use of clinical and impairment-based tests to predict falls by community-swelling older adults, *Phys Ther* 2003;83(40):328-339.

19. Condron J, Hill K: Reliability and validity of a dual-task force platform assessment of balance performance; effect of age, balance impairment, and cognitive task, *J Am Geriatr Soc* 2002;50:157-162.

20. Koepsell TD, Wolf ME, Buchner DM, et al: Footwear style and risk of falls in older adults, *J Am Geriatr Soc* 2004;52(9):1495-1501.

21. American Physical Therapy Association: Guide to physical therapist practice, second edition, *Phys Ther* 81:277-294, 2001.

22. Shumway-Cook A, Gruber W, Baldwin M, et al: The effect of multidimensional exercise on balance, mobility, and fall risk in community-living older adults, *Phys Ther* 77:46-57, 1997.

23. Rossiter-Fornoff JE, Wolf SL, Wolfson LI, et al: A cross-sectional validation study of the FICSIT common data base static balance measures, *J Gerontol* 50A(6):M291-M297, 1995.

24. Herdman SJ: *Vestibular Rehabilitation*, ed 2, Philadelphia, 2000, FA Davis.

25. Whitney SL, Blatchly CA: Dizziness and balance disorders, *Clin Manag* 11(1):42-44, 46-48, 1991.

26. Whitney SL: Management of the elderly person with vestibular dysfunction. In Herdman SJ: *Vestibular Rehabilitation*, ed 2, Philadelphia, 2000, FA Davis.

27. Schubert MC, Herdman SJ: Vestibular rehabilitation. In O'Sullivan SB, Schmitz TJ (eds): *Physical Rehabilitation: Assessment and Treatment*, ed 4, Philadelphia, 2001, FA Davis.

28. DiFabio RP, Badke MB: Relationship of sensory organization to balance function in patients with hemiplegia, *Phys Ther* 70:543-548, 1990.

29. Anacker SL, Di Fabio RP: Influence of sensory inputs on standing balance in community-dwelling elders with a recent history of falling, *Phys Ther* 72:575-584, 1992.

30. Maki BE, McIlroy WE: The role of limb movements in maintaining upright stance: the "change-in-support" strategy, *Phys Ther* 77(5):488-507, 1997.

31. Horak F, Shupert C: Role of the vestibular system in postural control. In Herdman SJ: *Vestibular Rehabilitation*, ed 2, Philadelphia, 2000, FA Davis.

32. Herdman SJ, Whitney SL: Treatment of vestibular hypofunction. In Herdman SJ: *Vestibular Rehabilitation*, ed 2, Philadelphia, 2000, FA Davis.

33. Horak FB, Nashner LM: Central programming of postural movements: adaptation to altered support-surface configurations, *J Neurophysiol* 55(6):1369-1381, 1986.

34. Mecagni C, Smith JP, Roberts KE, et al: Balance and ankle range of motion in community-dwelling women aged 64 to 87 years: A correlational study, *Phys Ther* 80(10):1004-1011, 2000.

35. Wolfson LI, Judge J, Whipple R, et al: Strength is a major factor in balance, gait, and the occurrence of falls, *J Gerontol A Biol Sci Med Sci* 50A:64-67, 1995.

36. Chu L-W, Pei CKW, Chiu A, et al: Risk factors for falls in hospitalized older medical patients, *J Gerontol* 54A(1):M38-M43, 1999.

37. Brown M, Sinacore DR, Host HH: The relationship of strength to function in the older adult. *J Gerontol A Biol Sci Med Sci* 50A:55-59, 1995.

38. Nevitt MC, Cummings SR, Kidd S, et al: Risk factors for recurrent nonsyncopal falls. A prospective study, *JAMA* 261(18):2663-2668, 1989.

39. Hines C, Mercer V: Anticipatory postural adjustments: An update, *Neurol Rep* 21(1):17-22, 1997.

40. Morris ME, Iansek R: Gait disorders in Parkinson's disease: a framework for physical therapy practice, *Neurol Rep* 21(4):125-131, 1997.

41. Roller P, Leahy P: Cerebellar ataxia, *Neurol Rep* 15(4):25-29, 1991.

42. Quinn L, Rao A: Physical therapy for people with Huntington Disease: Current perspectives and case report, *Neurol Rep* 26(3):145-153, 2002.

43. Hauer K, Pfisterer M, Weber C, et al: Cognitive impairment decreases postural control during dual tasks in geriatric patients with a history of severe falls, *J Am Geriatr Soc* 51:1638-1644, 2003.

44. Jensen J, Nyberg L, Gustafson Y, et al: Fall and injury prevention in residential care—effects in residents with higher and lower levels of cognition, *J Am Geriatr Soc* 51(5):627-635, 2003.

45. Morris M, Iansek R, Matyas T, et al: The pathogenesis of gait hypokinesia in Parkinson's disease, *Brain* 117:1169-1181, 1994.

46. Morris M, Iansek R: Characteristics of motor disturbance in Parkinson's disease and strategies for movement rehabilitation, *Human Move Sci* 1996:649-669, 1996.

47. Morris M, Iansek R, Matyas T, et al: Abnormalities in the stride length-cadence relation in parkinsonian gait, *Movement Dis* 13:61-69, 1998.

48. Geiger RA, Allen JB, O'Keefe J, et al: Balance and mobility following stroke: Effects of physical therapy interventions with and without biofeedback/forceplate training, *Phys Ther* 81(4):995-1005, 2001.

49. Garland SJ, Willems DA, Ivanova TD, et al: Recovery of standing balance and functional mobility after stroke, *Arch Phys Med Rehabil* 84:1753-1759, 2003.

50. Cecchini AS: Functional assessment after traumatic brain injury, *Neurol Rep* 22(4):136-143, 1998.

51. Frzovic D, Morris ME, Vowels L: Clinical tests of standing balance: Performance of persons with multiple sclerosis, *Arch Phys Med Rehabil* 81:215-221, 2000.

52. Asher A: Disequilibrium in the elderly: two case studies, *Neurol Rep* 21(1):11-16, 1997.

53. Agostini JV, Han L, Tinetti ME: The relationship between number of medications and weight loss or impaired balance in older adults, *J Am Geriatr Soc* 52(10):1719-1723, 2004.

54. Shumway-Cook A, Baldwin M, et al: Predicting the probability for falls in community-dwelling older adults, *Phys Ther* 77:812-819, 1997.

55. Stuart ME, Rose DJ: The effectiveness of the Balance Efficacy Scale to measure changes in confidence associated with the completion of a balance intervention program, *J Aging Phys Act* 26, 1995.

56. Powell LE, Myers AM: The activities-specific balance confidence (ABC) scale, *J Gerontol* 50A(1):M28-M34, 1995.

57. Myers AM, Powell LE, Maki BE, et al: Psychological indicators of balance confidence: relationship to actual and perceived abilities, *J Gerontol* 51A(1):M37-M13, 1995.

58. Myers AM, Fletcher PC, Myers AH, et al: Discriminative and evaluative properties of the activities-specific balance confidence (ABC) scale, *J Gerontol* 53A:M287-M294, 1998.

59. Whitehead C, Miller M, Crotty M: Falls in community-dwelling older persons following hip fracture: impact on self-efficacy, balance and handicap, *Clin Rehabil* 17(8):899-906, 2003.

60. Riolo L, Satterwhite LG, Pickelsimer KD: Using the dynamic gait index and activities specific balance confidence scale to identify older adults at risk for falls. Veterans Affairs Administration, Research and Development [abstract]. January 5, 2005. Available at: http://www.vard.org/va/02/htm/rrds_teb_2002_confriolo1.htm.

61. Jacobson GP, Newman CW: The development of the dizziness handicap inventory, *Arch Otolaryngol Head Neck Surg* 116:424, 1990.

62. Jacobson GP, Newman CW, Hunter L, et al: Balance function test correlates of the Dizziness Handicap Inventory, *J Am Acad Audiol* 2(4):253-260, 1991.

63. Whitney SL, Herdman SJ: Physical therapy assessment of vestibular hypofunction. In Herdman SJ (ed): *Vestibular Rehabilitation*, ed 2, Philadelphia, 2000, FA Davis.

64. Robertson DD, Ireland DJ: Dizziness Handicap Inventory correlates of computerized dynamic posturography, *J Otolaryngol* 24(2):118-124, 1995.

65. Tusa RJ: Psychological problems and the dizzy patient. In Herdman SJ: *Vestibular Rehabilitation*, ed 2, Philadelphia, 2000, FA Davis.

66. Horn LB: Differentiating between vestibular and nonvestibular balance disorders, *Neurol Rep* 21(1):23-27, 1997.

67. Danis CG, Krebs DE, Gill-Body KM, et al: Relationship between standing posture and stability, *Phys Ther* 78(5):502-517, 1998.

68. Haase B: Cognition. In Van Deusen J, Brunt D (eds): *Assessment in Occupational Therapy and Physical Therapy*, Philadelphia, 1997, WB Saunders.

69. Folstein MF, Folstein SE, McHugh PR: Mini-mental state: a practical method for grading the cognitive state of patients for the clinician, *J Psychiatr Res* 12:189-198, 1975.

70. Cornali C, Franzoni S, Stofler PM, et al: Mental functions and physical performance abilities as predictors of falling in a geriatric evaluation and rehabilitation unit, *J Am Geriatr Soc* 52(9):1591-1592, 2004.

71. Lundin-Olsson L, Nyberg L, Gustafson Y: "Stops walking when talking" as a predictor of falls in elderly people, *Lancet* 349:617, 1997.

72. Gill-Body KM: Current concepts in the management of patients with vestibular dysfunction, *Phys Ther* 9(12):40-58, 2001.

73. Schubert MC, Tusa RJ, Grine LE, et al: Optimizing the sensitivity of the head thrust test for identifying vestibular hypofunction, *Phys Ther* 84(2):151-158, 2004.

74. Honrubia V: Quantitative vestibular function tests and the clinical examination. In Herdman SJ: *Vestibular Rehabilitation*, ed 2, Philadelphia, 2000, FA Davis.

75. Fugl-Meyer AR, Jaasko L, et al: The post-stroke hemiplegic patient. I. A method for evaluation of physical performance, *Scand J Rehab Med* 7:13-31, 1975.

76. Fugl-Meyer AR: Post-stroke hemiplegia. Assessment of physical properties, *Scand J Rehab Med Suppl* 7:85-93, 1980.

77. Fugl-Meyer AR, Jaasko L: Post-stroke hemiplegia and ADL-performance, *Scand J Rehab Med Suppl* 7:140-152, 1980.

78. Duncan PW, Propst M, Nelson SG: Reliability of the Fugl-Meyer assessment of sensorimotor recovery following cerebrovascular accident, *Phys Ther* 63:1606-1610, 1983.

79. Buchner DM, Hornbrook MC, Kutner NG, et al: Development of the common data base for the FICSIT trials, *J Am Geriatr Soc* 41:297-308, 1993.

80. Weber PC, Cass SP: Clinical assessment of postural stability, *Am J Otolaryngol* 14:566-569, 1993.

81. Clendaniel RA: Cervical vertigo. In Herdman SJ: *Vestibular Rehabilitation*, ed 2, Philadelphia, 2000, FA Davis.

82. Woollacott MH, Tang P-F: Balance control during walking in the older adult: research and its implications, *Phys Ther* 77(6):646-660, 1997.

83. Tinetti ME: Performance-oriented assessment of mobility problems in elderly patients, *J Am Geriatr Soc* 34(2):119-126, 1986.

84. Trueblood PR: Partial body weight treadmill training in persons with chronic stroke, *NeuroRehabilitation* 16(3):141-153, 2001.

85. Behrman AL, Light KE, Miller GM: Sensitivity of the Tinetti Gait Assessment for detecting change in individuals with Parkinson's disease, *Clin Rehabil* 16(4):399-405, 2002.

86. VanSwearingen JM, Brach JSV: Making geriatric assessment work: Selecting useful measures, *Phys Ther* 81(6):1233-1252, 2001.

87. Tinetti ME, Williams TF, Mayewski R: Fall risk index for elderly patients based on number of chronic disabilities, *Am J Med* 80:429-434, 1986.

88. Galindo-Ciocon DJ, Ciocon JO, Galindo DJ: Gait training and falls in the elderly, *J Gerontol Nurs* 21(6):10-17, 1995.

89. Thapa PB, Gideon P, Brockman KG, et al: Clinical and biomechanical measures of balance as fall predictors in ambulatory nursing home residents, *J Gerontol A Biol Sci Med Sci* 51A(5):M239-246, 1996.

90. Tinetti ME: Yale FICSIT: Risk factor abatement strategy for fall prevention, *J Am Geriatr Soc* 41:315, 1993.

91. Whitney SL, Hudak MT, Marchetti GF: The dynamic gait index relates to self-reported fall history in individuals with vestibular dysfunction, *J Vestib Res* 10(2):99-105, 2000.

92. Wrisley DM, Walker ML, Echternach JL, et al: Reliability of the dynamic gait index in people with vestibular disorders, *Arch Phys Med Rehabil* 84(10):1528-1533, 2003.

93. Podsiadlo D, Richardson S: The timed "Up & Go": A test of basic functional mobility for frail elderly persons, *J Am Geriatr Soc* 39(2):142-148, 1991.

94. Mathias S, Nayak U, Isaacs B: Balance in elderly patients: The "Get-up and Go" test, *Arch Phys Med Rehabil* 67:387-389, 1986.

95. Shumway-Cook A, Brauer S, Woollacott MH: Predicting the probability for falls in community-dwelling older adults using the timed up & go test, *Phys Ther* 80(9):896-903, 2000.

96. Freter SH, Fruchter N: Relationship between timed 'up and go' and gait time in an elderly orthopaedic rehabilitation population, *Clin Rehabil* 14(1):96-101, 2000.

97. Stack E, Jupp K, Ashburn A: Developing methods to evaluate how people with Parkinson's Disease turn 180 degrees: An activity frequently associated with falls, *Disabil Rehabil* 26(8):478-484, 2004.

98. Sharp SA, Brouwer B: Isokinetic strength training of the hemiparetic knee: Effects on function and spasticity, *Arch Phys Med Rehabil* 78(11):1231-1236, 1997.

99. Hiroyuki S, Uchiyama Y, Kakurai S: Specific effects of balance and gait exercises on physical function among the frail elderly, *Clin Rehabil* 17(5):472-479, 2003.

100. Berg K, Wood-Dauphinee S, Williams JI: Measuring balance in the elderly: Preliminary development of an instrument, *Physiother Canada* 41:304, 1989.

101. Berg K, Wood-Dauphinee SL, Williams JI, et al: Measuring balance in the elderly: Validation of an instrument, *Can J Pub Health* 83:S7-11, 1992.

102. Thorbahn LDB, Newton RA: Use of the Berg Balance Test to predict falls in elderly persons, *Phys Ther* 76(6):576-585, 1996.

103. Kornetti DL, Fritz SL, Chiu Y-P, et al: Rating scale analysis of the Berg Balance Scale, *Arch Phys Med Rehabil* 85:1128-1135, 2004.

104. Harada N, Chiu V, Fowler E, et al: Physical therapy to improve functioning of older people in residential care facilities, *Phys Ther* 75(9):54-62, 1995.

105. Badke MB, Shea TA, Miedaner JA, et al: Outcomes after rehabilitation for adults with balance dysfunction, *Arch Phys Med Rehabil* 85(2):227-233, 2004.

106. Schenkman M, Cutson TM, Kuchibhatla M, et al: Reliability of impairment and physical performance measures for persons with Parkinson's Disease, *Phys Ther* 77(1):19-27, 1997.

107. Brauer S, Burns Y, Galley P: Lateral reach: A clinical measure of medio-lateral postural stability, *Physiother Res Int* 4(2):81-88, 1999.

108. Reuben DB, Siu AL: An objective measure of physical function of elderly outpatients: The physical performance test, *J Am Geriatr Soc* 38:1105-1112, 1990.

109. Van Swearingen JM, Paschal KA, et al: Assessing recurrent fall risk of community-dwelling, frail older veterans using specific tests of mobility and the physical performance test of function, *J Gerontol* 53A(6):M457-464, 1998.

110. Rose DJ: Balance and mobility disorders in older adults: Assessing and treating the multiple dimensions of balance, *Rehab Manag* 10(1):38, 40-41, 1997.

111. Schenkman M, Cutson TM, Kuchibhatla M, et al: Exercise to improve spinal flexibility and function for people with Parkinson's disease: A randomized, controlled trial, *J Am Geriatr Soc* 46:1207-1216, 1998.

112. Andersson C, Grooten W, Hellsten M, et al: Adults with cerebral palsy: Walking ability after progressive strength training, *Develop Med Child Neurol* 45(4):220-228, 2003.

113. Barnett A, Smith B, Lord SR, et al: Community-based group exercise improves balance and reduces falls in at-risk older people: A randomized controlled trial, *Age Ageing* 32(4):407-414, 2003.

114. Chang JT, Morton SC, Rubenstein LZ, et al: Interventions for the prevention of falls in older adults: A systematic review and meta-analysis of randomized clinical trials, *Br Med J* 328(7441):680-686, 2004.

115. Buchner DM, Cress ME, de Lateur BJ, et al: The effect of strength and endurance training on gait, balance, fall risk, and health services use in community-living older adults, *J Gerontol A Biol Sci Med Sci* 52A(4):M218-M224, 1997.

116. Douris P, Southard V, Varga C, et al: The effect of land and aquatic exercise on balance scores in older adults, *J Geriatr Phys Ther* 26(1):3-6, 2003.

117. Hart-Hughes S, Quigley P, Bulat T, et al: An interdisciplinary approach to reducing fall risks and falls, *J Rehabil Res Dev* 70(4):46-51, 2004.

118. Islam MM, Nasu E, Rogers ME, et al: Effects of combined sensory and muscular training on balance in Japanese older adults, *Prev Med* 39(6):1148-1155, 2004.

119. Sihvonen SE, Sipilä S, Era PA: Changes in postural balance in frail elderly women during a 4-week visual feedback training: A randomized controlled trial, *Gerontology* 50:87-95, 2004.

120. Walker C, Brouwer BJ, Culham EG: Use of visual feedback in retraining balance following acute stroke, *Phys Ther* 80(9):886-895, 2000.

121. Gentile AM: Skill acquisition: action, movement, and neuromotor processes. In Carr JH, Shepherd RB (eds): *Movement Science: Foundations for Physical Therapy in Rehabilitation*, ed 2, Gaithersburg, Md, 2000, Aspen.

122. Steadman J, Donaldson N, Kalra L: A randomized controlled trial of an enhanced balance training program to improve mobility and reduce falls in elderly patients, *J Am Geriatr Soc* 51:847-852, 2003.

123. Shimada H, Obuchi S, Furuna T, et al: New intervention program for preventing falls among frail elderly people: the effects of perturbed walking exercise using a bilateral separated treadmill, *Am J Phys Med Rehabil* 83:493-499, 2004.

124. Bateni H, Heung E, Zettel J, et al: Can use of walkers or canes impede lateral compensatory stepping movements? *Gait Posture* 20(1):74-83, 2004.

125. Laufer Y: The effect of walking aids on balance and weight-bearing patterns of patients with hemiparesis in various stance positions, *Phys Ther* 83(2):112-122, 2003.

126. Horak FB, Jones-Rycewicz C, Black FO, et al: Effects of vestibular rehabilitation on dizziness and imbalance, *Otolaryngol Head Neck Surg* 106(2):175-180, 1992.

127. Shepard NT, Telian SA, Smith-Wheelock M, et al: Vestibular and balance rehabilitation therapy, *Ann Otol Rhinol Laryngol* 102(3 Pt 1):198-205, 1993.

128. Herdman SJ, Clendaniel RA, Mattox DE, et al: Vestibular adaptation exercises and recovery: Acute stage after acoustic neuroma resection, *Otolaryngol Head Neck Surg* 113(1):77-87, 1995.

129. Hansson EE, Månsson N, Håkansson A: Effects of specific rehabilitation for dizziness among patients in primary health care. A randomized controlled trial, *Clin Rehabil* 18(5):558-565, 2004.

130. Kasai T, Zee DS: Eye-head coordination in labyrinthine-defective human beings, *Brain Res* 144(1):123-141, 1978.

131. Ireland DJ: The Semont maneuver. Paper presented at Barany Society Meeting, Prague, Czechoslovakia, 1994.

132. Semont A, Freyss G, Vitte E: Curing the BPPV with a liberatory maneuver, *Adv Otorhinolaryngol* 42:290-293, 1988.

133. Brandt T, Daroff R: Physical therapy for benign paroxysmal positional vertigo, *Arch Otolaryngol* 8:151-158, 1980.

134. Herdman SJ: Treatment of benign paroxysmal positional vertigo, *Phys Ther* 70(6):381-388, 1990.

135. Moncada LV: Diagnosis and treatment of falls in the elderly, *Resident Staff Physician* 50(8):28-30, 2004.

136. van Schoor NM, Smit JH, Twisk JW, et al: Prevention of hip fractures by external hip protectors: A randomized controlled trial, *JAMA* 289(15):1957-1962, 2003.

Chapter 14

Impaired Neuromotor Development

Debra Clayton-Krasinski, Susan Klepper

CHAPTER OUTLINE

OBJECTIVES

After reading this chapter, the reader will be able to:
1. Define impaired neuromotor development.
2. Discuss the core concepts of development and principles of motor development.
3. Apply the International Classification of Functioning, Disability, and Health and the *Guide to Physical Therapist Practice* to the examination and evaluation of a child with impaired neuromotor development.
4. Identify appropriate tests and measures of participation and activity for pediatric patients for a given purpose, age, and diagnosis.
5. Identify specific measures of body structure and function in the musculoskeletal, neuromuscular, and cardiovascular/pulmonary systems for pediatric patients.
6. Differentiate between typical and atypical motor development.
7. Evaluate findings to guide intervention planning.

INTRODUCTION

Children are different than adults. The clinician working with pediatric patients must be aware of the many unique characteristics of children and apply that knowledge to accurately diagnose and appropriately manage the young. Three important attributes that differentiate children from adults are rapid growth and maturation of multiple organ systems, rapid accession of *developmental milestones,* and

an ever-increasing range of functional capacities. Appreciation of normal growth and *development* is needed to understand what are normal, normal variants, and deviations from normal. Knowledge of growth and development provides the fundamental theoretical basis for rehabilitation examination, evaluation, and intervention for pediatric patients. Age-specific variations from normal remain some of the best early indicators of childhood disorders, particularly neuromotor disorders, and provide the basis for patient evaluation and for planning of therapeutic intervention.

This chapter provides the knowledge base needed to examine and evaluate a pediatric client with a neuromotor disorder, regardless of pathology. It includes an overview of typical development and sequential acquisition of important functional skills. Salient developmental concepts, principles of motor development, and a model for the examination and evaluation of body structure and function, activities, and participation are also presented. Specific standardized pediatric tests and measures and their contribution to the evaluative process are discussed. The next chapter, Chapter 15, applies the information from this chapter to guide the evaluation, diagnosis, prognosis, and intervention for pediatric patients with specific conditions.

DEVELOPMENT TERMINOLOGY

Development is the process of change in behavior or capacity that relates to the age of the individual.[1] Neuromotor development is development in the domains of physical or motor behaviors. Thus *impaired neuromotor development* infers the opposite of "normal or typical" and denotes a problem with the acquisition of motor skills and/or the occurrence of atypical movements. Impaired neuromotor development is generally caused by central and/or peripheral nervous system damage or dysfunction. However, the focus on nervous system damage or dysfunction as the cause for impaired neuromotor development does not clearly express the dynamic interplay between the complex and diverse systems responsible for development. Neuromotor damage can profoundly affect the development of musculoskeletal, cardiopulmonary, and other systems, which may in turn affect neuromotor development. Additionally, development emerges from an interplay between the child, his or her tasks, and the environment in which the tasks are being performed.[2]

DELAY, DISSOCIATION, AND DEVIANCE

Aylward describes three manifestations of impaired development: Delay, dissociation, and deviance.[3] *Delay* is when a child does not reach a developmental milestone at the appropriate age. *Dissociation* is when two or more developmental domains develop at different rates. For example, in a child with cerebral palsy (CP), cognitive skills may develop faster than motor skills. Unevenness can also occur within a domain. For example, fine motor abilities (reach, grasp, and manipulation) may be more advanced than gross motor abilities (mobility and postural control). *Deviance* is a clinically significant unevenness in the achievement of milestones or the appearance of an atypical developmental indicator. Deviance is abnormal at any age. Commonly used synonyms for deviance include atypical, abnormal, and dysfunctional. Examples of atypical indicators include altered muscle tone; stereotypic movement patterns; muscle weakness, including paresis and paralysis; and incoordination of the timing, grading, or sequencing of multiple muscle groups.[4] Although Aylward's system distinguishes types of impaired development, it is not uncommon for a child to display characteristics of two of more of these categories.[3] For example, a child may be delayed in the acquisition of motor milestones and display atypical movement characteristics.

CORE DEVELOPMENTAL CONCEPTS

Human development refers to changes that occur over the entire spectrum of a person's life, from conception to death. Development is generally divided into age-related segments of childhood, adolescence, and adulthood (Table 14-1).[5] Adolescence is described by changes in physical growth and sexual maturation rather than by age alone.

Tanner's classic scales describe five stages of physical development in adolescence.[6] In girls, Tanner's stages are based on breast size and pubic hair distribution. In boys, Tanner's stages are based on penis and scrotum size and shape and pubic hair development.

The Committee on Integrating the Science of Early Childhood Development[7] (CISECD) generated a 10-item list of core concepts that structure the overall understanding of the nature of early development (Box 14-1). (The CISECD is a multidisciplinary committee charged to keep up-to-date on the scientific literature and knowledge about early development and discuss the implications of this knowledge for early childhood policy, practice, professional development, and research. The comprehensive findings are a highly recommended source for pediatric specialists.)[8] The core concepts particularly relevant to neuromotor development are summarized next.

Development Is Multidimensional. Human development is complex and can be divided into four dimensions: Physical, cognitive, emotional, and social (Table 14-2). Although each dimension concentrates on a particular aspect of development, all of them are closely intertwined. For example, mobility can be thought of as only encompassing the physical dimension when one looks at activities such as rolling, crawling, creeping, or walking. However, mobility may also involve other dimensions. For example, walking across a busy intersection requires the interaction of cognitive and physical, as well as possibly social, skills for the child to decide when, where, and how to proceed so that the task is safely executed.

Development Is Influenced by Heredity and Environment. Both nature (heredity, genetic endowment) and nurture (environment, personal life experiences) influence development.[7] Some aspects of development seem to be influenced more by heredity, particularly growth parameters such as body size, whereas other aspects of development seem more influenced by environment.

TABLE 14-1	Pediatric Developmental Periods	
Developmental Period	**Stage**	**Time Frame**
Prenatal: Conception to birth	Embryonic	First 8 weeks
	Middle fetal	9 to 24 weeks
	Late fetal	25 weeks to birth (38-40 weeks)
Infancy: Birth to 2 years	Neonate	Birth to 1 month
	Infancy	1 month to 1 year
	Late infancy	1-2 years
Childhood:	Early childhood/toddler/preschool	2-5 years
Ages 2-10 years, girls	Middle childhood/elementary school age	6-10 years, girls
Ages 1-12 years, boys		6-12 years, boys
Adolescence:	Early adolescence (prepubescence): Tanner stage 1	10-13 years, girls
Ages 10-18, girls	Middle adolescence (pubescence): Tanner stage 3	10.5-14 years, boys
Ages 12-20, boys	Late adolescence (postpubescence): Tanner stage 5	11.8-14 years, girls
		12.8-15 years, boys
		14-17 years, girls
		14.8-16 years, boys

From Valadian I, Porter D: *Physical Growth and Development: From Conception to Maturity,* Boston, 1977, Little, Brown; Solorio MR, Wyatt-Henriques L: Health care of the adolescent. In David AK, Johnson TA, Phillips M, et al (eds): *Family Medicine: Principles of Practice,* ed 6, New York, 2003, Springer-Verlag; STAT!Online Electronic Medical Library, http://online.statref.com/document.aspx?fxid=32&docid=113; posted 8/26/2003; date accessed 3/18/2004.

BOX 14-1	Ten Core Concepts of Development

1. Human development is shaped by a dynamic and continuous interaction between biology and experience.
2. Culture influences every aspect of development and is reflected in child-rearing beliefs and practices designed to promote healthy adaptation.
3. The growth of self-regulation is a cornerstone of early childhood development that cuts across all domains of behavior.
4. Children are active participants in their own development, reflecting the intrinsic human drive to explore and master one's environment.
5. Human relationships are the building blocks of healthy development.
6. The broad range of individual differences among young children often makes it difficult to distinguish normal variations and maturational delays from transient disorders and persistent impairments.
7. The development of children unfolds along individual pathways whose trajectories are characterized by continuities and discontinuities, as well as by a series of significant transitions.
8. Human development is shaped by the ongoing interplay among sources of vulnerability and sources of resilience.
9. The timing of early experiences can matter, but, more often than not, the developing child remains vulnerable to risks and open to protective influences throughout the early years of life and into adulthood.
10. The course of development can be altered in early childhood by effective interventions that change the balance between risk and protection, thereby shifting the odds in favor of more adaptive outcomes.

From Committee on Integrating the Science of Early Childhood Development: Ten core concepts of development. In Shonkoff JP, Phillips DA (eds): *From Neurons to Neighborhoods: The Science of Early Childhood Development,* Washington, DC, 2000, National Academy Press.

TABLE 14-2	Dimensions of Human Development

Physical	Cognitive	Emotional	Social
Physical body growth	Intellectual processing	Attachment	Family
Skeletal	Thinking	Trust	Socialization
Muscle	Learning	Security	Relationships
Cardiopulmonary	Memory	Love	Peers
Nervous system	Problem solving	Affection	Family members
Sensory system	Language	Affect	Work
Motor development	Communication	Emotions	Play
Mobility	Reasoning	Feelings	Social norms
Postural control		Temperament	Cultural norms
Reach, grasp, manipulation		Motivation	
Reproduction		Interest	
Vision		Desire	
Hearing			
Endocrine			

Environmental influences that can impact development include illness, poverty, lack of opportunity or experience, and poor nutrition. The nature and quality of life experiences continuously and dynamically interact with genetic predispositions to shape individual development.

Development Reflects Individual Differences. The timing and rates of development of many factors, including height, weight, and physical abilities, vary among children, making it difficult to distinguish normal variations from maturational delays and transient disorders from persistent activity limitations.[7] There are many possible causes for individual differences in development, including cultural differences in child-rearing beliefs and practices, environmental factors that affect the opportunity to practice movements and skills, and gender. Although rates of development vary from child to child, there is a range of normal progression and timing for development, and a number of *norm-referenced tests* try to take into account this variability while also identifying delays in development, activity limitations, and partici-

pation restrictions. For example, the Denver Developmental Screening Test II illustrates typical variability for all test items graphically with a bar spanning the ages at which a percentage of the standardization sample passes that item. Thus the test item "walks well," which is defined as the child has good balance, rarely falls, and does not tip from side to side, has the ages at which 25%, 50%, 75%, and 90% of children can perform this task (11.1, 12.3, 13.6, and 14.9 months, respectively) on the graph (Fig. 14-1).

Developmental Influences Are Reciprocal. Researchers have traditionally emphasized the influence of adults and the environment on a child's development.[5] However, recent emphasis has shifted to include the influence of the child on its own development. Children are active participants in their own development as a result of the intrinsic human drive to explore and master the environment.[5] Human development is shaped by the ongoing interplay of all participants. The CISECD categorically concludes that children's early development is influenced most significantly by the health and well being of their

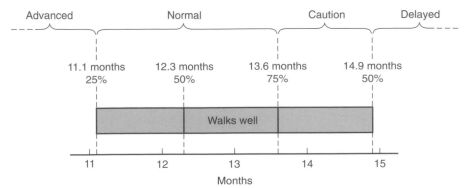

FIG. 14-1 "Walks well" test item of the Denver Developmental Screening Test II. Interpretation: *Advanced* = Child passes an item that 25% of the standardized sample failed (age equivalent—prior to 11.1 months); *Normal* = Child passes an item that 25% through 75% of the standardized sample passes (age equivalent between 11.1 to 13.6 months); *Caution* = Child fails an item that 75% of children in the standardized sample passed at an earlier age (age equivalent—between 13.6 and 14.9 months); and *Delayed* = Child fails and item that 90% of children in the standardized sample passed at an earlier age (age equivalent—after 14.9 months). *Modified from Frankenburg WK, Dodds J, Archer P, et al:* Denver II Training Manual, *Denver, 1992, Denver Developmental Materials.*

parents.[7] Children thrive in relationships that provide love, stability, responsive interaction, and encouragement of exploration and learning. Reciprocal influence can be seen when a child who exhibits shy, passive, cautious characteristics when exploring a playground may be protected by the concerned caregiver. The child's behavior triggers a reactive restriction in exploration and experimentation in a novel environment. Additionally, early experiences influence the development of the brain: The brain itself is molded through experience.[8,9]

Culture Influences Development. Culture exerts a profound effect on human development.[5,8] Values, aspirations, expectations, and practices shape developmental experiences. Culture affects parents and influences how disability and illness are perceived. The influence of culture on development can interfere with interpretation of standardized developmental tests because most of these are based on middle-class, European-American norms and reflect their values. A straightforward example is the use of utensils for eating. Developmental tests value the use of the spoon, fork, and knife rather than the use of chopsticks or the fingers for eating.

PRINCIPLES OF MOTOR DEVELOPMENT

Observing movement and remembering the progression of milestones becomes easier when general principles of motor development are applied.

Movements Progress from Generalized to Specific. One of the first principles to keep in mind is that movements develop from generalized, with a whole limb moving together, to specific, with delicate specific movements of each individual parts.

Movement Is an Interplay Between Stability and Mobility. In the 1960s, Margaret Rood, a physical therapist, proposed a four-stage sequence of motor development: Mobility, followed by stability, followed by combined mobility and stability in a weight-bearing position, followed by skill (Fig. 14-2).[10] Mobility encompasses

the range and speed of movements that translate a body part in space and is characterized by the development of antigravity movement. Stability is the ability to maintain weight-bearing postures against gravity. Combined mobility and stability in a weight-bearing position is when there is a proximal movement on a fixed distal extremity. An example of this is when a child is in the quadruped position, the extremities are "fixed," and the trunk rocks forward and backward over the supporting extremities. Combined mobility and stability in a weight-bearing position is analogous to the term "closed chain." Skill refers to combined mobility and stability in a non–weight-bearing position. An extremity is free from the supporting surface (lower extremity is lifted from the floor), and movements are superimposed on a stable proximal part (trunk holds lifted lower extremity). Examples of this pattern are reaching in sitting, creeping, cruising, and walking. Skill is analogous to the term "open chain." Rood's sequence seems rudimentary by today's developmental knowledge base and is not well studied, yet it provides a simple and straightforward method to categorize movement: Can the child move into a position (get to sitting), can the child hold the position (maintain sitting for a period of time), can the child move in the position with extremity support (move forward and backward, turn the head from side to side), and can the child move in the position without extremity support (sit without arm support, sit and reach for a toy)?

There Is More than One Right Way to Move. In studying the descriptions of important milestones and scrutinizing the criteria for passing standardized motor tests, one could think that there is only one typical way a specific movement is or should be performed. Take, for example, "sitting without arm support." The criteria could outline the proper posture, weight-bearing position, and position of the upper and lower extremities for this activity within a specified age range. But children can sit without arm support in many different ways, including with the

Mobility	Stability	Combined mobility and stability in weight-bearing	Skill

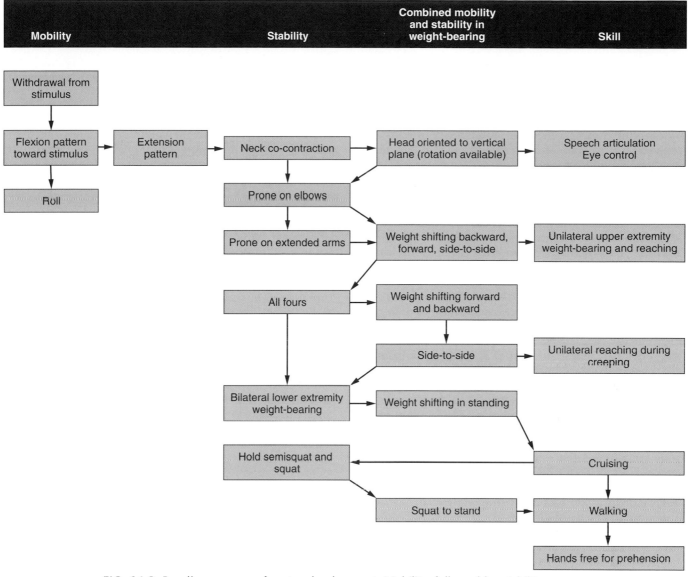

FIG. 14-2 Rood's sequence of motor development: Mobility, followed by stability, followed by combined mobility and stability in a weight-bearing position, followed by skill. *Redrawn from Case-Smith J (ed): Occupational Therapy for Children, ed 4, St. Louis, 2001, Mosby.*

lower extremities crossed, side-sitting to either side, long-sitting, or W-sitting, each of which would alter the criteria.

VanSant has described the ability to rise independently from supine to stand in toddlers, young children, and young adults.[11-14] She detailed a number of movement patterns for the rising task for three body regions: Six upper extremity, five axial, and seven lower extremity movement patterns and described the rising task in terms of various combinations of these movement patterns. Mathematically, although not all are biomechanically feasible, there are 210 different movement combinations that one could use to achieve this task. VanSant found, after observing 120 children aged 4 through 7 performing the rising task, that although the frequency of movement patterns of each body region varied among age groups, it also varied among subjects of the same age and within each individual child.[12]

Normalcy or typical movement may be thought of as a child's ability to perform a variety of movement patterns to achieve a given motor task, although the child may prefer a specific pattern under certain circumstances.[9] The movement pattern chosen may be affected by the constraints of the task, the environment, and the individual. Clinically, it is important to encourage a repertoire of movement choices for a single motor task when planning an intervention program.

Movement Is the Product of Multiple Developing Elements. Movement arises from a confluence of interdependent processes and from constraints in the person and within the environment.[9] Multiple elements developing together, potentially at different rates, promote movement. These include the following:

Sensation: The senses of touch, vision, hearing, and smell to obtain information about the environment and receptors within muscles, skin, joints, and the vestibular system to detect body position, force, and movement.

Biomechanics of skeletal muscles, including movement production, force production, and endurance.

Energy, including cardiopulmonary parameters.

Motivation.

Cognition.

Anthropometric measures, including height, weight, height : weight ratio, and head circumference.

Perception: Coordinating movements with concurrent perceptual information.

Central and peripheral nervous system processing.

Each of these is essential for typical movement. Since so many factors can affect motor task performance, multidimensional examination of each child is essential, and casual inferences as to why a child can or cannot perform a given task should be avoided.

ACQUISITION OF MOTOR MILESTONES

A milestone is a significant point in development or a significant functional ability achieved during the development process. A developmental progression can be described for individual motor components including postural *reflexes,* postural control, mobility function, reach, grasp, and manipulation. Age-related norms for important motor milestones are summarized in Table 14-3.

Functional Skills. The acquisition of motor milestones emphasizes the attainment of specific motor skills such as an infant learning to roll, sit, creep, and walk. Over time, the emphasis on milestones is translated into addressing a child's ability to function within their environment. *Functional activities* include age-expected day-to-day functional skills the children can perform within their natural environments of home, school, and community.[15] Functional activities allow the child to access their environment and independently meet their own needs. Some functional activities common to all children include independence in self-care, mobility, and social function.[16] Specific examples of functional activities include basic activities of daily living (BADLs), such as feeding, dressing, and grooming, and instrumental activities of daily living (IADLs), such as play skills and school performance. It is important for a child to perform essential functional activities as safely and independently as possible.[16]

EXAMINATION

The examination of a child is a process designed to deepen the understanding of the individual's competencies and resources for the purpose of evaluation and intervention planning.[17] An examination is performed to confirm the presence and extent of an impairment, determine activity limitation or participation restriction in neuromotor development, determine appropriate remediation (intervention planning), and monitor the child's neuromotor progress.

An initial examination is a sampling of the child's neuromotor skills taken at a particular point in time, from a particular vantage point, and with particular tests and measures.[17] The examination process, however, is cyclical and ongoing; the examination influences intervention and intervention influences the examination.

Coster et al encourage therapists to begin the examination using a use a "top-down" process.[18] This involves starting the examination with investigating the child's current level of participation at home, school, and community and following with measures of activity and body structure and function to clarify causes for gaps between current participation restrictions and the desired level of participation. This process assures that the examination focuses on functional motor skills that are meaningful and relevant to the child, family, and teacher.[19]

Neuromotor development is not unidimensional but rather a multidimensional concept requiring a core set of tests and measures to capture the intricacies of the child's motor performance. Ideally, a comprehensive examination includes valid and reliable tests and measures that assess all levels of the International Classification of Functioning, Disability and Health (ICF) model:[20] Participation, activity, body structure and function, and environmental and personal contextual factors. Additionally, specific structural and functional constraints may require one or more separate measures of the musculoskeletal, neuromuscular, cardiopulmonary, and integumentary systems. Determining which tests and measures to use for a specific individual requires consideration of the child's age, diagnosis, purpose of the referral, cultural context, the environment(s) in which function is expected to occur, and current health status. The policies, practices, and mandates of the supporting agency, as well as the strengths and limitations of the individual tests and measures, must also be taken into account.

Information obtained from a variety of sources and by a variety of methods can expand the examiners understanding of the child's optimal and typical performance. Sources of information can include parents; caregivers; school personnel, including teachers and assistants; day care providers; and health care professionals.

PATIENT HISTORY

The patient history for a child with impaired neuromotor development may be obtained by reviewing medical and educational records and interviewing the child, parents, caregivers, and/or teachers. One should establish a working alliance with the parents and listen to their views of the child's strengths and challenges and understand their concerns.[17] The parents can generally provide information on personal and environmental contextual factors, including a developmental and medical history, environmental demands, and formal and informal support structures.

SYSTEMS REVIEW

The systems review is used to target areas requiring further examination and to define areas that may cause complications or indicate a need for precautions during the examination and intervention processes. See Chapter 1 for details of the systems review.

TESTS AND MEASURES

Standardized Tests of Participation and Activity. A number of *standardized tests* can be used to examine a child's activity and participation developmental status.

TABLE 14-3	Motor Developmental Milestones*		
Position	**Milestone**	**Age When 50% of Infants Can Perform**	**Age When 90% of Infants Can Perform**
Prone	Lifts head to 45° (asymmetrically, holds momentarily)	0.5 months	2 months
	Prone prop, (weight on hands, forearms, and chest; elbows behind shoulders)	1.5 months	3 months
	Extended arm support (weight on hands, lower abdomen, and thighs)	4.5 months	6 months
	Rolling prone to supine without rotation	6 months	8.5 months
	Reaching from forearm support	5 months	7 months
	Pivoting	5.5 months	8 months
	Rolling prone to supine with rotation	7 months	9.5 months
	Reciprocal crawling (stomach touching floor)	7.5 months	9.5 months
	Reciprocal creeping (stomach off floor, mature posture of LE and trunk rotation)	8.5 months	11 months
Supine	Moves head toward midline	Birth	0.5 months
	Brings hands to midline	2.5 months	4 months
	Hands to feet	4.5 months	6 months
	Rolling supine to prone without rotation	5.5 months	9 months
	Rolling supine to prone with rotation	6.5 months	9 months
Sit	Sitting with propped arms (momentarily)	2.5 months	4.5 months
	Pull to sit (chin tuck)	3.5 months	5 months
	Sitting with arm support	4.5 months	6 months
	Sits without arm support	6 months	8 months
	Reach with rotation in sitting	7 months	8 months
	Get to sitting (from supine or prone)	8.4 months	9.9 months
	Sitting to prone	8 months	12 months
	Sitting to four-point kneeling	7.5 months	9.5 months
Stand	Supported standing (intermittently bears weight)	Birth	1 months
	Pulls to stand with support (external object-crib, chair)	8 months	9.5 months
	Stand 2 seconds	10.2 months	11.6 months
	Stand alone (10 seconds or more)	11.5 months	13.7 months
	Stand from modified squat	11.5 months	14 months
	Stand from quadruped position	11.5 months	15 months
Walk/run	Cruising without rotation	9 months	13 months
	Early stepping (5 independent steps)	11 months	13.5 months
	Walks alone (main mode of mobility)	11.5 months	14 months
	Walks backward	13.8 months	16.6 months
	Runs	15.8 months	19.9 months
Static standing balance	Balance each foot: 1 second	2.5 years	3.4 years
	Balance each foot: 2 seconds	3.1 years	4.0 years
	Balance each foot: 3 seconds	3.3 years	4.7 years
	Balance each foot: 4 seconds	4.0 years	5.1 years
	Balance each foot: 5 seconds	4.3 years	5.4 years
Curbs/stairs	Walk up steps	16.6 months	21.6 months
	Up/down curbs	1.5-2.0 years	2.0-2.5 years
	Climbs in/out of bed (using arms)	1.5-2.0 years	2.0-2.5 years
	Walks up full flight of stairs no difficulty	2.0-2.5 years	3.0-3.5 years
	Walks down full flight of stairs no difficulty	2.0-2.5 years	3.0-3.5 years
	Steps in/out of tub	2.5-3.0 years	4.0-4.5 years
Kick	Kick ball forward	18.3 months	23.2 months
	Coordinated kick (backward and forward LE motion)	—	4 years
	Runs forward, kicks ball	—	6 years
Jump/hop/skip	Gallops: Leading with one foot	—	6-7 years
	Jumps up (both feet off floor)	23.8 months	2.4 years
	Broad jump (approximately 8 inches)	2.7 years	3.2 years
	Hops (on 1 foot, 2 or more times in a row)	3.5 years	4.2 years
	Jump rope (3 consecutive times)	—	5-6 years

Data from Piper MC, Darrah J: *Motor Assessment of the Developing Infant,* Philadelphia, 1994, WB Saunders; Frankenburg WK, Dodds J, Archer P, et al: *DENVER II Training Manual,* Denver, 1992, Denver Developmental Materials; PEDI Research Group: *Pediatric Evaluation of Disability Inventory (PEDI) Development, Standardization and Administration Manual,* Boston, 1992, PEDI Research Group; Brigance AH: *Brigance Inventory of Early Development-II,* North Billerica, Mass, 2004, Curriculum Associates.

LE, Lower extremity.

*Norms should be used as guidelines only. Clinically significant variations in rates of development exist between subgroups because of variables such as race, sex, maternal education, and place of residence.

These tests assess different levels of the ICF model, use a variety of examination approaches, appraise different neuromotor components, and produce a variety of outcome scores and descriptions to aid in interpretation of the child's performance. There is no single "best" test. Each test must be analyzed for its appropriateness based on the needs of the child. A more detailed description of the commonly used tests that have good reliability and validity and represent various ICF levels (participation and/or activity), examination approaches (norm-referenced and/or criterion-referenced), and age targets is included in the next section. These tests are all measures in the categories of self-care and home management or of work, community, and leisure integration, as described in the *Guide to Physical Therapist Practice*.[21]

Pediatric Evaluation of Disability Index. The Pediatric Evaluation of Disability Index (PEDI), introduced in 1992, is a statistically sophisticated, innovative, comprehensive, and norm-referenced diagnostic test.[16] The test is remarkable for two reasons. First, it focuses exclusively on what a child can accomplish and excludes information on how the child accomplishes the task. Second, the test relies on information gathered from the child's caregiver rather than on direct observation of the child. The PEDI was standardized on a sample from the Northeast region (Massachusetts, Connecticut, and New York), representative of the 1980 United States (US) Census population. The sample was stratified by age, gender, race, parental educational levels, and community size. The sample included 412 typically developing children, with a range of children (n = 16 to 39) in each of 14 age groups of 6-month intervals between 5 months and 7.5 years of age. The PEDI is intended to (1) detect if a functional deficit or delay exists, and if so, (2) determine the extent and content area of the delay or deficit, and (3) monitor individual progress and assess outcomes for program evaluation. The test can be administered to children ranging in age from 6 months to 7.5 years of age and to older children whose functional abilities fall within those expected for this age range. The major attribute measured is functional abilities, defined as the ability of the child to perform daily activities independently and safely within the environment. The Nagi model provides the theoretical framework for the PEDI.

The PEDI measures (1) capacity, rated on the Functional Skills Scales, and (2) performance, rated on the Caregiver Assistance Scale in three content domains: Self-care, mobility, and social function. Capacity, a measure of activity limitations, assesses mastery of 197 specific functional skills. Performance, a measure of participation restrictions, consists of 20 items and assesses the extent of help the caregiver provides in typical daily situations. Participation is an indirect measure of the child's function in the self-care, mobility, and social function domains. Environmental alterations and equipment used by the child in routine daily functional activities is rated on the Modification Scale. The modifications are categorized into child-oriented (step stool, sippy cup), rehabilitation equipment (walker, orthoses, splints), or extensive modifications (manual or powered wheelchair, lift device). Table 14-4 shows the rating criteria for each section of the PEDI.

The PEDI can be administered in a variety of ways, including a structured interview with parents; observations of the child by parents, caregivers, teachers, or therapists; or an unstructured interview with parents. Separate summary scores are calculated for Functional Skills and the Caregiver Assistance Scales in each of the three content domains (self-care, mobility, and social function), yielding a total of six standard scores and six scaled scores. An example of the PEDI mobility domain and score summary for the child in Case Study 14-1 is shown in Figs. 14-3 and 14-4. A goodness-of-fit score that indicates the degree to which this child's pattern of item responses matches the pattern expected, based on normative data, can also be calculated. The PEDI manual contains a wealth of information that can augment the interpretation of a child's performance including age ranges at which functional skill items are mastered by 10%, 25%, 50%, 75%, and 90% of the sample; hierarchical scales that arrange the items in order of difficulty from easy to hard; and item maps that provide a visual display of individual items according to difficulty across content domains.

School Function Assessment. The School Function Assessment (SFA), introduced in 1998, offers a seminal, comprehensive, and sophisticated method for examining a child within the context of the school environment.[18] One major contribution of the SFA is its extensive analysis of the physical requirements needed to participate effectively in an educational program. The SFA is a criterion-referenced, transdisciplinary-focused, and judgment-based instrument for children in kindergarten through

TABLE 14-4	Rating Criteria for the Pediatric Evaluation of Disability Index (PEDI)

Self-Care, Mobility, Social Function		
Part I: Functional Skills (197 Discrete Items of Functional Skills)	**Part II: Caregiver Assistance (20 Functional Activities)**	**Part III: Modifications (20 Complex Functional Activities)**
0 = Unable, or limited in capability to perform item in most situations. 1 = Capable of performing item in most situations, or item has been previously mastered and functional skills have progressed beyond this level.	5 = Independent 4 = Supervise/prompt/monitor 3 = Minimal assistance 2 = Moderate assistance 1 = Maximal assistance 0 = Total assistance	N = No modifications C = Child-oriented (nonspecialized) R = Rehabilitation equipment E = Extensive modifications

From PEDI Research Group: Pediatric Evaluation of Disability Inventory (PEDI) Development, Standardization and Administration Manual, Boston, 1992, PEDI Research Group.

Mobility Domain   Place a check corresponding to each item:
Item score 0 = unable: 1 = capable

	0 Unable	1 Capable
A. Toilet Transfers		
1. Sits if supported by equipment or caregiver		✓
2. Sits unsupported on toilet or potty chair		✓
3. Gets on and off low toilet or potty		✓
4. Gets on and off adult-sized toilet		✓
5. Gets on and off toilet, not needing own arms	✓	
B. Chair/Wheelchair Transfers		
6. Sits if supported by equipment or caregiver		✓
7. Sits unsupported on chair or bench		✓
8. Gets on and off low chair or furniture		✓
9. Gets in and out of adult-sized chair/wheelchair	✓	
10. Gets in and out of chair, not needing own arms	✓	
C. Car Transfers		
11. Moves in car; scoots on seat or gets in and out of car seat	✓	
12. Gets in and out of car with little assistance or instruction	✓	
13. Gets in and out of car with no assistance or instruction	✓	
14. Manages seat belt or chair restraint	✓	
15. Gets in and out of car and opens and closes car door	✓	
D. Bed Mobility/Transfers		
16. Raises to sitting position in bed or crib		✓
17. Comes to sit at edge of bed; lies down from sitting at edge of bed		✓
18. Gets in and out of own bed	✓	
19. Gets in and out of own bed, not needing own arms	✓	
E. Tub Transfers		
20. Sits if supported by equipment or caregiver in a tub or sink		✓
21. Sits unsupported and moves in tub		✓
22. Climbs or scoots in and out of tub	✓	
23. Sits down and stands up from inside tub		✓
24. Steps/transfers into and out of an adult-sized tub	✓	
F. Indoor Locomotion Methods (Score = 1 if mastered)		
25. Rolls, scoots, crawls, or creeps on floor		✓
26. Walks, but holds onto furniture, walls, caregivers or uses devices for support		✓
27. Walks without support	✓	
G. Indoor Locomotion: Distance/Speed (Score = 1 if mastered)		
28. Moves within a room but with difficulty (falls; slow for age)		✓
29. Moves within a room with no difficulty		✓
30. Moves between rooms but with difficulty (falls; slow for age)		✓
31. Moves between rooms with no difficulty	✓	
32. Moves indoors 50 feet; opens and closes inside and outside doors	✓	
H. Indoor Locomotion: Pulls/Carries Objects		
33. Changes physical location purposefully		✓
34. Moves objects along floor		✓
35. Carries objects small enough to be held in one hand		✓
36. Carries objects large enough to require two hands	✓	
37. Carries fragile or spillable objects	✓	

	0 Unable	1 Capable
I. Outdoor Locomotion Methods		
38. Walks, but holds onto objects, caregiver, or devices for support		✓
39. Walks without support	✓	
J. Outdoor Locomotion: Distance/Speed (Score = 1 if mastered)		
40. Moves 10–50 feet (1–5 car lengths)		✓
41. Moves 50–100 feet (5–10 car lengths)		✓
42. Moves 100–150 feet (35–50 yards)		✓
43. Moves 150 feet and longer, but with difficulty (stumbles; slow for age)		
44. Moves 150 feet and longer with no difficulty	✓	
K. Outdoor Locomotion: Surfaces		
45. Level surfaces (smooth sidewalks, driveways)		✓
46. Slightly uneven surfaces (cracked pavement)		✓
47. Rough, uneven surfaces (lawns, gravel driveway)		✓
48. Up and down incline or ramps	✓	
49. Up and down curbs	✓	
L. Upstairs (Score = 1 if child has previously mastered skill)		
50. Scoots or crawls up partial flight (1–11 steps)	✓	
51. Scoots or crawls up full flight (12–15 steps)	✓	
52. Walks up partial flight	✓	
53. Walks up full flight, but with difficulty (slow for age)		
54. Walks up entire flight with no difficulty	✓	
M. Downstairs (Score = 1 if child has previously mastered skill)		
55. Scoots or crawls down partial flight (1–11 steps)		✓
56. Scoots or crawls down full flight (12–15 steps)		✓
57. Walks down partial flight	✓	
58. Walks down full flight, but with difficulty (slow for age)	✓	
59. Walks down full flight with no difficulty	✓	
Mobility Domain Sum	**30**	

Please be sure you have answered all items.

FIG. 14-3 Pediatric Evaluation of Disability Inventory (PEDI): Mobility domain performance of child described in Case Study 14-1. *Redrawn from Pediatric Evaluation of Disability Inventory (PEDI) Development, Standardization and Administration Manual, Score sheet, Boston, 1992, PEDI Research Group.*

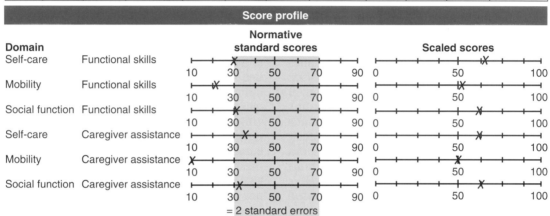

FIG. 14-4 Summary scores from the Pediatric Evaluation of Disability Inventory (PEDI) for the child described in Case Study 14-1. *Redrawn from Pediatric Evaluation of Disability Inventory (PEDI) Development, Standardization and Administration Manual, Score sheet, Boston, 1992 PEDI Research Group.*

sixth grade. The Nagi model provides the theoretical framework for the SFA.

The SFA consists of three parts: Participation, task supports, and activity performance. The participation scale examines the student's level of participation in six major school settings: Regular or special education classroom, playgroup, or recess; transportation to and from school; bathroom and toileting activities; transitions to and from class; and mealtime or snack time. Task support is composed of four scales and examines two separate types of support provided to the student when he or she performs school-related functional tasks: Assistance (adult help) and adaptations (modifications to the environment or program such as specialized equipment or adapted materials). Activity performance is composed of 21 separate scales and examines the student's performance of specific school-related functional activities. Each scale includes a comprehensive set of activities that share a common functional demand.

The SFA is completed by an individual or group of individuals who are familiar with the student's typical performance, have observed the student in a variety of school contexts on multiple occasions, and know the type and level of supports typically provided to the student. The SFA is similar to the PEDI in that items are rated on what the child can do and not on how the child performs the task. Ratings reflect the student's participation, need for supports, and activity performance compared to typical students in the same grade as the assessed child.

The SFA yields raw scores that are converted to criterion scores. Criterion scores range from 0 through 100, where 100 represents the highest measurable point and 0 represents the lowest measurable point. Achieved-criterion scores can be compared with derived-criterion cut-off scores to determine whether a child's performance is below the level of his or her typically developing peers (i.e., students in a regular education class). Scores are graphically displayed on the SFA Summary Score Form. Item maps can also be generated to assist the examiner in identifying the child's strengths and limitations and to note any unusual or unexpected performance.

Alberta Infant Motor Scale. The Alberta Infant Motor Scale (AIMS), introduced in 1992, is an individually administered, norm-referenced instrument designed to evaluate the motor development of infants between birth and 18 months of age.[22] The AIMS, a measure of activity level of the ICF, provides a model for examining the sequence of motor maturation in infants. The test highlights what the child can do and notes any deviations from the normal pattern of motor maturation. The AIMS was standardized on a cross-sectional sample of 2,202 sex- and age-stratified, full-term Albertan infants aged 0-18 months. Breakdowns on racial/ethic characteristics of the sample are not reported.

The two primary uses of the AIMS are to (1) identify infants with immature, delayed, or abnormal patterns of motor development and (2) evaluate motor development over time. The AIMS was developed to be used with infants who exhibit normal motor development and who are being monitored over time, have identified risk factors for developmental delay, have disorders that present with immature motor development, and are either immature or suspect in motor development. Examples of patient diagnoses where using the AIMS would be appropriate include Down syndrome, fetal alcohol syndrome, failure to thrive, seizure disorders, and developmental delay. The test is not designed to evaluate progress of infants with abnormal movement patterns, such as those caused by CP or spina bifida, nor is it intended for older children whose motor skills remain at an infantile level.

The AIMS contains 58 items divided into four subscales: Prone (21 items), supine (9 items), sit (12 items), and stand (16 items). Each item is accompanied by a photograph(s), caricature sketch, normative graph showing the age at which 50% and 90% of infants are credited for the item, and a qualitative description of the weight-bearing, posture, and antigravity movements the infant must exhibit to receive credit (Fig. 14-5). Administration of this test is quick, easy, and noninvasive and uses an observational approach. The examiner observes the infant's spontaneous movements, limiting the actual handling of the infant, although encouraging the infant to move spontaneously on items in the range of the infant's developmental level. Each of these items is scored using outlined criteria (observed, not observed). The least and most mature item in the infant's skill repertoire is noted for each of the four positions (Fig. 14-6). The AIMS yields a percentile rank score. The child's performance can be classified as: Normal (percentile rank above 1 SD below the mean), suspect (percentile rank between 1 SD and 2 SD below the mean), or abnormal (percentile rank below 2 SD below the mean).

Peabody Developmental Motor Scales-2. Folio and Fewell published the original Peabody Developmental Motor Scales (PDMS) in 1983 to provide physical education instructors with a way to assess and program motor patterns and skills within the physical education segment of a school program.[23] The second edition (PDMS-2) was revised and restandardized in 2000. The PDMS-2 is a widely used, individually administered, norm-referenced pediatric diagnostic instrument with examination and treatment (motor activities program) components.

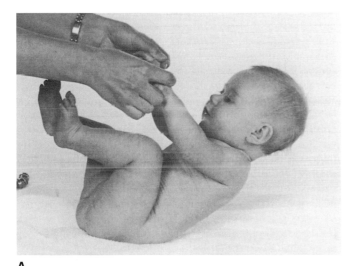

A

B

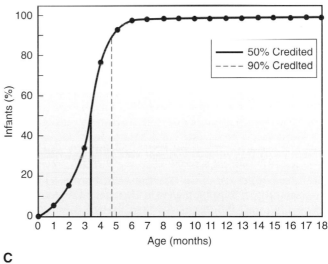

C

FIG. 14-5 "Pull to sit" item from the Alberta Infant Motor Scale (AIMS). **A,** Photo; **B,** caricature sketch; **C,** normative graph showing the age at which 50% and 90% of infants are credited for the item. *A From Piper MC, Darrah J: Motor Assessment of the Developing Infant, Philadelphia, 1994, WB Saunders; B and C redrawn from Piper MC, Darrah J: Motor Assessment of the Developing Infant, Philadelphia, 1994, WB Saunders.*

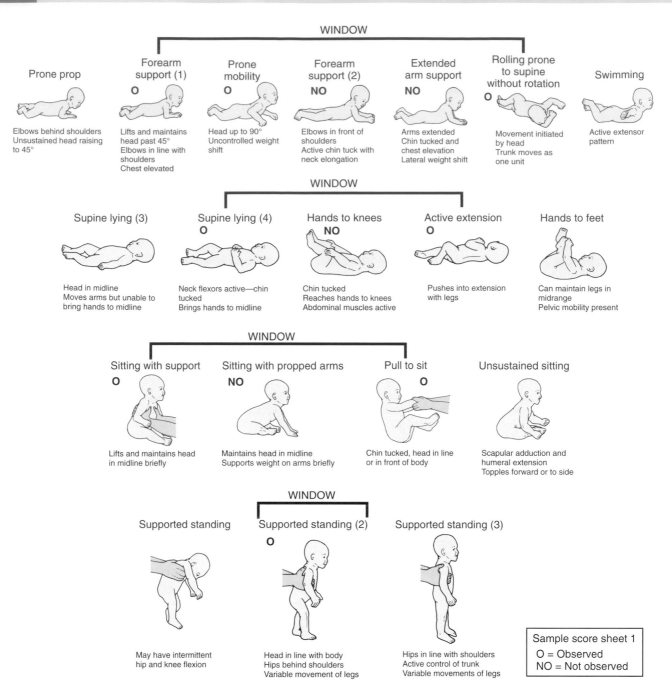

WINDOW

| Prone prop | Forearm support (1) O | Prone mobility O | Forearm support (2) NO | Extended arm support NO | Rolling prone to supine without rotation O | Swimming |

Prone prop — Elbows behind shoulders / Unsustained head raising to 45°

Forearm support (1) O — Lifts and maintains head past 45° / Elbows in line with shoulders / Chest elevated

Prone mobility O — Head up to 90° / Uncontrolled weight shift

Forearm support (2) NO — Elbows in front of shoulders / Active chin tuck with neck elongation

Extended arm support NO — Arms extended / Chin tucked and chest elevation / Lateral weight shift

Rolling prone to supine without rotation O — Movement initiated by head / Trunk moves as one unit

Swimming — Active extensor pattern

WINDOW

Supine lying (3) — Head in midline / Moves arms but unable to bring hands to midline

Supine lying (4) O — Neck flexors active—chin tucked / Brings hands to midline

Hands to knees NO — Chin tucked / Reaches hands to knees / Abdominal muscles active

Active extension O — Pushes into extension with legs

Hands to feet — Can maintain legs in midrange / Pelvic mobility present

WINDOW

Sitting with support O — Lifts and maintains head in midline briefly

Sitting with propped arms NO — Maintains head in midline / Supports weight on arms briefly

Pull to sit O — Chin tucked, head in line or in front of body

Unsustained sitting — Scapular adduction and humeral extension / Topples forward or to side

WINDOW

Supported standing — May have intermittent hip and knee flexion

Supported standing (2) O — Head in line with body / Hips behind shoulders / Variable movement of legs

Supported standing (3) — Hips in line with shoulders / Active control of trunk / Variable movements of legs

Sample score sheet 1
O = Observed
NO = Not observed

FIG. 14-6 Sample items from the AIMS score sheet. The least mature and most mature observed item is identified. The items between these two observed items are considered the motor window. *From Piper MC, Darrah J:* Motor Assessment of the Developing Infant, *Philadelphia, 1994, WB Saunders.*

The PDMS-2 was standardized on a sample stratified for age, gender, race/ethnicity, geographic region, community size, family income, parent education, and disability, representative of the 1997 US Census population for children under 5 years of age. The sample consisted of 2,003 typically developing children, with children in each of six age groups between birth and 71 months of age (n = 210 for the oldest age group to n = 557 for the youngest age group).

The purpose of the PDMS-2 is fivefold: (1) to estimate motor competence relative to the child's peers, (2) to compare the gross motor quotient (GMQ) and fine motor quotient (FMQ) to determine if there is disparity in motor abilities, (3) to assess qualitative and quantitative aspects of individual skills, (4) to evaluate progress, and (5) to study the nature of motor development in various populations. The PDMS-2 is predominately a measure of the activity level of the ICF model.

The gross motor scale consists of four subtests: Reflexes (8 items), stationary (30 items), locomotion (89 items), and object manipulation (24 items). The fine motor scale consists of two subscales: Grasping (26 items) and visual-

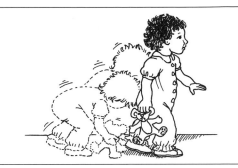

Item 36:	Standing and Moving Balance
Age:	13 Months
Position:	Standing
Stimulus:	Toy
Procedure:	Place the child in a standing position. Place a toy on the floor 2 ft. in front of the child. Say, "Get the toy and bring it to me."
Criteria:	2 Child picks up toy, returns to standing, and takes 3 steps without losing balance.
	1 Child picks up toy, returns to standing, and takes 1 or 2 steps before losing balance.
	0 Child remains stationary or loses balance when picking up toy.

FIG. 14-7 Item 36, standing and moving balance from the Peabody Developmental Motor Scales-2. *From Folio MR, Fewell RR: PDMS-2 Examiner's Manual, ed 2, Austin, 2000, Pro-Ed.*

motor integration (72 items). Test administration uses strictly standardized procedures. Entry points, based on chronological age, and basal and ceiling levels are used to minimize the number of items administered. The test manual describes the administration procedures for each item, provides an illustration of the activity, and lists the scoring criteria (Fig. 14-7). The type of instruction, demonstration, verbal instruction, or both, are specifically outlined and vary by item. The PDMS-2 yields multiple standard scores: GMQ; FMQ; total motor quotient (TMQ), which is a composite gross and fine motor score; six individual subscale scores; as well as age equivalents and percentiles. The child's fine and gross motor performance can be classified as below average (80-89), poor (70-79), or very poor (35-69).

Gross Motor Function Measure. The Gross Motor Function Measure (GMFM), introduced in 1993, is a measure of gross motor function published by an ongoing, active research group, the CanChild Centre for Childhood Disability Research.[24] The GMFM is the first validated evaluative measure of gross motor function for children with CP. The two versions of the GMFM are the original 88-item measure (GMFM-88) and the more recent (2002) 66-item measure (GMFM-66).[25] The GMFM-88 and GMFM-66 are individually administered, diagnosis-specific, criterion-referenced pediatric evaluative tests. The purposes of the GMFM are to measure gross motor function in children with CP and to evaluate the magnitude of change in gross motor function over time or after treatment in these children. The test can be administered to children ranging in age from birth to 5 years of age and can be used for older children whose functional abilities fall within the norms for this age range. The test is designed so that all items can be completed by a 5-year-old child with normal gross motor function.

The GMFM measures "gross motor function," which is defined as "how much a child can do." The two basic types of items are dynamic items and static items. Dynamic items require movement from one position to another. Static items require a position be maintained for a specific length of time. There are also items that involve a combination of dynamic movements and static positions. The developmental model is the theoretical framework of the GMFM. The GMFM is a measure of the activity level of the ICF.

Gross Motor Function Measure-88. The GMFM-88 is divided into five dimensions: Lying and rolling (17 items), sitting (20 items), crawling and kneeling (14 items), standing (13 items), and walking, running, and jumping (24 items). Items in each dimension are arranged in a developmental sequence, from easy to hard, based on clinical judgment. The test requires standardized administration with the test manual fully describing the child's starting position, instructions, and scoring criteria. The instructions allow for flexibility in the toys used to encourage movement, demonstrations, and verbal instruction. Items are individually scored on a 4-point ordinal scale, which range from "does not initiate" to "completes 100%"; however, more precise scoring criteria accompany many of the items. The GMFM yields five dimension percentage scores and a total percentage score. Each of the dimensions contributes equal weight to the total score, and the total score is calculated by adding all dimension percent scores and dividing by five.[25] The scores reflect how much as well as how well the child functioned on the GMFM. The GMFM-88 has been used extensively, both clinically and in research, to evaluate change in children with CP.[25] While the test was developed specifically for children with cerebral palsy, it has also been used in children with other diagnoses such as Down syndrome,[26] osteogenesis imperfecta,[27] and acute lymphoblastic leukemia.[28] The GMFM-88 is the instrument of choice when measuring (1) young children functioning primarily in the lying and rolling dimension, (2) children with severe motor disability, (3) the change in gross motor function with and without use of aids or orthoses, (4) a child's ability where the interval nature of the scale is not of concern, and (5) in the absence of computer access. Specific limitations of the GMFM-88 are: (1) individuals with identical percent scores could have very different scoring profiles limiting comparability; (2) the time it takes to administer, observe, and score all 88 test items; and (3) reduced responsiveness for children with very low or very high scores.[25]

Gross Motor Function Measure-66. The GMFM-66 consists of a subset of the original 88 items of the GMFM-88 divided into five dimensions: Lying and rolling (4 items), sitting (15 items), crawling and kneeling (10 items), standing (13 items), and walking, running, and jumping (24 items). The GMFM-66 was developed to improve the interpretability and clinical utility of the GMFM-88. The purpose, administration procedures, item scoring, testing equipment, examiner qualifications, theoretical background, and age-range tested are the same for both GMFM versions. The principal difference between the two versions is the number of items tested (22 fewer items), scoring of items that are refused or not tested, and how the collected data are analyzed. Additionally, the GMFM-66 is intended for use only with children with CP. On the GMFM-88, any item not observed scores zero. In contrast, on the GMFM-66, items not observed score as "not tested" or missing. Rasch analysis was applied to the GMFM-88 to produce the GMFM-66, converting the ordinal-level scale to an interval-level scale that arranges the items in terms of relative difficulty, from easy to hard. Additionally, the distance (i.e., difficulty level of each step) between the 0, 1, 2, and 3 score was determined. In the GMFM-88, item difficulty is arranged by expert opinion and the distance between the scores is assumed to be equal. A computer program, the Gross Motor Ability Estimator (GMAE), is required to calculate the GMFM-66 score. This program is supplied with the test manual. The GMAE calculates a score that estimates the child's gross motor ability. Along with the GMAE total score and standard error, item maps can be generated. Item maps provide a visual display of the difficulty estimates for test items and "steps" between scoring options.[25] The GMFM-66 score will differ from the GMFM-88 score because of the interval-level scale conversion.

The GMFM-66 is the measure of choice when the examiner wants to compare, on a common scale, changes in different children, or to follow a single child over time to compare the amount of change in common time frames. This common scale also makes it the test of choice for research involving children with CP. The test manual includes helpful information on patterns of motor development and change in motor function in children with CP across a range of ages and severity levels.

Criterion-Referenced Scales. An array of curriculum-based, interdisciplinary, informal, criterion-referenced instruments is available for therapists to examine motor performance. The Brigance Inventory of Early Development-II (IED-II)[29]; Early Intervention Developmental Profile (EIDP) [30]; Assessment, Evaluation, and Programming System (AEPS) for Infants and Children[31,32]; Hawaii Early Learning Profile (HELP)[33]; and the Carolina Curriculum for Infants and Toddlers with Special Needs (CCITSN)[34] are all examples of curriculum-based assessment tools. The scales often have a checklist of milestones in several developmental areas, including perceptual or fine motor, cognition, language, social or emotional, self-care, and gross motor development. The tests are intended for administration by multiple examiners to provide a comprehensive description of relative strengths and limitations. The test items for these instruments are selected from well-known standardized instruments, and an age is assigned at which the average typical child can successfully perform the item. Unfortunately, these tests are often misused in that age equivalents are generated, and children receive a motor diagnosis and referral for rehabilitation services based on information without proven norms. These *criterion-referenced tests* were never intended to be used as the primary source for motor diagnosis. They are intended to provide a structured procedure to examine a large number of physical tasks, analyze and synthesize individual strengths and weaknesses, and generate an appropriate intervention program.

Musculoskeletal

Posture and Postural Control. Postural control is fundamental to movement and is essential for the emergence and refinement of motor milestones.[4] Postural control allows an individual to (1) maintain a position (stability), (2) move into and out of positions (mobility), (3) recover from instability, and (4) anticipate and prepare for instability. Postural control is described under three conditions: Steady-state, anticipatory, and reactive. Steady-state adjustments require movement strategies that control a stable, quiet position in which the center of body mass is kept within the base of support. Anticipatory postural control adjustments require movement strategies that recover stability in response to a planned, voluntary movement. Reactive postural adjustments require movement strategies that recover stability in response to an unexpected, external disturbance, such as when an individual steps on ice, is jostled, or negotiates unsteady terrain. (See Chapters 4 and 13 for further discussion of posture and postural control.)

Postural control shows a distinct, continuous developmental progression and is a critical component of skill acquisition.[4] At birth, an infant's movement repertoire and control is limited. Over time, head control emerges, motor milestones are acquired, and the child gains the ability to sit and stand independently. The development of postural control appears to follow a cephalocaudal sequence starting with the head. Infants have limited head postural control at birth and do not develop good head control in response to positional perturbation until about 2 months of age (Fig. 14-8).[35] Over time, sensory inputs about the body's position with respect to the environment are integrated to produce motor actions that control the body's position. Vision seems to be the first step that is mapped to head control. Infants born at 32-34 weeks of gestation control head position in a simplified fashion that uses vision to keep the head in midline.[36]

Infants begin to sit independently at about 6-8 months of age when they can control spontaneous body sway sufficiently to stay upright. Directionally appropriate motor responses to sitting platform perturbations develop slowly. Two-month-old infants show no directionally appropriate responses; 3- to 4-month-olds coordinate responses in the neck 40% to 60% of the time; 5-month-olds coordinate trunk muscles 40% of the time; and by 8 months of age, neck and trunk responses are coordinated into effective patterns for controlling forward and backward sway (Fig. 14-9).[37]

Infants begin to stand independently at about 9-11 months of age when they can control many degrees of freedom over a small base of support (Fig. 14-10). As with sitting, directionally appropriate motor responses to platform perturbations when standing develop gradually. In response to a backward fall, 2- to 6-months-olds show no directionally appropriate responses, 7- to 9-month-olds

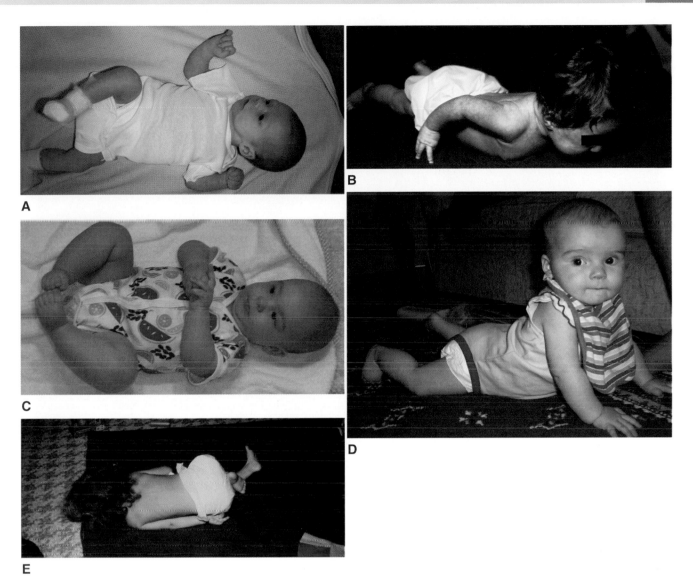

FIG. 14-8 Head control development. **A,** Supine, a newborn infant tends to keep her head rotated to one side. **B,** Prone, a 2-month-old infant can lift his head momentarily just high enough to clear his airway. **C,** Supine, a 4-month-old infant can maintain his head in midline. **D,** Prone, a 5-month-old can raise and maintain her head upright. **E,** Prone, a 3-year-old with athetoid cerebral palsy is only able to momentarily lift and turn her head.

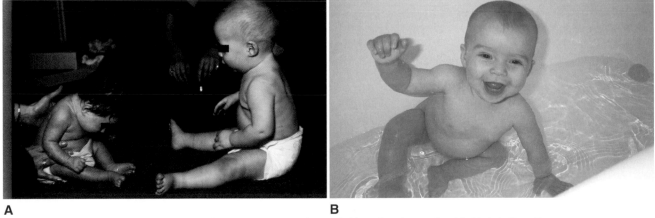

FIG. 14-9 Sitting development. **A,** Newborn *(left)* and a 6-month-old *(right);* **B,** a 5-month-old requires one hand support when reaching forward on a slippery surface.

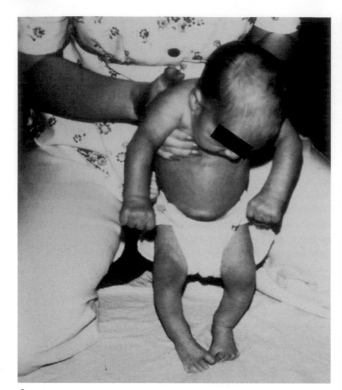

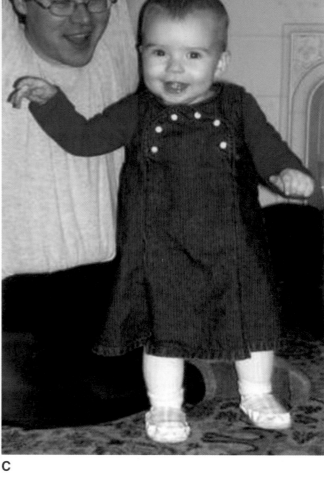

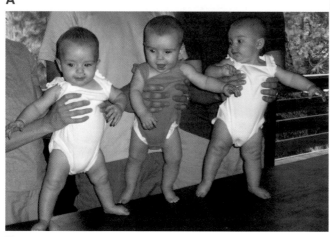

FIG. 14-10 Standing development. **A,** Newborn requires total support to stand; she bears some body weight intermittently on her flexed lower extremities. **B,** Three 8-month-olds all require support to stand, bear full body weight, and have an upright trunk and head. **C,** 12-month-old stands independently but cannot take a step forward without losing her balance.

begin to show directional responses at the ankle, and 9- to 11-month-olds show a complete postural standing synergy pattern, with responses at the ankle, thigh, and trunk in a distal to proximal sequence.[38,39] Visual maps to muscles controlling standing posture occur at approximately 5-6 months of age; followed by somatosensory maps at around 8-9 months of age.[40] A stepping strategy emerges at around 12-15 months of age as an adaptation to maintain standing in response to a perturbation. Hip strategies with minimal abdominal activity develop in new walkers with 3-6 months of walking experience, and a consistent hip strategy with active abdominal activity develops by 7-10 years of age.[41]

Postural control has been investigated in children in steady-state, anticipatory, and reactive states. The anthropometric characteristics of children make their postural responses different from those of adults. Children are shorter and have a larger head relative to their lower extremities. This places their center of mass higher than in adults, at about T12, making static balance more difficult.[4] Children compensate for this by swaying faster and further than adults. In quiet stance, amplitude and variability of sway decrease with age. Spontaneous sway in children reaches adult levels by 9-12 years of age for eyes-open conditions and by 12-15 years of age for eyes-closed conditions.[42]

In anticipatory postural control, a 9-month-old infant sitting on a parent's thigh activate trunk postural muscles before most reaching activities.[4] In standing, 12- to 15-month-olds activate postural control muscles before arm movements.[43] By the age of 4-6 years, standing anticipatory postural responses are essentially mature.[44,45]

Studies of postural adjustments to reactive perturbations show that $1\frac{1}{2}$ to 3 year olds produce well-organized muscle responses but with larger amplitudes and longer latencies and durations than adults.[46] Postural control develops gradually over time, and by the age of 7-10 years, reactive postural responses are similar to adult responses. The progression of postural control is not linear, in that 4- to 6-year-olds show postural responses that are generally slower and more variable than those found in the 15 month to 3 year old age group.[46] These discontinuous postural adjustments may be the result of the changes in body dimensions that occur in a growing child.

Atypical Postural Control. Delayed or abnormal development of postural control limits a child's ability to develop age-appropriate motor skills, including independent mobility and manipulation skills.[4] A wide range of problems can contribute to poor postural control, including insults to the motor or sensory components of the central and peripheral nervous system involved in postural control. Problems with sequencing, timely activation, and scaling of postural responses and poor adaptation of motor responses to task conditions are associated with motor coordination disturbances.[4] Abnormal sequencing of muscle recruitment in response to perturbations occurs in children with spastic hemiplegic and spastic diplegic CP.[44] Children with spastic diplegia tend to recruit muscles in a proximal to distal sequence, beginning at the neck and progressing downward in contrast to neurologically intact children who recruit muscles in a distal to proximal sequence, beginning with the muscles closest to the support surface. This abnormal pattern of muscle activation produces significantly less torque and larger lateral shifts of the body's center of mass.[44]

Spasticity is also associated with delayed muscle activation and poor recruitment and regulation of motor neuron firing.[47] Recruitment of proximal muscle synergies following a platform perturbation is delayed in children with Down syndrome (60-80 msec) when compared with normal children (36 msec).[48] Postural muscles are also not appropriately activated in anticipation of voluntary arm movements in children with CP and Down syndrome.[44,48] Normally, postural muscle activity in the trunk and lower extremities precedes activity in the prime movers of the arm. This pattern is reversed in children with CP. Inappropriate muscle coactivation is also reported in children with CP[41,44] and Down syndrome.[48]

Secondary musculoskeletal problems, such as poor postural alignment, abnormalities of muscle structure and function, and decreased strength, commonly observed in children with CNS damage can also limit postural control responses.[4] Additionally, solid ankle-foot orthoses (AFO), used to control the position and motion of the ankle joint, limit the use of ankle strategies and distal-to-proximal response sequencing.[49]

Children with sensory disturbances may also have difficulties with postural control. Sensory problems can affect a child's ability to adapt visual, somatosensory, and vestibular inputs to changes in task demands and prevent the development of accurate internal body models for postural control.

Examination of Postural Control. Examination of postural control requires testing musculoskeletal and neural systems. Musculoskeletal constraints, poor postural alignment, changes in muscle structure, function, and strength must also be integrated with motor and sensory findings. Postural control can be examined together with examination of milestones and functional skills. Head control and sitting and standing milestones can be described under steady-state, anticipatory, and reactive conditions. Although several tests and measures of postural control exist, all are limited in scope and only examine one small component of the postural system. There are few tests to assess functional balance in typical children and there are even fewer for children with neuromuscular impairments.[50] Common measures of postural control are tests of reflexes and *reactions,* balance as a component of a multidimensional test, and adult measures (see Chapter 13) adapted for children.

Adult Postural Control Tests and Measures Adapted For Children. Three adult measures of postural control have been used in the pediatric population: the Clinical Test for Sensory Interaction and Balance (CTSIB) fondly referred to as the "foam and dome," (see Fig. 13-14) the Functional Reach test (see Fig. 13-18), and the Berg Balance Scale (BBS) (see Chapter 13 for detailed descriptions of these tests).

A modified version of the foam and dome test can be used in children as young as 2 years of age.[46] A pediatric version of the CTSIB, the Pediatric CTSIB (P-CTSIB), has also been developed and performance described for two foot positions, feet-together and heel-toe, in typically developing children aged 4-9 years old.[51-53] In children 4-5 years of age (n = 40) the P-CTSIB in the feet-together position can discriminate between children with and without balance deficits, but the heel-toe position is too difficult for young children and therefore has limited discriminative value for this age group.[53] Typically developing children aged 6-9 years (n = 109) could generally maintain balance in all sensory conflict situations on the P-CTSIB in the feet-together position, but again the heel-toe position produced more variability without a clear developmental progression.[52]

The Functional Reach test (see Fig. 13-18) measures the maximum distance one can reach forward beyond arm's length while maintaining a fixed standing position. Subjects are instructed to reach forward with their shoulder at 90 degrees of flexion, without losing their balance. This test was developed on subjects aged 20-87 years.[54] Mean reach and critical reach values have also been determined for functional reach in typical children between the ages of 5 and 15 years.[55] The developers of this test state that it can reliably quantify (interrater reliability, ICC 0.98) balance in children within this age range. However, the group size in the reliability study (n = 116) was small and may not be representative of the entire population. In general, functional reach increases with age up to 11-12 years and then plateaus. Mean reach ranges from 21.1 cm in children 5-6 years old to 36.18 in 11-12-year-old children.[55]

The BBS is a functional measure of balance developed for use in the elderly and in individuals with neurological impairments.[56] The BBS emphasizes function and quantifies performance of activities such as moving from sitting to standing, standing with eyes closed, standing on one foot and picking up an object from the floor from a standing position. The BBS has also been used to examine balance in children ages 8 to 12 years with spastic hemiplegic or spastic diplegic CP, with and without aids.[50] The BBS is not sensitive enough for use with children with minimal motor deficits or only mild balance impairments but can be useful in ambulatory children with cerebral palsy with moderate balance impairments and has been shown to distinguish between groups of children with differing functional abilities.[50]

Postural Control as One Component in a Multidimensional Test. Postural control, which is called balance in this circumstance, is a component of the Bruininks-Oseretsky Test of Motor Proficiency (BOT).[57] The BOT balance subscale contains the following eight items:

1. Standing on preferred lower extremity on floor.
2. Standing on preferred lower extremity on balance beam.
3. Standing on preferred lower extremity on balance beam, eyes closed.
4. Walking forward on walking line.

5. Walking forward on balance beam.
6. Walking forward heel-to-toe on walking line.
7. Walking forward heel-to-toe on balance beam.
8. Stepping over response speed stick on balance beam.

Each task is administered and scored using specified criteria. Scoring criteria include amount of time (items 1-3), number of steps (items 4-7), or ability to perform, fail, or pass (item 8). The balance subtest score can be compared to an age-matched standardization sample.

Anthropometric Characteristics

Skeletal Development. Cartilage models of the long bones appear by the sixth week of gestation and primary centers of ossification appear in almost all bones of the limbs by the twelfth week, and in the vertebrae by the seventh or eighth week. At birth, the diaphyses of the long bones are ossified, although the epiphyses are still cartilaginous. Ossification continues up to the age of 25 years. Fig. 14-11 shows the age periods for appearance of the primary and secondary ossification centers and fusion of the epiphyses.

Body Composition. Body composition, the ratio of fat mass (FM) to fat-free mass (FFM), impacts performance on tests of aerobic and muscular fitness, including the 1-mile

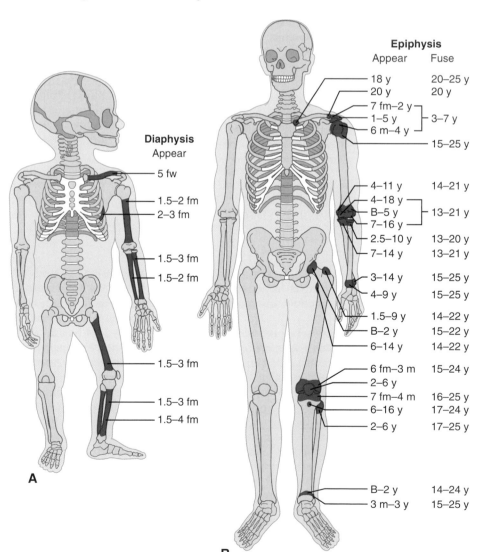

FIG. 14-11 Appearance of primary and secondary ossification centers. **A,** Appearance of diaphyses. **B,** Appearance and fusion of epiphyses. *Fw,* Fetal weeks; *fm,* fetal months; *m,* postnatal months; *y,* years; *B,* birth. *Modified from Anson B:* Morris' Human Anatomy, *ed 12, New York, 1966, McGraw-Hill. In Cech D, Martin S:* Functional Movement Development Across the Life Span, *ed 2, Philadelphia, 2002, WB Saunders.*

run-walk test (MRWT)[58] and tests of upper body strength.[59] Although absolute $\dot{V}O_{2max}$ values are often the same or even higher in children with mild to moderate obesity compared to normal weight children, $\dot{V}O_{2max}/kg$ and performance on weight-bearing endurance tests are poorer, probably a result of the increased inert load from excess body fat.[60] Children with neuromotor impairments, whose physical activity is limited, may become overweight as a result of the imbalance between energy intake and expenditure. It is important to identify and address excess weight in children because childhood obesity may continue into adulthood, increasing the risk for a wide range of serious health problems.[61]

Laboratory methods of measuring body composition include underwater weighing or doubly labeled water. Although these tests provide accurate measures of body composition, they are expensive and labor intensive and are therefore rarely used in practice. The most common clinical measures of body composition are measurement of skinfold thickness and calculated *body mass index* (BMI). Although skinfold thickness can be measured at up to seven sites, the standardized fitness test batteries listed in Table 14-5 use the sum of two sites (triceps and either calf or subscapular) to estimate body fat. The test manuals provide age- and gender-based standards for percentage of body fat. Fig. 14-12 shows skinfold thickness measures and corresponding body fat percentages for boys and girls.

BMI is a person's weight divided by their height in meters squared (kg/m²). Since BMI does not take into account that muscle:fat ratios may be different in children than in adults and measures of skinfold thickness are found to correlate better with laboratory measures of body density in both children and adults,[62] it is recommended that BMI only be used when other methods are not possible.[63]

Range of Motion. Because of the uterine molding of the fetus, especially during the last weeks of gestation, the neonate has a strong flexion bias and torsional deviations of the lower limbs. In the typically developing infant, these resolve over time as routine handling, gravity, and muscle action elongate the shortened flexor muscles and activate the extensor muscles of the trunk and lower limbs.[64] Joint range of motion (ROM) changes significantly from birth through the growing years. Table 14-6 shows reported values for lower limb joint ROM in the typically developing infant and child. In children born full term, upper extremity ROM is similar to adults, although elbow extension can be limited by as much as 30 degrees in some infants at birth.[64]

The basic shape of the skeleton and individual bones remains the same throughout life; however, bones increase in length, width, and girth because of postnatal skeletal modeling of the cartilage models. Intermittent compressive forces within a physiological range, the result of normal muscle pull and loading during weight bearing, stimulate longitudinal bone growth. The degree of modeling is greatest in young bone because it is highly compliant and responsive to dynamic strain from mechanical forces.[61,65] For examples, the angle of inclination between the femoral neck and shaft changes from approximately 135-145 degrees in the infant to approximately 125 degrees in the adult and the angle of femoral anteversion changes from a range of 25-30 degrees at birth to 10-15 degrees in the middle adult years.

The shape and joint angles of the knees also change throughout childhood (Fig. 14-13). The knee joint in the newborn has a mean of 16 degrees of tibiofemoral varum,[66] and this gradually decreases to approximately 0 degrees by the first or second year of life, then progresses to a valgus angle that peaks at approximately 11 degrees between the ages of 3-5 years. The mature angle of 5-7 degrees valgus is achieved between the ages of 6-12 years. There are slight gender differences by approximately age 15 on, with females having 5.5 degrees of valgum and males having on average 4.4 degrees.[67] The degree of tibiofemoral valgus can be estimated clinically by measuring the intermalleolar distance with the child positioned with the knees extended, patellae aligned in the sagittal plane, and medial femoral condyles touching. Cusick suggests that a tibiofemoral angle >10 degrees valgum or an intermalleolar distance >10 cm in a child older than 8 years is abnormal and may contribute to mechanical problems and pain in adolescence or adulthood.[65]

Atypical neuromuscular activity during the years of musculoskeletal growth can result in modeling errors that can cause joint dysfunction and disability. For example, in children with CP the configuration of the acetabulum often remains immature and the infantile femoral anteversion and neck to shaft angle fail to resolve, increasing the risk for hip subluxation or dislocation. Most newborns undergo screening for hip instability by a pediatrician using either the Barlow or Ortolani techniques.[68] Leg-length discrepancy, asymmetry of the lower extremity skin creases, limited hip abduction, or a positive Trendelenburg sign in an older child should arouse suspicion of unilateral hip dysplasia that should be further evaluated by an orthopedist. Bilateral hip dislocation is more difficult to detect because there is no asymmetry; however, there may be excessive lumbar lordosis, limited hip abduction, and a wide perineal gap.

Lower limb rotational deformities are also common in children with neuromuscular disorders and often present as an "in-toeing" or "out-toeing" gait. These conditions may result from persistent torsional deformities in the lower limbs, abnormal muscle activity, or habitual sitting and sleeping postures. For example, sitting in the reversed tailor or W position, with the feet internally rotated and beneath the buttocks encourages medial rotation contracture of the hips, medial tibial torsion, and adduction of the forefoot.[69,70] These complex conditions require careful and systematic examination to pinpoint the location and cause of the problem.

Staheli developed a test involving six different measures to help assess for the presence and cause of rotational deformities in children.[71] The six measures in this test are foot progression angle, hip medial and lateral rotation, thigh-foot angle, angle of the transmalleolar axis, and shape of the sole of the foot. The latter two tests are performed with the child lying prone with the hip extended and knee flexed to 90 degrees. Normative means and

TABLE 14-5   Physical Fitness Test Batteries Appropriate for Children with Neuromotor Impairments

Target Age	Fitness Component	Test Item	Modifications for Children with Disabilities?	Standards/Reporting Method	Training Program
PRUDENTIAL FITNESSGRAM[81]					
5-17+ years	Aerobic fitness	MRWT, PACER— 20 meter.	Swimming Stationary bicycle Wheelchair propulsion Walking	Criterion-referenced standards for the general population.* Child's performance is classified as in the "healthy fitness zone" or "needs improvement." Computer software program for report for typically developing population. Use paper form to report results for children with disabilities.	Minimal general guidelines for fitness training are provided in the test manual.
	Body composition	Skinfold measurements (triceps and calf), BMI.	Measure skinfolds on either side of body		
	Muscle strength and endurance	Abdominals: Curl-up. Upper body: Trunk lift, push-up, pull-up, modified pull-up, flexed arm hang.	Use any movement child can perform to measure strength; perform multiple repetitions to measure endurance		
	Flexibility	Back saver sit and reach (hamstrings). Shoulder stretch (upper body/ shoulder girdle).			
BROCKPORT PHYSICAL FITNESS TEST[82]					
10-17 years	Aerobic capacity	MWRT PACER—20 meter.	PACER—16 meter TAMT	Criterion-referenced standards for the typically developing child (minimum, preferred performance).† Specific standards for child with sensory, neuromotor, and orthopedic impairments. Software program for reporting individual or group test profiles. Paper test forms and fitness profile are available in the test manual.	Complete training manual included with test kit. Some condition-specific guidelines are provided.
	Body composition	Skinfold measurements (triceps and subscapular or triceps and calf), BMI.			
	Muscle strength and endurance	Recommended items for the general population include push-up, curl-up, trunk lift. Optional test items include flexed arm hang, pull-up, modified pull-up.	Reverse curl Seated push-up 40-meter push/walk Bench press Grip strength Dumbbell press		
	Flexibility	Recommended test item is the back-saver sit and reach. Optional test item is the shoulder stretch.	Modified Apley Test‡ Modified Thomas Test§ Target Stretch Test‖		

*Criterion-referenced standards, determined by research or expert opinion, to indicate the level of performance believed to be compatible with good health and prevention of chronic diseases related to a sedentary lifestyle.

†The BPFT manual lists optional test items for each component based on the child's diagnosis and capabilities, impairments, and activity restrictions.

‡The Modified Apley test assesses the flexibility of the shoulder girdle.

§The Modified Thomas Test assesses length of hip flexor muscles.

‖In the Target Stretch Test, the examiner scores joint motion on an ordinal scale by comparing the subject's active range of motion to expected values.

MRWT, 1-mile run-walk test; *PACER*, Progressive Aerobic Cardiovascular Endurance Run; *BMI*, body mass index (based on the formula weight [kg]/height [m^2]); *TAMT*, Target Aerobic Movement Test (measures child's ability to exercise at or above a recommended target heart rate for 15 minutes).

standard deviations (SD) have been determined for these tests and values within 2 SD from the mean are considered to be normal variations, whereas those outside this range are considered to indicate a torsional deformity. If the child is found to have a torsional deformity, the specific abnormal test scores may help to identify the cause of the abnormality and be used to guide interventions.

Muscle Performance. Many factors contribute to the development of strength during childhood and adolescence, including gender, age, body size and type, muscle

BOYS
TRICEPS PLUS CALF SKINFOLDS

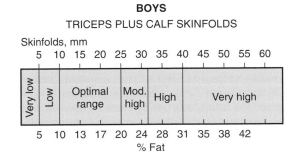

GIRLS
TRICEPS PLUS CALF SKINFOLDS

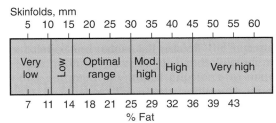

TRICEPS PLUS SUBSCAPULAR SKINFOLDS

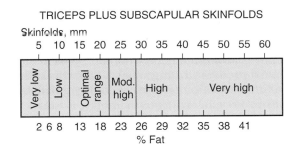

TRICEPS PLUS SUBSCAPULAR SKINFOLDS

FIG. 14-12 Skinfold thickness measures and corresponding percentage of body fat charts for boys and girls. *From Lohman TG: Measuring body fat using skinfolds (videotape), Champaign, Ill, 1987, Human Kinetics.*

TABLE 14-6	Lower Extremity Passive Range of Motion at Selected Ages Through the Lifespan

Motion/Average PROM ± 2 SD (Range)	Newborn	12 Months	24 Months	3-5 Years	5-12 Years	Adult
Hip extension limitation	46° ± 8.2° (21.7°-68.3°)	9° ± 4.8°	3° ± 3.0°	0° ± 5.0°	No limitation	No limitation
Hip abduction with hips flexed	79.3° ± 4.34° (63°-80°)					
With hips extended	39° ± 5.11° (27-58)	59° ± 7.3°	54° ± 7.5°	60° ± 7.1°	45°-55°	Male: 45° Female: 50°
Hip medial rotation	40° (20°-60°)	44° + 9.1°	52° ± 10.1°	50°	Male: 50° Female: 55°	Male: 35°-45° Female: 40°-45°
Hip lateral rotation	63° (45°-89°)	58° ± 8.8°	No data	No data	No data	45°-60°
Knee extension limitation	21.5° ± 4.7° (15°-30°)	Progressive ↑ in ROM until full at ≈12 months	<15° hyper-extension between 2-3 years of age	Incidence of knee hyperextension decreases by 4-7 years of age	No data	No limitation
Ankle dorsiflexion	58.9° + 7.9° (36.7°-71.7°)	25°-45°	38° (mean)	15°-30°	No data	20°-30°
Ankle plantarflexion	25.7° ± 6.3° (10.0°-41.7°)	45°-50°	No data	No data	No data	40°-65°

Data from Cusick, 2000; Forero et al., 1989; Giannestras et al, 1973; Katz et al, 1992; Kendal et al, 1993; Klevin et al, 1989; Phelps et al, 1985; Reade et al, 1984; Staheli, 1987; Stout, 2000; Sutherland et al, 1988; Tardieu and Tardieu, 1987; Waugh et al, 1983; Wong et al, 1998. *PROM,* Passive range of motion; *SD,* standard deviation; *ROM,* range of motion.

cross-sectional area, and fiber type proportions. Strength increases throughout childhood, and gains in strength generally parallel the typical growth curves for height and weight. There are gender differences in strength in children as young as 3 years of age that continue throughout development.[61] Strength increases linearly in boys until puberty, at which time, strength increases sharply, probably a result of the influence of androgenic hormones. Smaller increases in strength continue through the adolescent years. In contrast, in girls the curve either plateaus or continues to increase linearly at puberty. Fig. 14-14 shows changes in scores on the curl-up test of abdominal strength in boys and girls during the growing years.

Muscle size accounts for much of the age and gender differences in strength during childhood and adolescence. Changes in muscle function follow increases in muscle size, but qualitative improvements also result from neural changes, including myelination, increased coordination of muscle synergists and antagonists, and improvements in motor unit recruitment.[72]

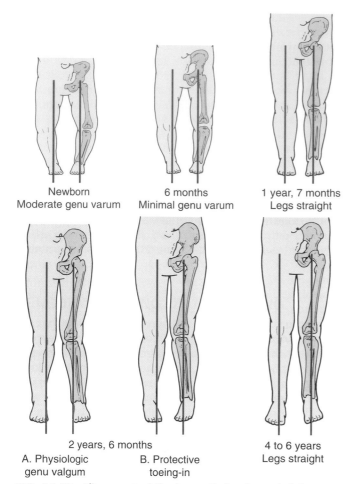

Newborn
Moderate genu varum

6 months
Minimal genu varum

1 year, 7 months
Legs straight

2 years, 6 months
A. Physiologic genu valgum

B. Protective toeing-in

4 to 6 years
Legs straight

FIG. 14-13 Alignment of the lower limbs through infancy and childhood. *Redrawn from Tachdjian MO: Pediatric Orthopedics, ed 2, Philadelphia, 1990, WB Saunders.*

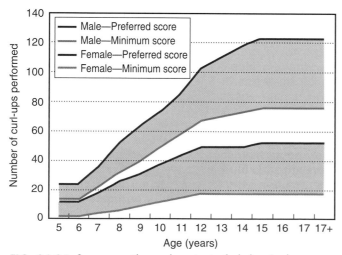

FIG. 14-14 Scores on the curl-up test of abdominal strength in boys and girls. *Data from Prudential Health Fitness Standards.*

Abnormalities in muscle structure or function may have a number of causes, including defects in neuromuscular development during gestation and deficits in blood supply, nutrition, or innervation after birth. Disease, immobilization, disuse, and postural imbalances also affect muscle function. Direct abnormalities in muscle tissue occur in conditions like muscular dystrophy or arthrogryposis multiplex congenita, whereas indirect changes, including hypertonia or hypotonia, may result from abnormal neuronal activity in conditions like CP. Alterations in the normal mosaic pattern or distribution of fiber types in muscles, with predominance of one fiber type or changes in fiber size as a result of atrophy or hypertrophy, can also change muscle strength and endurance. For example, type I muscle fibers atrophy more in children with hypotonia[73] and congenital myotonic dystrophy,[65] whereas type II muscle fibers atrophy more in chronic inflammatory conditions such as rheumatoid arthritis.[74]

Measuring Muscle Strength in Children. Measurement of muscle strength in children with neuromotor disorders helps to identify deficits that may contribute to activity restrictions. Observation of antigravity movements can be used to determine functional strength in infants and very young children. Fig. 14-15 shows tests for assessing strength of the neck extensor muscles in an infant.

In older children, manual muscle testing (MMT) is usually used to test strength in the clinic (see Chapter 5). Florence et al demonstrated that MMT scores had fair reliability in children with Duchenne muscular dystrophy with standardization of the procedure and training of the testers.[75] Although the one repetition maximum (1 RM; i.e., maximal weight the child can move through the available range for one repetition) can also be used to estimate strength, the 6 RM is preferred in prepubertal children because it is safer.[76]

Instruments for measuring strength, including handheld or isokinetic dynamometers, provide reliable results in most children.[77] Wiley and Damiano found strength deficits in children with cerebral palsy based on testing with an isokinetic dynamometer, although the effect of spasticity on isokinetic measures of strength is debated.[78] Bar-Or reported good reliability of measures of peak force in children with CP, using the 30-second Wingate anaerobic test, an all-out cycling test.[79] In contrast, van der Berg-Emons et al found that reliability decreased at higher speeds of muscle contraction in children with neurological impairments.[80]

Field tests that measure relative strength, using the body as resistance, are commonly used in schools. Two such tests are the Prudential FITNESSGRAM[81] and the Brockport Physical Fitness Test (BPFT) (see Table 14-5).[82] In typically developing children, height, weight, percentage of body fat, and gender impact performance on field tests of upper body strength, including the pull-up, modified pull-up, flexed arm hang, and push-up. Most health-related fitness tests provide age- and gender-based criterion-referenced standards to determine if a child's test scores are consistent with good health. The BPFT also provides specific standards for several tests in children with cerebral palsy and spinal cord injury.[82]

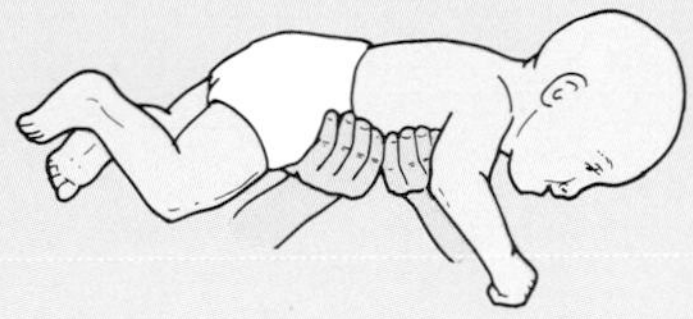

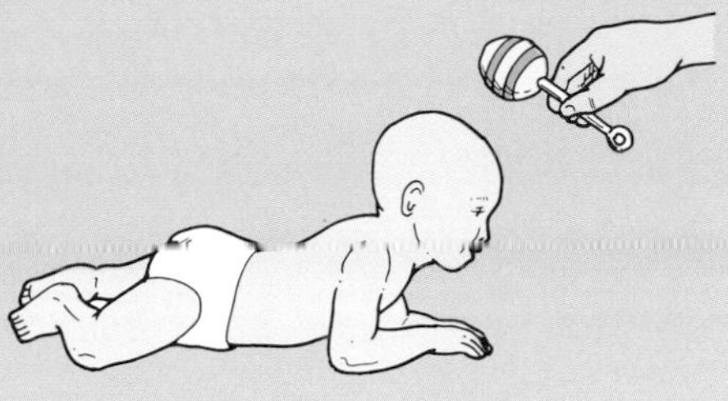

FIG. 14-15 Assessing neck extensor strength in an infant. *Redrawn from Connelly B: Testing in infants and children. In Hislop H, Montgomery J (eds): Daniels and Worthingham's Muscle Testing, ed 6, Philadelphia, 1995, WB Saunders.*

Test position:	Child is suspended by the therapist's hands placed under the chest.
Expected response:	2 months — Child raises head to midline and holds it for 2 to 3 seconds
	3 months — Child lifts head beyond plane of body.

Test position:	Child is placed on stomach, and the therapist shakes a rattle above the childs head.
Expected response:	2 months — Child actively extends head to 45°.
	3 months — Child actively extends head to 90° and maintains position.

Neuromuscular

Reflex Integrity. Traditionally, developmental reflexes are examined as part of the assessment of postural control. Developmental reflexes consist of attitudinal reflexes, righting reactions, and balance and protective reactions.[83] A developmental reflex is a stereotyped response to a specific stimulus and is categorized as primitive or reactive. A primitive reflex appears during fetal development or at birth and is difficult to elicit after approximately 6 months of age in children with typical development. A reactive reflex appears in infancy or childhood and persists throughout life. Developmental reflexes are evaluated in terms of when they appear and disappear in relation to typically developing children. For example, the reaction "forward protective extension" should appear at 6 months of age and persist thereafter. It would therefore be considered normal if this response was absent at 4 months of age, but abnormal or delayed if still absent at 12 months. However, since the reported norms for age of onset for developmental reflexes are broad and variable, they must be used judiciously in assigning a label of normal or abnormal.[84]

Examination of developmental reflexes also provides a standardized format for observing symmetry, comparing upper and lower body responses, responses of the head and trunk, and association of the intensity of the stimulus to the size of the response and can also be useful in young infants in whom the expected movement repertoire is limited. Table 14-7 outlines reported developmental reflexes, and Figs. 14-16, 14-17, and 14-18 show responses of forward upper extremity protective extension, asymmetrical tonic neck reflex, and Landau righting reaction, respectively.

Motor Function—Control and Learning. Muscle tone abnormalities are common in children with impaired neuromotor development and range from hypertonicity, spasticity, and rigidity to hypotonicity, hypotonia, and flaccidity. Tone abnormalities are associated with a wide variety of conditions including Down syndrome, Prader-Willi syndrome, and cognitive impairments such as mental retardation. Abnormalities in tone are consistent

and predictive findings in young children at risk for CP and are hallmarks of children described as having CP.[85,86] Spasticity is the most common impairment in children with CP and is associated with limited selective motor control, abnormal and limited movement synergies, limited active ROM, and abnormal timing of muscle activation and postural responses.[87] Hypotonicity in infants may also herald a neuromuscular condition. The tonal pattern can gradually change over time from low tone to high tone. Muscle tone normally changes in the premature infant during the first year of life.[88]

Abnormal tone can be described by the tonal level (hypotonic to spastic), intensity (severity) and distribution.[89] No single clinical instrument measures all of these. Hyperactive stretch reflexes, abnormal posturing of the extremities, associated movements, clonus, and stereotyped movement synergies are all measurable behaviors associated with spasticity. The Modified Ashworth Scale (MAS) is a frequently cited instrument used to describe alterations in muscle tone in adults.[90,91] The MAS focuses only on the "increased" portion of the tone continuum; thus decreased tone can not be assessed. Howle proposed a muscle tone scale that expands on the MAS to cover the entire spectrum of tonal levels (−3: severe hypotonia to +3: severe hypertonia) and allow description of both resistance to passive movement and constraints on active movement by the child.[85]

Tone assessment is also sometimes a component of a multidimensional test. In general, there is little consistency in the operational definition, administration procedures, or scoring methods used by the various tests, resulting in suspect validity and modest reliability. Tone is incorporated in the Movement Assessment of Infants (MAI),[92] Neonatal Behavioral Assessment Scale (NBAS),[93] and Bayley Scales of Infant Development-II (BSID-II).[94] The MAI refers to muscle tone as the readiness of muscles to respond to gravity. The NBAS rates two tonal items: general tonus and balance of motor tone. The Behavioral Rating Scale of the BSID-II has a motor quality factor in which hypotonicity and hypertonicity are individually rated on a 5-point ordinal scale. The hypotonicity scale, for example, ranges from "consistently hypotonic, like a

TABLE 14-7	Selected Developmental Reflexes and Reactions		
Time Course	**Position**	**Test Procedure**	**Response**
ATTITUDINAL REFLEXES			
Asymmetrical Tonic Neck			
Birth to 6 months	Supine	Rotate head, actively or passively, to one side.	"Bow and arrow position." UE and LE extension on "chin side." UE and LE flexion on "skull" side.
Symmetrical Tonic Neck			
4/6 months to 8/12 months	Prone, overlap	1. Flex the head. 2. Extend the head.	1. UE flexion and LE extension. 2. UE extension and LE flexion.
Tonic Labyrinthine			
Birth to 6 months	1. Prone 2. Supine	1. Position in prone. 2. Position in supine.	1. Increased flexion of all limbs. 2. Increased extension of all limbs.
RIGHTING REACTIONS			
Optical Righting			
Birth-Persists	Body held vertical in space	Tilt body: Forward. Backward. Left. Right.	Head orients to vertical position. Head extension. Head flexion. Head laterally flexes right. Head laterally extends left.
Labyrinthine Righting			
Birth-Persists	Body held vertical in space	Obscure vision, tilt body: Forward. Backward. Left. Right.	Head orients to vertical position. Head extension. Head flexion. Head laterally flexes right. Head laterally flexes left.
Body-on-Head Righting			
Birth/2 months to 5 years	Prone	Place prone.	Head extends and rotates to one side.
Neck-on-Body Righting			
Neonatal: 34 weeks' gestation to 2 months Mature: 4/6 months to 5 years	Supine	Rotate head passively to one side.	Neonatal: Body rotates as a whole (log rolls, no rotation) to align body with head. Mature: Body rotates with rotation to align body with head.
Body-on-Body Righting			
Neonatal: 34 weeks' gestation to 4/5 months Mature: 4/6 months to 5 years	Supine	Flex and rotate LE across body.	Neonatal: Body rotates as a whole (log rolls, no rotation) to align body with head. Mature: Body rotates with rotation to align body with head.
Landau Righting			
3 months to 12/24 months	Prone	Hold in horizontal suspension.	Head, limbs, and trunk extend.
BALANCE AND PROTECTIVE RESPONSES			
Protective Extension: UE			
Forward: 6 months-Persists	1. Support body in space	Plunge body downward.	UEs extend, abduct to support and protect the body from falling:
Left/right side: 7 months-Persists	2. Sitting	Push sideways.	Forward. To the left and right side. Backward.
Backward: 9/10 months-Persists	3. Sitting	Push backward.	
Tilting Reactions			
Prone: 5 months-Persists	Prone	Place on tilt board in one of the four positions, tilt board.	Preserve the equilibrium of the body under conditions of instability. Head rotates, trunk curvature, extension and abduction of limbs toward upward side of board.
Supine: 7/8 months-Persists	Supine		
Sit: 7/8 months-Persists	Sit		
Stand: 12/21 months-Persists	Stand		

Data from Barnes MR, Crutchfield CA, Heriza CB: *The Neurophysiological Basis of Patient Treatment,* Morgantown, WVa, 1978, Stokesville.
UE, Upper extremity; *LE,* lower extremity.

rag doll" to "absence of hypotonicity."[94] Tone is also incorporated into the Clinical Assessment of Gestational Age in the Newborn.[95] This is based on 10 criteria, including posture, ROM of popliteal angle and ankle dorsiflexion, and prone suspension.

Quality of Movement. It is important to examine how a child moves to guide rehabilitation evaluation and interventions. The quality of a child's movement is emphasized by the neurodevelopment treatment (NDT) approach introduced by the Bobaths and remains important today.

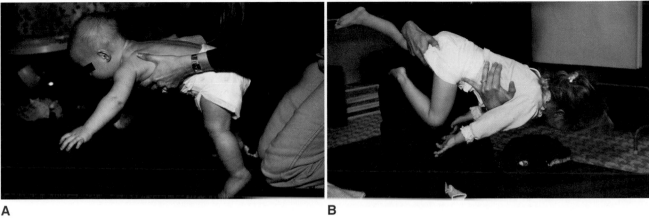

A   **B**

FIG. 14-16 Forward protective extension of the upper extremities. **A,** Normal response by an 8-month-old with arms outstretched to protect the body. **B,** Absent response in a 3-year-old child with athetoid cerebral palsy.

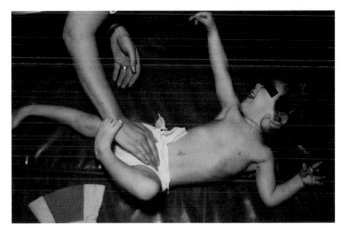

FIG. 14-17 Asymmetrical tonic neck reflex response in a 3-year-old child with athetoid cerebral palsy.

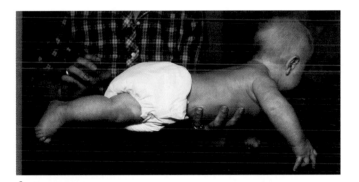

A

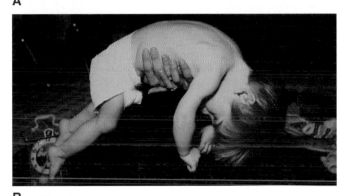

B

FIG. 14-18 Landau righting reaction. **A,** Normal response by 6-month-old (head, trunk, and limbs extending); **B,** Absent response in a 1-year-old child with spastic diplegic cerebral palsy.

Unfortunately, there is no consensus on what movement components should be observed and analyzed to assess movement quality. This is further complicated by the fact that typical movements change with age; infant movement is not as smooth and coordinated as that of an adult. Movements performed with age-appropriate quality are thought to be the most efficient and least likely to be associated with future secondary complications.[96]

The concepts of consistency, flexibility, and efficiency have been used to describe how one moves.[97] Consistency is the ability to successfully perform a skill repeatedly over multiple days. Flexibility is the ability to perform a skill under a variety of environmental conditions. Efficiency is the ability to perform a skill within a certain level of cardiopulmonary and musculoskeletal energy expenditure.

Atypical or poor quality movement descriptions fall under the ICF category of impairment. Poor quality movements may be immature or atypical. Immature movements are those observed in typically developing children at a younger age. Atypical movements are not observed in typically developing children. Movement components that contribute to immature or atypical quality include paresis, abnormal muscle tone, abnormal synergies, coordination problems (poor motor activation and sequencing, coactivation, impaired interjoint coordination, delayed reaction time), slow or fast movement, inability to terminate a movement, involuntary movements, associated movements, somatosensory deficits, and perceptual disorders. Children with impaired neuromotor development show fixed movement strategies, losing movement flexibility and adaptability.[98]

There is no well-accepted procedure for examining movement quality. Quality is generally documented with a detailed, narrative description. Standardized tests often include a qualitative component within an individual test item. The test item describes how the movement must be performed in order to receive credit for the particular item. For example, the "pull to sit" item on the AIMS states that arms, hips, and knees are flexed, weight is on buttocks and lumbar spine, the chin is tucked, and the head is in line or in front of the body (see Fig. 14-5).

The GMPM was developed as an observational instrument to measure changes in quality of movement in children with CP.[99] Alignment, coordination, dissociated movement, stability, and weight shift are individually scored while the child performs designated items on the GMPM.[100]

The Toddler and Infant Motor Evaluation (TIME) includes three subtests that quantify how the child moves: component analysis, quality rating, and atypical positions.[86] This test is intended for use with children from 4 months to $3\frac{1}{2}$ years of age. The component analysis subtest measures the degree of developmental maturity of movement of each segment of the body, including the head and neck, trunk, upper extremities, lower extremities, with weight bearing and weight shifting, and movement in each position. The component analysis is completed separately for each of seven situations: Supine, prone, quadruped, kneeling, standing, balance, and running. The quality rating subtest is a detailed description of deviations in tone, reflex integration, balance, and balance between flexion and extension. The atypical positions subtest records the number and severity of abnormal movement patterns. Pictorial representations of atypical patterns are included in the manual.

Cardiovascular/Pulmonary.

A basic examination of vital functions and exercise performance are essential components of the assessment of a child with impaired neuromotor development. The examination should include measurements of heart rate (HR), respiratory rate (RR), and blood pressure (BP) (see Chapter 22).

Circulation. The infant's pulse is measured at the femoral or brachial artery and should be counted for a full minute. Pain, crying, cardiac abnormalities, and some medications may cause tachycardia or a rapid heart rate. A slow heart rate, or bradycardia, may result from hypoxia, cardiac disease, and some medications.[101]

Ventilation and Respiration/Gas Exchange. Respiratory rate can be measured in an infant or very young child by counting chest expansions for one full minute. Newborn infants, especially those who are premature, often demonstrate an irregular breathing pattern with short periods (5-10 seconds) of apnea.[102] Apnea lasting longer than 20 seconds is abnormal and may indicate CNS hemorrhage, sepsis, or respiratory distress.[101] It is not uncommon to see slight intercostal retractions during inspiration in healthy infants; however, paradoxical breathing, in which the abdomen is drawn inward on inspiration while the thorax expands outward, suggests fatigue of the respiratory muscles. In this situation the infant should be referred to the pediatrician for further examination.[102]

The therapist should assess the infant's ability to sneeze spontaneously to clear the airway. Toddlers and older children should demonstrate an effective cough in order to clear secretions. Auscultation of the lungs is necessary to determine the presence of adventitious breath sounds, including crackles and rales (indicate excess fluid in the lungs), wheezing (a sign of restricted air flow from constricted or obstructed airways), or decreased breath sounds (poor airflow from narrowing or atelectasis) (see Chapters 24 and 26). The examination of respiratory function should include postural screening for scoliosis or kyphosis that may limit thoracic mobility (see Chapter 4) and for limited shoulder mobility from soft tissue contractures or muscle weakness because these may contribute to impaired chest expansion.[101]

Aerobic Capacity and Endurance. Periodic examination of the child's aerobic fitness and energy expenditure during exercise is useful for planning and monitoring the effects of interventions. Absolute $\dot{V}O_{2max}$ increases linearly with growth in both boys and girls, paralleling the increasing dimensions of the heart, lungs, and vascular system.[103] Expressed relative to body mass ($\dot{V}O_{2max}$/kg), aerobic capacity remains stable in males from 6-16 years of age, with an average of 50-53 ml/kg^{-1}/min^{-1}. In contrast, relative $\dot{V}O_{2max}$ in females declines throughout childhood and adolescence. Despite the relative stability of weight-adjusted $\dot{V}O_{2max}$, submaximal running economy progressively improves throughout childhood. Time to complete the MRWT field test of aerobic endurance also decreases in boys and girls from the ages of 5-13 years, although run times increase in females at puberty.[104]

Examination of aerobic performance in the field usually includes tests that measure the time it takes the child to run or walk a given distance, as with the MRWT, or the distance run or walked in a specified time, as with the 9-minute run-walk test (9MRWT) or 12-minute run-walk test (12MRWT). Both the MRWT and the 12MRWT demonstrate acceptable concurrent validity with laboratory measures of $\dot{V}O_{2max}$, although distance run times have been shown to be influenced in children by factors other than $\dot{V}O_{2max}$, including body composition and peak muscle power.[105] The typically developing child shows progressive improvement in MRWT time and 9MRWT distance between the ages of 5-13 years, a period when both muscle mass and strength increase.

Studies indicate that children with CP[91] and muscular dystrophy[106] have reduced aerobic capacity and use a higher percentage of their available aerobic function during routine activities, resulting in poor mechanical efficiency. Multiple factors may be involved, including abnormalities in structures (heart, lung, muscle tissue) or physiological function, resulting in poor delivery or uptake of oxygen by tissues, as well as increased energy use for maintaining postural stability as a result of impaired muscle tone or motor control. Exercise tolerance may also be limited by poor muscle endurance in children with neuromuscular impairments. Bar-Or found that peak muscle power and muscle endurance are lower in children with cerebral palsy and neuromuscular disorders than in healthy controls.[79]

Several standardized fitness test batteries (see Table 14-5) include the MRWT as the primary measure of aerobic endurance performance, whereas some provide optional

TABLE 14-8	Sample Physical Fitness Test Profile for a 10-Year-Old Girl with Cerebral Palsy			
Attribute	**Test Item**	**Unit of Measure**	**Score**	**Health Fitness Standards***
Aerobic function	9MRWT	Yards	900 yards	1,480 yards
Body composition	Sum of triceps and subscapular skinfold thickness	Millimeters (mm)	36 mm	18-41 mm
	BMI	Weight (kg)/height (m²)	26	16.6-23.5
Muscle strength	Upper body: Modified pull-up	Number of pull-ups performed correctly	2	4 (minimal standard)
	Trunk: Curl-up	Number of curl-ups performed correctly	8	13 (preferred standard)
	Lower body: 40-meter walk	Time in seconds HR (bpm): Score as pass/fail	90 seconds HR: 150 bpm	60 seconds HR <125 bpm
Flexibility	Back-saver sit and reach	Inches	5 inches	9 inches
	Shoulder stretch	Inches (score as pass/fail)	Fingertips meet behind back	Fingertips meet behind back

*Standards from *Physical Best: The AAHPERD Guide to Physical Fitness Education and Assessment,* Reston, Va, 1990, AAHPERD; Winnick J, Short F: *The Brockport Physical Fitness Test Manual,* Champaign, IL, 1999, Human Kinetics. General standards are shown for all measures except the 40-meter walk, for which specific standards for a child with CP are shown.
9MRWT, 9-minute run-walk test; *BMI,* body mass index; *HR,* heart rate; *bpm,* beats per minute.

tests for younger children or for those with significant movement limitations. The child's score is compared to the age- and gender-based criterion-referenced health fitness standards established by research or expert opinion to indicate the level of aerobic fitness believed to be consistent with good cardiopulmonary health.[79]

The physiological cost index (PCI), also referred to as the energy cost index, is another measure of aerobic performance often used in children with impaired neuromotor development. In this test the child, wearing a portable HR monitor, rests quietly for 5 minutes, while resting HR (RHR) is measured. The child then walks at a self-selected pace for a specified distance while walking HR (WHR) is recorded. The formula for the PCI is WHR−RHR/average speed to walk the distance. An average energy expenditure index (EEI), using the same formula as the PCI, of 0.47 beats per meter has been reported for healthy children and adolescents.[107] Children with CP often exhibit much higher values because of higher WHR and slower walking speeds.[108] Table 14-8 illustrates a physical fitness profile for a 10-year-old girl with CP, using standards for the general population and specific standards for children with CP.

CASE STUDY 14-1

CEREBRAL PALSY

The following case study illustrates the application of the principles discussed in this chapter. The case is presented as a written report to provide an example of how examination is translated into a report and leads to intervention. The case has four significant decision-making points: (1) what tests and measures are best to administer given the parents' complaints; (2) specific problems identified from the examination at the participation, activity, and impairment level and of those, which are priorities; (3) the

probable constraints from the child, task, and environment that hinder the child's performance; and (4) risk factors for the future.

Examination
Patient History
ST is a 5-year, 8-month-old girl with Level III, spastic diplegic CP and periventricular leukomalacia, with CNS findings greater on the left than the right side. She is a first grader at a regular public school and has a full-time aide to help her physically negotiate the school. She currently receives home physical therapy 3 days a week, school-based physical therapy 2 days a week, and school-based occupational therapy 3 days a week for 1-hour sessions each. ST was born prematurely at 32 weeks' gestation, weighing 3 lb 7 oz. She remained in the neonatal intensive care unit (NICU) for her first 5 weeks of life where she experienced episodes of apnea and bradycardia. No ventilator support was required. She had delayed developmental milestones, rolling from her stomach to her back at 6 months of age and sitting independently at 16 months of age. ST had a selective dorsal rhizotomy at 4 years of age for severe lower extremity spasticity. She is medically stable and takes no medications. She has bilateral astigmatism and wears corrective eyeglasses.

ST ambulates with a posterior walker at school and outdoors. Indoors, she uses bilateral quad canes. For long distances, the family uses a stroller. She tires easily with physical tasks. She moves only when required, preferring sedentary activities. Despite the physical challenges, ST is cooperative, well behaved, and able to complete her academic work.

Parental Concerns: ST's parents have two primary concerns. First, it is getting increasingly difficult for the mother to physically lift and carry ST up and down stairs, in and out of the car, bed, and tub, and on and off living or dining room furniture. Second, ST is having difficulty getting around school in a safe and timely manner, and school personnel have requested that she transfer to a handicap accessible school. ST's parents are strongly opposed to the transfer.

School History: The classroom teacher and the PT report that ST has great difficulties in school. She is the first child with a physical disability to ever attend the school, and the school is not handicap accessible. It has an entrance with four steps with no handrail, a bathroom 60 feet away from the classroom with no handrails, an art classroom and cafeteria downstairs, long congested hallways, and playground equipment in an elevated sandbox about 300 feet from ST's classroom. Although ST is able to complete her academic work, her teacher is concerned about ST's loss of time in classroom instruction, safety on the school grounds, especially the stairs, and social isolation. ST takes about an hour to go to the bathroom and 10-20 minutes to change classrooms. She does not participate in physical education, outdoor recess, or field trips. Table 14-9 shows the tests and measures selected and administered based on the findings from the patient history.

Tests and Measures

Function

Pediatric Evaluation of Disability Inventory Normative standard scores on the functional skills and caregiver assistance mobility domain on the PEDI indicate that ST is performing significantly below the level expected for her age and that she requires significantly more assistance from her caregivers. She uses a posterior walker, bilateral quad canes, bilateral straight canes, and bilateral dynamic

AFOs. She can maintain good hygiene, manage toileting tasks, and use utensils and drinking containers. She can brush her teeth and wash her body but has limitations in hair brushing and dressing. ST can put on and take off pullover garments and front-opening shirts, but she is unable to manage fasteners (buttons, zippers, belt buckles, snaps, and shoes). She cannot remove or put on pants. She can remove her shoes, but she cannot put on her shoes over the AFOs. She cannot tie shoelaces, but she can open and close Velcro straps.

Transfers ST climbs on and off an adult-sized toilet independently, using her arms for support. She can sit down and stand up from low furniture, using an assistive device. She requires maximal assistance for all car transfers, including scooting to her seat, fastening or unfastening the seatbelt, or opening and closing the car door. She can move in her bed, sit on the edge, and lie down from sitting, but she cannot get in and out by herself. She can move around in the bathtub safely without help and sit down and stand up from inside the tub; however, she cannot safely step in and out of the tub by herself. Her parents lift her in and out.

Indoor Locomotion ST walks throughout the apartment independently using bilateral quad canes at a slow pace, with no limitation in distance. She is unable to open and close doors in the house. She is able to carry a small object in one hand as long as she can also hold onto the assistive device.

Outdoor Locomotion ST can walk independently outdoors with either her quad canes or posterior walker. She can move at a quicker pace and for longer distances

TABLE 14-9	Decision-Making Point One: What Tests and Measures to Administer Given the Parents' Concerns?		
Concern	**Domain of Inquiry**	**Tests**	**Source of Information**
1. Parent unable to lift and transfer patient.	**Participation:** Type and amount of caregiver assistance and required modifications	PEDI caregiver assistance and modification scale	Parent interview
	Activity: Capabilities at home	1. PEDI functional skills: Self-care, mobility, and social function 2. GMFM-88	1. Parent interview 2. PT
	Body structure and function: Musculoskeletal system Neuromuscular system	1. ROM screening exam 2. Field tests of strength and flexibility (Prudential FITNESSGRAM: Curl-up, modified pull-up, trunk lift, 40-meter walk, and sit and reach) 3. Assessment of muscle tone (Howle[85]) 4. Postural control checklist	PT
2. Inability to negotiate school building and grounds.	**Participation:** Type and amount of assistance and required modifications	SFA: Participation, task supports (assistance and adaptations)	School personnel (teacher, assistant, PT, OT)
	Activity: Capabilities at school	SFA: Activity performance, physical tasks, cognitive/behavioral tasks	School personnel (teacher, assistant, PT, OT)
	Body structure and function: Musculoskeletal system Neuromuscular system Cardiopulmonary system	Same tests as above plus the following: 1. 9MRWT 2. PCI 3. BMI: Health fitness standards 4. Skin-fold measures: Triceps and subscapular	PT

PEDI, Pediatric Evaluation of Disability Index; *GMFM,* Gross Motor Function Measure; *ROM,* range of motion; *SFA,* School Function Assessment; *PT,* physical therapist; *OT,* occupational therapist; *9MRWT,* 9-minute run-walk test; *PCI,* physiological cost index; *BMI,* body mass index.

with the walker. She can walk on uneven surfaces and go up and down inclines, but her speed is greatly reduced.

Stairs ST can independently crawl up and down a partial flight of stairs at an extremely slow pace and with great trepidation. She can slowly ascend a full flight of stairs with two hands held if given multiple breaks. She is fearful of descending a flight of stairs and prefers to be carried.

Social Function ST comprehends complex sentences and commands. She effectively verbalizes her thoughts and opinions. When ST encounters a problem, she needs help right away. She enjoys playing with adults and prefers their company over that of her peers. She does not really interact with other children, but she is interested in watching them play.

School Function Assessment

Participation ST's participation level is highest at mealtimes, when she participates with modified full participation. In contrast, during recess on the playground, her participation is extremely limited. ST sits in the sandbox and watches the other children play. In all other areas (classroom, transportation, bathroom, and transitions), she participates in all aspects with constant supervision.

Task Supports ST is rated as having very high needs for assistance (a one-on-one aide) and a high level of adaptations for physical tasks. ST needs less support for cognitive and behavioral tasks.

Activity Performance ST has great variability in her performance. Her strengths are in the areas of hygiene, feeding, material use, communication, and maintaining and changing positions. ST has good manners, understands social boundaries, is well behaved, and follows social norms. ST can use paper, paint brushes, markers, and scissors. ST's limitations are in recreational movement, negotiating stairs, and manipulation with movement.

Peer Interactions ST has little peer interaction. She does not initiate conversations nor does she join in play with peers. Her classmates are interested in physically assisting her (bringing her materials, opening doors).

Travel and Recreational Movement ST takes an extraordinary amount of time traveling about school, which takes away from both instructional and social time, especially during lunch and recess. There is great concern for her safety in the event of an evacuation because she cannot exit the building within the required time frame and there is currently no contingency plan. ST does not participate in any games involving walking, running, kicking, or throwing, and she cannot play on the playground equipment.

Manipulation with Movement ST cannot carry sizeable objects in one hand or carry large objects with two hands because of her need for assistive equipment. She cannot carry her books, lunch box, or lunch tray. She cannot open or close any of the doors in the school, most of which are heavy and have a push bar and pneumatic closure spring.

Stairs ST ascends and descends the stairs with her aide holding her two hands. Another person must carry her walker. Although there are several stairwells in the school,

ST will only negotiate one of them. This staircase is rather narrow, has handrails on both sides, and a midway landing. Unfortunately, the staircase is not always the closest for her destination, requiring significantly increased walking time and distance. ST asks to be carried up and down the stairs, but this is against school policy.

Musculoskeletal

Posture ST sits with a posterior pelvic tilt; trunk flexion; anteriorly rounded shoulders; protracted scapulae; forward, right laterally flexed head; and neck hyperextension. In addition, ST stands with an elevated right pelvis, bilateral hip flexion, internal rotation, and adduction and genu recurvatum. The AFOs correct ankle plantarflexion.

Range of Motion ST has hypoextensible hamstrings (sit and reach test score = 5 inches, health standard = 9 inches) and decreased upper extremity flexibility on shoulder stretch test (3-inch gap, health standard is fingertips touch).

Muscle Performance

Muscle Strength ST has bilateral lower extremity weakness, right greater than left, estimated by observation but not formally tested. Overall, lower extremity strength is grossly 3/5 except for bilateral hip and knee extensors, which she cannot move against gravity. ST demonstrates substitutions, using external rotation with abduction to accomplish hip flexion and compensations, locking her knees in extension for stability and using her upper extremities to lift her lower extremities when sitting. ST's scores on the trunk lift (1), modified pull-up (1), and curl-up (1) on the Prudential FITNESSGRAM tests are below the health fitness standards for her age.

Endurance ST's score on the 9MRWT was 450 yards, well below that of other children her age. Her PCI was 3.65 beats per minute indicating that ST expends much more energy than her peers to perform usual tasks. Her BMI is 18, which is on the higher end of the normal range. ST performs tasks in prone, supine, and sitting and moves into quadruped without signs or complaints of fatigue.

Neuromuscular

Reflex Integrity Head and trunk righting reactions are present in all directions, but the response time is increased with a poorly graded muscle response; small perturbations yield large sway. Upper extremity protective extension is present anteriorly and sideways (left and right) but is absent posteriorly. ST primarily depends on upper extremity protective responses rather than righting reactions to keep herself upright. In standing, she uses a stepping strategy or fixation to maintain the upright position. Response time is slow and inadequate when the perturbation is large.

Motor Function

Gross Motor Function Measure-88 Scores on the GMFM-88 are 96.08% lying and rolling, 93% sitting, 78.57% crawling and kneeling, 28.21% standing, and 16.67% walking, running, and jumping. The total GMFM-88 score is 62.57%, and the total GMFM-66 score is 50.62% (95% confidence interval = 48.33% to 52.91%).

Lying and Rolling ST is able to quickly and efficiently complete all but two of the 17 items: Flex her right and left lower extremities through full range. She projects a happy, confident, and enthusiastic demeanor when moving in the supine and prone positions.

Sitting ST completed all but 3 of the 37 sitting items: (1) sit, lower herself with control prone, (2) sit, pivot 90 degrees without arm use, and (3) sit on a large bench. She maintains various floor sitting positions without arm use including: W-sit, left and right side-sit, long-sit, and cross-leg sit and she can easily transfer into and out of sitting. She is most stable with a wide base of support and prefers W sitting. She requires arm support to maintain her position when reaching outside of her base of support. When placed, ST can sit on a small and large bench, with and without arm and foot support. She struggles to independently sit on the small bench, requiring four separate attempts before finding a successfully strategy. Once successful, she is able to quickly repeat the task. ST is unable to independently sit herself in an adult-sized chair. She relies solely on upper extremity strength to pull herself up.

Crawling and Kneeling ST is comfortable moving in and out of the quadruped position, and she can swiftly crawl within and between rooms. Her quadruped posture is poor, exhibiting wide abducted lower extremities, large posterior weight shift so that her buttocks almost touch the back of her legs, and increased lumbar lordosis. She uses two crawling techniques: Reciprocal (alternately moving extremities) and nonreciprocal (upper extremities to pull body and lower extremities forward). In a slow but steady pace, ST can crawl up four steps. She timidly can crawl backward down the steps, carefully lowering herself with her arms. Both ascent and descent are exceedingly time consuming and not functional either at home or school. ST approximates kneeling with her hips in extreme internal rotation. She is unable to transition from high-kneel to half-kneel.

Standing Standing is extremely challenging for ST; she completed only one item at the highest difficulty level. She repeatedly verbalizes her discontent ("I can't" or "Help me"). ST can stand independently over extended time with support from either her posterior walker or quad canes and her AFOs. She slowly and laboriously pulls herself up with her upper extremities on furniture. Her lower extremities extend simultaneously, producing an inefficient narrow base of support. She can stand up using her posterior walker and quad canes; however, it can take several attempts before she is successful. Once standing, she has difficulty controlling any movements, including lifting a foot off the floor, releasing her hand from the assistive device and reaching forward, and picking up an object from the floor. Her only strategy to pick up a toy placed on the floor is to "fall" to her knees.

Walking, Running, and Jumping ST is only able to partially perform 5 of this section's 24 items. ST can cruise around a small table, holding on with both hands, and at times resting her entire upper body on the table. She is proficient walking long distances with her posterior walker, on both even and uneven surfaces, indoors and outdoors. She is less proficient with the quad canes, and she therefore uses these only for short, indoor distances. She relies heavily on her arms to allow for unweighting and subsequent progression of her lower extremities. She can walk well with two hands held but can only walk 4-5 steps with one hand held.

Tone Tone is rated 1+ on the Modified Ashworth Scale and 2+ on Howe's assessment of muscle tone.

Motor Control ST's movement quality is poor. She demonstrates impaired selective motor control (abnormal upper and lower extremity extensor synergies, and difficulty with lower extremity reciprocal movements), poor coordination (slow movements, delayed motor responses, weak force production, and large muscle amplitudes), and an inability to grade muscle responses, especially in midrange, and she lacks a rotation component to many of her movements.

Neuromotor Development

Steady-State ST can maintain a steady, wide-based sitting position indefinitely, even with hands free. She cannot maintain standing, even momentarily, without external support (two hands support, assistive device). Her poor postural alignment results in a small lower extremity base of support. Likewise, her shoulder internal rotation and adduction result in a small base of support with her quad canes as the canes actually touch.

Anticipatory State ST can maintain a sitting position when reaching within arms length in all directions. When reaching beyond arms length, she maintains the sitting position by putting one hand on the supporting surface and/or widening her base of support. In standing, she is quite hesitant to release one hand from her device, even momentarily, and she does not voluntarily reach outside her base of support. In walking, she does not adequately shift her weight to the supported side, so she has difficulty advancing her opposite lower extremity. When she experiences a loss of balance, she relies on the external device, large sway in her trunk, hip strategy, lower extremity fixation, and a stepping response to maintain upright stance. Two falls occurred during the assessment. She fell backward once when she attempted to reach behind to retrieve a toy while sitting. The other fall occurred when she attempted to stand up using her walker.

Reactive Reactive postural control is tested cautiously. In sitting, she can maintain an upright position only with a small, unexpected perturbation. In standing, a small unexpected perturbation causes acute fear and hesitancy to continue with the examination, but she remains upright. In a crowded hallway, she prevents jostling by standing still, moving very slowly, and/or telling people to move out of her way.

Table 14-10 shows the evaluation of test results and the synthesis of these findings into a problem list. Table 14-11 shows the final prioritized problems and probable constraints. This analysis is used to devise an intervention program.

CHAPTER SUMMARY

Children with impaired neuromotor development frequently exhibit participation restrictions, activity limitations, and *primary* and/or *secondary impairments* in one or more of the musculoskeletal, neuromuscular, cardiovascular/pulmonary, and integumentary systems. This chapter reviewed typical and atypical neuromotor development and methods of examination using norm-referenced and

TABLE 14-10	Decision-Making Point Two: What Specific Problems Are Evident from the Examination on the Participation, Activity, and Body Structure/Function Level?

Test Result	Problem List
Participation: PEDI, SFA, social history Needs minimal or no assistance or modifications in cognitive/behavioral and social tasks and when using school materials sitting in a chair. **Participation Restrictions:** 1. Needs significantly more caregiver assistance for mobility in both home and school in comparison to same age peers. 2. Requires a number of modifications for mobility and other physical tasks (basic and instrumental activities of daily living) at home and in school.	1. Number and type of family outings are limited by excessive need for caregiver assistance. 2. Amount and quality of peer interactions are limited in school and community. 3. Missing large block of academic instructional time due to excessive time needed for mobility and ADLs. 4. Access to school and community activities limited by environmental constraints. 5. Lack of understanding by school personnel about her diagnosis, abilities, and needs. 6. Concerns for physical safety in school setting as a result of lack of adequate evacuation procedures.
Activity: PEDI, GMFM-88, SFA, school interview 1. Mobility is good when performing physical tasks in prone, supine, sitting, and quadruped positions. 2. When given postural support, she can perform many self-care and manipulative tasks. **Activity Restrictions:** 1. Significantly below the level expected for her age in mobility tasks. 2. Limitations in recreational activities during recess, free time, and physical education class. 3. Mobility is limited when performing physical tasks in kneeling, standing, and walking.	1. Unable to kneel, ½ kneel, stand, and walk independently without assistive device. 2. Unable to transfer to car, bed, tub, and adult-sized furniture. 3. Unable to negotiate stairs. 4. Unable to manipulate door knobs or open and close doors. 5. Unable to get on and off playground equipment. 6. Unable to play games involving walking, running, kicking, or throwing. 7. Unable to carry personal or school belongings while walking.
Body Structure and Body Function: 1. BMI: 18 2. Skin-fold measures: Triceps + subscapular: 26 mm 3. Head and trunk righting reactions present in all directions. 4. Present UE protective extension, forward and sideways. 5. Steady-state sitting postural control is good. 6. Impaired standing anticipatory and reactive postural control. 7. All joint PROM is WFL, but hamstring length is reduced. Sit and reach: 5 inches (norm: 9 inches). 8. Strength: UE 4+/5, LE 3/5 on right, 4+/5 on left. Modified pull up: 1 (norm: 2 to 7). Curl-up: 1 (norm: 2 to 10). Trunk lift: 4 inches (norm: 6-12 inches). 9. Muscle tone: 2+ (Howle[85]). 10. 9MRWT: 450 yards (norm: 1,200 yards). PCI: 3.65 bpm.	1. Increased weight for height and age. 2. Impaired body alignment. 3. Impaired steady-state, anticipatory, and reactive postural control, especially in standing. 4. Hypoextensible hamstrings. 5. Muscle weakness, right LE most affected. 6. Decreased muscle endurance. 7. Moderate hypertonia. 8. Impaired selective motor control. 9. Impaired aerobic endurance performance. 10. High energy cost for submaximal activities.

PEDI, Pediatric Evaluation of Disability Index; *SFA,* School Function Assessment; *ADLs,* activities of daily living; *GMFM-88,* Gross Motor Function Measure-88; *BMI,* body mass index; *UE,* upper extremity; *LE,* lower extremity; *PROM,* passive range of motion; *WFL,* within functional limits; *9MRWT,* 9-minute run walk test; *PCI,* physiological cost index.

TABLE 14-11	Decision-Making Point Three: What Are the Probable Constraints from the Child, Task, and Environment That Hinder ST's Performance?		
Prioritized Problem	**Child**	**Task Requirement**	**Environment**
Excessive time out of the classroom for ADLs.	1. Decreased walking speed 2. LE and trunk muscle weakness 3. Decreased muscle endurance 4. Impaired selective motor control 5. Poor aerobic endurance 6. High energy cost walking 7. Impaired postural control	1. Walk in crowded hallway. 2. Open and close heavy doors. 3. Don and doff clothing while standing for toileting.	1. School not handicap accessible 2. 60 feet distance from classroom to bathroom 3. Congested hallway 4. Heavy doors to open
Caregiver assistance is needed to access school, home, and community activities.	Same as above	1. Negotiate stairs. 2. Climb on and off playground equipment. 3. Walk long distances.	1. 300 feet to playground 2. Elevated sandbox 3. Stairs with no handrails 4. Crowded stairways
Increased caregiver assistance for transfers.	1. LE and trunk muscle weakness 2. Impaired postural control 3. Impaired selective motor control	1. Climb on and off high surfaces. 2. Adjust body position and control posture while moving.	1. Size, shape, and height of furniture, tub, and car

ADLs, Activities of daily living; *LE,* lower extremity.

criterion-referenced standardized tests and measures. Therapists perform an examination by hypothesizing about the child's problems, selecting and administering the most appropriate tests to directly measure the perceived issues, and evaluating the test results. The evaluation forms the basis for determining the specific problems that can be effectively addressed with evidence-based interventions.

ADDITIONAL RESOURCES

Useful Forms

Pediatric Evaluation of Disability Inventory (PEDI)
Alberta Infant Motor Scale (AIMS)
School Function Assessment (SFA)
Peabody Developmental Motor Scales-2 (PDMS-2)
Gross Motor Function Measure (GMFM), (GMFM-66), (GMFM-88)

Web Sites

National Institute of Neurological Disorders and Stroke (NINDS): www.ninds.nih.gov/disorders/
Children's Hemiplegia and Stroke Association (CHASA): www.chasa.org
National Dissemination Center for Children with Disabilities: www.nichcy.org
National Downs Syndrome Society: www.ndss.org

GLOSSARY

Body mass index: A person's weight (kg) divided by his or her height squared (meters^2). An estimate of body composition.
Criterion-referenced test: A type of test that indicates an individual's level of performance or degree of mastery of specific skills that reflect a particular domain. Curriculum-based and performance measurements are sub-category of these tests.
Delay: A significant lag in achieving age-appropriate developmental milestones. Delay can occur in one or more dimensions including physical, cognitive, emotional, and social.
Development: Changes that occur over a person's life from conception to death.
Developmental milestones: Skills, abilities, or physical attributes specific to age.
Deviance: Atypical or abnormal appearance of a motor milestone.

Dissociation: A difference or unevenness between the rates of development of two or more dimensions (e.g., cognitive level is more advanced than the physical level).
Functional activities: Age-expected day-to-day skills performed within an individual's natural environments of home, school, and/or community.
Impaired neuromotor development: A delay in the acquisition of motor skills, and/or the occurrence of atypical movements
Norm-referenced test: A type of test that ranks an individual numerically and compares their score with a set of external standards. These tests allow comparison of an individual's performance to test scores from a defined population.
Primary impairments: Direct effects of the disease or pathology on the body's particular structures and function. Examples of primary impairments in children with CP include insufficient muscle force generation, spasticity, and hyperactive reflexes.
Reaction: Stereotyped response to specific stimuli.
Reflex: An involuntary response to a stimulus applied to the periphery and transmitted to the brain or spinal cord.
Secondary impairments: Changes in body structures and functions that are indirect consequences of the primary impairments. For example, decreased aerobic capacity may occur in children with CP as a consequence of a sedentary lifestyle as a result of the primary impairments of spasticity, muscle weakness, and joint stiffness.
Standardized test: Uniform testing procedure.

References

1. VanSant A, Goldberg C: Normal motor development. In Tecklin JS (ed): *Pediatric Physical Therapy,* ed 3, Philadelphia, 1999, JB Lippincott.
2. Shumway-Cook A, Woollacott MH: Motor control: Issues and theories. In Shumway-Cook A, Woollacott MH (eds): *Motor Control: Theory and Practical Applications,* ed 2, Philadelphia, 2001, Lippincott Williams & Wilkins.
3. Aylward GP: Conceptual issues in developmental screening and assessment, *J Dev Behav Pediatr* 18(5):340-349, 1997.
4. Shumway-Cook A, Woollacott MH. Constraints on motor control: An overview of neurological impairments. In Shumway-Cook A, Woollacott MH: *Motor Control: Theory and Practical Applications,* ed 2, Philadelphia, 2001, Lippincott Williams & Wilkins.
5. Rice FP: Human Development, Upper Saddle River, NJ, 2001, Prentice Hall.
6. Tanner J: Growth at adolescence, London, 1962, Blackwell.
7. Committee on Integrating the Science of Early Childhood Development: Ten core concepts of development. In Shonkoff JP, Phillips DA (eds): *From Neurons to Neighborhoods: The Science of Early Childhood Development,* Washington, DC, 2000, National Academy Press.
8. Shonkoff JP: From neurons to neighborhoods: Old and new challenges for developmental and behavioral pediatrics, *J Devel Behav Pediatr* 24(1):70-76, 2003.

9. Thelen E: Motor development: A new synthesis, *Am Psychologist* 50(2):79-95, 1995.
10. Stockmeyer SA: An interpretation of the approach of Rood to the treatment of neuromuscular dysfunction. Paper presented at the Proceedings of Northwestern University Special Therapeutic Exercise Project (NUSTEP): An exploratory and analytical survey of therapeutic exercise, Evanston, Ill, 1967.
11. VanSant A: Rising from a supine position to erect stance: description of adult movement and a developmental hypothesis, *Phys Ther* 68:185-192, 1988.
12. VanSant A: Age differences in movement patterns used by children to rise from a supine position to erect stance, *Phys Ther* 68:1330-1339, 1988.
13. Marsala G, VanSant A: Age-related differences in movement patterns used by toddlers to rise from a supine position to erect stance, *Phys Ther* 78:149-159, 1998.
14. VanSant A: Life-span development in functional tasks, *Phys Ther* 70:788-798, 1990.
15. Hinojosa J, Kramer P: Developmental perspective: Fundamentals of developmental theory. In Kramer P, Hinojosa J (ed): *Frames of Reference for Pediatric Occupational Therapy*, ed 2, New York, 1999, Lippincott Williams & Wilkins.
16. Haley SM, Coster WJ, Ludlow LH, et al: *Pediatric Evaluation of Disability Inventory (PEDI): Development, Standardization, and Administration Manual*, Boston, 1992, New England Medical Center Hospital, PEDI Research Group.
17. Greenspan SI, Meisels SJ: Towards a new vision for the developmental assessment of infants and young children. In Meisels SJ, Fenichel E (eds): *New Visions for the Developmental Assessment of Infants and Young Children*, Washington, DC, 1996, Zero to Three.
18. Coster WJ, Deeney T, Haltiwanger J, et al: *School Function Assessment*, San Antonio, Tex, 1998, The Psychological Corporation.
19. Campbell SK: Models for decision making in pediatric neurologic physical therapy. In Campbell SK (ed). *Decision Making in Pediatric Neurologic Physical Therapy*, New York, 1999, Churchill Livingstone.
20. The International Classification of Functioning, Disability and Health (ICF): Geneva, Switzerland, 2001, World Health Organization.
21. American Physical Therapy Association: Guide to Physical Therapist Practice, second edition, *Phys Ther* 81(1):6-746, 2001.
22. Piper M, Darrah J: *Motor Assessment of the Developing Infant*, Philadelphia, 1994, WB Saunders.
23. Folio M, Fewell R: *Peabody Developmental Motor Scales and Activity Cards*, Austin, Tex, 1983, Pro-Ed.
24. Russell D, Rosenbaum P, Gowland C, et al: *Gross Motor Function Measure Manual*, ed 2, Hamilton, Ontario, 1993, McMaster University/CanChild.
25. Russell D, Rosenbaum P, Avery L, et al: *Gross Motor Function Measure (GMFM-88 & GMFM-66) User's Manual*, New York, 2002, Mac Keith Press.
26. Russell D, Palisano RJ, Walter S, et al: Evaluating motor function in children with Down syndrome: Validity of the GMFM, *Dev Med Child Neurol* 40:693-701, 1998.
27. Ruck-Gibis J, Rosenbaum P, Lane M, et al: Reliability of the Gross Motor Function Measure for children with osteogenesis imperfecta, *Physiother Canada* 53(1):S16, 2001.
28. Wright M, Halton J, Matrin R, et al: Long-term gross motor performance following treatment for acute lymphoblastic leukemia, *Med Pediatr Oncol* 31:86-90, 1998.
29. Brigance AH: *Brigance Inventory of Early Development-II*, North Billerica, Mass, 2004, Curriculum Associates.
30. Rogers S, D'Eugenio D: Assessment and application. In Schafer D, Moersch M (eds): *Developmental Programming for Infants and Young Children*, vol 3, Ann Arbor, Mich, 1977, The University of Michigan Press.
31. Bricker D, Pretti-Frontezak K: *Assessment, Evaluation, and Programming System (AEPS) for Infants and Children: AEPS Measurement for Three to Six years*, vol 3, Baltimore, 1996, Paul H. Brooks Publishing.
32. Bricker D, Wadell M: *Assessment, Evaluation, and Programming System (AEPS) for Infants and Children: AEPS Curriculum for Three to Six Years*, vol 4, Baltimore, 1996, Paul H. Brooks Publishing.
33. Corporation V: Hawaii Early Learning Profile (HELP): *HELP for Preschoolers (3-6)*, Palo Alto, Calif, 1992, VORT Corporation.
34. Johnson-Martin N, Jens K, Attermeier S, et al: *The Carolina Curricula: The Carolina Curriculum for Infants and Toddlers with Special Needs*, vol 2, Baltimore, 1991, Paul H. Brooks Publishing.
35. Prechtl H: Prenatal motor development. In Wade M, Whiting H (eds): *Continuity of Neural Functions from Prenatal to Postnatal Life*, vol 94, Oxford, 1986, Blackwell Scientific.
36. Jouen F: Early visual-vestibular interactions and postural development. In Bloch H, Bertenthal B (eds): *Sensory-Motor Organizations and Development in Infancy and Early Childhood*, Dordrecht, 1990, Kluwer.
37. Woollacott M, Debu B, Mowatt M: Neuromuscular control of posture in the infant and child: is vision dominate? *J Motor Behav* 19:167-186, 1987.
38. Woollacott M, Sveistrup H: Changes in the sequencing and timing of muscle response coordination associated with developmental transitions in balance activities, *Hum Mov Sci* 11:23-36, 1992.
39. Sveistrup H, Woollacott M: Longitudinal development of the automatic postural response in infants, *J Motor Behav* 28:58-70, 1996.
40. Foster E, Sveistrup H, Woollacott M: Transitions in visual proprioception: a cross-sectional developmental study of the effect of visual flow on postural control, *J Motor Behav* 28:101-112, 1996.
41. Woollacott M, Burtner P, Jensen J, et al: Development of postural responses during standing in healthy children and in children with spastic diplegia, *Neurosci Biobehav Rev* 22:583-589, 1998.
42. Taguchi K, Tada C: Change of body sway with growth of children. In Amblard B, Beerthoz A, Clarac F (eds): *Posture and Gait: Development, Adaptation, and Modulation*, Amsterdam, 1988, Elsevier.
43. Forssberg H, Nashner L: Ontogenetic development of postural control in man: Adaptation to alter support and visual conditions during stance, *J Neurosci* 2:545-552, 1982.
44. Nashner L, Shumway-Cook A, Marin O: Stance posture control in select groups of children with cerebral palsy: Deficits in sensory organization and muscular coordination, *Exp Brain Res* 49:393-409, 1983.
45. Woollacott M, Shumway-Cook A, Nashner L: Aging and posture control: changes in sensory organization and muscular coordination, *Int J Aging Hum Dev* 23:97-114, 1986.
46. Shumway-Cook A, Woollacott M: The growth of stability: postural control from a developmental prospective, *J Motor Behav* 17:131-147, 1985.
47. Sahrmann S, Norton B: The relationship of voluntary movement to spasticity in the upper motor neuron syndrome, *Arch Neurol* 2:460-465, 1977.
48. Shumway-Cook A, Woollacott M: Postural control in the Down's syndrome child, *Phys Ther* 9:211-235, 1985.
49. Burtner P, Woollacott M, Qualls C: Stance balance control with orthoses in a select group of children with and without spasticity, *Dev Med Child Neurol* 41:748-757, 1999.
50. Kembhavi G, Darrah J, Magill-Evans J, et al: Using the Berg balance Scale to distinguish balance abilities in children with cerebral palsy, *Pediatr Phys Ther* 14(2):92-99, 2002.
51. Crowe T, Deitz J, Richardson P, et al: Interrater reliability of the Pediatric Clinical Test of Sensory Integration for Balance, *Phys Occup Ther Pediatr* 10(4):1-27, 1990.
52. Deitz J, Richardson P, Atwater S, et al: Performance of normal children on the Clinical Test of Sensory Interaction for Balance, *Occup Ther J Res* 11:336-356, 1991.
53. Richardson P, Atwater S, Crowe T, et al: Performance of preschoolers on the Pediatric Clinical Test of Sensory Interaction for Balance, *Am J Occup Ther* 46(9):793-800, 1992.
54. Duncan PW, Weiner DK, Chandler J, et al: Functional reach: A new measure of balance, *J Gerontol* 45:192-197, 1990.
55. Donohue B, Turner D, Worell T: The use of functional reach as a measurement of balance in typically developing boys and girls ages 5-15 years, *Pediatr Phys Ther* 6:189-193, 1994.
56. Berg K, Maki B, Williams J: Clinical and laboratory measures of postural balance in an elderly population, *Arch Phys Med Rehabil* 73:1073-1083, 1992.
57. Bruininks R: *Examiner's Manual for Bruininks-Oseretsky Test of Motor Proficiency*, Circle Pines, Minn, 1978, American Guidance Service.
58. Boileau R, Lohman T: The measurement of human physique and its effect on physical performance, *Orthop Clin North Am* 8:563-572, 1977.
59. Woods J, Pate R, Burgess M: Correlates to performance on field tests of muscular strength, *Pediatr Exerc Sci* 1:302-311, 1992.
60. Rowland T: Effects of obesity on aerobic fitness in adolescent females, *Am J Dis Child* 145:464-468, 1991.
61. Rowland T: *Developmental Exercise Physiology*, Champaign, Ill, 1990, Human Kinetics.
62. Roche A, Siervogel R, Chumlea W, et al: Grading fatness from limited anthropometric data, *Am J Clin Nutr* 34:2831-2838, 1981.
63. Lohman T: Assessment of body composition in children, *Pediatr Exerc Sci* 1:19-30, 1989.
64. Long T, Toscano K: *Handbook of Pediatric Physical Therapy*, ed 2, New York, 2002, Lippincott Williams & Wilkins.
65. Cusick B: Lower extremity musculoskeletal development. In Wadsworth C (ed): *Orthopedic Interventions in Pediatric Patients: Home Study Course 10.2.1*, LaCrosse, Wis, 2000, Orthopedic Section, American Physical Therapy Association.
66. Salenius P, Vankka E: The development of the tibiofemoral angle in children, *J Bone Joint Surgery Am* 57:259-261, 1975.
67. Morley A: Knock-knee in children, *BMJ* 976-977, 1957.
68. Staheli L: *Fundamentals of Pediatric Orthopedics*, New York, 1998, Lippincott Williams & Wilkins.
69. Tachdjian M: *Pediatric Orthopedics*, vol IV, ed 2, Philadelphia, 1990, WB Saunders.
70. Farkas-Bargeton E, Barbet J, Dancea S, et al: Immaturity of muscle fibers in the congenital form of myotonic dystrophy: Its consequences and its origin, *J Neurol Sci* 83:145-159, 1998.
71. Staheli L: Torsional deformity, *Pediatr Clin North Am* 33:1373-1383, 1986.
72. Blimkie C: Age and sex-associated variation in strength during childhood: Anthropometric, morphological, neurologic, biomechanical, endocrinologic, genetic, and physical activity correlates. In *Perspectives in Exercise Science and Sport*, Indianapolis, 1989, Benchmark Press.

73. Brooke M, Engel W: The histographic analysis of human muscle biopsies with regard to fiber types: Children's biopsies, *Neurology* 19:591-605, 1969.

74. Edstrom L, Nordemar R: Differential changes in type I and type II muscle fibers in rheumatoid arthritis, *Scand J Rheumatol* 3:155-160, 1974.

75. Florence J, Pandya S, King W, et al: Clinical trials in Duchenne dystrophy: standardization and reliability of evaluation procedures, *Phys Ther* 64:41-45, 1984.

76. Kraemer W, Fleck S: *Strength Training for Young Athletes,* Champaign, Ill, 1993, Human Kinetics.

77. Effgen S, Brown D: Long-term stability of hand-held dynamometric measurements in children who have myelomeningocele, *Phys Ther* 72:458-465, 1992.

78. Wiley M, Damiano D: Lower-extremity strength profiles in spastic cerebral palsy, *Dev Med Child Neurol* 40:100-107, 1998.

79. Bar-Or O: Pathophysiological factors which limit the exercise capacity of the sick child, *Med Sci Sports Exerc* 18:276-282, 1986.

80. van der Berg-Emons R, van Baak M, de Barbanson D, et al: Reliability of tests to determine peak aerobic power, anaerobic power and isokinetic muscle strength in children with spastic cerebral palsy, *Dev Med Child Neurol* 38:1117-1125, 1996.

81. *The Prudential FITNESSGRAM Test Administration Manual,* Dallas, 1994, The Cooper Institute for Aerobics Research.

82. Winnick J, Short F: *The Brockport Physical Fitness Test Manual,* Champaign, IL, 1999, Human Kinetics.

83. Barnes M, Crutchfield C, Heriza C: *The neurophysiological basis of patient treatment. Vol II: Reflexes in motor development,* Morgantown, W Va, 1978, Stokesville.

84. Capute A, Accardo P, Vining E: *Primitive Reflex Profile,* Baltimore, 1978, University Park.

85. Howle JMW: Cerebral palsy. In Campbell SK (ed): *Decision Making in Pediatric Neurologic Physical Therapy,* New York, 1999, Churchill Livingstone.

86. Miller LJ, Roid GH: *The T.I.M.E. Toddler and Infant Motor Evaluation: A Standardized Assessment,* San Antonio, 1994, Therapy Skill Builders.

87. Holt KG, Butcher R, Fonseca S: Limb stiffness in active leg swinging of children with spastic hemiplegic cerebral palsy, *Pediatr Phys Ther* 12(2):50-61, 2000.

88. Amiel-Tison C: Neurological examination of the maturity of newborn infants, *Arch Dis Child* 43:89, 1968.

89. Pierson SH: Outcome measures in spasticity management. In Brin M (ed): *Spasticity: Etiology, Evaluation, Management, and the Role of Botulinum Toxin Type A,* New York, 1997, John Wiley & Sons.

90. Bohannon R, Smith M: Inter-rater reliability of a modified Ashworth scale of muscle spasticity, *Phys Ther* 67:206-207, 1987.

91. Hoofwijk M, Unnithan V, Bar-Or O: Maximal treadmill performance of children with cerebral palsy, *Pediatr Exerc Sci* 7:305-313, 1995.

92. Chandler L, Andrews M, Swanson M: *Movement Assessment of Infants—A Manual,* Rolling Bay, Wash, 1980, Chandler, Andrews, and Swanson.

93. Brazelton T: Neonatal behavioral assessment scale, *Clin Dev Med* 50, 1973.

94. Bayley N: *Bayley Scales of Infant Development,* ed 2, San Antonio, 1993, Psychological Corporation.

95. Dubowitz L, Dubowitz V, Goldberg C: Clinical assessment of gestational age in the newborn infant, *J Pediatr* 77, 1985.

96. Schoen SA, Anderson J: Neurodevelopmental treatment frame of reference. In Kramer P, Hinojosa J (eds): *Frames of Reference for Pediatric Occupational Therapy,* ed 2, New York, 1999, Lippincott Williams & Wilkins.

97. Quinn L, Gordon J: *Functional Outcomes: Documentation for Rehabilitation,* St. Louis, 2003, WB Saunders.

98. Kamm K, Thelan E, Jenson J: A dynamical systems approach to motor development. In Rothstein J (ed): *Movement Science,* Alexandria, Va, 1991, American Physical Therapy Association.

99. Gowland C, Boyce W, Wright V, et al: Reliability of the Gross Motor Performance Measure, *Phys Ther* 75:597-602, 1995.

100. Boyce W, Gowland C, Rosenbaum P, et al: The gross motor performance measure: Validity and responsiveness of a measure of quality of movement, *Phys Ther* 75:603-613, 1995.

101. Gould A: Cardiopulmonary evaluation of the infant, toddler, child, and adolescent, *Pediatr Phys Ther* 3:9-13, 1991.

102. Tecklin J: Pulmonary disorders in infants and children and their physical therapy management. In Tecklin J (ed): *Pediatric Physical Therapy,* ed 3, New York, 1999, Lippincott Williams & Wilkins.

103. Krahenbuhl G, Skinner J, Kohert W: Developmental aspects of maximal aerobic power in children, *Exerc Sport Sci Rev* 13:503-538, 1985.

104. Rowland T: *Exercise and Children's Health,* Champaign, Ill, 1990, Human Kinetics.

105. Mahon A, Del Corral P, Howe C, et al: Physiological correlates of 3-kilometer running performance in male children, *Int J Sports Med* 580-584, 1996.

106. Carroll J, Hagberg J, Brooke G, et al: Bicycle ergometry and gas exchange measurements in neuromuscular diseases, *Arch Neurol* 36:457-461, 1979.

107. Rose J, Gamble J, Lee J, et al: A method to quantitate and compare walking energy expenditure for children and adolescents, *J Pediatr Orthop* 11:571-578, 1991.

108. Rose J, Mederios J, Parker R: Energy cost index as an estimate of energy expenditure of cerebral palsied children during assisted ambulation, *Dev Med Child Neurol* 27:485-490, 1985.

Chapter 15

Pediatric Nonprogressive Central Nervous System Disorders

Debra Clayton-Krasinski, Linda Fieback

OBJECTIVES

After reading this chapter, the reader will be able to:
1. Explain the pathology and natural history of cerebral palsy and describe how cerebral palsy influences typical development and motor control.

2. Describe the essential musculoskeletal, neuromuscular, cardiovascular/pulmonary, and integumentary clinical manifestations in children with cerebral palsy that impact a child's motor performance.
3. Select appropriate evidence-based interventions for pediatric clients with cerebral palsy and indicate how the treatment outcomes address specific impairments, functional limitations, and/or disability.
4. Explain the pathology and natural history of one type of open spinal dysraphism, myelomeningocele, and describe how myelomeningocele influences typical development and motor control.
5. Describe the essential musculoskeletal, neuromuscular, cardiovascular/pulmonary, and integumentary clinical manifestations in children with myelomeningocele that impact a child's motor performance.
6. Select appropriate evidence-based interventions for pediatric clients with myelomeningocele and indicate how the treatment outcomes address specific impairments, functional limitations, and/or disability.

*P*ediatric nonprogressive central nervous system (CNS) disorders consist of an array of diagnoses, including cerebral palsy, genetic syndromes such as Down syndrome, open and closed spinal dysraphism, meningitis, and traumatic brain injury. Each diagnosis results in a unique combination of disability, functional limitations, and impairments that may benefit from rehabilitation services. *The Guide to Physical Therapy Practice*[1] preferred practice pattern 5C: Impaired motor function and sensory integrity associated with nonprogressive disorders of the CNS—congenital origin or acquired in infancy or childhood outlines the generally accepted elements of physical therapy management for this group of conditions.

This chapter focuses on the two most common pediatric nonprogressive CNS disorders encountered by rehabilitation clinicians: cerebral palsy and myelomeningocele, which is a type of spinal dysraphism (spina bifida). Cerebral palsy is the most common neurological condition encountered by therapists treating pediatric patients and the most common form of chronic motor disability in children.[2,3] Patients with cerebral palsy may present with a spectrum of delayed motor development and impaired motor function. Myelomeningocele directly causes motor paralysis and produces secondary complications involving multiple body systems that challenge therapists to use and integrate many facets of their knowledge and skill throughout the patient's lifespan.[4] This chapter applies concepts for patient examination presented in Chapter 14 and focuses on the pathology, evaluation, and interventions for pediatric patients with cerebral palsy and myelomeningocele and provides a model for clinical decision making for children with these and other disorders.

CEREBRAL PALSY
PATHOLOGY

Cerebral palsy (CP) is not a single disease but rather a clinically defined complex of static, nonprogressive posture and movement abnormalities caused by damage to the developing CNS in which the motor impairment occurs before, during, or soon after birth.[5,6] Although the clinical manifestations of CP often change over time, these changes are not due to additional CNS damage. CP is cerebral in origin and is associated with life-long, chronic motor impairments. Although motor dysfunction is the hallmark of CP, CP is also associated with other disabilities, including mental retardation or learning disabilities (50% to 75%), speech and language disorders (65%), hearing impairments (25%), epilepsy (25% to 35%), and visual disorders (25%).[7] Currently, there is a trend toward fewer coexisting disabilities, which may be due to improvements in perinatal and postnatal medical care.[8] Children with one or more coexisting disabilities may require more and more varied services.[8] The prevalence of CP is estimated at approximately 2 to 3 per 1,000 live births.[8] There is conflicting evidence regarding changes in rates over time. Data from Sweden and the United States (US) indicate that the rate of CP increased from the late 1960s to the mid-1980s, from 1.3 to 2.5 per 1,000 live births in Sweden and from 1.7 to 2.0 per 1,000 in 1-year survivors in the Atlanta area in the US.[8-10] In contrast, data from Western Australia indicate that the overall prevalence of CP did not change over this time period.[11] Differences in prevalence estimates among studies may reflect true differences in prevalence, be the result of changes in diagnostic methods or criteria or, be a result of differences or changes in obstetric and neonatal care.

RISK FACTORS

Although CP has a wide range of causes, all are thought to be related to aberrations in CNS maturation or to CNS injury.[2,5,12] The pathogenesis of CP is complex, and uncertainty regarding the range and relative contributions of different etiological factors has made prevention elusive.[5,13] Technological advances in imaging techniques, especially computed tomography (CT) and magnetic resonance imaging (MRI), have helped identify possible causes of CP and increased the recognition of developmental malformations of the brain.[14,15] Risk factors for CP are often broadly categorized according to the timing of the insult as prenatal (antepartum), perinatal (intrapartum), or postnatal. In the past, isolated perinatal events or difficulties during labor or delivery were thought to be the most common cause of brain injury.[14] However, recent findings indicate that children with CP often develop encephalopathy long before birth which makes them less able to tolerate problems during delivery.[16] *Neonatal encephalopathy*, which is clinically defined as including a combination of abnormal consciousness, deviant tone and reflexes, feeding and respiration difficulties; and/or seizures, may or may not result in permanent neurological impairment; however, a diagnosis of neonatal encephalopathy is a common precursor to a diagnosis of CP.

Premature Birth and Low Birth Weight. Although term and near-term infants are at relatively low risk for CP, because they constitute the majority of live births, they still represent approximately half of all births of children with CP.[2] Evidence shows that the risk of CP is greater with premature birth (>37 weeks) and *low birth weight* (>2,500 gm)[2,17,18] and that 25% to 35% of children with CP are born with a birth weight of less than 1,500 gm.[8] Prematurity predisposes the fetus to pathological events that can directly injure the brain and interrupt the normal process of intrauterine brain development.[19]

Perinatal Stroke. In addition to prematurity and low birth weight, perinatal stroke is also associated with an increased risk of CP.[2] Arterial ischemic stroke before birth or within the first month after birth occurs in approximately 1 in 4,000 term infants,[20] and CP develops in more than 50% of infants who have strokes. This is probably the most common cause of hemiparetic CP and a significant proportion of spastic quadriplegic CP.[2,14] Five subtypes of intrapartum hypoxic-ischemic cerebral injury, based on neuroanatomical distribution, are described. These subtypes are (1) parasagittal, (2) basal ganglia, (3) periventricular white matter, (4) focal/multifocal, and (5) selective neuronal necrosis.[14] These subtypes may occur alone or in combination. The nature of the insult (acute versus intermittent ischemia) and the stage of vascular and neurological development affect the extent of the lesion and the resulting functional impairments. Parasagittal injuries are most common in infants delivered after 34 weeks of gestation, whereas periventricular white matter injury is most common in infants delivered earlier.[14]

Intrauterine Infection. Placental infection during pregnancy is also associated with an increased risk of CP in near-term and *full-term infants*.[21] Intrauterine infection may be established before or during the pregnancy. Certain maternal infections, particularly toxoplasmosis, rubella, cytomegalovirus, and herpes simplex virus among others, can affect the fetus in the uterus and are also associated with premature birth and an increased risk of CP.[18] Infection is the most commonly identified cause of preterm birth at the lowest viable gestational age, and it is estimated that maternal infection accounts for 12% of spastic CP.[17] Spastic quadriplegia is the most common finding in infants with evidence of placental infection who later develop CP.[17] Infection, along with thrombosis and coagulopathy, are particularly associated with white matter damage and CP.[22]

Common aerobic bacteria, such as group B streptococci, *Escherichia coli*, and *Listeria monocytogenes*, can also cause CNS infections in the fetus or neonate, including meningitis, meningoencephalitis, cerebritis, and vasculitis. These can also result in long-term neurological deficits including CP.

Multiple Births. The incidence of CP is higher among twins and triplets than among singletons, and although multiple births are uncommon, they account for about 10% of cases of CP.[23] Multiple gestation is an independent risk factor for CP, and the risk is significantly higher for monochorionic twins, in which a single membrane encloses both of the fetuses, than for dichorionic twins.[14] The increased risk associated with multiple gestation appears to be chiefly related to the higher rate of premature delivery.[2] The risk of producing at least one child with CP is 15 per 1,000 for twins, 80 per 1,000 for triplets, and 429 per 1,000 for quadruplets.[22,23] In vitro fertilization (IVF) and other embryo implantation procedures are associated with a higher frequency of multiple births. Children born after IVF have an increased risk of developing neurological problems, especially CP, and these risks are largely attributed to the high risk of twin pregnancies, low birth weight, and prematurity.[24]

Birth Asphyxia. Birth asphyxia is another commonly implicated risk factor for CP. Alterations in the delivery of blood and oxygen to the fetus via maternal, uteroplacental, or umbilical circulation can result in fetal hypoxia.[14] For example, placental abruption, a tight or prolapsed nuchal cord, maternal shock, or a large placental infarct can all acutely interrupt fetal oxygen delivery.[2] In a population-based, case-control study of birth records, Nelson and Grether found that a tight nuchal cord was more common in children with CP than in children in the control group.[25] Furthermore, a tight nuchal cord was associated with spastic quadriplegic CP and accompanying dyskinesia.[26] There appears to be a narrow margin between the level of hypoxia that results in CP and the level that results in perinatal death, and of the infants who survive a hypoxic event, only a few develop CP. There is also no consistent dose-response association between the magnitude of hypoxia and neurological damage.[14]

Prevention of CP caused by intrapartum hypoxia remains a distant goal despite multiple innovations and substantial research. The prevalence of CP has not decreased with increased cesarean section operations or fetal monitoring aimed at detecting adverse events during labor.[7]

Postnatal Risk Factors. The postnatal period refers to the first few hours or days after birth to the first few years of life.[27] The Metropolitan Atlanta Developmental Disabilities Study reported that approximately 16% of children with CP acquire it postnatally.[28] Children who acquired CP postnatally were more likely to be black and male in comparison to children with congenital CP. Acquired CP can result from brain infections, such as bacterial meningitis or viral encephalitis; from head injuries caused by falls, motor vehicle accidents, or child abuse; or from near-drowning. The risk of neurological injury to infants and children has been reduced through a range of interventions, including the requirement in many areas for proper use of helmets and car seats for infants and older children.[2] The Centers for Disease Control and Prevention (CDC) analyzed data from its ongoing Metropolitan Atlanta Developmental Disabilities Surveillance Program and found that in 1991 bacterial meningitis and child battering were the chief postnatal causes of developmental disabilities in children aged 3 to 10 years.[29]

CLASSIFICATION

CP is heterogeneous in its manifestations.[2] It is generally classified by severity (mild, moderate, or severe and/or Gross Motor Disability Classification System), clinical type (spastic, dyskinetic, ataxic, and hypotonic), and topographic distribution of movement impairment (hemiplegia, diplegia, and quadriplegia).[30] A complete diagnosis includes findings in each domain to best describe the individual's condition. For example, a diagnosis could be recorded as level V (severe), spastic (type) diplegic (topographic distribution) CP.

CLINICAL TYPES

In 1956, Minear developed a system for classifying CP that was endorsed by the American Academy for Cerebral Palsy, now the American Academy for Cerebral Palsy and Developmental Medicine (AACPDM).[31] This system continues to be widely used and cited in current literature. It describes seven physiological (motor) types of CP: Spastic, athetotic, rigid, tremor, hypotonic, mixed, and unclassified. Additionally, the spastic type of CP is further classified by topographic region. Among the major CP types, each exhibits a different etiologic spectrum.[5]

Spastic Cerebral Palsy. The hallmark of spastic CP is hypertonicity; muscles are perceived as excessively stiff especially during movement.[3] Children with spastic CP have upper motor neuron signs including hypertonicity, hyperreflexia, clonus, and positive Babinski reflex; abnormal posturing of the extremities (abnormal flexor or extensor synergy patterns), limited selective control, coactivation of muscular activity, abnormal timing of muscle activation and abnormal postural responses.[17,30] The spastic CP type results from involvement of the motor cortex or white matter projections to and from cortical sensorimotor areas of the CNS. Spastic CP is the most common type of CP and accounts for about 75% of all children with CP.[30]

Topographic Distribution. Spastic CP can be classified as hemiplegia, diplegia, or quadriplegia according to the area of the body affected. *Spastic hemiplegia* chiefly involves one side of the body. A typical clinical presentation for spastic hemiplegia includes atypical posturing, such as upper extremity forearm pronation; elbow, wrist, and finger flexion; lower extremity hip internal rotation, adduction, and flexion; knee flexion; and ankle plantarflexion (Fig. 15-1). The most common etiologies of spastic hemiplegia are vascular (26.5%), periventricular leukomalacia (PVL) (14.7%), cerebral dysgenesis (13.2%), asphyxia (11.8%), and unknown (19.1%).[5] When the pathology involves the vascular territory of the middle cerebral artery, the upper extremity is more affected than the lower extremity and the distal portions are more involved than the proximal portions.[17] Spastic hemiplegia resulting from periventricular hemorrhage (i.e., bleeding in and around the ventricles) in the *premature infant* may

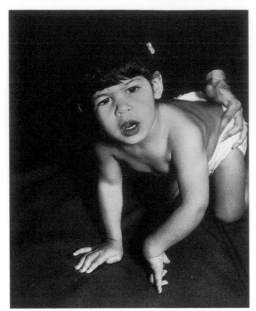

FIG. 15-1 A child with left-sided spastic hemiplegic, cerebral palsy. Note the left forearm pronation; elbow, wrist, and finger flexion; and hip adduction and flexion.

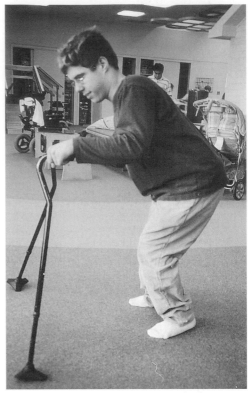

FIG. 15-2 A young man with spastic diplegic cerebral palsy. Note crouched stance with flexion, adduction, and internal rotation of the hips; flexion of the knees; and equinus feet.

present with the lower extremity being more involved than the upper extremity, since the descending motor tract for the lower extremity is closer to the ventricle.[17]

Spastic diplegia involves the entire body, but the lower extremities are more involved than the upper extremities. Children with spastic diplegia are frequently premature, and the underlying pathology is often PVL. Children with spastic diplegia often have trunk weakness and varying degrees of mobility and posture difficulties. Children with severe mobility restrictions may require a wheelchair, and those with moderate mobility difficulties may require assistive devices such as a walker or quad canes. Children with mild mobility difficulties require no assistance but may have difficulties performing more advanced gross motor skills such as running, jumping, and skipping. Standing and walking gait in severely and moderately involved children is frequently "crouched" and characterized by flexion, adduction, and internal rotation of the hips, flexion of the knees, and equinus feet[32] (Fig. 15-2). Upper extremity impairments can result in difficulties with fine motor tasks and cause difficulty with school work such as handwriting. Shevell et al report the most commonly identified etiologies of spastic diplegia are PVL (53.9%), intracranial hemorrhage (15.4%), asphyxia (12.8%), and toxins (7.7%), however, no specific cause was identified for 41% of cases.[5]

Spastic quadriplegia involves the entire body with all four extremities relatively equally involved (Fig. 15-3). Children with spastic quadriplegia tend to have more severe impairments than children with hemiplegia and diplegia. Hip subluxation or dislocation, contractures, and scoliosis can all occur in this population. Bilateral corticobulbar fiber involvement can also lead to poor control of the mouth, tongue, and pharynx resulting in swallowing and respiratory difficulties, drooling and dysarthric speech.[17,33] Spastic quadriplegia is the only type of CP asso-

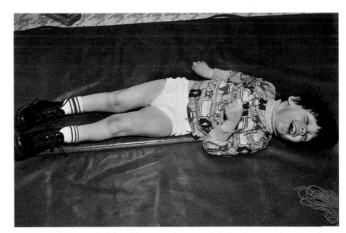

FIG. 15-3 A child with spastic quadriplegic cerebral palsy.

ciated with but not specific to acute interruption of the cerebral blood supply and is commonly associated with a parasagittal CNS injury.[14] The most common causes of spastic quadriplegia are asphyxia (32.5%), PVL (29.9%), intracranial hemorrhage or infection (14.3%), and unknown (9.1%).[5]

Dyskinetic Cerebral Palsy. The hallmark of *dyskinetic CP* is impaired volitional activity perceived as uncontrolled and purposeless movements that affect the entire body. Dyskinesias associated with this type of CP include athetosis, rigidity, and tremor. Athetosis refers to involuntary slow, irregular, writhing movements of the extremities, face, neck, and trunk.[17] Athetosis can impair postural control, increase latency of movement onset and cause oral-motor dysfunction leading to dysphagia and dysarthria. Muscle tone may or may not be abnormal.[30,34,35] Athetosis, which occurs in about 20% of all people with CP, is the most common type of dyskenesia.[30] Rigidity involves constant resistance throughout a movement in both the agonist and antagonist muscles. This type of hypertonicity is commonly referred to as "lead pipe" rigidity. Rigidity is much less common in people with CP than athetosis.[30] Tremor, a rhythmic involuntary small amplitude motion, is the least common type of CP.[30] Dyskinesias are associated with damage to the basal ganglia and their connections to the prefrontal and premotor cortex. Dyskinesia, especially when associated with learning difficulty, commonly has a genetic origin and is rarely caused by intrapartum or peripartum injury.[5,14]

Ataxic Cerebral Palsy. The hallmarks of ataxic CP are dysfunction in coordination, gait, and rapid distal movements of the extremities.[17] Ataxic CP is primarily a disorder of postural control and timing of coordinated movement.[30] Ataxia results from damage to the cerebellum and is characterized by dysarthria, dysmetria, and dysdiadochokinesia. Ataxia is also usually associated with hypotonia. Ataxia accounts for less than 10% cases of CP and commonly has a genetic origin (91.7%).[14]

Hypotonic Cerebral Palsy. Diminished resting muscle tone is the hallmark of hypotonic CP. Children with hypotonic CP present with excessive joint range of motion (ROM), postural instability, and a decreased ability to generate voluntary muscle force.[36] Hypotonia is often seen temporarily during development and can be the precursor to either spasticity or athetosis. It is not associated with a particular neurological lesion and commonly has a genetic origin.[14]

Mixed Cerebral Palsy. It is not unusual for a child to have signs of more than one of the previously described types of CP. The most common mixed type of CP is spastic with athetoid but other combinations can also occur. The most common etiologies of mixed types of CP are asphyxia (50%) and toxin exposures (16.7%).[5]

SEVERITY OF CEREBRAL PALSY

The severity of impairments caused by CP may vary and may be described as mild, moderate, or severe; however, these terms are generally poorly defined, with no universally agreed upon meaning, and are based primarily upon individual examiner knowledge, with resulting questionable reliability and validity.[30,37] Minear categorizes four levels of severity for patients with CP:[31]

Class I: No practical limitation of activity
Class II: Slight to moderate limitation of activity
Class III: Moderate to great limitations of activity
Class IV: Unable to carry on any useful physical activity.

This system relies heavily on clinical judgment and therefore also has questionable reliability and validity.

The *Gross Motor Function Classification System* for CP (GMFCS) is a new system for categorizing the severity of CP and includes 5 levels of severity:[38]

Level I: Walks without restrictions; limitations in more advanced gross motor skills.
Level II: Walks without assistive devices; limitations walking outdoors and in the community.
Level III: Walks with assistive mobility devices; limitations walking outdoors and in the community.
Level IV: Self-mobility with limitations; children are transported or use power mobility outdoors and in the community.
Level V: Self-mobility is severely limited even with the use of assistive technology.

Each level has separate descriptions for four separate age groups: 1-2 years, 2-4 years, 4-6 years, and 6-12 years of age (see CD for full descriptions). The GMFCS has clearly established itself as the principal classification system of functional ability for children with CP.[39] It is used across the spectrum of health professions and throughout the world. The GMFCS has been shown to be a valid and reliable measure when used by various professionals for children between 2 and 12 years of age.[39]

EXAMINATION

PATIENT HISTORY

The patient history for the pediatric client should include comprehensive assessment of all levels of the International Classification of Functioning, Disability, and Health (ICF) model, with a focus on the development of the patient's problem and their experience of its impact on activity and participation.

SYSTEMS REVIEW

The systems review is used to target areas requiring further examination and to define areas that may cause complications or indicate a need for precautions during the examination and intervention processes. See Chapter 1 for details of the systems review.

TESTS AND MEASURES

The final step in the examination process is the selection and implementation of appropriate tests and measures. Guided by the history and systems review, tests and measures are selected to assist the therapist in determining a diagnosis, prognosis, and plan of intervention. Chapter 14 includes detailed examination procedures for patients with CP that can assist the therapist in determining which tests and measures are best to administer for each individual child.

EVALUATION, DIAGNOSIS, AND PROGNOSIS

The probability of long-term survival for children with CP has increased, even among those with severe disabilities,[40] and most persons with CP can expect to survive well into adulthood.[41] Evans et al report the survival rate for persons with CP to be close to average[42]; however, the severity of disability strongly influences survival.[43,44] Mortality risk increases with increasing intellectual impairment, severity of motor impairment, and number of severe impairments.[41] Respiratory problems, especially aspiration pneumonia, are the leading cause of death.[41]

The severity of gross motor disability in children with CP, as defined by the GMFCS, is a strong indicator of future level of disability.[45] The greater the limitation in achievement of activities, the greater the need for caregiver assistance, and the greater the restrictions in participation in day-to-day activities.[45] Assistive devices can promote the achievement and performance of activities and lighten the burden of care.[46] Bottos et al studied 72 individuals with CP in Italy born between 1934 and 1980 from childhood to adulthood.[47] They found that, as adults, 75% of the subjects lived with their parents, 88% were not married, 66% were unemployed, and 16% had sheltered employment. Independent ambulation or other forms of supported ambulation was lost in 44.8% of previously ambulatory participants by the time they reached adulthood. Nine of the 13 participants who lost independent ambulation did so between the ages of 20 and 40 years, two did so after the age of 40, while the remaining two lost function before the age of 20. Maintenance of walking was related to diagnosis and motor impairment. Additionally, Bottos et al reported much reduced contact with health and rehabilitation services once individuals reached adulthood, although there was an increase in the frequency and severity of deformity in participants in all levels of motor impairment.[47] Murphy et al suggested that abnormal biomechanical forces and immobility leading to excessive physical stress and strain, overuse syndromes, and possibly early joint degeneration are likely responsible for later musculoskeletal problems and functional decline in patients with CP.[48]

A study of adults with CP performed using the California Developmental Disabilities database (n = 904 subjects) reported similar findings.[49] They noted a marked decline in ambulation in adults with CP, especially in later adulthood. Older subjects also frequently lost the ability to dress themselves, although speech, self-feeding, and the ability to order meals in public were well preserved. Most young adults lived in their families' homes or in small private group homes. Only 18% of the 60-year-olds lived independently or semi-independently, and 41% resided in facilities providing a higher level of medical care.

MEDICAL AND SURGICAL INTERVENTION FOR CHILDREN WITH CEREBRAL PALSY

There are a range of medical and surgical interventions available to help improve function in children with CP. These are discussed briefly in this section. Rehabilitation interventions for children with CP are discussed later in this chapter, together with interventions for children with *myelomeningocele* (MM).

MEDICAL MANAGEMENT

Children with CP often have spasticity that results in abnormal patterns of muscle coordination, abnormal muscle co-contraction during volitional movement, hypersensitivity to various sensory input, paresis, and delays in automatic postural reactions.[50,51] Although spasticity is not necessarily the primary factor limiting voluntary movement, spasticity will compromise transitional

movements and temporal sequencing of muscle activation that can affect postural control (righting, equilibrium, and protective reactions) and body alignment.[51,52] Medical management of spasticity in children includes both pharmacological (oral medications, intrathecal infusion, and muscle injections) and neurosurgical interventions (selective dorsal rhizotomy).

Pharmacological Management of Spasticity. A few oral medications are commonly used to reduce spasticity in children and adults. The most common are diazepam (Valium) and *baclofen* (Lioresal). Diazepam acts both centrally and at spinal polysynaptic pathways, stimulating the release of gamma-aminobutyric acid (GABA), an inhibitory neurotransmitter, from presynaptic neurons.[51,53] Baclofen mimics the action of GABA at postsynaptic motor neurons in the spinal cord.[51] Oral baclofen and diazepam have variable effects in reducing spasticity and often cause sedation.[54] Diazepam use should not be stopped suddenly because of the risk of withdrawal seizures.

Baclofen can also be administered by continuous intrathecal infusion (CIBI). With CIBI, baclofen is delivered in small, controlled doses from a pump to the spinal fluid via a catheter inserted into the intrathecal space at L1-L2 and threaded up to as high as T6 (Fig. 15-4). The primary indication for CIBI therapy is spasticity severe enough to impair motor function and self-care.[55] CIBI has the advantage of localizing the effects of the drug but is associated with infection at the site of pump implantation.

The usefulness of antispasticity medications in children with CP remains controversial. The Cochrane Database of Systematic Reviews is currently reviewing the effectiveness of these therapies in children with CP. Reducing spasticity does not necessarily improve function, and in some children, spasticity may actually allow for certain functional abilities. Reducing spasticity in the limbs may

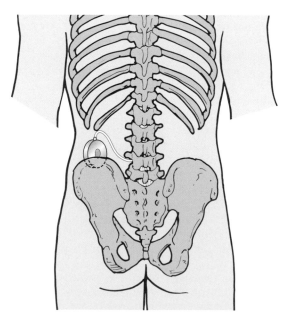

FIG. 15-4 Baclofen administration by continuous intrathecal infusion.

improve function, but reduction of spasticity in the trunk is often counterproductive.

Botulinum toxin A (BtA) can also be used to reduce muscle tone and spasticity and thereby increase ROM and improve function in children with CP. BtA, a purified form of the neurotoxin of *Clostridium botulinum,* paralyses muscles by inhibiting the release of acetylcholine at the neuromuscular junction.[51,56] In patients with CP, BtA is injected into selected muscle groups to produce a dose-dependent reduction in muscular activity. For example, BtA is injected in the gastrocnemius to treat dynamic equinus or into the hamstrings to treat crouch gait. The effect of BtA lasts about 12-16 weeks, during which time physical therapy, orthoses, and orthopedic surgery may be helpful.[57,58] Targeted motor training, such as strengthening of nonspastic antagonist muscle groups, and biofeedback may enhance the effects of BtA injection.[51] Fixed contractures can be addressed by combining BtA with serial casting. A systematic review of the effectiveness and safety of BtA for lower limb spasticity (dynamic calf equinus) in children aged 2-11 years with CP found three randomized controlled trials each involving a short-term, single course of intramuscular calf injections with different doses and preparations of BtA.[58-62] The reviewers found only weak evidence to support the effectiveness of BtA for improving function. BtA was found to be safe, at least in the short run; only a mild adverse effect of calf pain at the injection site was reported.[59] A systematic review of the effectiveness of BtA for the upper extremity in children with CP found only two studies that met the inclusion criteria of the review. Therefore the reviewers concluded that there was not enough evidence to support or refute the efficacy of BtA in improving upper extremity function in children with CP.[63]

Neurosurgical Management of Spasticity. Surgical interventions, as opposed to pharmacological interventions, generally cause permanent, irreversible changes in spasticity. *Selective dorsal rhizotomy* (SDR), where selective sensory nerve roots in the lumbar and sacral region are transected, can reduce lower extremity spasticity. In this procedure, sensory nerve rootlets with abnormal responses to testing are cut. This results in decreased spasticity and temporary or permanent muscle weakness. SDR was popular during the mid-1980s but has fallen from favor with the advent of a greater selection of reversible pharmacological interventions. An intense therapy program focusing on improving lower extremity antigravity strength and motor function typically follows this type of surgery. A meta-analysis of three randomized clinical trials found a clinically important change in spasticity 9-12 months after SDR surgery.[64] A small but statistically significant advantage to SDR plus physical therapy was shown on the Gross Motor Function Measure (GMFM) when compared with physical therapy alone. The researchers concluded that the decision as to whether or not to perform SDR on a similar child (between 3-8 years of age, GMFCS level III to IV) rests on whether or not an anticipated mean GMFM change score increment of 4 percentage points above the amount of change with non-invasive care justifies the time, effort and risks involved.

ORTHOPEDIC MANAGEMENT

Orthopedic surgery can alter bony mechanical alignment and deformities, control effects of spasticity on individual joints, correct dislocation or contraction, or control scoliosis for the purpose of maximizing function in patients with CP.[65] Typical orthopedic procedures in children with CP include correction of bony abnormalities such as excessive femoral anteversion or tibial torsion or hip subluxation or dislocation.[51] Surgery may also be used to release, lengthen, or transfer muscles. These procedures alter tension on the intrafusal muscle spindle and should therefore decrease the stimulus for stretch responses. A muscle lengthening procedure may also reduce spasticity by placing the joint in a more effective position for muscle activation or by altering the balance of muscle forces at a joint. Single operative procedures used to be common, but recently, single-event multilevel surgery correcting all existing soft tissue and bony deformities at the same time has gained popularity.[66] For example, a 10-year-old child with spastic diplegic CP may undergo a bilateral femoral derotation osteotomy and distal hamstring lengthening, left psoas intramuscular lengthening, and left gastrocnemius slide all at one time. This type of procedure offers the advantages of lower incidence of recurrence of deformities than with single operative procedures and improvements in ambulatory status and joint ROM at the cost of longer operating times and more intraoperative blood loss.[67,68] Postoperatively, the limb is generally immobilized with a cast for 3-6 weeks, after which an orthosis may be used. Postoperative rehabilitation generally includes passive and active ROM, strengthening, functional training, and gait training, depending on the examination findings at the time. Gross motor function tends to deteriorate immediately after surgery because of weakness of the released muscle, decreased physical fitness, and immobility, and functional abilities may take months to recover.[69] Improvements are generally greatest in the first 6 months after surgery, with continued, although slower, improvements reported to occur up to 12 months after muscle release surgery.[69]

The effectiveness of orthopedic surgery in children with CP remains controversial. An AACPDM evidence report[70] reviewed 27 research articles on the effects of surgical adductor releases for hip subluxation in children with CP and concluded that the published evidence was preliminary at best. Outcome measures generally assessed more for correction of the deformity than for improvement of function.

SPINAL DYSRAPHISM
PATHOLOGY

Spinal dysraphisms (Greek = bad + suture), also known generically as *spina bifida,* are congenital malformations of the spine and spinal cord, including anomalies of the skin, muscles, vertebrae, meninges, and nervous tissue. The incidence of spinal dysraphism is estimated at 0.5 to 0.25 per 1,000 births.[73] Dysraphism occurs within the first 2 months of pregnancy if the spine fails to fuse. It is the most frequent permanently disabling *neural tube defect* with a prevalence of approximately 70,000 in the US in

2001 (20.09 per 100,000 live births).[74,75] During 1996-2001 the incidence of spinal dysraphisms decreased by 24%, largely as a result of increased maternal prenatal intake of folic acid.[76]

The abnormalities usually involve the lumbosacral spine although lesions can occur in the cervical and thoracic regions. Spinal dysraphisms are categorized as either *open spinal dysraphisms* (OSD) or *closed spinal dysraphisms* (CSD) (Fig. 15-5). In OSD, the nervous tissue and/or meninges are exposed through a congenital bony defect. In CSD, neural tissue is covered by skin, although cutaneous stigmata, such as a hairy nevus, capillary hemangioma, dimples, dystrophy, and subcutaneous masses, indicate the presence of, or suggest dysraphism in as many as 50% of cases.[77] CSDs are more common than OSDs, accounting for 64.2% of cases.[78]

OPEN SPINAL DYSRAPHISMS

There are four types of OSDs: Myelomeningocele (MM), myeloschisis, hemimyelomeningocele, and hemimyelocele.[71] MM is the most common, accounting for more than 98% of all OSDs. OSDs are typically located at the lumbar or lumbosacral level. OSDs can be detected during pregnancy by maternal serum biochemical tests and ultrasound assessments.

Myelomeningocele. MM is an OSD that occurs when a segment of the spinal cord and meninges protrudes through a bony defect in the midline of the back and is exposed to the environment (see Fig. 15-5, *A*). MM occurs in 0.6 per 1,000 live births and is slightly more frequent in females than in males.[71] Serum alpha-fetoprotein (AFP) levels and ultrasonography are used to identify fetuses with MM at 16-20 weeks of gestation. The incidence of MM in infants has been reduced in western countries by maternal folic acid supplementation before and during pregnancy and by parents choosing to interrupt pregnancy if MM is diagnosed prenatally.[71,74] Should MM be diagnosed prenatally and the parents elect to complete the pregnancy, delivery by cesarean operation is recommended to reduce the risk of injury to the exposed neural tissue.

Shortly after birth, the open area of the back is surgically repaired to avoid ulceration and infection of the exposed tissue. Closure of the dural defect can change cerebrospinal fluid (CSF) dynamics, resulting in insufficient drainage and hydrocephalus. Hydrocephalus occurs in 70% to 90% of children with MM and may occur prenatally or 48-72 hours after surgical repair of the spinal malformation. Hydrocephalus may be treated by ventriculoperitoneal (VP) shunting. Intrauterine repair of MM has been performed since 1994.[78] It has been suggested that the fetal surgery is associated with a reduction in hindbrain herniation and a decrease in the need for VP shunting for hydrocephalus during the first year of life.[74] Hydromyelia, an increase in fluid in the dilated central canal of the spinal cord, may also occur in as many as 80% of infants who have surgery for a MM and is a leading cause of neurological deterioration.[71] Children may have intellectual and psychological disturbances as the result of brain damage caused by hydrocephalus.

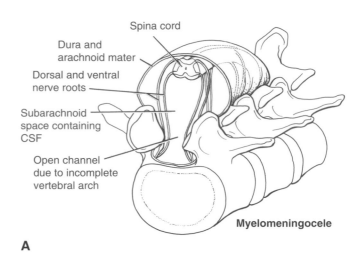

A

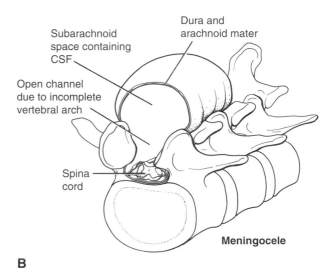

B

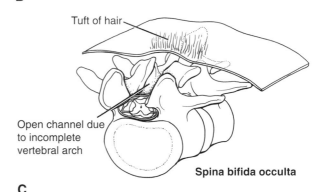

C

FIG. 15-5 Spinal dysraphisms. **A,** Myelomeningocele: An open spinal dysraphism with a cyst-like pouch containing spinal cord (myelo-) and meninges. **B,** Meningocele: A closed spinal dysraphism with a cyst-like pouch lined with meninges. **C,** Spina bifida occulta: A closed spinal dysraphism with posterior spinal boney defect and a hairy tuft on the skin. *From Larsen W: Human Embryology, ed 3, Philadelphia, 2001, Churchill Livingstone.*

Findings on examination of children with MM may include sensorimotor deficits of the lower extremities, bowel and bladder incontinence and hindbrain dysfunction. Children with MM differ from children with spinal cord injury in that they often have impairments of both

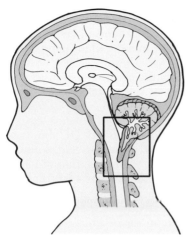

FIG. 15-6 Chiari II malformation. Note the downward displacement of the cerebellum through the foramen magnum.

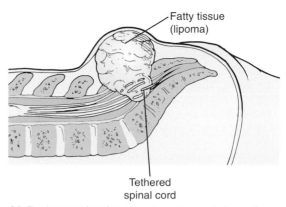

FIG. 15-7 Lipomyeloschisis, a closed spinal dysraphism. Note the lipoma is attached to a tethered spinal cord and there is obvious soft tissue swelling over the spine in the lumbosacral region.

the spinal cord and the brain. Each child has a different spectrum and severity of impairments, functional limitations, and disability. Some children will be near normal, whereas others will be severely involved with complete lower extremity paralysis and very impaired cognition.

Chiari II Malformation. There is a 100% association between OSD and the *Chiari II malformation*. This malformation is an anomaly of the hindbrain characterized by: (1) Downward displacement of the cerebellum through the foramen magnum; (2) resulting changes in the fourth ventricle, (3) downward displacement of the brainstem with potential for altered pressures on the lower cranial nerves, and (4) a smaller, tighter posterior fossa and a somewhat larger foramen magnum than is usual (Fig. 15-6).[73,79] The severity of the Chiari II malformation can range from a nearly normal-sized posterior fossa to a severe abnormality that can produce life-threatening symptoms such as respiratory failure as a result of brainstem dysfunction. The most common early symptom is respiratory stridor, especially with inspiration, occurring within 1-2 weeks of birth. Stridor is a high-pitched, noisy respiration associated with obstruction commonly of the trachea or larynx (see Chapter 26). The stridor usually disappears spontaneously within a few days but may persist until up to 3 months of age. Stridor caused by lower brainstem dysfunction is associated with difficulties swallowing and intermittent apnea (cessation of breathing). In these cases, serious consideration is given to decompression of the hindbrain by surgical removal of the posterior arch of the upper spine.

CLOSED SPINAL DYSRAPHISMS

Many spinal dysraphisms are CSDs. Some CSDs, such as tethered cord syndrome (TCS), are not clinically evident at birth; however, cutaneous stigmata, such as an area of abnormal hair growth over the thoracic or lumbar spine, often indicate the presence of an underlying spinal malformation[72] (see Fig. 15-5, *C*). A subcutaneous mass in the lumbar or lumbosacral region can also be associated with two common malformations: Lipomyeloschisis and

lipomyelomeningocele. Meningocele and terminal myelocystocele are two other rare forms of CSD.

Lipomyeloschisis and Lipomyelomeningocele. Lipomyeloschisis and lipomyelomeningocele are forms of CSD that occur in conjunction with lipomas (subcutaneous fat masses) derived from epidermal and mesodermal tissue located in the lumbosacral region. With lipomyeloschisis, the lipoma is inside the spinal canal, whereas with lipomyelomeningocele the lipoma is outside the spinal canal inside a meningeal outpouching. The lipoma grows through the vertebral defect and attaches to an elongated and tethered spinal cord and often disturbs the formation of neural elements by adhesion or pressure (Fig. 15-7). Lipomas with dural defects account for 87.4% of all CSDs.[71] More than 90% of infants with these disorders will have an obvious soft tissue swelling over the spine in the lumbosacral region, and most will develop neurological symptoms within the first few months to years of life.[80] Neurological symptoms are caused by tethering of the spinal cord, especially during growth spurts, and compression that results from progressive deposition of fat, especially during periods of rapid weight gain.[80] Clinical manifestations include deformity and weakness of one or both lower extremities and bowel and bladder dysfunction. The weakness may be symmetrical or asymmetrical and may result in atrophy of the lower extremities. Surgery to release the attachment of the fat to the spinal cord and debulk the lipoma is recommended when the infant reaches 2 months of age or at the time of diagnosis, if the individual presents at a later age, although this does not always improve functional outcome.[80] One study reported that surgery for spinal lipomas was associated with improved outcome in 19%, worsened outcome in 6%, and no change in 75% of patients.[80]

Meningocele. Meningocele is characterized by herniation of a CSF-filled sac lined with dura and arachnoid (meninges) through a posterior spinal bony defect (see Fig. 15-5, *B*). The deficit, most commonly of lumbar or sacral origin,[71] results from splitting of one or more spinous processes, causing widening of the space between pedicles.[81] The spinal cord itself is structurally normal, and the lesion is not associated with nerve damage or paralysis.

Spinal meningoceles are uncommon, representing only 2.4% of all CSDs.[73]

EMBRYOLOGY

Spinal dysraphisms result from a disturbance in embryonic development between the second and sixth weeks of gestation when gastrulation (weeks 2-3), primary neurulation (weeks 3-4), and secondary neurulation and retrogressive differentiation (weeks 5-6) occur. Gastrulation transforms the two-layered embryo into a three-layered structure of ectoderm, mesoderm, and endoderm.[82] Primary neurulation results in the formation of the neural tube, the future brain, and the spinal cord as far as S2. Primary neurulation starts at the future craniocervical junction and then proceeds cephalad and caudad with the cranial end of the neural tube closing at about day 25 and the caudal end closing at about day 27 (Fig. 15-8).[71] After the caudal portion of the neural tube closes, the entire nervous system is covered with skin and the more caudal neural development, S3 through S5, occurs by secondary neurulation. Retrogressive differentiation is a combination of regression, degeneration, and further differentiation that eventually results in formation of the tip of the conus medullaris and filum terminale.[71] The conus medullaris moves caudally with respect to the adjacent vertebral column from postovulatory days 43-48 onward throughout fetal development or possibly even for the first months after birth.[83]

Neural tube defects (NTDs) can cause incomplete development of the brain, spinal cord, and/or meninges because of errors or disturbances in any of the embryo-genic processes described (Fig. 15-9). Three types of neural tube defects can occur: Anencephaly, encephalocele, and spinal dysraphisms. Anencephaly is a closed NTD that results in small or missing brain hemispheres. Encephalocele is an open NTD resulting in a portion of brain protruding out from the occipital region in a skin covered sac. MM, a disorder of the spinal cord as described earlier in this chapter, is thought to be a disorder of primary neurulation caused by failure of the developing neural tube to fully close and development of abnormal mesodermal tissue. It has been proposed that some cervicothoracic MMs are caused by disordered midline integration during gastrulation.[83] Spinal lipomas with dural defects are also thought to result from abnormalities during primary neurulation. The cutaneous ectoderm fails to separate from the neuroectoderm. The embryogenic origin of meningoceles is unknown.

ETIOLOGY

The causes of NTDs remain unknown but are likely heterogeneous. The forces underlying neural development from conception to the ascent of the conus medullaris, the mechanical and molecular biology of neural tube closure, and genetic and environmental influences are not well understood.[82] NTDs may result from a number of embryonic insults and may have a variety of mechanisms.

Four lines of evidence point to interactions between genetic and environmental factors.[82] First, the incidence of neural tube defects is higher in first-degree relatives; the risk of the parents of a child with a NTD giving birth to a second child with a NTD is 2% to 3% and of giving birth

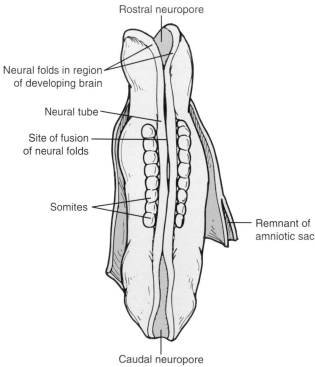

FIG. 15-8 Dorsal view of an 8-somite embryo. The neural tube is in open communication with the amniotic cavity at the cranial and caudal ends.

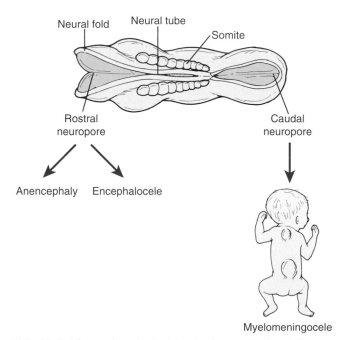

FIG. 15-9 The embryological basis of neural tube defect. Myelomeningocele from defective closure of the caudal neuropore. *From Moore KL, Persaud TVN:* The Developing Human: Clinically Oriented Embryology, *ed 7, Philadelphia, 2003, WB Saunders.*

to a third child with a NTD is 10% or more.[84] Second, the incidence of NTDs varies widely between populations. African blacks have the lowest incidence at 1 in 10,000, whereas Celts (Eastern Irish, Western Scots, and Welsh) have had an incidence as high as 1 in 80.[85] Third, in 3.7% to 18% of monozygotic twins, both have NTDs.[86] Fourth, NTDs are associated with genetic syndromes (Waardenburg syndrome) and chromosomal anomalies (trisomy 13 and 18).[82]

More than 60 genetic mouse mutants with NTDs have been identified and mutants may be specific to a certain type of NTD.[87] The role of nutrition in the etiology of NTDs, especially deficiencies in folic acid (a common water-soluble B vitamin), is well described. Administration of supplemental folate before conception has been shown in randomized placebo-controlled studies to reduce the recurrence rate of NTDs in women with a previously affected pregnancy and the incidence of NTDs in women who had never had an affected pregnancy.[78,88,89] However, as many as 30% to 50% of NTDs appear to be caused by factors that are not responsive to folate administration.[82] A number of teratogens, including certain medications and alcohol, are known to increase the risk of NTDs in humans.

PRENATAL TESTING AND PREVENTION

It is estimated that 50% to 70% of spinal dysraphisms can be prevented if a woman consumes sufficient folic acid (400 µg [i.e., 0.4 mg] daily) before conception and throughout the first trimester of pregnancy.[90] Therefore the US Public Health Service recommends that all women of reproductive age consume the suggested dosage of folic acid daily. Additionally, a healthy diet rich in folic acid that emphasizes fresh fruits, green leafy vegetables (spinach, broccoli, asparagus), orange juice, enriched whole grain foods, and fortified cereals is recommended. In January 1998, all enriched cereal grain products were fortified with folic acid by mandate of the Food and Drug Administration (FDA).[91] After folic acid fortification, spinal dysraphism incidence decreased by 24% and anencephaly incidence decreased by 21%.[78]

Early intrauterine detection followed by pregnancy termination is the only other option for preventing the birth of children with spinal dysraphisms. The majority of NTDs occur in families with no prior history of birth defects, thus screening tests are used to identify individuals at sufficient risk to warrant further evaluation. A simple "triple screen" blood test that measures alpha-fetoprotein (AFP), estriol, and human chorionic gonadotropin levels can be performed between 15-22 weeks of pregnancy to check for abnormalities common with NTDs and certain chromosomal defects.[92]

When an elevated serum AFP level is detected, the fetus is then evaluated for NTDs by targeted ultrasound. OSDs, anencephaly, and other cranial defects are usually readily visualized. The risk of an NTD is reduced by 95% if no spine defects or cranial abnormalities are visualized by ultrasound in women with an elevated serum AFP level.[93] When the diagnosis by ultrasound is uncertain, AFP in amniotic fluid is measured by amniocentesis. The presence of acetylcholinesterase and elevated levels of AFP in the amniotic fluid support the diagnosis of NTD.[93] CSDs cannot be detected by maternal serum or amniotic fluid tests.

EXAMINATION

PATIENT HISTORY

Children with MM present with a broad spectrum of impairments, functional limitations, and disabilities. The nonprogressive spinal cord injury preferred practice pattern 5H of the *Guide*[1] can serve as a template for physical therapy practice for children with MM (see Chapter 20). However, children with MM differ substantially from children with spinal cord injury because of the potential multifocal involvement of the CNS, including not only the spinal cord but also the brain and the brainstem. The complex and challenging problems of MM require a multidisciplinary team approach and age-specific, life-long medical and rehabilitation management. The list of impairments in individuals with MM includes paralysis, musculoskeletal deformities, sensory deficits, cranial nerve deficits, cognitive and language dysfunction, visuoperceptual deficits, seizures, neurogenic bowel and bladder, osteoporosis, obesity, and skin breakdown. Ongoing, objective monitoring is essential for proper medical management as the degree of impairment may increase over time. The deterioration can be due to CSF shunt obstruction, hydromyelia, growth of a lipoma at the site of repair, subarachnoid cysts of the cord, spinal cord tethering, or other unknown causes. Progressive deterioration that results from some of these causes may be amenable to neurosurgical interventions.

SYSTEMS REVIEW

The systems review is used to target areas requiring further examination and to define areas that may cause complications or indicate a need for precautions during the examination and intervention processes. See Chapter 1 for details of the System Review.

TESTS AND MEASURES
Musculoskeletal

Posture. Spinal and lower extremity deformities and joint contractures frequently occur in individuals with MM.[4] A combination of hip flexion, adduction, and internal rotation contractures leading to hip subluxation or dislocation is common. Many of the musculoskeletal deformities are present at birth and are exacerbated by the effects of gravity as the child grows.[94] Musculoskeletal deformities observed in MM may result from an imbalance between muscle groups; the effect of stress, posture and gravity; lack of mobility; and coexisting congenital malformations.[94] The type and extent of lower extremity deformity depends on the degree of imbalance between active and inactive muscle groups, which depend largely on the level of spinal cord disruption. For example, if the cord is affected in the midlumbar region, when supine the infant's hips will be flexed and adducted because the iliopsoas and adductors are strong, while the hip extensors and abductors are weak.[95] This may result in extreme tightness of the hip flexors and hip adductors.[96]

Patients with MM commonly have musculoskeletal deformities in all lower extremity joints and the spine. These deformities can affect activities, especially in sitting and standing, and can alter postural control mechanisms. Foot deformities occur in 60% to 90% of children with low level MM.[97] 41% of children with L4-L5 spinal lesions have calcaneus deformities. This is caused by strong ankle dorsiflexion from the anterior tibialis and toe extensors with weak or absent plantar flexion resulting from denervation of the toe flexors and the gastrocnemius/soleus group. Surgically transferring the tibialis anterior muscle to the calcaneus can improve this deformity, with outcomes being best when the surgery is performed when the child is 4-7 years of age.[79] Lower sacral lesions can result in cavus foot deformities. When the deformity is mild, orthotic shoe inserts may assist with balance and comfort; however, for more severe cases, metatarsal osteotomies or triple arthrodesis of the hindfoot may be required.

Knee contractures, in both flexion and extension, are also common in this population and are seen with all levels of cord involvement. Knee flexion contractures occur in children who primarily use a wheelchair for mobility. Knee extension contractures occur after periods of immobilization in bed necessitated by pressure ulcers or surgical procedures.[98] The frequency and severity of knee contractures vary with age and level of involvement: 65% to 70% in thoracic and high level lumbar groups have knee contractures by age 6 to 8, 20% to 25% of the L4-L5 group have knee contractures by age 9 to 12, and a few children with sacral level lesions also develop knee contractures.[99] Up to a quarter of young to middle-aged adults with MM report chronic knee pain or have instability.[79]

Hip dislocations are seen in about a quarter to a third of individuals with thoracic to L2 level lesions, in up to half of those with L4 level lesions, and infrequently with lower lesions. It is uncommon for hips that are stable through the first decade of life to subsequently dislocate. Hip dislocations do not usually cause pain or interfere with seating, and surgical hip reduction is not a requirement for ambulation in children with MM.[79] Surgical

management of hip dislocations differs among surgeons and medical centers and may be based on whether the dislocation is unilateral or bilateral, where the spinal lesion is located, and the strength of the quadriceps muscles. Potential adverse outcomes from such surgeries include postoperative contractures (stiff hip) that can affect seating, wound complications, and redislocation.

The spinal deformities most frequently associated with MM are scoliosis, kyphosis, and lordosis (Fig. 15-10) (see Chapter 4). The obvious malformation of vertebrae at the site of the lesion, hemivertebrae and their corresponding ribs contribute to spinal instability. A lumbar kyphosis may also be present as a result of the original deformity.[94] Scoliosis may be present at birth as a result of the vertebral abnormalities or may be acquired later because of muscle imbalance. Progressive scoliosis is one of the most severe complications of MM.[95] Scoliosis frequently occurs in children with higher spinal lesions, and curves tend to progress with age.[4] Excessive lordosis or lordoscoliosis is common in the adolescent and is associated with hip flexion deformities and a large spinal defect. Spinal orthoses, a custom molded thoracolumbosacral orthosis (TLSO) or total contact body jacket, may support the spine during growth or after surgical spinal procedures (see Chapter 34).

An uncorrected postural deformity can cause joint contractures and deformities, muscle weakness, poor joint alignment, and musculoskeletal pain, ultimately leading to functional limitations.[4] Additionally, musculoskeletal deformities can adversely affect positioning, body image, sitting and standing weight bearing, activities of daily living (ADLs), energy expenditure, and mobility throughout the lifespan.[4]

Management of musculoskeletal deformities associated with MM requires good coordination between all members of the rehabilitation team, including the physical therapist (PT), occupational therapist (OT), orthotist, and orthopedic surgeon. Interventions are directed at decreasing the impact of congenital malformations, when possible, and preventing the development of secondary

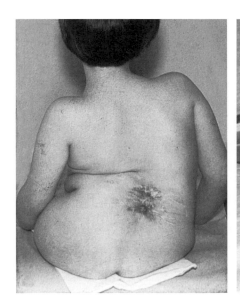
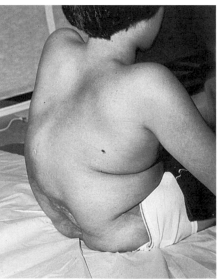

FIG. 15-10 Musculoskeletal deformities in patients with myelomeningocele. Note scoliosis and kyphosis. *From Hinderer KA, Hinderer SR, Shurtleff DB: Myelodysplasia. In Campbell S, Vander Linden D, Palisano RJ (eds):* Physical Therapy for Children, *ed 3, St. Louis, 2006, WB Saunders.*

deformities. A regular, diligent program combines positioning and handling, passive ROM exercises, stretching, adaptive functional training, and parent education and instruction in following through with these activities when away from therapy. Older children with MM must collaborate in and become responsible for their own care once they understand the exercise protocols.

Anthropometric Characteristics

Osteoporosis. Osteoporosis can occur in children with MM. Paralysis, disuse, immobility, and decreased loading of long bones of the lower extremities contribute to decreased bone mineral density and increased risk of osteoporotic fractures. Parsch reported a fracture rate of 12.2% in 1,400 children with spina bifida.[100] Fractures can occur after minor, painless trauma (as a result of sensory deficit); postsurgical immobilization; or prolonged bed rest for skin breakdown.[95] Breaks are frequent after operations that require cast immobilization; thus early standing and short immobilization times are recommended.[100] There is often redness and swelling around the fracture site, but the child will not complain of pain because of a lack of sensation. A passive weight-bearing standing program does not seem to decrease the risk of fracture in children with MM, probably because maintenance of bone density depends on torque generated from volitional muscle activity.[4,101] Nonetheless, upright positioning and mobility is important and restricting physical activity for fear of a fracture is not indicated.[4]

Obesity. About two thirds of children with MM are significantly overweight.[98] Children with MM, especially those with higher level lesions (thoracic to L2), are at increased risk for obesity because of decreased physical activity and decreased lower extremity muscle mass.[4] The most appropriate screening measurements for obesity in this population are arm span to weight ratio and subscapular skinfold thickness.[85] A height to weight ratio is not recommended because children with MM tend to be short. To help control body weight, in addition to supporting nutritional control, the clinician can help the child find age-appropriate physical activities that they can perform and enjoy. A physical fitness program tailored to the needs of the individual child can be developed and implemented at home and/or at school.

Muscle Performance. The most obvious impairment of MM is paralysis of the lower extremities, paraplegia, that results from the spinal cord malformation.[4] Upper extremity weakness can also occur with lesions in the cervical spine. Paralysis may follow the distribution of a complete cord transection, an incomplete lesion, or a skip lesion. Patients with complete cord transections have normal function down to a specific spinal level, below which there is flaccid paralysis, loss of sensation, and absent reflexes. Incomplete lesions present with mixed upper and lower motor findings, spasticity and flaccidity. Skip lesions manifest either with isolated muscle function below the last functional level or with inadequate muscle strength of muscle groups that have innervation higher than the lowest functioning group. Children with MM may also present with asymmetrical signs (right differing from the left side), and with both upper and lower motor neuron findings that change over time. They may also have discordant motor and sensory levels.[95] The International Myelodysplasia Study Group (IMSG) provides criteria for assigning motor levels from manual muscle test results.[103] The motor level is the lowest intact functional neuromuscular segment, with segments below this level not being intact. Table 15-1 shows the motor levels and commonly associated muscle dysfunctions observed in children with MM.

Muscle strength is tested to determine the extent of paralysis; however, the testing method varies according to the child's age and cognitive ability. In the newborn period through early childhood, muscle strength is assessed through observation and muscle palpation during spontaneous movements and postural attitude. Manual muscle testing and assignment of muscle grades (see Chapter 5) is used when the individual can follow the instructions of the testing procedure, which is typically at around 4-5 years of age.[94] Key movements to observe are hip flexion and adduction, knee flexion and extension, and dorsiflexion and plantarflexion at the ankle.[95] Detailed muscle testing should be performed every 6 months to 1 year and before and after any surgical procedure.[94]

Neuromuscular

Arousal, Attention, Cognition. Specific and general learning problems and mental retardation are commonly associated with MM. These have a range of causes, including complications of untimely treatment of hydrocephalus, cerebral infection from an infected shunt, and prenatal hydrocephalus.[104,105] Approximately three quarters of children with MM without hydrocephalus or with uncomplicated hydrocephalus have intelligence within the normal range.[106] Children who have had significant CNS infections tend to have lower intelligence than those who have not.[107] Intelligence tends to be higher in children with lumbar and sacral level lesions than in children with higher level lesions.[107] However, children with normal intelligence with MM still tend to have learning problems and poor academic achievement that are thought to result from deficits in perceptual skills, organizational abilities, attention, sequencing, reasoning, speed of motor response, memory, and hand function.[94,108,109]

Language dysfunction observed in children with MM and hydrocephalus is characterized by deficits in discourse (high frequency of irrelevant content), excessive chatter, and poorer performance, with abstract rather than concrete language.[4,110] Ten percent of children with MM have speech deficits and the incidence of hearing loss as a result of conductive or sensorineural impairment has been found to be as high as 13.4%.[95]

Cranial Nerve Integrity. Cranial nerve deficits can result from the Chiari II malformation, hydrocephalus, and/or brainstem dysplasia.[4] Gaston reported that only 27% of 322 children with MM monitored for 6 years had normal vision, 42% of children with MM had a manifest squint, 29% had an oculomotor nerve palsy or musculoparetic nystagmus, 14% had papilledema, and 17% had optic nerve atrophy.[111] Pharyngeal and laryngeal dysfunction including a croupy, hoarse cry and swallowing difficulties can occur with damage to cranial nerve IX

TABLE 15-1	Motor Levels and Commonly Associated Muscle Dysfunctions in Children with Myelomeningocele			

Motor Level	Muscle Function	Musculoskeletal Deformities	Mobility Options	Equipment Needs
T10	*Functional:* Neck, upper extremity, shoulder girdle, upper trunk musculature *Absent or weak (> grade 3):* Weak lower trunk musculature No volitional lower extremity movements	Kyphoscoliosis; congenital hip subluxation or dislocation, often bilateral; hip abduction and external rotation contractures; club feet	Exercise ambulation Household (short distances) ambulation in young children Wheeled mobility for functional household and community	Parapodium, THKAO, TLSO, night splints
T12	*Function:* Some pelvic control in supine and sitting (abdominals or paraspinal muscles) *Absent or weak (> grade 3):* Hip hiking (quadratus lumborum, grade 2)			
L2	*Function as above plus:* Hip hiking Hip flexion (iliopsoas, sartorius, grade 3 or better) Hip adduction (grade 3 or better)	Congenital hip subluxation or dislocation (L1, L2), scoliosis, calcaneus-valgus, hip flexion contracture	Exercise ambulation Household (short distances) ambulation in young children Wheeled mobility for functional household and community	Parapodium, THKAO, RGO, KAFO, upper extremity support (crutches, walker)
L3	*Function as above plus:* Strong hip flexion and adduction Some knee extension (quadriceps; grade 3 or better)	Congenital hip subluxation or dislocation (L1, L2), scoliosis, calcaneus-valgus, hip flexion contracture	Household and community (short distance) ambulation Wheeled mobility for community	RGO or HKAFOs, upper extremity support (forearm crutches)
L4	*Function as above plus:* Stronger knee extension (medial hamstrings; grade 3 or better) Some ankle dorsiflexion and inversion (tibialis anterior; grade 3 or better) Weak peroneus tertius	Calcaneal foot deformities, ankle-knee valgus deformities	Household and community ambulation Wheeled mobility for distance, sports, etc	Standard or ground reaction force (AFO) or KAFOs RGO Upper extremity support (crutches)
L5	*Function as above plus:* Stronger dorsiflexion with inversion Stronger knee flexion (lateral hamstring; grade 3 or better) Plus one of the following: • Stronger plantarflexion with inversion (peroneus tertius; grade 4 or better) • Tibialis posterior (grade 3 or better) Weak hip extension and abduction (gluteus minimus; grade 2)	Calcaneal foot deformities, hindfoot valgus, late hip dislocation, lumbar lordosis	Household and community ambulation Wheeled mobility for distance, sports, etc	Standard or ground reaction force AFO Bilateral upper extremity support
S1	*Function as above plus:* At least 2 of the following: Improved hip stability Gastrocnemius/soleus (grade 2 or better) Gluteus medius (grade 3 or better) Gluteus maximus (grade 2 or better)	Calcaneal varus	Community ambulation	AFO, SMO, or shoe insert for proper foot alignment and/or medial/ lateral ankle stability
S2	*Function as above plus:* Gastrocnemius/soleus (grade 3 or better) Gluteus medius and maximus (grade 4 or better)	Toe-clawing	Community ambulation	AFO, SMO, or shoe insert for proper foot alignment and/or medial/ lateral ankle stability
S2-S3	All muscles grade 5 except for one or two groups with grade 4	None	Community ambulation	AFO, SMO, or shoe insert for proper foot alignment and/or medial/ lateral ankle stability

THKAO, Thoracic hip-knee-ankle-foot orthoses; *TLSO,* thoracolumbosacral body orthoses; *KAFO,* knee-ankle-foot orthroses; *AFO,* ankle-foot orthroses; *SMO,* supramalleolar orthoses; *RGO,* reciprocating gait orthoses; *HKAFO,* hip-knee-ankle-foot orthoses.

(glossopharyngeal) and cranial nerve X (vagus).[4] Other symptoms associated with Chiari II malformation include vocal cord paralysis, stridor (especially with inspiration), apnea when crying or at night, and/or bronchial aspiration.[96]

Sensory Integrity. MM causes sensory deficits as well as paralysis. Although sensory levels often do not coincide with motor levels, findings from sensory and motor testing can help to establish the spinal lesion level.[96] Because sensory deficits may be complete, incomplete, or skip areas, it is important to test all dermatomes, as well as multiple sites within each dermatome.[4] Additionally, different sensory modalities (light touch, pain, proprioception, kinesthetic, vibration, and thermal) should be tested because these are transmitted by different parts of the spinal cord. Results are recorded on a dermatome chart indicating areas of absent and altered sensitivity.

Sensory testing differs according to the age and cognitive level of the child. In infancy, reactions to pain sensation, such as facial grimace or cry, are observed. The order of testing can begin with the lowest to highest level of innervation: Anal area, across the buttocks, down the posterior thigh and leg, anterior surface of the leg and thigh, and abdominal muscles.[94] In young children, from 2-7 years of age, light touch and proprioception can be tested along with pain sensation when child-friendly testing procedures are used.[94] Schneider and Gabriel give the example of using games, such as "Tell me when the puppet touches you," or "Put your hand out for a sticker when I touch you," to elicit accurate and reliable responses.[94] From ages 7 years on, thermal and 2-point discrimination sensory testing may be reliably performed.[94]

Educating the family and individual with MM about the sensory deficit is an important component of management. Insensitive areas require vigilant attention and protection from skin breakdown, abrasions, and burns. Shurtleff reported that 95% of children with spina bifida experience some form of skin breakdown before they reach adulthood.[112] Persons with insensitivity may develop skin problems from sitting because they do not shift their weight, change their position, or relieve pressure.[96] Skin breakdown commonly occurs over bony prominences such as the greater trochanter, ischii, sacrum, or heels. Bowel and bladder deficits contribute to skin maceration in the diaper area. Skin abrasions of the knees and feet can occur as the child moves by crawling or creeping. Proper shoe and orthotic fit is also essential to avoid pressure sores and abrasions. Bath water temperature must always be tested before placing the child in the tub. Serious burns can and do occur because of the inability to sense temperature. Pressure relief and skin inspection should be taught early on, so they are incorporated into the daily routine.[4]

Motor Function—Control and Learning

Neurogenic Bowel and Bladder. The bladder, urinary outlet, and rectum are innervated by spinal segments S2-S4. Because these nerves leave the spinal cord in the lower sacrum, bowel and bladder dysfunction occurs in most children with MM and fewer than 5% develop voluntary urinary and anal sphincter control.[113] Even children with sacral level lesions with normal leg movement often have bowel and bladder problems.[102] The two major functions of the bladder are storing urine produced by the kidneys and emptying urine once the bladder is full. Children with MM have problems with both functions, resulting in incontinence.[114] Incomplete emptying of the bladder is of concern and may predispose the child to urinary tract infections and kidney damage; therefore regular urological evaluations are necessary throughout life. Various types of bladder dysfunction can occur, depending on the spinal cord lesion affecting lower motor neuron and upper motor neuron loops.[79] An areflexic system results in constant dribbling, whereas an excessively tight urinary sphincter results in frequent small volume urination. Urological management objectives are prevention of renal damage and socially acceptable control of incontinence.[95] Bladder training programs include regularly scheduled clean intermittent catheterization. Six- to eight-year-old children can usually master the catheterization technique.[4] An appendicovesicostomy (catheterizing the bladder through an abdominal stoma) is a recent method used to empty the bladder and has the added benefit of not requiring clothing removal and wheel-chair transfers.[79]

Neurogenic bowel dysfunction is closely associated with neurogenic bladder dysfunction. Bowel problems are related to uncoordinated propulsive action of the intestines, an ineffective anal sphincter, and a lack of rectal sensation.[102] The anal sphincter can be flaccid, hypotonic, or spastic, causing different types of dysfunction during defecation. The lack of anorectal sensation prevents the individual from receiving sensory information of an imminent bowel movement and frequently results in bowel incontinence.[4] Constipation and impaction are also common and may be interspersed with periods of overflow diarrhea.[102] Lower motor neuron innervation of the sphincter, tested by the presence of a bulbocavernosus or anal cutaneous reflex, is highly predictive of a successful bowel training program.[115] Bowel training programs can be highly successful and bowel continence should be a goal for the preschool or early elementary school-aged child with MM.[79]

Rehabilitation management to facilitate bowel continence may include abdominal strengthening and wheelchair push-ups to assist bowel motility; education about skin inspection; ADL functional training for bathing, dressing, and toileting; recommendations for adaptive equipment, including wheelchair cushions and bathroom modifications; and functional transfer training.

Function

Gait, Locomotion, and Balance. Mobility achievement by children with MM has received much attention in the literature with most of the focus being on bipedal ambulation (Fig. 15-11). In this population, mobility must be expanded from the concept of walking to include any efficient and effective means of moving about that enables the individual to easily traverse and explore the environment and independently pursue an education, vocation, or avocation.[99] Endurance, efficiency, effectiveness, safety, degree of independence, and accessibility can all be monitored for the different types of mobility, including

generally delivered 2 or 3 times per week for 30 minutes, whereas in the acute care hospital setting, therapy is generally delivered daily for 30 minutes. The intensity recommended is also often related to the severity of involvement of the child; infants with more delayed development tend to receive more therapy.[140] To date, studies in which therapy has been provided in variable intensities have not been conclusive. Some studies show that greater frequency of treatments yields better results, including improvement in motor function,[141-144] whereas other studies have not shown such an advantage.[139] The interventional intensity considered by the therapist should take into account the child's age, type and severity of impairments, task demands, and skill level.

HEALTH PROMOTION AND PREVENTION OF SECONDARY COMPLICATIONS

One goal for habilitation of children is to promote the attainment and long-term maintenance of functional goals and community participation. Life-long, early-onset chronic disabilities cause primary impairments, as well as secondary conditions that develop with age. Secondary conditions develop for a variety of reasons, including (1) overuse of an already weakened neuromuscular system; (2) underuse or misuse because of poor movement quality, immobility, or deconditioning; (3) poor lifestyle behaviors, such as lack of exercise and/or poor nutrition; and (4) environmental and attitudinal barriers that may limit access to preventive services and opportunities for social participation and health-promoting activities.[145] A child who acquires movement of poor quality may develop compensatory patterns that over time lead to musculoskeletal deformities (e.g., scoliosis), skin breakdown, joint pain, and osteoporosis. Intervention strategies must weigh the inherent trade-offs between facilitating function despite poor movement quality and restricting function with a goal of higher movement quality.[146] Neither of these is ideal nor is it currently possible to totally resolve the neuromuscular impairments that contribute to atypical movement quality. Campbell advises therapists to wisely and judiciously consider the child's use of compensations and work toward goals that promote both current and future needs.[128]

It has been suggested that individuals with neuromuscular impairments should maintain higher levels of physical fitness than the general population to offset the decline in function associated with the disorder in addition to the changes related to typical ageing.[147] The *Guide* emphasizes the importance of primary prevention and risk reduction strategies within a complete physical therapy intervention program.[1] Promotion of physical fitness and life-long habits of physical activity can enhance health and prevent diseases in adulthood.[148] Physical fitness programs for children with neuromuscular disorders should include activities that promote cardiorespiratory endurance, muscular strength and endurance, flexibility, and ideal body composition. The principles of an effective conditioning program, including specificity of training, intensity, frequency, and duration, should also be incorporated in an intervention program for children with neuromuscular disorders (see Chapter 23).

FOCUSED INTERVENTIONS

When selecting an intervention for a child with a neuromuscular disorder, it is essential to analyze why the child has greater difficulties moving in and out of their environments and participating in life tasks than a child without deficits. The overall goal is for the child to participate in a variety of venues (e.g., home, school, playground) using their upper extremities freely while engaging in body transport or movement with a stable posture while being able to pay attention to the environment. The intervention program should address goals that can be maintained over the lifetime of the client. Box 15-1 outlines commonly overlooked areas when designing an intervention program that has effects that last a lifetime.[146]

Valvano[149] describes two intervention models for children with neuromuscular disorders: *Activity-focused intervention* and *impairment-focused intervention*. Activity-focused interventions involve structured practice and repetition of functional actions. Impairment-focused interventions address impairments in body structure and functions that affect the process of motor learning and may cause secondary impairments.

Activity-focused interventions are system-based and include the task-oriented approach and constraint-induced movement therapy. An activity-focused intervention often adapts the physical environment by using therapeutic equipment, such as balls and bolsters, and adaptive equipment, such as seating and mobility aids.

Impairment-focused interventions include *neurodevelopmental treatment* (NDT), strength training, electrotherapeutic modalities, biofeedback, and aerobic conditioning.

Passive impairment-focused interventions are aimed at reducing primary or secondary musculoskeletal impair-

---

BOX 15-1	**Characteristics of an Intervention Program That Produces Life-Long Results**

- Promotes engagement in life-long fitness activities, including exercise, proper nutrition and hydration, weight control, stress management, and energy conservation for meaningful pursuits.
- Promotes the individual's ability to take personal responsibility for personal health, to be knowledgeable about one's own condition, and to be assertive in addressing needs: Is the individual encouraged to speak, or otherwise communicate, for himself or herself?
- Program supports the child's motivation to persist in attaining difficult goals, despite failure along the way.
- Program develops the individual's perception of self-control and successful accomplishment of personally meaningful goals that are likely to foster self-esteem.
- Program uses activities that over the short and long term are not likely to lead to chronic musculoskeletal problems and excess fatigue to the detriment of engagement in meaningful activities.
- Program fosters prevention of increasing impairment rather than promoting function at all costs.

Data from Campbell SK: *Phys Occup Ther Ped* 17(1):10-15, 1997.

ments. Passive impairment-focused interventions include manual therapy techniques, therapeutic electrical stimulation administered while the child sleeps, positioning equipment (stander, long-sitter, orthoses, splints, and casts), and therapeutic exercises such as ROM and flexibility procedures not administered in the context of a purposeful task.

Sensory integration (SI) is a commonly described intervention approach that is primarily used by occupational therapists working with patients with neuromuscular disorders. Conductive education (CE) and Mobility Opportunities Via Education (MOVE) are adaptive education programs designed for children with neuromotor impairments. CE and MOVE programs are generally applied by teachers rather than by habilitation clinicians; therapists may provide input to teachers regarding their use for a particular child.

Currently, few systematic reviews, meta-analyses, or randomized clinical trials exist on interventions used with children with CP. There are a number of articles pertaining to prevention and medical treatment of various conditions in children with MM, but there are no evidence-based habilitation studies recorded in the Cochrane Library, including the Cochrane Database of Systematic Reviews.

Activity-Focused Interventions

Task-Oriented Approach. Task-oriented motor approaches emphasizing the learning of motor tasks that increase independence and participation in daily tasks are currently emphasized in interventions for children with neuromuscular disorders such as CP; however, the evidence supporting this practice is currently in its infancy and there are no systematic studies regarding the effectiveness of this intervention approach. There is also no single, generally accepted task-oriented approach for children with CP. Rather, therapists individually combine the concepts of motor learning, motor control, motor development, and learning theory in their clinical practice. The concepts emphasized are the therapeutic use of purposeful, functional skills; active role of the learner; role of feedback in learning; type and amount of practice and experimentation; promotion of flexible strategies through variation of practice; and the transfer of learning from one skill to another and among different environments (see Chapter 16). Task-oriented approaches have limited application for children with MM because most assume that spinal cord and peripheral innervation are intact and therefore the patient can learn to use affected body parts through extensive and appropriate practice. Box 15-2 lists general guidelines for applying the principles of a task-oriented approach to clinical practice.[150]

Valvano's model of activity-based interventions involves developing activity-related goals and objectives, planning activity-focused interventions (AFI) based on the environment and tasks to be accomplished, and integrating these with impairment-focused interventions (IFI) to develop a complete intervention plan (Fig. 15-12).[151] The goals focus on outcomes that allow the child to increase function and/or participation at home, school, or in the community. Components that limit achievement of these

---

BOX 15-2	**General Guidelines for Applying a Task-Oriented Approach to Clinical Practice**

- Identify important, meaningful tasks that the child has difficultly performing.
- Select tasks that are the focus of intervention reasonably within the child's capabilities to learn.
- Observe the child perform the task in the environment where it is naturally performed, when possible, and document current level of abilities.
- Analyze the requirements and characteristics of the task.
- Analyze the demands and characteristics of the environment in which the task is performed. Consider physical characteristics, regulatory conditions, and the sociocultural context.
- Examine and evaluate the child's performance on the task and determine what the child is able to do, what the child is unable to do, task and environmental constraints that interfere with successful performance, and task and environmental factors that support the success of the performance.
- Identify possible intervention strategies directed toward reducing the constraints considering the influence of the musculoskeletal, neuromuscular, cardiovascular/pulmonary, and integumentary systems; possible modifications of the task and environment; type of feedback; and practice schedule.
- Allow the child to practice the task under the specific conditions, provide feedback, and document performance level.

Data from Kaplan M, Bedell G: Motor skill acquisition frame of reference. In Kramer P, Hinojosa J (eds): *Frames of Reference for Pediatric Occupational Therapy*, ed 2, New York, 1999, Lippincott Williams & Wilkins.

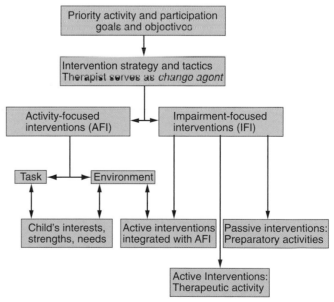

FIG. 15-12 Model of activity-based intervention for children with neurological conditions. *Adapted from Valvano J: Phys Occup Ther Ped 24: 82, 2004.*

goals, including impairments such as decreased strength and ROM, are then assessed. Activity-focused interventions involve practice of actions that produce results related to the overall goals rather than on patterns or quality of movement. The intervention is planned according to motor learning guidelines, taking into consideration the strengths and learning needs of the child. Practice may be variable (rehearsal of a number of variations) or constant (rehearsal of only one variation) and generally includes augmented instruction (physical guidance, focus of attention to the task requirements, setting of goals for the child) and feedback about the results and performance of the task. Impairment-level interventions are integrated with activity-focused interventions so that impairments that critically limit performance are addressed within the context of active practice.

Research on the effectiveness of the task-oriented approach for children with neuromuscular disorders remains scarce and interpretation of findings is complex,[152] as demonstrated by the following two studies.[153,154] Thorpe and Valvano examined the effects of presenting augmented information to children with CP during practice of a novel motor skill.[153] Thirteen children with level III CP aged 6-12 years (mean = 8.6 years) were randomly assigned to one of three practice protocols (no augmented information, knowledge of performance, and knowledge of performance enhanced by a cognitive strategy) while performing 36 10-second trials to learn to move a therapeutic exercise vehicle (Pedalo) backwards. Knowledge of performance was verbally provided to the child ("your body was too bent over" or "your knees were too close together"). Cognitive strategies were provided by presenting the child with a picture of images of actions along with a corresponding verbal label. For example, a picture of a toy soldier standing straight was labeled "standing straight like a soldier." All subjects improved their performance during treatment sessions; however, only eight subjects maintained a significant improvement. One of these eight subjects demonstrated significant improvement in performance with practice alone, two when provided with knowledge of performance, and five when provided with knowledge of performance enhanced by a cognitive strategy. The researchers concluded that children with CP benefit from practice of the motor task and that some children may benefit from knowledge of performance enhanced by a cognitive strategy. Augmented information may have had a small effect because of the amount and content of the verbal instruction or disparity in subject characteristics (age, degree of motor impairment).

Ketelaar et al compared a functional physical therapy program with a standard physical therapy program in 55 Dutch children aged 2-7 years (median = 55 months) with mild or moderate spastic CP.[154] A modified randomized block design was used, and children were assessed before the intervention and at 6, 12, and 18 months after the intervention. Outcome measures were GMFM scores and the self-care, mobility and caregiver assistance domains of the Pediatric Evaluation of Disability Index (PEDI). Interventions were based on a task-specific individual plan designed to help the child master important functional skills. The main features of this approach were the estab-

lishment of functional goals, repetitive practice of the problematic motor abilities in functional situations, an active role for the child, and active involvement of parents throughout the program. Standard physical therapy was only described as a neurophysiological treatment method (NDT or Vojta method), with the assumption that attention was directed at promoting normalization of movement. Neither of the two treatment programs was standardized because of variability among the subjects' impairments and functional limitations. Precise intensity of the interventions was difficult to ascertain and was not constant throughout the study. Frequency of therapy for the standard physical therapy group was reported to gradually increase from a mean of 3.8 times per month at the time of the initial measurements to a mean of 4.3 times per month (standard deviation [SD] = 1.3, n = 19) on the last follow-up assessment. Frequency of functional training gradually decreased from a mean of 3.4 times per month to a mean of 2.4 times per month (SD = 1.3, n = 19) on the last follow-up assessment. There was a significant difference (t[37] = 4.44, $p > 0.001$) between the groups' frequency on the last follow-up assessment. All sessions lasted an average of 45 minutes. Both treatment groups improved on all domains of the GMFM; the groups did not differ with respect to the degree of improvement. The functional group showed significantly higher gains in function as measured by the self-care and mobility domains of the PEDI. The researchers conclude that physical therapy treatment that focuses on function, rather than on normalization of movement, leads to a greater increase in daily functional skill and independence in children with mild to moderate CP.

In general, studies have shown that children who participate in task-oriented therapy do show improvements in their ability to perform functional skills; however, there is insufficient data from well-controlled trials to definitively conclude that this type of intervention is superior to others or exceeds the effects of time and maturation alone.

Therapeutic Equipment. The clinician may use various equipment, such as mats, benches, bolsters, balls, "eggs" (egg-shaped balls), and "peanuts" (peanut-shaped balls) (Fig. 15-13), to alter the physical environment during practice to support the performance of motor skills such as rolling from prone to supine, moving from prone to sitting, or from half-kneeling to standing.[149] Equipment can allow the therapist to control the degree and direction of movement within the context of the environment, introduce instability to the movement, and control the degree to which a movement is assisted by or performed against gravity.[155]

Assistive Mobility Devices. The success of activity-based interventions often depends on the use of appropriate assistive devices to help the child with functional, energy-efficient mobility (bed, floor, wheelchair, ambulation, and transfer). These devices include items such as walkers, crutches, canes, wheelchairs, bicycles, and tricycles (see Chapter 33). Once the child is identified as needing an assistive device, the therapist must decide which devices provide the appropriate support, minimize secondary complications such as overuse syndromes, support energy

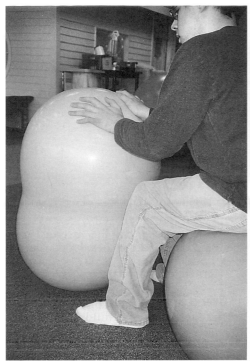

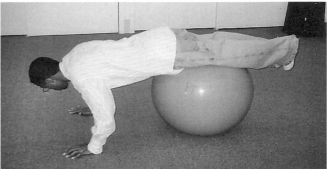

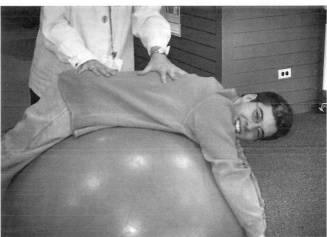

FIG. 15-13 Interventions using balls of various shapes and sizes.

efficient mobility for needed distances, and are useful in the child's home, school, outdoor, and community settings. Changes in body proportions and environmental demands necessitate reevaluating mobility options across the lifespan.[4]

Walker configurations (anterior versus posterior), number and placement of wheels, and upper extremity placement (turned-up handles, forearm trough support) are evaluated to determine the effect on the child's upright posture, body alignment, and center of gravity. Park and colleagues compared gait pattern and energy consumption in 10 children with spastic CP (mean age – 9 years) when using anterior and posterior walkers.[156] Energy expenditure, as measured by oxygen consumption and oxygen cost, was significantly lower with the posterior walker than with the anterior walker, although walking speed was not significantly different between the walker types. Prior studies had not reached consensus on which type of walker was preferred[157-159]; however, Park also found that the posterior walker facilitated a more upright walking position and decreased the amount of double support time.[156]

Less restrictive devices, such as canes or crutches, have the advantage of allowing children to negotiate smaller spaces. Their weight and height will affect how much support they give, upper extremity orientation, and the child's center of gravity. Support may be reduced gradually from Lofstrand crutches, quad canes, tripod canes, or offset handle straight canes to encourage more weight

bearing through the lower extremities as the child develops better control (Fig. 15-14).

Tricycles and bicycles can be a fun adjunct to any intervention program and provide a means of mobility for children who cannot walk. The cycle should be evaluated for fit and alignment. The ease with which the cycle can be pedaled, as well as the effort it takes to move the wheels, should be considered in cycle selection. Cycling promotes weight shift through the pelvis, lower extremity dissociation, upright posture with bilateral hand use, an age-appropriate means of negotiating the environment, and provides an opportunity to socialize with peers.

Palisano and colleagues[160] described the usual mobility methods of 636 children with CP living in Ontario, Canada, in home, school, outdoor, and community settings. The children were stratified by age and GMFCS level. The study found that mobility methods varied by age, severity of involvement and environmental setting. For example, children with GMFCS level I CP aged 2-3 years old generally could walk alone in all settings. Children with GMFCS level II CP of the same age sometimes could walk alone but often were carried by an adult; pushed by an adult in a stroller or wheelchair; rolled, crept, or crawled on the floor; or walked with support. Children were more dependent on adult assistance for mobility when outdoors and in the community than at home. This study suggests that the clinician should consider mobility in all settings, physical and social features of the

activities is performed to determine his ability level, and techniques for practicing missing components were implemented. When working on these activities, weight shifting, hip stability, and active isolated muscle control of lower extremities are emphasized. A modified adult tricycle was introduced so that he could work on the scouting cycling merit badge. He prefers using the modified tricycle rather than the alternative of not participating. TQ is exploring motor skills that will be necessary for him to fully participate in the college environment and skills that will maintain his mobility.

CASE STUDY 15-2

MYELOMENINGOCELE

Examination at Birth to 6 Months of Age
Patient History
JM is a 6-month-old boy with a diagnosis of MM at T12, arrested hydrocephalus, and resolved hydronephrosis (internal dilation of the kidney). He has a VP shunt and vesicotomy (surgical creation of a stoma between the anterior bladder wall and the skin of the lower abdomen). His history is significant for the presence of Chiari II malformation, right subluxed hip, and bilateral equinovalgus with calcaneus deformities. He was born 1 month premature, and his MM was repaired at birth.

Tests and Measures at 6 Months of Age
Musculoskeletal

Range of Motion JM's upper extremity ROM is within normal limits. His lower extremities have a tendency to be in a "windswept" (hip flexion and adduction) position to the right. He has minor limitations in hip abduction and external rotation. Ankle plantarflexion is limited as a result of his bilateral foot deformity.

Neuromuscular: JM has flaccid paralysis at the thoracic level 12 and below, with slightly more motor innervation on the right than on the left side. Toe fasciculations are present. LE postural control responses are absent.

Integumentary: Scars from the surgical repair of the MM, shunt insertion and vesicotomy procedure are all well healed.

Function: JM can prop himself on flexed arms in the prone position and commando crawl. He cannot sit independently.

Evaluation, Diagnosis, and Prognosis
JM presents with delay in acquisition of age appropriate motor milestones, flaccidity (T12 and below), asymmetrical findings, delayed postural control, and abnormal body alignment. The diagnosis is preferred practice pattern 5C: Impaired motor function and sensory integrity associated with nonprogressive disorders of the CNS.

Intervention
JM began receiving early intervention services at 6 months of age. He was treated at home (1 hour once per week) and in an outpatient early intervention program (3 times a week, morning session). The rehabilitation program used both activity and impairment-level interventions to promote gross motor skills and maintain and improve lower extremity ROM. Because of some residual muscle activity of the right hip, therapy focused on keeping the hip muscles balanced with the goal of preventing future hip contractures. Activity-level intervention focused on promoting independent sitting balance with the trunk over the pelvis and activation of innervated abdominal muscles while JM engaged in reaching and bimanual hand skills. To maintain lower extremity ROM, JM wears Aquaplast SAOs during the day. An A-frame with SAOs are used for night time positioning. A parapodium was used as JM's first standing device to promote static standing, as well as beginning ambulation, skills. The parapodium is introduced at the time when a child would normally pull to stand, approximately 8-10 months of age.

Examination at 5 to 6 Years of Age
Patient History
JM underwent a right iliopsoas and percutaneous adductor longus tenotomy, varus osteotomy, and acetabular shelf procedure at $1\frac{1}{2}$ years of age.

Tests and Measures
Musculoskeletal: Upper extremity mobility and strength are within normal limits for his age. Lower extremity ROM is within normal limits except for the bilateral calcaneal deformity.

Neuromuscular: JM's intact muscle strength has been maximized. Righting and equilibrium responses are intact for his upper extremities and trunk above the T12 level. Upper extremity protective extension responses are intact in all directions (forward, sideways, and backward).

Integumentary: JM's skin is intact; however, he had a pressure ulcer on his right knee that occurred during his inpatient hospital stay.

Function: JM can complete many fundamental motor skills. He can roll, sit independent with arms free, transition from the floor to sitting, and maintain tall kneeling with upper extremity support. He ambulates using RGOs and Lofstrand crutches He can don/doff his orthosis independently and can lock his orthosis and come to standing independently. He is a community walker. He can safely cross a busy intersection in the allotted time frame.

Intervention
JM attends a school program housed in a rehabilitation center. He receives therapy 5 days per week. The rehabilitation program emphasizes maintaining and improving ROM and muscle strength, improving functional skills, progressing adaptive devices for mobility, and education in skin protection. Ambulation initially required an anterior walker. He progressed to using a reversed walker, then heavy Lofstrand crutches and then lightweight Lofstrand crutches. Treatment addresses ascending and descending stairs and curbs. This activity is difficult for JM and requires much practice. Throughout this time, improvement and maintenance of ROM and strength were emphasized through daily ROM and strengthening exercises of

the intact muscles during practice of functional skills. Scar tissue was kept mobile through massage. JM will be trained in skin inspection and monitoring.

Examination at 14 to 15 Years of Age
Patient History
JM's vesicostomy was closed. A clean catheterization procedure is now used for bladder management. JM developed an allergy to latex.

Tests and Measures
Musculoskeletal: Lower extremity malalignment is developing due to lack of orthosis use, uneven muscle innervation, and prolonged effects of gravity. JM has tibial valgum on the left and bilateral knee and hip flexion contractures, although currently his lower extremity ROM is within functional range.

Neuromuscular: Status is unchanged.

Integumentary: There is a small healed scar on the right knee as a result of a staphylococcal infection during an earlier hospitalization.

Function: JM continues to use lightweight Lofstrand crutches for mobility, but he no longer wears any type of orthosis.

Intervention
JM receives rehabilitation services at home because therapy was not consistently delivered at his high school to avoid interference with his academic instruction. Mobility is augmented with a wheelchair, which he currently uses full time. Prior ambulation training was successful in development of postural control and mastering transfer skills. JM is interested in practicing ambulation for possible future use of this skill. At home, his primary mode of mobility is scooting on his bottom; however, this has lead to some adverse secondary compensations (left tibial valgum).

The focus of therapy is to maintain integrity of the shoulder girdle, ensure that full mobility and strength are maintained, alternate positions from the wheelchair during the day, and maintain trunk and lower extremity alignment and mobility. A greater proportion of the therapy session is spent on soft tissue mobility. JM competes competitively in swimming, preferring the backstroke. Currently, he is interested in preparing for competitive wheelchair racing, so endurance and strength training have become a self-driven goal. He is active in scouting. Some adaptations are necessary for him to participate in camping events; he requires an air mattress for skin protection and must bring extra water to ward off dehydration.

CHAPTER SUMMARY
This chapter addresses the management of children with nonprogressive CNS disorders. CP and MM, two disorders representing these practice patterns, are presented to illustrate how their pathology and natural history are linked to the clinical judgments regarding rehabilitation interventions aimed at improving motor performance and promoting the attainment and maintenance of functional goals and community participation. The evidence supporting or refuting clinical interventions is reviewed. Further studies are needed to evaluate the plethora of therapeutic approaches addressing multiple neuromuscular conditions across the lifespan. To paraphrase the Committee on Integrating the Science of Early Childhood Development,[19] "successful interventions are determined by sound strategies, acceptability to the child and caregivers, and quality implementation."

ADDITIONAL RESOURCES

Useful Forms
Gross Motor Function Classification System (GMFCS) for Cerebral Palsy
Gross Motor Function Measure (GMFM)
Pediatric Evaluation of Disability Index (PEDI)

Books
Campbell SK: *Decision Making In Pediatric Neurologic Physical Therapy,* New York, 1999, Churchill Livingstone.
Campbell SK, Vander Linden DW, Palisano RJ (eds): *Physical Therapy for Children,* ed 2, Philadelphia, 2000, WB Saunders.
Effgen SK (ed): *Meeting the Physical Therapy Needs of Children,* Philadelphia, 2005, FA Davis.
Long T, Cintas H: *Handbook of Pediatric Physical Therapy,* Baltimore, 1995, Williams & Wilkins.
Shumway-Cook A, Woollacott MH: *Motor Control: Theory and Practical Applications,* ed 2, New York, 2001, Lippincott Williams & Wilkins.

Web Sites
Pedi Links: www.uvm.edu
Spina Bifida Association of America: www.sbaa.org
United Cerebral Palsy (UCP): www.ucp.org

GLOSSARY

Activity-focused intervention: Plan of care that incorporates structured practice and repetition of functional activities that emphasizes a child's ability to learn motor tasks that increase independence and participation in daily responsibilities.

Baclofen: Pharmacological agent, administered either orally or intrathecally, to reduce spasticity.

Botulinum toxin A (BtA): A toxin that paralyzes muscles by interfering with transmission at the neuromuscular junction. BtA can be administered by injection into selected muscles to temporarily reduce muscle tone and spasticity and thereby promote increased ROM and improved function in children with neuromuscular disorders.

Cerebral palsy (CP): A symptom complex of static, nonprogressive posture and movement abnormalities caused by damage to the developing CNS in which motor impairment occurs before, during, and/or soon after birth.

Chiari II malformation: Anomaly of the hindbrain associated with open spinal dysraphism.

Closed spinal dysraphism (CSD): Congenital malformation of the spine and spinal cord where the neural tissue is covered by skin, although cutaneous stigmata, such as hairy nevus, capillary hemangioma, dimples, and subcutaneous masses, may exist.

Constraint-induced movement therapy (CIMT): A task-oriented intervention involving restraining the nonparetic upper extremity in conjunction with highly intensive, repetitive, and structured functional activities for the hemiparetic upper extremity.

Dyskinetic CP: A type of CP characterized by impaired volitional activity (athetosis, rigidity, and tremor) with uncontrolled and purposeless movements affecting the entire body.

Full-term infant: A baby born between 37-42 weeks of gestation.

Gross Motor Function Classification System (GMFCS): An ordinal, five-level system for categorizing the severity of CP based on self-initiated movement, need for assistive technology, and movement quality at a given age.

Impairment-focused intervention: A plan of care that addresses impairments in body structure and functions.

Low birth weight: A baby who weighs less than 2,500 gm (5 lb, 7½ oz) at birth.

Myelomeningocele (MM): An OSD that occurs when a segment of the spinal cord and meninges protrudes through a bony defect in the midline of the back and is exposed to the environment.

Neonatal encephalopathy: A clinically defined syndrome of disturbed neurological function in the earliest days of life in the full-term infant, manifested by abnormal consciousness, depression of tone and reflexes, feeding and respiratory difficulties, and/or seizures.

Neural tube defect (NTD): Incomplete development of the brain, spinal cord and/or meninges as a result of errors or disturbances in any of the embryogenic process.

Neurodevelopmental treatment (NDT): Impairment-focused intervention that uses a developmental framework emphasizing a child's ability to learn functional skills and typical movement patterns.

Open spinal dysraphism (OSD): Congenital malformation of the spine and spinal cord where nervous tissue and/or meninges are exposed to the environment through a congenital bony defect of the vertebrae.

Premature infant: A baby born at less than 37 weeks of gestation.

Selective dorsal rhizotomy (SDR): Neurosurgical intervention where selective sensory nerve roots in the lumbar and sacral region are transected to reduce spasticity.

Spastic diplegia: A clinical type of CP characterized by paresis and hypertonicity of the entire body, with the legs being more involved than the arms.

Spastic hemiplegia: A clinical type of CP with paresis and hypertonicity on one side of the body, including the arm, trunk, and leg.

Spastic quadriplegia: A clinical type of CP with paresis and hypertonicity of the entire body with all four extremities relatively equally involved.

Spina bifida: Generic term used to describe spinal dysraphism.

Spinal dysraphism: Congenital malformations of the spine and spinal cord, including anomalies of the skin, muscles, vertebrae, meninges, and nervous tissue.

References

1. American Physical Therapy Association: Guide to Physical Therapist Practice, second edition, *Phys Ther* 81(1):6-746, 2001.
2. Nelson K: Can we prevent cerebral palsy? *N Engl J Med* 349(18):1765-1769, 2003.
3. Olney S, Wright M: Cerebral palsy. In Campbell S, Vander Linden D, Palisano RJ (eds): *Physical Therapy for Children,* ed 2, New York, 2000, WB Saunders.
4. Hinderer K, Hinderer S, Shurtleff D: Myelodysplasia. In Campbell S, Vander Linden D, Palisano RJ (eds): *Physical Therapy for Children,* ed 2, New York, 2000, WB Saunders.
5. Shevell M, Majnemer A, Morin I: Etiologic yield of cerebral palsy: A contemporary case study, *Pediatr Neurol* 28(5):352-359, 2003.
6. Kuban K: Cerebral palsy, *N Engl J Med* 330:188-195, 1994.
7. Batshaw M, Perret Y: *Children with Disabilities: A Medical Primer,* ed 3, Toronto, 1992, Paul H. Brookes.
8. Boyle C, Yeargin-Allsopp M, Doernberg N, et al: Prevalence of selected developmental disabilities in children 3-10 years of age: The Metropolitan Atlanta Developmental Disabilities Surveillance program, *MMWR CDC Surveill Summ* 45:1-14, 1996.
9. Hagberg V, Hagberg G, Olow I, et al: The changing panorama of cerebral palsy in Sweden. V. The birth year period 1979-82, *Acta Paediatr Scand* 78:283-290, 1989.
10. Hagberg B, Hagberg G, Olow I: The changing panorama of cerebral palsy in Sweden. VI. Prevalence and origin during the birth year period 1983-1986, *Acta Paediatr* 82:387-393, 1993.
11. Stanley F, Watson L: The cerebral palsies in Western Australia: 1968-1981, *Am J Obstet Gynecol* 158:89-93, 1988.
12. Paneth N: Etiologic factors in cerebral palsy, *Pediatr Ann* 15:191-201, 1986.
13. Hankins G: Neonatal encephalopathy and cerebral palsy: Defining the pathogenesis and pathophysiology, Washington, DC, 2003, American College of Obstetricians and Gynecologists.
14. Freeman J, Nelson K: Intrapartum asphyxia and cerebral palsy, *Pediatrics* 82:240-249, 1988.
15. Lequin M, Barkovich A: Current concepts of cerebral malformation syndromes, *Current Opin Pediatr* 11:492-496, 1999.
16. Badawi N, Kurinczuk J, Keogh J, et al: Intrapartum risk factors for newborn encephalopathy: the Western Australian case-control study. BMJ. 1998;317:1554-1558
17. Wollack J, Nichter C: Static encephalopathies. In: Rudolph A, Rudolph C (eds): Rudolph's Pediatrics. 21st ed, New York, McGraw-Hill; 2002.
18. National Institute of Neurological Disorders and Stroke: Cerebral palsy: Hope through research, National Institute of Health. Accessed October 26, 2004.
19. Shonkoff JP: From neurons to neighborhoods: Old and new challenges for developmental and behavioral pediatrics, *J Devel Behav Pediatr* 24(1):70-76, 2003.
20. Lynch J, Nelson K: Epidemiology of perinatal stroke, *Curr Opin Pediatr* 13:499-505, 2001.
21. Grether J, Nelson K: Maternal infection and cerebral palsy in infants of normal birth weight, *JAMA* 278:207-211, 1997.
22. Hankins G: The long journey: Defining the true pathogenesis and pathophysiology of neonatal encephalopathy and cerebral palsy, *Obstet Gynecol Surv* 58(7):435-437, 2003.
23. Petterson B, Nelson K, Watson L, et al: Twins, triplets, and cerebral palsy in births in Western Australia in the 1980s, *BMJ* 307:1239-1243, 1993.
24. Stromberg B, Dahlquist G, Ericson A, et al: Neurological sequelae in children born after in-vitro fertilisation: A population-based study, *Lancet* 359:461-465, 2002.
25. Nelson K, Grether J: Potentially asphyxiating conditions and spastic cerebral palsy in infants of normal birth weight, *Am J Obstet Gynecol* 179(2):507-513, 1998.
26. Thacker S, Stroup D, Chang M: Continuous electronic heart rate monitoring for fetal assessment during labor, *Cochrane Database Syst Rev* 2:CD000063, 2001.
27. Dormans J, Pellegrino L: Caring for children with cerebral palsy, Baltimore, 1998, Paul H. Brookes.
28. Murphy C, Yeargin-Allsopp M, Decoufle P, et al: Prevalence of cerebral palsy among ten-year-old children in metropolitan Atlanta, 1985 through 1987, *J Pediatr Orthop* 123(5):S13-20, 1993.
29. Postnatal causes of developmental disabilities in children aged 3 to 10 years: Atlanta, Georgia 1991, *MMWR Morb Wkly Rep* 16 45(6):130-134, 1996.
30. Wilson-Howle J: Cerebral palsy. In Campbell S (ed): *Decision Making in Pediatric Neurologic Physical Therapy,* New York, 1999, Churchill Livingstone.
31. Minear W: A classification of cerebral palsy, *Pediatrics* 18:841-852, 1956.
32. Ratliffe K: *Clinical Pediatric Physical Therapy: A Guide for the Physical Therapy Team,* St. Louis, 1988, Mosby.
33. Pellegrino L: Cerebral palsy. In Batshaw M (ed): *Children with Disabilities,* ed 4, Baltimore, 1997, Paul H. Brookes.
34. Fletcher N, Marsden C: Dyskinetic cerebral palsy: A clinical and genetic study. *Dev Med Child Neurol* 38:873, 1996.
35. Yokochi K, Aiba K, Kodama M, et al: Motor function of infants with athetoid cerebral palsy. *Dev Med Child Neurol* 35:909, 1993.
36. Lesny I: Follow-up study of hypotonic forms of cerebral palsy, *Brain Dev* 1:87, 1979.
37. Russell D, Rosenbaum P, Avery L, et al: Gross Motor Function Measure (GMFM-66 & GMFM-88) User's Manual, New York, 2002, Mac Keith Press.
38. Palisano RJ, Rosenbaum P, Walter S, et al: Development and reliability of a system to classify gross motor function in children with cerebral palsy, *Dev Med Child Neurol* 39:214-223, 1997.
39. Morris C, Bartlett D: Gross motor function classification system: Impact and utility, *Dev Med Child Neurol* 46:60-65, 2004.
40. Beckung E, Hagberg G: Correlation between the ICIDH handicap code and Gross Motor Function Classification System in children with cerebral palsy, *Dev Med Child Neurol* 42:669-673, 2000.
41. Blair E, Watson L, Badawi N, et al: Life expectancy among people with cerebral palsy in Western Australia, *Dev Med Child Neurol* 43:508-515, 2001.
42. Evans P, Evans S, Alberman E: Cerebral palsy: Why we plan for survival, *Arch Dis Child* 65:1329-1333, 1990.
43. Hutton J, Colver A, Mackie P: Effect of severity of disability on survival in north east England cerebral palsy cohort, *Arch Dis Child* 83:469-474, 2000.
44. Hutton J, Pharoah P: Effects of cognitive, motor, and sensory disabilities on survival in cerebral palsy, *Arch Dis Child* 86:84-90, 2002.
45. Ostensjo S, Carlberg E, Vellestad N: Everyday functioning in young children with cerebral palsy: Functional skills, caregiver assistance, and modifications of the environment, *Dev Med Child Neurol* 45:603-612, 2003.

46. Hammel J: What's the outcome? Multiple variables complicate the measurement of assistive technology outcomes, *Rehabil Manag* 9:97-99, 1996.

47. Bottos M, Feliciangeli A, Sciuto L, et al: Functional status of adults with cerebral palsy and implications for treatment of children, *Dev Med Child Neurol* 2001;43:516-528.

48. Murphy K, Molnar G, Lankasky K: Medical and functional status of adults with cerebral palsy, *Dev Med Child Neurol* 37(12):1075-1084, 1995.

49. Strauss D, Ojdana K, Shavelle R, et al: Decline in function and life expectancy of older persons with cerebral palsy, *NeuroRehabilitation* 19(1):69-78, 2004.

50. Leonard C, Hirschfeld H, Forssberg H: Deficits in reciprocal inhibition in children with CP as revealed by H-reflex testing, *Dev Med Child Neurol* 32:974-984, 1990.

51. Bjornson K: Role of the physical therapist in the management of children with spasticity. In *Topics in Physical Therapy—Pediatrics: Lesson 8*, Alexandria, Va, 2001, American Physical Therapy Association.

52. Charness A: *Stroke/Head Injury: A Guide to Functional Outcomes in Physical Therapy Management*, Rockville, Md, 1986, Aspen Publications.

53. Gracies J, Elovic E, McGuire J, et al: Traditional pharmacological treatments for spasticity. II. General and regional treatments, *Muscle Nerve Suppl* 6:S92-S121, 1997.

54. Knuttson E, Lindblom U, Beissinger R, et al: Plasma and cerebrospinal fluid levels of baclofen (Lioresal) at optimal therapeutic responses in spastic paresis, *J Neurolog Sci* 23:473-484, 1974.

55. Gianino J: Intrathecal baclofen for spinal spasticity: implications for nursing practice, *J Neurosci Nurs* 25:254-264, 1993.

56. Hambleton P, Moore A: Botulinum neurotoxins. In Moore P (ed): *Handbook of Botulinum Toxin Treatment*, Oxford, 1995, Blackwell Science Ltd.

57. Graham H: Botulinum toxin A in cerebral palsy: Functional outcomes, *J Pediatr* 137(3):300-303, 2000.

58. Boyd R, Graham H: Botulinum toxin A in the management of children with CP: Indications and outcome, *Europ J Neuro* 4(2):15-22, 1997.

59. Ade-Hall R, Moore A: Botulinum toxin type A in the treatment of lower limb spasticity in cerebral palsy: Review, *Cochrane Database Syst Rev* 2:CD001408, 2000.

60. Koman L, Mooney J, Smith B, et al: Management of spasticity in cerebral palsy with botulinum toxin A: Report of a preliminary, randomized, double-blind trial, *J Pediatr Orthop* 14:299-303, 1994.

61. Corry I, Cosgrove A, Duffy C, et al: Botulinum toxin A compared with stretching casts in the treatment of spastic equinus: A randomized prospective trial, *J Pediatr Orthop* 18:304-311, 1998.

62. Flett P, Stern L, Waddy H, et al: Botulinum toxin A versus fixed cast stretching for dynamic calf tightness in cerebral palsy, *J Pediatr Orthop* 35:71-77, 1999.

63. Wasiak J, Hoare B, Wallen M: Botulinum toxin A as an adjunct to treatment in the management of children with spastic cerebral palsy, *Cochrane Database Syst Rev* 18(4):CD003469, 2004.

64. McLaughlin J, Bjoronson K, Temkin N, et al: Selective dorsal rhizotomy: meta-analysis of three randomized controlled trials, *Dev Med Child Neurol* 44:17-25, 2002.

65. Skinner H: *Current Diagnosis and Treatment in Orthopedics*, ed 3, New York, 2003, McGraw-Hill.

66. Saraph V, Zwick E, Zwick G, et al: Multilevel surgery in spastic diplegia: evaluation by physical examination and gait analysis in 25 children, *J Pediatr Orthop* 22:150-157, 2002.

67. Browne A, McManus F: One-session surgery for bilateral correction of lower limb deformities in spastic diplegia, *J Pediatr Orthop* 7:259-261, 1987.

68. Norlin R, Tkaczuk H: One-session surgery for correction of lower extremity deformities in children with cerebral palsy, *J Pediatr Orthop* 5:208-211, 1985.

69. Kondo I, Hosokawa K, Iwata M, et al: Effectiveness of selective muscle-release surgery for children with cerebral palsy: longitudinal and stratified analysis, *Dev Med Child Neurol* 46:540-547, 2004.

70. Stott N, Piedrahita L: Effects of surgical adductor releases for hip subluxation in cerebral palsy: An AACPDM evidence report, *Dev Med Child Neurol* 46:628-645, 2004.

71. Tortori-Donati P, Rossi A, Biancheri R, Cama A: Magnetic resonance imaging of spinal dysraphism, *Top Magn Reson Imaging* 12(6):375-409, 2001.

72. Drolet B: Birthmarks to worry about. Cutaneous markers of dysraphism, *Dermatol Clin* 16:447-453, 1998.

73. Tortori-Donati P, Rossi A, Cama A: Spinal dysraphism: A review of neuroradiological features with embryological correlations and proposal for a new classification, *Neuroradiology* 42:471-491, 2000.

74. The facts about Spina Bifida, Spina Bifida Association of America: www.sbaa.org. Accessed March 22, 2004.

75. Centers for Disease Control: Spina bifida and anencephaly prevalence—United States, 1991-2001, *MMWR* 51(RR13):9-11, 2002.

76. Smithells R, Sheppard S, Schorah C, et al: Possible prevention of neural tube defects by periconceptional vitamin supplementation, *Lancet* 1:339-340, 1980.

77. Shinjiro H, Farmer D, Albanese C: Fetal surgery for myelomeningocele, *Curr Opin Ob Gyn* 13:215-222, 2001.

78. Bruner J, Tulipan N, Reed G, et al: Intrauterine repair of spina bifida: preoperative predictors of shunt-dependent hydrocephalus, *Am J Obstet Gynecol* 190:1305-1312, 2004.

79. Adams R: Spina Bifida: Life Span Management, *Orthopedic Interventions for Pediatric Patients*, Home Study Course 10.2.2, Orthopaedic Section, LaCrosse, Wis, 2000, APTA.

80. Lazareff J: Lipomas and lipomyelomeningoceles, Spina Bifida Association: www.sbaa.org Accessed March 22, 2004.

81. Samuel M, Boddy S: Is spina bifida occulta associated with lower urinary tract dysfunction in children? *J Urology* 171:2664-2666, 2004.

82. Dias M, Partington M: Embryology of myelomeningocele and anencephaly, *Neurosurg Focus* 16(2):1-16, 2004.

83. Dias M, Walker M: The embryogenesis of complex dysraphic malformations: A disorder of gastrulation? *Pediatr Neurosurg* 18:229-253, 1992.

84. Luo J, Nye J: Evidence for genetic etiologies of neural tube defects. In Sarwark J, Lubicky J (eds): *Caring for the Child with Spina Bifida*, Rosemont, Ill, 2001, American Academy of Orthopaedic Surgeons.

85. Shurtleff D, Lemire R, Warkany J: Embryology, etiology and epidemiology. In Shurtleff D (ed): *Myelodysplasias and Exstrophies: Significance, Prevention, and Treatment*, Orlando, Fla, 1986, Grune & Stratton.

86. McLone D, George T, Worley G, et al: Genetic studies in neural tube defects. NTD Collaborative group, *Pediatr Neurosurg* 32:1-9, 2000.

87. Juriloff D, Harris M: Mouse models for neural tube closure defects, *Human Mol Genet* 9:993-1000, 2000.

88. Prevention of neural tube defects: Results of the Medical Research Council Vitamin Study, MRC Vitamin Study Research Group, *Lancet* 338:131-137, 1991.

89. Mersereau P: Spina bifida and anencephaly before and after folic acid mandate—United States, 1995-1996 and 1999-2000, *MMWR* 53(17):362-365, 2004.

90. Centers for Disease Control: Recommendations for the use of folic acid to reduce the number of cases of spina bifida and other neural tube defects, *MMWR* 41(No.RR-14), 1992.

91. Food and Drug Administration: Food standards, *Federal Register* 61:8781-8797, 1996.

92. Cunningham F: *Williams Obstetrics*, ed 21, New York, 2001, McGraw-Hill.

93. Morrow R, McNay M, Whittle M: Ultrasound detection of neural tube defects in patients with elevated maternal serum alpha-fetoprotein, *Obstet Gynecol* 78:1055, 1991.

94. Schneider J, Gabriel K: Congenital spinal cord injury. In Umpred D (ed): *Neurological Rehabilitation*, ed 3, St. Louis, 1994, Mosby.

95. Badell-Ribera A: Myelodysplasia. In Molnar G (ed): *Pediatric Rehabilitation*, Baltimore, 1985, Williams & Wilkins.

96. Tappit Emas E: Spina bifida. In Tecklin JS (ed): *Pediatric Physical Therapy*, ed 3, New York, 1999, Lippincott Williams & Wilkins.

97. Frawley P, Broughton N, Menelaus M: Incidence and type of hindfoot deformities in patients with low-level spina bifida, *J Pediatr Orthop* 18:312-313, 1998.

98. Liptak G, Shurtleff D, Bloss J, et al: Mobility aids for children with high-level myelomeningocele. Parapodium versus wheelchair, *Dev Med Child Neurol* 34:787-796, 1992.

99. Shurtleff D: Mobility. In Shurtleff D (ed): *Myelodysplasias and Exstrophies: Significance, Prevention, and Treatment*, Orlando, Fla, 1986, Grune & Stratton.

100. Parsch K: Origins and treatment of fractures in spina bifida, *Eur J Pediatr Surg* 1(5):298-305, 1991.

101. DeSouza L, Carroll N: Ambulation of the braced myelomeningocele patient, *J Bone Joint Surg Am* 58:1112-1118, 1976.

102. Liptak G: Neural tube defects. In Batshaw M (ed): *Children with Disabilities*, ed 4, Baltimore, 1997, Paul H Brookes.

103. International Myelodysplasia Study Group Database, Seattle, 1993, Department of Pediatrics, University of Washington.

104. McLone D, Czyzewski D, Raimondi A, et al: Central nervous system infections a limiting factor in the intelligence of children with myelomeningocele, *Pediatrics* 70:338-342, 1982.

105. Brumfield C, Aronin P, Cloud G, et al: Fetal myelomeningocele: Is antenatal ultrasound useful in predicting neonatal outcome? *J Reproductive Med* 40:26-30, 1995.

106. Friedrich W, Lovejoy M, Shaffer J, et al: Cognitive abilities and achievement status of children with myelomeningocele: A contemporary sample, *J Pediatr Psych* 16:423-428, 1991.

107. Shaffer J, Wolfe L, Freidrich W, et al: Developmental expectations: Intelligence and fine motor skill. In Shurtleff D (ed): *Myelodysplasias and Exstrophies: Significance, Prevention, and Treatment*, Orlando, Fla, 1986, Grune & Stratton.

108. Snow J: Memory functions for children with spina bifida: Assessment in rehabilitation and exceptionality, *Pediatrics* 1:20-27, 1994.

109. Lollar D: Learning among children with spina bifida, Spina Bifida Association: www.sbaa.org.

110. Culatta B, Young B: Linguistic performance as a function of abstract task demands in children with spina bifida, *Dev Med Child Neurol* 34(5):434-440, 1992.

111. Gaston H: Ophthalmic complications of spina bifida and hydrocephalus, *Eye* 5:279-290, 1991.
112. Shurtleff D: Decubitus formation and skin breakdown. In Shurtleff D (ed): *Myelodysplasias and Exstrophies: Significance, Prevention, and Treatment*, Orlando, Fla, 1986, Grune & Stratton.
113. Reigel D: Spina bifida from infancy through the school years. In Rowley-Kelly F, Reigel D (eds): *Teaching the Students with Spina Bifida*, Baltimore, 1993, Paul H. Brooks.
114. Vereecken R: Bladder pressure and kidney function in myelomeningocele, *Paraplegia* 30:153-159, 1992.
115. King J, Currie D, Wright E: Bowel training in spina bifida: Importance of education, patient compliance, age, and anal reflexes, *Arch Phys Med Rehabil* 75:243-247, 1994.
116. Centers for Disease Control and Prevention: *Evidence-based practice in spina bifida: Developing a research agenda*, Conference held in Washington, DC, May 9-10, 2003.
117. McDonald C, Jaffe K, Mosca V, et al: Ambulatory outcome of children with myelomeningocele: Effect of lower-extremity muscle strength, *Dev Med Child Neurol* 33:482-490, 1991.
118. Duffy C, Hill A, Cosgrove A, et al: The influence of abductor weakness on gait in spina bifida, *Gait Posture* 4:34-38, 1996.
119. Vanoski S, Bare A, Dias L, et al: Energy expenditure in myelomeningocele: what's the cost of walking? *Dev Med Child Neurol* 75(Suppl):18-19, 1997.
120. Bartonek A, Eriksson C, Saraste H: Heart rate and walking velocity during independent walking in children with low and midlumbar myelomeningocele, *Pediatr Phys Ther* 14:185-190, 2002.
121. Sousa J, Gordon L, Shurtleff D: Assessing the development of independence of daily living skills in patients with spina bifida, *Dev Med Child Neurol* 18(suppl 37):134-142, 1976.
122. Sousa J, Telzrow R, Holm R, et al: Developmental guidelines for children with myelodysplasia, *Phys Ther* 63(1):21-29, 1983.
123. Bowman R, McLone D, Grant J, et al: Spina bifida outcome: A 25-year prospective, *Pediatr Neurosurg* 34(3):114-120, 2001.
124. Centers for Disease Control: Current trends economic burden of spina bifida—United States, 1980-1990, *MMWR Morb Mortal Wkly Rep* 38(15):264-267, 1989.
125. Brown M, Gordon W: Impact of impairment on activity patterns of children, *Arch Phys Med Rehabil* 68(12):828-832, 1987.
126. Conner-Kuntz F, Dummer G, Paciorek M: Physical education and sport participation of children and youth with spina bifida myelomeningocele, *Adap Phys Activity Q* 12(3):228-238, 1995.
127. Committee on Integrating the Science of Early Childhood Development: *From Neurons to Neighborhoods: The Science of Early Childhood Development*, Washington, DC, 2000, National Academy Press.
128. Campbell SK: The child's development of functional movement. In Campbell SK, Linden DWV, Palisano RJ (eds): *Physical Therapy for Children*, ed 2, New York, 2000, WB Saunders.
129. Croce R, DePaepe J: A critique of therapeutic intervention programming with reference to an alternative approach based on motor learning theory, *Phys Occup Ther Pediatr* 9(3):5-33, 1989.
130. Bernstein N: *The Co-Ordination and Regulation of Movements*, Oxford, 1967, Pergamon Press.
131. Larin H: Motor learning: Theories and strategies for the practitioner. In Campbell SK, Linden DWV, Palisano RJ (eds): *Physical Therapy for Children*, ed 2, New York, 2000, WB Saunders.
132. Edwards R: The effects of performance standards on behavior patterns and motor skill achievement in children, *J Teach Phys Educ* 7:90-120, 1988.
133. Shumway-Cook A, Woollacott MH: Motor control: Issues and theories. In Shumway-Cook A, Woollacott MH (eds): *Motor Control: Theory and Practical Applications*, ed 2, Philadelphia, 2001, Lippincott Williams & Wilkins.
134. Adolph K: Learning to keep balance. In Kail R (ed): *Advances in Child Development and Behavior*, vol 30, Amsterdam, 2002, Elsevier Science.
135. Adolph K, Eppler M: Flexibility and specificity in infant motor skill acquisition. In Fagen J (ed): *Progress in Infancy Research*, vol 2, Norwood, NJ, 2002, Ablex.
136. Adolph K, Vereijken B, Shrout P: What changes in infant walking and why, *Child Devel* 74(2):475-497, 2003.
137. Edwards J, Elliott D, Lee T: Contextual interference effects during skill acquisition and transfer in Down's syndrome adolescents, *Adap Phys Activity Q* 3:250-258, 1986.
138. Chan M, Lu Y, Martin L, et al: A baby's day: Capturing crawling experience. In Grealy MA, Thompson JA (eds): *Studies in Perception and Action V*, Mahwah, NJ, 1999, Lawrence Erlbaum Publishers.
139. Bower E, Michell D, Burnett M, et al: Randomized controlled trial of physiotherapy in 56 children with cerebral palsy followed for 18 months, *Dev Med Child Neurol* 43:4-15, 2001.
140. Haley SM: Patterns of physical and occupational therapy implementation in early motor intervention, *TECSE* 7:46-63, 1988.
141. Trahan J, Malouin F: Intermittent intensive physiotherapy in children with cerebral palsy: A pilot study, *Dev Med Child Neurol* 44:233-239, 2002.
142. Mayo N: The effect of physical therapy for children with motor delay and cerebral palsy. A randomized clinical trial, *Am J Phys Med Rehabil* 70:258-267, 1991.
143. Bower E, McLellan D: Effect of increased exposure of physiotherapy on skill acquisition of children with cerebral palsy, *Dev Med Child Neurol* 34:25-39, 1992.
144. Bower E, McLellan D, Arney J, et al: A randomized controlled trial of different intensities of physiotherapy and different goal-setting procedures in 44 children with cerebral palsy, *Dev Med Child Neurol* 38:226-237, 1996.
145. Campbell M, Sheets D, Strong P: Secondary health conditions among middle-aged individuals with chronic physical disabilities: Implications for unmet needs for services, *Asst Technol* 11:105-122, 1999.
146. Campbell S: Therapy programs for children that last a lifetime, *Phys Occup Ther Pediatr* 17(1):10-15, 1997.
147. Rimmer J: Physical fitness levels of persons with cerebral palsy, *Dev Med Child Neurol* 2001;43:208-212.
148. Strong W: Physical activity and children, *Circulation* 81:1697-1701, 1990.
149. Valvano J: Neuromuscular system: The plan of care. In Effgen S (ed): *Meeting the Physical Therapy Needs of Children*, Philadelphia: 2005, FA Davis.
150. Kaplan M, Bedell G: Motor skill acquisition frame of reference. In Kramer P, Hinojosa J (eds): *Frames of Reference for Pediatric Occupational Therapy*, ed 2, New York, 1999, Lippincott Williams & Wilkins.
151. Valvano J: Activity-focused motor interventions for children with neurological conditions, *Phys Occup Ther Pediatr* 24:79-107, 2004.
152. Duff S, Quinn L: Motor learning and motor control. In Cech D, Martin S (eds): *Functional Movement Development Across the Life Span*, Philadelphia, 2000, WB Saunders.
153. Thorpe D, Valvano J: The effects of knowledge of performance and cognitive strategies on motor skill learning in children with cerebral palsy, *Pediatr Phys Ther* 14:2-15, 2002.
154. Ketelaar M, Vermeer A, Hart H, et al: Effects of a functional therapy program on motor abilities of children with cerebral palsy, *Phys Ther* 81(9):1534-1545, 2001.
155. Styer-Acevedo J: Physical therapy for the child with cerebral palsy. In Tecklin JS (ed): *Pediatric Physical Therapy*, ed 3, New York, 1999, Lippincott Williams & Wilkins.
156. Park E, Park C, Kim J: Comparison of anterior and posterior walkers with respect to gait parameters and energy expenditure of children with spastic diplegic cerebral palsy, *Yonsei Med J* 42(2):180-184, 2001.
157. Levangie P, Chimera M, Johnston M, et al: The effects of posterior rolling walkers on gait characteristics of children with spastic cerebral palsy, *Phys Occup Ther Ped* 9:1-17, 1989.
158. Mattsson E, Andersson CP: Oxygen cost, walking speed, and perceived exertion in children with cerebral palsy when walking with anterior and posterior walkers, *Dev Med Child Neurol* 39:671-676, 1997.
159. Logan L, Byers-Hinkley K, Ciccone C: Anterior versus posterior walkers: a gait analysis study, *Dev Med Child Neurol* 32:1044-1048, 1990.
160. Palisano RJ, Tieman B, Walter S, et al: Effect of environmental setting on mobility methods of children with cerebral palsy, *Dev Med Child Neurol* 45:113-120, 2003.
161. Taub E, Ramey S, DeLuca S, et al: Efficacy of constraint-induced movement therapy for children with cerebral palsy with asymmetric motor impairment, *Pediatrics* 113:305-312, 2004.
162. Schoen SA, Anderson J: Neurodevelopmental treatment frame of reference. In Kramer P, Hinojosa J (eds): *Frames of Reference for Pediatric Occupational Therapy*, ed 2, New York, 1999, Lippincott Williams & Wilkins.
163. Butler C, Darrah J: Effects of neurodevelopmental treatment for cerebral palsy: An AACPDM evidence report, *Dev Med Child Neurol* 43:778-790, 2001.
164. Dodd K, Taylor N, Damiano D: A systematic review of the effectiveness of strength-training programs for people with cerebral palsy, *Arch Phys Med Rehabil* 83(8):1157-1164, 2002.
165. Kerr C, McDowell B, McDonough S: Electrical stimulation in cerebral palsy: a review of effects on strength and motor function, *Dev Med Child Neurol* 46:205-213, 2004.
166. Aubert E: Adaptive equipment for physically challenged children. In Tecklin JS (ed): *Pediatric Physical Therapy*, ed 3, New York, 1999, Lippincott Williams & Wilkins.
167. Jones M, Gray S: Assistive technology: Positioning and mobility. In Effgen S (ed): *Meeting the Physical Therapy Needs of Children*, Philadelphia: 2005, FA Davis.
168. Stuberg W: Considerations related to weight-bearing programs in children with cerebral palsy, *Phys Ther* 72:35-40, 1992.
169. Edelstein J: Orthotic assessment and management. In O'Sullivan S, Schmitz T (eds): *Physical Rehabilitation: Assessment and Treatment*, ed 4, Philadelphia, 2001, FA Davis.
170. Brown J: Orthopaedic care of children with spina bifida, *Orthop Nurs* 20(4):51-58, 2001.
171. Morris C: A review of the efficacy of lower-limb orthoses used for cerebral palsy, *Dev Med Child Neurol* 44:205-211, 2002.

Chapter 16

Adult Nonprogressive Central Nervous System Disorders

Lisa L. Dutton

OBJECTIVES

After completing this chapter, the reader will be able to:
1. Describe and differentiate between different types of adult nonprogressive central nervous system disorders.
2. Understand and apply tests and measures appropriately for adult patients and clients with nonprogressive central nervous system disorders.
3. Accurately evaluate, diagnose, and provide an evidence-based prognosis for individuals who have sustained a stroke or traumatic brain injury.
4. Discuss the theoretical principles underlying neurodevelopmental treatment, proprioceptive neuromuscular facilitation, and task-oriented approaches to rehabilitation intervention.
5. Select appropriate evidence-based interventions to address common impairments, functional limitations, and disabilities observed in individuals included in this practice pattern.
6. Apply knowledge of patient/client management for the individual who has sustained a stroke or traumatic brain injury to case studies.

This chapter addresses the rehabilitation of adults with impaired motor function and sensory integrity associated with nonprogressive central nervous system (CNS) disorders. The most common of these disorders are cerebrovascular accident (stroke) and traumatic brain injury. Patients with nonprogressive CNS disorders may exhibit a range of impairments, functional limitations, and disabilities that include:

- Altered cognition and behavior
- Impaired motor control and performance, including weakness, abnormal tone, abnormal reflexes, and altered movement patterns
- Disturbances in postural control and balance
- Decreased endurance
- Impaired sensory and perceptual integrity including altered proprioception, vision, and unilateral neglect
- Decreased ability to perform functional activities such as bed mobility, transfers, and ambulation
- Decreased ability to function in work or home environments and fulfill social roles.

In addition to the influence of varied pathology, all of these impairments, functional limitations, and disabilities are uniquely expressed in each patient based on the impact of individual and environmental factors. Individual factors include demographics, culture, lifestyles, psychological traits, and social support. Environmental factors are composed of influences such as social, political, and economic structures; the physical environment; available medical and/or rehabilitation care; and societal views of disability.[1]

Using the frameworks provided by Nagi's disablement model[2] and the *Guide to Physical Therapist Practice*,[1] this chapter discusses pathologies commonly linked with preferred practice pattern 5D: Impaired motor function and sensory integrity associated with nonprogressive disorders of the CNS—acquired in adolescence or adulthood. This is followed by consideration of appropriate examination procedures, including tests and measures for impairments and functional limitations often observed in patients with nonprogressive CNS disorders. This examination provides the basis for evaluation and determination of a physical therapy diagnosis and prognosis. Based on the plan of care, a variety of intervention approaches for these patients are then discussed. All of these are considered within the context of "the conscientious, explicit, and judicious use of current best evidence in making decisions about the care of individual patients."[3]

PATHOLOGY

CEREBROVASCULAR ACCIDENT

Stroke or cerebrovascular accident (CVA) has been defined as an "acute neurologic dysfunction of vascular origin . . . with symptoms and signs corresponding to the involvement of focal areas of the brain."[4] As the third leading cause of death and the number one cause of serious disability in the United States (US), stroke poses a significant public health concern.[5] Strokes are typically classified as occlusive or hemorrhagic. Occlusive strokes are associated with a restriction in blood flow to the brain that results in ischemia. Occlusive strokes account for 80% of all CVAs[6] and may be thrombotic or embolic in origin. A thrombotic stroke is caused by the development of a blood clot or thrombus in a vessel in the brain. Thrombus formation is associated with endothelial injury, slowed or turbulent blood flow, and increased blood coagulability. These factors lead to smooth muscle and endothelial proliferation that in turn can result in narrowing and eventual occlusion of blood vessels. An embolic stroke is caused by material from another area of the body moving to a blood vessel in the brain and occluding it. Emboli that go to the brain are typically blood clots that detach from blood vessels, or from within the heart, that travel through the bloodstream to suddenly occlude a cerebral artery.[7] Emboli may also be composed of other materials such as fat, which occurs occasionally after fractures of long bones, or necrotic material, which can occur with infection of the heart valves (endocarditis).

The clinical syndromes associated with occlusive strokes vary according to the cerebral artery involved (Fig. 16-1). For example, occlusion of the middle cerebral artery, the most common site of stroke,[8] typically results in contralateral paralysis and sensory deficits in the face and upper extremities that is greater than in the lower extremities, as well as motor speech impairment and aphasia if the dominant hemisphere is involved. When the anterior cerebral artery is occluded, contralateral paralysis and sensory loss is generally greater in the lower extremity than the upper extremity. In addition, ischemia in the frontal lobe may cause declarative memory loss and behavioral impairments. When the posterior cerebral artery is involved, homonymous hemianopsia (a loss of vision in the half of the visual field contralateral to the lesion), cortical blindness, and memory deficit can ensue. In addition, with loss of blood supply to the thalamus, patients often develop choreoathetosis, spontaneous pain and dysesthesias, sensory loss, and intention tremor.

Hemorrhagic strokes, which are those associated with the rupture of a blood vessel, account for approximately 20% of strokes.[6] They are often associated with hypertension or vascular malformations such as cerebral aneurysms and arteriovenous malformations (AVM). With this type of stroke, brain tissue death occurs because of ischemia and mechanical and chemical injury associated with the release of blood into the extravascular space. The mortality rates for hemorrhagic stroke are much higher than for occlusive strokes.[9] Eighty percent of hypertensive hemorrhages involve the cerebral hemispheres, they are often large, and common sites of involvement include the basal

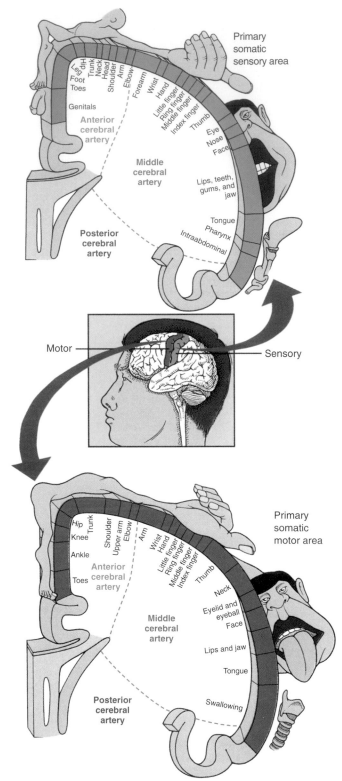

FIG. 16-1 Arterial blood supply of the motor and sensory cortex. *Adapted from Thibodeau GA, Patton KT:* Anatomy and Physiology, *ed 6, St. Louis, 2006, Mosby.*

ganglia, thalamus, cerebellum, and the pons.[10] Subarachnoid hemorrhages are often seen in normotensive individuals, with 85% arising from congenital berry aneurysms, and they frequently occur in the circle of

Willis. The clinical syndromes associated with hemorrhagic stroke tend to be more varied as they are related to the size and extent of damage associated with the bleed. Cases can range from mild, where only a small amount of blood is released and then reabsorbed, to severe in which there is a rapid accumulation of blood that compresses the brain tissues and can push the brainstem through the foramen magnum, generally resulting in death.

TRAUMATIC BRAIN INJURY

According to the Centers for Disease Control and Prevention (CDC), each year 1.5 million people in the US sustain a traumatic brain injury (TBI); 50,000 of these individuals die and 80,000-90,000 experience long-term disability.[11] The leading causes of TBI are motor vehicle accidents, gunshot wounds, and falls.[12] TBI has been defined as "an insult to the brain, not of a degenerative or congenital nature, but caused by an external physical force."[13] Such insults can be classified as penetrating or blunt and may result in either an open or closed injury.[14] Penetrating injuries tend to cause more focal damage along the path of impact, whereas blunt injuries can cause cortical contusions and damage in areas away from the point of original contact.[15] Damage in areas distant from the site of trauma is common when the brain is subjected to rapid acceleration and deceleration. In addition, high velocity movement may also result in diffuse axonal injury in the cerebral cortex as a result of shearing forces exerted on the brain when it moves rapidly within the skull. Secondary brain damage can also occur after TBI because bleeding into the cranium and edema may result in progressive compression and distortion of brain tissue and impingement of major arteries. The clinical syndromes associated with TBI vary in severity and typically involve a broader spectrum of physical, cognitive, and behavioral sequelae than stroke because of the wide distribution of brain structures associated with this type of injury.

EXAMINATION

PATIENT HISTORY

Taking the patient's history allows the clinician to gather information regarding past and current health status, primary complaints, social history, living environment, health habits, lifestyle, employment and work, current functional status, and personal goals. This information enables the therapist to begin to assess co-morbidities that may impact the rehabilitation process and to develop hypotheses to guide further examination, evaluation, diagnosis, prognosis, and interventions. For patients receiving inpatient services, information from the patient's history is used to begin discharge planning. For example, initial information about the severity of a stroke or TBI, combined with knowledge of the patient's home environment and level of family support, give the therapist early insight into potential needs for equipment and support services on discharge.

SYSTEMS REVIEW

The systems review is used to target areas requiring further examination and to define areas that may cause complications or indicate a need for precautions during the examination and intervention processes. See Chapter 1 for details of the systems review.

TESTS AND MEASURES

The final step in the examination process is the selection and implementation of appropriate tests and measures. Guided by the history and systems review, tests and measures are selected to assist the therapist in determining a diagnosis, prognosis, and plan of care. In addition, they allow the therapist to specifically document impairments, functional limitations, and disabilities that may be impacted by rehabilitation services. When selecting a test or measure, it is important to consider its reliability and validity, the purpose for which it was established, and the patient population for which it is most appropriate. For example, there are multiple tests and measures available for balance. Some of these assess steady state or static balance and others assess dynamic postural control. The appropriate test and measure must be selected with both the purpose of the test and the abilities of the patient in mind. For example, a balance assessment that requires the patient to be ambulatory for completion may be appropriate in regard to purpose but inappropriate based on the functional level of the patient. Tests and measures that may be appropriate for adults with nonprogressive neuromuscular disorders are discussed in the next section. This discussion is not comprehensive but rather highlights well-validated and commonly used tests and measures for this patient population that are not covered in detail elsewhere in this text.

Musculoskeletal

Muscle Performance. In patients with neurological disorders, one accepted definition of strength is "the capacity of a muscle or group of muscles to produce the force necessary for initiating, maintaining, and controlling movement."[16] Strength can be assessed as reliably through isometric, isokinetic, and functional measures in individuals with neurologic dysfunction as in those with musculoskeletal dysfunction[17-19] (see Chapter 5). Historically, it has been suggested that *spasticity* may prevent reliable and valid assessments of strength in individuals with upper motor neuron disorders.[20,21] Specifically, it was proposed that excessive co-contraction by spastic antagonists masked true agonist muscle strength and resulted in the appearance of weakness, when in fact, muscle strength was intact. Despite this persistent clinical belief, it has been demonstrated in patients with strokes that inadequate recruitment of agonist muscles is not related to spasticity in the antagonist.[22] Furthermore, in a study of 20 individuals with diagnoses of stroke and TBI who had spastic hemiparesis, the test-retest reliability of isokinetic testing of knee extension and flexion torque was found to be excellent for both the involved and noninvolved lower extremity (ICC > 0.91).[18] Similar results were also reported in a study of 14 subjects with stroke (ICC > 0.92).[23]

Neuromuscular

Arousal, Attention, and Cognition. One frequently used measure of arousal, particularly in the case of individuals with TBI, is the Glasgow Coma Scale (GCS) (see Chapter 21).[24] This scale was designed to provide a measure of altered consciousness through assessment of eye opening, best motor response, and a verbal score. The GCS score within the first 24 hours after injury has also been used as an indicator of severity and a predictor of outcome after TBI.

One commonly observed attentional deficit after stroke is unilateral spatial neglect. Individuals with this behavioral syndrome fail to "report or respond to people or objects presented to the side opposite a brain lesion."[25] This lack of response cannot be attributed to sensory or motor deficits.[26] Some researchers have reported the incidence of unilateral neglect after stroke to be as high as 82% for strokes in the right hemisphere and 65% for strokes in the left hemisphere.[27] When classifying unilateral neglect, it is important to consider whether it is sensory (e.g., auditory, visual, tactile), motor, or representational in nature and whether the behavior involves personal and/or spatial neglect.[25] Understanding the type of neglect allows the therapist to more appropriately structure patient intervention. Types of neglect are more specifically described in Table 16-1.[28-30]

Cognition includes *skills* such as the ability to discriminate between relevant and irrelevant information, understanding and retention, and the ability to appropriately apply knowledge.[32] Deficits in cognitive function are a significant cause of disability after TBI and stroke and can decrease patients' capacity to complete routine daily tasks and impair their ability to respond to new or challenging situations.

The most common screening test used for cognition is the Mini-Mental State Examination (MMSE).[33] This examination can be completed in 10 minutes or less and addresses: orientation to time and place, registration of words, attention, calculation, recall, language, and visual construction. Although designed for patients with dementia, it has been shown to be a valid and reliable tool in a range of populations, including patients with stroke.[33-35] In one study, concurrent validity of MMSE with the cognitive subscale of the Functional Independence Measure (FIM) and the Loewenstein Occupational Therapy Cognitive Assessment was established with a sample of 66 stroke patients undergoing inpatient rehabilitation.[36] In addition, this study supported the predictive validity of this measure through documentation of a correlation between the MMSE at admission and functional outcomes at discharge.

A second test of cognition that is recommended by the Agency for Health Care Policy and Research (AHCPR) in their clinical practice guideline for stroke[5] is the Neurobehavioral Cognitive Status Examination (NCSE).[36] This examination takes slightly longer to administer than the MMSE and addresses ten domains: Orientation, attention, comprehension, naming, construction, memory, calculation, similarities, judgment, and repetition. The test starts with a difficult item in each domain as an initial screen. If a patient fails this screening item he or she completes additional items, progressing from easy to more difficult, to identify the extent of his or her deficit. If a patient passes the screening item, he or she is considered to have no deficit in that domain. The NCSE has been validated in samples of neurosurgical patients,[37] patients with TBI,[38,39] and patients with stroke.[40] In addition, the NSCE was found to be more sensitive than the MMSE at detecting cognitive dysfunction in a sample of 30 neurosurgical patients.[41] Similarly, another study with 38 patients with stroke entering inpatient rehabilitation found the NSCE to be more a more sensitive predictor of discharge outcomes related to personal care and mobility.[42]

Finally, while the GCS is primarily used as an acute measure of arousal, the Rancho Los Amigos Levels of Cognitive Functioning Scale (LCFS) is the most commonly used measure of arousal and cognitive functioning in the TBI population (Table 16-2).[43] This scale classifies individuals recovering from TBI into one of eight possible categories. These categories range from no response to purposeful and appropriate responses. Although commonly used as a means of quantifying improvement in individuals with TBI, no literature supports the validity or reliability of this tool.

When evaluating the impact of cognitive deficits on a patient's ability to participate in rehabilitation, one must consider the roles and functioning of the implicit and the explicit learning systems. Declarative memory is considered to be part of the explicit learning system and typically involves the conscious recall of knowledge or information.[44] In contrast, procedural memory is unconscious and is generally considered part of the implicit learning system. This learning occurs with practice and

TABLE 16-1	**Classification of Neglect**[31]
Classification	**Definition**
Sensory neglect	Decreased awareness of sensory stimulation on the involved side of the body. Can include decreased awareness of auditory, visual, or somatosensory input.
Motor neglect	Decreased ability to generate a movement response despite awareness of a stimuli. This type of neglect may be observed throughout the body including the eyes, head, neck, trunk and limbs.
Representational neglect	Failure to construct one side of a visual memory or image. This may be observed when a patient is asked to describe a familiar place from a particular orientation (e.g., if asked to describe the front of his/her home only one side is described, but if the orientation is changed by having the patient imagine he/she is facing a different direction, then the previously omitted side of the image is included).
Personal neglect	Decreased awareness of the limb or side of the body opposite the brain lesion.
Spatial neglect	Decreased awareness of space on the side of the body opposite the brain lesion.

TABLE 16-2	Rancho Los Amigos Levels of Cognitive Functioning	
Level	**Response**	**Characteristics**
I	No response	Unresponsive to any stimulus
II	Generalized response	Limited, inconsistent, nonpurposeful responses, often to pain only
III	Localized response	Purposeful responses May follow simply commands May focus on presented object
IV	Confused, agitated	Heightened state of activity Confusion, disorientation Aggressive behavior Unable to do self-care Unaware of present events Agitation appears related to internal confusion
V	Confused, inappropriate	Nonagitated Appears alert Responds to commands Distractable Does not concentrate on task Agitated responses to external stimuli Verbally inappropriate Does not learn new information
VI	Confused, appropriate	Goal directed behavior, needs cueing Can relearn old skills as ADLs Severe memory problems Some awareness of self and others
VII	Automatic, appropriate	Appears appropriate Oriented Frequently robot-like in daily routine Minimal or absent confusion Shallow recall Increased awareness of self, interaction in environment Lacks insight into condition Decreased judgment and problem solving Lacks realistic planning for future
VIII	Purposeful, appropriate	Alert, oriented Recalls and integrates past events Learns new activities and can continue without supervision Independent in home and living skills Defects in stress tolerance, judgment, abstract reasoning persist May function at reduced levels in society

From Hagan C, Malkmus D, Durham P: Levels of cognitive functions. In *Rehabilitation of the Head Injured Adult: Comprehensive Physical Management*, Downey, Calif, 1979, Professional Staff Association of Rancho Los Amigos Hospital.
ADLs, Activities of daily living.

TABLE 16-3	Modified Ashworth Scale
Muscle Tone Grade	**Definition**
0	No increase in muscle tone.
1	Slight increase in muscle tone, manifested by a slight catch and release or by minimal resistance at the end of the ROM when the affected part(s) is moved in flexion or extension.
1+	Slight increase in muscle tone, manifested by a catch, followed by minimal resistance throughout the remainder (less than half) of the ROM.
2	More marked increase in muscle tone through most of the ROM, but affected part(s) easily moved.
3	Considerable increase in muscle tone, passive movement difficult.
4	Affected part(s) rigid in flexion or extension.

From Bohannon RW, Smith MB: *Phys Ther* 67:206-207, 1987.
ROM, Range of motion.

does not require conscious thought or direct attention.[45] A number of research studies support the idea that individuals with diagnoses of stroke and TBI, who also have declarative memory deficits, can demonstrate procedural learning of motor tasks with practice over time.[46-50] Furthermore, individuals who have sustained a stroke can learn rapid motor tasks requiring feedforward processes, such as catching a ball or performing rapid repetitive motions, as well as age-matched controls.[51] As such, even when declarative memory is significantly impaired, a patient's ability to learn motor tasks may not be affected.

Sensory Integrity. Patients within the adult nonprogressive CNS disorder practice pattern typically present with sensory and in some cases, perceptual deficits. Sensory deficits can include impairments in discriminative touch, proprioception, and sensation of pain and temperature (see Chapter 18 for further details of tests and measures of sensation). The ability to discriminate light touch can be grossly assessed with the patient's eyes closed by asking her to indicate whether or not she feels the stimulus. Proprioception, including joint position and joint motion, can be assessed with the patient's eyes closed by asking the patient to indicate the position of a limb or the direction of movement.[52]

Spasticity and Muscle Tone. Spasticity is characterized by a velocity dependent increase in tonic stretch reflexes accompanied by exaggerated tendon jerks.[53] *Muscle tone* has been defined as resistance to passive stretch[54] and increased muscle tone in individuals with neuromuscular disorders can be related to both changes in the intrinsic properties of muscle, tendon, and connective tissue, as well as hyperactive stretch reflexes. The most commonly used clinical measure of muscle tone is the Modified Ashworth Scale.[55] This 6-point scale allows the therapist to grade muscle tone based on resistance to passive movement. Specifically, the test is conducted by passively moving the muscle or muscle group under consideration through its full range of motion (ROM). The definitions for each grade are provided in Table 16-3. Reported reliability for the Modified Ashworth Scale is variable. Bohannon and Smith reported a Kendall tau-b of 0.847 for interrater reliability at the elbow with a sample of patients with diagnoses of stroke, multiple sclerosis, and closed head injury.[55] In contrast, Blackburn, van Vliet, and Mockett reported moderate intrarater reliability (Kendall tau-b = 0.567) and poor interrater reliability (Kendall tau-b = 0.062) for the lower extremity in patients with stroke.[56] Although a more reliable measure of spasticity and tone is desirable, the Modified Ashworth Scale is the most commonly used and has the most data evaluating its reliability and validity.

Coordination. Nonequilibrium coordination tests are typically used to assess motor performance deficits related to cerebellar dysfunction. For example, they may be used to identify impairments such as *dysdiadochokinesia, dysmetria,* or *dyssynergia.*[57] Common coordination tests include examination of alternating finger to nose move-ment, rapid finger opposition, pronation/supination, tapping of the hand or foot, and moving the heel up and down the shin (Table 16-4).

Movement Patterns. Abnormal movement patterns, or synergies, have been described after CNS disorders such as stroke or TBI.[20,57] Abnormal synergies are stereotyped patterns of movement that limit an individual's ability to dissociate movement at one joint from movement at another and generate a variety of movement patterns in response to task demands.[45] For example, when asked to raise his arm, the patient with an abnormal flexor synergy in the upper extremity may be unable to flex his

TABLE 16-4	Nonequilibrium Coordination Tests
Test	**Description**
Finger to nose	The shoulder is abducted to 90° with the elbow extended. The patient is asked to bring the tip of the index finger to the tip of the nose. Alterations may be made in the initial starting position to assess performance from different planes of motion.
Finger to therapist's finger	The patient and therapist sit opposite each other. The therapist's index finger is held in front of the patient. The patient is asked to touch the tip of the index finger to the therapist's index finger. The position of the therapist's finger may be altered during testing to assess ability to change distance, direction, and force of movement.
Finger to finger	Both shoulders are abducted to 90° degrees with the elbows extended. The patient is asked to bring both hands toward the midline and approximate the index fingers from opposing hands.
Alternate nose to finger	The patient alternately touches the tip of the nose and the tip of the therapist's finger with the index finger. The position of the therapist's finger may be altered during testing to assess ability to change distance, direction, and force of movement.
Finger opposition	The patient touches the tip of the thumb to the tip of the fingers in sequence. Speed may be gradually increased.
Mass grasp	An alternation is made between opening and closing fist (from finger flexion to full extension). Speed may be gradually increased.
Pronation/supination	With elbows flexed to 90° and held close to body, the patient alternately turns the palms up and down. This test also may be performed with shoulders flexed to 90° and elbow extended. Speed may be gradually increased. The ability to reverse movements between opposing muscle groups can be assessed at many joints. Examples include active alternation between flexion and extension of the knee, ankle, elbow, fingers, and so forth.
Rebound test	The patient is positioned with the elbow flexed. The therapist applies sufficient manual resistance to produce an isometric contraction of biceps. Resistance is suddenly released. Normally, the opposing muscle group (triceps) will contract and "check" movement of the limb. Many other muscle groups can be tested for this phenomenon such as the shoulder abductors or flexors, elbow extensors, and so forth.
Tapping (hand)	With the elbow flexed and the forearm pronated, the patient is asked to "tap" the hand on the knee.
Tapping (foot)	The patient is asked to "tap" the ball of one foot on the floor without raising the knee; heel maintains contact with floor.
Pointing and past pointing	The patient and therapist are opposite each other, either sitting or standing. Both patient and therapist bring shoulders to a horizontal position of 90° of flexion with elbow extended. Index fingers are touching or the patient's finger may rest lightly on the therapist's. The patient is asked to fully flex the shoulder (fingers will be pointing toward ceiling) and then return to the horizontal position such that index fingers will again approximate. Both arms should be tested, either separately or simultaneously. A normal response consists of an accurate return to the starting position. In an abnormal response, there is typically a "past pointing," or movement beyond the target. Several variations to this test include movements in other directions such as toward 90° of shoulder abduction or toward 0° of shoulder flexion (finger will point toward floor). Following each movement, the patient is asked to return to the initial horizontal starting position.
Alternate heel to knee; heel to toe	From a supine position, the patient is asked to touch the knee and big toe alternately with the heel of the opposite extremity.
Toe to examiner's finger	From a supine position, the patient is instructed to touch the great toe to the examiner's finger. The position of finger may be altered during testing to assess ability to change distance, direction, and force of movement.
Heel on shin	From a supine position, the heel of one foot is slid up and down the shin of the opposite lower extremity.
Drawing a circle	The patient draws an imaginary circle in the air with either upper or lower extremity (a table or the floor also may be used). This also may be done using a figure-eight pattern. This test may be performed in the supine position for lower extremity assessment.
Fixation or position holding	Upper extremity: The patient holds arms horizontally in front (sitting or standing). Lower extremity: The patient is asked to hold the knee in an extended position (sitting).

From Schmitz TJ: Coordination assessment. In O'Sullivan SB, Schmitz TJ (ed): *Physical Rehabilitation: Assessment and Treatment,* ed 4, Philadelphia, 2001, FA Davis.

shoulder without shoulder elevation, shoulder abduction, and elbow flexion accompanying the movement. The full *abnormal synergy* patterns for the upper and lower extremity are shown in Fig. 16-2.

The most common measure of motor recovery in stroke patients is the Fugl-Meyer Assessment.[58] This test is based on the motor recovery sequence described by Brunnstrom in which reflexes reoccur first, followed by volitional movement dominated by abnormal synergy patterns, and subsequent progressive isolation of movement outside of the synergy pattern. Thus the motor recovery portion of the Fugl-Meyer Assessment includes measurement of the patient's ability to move in and out of synergy with the upper and lower extremities. The validity[58,59] and reliability[60,61] of this assessment tool are well established in patients with stroke. This tool is not typically used for patients with TBI as their patterns of motor recovery tend to be more variable.

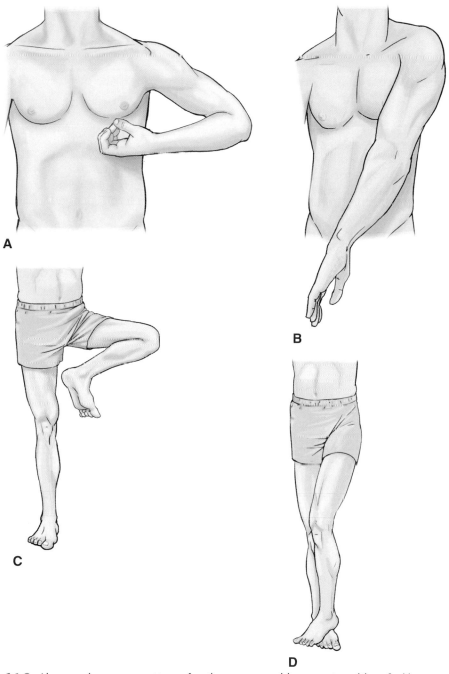

FIG. 16-2 Abnormal synergy patterns for the upper and lower extremities. **A,** Upper extremity flexion—shoulder abduction, elbow flexion, forearm supination, wrist and finger flexion; **B,** upper extremity extension—shoulder adduction, elbow extension, forearm pronation, wrist and finger extension; **C,** lower extremity flexion—hip abduction, hip and knee flexion, ankle dorsiflexion; **D,** lower extremity extension—hip adduction, hip and knee extension, ankle plantar flexion.

Cardiovascular/Pulmonary

Aerobic Capacity and Endurance. Tests and measures commonly associated with the assessment of aerobic capacity and endurance in adults with nonprogressive CNS disorders include measures such as heart rate, blood pressure, and respiratory rate at rest and during and after functional activities and exercise, as well as standardized tests such as the 6-minute walk test (6MWT). The 6MWT involves the measurement of the distance that an individual can walk in 6 minutes[62] and is considered a submaximal test of aerobic capacity.[63] This test has been validated through correlations between the distance walked in 6 minutes with peak oxygen consumption for individuals with heart failure[64] and individuals with pulmonary disease.[65] In a sample of 86 adults 65 years and older, 1 week test-retest reliability for the 6MWT was high (r = 0.95) and older adults from community centers walked significantly further than less active older adults living in retirement homes (t = 10.1, p < .0001), indicating that the test demonstrated known-groups validity.[66] In this study, moderate correlations were also found between the distance walked in 6 minutes and body strength (r = 0.67), tandem balance (r = 0.52), and gait speed (r = 0.73). One study examining 46 individuals with diagnoses of stroke reported statistically significant differences in pulse and systolic blood pressure before and after the 6MWT.[67] No reported studies were located that documented the validity of this test for individuals with TBI. It is important to realize that the 6MWT may be impacted by impairments in lower limb motor ability and balance, as well as endurance.[67] In addition, its applicability is limited to those who can ambulate for 6 minutes. Despite these limitations, for patients who are able to complete the test, changes in systolic blood pressure and pulse before and after the test do provide a means of assessing aerobic fitness in this population.

Function

Balance. Balance is a multidimensional construct which has been described as including the ability to maintain one's position in space, stabilize in anticipation of voluntary movement, and respond to external perturbations.[68,69] In addition, one's ability to demonstrate symmetry or equal weight distribution in sitting or standing is also often included as an important aspect of balance.[70-72] Accordingly, a variety of tests and measures have been developed that examine one or more of these different components. These include scales such as the Berg Balance Scale (BBS), Tinetti's Performance-Oriented Mobility Assessment (POMA), Timed Up and Go, and Functional Reach Test (see Fig. 13-18). Of these, the BBS addresses all three components of balance: Maintenance of position, postural adjustment to voluntary movement, and reaction to external disturbances. In addition, it has well-established validity and reliability.[68,73]

Gait. For adults with neuromuscular disorders, one of the most clinically practical measures of gait ability is gait speed. This measure has been shown to be valid, reliable and sensitive to change in a wide range of populations.[74-80] Although gait speed does not give the therapist specific information about where to direct interventions,

comfortable walking speed in individuals with neuromuscular disorders has been shown to be significantly correlated with maximum hip extension angle,[76] hip flexor strength,[75] and plantarflexor power burst at push-off.[81] Maximal walking speed has also been associated with hip flexor strength, lower extremity sensation, and plantarflexor strength.[75] Normative values for comfortable gait speed for individuals between the ages of 60 and 89 have been reported to range, based on age and gender, from 1.59 meters/second (m/sec) to 1.15 m/sec.[63] It has been suggested that a minimum walking speed of 0.8 ± 0.18 m/sec is required for community independence.[82] In addition to measures of gait speed, it is also important to consider the patient's ability to negotiate different types of surfaces and obstacles.

Measures of gait speed are only appropriate for individuals who are able to ambulate without significant manual assistance. For individuals who require assist for ambulation, other tests and measures may be preferable. For instance, the mobility sections of the Barthel Index[83] and the FIM[84] include assessments of gait and locomotion that are based on how independent the individual is with tasks such as ambulating on level surfaces. Specifically, on the FIM, ambulation is rated from dependent (level 1) when the patient is unable to assist at all to fully independent (level 7) when the patient is able to ambulate without physical assistance or an assistive device (see Chapter 32 for further information on gait assessment).

Self-Care and Home-Management. There are a number of global measures of function that can be used for adults with nonprogressive CNS disorders. These include previously mentioned measures such as the FIM and the Barthel Index. The FIM is probably the most widely used outcome measure for individuals with neuromuscular disorders, particularly for those receiving inpatient rehabilitation services. The FIM measures function in the areas of self-care, sphincter control, mobility, locomotion, communication, and social cognition and is reported to be valid, reliable, and generally sensitive to change for most individuals, including those with stroke and TBI, with the exception of those functioning at the lowest and highest levels.[85,86] This measure has also been shown to be a good predictor of level of disability and discharge status in patients who have sustained strokes.[87] A threshold FIM score of 80 has been reported as indicative of a functional level associated with discharge to home.[88,89]

The Barthel Index is primarily intended for patients after stroke. This index assesses activities in two major categories: Personal care and mobility. The personal care items include tasks such as drinking from a cup, dressing, grooming, bathing, and bowel and bladder continence. The mobility items include wheelchair maneuvering, walking, stairs, and transfers. This measure also has well-documented reliability,[90] validity,[83] and sensitivity[91] when used for individuals diagnosed with stroke.

EVALUATION, DIAGNOSIS, AND PROGNOSIS

On completion of the examination, the therapist must make clinical judgments about the collected data to determine a diagnosis, prognosis, and appropriate plan of care.

The appropriate diagnostic category for most adults after stroke or TBI is preferred practice pattern 5D: Impaired motor function and sensory integrity associated with nonprogressive disorders of the CNS.

When considering outcomes, there are a variety of individual, environmental, and social factors that impact the prognosis for individuals who have experienced a stroke or TBI. In general, greater sensory and motor deficits one week after onset are associated with poorer overall prognosis for functional recovery. For example, individuals with higher levels of sitting balance and bowel and bladder control one week after stroke are more likely to be ambulating at discharge.[92] After TBI, cognitive and behavioral impairment levels are of particular prognostic importance.[32] For individuals who have experienced a stroke, those who are married, have family members that do not work outside the home and have higher total Barthel Index scores are more likely to be discharged home.[89,93] Finally, as previously mentioned, a total score of 80 is the reported FIM threshold for discharge to home.[88,89]

INTERVENTION

There are a variety of approaches to intervention for adults with nonprogressive CNS disorders. These approaches can be classified according to the motor control theories that support them. The more traditional neurofacilitation techniques, such as proprioceptive neuromuscular facilitation (PNF) and neurodevelopmental treatment (NDT), have historically been associated with the reflex and hierarchical models of motor control.[54] In these models, sensory input is used to influence motor output and the CNS is considered to be organized hierarchically, beginning with the spinal level as the lowest level of integration and extending upward to the prepontine, midbrain, and cortical levels, respectively. It should be noted that NDT in particular has begun to move away from its historical theoretical base to incorporate tenets of the systems model into its underlying assumptions.[94] The emphasis of intervention in these approaches is on facilitation of normal movement patterns while inhibiting abnormal synergies and motor recovery is assumed to follow a predictable sequence.[54,95] In contrast, the task-oriented approaches[45,96,97] are supported by the systems theory of motor control. The theoretical basis for these approaches was originally proposed by Nicoli Bernstein and suggests that movement emerges as the result of the interaction of multiple systems.[98] Furthermore, this theory posits that in the case of motor control, these systems are organized around the goal of accomplishing a particular motor task as opposed to the generation of a selected movement pattern.[54,95] Also associated with the task-oriented approaches are more recently introduced interventions such as constraint-induced movement therapy and body weight–supported (BWS) ambulation (see later).

In general, the evidence supporting the use of NDT and PNF for adults with nonprogressive neuromuscular disorders is limited. A Medline abstract search using the terms "neurodevelopmental treatment" and "Bobath" from 1966 to the present generated 35 articles related to the nonpediatric population. Of these, fourteen examined NDT as an intervention technique through an experimental, quasi-experimental, or case study design. Eleven concluded that NDT was no better or was worse than the control or comparison treatment and three reported that NDT was superior. Of those reporting positive effects associated with NDT, one related immediate but not sustained outcomes,[99] one was a study of the application of NDT in nursing,[100] and one was a case report.[101]

Similarly, a Medline abstract search from 1966 to the present using the term "proprioceptive neuromuscular facilitation" produced 26 references. Only five of these studies addressed individuals with diagnoses of stroke and one of those five was a review paper.[102-106] In addition, one each addressed individuals with lower extremity amputations,[107] older adults,[108] individuals with spinocerebellar degeneration,[109] and individuals with chronic obstructive pulmonary disease.[110] The remainder primarily involved healthy individuals and athletes. No studies were identified that included subjects with TBI. Of the research that addressed individuals with stroke, one study included a sample of 131 patients and found no significant difference between groups receiving conventional intervention (defined as including straight plane exercises, compensation techniques, and early introduction of functional activities), NDT, or PNF.[102] Another study with 22 subjects found PNF to be less effective than electromyographic (EMG) biofeedback combined with electrical stimulation in improving upper extremity motor function both immediately posttreatment and after 3 and 9 months.[105] In contrast, Trueblood et al found that a single 15-minute PNF intervention resulted in improved gait characteristics in 20 subjects who had had a stroke but that these improvements no longer remained after 30 minutes.[103] Finally, a small study applied 12 PNF treatments to two groups of 10 subjects: Those who were an average of 4.4 months poststroke and those who were an average of 15.4 months poststroke.[106] These researchers reported that gait speed and cadence improved in both groups, although more quickly in the less chronic group. No follow-up measures beyond those taken at the conclusion of the intervention period were reported. Thus both of the studies reporting positive effects for PNF failed to demonstrate carry-over beyond immediate posttreatment effects and are weakened by the absence of control groups or baseline measurements.

Although there are very few studies evaluating their effectiveness, PNF and NDT continue to be widely used approaches in clinical practice and therefore are discussed in some detail in the next section. In contrast, more recent task-oriented approaches, such as BWS gait training and constraint-induced movement therapy (CIMT), are less commonly used in clinical practice but have been more extensively studied. These approaches have good scientific evidence demonstrating efficacy and are also described later.

NEURODEVELOPMENTAL TREATMENT

The NDT approach was originally developed by Berta Bobath and Dr. Karel Bobath in the 1940s.[20] The Bobaths described their approach as "not a method but a living concept . . . a management."[111] As such, the approach has changed and adapted over the years to accommodate emerging knowledge in neuroscience.[112] A key element of this approach is its foundation in normal movement.[20,21] Mrs. Bobath described normal movement as including normal postural control upon which coordinated and isolated movements could be superimposed. Thus intervention is focused on the inhibition of abnormal synergies and tone and the facilitation of normal movement patterns with the ultimate goal of optimizing function.[20,21,94,113] This is accomplished in part through the use of key points of control or the use of therapist-generated proximal or distal input to the patient. For example, the therapist might provide input to the patient's left paraspinal muscles by lightly and quickly touching the skin and musculature in that area while simultaneously providing a lateral and superiorly directed cue at the right shoulder by gently holding the glenohumeral joint and lifting up and over to encourage trunk shortening on the left with weight shifting to the right. In addition, therapists practicing this approach overlap assessment and treatment so that the therapist continually reassesses the patient's movement patterns and then intervenes and reassesses again.

As previously noted, there is limited evidence supporting the effectiveness of NDT as a neurological treatment intervention. In one study, Hesse et al examined the impact of therapeutic facilitation as used in the NDT approach on functional movement in 22 patients with diagnoses of stroke and TBI.[99] In this study, the authors found immediate benefits of NDT facilitation on gait as compared to nonfacilitated ambulation with or without a cane. These benefits included faster walking speed, longer stance time on the hemiparetic limb, greater gait symmetry and hip extension, and faster muscle activation. Five of the subjects were also assessed 1 hour after gait training, and none of the effects related to the NDT facilitation remained. Thus no strong conclusions could be drawn regarding whether the observed effects were sustained after the intervention ended. In 2001, Lennon published a case report describing two individuals poststroke who received therapy based on NDT concepts.[101] Evaluation of angular displacements and joint moments in the sagittal plane indicated that these individuals demonstrated more normal movement patterns at the pelvis, knee, and ankle after completing 28-30 therapy sessions. Despite this, it should be noted that these changes, as well as changes reported in step length, single-leg support time, and walking speed, were quite small. This study is also limited by its restricted sample size, lack of a control or comparison group, and lack of blinding.

As mentioned in the context of PNF, in an early study examining different intervention approaches in neurological physical therapy, 131 adult inpatients with stroke were randomly assigned to receive conventional physical therapy (defined as including straight plane exercises, compensatory techniques, and early functional training), NDT, or PNF.[102] After 6 weeks there were no differences between groups in improvement on any of the identified outcome measures. In a similar study, Gelber et al also found no advantage for NDT over a treatment approach including resistive exercise, compensatory techniques, and early introduction of functional activities.[114] When compared with EMG biofeedback, NDT intervention did not produce superior upper extremity function, finger oscillation ability, health beliefs, or overall effect.[115]

In another study with inconclusive results, Mudie et al randomly assigned 40 patients with recent diagnoses of stroke and asymmetrical sitting posture to one of four groups.[116] The first group received visual feedback from a Balance Performance Monitor (BPM) regarding their postural symmetry in sitting and during reaching activities. The second group participated in task-related reach training in which they reached for grocery items on the floor and placed them into a cupboard. No feedback or guidance was provided to this group. The third group participated in NDT activities focused on normalizing muscle tone in the trunk and facilitating appropriate postural control and balance responses. The control group and the three treatment groups also received "standard physiotherapy and occupational therapy," which was not further defined. At the conclusion of the study, the authors reported a significant improvement in sitting weight distribution from pretreatment to posttreatment for the NDT group, the BPM group, and the control group. Results at 2 and 12 weeks posttreatment were no longer significantly different between groups. Thus the authors suggested that NDT, visual feedback training with a force platform, and conventional physical therapy can produce changes in static sitting symmetry from pretreatment to posttreatment. They were not able to conclude that one approach was superior to the others. Similarly, a recent systematic review of studies related to the effectiveness of the NDT approach for individuals after stroke identified 15 trials suitable for inclusion and concluded that there was no evidence to support NDT as an optimal approach to treatment.[117]

In contrast to this literature, a few studies have suggested that NDT may be inferior for at least some outcome measures when compared to other approaches. In one study, 27 hemiparetic patients were randomly assigned to one of two groups.[118] Both groups participated in a 2-week baseline phase during which the participants received NDT based therapy, and this continued throughout the intervention phases. Following the baseline phase, the second group received transcutaneous electrical nerve stimulation (TENS) for a 2-week period for 15 minutes twice per day. Then both groups participated in an exercise program 2 times per day for 15 minutes each time that included grip, rapid wrist extension, and finger flexion exercises. Measures of grip strength, rapid isometric and isotonic hand extension, and the arm section of the Rivermead Motor Assessment showed no significant change during the baseline NDT or the TENS plus NDT phases of the study. In contrast, all of these measures significantly improved after the addition of repetitive training to the NDT-based intervention. In a study with a similar design, Hesse et al conducted an A-B-A case series in which 7 subjects poststroke participated in 3 weeks of treadmill training with partial BWS, 3 weeks of NDT, and another 3 weeks of partial BWS treadmill training.[119] Functional Ambulation Category (FAC) levels and gait velocity improved only during the treadmill phases of the study and not during the NDT intervention phase. NDT was also found to be less effective than CIMT when assessed by measures of dexterity and self-reports of how well and how much subjects used the involved extremity in every day activities.[120] Similarly, in another study, 61 individuals with diagnoses of stroke were randomized into two groups: One group received physical therapy in accordance with a Motor Relearning Programme (MRP), briefly described as a task-oriented approach to intervention, and another group received NDT-based interventions.[121] Intervention was provided 5 days per week for a minimum of 40 minutes per session throughout the individual's inpatient hospital stay and continued for the duration of any prescribed outpatient physical therapy. Although there were no differences reported between groups in total Barthel Index score at 2 weeks or 3 months posttreatment initiation, at 2 weeks the MRP group showed greater improvement than the NDT group on the Motor Assessment Scale. In addition, the length of stay in the hospital was significantly longer for the NDT group (34 days versus 21 days). In a follow-up to this study, these same patients were reexamined at 1 year and 4 years poststroke.[122] Scores for both groups declined on the Motor Assessment Scale and the Barthel Index at the 1-year and 4-year follow-up assessments, and there were no longer significant differences on these outcome measures between the two groups.

In conclusion, as indicated by the evidence above, aside from possible immediate effects related to NDT facilitation, there is limited evidence to suggest that NDT is superior to other neurorehabilitation approaches as measured by short- or long-term outcomes. Table 16-5 summarizes evidence on the effectiveness of NDT.

PROPRIOCEPTIVE NEUROMUSCULAR FACILITATION

PNF is based on concepts first introduced by Dr. Herman Kabat in the 1950s and later expanded on by Margaret Knott and Dorothy Voss. This intervention approach was described by Voss as including "methods of promoting or hastening the response of the neuromuscular mechanism through stimulation of proprioceptors."[123] PNF is carried out using defined combinations of movement that include diagonal and spiral components. The use of these movement combinations takes into consideration Dr. Kabat's observations that (1) normal coordinated activities are accomplished through complex movement patterns that do not occur in straight planes; (2) the stretch reflex is most effectively elicited when the extremity is elongated in a specific diagonal; and (3) the muscular response is more coordinated and forceful when resisted within a specific diagonal. In addition, PNF incorporates the use of a variety of sensory inputs, such as traction, approximation, resistance, quick stretch, verbal stimuli, and visual stimuli to facilitate a desired motor response.[124] The goals of this facilitation may include either increased contraction or relaxation of various muscle groups.

In PNF, specific techniques are generally imposed upon diagonal patterns for the trunk, pelvis, shoulder girdle, and extremities. They may also be applied to developmental positions such as prone on elbows, quadruped, or tall kneeling. It has been suggested that these techniques and patterns should be progressed in a manner that supports the concept of a developmental progression of motor control, moving from *initial mobility*, then to *stability*, and finally to *controlled mobility*, and skill.[125] Thus, this sequence implies that after developing some initial ability to move, proximal stability is needed prior to movement of either the trunk on stable extremities or skilled open chain movement of the extremities on the trunk. Despite the continued use of this sequencing in practice, there is limited research to support that such a progression occurs during normal motor development. In fact, there is some evidence that proximal and distal skills develop concurrently in infants.[126,127]

There are four upper extremity and lower extremity diagonal patterns of motion used in PNF. They are labeled by diagonal number (1 or 2) and direction (flexion or extension). The upper extremity patterns are as follows (Fig. 16-3):[124]

- Diagonal 1 flexion (D1F): Shoulder flexion, adduction, and external rotation; forearm supination; wrist and finger flexion and radial deviation
- Diagonal 1 extension (D1E): Shoulder extension, abduction, and internal rotation; forearm pronation; wrist and finger extension and ulnar deviation
- Diagonal 2 flexion (D2F): Shoulder flexion, abduction, and external rotation; forearm supination; wrist and finger extension and radial deviation
- Diagonal 2 extension (D2E): Shoulder extension, adduction, and internal rotation; forearm pronation; wrist and finger flexion and ulnar deviation

Similarly, the lower extremity patterns are listed as follows (Fig. 16-4):

- Diagonal 1 flexion (D1F): Hip flexion, adduction and external rotation; ankle/foot dorsiflexion and inversion; toe extension
- Diagonal 1 extension (D1E): Hip extension, abduction, and internal rotation; ankle/foot plantar flexion and eversion; toe flexion
- Diagonal 2 flexion (D2F): Hip flexion, abduction, and internal rotation; ankle/foot dorsiflexion and eversion; toe extension
- Diagonal 2 extension (D2E): Hip extension, adduction, and external rotation; ankle/foot plantarflexion and inversion; toe flexion.

When applying these diagonals specifically to the shoulder girdle or pelvis, there are generally two diagonals considered: Anterior-elevation/posterior-depression and posterior-elevation/anterior-depression, and intervention is generally conducted with the patient in sidelying (Fig. 16-5). In addition, the extremity, shoulder girdle, and pelvic diagonals can also be applied with the patient in various developmental postures. For example, in quadruped a patient could be asked to shift weight down and back to the right and up and forward to the left, thus incorporating pelvic, shoulder, and portions of the extremity diagonals.

A number of techniques associated with PNF are superimposed on these diagonals as applied to the extremities, trunk, or in developmental postures. These techniques are based on neurophysiological evidence that sensory inputs can influence motor output[128,129] and they are described in Table 16-6.[123,124]

Text continued on p. 420.

TABLE 16-5	Summary of the Evidence on the Effectiveness of Neurodevelopmental Therapy	
Reference/Subjects	**Design/Interventions/Outcomes**	**Results/Conclusions**
Dickstein et al[102] 131 subjects status poststroke Mean age: 70.5 Mean time after onset: 8 days	*Design:* RCT Intervention 5 days/week, 30-45 minutes/day for 6 weeks *Group 1:* Conventional (straight plane exercises, compensation techniques, and early introduction of functional activities) *Group 2:* PNF *Group 3:* NDT *Outcomes:* Barthel Index, muscle tone, active ROM and strength in ankle dorsiflexion and wrist extension and ambulatory status assessed on admission and every 2 weeks.	*Results:* No differences between groups on any of the outcome measures. *Conclusions:* ± No advantage of one approach over the other relative to these outcomes.
Basmajian et al[115] 29 subjects status poststroke Mean age: 62 Mean time after onset: 16.19 weeks	*Design:* RCT Intervention 3 times/week, 45 minutes/ session for 5 weeks *Group 1:* EMG biofeedback *Group 2:* NDT *Outcomes:* Blinded pretest, posttest, and 9 month assessment of UEFT, finger oscillation, Health Belief Survey, mood and affect.	*Results:* No difference between groups on any of the outcome measures at any testing point. *Conclusions:* +/− No advantage of one approach over the other relative to these outcomes.
Butefisch et al[118] 27 subjects status poststroke Mean age: 62 Mean time after onset: 8.37 weeks	*Design:* Multiple baseline design NDT (OT/PT): 1-2 hours/day throughout study Experimental intervention (C) 2 times/day, 15 minutes/session for 4 weeks *Conditions:* *A:* NDT (baseline) *B:* TENS (2 weeks for $\frac{1}{2}$ the group as a control for effect of additional treatment) *C:* Grip and repetitive wrist and finger flexion and extension exercises. *Outcomes:* Weekly assessment of grip strength, isometric and isotonic hand extension, Rivermead motor assessment.	*Results:* Minimal or no change in any outcome measure during baseline (NDT only) or baseline + TENS phases. Significant improvement in outcome measures from beginning to end of C phase. *Conclusions:* − NDT was less effective than grip strengthening and repetitive wrist and finger flexion and extension exercises.
Gelber et al[114] 27 subjects status post pure motor stroke Mean age: 71.8 Mean time after onset: 12.55 days	*Design:* RCT Intervention duration/frequency not reported *Group 1:* NDT *Group 2:* TFR (early introduction of functional activities, resistive exercise, compensation allowed) *Outcomes:* FIM, gait parameters, gross and fine motor upper extremity dexterity measured at admission, discharge, 6-month, and 12-month follow-ups.	*Results:* No significant differences between NDT and TFR group on any outcome measure. *Conclusions:* ± No advantage of one approach over the other relative to these outcomes.
Hesse et al[119] 7 subjects status poststroke Mean age: 60.3 Mean time after onset: 176.8 days	*Design:* A-B-A Case Series Intervention 3 weeks for each phase (9 weeks total) *Intervention A:* Treadmill training with partial BWS; 30 minutes sessions 5 times/week *Intervention B:* NDT; 45 minute sessions, 5 times/week *Outcomes:* Weekly assessments included FAC, gait velocity Rivermead Motor Assessment Motricity Index, and Modified Ashworth Scale.	*Results:* FAC levels and gait velocity improved only during the treadmill phases. Rivermead scores improved equally across both interventions. Motricity Index did not change for either group and the Modified Ashworth Scale scores were variable for both groups. *Conclusions:* − Treadmill training was superior to NDT for outcomes related to gait.

TABLE 16-5	Summary of the Evidence on the Effectiveness of Neurodevelopmental Therapy—cont'd	
Reference/Subjects	**Design/Interventions/Outcomes**	**Results/Conclusions**
Hesse et al[99] 22 subjects status poststroke (n = 16) and TBI (n = 6) Mean age: 56 Mean time after onset: 2.2 months	*Design:* Pretest, posttest design In random order, all subjects engaged in walking (1) without assistance, (2) with a cane, and (3) with NDT facilitation. Five subjects received 30 minutes of NDT facilitated gait training and retested after 1 hour. *Outcomes:* Gait cycle parameters and lower extremity EMG	*Results:* NDT facilitation condition resulted in improved gait velocity, symmetry, and activation of weight-bearing muscles versus walking with or without a cane. No sustained effect of the NDT facilitated gait training after 1 hour when walking with or without a cane. *Conclusions:* ± Confirmed that during the application of NDT facilitation improvements in gait parameters and muscle activation are observed. Failed to confirm any carry-over 1 hour after treatment.
van der Lee et al[120] 66 subjects status poststroke Mean age: 61 Mean time after onset: 3 years	*Design:* RCT Intervention 6 hours/day, 5 days/week for 2 weeks. *Group 1:* NDT *Group 2:* CIMT *Outcomes:* ARA test, RAP, Fugl-Meyer Assessment, and MAL assessed 2 weeks before treatment, pretreatment, and 3 months, 6 months, and 1-year posttreatment.	*Results:* CIMT group performed significantly better on ARA and MAL than NDT group. No differences between groups noted on RAP or Fugl-Meyer Assessment. *Conclusions:* – CIMT resulted in superior outcomes on ARA and MAL when compared with NDT intervention of equal intensity.
Langhammer and Stanghelle[121] 61 subjects status poststroke Mean age: 78 Mean time after onset: Not reported (hospital inpatients)	*Design:* RCT Intervention 5 times/week, 40 minute sessions for duration of inpatient stay *Group 1:* MRP (task-oriented) *Group 2:* NDT *Outcomes:* Blinded assessments 3 days postadmission, after 2 weeks and 3 months poststroke included the Motor Assessment Scale, Sodring Motor Evaluation Scale, and Barthel Index. Other outcomes included length of stay, discharge destination, and use of assistive devices.	*Results:* Significant differences in favor of the MRP group were found on the MAS and SMES part 2 (arm function). The length of stay for the MRP group was also less (21 v. 34 days). *Conclusions:* – Patients treated with the task-oriented approach (MRP) had shorter hospital stays and superior motor function at 2 weeks and 3 months poststroke than those in the NDT group.
Mudie et al[116] 40 subjects status poststroke Mean age: 72.4 Mean time after onset: Not reported (subjects had been admitted to a rehabilitation center)	*Design:* RCT Intervention 3 times/week, 30 minute sessions for 2 weeks *Intervention 1:* BPM *Intervention 2:* Task-related reaching w/out feedback *Intervention 3:* NDT *Intervention 4:* Nonspecific OT/PT (control) *Outcomes:* Blinded pretest, posttest, 2 week, and 12 week assessment of symmetry of weight distribution in sitting and standing.	*Results:* Posttreatment the BPM, NDT, and control group demonstrated greater improvement in symmetrical sitting than the task-specific group. No differences between groups remained at 2 or 12 weeks after. *Conclusions:* ± NDT may be better than task specific reaching for training static sitting symmetry in the short term. No advantage of this approach in the long term.

RCT, Randomized controlled trial; *PNF,* proprioceptive neuromuscular facilitation; *NDT,* neurodevelopmental therapy; *EMG,* electromyography; *OT,* occupational therapy; *PT,* physical therapy; *TENS,* transcutaneous electrical nerve stimulation; *FIM,* Functional Independence Measure; *UEFT,* Upper Extremity Function Test; *TFR,* Traditional Functional Retraining; *FAC,* Functional Ambulation Category; *CIMT,* constraint-induced movement therapy; *ARA,* Action Research Arm test; *RAP,* Rehabilitation Activities Profile; *MAP,* Motor Activity Log; *MRP,* Motor Relearning Program; *BPM,* Balance Performance Monitor.

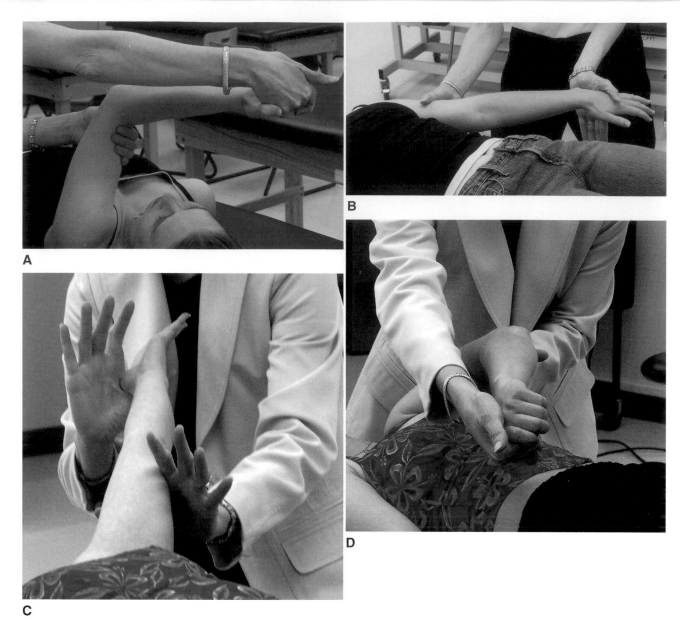

FIG. 16-3 Upper extremity diagonal patterns. **A,** Diagonal 1 flexion (D1F); **B,** diagonal 1 extension (D1E); **C,** diagonal 2 flexion (D2F); **D,** diagonal 2 extension (D2E).

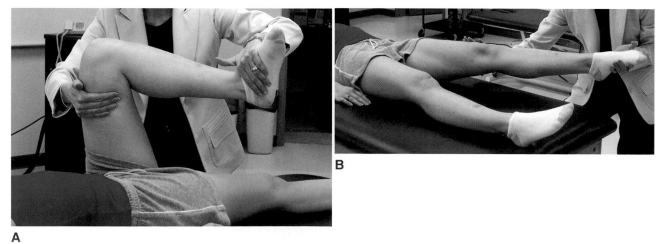

FIG. 16-4 Lower extremity diagonal patterns. **A,** Diagonal 1 flexion (D1F); **B,** diagonal 1 extension (D1E).

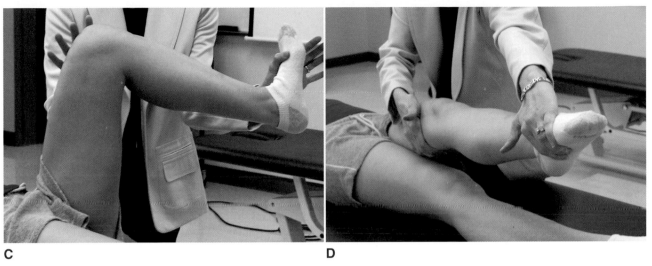

C   **D**

FIG. 16-4, cont'd   **C,** Diagonal 2 flexion (D2F); **D,** diagonal 2 extension (D2E).

FIG. 16-5 Anterior-elevation/posterior-depression of the shoulder girdle. *From Waddington PJ: PNF head and neck, scapular, and trunk patterns. In Hollis M, Fletcher-Cook P: Practical Exercise Therapy, ed 4, Oxford, 1999, Blackwell Science.*

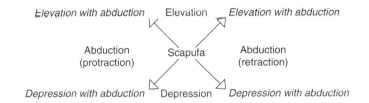

TABLE 16-6	PNF Techniques
Technique	**Method**
Hold-relax active motion	An isometric contraction in the shortened range of the diagonal, followed by passive movement into the lengthened range and then followed by active contraction into the shortened range.
Repeated contractions	Repeated use of the stretch reflex to initiate a contraction or reinforce and strengthen an existing contraction.
Rhythmic initiation	Progression of movement in diagonal from passive to active assistive to active to resisted.
Timing for emphasis	Maximal isometric resistance applied to stronger components of the diagonal to allow for facilitation or irradiation to weaker components.
Rhythmic rotation	Active or passive rotation around the longitudinal axis with the extremity positioned in the desired diagonal.
Alternating isometrics	Alternating isometric contractions of the agonist and antagonist.
Rhythmic stabilization	An extension of alternating isometrics in which the manual contacts are on opposite joint surfaces simultaneously.
Contract-relax	Movement into agonist pattern until a point of limitation, followed by isometric contraction of all components of the antagonist pattern except for the rotation component, which is allowed to contract isotonically; repeated with passive movement into any newly gained range after each trial.
Hold-relax	Isometric contraction of the agonist or antagonist musculature in the desired diagonal at the point of range limitation; repeated with passive movement into any newly gained range after each trial.
Slow reversals	Slow concentric contractions alternating between the agonist and antagonist muscle groups.
Slow reversal-hold	Slow concentric contractions alternating between the agonist and antagonist muscle groups with an isometric contraction applied at the end of each diagonal.
Agonist reversals	Isotonic contraction in the diagonal followed by an eccentric contraction of the same muscle groups.

For initial mobility, techniques such as *rhythmic initiation, repeated contractions,* and *timing for emphasis* are used. For stability, *rhythmic stabilization* and *alternating isometrics* are suggested. For controlled mobility and skill, therapists may utilize *hold-relax active motion, slow reversal-hold, slow reversals,* and *agonistic reversals.* Hold-relax and *contract-relax* are intended to improve ROM and flexibility.

Few studies address the application of PNF to individuals with diagnoses of stroke or TBI and only two, without the use of a control group or baseline measures, reported positive immediate effects of PNF on gait characteristics.[103,106] Neither of these studies demonstrated carry-over of these effects after treatment. A few studies, conducted with athletes or individuals without known impairment, have attempted to examine the theoretical rationale for some of the PNF techniques. For example, a number of studies with small samples of healthy individuals have demonstrated reduced Hoffman reflexes (H-reflexes) following modified or redefined PNF techniques (study specific definitions are included later for clarity), such as contract-relax (isometric contraction of the shortened muscle), contract-relax active-contraction (isometric contraction of the shortened muscle followed by active contraction into the limited range), and agonist contraction (contraction into the limited range), indicating that these techniques do produce some level of reflex inhibition in the shortened muscle.[130,131] Despite this, a number of studies have also demonstrated that although H-reflexes may be depressed, EMG activity is actually increased during some of the PNF techniques.[132-135] In general, these studies concluded that the PNF techniques that produced the greatest increases in ROM were also associated with the highest levels of EMG activity during application of the technique. Thus although there is evidence supporting the theoretical suggestion that PNF stretching techniques impact reflex responses, documented increases in EMG activity in the shortened muscle indicate that these techniques do not appear to relax the shortened muscle nor does such relaxation seem to be necessary for subsequent gains in ROM. Furthermore, it should be noted that these studies were conducted with relatively small samples and did not include individuals with diagnoses such as stroke or TBI. Thus one must be cautious in assuming that these results would carry over to individuals with neuromuscular disorders.

In addition to the evidence examining the neurophysiological basis for PNF, these and other studies have also focused more specifically on comparisons of different techniques designed to increase ROM and flexibility. In terms of hamstring flexibility, a number of studies have concluded that PNF techniques, such as hold-relax and contract-relax, are superior to passive stretching techniques.[133-136] In an extension of this line of research, it has also been suggested that the application of PNF techniques after exercise results in greater hamstring flexibility than static stretching before or after exercise or PNF before exercise.[137] Finally, the superiority of PNF to static stretching has also been established for muscle groups other than the hamstrings.[136,138] Thus there does appear to be evidence that the stretching techniques associated with PNF are generally more effective than passive stretching. However, one specific PNF technique does not appear to better than another. This evidence is limited in that it is generally, with the exception of one study, restricted to individuals who are college age and without impairment. No evidence suggesting that PNF techniques were superior to other approaches in addressing impairments related to strength, coordination, or function in any populations was found. A summary of the evidence on the effectiveness of PNF can be found in Table 16-7.

TASK-ORIENTED APPROACHES

The task-oriented approaches suggested by Carr and Shepherd[96,97,139] and Shumway-Cook and Woollacott[45] are based on scientists' current understanding of how movement arises from the interaction between systems at the level of the individual, the environment, and the task. In addition, these approaches more fully incorporate emerging knowledge regarding neural plasticity and *motor learning* and take into consideration the implications of research in the areas of environmental and task analysis, feedback, and practice. Gentile's Taxonomy of Movement Tasks is often used as the framework for environmental and task analysis for the purpose of guiding examination and intervention.[140] In this taxonomy, functional activities are evaluated based on the environmental context of the task and its functional role. Specifically, *regulatory conditions*, or those elements of the environment to which a task must conform, are conceptualized as being either stationary or in motion and presenting with or without intertrial variability. For example, if one were to practice a sit-to-stand transfer from a kitchen chair in the patient's home, the regulatory conditions (the chair) would be stationary and assuming that the person only practiced from one specific chair, present no intertrial variability. This is considered a closed task. On the other hand, if the patient were to practice sit-to-stand from a therapy ball, the regulatory conditions (the ball) would be in motion and that motion would be variable from trial to trial. This is considered an open task. This taxonomy is described in Table 16-8.

One can also analyze the function of the task. From this perspective, Gentile suggested considering whether or not the task required body stability or transport and whether the upper extremities were used primarily for stability or manipulation. In this case, if an individual was practicing sitting balance with the upper extremities providing support on the mat, the task would be stable with the upper extremities yoked into the postural system. If the person was ambulating while looking for a pencil in his or her pocket, the task would be more difficult and require both transport and manipulation. This taxonomy is provided in Table 16-9. From these two taxonomies, a full 16-cell taxonomy, combining both analysis of the environment and the task, can be created that allows one to structure interventions based on the inclusion of appropriately challenging activities. For example, a task such as ambulating through a busy shopping mall while carrying a wiggling baby would be at the highest level of the full taxonomy and includes regulatory conditions that are variable and in motion, as well as transport and upper extremity manipulation.

Feedback and its use to enhance motor learning, recovery, and control is also an important component of the

TABLE 16-7	Summary of the Evidence on the Effectiveness of Proprioceptive Neuromuscular Facilitation

Reference/Subjects	Design/Interventions/Outcomes	Results/Conclusions
GENERAL EFFECTIVENESS OF PNF AS AN INTERVENTION FOR INDIVIDUALS STATUS POSTSTROKE		
Dickstein et al[102] 131 subjects status poststroke Mean age: 70.5 Mean time after onset: 8 days	*Design:* RCT Intervention: 5 days/week, 30-45 minutes/day for 6 weeks *Group 1:* Conventional (straight plane exercises, compensation techniques, and early introduction of functional activities). *Group 2:* PNF. *Group 3:* NDT. *Outcomes:* Barthel index, muscle tone, active range of motion and strength in ankle dorsiflexion and wrist extension and ambulatory status assessed on admission and every 2 weeks thereafter.	*Results:* No differences between groups on any of the outcome measures. *Conclusions:* ± No advantage of one approach over the other relative to these outcomes.
Trueblood et al[103] 20 subjects status poststroke Mean age: 48 Mean time after onset: 2 months	*Design:* Pretest, posttest design Intervention: Single 15 minute PNF treatment (resisted pelvic diagonals). *Outcomes:* Gait characteristics assessed pretreatment, immediately posttreatment, and 30 minutes posttreatment.	*Results:* Gait characteristics improved immediately posttreatment but differences were no longer evident 30 minutes posttreatment. *Conclusions:* ± Some immediate improvement in gait characteristics but no carry-over noted.
Kraft et al[105] 22 subjects status poststroke Mean age: 63.2 Mean time after onset: 24.2 months	*Design:* RCT Intervention for 3 months *Group 1:* EMG biofeedback and stimulation to wrist extensors 60 minutes sessions, 3 times/week. *Group 2:* Low intensity stimulation combined with voluntary wrist extension, 30 minutes sessions, 5 times/week. *Group 3:* PNF to upper extremity 60 minutes sessions, 3 times/week. *Group 4:* Control. *Outcomes:* Assessments pretreatment and posttreatment and at 3- and 9-month follow-up included the Fugl-Meyer Assessment and grip strength.	*Results:* Treated subjects, regardless of group, improved more on the Fugl-Meyer Assessment than the control group. Of the treatment groups. *Group 1:* (EMG-stim) improved significantly more than *Group 3:* (PNF). Grip strength did not improve significantly in any group. *Conclusions:* – EMG biofeedback and stimulation to wrist extensors resulted in greater improvements in upper extremity motor control than PNF.
Wang[106] 28 subjects status poststroke Mean age: 55.7 Mean time after onset: 4.4 months (short duration group) and 15.4 months (long duration group)	*Design:* Pretest, posttest design Intervention: PNF 3 days/week, 30 minutes/day for 12 weeks. *Group 1:* <6 months poststroke. *Group 2:* >12 months poststroke. *Outcomes:* Cadence and gait speed assessed before treatment, after 1 treatment, and after 12 treatments.	*Results: Group 1:* Increased gait speed and cadence after 1 and 12 PNF treatments. *Group 2:* Decreased after 1 and then increased after 12 treatments on measures of gait speed and cadence. *Conclusions:* ± Although limited by lack of a control group, improvements in cadence and gait speed noted after PNF intervention.
EFFECTIVENESS OF INCREASING ROM AND FLEXIBILITY		
Sady, Wortman, Blanke[138] 65 males; no known impairment Mean age: 22.9 years	*Design:* RCT Intervention: 3 days/week for 6 weeks. *Group 1:* Control. *Group 2:* Ballistic stretch. *Group 3:* Static stretch. *Group 4:* (PNF) Passive stretch, isometric contraction of muscle being stretched, passive stretch. *Outcomes:* 2-day baseline and posttreatment ROM measurements to assess shoulder, hamstring, and trunk flexion flexibility.	*Results:* PNF group was the only group to increase flexibility in comparison to the control group (10.6 versus 3.4 degrees). *Conclusions:* + PNF was more effective in increasing shoulder, hamstring, and trunk flexibility than no stretch, ballistic, or static stretch. Greatest gains were observed in hamstring flexibility.
Osternig et al[133] 10 subjects; no known impairment Mean age: Not reported (range 32-36)	*Design:* Pretest, posttest design All subjects engaged in 3 conditions: 1. Passive stretch of the hamstrings. 2. Contract relax (CR = maximal contraction of hamstrings followed by passive stretch). 3. Agonist contract relax (ACR = maximal contraction of quadriceps followed by passive stretch). *Outcomes:* EMG activity of hamstrings and knee extension ROM.	*Results:* Greatest range achieved in the ACR condition. EMG activity in hamstrings was increased in the CR and ACR conditions and reduced during passive stretching. *Conclusions:* + Increase in muscle tension in the hamstrings (versus relaxation) associated with ACR condition may increase potential for muscle strain or soreness.

Continued

TABLE 16-7	Summary of the Evidence on the Effectiveness of Proprioceptive Neuromuscular Facilitation—cont'd	
Reference/Subjects	**Design/Interventions/Outcomes**	**Results/Conclusions**
Osternig et al[134] 30 subjects (endurance athletes, high intensity athletes, control); no known impairment Mean age: 24.6	*Design:* Pretest, posttest design All subjects engaged in 3 conditions: 1. Passive stretch of the hamstrings. 2. Contract relax (CR = maximal contraction of hamstrings followed by passive stretch). 3. Agonist contract relax (ACR = maximal contraction of quadriceps followed by passive stretch). *Outcomes:* EMG activity of hamstrings and knee extension ROM.	*Results:* Greatest range achieved in ACR condition (9%-13% more than CR or passive stretch conditions). ACR condition also resulted greatest hamstring EMG activity. *Conclusions:* + Although ACR was the most effective technique, increases in hamstring muscle tension associated with the ACR condition may increase potential for muscle strain or soreness.
Cornelius et al[136] 120 male college students; no known impairment Mean age: 21.5	*Design:* RCT All interventions began and ended with passive stretch. *Group 1:* Passive stretch. *Group 2:* Concentric contraction of hip flexors. *Group 3:* Isometric contraction of hip extensors, concentric contraction of hip flexor. *Group 4:* Isometric contraction of hip flexors, concentric contraction of hip flexors. *Group 5-8:* Each of the above conditions preceded by 10 minutes of icing. *Outcomes:* Pretreatment and posttreatment assessment of hip flexion ROM.	*Results:* No difference between conditions with or without icing. Groups receiving PNF intervention *(Groups 2-4)* demonstrated greater hip flexion ROM. *Conclusions:* + PNF techniques resulted in greater increases in ROM than passive stretching. No advantage of one PNF technique over the other.
Ferber, Osternig, Gravelle[135] 26 male subjects; no known impairment Mean age: Not reported (range: 55-75 years)	*Design:* Pretest, posttest counterbalanced design Each subject participated in 3 conditions presented in random order: (1) static stretch; (2) contract relax (CR = isometric contraction of knee flexors); (3) agonist contract relax (ACR = isotonic contraction of quadriceps). *Outcomes:* Pretreatment and posttreatment assessment of knee extension ROM and hamstring EMG activity.	*Results:* ACR condition resulted in greatest gains in range and greatest hamstring EMG activity. *Conclusions:* + ACR condition was better than both CR and passive stretch.
Funk et al[137] 40 undergraduate student athletes; no known impairment Mean age: 19.7	*Design:* RCT Subjects were randomly assigned to 2 conditions: 1. 5 minutes of contract-relax 2. 5 minutes of static stretching As a counterbalance, within 7 days subjects participated in the alternate condition. *Outcomes:* Hamstring flexibility assessed at baseline, posttreatment, and post-treatment plus 60 minutes of cycling and upper extremity conditioning.	*Results:* Contract relax followed by exercise resulted in greater hamstring flexibility than static stretching with or without exercise or CR without exercise. *Conclusions:* + Contract relax condition followed by exercise resulted in greatest gains in hamstring flexibility.

RCT, Randomized controlled trial; *NDT,* neurodevelopmental therapy; *PNF,* proprioceptive neuromuscular facilitation; *ROM,* range of motion; *EMG,* electromyography.

task-oriented approaches. A variety of types of feedback are available to patients as they learn and refine motor skills. For example, patients have access to *intrinsic feedback* about both the outcome of a functional task, as well as the movement used to accomplish that outcome.[140] Intrinsic feedback includes any type of feedback that is naturally available to the individual such as somatosensory, proprioceptive, or visual input. External or *augmented feedback* related to *knowledge of results* (KR) or *knowledge of*

performance (KP) is also often provided to patients by therapists with the goal of improving motor control. Examples of augmented feedback include verbal or tactile cues and such feedback may be provided concurrently, immediately following, or be delayed in relation to the action.[141] The impact of augmented feedback on both the performance of motor skills and motor learning has been studied in individuals with and without neurological deficit. Motor learning has typically been defined as a process

TABLE 16-8	Environmental Context: Task Categories and Examples

Regulatory Conditions	Intertrial Variability: Absent	Intertrial Variability: Present
Stationary	*Closed tasks:* Climbing stairs at home Brushing teeth Unlocking the front door Stepping on the bathroom scale	*Variable motionless tasks:* Walking on different surfaces Climbing stairs of different heights Drinking from mugs, glasses, cups
Motion	*Consistent motion tasks:* Stepping onto an escalator Lifting luggage from an airport conveyor Moving through a revolving door	*Open tasks:* Sitting in a moving automobile Catching a ball Walking down a crowded hallway Carrying a wiggling child

From Gentile A: Skill acquisition: Action, movement, and neuromotor processes. In Carr J, Shepherd R (eds): *Movement Science: Foundations for Physical Therapy in Rehabilitation,* ed 2, Gaithersburg, Md, 2000, Aspen.

TABLE 16-9	Function of the Action: Task Categories and Examples

Body Orientation	Manipulation: Absent	Manipulation: Present
Stability	*Body stability:* Sit Stand Lean on table	*Body stability plus manipulation:* Hold object while standing Reach for glass while sitting Writing at a desk
Transport	*Body transport:* Run Walk Crawl	*Body transport plus manipulation:* Carry child while walking Run to catch a ball Drive an automobile

From Gentile A: Skill acquisition: Action, movement, and neuromotor processes. In Carr J, Shepherd R (eds): *Movement Science: Foundations for Physical Therapy in Rehabilitation,* ed 2, Gaithersburg, Md, 2000, Aspen.

associated with practice that leads to a relatively permanent change in performance of motor skills.[142,143] As such, changes in performance observed immediately after a treatment session are not generally considered evidence of motor learning unless these changes are retained over time. For example, if a patient moved from sit-to-stand asymmetrically and with assistance at the beginning of a treatment session and demonstrates the ability to move from sit-to-stand symmetrically and independently at the end of the session, this would be evidence of improved performance. If the patient continues to be able to demonstrate a symmetrical and independent sit-to-stand at the beginning of his or her next treatment session, this would be evidence of retention of that skill and thus motor learning.

In general, although more research has been conducted on the use of feedback with people without neurological conditions than in people with neurological impairments, the evidence suggests that both the timing and frequency of feedback may significantly influence its effects on motor performance and learning. Explicit knowledge of the task goals before practice for individuals poststroke appears to improve implicit learning of motor skills. For example, in a study by Boyd and Winstein, 12 individuals with diagnoses of chronic stroke were randomly assigned to one of three practice conditions for a serial reaction-time task in which subjects were asked to press buttons in response to a 9-element light sequence.[144] The conditions included (1) unaware of the light pattern and practiced for 1 day, (2) unaware of the light pattern and practiced for 3 days, and (3) aware of the light pattern and practiced for 1 day. Reaction time did not improve in either of the conditions in which subjects were not made explicitly aware of the pattern. In contrast, the group with explicit knowledge performed significantly better over the practice blocks. These results suggest that explicit knowledge before practice facilitated improved motor learning. For more complex tasks, in studies with individuals without neurological deficits, there is evidence that motor learning is enhanced with instructions that focus on the effects of movement (external focus) rather than the movement itself (internal focus).[145,146] For example, in one study, 22 college students without prior experience playing golf were taught to drive a golf ball.[147] Both groups received the same information regarding grip, stance, and posture, but one group received instructions on the swing that were focused on the motion of the arms and the other received instruction focused on the movement of the golf club. Accuracy in hitting the golf ball was significantly better during both the practice phase and the retention test 1 day later for the group that received the externally-focused instructions, which emphasized the movement of the golf club. Although not empirically supported for individuals with neuromuscular disorders, this body of evidence has led some researchers to suggest that if the goal of an intervention session is to increase step length, it may be more effective to focus on having the patient move her cane further in front of her (external focus) in order to "force" a longer step than having her focus on more fully extending the knee (internal focus).[148]

In terms of the timing and amount of feedback provided, a number of research studies have found that providing knowledge of results in a summary form (e.g., after 10 trials) is detrimental to initial performance but enhances learning on retention tests.[149,150] In these studies, groups of 60-70 college students were trained in an upper extremity task that involved using a lever to backswing, intersect a moving light at a specific point, and follow through (similar to the motion required for batting). Skill in the task was judged based on the velocity of the lever or "bat" at the time of contact with the light and minimization of spatial errors (e.g., how solid the contact was between the "bat/lever" and the "ball/light"). The knowledge of results provided to the subjects was a score that reflected both velocity and spatial accuracy. In these studies, subjects receiving summary feedback made more errors while learning the motor task than did subjects who received knowledge of results after every trial. But when they were tested for retention at a later date, the subjects who had received summary feedback made fewer errors than those who had received constant feedback. Supporting these results, another study with 25 adults without disabilities that compared feedback during every trial, feedback after every trial (100%), and feedback after every other trial (50%) on a task requiring modulation of isometric elbow extension force found that while performance was best during acquisition in the concurrent group, on retention tests the 50% feedback group made the fewest errors.[151] Furthermore, in a study with 136 graduate students when KR was provided on a faded schedule, with more feedback provided in the early phases of learning and gradually less feedback provided in the later phases, superior motor learning occurred than in a 100% KR practice condition.[152] Similar results have been found with physical guidance feedback (e.g., providing a physical block to assist the individual in learning where to target a movement).[153] Specifically, 40 individuals learning an upper extremity motor task had the poorest retention when they received high frequency physical guidance as opposed to faded physical or verbal feedback. Furthermore, high frequency physical guidance resulted in poorer learning outcomes than verbal knowledge of results feedback provided with the same frequency. These findings indicate that in addition to the frequency of feedback, the type of feedback may also affect motor learning and more specifically, that physical guidance provided at high frequencies may be more detrimental to learning than verbal feedback. In addition, research with subjects without neuromuscular disorders also suggests that instantaneous KR feedback adversely impacts motor learning because it interferes with the individual's self-assessment of performance.[154]

In terms of practice, although initial acquisition and performance of a motor skill may be best when a blocked practice paradigm is incorporated, learning, as measured by retention of the motor skill, is improved when healthy subjects engage in random practice.[155] This has also been demonstrated in individuals with neuromuscular disorders.[156] Specifically, in a randomized controlled trial with 24 individuals poststroke, the group that alternated practice of the experimental task with other tasks (random practice) performed better on retention tests than the group that practiced the experimental task for multiple consecutive repetitions (blocked practice). As with the studies on feedback, the number of errors while the participant is acquiring the motor skill is reduced with a blocked practice paradigm. Although most of this research was conducted in individuals without neuromuscular disorders, it appears that the conditions that improve performance within a treatment session are not the same practice or feedback conditions that improve learning and retention of motor skills.

One of the more promising task-oriented approaches for facilitating function of the hemiplegic upper extremity is CIMT (Fig. 16-6). In this approach the nonparetic upper extremity is typically restrained for most of the patient's waking hours, and the patient spends 6 hours per

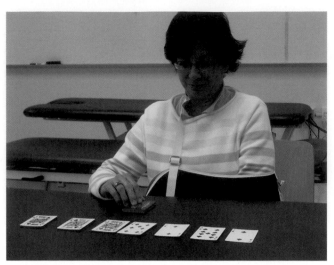

FIG. 16-6 Constraint-induced movement therapy.

day for 2 weeks performing repetitive and structured functional activities that require use of the hemiparetic upper extremity.[157] An important component of CIMT is shaping. Shaping is an operant conditioning method in which the difficulty of the movement task is progressively increased, and individuals are given regular positive reinforcement and feedback regarding their performance. Positive results associated with CIMT have been documented in individuals with chronic stroke and have been shown to be sustained over time.[157-159] In the only larger scale randomized clinical trial (RCT) evaluating CIMT, forced use was compared with NDT in a sample of 66 chronic stroke patients.[120] The forced-use group received intervention for 6 hours per day, 5 days per week for 2 weeks, with the stronger arm immobilized. The subjects in the NDT group received the same intensity of treatment and practiced bimanual activities, with an emphasis on postural symmetry and normal movement. To meet the inclusion criteria for this study, all of the subjects had at least 20 degrees of active wrist extension and 10 degrees of finger extension in the affected arm. The authors found that the CIMT group had better outcomes on the Action Research Arm (ARA) test, a measure of dexterity, than the NDT group. In addition, there was a differential effect based on treatment group for those with and without sensory deficits. For those with sensory deficits, the forced-use group experienced greater mean improvement on the ARA (6.7 points) than those receiving the NDT treatment. These treatment effect differences were sustained at 3 weeks, 6 weeks, and 1 year after completion of treatment. At 3 weeks after completion of treatment, there were also significant differences between the treatment groups on the Motor Activity Log (MAL), a measure of how well and how much patients use an extremity for normal daily activities. Again, there was a differential effect: In this case, the forced-use treatment was of particular benefit for those patients with hemineglect. There were no differences between groups on the Fugl-Meyer Assessment scale.

Other researchers have also begun to investigate modified approaches to CIMT. In a case series, Page et al assigned 6 patients, who were able to actively extend the hemiparetic wrist 20 degrees, the fingers 10 degrees, and move the affected arm outside of synergy, to one of 3 groups.[160] Two patients participated in CIMT and two patients participated in traditional rehabilitation, defined as incorporating PNF techniques and functional tasks with 20% of the time devoted to compensatory techniques with the nonaffected extremity. The final two patients were assigned to a control group in which no therapy was offered. The patients in the two treatment groups participated in their assigned intervention for 1 hour sessions, 3 times per week for 10 weeks. Outcome measures included the Fugl-Meyer Assessment, ARA test, Wolf Motor Function Test (WMFT), and the MAL, which were assessed on conclusion of the 10-week program. Across two pretesting trials, the Fugl-Meyer and ARA measures remained stable. The individuals in the CIMT group demonstrated greater change on the Fugl-Meyer, ARA test, and MAL than those in either the traditional or control group, but minimal differences between groups were noted on the WMFT. Given the case series design, the statistical significance of these reported differences was not assessed. While potentially promising, this study is limited by small group sizes and lack of posttreatment follow-up.

In another study that examined the amount of time per day needed for CIMT, Sterr et al randomly assigned 15 individuals with diagnoses of chronic (greater than 1 year) stroke and TBI to a group that received CIMT 6 hours per day or a group that received CIMT 3 hours per day, 5 days per week for 2 weeks.[161] These subjects met the same active movement criteria as required for previous studies (20 degrees of active wrist extension and 10 degrees of active finger extension). Outcome measures included the MAL and the WMFT. These were completed twice before intervention, directly after the intervention, and at four additional follow-up points over a period of 1 month. The authors reported that both groups showed significant and sustained improvements in the outcome measures when compared to the baseline measurement. There was a stronger effect for the group that received the 6 hour per day intervention.

Very few studies have examined the effects of CIMT in an acute population. In one study by Dromerick et al, researchers randomly assigned 20 patients with diagnoses of stroke within the previous 14 days to either a traditional occupational therapy group or a CIMT group.[162] Patients in both groups received equivalent time and intensity of treatment: In this case, 2 hours per day, 5 days per week for 2 weeks. In addition, patients in the CIMT group wore a restraint on the noninvolved extremity at least 6 hours per day. Posttreatment measures were performed by a blinded evaluator and included the ARA test, Barthel Index, and the FIM. After treatment, the total ARA score was significantly higher in the CIMT group. The Barthel Index and FIM results were not significantly different between groups. Although this study suggested that CIMT for patients in the acute rehabilitation setting may be feasible and beneficial for some outcomes, it is limited by the lack of long-term follow-up, the reduced intensity of the CIMT protocol, and the choice of outcome measures. More specifically, the Barthel Index and FIM may not be sensitive enough to detect meaningful change in upper extremity function.

Thus it appears that CIMT may benefit some patients with neuromuscular disorders. In general, it appears that CIMT is most beneficial for subjects with intact cognition and moderate active movement in the involved upper extremity. In addition, there may be different effects for those with sensory disorders. In general, the intensity of training appears to be a key factor in this approach, with greater intensity (e.g., 6 hours per day) producing more substantial and clinically meaningful results.

In a related study, Winstein et al randomly assigned 64 patients admitted for rehabilitation with recent stroke diagnoses to one of three groups: Functional training, strengthening and motor control, and standard care.[163] The functional training group participated in repetitive task-specific functional activities that were progressed in accordance with the patient's ability. The authors differentiated this approach from the shaping included in CIMT and described it as incorporating active problem-solving of movement problems within the context of functional task practice. In the strengthening and motor control group, patients used a variety of exercise approaches to increase upper extremity strength. Finally, all groups received the control group treatment, which included an NDT approach, neuromuscular electrical stimulation, and activities of daily living (ADLs). In total, the experimental groups participated in their intervention 1 hour per day, 5 days per week, over a 4-6 week period for a total of 20 additional hours of therapy. Subjects were stratified into two groups based on severity using the Orpington Prognostic Scale and were assessed pretreatment, immediately posttreatment, and 6 and 9 months poststroke on the FIM, the upper-extremity subsection of the Fugl-Meyer Assessment, and the Functional Test of the Hemiparetic Upper Extremity (FTHUE). Isometric torque and grip and pinch force were also assessed at these measurement points. These authors found that for those subjects categorized as less severe based on their Orpington Prognostic Scale score, the functional training and strengthening groups performed significantly better than the standard care group on the motor function portion of the Fugl-Meyer Assessment and the isometric torque measurements. There were no differences between groups for those categorized as more severe. For the long-term follow-up, persistent differences remained for the less severe group in isometric torque, with the functional training group performing better than the other groups. Thus this study suggests that both the type of intervention and stroke severity affect short- and long-term motor recovery.

Finally, another promising task-oriented approach to rehabilitation for individuals with nonprogressive neuromuscular disorders is treadmill training with partial BWS. A growing body of evidence indicates that this intervention is an effective means of gait rehabilitation for individuals after a stroke (Fig. 16-7). Hesse et al used an A-B-A single case study design to compare BWS treadmill training with an NDT approach to rehabilitation.[119] Specifically, seven individuals with diagnoses of stroke within the previous 3 months participated in 3 weeks, 30 minutes per day, 5 days per week of (1) BWS treadmill training; (2)

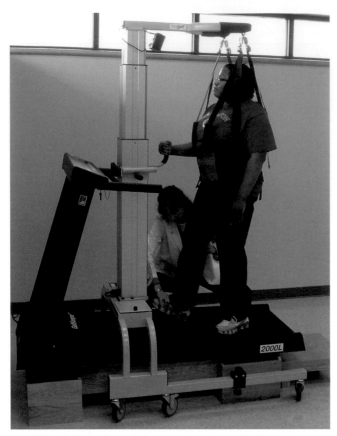

FIG. 16-7 Body weight–supported treadmill training.

NDT-based physical therapy; and (3) BWS treadmill training in random order. Outcome measures included the Functional Ambulation Category (FAC), Rivermead Motor Assessment, Motricity Index, and Modified Ashworth Scale (see Table 16-3), which were assessed before intervention and once a week for the duration of the 9-week study. In addition, gait speed, cadence, and stride length were assessed. BWS treadmill training was superior to the NDT approach for functional gait ability (FAC) and gait velocity. No differences between phases were noted for any of the other outcome measures.

Visintin and Barbeau conducted a RCT with 100 subjects admitted for inpatient stroke rehabilitation.[164] Subjects were stratified based on initial ambulatory status (low being defined as requiring maximal assistance to walk) and randomly assigned to one of two groups: A group that started with 40% BWS and gradually progressed to 0% BWS and a group that did not receive BWS during treadmill training. Both groups participated in treadmill training for up to 20 minutes per day, 4 days per week for 6 weeks. Forty-three subjects in the BWS group and thirty-six subjects in the no-BWS group completed the training. Subjects who did not complete the training were more likely to be female, older, and have more co-morbidities. Outcomes were assessed pretraining, immediately posttraining, and at a 3-month follow-up session. Significant differences were found between groups, with the BWS group performing better on measures of balance (BBS), lower extremity motor recovery (Stroke Rehabilitation Assessment of Movement [STREAM] scale), over ground walking speed, and over ground endurance. These differences persisted at the 3-month follow-up in all areas except for balance and over ground endurance. Barbeau and Visintin extended this study and examined possible differential treatment effects for the BWS training associated with pretraining scores.[165] Their analysis suggested that individuals who were more functionally impaired initially, based on lower over ground walking speed, over ground endurance, balance, and lower extremity motor control, experienced a greater training effect. In contrast, training effects were not significantly different between groups for those patients with higher initial scores. This differential effect may be due to the limited range for demonstrating improvement in higher functioning patients or inability of the outcome measures to detect small changes.

In a study by Nilsson et al, researchers randomly assigned 73 patients with hemiparesis after stroke to either a BWS treadmill training group or an over ground walking group.[166] Both groups participated in the intervention for 30 minutes per day, 5 days per week. Both groups also received other rehabilitation during the intervention phase. Treatment duration varied based on the patient's length of stay on the rehabilitation unit from 3-19 weeks (median of 68 days in the control group and 68 days in the treatment group). Outcome measures included the FIM, Fugl-Meyer Assessment, FAC, walking speed, and BBS. Both groups improved on all measures, and no significant differences were noted between groups at discharge or at the 10-month follow up. The results of this study may have varied from those discussed previously because of differences in the patient population (the patients in the Nilsson study were an average 55 years of age), as well as the intensity and type of training provided to the control group.

BWS treadmill training may improve functional gait and velocity, particularly for those individuals who are either unable to walk or require maximal assistance of one or more individuals for ambulation (see Chapter 32). For this patient population, reported advantages of BWS treadmill training include the ability to begin gait training earlier in the recovery process and its repetitive, task-specific nature.[167] Although no studies were identified that included individuals with TBI as subjects, given the effectiveness of this approach in patients with stroke and the similarities in impairments and functional limitations associated with both pathologies, this approach also holds promise for patients with TBI.

THERAPEUTIC EXERCISE

Aerobic and Endurance Conditioning/Reconditioning. Many of the impairments associated with stroke and TBI, such as abnormal motor control, reduced strength and power, impaired sensation, and hypertonicity or hypotonicity, may lead to inefficient motor control that results in increased energy expenditure during ambulation and other functional activities.[168,169] In addition, individuals with stroke are often physically deconditioned and have reduced aerobic capacity compared to age-matched controls.[170] As such, there is good evidence that individuals with nonprogressive CNS disorders may benefit from aerobic exercise and endurance training.

A number of different aerobic exercise training regimens, particularly for individuals at least 6 months post stroke, have been evaluated in the literature.[168,170-172] Positive effects have been reported for submaximal training programs involving 6 months of treadmill ambulation 2-3 times per week for 40-minute sessions.[168,171] Specifically, in these studies, individuals who exercised at 50% to 60% of their heart rate reserve significantly improved their fitness reserve or their percentage of peak oxygen consumption during submaximal exercise. These programs were conducted without BWS on the treadmill. Although treadmill training can be conducted with BWS, not surprisingly, oxygen uptake and heart rate measures have been found to be lower under these conditions.[172] It should be noted that almost 25% of the patients screened for this treadmill training study could not participate either because of co-morbidities or neurological deficits that prevented full weight-bearing treadmill walking.[168] It is possible that more individuals could have participated if some percentage of BWS had been allowed. While these studies provide preliminary support for the effectiveness of treadmill exercise training programs after stroke, they are all limited by small sample sizes, ranging from 9 to 23 subjects, and no meta-analyses of these studies has been published.

Balance, Coordination, and Agility Training. Individuals with diagnoses of stroke or TBI often present with perceptual, sensory, and motor impairments that impact balance and coordination. In addition, balance status has been associated with length of stay and other rehabilitation outcome measures.[173] As such, significant attention is often given to addressing these functional limitations and interventions to improve balance or postural control may take various approaches. Interventions can be designed to improve postural control in either sitting or standing, and they may be focused on symmetry, stability, anticipatory, or reactionary control.

Postural Symmetry. From an NDT perspective, postural symmetry, or the ability to evenly bear weight in sitting or standing, is a key indicator of improved motor control.[20,113] A symmetrical base of support allows individuals to appropriately prepare for movement and provides a foundation for normal equilibrium reactions, as well as other functional activities. For example, by establishing equal weight bearing with a neutral pelvis in sitting, a patient with a stroke or TBI can better activate his or her trunk musculature to move from a sitting position to standing.

In preparation for sitting, therapists using an NDT approach should first work to establish symmetrical alignment and a neutral pelvis. This would include even weight bearing on the ischial tuberosities, lower extremities, and feet.[21] In addition, the shoulders and head should be positioned symmetrically and there should be no rotation in the trunk. From this position, the therapist can facilitate anterior and posterior tilts of the pelvis, as well as lateral weight shifting. To facilitate an anterior pelvic tilt, while sitting in front of the patient, the therapist's hands are positioned around the patient's trunk to the back, aiming

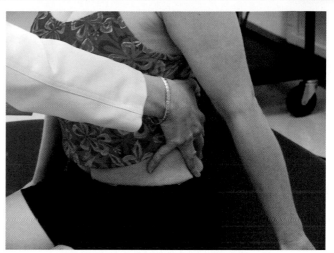

FIG. 16-8 Neurodevelopmental treatment facilitation of sitting posture.

down and in. The hands then give a cue forward and up and the fifth digit can be used to cue the abdominal musculature (Fig. 16-8). For a posterior pelvic tilt, similar hand holds are used, but the fifth digit is used to cue the patient's trunk down and back.

From a PNF perspective, to achieve good sitting balance and symmetry, repeated contractions or resistance in a diagonal through the anterior superior iliac spines can be used to facilitate an anterior pelvic tilt. Once a neutral pelvic position is achieved, rhythmic stabilization or alternating isometrics can be applied to the trunk to promote a stable posture.

In standing, postural symmetry can be encouraged through NDT techniques by facilitating alignment of the trunk and lower extremities. Important key points of control to achieve this alignment include the trunk, pelvis, and knees. As with sitting, PNF stability techniques, such as rhythmic stabilization and alternating isometrics, can be superimposed at the shoulders or pelvis to encourage symmetry and stability in standing. As discussed earlier, there is limited evidence to support the effectiveness of these approaches to postural control.

Another approach to retraining symmetry is through the use of postural biofeedback. For this method, patients typically sit or stand on a force platform and perform activities with or without visual and auditory feedback regarding the symmetry of their position. This training can also involve weight shifting either laterally or in an anterior/posterior direction. In this case, the patient may be provided with visual feedback about the position of his center of mass (Fig. 16-9). There is evidence that this intervention approach is more effective than others in improving stance symmetry. In one study, sixteen individuals with stroke were randomly assigned to force-platform biofeedback training or a control group that participated in standing balance training without the use of force-platform biofeedback.[71] Both groups received the assigned intervention for 15 minutes of their regular therapy session, 2 times per day for 2 weeks. Patients in the experimental group showed greater improvements in stance symmetry than the control group. Similarly, in another study, 42 subjects matched, based on factors such as motor

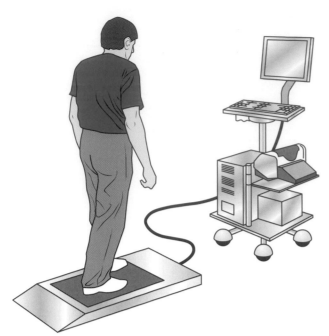

FIG. 16-9 Force-plate biofeedback training for postural symmetry.

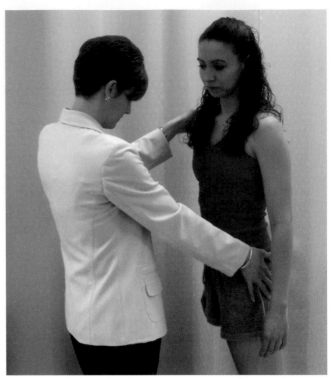

FIG. 16-10 Neurodevelopmental treatment facilitation of weight shifting in standing.

control, functional status, time since stroke, and age, were assigned to either a force-platform biofeedback group or a control group that participated in standing balance and weight-shifting activities.[72] The group that received force-platform biofeedback training demonstrated greater improvements in stance symmetry; however, there were no differences between groups on measures of gait velocity, cadence, or stride length.

Dynamic Balance/Stability. After symmetry has been established, NDT theory suggests that the therapist begin to work on dynamic postural control. Activities that may be incorporated at this stage include facilitated weight shifting that is progressed to stepping forward and back with the nonparetic leg and weight shifting in a stride position (Fig. 16-10). This can then be progressed to include lifting and stepping with the paretic lower extremity. NDT facilitation is structured based on the needs of the patient and possible hand placements to facilitate dynamic postural control, including bilateral control at the pelvis, control at the pelvis on the nonparetic side and control at the paretic shoulder or upper extremity, control at the nonparetic shoulder with support for the involved upper extremity, and control from the side at the paretic pelvis and knee.

From a PNF perspective, the recommended activities to facilitate dynamic postural control are similar to those that would be used with an NDT approach, but the facilitation techniques differ. For example, the therapist working from this perspective might start by applying rhythmic initiation and repeated contraction to weight shifting in stride to assist with initiation of movement. This can be progressed to the application of slow reversals and agonistic reversals (Fig. 16-11). From this point, the patient can begin to work on pre-gait activities such as repeated stepping with one lower extremity. This is typi-

cally facilitated by providing approximation through the stance leg at midstance and applying repeated contractions down and back through the anterior superior iliac spine during swing.

From a task-oriented perspective, dynamic postural control in sitting and standing is addressed through specific tasks designed to facilitate lateral and anterior/posterior control. For example, patients may be asked to reach for objects in different directions or catch objects while sitting or standing on different surfaces.[96] The principles of feedback and practice previously discussed would be superimposed on these activities.

Flexibility. Bobath suggested that reducing spasticity is a key step in moving patients with CNS disorders toward increased flexibility and more normal motor control.[20] Specific techniques that may assist with this include gentle stretching of spastic muscles and approximation of proximal joint structures. However, there are no RCTs that indicate that either of these approaches has any more than a transient effect on hypertonicity. In one study of 20 subjects with multiple sclerosis, the author reported a differential effect: in one group of patients, muscle firing rates were unaffected by stretch of the muscle, and in another group, firing rates gradually reduced and disappeared in response to continuous stretch.[174]

When severe, splints or casts may be recommended to reduce spasticity and increase joint ROM. These are most commonly applied to the ankle, knee, or elbow. It has been proposed that casts are effective because they provide prolonged stretch, warmth, and pressure.[175-177] A recent systematic review on this topic concluded that there was limited support in nonrandomized studies for the reduc-

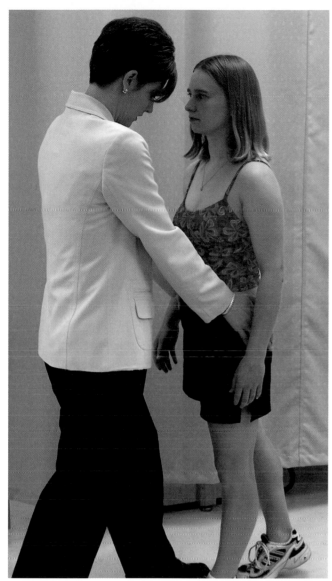

FIG. 16-11 Application of slow reversals to weight shifting in standing.

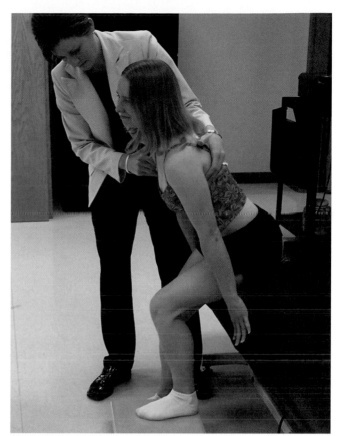

FIG. 16-12 Task-oriented approach to improve ankle dorsiflexion range of motion.

tion of spasticity through the use of serial casting but good support for improved ROM through use of this technique.[178]

The two most common PNF techniques that address flexibility in patients with neuromuscular disorders are hold-relax and contract-relax. The evidence related to these techniques has been previously discussed and supports their use over passive stretching for the improvement of flexibility in individuals without neuromuscular disorders.

The task-oriented approaches recognize the importance and impact of impairments in flexibility on motor control and function.[96,97] In addition to standard stretching and joint mobilization, therapists employing this approach use functional activities to improve flexibility and ROM. For example, sit-to-stand activities can be structured to use more dorsiflexion range based on foot placement and

surface height (Fig. 16-12). Similarly, reaching activities can be structured so that they demand more hip or knee extension. No evidence in support of the efficacy of this approach to improving flexibility was found.

Gait and Locomotion Training. From an NDT perspective, gait rehabilitation involves both pre-gait and gait activities. Pre-gait activities related to dynamic postural control were addressed previously and are believed to provide a foundation for gait activities.[113] Despite the belief that pre-gait activities influence gait, there is some evidence that this is not the case. For example, as previously mentioned, Winstein failed to demonstrate carry over of improved symmetry in standing to gait velocity, cadence, stride length, or gait cycle duration.[72] Direct gait training activities may include facilitation through the use of key points of control at the shoulders, trunk, hip, knee, ankle, or foot, depending on the gait deviations observed. The objective is to facilitate biomechanical alignment and muscle activation that is as close to normal as possible. As previously discussed, there are no RCTs supporting the effectiveness of NDT techniques over other approaches for the improvement of gait in individuals with neuromuscular disorders. A recent case description of two subjects status poststroke treated from an NDT perspective reported small improvements in movement patterns, reduced tone, and improved mobility.[101] However, in another A-B-A single-case design, the NDT approach was significantly less effective than BWS treadmill training in improving parameters of gait.[119]

With PNF, gait is typically facilitated by applying approximation through the weight-bearing limb and repeated contractions to the pelvis during swing phase. As with the NDT approach, pre-gait activities typically precede facilitation of gait. No studies documenting the effectiveness of these techniques for the rehabilitation of gait were located in a recent Medline abstract search from 1966 to the present using the term "proprioceptive neuromuscular facilitation."

Strength, Power, and Endurance Training. A positive relationship between hip flexor, knee flexor, and ankle plantarflexor torque on both the paretic and nonparetic side and speed of gait and stair climbing has been documented for individuals with stroke.[179] Knee extension force has also been correlated to sit-to-stand ability for patients with a variety of diagnoses receiving inpatient rehabilitation.[180] Furthermore, a number of studies indicate that strength training benefits individuals with non-progressive CNS disorders and that this training does not adversely affect muscle tone or spasticity. For example, as previously described, Butefisch et al compared NDT based treatment to repetitive resistance training for the hand in 27 individuals with hemiplegia and found that improvements in strength and hand function were limited to the repetitive resistance training group.[118] In another study, 15 subjects with poststroke hemiplegia attempted 12 randomly ordered workload and cadence combinations on a lower extremity cycle ergometer.[181] Results indicated that individuals with stroke could increase the strength of their hemiplegic leg using increased workload conditions without increasing spasticity.

The NDT approach only addresses strength as it relates to normal movement patterns and functional activities due to concern that the excessive effort associated with resisted strength training may worsen hypertonicity and subsequently interfere with normal movement.[21] One NDT method used to improve lower extremity strength is the facilitation of bridging (Fig. 16-13). For this activity, the therapist uses key points of control on both thighs or at the pelvis to assist the patient to bridge. Bridging can be progressed to single leg bridging and single leg bridg-

ing with the leg over the edge of the mat and supported on a stool or step. A proposed advantage of this activity is that it facilitates hip extension strength with knee and ankle flexion and therefore does not encourage an abnormal synergy pattern.

A number of PNF techniques are designed to increase strength through the use of manual resistance. Strength training in the extremity diagonals using rhythmic initiation, slow reversal hold, and slow reversals are suggested for individuals after stroke or TBI.[124] In addition, these techniques can be applied to the pelvis, shoulder girdle, and trunk and in a variety of positions such as prone on elbows, quadruped, kneeling, or half-kneeling. Although limited evidence exists, it is suggested that this approach can improve strength, ROM, and motor control.[123] As previously discussed, one nonrandomized trial with 20 subjects with diagnoses of stroke was located which addressed this topic.[106] This study found that application of the PNF techniques rhythmic initiation, slow reversals, and agonistic reversals to the pelvic region of individuals with hemiplegia (3 times per week for 4 weeks) resulted in significantly improved gait speed and cadence immediately after the intervention. Limitations of this research included the absence of a control group or long-term follow-up testing.

The task-oriented approaches include a number of strategies designed to strengthen muscles in patients with hemiparesis. For example, patients may be asked to step up and down from surfaces of different heights and in different directions, raise and lower the foot while standing on steps of different heights, or complete other activities requiring single leg stance on the hemiplegic extremity.[96] No evidence was found supporting the effectiveness of these activities for strengthening in individuals with non-progressive neuromuscular disorders.

FUNCTIONAL TRAINING IN SELF-CARE AND HOME MANAGEMENT

Functional training can include a variety of activities such as bed mobility, transfers and activities of daily living. When facilitating rolling using NDT principles, the therapist is encouraged to pay close attention to the positioning of the involved upper extremity, particularly if it is flaccid, to ensure that the scapula maintains a protracted position and that the extremity is protected. The patient can also be taught to use the nonparetic extremity to support the paretic lower extremity during rolling to facilitate this motion. When training the patient to move from sidelying on the hemiparetic side to sitting upright, it is suggested that the therapist facilitate lateral trunk flexion on the paretic side and weight shift through the pelvis on the nonparetic side. In addition, the therapist may support the hemiparetic scapular region and incorporate weight bearing through the hemiparetic arm. This can assist with muscle activation, reduce tone, and increase stability in the involved extremity. In transfers, the goal is to facilitate symmetrical, normal movement during the activity. Special attention is given to trunk activation, symmetrical lower extremity weight bearing, and activation of the involved extremity. The therapist can use key points of control at the trunk or lower extremity or both. If the

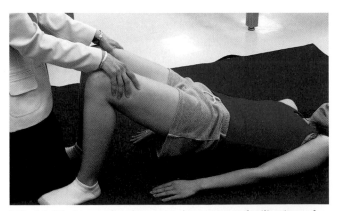

FIG. 16-13 Neurodevelopmental treatment facilitation of bridging with key points of control on the distal femurs.

involved upper extremity is flaccid, it should be supported on the patient's knee or by the therapist to avoid shoulder or upper extremity injury.

With a PNF approach, rolling can be encouraged with techniques that promote either mass or reciprocal trunk patterns. With mass rolling patterns the upper and lower trunk move simultaneously to complete the roll. To facilitate mass flexion or extension, techniques, such as rhythmic initiation, slow reversals and agonistic reversals of the pelvis and shoulder, can be used. For example, in sidelying, mass flexion can be facilitated through simultaneous resistance of anterior depression at the shoulder girdle and anterior elevation at the pelvis. Reciprocal trunk patterns in rolling occur when the roll is initiated by either the upper or lower trunk. This can be facilitated in sidelying by applying rhythmic initiation to anterior elevation at the shoulder girdle with posterior depression at the pelvis. This can be followed by rhythmic initiation to posterior depression at the shoulder and anterior elevation at the pelvis. The verbal cue, "twist," can be used to assist the patient with this activity.

In the task-oriented approach, functional activities are facilitated through the therapist's design of the task, structure of the environment, feedback, and practice. For example, the therapist can structure transfers from sitting to standing to incorporate different seat heights or surfaces. A higher seat height makes the task easier as the patient does not need to raise his or her center of gravity as far. This activity can be progressed by reducing the seat height or by asking the patient to perform an upper extremity task, such as picking up a glass, while moving from sitting to standing. Feedback can also be provided in summary form after three to five trials. In addition, the therapist should withhold feedback for a short period to allow the patient to reflect on his or her performance and engage him or her in active problem solving. Rolling can also incorporate functional reaching activities. For example, the patient could be asked to reach for items located in a variety of spatial positions at the bedside.

CASE STUDY 16-1

STROKE

Examination
Patient History
Three weeks ago, MF, a 72-year-old man, presented to the emergency room 3 hours after sudden onset of slurred speech and weakness of the right upper and lower extremity. MF was diagnosed with a left CVA in the distribution of the anterior cerebral artery and was admitted to the hospital. Since that time, he has progressed well, with improvements in right upper and lower extremity motor control and functional status. MF's past medical history includes hypertension. He was recently discharged home with his wife and has been referred for outpatient services.

Tests and Measures
Musculoskeletal: MF has 3/5 strength throughout the right lower extremity. Other strength is 5/5.

Neuromuscular: MF is alert and oriented and he scored 27/30 on the MMSE. Light touch sensation is intact, but proprioception is decreased at the right ankle (he is able to correctly identify the position of his right ankle 2/3 times). When examining lower extremity motor control, he achieves a score of 1 for hip, knee, and ankle motion (total score of 3/6) on the Fugl-Meyer Assessment when asked to flex his right knee and dorsiflex his ankle in standing while maintaining his hip in a neutral position.

Function: MF can stand for less than 1 minute without support, and he has increased postural sway when standing. Minimal assistance is required for standing pivot transfers. MF can ambulate 50 feet with minimal to moderate assistance (score of 3-4 on the FIM) and use of a cane. Gait deviations include decreased right hip extension in terminal stance, right knee hyperextension in midstance, and decreased right ankle push-off.

Evaluation, Diagnosis, and Prognosis
MF presents with impaired proprioception, strength, motor control, and balance. These impairments have resulted in decreased transfer and gait ability. Diagnosis is in the preferred practice pattern 5D: Impaired motor function and sensory integrity associated with nonprogressive disorders of the CNS—acquired in adolescence or adulthood.

Goals
Goals include improving strength, motor control, balance, transfer, and gait ability so that this patient can function independently in his home and in most community activities. The plan is for outpatient treatment to include aerobic conditioning and endurance exercises, therapeutic exercise and functional training 3 times per week for 3-6 weeks with reassessment for consideration of need for continued therapy bi-weekly at the end of this period.

Interventions
Interventions for MF would include PNF beginning with slow reversals of the right lower extremity in the D1F/D1E diagonal. This diagonal would promote strengthening and isolated control of the lower extremity emphasizing terminal hip extension and ankle dorsiflexion. In addition, from a task-oriented perspective, MF would be asked to stand with his right lower extremity on steps of varying heights and raise and lower his left heel from the ground in a controlled manner. This would also encourage strengthening and isolated control of the right lower extremity. To address MF's balance deficits, a task-oriented approach including static standing activities and activities during which he must reach outside of his base of control (such as reaching for objects at a counter) would also be incorporated. In addition, during each session he would practice treadmill ambulation to improve gait and increase strength and endurance.

Please see the CD that accompanies this book for case studies describing the examination, evaluation, and interventions for a patient undergoing rehabilitation after traumatic brain injury and for another patient undergoing rehabilitation after stroke.

CHAPTER SUMMARY

This chapter addresses the management of adult patients with impaired motor function and sensory integrity secondary to nonprogressive CNS disorders. Common pathologies related to this practice pattern, as well as tests and measures for aerobic capacity and endurance; arousal, attention and cognition; gait, locomotion and balance; motor function; muscle performance; self-care and home management; and sensory integrity, were introduced. Evaluation, diagnosis, and prognosis were then discussed along with research related to outcomes for these patient populations. Finally, interventions associated with NDT, PNF, and task-oriented approaches were discussed, and the evidence available to support or refute these interventions was presented. The chapter concludes with case study examples of the application of the above information related to the rehabilitation of individuals with nonprogressive CNS disorders.

ADDITIONAL RESOURCES

Useful Forms

Berg Balance Scales (BBS)
Fugl-Meyer Assessment
Performance-Oriented Mobility Assessment (POMA)

Web Sites

American Heart Association: www.americanheart.org
Brain Injury Association of America: www.biausa.org
National Resource Center on Traumatic Brain Injury: www.neuro.pmr.vcu.edu/
Neuro-Developmental Treatment Association: www.ndta.org

Books

Adler SS, Beckers D, Buck M: *PNF in Practice: An Illustrated Guide,* Berlin, 1993, Springer-Verlag.

Bobath B: *Adult Hemiplegia: Evaluation and Treatment,* ed 3, Oxford, 1990, Heinemann Medical Books.

Carr J, Shepherd R: *Neurological Rehabilitation: Optimizing Motor Performance,* Oxford, 1998, Butterworth Heinemann.

Carr J, Shepherd R: *Stroke Rehabilitation: Guidelines for Exercise and Training to Optimize Motor Skill,* Edinburgh, 2003, Butterworth Heinemann.

Davies PM: *Steps to Follow: A Guide to the Treatment of Adult Hemiplegia,* New York, 1984, Springer-Verlag.

Davies PM: *Right in the Middle: Selective Trunk Activity in the Treatment of Adult Hemiplegia,* New York, 1990, Springer-Verlag.

Howle JM: *Neuro-Developmental Treatment Approach: Theoretical Foundations and Principles of Clinical Practice,* Laguna Beach, Calif, 2002, NDTA.

Voss DE, Ionta MK, Myers BJ: *Proprioceptive Neuromuscular Facilitation: Patterns and Techniques,* ed 3, Philadelphia, 1985, JB Lippincott.

GLOSSARY

Abnormal synergy: Stereotyped patterns of movement that cannot be changed or adapted in response to task or environmental demands.

Agonistic reversals: Isotonic contraction in the diagonal, followed by an eccentric contraction of the same muscle groups.

Alternating isometrics: Alternating isometric contractions of the agonist and antagonist.

Augmented feedback: External feedback provided to the patient by the therapist; examples include verbal, visual, or tactile cues.

Contract-relax: Movement into agonist pattern until point of limitation followed by isometric contraction of all components of the antagonist pattern except for the rotation component, which is allowed to contract isotonically; repeated with passive movement into any newly gained range after each trial.

Controlled mobility: Ability to alter a position or move in a weight-bearing position while maintaining postural stability.

Dysdiadochokinesia: Impaired ability to perform rapidly alternating movements.

Dysmetria: Impaired ability to judge the distance or range of a movement.

Dyssynergia: Impaired interjoint coordination.

Hold-relax: Isometric contraction of the agonist or antagonist musculature in the desired diagonal at the point of range limitation; this is repeated with passive movement into any newly gained range after each trial

Hold-relax active motion: An isometric contraction in the shortened range of the diagonal, passive movement into the lengthened range followed by active contraction into the shortened range.

Initial mobility: Discrete movements that are not well controlled; postural or antigravity control is lacking.

Intrinsic feedback: Any type of feedback that is naturally available to the individual such as somatosensory, proprioceptive, or visual input.

Knowledge of performance (KP): Augmented feedback about the individual's movement performance.

Knowledge of results (KR): Verbal, terminal, augmented feedback about the outcome of a motor task.

Motor learning: Process associated with practice that leads to a relatively permanent change in one's ability to produced skilled movement.

Muscle tone: Resistance to passive stretch.

Regulatory conditions: Elements of the environment to which a task must conform.

Repeated contractions: Repeated use of the stretch reflex to initiate a contraction or reinforce and strengthen an existing contraction.

Rhythmic initiation: Progression of movement in diagonal from passive to active assistive to active to resisted.

Rhythmic stabilization: An extension of alternating isometrics in which the manual contacts are on opposite joint surfaces simultaneously.

Skill: Highly coordinated movement that allows for adaptability to meet the demands of the individual and the environment.

Slow reversals: Slow concentric contractions alternating between the agonist and antagonist muscle groups.

Slow reversal-hold: Slow concentric contractions alternating between the agonist and antagonist muscle groups with an isometric contraction applied at the end of each diagonal.

Spasticity: A motor disorder characterized by a velocity-dependent increase in tonic stretch reflexes accompanied by exaggerated tendon jerks.

Stability: Ability to maintain a steady position in a weight-bearing, antigravity posture.

Timing for emphasis: Maximal isometric resistance applied to stronger components of the diagonal to allow for facilitation or irradiation to weaker components.

References

1. American Physical Therapy Association: *Guide to Physical Therapist Practice,* ed 2, Alexandria, Va, 2001, APTA.
2. Guccione AA: Arthritis and the process of disablement, *Phys Ther* 1994; 74:410, 1994.
3. Sackett DL, Rosenberg WMC, Gray JA, et al: Evidence based medicine: What it is and what it isn't, *BMJ* 312:71-72, 1996.
4. World Health Organization: Stroke—1989: Recommendations on stroke prevention, diagnosis, and therapy: Report of the WHO task

force on stroke and other cerebrovascular disorders, *Stroke* 20:1407-1431, 1989.

5. Agency for Health Care Policy and Research: *Post-Stroke Rehabilitation: Clinical Practice Guideline*, Rockville, Md, 1995, Aspen.

6. Wolf PA, D'Agostino RB, Belanger AJ, et al: Probability of stroke: a risk profile from the Framingham Study, *Stroke* 22:312-318, 1991.

7. Mitchell RN, Cotran RS: Hemodynamic disorders, thrombosis, and shock. In Cotran RS, Kumar V, Collins T (eds): *Robbins Pathologic Basis of Disease*, ed 6, Philadelphia, 1999, WB Saunders.

8. Saladin LK: Cerebrovascular disease: Stroke. In Fredericks CM, Saladin LK (eds): *Pathophysiology of the Motor Systems*, Philadelphia, 1996, FA Davis.

9. Broderick JP, Phillips SJ, Whisnant JP, et al: Incidence rates of stroke in the eighties: the end of the decline in stroke, *Stroke* 20:577-582, 1989.

10. Andreoli TE, Bennett JC, Carpenter CC, et al: *Cecil Essentials of Medicine*, ed 4, Philadelphia, 1997, WB Saunders.

11. Kegler S, Coronado V, Annest J, et al: Estimating nonfatal traumatic brain injury hospitalizations using and urban/rural index, *J Head Trauma Rehabil* 18:469-478, 2003.

12. Thurman D, Alverson C, Dunn K, et al: Traumatic brain injury in the United States: A public health perspective, *J Head Trauma Rehabil* 14:602-615, 1999.

13. Harrison CL, Dijkers M: Traumatic brain injury registries in the United States, *Brain Inj* 6:206, 1992.

14. De Girolami U, Anthony DC, Frosch MP: The central nervous system. In Cotran RS, Kumar V, Collins T (eds): *Robbins Pathologic Basis of Disease*, ed 6, Philadelphia, 1999, WB Saunders.

15. Campbell M. *Rehabilitation for Traumatic Brain Injury: Physical Therapy Practice in Context*, Edinburgh, 2000, Churchill Livingstone.

16. Guiliani C: Strength training for patients with neurological disorders, *Neurology Rep* 19:29-34, 1995.

17. Armstrong LE, Winant DM, Swasey PR, et al: Using isokinetic dynamometry to test ambulatory patients with multiple sclerosis, *Phys Ther* 63:1274-1279, 1983.

18. Tripp EJ, Harris SR: Test-retest reliability of isokinetic knee extension and flexion torque measurements in persons with spastic hemiparesis, *Phys Ther* 71:290-296, 1991.

19. Watkins MP, Harris BA, Kozlowski BA: Isokinetic testing in patients with hemiparesis, *Phys Ther* 2:1185-1189, 1984.

20. Bobath B: *Adult Hemiplegia: Evaluation and Treatment*, ed 3, Oxford, 1990, Heinemann Medical Books.

21. Davies PM: *Steps to Follow: A Guide to the Treatment of Adult Hemiplegia*, New York, 1985, Springer-Verlag.

22. Sahrmann SA, Norton BS: The relationship of voluntary movement to spasticity in the upper motor neuron syndrome, *Ann Neurol* 2:460-465, 1977.

23. Bohannon RW, Walsh S: Nature, reliability, and predictive value of muscle performance measures in patients with hemiparesis following stroke, *Arch Phys Med Rehabil* 73:721-725, 1992.

24. Teasdale G, Jennett B: Assessment of coma and impaired consciousness: A practical scale, *Lancet* 2:81-84, 1974.

25. Plummer P, Morris ME, Dunai J: Assessment of unilateral neglect, *Phys Ther* 83:732-740, 2003.

26. Heilman KM, Watson RT, Valenstein E: Neglect and related disorders. In Heilman KM, Valenstein E (eds): *Clinical Neuropsychology*, New York, 1993, Oxford University Press.

27. Stone SP, Halligan PW, Greenwood RJ: The incidence of neglect phenomena and related disorders in patients with an acute right or left hemisphere stroke, *Age Ageing* 22:46-52, 1993.

28. Bisiach E, Luzzatti C: Unilateral neglect of representational space, *Cortex* 14:129-133, 1978.

29. Beschin N, Robertson IH: Personal versus extrapersonal neglect: A group study of their dissociation using a reliable clinical test, *Cortex* 33:379-384, 1997.

30. Bisiach E, Perani D, Vallar G: Unilateral neglect, *Neuropsychologia* 24:759-767, 1986.

31. Schmidt RA: *Motor Control and Learning: A Behavioral Emphasis*, Champaign, Ill, 1982, Human Kinetics.

32. Cicerone KD, Dahlberg C, Kalmar K, et al: Evidence-based cognitive rehabilitation: recommendations for clinical practice, *Arch Phys Med Rehabil* 81:596-615, 2000.

33. Folstein MF, Folstein SE, McHugh PR: Mini-mental state: A practical method for grading the cognitive state of patients for the clinician, *J Psychiatr Res* 12:189-198, 1975.

34. Agrill B, Dehlin O: Mini Mental State Examination in geriatric stroke patients. Validity, differences between subgroups of patients, and relationships to somatic and mental variables, *Aging Clin Exp Res* 12:439-444, 2000.

35. Tombaugh TN, McIntyre NJ: The Mini-Mental Status Examination: A comprehensive review, *J Am Geriatr Soc* 40:922-935, 1992.

36. Zwecker M, Levenkrohn S, Fleisig Y, et al: Mini-Mental State Examination, Cognitive FIM Instrument and the Loewenstein Occupational Therapy Cognitive Assessment: Relation to functional outcome of stroke patients, *Arch Phys Med Rehabil* 82:342-345, 2002.

37. Kiernan RJ, Mueller J, Langston JW, et al: The Neurobehavioral Cognitive Status Examination: A brief but differentiated approach to cognitive assessment, *Ann Int Med* 107:481-485, 1987.

38. Nabors NA, Millis SR, Rosenthal M: Use of the Neurobehavioral Cognitive Status Examination (Cognistat) in traumatic brain injury, *J Head Trauma Rehabil* 12:79-84, 1997.

39. Blostein PA, Jones SJ, Buecheler CM, et al: Cognitive screening in mild traumatic brain injuries: Analysis of the Neurobehavioral Cognitive Status Examination when utilized during initial trauma hospitalization, *J Neurotrauma* 14:171-177, 1997.

40. Osmon DC, Smet IC, Winegarden B, et al: Neurobehavioral Cognitive Status Examination: Its use with unilateral stroke patients in a rehabilitation setting, *Arch Phys Med Rehabil* 73:414-418, 1992.

41. Schwamm LH, Van Dyke C, Kiernan RJ, et al: The Neurobehavioral Cognitive Status Examination: Comparison with the Cognitive Capacity Screening Examination and the Mini-Mental State Examination in a neurosurgical population, *Ann Int Med* 107:486-491, 1987.

42. Mysiw WJ, Beegan JG, Gatens PF: Prospective cognitive assessment of stroke patients before inpatient rehabilitation, *Am J Phys Med Rehabil* 68:168-171, 1989.

43. Hagan C, Malkmus D, Durham P: Levels of cognitive functions. In Rehabilitation of the Head Injured Adult: Comprehensive Physical Management, Downey, Calif, 1979, Professional Staff Association of Rancho Los Amigos Hospital.

44. Squire LR: Declarative and nondeclarative memory: Multiple brain systems supporting learning and memory, *J Cogn Neurosci* 4:232-243, 1992.

45. Shumway-Cook A, Woollacott MH (eds): *Motor Control: Theory and Practical Applications*, ed 2, Philadelphia, 2001, Lippincott Williams & Wilkins.

46. Bondi MW, Kaszniak AW, Rapcsak SZ, et al: Implicit and explicit memory following anterior communicating artery aneurysm rupture, *Brain Cogn* 22:213-229, 1993.

47. Cushman L, Caplan B: Multiple memory systems: Evidence from stroke, *Percep Motor Skills* 64:571-577, 1987.

48. Platz T, Denzler P, Kaden B, et al: Motor learning after recovery from hemiparesis, *Neuropsychologia* 32:1209-1233, 1994.

49. Ewert J, Levin IIS, Watson MG, et al: Procedural memory during post-traumatic amnesia in survivors of severe closed head injury, *Arch Neurol* 45:911-916, 1989.

50. Mutter SA, Howard JH, Howard DV: Serial pattern learning after head injury, *J Clin Exp Neuropsychol* 15:271-288, 1994.

51. Winstein CJ, Merians AS, Sullivan KJ: Motor learning after unilateral brain damage. *Neuropsychologia* 37:975-987, 1999.

52. Bentzel K: Evaluation of sensation. In Trombly CA (ed): *Occupational Therapy for Physical Dysfunction*, ed 4, Baltimore, 1995, Lippincott Williams & Wilkins.

53. Lance JW: What is spasticity? *Lancet* 335.606, 1990.

54. Horak FB: Assumptions underlying motor control for neurologic rehabilitation. In Lister MJ (ed): *Contemporary Management of Motor Control Problems: Proceedings of the II STEP Conference*, Fredricksberg, Va, 1991, Foundation for Physical Therapy.

55. Bohannon RW, Smith MB: Interrater reliability of a Modified Ashworth Scale of muscle spasticity, *Phys Ther* 67:206-207, 1987.

56. Blackburn M, van Vliet P, Mockett SP: Reliability of measurements obtained with the Modified Ashworth Scale in the lower extremities of people with stroke, *Phys Ther* 82:25-34, 2002.

57. Sawner K, LaVigne J: *Brunnstrom's Movement Therapy In Hemiplegia: A Neurophysiological Approach*, ed 2, Philadelphia, 1992, JB Lippincott.

58. Fugl-Meyer AR, Jaasko L, Leyman I, et al: The post-stroke hemiplegic patient. I. A method for evaluation of physical performance, *Scand J Rehabil Med* 7:13-31, 1975.

59. Wood-Dauphinee S, Williams J, Shapiro S: Examining outcome measures in a clinical study of stroke, *Stroke* 21:731-739, 1990.

60. Duncan PW, Propst M, Nelson SG: Reliability of the Fugl-Meyer Assessment of sensorimotor recovery following cerebrovascular accident, *Phys Ther* 63:1606-1610, 1983.

61. Sanford J, Moreland J, Swanson L, et al: Reliability of the Fugl-Meyer Assessment for testing motor performance in patients following stroke, *Phys Ther* 73:447-454, 1993.

62. Van Swearingen JM, Brach JS: Making geriatric assessment work: Selecting useful measures, *Phys Ther* 81:1233-1252, 2001.

63. Steffen TM, Hacker TA, Mollinger L: Age- and gender-related test performance in community dwelling elderly people: SMWT, Berg Balance Scale, Timed Up & Go Test, and gait speeds, *Phys Ther* 82:128-137, 2002.

64. Cahalin LP, Mathier MA, Semigran MJ, et al: The six-minute walk test predicts peak oxygen uptake and survival in patients with advanced heart failure, *Chest* 110:325-332, 1996.

65. Cahalin LP, Pappagianopoulos P, Prevost S, et al: The relationship of the 6-minute walk test to maximal oxygen consumption in transplant candidates with end-stage lung disease, *Chest* 108:452-459, 1995.

66. Harada ND, Chiu V, Stewar AL: Mobility-related function in older adults: assessment with a 6-minute walk test, *Arch Phys Med Rehabil* 80:837-841, 1999.

67. Pohl PS, Duncan PW, Perera S, et al: Influence of stroke-related impairments on performance in 6-minute walk test, *J Rehabil Res Dev* 39:439-444, 2002.

68. Berg KO, Maki BE, Holliday PJ, et al: Clinical and laboratory measures of postural balance in an elderly population, *Arch Phys Med Rehabil* 73:1073-1080, 1992.

69. Horak FB, Henry SM, Shumway-Cook A: Postural perturbations: new insights for treatment of balance disorders, *Phys Ther* 77:517-533, 1997.

70. Goldie PA, Bach TM, Evans OM: Force platform measures for evaluating postural control: Reliability and validity, *Arch Phys Med Rehabil* 70:510-517, 1989.

71. Shumway-Cook A, Anson D, Haller S: Postural sway biofeedback: Its effect on reestablishing stance stability in hemiplegic patients, *Arch Phys Med Rehabil* 69:395-400, 1988.

72. Winstein CJ, Gardner ER, McNeal DR, et al: Standing balance training: Effect on balance and locomotion in hemiparetic adults, *Arch Phys Med Rehabil* 70:755-762, 1989.

73. Berg K, Wood-Dauphinee S, Williams JI, et al: Measuring balance in the elderly: preliminary development of an instrument, *Physiother Can* 41:304-311, 1989.

74. Andriacchi TP, Ogle JA, Galante JO. Walking speed as basis for normal and abnormal gait measurements, *J Biomech* 10:261-268, 1977.

75. Nadeau S, Arsenault AB, Gravel D, et al: Analysis of the clinical factors determining natural and maximal gait speeds in adults with a stroke, *Am J Phys Med Rehabil* 78:123-130, 1999.

76. Olney SJ, Griffin MP, McBride ID: Temporal, kinematic, and kinetic variables related to gait speed in subjects with hemiplegia: A regression approach, *Phys Ther* 74:872-885, 1994.

77. Olney SJ, Griffin MP, McBride ID: Multivariate examination of data from gait analysis of persons with stroke, *Phys Ther* 78:814-828, 1998.

78. Bohannon RW: Comfortable and maximum walking speeds of adults aged 20-79 years: Reference values and determinants, *Age Ageing* 26:15-19, 1997.

79. Wade DT, Wood VA, Heller A, et al: Walking after stroke: measurement and recovery over the first 3 months, *Scand J Rehabil Med* 19:25-30, 1987.

80. Holden MK, Gill KM, Magliozzi MR, et al: Clinical gait assessment in the neurologically impaired: reliability and meaningfulness, *Phys Ther* 64:35-40, 1984.

81. Olney SJ, Griffin MP, Monga TN, et al: Work and power in gait of stroke patients, *Arch Phys Med Rehabil* 72:309-314, 1991.

82. Richards CL, Malouin F, Dean C: Gait in stroke: Assessment and rehabilitation, *Clin Geriatr Med* 15:833-855, 1999.

83. Wade DT, Collin C: The Barthel ADL Index: A standard measure? *Int Disabil Stud* 10:64-67, 1988.

84. Granger CV, Hamilton BB, Keith RA, et al: Advances in functional assessment for medical rehabilitation, *Top Geriatr Rehabil* 1:59-74, 1986.

85. Granger CV, Hamilton BB: Measurement of stroke rehab outcome in 1980s, *Stroke* 21(suppl II):II:46-47, 1990.

86. Granger CV, Hamilton BB: UDS Report: The uniform data system for medical rehabilitation report on the first admissions for 1990, *Am J Phys Med Rehabil* 71:108-113, 1992.

87. Oczkowski WJ, Barreca S: The Functional Independence Measure: Its use to identify rehabilitation needs in stroke survivors, *Arch Phys Med Rehabil* 12:1291-1294, 1993.

88. Granger CV, Clark GS: Functional outcomes of stroke rehabilitation, *Top Geriatr Rehabil* 9:72-84, 1994.

89. Black TM, Soltis T, Bartlett C: Using the Functional Independence Measure instrument to predict stroke rehabilitation outcomes, *Rehabilitation Nurs* 24:109-114, 1999.

90. Wade DT, Hewer RL: Functional abilities after stroke: Measurement, natural history, and prognosis, *J Neurol Neurosurg Psychiatr* 50:177-182, 1987.

91. Granger CV, Albrecht GL, Hamilton BB: Outcome of comprehensive medical rehabilitation: measurement by PULSES Profile and the Barthel Index, *Arch Phys Med Rehabil* 60:145-154, 1979.

92. Loewen SC, Anderson BA: Predictors of stroke outcome using objective measure scales, *Stroke* 21:78-81, 1990.

93. DeJong G, Branch LG: Predicting the stroke patient's ability to live independently, *Stroke* 13:648-655, 1982.

94. Howle JM: *Neuro-Developmental Treatment Approach: Theoretical Foundations and Principles of Clinical Practice*, Laguna Beach, Calif, 2002, NDTA.

95. Gordon J: Assumptions underlying physical therapy intervention: theoretical and historical perspectives. In Carr J, Shepherd R: *Movement Science: Foundations for PT Rehabilitation*, Gaithersburg, Md, 2000, Aspen.

96. Carr J, Shepherd R: *Neurological Rehabilitation: Optimizing Motor Performance*, Oxford, 1998, Butterworth Heinemann.

97. Carr J, Shepherd R: *Stroke Rehabilitation: Guidelines for Exercise and Training to Optimize Motor Skill*, Edinburgh, 2003, Butterworth Heinemann.

98. Bernstein NA: *The Coordination and Regulation of Movements*, New York, 1967, Pergamon.

99. Hesse S, Jahnke MT, Schaffrin A, et al: Immediate effects of therapeutic facilitation on the gait of hemiparetic patients as compared with walking with and without a cane, *Electroencephalorg Clin Neurophysiol* 109:515-522, 1998.

100. Passarella PM, Lewis N: Nursing application of Bobath principles in stroke, *J Neurosci Nurs* 19:106-109, 1987.

101. Lennon S: Gait re-education based on the Bobath concept in two patients with hemiplegia following stroke, *Phys Ther* 81:924-935, 2001.

102. Dickstein R, Hocherman S, Pillar T, et al: Stroke rehabilitation. Three exercise therapy approaches, *Phys Ther* 66:1233-1238, 1986.

103. Trueblood PR, Walker JM, Perry J: Pelvic exercise in gait in hemiplegia, *Phys Ther* 1989; 69:18-26.

104. Anderson TP: Studies up to 1980 on stroke rehabilitation outcomes, *Stroke* 21:1143-1145, 1990.

105. Kraft GH, Fitts SS, Hammond MC: Techniques to improve function of the arm and hand in chronic hemiplegia, *Arch Phys Med Rehabil* 73:220-227, 1992.

106. Wang RY: Effect of proprioceptive neuromuscular facilitation on the gait of patients with hemiplegia of long and short duration, *Phys Ther* 74:1108-1115, 1994.

107. Yigiter K, Sner G, Erbahceci F, et al: A comparison of traditional prosthetic training versus proprioceptive neuromuscular facilitation resistive gait training with trans-femoral amputees, *Prosthet Orthot Int* 26:213-217, 2002.

108. Ferber R, Osternig L, Gravelle D: Effect of PNF stretch techniques on knee flexor muscle EMG activity in older adults, *J Electromyogr Kinesiol* 12:391-397, 2002.

109. Nakamura R, Kosaka K: Effect of proprioceptive neuromuscular facilitation on EEG activation induced by facilitating position in patients with spinocerebellar degeneration, *Tohoku J Exp Med* 148:159-161, 1986.

110. Ries AL, Ellis B, Hawkins RW: Upper extremity exercise training in chronic obstructive pulmonary disease, *Chest* 93:688-692, 1988.

111. Bohman I: *The Philosophy and Evolution of the NDT (Bobath) Approach*, Oak Park, Ill, 1984, NDTA.

112. Bly L: A historical and current view of the basis of NDT, *Pediatr Phys Ther* 3:131-135, 1991.

113. Davies PM: *Right in the Middle: Selective Trunk Activity in the Treatment of Adult Hemiplegia*, New York, 1990, Springer-Verlag.

114. Gelber DA, Josefczyk PB, Herrman D, et al: Comparison of two therapy approaches in the rehabilitation of the pure motor hemiparetic stroke patient, *J Neuro Rehab* 9:191-196, 1995.

115. Basmajian JV, Gowland CA, Finlayson AJ, et al: Stroke treatment: comparison of integrated behavioral physical therapy vs traditional physical therapy programs, *Arch Phys Med Rehabil* 68:267-272, 1987.

116. Mudie MH, Winzeler-Mercay U, Radwan S, et al: Training symmetry of weight distribution after stroke: A randomized controlled pilot study comparing task-related reach, Bobath and feedback training approaches, *Clin Rehabil* 16:582-592, 2002.

117. Paci M: Physiotherapy based on the Bobath concept for adults with post-stroke hemiplegia: a review of effectiveness studies, *J Rehabil Med* 35:2-7, 2003.

118. Butefisch C, Hummelsheim H, Denzler P, et al: Repetitive training of isolated movement improves the outcome of motor rehabilitation of the centrally paretic hand, *J Neurol Sci* 130:59-68, 1995.

119. Hesse S, Bertelt C, Jahnke MT, et al: Treadmill training with partial body weight support compared with physiotherapy in nonambulatory hemiparetic patients, *Stroke* 26:976-981, 1995.

120. van der Lee JH, Wagenaar RC, Lankhorst G, et al: Forced use of the upper extremity in chronic stroke patients: Results from a clinical trial, *Stroke* 30:2369-2375, 1999.

121. Langhammer B, Stanghelle JK: Bobath or Motor Relearning Programme? A comparison of two different approaches of physiotherapy in stroke rehabilitation, *Clin Rehabil* 14:361-369, 2000.

122. Langhammer B, Stanghelle JK: Bobath or Motor Relearning Programme? A follow-up one and four years post stroke, *Clin Rehabil* 17:731-734, 2003.

123. Voss DE, Ionta MK, Myers BJ: *Proprioceptive Neuromuscular Facilitation: Patterns and Techniques*, ed 3, Philadelphia, 1985, JB Lippincott.

124. Adler SS, Beckers D, Buck M: *PNF in Practice: An Illustrated Guide*, Berlin, 1993, Springer-Verlag.

125. O'Sullivan SB, Schmitz TJ: *Physical Rehabilitation Laboratory Manual: Focus on Functional Training*, Philadelphia, 1999, FA Davis.

126. Case-Smith J, Fisher AG, Bauer D: An analysis of the relationship between proximal and distal motor control, *Am J Occup Ther* 43:657-662, 1989.

127. Shumway-Cook A, Woollacott MH: The growth of stability: postural control from a developmental perspective, *J Motor Behav* 17:131-147, 1985.

128. Johansson CA, Kent BE, Shepard KF: Relationship between verbal command volume and magnitude of muscle contraction, *Phys Ther* 63:1260-1265, 1983.

129. Chan CWY: Neurophysiological basis underlying the use of resistance to facilitate movement, *Physiother Canada* 36:335-341, 1984.

130. Etnyre BR, Abraham LD: H-reflex changes during static stretching and two variations of proprioceptive neuromuscular facilitation techniques, *Electroencephalogr Clin Neurophsiol* 63:174-179, 1986.

131. Moore MA, Kukulka CG: Depression of Hoffmann reflexes following voluntary contraction and implications for proprioceptive neuromuscular facilitation therapy, *Phys Ther* 71:321-333, 1991.

132. Condon SM, Hutton RS: Soleus muscle electromyographic activity and ankle dorsiflexion range of motion during four stretching procedures, *Phys Ther* 67:24-30, 1987.

133. Osternig LR, Robertson R, Troxel R, et al: Muscle activation during proprioceptive neuromuscular facilitation (PNF) stretching techniques, *Am J Phys Med* 66:298-307, 1987.

134. Osternig LR, Robertson RN, Troxel RK, et al: Differential responses to proprioceptive neuromuscular facilitation (PNF) stretch techniques, *Med Sci Sports Exerc* 22:106-111, 1990.

135. Ferber R, Osternig LR, Gravelle DC: Effect of PNF stretch techniques on knee flexor muscle EMG activity in older adults, *J Electromyogr Kinesiol* 12:391-397, 2002.

136. Cornelius WL, Ebrahim K, Watson J, et al: The effects of cold application and modified PNF stretching techniques on hip joint flexibility in college males, *Res Q Exerc Sport* 63:311-314, 1992.

137. Funk DC, Swank AM, Mikla BM, et al: Impact of prior exercise on hamstring flexibility: Comparison of PNF and static stretching, *J Strength Cond Res* 17:489-492, 2003.

138. Sady SP, Wortman M, Blanke D: Flexibility training: Ballistic, static or proprioceptive neuromuscular facilitation? *Arch Phys Med Rehabil* 63:261-263, 1982.

139. Carr J, Shepherd R: *Movement Science: Foundations for Physical Therapy in Rehabilitation,* ed 2, Gaithersburg, Md, 2000, Aspen.

140. Gentile A: Skill acquisition: Action, movement, and neuromotor processes. In Carr J, Shepherd R (eds): *Movement Science: Foundations for Physical Therapy in Rehabilitation,* ed 2, Gaithersburg, Md, 2000, Aspen.

141. Winstein CJ: Knowledge of results and motor learning—implications for PT, *Phys Ther* 71:140-149, 1991.

142. Schmidt RA: *Motor Control and Learning,* Champaign, Ill, 1988, Human Kinetics.

143. Salmoni AW, Schmidt RA, Walter CB: Knowledge of results and motor learning: A review and critical reappraisal, *Psychol Bull* 95:355-386, 1984.

144. Boyd LA, Winstein CJ: Implicit motor-sequence learning in humans following unilateral stroke: The impact of practice and explicit knowledge, *Neurosci Lett* 298:65-69, 2001.

145. Wulf G, Weigelt C: Instructions about physical principles in learning a complex motor skill, *Res Q Exerc Sport* 68:362-367, 1997.

146. Wulf G, Hob M, Prinz W: Instructions for motor learning: differential effects of internal vs external focus of attention, *J Motor Behav* 30:169-179, 1998.

147. Wulf G, Lauterbach B, Toole T: The learning advantages of an external focus of attention in golf, *Res Q Exerc Sport* 70:120-126, 1999.

148. McNevin NH, Wulf G, Carlson C: Effects of attentional focus, self-control, and dyad training on motor learning: implications for physical rehabilitation, *Phys Ther* 80:373-385, 2000.

149. Schmidt RA, Young DE, Swinnen S, et al: Summary of knowledge of results for skill acquisition: Support for the guidance hypothesis, *J Exp Psych* 15:352-359, 1989.

150. Schmidt RA, Lange C, Young DE: Optimizing summary knowledge of results for skill learning, *Human Mov Sci* 9:325-348, 1990.

151. Vander Linden DW, Cauraugh JH, Green TA: The effect of frequency of kinetic feedback on learning an isometric force production task in nondisabled subjects, *Phys Ther* 73:79-87, 1993.

152. Winstein CJ, Schmidt RA: Reduced frequency of knowledge of results enhances motor skill learning, *J Exp Psychol* 16:677-691, 1990.

153. Winstein CJ, Pohl PS, Lewthwaite R: Effects of physical guidance and knowledge of results on motor learning: Support for the guidance hypothesis, *Res Q Exerc Sport* 65:316-323, 1994.

154. Swinnen SP, Schmidt RA, Nicholson DE, et al: Information feedback for skill acquisition: Instantaneous knowledge of results degrades learning, *J Exp Psychol* 16:706-716, 1990.

155. Shea JB, Morgan RL: Contextual interference effects on the acquisition, retention, and transfer of a motor skill, *J Exp Psychol Hum Learn Mem* 4:179-187, 1979.

156. Hanlon RE: Motor learning following unilateral stroke, *Arch Phys Med Rehabil* 77:811-815, 1996.

157. Blanton S, Wolf SL: An application of upper-extremity constraint-induced movement therapy in a patient with subacute stroke, *Phys Ther* 79:847-853, 1999.

158. Bonifer N, Anderson KM: Application of constraint-induced movement therapy for an individual with severe chronic upper-extremity hemiplegia, *Phys Ther* 83:384-398, 2003.

159. Kunkel A, Kopp B, Muller G, et al: Constraint-induced movement therapy for motor recovery in chronic stroke patients, *Arch Phys Med Rehabil* 80:624-628, 1999.

160. Page SJ, Sisto SA, Levine P, et al: Modified constraint induced therapy: A randomized feasibility and efficacy study, *J Rehab Res Dev* 38:583-590, 2001.

161. Sterr A, Elbert T, Berthold I, et al: Longer versus shorter daily constraint-induced movement therapy of chronic hemiparesis: An exploratory study, *Arch Phys Med Rehabil* 83:1374-1377, 2002.

162. Dromerick AW, Edwards DF, Hahn M: Does the application of constraint-induced movement therapy during acute rehabilitation reduce arm impairment after ischemic stroke? *Stroke* 31:2984-2988, 2000.

163. Winstein CJ, Rose DK, Tan SM: A randomized controlled comparison of upper-extremity rehabilitation strategies in acute stroke: A pilot study, *Arch Phys Med Rehabil* 85:620-628, 2004.

164. Visintin M, Barbeau H, Korner-Bitensky N, et al: A new approach to retrain gait in stroke patients through body weight support and treadmill stimulation, *Stroke* 29:1122-1128, 1998.

165. Barbeau H, Visintin M: Optimal outcomes obtained with body-weight support combined with treadmill training in stroke subjects, *Arch Phys Med Rehabil* 84:1458-1465, 2003.

166. Nilsson L, Carlsson J, Danielsson A, et al: Walking training of patients with hemiparesis at an early stage after stroke: A comparison of walking training on a treadmill with body weight support and walking training on the ground, *Clin Rehab* 15:515-527, 2001.

167. Richards CL, Malouin F, Wood-Dauphinee S, et al: Task-specific physical therapy for optimization of gait recovery in acute stroke patients, *Arch Phys Med Rehabil* 74:612-620, 1993.

168. Macko RF, Smith GV, Dobrovolny CL, et al: Treadmill training improves fitness reserve in chronic stroke patients, *Arch Phys Med Rehabil* 82:879-884, 2001.

169. Potempa K, Braun TL, Tinknell T: Benefits of aerobic exercise after stroke, *Sports Med* 21:337-346, 1996.

170. Potempa K, Lopez M, Braun L, et al: Physiological outcomes of aerobic exercise training in hemiparetic stroke patients, *Stroke* 26:101-105, 1995.

171. Macko RF, De Souza CA, Tretter LD, et al: Treadmill aerobic exercise training reduces the energy expenditure and cardiovascular demands of hemiparetic gait in chronic stroke patients: a preliminary report, *Stroke* 28:326-330, 1997.

172. Danielsson A, Sunnerhagen KS: Oxygen consumption during treadmill walking with and without body weight support in patients with hemiparesis after stroke and in healthy subjects, *Arch Phys Med Rehabil* 81:953-957, 2000.

173. Franchignoni FP, Tesio L, Ricupero C, et al: Trunk control test as an early predictor of stroke rehabilitation outcome, *Stroke* 28:1382-1385, 1997.

174. Petajan JH: Spasticity: effects of physical interventions. *J Neuro Rehab* 4:219-225, 1990.

175. Carlson SJ: A neurophysiological analysis of inhibitive casting, *Phys Occup Ther Pediatr* 4:31-41, 1984.

176. Watkins CA: Mechanical and neurophysiological changes in spastic muscles: serial casting in spastic equinovarus following traumatic brain injury, *Physiotherapy* 85:603-609, 1999.

177. Stoeckmann T: Casting for the person with spasticity, *Top Stroke Rehabil* 8:27-35, 2001.

178. Mortenson PA, Eng JJ: The use of cases in the management of joint mobility and hypertonia following brain injury in adults: a systematic review, *Phys Ther* 83:648-658, 2003.

179. Kim CM, Eng JJ: The relationship of lower-extremity muscle torque to locomotor performance in people with stroke, *Phys Ther* 83:49-57, 2003.

180. Eriksrud O, Bohannon RW: Relationship of knee extension force to independence in sit-to-stand performance in patients receiving acute rehabilitation, *Phys Ther* 83:544-551, 2003.

181. Brown DA, Kautz SA: Increased workload enhances force output during pedaling exercise in persons with poststroke hemiplegia, *Stroke* 29:598-606, 1998.

Chapter 17

Progressive Central Nervous System Disorders

Lori Quinn, Vanina Dal Bello-Haas

OBJECTIVES

After reading this chapter, the reader will be able to:
1. Describe and differentiate different types of adult progressive central nervous system disorders, including Alzheimer's disease, amyotrophic lateral sclerosis, Huntington's disease, multiple sclerosis, and Parkinson's disease.
2. Describe the underlying pathology and common presentation of impairments and functional limitations for adults with progressive central nervous system disorders.
3. Discuss factors that may affect the examination of an individual with an adult progressive central nervous system disorder.
4. Discuss commonly used tests and measures for individuals with an adult progressive central nervous system disorder.
5. Identify and provide a rationale for rehabilitation interventions for adults with progressive central nervous system disorders.

$\mathcal{T}$his chapter concerns the examination, evaluation, and treatment of patients with progressive central nervous system (CNS) disorders that result in impaired motor function and sensory integrity. These include such commonly known diseases as Alzheimer's disease, Parkinson's disease, and multiple sclerosis, as well as a range of other disabling disorders, such as amyotrophic lateral sclerosis, Huntington's disease, cerebellar disorders (including cerebellar ataxia), and progressive muscular atrophy. Other disorders that have progressive effects on the CNS include acquired immune deficiency syndrome (AIDS), basal ganglia disease, idiopathic progressive cortical disease, neoplasms, primary lateral palsy, and progressive muscular atrophy. These disorders or conditions and suggested readings are summarized in Table 17-1.

Patients affected by progressive CNS disorders face many challenges. Therapists working with such patients must plan not just for the immediate problems but anticipate impairments and functional limitations as the disorder progresses. Therapists play an integral role in helping these patients maintain independent functioning for as long as possible and in helping patients and their families achieve and maintain a good quality of life.

PATHOLOGY

ALZHEIMER'S DISEASE

Dementia is an acquired syndrome of progressive deterioration in global intellectual abilities that interferes with the person's usual occupational and social performance, excluding impairments in consciousness. Alzheimer's disease (AD) accounts for 45% to 75% of patients with dementia,[1,2] and it has been estimated that prevalence rates double every 4.5 years until at least age 90.[3]

The pathological hallmark of AD is the development of neurofibrillary tangles (tangled masses of neurofilaments partly made up of a protein called tau) within neurons and plaques (deposits of amyloid matter).[4,5] The density of the filaments within neurons in the brain is directly related to the severity of dementia. The ultimate effect of these tangles is compromise of microtubular function and eventual destruction of the neuron.[5-7] Plaques, which are composed of beta-amyloid polypeptides, seem to form as a

| TABLE 17-1 | Other Disorders That May Cause Progressive Central Nervous System Dysfunction |

Disorder	Pathology	Common Impairments and Disabilities	Resources for Additional Reading
Acquired immunodeficiency syndrome (AIDS)	Direct insult, opportunistic infections, autoimmune reactions and neoplasms associated with HIV infection resulting in HIV leukoencephalopathy, astrogliosis, CNS lesions, hemorrhagic or coagulative CNS necrosis, abscesses, inflammation, demyelination, and intramyelinic and periaxonal vacuoles	Dementia Altered mental status Focal neurological deficits Paresthesia and diminished sensation Progressive muscle weakness Hemiparesis Aphasia Visual disturbances Spastic paresis Autonomic nervous system dysfunction	Berger JR, Levy RM: *AIDS and the Nervous System,* Philadelphia, 1997, Lippincott-Raven. Kietrys D, Gillardon P, Galantino ML: Contemporary issues in rehabilitation of patients with HIV disease. Part I: The team approach to rehabilitation of patients with HIV disease. Part II: Complications of HIV disease, *Rehabil Oncol* 20(1):21-26, 2002. Hobbs J, Galantino ML: HIV rehabilitation strategies: Clinical manifestations and rehabilitation management, *Rehabil Oncol* 16(3):15-19, 1998.
Basal ganglia diseases	Wilson's disease: Copper toxicity leading to degeneration of the globus pallidus, putamen, and caudate nucleus	Dystonia, incoordination, dysphagia, dysarthria, personality changes	Ferenci P: Pathophysiology and clinical features of Wilson disease, *Metab Brain Dis* 19(3-4): 229-239, 2004.
	Tardive dyskinesia: Occurs from long-term neuroleptic use	Choreoathetoid or dystonic movements, postural tone and control abnormalities	Fernandez HH, Friedman JH: Classification and treatment of tardive syndromes, *Neurologist* 9(1):16-27, 2003. World Federation of Neurology: *Seminars in Clinical Neurology: Dystonia,* vol 3, New York, 2005, Demos.
	Dystonia	Involuntary, sustained muscle contraction in the extreme end range of movement, impaired timing and execution of movement, loss of ROM	www.wfneurology.org/docs/pdf/wfn_demos_dystonia.pdf
Cerebellar ataxia/disease	Alcoholism, developmental disorders, genetic mutations, neoplasm, stroke, inflammation, vitamin deficiency, metabolic disorders resulting in, e.g., loss of Purkinje cells, atrophy of cerebellar cortex, axonal demyelination and degeneration	Dysmetria, ataxia, asthenia, tremor, impaired postural control, hypotonicity, impaired execution of movement	Klockgehter T: *Handbook of Ataxia Disorders,* New York, 2000, Marcel Dekker.
Neoplasm	Neoplasm	Depends on the location of the tumor within the CNS	
Primary lateral sclerosis	Degeneration of the corticospinal tracts and motor neurons	Early stage: LE spasticity and muscle weakness, gait abnormalities. Later stages: UE muscle weakness and spasticity, bulbar dysfunction	Pringle CE, Hudson AJ, Munoz DG: Primary lateral sclerosis. Clinical features, neuropathology and diagnostic criteria, *Brain* 115 (Pt 2):495-520, 1992. Swash M, Desai J, Misra V: What is primary lateral sclerosis? *J Neurol Sci.* 170(1):5-10, 1999. Donaghy M: Classification and clinical features of motor neuron diseases and motor neuropathies in adults, *J Neurol* 246(5): 331-333, 1999.
Progressive muscular atrophy	Loss or chromatolysis of the motor neurons of the spinal cord and brainstem	Progressive muscle weakness	Van Den Berg-Vos RM, Van Den Berg LH, Visser J, et al: The spectrum of lower motor neuron syndromes, *J Neurol* 250(11):1279-1292, 2003. Munsat TL: The spinal muscular atrophies. In Munsat TL (ed): *Current Neurology,* vol 14, St Louis, 1994, Mosby. Talbot K, Davies KE: Spinal muscular atrophy, *Semin Neurol* 21:189-197, 2001.

HIV, Human immunodeficiency virus; *CNS,* central nervous system; *LE,* lower extremity; *PNS,* peripheral nervous system; *ROM,* range of motion; *UE,* upper extremity.

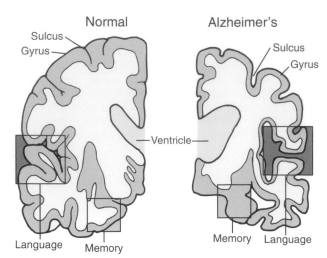

FIG. 17-1 Typical changes in the brain with Alzheimer's disease. Note that there is loss of cortex, particularly in the areas controlling memory and language, widening of the sulci, and enlargement of the ventricles.

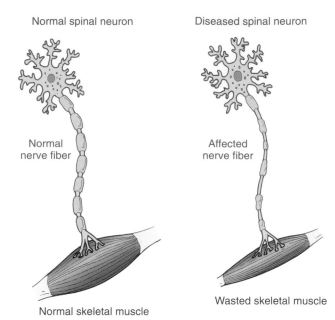

FIG. 17-2 Motor nerve degeneration and its effect on the muscle fibers it innervates

result of disordered processing of beta-amyloid and its precursors, and it is thought that inflammation around plaques destroys neighboring neurons.

Synaptic degeneration and neuronal death in the cortex and limbic brain regions (limbic cortex, anterior and medial nuclei of the thalamus, hippocampus, amygdala, and basal forebrain) result in cognitive and behavioral abnormalities (Fig. 17-1). AD is manifested by impairments in memory and one or more of the following: Aphasia, apraxia, agnosia, or disturbances in executive abilities such as abstracting, organizing, planning, and sequencing.[8] In addition to memory loss, individuals with AD may have dramatic personality changes, disorientation, declining physical coordination, and an inability to care for themselves.[9] In the final stages of the disease, patients are bedridden, lose urinary bladder and bowel control, and are completely dependent on the care of others. Death is usually due to pneumonia or urinary tract infection. Studies have found survival after a diagnosis of AD depends on age at diagnosis. Median survival was almost 9 years for persons diagnosed at age 65, whereas survival was approximately 3 years for persons diagnosed at age 90.[10]

AMYOTROPHIC LATERAL SCLEROSIS

Amyotrophic lateral sclerosis (ALS), commonly known as Lou Gehrig's disease, is the most common and devastatingly fatal *motor neuron disease* among adults. The prevalence of ALS is 5-7 per 100,000 in the United States, and the disease affects men slightly more than women. The average age of onset is 58 years, with a range of 40-70 years.[11-14]

ALS is characterized by degeneration and loss of upper motor neurons in the cortex, brainstem nuclei for cranial nerves (CNs) V, VII, IX, X, and XII, and anterior horn cells (lower motor neurons) in the spinal cord. As motor neurons degenerate, they can no longer control the muscle fibers they innervate (Fig. 17-2). Healthy, intact surrounding axons sprout and reinnervate the partially denervated muscle,[15] thereby preserving strength and function early in the disease. This reinnervation can compensate for the progressive degeneration until about 50% of motor units are lost.[16,17] With disease progression reinnervation can no longer compensate for the degeneration,[18] resulting in a combination of upper motor neuron (UMN) and lower motor neuron (LMN) signs and symptoms. These include weakness, muscle *atrophy*, hyperreflexia or areflexia, and muscle *fasciculations*.

The most frequently presenting symptom, occurring in more than 70% of patients with ALS, is focal weakness beginning in the leg, arm, or bulbar muscles.[19] Patients gradually become weaker all over, eventually having difficulty breathing because of diaphragmatic weakness. Most patients remain relatively intact cognitively, although speech production becomes difficult and alternative communication methods are required. Although disease progression varies between individuals, death usually results from respiratory failure, and the 50% survival after the first symptom appears is about 3 years, unless mechanical ventilation is used to sustain breathing.[20]

HUNTINGTON'S DISEASE

Huntington's disease (HD) is a fatal, autosomal dominant hereditary disorder affecting 5-10 per 100,000 people.[21] The disease has an insidious onset, generally manifests when the patient is in the mid-thirties to mid-forties, and causes cognitive and emotional disturbances, in addition to problems with voluntary and involuntary movement.[22] The disease typically progresses over 15-20 years, although progression is faster in individuals with an earlier age of onset.[22]

HD is caused by an increased number of cytosine-adenine-guanine (CAG) triplet repeats in the HD gene. Individuals without HD have 9-34 repeats of this triplet.

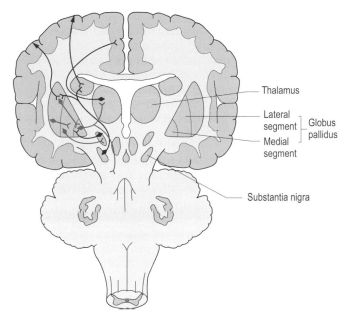

FIG. 17-3 Areas of degeneration in Huntington's disease (frontal cortex, globus pallidus, and thalamus) and Parkinson's disease (substantia nigra). *From Crossman AR, Neary D: Neuroanatomy: An Illustrated Colour Text, ed 3, Philadelphia, 2006, Churchill Livingstone.*

Huntington's disease occurs when there are more than 37 CAG triplet repeats.[23-25] How this defect is translated into pathogenesis has yet to be determined; however, the leading hypothesis centers around excitotoxicity and apoptosis induced by a defect in energy metabolism caused by oxidative stress.[23] Degeneration of the caudate and putamen are most characteristic of HD, but the frontal cortex, globus pallidus, and thalamus also degenerate as the disease progresses (Fig. 17-3).[25]

Chorea, abnormal extraocular movements, hypertonic reflexes, and abnormal rapid alternating movements are the most consistent early manifestations of HD.[26] As the disease progresses, other functionally limiting motor symptoms, such as dystonia,[27] athetosis, *akinesia*, and *bradykinesia*, develop.[21,25,26] In addition to motor problems, depression, cognitive decline, and personality changes occur, progressing from deficits in executive function, short-term memory, and visuospatial functioning in the early stage of the disease to dementia in the later stages.[26,28] Cognitive impairments and depression are associated with more rapid functional decline.[29,30] The most common cause of death is respiratory complications.[31]

PARKINSON'S DISEASE

Parkinson's disease (PD) is an idiopathic, hypokinetic movement disorder of the basal ganglia. It affects men slightly more often than women, and approximately 1.5 million Americans are currently diagnosed with the disease. The typical age of onset is 60, however, 15% of those diagnosed are under age 50. The risk of PD increases with age. In certain cases, there is a strong genetic predisposition, but PD is not an inherited disease. Although the cause of PD is unknown, researchers believe that several factors may be involved, including accelerated aging,

exposure to environmental toxins, and free radical oxidative damage.[32,33]

The primary pathology in PD is degeneration of neurons that produce dopamine and degeneration within the dopaminergic nigrostriatal pathway (primarily those in the substantia nigra; see Fig. 17-3). Changes are also seen in other CNS structures, such as the locus coeruleus, the hypothalamus, the dorsal vagal nucleus, and the cerebral cortex; in addition, there are deficiencies in other neurotransmitters such as serotonin and norepinephrine.[32-34] Symptoms do not generally appear until approximately 80% of dopaminergic cells in the substantia nigra are lost. First symptoms typically include resting tremor, bradykinesia, *rigidity*, and impaired balance or postural control. Disease progression is quite variable: Some patients are able to live for many years with PD, whereas others decline rapidly. Medications (particularly those containing combinations of levodopa and carbidopa) can control symptoms for many years by increasing levels of dopamine in the brain. But as the disease progresses, medications are less effective and produce more side effects, particularly bradykinesia and rigidity as they wear off, and dyskinesias at peak dose. Many patients also experience varying degrees of dementia. In the endstages of the disease, patients are generally totally dependent for physical care and have problems communicating. The cause of death is typically respiratory failure.

MULTIPLE SCLEROSIS

Multiple sclerosis (MS) is a demyelinating disease of the CNS.[35] The typical age of onset of symptoms is between 20-50 years of age, and the disease affects women almost 3 times more often than men. The prevalence of the disease in the United States is 1 in 700. Although the exact cause of MS is unknown, studies suggest that genetics may play a role; however, MS is not a directly inherited disease.[36,37] MS has been found to occur more frequently in people with northern European ancestry and those who live in more northern areas of the world. The proposed pathogenic mechanisms for the onset for MS include (1) an autoimmune response causing a wide-spread attack on the neural tissue, (2) a slow-acting or latent viral infection that triggers an immune response, or (3) environmental factors.[37]

Demyelination can occur almost anywhere in the brain or spinal cord and manifests as a variety of physical, cognitive, or psychological impairments. Recent evidence suggests MS may also cause irreversible CNS axonal damage early in the disease,[38] and this may contribute to the development of persistent impairments and disability in the later stages of the disease.[39] The clinical course of MS typically falls into one of the following 4 categories:

1. Relapsing-remitting (85% to 90% of patients): Characterized by episodes of acute attacks followed by recovery and disease stability between relapses. Recovery after a relapse may be full but is usually characterized by some residual deficits. Over time, the degree of disability increases.
2. Primary progressive (10%): Characterized by steady progression of the disease and continuous worsening over time. There may be occasional plateaus and

temporary minor improvements in impairments and functional limitations.

3. Secondary progressive (40% to 50% of people with relapsing-remitting develop this form within 10 years of initial diagnosis): Characterized by relapsing-remitting disease for a period of time followed by progressive disease with or without occasional minor relapses, remission, or plateau.

4. Progressive relapsing (rare): Characterized by progressive disease from the onset, with periods of acute relapses, with or without recovery; between relapses there is progressive worsening of the disease.[42]

In newly diagnosed cases of MS, most experience a relapsing-remitting course, with relapses occurring usually a little less than once a year.[40-41] A typical relapse increases in severity over a few weeks, begins to remit after 4 weeks, and resolves over 2-3 months.[42] In the early stages, clinical recovery is virtually complete, although persistent structural and conduction abnormalities can be detected. Although the course of the disease is variable, after a number of years, neurological impairments begin to accumulate after each relapse.[42] After 10 years, 40% to 50% of patients with a relapsing-remitting disease will develop a progressive course in which there is a continuous accrual of impairments and functional limitations, with or without relapses.[42] Approximately 50% of patients are unable to work 5 years after disease onset,[43] and approximately 50% of patients require an assistive device or wheelchair within 15 years of diagnosis.[44] Respiratory complications are the most common cause of death in patients with MS.[45]

STAGES OF PROGRESSIVE CENTRAL NERVOUS SYSTEM DISORDERS

A commonality among progressive CNS disorders is their progressive and deteriorating trajectory. Although the course of some diseases (such as MS) can be altered or slowed by disease-modifying agents (typically medications), there is currently no cure for any of the progressive CNS disorders discussed in this chapter.

Most progressive CNS diseases can be viewed in three functional stages: Early, middle, and late (Fig. 17-4). In the early stage of the disorder, the pathology manifests as a variety of signs and symptoms recognized by the individual as abnormal. At this stage, resultant impairments may or may not cause minor functional limitations, and the individual's ability to perform typical roles is usually not affected. In the middle stage of the progressive CNS disorder, an individual experiences increasing signs and symptoms and develops an increasing number of impairments or more severe impairments. The individual is minimally to moderately functionally limited and experiences disabilities. In the late stage, progression of the disease leads to numerous and increasingly more severe impairments. The individual becomes increasingly more limited functionally because of the lack of voluntary motor control and numerous disabilities ensue. The individual becomes dependent in essentially all aspects of mobility and self-care, and depending on the disease process, speech, swallowing, pulmonary, bowel, bladder, and cognitive function may also be significantly compromised, if not already affected.[46]

Common impairments and functional limitations in the early, middle, and late stages of AD, ALS, HD, MS and PD are summarized in Table 17-2.

EXAMINATION

The purpose of examination in patients with progressive CNS disorders is to (1) identify impairments that can be causing functional problems, (2) identify specific functional problems and disabilities, and (3) identify the stage of the disease to determine prognosis through both impairment and functional testing.

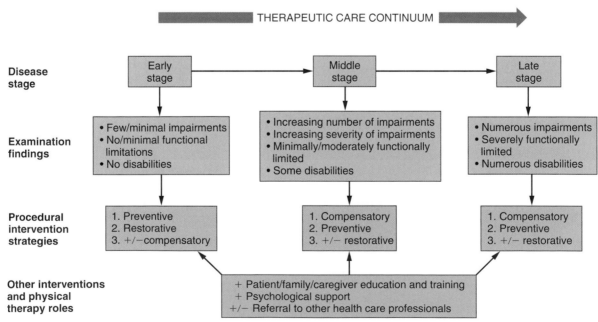

FIG. 17-4 Framework for planning care for patients with progressive CNS disorders. *From Dal Bello-Haas V: Neuro Rep 2:116, 2002.*

TABLE 17-2	Common Impairments and Disabilities at Different Disease Stages		
Disease	**Early Stage**	**Middle Stage**	**Late Stage**
Alzheimer's disease	Mild memory problems Difficulty with word finding Attention and comprehension problems Mild gnosis or praxis Mild problems with job performance	Moderate memory loss Decreased concentration Difficulty with complex information and problem solving Difficulty with new learning Increasing visuospatial deficits throughout stage Moderate impairment in complicated IADL in early part of stage Mild impairment in ADL in early part of stage Disorientation to time, place, and extended family toward end of stage Progressively impaired concentration toward end of stage Unable to perform most IADL, assistance with ADL toward end of stage Gait and balance disturbances Urinary and fecal incontinence toward end of stage	Severe memory loss Gait and balance disturbances Slowing of motor function and deterioration of psychomotor skills Dependence in mobility, self-care, and ADLs Anarthria Lack of bowel and bladder control Dysphagia
Amyotrophic lateral sclerosis	Mild to moderate weakness in specific muscle groups Difficulty with ADLs and mobility towards the end of this stage	Progressive decrease in mobility throughout stage Increasing fatigue throughout stage Wheelchair needed for long distances; increased wheelchair use toward end of stage Severe muscle weakness in some groups; mild to moderate weakness in other groups Progressive decrease in ADLs Pain	Wheelchair dependent or restricted to bed Complete dependence with ADLs Severe weakness of UE, LE, neck, and trunk muscles Dysarthria, dysphagia Respiratory compromise Pain
Huntington's disease	Weakness of neck extensors, trunk muscles, intrinsic muscles of the hands and feet Chorea, often limited to hands Balance problems with turning and changing directions quickly, wearing unsupportive footwear Postural changes Mild visuospatial deficits (e.g., spatial awareness, perception) Mild cognitive deficits	Memory, concentration, decision-making, thought processing problems Irritability, depression Moderate to severe chorea Bradykinesia, akinesia, dystonia Postural instability Gait problems Decreased spatial awareness Fatigue Incoordination Changes in sleep patterns Delusions, hallucinations, paranoia Difficulties with self-care	Bradykinesia Hypertonicity Chorea (may be decreased) Decreased eye movements Dependence in mobility, self-care, and ADLs Dementia Dysarthria and dysphagia Weight loss Lack of bowel and bladder control
Multiple sclerosis	Visual impairments Sensory impairments Fatigue Unilateral muscle weakness Mild gait disturbances Mild balance impairments	Increasing muscle weakness Progressive loss of mobility and ADLs Impaired balance Spasticity Ataxia, tremor Sensory loss Cognitive impairments	Severe muscle weakness Wheelchair bound or restricted to bed Respiratory compromise Dysarthria, dysphagia Dependent in mobility, self-care, and ADLs Bladder dysfunction, incontinence Severe visual impairments Cognitive deficits
Parkinson's disease	Unilateral tremor Rigidity Mild gait hypokinesia Micrographic handwriting Reduced speech volume	Some functional limitations Speech impairments Bilateral bradykinesia, rigidity Axial rigidity Postural instability Gait impairments Balance problems May require assistance toward end of stage	Severely impaired, disabled Pulmonary function and swallowing compromised Dependent in mobility, self-care, and ADLs Bladder dysfunction, incontinence

ADLs, Activities of daily living; *IADLs,* instrumental ADLs; *LE,* lower extremity; *UE,* upper extremity.

Progressive CNS disorders can affect many regions of the CNS at any one time, and for some diseases, in various combinations. Impairments may occur as (1) a direct result of the CNS pathology (primary impairment), (2) a sequela to the primary pathology (secondary impairment), (3) a result of preexisting pathology (co-morbid condition), and (4) as a result of habits independent of a specific disease process (disuse and abuse).[47] Therefore a careful and comprehensive examination is required to determine the extent of involvement and the impact of involvement on functional limitations and disabilities.

Reexamination at regular intervals is necessary to determine the extent and rate of progression of the disorder and the effectiveness of interventions; however, it may be difficult to differentiate between the progressive course of the disorder and ineffectiveness of the interventions. In considering the tests and measures to include in reexamination and the timing of reexaminations, the therapist needs to weigh the benefits versus the psychological impact of repeating tests and measures when the individual is progressively deteriorating. This is especially true in the late-middle and late stages of the disease. Regardless, reexamining, monitoring, and evaluating changes at regular intervals are essential for planning ongoing care and intervention.

Most individuals who have been diagnosed with a progressive CNS disorder will have a complex array of examination findings. Even patients with the same diagnosis can present with a significantly different presentation of symptoms. Thus a thorough screening of all areas is imperative to assure that nothing is overlooked. The patient's goals and individual factors, rate of disease progression, extent and area of involvement, stage of the disease, and respiratory factors that may impact the individual's ability to participate in the examination must all be considered when structuring the examination.

PATIENT HISTORY

One of the key elements when collecting data from patients with a progressive CNS disorder is to determine what is most important, relevant, and valued by the individual. Because of the progressive nature of the disorder, there may be many immediate problems and future potential impairments and functional limitations as the disease progresses. The patient's goals, needs, and priorities will help structure the examination.

Reviewing the patient's history of symptoms since diagnosis provides the clinician with an indication of the course of the disease (e.g., slow versus fast deteriorating course) and may help the therapist narrow down what tests are likely to be relevant to the patient's problems and goals. In addition, the history can provide hints of cognitive deficits that may impact the implementation of interventions. A thorough understanding of the roles of the spouse, caregiver, and family members is important, as their participation is frequently crucial to the viability and success of any intervention program.

SYSTEMS REVIEW

The systems review is used to target areas requiring further examination and to define areas that may cause complications or indicate a need for precautions during the examination and intervention processes. See Chapter 1 for details of the systems review.

TESTS AND MEASURES
Musculoskeletal

Posture. Examination and evaluation of posture (see Chapter 4) in patients with progressive CNS disorders can reveal muscle imbalances caused by dystonia, *spasticity*, disuse, or compensatory behaviors.

In patients with PD, postural impairments become noticeable in the early to middle stages. Patients begin to develop a flexed (or stooped) posture, with a forward head, increased thoracic kyphosis, decreased lumbar lordosis, and flexed hips and knees in static stance (Fig. 17-5). A similar flexed posture is also common in individuals with middle to late stage AD or other types of dementia.[48]

ALS may alter sitting and standing postures because of cervical or trunk extensor muscle weakness, causing the head to droop forward. When the patient becomes so weak they cannot lift their chin off the chest wall, the forward field of vision will be severely restricted during gait, speech, swallowing, and potentially breathing. To compensate, the patient will use their hands to support the chin and will adopt an exaggerated lumbar lordosis in the upright position.

In HD, more than 95% of patients develop dystonia,[27] which can lead to muscle imbalances, and abnormal posturing. The most prevalent types of dystonia in HD are internal rotation of the shoulder, sustained fist clenching, and excessive knee flexion and foot inversion during

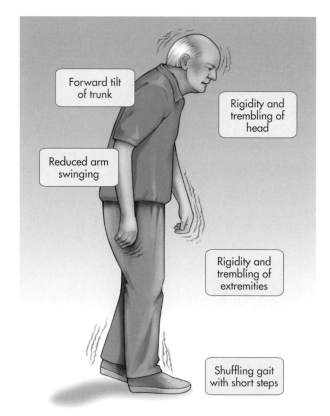

Forward tilt of trunk

Rigidity and trembling of head

Reduced arm swinging

Rigidity and trembling of extremities

Shuffling gait with short steps

FIG. 17-5 Typical posture of a person with Parkinson's disease. *From Thibodeau GA, Patton KT:* The Human Body in Health & Disease, *ed 4, St. Louis, 2002, Mosby.*

ambulation, with the dystonia becoming more severe over time. Patients with HD who take antidopaminergic medications, which can decrease choreiform movements, also have more severe dystonia. Severity of dystonia has been found to correlate inversely with independence in patients with HD, indicating that dystonia can contribute to loss of physical independence in these patients.[27]

Anthropometric Characteristics. Flaccid muscle weakness that results from progressive CNS diseases, such as ALS and MS, can result in swelling of the distal extremity as a result of the failure of muscle pumping in a weakened limb. Standard measures of edema, such as girth, volumetric measurements, and palpation (see Chapter 27), should be used to measure edema in these patients. Muscle disuse can also lead to atrophy, particularly in diseases such as ALS that affect the peripheral nervous system, as well as the CNS.

Range of Motion and Muscle Length. Functional range of motion (ROM); active, active-assisted, and passive ROM; muscle length; and soft tissue flexibility and extensibility should be examined in all patients using standard methods. Patients with progressive CNS disorders are at risk for loss of ROM for several reasons. Most patients have impairments in reflexes and muscle tone (see section on Reflex Integrity). *Hypertonicity,* specifically rigidity (seen in PD) and hyperreflexia (seen in ALS, MS, and HD), can result in muscle shortening over time. Risk of contractures is one of the key reasons why one tries to control spasticity and rigidity in patients. Furthermore, patients with HD frequently have dystonia, which can cause muscle length imbalances, typically in the trunk and lower extremities.[27]

Muscle Performance. Any patient with a progressive CNS disorder is at risk for strength deficits because of lack of activity and subsequent muscle disuse. Therefore, at a minimum, therapists should perform a screening examination of the strength of the upper extremities, lower extremities, and the trunk musculature, using manual muscle tests or functional tests (see Chapter 5). Functional testing, such as checking if a person can get out of a chair or reach for an object, may be more appropriate in patients with significant cognitive impairments (e.g., patients with AD or PD-related dementia) because these patients may have difficulty following the commands for manual muscle testing. If areas of weakness are found, more detailed testing should be attempted.

Maximum voluntary isometric contraction (MVIC) has proven to be reliable, accurate, and sensitive for quantitative testing of muscle strength in patients with ALS and has been used in patients with MS.[49] Hand-held dynamometry has also been used to measure strength in patients with ALS and MS.[50,51] However, one study found that hand-held dynamometry was less sensitive than MVIC for detecting below normal muscle strength in very strong muscle groups in patients with ALS because of the limited strength of the tester.[50]

Amyotrophic Lateral Sclerosis. Muscle strength is an important measure of disease progression in ALS. Patients with ALS develop muscle atrophy and weakness as a result of involvement of the LMNs. The weakness generally starts in a distal muscle group of one arm or leg, or in the bulbar muscles, and then progresses in distribution and severity.

Muscle strength, particularly of the knee flexors and hip extensors, impacts the ability to ambulate in the community and at home, whereas bulbar weakness affects the ability to swallow.[52]

Parkinson's Disease. Muscle weakness can occur in individuals with PD at all stages of the disease,[53-56] although it is more pronounced at later stages and at faster movement speeds.[54,57] Muscle weakness appears to be a primary symptom of PD contributing to a patient's functional status.[56,57]

Multiple Sclerosis. Patients with MS demonstrate muscle weakness because of impaired CNS nerve conduction. They can be weak in almost any part of the body but most frequently in the trunk and lower extremities.[49,58,59] Impairment of muscle performance in MS is more often related to muscle fatigue than reduced strength or power. The Fatigue Index (FI), the ratio of maximal isometric torque at 5 and 30 seconds, has been found to be a reliable quantitative measure of muscle fatigue in patients with MS.[51]

Huntington's Disease and Alzheimer's Disease. Strength deficits are not primary impairments associated with HD or AD, and their presence has not been specifically reported in the literature to date. However, with progression of all degenerative diseases, weakness often develops as a secondary impairment because of disuse. In addition, since some progressive CNS disorders tend to disproportionately affect the elderly, age-related decreases in muscle strength may also develop.

Neuromuscular

Arousal, Attention, and Cognition. Examination of cognition, communication, language, and learning style is important in patients with progressive CNS disorders, particularly those with AD and HD, which are associated with significant impairments in cognition and behavior. Cognition should also be examined in patients in the later stages of MS and PD, where cognitive deficits are common, and communication should be examined in the later stages of ALS, where bulbar and respiratory weakness can impair speech production. Although physical therapists (PTs) are often primarily concerned with motor impairments, the patient's ability to communicate and reason can significantly impact their rehabilitation potential.

Alzheimer's Disease. Diagnostic criteria for AD include memory impairment and one or more of the following cognitive disturbances: Aphasia (language disturbance), apraxia (impaired ability to carry out motor activities despite intact motor function), agnosia (failure to recognize or identify objects despite intact sensory function), or disturbances in executive functioning, such as planning, organizing, sequencing, and abstracting.[8]

AD is characterized by progressive memory loss. In the early stages, patients typically have difficulty recalling information after more than a few minutes and difficulty learning new information. Semantic memory, which is related to understanding the meanings and representations of words, objects, concepts, and facts, may also be impaired early in the course of AD. As the disease progresses, learning and recall decline further and other cognitive deficits develop and progressively worsen[60] (see Table 17-2).

Amyotrophic Lateral Sclerosis. ALS, traditionally considered to be a disease affecting only motor performance, has also been found to be associated with cognitive impairments. Mild cognitive deficits to severe frontotemporal dementia (FTD) have been reported in patients with ALS, and it has been suggested that FTD be considered a component of the pathological spectrum of ALS.[61] ALS-associated FTD is characterized by cognitive decline; executive functioning impairments; difficulties with planning, organization, and concept abstraction; and personality and behavior changes.[62-64] Individuals with ALS but without FTD may also have some cognitive impairment, including difficulties with verbal fluency, language comprehension, memory, abstract reasoning, and generalized impairments in intellectual function.[64,65]

Huntington's Disease. In HD, cognitive symptoms are an early sign and are found in some otherwise asymptomatic at-risk individuals.[66,67] Early cognitive problems include slowed thinking, impaired ability to manipulate information,[68] and impaired attention.[69] Patients also may have difficulties switching from one task to another.[69] As the disease progresses, patients have difficulty with short-term memory and visuospatial abilities, and eventually global dementia develops.[70,71] However, many people with HD maintain good distant long-term recall until late in the disease.[72]

Parkinson's Disease. Many patients with PD have some degree of cognitive impairment early in the disease.[73] Patients tend to have impairments in executive functioning, such as initiation, reasoning, and planning,[74] and demonstrate interference effects when performing dual-motor and dual-cognitive tasks.[75] In about 20% to 40% of patients with PD, cognitive impairments progress to dementia.[76,77] Dementia in PD is characterized by progressive impairments in executive functioning and attention and is often accompanied by psychotic symptoms, particularly visual hallucinations.

Multiple Sclerosis. Cognitive impairments are common in all types of MS[78] and have been reported to occur in 43% to more than 80% of a patient sample.[79,80] In the early stages of the disease, many aspects of cognition remain relatively intact, but patients may have slowed motor execution and cognitive processing.[81] Cognitive impairments in MS usually affect short-term memory, attention, verbal fluency, and working memory.[79,82]

Tests of Cognition. If dementia or cognitive impairments are suspected in a patient with a progressive CNS disorder, referral for neuropsychological evaluation to thoroughly examine performance across different domains of cognition may be beneficial. PTs may administer simple cognitive tests such as the Mini-Mental Status Examination (MMSE).[83] The MMSE is intended for examination of patients with or at risk for dementia. Scores range from 0-30, with scores of 24 indicating very mild dementia, 20-23 mild dementia, 10-19 moderate dementia, and 0-9 severe dementia.[83,84] The MMSE lacks sensitivity to early changes in cognition associated with dementia and has a floor effect late in the course of dementia.

Several cognitive tests have been developed for specific patient populations. Cognitive ability in AD can be tested with the cognitive subscale of the Alzheimer's Disease Assessment Scale (ADAS-cog).[85] This subscale includes 11 items that assess receptive and expressive language ability; orientation to person, time, and place; constructional and ideational praxis; and word-list recall and recognition. Total scores can range from 0-70, with higher scores reflecting greater dysfunction. The ADAS-cog is frequently used in clinical trials of AD, and although it is useful for cognitive assessment in most patients with AD, it is less sensitive in those with very mild or very severe involvement.[86]

Screening for cognitive impairments in patients with MS can be done using the MS Neuropsychological Screening Questionnaire (MSNQ). The MSNQ is a brief, 15-item questionnaire that evaluates neuropsychological competence with activities of daily living (ADLs) in patients with MS.[87] This test appears to be sensitive to cognitive impairments in patients with MS and has good test-retest reliability.[87]

No disease-specific measures exist for measuring cognitive function in HD, ALS, or PD. In addition to the MMSE, alternative screening measures that may be utilized in these patients include the Quick Cognitive Screening test[88] and the AB Cognitive Screen (ABCS), which has been found to be more sensitive than the MMSE in differentiating normal cognition from mild cognitive impairment.[89]

Pain. Pain is common in individuals with ALS, MS, and PD.[90-92] Although sensory pathways are mostly spared in ALS and PD, patients often have vague, ill-defined paresthesias or pain. In ALS, muscle cramps and spasticity may also cause pain; whereas in PD, severe rigidity or off-period dystonia can be the source of pain.[93,94] In MS, demyelination of the sensory tracts often causes *dysesthesia* and stabbing, aching, or burning sensations.[91,92] Posterior column involvement can also cause *Lhermitte's sign,* a sudden electric-like sensation radiating down the spine or extremities that usually occurs with neck flexion.[95] Demyelination of the sensory division of the trigeminal nerve in MS can also cause *trigeminal neuralgia,* in which short periods of stabbing facial pain are triggered by tactile stimulation of the face.[96] Similar to individuals with ALS, spasticity may also cause pain in individuals with MS.

In addition to pain caused by direct effects of progressive CNS disorders, individuals with any of these disorders may develop pain as a result of indirect (e.g., decreased ROM or contractures secondary to muscle weakness, spasticity, or rigidity), or composite impairments (e.g., joint malalignment secondary to spasticity). Thus pain should be examined closely in all patients with progressive CNS disorders who report pain in the patient history (see Chapter 22).

Cranial Nerve Integrity. Many patients with progressive CNS disorders have impairments in CN integrity, particularly in the nerves that control eye movements and the bulbar muscles. Examination of eye movements requires testing of extraocular movements in all directions. These tests may be performed by the PT or another qualified clinician. General oral motor and speech function, phonation, and speech production can be assessed during the interview and through observation. Referral to a nutritionist and speech language pathologist for further evaluation and consultation is recommended.

Up to 85% of individuals with MS have visual symptoms, including *diplopia,* visual field deficits, and altered visual acuity in one or both eyes. Altered visual acuity, blurring, or partial or total loss of vision in one eye in patients with MS is usually caused by *optic neuritis* (inflammation of the optic nerve; Fig. 17-6).[97]

Most patients with HD have some impairment in oculomotor function, most commonly difficulties with initiation of eye movement, slowness of pursuit and volitional saccadic movements, and inability to initiate a volitional saccade without movement of the head.[98-100] Patients with PD also often have impaired saccadic and smooth ocular pursuit, hypometric ocular saccades, up gaze and convergence limitations, spontaneous and reflex *blepharospasm* (spasmodic contraction of the eyelid muscles), and apraxia of eyelid opening (a result of involuntary levator inhibition) and closing.[101-103]

Oculomotor function is also impaired in MS. *Nystagmus* (rapid involuntary oscillations of the eye), most often horizontal, is very common and is caused by cerebellar and central vestibular pathway lesions. Patients with nystagmus may complain of blurred vision or *oscillopsia* (jumping images).[104] Bilateral or unilateral internuclear *ophthalmoplegia* (INO) is also common in MS and occurs as a result of lesions in the medial longitudinal fasciculus (MLF), which connects CNs III and VI. Signs of internuclear ophthalmoplegia are elicited by asking the patient to look laterally to one side. Adduction of the adducting eye will be slow or absent, and horizontal nystagmus of the abducting eye will be seen (Fig. 17-7). Lesions affecting

CNs III, IV, or VI may also cause additional impairments in conjugate gaze and control of eye movements. Diplopia (double vision) occurs when the muscles controlling eye movements are not coordinated as a result of an INO or involvement of other CNs that control extraocular mucles.[97]

Lesions in the vestibular nerve (CN VIII), vestibular nucleus in the lateral medulla, and in the pathways from the vestibular nucleus to the vestibular cortex commonly produce vertigo, nausea, and *ataxia* in patients with MS.[104]

In ALS, CNs V, VII, IX, X, and XII are commonly affected, causing spastic and/or *flaccid bulbar palsy,* which results in difficulties with speech and swallowing.[19] *Dysarthria* and *dysphagia* are also common in the later stages of MS, PD, and HD. With spastic dysarthria, the voice sounds forced because more effort is needed to move air through the upper airway; whereas, with flaccid dysarthria, the voice sounds hoarse or breathy. Pharyngeal weakness also causes air in the mouth to leak into the nose during enunciation, producing a nasal tone. As ALS progresses, speech becomes more difficult to produce and less intelligible, and eventually the individual becomes

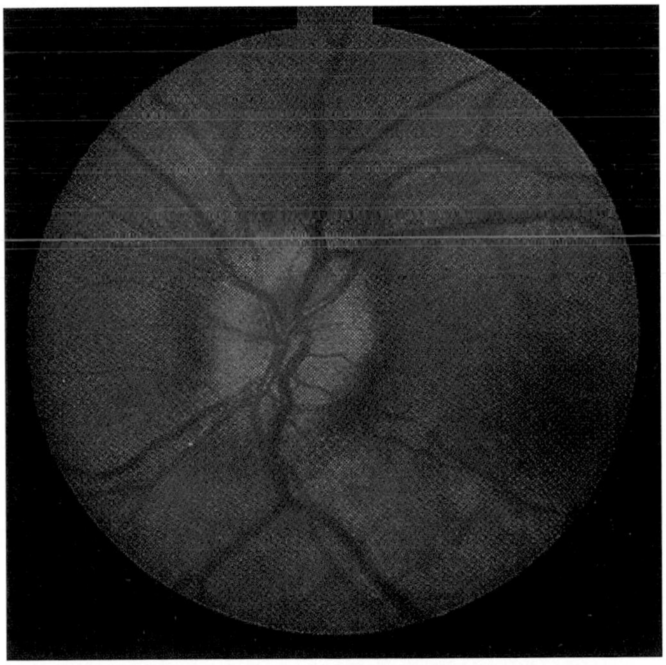

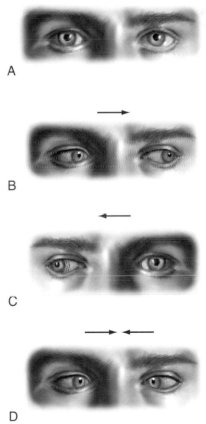

A

B

C

D

FIG. 17-7 Internuclear ophthalmoplegia on the *left.* **A,** Patient looking ahead. **B,** Patient looking to the left. Normal eye movements, left eye abducts and right eye adducts. **C,** Patient looking to the right. The right eye abducts/moves to the right but develops nystagmus at end gaze. The left eye cannot adduct beyond midline. **D,** Patient looking at a close object in midline. Both eyes adduct.

FIG. 17-6 Optic neuritis with mild swelling of the optic disk. *From Yanoff M, Duker J, Augsburger J:* Opthalmology, *ed 2, St. Louis, 2003, Mosby.*

anarthric (completely unable to speak).[19,106] In MS, spastic dysarthria, impaired articular agility, and *scanning speech,* in which each word or syllable is emphasized, may also occur.[97,105]

Dysphagia, which can occur with spastic or flaccid bulbar paralysis, increases the risk for aspiration pneumonia, poor nutritional intake, weight loss, and dehydration. In ALS and MS, sealing the lips, keeping food inside the mouth, or moving food into the esophagus can become difficult, impairing the ability to swallow. Flaccid bulbar palsy also results in regurgitation of liquids into the nose because of pharyngeal weakness, and *spastic bulbar palsy* causes uncoordinated epiglottis closure, which may allow liquids or solids to pass to the larynx and cause choking.[19]

Individuals with ALS also frequently experience *sialorrhea* (drooling) because of an absence of automatic, spontaneous swallowing to clear excessive saliva or because the lower facial muscles are too weak to close the lips tightly to prevent leakage.[19] *Pseudobulbar affect,* in which there is expression of emotion, such as spontaneous crying or laughing, in the absence of emotional triggers or feelings, is also sometimes seen in individuals with spastic bulbar palsy, including those with ALS and MS.[104] In contrast, the orofacial-laryngeal bradykinesia and rigidity caused by PD leads to *hypomimia,* a loss of facial expression also known as masked facies, as well as *hypophonia.*[107,108]

Reflex Integrity. In addition to the hyperreactive stretch reflexes generally found in patients with progressive CNS disorders, many of these disorders also cause a variety of other typical motor impairments[109,110] (Table 17-3).

Myoclonus, a sudden, very brief, and shock-like involuntary movement caused by muscular contractions or loss of normal inhibitory influences, can occur in the later stages of AD. Rigidity, non-velocity–dependent resistance to passive movement, and *clonus* may also occur in the late stages of the disease. In addition, primitive reflexes, such as glabellar, snout, and grasp reflex, may be common; it is important to note that primitive reflexes are also common in healthy elderly and thus alone are not indicative of AD (see Chapter 14 for further information on primitive reflexes).

Rigidity is a clinical hallmark of PD. Rigidity may be *"lead-pipe,"* which is a uniform increased resistance to passive stretch, or *"cog-wheel,"* which is jerky resistance, where tremor is superimposed on rigidity and causes rhythmic interruptions in resistance. Deep tendon reflexes are usually normal in PD, and the plantar responses are flexor.

In the early stages of HD, muscle tone can be normal or decreased (hypotonia). During the later stages of the disease, most patients develop hypertonia, which may present as extrapyramidal rigidity or spasticity. Rigidity occurs most commonly in patients at the extremes of age (e.g., very young or old patients with HD). Spasticity, hyperreflexia, positive Babinski's sign, and clonus may also be seen.[109,110]

In ALS, both UMN and LMN signs may be seen. Thus on examination one may find spasticity, hyperreflexia, clonus, and pathological reflexes, such as a Babinski's or Hoffmann's sign, and hyporeflexia, decreased or absent reflexes, decreased muscle tone or *flaccidity.* As the disease progresses, UMN signs may decrease.[19] Because MS is a disease of the CNS, spasticity, hyperreflexia, clonus, Babinski's sign, and exaggerated cutaneous reflexes will be found on examination.

Muscle tone can be graded using the Modified Ashworth Scale (see Chapter 16),[111] and deep tendon and pathological reflexes should be assessed to determine the extent of UMN, LMN, and extrapyramidal involvement.

Sensory Integrity. Tactile sensation is spared in most progressive CNS diseases. However, patients with MS often have focal sensory loss and paresthesias (pins and needles sensation), numbness, hypersensitivity to minor sensory stimuli, and deficits in position and vibratory sense, especially in the lower extremities.[97] In addition, because of involvement of the thalamus and spinal dopaminergic pathways, patients with PD may experience burning-tingling parasthesias.[94] If the patient complains of sensory symptoms or if sensory involvement is suspected, a thorough sensory examination should be completed (see Chapter 18).

Impairments in Motor Control and Motor Learning. Accurate examination of motor control and motor learning abilities is a critical component of the physical therapy evaluation for individuals with progressive CNS disorders because deficits in these areas can significantly impact functional abilities (see Table 17-3).

Motor learning is typically examined by observing the ability of a patient to learn a new skill (acquisition), the ability to retain that skill (retention), and the ability to transfer the skill to a similar (but slightly different) task (transfer). Gentile has suggested that motor skill learning involves two parallel yet distinct learning processes: implicit and explicit.[112] Explicit learning is supported by declarative memory and involves the conscious focus on attainment of a skill or action goal. Implicit learning is supported by procedural memory and involves the learning of complex information in an incidental manner, without awareness of what has been learned.[113]

Patients with AD have significant impairments in declarative memory, reducing explicit learning, while procedural memory and thus implicit learning of motor skills are relatively preserved.[114] In contrast, individuals with HD, and even more so those with PD, tend to have impaired procedural memory and implicit learning and only develop deficits in declarative memory later in the disease as dementia becomes prominent.[115,116]

Amyotrophic Lateral Sclerosis. Patients with ALS typically present with a combination of UMN and LMN signs, resulting in spasticity and hyperreflexia (UMN signs) and muscle weakness and atrophy (LMN signs).

Huntington's Disease. Individuals with HD typically present with chorea, which are involuntary writhing movements of the body. These can begin as relatively small twitches of the hands, feet, and face and progress to larger movements of more proximal joints. People with HD can also present with motor restlessness, which results in an inability to suppress unwanted movements. Dystonia, an abnormal posturing of a part of the body, has been reported in a 90% of patients with HD[27] and is believed to be more functionally disabling than the chorea.[117] Feigin

TABLE 17-3	**Common Motor Impairments in Patients with Progressive CNS Disorders**	
Motor Impairment	**Typically Seen in These Diseases**	**Assessment Method**
Akinesia: Impaired initiation of movement	PD, HD	Record time for a patient to initiate an action. Use stopwatch to record the difference between instruction to move (e.g., "GO") and the observable onset of movement. This may not be sensitive for very fast movements.
Bradykinesia, hypokinesia: Slowness of movements; reduced movement speed and amplitude	PD, HD	Record time to perform a task (e.g., walking from point-to-point, or performing a reach-to-grasp task. Record time with stopwatch.
Spasticity: Increased resistance to passive stretch of a muscle that is velocity dependent	ALS, HD, MS	Position patient in comfortable position and perform passive ROM of specific joint. Gradually increase velocity at which passive ROM is performed. If patient has spasticity, there will be an increase in resistance to movement at higher velocities. Measured with Modified Ashworth Scale* (see Chapter 16)
Rigidity: Excessive muscle activity involving agonist and antagonist muscle groups	PD	Position patient in comfortable position and perform passive ROM of specific joint. Joint will be resistant toward movement in both directions. Occasionally, there will be sudden brief relaxation followed by resumption of contraction (cogwheel rigidity).
Chorea: Involuntary writhing movements of varying amplitude of almost any part of the body	HD	Observe patient while sitting and standing at rest. Note presence of involuntary movements; typically seen in early stages in face, fingers, hands, toes, and feet.
Tardive dyskinesia: Involuntary movements of the face, trunk, or limbs	Patients who have been treated with long-term dopaminergic-antagonist medications	Observe patient while sitting and standing at rest. Note presence of involuntary movements.
Dystonia: Involuntary, sustained contractions of the muscles of the head, limbs, or trunk, producing abnormal postures	PD, HD	Observe patient while sitting and standing, from front, back and side. Note any asymmetries in posture, or sustained posturing of any part of the body (e.g., one shoulder elevated; arm maintained in internal rotation; head tilted or turned to one side). Observe patient while walking 50 ft (minimum 3 trials). Note any change in postures.
Tremor: Involuntary, rhythmic contractions of agonist/antagonist muscles, producing the appearance of trembling. May be present at rest (resting tremor), during specific postures (postural tremor), or during a voluntary movement (intention tremor)	PD	*Resting tremor:* Observe patient's limbs at rest. Note if tremor is present at rest (resting tremor). *Postural tremor:* Observe patient's hands during the following postures: (1) the arms outstretched and the hands pronated, and (2) the arms flexed at the elbows, and abducted at the shoulders to 90° with the hands pronated and the fingers held near the nose ("the batswing" position).† *Intention tremor:* Observe finger and hand while patient performs finger-nose-finger test. Patient begins by touching examiner's finger, which is held just within arm's reach, then touches their nose, and then touches the examiner's finger, continuing to alternate between the two. Note if tremor is present, particularly as finger approaches target (either finger or nose).
Freezing: Sudden inability to move during the execution of a motor sequence	PD	Observe patient walking down a corridor at least 100 feet, 3 trials. Note any episodes where patient stops movement suddenly and has difficulty restarting movement.
Dysmetria: Inability to control the direction and amplitude of muscle force during a purposeful movement	MS, HD, PD	Ask the patient reach to touch a target (typically the examiner's fingertip, position just at the end of arm's length). Rate according to the following scale:† 0 = No impairment 1 = Mild dysmetria but reaches the target 2 = Moderate dysmetria, reaches target after several attempts 3 = Severe dysmetria, short of target after many attempts 4 = Cannot use hands
Dysdiadochokinesia: Inability to alternately contract and relax agonist and antagonist muscles or muscle groups	MS, HD, PD	Observe patient performing rapid alternating movement of pronation/supination of both arms simultaneously. Rate according to following scale:† 0 = No problem 1 = Mild but detectable clumsiness and slowing of pronation/supination rate 2 = Moderate clumsiness and slowing of pronation/supination rate 3 = Severe clumsiness and slowing of pronation/supination rate 4 = Unable to perform repetitive sequential movements

Adapted from Nolan MF: *Introduction to the Neurologic Examination,* Philadelphia, 1994, FA Davis and Morris ME: *Phys Ther* 80(6):578-597, 2000.
PD, Parkinson's disease; HD, Huntington's disease; ALS, amyotrophic lateral sclerosis; MS, multiple sclerosis.
*From Bohannon R, Smith M: *Phys Ther* 67:207, 1987.
†From Alusi SH, Worthington J, Glickman S, et al: *J Neurol Neurosurg Psychiatry* 68:756-760, 2000.

and colleagues have found that as functional capacity worsened in patients with HD, chorea lessened and dystonia intensified.[117]

Bradykinesia is also prevalent in patients with HD, despite the fact that HD is considered a hyperkinetic disorder. Quinn et al found that bradykinesia in HD was task dependent, rather than a general slowness of movement.[118] In comparing the kinematics and force coordination during transport of a grip instrument in 12 individuals with HD to age-matched controls, the authors found that although bradykinesia was present, the slowness occurred in certain phases of the movement, suggesting that the slowness of movement was due to impairments in sequencing and movement strategies selection.[118] In addition, with a heavier instrument, movement trajectory and grip force variability improved.

The motor control deficits seen in HD can be assessed systematically using the Unified Huntington's Disease Rating Scale (UHDRS) motor subscale.[119] This scale is very similar in design to the Unified Parkinson's Disease Rating Scale (UPDRS) used in patients with Parkinson's disease. It includes such items as saccadic eye movement and smooth pursuit, bradykinesia, gait, presence of chorea and dystonia postural control (pull test), and rapid alternating movements. The scale assesses relevant clinical features of HD and has been found have high interrater reliability for the motor scores.[119]

Parkinson's Disease. Patients with PD exhibit akinesia (difficulty initiating movements), bradykinesia (reduced speed and amplitude of movement), tremor (usually at rest), muscle rigidity (hypertonicity and hyperreflexia in agonist and antagonist muscle groups), impaired postural control and balance, and episodes of *freezing* (sudden inability to move). Akinesia and bradykinesia appear to be the two factors that most affect patient's functional abilities. Individuals with PD have significantly delayed onset of movement and overall slowness of movement compared to healthy individuals.

Bradykinesia and akinesia in patients with PD can be seen in all types of tasks and often from relatively early in the disease. Complex movements, such as repetitive or sequential movements, are most impaired[120] and patients have particular difficulty with performing dual tasks.[121] Patients with PD also demonstrate *hypokinesia* (abnormally decreased motor function or activity), as evidenced during handwriting and walking. In both tasks, the movement amplitude typically decreases as the duration of the task increases. Handwriting becomes increasing smaller as a paragraph is written,[122] and steps often become shorter and shorter as walking distance increases.

The UPDRS is a scale designed specifically for the examination and evaluation of patients with Parkinson's disease. The motor subscale of the UPDRS is designed to evaluate impairments in motor control. It ranks patient's motor impairments on a scale of 0-4, with 0 typically indicating no observed abnormality. This scale is useful during initial examination and for tracking changes in motor function over time.

Multiple Sclerosis. Patients with MS have weakness and hyperreflexia primarily as a result of damage to the corticospinal tracts. This may result in impaired dexterity and coordination of large movement patterns and gross and fine motor control. Lesions in the cerebellum may also cause impairments in coordination, such as dysmetria and dysdiadochokinesia (see Table 17-3), as well as in proactive and reactive balance control.

Cardiovascular and Pulmonary

Ventilation and Respiration/Gas Exchange. A variety of ventilatory impairments may be seen in patients with progressive CNS disorders, and the incidence and severity of these impairments vary. In all patients with progressive CNS disorders, respiratory and ventilation impairments may lead to atelectasis, pneumonia, and ventilatory failure (see Chapters 24 and 26). Respiratory complications are a major cause of morbidity and mortality in many patients with these disorders.[25,123,124]

In patients with ALS, respiratory impairments are caused by loss of respiratory muscle strength, and although the rate of respiratory muscle weakening varies among individuals, for the most part it tends to progress linearly.[125] Early signs and symptoms of respiratory muscle weakness include fatigue, *dyspnea* on exertion, difficulty sleeping in a supine position and frequent awakening at night, frequent sighing, excessive daytime sleepiness, and morning headaches that result from hypoxia.[13,126,127]

Individuals with a gradual progression of respiratory muscle weakness may not complain of respiratory symptoms because they tend to decrease their overall level of physical activity due to concomitant muscle weakness in the extremities. As weakness progresses, truncated speech, *orthopnea* (shortness of breath when lying supine), dyspnea at rest, paradoxical breathing, accessory muscle use, and a weak cough occur. If an individual does not receive ventilatory support, eventually carbon dioxide (CO_2) retention will lead to acidosis, coma, respiratory failure, and death.[124]

Rigidity of the respiratory muscles, flexed posture, and kyphosis in PD tend to produce a restrictive pattern of respiratory dysfunction. Upper airway obstruction due to involvement of the upper airway muscles and obstructive pulmonary disease are also associated with PD.[128-130] Levodopa may also induce respiratory *dyskinesia*, which may produce restrictive and dyskinetic ventilation patterns as well as abnormal control of ventilation.[131,132]

In patients with MS, ventilatory impairments may be caused by immobility which reduces lung volume and by direct involvement of the respiratory motor pathways causing inspiratory and expiratory muscle weakness.[133-135] As a result, patients with MS have poor exercise tolerance, fatigue, and dyspnea on exertion.[134]

Examination of respiratory status and function for patients with progressive CNS disorders should include assessment of respiratory symptoms, respiratory muscle function and strength, breathing pattern, chest expansion, auscultation, cough effectiveness, and standard pulmonary function tests, such as vital capacity or forced vital capacity, forced expiratory volume, and flow rate, as described in Chapters 24 and 26.

Aerobic Capacity and Endurance. Little has been documented about deconditioning and decreased endurance in individuals with progressive CNS disorders, although these impairments are often seen clinically. Impaired aerobic capacity and endurance occur because of direct or indirect impairments, or disuse and abuse. For example, in patients with PD, rigidity and flexed posture (direct impairments) and resultant kyphosis (indirect impairment) leads to decreased lung capacity and a restrictive pulmonary disease pattern; in addition, a sedentary lifestyle may also lead to decreased endurance (disuse).

Studies of patients with PD, using cycle or upper extremity ergometry, have found that peak cardiovascular and metabolic responses are comparable to those of healthy controls, although those with PD do tend to have higher oxygen consumption rates (VO_2) and submaximal heart rates and may not be able to exercise for as long as healthy normals before reaching VO_{2max}, suggesting that individuals with PD may exercise less efficiently.[136-138]

Although the maximal aerobic capacity of patients with MS has been found to be significantly lower than that of matched healthy controls,[139-141] indicating deconditioning and disuse, studies have found that a graded maximal exercise test[139] or a modified (e.g., discontinuous) exercise test[140,141] can safely be performed in this patient population. A small study of 10 patients with MS compared metabolic and cardiopulmonary responses during maximal exercise using three modes of ergometry: Arm cranking, leg cycling, and combined arm and leg cycling (Fig. 17-8). The combined arm and leg mode elicited greater metabolic and cardiopulmonary responses, indicating that this mode may be better for fitness testing and training because the exercise load can be distributed over a larger muscle mass, thereby reducing the load placed on an individual group of muscles.[140]

Aerobic capacity and cardiovascular/pulmonary endurance can be examined in individuals with early stage ALS or HD using standardized protocols (see Chapter 23); however, decreased muscular strength and endurance and abnormal muscle tone and control may limit testing.

For ambulatory patients, the 6-minute walk test (6MWT), in which the total distance walked as fast as possible in 6 minutes is recorded, is often a useful functional measure of aerobic capacity and endurance. This test reflects cardiorespiratory endurance, speed, balance, and agility during ambulation, and its results correlate with maximal oxygen uptake and disease prognosis in several clinical populations.[142-145] To increase the reliability and eliminate the effects of practice for the 6MWT, three trials are recommended (two initial practice trials, with the third being the trial that is recorded), but this may be too fatiguing for many patients with progressive CNS disorders. For this reason, a 2-minute walk test (2MWT) is recommended. The 2MWT has been found to be reliable and valid measure of endurance and has been found to be sensitive for detecting endurance problems in patients with stage III and stage IV PD.[146]

Fatigue is common in individuals with PD, MS, and ALS. Fatigue is one of the most disabling symptoms in MS and is the most likely of all primary symptoms to interfere with ADLs.[147] A diurnal pattern of fatigue, least in the morning and greatest in the afternoon, is common, although fatigue can occur with minimal activity and lead to a sense of continuous exhaustion.[147] Patients with PD

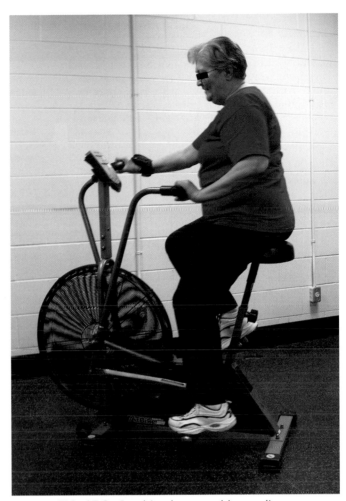

FIG. 17-8 Combined arm and leg cycling.

also report that fatigue is among their most severe and disabling symptoms.[148-150]

The cause of fatigue in progressive CNS disorders may be related to peripheral or central mechanisms or both. In ALS, as motor neurons die, the remaining weakened muscles have to work at a higher percentage of their maximal strength, accelerating muscle fatigue.[151,152] In MS, widespread axonal dysfunction and increased recruitment of cortical areas and pathways are thought to be associated with fatigue and a patient's sense that a great effort is required to perform actions.[153] In addition, reduced efficiency of action-potential propagation in partially demyelinated or degenerated central motor axons or intracortical circuits[154] and increased energy demands for muscle activation due to impaired recruitment of alpha motor neurons because of corticospinal involvement or spasticity[155,156] may be responsible for MS-related fatigue. Central dopamine deficiency[157] and mitochondrial dysfunction[158] are thought to play a role in fatigue in patients with PD. Fatigue may also be related to deconditioning secondary to decreased activity levels, sleep disturbances, respiratory impairments, hypoxia (in the case of ALS), ataxia, dyskinesias, spasticity, emotional stress, and depression.

The Modified Fatigue Impact Scale (MFIS) is the tool of choice for measuring fatigue in MS.[159] The MFIS consists of 21 questions, grouped by cognitive functioning, physical functioning, and psychosocial functioning domains. The subject rates the extent to which fatigue causes problems, from 0 for no problem to 4 for extreme problem so that a higher score indicates that fatigue is having a greater impact.[159] The Fatigue Severity Scale (FSS) is an alternative tool for assessing fatigue. It has nine statements that are each rated on 7-point scale. The average score for all of the items is the final score on the FSS, with a higher score indicating more severe fatigue.[160] The MFIS and FSS are both valid and reliable for assessing fatigue in people with MS and may also be used in patients with other progressive CNS disorders.[160-164]

Integumentary

Integumentary Integrity. Examination of integumentary integrity in patients with progressive CNS disorders focuses on the skin. In general, skin breakdown tends to develop in individuals with conditions that impair sensation, such as MS, and in those who become incontinent. Contact points between the patient's skin and any devices and the patient's bed should be examined, especially when the patient's mobility becomes increasingly dependent. In patients with HD, bruising and skin abrasions on the feet, shins, forearms, and elbows can occur because of frequent choreiform movements.

Function

Gait, Locomotion, Balance, and Postural Control. Problems with gait and balance are common in patients with progressive CNS disorders. Gait or balance impairments are often one of first signs in individuals with these types of disorders (see Chapter 32).

Alzheimer's Disease. Gait abnormalities,[165,166] impaired tandem gait,[167] postural instability,[166,168,169] decreased gait speed,[166,170-174] decreased stride length,[175] decreased step length,[176] increased cadence,[170] and stride length variability[169,175] have been described in the dementia sub-types, including AD, vascular dementia (VaD), and normal pressure hydrocephalus (NPH). Postural sway, decreased gait speed, and stride length have been found to be associated with reduced cerebral blood flow in the frontal lobes and basal ganglia in patients with AD.[176] A recent, prospective study of moderately to severely affected people with AD found that those who fell had significantly higher UPDRS motor scores, an indicator of motor impairments.[177] It has been proposed that gait apraxia, rather than extrapyramidal deficits, may underlie gait abnormalities in some patients with AD.[178]

The annual incidence of falls in persons with dementia is 40% to 60%, twice the rate in cognitively normal elderly[179-181]; however, few studies have examined specific gait impairments and fall risk in people with dementia. Nakamura, Meguro, and Saskai found falls were significantly more common in institutionalized adults with moderately severe AD than in those with mild AD and that stride-length variability was an important independent predictor for falls.[168] O'Keefe and colleagues found that gait disturbance was a predictor of falls in patients with moderate and severe AD,[175] and a recent study of individuals with moderate to severe AD living in specialized AD care units found decreased cadence to be predictive of falls.[177]

Amyotrophic Lateral Sclerosis. In ALS, ambulation difficulties and impaired postural control and balance are caused by muscle weakness and/or spasticity. Almost 50% of people with ALS are reported to fall.[182] Difficulties with swing phase because of lower extremity spasticity, decreased balance because of generalized spasticity, foot drop because of distal weakness, and instability because of proximal weakness are all common. As the disease progresses, cadence, stride length, and gait velocity all decrease, and patients tend to spend less time in single-leg stance.[183] Jette and colleagues found that in patients with ALS, decreases in walking ability from independent walking to walking in the community with assistance to walking only at home to being unable to walk were precipitated by relatively small changes in muscle force.[184]

Huntington's Disease. In HD ambulation is characterized by a wide-based staggering gait, sometimes in a zigzag pattern of progression, with the arms fixed. Individuals with HD have decreased stride length and stepping rate, poorly modulated cadence, and increased variability in velocity, stride length, and cadence.[185-187] In addition, individuals with HD have difficulties performing simultaneous and sequential movements,[188,189] running a sequence of motor programs in the absence of advance information, and planning and performing movements.[190,191] Individuals with HD also have difficulties maintaining balance in response to sudden perturbations particularly when sensory cues are eliminated.[192]

Early in the progression of HD, chorea, weakness of specific muscle groups (often the upper back and trunk), and mild cognitive and visuospatial impairments may all contribute to balance problems, difficulty walking, and falls. Patients may lose their balance when turning quickly, especially while carrying a load, changing directions suddenly, or wearing unsupportive footwear.[193] As HD progresses, the early stage impairments become more pronounced, and changes in muscle tone are common. Weakness of the postural muscles increases, and proximal stability decreases. Balance impairments become more severe, and spatial awareness deficits can compound the balance problems, making everyday tasks dangerous.[193]

Parkinson's Disease. Akinesia (lack of movement), bradykinesia (slowed speed and amplitude of movement), rigidity (resistance to passive movement), dyskinesia (extraneous movement), and postural instability are associated with the loss of neurons in the substantia nigra and decreased levels of dopamine and cause the balance and gait impairments seen in individuals with PD.[194] Preambulation is marked by a lack of normal preparatory trunk and extremity movements. Patients may have difficulty transferring their weight from one foot to the other to initiate gait ("ignition disorder"). In most patients, ambulation is initially characterized by a shortened stride, with intact cadence,[195-197] producing short shuffling steps with a narrowed base of support.

As the disease progresses, cadence increases and stride further shortens resulting in *festinating gait.*[197-199] This gait pattern attempts to keep the center of gravity (COG) between the feet while the trunk leans forward involuntarily and shifts the COG forward. In an attempt to correct balance, instead of making one or two large corrective steps, the patient can only make short (hypometric) steps, which still leaves the COG in front of the feet. To compensate for the hypokinesia and in an attempt to prevent falling, stepping velocity increases.[200]

Arm swing, trunk rotation, and pelvic movement are often decreased or absent in patients with PD. The patient also has great difficulty stopping movement, changing directions, and stepping over or walking around objects because of freezing ("motor block"). Freezing, a sudden transient inability to move, commonly occurs when walking in crowded areas with competing auditory and visual stimuli, walking down a narrow hallway, changing tasks, or when the support surface changes.[194,201,202]

Postural control impairments and balance problems are common in patients with late stage PD and have many causes, as demonstrated in Fig. 17-9. Patients with PD can usually maintain balance in static standing or sitting postures or with self-generated perturbations to their center of mass but have great difficulty maintaining balance when there is an unexpected perturbation or when they do not have sufficient time to prepare in advance for threats to balance.[121,203]

In PD, impairments in automatic postural reflexes and equilibrium reactions caused by dopamine loss result in the patient being unable to correct for mild perturbations.[204-206] Lack of trunk and pelvic mobility may mechanically limit the patient's ability to respond to perturbations,[207] and decreased or absent vestibular responses may also impact balance control.[208] Although individuals with PD can generally use visual, somatosensory, and vestibular information during quiet stance,[209]

when they need to simultaneously perform cognitive or motor tasks, postural control becomes impaired, particularly in patients with a history of falls.[210-212]

Individuals with PD also have difficulty activating feedforward mechanisms and shaping the pattern and magnitude of postural muscle responses in response to changes in perturbation direction and stance position and have absent or decreased ankle, hip, arm, and stepping strategies.[209,213] Because they cannot activate appropriate postural responses, when perturbed, patients with PD may take several steps to recover stability or may fall. The incidence of falls in PD is reported to be as high as 68%.[214-216] Previous falls, disease duration, dementia, and loss of arm swing are predictors of falling in this population, and there are significant associations between disease severity, balance impairment, depression, and falling.[216]

Multiple Sclerosis. Patients with MS may have gait problems because of lower extremity weakness, spasticity, or ataxia. Common impairments include weakness of the hip flexor muscles, resulting in difficulty lifting the lower extremity; weakness of the hip abductors, resulting in a Trendelenburg gait pattern; and weakness of the dorsiflexors and evertors of the foot, resulting in foot drop. Patients with spasticity (usually increased extensor tone) will ambulate stiffly and will drag the toes and circumduct the hip during swing phase.

Ataxia, which is uncoordinated movement, occurs when there are lesions in the cerebellum, the cerebellar pathways, or the sensory pathway and is common in MS. Cerebellar ataxia produces a gait characterized by a broad-based, staggering pattern. The patient appears to stagger from side to side with bilateral involvement or will drift to one side with unilateral involvement. Reciprocal lower extremity movement is slow and uncoordinated, and patients have difficulty with foot placement. Sensory ataxia is characterized by a wide-based gait with the heel striking the ground first and then the foot slapping down. Patients tend to watch their feet during ambulation to compensate for the sensory loss.

Clinical Measurement of Balance and Gait Disturbances. Parameters and characteristics of gait (speed, stride length, step width, episodes of freezing) during forward, backward, and sideward walking should be examined and documented (see Chapter 32), as should overall stability, safety, and endurance (see Chapter 13). Gait and walking ability should be analyzed in a variety of contexts and during complex, functional walking tasks,[77,217] including during performance of dual tasks, such as walking and talking[218] or walking while performing a cognitive task.[219] Energy expenditure, alignment, fit, practicality, and safety and ease of orthotic and assistive devices used during gait should also be examined. Postural orientation, postural stability, reactive control, anticipatory control, and adaptive postural control should be assessed. It is also important to document any falls and related injuries that have occurred.

A variety of tests and measures are available to examine balance and gait in patients with specific progressive CNS disorders (see Chapter 13). The Berg Balance Scale[220] and the Functional Ambulation Performance/Gait Rite have been used to test populations with PD and HD.[221-226]

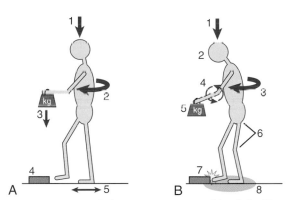

FIG. 17-9 A, Postural threats encountered in daily life. *1,* Gravity; *2,* self-generated movement; *3,* external postural perturbations; *4,* obstacles; *5,* moving or slippery support surface. **B,** Postural control impairments and balance problems in patients with late stage PD. *1,* Orthostatic hypotension and abnormal perception of gravity; *2,* visual and occulomotor disturbances; *3,* impaired automatic peripherally triggered postural responses; *4,* dyskinesias; *5,* abnormal anticipatory postural responses; *6,* stiffness; *7,* reduced step height and abnormal stepping responses; *8,* narrowed limit of stability. *From Horak FB, Henry SM, Shumway-Cook A: Phys Ther 77(5):517-533, 1997.*

Patients with MS have been tested with the Dynamic Gait Index,[227,228] and patients with PD have been tested with the Timed Up and Go[229] and the Functional Reach Test[230] (see Fig. 13-18)

Assistive and Adaptive Devices. At some point during the disease course, most patients with progressive CNS disorders will require some sort of assistive or adaptive device (see Chapter 33) to maintain or assist with function. In fact, many patients will require several different types of devices over the course of their disease. For example, a patient with HD may initially walk independently but soon may need a straight cane for help with balance. Later on, a rolling walker may be prescribed, and later still, as the disease progresses, a customized wheelchair is likely to be required. Because of the expense of adaptive equipment, therapists must consider not just the current needs of a patient but also their needs as the disease progresses. In addition, one should keep in mind the cognitive skills needed to use a device when considering a device for a patient with a dementing disorder, such as AD, and in the later stages of HD, PD, and often MS.

Patients with progressive CNS disorders should be evaluated for assistive devices for ambulation, such as canes, walkers, or rolling walkers, and for the use of wheelchairs. For ambulation, a straight cane or quad cane can help patients with mild balance disorders or lower extremity weakness. A walker can provide even more assistance for lower extremity weakness and poor balance. However, patients with spasticity of the upper extremities or movement disorders, such as tremor from PD or chorea from HD, may find it difficult to manage any hand-held assistive device. In addition, because a walker interrupts the normal rhythm and pattern of ambulation, it can cause more problems than it solves for certain patients. For example, patients with PD who have akinesia may have difficulty with the starting and stopping of movement required with a walker. For such patients, wheeled walkers may be more helpful, although a study of nineteen patients with PD found that patients walked more slowly during a trial with a wheeled or standard walker than unassisted. They also had more episodes of freezing using the standard walker. These findings suggest that, at least at first, assistive devices should be used with caution in patients with PD because they are associated with slower walking and no reduction in freezing. However, with continued practice, patients may improve their walking speed with an assistive device and these devices may prevent falls.

As patients progress to the end stages of a neurodegenerative disease, it is likely that they will want to or need to use some form of wheeled mobility. Many individuals with MS, even in the early midstages of the disease, find a motorized scooter a good way to conserve energy and prevent fatigue during long distance mobility. Although a standard manual wheelchair may be useful briefly for patients with midstage ALS, if strength impairments are more pronounced in the lower extremities, it is likely that such a patient would soon not be able to propel the wheelchair due to upper extremity weakness, or may need more trunk support due to trunk weakness and would therefore need a motorized wheelchair.[231] This patient may instead benefit from a tilt-in-space or motorized wheelchair, even though he may initially not require all of these components. Individuals in the later stages of disease may require more significant postural support in a wheelchair. Patients with HD, for example, have very limited motor control at this stage and benefit from padded, reclining wheelchairs, such as a Broda chair. This chair provides soft padding to prevent skin damage from involuntary movements and also allows the patient to be fully reclined or tilted back.

Orthotic, Protective, and Supportive Devices. As most individuals with a progressive CNS have primary or secondary impairments in muscle strength or secondary impairments in joint integrity, the need for devices and equipment that may enhance function or performance should be assessed (see Chapter 34).

For example, in individuals with ALS and MS, foot drop is common and an ankle-foot orthosis (AFO) may be prescribed to increase safety during gait. Cattaneo and colleagues found that a dynamic AFO that allowed plantarflexion improved standing balance in individuals with MS with mild strength and balance problems, while static AFOs reduced gait speed without improving balance.[232] This study provides preliminary evidence that AFOs may improve standing balance in patients with MS who have mild strength and balance deficits but that therapists should be cautious in prescribing AFOs as they can also adversely affect motor performance.

Individuals with HD with dystonic posturing may benefit from a shoe insert to control the position of the foot during ambulation. When selecting an orthosis, one must balance the benefits of support against the potential costs of increased energy expenditure associated with additional weight of a device and the financial expense of a device that may only be useful for a short period of time, depending on the rate of disease progression.

Individuals with ALS often develop cervical extensor muscle weakness, making it difficult to keep the head up for prolonged periods or with unexpected movements. To address this, a soft, foam neck collar may help initially when weakness is mild, and a semirigid collar may help when weakness becomes more severe.

Protective devices, such as helmets or elbow and knee protectors, may be prescribed for individuals at risk of falling or for individuals with HD who are prone to injuries because of chorea. Not surprisingly, it is often difficult to persuade an individual to wear protective devices.

Environmental Barriers at Home and Work. The patient's home and work environments should be examined for current and potential barriers, including access and safety issues (see Chapter 35). In the initial stages of a degenerative disease, the therapist may evaluate the home and work (if applicable) environments and make recommendations to allow the patient maximal access to his or her environment. Since it is expected that a patient's condition will change and deteriorate over time, therapists must also try to anticipate a patient's future needs (see Table 17-2). For example, a patient with ALS may initially be able to ascend and descend stairs with minimal difficulty, but within a short time (months to a few years), this task will become impossible. The patient will then require either a single-level home, a home with their bedroom and living facilities on one floor, or a stair lift/elevator in the home. These issues should be considered as early as possible so that the appropriate modifications are in place when needed.

In the later stages of progressive CNS disorders, therapists may evaluate a patient's home and work environment for accessibility of assistive and adaptive devices such as walkers, wheelchairs, and scooters. This may also include assessing the patient's ability to access transportation, including public transportation. For individuals with MS, it is also important to consider the environment with respect to energy conservation. Therapists can assist patients in structuring a living and work environment (by arranging furniture or organizing desktop equipment, for example) so that everyday tasks are completed with minimal energy expenditure.

Self-Care and Home Management. Loss of independence in ADLs and instrumental ADLs (IADLs) can be the result of physical and/or cognitive impairments. Physical impairments, such as weakness, decreased ROM, spasticity, impaired coordination and balance, can limit independence or impair performance of ADLs. Cognitive impairments, resulting from dementia, can also significantly impact functional abilities. This decline in functional abilities, which is inevitable for patients with progressive CNS disorders, is one of the most troubling aspects of dementia for patients[233] and their caregivers.[234] Early in the dementing process, the loss of ability to function may cause the patient to feel useless, dependent, and burdensome.[233] For families of persons with more advanced stages of dementia, such as seen in AD, HD, and PD, the major problems of care include impairments of communication, eating, and bathing and wandering.[235] Incontinence is also a significant problem that causes stress for the patient and caregiver.

A number of ADL and IADL scales used in the general population, including the Index of Activities of Daily Living,[236] the Physical Self-Maintenance Scale (PSMS), the Lawton-Brody Instrumental Activities of Daily Living Scale,[237] the Functional Activities Questionnaire (FAQ),[238] and the Structured Assessment of Independent Living Skills (SAILS)[239] are appropriate for use with patients with progressive disorders.

Daily functioning in patients with severe AD can also be assessed with the Alzheimer's Disease Cooperative Study ADL–severe scale (ADCS/ADL–severe scale). This scale uses information provided by caregivers to rate performance of 19 daily activities. Activity performance is rated from 0-1 to 0-5, depending on the question, with a possible total score of 54. Higher scores indicate higher functioning.[240] An additional useful tool is the Disability Assessment in Dementia scale. This 10-domain, 40-item instrument measures instrumental and basic ADL.[241]

The Schwab and England Rating Scale (SERS) is an 11-point global measure of functioning that asks the rater to report ADL function from 100% (normal) to 0% (vegetative functions only). The scale was originally designed to evaluate function in people with PD but has also been found to have excellent test-retest reliability, to correlate well with qualitative and quantitative changes in function

and to be sensitive to changes over time in individuals with ALS.[242]

The HD-ADL scale is a scale developed to evaluate ADL functions in patients with HD.[243] It consists of 5 general categories—personal care, household, work and finances, social relationships, and communications. This scale can provide an overall level of ADL functioning but may not be sensitive enough to detect subtle changes (either improvements or decline) in ADL abilities.

The UPDRS, for use with patients with PD, includes an ADL component to assess the impact of PD on various ADL functions. These include speech, salivation, swallowing, handwriting, cutting food and handling utensils, dressing, hygiene, turning in bed and adjusting bedclothes, falling, freezing when walking, walking, left-sided tremor, right-sided tremor, and sensory complaints. This scale, however, does not measure pure ADL function but rather contains a mixture of impairment- and disability-related items.[244] Thus, to measure only ADL function in patients with PD, a more generic ADL measure may be more appropriate.

In addition to use of generic ADL scales, the Assessment of Motor and Process Skills (AMPS) and the Functional Independence Measure (FIM) have been used to assess ADL function in patients with MS.[245] Researchers have advocated for evaluation of both ADLs and IADLs in patients with MS. Mansson and Lexell[245] have found that individuals with MS can be independent in ADLs (as measured by the FIM) but still have limitations in IADL (as measured by the AMPS).

Work, Community, and Leisure Integration. Examination of a patient's ability to work and be involved in their community and leisure activities is very important for patients with progressive CNS disorders. These disorders often cause progressive loss of independence and reduced involvement in activities that are central to a fulfilling life. These issues are often most effectively assessed by asking the patient about their ability to participate in school, work, sport, leisure, and community activities. Some sample interview questions for an older patient with PD (being examined in an outpatient setting) might be the following:

Work*
- Describe your current job.
- To what extent have you recently been involved in your work?
- To what degree are you limited in your ability to work?

Community
- Are you involved in any activities within your community?
- If so, are you having any difficulty or limitations performing those activities now?

Leisure
- What recreational activities (e.g., sports, hobbies, leisure activities) did you engage in prior to your diagnosis? What activities do you engage in now? Are you having any difficulty or limitations performing those activities now?

- Has your social activity (for example, time spent with family and friends) changed at all because of your current condition?

*Adapted with permission from Quinn L, Gordon J: *Functional Outcomes Documentation for Rehabilitation,* Philadelphia, 2003, WB Saunders.

There are also several generic measures designed to formally assess the ability to participate in work, community, and leisure activities. The SF-36 and the Sickness Impact Profile[246] are general health status measures that have been used in a variety of patient populations. Although these scales measure general well being and participation in daily living, social, and recreational activities, the test items are not all applicable for patients with chronic degenerative diseases.

The Parkinson's Disease Questionnaire (PDQ-39) was designed to measure health-related quality of life in patients with PD. It consists of 39 items with eight subscales: Mobility (10 items), ADLs (6 items), emotional well being (6 items), stigma (4 items), social support (3 items), cognition (4 items), communication (3 items), and bodily discomfort (3 items).[247] Items in each subscale[248] and the total scale[249] can be summarized into an index and transformed to a score on a 0-100 scale, with higher scores reflecting lower health-related quality of life. This questionnaire is available in several languages, including Spanish, and has been found to have good internal consistency and test-retest reliability.[250,251] A shorter summary index (PDQ-8 SI) can also be calculated.[252]

The MS Quality of Life-54 (MSQOL-54) is a quality of life, self-report questionnaire designed for people with MS.[253] This 54-item scale has 12 subscales (physical function, role limitations-physical, role limitations-emotional, pain, emotional well being, energy, health perceptions, social function, cognitive function, health distress, overall quality of life, and sexual function) and 2 additional single-item measures. Two summary scores are then calculated: One for physical health and one for mental health. The MSQOL-54 has been found to have good test-retest reliability.[253]

The ALS Assessment Questionnaire-40 (ALSAQ-40), an ALS-specific quality of life measure, contains 40 items that form 5 subscales representing 5 areas of health: Mobility, ADLs, eating and drinking, communication, and emotional functioning. The questions refer to the patient's condition during the past 2 weeks, and responses are recorded on a 5-point Likert scale. The ALSAQ-40 indicates the amount of ill health in each domain assessed, using a summary score from 0 (best health status) to 100 (worst health status). This instrument has demonstrated validity and reliability.[254,255]

A relatively new tool has been developed for assessing quality of life in patients with AD. The Quality Of Life-AD (QOL-AD) consists of 13 items that measure physical condition, mood, memory, functional abilities, interpersonal relationships, ability to participate in meaningful activities, financial situation, and global assessments of self as a whole and quality of life as a whole.[256,257] Ratings for each item are scored on a scale of 1-4 (1 = poor, 4 = excellent). Total sum scores range from 13-52, with higher scores indicating better quality of life. This scale is relatively quick to administer and can be administered to patients, caregivers, or both. The QOL-AD seems to be most useful for individuals with MMSE scores greater than 10. Individuals with MMSE scores less than 10 may not be able to complete the test because of the severity of their dementia.

Psychosocial Function. Although this category of examination is not listed in the *Guide to Physical Therapist Practice,* it is an essential component of a physical therapy examination for adults with progressive CNS disorders. Depression and anxiety are common in individuals with neurodegenerative disorders,[258,259] thus screening is important and referral to a psychologist or psychiatrist for further evaluation may be warranted. The Beck Depression Inventory,[260] the Center of Epidemiologic Study-Depression (CES-D) scale,[261] the Hospital Anxiety and Depression Scale,[262] and the State-Trait Anxiety Inventory (STAI)[263] may be used to examine the psychosocial function of patients with progressive CNS disorders.

Disease-Specific Measures of General Physical Functioning. The measures previously described can be used to examine specific or general physical functioning in patients with progressive CNS disorders. However, disease-specific measures of general physical functioning, often initially designed for research purposes, can also be used in a clinical setting to classify patients with the same disease into a certain category or disease stage and to evaluate impairments and functional abilities specific to a disorder, thereby minimizing unnecessary testing.

Alzheimer's Disease. The two tools commonly used to stage AD are the Clinical Dementia Rating Scale (CDRS) and the Global Deterioration Scale (GDS) staging system. The CDRS is based on an interview with the patient and an appropriate informant or caregiver and is used to stage and assess progression of AD.[264] Scores of 0 (none) to 5 (terminal) are given in six cognitive areas: Memory, orientation, judgment and problem solving, community affairs, home and hobbies, and personal care. Although the original scale had a floor effect that made it not particularly useful in patients with severe AD, higher scores on the new extended version do correlate with increasing functional impairment, decreasing independence, and nursing home residence, and both the profound (stage 4) and terminal (stage 5) stages have been shown to predict shortened survival.[265]

The GDS is used in conjunction with the Brief Cognitive Rating Scale (BCRS) axes I through IV and the Functional Assessment Staging (FAST) measure to assess AD severity and progression. The GDS is a 7-stage rating system based on a clinical interview with the patient and informant or caregiver. Stage 1 indicates no cognitive decline, and stage 7 indicates very severe cognitive decline.[266] The BCRS uses semistructured clinical assessments to evaluate concentration, recent memory, remote memory, and orientation, and the FAST assesses functional impairment associated with changes in cognition. The FAST is derived from the 7-point functioning and self-care axis (axis V) of the BCRS and identifies 10 successive stages of functional impairment. The FAST is especially useful in patients with greater disability because stages 6 and 7 include several substages that describe the level of impairment very specifically.[267]

While the GDS and CDRS consider the impact of cognition on functional abilities, the Dependence Scale measures the amount of assistance required by people with AD.[268] This scale consists of 13 questions, and items are rated according to frequency with which assistance is needed.

Amyotrophic Lateral Sclerosis. The ALS Functional Rating Scale-Revised (ALSFRS-R) assesses functional status and change in patients with ALS.[269] Individuals are asked to rate their function for 12 items on a scale from 4 (normal function) to 0 (unable to attempt the task). Scores on the original scale, the ALSFRS, correlate positively with objective measures of upper and lower extremity muscle strength (r = 0.88; r = 0.86) and is valid and reliable for measuring the decline in function associated with loss of muscular strength in patients with ALS.[270] The ALSFRS-R was expanded to include additional items related to respiratory function. Other disease specific scales include the Appel ALS Scale (AALS), the ALS Severity Scale (ALSSS), and the Norris Scale.

Huntington's Disease. The stages of HD are typically measured using the Total Functional Capacity (TFC) scale, which is a component of the UHDRS.[271] The TFC lists five stages of HD (I-V) and five levels of function in occupation, finances, domestic responsibilities, ADLs, and living situation.

Parkinson's Disease. The Hoehn and Yahr scale has been used for many years to categorize patients into one of five stages of PD. While the scale is widely recognized and used in the PD medical community, it mixes impairment and disability information and is heavily weighted towards postural impairments.[272] A "modified" Hoehn and Yahr scale, which incorporates $\frac{1}{2}$-point increments, is currently used by many clinicians, but the psychometric properties of this version have not been evaluated.

Multiple Sclerosis. The most commonly used disability scale for patients with MS is the Expanded Disability Status Scale (EDSS).[273] Although this scale is not comprehensive, it does provide a general measure of disability and allows for the classification of patients, and for tracking progression of the disease. The scale has a strong emphasis on ambulation, particularly in the mid-range, making it particularly relevant for physical therapists. However, it is not sensitive to changes in cognitive functioning, which can significantly affect disability in people with MS.

The Multiple Sclerosis Impact Scale (MSIS-29)[274] was designed to measure the impact of MS on normal daily life. It consists of 29 questions, 20 of which address physical impact and nine of which address the psychological impact of the disease. A combined score can be generated, or both components can be reported separately, which is useful for comparing the differing impacts of physical and psychological impairments in patients with MS.

EVALUATION, DIAGNOSIS, AND PROGNOSIS

According to the *Guide to Physical Therapy Practice*,[275] the preferred practice pattern for patients with progressive CNS disorders is 5E: Impaired motor function and sensory integrity associated with progressive disorders of the CNS. With progressive CNS disorders, progression of pathology, impairments, functional limitations, and disabilities is inevitable. It is imperative that clinicians understand the nature and progression of the disease and the stage of the disease to not only address an individual's immediate problems but to also plan ahead for future problems.

Adults with progressive CNS disorders will have a number of different abnormal examination findings that will vary considerably in severity and in their impact on prognosis. Many factors can affect a patient's functional prognosis (Fig. 17-10).

The *Guide to Physical Therapist Practice* states that the expected range of number of visits per episode of care for patients with progressive CNS disorders is 6 to 50.[275] Over the course of a disease, patients are likely to require multiple episodes of care. Ideally, patients would receive ongoing consultation with a PT. In many major medical centers, clinics focused on caring for patients with specific progressive CNS disorders (e.g., PD, MS) include a variety of clinicians, including PTs and occupational therapists, specially trained in working with patients with that disorder. Patients are typically seen by the physician and other clinicians at set intervals (e.g., 3 or 6 months) for ongoing management. Therapists can then make

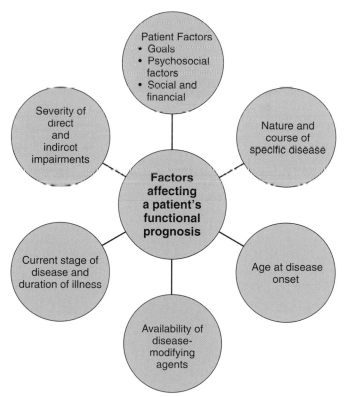

FIG. 17-10 Factors affecting functional prognosis for a patient with a progressive CNS disorder. *Redrawn from* Phys Ther, *2004.*

recommendations for initiating new episodes of therapy, if warranted.

INTERVENTION

Interventions for individuals with progressive CNS disorders are influenced by numerous factors, including the examination findings, the patient's goals, financial and human resources, the nature and course of the disease, individual variability throughout the disease course, age at disease onset, disease stage, and the availability of disease modifying agents.

Therapeutic management for individuals with a neurodegenerative disease should occur along a care continuum (Fig. 17-11). The care continuum suggests the disease process has a trajectory that varies and changes over time, as a result of progression and deterioration. Along the continuum, resultant impairments, functional limitations, and disabilities are managed through interventions tailored to the stage of the disease and grounded in evidenced-based research whenever possible. Even though the course of the disease itself cannot be altered, appropriate rehabilitation can help an individual maintain his or her independence and function for as long as possible, within the context of his or her goals and resources, throughout the stages of the disease and in different health care settings (acute care, rehabilitation, outpatient, long-term care, home care, and hospice settings).

AEROBIC EXERCISE

Depending on the disease pathology and stage, an aerobic exercise program may be indicated to address deconditioning, decreased endurance, or fatigue. Four factors should be considered when prescribing aerobic exercise: Frequency, duration, intensity, and mode of exercise (see Chapter 23). For patients with progressive CNS disorders,

frequency and duration will depend on the overall cardiovascular fitness of the individual and any undesirable effects associated with over exercising. Some patients will find shorter periods of exercise more frequently throughout the week to be less fatiguing. Submaximal exercise, usually at 50% to 65% of heart rate reserve, or intermittent exercise with repetitive exercise-rest periods tends to be safer and is therefore recommended. Mode of exercise depends on the ability of the patient. For example, patients with severe lower extremity spasticity will do better with an upper extremity cycle ergometer than with walking or bicycling.

In addition to considering frequency, duration, intensity, and mode of exercise, careful monitoring may be necessary to ensure patient safety. For example, HD, MS AD, and PD can all cause autonomic dysfunction, resulting in orthostatic hypotension, excessive sweating, heat intolerance, and abnormal cardiovascular responses.[276-280] Vital signs; symptoms of exertion, such as dyspnea, excessive fatigue, pallor, and dizziness; and signs and symptoms specific to the disorder should be monitored and documented, at rest and during and after exercise. The Borg Rating of Perceived Exertion (RPE) Scale (see Chapter 23) can also be used to objectively record perceived exertion.

Amyotrophic Lateral Sclerosis. When prescribing exercise for patients with ALS, the PT must consider the possibility of overwork damage or overuse fatigue. Patients should be advised not to carry out any activities to the point of extreme fatigue and should keep track of symptoms of overuse, such as the inability to perform daily activities following exercise because of exhaustion or pain, increased fasciculations, or muscle cramping.

Pinto et al evaluated the effects of exercise in eight patients with ALS and respiratory insufficiency, using bidirectional positive airway pressure (BiPAP) ventilation

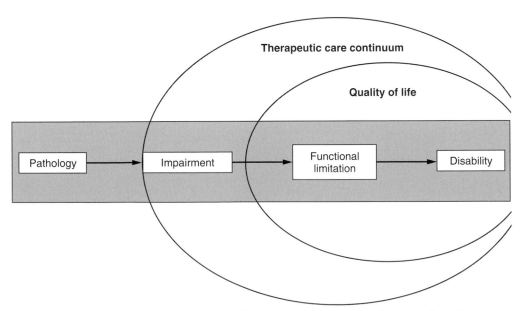

FIG. 17-11 Management for individuals with progressive CNS disorders should occur along a therapeutic care continuum. *Adapted from Jette AM: Phys Ther 74(5):380-386, 1994.*

during exercise.[281] Compared to 12 control patients with ALS who did not exercise, after one year, patients in the exercise group had significantly higher FIM scores, a slower disease course as demonstrated by Spinal Norris score decline and a significant difference in the slope of forced vital capacity decline.

Animal studies using SOD1 transgenic mice, an animal model of ALS, have demonstrated that endurance exercise training at moderate intensity slowed disease progression and may prolong survival in affected animals,[282,283] although high endurance exercise training can shorten survival.[284]

Parkinson's Disease. While several studies have investigated the benefits of general exercise in patients with PD (see section on Strength Training later in this chapter), only a few have specifically assessed the benefits of aerobic conditioning. Bridgewater and colleagues found that 12 weeks of twice weekly aerobic exercise increased cardiorespiratory fitness and habitual activity level and marginally improved mood in a group of 13 people with early PD.[287] No differences were found in severity of PD signs between the control group and the exercise group, but while functional ability decreased in the control group, it remained stable in the exercise group.

A small study of four patients with PD, Hoehn and Yahr Stage 2, who completed a 16-week exercise program of cycling and treadmill walking at 60% to 70% of heart rate reserve found peak VO_2 significantly increased by 26% compared to a control group, suggesting that aerobic exercise may improve cardiovascular conditioning, which can be impaired at all stages of PD.[286]

Multiple Sclerosis. In patients with MS, Uthoff's phenomenon, an adverse reaction to external heat or increased body temperature, can occur with exercise, resulting in extreme fatigue and worsening of symptoms. An ear thermometer can therefore be used to monitor temperature before, during, and after exercise in patients with MS. Precooling with cold water immersion,[287] cooling garments,[288] ice packs, or by the patient consuming iced drinks or having the patient exercise in an air-conditioned room can prevent excessive gains in core temperature with physical work and may allow heat-sensitive individuals with MS to exercise without adverse effects. A randomized controlled study of 84 patients with MS found that wearing a liquid cooling garment (Fig. 17-12) for 1 hour a day for a month resulted in significant improvements in functional abilities as measured by the MS Functional Composite scale.[289] Patients also reported less fatigue during the month of daily cooling. Because core body temperature is lowest in the morning, patients with MS may tolerate exercise better in the morning.

A few studies have examined the effects of aerobic exercise in patients with MS.[139,258,290-292] Petajan and colleagues evaluated the impact of 15 weeks of aerobic training (40 minutes of exercise 3 times per week) on fitness and quality of life in a group of individuals with MS with an EDSS score of less than 6.0.[292] This training program resulted in a 22% increase in VO_2 max, a 48% increase in maximal power output, and significant improvements in body composition and serum triglyceride levels for the exercise group. Depression and anger scores as measured

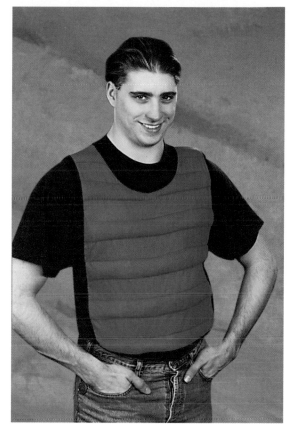

FIG. 17-12 Patient using a cooling vest. *Image of Miracool Cooling Vest courtesy OccuNomix International.*

by the Profile of Mood States (POMS) were reduced at weeks 5 and 10. Furthermore, quality of life as measured by Sickness Impact Profile (SIP) scores improved, with the exercise group having significantly improved physical dimension scores and significant improvements in social interaction, emotional behavior, home management, and recreation and pastime scores.

Alzheimer's Disease and Huntington's Disease. There are limited studies evaluating the effects of aerobic training in patients with AD or HD. One study found that student-led exercise sessions combined with cognitive and social stimulation improved fitness in patients with AD.[293] Several studies have reported benefits of general exercise in these populations (see section on Strength Training).

BALANCE, COORDINATION, AND AGILITY TRAINING

Selection of interventions for retraining balance in individuals with progressive disorders depends on the underlying neural, motor, and sensory impairments that contribute to postural instability and balance problems. In addition, postural control impairments are closely tied to gait abnormalities, so interventions for gait problems may also indirectly or directly affect balance (see section on Gait Intervention). In general, balance interventions should focus on (1) restoring underlying impairments whenever possible, (2) preventing secondary impairments that may affect postural instability, (3) facilitating task-specific sensory and motor strategies necessary for meeting postural control demands, and (4) practicing the maintenance of postural control in a variety of tasks and environments.[294]

Balance training activities in general are progressed from a wide to narrower base of support, from static to dynamic activities, from a low to a high center of gravity, and with increasing degrees of freedom that must be controlled (see Chapter 13). When restoration is not possible, compensatory interventions may be needed to address sensory, visual, vestibular, and motor impairments and promote balance safety. Modifications of the home, work, and community environments and recommendations for assistive and adaptive devices may also be required for balance safety.

Huntington's Disease. For patients with HD, strategies found to be useful in individuals with PD described directly below, such as attentional strategies and avoiding dual-task performance, may be useful.[210] Balance retraining, strengthening of the postural muscles to enhance postural stability, and increasing the base of support of footwear is recommended in the early stage of HD.[216] As the disease progresses, compensatory strategies, such as teaching the patient the Touch-Turn-Sit maneuver are implemented. The Touch-Turn-Sit maneuver involves instructing the patient to touch the chair initially and then turn before sitting down (i.e., a sensory cue attentional strategy). Assistive devices (walker with wheels is preferred) and safety equipment, such as a helmet or elbow and knee protectors, may be recommended. Because cognitive impairments also increase in number and severity as the disease progresses, additional compensatory strategies, such as providing cues, teaching skills using one-step commands, and providing treatment in a quiet, nondistracting environment should also be incorporated into treatment.[216]

Parkinson's Disease. Because balance is often affected in the early stages of PD, balance training should begin early.[295] This training should take place in the environment where the individual's problems are the worst. Patients with PD have difficulty maintaining stability when they do not have sufficient time to prepare for threats to balance. They should therefore be taught to deliberately prepare in advance for forthcoming threats to balance, or to focus their attention on maintaining balance before a task in which equilibrium is challenged.[296] This strategy may allow patients to use intact frontal cortical systems to regulate stability to substitute for impaired basal ganglia mechanisms.[296] Training the patient to step in response to perturbations, with an emphasis on speed and accuracy of the stepping strategy, is also recommended.[297] Balance training may also be enhanced through the use of auditory and visual cueing (Fig. 17-13) (see section on Gait Interventions for more details).[298]

Dancing, particularly ballroom dancing, and karate, both of which incorporate changes in direction, rhythmical movement, rotation, balance, and coordination may be useful in addressing several impairments.[299,300] To address the inability to attend to more than one task at a time patients should be taught to break down complex

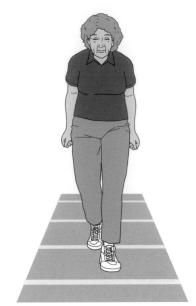

FIG. 17-13 Visual cueing for a patient with Parkinson's disease.

activities into simple tasks and to focus their attention on performing each task separately, and to practice performing two activities at the same time under various practice and context conditions.

In a randomized, single-blind, cross-over study, 16 individuals with PD (Hoehn and Yahr stage 2 or 3) performed a series of 69 repetitive exercises for 1 hour, 3 times per week for 4 weeks.[301] Exercises included ROM, endurance, balance, walking, and fine motor dexterity exercises. Significant improvements on the motor and ADL subsections of the UPDRS were found. However, despite patients being instructed to continue the exercises at home, all measures returned to baseline 6 months after completing the exercise program because the patients resumed a more sedentary lifestyle.

A second randomized controlled trial of 15 individuals with PD compared the effects of 10 weeks of balance and resistance training with the effects of balance training alone.[302] Resistance training consisted of high-intensity resistance exercises of the knee extensors and flexors and ankle plantarflexors, and balance training occurred under altered visual and somatosensory conditions. Both groups improved in their ability to respond to reduced or altered visual and somatosensory orientation cues, and this effect was larger in the combined activity group. Both groups could balance longer before falling and muscle strength increased marginally in the balance group and significantly in the combined group. These effects persisted for at least 4 weeks.[302]

Multiple Sclerosis. In MS, sensory and vestibular disorders, ataxia, dysmetria, muscle weakness, spasticity, and tremor may cause balance impairments and incoordination. Where possible, interventions should first be directed toward the cause of these specific problems and then toward improving postural stability and accuracy of upper and lower extremity movements through balance and coordination training during functional activities. For example, if the patient has weak trunk muscles, strengthening exercises should be prescribed to increase strength and stability before coordination and balance problems are addressed.

Light weights (cuff weights, weight belt, weighted jacket) and weighted ambulation devices, which provide proprioceptive loading and can stabilize movements, are sometimes used clinically to control the incoordination of ataxic and dysmetric movements in patients with MS. However, research studies have not consistently found these interventions to be beneficial.[303-306] Frenkel's exercises, a series of exercises that emphasize normal daily activates, increase in difficulty and are performed in four positions: Lying, sitting, standing, and walking,[307] have also been suggested as an intervention for MS-related ataxia and dysmetria, although there are no published studies examining these exercises. Incoordination caused by poor proximal joint control may be addressed by proprioceptive neuromuscular facilitation (PNF) techniques including rhythmic stabilization, alternating isometrics and slow reversal hold, and by activities that emphasize weight-bearing activities through proximal joints (e.g., 4-point kneeling).

Frenkel's exercises

Exercises while lying *Starting position:* Lie on bed or couch with a smooth surface along which the feet may be moved easily. Your head should be raised on a pillow so that you can watch every movement.
1. Bend one leg at the hip and knee sliding your heel along the bed. Straighten the hip and knee to return to the starting position. Repeat with the other leg.
2. Bend one leg at the hip and knee as in #1. Then slide the same leg out to the side leaving your heel on the bed. Slide your leg back to the center and straighten your hip and knee to return to the starting position. Repeat with the other leg.
3. Bend one leg at the hip and knee with the heel raised from the bed. Straighten your leg to return to the starting position. Repeat with the other leg.
4. Bend and straighten one leg at the hip and knee sliding your heel along the bed stopping at any point of command. Repeat with the other leg.
5. Bend the hip and knee of one leg and place the heel on the opposite knee. Then slide your heel down the shin to the ankle and back up to the knee. Return to starting position and repeat with the other leg.
6. Bend both hips and knees sliding heels on the bed keeping your ankles together. Straighten both legs to return to starting position.
7. Bend one leg at the hip and knee while straightening the other in a bicycling motion.

Exercises while sitting *Starting position:* Sit on a chair with feet flat on the floor.
1. Mark time, raising just the heel. Then, mark time lifting the entire foot and placing the foot firmly on the floor on a traced foot print.
2. Make two cross marks on the floor with chalk. Alternately glide the foot over the marked cross: forward, backward, left and right.
3. Rise from the chair and sit again to a counted cadence. At one, bend knees and draw feet under the chair; at two, bend trunk forward; at three, rise by straightening the hips and knees and then the trunk. Reverse the process to sit down.

Exercises while standing and walking
Starting position: Stand erect with feet 4-6 inches apart.
1. Walk sideways beginning with half steps to the right. Perform this exercise in a counted cadence: At one, shift the weight to the left foot; at two, place the right foot 12 inches to the right; at three, shift the weight to the right foot; at four, bring the left foot over to the right foot. Repeat exercise with half steps to the left. The size of the step taken to right or left my be varied.
2. Walk forward between two parallel lines 14 inches apart placing the right foot just inside the right line and the left foot just inside the left line. Emphasize correct placement. Rest after 10 steps.
3. Walk forward placing each foot on a footprint traced on the floor. Footprints should be parallel and 2 inches from a center line. Practice with quarter steps, half steps, three-quarter steps and full steps.
4. Turn to the right in a counted cadence. At one, raise the right toe and rotate the right foot outward, pivoting on the heel; at two, raise the left heel and pivot the left leg inward on the toes; at three, completing the full turn, and then repeat to the left.
5. Walk up and down the stairs one step at a time. Place the right foot on one step and bring the left up beside it. Later practice walking up the stairs placing one foot on each step. At first use the railing, then as balance improves, do not use the railing.

Individually tailored occupational and physical therapy consisting of (1) promoting normal posture and movement with weight bearing, joint approximation, co-contraction, and compression; (2) providing equipment and ADL advice; (3) proximal stabilization and equilibrium reaction exercises; and (4) use of weighed items was found to significantly improve the ability and speed of performance for all items of the modified Northwick Park ADL Index,[308] except for stair climbing ability, in patients with MS and ataxia of the upper limb and trunk.[309]

A small randomized controlled trial found that a 10-week program of Awareness Through Movement classes reduced falls by 34% from baseline and increased scores on the activities balance confidence (ABC) scale in subjects with MS.[310] Another small study with 4 patients with MS found that 12 weeks of a balance training on the Pro Balance Master 2 days per week improved postural control and dynamic balance as measured by the Limits of

Stability (LOS) test and the four condition Sensory Organization Test (SOT).[311] The subjects also reported they were more confident performing ADLs and were more active than before the intervention.

STRENGTH TRAINING

Alzheimer's Disease. Dementia is commonly associated with reduced activity which is thought to contribute to weakness as well as gait abnormalities and falls. Therefore exercise programs are often recommended to minimize the functional impact of any type of dementia including AD.

Moderate intensity lower extremity strengthening exercise 2-3 times per week was found in one study to increase gait speed but not strength in patients with dementia,[312] whereas in another study using similar exercises, patients demonstrated improvements in quadriceps strength, handgrip strength, sit-to-stand time, usual gait time, as well as fast gait time.[313] An individualized exercise program, which was most often walking, also improved nutritional status and MMSE scores and reduced the number of behavioral problems in patients with moderate to severe AD, while not increasing caregiver burden.[314] These studies suggest that exercise, including strengthening exercises, can reduce impairments and improve functional performance in patients with AD.

Amyotrophic Lateral Sclerosis. The benefit of muscle strength training in patients with ALS is controversial and there is a concern that strength training may cause muscle damage in these patients. However, one randomized controlled trial found that patients with ALS can derive short-term benefits from muscle strengthening exercises.[315] In this trial, 14 patients participated in a 3-month daily program of individualized, moderate intensity, endurance type exercises for the trunk and limbs. At 3 months, patients who participated in this program had less decline in function (measured by the ALS functional rating scale), and less spasticity (measured on the Modified Ashworth scale) but similar muscle strength, fatigue severity, pain, and quality of life (SF-36) as patients with ALS who did not participate in the program. At 6 months, there were no significant differences between the groups and at 9 and 12 months, there were too few patients still alive for statistical evaluation of the results. The authors concluded that moderate intensity exercise can have short-term benefits for patients with ALS.[315]

Huntington's Disease. Relatively few studies have examined the effects of any type of physical therapy for people with HD. Peacock and Imbriglio have documented the benefits of physical therapy based on their extensive experience working with people with HD. In an informal study, Peacock reported improvements in flexibility, coordination and balance following a 12-week exercise class (once a week) that included exercises designed for relaxation, flexibility, coordination, balance, breath control and strength.[316] In an overview article, Imbriglio provided a framework for physical therapy evaluation and intervention for patients with HD with aims of maximizing independence while minimizing risk.[317] Both authors stressed the importance of routine exercises including strengthening, flexibility and endurance training.

Quinn and Rao reported on a case study of a patient with midstage HD, who was experiencing falls and impaired balance control.[224] Intervention consisted of a home exercise program that was instructed in person and by videotape (Table 17-4) 5 days per week. The patient consistently performed the exercises with the assistance of a home health aide, and at 14 weeks, demonstrated improvements in disability (SF-36), balance (Berg Balance Scale), gait speed, and UHDRS motor score, and the patient did not fall at all during the 14-week intervention.

These reports provide preliminary evidence to support the use of physical therapy interventions, in particular exercise involving strengthening and balance training, to improve function in patients with HD.

Parkinson's Disease. Strength training has been found to be particularly beneficial for patients with PD. A study with 14 patients with mild to moderate PD and 6 age-matched controls, found that 8 weeks of resistance training twice a week focusing on lower extremity strengthening produced significant increases in strength in both groups and improved stride length, walking velocity, and postural angles in the patients with PD.[318] Intensive exercise training over 14 weeks was also found to

TABLE 17-4	Home Exercise Program
Exercise Type	**Specific Exercise**
Warm-up: *Each exercise performed 10 times*	Deep breathing Neck flexion, extension, rotation Arm circles forward and backward Squatting Reaching up to "sky," alternating arms Reaching to each side, crossing arms across body Reach to floor, keeping knees slightly bent
Leg exercises (standing): *Each exercise performed 10-15 times*	Knee lifts both legs* Kicks to front both legs* Squats* Walk forwards and back Walk to side (side step) Jump in place*

Arm exercises (standing): *Each exercise performed 10-15 times both arms*	Using 2 lb weights, or heavy cans:
	  Overhead press
	  Large arm circles
	  Biceps curls
	Thera-Band exercises
	  Horizontal abduction
	  Shoulder flexion/extension

Floor exercises: Stretching and strengthening	Hamstring stretch (hold 30 seconds × 3 each leg) Inner thigh stretch (hold 30 seconds × 3) Sit ups (20 times) Straight leg raises (15 each leg) Prone press ups (10 times) Push ups (15 times) Cat camel
Cool down	Repeat warm-up

*Participants are instructed to hold onto a chair for support if needed.

improve motor disability, mood, and well being in patients with mild to moderate PD.[319]

Strengthening exercises can also improve impairments in areas other than strength, flexibility and coordination. For example, a 10-week program of therapeutic exercise and relaxation for patients with PD (Hoehn and Yahr stage 2-3) improved spinal flexibility and performance on the Functional Reach test[320] (see Fig. 13-18) and an 8-week general exercise program, also for patients at Hoehn and Yahr stage 2-3, improved coordination of sequential movements and improved postural control during a box lifting task.[321] Two studies have demonstrated that a general program of physical therapy, which may include strengthening and stretching exercises, balance and gait activities, recreational games, and relaxation and ADL training, can improve scores on the UPDRS (total and ADL and motor sections), the Self-Assessment PD Disability Scale, a 10-minute walk test (10MWT), the SIP mobility measure, and the Zung scale for depression in patients with all stages of PD.[322,323]

Multiple Sclerosis. Several studies show that strengthening exercises and general physical therapy interventions help patients with varying stages of MS.[324-329] It appears that resistance training of the lower extremities at submaximal levels (e.g., 5% to 50% of maximum voluntary contraction), is safe for patients with MS, as long as fatigue is appropriately monitored. Although research suggests that strengthening improves various impairments, such as strength[325,327] and fatigue,[329] and functional abilities, such as walking,[324,326] in patients with MS, improvements in disability have only been demonstrated when strengthening exercises are components of a more comprehensive rehabilitation program.[330,331]

Aquatic exercise, in which patients perform strengthening and endurance exercises in a pool, has been found to improve lower extremity fatigue and strength[332] and health-related quality of life in patients with MS.[333] Ideally, aquatic exercise should be performed in cooler water (less than 85° F), although one case study demonstrated benefits without excessive fatigue or heat sensitivity in a pool at 94° F.[334]

Several studies have also demonstrated that respiratory muscle training produces significant improvements in measures of respiratory function (maximal expiratory pressure or maximal inspiratory pressure) in individuals in the middle and late stages of MS.[334-336]

GAIT AND LOCOMOTION TRAINING

Gait impairments are common in individuals with progressive CNS disorders and many patients hope that physical therapy interventions will improve their walking ability (speed, coordination, balance, and safety) or allow them to continue walking for as long as possible. Gait training should focus on ameliorating or compensating for impairments which most contribute to functional gait limitations to help patients reach their ambulation goals.

Patients with progressive CNS disorders can benefit from task specific gait training, including extended practice of walking. In addition, for best results, since the practice environment can influence carryover, walking practice should occur in an environment that is similar to

the patient's current life situation (e.g., including obstacles or timing constraints). Although limited research supports specific approaches to gait training in this population, several models for task-based intervention have been developed.[337] Box 17-1 outlines a plan for task-based intervention to enhance skill learning that can be applied to gait training for individuals with progressive CNS disorders. For patients with cognitive impairments, practice with much contextual interference (random practice) and extensive verbal feedback should be avoided as this may interfere with task performance.[295]

Treadmill Training. Within the past 10 years, many studies have examined the effects of treadmill gait training in patients with CNS disorders. This work began primarily in patients with stroke and spinal cord injury but is now continuing in patients with PD and MS.

BOX 17-1	Clinical Implications: Task-Based Intervention to Enhance Skill Learning

The steps describe the components to consider before task practice is initiated. Practice can incorporate methods to structure practice, set up the environment, or provide augmentative input to the learner before, during, and after performance of the task.

Step 1: Determine the goal and define the task to be learned:
- Consider type of task: serial, discrete, or continuous
- Analyze environmental conditions by identifying regulatory features of the environment and recognizing the task as closed or open.

Step 2: Determine level of skill learning.
- Cognitive, associative, or automatic stage of learning
- Explicit versus implicit processes

Step 3: Choose method of intervention based on task, environment, and performer characteristics.

Task Level—Structuring Practice
- Task-specific practice
- Amount of practice
- Schedule of practice
  - Massed versus distributed practice
  - Contextual interference-random versus blocked practice
- Transfer of training
  - Whole versus part practice

Environment Level—Structuring the Environment
- Closed versus open environment
- Consider what is available

Performer Level—Before, During, and After Performance
- Before task performance
  - Demonstration and modeling
  - Mental practice and imagery
- During task performance-concurrent feedback
  - Manual assistance and manual guidance (manual facilitation, physical assistance, braces, assistive devices)
  - Verbal information
- After task performance-terminal feedback
  - Knowledge of results (KR)
  - Knowledge of performance (KP)

Miyai and colleagues conducted two studies testing the effectiveness of body weight–supported treadmill training (BWSTT) for individuals with PD. In the first study, 10 individuals with midstage PD (Hoehn and Yahr stage 2.5-3.0) were randomized into 2 groups of 5 patients.[338] Both groups received 4 weeks BWSTT, with up to 20% of their body weight supported, and 4 weeks of typical physical therapy, but the groups received the interventions in reverse order. Significant improvements in UPDRS scores, ambulation speed, and number of steps were found immediately after the BWSTT sessions compared to typical physical therapy (Fig. 17-14).

The second study by these authors was a randomized controlled trial including 24 patients with PD.[339] Patients in one group received BWSTT (with up to 20% body weight support), whereas patients in the other group received conventional physical therapy that consisted of general conditioning, ROM, ADL, and gait training. Both groups practiced walking for 45 minutes 3 days per week for 1 month. Twenty patients completed the study and were included in the final analysis. The BWSTT group had significantly faster ambulation speed than the conventional PT group at 1 month and took longer steps when evaluated 1, 2, 3, and 4 months after the intervention. The authors concluded that treadmill training specifically improved short-step gait in patients with PD.

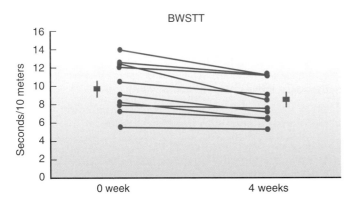

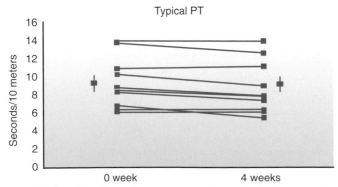

FIG. 17-14 Significant improvements in ambulation speed were found immediately after the body weight–supported treadmill training *(BWSTT)* sessions compared to typical physical therapy *(PT)*. From Miyai I, Fujimoto Y, Ueda Y, et al: *Arch Phys Med Rehabil 81(7):849-852, 2000.*

A later study with 17 patients with PD (Hoehn and Yahr stages 1-3) evaluated the effects of regular unsupported treadmill training and the effects of speed of training on walking performance in patients with PD.[340] The patients were randomly assigned to one of four single-session interventions: Structured speed-dependent treadmill training (STT); limited progressive treadmill training; conventional gait training; and a control intervention. Significantly greater improvements occurred in all basic gait parameters following the two treadmill interventions than with conventional gait training or the control intervention, and there were no significant differences between any gait parameters for the two types of treadmill training. The authors concluded that even a single-session of treadmill training can improve many of the main gait impairments in PD, at least in the short-term. They did not examine the long-term effects of this single session of training.

SENSORY CUEING

Sensory cueing involves the use of augmented sensory information, typically in the form of external visual,[341] auditory, or manual cueing, to improve task performance. Visual or auditory sensory cueing is commonly used in patients with PD to facilitate movement and overcome episodes of freezing and akinesia during gait. This approach is thought to work by using frontal pathways that respond to visual or auditory input to bypass damaged basal ganglia structures that are usually involved in self-initiating movement.[342] Use of visual cues, such as brightly colored objects or lines at consistent intervals along a walkway, during a walking task has been shown to improve walking performance (stride length and step length) in patients with PD[196,197,341,343] (see Fig. 17-13). Auditory cues, such as a series of tones or a metronome, to which a patient can entrain the tempo of their walking have also been found to improve gait cadence,[198,199,343] velocity, and stride length[198,199] in patients with PD. Synchronizing gait to rhythmic beats has also been shown to help modulate gait speed in people with HD.[344] Although training effects may not be long lasting when training is brief,[197] a recent case report of a patient who performed visually cued gait training for 30 minutes, 3 times per week for 4 weeks, found that the patient increased her gait speed and stride length directly after completing the training and that this effect was retained 1 month after the training was discontinued.[345]

Although, in general, sensory cueing improves parameters of gait performance, one study found that while auditory and cutaneous cueing improved gait by decreasing double limb support time and increasing center or pressure displacement and velocity in patients with PD, it also had the adverse effects of reducing the displacement and velocity of the swing limb and sacrum.[346] The authors of this study suggest that sensory cueing that focuses the patient on walking faster may interfere with a patient's walking pattern.

RELAXATION

Although there are no published studies examining the effects of relaxation on spasticity and rigidity, clinical observations demonstrate that slow, rhythmic rotational movements through small ranges of movement can temporarily reduce hypertonicity. For example, lower trunk rotation in hook or sidelying can decrease tone in patients with ALS or MS with increased lower extremity extensor muscle tone.

Schenkman et al also recommend that relaxation be used initially in a treatment session to decrease rigidity and increase flexibility in patients with PD.[347] The patient should focus on differentiating between body segments (e.g., thorax on pelvis, shoulder complex on thorax) when performing slow, rhythmic rotational movements. Deep breathing during rotational movements may further enhance relaxation.[347]

PNF, especially the technique of contract-relax, and biofeedback may also promote relaxation. In addition, a generalized decrease in muscle tone and overall increased well being may be achieved through cognitive relaxation techniques such as Jacobsen's progressive relaxation exercises.[348] Because stress can induce fatigue and anxiety, effective recognition and management of stress are also important in an overall rehabilitation program.

FUNCTIONAL AND TASK-SPECIFIC TRAINING

Functional training is often essential for patients with progressive CNS disorders. Functional training refers to strategies to improve the ability to perform daily functional tasks, such as dressing, bathing, and climbing stairs, as well as training in the use of devices and equipment (see section on Orthotic, Protective, and Supportive Devices), training in IADLs (using the phone, for example), and in injury prevention or reduction. Task-specific training, such as working on the speed of reaching, may be particularly helpful for patients with movement disorders, such as those caused by PD, because motor disturbances are typically context-dependent, and occur during complex, well-learned tasks such as walking and reaching.[295,349] A task-based model of intervention (see section on Gait Training) can enhance skill learning through identification of tasks to be learned, followed by appropriately sequenced practice of these tasks within a structured environment and with augmented information before, during, and after task performance[202,337] (see Box 17-1).

PRESCRIPTION, APPLICATION, AND FABRICATION OF DEVICES AND EQUIPMENT

Patients with progressive CNS disorders frequently benefit from use of assistive and adaptive devices, with changing needs as their condition progresses (see section on Assistive and Adaptive Devices). Keep in mind that while some equipment, such as a cane or a walker, is usually quickly and readily available, customized equipment, such as a customized wheelchair, may take many months to be made, by which time a patient's needs may have changed. One should therefore try to anticipate patient's needs and order more complex devices in advance.

VENTILATORY SUPPORT AND AIRWAY CLEARANCE TECHNIQUES

Respiratory problems may develop at any stage of a progressive CNS disorder but are more common in the late-middle and late stages as respiratory muscle weakness increases (with ALS and MS) and/or as mobility becomes more and more limited (in AD, ALS, MS, HD and PD). Various interventions, including ventilatory support, deep breathing exercises, body positioning to optimize secretion drainage and ventilation-perfusion matching, and other airway clearance techniques may help alleviate functional limitations caused by respiratory impairments (see Chapters 24 and 26 for further details).

Amyotrophic Lateral Sclerosis. Respiratory failure is common in the late stage of ALS. Health care professionals should therefore discuss options for ventilatory support with all patients with ALS early on, well before the development of respiratory insufficiency.[350] Many patients with ALS will choose to use some type of assisted ventilation to prolong life and hopefully improve quality of life. Therefore it is highly likely the physical therapist will treat an individual with ALS who is mechanically ventilated. Symptoms of respiratory difficulties typically occur in ALS when forced vital capacity (FVC) reaches about 50% of the predicted value, or when there is a rapid decline in FVC over a short period of time.[351] Even in the absence of symptoms, when the FVC reaches 50% of predicted, ventilatory support will likely be considered.

Ventilatory support may be provided using noninvasive or invasive approaches. Noninvasive ventilatory support is usually accomplished with bi-level positive airway pressure (BiPAP). BiPAP is a type of pressure-cycled ventilator in which inspiratory and expiratory pressure can be set independently. Patients with ALS usually use a higher inspiratory pressure and a lower expiratory pressure to particularly support the inspiratory muscles. BiPAP may decrease symptoms while it is being used and because it allows the muscles to rest while it is on, may also reduce muscle fatigue and thus help even between periods of use. Patients usually initially use the device only at night while asleep and intermittently during the day and then for a greater proportion of the day as the condition progresses.

Permanent invasive ventilatory support is chosen by some, but not most, patients with ALS.[352] Although this intervention can prolong survival, patient satisfaction with this is poorer than with noninvasive ventilation.[353] This is often because use of invasive ventilatory support generally prevents the patient from speaking and because by the time the patient requires invasive ventilatory support, their muscles are so weak that they cannot participate in other activities that would enhance quality of life.[354] Noninvasive ventilation is preferred by most patients and has been shown to improve symptoms of hypoventilation,[355,356] and prolong life in patients with ALS by several months.[357] As ALS progresses, the patient is likely to become completely dependent on ventilatory support and may eventually not be able to communicate at all. Therefore it is essential that the patient, family/caregiver, and physician agree, before this point, which circumstances will trigger withdrawal of ventilatory support.[358,359]

Caregivers of patients with expiratory muscle weakness should be taught how to assist the patient with coughing, and a suction machine should be made available for those patients who have difficulty clearing secretions. Mechanical insufflation-exsufflation devices to mechanically assist coughing can help patients with ALS generate enough expiratory flow for airway clearance.[360-362] Educating care-givers regarding the signs of aspiration and choking and the application of the Heimlich maneuver may also help because many patients with ALS, as well as other progressive CNS disorders, have difficulty with swallowing.

INTEGUMENTARY REPAIR AND PROTECTIVE TECHNIQUES

Integumentary protection is indicated for patients who have very limited ability to move, which is common in the late stages of most progressive CNS disorders and for patients who have an increased risk of bruising and fractures because of involuntary movements, such as those with HD. Patients may benefit from pressure relief interventions, including positioning, turning, and appropriate support surfaces (see Chapter 28) and if mobile, from protective padding on the elbows, forearms, knees and shins. For added safety in the ambulatory patient with poor movement control, a helmet, hip protectors, and other body padding, may be used to prevent more serious injuries, including fractures and head injury.

CASE STUDY 17-1

EARLY-MID STAGE MULTIPLE SCLEROSIS

Examination
Patient History

RC is a 45-year-old woman who was diagnosed with MS 5 years ago. She has had three relapses over the last five years. During each episode her legs became weak and she had visual problems. After each episode, she recovered most but not all of her strength. Her most recent episode was 2 months prior to this evaluation. RC requested physical therapy to address balance difficulties, weakness, and fatigue that have worsened over the past few months.

RC requires assistance for heavy lifting, putting away heavy groceries and other items, and activities that require her to walk for extended distances ($>\frac{1}{4}$ mile). She is independent with all ADLs, but it takes her longer to get dressed and finish her grooming routine because of fatigue and leg weakness (approximately 30 minutes after showering). She stopped driving about 6 months prior to this evaluation. She expressed frustration about her progressive loss of independence and her inability to completely care for her family. She had enjoyed playing tennis and running until about 1 year ago, when she found these activities too difficult because of her balance problems. RC reports occasionally being depressed and frustrated with the lack of available interventions for MS.

RC has no other significant past medical history. She was hospitalized for the birth of her 3 children, one by cesarean section. Her current medications are glatiramer acetate (Copaxone), a disease-modifying agent, and baclofen, to address hamstring spasticity. She had been taking both of these drugs for 18 months.

Tests and Measures
Musculoskeletal

Posture Stands with a wide base of support and slightly forward head.

TABLE 17-5	Muscle Performance of Patient in Case Study 17-1	
Strength (MMT)	**Left**	**Right**
Hip flexion	4/5	4/5
Hip extension	4/5	4/5
Hip abduction	4/5	4/5
Hip adduction	3/5	3/5
Knee extension	3/5	4/5
Knee flexion	4/5	4/5
Ankle dorsiflexion	2/5	3/5
Ankle plantarflexion	3/5	4/5

Range of Motion Passive ROM hip abduction left 0-35 degrees, right 0-40 degrees, ankle dorsiflexion left 0 degrees, right 0-5 degrees, all others within normal limits (WNL).

Muscle Performance See Table 17-5.

Neuromuscular

Arousal, Attention, and Cognition RC was conversant and able to understand multi-step directions. She had some limitations in short term recall (2/4 items correct). RC reported that she had been having problems with short-term memory (e.g., what she ate for breakfast) but not with long-term memory.

Pain No reports of pain.

Cranial Nerve Integrity RC reports diplopia, particularly when looking at close objects. She had mild lateral nystagmus on the right more than the left and slight ptosis bilaterally. Smooth tracking was intact in all 4 quadrants.

Reflex Integrity Deep tendon reflexes: 2/4 in all extremities except for the following: Bilateral hamstrings 3/4; left Achilles 4/4 with multibeat clonus, right Achilles 3/4.

Muscle Tone Moderate spasticity in both lower extremities rated 2/4 on the Modified Ashworth Scale in both hamstrings, adductors, and calf muscles.

Sensory Integrity Impaired sensation to light touch (5/8 correct responses) and pinprick (4/8 correct responses) below the knees bilaterally. Proprioception impaired in both ankles (right 4/8 correct responses, left 2/8 correct responses) and knees (right 4/8 correct responses, left 0/8 correct responses).

Cardiovascular/Pulmonary

Aerobic Capacity and Endurance 6MWT: Distance walked: 850 ft. Surface: Outdoor/level/pavement. Borg RPE during the test: 5 (RC was requested to report when fatigue level was greater than 6 at any point during the test, and a rest was taken. RC took 3 rests during the entire test). After test: HR 80 bpm, BP 142/70 mmHg, RR 18 bpm.

Fatigue: RC reported fatigue as averaging 3/7 on the Fatigue Severity scale (scale 1-7, 7 = highest severity). RC reports that her fatigue has worsened since her most recent exacerbation 2 months ago.

Integumentary

Integumentary Integrity Intact, no erythema or skin breakdown.

Function

Gait, Locomotion, and Balance RC walked independently without an assistive device. She could ascend and descend the 12 stairs she had at home with a step over step gait, while holding the railing, in 16 seconds. She lost her balance twice when she tried to manage the stairs without holding the railing and caught herself by holding onto the railing. RC reported that she only carried very small items in one hand up and down the stairs because of fear of falling or dropping items.

Gait: RC had a slight steppage gait on the left, likely to compensate for the profound left DF weakness. She also had a wide-based gait and decreased arm swing.

Balance: Sitting: RC could sit erect on the edge of the bed for 10 minutes without UE support but could not do this for longer due to self-reported fatigue. Standing: RC could stand independently for up to 5 minutes, limited by self-reported fatigue. She could reach for objects within about 2 inches from arm's length in all directions and could squat to the floor to retrieve a 2 lb object without loss of balance.

Berg Balance Scale: 40/56. Most difficulty standing with eyes closed, turning 360 degrees, placing alternate foot on step, standing in tandem, and standing on one foot.

Self Care and Home Management *Bed mobility:* RC had no difficulty getting in and out of bed at home. She could roll independently to both sides and move from supine to sitting on a mat table, although she moved her legs off the table slowly when coming to sit.

Transfers: RC could move from sitting to standing independently, using both arms to assist with push off.

Dressing/bathing: RC dresses and bathes independently, but it takes her at least 15 minutes to get dressed and, although she has not fallen, she is worried about falling while in the shower.

Disability: EDSS rating for individuals with MS score = 3.5, indicating moderate disability.

Evaluation, Diagnosis, and Prognosis

RC exhibits limitations in ambulation and standing balance which affect her quality of life and limit her independence in daily life responsibilities. These functional limitations are a result of lower extremity weakness, spasticity, and impaired postural control. RC's physical therapy diagnosis is preferred practice pattern 5E: Impaired motor function and sensory integrity associated with progressive disorders of the CNS. RC's prognosis is positively affected by her young age, her healthy lifestyle before diagnosis, and her use of a disease-modifying medication (glatiramer acetate).

Goals

The goals of intervention are focused on secondary and tertiary prevention and on reducing current disability.

1. RC will walk 1200 feet in 6 minutes, with Borg RPE < 3.
2. RC will be able to ascend/descend 12 stairs while carrying an item in both hands without loss of balance for 3/3 trials.
3. RC will know fatigue management strategies to minimize her fatigue throughout the day.
4. Hip abduction passive ROM will increase to 0-45 degrees bilaterally.

Intervention

RC received physical therapy 2 times per week for 8 weeks and received the following interventions:

- Instruction in energy conservation techniques and fatigue management.
- Strengthening exercises: Isokinetic strengthening of the hamstring and quadriceps muscle groups. Hip strengthening exercises while lying on a mat using 1 lb weights.
- Cardiovascular training (RC was trained to monitor fatigue) on a treadmill, stationary bicycle, and elliptical trainer to improve cardiovascular endurance.
- AFO for the left ankle to compensate for ankle dorsiflexion weakness and improve foot clearance during ambulation and prevent steppage gait.
- Gait training with a straight cane for long distance ambulation.
- Recommendations for installing grab bars and nonslip matting in RC's shower.
- Instruction in an ongoing daily exercise routine including: Lower extremity stretching and strengthening; coordination activities (Frenkel's exercises); additional balance exercises including practice of standing with eyes closed, turning 360 degrees, placing alternate foot on step, standing in tandem, and standing on one foot; aerobic exercise to be performed only on days RC felt fatigue was low (ideally at least 3 times per week).
- Referral to a rehabilitation psychologist who specializes in depression and coping with disease exacerbations.

Outcomes

Following 8 weeks of physical therapy intervention, the following outcomes were achieved:

1. 6MWT: Distance walked 1300 feet, Borg RPE 3 (with 2 rests); post test: HR 86 bpm, BP 140/80, RR 18 bpm (Goal 1 achieved).
2. Goals 2 and 3 achieved.
3. Hip abduction passive ROM 0-45 degrees right, 0-40 degrees left. (Goal 4 partially achieved.)
4. Strength (MMT): Ankle dorsiflexion left 3/5, right 4/5; knee flexion and extension 4/5 bilaterally.
5. Fatigue severity scale: 1/7. RC reports being able to manage fatigue more effectively throughout the day.
6. Berg Balance Scale: 46/58; with improvements in single leg stance, tandem stance, and standing with eyes closed.
7. RC was independent in a home exercise program. She walked 3 times per week with her husband in the evenings and weekends. RC paid for PT herself 1 time per week to assist with balance training and strengthening exercises.

Please see the CD that accompanies this book for case studies describing the examination, evaluation, and interventions for a patient with Huntington's disease midstage and a patient with middle-late stage Parkinson's disease.

CHAPTER SUMMARY

Patients with progressive CNS disorders present with a variety of impairments and functional limitations. There is currently no cure for any of the disorders presented here, although for some there are medications that alter symptoms or the course of the disease. All of these disorders progress over time, ultimately leading to disability and change in a patient's quality of life. And, all of these disorders involve the neurological system, often causing an array of cognitive and emotional changes that can compound the devastating effects on the motor and sensory systems.

Therapists need to keep in mind that these disorders do progress and that intervention should therefore address both current and expected future needs. Appropriate rehabilitation intervention can improve quality of life, functional abilities and, possibly, disease progression. While we wait for a cure, therapists can help patients maintain functional independence and optimize quality of life.

ADDITIONAL RESOURCES

Useful Forms

ALS Functional Rating Scale-Revised (ALSFRS-R)
Berg Balance Scale (BBS)
Dynamic Gait Index (DGI)
Expanded Disability Status Scale (EDSS)
Global Deterioration Scale for Assessment of Primary Degenerative Dementia (GDS)
Hoehn and Yahr Staging of Parkinson's Disease
Mini-Mental Status Examination (MMSE)
Modified Fatigue Impact Scale (MFIS)
Total Functional Capacity (TFC) Scale
Unified Parkinson's Disease Rating Scale (UPDRS)

Web Sites

Alzheimer's Association: www.alz.org
Alzheimer's Disease Education and Referral Center: www.alzheimers.org/adear
American Parkinson's Disease Association: www.parkinsonsapda.org/
Amyotrophic Lateral Sclerosis Association: www.alsa.org
National Institute of Neurological Disorders and Stroke: www.ninds.nih.gov/index.htm
National Parkinson Foundation Inc.: www.parkinson.org
Parkinson's Disease Foundation: www.parkinsons-foundation.org/
Worldwide Education and Awareness for Movement Disorders (WEMOVE): www.wemove.org/

GLOSSARY

Akinesia: Lack of movement.
Ataxia: Uncoordinated movement.
Atrophy: Wasting or loss of muscle tissue resulting from disease or lack of use.
Blepharospasm: Spasmodic contraction of the eyelid muscles.
Bradykinesia: Slowed speed and amplitude of movement.
Clonus: Alternate muscular contraction and relaxation in rapid succession.
Cog-wheel rigidity: Jerky resistance, where tremor is superimposed on rigidity.
Diplopia: Double vision.
Dysarthria: Impaired speech.
Dysesthesia: Stabbing, aching, or burning sensation.
Dyskinesia: Extraneous movement.
Dysphagia: Impaired chewing or swallowing.
Dyspnea: Shortness of breath.
Fasciculations: Involuntary contraction, or twitching, of groups of muscle fibers.
Festinating gait: A gait pattern seen in patients with PD, characterized by increased speed, shortened stride, and increased stepping velocity.

Flaccid bulbar palsy: Degeneration of the LMNs of the bulbar muscles.
Flaccidity: Loss of muscle tone.
Freezing: A sudden transient inability to move.
Hypertonicity: Increase in muscle tone.
Hypokinesia: Abnormally decreased motor function or activity.
Hypomimia: Loss of facial expression or masked face.
Hypophonia: Decreased voice volume.
Lead-pipe rigidity: A uniform increased resistance to passive stretch.
Lhermitte's sign: A sudden electric-like sensation radiating down the spine or extremities that usually occurs with neck flexion; a sign of posterior column pathology.
Motor neuron disease: A heterogeneous spectrum of inherited and sporadic clinical disorders of the upper motor neurons, lower motor neurons or both.
Myoclonus: A sudden, very brief, shock-like involuntary movement caused by muscular contractions or loss of normal inhibitory influences.
Nystagmus: Rapid involuntary oscillations of the eye.
Ophthalmoplegia: Ocular paralysis.
Optic neuritis: Inflammation of the optic nerve causing altered visual acuity, blurring, partial or total loss of vision in one eye.
Orthopnea: Shortness of breath in supine.
Oscillopsia: Continuous, involuntary, and chaotic eye movements that result in a visual disturbance in which objects appear to be jumping or bouncing.
Pseudobulbar affect: Spontaneous crying or laughter or other emotional expressions that occurs without emotional triggers.
Rigidity: Non-velocity–dependent resistance to passive movement.
Scanning speech: Speech in which each word or syllable is emphasized. There is a pause after every syllable and the syllables are pronounced slowly, creating a particular rhythm and cadence.
Sialorrhea: Excessive saliva; drooling.
Spastic bulbar palsy: Degeneration of the UMNs of the bulbar muscles.
Spasticity: Velocity dependent resistance to passive movement.
Trigeminal neuralgia: Short periods of stabbing facial pain that is triggered by tactile stimulation; caused by demyelination of the sensory division of the trigeminal nerve.

References

1. Gorelick PB, Mangone C, Bozzola F: Epidemiology of vascular dementia. In Gorelick PB (ed): *Atlas of Cerebrovascular Disease*, Chicago, 1996, Churchill-Livingstone.
2. Small GW, Rabins PV, Barry PP, et al: Diagnosis and treatment of Alzheimer's disease and related disorders. Consensus statement of the American Association of Geriatric Psychiatry, the Alzheimer's Association and the American Geriatrics Society, *JAMA* 278(16):1363-1371, 1997.
3. Jorm AF, Korten AE, Henderson AS: The prevalence of dementia: A quantitative integration of the literature, *Acta Psychiatr Scand* 76:465-479, 1987.
4. Arnold SE, Hyman BT, Flory J, et al: The topographical and neuroanatomical distribution of neurofibrillary tangles and neuritic plaques in the cerebral cortex of patients with Alzheimer's disease, *Cereb Cortex* 1:103-116, 1991.
5. Clark CM, Trojanowski JQ, Lee M-YL: Neurofibrillary tangles in Alzheimer's disease: clinical and pathological implications. In Brioni JD, Decker MW (eds): *Pharmacological Treatment of Alzheimer's Disease: Molecular and Neurobiological Foundations*, New York, 1997, Wiley-Liss.
6. Cotman CW, Anderson AJ: Selective vulnerability of the brain to Alzheimer's disease pathology. In Clark CM, Trojanowski JQ (eds): *Neurodegenerative Dementias*, New York, 2000, McGraw-Hill.
7. Bayer TA, Wirths O, Majtényi K, et al: Key factors in Alzheimer's disease: Beta-amyloid precursor protein processing, metabolism and intraneuronal transport, *Brain Pathol* 11:1-11, 2001.
8. American Psychiatric Association: *Diagnostic and Statistical Manual of Mental Disorders*, ed 4, Washington, DC, 1994, American Psychiatric Association.
9. Mega M, Cummings J, Fiorello T, et al: The spectrum of behavioral changes in Alzheimer's disease, *Neurology* 46(1):130-135, 1996.
10. Brookmeyer R, Corrada MM, Curriero FC, et al: Survival following a diagnosis of Alzheimer disease, *Arch Neurol* 59(11):1764-1767, 2002.
11. Norris F, Sheperd R, Denys E, et al: Onset, natural history and outcome in idiopathic adult motor neuron disease, *J Neurol Sci* 118(1):48-55, 1993.

12. Pradas J, Finison L, Andres PL, et al: The natural history of amyotrophic lateral sclerosis and the use of natural history controls in therapeutic trials, *Neurology* 43(4):751-755, 1993.
13. Ringel SP, Murphy JR, Alderson MK, et al: The natural history of amyotrophic lateral sclerosis, *Neurology* 43(7):1316-1322, 1993.
14. Worms PM: The epidemiology of motor neuron diseases: A review of recent studies, *J Neurol Sci* 191:3-9, 2001.
15. Wohlfart G: Collateral regeneration in partially denervated muscles, *Neurology* 8:175-180, 1958.
16. Hansen S, Ballantyne JP: A quantitative electrophysiological study of motor neuron disease, *J Neurol Neurosurg Psychiatry* 41:773-783, 1978.
17. McComas AJ, Sica REP, Campbell MJ, et al: Functional compensation in partially denervated muscles, *J Neurol Neurosurg Psychiatry* 34:453-460, 1971.
18. Swash M, Schwartz MS: A longitudinal study of changes in motor units in motor neuron disease, *J Neurol Sci* 56:185-197, 1982.
19. Mitsumoto H, Chad DA, Pioro EK: *Amyotrophic Lateral Sclerosis,* Philadelphia, 1998, FA Davis.
20. Haverkamp LJ, Appel V, Appel SH: Natural history of amyotrophic lateral sclerosis in database population. Validation of a scoring system and a model for survival prediction, *Brain* 118:707-719, 1995.
21. Harper PS: The natural history of Huntington's disease. In Harper PS (ed): *Huntington's Disease,* London, 1996, WB Saunders.
22. Folstein S: *Huntington's Disease: A Disorder of Families,* Baltimore, 1989, Johns Hopkins University Press.
23. Huntington's Disease Collaborative Research Group: A novel gene containing a trinucleotide repeat that is expanded and unstable on Huntington's disease chromosomes, *Cell* 72:971-983, 1993.
24. Gusella JF, Wexler NS, Conneally PM, et al: A polymorphic DNA marker genetically linked to HD, *Nature* 306:234-238, 1983.
25. Penny JB, Young AB: Huntington's disease. In Jankovic J, Tolosa E (eds): *Parkinson's Disease and Movement Disorders,* Baltimore, 1998, Williams & Wilkins.
26. Kirkwood SC, Su JL, Conneally M, et al: Progression of symptoms in the early and middle stages of Huntington disease, *Arch Neurol* 58(2):273-278, 2001.
27. Louis ED, Quinn L, Marder K: Dystonia in Huntington's disease: Prevalence and clinical characteristics, *Mov Disord* 14(1):95-101, 1991.
28. Kirkwood SC, Siemers E, Bond C, et al: Confirmation of subtle motor changes among presymptomatic carriers of the Huntington gene, *Arch Neurol* 57:1040-1044, 2000.
29. Mayeux R, Stern Y, Herman A, et al: Correlates of early disability in Huntington's disease, *Ann Neurol* 20:727-731, 1986.
30. Marder K, Shao H, Myers RH, et al: Rate of functional decline in Huntington's disease, *Neurology* 54(2):452-458, 2000.
31. Hayden MR: *Huntington's Chorea,* New York, 1981, Springer-Verlag.
32. Tanner CM, Hubble JP, Chan P: Epidemiology and genetics of Parkinson's disease. In Watts RL, Koller WE (eds): *Movement Disorders. Neurologic Principles and Practice,* New York, 1997, McGraw-Hill.
33. Barker R, Rosser A: Disorders of the basal ganglia. In Scolding N (eds): *Contemporary Treatments in Neurology,* Oxford, 2001, Butterworth-Heinemann.
34. Fearnley J, Lees AJ: Parkinson's Disease: Neuropathology. In Watts RL, Koller WE (eds). *Movement Disorders: Neurologic Principles and Practice,* New York, 1997, McGraw-Hill.
35. Martin R, Dhib-Jalbut S: Immunology and etiologic concepts. In Burks JS, Johnson KP (eds): *Multiple Sclerosis: Diagnosis, Medical Management, and Rehabilitation,* New York, 2000, Demos.
36. Compston A: Genetic susceptibility to multiple sclerosis. In Compston A, Ebers G, Lassman H, et al (eds): *McAlpine's Multiple Sclerosis,* ed 3, London, 1998, Churchill-Livingstone.
37. Kurtzke JF, Wallin MT: Epidemiology. In Burks JS, Johnson KP (eds): *Multiple Sclerosis: Diagnosis, Medical Management, and Rehabilitation,* New York, 2000, Demos.
38. DeStefano N, Sridar N, Gordon FS, et al: Evidence of axonal damage in the early stages of multiple sclerosis and its relevance to disability, *Arch Neurol* 58(1):65-70, 2001.
39. Silber E, Sharief MK: Axonal degeneration in the pathogenesis of multiple sclerosis, *J Neurol Sci* 170:11-18, 1999.
40. Lublin FD, Reingold SC: Defining the clinical course of multiple sclerosis: results of an international survey, *Neurology* 46:907-911, 1996.
41. Coles A: Multiple sclerosis. In: Scolding N (eds): *Contemporary Treatments in Neurology,* Oxford, 2001, Butterworth-Heinemann.
42. McDonald WI, Ron MA: Multiple sclerosis: The disease and its manifestations, *Philos Trans R Soc Lond B Biol Sci* 354(1390):1615-1622, 1999.
43. Ebers GC: The natural history of multiple sclerosis. In Compston A, Ebers G, Lassmann H, et al (eds): *McAlpine's Multiple Sclerosis,* London, 1998, Churchill-Livingstone.
44. Weinshenker BG, Bass B, Rise GP, et al: The natural history of multiple sclerosis: a geographically based study. Predictive value of the early clinical course, *Brain* 112:1419-1428, 1989.
45. Sadovnik AD, Eisen K, Ebers GC, et al: Cause of death in patients attending multiple sclerosis clinics, *Neurology* 41:1193-1196, 1991.
46. Dal Bello-Haas V: A framework for rehabilitation in degenerative diseases: planning care and maximizing quality of life, *Neurol Rep* 26(3):115-129, 2002.
47. Schenkman M, Bliss ST, Day L, et al: Multisystem model for management of neurologically impaired adults—an update and illustrative case, *Neurol Rep* 23:145-157, 1999.
48. Waite LM, Broe GA, Grayson DA, et al: Motor function and disability in the dementias, *Int J Geriatr Psychiatr* 15(10):897-903, 2000.
49. Schwid SR, Thornton CA, Pandya S, et al: Quantitative assessment of motor fatigue and strength in MS, *Neurology* 53(4):743-750, 1999.
50. Visser J, Mans E, de Visser M, et al: Comparison of maximal voluntary isometric contraction and hand-held dynamometry in measuring muscle strength of patients with progressive lower motor neuron syndrome, *Neuromuscul Disord* 13(9):744-750, 2003.
51. Surakka J, Romberg, A, Ruutiainen J, et al: Assessment of muscle strength and motor fatigue with a knee dynamometer in subjects with multiple sclerosis: A new fatigue index, *Clin Rehabil* 18(6):652-659, 2004.
52. Slavin MD, Jette DU, Andres PL, et al: Lower extremity muscle force measures and functional ambulation in patients with amyotrophic lateral sclerosis, *Arch Phys Med Rehabil* 79(8):950-954, 1998.
53. Koller W, Kase S: Muscle strength testing in Parkinson's disease, *Eur Neurol* 25(2):130-133, 1986.
54. Nogaki H, Kakinuma S, Morimatsu M: Movement velocity dependent muscle strength in Parkinson's disease, *Acta Neurol Scand* 99(3):152-157, 1999.
55. Pedersen SW, Oberg B, Larsson LE, et al: Gait analysis, isokinetic muscle strength measurement in patients with Parkinson's disease, *Scand J Rehabil Med* 29(2):67-74, 1997.
56. Paasuke M, Ereline J, Gapeyeva H, et al: Leg-extension strength and chair-rise performance in elderly women with Parkinson's disease, *J Aging Phys Act* 12(4):511-524, 2004.
57. Corcos DM, Chen CM, Quinn NP, et al: Strength in Parkinson's disease: relationship to rate of force generation and clinical status, *Ann Neurol* 39(1):79-88, 1996.
58. Lambert CP, Archer RL, Evans WJ: Muscle strength and fatigue during isokinetic exercise in individuals with multiple sclerosis, *Med Sci Sports Exerc* 33(10):1613-1619, 2001.
59. Armstrong LE, Winant DM, Swasey PR, et al: Using isokinetic dynamometry to test ambulatory patients with multiple sclerosis, *Phys Ther* 63(8):1274-1279, 1983.
60. Morris JC: Clinical presentation and course of Alzheimer disease. In Terry RD, Katzman R, Bick KL, et al (eds): *Alzheimer Disease,* ed 2, Philadelphia, 1999, Lippincott Williams & Wilkins.
61. Wilson CM, Grace GM, Munoz DG, et al: Cognitive impairment in sporadic ALS. A pathological continuum underlying a multisystem disorder, *Neurology* 57:651-657, 2001.
62. Lomen-Hoerth C, Murphy J, Langmore S, et al: Are amyotrophic lateral sclerosis patients cognitively normal? *Neurology* 60(7):1094-1097, 2003.
63. Neary D, Snowden JS, Mann DMA, et al: Frontal lobe dementia and motor neuron disease, *J Neurol Neurosurg Psychiatry* 53:23-32, 1990.
64. Strong MJ, Grace GM, Orange JB, et al: A prospective study of cognitive impairment in ALS, *Neurology* 53:1665-1670, 1999.
65. Abrahams S, Leigh P, Harvey A, et al: Verbal fluency and executive dysfunction in amyotrophic lateral sclerosis, *Neuropsychologia* 38(6):734-737, 2000.
66. Hahn Barma V, Deweer B, Durr A, et al: Are cognitive changes the first symptoms of Huntington's Disease? A study of gene carriers, *J Neurol Neurosurg Psychiatry* 64:172, 1998.
67. Paulson J, Ready, R, Hamilton J, et al: Neuropsychiatric aspects of Huntington's disease, *J Neurol Neurosurg Psychiatry* 71:310-314, 2001.
68. Brandt J: Cognitive impairments in Huntington's Disease: Insights into the neuropsychology of the striatum. In Corkin S, Grafmaan J, Boller F (eds): *Handbook of Neuropsychology,* Amsterdam, 1991, Elsevier.
69. Rothlind J, Bylsma F, Peyser C, et al: Cognitive and motor correlates of everyday functioning in early Huntington's disease, *J Nerv Ment Dis* 181:194-199, 1993.
70. Brandt J, Strauss M, Larus J, et al: Clinical correlates of dementia and disability in Huntington's disease, *J Clin Neuropsychol* 6:401-412, 1984.
71. Brandt J, Butters N: The neuropsychology of Huntington's disease, *Trends Neurosci* 9:118-120, 1986.
72. Butters N, Wolfe J, Granholm E: An assessment of verbal recall, recognition and fluency abilities in patients with Huntington's disease, *Cortex* 22:11-32, 1986.
73. Henry JD, Crawford JR: Verbal fluency deficits in Parkinson's disease: A meta-analysis, *J Int Neuropsychol Soc* 10(4):608-622, 2004.
74. Uekermann J, Daum I, Bielawski M, et al: Differential executive control impairments in early Parkinson's disease, *J Neural Transm Suppl* 68:39-51, 2004.
75. Rochester, L, Hetherington V, Jones D, et al: Attending to the task: interference effects of functional tasks on walking in Parkinson's disease

and the roles of cognition, depression, fatigue, and balance, *Arch Phys Med Rehabil* 85(10):1578-1585, 2004.

76. Bosboom JL, Stoffers D, Wolters EC: Cognitive dysfunction and dementia in Parkinson's disease, *J Neural Transm* 111(10-11):1303-1315, 2004.

77. Anderson KE: Dementia in Parkinson's disease, *Curr Treat Options Neurol* 6(3):201-217, 2004.

78. Heaton RK: Neuropsychological findings in relapsing-remitting and chronic-progressive multiple sclerosis, *J Consult Clin Psychol* 53:103-110, 1985.

79. Rao SM, Leo GJ, Bernardin L, et al: Cognitive dysfunction in multiple sclerosis. I. Frequency, patterns and prediction, *Neurology* 41(5):685-691, 1991.

80. Fraser C, Stark S: Cognitive symptoms and correlates of physical disability in individuals with multiples sclerosis, *J Neurosci Nurs* 35(6):314-320, 2003.

81. Olivares T, Nieto A, Sanchez MP, et al: Pattern of neuropsychological impairment in the early phase of relapsing-remitting multiple sclerosis, *Mult Scler* 11(2):191-197, 2005.

82. Huijbregts SC, Kalkers NJF, de Sonneville LM, et al: Differences in cognitive impairment of relapsing remitting, secondary and primary progressive MS, *Neurology* 63(2):335-339, 2004.

83. Folstein MF, Folstein SE, McHugh PR: Mini-Mental State: a practical method for grading the cognitive state of patients for the clinician, *J Psychiatr Res* 12:189-198, 1975.

84. Zec RF, Landreth ES, Vicari SK, et al: Alzheimer disease assessment scale: useful for both early detection and staging of dementia of the Alzheimer type, *Alzheimer Dis Assoc Disord* 6:89-102, 1992.

85. Rosen WG, Mohs RC, Davis KL: A new rating scale for Alzheimer's disease, *Am J Psychiatry* 141:1356-1364, 1984.

86. McLendon BM, Doraiswamy PM: Defining meaningful change in Alzheimer's disease trials: The donepezil experience, *J Geriatr Psychiatry Neurol* 12:39-48, 1999.

87. Benedict RHB, Cox D, Thompson LL, et al: Reliable screening for neuropsychological impairment in multiple sclerosis, *Mult Scler* 10:675-678, 2004.

88. Mate-Kole CC, Major A, Lenzer I, et al: Validation of the quick cognitive screening test, *Arch Phys Med Rehabil* 75(8):867-875, 1994.

89. Molloy DW, Standish TI, Lewis DL: Screening for mild cognitive impairment: Comparing the SMMSE and the ABCS, *Can J Psychiatry* 50(12):52-58, 2005.

90. Goetz CG, Tanner CM, Levy M, et al: Pain in Parkinson's disease, *Mov Disord* 1:45-49, 1996.

91. Clifford DB, Trotter JL: Pain in multiple sclerosis, *Arch Neurol* 41:1270-1272, 1984.

92. Moulin DE, Foley KM, Ebers GC: Pain syndromes in multiple sclerosis, *Neurology* 38:1830-1834, 1988.

93. Hillen ME, Sage JI: Non-motor fluctuations in patients with Parkinson's disease, *Neurology* 47:1180-1183, 1996.

94. Witjas T, Kaphan E, Azulay JP, et al: Nonmotor fluctuations in Parkinson's disease: frequent and disabling, *Neurology* 59(3):408-413, 2002.

95. Kanchandani R, Howe JG: Lhermitte's sign in multiple sclerosis: A clinical survey and review of the literature, *J Neurol Neurosurg Psychiatry* 45:308-312, 1982.

96. Gass A, Kitchen N, MacManus DG, et al: Trigeminal neuralgia in patients with multiple sclerosis: Lesion localization with magnetic resonance imaging, *Neurology* 49(4):1142-1144, 1997.

97. Miller JR: Multiple Sclerosis. In Rowland LP (ed): *Merritt's Neurology*, ed 10, Philadelphia, 2000, Lippincott, Williams & Wilkins.

98. Leigh RJ, Newman SA, Folstein SE, et al: Abnormal ocular motor control in Huntington's disease, *Neurology* 33:1268-1275, 1983.

99. Lasker AG, Zee DS, Hain TC, et al: Saccades in Huntington's disease: Initiation defects and distractibility, *Neurology* 37:364-370, 1987.

100. Lasker AG, Zee DS, Hain TC, et al: Saccades in Huntington's disease: slowing and dysmetria, *Neurology* 38(3):427-431, 1988.

101. Leport FE, Duvoisin RC: Apraxia of eyelid opening: An involuntary levator inhibition, *Neurology* 1985;35:423-427, 1985.

102. White OB, Saint-Cyr JA, Tomlinson RD, et al: Ocular motor deficits in Parkinson's disease II. Control of the saccadic and smooth pursuit systems, *Brain* 106:571-587, 1983.

103. Vidailhet M, Rivaud S, GouiderKhouja N, et al: Eye movements in parkinsonian syndromes, *Ann Neurol* 35:420-426, 1994.

104. Mathews B: Symptoms and signs of multiple sclerosis. In Compston A, Ebers G, Lassmann H, et al (eds): *McAlpine's Multiple Sclerosis*, ed 3, London, 1998, Churchill-Livingstone.

105. Dailey FL, Brown JR, Goldstein FJ: Dysarthria in multiple sclerosis, *Speech Hear Res* 15:725-728, 1972.

106. Gallagher JP: Pathologic laughter and crying in ALS: A search for their origin, *Acta Neurol Scand* 80:114-117, 1989.

107. Critchley M: Speech disorders of parkinsonism: A review, *J Neurol Neurosurg Psychiatry* 44:757-758, 1981.

108. Hunker CJ, Abbs JH, Barlow SW: The relationship between parkinsonian rigidity and hypokinesia in the orofacial system: A quantitative analysis, *Neurology* 32:749-755, 1982.

109. Bruyn GW, Went LN: Huntington's chorea. In Vinken PJ, Bruyn GW, Klawans HL (eds): *Extrapyramidal Disorders*, Amsterdam, 1996, Elsevier Science.

110. Fahn S: Huntington's disease. In Rowland LP (ed): *Merritt's Neurology*, ed 10, Philadelphia, 2000, Lippincott Williams & Wilkins.

111. Bohannon RW, Smith MB: Interrater reliability of a modified Ashworth scale of muscle spasticity, *Phys Ther* 67:206-207, 1987.

112. Gentile AM: Implicit and explicit processes during acquisition of functional skills, *Scand J Occup Ther* 5:7-16, 1998.

113. Segar CA: Implicit learning, *Psychol Bull* 115:163-196, 1994.

114. Eslinger PJ, Damasio AR: Preserved motor learning in Alzheimer's disease: Implications for anatomy and behavior, *J Neurosci* 6(10):3006-3009, 1986.

115. Bylsma FW, Brandt J, Strauss ME: Aspects of procedural memory are differentially impaired in Huntington's disease, *Arch Clin Neuropsychol* 5(3):287-297, 1990.

116. Sprengelmeyer R, Canavan AG, Lange HW, et al: Associative learning in degenerative neostriatal disorders: Contrasts in explicit and implicit remembering between Parkinson's and Huntington's diseases, *Mov Disord* 10(1):51-65, 1995.

117. Feigin A, Kieburtz K, Bordwell K, et al: Functional decline in Huntington's disease, *Mov Disord* 10(2):211-214, 1995.

118. Quinn L, Gordon A, Reilmann R, et al: Altered movement trajectories and force control during object transport in Huntington's disease, *Mov Disord* 16(3):469-480, 2001.

119. Huntington Study Group: Unified Huntington's Disease Rating Scale: Reliability and consistency, *Mov Disord* 11(2):136-142, 1996.

120. Marsden CD: Parkinson's disease, *J Neurol Neurosurg Psychiatry* 57:173-211, 1994.

121. Morris ME, Iansek R: Characteristics of motor disturbance in Parkinson's disease and strategies for movement rehabilitation, *J Hum Mov Sci* 3:9, 1996.

122. Oliveira RM, Gurd JM, Nixon P, et al: Micrographia in Parkinson's disease: The effect of providing external cues, *J Neurol Neurosurg Psychiatry* 63:429-433, 1997.

123. Beyer MK, Herlofson K, Arsland D, et al: Causes of death in a community-based study of Parkinson's disease, *Acta Neurol Scand* 103(1):7-11, 2001.

124. Krivickas L: Pulmonary function and respiratory failure. In Mitsumoto H, Chad DA, Pioro EK (eds): *Amyotrophic Lateral Sclerosis*, Philadelphia, 1998, FA Davis.

125. Schiffman PL, Belsh JM: Pulmonary function at diagnosis of amyotrophic lateral sclerosis. Rate of deterioration, *Chest* 103:508-513, 1993.

126. Rochester DF, Esau SA: Assessment of ventilatory function in patients with neuromuscular disease, *Clin Chest Med* 14:751-763, 1994,

127. Vitacca M, Clini E, Facchetti D, et al: Breathing pattern and respiratory mechanics in patients with amyotrophic lateral sclerosis, *Eur Respir J* 10:1614-1621, 1997.

128. Vincken WG, Gauthier MD, Dollfuss RE, et al: Involvement of the upper airway muscles in extrapyramidal disorders. A cause of airflow limitation, *N Engl J Med* 311:348-442, 1984.

129. Sabaté M, Rodríguez M, Méndez E, et al: Obstructive and restrictive pulmonary dysfunction increases disability in Parkinson's disease, *Arch Phys Med Rehabil* 77:29-34, 1996.

130. Hovestadt A, Bogaard JM, Meerwaldt JD, et al: Pulmonary function in Parkinson's disease, *J Neurol Neurosurg Psych* 52:329-333, 1989.

131. Jankovic J: Respiratory dyskinesia in Parkinson's disease, *Neurology* 36:303-304, 1986.

132. Rice JE, Antic R, Thompson PD: Disordered respiration as a levodopa-induced dyskinesia in Parkinson's disease, *Mov Disord* 17:524-527, 2002.

133. Smeltzer SC, Utell MJ, Rudick RA, et al: Pulmonary function and dysfunction in multiple sclerosis, *Arch Neurol* 45:1245-1249, 1988.

134. Foglio K, Clini E, Facchetti D, et al: Respiratory muscle function and exercise capacity in multiple sclerosis, *Eur Respir J* 7:23-28, 1994.

135. Buyse B, Demedts M, Meekers J et al: Respiratory dysfunction in multiple sclerosis: a prospective analysis of 60 patients, *Eur Respir J* 10:139-145, 1997.

136. Protas EJ, Stanley RK, Jankovic J, et al: Cardiovascular and metabolic responses to upper- and lower-extremity exercise in men with idiopathic Parkinson's disease, *Phys Ther* 76(1):34-40, 1996.

137. Stanley RK, Protas EJ, Jankovic J: Exercise performance in those having Parkinson's disease and healthy normal, *Med Sci Sports Exerc* 31(6):761-766, 1999.

138. Canning CG, Alison JA, Allen NE, et al: Parkinson's disease: An investigation of exercise capacity, respiratory function, and gait, *Arch Phys Med Rehabil* 78(2):199-207, 1997.

139. Mostert S, Kesselring J: Effects of a short-term exercise training program on aerobic fitness, fatigue, health perception and activity level of subjects with multiple sclerosis, *Mult Scler* 8:161-168, 2002.

140. Pontichera-Mulcare JA, Mathews T, Glaser RM, et al: Maximal aerobic exercise of individuals with multiple sclerosis using three modes of ergometry, *Clin Kines* 49:4-13, 1995.

141. Pontichtera-Mulcare JA, Glaser RM, Mathews T, et al: Maximal aerobic exercise in persons with multiple sclerosis, *Clin Kines* 46:12-21, 1993.

142. Cahalin LP, Mathier MA, Semigran MJ, et al: The 6-minute walk test predicts peak oxygen uptake and survival in patients with advanced heart failure, *Chest* 110:325-332, 1996.

143. Redelmeier DA, Bayoumi AM, Goldstein RS, et al: Interpreting small differences in functional status: The 6-minute walk test in chronic lung disease patients, *Am J Respir Crit Care Med* 155:1278-1282, 1997.

144. Montgomery PS, Gardner AW: The clinical utility of a 6-minute walk test in peripheral arterial occlusive disease, *J Am Geriatr Soc* 46:706-711, 1998.

145. Garber CE, Rourke SL, Choulba S, et al: Functional ability and functional capacity in patients with Parkinson's disease, *Med Sci Sports Exerc* 33:S312, 2001.

146. Light KE, Behrman AL, Thigpen M, et al: The 2-minute walk test: A tool for evaluating walking endurance in clients with Parkinson's disease, *Neurol Rep* 21(4):136-139, 1997.

147. Freal JE, Kraft GH, Coryell JK: Symptomatic fatigue in multiple sclerosis, *Arch Phys Med Rehabil* 65:135-138, 1984.

148. Friedman JH, Friedman H: Fatigue in Parkinson's disease: a nine-year follow-up, *Mov Disord* 16:1120-1122, 2001.

149. Friedman JH, Friedman H: Fatigue in Parkinson's disease, *Neurology* 43:2016-2018, 1993.

150. Karlsen K, Larsen JP, Tandberg E, et al: Fatigue in patients with Parkinson's disease, *Mov Disord* 14:237-241, 1999.

151. Kilmer DD: The role of exercise in neuromuscular disease, *Phys Med Rehabil Clin N Am* 9(1):115-125, 1998.

152. Sharma KR, Kent-Braun JA, Majumdar S, et al: Physiology of fatigue in amyotrophic lateral sclerosis, *Neurology* 45:733-740, 1995.

153. Krupp LB, Pollina DA: Mechanisms and management of fatigue in progressive neurological disorders, *Curr Opin Neurol* 9:456-460, 1996.

154. Sandroni P, Walker C, Starr A: "Fatigue" in patients with multiple sclerosis: motor pathway conduction and event-related potentials, *Arch Neurol* 49:517-524, 1992.

155. Patten BM, Hart A, Lovelace R: Multiple sclerosis associated with defects in neuromuscular transmission, *J Neurol Neurosurg Psychiatry* 35:385-394, 1972.

156. Olgiati R, Burgunder JM, Mumenthaler M: Increased energy cost of walking in multiple sclerosis: effect of spasticity, ataxia, and weakness, *Arch Phys Med Rehabil* 69:846-849, 1988.

157. Ziv I, Avraham M, Michaelov Y, et al: Enhanced fatigue during motor performance in patients with Parkinson's disease, *Neurology* 51(6):1583-1586, 1998.

158. Schapira AH: Evidence for mitochondrial dysfunction in idiopathic Parkinson's disease. A critical appraisal, *Mov Disord* 9:125-138, 1994.

159. Multiple Sclerosis Council for Clinical Practice Guideline: Fatigue and Multiple Sclerosis: Evidence-Based Management Strategies for Fatigue in Multiple Sclerosis, Washington, DC, 1999, Paralyzed Veterans of America.

160. Schwartz JE, Jandorf L, Krupp LB: The measurement of fatigue: A new instrument, *J Psychosom Res* 37:753-762, 1993.

161. Krupp LB, Alvarez LA, LaRocca NG, et al: Fatigue in multiple sclerosis. *Arch Neurol* 45:435-437, 1988.

162. Krupp LB, Elkins LE: Fatigue and declines in cognitive functioning in multiple sclerosis, *Neurology* 55:934-938, 2000.

163. Krupp LB, LaRocca NG, Muir-Nash J, et al: The fatigue severity scale. Application to patients with multiple sclerosis and systemic lupus erythematosus, *Arch Neurol* 46:1121-1123, 1989.

164. Herlofson K, Larsen JP: Measuring fatigue in patients with Parkinson's disease: The Fatigue Severity Scale, *Euro J Neurol* 9:595-600, 2002.

165. Hennerici JG, Oster J, Cohen S, et al: Are gait disturbances and white matter degeneration early indicators of vascular dementia? *Dementia* 5.197-202, 1994.

166. Thajeb P: Gait disorders of multi-infarct dementia, *Acta Neurol Scand* 87:239-242, 1993.

167. Buchner DM, Larson EB: Falls and fractures in patients with Alzheimer-type dementia, *JAMA* 257:1492-1495, 1987.

168. Nakamura T, Meguro K, Saskai H: Relationship between falls and stride length variability in senile dementia of the Alzheimer type, *Gerontology* 42:108-113, 1996.

169. Stolze H, Kuhtz-Buschbeck JP, Drucke H, et al: Comparative analysis of the gait disorder of normal pressure hydrocephalus and Parkinson's disease, *J Neurol Neurosurg Psych* 70(3):289-297, 2001.

170. Visser H: Gait and balance in senile dementia of Alzheimer's type, *Age Ageing* 12:296-301, 1983.

171. Pettersson AF, Engardt M, Wahlund L: Activity level and balance in subjects with mild Alzheimer's disease, *Dement Geriatr Cogn Disord* 13(4):213-216, 2002.

172. Alexander NB, Mollo JM, Giordani B, et al: Maintenance of balance, gait patterns, and obstacle clearance in Alzheimer's disease, *Neurology* 45:908-914, 1995.

173. Goldman WP, Baty JD, Buckles VD, et al: Motor dysfunction in mildly demented AD individuals without extrapyramidal signs, *Neurology* 53(5):956-962, 1999.

174. Tanaka A, Hideyuki O, Kobayashi I, et al: Gait disturbance of patients with vascular and Alzheimer-type dementias, *Percep Mot Skills* 80:735-738, 1995.

175. O'Keeffe ST, Kazeem H, Philpot RM, et al: Gait disturbance in Alzheimer's disease: A clinical study, *Age Ageing* 25(4):313-316, 1996.

176. Nakamura T, Meguro K, Yamazaki H, et al: Postural and gait disturbance correlated with decreased frontal cerebral blood flow in Alzheimer disease, *Alzheimer Dis Assoc Disord* 11(3):132-139, 1997.

177. Camicioli R, Licis L: Motor impairment predicts falls in specialized Alzheimer care units, *Alzheimer Dis Assoc Disord* 18(4):214-218, 2004.

178. Della Sala S, Spinnler H, Venneri A: Walking difficulties in patients with Alzheimer's disease might originate from gait apraxia, *J Neurol Neurosurg Psych* 75:196-201, 2004.

179. Tinetti ME, Speechley M, Ginter SE: Risk factors for falls among elderly persons living in the community, *N Engl J Med* 319:1701-1707, 1988.

180. Morris JC, Rubin EH, Morris EJ, et al: Senile dementia of the Alzheimer's type: An important risk factor for serious falls, *J Gerontol* 42:412-417, 1987.

181. van Dijk PT, Meulenberg OG, van de Sande HJ, et al: Falls in dementia patients, *Gerontologist* 33:200-204, 1993.

182. Dal Bello-Haas V, Andrews-Hinders D, Balsdon Richer C, et al: Development, analysis, refinement and utility of an interdisciplinary amyotrophic lateral sclerosis database, *Amyotroph Lateral Scler Other Motor Neuron Disord* 2(1):39-46, 2001.

183. Goldfarb BJ, Simon SR: Gait patterns in patients with amyotrophic lateral sclerosis, *Arch Phys Med Rehabil* 65(2):61-65, 1984.

184. Jette DU, Slavin MD, Andres PL, et al: The relationship of lower-limb muscle force to walking ability in patients with amyotrophic lateral sclerosis, *Phys Ther* 79(7):672-681, 1999.

185. Hausdorff JM, Cudkowica ME, Firtion R, et al: Gait variability and basal ganglia disorders: Stride-to-stride variations of gait cycle timing in Parkinson's disease and Huntington's disease, *Mov Disord* 13:428-437, 1998.

186. Reynolds NC, Myklebust JB, Prietro TE, et al: Analysis of gait abnormalities in Huntington disease, *Arch Phys Med Rehabil* 80:59-65, 1999.

187. Churchyard ME, Morris ME, Georgiou N, et al: Gait dysfunction in Huntington's disease: Parkinsonism and a disorder of timing, *Adv Neurol* 87:335-385, 2001.

188. Thompson PD, Berardelli A, Rothwell JC, et al: The coexistence of bradykinesia and chorea in Huntington's disease and its implications for theories of basal ganglia control of movement, *Brain* 111:223-244, 1988.

189. Agostino R, Berardelli A, Formica A, et al: Sequential arm movements in patients with Parkinson's disease, Huntington's disease and dystonia, *Brain* 115:1481-1495, 1992.

190. Georgiou N, Bradshaw JL, Philips JG, et al: Reliance on advance information and movement sequencing in Huntington's disease, *Mov Disord* 10:477-481, 1985.

191. Hefter H, Homberg V, Lange HW, et al: Impairment of rapid movements in Huntington's disease, *Brain* 110:585-612, 1987.

192. Tian J, Herdman SJ, Zee DS, et al: Postural instability in patients with Huntington's disease, *Neurology* 42:1232-1238, 1992.

193. Imbriglio S: *Physical and Occupational Therapy for Huntington's Disease*, New York, 1997, Huntington's Disease Society of America.

194. Morris ME, Iansek R: Gait disorders in Parkinson's disease: A framework for physical therapy practice, *Neurol Rep* 21(4):125-131, 1997.

195. Morris ME, Iansek R, Matyas TA, et al: Stride length regulation in Parkinson's disease: Normalization strategies and underlying mechanisms, *Brain* 119:551-568, 1996.

196. Morris ME, Iansek R, Matyas TA, et al: The ability to modulate walking cadence remains intact in Parkinson's disease, *J Neurol Neurosurg Psych* 57:1532-1534, 1994.

197. Morris ME, Iansek R, Matyas TA, et al: The pathogenesis of gait hypokinesia in Parkinson's disease, *Brain* 117:1161-1182, 1994.

198. Thaut MH, McIntosh GC, Rice RR, et al: Rhythmic auditory stimulation in gait training for Parkinson's disease patients, *Mov Disord* 11:193-200, 1996.

199. McIntosh GC, Brown SH, Rice RR, et al: Rhythmic auditory-motor facilitation of gait patterns in patients with Parkinson's disease, *J Neurol Neurosurg Psychiatry* 62:22-26, 1997.

200. Brown P, Steiger M: Basal ganglia gait disorders. In Bronstein A, Brandt T, Woolacott M (eds): *Balance Posture and Gait*, New York, 1996, Oxford University Press.

201. Giladi N, McMahon D, Przedborski S, et al: Motor blocks in Parkinson's disease, *Neurology* 42:333-339, 1992.

202. Giladi N, Kao R, Fahn S: Freezing phenomenon in patients with parkinsonian syndromes, *Mov Disord* 12:302-305, 1997.

203. Smithson F, Morris ME, Iansek R: Performance on clinical tests of balance in Parkinson's disease, *Phys Ther* 78:577-592, 1998.

204. Dietz V, Berger W, Horstmann GA: Posture in Parkinson's disease: Impairment of reflexes and programming, *Ann Neurol* 24:660-669, 1988.

205. Schieppati M, Nardone A: Free and supported stance in Parkinson's disease, *Brain* 144:1227-1244, 1991.

206. Bloem BR, Beckley DJ, Remler MP, et al: Postural reflexes in Parkinson's disease during "resist" and "yield" tasks, *J Neurol Sci* 129:109-119, 1995.

207. Schenkman M, Butler RB: A model for multisystem evaluation treatment of individuals with Parkinson's disease, *Phys Ther* 69(11):932-943, 1989.

208. McDowell FH, Reicher WH, Doolittle K: Vestibular dysfunction in Parkinson's disease, *Ann Neurol* 10:94, 1981.

209. Horak FB, Nutt JG, Nashner LM: Postural inflexibility in Parkinson's subjects, *J Neurol Sci* 111:46-58, 1992.

210. Bond JM, Morris ME: Goal-directed secondary motor tasks: Their effects on gait in subjects with Parkinson's disease, *Arch Phys Med Rehabil* 81:110-116, 2000.

211. Marchese R, Bove M, Abbruzzese G: Effect of cognitive and motor tasks on postural stability in Parkinson's disease: A posturographic study, *Mov Disord* 8(6):652-658, 2003.

212. Morris M, Iansek R, Smithson F, Huxham F: Postural instability in Parkinson's disease: a comparison with and without concurrent task, *Gait Posture* 12:205-216, 2000.

213. Dimitrova D, Horak FB, Nutt JG: Postural muscle responses to multidirectional translations in patients with Parkinson's disease, *J Neurophys* 91(1):489-501, 2004.

214. Bloem BR, Grimbergen YA, Cramer M, et al: Prospective assessment of falls in Parkinson's disease, *J Neurol* 248:950-958, 2001.

215. Gray P, Hildebrand K: Fall risk factors in Parkinson's disease, *J Neurosci Nurs* 32:222-228, 2000.

216. Wood BH, Bilclough JA, Bowron A, et al: Incidence and prediction of falls in Parkinson's disease: a prospective multidisciplinary study, *J Neurol Neurosurg Psych* 72(6):721-725, 2002.

217. Morris ME, Huxham F, McGinley J, et al: The biomechanics and motor control of gait in Parkinson disease, *Clin Biomech* 16(6):459-470, 2001.

218. Verghese J, Buschke H, Viola L, et al: Validity of divided attention tasks in predicting falls in older individuals: a preliminary study, *J Am Geriatr Soc* 50(9):1572-1576, 2002.

219. Pettersson AF, Olsson E, Wahlund LO: Motor function in subjects with mild cognitive impairment and early Alzheimer's disease, *Dement Geriatr Cogn Disord* 19(5-6):299-304, 2005. Epub 2005 Mar 22.

220. Berg KO, Wood-Dauphinee SL, Williams JI, et al: Measuring balance in the elderly: validation of an instrument, *Can J Public Health* 83-S7-11, 1992.

221. Lim LI, van Wegen EE, de Goede CJ, et al: Measuring gait and gait-related activities in Parkinson's patients own home environment: a reliability, responsiveness and feasibility study, *Parkinsonism Relat Disord* 11(1):19-24, 2005.

222. Qutubuddin AA, Pegg PO, Cifu DX, et al: Validating the Berg Balance Scale for patients with Parkinson's disease: a key to rehabilitation evaluation, *Arch Phys Med Rehabil* 86(4):789-792, 2005.

223. Brusse, KJ, Zimdars, S: Testing functional performance in people with Parkinson's disease, *Phys Ther* 85(2):134-141, 2005.

224. Quinn L, Rao A: Physical therapy for people with Huntington Disease: current perspectives and case report, *Neurology Report* 26(3):145-153, 2002.

225. Nelson AJ, Zwick D, Brody S, et al: The validity of the GaitRite and the Functional Ambulation Performance scoring system in the analysis of Parkinson gait, *Neurorehabilitation* 17(3):255-262, 2002.

226. Rao AK, Quinn L, Marder KS: Reliability of spatiotemporal gait outcome measures in Huntington's disease, *Mov Disord* 20(8):1033-1037, 2005.

227. Shumway-Cook A, Baldwin M, Polissar N, et al: Predicting the probability for falls in community-dwelling older adults, *Phys Ther* 77:812-819, 1997.

228. McConvey J, Bennett SE: Reliability of the dynamic gait index in individuals with multiple sclerosis, *Arch Phys Med Rehabil* 86(1):130-133, 2005.

229. Podsiadlo D, Richardson S: The timed "Up & Go": a test of basic functional mobility for frail elderly persons, *J Am Geriatr Soc* 39(2):142-148, 1991.

230. Duncan PW, Weiner DK, Chandler J, et al: Functional reach: a new clinical measure of balance, *J Gerontol* 45(6):M192-M197, 1990.

231. Dal Bello-Haas V, Kloos AD, Mistumoto H: Physical therapy for a patient through six stages of amyotrophic lateral sclerosis, *Phys Ther* 78:1312-1324, 1998.

232. Cattaneo D, Marazzini F, Crippa A, et al: Do static or dynamic AFOs improve balance? *Clin Rehabil* 16(8):894-899, 2002.

233. Cotrell V, Schulz R: The perspective of the patient with Alzheimer's disease: a neglected dimension of dementia research, *Gerontologist* 33(2):205-211, 1993.

234. Green, Mohs, Schmeidler, et al: 1993 Functional decline in Alzheimer's disease: a longitudinal study, *J Am Geriatr Soc* 41(6):654-661, 1993.

235. Rabins PV, Mace NL, Lucas MJ: The impact of dementia on the family, *JAMA* 248(3):333-335, 1982.

236. Katz S, Ford AB, Moskowitz RW, et al: Studies of illness in the aged. The index of ADL: a standardized measure of biological and psychosocial function, *JAMA* 185:914-919, 1963.

237. Lawton MP, Brody EM: Assessment of older people: self-maintaining and instrumental activities of daily living, *Gerontologist* 9:179-186, 1969.

238. Pfeffer RI, Kurosaki TT, Harrah CH, et al: Measurement of functional activities in older adults in the community, *J Gerontol* 37(3):323-329, 1982.

239. Mahurin RK, DeBettignies BF, Pirozzolo HJ: Structured assessment of independent living skills: preliminary report of a performance measure of functional abilities in dementia, *J Gerontol* 46(2):P58-66, 1991.

240. Galasko D, Bennett D, Sano M, et al: An inventory to assess activities of daily living for clinical trials in Alzheimer's disease: the Alzheimer's Disease Cooperative Study, *Alzheimer Dis Assoc Disord* 11(suppl 2):33-39, 1997.

241. Gélinas I, Gauthier L, McIntyre M, et al: Development of a functional measure for persons with Alzheimer's disease: the Disability Assessment for Dementia, *Am J Occup Ther* 53:471-481, 1999.

242. Schwab R, England A: Projection technique for evaluating surgery in Parkinson's disease. In Gillingham J, Donaldson I: *Third Symposium on Parkinson's Disease*, Edinburgh, 1969, Livingstone.

243. Bylsma FW, Rothlind J, Hall MR, et al: Assessment of adaptive functioning in Huntington's disease, *Mov Disord* 8(2):183-190, 1993.

244. Hariz GM, Lindberg M, Hariz MI, et al: Does the ADL part of the unified Parkinson's disease rating scale measure ADL? An evaluation in patients after pallidotomy and thalamic deep brain stimulation, *Mov Disord* 18(4):373-381, 2003.

245. Mansson E, Lexell J: Performance of activities of daily living in multiple sclerosis, *Disabil Rehabil* 26(10):576-585, 2004.

246. Bergner M, Bobbitt RA, Kressel S, et al: The sickness impact profile: conceptual formulation and methodology for the development of a health status measure, *Int J Health Serv* 6(3):393-415, 1976.

247. Peto V, Jenkinson C, Fitzpatrick R, et al: The development and validation of a short measure of functioning and well being for individuals with Parkinson's disease, *Qual Life Res* 4:241-248, 1995.

248. Peto V, Jenkinson C, Fitzpatrick R: PDQ-39: a review of the development, validation and application of a Parkinson's disease quality of life questionnaire and its associated measures, *J Neurol* 245 Suppl 1:S10-14, 1998.

249. Jenkinson C, Fitzpatrick R, Peto V, et al: The Parkinson's disease questionnaire (PDQ-39): development and validation of a Parkinson's disease summary index score, *Age Ageing* 26:353-357, 1997.

250. Bushnell DM, Martin ML: Quality of life and Parkinson's disease: translation and validation of the US Parkinson's Disease Questionnaire (PDQ-39), *Qual Life Res* 8(4):345-350, 1999.

251. Martinez MP, Frades B, Jimenez FJ, et al: The PDQ-39 Spanish version: reliability and correlation with the short-form health survey (SF-36), *Neurologia* 14(4):159-163, 1999.

252. Jenkinson C, Fitzpatrick R, Peto V, et al: The PDQ-8: development and validation of a short-form Parkinson's disease questionnaire, *Psychology and Health* 12:805-814, 1997.

253. Vickrey BG, Hays RD, Harooni R, et al: A health-related quality of life measure for multiple sclerosis, *Qual Life Res* 4(3):187-206, 1995.

254. Jenkinson C, Fitzpatrick R, Brennan C, et al: Development and validation of a short measure of health status for individuals with amyotrophic lateral sclerosis/motor neuron disease: The ALSAQ-40, *J Neurol* 246:16-21, 1999.

255. Jenkinson C, Fitzpatrick R, Brennan M, et al: Evidence for the validity and reliability of the ALS assessment questionnaire: the ALSAQ-40, *Amyotroph Lateral Scler Other Motor Neuron Disord* 1:33-40, 1999.

256. Logsdon RG, Gibbons LE, McCurry SM, et al: Quality of life in Alzheimer's disease: Patient and caregiver reports, *Journal of Mental Health and Aging* 5:21-32, 1999.

257. Logsdon RG, Gibbons LE, McCurry SM, et al: Assessing quality of life in older adults with cognitive impairment, *Psychosom Med* 64(3):510-519, 2002.

258. Cummings JL: Behavioral and psychiatric symptoms associated with Huntington's disease, *Adv Neurol* 65:179-186, 1995.

259. Sadovnik AD, Remick RA, Allen J, Swartz E, Yee IML, Eisen K, et al: Depression and multiple sclerosis, *Neurology* 46:628-632, 1996.

260. Beck AT, Ward CH, Mendelson M: An inventory for measuring depression, *Arch Gen Psych* 4:561-571, 1961.

261. Radloff LS: CES-D scale: A self-report depression scale for research in the general population, *Appl Psychol Meas* 1:385-401, 1977.

262. Zigmond AS, Snaith RP: The Hospital Anxiety and Depression Scale, *Acta Psychiatr Scand* 67:361-370, 1983.

263. Spielberger CS, Gorsuch RL, Lushene RE: Manual for the State Trait Anxiety Inventory, Palo Alto, Calif, 1970, Consulting Psychologists Press.

264. Heyman A, Wilkinson W, Hurwitz B, et al: Early-onset Alzheimer's disease: Clinical predictors of institutionalization and death, *Neurology* 37:980-984, 1987.

265. Dooneief G, Marder K, Tang MX, et al: The Clinical Dementia Rating scale: community-based validation of "profound" and "terminal" stages, *Neurology* 46:1746-1749, 1996.

266. Reisberg B, Ferris SH, de Leon MJ, et al: The Global Deterioration Scale for assessment of primary degenerative dementia, *Am J Psychiatry* 139:1136-1139, 1982.

267. Sclan SG, Reisberg B: Functional assessment staging (FAST) in Alzheimer's disease: Reliability, validity, and ordinality, *Int Psychogeriatr* 4(suppl 1):55-69, 1992.

268. Brickman AM, Riba A, Bell K, et al: Longitudinal assessment of patient dependence in Alzheimer Disease, *Arch Neurol* 59:1304-1308, 2002.

269. Cedarbaum JM, Stambler N, Malta E, et al: The ALSFRS-R: A revised ALS functional rating scale that incorporates assessments of respiratory function. BDNF ALS Study Group (Phase III), *Neurol Sci* 169(1-2):13-21, 1999.

270. The Amyotrophic Lateral Sclerosis Functional Rating Scale: Assessment of activities of daily living in patients with amyotrophic lateral sclerosis. The ALS CNTF treatment study (ACTS) phase I-II Study Group, *Arch Neurol* 53(2):141-147, 1996.

271. Unified Huntington's Disease Rating Scale: Reliability and consistency: Huntington Study Group, *Mov Disord* 11(2):136-142, 1996.

272. Goetz CG, Poewe W, Rascol O, et al: Movement Disorder Society Task Force on Rating Scales for Parkinson's Disease. Movement Disorder Society Task Force report on the Hoehn and Yahr staging scale: Status and recommendations, *Mov Disord* 19(9):1020-1028, 2004.

273. Kurtzke, JF: Rating neurologic impairment in multiple sclerosis: an expanded disability status scale (EDSS), *Neurology* 33(11):1444-1452, 1983.

274. Hobart J, Lamping D, Fitzpatrick R, et al: The Multiple Sclerosis Impact Scale (MSIS-29): A new patient-based outcome measure, *Brain* 124(Pt 5):962-973, 2001.

275. American Physical Therapy Association: *Guide to Physical Therapist Practice*, Alexandria, Va, 1998, American Physical Therapy Association.

276. Appenzeller O, Goss JE: Autonomic deficits in Parkinson's disease, *Arch Neurol* 24(1):50-57, 1971.

277. Ponichtera-Mulcare J: Exercise and multiple sclerosis, *Med Sci Sports Exerc* 25:451-465, 1993.

278. Senaratne M, Carroll D, Warren K, Kappagoda T: Evidence for cardiovascular autonomic nerve dysfuncion in multiple sclerosis. *J Neurol Neurosurg Psychiatry* 47:947-952, 1984.

279. Den Heijer JC, Bollern WLE, Reulen JP, et al: Autonomic nervous function in Huntington's disease, *Arch Neurol* 45:309-312, 1988.

280. Passant U, Warkentin S. Gustafson L: Orthostatic hypotension and low blood pressure in organic dementia: A study of prevalence and related clinical characteristics, *Int J Geriatr Psychiatry* 12(3):395-403, 1997.

281. White AT, Wilson TE, Davis SL, et al: Effect of precooling on physical performance in multiple sclerosis. *Mult Scler* 6(3):176-180, 2000.

282. Webbon B, Montgomery L, Miller L, et al: A comparison of three liquid-ventilation cooling garments during treadmill exercise, *Aviat Space Environ Med* 52:408-415, 1981.

283. Schwid SR, Petrie MD, Murray R, et al: A randomized controlled study of the acute and chronic effects of cooling therapy for MS, *Neurology* 60(12) 1955-1960, 2003.

284. Ponichtera-Mulcare JA, Mathews T, Barrett PJ, et al: Change in aerobic fitness of patients with multiple sclerosis during a 6-month training program. *Sports Med Train Rehabil* 7:265-272, 1997.

285. Rodgers MM, Mulcare JA, King DL, et al: Gait characteristics of individuals with multiple sclerosis before and after a 6-month aerobic training program, *J Rehabil Res Dev* 36(3):183-188, 1999.

286. Petajan JH, Gappmaier E, White AT, et al: Impact of aerobic training on fitness and quality of life in multiple sclerosis, *Ann Neurol* 39(4):432-441, 1996.

287. Bridgewater KJ, Sharpe MH: Aerobic exercise and early Parkinson's disease, *J Neurol Rehabil* 10(4):233-241, 1996.

288. Bergen JL, Toole T, Elliott RG, et al: Aerobic exercise intervention improves aerobic capacity and movement initiation in Parkinson's disease patients, *Neurol Rehabil* 17:161-168, 2002.

289. Pinto AC, Alves M, Nogueira A: Can amyotrophic lateral sclerosis patients with respiratory insufficiency exercise? *J Neurol Sci* 169:69-75, 1999.

290. Kirkinezos IG, Hernandez D, Bradley WG, et al: Regular exercise is beneficial to a mouse model of amyotrophic lateral sclerosis, *Ann Neurol* 53:804-807, 2003.

291. Veldink JH, Bar PR, Joosten EA, Mahoney DJ, et al: Sexual differences in onset of disease and response to exercise in a transgenic model of ALS, *Neuromuscul Disord* 13:737-743, 2003.

292. Mahoney DJ, Rodriguez C, Devries M, et al: Effects of high-intensity endurance exercise training in the G93A mouse model of amyotrophic lateral sclerosis, *Muscle Nerve* 29:656-662, 2004.

293. Arkin SM: Student-led exercise sessions yield significant fitness gains for Alzheimer's patients, *Am J Alzheimers Dis Other Demen* 18(3):159-170, 2003.

294. Shumway-Cook A, Woollacott MH: *Motor Control: Theory and Practical Applications*, ed 2, Philadelphia, 2001, Lippincott Williams & Wilkins.

295. Morris ME: Movement disorders in people with Parkinson disease: A model for physical therapy, *Phys Ther* 80(6):578-597, 2000.

296. Morris ME, Bruce M, Smithson F, et al: Physiotherapy strategies for people with Parkinson's disease. In Morris ME, Iansek R (eds): *Parkinson's Disease: A Team Approach*, Blackburn, Victoria, Australia, 1997, Buscombe-Vicprint.

297. Morris M, Huxham F, McGinley J: Strategies to prevent falls in people with Parkinson's disease, *Physiotherapy Singapore* 2:135-141, 1999.

298. Dibble LE, Nicholson DE: Sensory cueing improves motor performance and rehabilitation in persons with Parkinson's disease, *Neurol Rep* 21:117-124, 1997.

299. Melnick ME: Basal ganglia disorders: Metabolic, hereditary, and genetic disorders in adults. In Umphred DA (ed): *Neurological Rehabilitation*, ed 4, St. Louis, 2001, Mosby.

300. Palmer SS, Mortimer JA, Webster DD, et al: Exercise therapy for Parkinson's disease, *Arch Phys Med Rehabil* 67:741, 1986.

301. Comella CL, Stebbins GT, Brown-Toms N, et al: Physical therapy and Parkinson's disease: a controlled clinical trial, *Neurology* 44:376-378, 1994.

302. Hirsch MA, Toole T, Maitland CG, et al: The effects of balance training and high-intensity resistance training on persons with idiopathic Parkinson's disease, *Arch Phys Med Rehabil* 84(8):1109-1117, 2003.

303. Morgan MH: Ataxia and weights, *Physiotherapy* 61:332-334, 1975.

304. Lucy SD, Hayes KC: Postural sway profiles: Normal subjects and subjects with cerebellar ataxia, *Physiother Can* 37:140-148, 1985.

305. Manto M, Godaux E, Jacquy J: Cerebellar hypermetria is larger when the inertial load is artificially increased, *Ann Neurol* 35:45-52, 1994.

306. Clopton N, Schultz D, Boren C, et al: Effects of axial weight loading on gait for subjects with cerebellar ataxia: Preliminary findings, *Neurol Rep* 27(1):15-21, 2003.

307. Cailliet R: Exercise in multiple sclerosis. In Basmajian IV (ed): *Therapeutic Exercise*, Baltimore, 1984, Williams & Wilkins.

308. Sheikh K, Smith DS, Meade TW, et al: Repeatability and validity of a modified activities of daily living (ADL) index in studies of chronic disability, *Int Rehabil Med* 1(2):51-58, 1979.

309. Jones L, Lewis Y, Harrison J, et al: The effectiveness of occupational therapy and physiotherapy in multiple sclerosis patients with ataxia of the upper limb and trunk, *Clin Rehabil* 20:277-282, 1996.

310. Stephens J, DuShuttle D, Hatcher C, et al: Use of awareness through movement improves balance and balance confidence in people with multiple sclerosis: A randomized controlled study, *Neurol Rep* 25:39-49, 2001.

311. Kasser SL, Rose DJ, Clark S: Balance training for adults with multiple sclerosis: Multiple case studies, *Neurol Rep* 23:5-12, 1999.

312. Hageman PA, Thomas VS: Gait performance in dementia: The effects of a 6 week resistance training program in and adult day-care setting, *Int J Geriatr Pyschiatry* 17:329-334, 2002.

313. Thomas VS, Hageman PA: Can neuromuscular strength and function in people with dementia be rehabilitated using resistance-exercise training? Results from a preliminary intervention study, *J Gerontol* 58A(8):746-751, 2003.

314. Rolland Y, Rival L, Pillard F, et al: Feasibility of regular physical exercise for patients with moderate to severe Alzheimer's disease, *J Nutr Health Aging* 4(2):109-113, 2000.

315. Drory VE, Goltsman E, Reznik JG, et al: The value of muscle exercise in patients with amyotrophic lateral sclerosis, *J Neurol Sci* 191:133-137, 2001.

316. Peacock IW: A physical therapy program for Huntington's disease patients, *Clin Management Phys Ther* 7:22-23, 34, 1987.

317. Imbriglio S: Huntington's disease at mid-stage, *Clin Manage* 12:62-72, 1992.

318. Scandalis TA, Bosak A, Berliner JC, et al: Resistance training and gait function in patients with Parkinson's disease, *Am J Phys Med Rehabil* 80(1):38-43, 2001.

319. Reuter I, Engelhardt M, Stecker K, et al: Therapeutic value of exercise training in Parkinson's disease, *Med Sci Sports Exerc* 31(11):1544-1549, 1999.

320. Schenkman M, Cutson TM, Kuchibhatla M, et al: Exercise to improve spinal flexibility and function for people with Parkinson's disease: a randomized, controlled trial, *J Am Geriatr Soc* 46(10):1207-1216, 1998.

321. Curtis CL, Bassile CC, Cote LJ, et al: Effects of exercise on the motor control of individuals with Parkinson's disease: case studies, *Neurology Rep* 25(1):2-11, 2001.

322. Pellecchia MT, Grasso A, Biancardi LG, et al: Physical therapy in Parkinson's disease: an open long-term rehabilitation trial, *J Neurol* 251(5):595-598, 2004.

323. Ellis T, De Goede CJ, Feldman RG, et al: Efficacy of a physical therapy program in patients with Parkinson's disease: A randomized controlled trial, *Arch Phys Med Rehabil* 86(4):626-632, 2005.

324. Romberg A, Virtanen A, Ruutiainen J: Long-term exercise improves functional impairment but not quality of life in multiple sclerosis, *J Neurol* 252(7):839-845, 2005.

325. DeBolt LS, McCubbin JA: The effects of home-based resistance exercise on balance, power and mobility in adults with multiple sclerosis, *Arch Phys Med Rehabil* 85(2):290-297, 2004.

326. Romberg A, Virtanen A, Ruutiainen J: Effects of a 6-month exercise program on patients with multiple sclerosis: A randomized study, *Neurology* 63(11):2034-2038, 2004.

327. White LJ, McCoy SC, Castellano V, et al: Resistance training improves strength and functional capacity in persons with multiple sclerosis, *Mult Scler* 10(6):668-674, 2004.

328. Harvey L, Smith AD, Jones R: The effect of weighted leg raises on quadriceps strength, EMG parameters and functional activities in people with multiple sclerosis, *Physiotherapy* 85(3):154-161, 1999.

329. Oken BS, Kishiyama S, Zajdel D, et al: Randomized controlled trial of yoga and exercise in multiple sclerosis, *Neurology* 62(11):2058-2064, 2004.

330. Patti F, Ciancio MR, Cacopardo M, et al: Effects of a short outpatient rehabilitation treatment on disability of multiple sclerosis patients—a randomized controlled trial, *J Neurol* 250(7):861-866, 2003.

331. Lui C, Playford ED, Thompson AJ: Does neurorehabilitation have a role in relapsing-remitting multiple sclerosis? *J Neurol* 250(10):1214-1218, 2003.

332. Gehlsen GM, Grigsby SA, Winant DM: Effects of an aquatic fitness program on the muscular strength and endurance of patients with multiple sclerosis, *Phys Ther* 64(5):653-657, 1984.

333. Roehrs TG, Karst GM: Effects of an aquatics exercise program on quality of life measures for individuals with progressive multiple sclerosis, *J Neurol Phys Ther* 28(2):63-71, 2004.

334. Peterson C: Exercise in 94 degrees F water for a patient with multiple sclerosis, *Phys Ther* 81(4):1049-1058, 2001.

335. Smeltzer SC, Lavietes MH, Cook SD: Expiratory training in multiple sclerosis, *Arch Phys Med Rehabil* 77:909-912, 1996.

336. Gosselink R, Kovacs L, Ketelaer P, et al: Respiratory muscle weakness and respiratory muscle training in severely disabled multiple sclerosis patients, *Arch Phys Med Rehabil* 81(6):747-751, 2000.

337. Duff S, Quinn L: Motor learning and motor control. In Cech D, Martin T: *Functional Movement Development Across the Lifespan*, ed 2, Philadelphia, 2002, WB Saunders.

338. Miyai I, Fujimoto Y, Ueda Y, et al: Treatmill training with body weight support: its efficacy on Parkinson's disease, *Arch Phys Med Rehabil* 81(7):849-852, 2000.

339. Miyai I, Fujimoto Y, Yamamoto H, et al: Long-term effect of body weight-supported treadmill training in Parkinson's disease: A randomized controlled trial, *Arch Phys Med Rehabil* 83(10):1370-1373, 2002.

340. Pohl M, Rockstroh G, Ruckriem S, et al: Immediate effects of speed-dependent treadmill training on gait parameters in early Parkinson's disease, *Arch Phys Med Rehabil* 84(12):1760-1766, 2003.

341. Bagley S, Kelly B, Tunnicliffe N, et al: The effect of visual cues on the gait of independently mobile Parkinson's disease patients, *Physiotherapy* 77(6):415-420, 1991.

342. Bilney B, Morris ME, Denisenko S: Physiotherapy for people with movement disorders arising from basal ganglia dysfunction, *N Z J Physiother* 31(2):94-100, 2003.

343. Suteerawattananon M, Morris GS, Etnyre BR, et al: Effects of visual and auditory cues on gait in individuals with Parkinson's disease, *J Neurol Sci* 219(1-2):63-69, 2004.

344. Thaut MH, Miltner R, Lange HW, et al: Velocity modulation and rhythmic synchronization of gait in Huntington's disease, *Mov Disord* 14:808-819, 1999.

345. Sidaway B, Anderson J, Danielson G, et al: Effects of long-term gait training using visual cues in an individual with Parkinson disease, *Phys Ther* 86(2):186-194, 2006.

346. Dibble LE, Nicholson DE, Shultz B, et al: Sensory cueing effects on maximal speed gait initiation in persons with Parkinson's disease and healthy elders, *Gait Posture* 19(3):215-225, 2004.

347. Schenkman M, Donovan J, Tsubota J, et al: Management of individuals with Parkinson's disease: Rationale and case studies, *Phys Ther* 69(11):944-955, 1987.

348. Jacobson E: *Progressive Relaxation*, Chicago, 1938, University of Chicago Press.

349. Platz T, Brown, RG, Marsden CD: Training improves the speed of aimed movements in Parkinson's disease, *Brain* 121:505-514, 1998.

350. Miller RG, Rosenberg JA, Gelinas DF, et al: ALS Practice Parameters Task Force: the care of the patient of amyotrophic lateral sclerosis (an evidence-based review): Report of the Quality Standards Subcommittee of the American Academy of Neurology: ALS Practice Parameters Task Force, *Neurology* 52:1311-1323, 1999.

351. Bach JR: Amyotrophic lateral sclerosis: Predictors for prolongation of life by noninvasive respiratory aids, *Arch Phys Med Rehabil* 76:828-832, 1995.

352. Moss AH, Casey P, Stocking CB, et al: Home ventilation for amyotrophic lateral sclerosis patients: Outcomes, costs and patient, family and physician attitudes, *Neurology* 38:409-413, 1993.

353. Cazzolli PA, Oppenheimer EA: Home mechanical ventilation for amyotrophic lateral sclerosis: Nasal compared to tracheostomy-intermittent positive pressure ventilation, *J Neurol Sci* 139(suppl):123-128, 1996.

354. Moss AH, Oppenheimer EA, Casey P, et al: Patients with amyotrophic lateral sclerosis receiving long-term mechanical ventilation: Advance care planning and outcomes, *Chest* 110:249-255, 1996.

355. Howard RS, Wiles CM, Loh L: Respiratory complications and their management in motor neuron disease, *Brain* 112:1155-1170, 1989.

356. Piper AJ, Sullivan CE: Effects of long-term nocturnal nasal ventilation on spontaneous breathing during sleep in neuromuscular and chest wall disorders, *Eur Respir J* 9:1515-1522, 1996.

357. Pinto AC, Evangelista T, Carvalho M, et al: Respiratory assistance with a non-invasive ventilator (Bipap) in MND/ALS patients: survival rates in controlled trials, *J Neurol Sci* 129(suppl):19-26, 1995.

358. Oppenheimer EA: Decision-making in the respiratory care of amyotrophic lateral sclerosis: should home mechanical ventilation be used? *Palliat Med* 5(suppl 2):49-64, 1993.

359. Goldblatt D, Greenlaw J: Starting and stopping the ventilator for patients with amyotrophic lateral sclerosis, *Neurol Clin* 7:789-806, 1989.

360. Sancho J, Servera E, Diaz J, et al: Efficacy of mechanical insufflation-exsufflation in medically stable patients with amyotrophic lateral sclerosis, *Chest* 125(4):1400-1405, 2004.

361. Lahrmann H, Wild M, Zdrahal F, et al: Expiratory muscle weakness and assisted cough in ALS, *Amyotroph Lateral Scler Other Motor Neuron Disord* 4(1):49-51, 2003.

362. Hanayama K, Yuka I, Bach JR: Amyotrophic lateral sclerosis: Successful treatment of mucous plugging by mechanical insufflation-exsufflation, *Am J Phys Med Rehabil* 76:338-339, 1997.

Peripheral Nerve Injuries

Ginny Gibson

OBJECTIVES

After reading this chapter, the reader will be able to:
1. Describe the mechanisms of and classification systems for peripheral nerve injuries and their relevance to functional outcomes.
2. Describe the etiology and resultant clinical picture of common peripheral nerve injuries.
3. Explain the physiological processes after nerve injury and repair.
4. Summarize current approaches to surgical and medical management of peripheral nerve injuries.
5. Explain the relevance and general methods of electromyographic and nerve conduction testing.
6. Determine and describe the examination specific to the client with peripheral nerve pathology.
7. Describe rehabilitation interventions for patients with traumatic peripheral nerve injury, nerve compression and nerve entrapment.

Depending on the nature and extent of peripheral nerve pathology, individuals with peripheral nerve injury* experience various degrees of recovery and in more advanced or severe injury, often do not return to their prior functional status. Appropriate interventions can reduce the extent of long-term dysfunction. This chapter describes the nature of peripheral nerve injury, reviews the examination shown to aid in determining a diagnosis and prognosis, and describes interventions shown to be effective in the rehabilitation of individuals with peripheral nerve injuries.

OVERVIEW OF THE PERIPHERAL NERVOUS SYSTEM

The nervous system is typically divided into central and peripheral components. Central components include nerves that are wholly contained within the brain and spinal cord. Peripheral components include nerves that originate in the brain or spinal cord and end peripherally, as well as cranial and spinal nerves. The *peripheral nervous system* (PNS) includes motor, sensory, sympathetic, and parasympathetic *neurons,* with most nerves containing a mixture of these types of neurons. *Efferent pathways* (those that send messages from the center to the periphery) include somatic motor nerves that innervate skeletal muscles and the *autonomic nervous system* (ANS) with sympathetic and parasympathetic divisions that regulate smooth muscle, cardiac muscle, and glandular activity (Fig. 18-1). *Afferent* pathways (those that send messages from the periphery towards the center) transmit a range of sensory modalities including touch, position, vibration and pain.[1,2]

---

*For clarity, this chapter will use the term injury to refer to all insults to peripheral nerves.

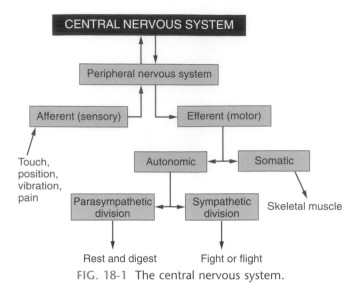

FIG. 18-1 The central nervous system.

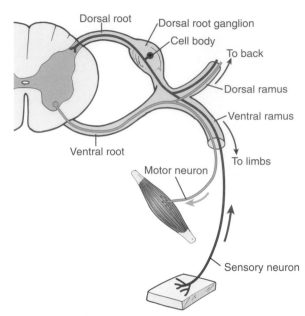

FIG. 18-2 Spinal nerves contain motor nerves that originate in the anterior horn of the spinal cord and sensory nerves that originate in the dorsal horn of the spinal cord.

Motor nerves originate in the anterior horn of the spinal cord, and sensory nerves originate in the dorsal root ganglia. Sympathetic nerves originate in the lateral horn of the thoracic spinal cord and continue in sympathetic ganglia. Parasympathetic nerves originate from the brain and lateral gray matter of the sacral spinal cord and continue in the parasympathetic ganglia. Motor neurons of *cranial nerves* extend from the brainstem, and sensory neurons of cranial nerves have their cell bodies in cranial nerve ganglia. Motor and sensory cranial nerves serve structures in the head and neck, with the exception of the vagus nerve, which also continues to the chest and abdomen. Spinal nerves, of which there are 31 pairs, extend from their cell bodies and provide sensory and motor functions to all of the body, except the head.[1,2]

Spinal nerves, with their contributory dorsal and ventral roots, exit the intervertebral foramen and divide into dorsal and ventral rami (Fig. 18-2). With exception of the thoracic region, the ventral rami combine to form the cervical, brachial, and lumbosacral *plexuses* (Fig. 18-3).[1,2] This chapter discusses the examination and management of clients with nerve damage distal to these plexuses, as well as injuries to cranial nerves.

ANATOMY OF A PERIPHERAL NERVE

Neural tissue includes excitable neurons (nerve cells) that propagate electrical impulses and *glia* cells that facilitate impulse conduction and support and protect the neurons.[1] All neurons have a cell body that contains a nucleus and organelles (mitochondria, rough endoplasmic reticulum, ribosomes, and Golgi apparatus). Almost all of a neuron's proteins, enzymes, and organelles are synthesized in the cell body. Most neurons have *dendrites,* an *axon,* and terminal branches. Dendrites are branching and tapering extensions of the axon that receive signals from other neurons, which the axon then carries to the cell body. Signals are then carried away from the cell body toward terminal branches, where electrical

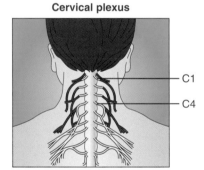

Cervical plexus

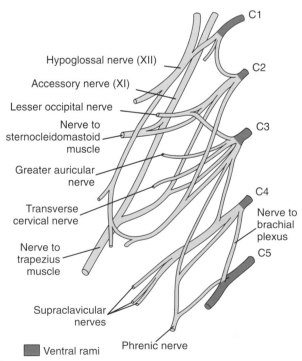

FIG. 18-3 **A,** Cervical plexus.

A

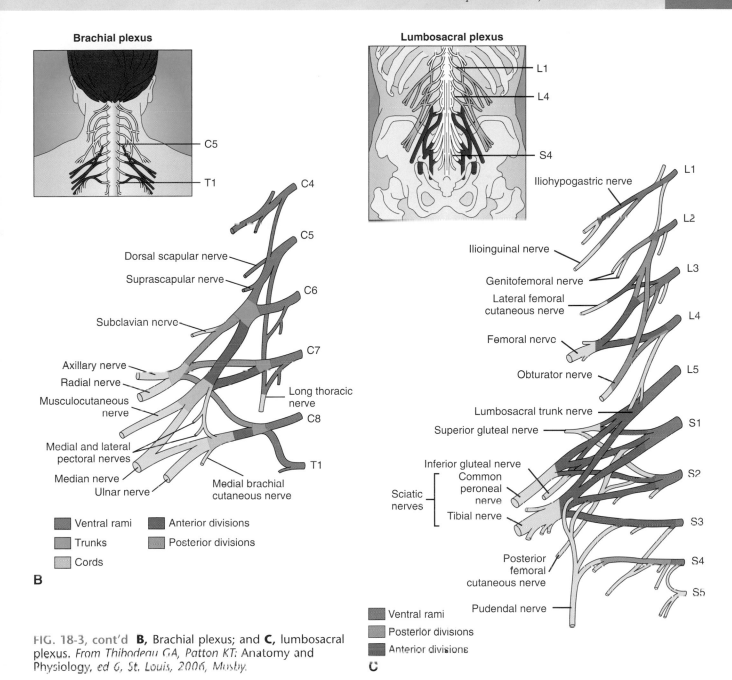

Brachial plexus

C5
T1

C4
C5
Dorsal scapular nerve
C6
Suprascapular nerve
Subclavian nerve
C7
Axillary nerve
Radial nerve
Long thoracic nerve
Musculocutaneous nerve
C8
Medial and lateral pectoral nerves
T1
Median nerve
Ulnar nerve
Medial brachial cutaneous nerve

Ventral rami	Anterior divisions
Trunks	Posterior divisions
Cords	

B

Lumbosacral plexus

L1
L4
S4

L1
Iliohypogastric nerve
L2
Ilioinguinal nerve
L3
Genitofemoral nerve
Lateral femoral cutaneous nerve
L4
Femoral nerve
Obturator nerve
L5
Lumbosacral trunk nerve
Superior gluteal nerve
S1
Inferior gluteal nerve
Common peroneal nerve
S2
Sciatic nerves
Tibial nerve
S3
Posterior femoral cutaneous nerve
S4
Pudendal nerve
S5

Ventral rami	
Posterior divisions	
Anterior divisions	

C

FIG. 18-3, cont'd **B**, Brachial plexus; and **C**, lumbosacral plexus. *From Thibodeau GA, Patton KT:* Anatomy and Physiology, *ed 6, St. Louis, 2006, Mosby.*

and chemical signals are transmitted to other nerves or end-organs.[1,2]

In the PNS axons are wrapped in *myelin* from *Schwann cells.* A single Schwann cell wraps around an axon in a spiral fashion with small gaps, known as *nodes of Ranvier,* approximately 1 mm apart. The segments of axon between the nodes of Ranvier are called the internodes (Fig. 18-4). The myelin sheath accelerates the propagation of signals along the axon because impulses can jump from node to node rather than traversing the entire length of the nerve. This is known as saltatory conduction. Unmyelinated neurons conduct more slowly because they do not have a myelin sheath, although there are some Schwann cells within bundles of unmyelinated neurons.[1,2]

A nerve consists of multiple neurons. Each neuron is surrounded by a semipermeable membrane called the *plasmalemma.* Groups of neurons are arranged in bundles, called *fascicles,* and groups of fascicles make up a nerve. Protective coverings of connective tissue, called endoneurium, perineurium, and epineurium, envelop individual neurons, fascicles, and groups of fascicles, respectively (Fig. 18-5). The endoneurium, which is composed primarily of loose connective tissue, provides electrical insulation between neurons and in part, prevents elongation of the nerve under tension. The perineurium, which is composed of multiple layers of dense connective tissue, resists tensile forces from stretching, helps to maintain intrafascicular pressure, and acts as a chemical barrier. The epineurium is composed of two layers of collagen and

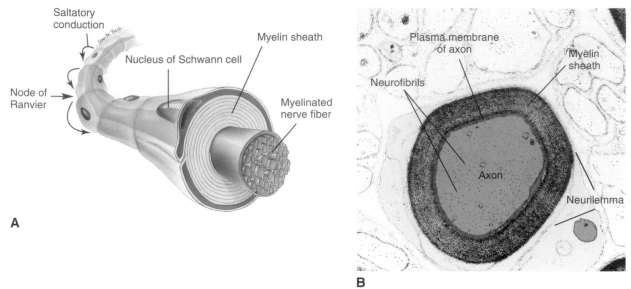

FIG. 18-4 A myelinated peripheral nerve. Note that the Schwann cell forms the myelin that wraps around the nerve axon and that the myelin promotes faster nerve transmission by allowing for saltatory conduction. *A Courtesy Brenda Russell, PhD, University of Illinois at Chicago; B from Thibodeau GA, Patton KT:* Anatomy and Physiology, *ed 6, St. Louis, 2006, Mosby.*

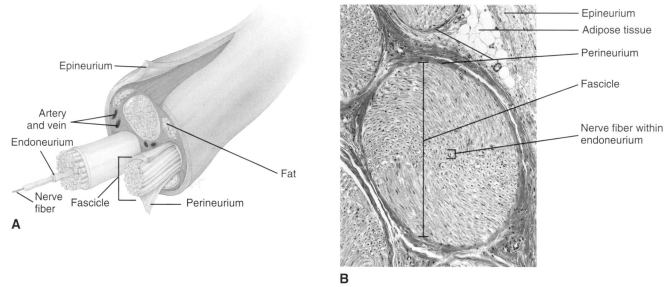

FIG. 18-5 Cross-section of a peripheral nerve showing the nerve fibers, fascicles, and groups of fascicles enveloped in endoneurium, perineurium, and epineurium, respectively. *From Thibodeau GA, Patton KT:* Anatomy and Physiology, *ed 6, St. Louis, 2006, Mosby.*

fibroblasts and accounts for much of a nerve's cross-sectional area.[2] The innermost layer is loose and fills space around groups of fascicles, and the outer layer surrounds the entire nerve. The epineurium provides tensile strength and cushions fascicles from external trauma. Surrounding the epineurium is a layer of loose areolar tissue called the mesoneurium.[3]

Along a nerve, the thickness and presence of connective tissue layers vary. Where nerves cross over joints there is more connective tissue. The epineurium thins distally and both perineurium and epineurium are absent proxi-mally at the spinal nerve root. Nerves may be more prone to injury at locations where the layers are thinner or absent.[3]

BLOOD SUPPLY OF PERIPHERAL NERVES

Peripheral nerves require oxygen to maintain the energy levels needed for axonal transport and cell viability. Nerves receive oxygen via extraneural and intraneural blood vessels.[4] The extraneural vessels lie next to the nerves and the intraneural vessels are within the endoneurium, perineurium, and epineurium (Fig. 18-6).

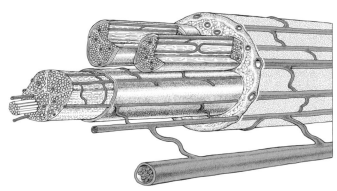

FIG. 18-6 *Vascular supply of the peripheral nerve. Adapted from Lundborg G:* Nerve Injury and Repair, *Edinburgh, 1988, Churchill Livingstone.*

The extraneural vessels connect to the intra-neural vessels through the mesoneurium. There are larger vessels in the epineurium and perineurium and only a fine capillary network in the endoneurium. This network of capillaries is susceptible to compression injury.[5]

Peripheral nerves are immunologically isolated from the rest of the body by a blood-nerve barrier, comprised of tightly packed endothelial cells of the endoneurium and the internal layers of the perineurium. Injury to a nerve and the blood-nerve barrier may result in exposure of the nerve and trigger an immunological response.[6]

PERIPHERAL NERVE END-ORGANS

Peripheral nerves connect distally to end-organs that are sensory receptors, muscles, or glands. Sensory end-organs include mechanoreceptors, thermoreceptors, nociceptors, chemoreceptors, photoreceptors, and free nerve endings. Different subtypes of sensory end-organs are listed and described in Table 18-1. Mechanoreceptors, thermoreceptors, and nociceptors detect sensory stimulation subsequent to chemical changes or physical deformation of the receptor.[1,2]

In the somatic motor system, a single alpha motor neuron and all of the muscle fibers it innervates are known as a *motor unit*. A single motor unit, when stimulated sufficiently, will cause all of the muscle fibers it innervates to contract. Within the ANS, efferent pathways signal secretions from glands, including sweat glands.[1,2]

PERIPHERAL NERVE CLASSIFICATION

Peripheral nerves can be classified by axon diameter or by speed of conduction (Table 18-2). When classified according to size or diameter of the axon, neurons are referred to as type I, II, III, or IV, with type I the largest and type IV the smallest. Only sensory neurons are classified by size. Type I, II, and III axons are myelinated, and type IV axons are unmyelinated. Large diameter axons conduct rapidly and have lower thresholds for electrical stimulation.[1,2]

When classified according to *nerve conduction velocity* (NCV), the speed at which electrical impulses can be propagated along the axon, neurons are classified as type A or B, which are myelinated, or type C, which are unmyelinated. Both sensory and motor neurons are classified according to speed of conduction. There are four subtypes of A fibers: A-alpha neurons, A-beta neurons, A-gamma neurons, and A-delta neurons.

PHYSIOLOGY OF THE PERIPHERAL NERVOUS SYSTEM

AXONAL TRANSPORT

Neurotransmitters, proteins, and organelles are transported along axons using a system of microtubules and neurofibrils. Anterograde flow provides transport away from the cell body and occurs either quickly or slowly. Neurotransmitters and structures necessary to replenish the plasmalemma are transported quickly, whereas proteins and organelles needed for new axoplasm or to replenish axoplasm in regenerating neurons or mature neurons are transported more slowly. Retrograde flow, toward the cell body, occurs at a constant slow rate and returns organelles

TABLE 18-1	Cutaneous Sensory End-Organ Receptors			
Type of Receptor	**Name of Receptor**	**Encapsulated or Free**	**Stimulation Detected**	**Adaptation**
Mechanoreceptor	Ruffini's corpuscle	Encapsulated (thin)	Deep pressure, stretch of skin	Slow
	Pacinian corpuscle	Encapsulated	Deep moving pressure, stretch, high frequency vibration (256 Hz)	Rapid
	Meissner's corpuscle	Encapsulated	Light pressure, light moving touch, low frequency vibration (30 Hz)	Rapid
	Root hair plexus	Free	Hair deflection	Rapid
	Merkel's disc	Encapsulated	Light pressure, constant touch	Slow
	Free nerve ending	Free	Pressure	Slow
	Muscle spindle	Encapsulated (thin)	Type Ia: Rate and degree of muscle stretch and tension	Slow and rapid
			Type II: Degree of stretch and tension	
	Golgi tendon organ		Tendon stretch, muscle tension	Slow
Thermoreceptors	Free nerve ending	Free	Temperature	
Nociceptors	Free nerve ending	Free	Pain	Slow and rapid

TABLE 18-2	Two Systems for Classifying Peripheral Nerves

By Diameter		Function
Fiber Classification	**Diameter (μm)**	
Ia	12-20	Muscle spindle primary endings
Ib	11-19	Golgi tendon organs
II	5-12	Touch, kinesthesia, muscle spindle secondary endings
III	1-5	Pain, crude touch, pressure, temperature
IV	0.1-2	Pain, touch, pressure, temperature

By Conduction Velocity		Function
Fiber Classification	**Conduction Velocity (m/sec)**	
A-alpha	70-120	Alpha-motoneurons, muscle spindle primary endings, Golgi tendon organs, touch
A-beta	40-70	Touch, kinesthesia, muscle spindle secondary endings
A-gamma	15-40	Touch, pressure, gamma-motoneurons
A-delta	5-15	Pain, crude touch, pressure, temperature
B	3-14	Preganglionic autonomic
C	0.2-2	Pain, touch, pressure, temperature, postganglionic autonomic

to the cell body for disposal and carries nerve growth factor toward the cell body. Both anterograde flow and retrograde flow require an energy source that is compromised if circulation is disrupted.[8]

ION CHANNELS AND NERVE CONDUCTION

Two ions, potassium (K+) and sodium (Na+), are primarily responsible for nerve conduction. At rest, there is more sodium outside and more potassium inside a neuron. These concentrations are maintained by chemical and electrical gradients together with the sodium-potassium adenosinetriphosphatase (ATPase) pumps that pump three sodium ions out of the cell for every two potassium ions they pump into the cell. At rest, a neuron is more negatively charged inside than outside and has a resting membrane potential of −60 to −90 mV.

When the nerve is stimulated sufficiently, sodium ions will enter the neuron, depolarizing it. The depolarization is quickly followed by repolarization, and this sequence of depolarization and repolarization is known as an *action potential* (Fig. 18-7, *A*). The action potential will then be propagated along the nerve until it reaches the end of the nerve (Fig. 18-7, *B*).

A *synapse* is the meeting point of the axon terminal of one neuron (the presynaptic neuron) and a dendritic ending or cell body of another neuron (the postsynaptic neuron). The presynaptic axon terminal has vesicles containing a neurotransmitter that is released into the synaptic cleft, the space between the presynaptic and postsynaptic nerve, in response to an electrical signal (Fig. 18-8). The neurotransmitter then binds to postsynaptic receptors causing the postsynaptic nerve to become excited (i.e., less negative), if more sodium ions enter the neuron, or inhibited (i.e., more negative), if chloride ions enter the neuron.[1,2] Each neuron can receive inputs from many other neurons and with a sufficient dominance of depolarizing inputs, an action potential will start in the postsynaptic neuron and propagate along the length of this nerve.

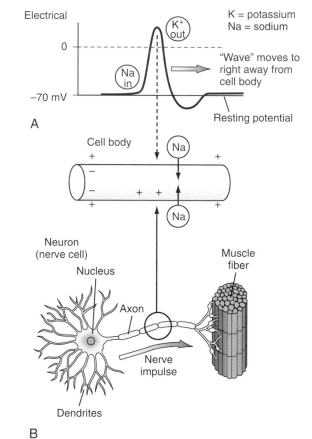

FIG. 18-7 An action potential propagating along a nerve. *Copyright Royal Society of Chemistry 2006.*

EFFECTS OF MOVEMENT ON PERIPHERAL NERVES

Movement and positioning of the limbs, head, neck, or trunk can cause nerves to slide, become elongated, or recoil.[9-11] The tissues around peripheral nerves, including

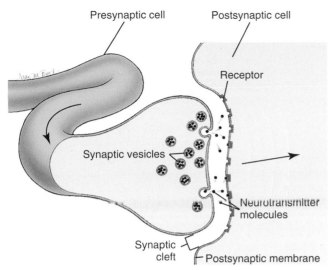

FIG. 18-8 Synaptic transmission. *From Thibodeau GA, Patton KT:* Anatomy and Physiology, *ed 6, St. Louis, 2006, Mosby.*

bone, cartilage, muscle, tendon, vessels, and fascia, form tunnels or passageways of various sizes through which the nerves pass. These tunnels may apply pressure to the nerves when the nerves move. Movement at one joint may require the nerve to lengthen at that joint and can pull on the nerve where it crosses other joints.[11] When a nerve is elongated it gets narrower,[12] intraneural pressure increases,[12-14] blood flow decreases,[15,16] and strain increases.[11,17] Strain on the median and ulnar nerves has also been shown to increase more with movement (activity) than with maintained postures that impose incremental strain.[10]

NERVE PATHOLOGY

Nerve pathology can be localized or diffuse and may be caused by acute or cumulative trauma. An isolated nerve lesion is termed a *mononeuropathy,* and a condition with asymmetrical lesions of multiple nerves is termed *mononeuropathy multiplex.* Symmetrical diffuse nerve dysfunction is termed *polyneuropathy.* Polyneuropathy generally presents initially with symmetric distal symptoms and is most often caused by a disease process rather than trauma (see Chapter 19).

MECHANISMS OF NERVE INJURY

The mechanism of a nerve injury influences its acute and long-term consequences and the selection of medical, surgical, and rehabilitation interventions. Nerves may be injured by excessive stretch or compression, inadequate blood supply, or exposure to excessive electric energy, radiation, or toxins. Inadequate blood supply is a feature of most mechanically-induced nerve injury. Regardless of the mechanism of injury, the clinical findings of pain, paresthesia, and motor impairment are similar for most nerve injuries.

Nerves may be injured by a single application of high force traction or by repeated application of lower levels of traction that would not cause injury if they occurred only

once.[18] Acute traction injuries are associated with fractures, either directly or secondary to reduction or fixation; joint dislocation; extreme limb or body segment positioning, as might occur during positioning for surgical access; and pulling on a limb segment, as seen in obstetrical brachial plexus injury. Traction injuries have also been reported during and subsequent to limb-lengthening procedures.[19] When nerves are stretched by more than 6% to 8% of their original length, intraneural circulation is impaired[15] and compound motor action potentials are reduced.[20] Stretching of a nerve by more than 10% to 20% of its original length is associated with structural failure[21,22] and changes in compound motor action potentials to complete conduction block.[20,23] With elongation by 20% to 30% or more, perineural sheaths begin to rupture.[24] After intraneural tearing, there is hemorrhage and consequently intraneural scarring as a result of proliferation of fibroblasts and production of collagen.[25]

Nerves may be compressed by a variety of mechanisms. Edema from acute and chronic inflammation,[26] inflammatory diseases, increased compartmental pressures, space-occupying lesions, contact against bones, and entrapment within soft tissues, as well as iatrogenic causes, such as tourniquet[27] and blood pressure cuff application, are all associated with compression neuropathies.[28,29] Koo and Szabo proposed that *ischemia* may underlie the nerve damage associated with compression neuropathies and that when secondary effects of ischemia, including segmental anoxia, capillary vasodilation, and edema, are managed early, good symptom resolution follows. However, with chronic compression, intraneural fibrosis appears to impede recovery.[30]

The amount of compression applied to a nerve affects the nature and degree of nerve damage. Under normal circumstances the pressure on the median nerve in the carpal tunnel is approximately 2.5 mm Hg.[31] Peripheral nerves have been shown to be damaged, with partial or complete blocking of axonal transport and increased vascular permeability resulting in edema,[32,33] when exposed to pressures of more than 30 mm Hg, and complete ischemia occurs at pressures over 60-70 mm Hg.[34,35] Because there are no lymphatic vessels in the endoneural space, intraneural edema can take a long time to resolve.

The nature of a nerve injury also depends on the duration of compression and how much of the nerve is compressed.[36] Acute and localized compression generally causes less severe injury than chronic and diffuse compression.[37] Szabo and Sharkey compared cyclic compression, as one might see in repetitive motion, with chronic compression in rats (in this case, chronic compression lasted 6 hours) and found that cyclic and chronic compression caused similar changes in nerve conduction velocity.[38]

Experimental studies of controlled vibration and studies with workers using vibrating tools have found that vibration can cause nerve demyelination and fibrosis.[39,40] Vibration is thought to cause damage directly and indirectly, by causing edema.[41] Vibration-induced nerve injury is common in workers using heavy machinery such as jack-hammers.[42]

Nerve ischemia may also be caused by vascular occlusion[43] and other vascular disorders. Chronic ischemia damages the blood-nerve barrier, causing an influx of proteinaceous fluid followed by a proliferation of fibroblasts and intraneural scarring. Since ischemic injury alone does not disturb the continuity of the plasmalemma, nerves recover more readily from this type of injury than from others. However, prolonged ischemia may lead to nerve *infarction,* which then has a similar prognosis to nerve injuries with other mechanisms.[44,45]

When a nerve is subjected to accidental injection, it may be damaged by the physical trauma of the needle and by exposure to the drug or agent. Accidental injection injuries occur most often during medication delivery,[46,47] with the sciatic nerve being the nerve most frequently injured by injection.[48] Needle-stick injuries to nerves during acupuncture are rare but have also been reported.[49] Injection of a nerve usually causes severe, radiating pain.

Nerve lacerations can occur as result of contact with a sharp object, such as a piece of glass, metal, knife, razor blade, or scalpel, or from contact with a blunt object, such as components of power tools or other machinery, and gunshot wounds. Sharp injuries may occur intraoperatively.[50] Blunt objects generally produce jagged, shredded injuries with ill-defined edges, whereas sharp objects produce injuries with a well-defined edge. Gunshot wounds may injure a nerve directly or secondarily as the result of shock, blast, or cavitation effects.[51,52]

Nerves may also be damaged by heat, either through direct exposure or by exposure to electrical current or radiation. Nerve tissue has the lowest electrical impedance of any body tissue, therefore electrical currents tend to travel along neurovascular bundles. Most neurovascular bundles run deep to the muscles they innervate, thus tissues lying close to this pathway may also be damaged. An electrical current can injure nerves directly by heating them and causing coagulation necrosis or by damaging the nerve cell membrane and increasing its permeability.[53] Radiation injury is associated with treatment for cancer, and when it occurs, the damage to irradiated nerves appears to be related to an increase in temperature and is generally permanent.[54]

DOUBLE-CRUSH SYNDROME

Double-crush syndrome is a phenomenon in which two or more lesions along the same nerve produce symptoms that would be less observable or severe if only one lesion existed.[55-57] Double-crush injury is thought to occur when one lesion disrupts axonal transport and thus impairs delivery of substances essential to the maintenance of membrane integrity and disposal of waste material in other parts of the nerve. Many doubt the existence of the double-crush syndrome[58,59] or suggest that it is over diagnosed.[60] For example, Chaudhry and Clawson conducted a small study of subjects with amyotrophic lateral sclerosis (ALS), a disease of motor nerves, to see if the presence of this nerve disease predisposed nerves to a second pathology.[59] The authors made three predictions that would support the concept of double-crush: (1) There would be a greater incidence of ulnar neuropathy at the elbow of the motor versus sensory nerve in subjects with ALS; (2) in subjects with ALS with an ulnar neuropathy at the elbow, the sensory fibers should have less involvement

than the motor fibers; and (3) motor nerves from patients with ALS and ulnar neuropathy at the elbow would have more axonal loss than motor nerves from patients with ALS without ulnar neuropathy. After establishing a definition of ulnar neuropathy at the elbow (a focal reduction in nerve conduction velocity [NCV] of ≥ 10 m/sec), the investigators compared nerves and found that there was no greater incidence of motor ulnar neuropathy than sensory ulnar neuropathy at the elbow in patients with ALS and that in those with ulnar neuropathy at the elbow there was not a significantly more motor nerve involvement than sensory nerve involvement. These findings did not support the concept of double-crush syndrome. The third prediction was supported but only demonstrated that ulnar neuropathy can affect the motor nerves.[59] Despite the paucity of evidence supporting the existence of double-crush injury, this concept continues to be popular among clinicians.

CLASSIFICATION OF NERVE INJURY

Several authors have proposed classifications systems for nerve injury (Table 18-3).[61-64] These systems describe the extent of nerve injury. Seddon describes three categories of nerve injury: Neurapraxia, axonotmesis, and neurotmesis,[61,63] whereas Sunderland describes five categories, numbered first through fifth degree, which are similar to Seddon's, but axonotmesis and neurotmesis are divided into two categories each.[62] A sixth category, which includes concurrent damage at all the levels described by Sunderland with some degree of injury to all five tissues, has been proposed by MacKinnon.[64]

SPECIFIC NERVE LESIONS

Although nerves may be injured at any location and by a variety of mechanisms, certain lesions are more common. The following section discusses the more common specific peripheral nerve injuries and includes examples of unique mechanisms of injury. This section is sequenced anatomically, starting cranially and proximally and moving caudally and distally.

Nerve Lesions Affecting the Head and Neck. Cranial nerves may be injured by external forces such as penetration from bullets or needles, or by blunt trauma causing fractures.[65] Injury may also occur from compression by edema, tumors, and entrapment. For example, pituitary tumors often compress the optic nerves,[65] the trigeminal nerve may be injured in association with mandibular or maxillary fractures,[65] mandibular surgery[66] or dental work,[67,68] and the facial nerve may be injured in association with mandibular condyle,[69] laterobasal fractures,[65] and parotidectomy.[70] Bell's palsy, the acute onset of idiopathic of facial nerve palsy, may occur subsequent to a viral infection[71] or may have a vascular cause.[65] Glossopharyngeal, vagus, and hypoglossal nerve injuries have been reported after subluxation of the cervical spine in subjects with rheumatoid arthritis.[72,73] Spinal accessory nerve injuries may occur during lymph node biopsy,[74-76] and the hypoglossal nerve may be injured by intubation.[77,78]

Nerve Lesions Affecting the Upper Extremity. Brachial plexus injuries can be caused by blunt trauma

TABLE 18-3	Classification of Peripheral Nerve Injury				
Seddon	**Sunderland**	**Injury**	**Symptoms**	**Mechanism of Injury**	**Recovery**
Neurapraxia	First degree	Structure of nerve intact, focal demyelination, localized area of conduction block	Pain Minimal to no muscle atrophy Numbness Diminished proprioception	Compression, ischemia, stretch, blunt trauma, metabolic derangement, toxins, diseases	Spontaneous and complete return within days to months
	Second degree	Interruption of axons, epineurium, perineurium, and endoneurium intact	Pain Some muscle atrophy Complete loss of motor, sensory and sympathetic function	Greater nerve compression or traction	Spontaneous and complete return within months
Axonotmesis	Third degree	Disruption of axons, injury to funiculi		Severe traction, crush with subsequent scarring causing entrapment	Spontaneous but faulty to no recovery
	Fourth degree	Disruption of perineurium	No pain Muscle atrophy Complete loss of motor, sensory, and sympathetic function	No conduction because of scar	Incomplete spontaneous recovery, surgery likely required for repair or grafting
Neurotmesis	Fifth degree	Complete transection of nerve		Complete laceration	No spontaneous recovery without surgical intervention

from falls and lacerations from penetrating injuries, as well as compression and traction. In a report of 100 consecutive cases of subjects undergoing surgical repair of brachial plexus injuries, most injuries included trauma (motorcycle accidents, gunshot wounds, and penetrating wounds) and nine were iatrogenic.[79] Positioning the shoulder in hyperabduction for surgical procedures, such as mammoplasty, can also be associated with brachial plexus traction injuries.[80]

Obstetrical brachial plexus palsy (OBPP) is a brachial plexus injury in the newborn. OBPP is associated with increased birth weight, operative vaginal delivery,[81] advanced maternal age, and maternal diabetes.[82] Patterns of injury for OBPP are described in Table 18-4. It has been proposed that this injury occurs when the infant presents in the vertex position, causing the infant's shoulder to be impeded by the mother's pubic symphysis.[83] However, a systematic review of the literature found that OBPP had a greater association with a very short duration of the second stage of delivery than with shoulder dystocia or forceps delivery, which are typical with vertex positioning.[84] Most infants with OBPP have complete neurological recovery,[85] and predictors of optimal recovery include intact active elbow flexion by 3 months of age, C7 involvement, and high birth weight.[86] Children with OBPP may develop secondary deformities about the shoulder because of muscle imbalance, which progress with suboptimal neural recovery.[87] In a study of 16 infants (17 shoulders) with OBPP without full recovery, nine demonstrated an irregular glenoid, retroversion of the glenoid, or subluxation of the humerus. The authors of this study suggest that even with neural recovery, children with OPPB may have functional deficits that are a result of structural irregularities.[88]

Peripheral nerves projecting off the trunks and cords of the brachial plexus include the long thoracic and suprascapular nerves. The long thoracic nerve is susceptible to injury during first rib resections,[89] and a single case report describes an incident of long thoracic nerve palsy after palpation along the first rib.[90] In studies of the long thoracic nerve in six fresh cadavers, investigators found a tight fascial band arising from the inferior aspect of the brachial plexus and extending to the first rib that caused bowstringing of the nerve when the shoulder was passively abducted and externally rotated and proposed that this band could damage the nerve because of intermittent dynamic tension.[91] The suprascapular nerve may be damaged where it passes underneath the superior transverse scapular ligament at the scapular notch[92] or where it passes under the inferior transverse scapular ligament at the spinoglenoid notch.[93] In a review of 88 cases of isolated suprascapular nerve injury, a ganglion or entrapment by the inferior transverse scapular ligament were the most frequent causes.[94] Some patients who have a wide transverse scapular ligament and a narrow spinoglenoid notch may be at increased risk for suprascapular nerve injury.[95] There are many injuries that may occur more distally in

TABLE 18-4	Patterns of Obstetrical Brachial Plexus Palsy	
Type	**Incidence***	**Pattern of Involvement**
Erb-Duchenne	73%	Upper plexus
Total plexus injury	25%	Total plexus
Klumpke's	2%	Lower plexus

*Data from Shenaq SM, Bullocks JM, Dhillon G, et al: *Clin Plast Surg* 32(1):79-98, 2005.

TABLE 18-5	Etiology of Upper Extremity Nerve Lesions
Nerve	**Mechanism of Injury**
Axillary	Anterior shoulder dislocation, trauma during anterior shoulder stabilization procedures, fracture of the humeral neck*
Musculocutaneous	Clavicular fracture†
Radial nerve	Humeral fractures,‡ compression in the radial tunnel§¶
Median nerve	Entrapment in pronator teres,‖ compression in the carpal tunnel
Ulnar	Cross pinning following supracondylar fractures,¶ entrapment in the cubital tunnel, entrapment in Guyon's canal

*Kline DG, Kim DH: *J Neurosurg* 99(4):630-636, 2003.
†Bartosh RA, Dugdale TW, Nielsen R: *Am J Sports Med* 20(3):356-359, 1992.
‡Ring D, Chin K, Jupiter JB: *J Hand Surg* 29(1):144-147, 2004.
§Portilla Molina AE, Bour C, Oberlin C, et al: *Int Orthop* 22:102-106, 1998.
‖Johnson RK, Spinner M, Shrewsbury MM: *J Hand Surg* 4A(1):48-51, 1979.
¶Skaggs DL, Hale JM, Bassett J, et al: *J Bone Joint Surg Am* 83(5):735-740, 2003; Taniguchi Y, Matsuzaki K, Tamaki T: *J Shoulder Elbow Surg* 9(2):160-162, 2000.

the upper extremity. Nerve injuries beyond the cords of the brachial plexus are summarized in Tables 18-5 and 18-6.

Nerve Lesions Affecting the Lower Extremity.

Peripheral nerve injuries of the lower extremities in women are often associated with labor and delivery and pelvic surgery. In a study of 6,057 women after childbirth, 56 reported a new onset of nerve injury.[96] Cardosi, Cox, and Hoffman described a 1.9% incidence of postoperative neuropathy involving (in order of decreasing frequency) the obturator, ilioinguinal/hypogastric, genitofemoral, femoral, or lumbosacral nerves in a group of women who underwent pelvic surgery.[97] Although rare, compression of the femoral nerve was reported in three cases to be associated with entrapment at the iliopectineal arch.[98] Traumatic femoral nerve injuries may occur as a result of displaced acetabular fractures,[99] total hip arthroplasty,[100-102] and anterior dislocation of the femur.[103] Iatrogenic injuries are associated with inguinal hernia repair, arterial bypass, appendectomy,[104] and hysterectomy.[105,106] In a systematic review of the literature pertaining to gynecological surgical procedures and nerve injuries, Irwin et al found that improper placement of retractors was the most common cause of femoral nerve injury subsequent to gynecological surgical procedures.[107] Sciatic nerve compression has been reported as a consequence of an anomalous course of the sciatic nerve between the two tendinous origins of the piriformis muscle.[108] Sciatic nerve lesions can occur after a blunt force to buttock region[109] or accidental injection[48] and as an iatrogenic consequence of hip arthroplasty.[101,110] Bradshaw et al described 32 cases of obturator nerve entrapment caused by thick fascia overlying the short adductor muscle.[111] Obturator nerve injuries are often associated with other nerve injuries, although isolated injuries have been reported with femur fracture fixation,[112]

hip replacement,[101] and cement extrusion (for hip replacement).[113] Other nerve injuries that occur more distally in the lower extremity are summarized in Tables 18-7 and 18-8.

NERVE DEGENERATION AND REGENERATION

Nerve recovery after complete nerve transection (neurotmesis) occurs if there is no damage to the cell body (Fig. 18-9). This process involves changes in the proximal and distal axon segments, as well as the nerve cell body. After neurotmesis, nonviable tissue must be removed and then the nerve must regenerate. First, within hours of the injury, chromatolysis, with breakdown of rough endoplasmic reticulum, occurs in the injured part of the nerve. The proximal axon degenerates from the site of injury up to at least the closest node of Ranvier. Following this degeneration, protein production accelerates to provide materials for nerve regeneration. These new proteins are transported to the stump of the proximal axon where they are assembled within approximately 24 hours from the initial injury. While more proteins are being made for nerve repair, the production of proteins for neurotransmission and the proliferation of Schwann cells decrease.[114] Axonal sprouting then occurs from the stump, just distal to the last intact node of Ranvier. Each axon forms up to 15 sprouts, collectively called a growth cone. These sprouts migrate, directed in part by signals received by projections of the basement membrane of the axon called filopodia. The filopodia are sensitive to growth factors, such as nerve growth factor (NGF), that act as targets, attracting regenerating axons.

Because the organelles required for protein synthesis are only located in the cell body, when a nerve is transected the proteins needed for its maintenance and repair can only reach the proximal nerve segment. Therefore the distal nerve segment degenerates. This type of degeneration is known as *Wallerian degeneration* and involves disintegration of the axoplasm and axolemma over the course of 1-12 weeks and degradation of the surrounding myelin. The remnants of these materials are cleared from the area by macrophages. Residual Schwann cells in the area of the distal portion of the injured nerve, responding to the Wallerian degeneration, stimulate the production of high levels of NGF for up to 2 weeks after nerve injury.[115] Although NGF promotes nerve regeneration, it has also been implicated in the development of *neuromas* and neuropathic pain after nerve injury.

Studies have shown that nerve axons preferentially grow toward distal nerve stumps rather than toward other soft tissues and toward their own distal stump rather than other distal nerve stumps and that motor neurons grow toward denervated muscle rather than toward innervated muscle.[116] There are several proposed mechanisms for these patterns of regeneration. The growth cone and filopodia are attracted to negatively charged proteins present in the basement membrane of the distal nerve stump, thus axon sprouts are directed toward the distal nerve segment, specifically the basement membrane. When one axon, from a single growth cone, reaches the basement membrane of the distal segment of the same

TABLE 18-6	Major Nerve Injuries of the Upper Extremity	
Nerve	**Muscles**	**Clinical Signs**
Dorsal scapular	Rhomboid major Rhomboid minor	Weakened scapular adduction.
Suprascapular	Supraspinatus Infraspinatus	Weakened shoulder abduction and external rotation.
Subscapular	Subscapularis Teres major	Weakened shoulder medial rotation.
Long thoracic	Serratus anterior	Weakened scapular abduction and upward rotation, incomplete shoulder elevation through flexion and abduction, scapular winging.
Thoracodorsal	Latissimus dorsi	Diminished ability to depress scapula against resistance.
Lateral pectoral	Pectoralis major	Weakened shoulder flexion, medial rotation, and horizontal adduction.
Medial pectoral	Pectoralis major (PMa) and minor (PMi)	*PMa:* Weakened shoulder flexion, medial rotation, and horizontal adduction. *PMi:* Weakened scapular downward rotation.
Axillary	Deltoid Teres minor	Weakened shoulder abduction, flexion, and/or extension, shoulder impingement.
Musculocutaneous	Coracobrachialis Biceps Brachialis	Significantly diminished elbow flexion. Requires abduction of shoulder to flex the elbow via brachioradialis.
Radial	Triceps Anconeus Brachioradialis Extensor carpi radialis longus Extensor carpi radialis brevis	Supination diminished, loss of wrist and MCP extension.
Posterior Interosseus	Supinator Extensor digitorum communis Extensor digiti minimi Extensor carpi ulnaris Abductor pollicis longus Extensor pollicis brevis Extensor pollicis longus Extensor indicis proprius	Full wrist extension but weak, weak ulnar deviation, unable to extend MCP joints.
Median	Pronator teres Flexor carpi radialis Palmaris longus Flexor digitorum superficialis Flexor pollicis brevis (superficial head) Opponens pollicis Lumbricales (1 and 2)	High (above or near elbow): Weakened pronation; weakened wrist flexion; loss of digital flexion of IF, MF; weakened flexion of RF and MF; weakened thumb MCP flexion, loss of thumb opposition, and palmar abduction. Benedictine hand: clawing of the index and middle finger.
Anterior interosseus	Flexor pollicis longus Flexor digitorum profundus (1 and 2) Pronator quadratus Abductor pollicis brevis	Weakened forearm pronation; weakened flexion of IF, MF; loss of thumb palmar abduction. Unable to make the "O" sign with thumb and index finger.
Ulnar	Flexor carpi ulnaris Flexor digitorum profundus (3 and 4) Palmaris brevis	High (at or above elbow): Weakened wrist flexion and ulnar deviation, loss of DIP flexion RF, SF; loss of MCP flexion SF; weakened MCP flexion RF; loss or significantly diminished IP extension IF, MF, RF, and SF; loss of lateral pinch; loss of SF opposition to thumb. *Froment's paper sign:* In presence of ulnar nerve palsy, client will flex the thumb IP joint instead of contracting the adductor pollicis muscle when asked to hold paper between the pads of the thumb and index finger. *Jeanne's sign:* The client may hyperextend the MCP joint in the above task. *Egawa's sign:* Client cannot radially and ulnarly abduct the MF.
Deep branch	Abductor digiti minimi Flexor digiti minimi Opponens digiti minimi Lumbricales (3 and 4) Palmar interosseus Dorsal interosseus Adductor pollicis	Weakened MCP flexion SF; loss or significantly diminished IP extension IF, MF, RF, and SF; loss of lateral pinch; loss of SF opposition to thumb. Froment's sign, Jeanne's sign, Egawa's sign, clawing of RF and SF.

MCP, Metacarpophalangeal; *IF,* index finger; *MF,* middle finger; *RF,* ring finger; *SF,* small finger; *DIP,* distal interphalangeal; *IP,* interphalangeal.

TABLE 18-7	Common Causes of Lower Extremity Nerve Lesions
Nerve	**Cause**
Peroneal	Fractures of the femur, tibia, and fibula;* knee dislocation;† leg crossing; positioning in persons who are mobility impaired or comatose; and positioning during surgical procedures
Deep peroneal	Compression beneath fibular fibrous arch‡ in the anterior tarsal tunnel, from constricting shoe laces and in the presence of pes cavus
Superficial peroneal nerve	Inversion sprain§
Tibial	Compression because of entrapment in the tarsal tunnel or in the popliteal fossa‖
Sural	Lateral malleolus fracture, calcaneus fracture, small saphenous vein stripping¶

*Data from Mont MA, Dellon AL, Chen F, et al: *J Bone Joint Surg Am* 78:863, 1996.
†Data from Goitz RJ, Tomaino MM: *Am J Orthop* 32(1):14-16, 2003.
‡Data from Fabre T, Piton C, Andre D, et al: *J Bone Joint Surg Am* 80(1):47-54, 1998.
§Data from Johnston EC, Howell SJ: *Foot Ankle Int* 20(9):576-582, 1999.
‖Data from Mastaglia FL: *Muscle Nerve* 23(12):1883-1886, 2000.
¶Data from Seror P: *Am J Phys Med Rehabil* 81(11):876-880, 2002.

TABLE 18-8	Signs and Symptoms of Lower Extremity Nerve Injuries		
Nerve	**Muscle(s)**	**Clinical Signs**	**Sensory Loss**
Superior gluteal *Inferior gluteal*	Tensor facia late	Trendelenburg gait	None
Sciatic	Abductor magnus	High steppage gait, inability to stand on heel or toes	Posterior thigh and calf
	Semimembranous		Entire foot with exception of medial malleolus and medial aspect
	Biceps femoris		
Common peroneal			
Superficial	Peroneus longus	Foot drop, inability to evert the foot	Lateral aspect of calf
	Peroneus brevis	Foot drop	Dorsum of foot
Deep	Tibialis anterior		First web space of toes
	Extensor digitorum longus		
	Extensor hallucis longus		
	Peroneus tertius		
	Extensor digitorum brevis		
	Extensor hallucis brevis		
Tibial	Gastrocnemius	Inability to plantar flex the ankle and invert the foot	Plantar aspect of foot and toes except medial border
	Soleus		
	Tibialis posterior	Toe flexion, abduction, and adduction lost	
	Flexor digitorum longus		
	Flexor hallucis longus		
	Intrinsics on plantar foot		
Femoral	Pectinius	Falling because of an unstable knee and difficulty with stair climbing	Medial distal thigh
	Sartorius		Medial aspect calf and foot
	Rectus femoris		
	Vastus medialis		
	Vastus intermedius		
	Vastus lateralis		
Obturator	Adductor brevis	—	Medial aspect of thigh
	Adductor magnus		
	Adductor longus		
	Gracilis		

nerve a protein known as actin, found in the growth cone, attaches to the basement membrane of that distal segment and the other nerve sprouts in that growth cone degenerate. In addition, a protein called neural cell adhesion molecule (NCAM) that is expressed by muscle attracts motor nerves, and for other nerves, axonal regeneration and myelinization are promoted by the nerve connecting with an end-organ.[114]

After repair of a transected nerve, the rate of regeneration is at the most 10 mm per day. However, regeneration rates differ among fibers, depending on their type and location (Table 18-9). Small fibers regenerate more quickly than larger diameter fibers. Therefore C fibers carrying information about dull, aching pain and temperature will regenerate more quickly than A-beta and A-delta fibers that carry information about discriminative touch, proprioception, and sharp pain.

Surgical repair of transected nerves does not ensure full functional return. Nerve cell viability, rate of recovery, and axonal direction all affect the degree of nerve regeneration and the viability of end-organs.[117] Additionally, neuroma development and neuropathic pain can contribute to poor

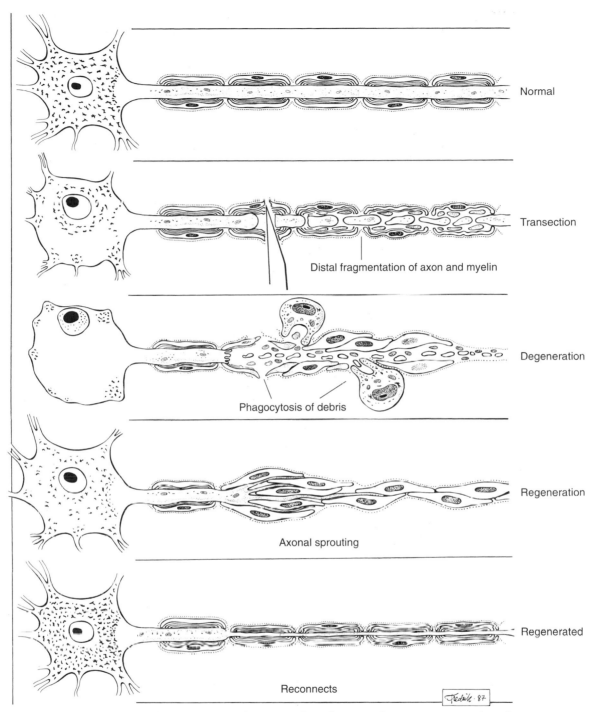

FIG. 18-9 Nerve degeneration and regeneration after complete nerve transection. *From Lundborg G: Nerve Injury and Repair, Edinburgh, 1988, Churchill Livingstone.*

functional outcomes despite optimal surgical repair and subsequent regeneration.

FUNCTIONAL RECOVERY FROM PERIPHERAL NERVE INJURY

For a peripheral nerve to successfully regenerate, four criteria must be met: Survival of the cell body; absence of barriers, such as scar or bone that would prevent axonal sprouting; accurate growth toward appropriate end-organs; and accommodation of the *central nervous system* (CNS) to reorganize mixed afferent signals.[118] In addition, functional recovery from peripheral nerve injury may be affected by the age and cognitive capacity of the patient, the circumstances or nature of the nerve injury, and the subsequent repair.[119]

Children tend to have better functional outcomes from peripheral nerve injury than adults.[120-122] Proposed reasons for this include that the nerves have less distance to cover

TABLE 18-9	Rate of Nerve Regeneration by Region
Location	**Rate of Regeneration (mm/day)**
Upper arm	2.5-8.5
Proximal forearm	2-6
Wrist	1-2
Hand	1-1.5
Upper leg	2
Lower leg	1.5
Ankle	1

to reach their end-organ[120] and that children have more cerebral plasticity[123,124] and better nerve regeneration.[125] The latter theory, however, is controversial with studies showing both better[120] and similar nerve regeneration in adults and children.[126,127] Whether age affects recovery from nerve injury beyond childhood is also controversial. One study found no difference in the improvements from carpal tunnel surgery between elderly patients (70-89 years) and younger adults (30-69 years).[128] However, another study with 84 subjects who underwent carpal tunnel release found that patients over the age of 60 fared less well than those between 31 and 59 years of age, with worse symptoms ($p = 0.003$), poorer functional outcomes ($p = 0.046$), and less improvement in nerve conduction study findings ($p = 0.027$).[129]

Patients with traumatic peripheral neuropathies have worse outcomes than patients with peripheral neuropathies from nontraumatic causes.[130] Functional outcomes after crush injuries are better than those after transection followed by repair or nerve grafting.[131] Nerves repaired sooner fare better, with less cell death, than those repaired later.[132] Generally, the more proximal a nerve injury is the poorer the outcome because of the length of nerve that needs to regrow for reinnervation.

EXAMINATION

PATIENT HISTORY

Information obtained from the medical record and patient interview includes the patient's name, gender, race/ethnicity, and primary language. Gender appears to be a risk factor for certain peripheral nerve injuries. For example, carpal tunnel syndrome (CTS) seems to be more common in women,[133] whereas cubital tunnel syndrome affects more men.[134] In the presence of OBPP, a developmental and birth history should be obtained.

Specific aspects of the patient history to be emphasized for patients with peripheral nerve pathology include employment status and sports activities. Since entrapment mononeuropathy may be caused by specific activities, the clinician should ask the patient about the nature of their activities at work, school, and home. Particular attention should be paid to repetitive activities and positions or activities where compression may be placed on a nerve by an external object. For example, suprascapular nerve entrapment has been reported to occur in newsreel cameramen as a result of compression of the nerve by the

weight of the camera on the shoulder.[135] Although work activities may affect the risk for nerve injury, there is evidence that other factors, such as body mass index, age, and anatomical variation, may play a greater role for industrial workers with abnormal nerve function.[136] Sports-related injuries, whether as employment or leisure activity, are commonly reported. Examples include suprascapular and dorsal scapular nerve injury in volleyball players[137] and cubital tunnel syndrome in throwing athletes.[138,139]

The medical chart should be reviewed for results of radiographs, computed tomography (CT), magnetic resonance imaging (MRI), nerve conduction studies, and diagnostic nerve blocks. Radiographic studies, particularly CT and MRI, may reveal presence of a soft tissue mass along nerves causing compression. Diagnostic nerve blocks and nerve conduction studies aid in localizing sources of noxious stimuli and pathways for transmission of noxious stimuli. Further discussion of nerve conduction studies follow later in this chapter.

The client's understanding of the current problem and reason for referral to rehabilitation therapy are recorded. Response to other therapies, including past and present, may help in determining prognosis. The mechanism of injury and date of injury or onset of symptoms are also crucial for diagnostic and prognostic determination. Since more proximal injuries have less favorable outcome, recording the level of injury is also essential.

SYSTEMS REVIEW

The systems review is used to target areas requiring further examination and to define areas that may cause complications or indicate a need for precautions during the examination and intervention processes. See Chapter 1 for details of the systems review.

TESTS AND MEASURES

There is no single test shown to accurately assess the presence and status of nerve pathology, thus a battery of tests should be used to evaluate subjects with suspected nerve lesions as in some cases this increases the probability of making a correct diagnosis.[140,141]

Musculoskeletal

Posture. Posture may play a role in the development or exacerbation of symptoms associated with peripheral nerve entrapment or compression (see Chapter 4).

Anthropometric Characteristics

Edema. Peripheral nerve injury may be associated with edema, heat, and redness when there is inflammation present and with edema, coolness, and pallor when active motion is significantly impaired. Limb volume can be estimated by water displacement using commercially available hand volumeters (Fig. 18-10) or by circumferential measurements. Hand volumeters have been found to be accurate within 1%,[142] and their standard error can be reduced from 10 ml to 3 ml by placing the device on a height-adjustable table, supporting the patient's trunk, and measuring the displaced water with a 1-ml micropipette.[143] Circumferential measurements and volumetry have both been found to have high interrater and

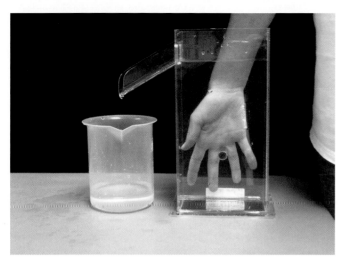

FIG. 18-10 Measurement of hand volume (edema) using a hand volumeter.

test-retest reliability coefficients of 0.99.[144] When estimating hand or foot volume with a tape measure, the figure-of-eight method has been found to be most reliable.[145-148]

There are no standards for these measurements, but comparison with the uninvolved limb and over time can be used to evaluate for abnormalities and changes. Note that it is not uncommon for the dominant hand to be larger than the nondominant hand by as much as 10-16.9 ml.[149,150]

Range of Motion and Muscle Length. Joint contractures and muscle shortening frequently occur after peripheral nerve injury as a result of unbalanced forces around a joint. For example, 52% of a sample of patients with cubital tunnel syndrome was found to have elbow flexion contractures.[151] Therefore both active and passive ROM, as well as muscle length, should be examined in patients with peripheral nerve injuries. These measurements should be performed at least for all areas that the involved nerve crosses.

Muscle Performance. Muscle strength testing is essential for patients with peripheral nerve injuries because a peripheral motor nerve injury will produce specific weakness in the muscles innervated by that nerve. Muscles should be tested individually rather than with others performing similar movements because muscles performing similar movements may have different innervations. Muscle weakness that results from peripheral nerve injury is examined using manual muscle tests. Prolonged weakness as a result of motor nerve injury may also be detectable by observation of muscle atrophy and loss of muscle bulk. Although changes in girth measurements over time have been shown to correlate with other measures of strength, the poor specificity of this method limits its utility (see Chapter 5).[152]

The British Medical Research Council (BMRC) developed a scale, later modified by Dellon (Table 18-10), for grading motor and sensory function after peripheral nerve injury.[153] This scale grades motor function based on the strength of proximal and peripheral muscles innervated by the nerve in question to indicate the degree of nerve function. Since distal weakness indicates less severe or more distal peripheral nerve involvement than proximal weakness, this scale is helpful for localizing and determining the severity of peripheral nerve injuries and in evaluating recovery.

Assessment of Muscle Function in Children with Obstetrical Brachial Plexus Palsy. Several tools are available to examine muscle performance in children with OBPP. The BMRC system as previously described is not suitable for measuring strength in infants and small children because it depends on cooperation for tests requiring manual resistance. A modified BMRC appropriate for children is described by Gilbert and Tassin.[154]

Bae et al recently evaluated the reliability of three movement scales for children with OBPP: The Mallet Classification, the Toronto Test, and the Active Movement Scale (AMS).[155] Based on examination of 80 children by two examiners two different times, each reported fair to excellent intraobserver and interobserver reliability for all 3 of these scales, with higher intraobserver agreement than interobserver agreement. They did not comment on the sensitivity or specificity of these tests.

The Mallet Classification is useful for defining recovery of upper trunk lesions and can be used with toddlers but

TABLE 18-10	British Medical Research Council Scale of Nerve Function		
Motor Function		**Sensory Function**	
M0	No contraction	S0	Absence of sensibility in the autonomous area
M1	Perceptible contraction in proximal muscles	S1	Recovery of deep cutaneous pain in the autonomous area
M2	Perceptible contraction in proximal and distal muscles	S1+	Recovery of superficial pain in the autonomous area
M3	Contraction of proximal and distal muscles with sufficient power to allow movement against resistance	S2	Return of some degree of superficial cutaneous pain and some tactile sensibility in the autonomous area
		S2+	S2 but with an overresponse
M4	Return of function as in stage 3 but synergistic and independent movements are possible	S3	Return of superficial cutaneous pain and tactile sensitivity throughout the autonomous area, with disappearance over response, static 2-point discrimination >15 mm
		S3+	S3, with localization and recovery of 2-point discrimination at 7-15 mm in the autonomous area
M5	Complete recovery	S4	Complete recovery with static 2-point discrimination at ≤6 mm

Modified by Dellon A, Curtis R, Edgerton M: *Plast Reconstr Surg* 53:297-305, 1974.

not infants. To perform this test the child is asked to place the hands on the back of the neck, on the low back (using shoulder internal rotation), and to the mouth. The movements are evaluated on a scale of I-V, with I being no movement and V being normal and symmetrical movement.[156]

The Toronto Test uses a 0-2 scale to assess elbow flexion, elbow extension, wrist extension, finger extension, and thumb extension with a maximum of 10 points available.[157] The AMS is a tool with 8 grades for quantifying motor function in infants and older children with OBPP.[158] The AMS, which was designed to elicit movements against gravity or with gravity minimized, examines joint movement rather than individual muscle function and does not require the child to be able to follow commands. In a study with 63 infants with OBPP, most components of the AMS were found to have high interrater reliability, with the exception of forearm rotation.[159]

Neuromuscular

Pain. Peripheral nerve injury is often associated with changes in sensation. Although decreased sensation, causing numbness and tingling, is most common, burning, shooting, and sharp electrical-type pains are also often associated with peripheral nerve injuries. In addition, tingling or paresthesias may also be described by the patient as pain.[160] The nature of the pain may help to distinguish nerve-related pain from pain of musculoskeletal origin. Pain associated with peripheral nerve injury may indicate normal nerve regeneration but is thought more often to be a result of irritation of small diameter nociceptive A-delta and C fibers.

Pain may also be caused by neuromas, which are benign tumors made up largely of nerve cells and nerve fibers, that often occur after peripheral nerve injury. Neuromas are thought to be formed when nerve regeneration is blocked by scar tissue, preventing further regeneration. Movement of adjacent tissues or direct application of pressure on neuromas often causes pain by stimulating the nerve enclosed by the neuroma. Standard pain assessment measures (see Chapter 22) may be used to measure pain in clients with peripheral nerve injury.

Cranial and Peripheral Nerve Integrity

Electrophysiological Testing. Electrodiagnostic studies are generally considered the gold standard for evaluating peripheral nerve integrity. There are electrodiagnostic studies that examine sensory and motor nerve conduction, known as nerve conduction studies (NCS) or NCV studies, and studies that examine muscle activity in response to stimulation or activation, known as an *electromyogram* (EMG). Together, these studies can help to localize peripheral nerve lesions, determine their severity, and distinguish between neuromuscular dysfunction caused by demyelination, axonal damage, motor endplate dysfunction, and muscle dysfunction. These tests are frequently used to assist with diagnosis and to evaluate recovery over time or in response to treatment. Therapists with specific advanced training and necessary certification may perform electrodiagnostic testing in many parts of the United States.

NCS can confirm the presence of both symptomatic and asymptomatic nerve pathology.[161] A joint literature review by three medical professional associations published in 2002 concluded that NCS has high sensitivity and specificity for identifying CTS,[162] despite the fact that these studies can produce negative results in the presence of clinical symptoms and positive results in the absence of symptoms or pathology.[163,164] Because of these limitations, some still recommend using clinical history and physical examination rather than NCS to diagnose CTS, and all recommend correlation of study findings with findings from the clinical examination.[140,165,166]

It has been suggested that NCS can also be used to identify and predict those at risk for developing CTS. A prospective study involving 77 subjects without CTS symptoms but with abnormal NCS at baseline and a similar number of asymptomatic subjects with normal NCS at baseline found that over a period of 70 months, 23% of those with abnormal NCS and only 6% of those with normal NCS developed symptomatic CTS ($p = 0.01$).[167] However, although Nathan et al's study of 289 workers over 11 years found a strong, direct linear correlation between initial severity of median nerve conduction slowing and subsequent development of CTS, they found that most workers who developed de novo slowing did not develop symptoms or CTS. They therefore concluded that changes in conduction status of the median nerve occur naturally with increasing age and do not necessarily lead to symptoms and CTS.[168] Additionally, in a study of 700 workers, abnormal median sensory NCS were not found to be predictive of future hand or finger complaints in asymptomatic workers.[169] Werner et al recommend that if the results of these tests are used for preplacement screening among active workers, it should be done with caution.[169]

Provocative Tests to Detect Nerve Injury. Clinicians often subject nerves to compression or traction in an attempt to detect nerve injury or dysfunction. Production of symptoms by these provocative testing maneuvers is thought to indicate nerve injury. Compression can be applied manually or with a device, and tension is generally applied by placing the client in positions that are thought to put the nerve on stretch and would not elicit symptoms in normal subjects. This latter type of maneuver is referred to as a neural tension test. When neural tension tests are performed by stretching the nerve along its course with a series of maneuvers, each subjecting the nerve to greater amounts of tension, the clinician may be able to detect the presence of nerve entrapment or double-crush syndrome. The following are examples of commonly used provocative tests for peripheral nerve pathology; most are tests for specific nerve lesions.

Tinel's Test. Tinel's test is used to detect Tinel's sign, which is a hyperirritability or response to mechanical inputs such as tapping, and is thought to be indicative of nerve injury. The presence of this finding may indicate the location of nerve injury. Although its presence and advancing presence (presence along a regenerating nerve) is not always a reliable indicator of nerve injury or of regeneration following injury,[170,171] the lack of an advancing Tinel's sign is thought to indicate poor nerve regeneration. Tinel's test is performed by tapping on the skin directly over the nerve in question (Fig. 18-11). The speci-

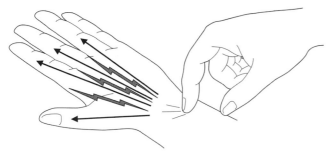

FIG. 18-11 Tinel's test of the median nerve at the carpal tunnel. *Adapted from Goodman CC, Boissonnault WG, Fuller KS: Pathology: Implications for the Physical Therapist, ed 2, Philadelphia, 2002, Saunders.*

ficity of this test is limited by the fact that even when a normal amount of force is applied, the Tinel's sign may be positive in 20% to 45% of subjects without nerve pathology[172,173] and that when excessive force is applied, there are even more false-positive outcomes.[174] Although many clinicians find the Tinel's sign to be a useful indicator of nerve injury, because of its poor sensitivity (0.63 in subjects with electrophysiologically confirmed CTS) and specificity, it should not be used alone.[173]

A study by Novack et al suggested that Tinel's test may be more reliable for identifying nerve compression in advanced rather than early stages.[175] In addition, Spicher et al proposed a standardizing the technique for eliciting and analyzing Tinel's sign through use of a vibrostimulator to improve standardization and quantification of the stimulation provided and thus possibly improve the utility of the Tinel's test.[176]

Roos Test. Roos test, also known as the elevated arm stress test (EAST), is a test of vascular and neurological function in the upper extremity and is used to screen for thoracic outlet syndrome. To perform this test, the client is asked to abduct and externally rotate the shoulder to 90 degrees, flex the elbow to 90 degrees, and maximally open and close the hand slowly and repetitively for 3 minutes. The test is considered positive if the client reports or demonstrates an inability to maintain the position because of a sensation of heaviness or weakness of the arm or reports tingling or numbness. No studies regarding the validity or reliability of the Roos test could be found from a MEDLINE search (1960-2005).

Neural Tension Tests. Neural tension tests can be performed on both the upper and lower extremities. Neural tension tests for the lower extremities include the straight leg raise test (SLR), the slump test, and the prone knee bend test. The SLR and slump test primarily apply tension to the sciatic nerve, whereas the prone knee bend test primarily applies tension to the femoral nerve (see Chapter 8).

A number of neural tension tests, collectively known as upper limb neural tension tests (ULNTTs), have been described for the upper extremities. The brachial plexus tension test, which was first described by Elvey, involves the patient being supine and the clinician sequentially passively moving the upper extremity into shoulder abduction, lateral rotation and slight extension posterior

to the frontal plane, elbow extension, forearm supination, wrist extension, and digital extension.[177] The ULNTTs, as described by Butler, include a series of four basic tests; the first and second tests selectively apply more tension to the median nerve, and the third and fourth selectively apply more tension to the radial and ulnar nerves, respectively (Figs. 18-12 to 18-15).[178] Hunter more recently developed two tests to evaluate the brachial plexus: The high abduction arm test and the low abduction arm test[179] (Table 18-11). For each of these tests, results are documented in terms of the ROM at which symptoms are provoked and the type of symptoms provoked. These tests are generally performed bilaterally for comparison.

The median nerve tension test, as described by Butler, has been shown in fresh cadavers to significantly and incrementally change the strain in the median nerve.[10,180,181] The ulnar nerve tension test has also been found to strain the ulnar nerve, although less than the median nerve test strains the median nerve, with the greatest strain noted at the cubital tunnel. Furthermore, the ulnar nerve test has also been found to increase strain in the median nerve.[10] In contrast, the radial nerve test has been found to produce minimal tension in any specific nerve and is therefore considered neither sensitive nor specific for radial nerve involvement.[181]

Although ULNTTs have been found to be reliable in both symptomatic and asymptomatic individuals (ICC 2.1 ≥0.98; standard error of measurement [SEM] ≤3.4 degrees for symptomatic and ICC 2.1 ≥0.95; SEM ≤4.9 degrees for asymptomatic),[182] the specificity of neural tension testing overall is called into question by the finding that ULNTTs produce symptoms or less than full ROM in many asymptomatic persons without nerve pathology.[183]

Elbow Flexion Test. Elbow flexion test is used in the examination and evaluation of suspected cubital tunnel syndrome. With the wrists in full extension, the client is asked to actively hold the elbow in maximal flexion for 3-5 minutes.[184] Reproduction of the patient's symptoms is considered a positive test. In a prospective, randomized control study of 44 extremities with cubital tunnel syndrome, 75% had a positive elbow flexion test. This increased with the addition of pressure on the ulnar nerve to 93%.[185] However, since no studies have evaluated the frequency of a positive elbow flexion test in individuals without cubital tunnel syndrome, the specificity of this test is not known.

Phalen's Test. Phalen's test is used in the evaluation of suspected CTS (Fig. 18-16). The client is asked to flex both wrists for 1 minute. Any numbness or tingling in the median nerve distribution during the 1-minute period is considered a positive test.[186] In a study of 127 patients with CTS and a control group of 20 without CTS, in whom both Phalen's test and NCS were performed, although there was statistically significant relationship between a positive Phalen's test and slowed NCV, 34% of those with CTS diagnosed by NCS had a negative Phalen's test and 20% of those without CTS by NCS had a positive Phalen's test, indicating that this test has a sensitivity of 66% and a specificity of 80%.[187]

Carpal Compression Test. Carpal compression test (CCT), another test for CTS, is performed by the examiner

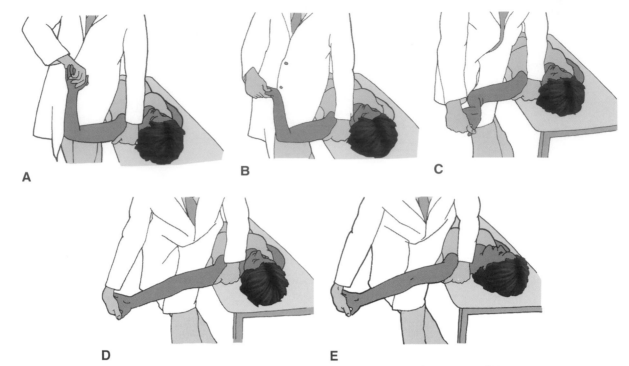

FIG. 18-12 Upper limb tension test 1 (ULTT1): Median nerve dominant utilizing shoulder abduction. **A,** Position the patient with the shoulder abducted to 90 degrees and in neutral rotation, the elbow flexed to 90 degrees, and the wrist in neutral. Then extend the shoulder to neutral. **B,** Extend the wrist and fingers. **C,** Externally rotate the shoulder. **D,** Extend the elbow. **E,** Side bend the neck away from the side being tested. *Adapted from Butler DS:* Mobilisation of the Nervous System, *Edinburgh, 1991, Churchill Livingstone.*

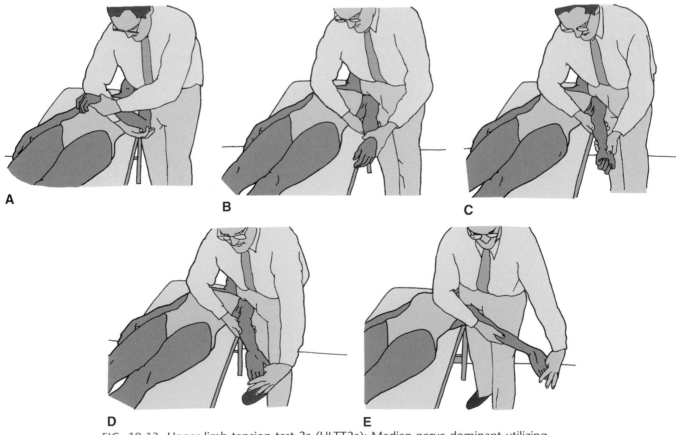

FIG. 18-13 Upper limb tension test 2a (ULTT2a): Median nerve dominant utilizing shoulder girdle depression and external rotation of the shoulder. **A,** Position the patient with the arm at the side, elbow slightly flexed. Then add shoulder girdle depression. **B,** Extend the elbow. **C,** Externally rotate the shoulder. **D,** Extend the wrist, fingers and thumb. **E,** Abduct the shoulder. *Adapted from Butler DS:* Mobilisation of the Nervous System, *Edinburgh, 1991, Churchill Livingstone.*

FIG. 18-14 Upper limb tension test 2b (ULTT2b), radial nerve dominant utilizing shoulder girdle depression plus internal rotation of the shoulder. **A,** Position the patient as in ULTT2a and extend the elbow. Then medially rotate the shoulder and pronate the forearm. **B,** Flex the wrist, fingers, and thumb. *Adapted from Butler DS:* Mobilisation of the Nervous System, *Edinburgh, 1991, Churchill Livingstone.*

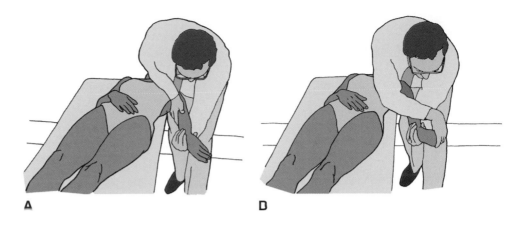

A   D

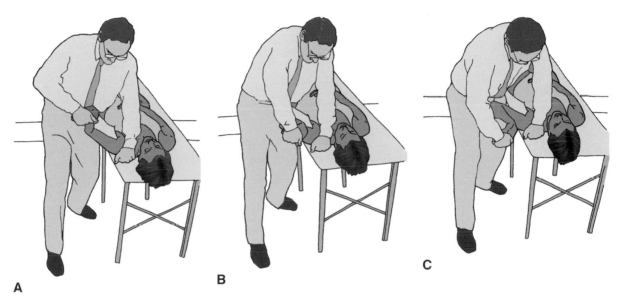

A   B   C

FIG. 18-15 Upper limb tension test 3 (ULTT3), ulnar nerve dominant utilizing shoulder abduction and elbow flexion. **A,** Position the patient as for ULTT1. Then extend the wrist and supinate the forearm. **B,** Fully flex the elbow. **C,** Depress the shoulder girdle and externally rotate the shoulder. **D,** Abduct the shoulder. **E,** Side bend the neck away from the side being tested. *Adapted from Butler DS:* Mobilisation of the Nervous System, *Edinburgh, 1991, Churchill Livingstone.*

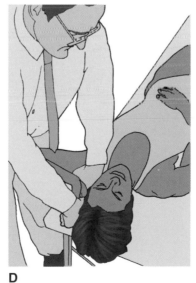
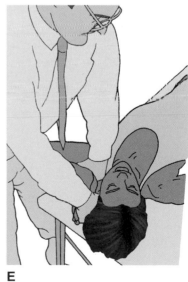

D   E

TABLE 18-11	Hunter Tests of the Brachial Plexus	
Test	**Sequential Maneuvers**	**Positive Test Findings**
High abduction arm test	1. Shoulder abduction, extension and internal rotation 2. Elbow flexion to 90° 3. Elbow extension 4. Forearm supination	Paresthesia: Ulnar nerve distribution, C8-T1 dermatomes
Low abduction arm test	1. Shoulder adduction and external rotation 2. Forearm supination (wrist neutral)	Paresthesia: Median nerve distribution, C6-C7 dermatomes

Data from Hunter JM, Whitenack SH: Entrapment neuropathies of the brachial plexus and its terminal nerves: Hunter traction tests for differential diagnosis. In Macklin EJ, Callahan AD, Osterman AL (eds): *Rehabilitation of the Hand and Upper Extremity*, ed 5, St. Louis, 2002, Mosby; Trotten PA, Hunter JA: *Hand Clinics* 7(3):505-520, 1991.

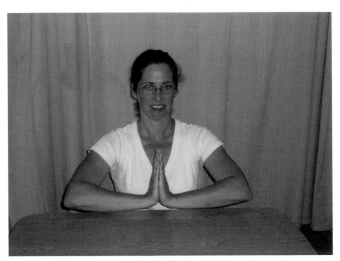

FIG. 18-16   Phalen's test.

applying direct pressure over the carpal tunnel for 30 seconds, with the patient's forearm held in supination. Reproduction of the patient's symptoms is indicative of CTS. Durkan found that this test had a sensitivity of 87% and specificity of 90%.[188] Furthermore, Williams et al found that this test was 100% sensitive in a group of 30 subjects with NCS-confirmed CTS and therefore recommended that this test be used in lieu of Phalen's test when clients are experiencing pain associated with wrist flexion.[189] Tetro et al found that adding 20 seconds of wrist flexion to the CCT flexion improved both the sensitivity and the specificity of this test in patients with and without electrodiagnostically-confirmed CTS.[190]

Piriformis Tests. Piriformis tests are performed in a subject presenting with sciatic pain and may be used to identify compression of the nerve by the piriformis muscle. A number of variations of these tests have been described. The flexion, adduction, and internal rotation (FAIR) test, which is intended to compress the sciatic nerve by stretching the piriformis muscle, is performed with the client sidelying on the uninvolved side with the involved hip in 60 degrees of flexion and the knee flexed. With the involved hip stabilized, the examiner places a hand on the lateral aspect of the knee and then applies a downward force as if to push the hip into adduction. This test is considered positive if it reproduces the patient's symptoms.

Beatty described a test that compresses the sciatic nerve in the piriformis muscle by contracting rather than stretching the muscle. For this test the client is positioned as for the FAIR test but is then asked to lift the knee off the table by abducting the hip. This test is considered positive if it produces pain in the buttock area.[191]

Fishman et al, in a study with 918 subjects (1,014 lower extremities) with complaints of low back pain or sciatica and 88 asymptomatic controls, found that the FAIR test was more than 96% sensitive and more than 68% specific for piriformis syndrome and that it was a better predictor of recovery than the current working definition of this syndrome.[192]

Comparison of Provocative Tests for Carpal Tunnel Syndrome. Many studies have compared the sensitivity and specificity of the various tests recommended for diagnosing CTS. Phalen's test has generally been found to be better than Tinel's test in identifying patients with CTS.[193,194] Gellman et al found that Phalen's test is more sensitive than the Tinel's test, but Tinel's test is more specific.[195] Priganc and Henry compared five tests used to diagnose CTS, including Tinel's test, the manual CCT, and Phalen's test, and found that Phalen's test is most effective for detecting the severity of CTS.[196] Koris et al recommended combining a Phalen's test with a sensory test (using Semmes-Weinstein monofilaments as described later) to achieve greater sensitivity and specificity.[197] Durkan compared the CCT with Phalen's test and Tinel's test. While assuring the amount of pressure being externally applied was maintained at 150 mm Hg for the CCT, he found that of 40 of 46 symptomatic hands had a positive CCT, and of these, 31 had a positive Phalen's test and 25 had a positive Tinel's test.[188] Szabo et al also found that the CCT was more sensitive (0.83) for CTS than either Phalen's test or Tinel's test and that abnormal findings on the hand diagram (see section on Pain Assessment), night pain, and abnormal sensibility as determined by the Semmes-Weinstein monofilaments (see section on Sensory Testing) slightly increased the sensitivity of the CCT (to 0.86).[198] A systematic review of clinical diagnostic tests for CTS found that both Phalen's test and the CCT were well supported,[199] and a more recent systematic review of clinical tests to diagnose CTS found that the CCT had the highest sensitivity (0.80) and specificity (0.92) overall.[200]

Autonomic Tests. Most noninvasive tests of peripheral nerve function depend on accurate sensory reporting by the patient. Two tests that do not rely on the patient's report that can objectively examine nerve function are the wrinkle test[201] and Moberg's ninhydrin test.[202] Both of these tests rely on autonomic nerve functions. When using the wrinkle test for hands, the hands are immersed in warm water at 40-42.2° C, with wrinkling of the skin occurring in approximately 3½ minutes if the nerve is intact and taking longer if the nerve is not intact.[203-204] A positive wrinkle test (i.e., wrinkling in more than 3½ minutes) has been found to be consistent in patients with recent and complete nerve transection but not in those with nerve compressions.[204] For the ninhydrin test, the client's hand is washed and gently warmed for 10-30 minutes. The hand is then pressed for 15-30 seconds onto previously untouched white bond paper to absorb any sweat from the hand. The paper is then sprayed with ninhydrin and dried. If there is sweat present, the ninhydrin will react with amino acids in the sweat and make the paper turn blue. If the paper does not change color, no sweat is indicated and there is impaired autonomic function in the hand, indicating probable nerve injury.[205]

Reflex Integrity. Deep tendon reflex (DTR) testing can help establish the presence of nerve pathology even in the absence of other clinical findings and is performed by tapping on tendons with a reflex hammer. With peripheral nerves injury, the DTRs will be hyporeactive. Although widely used as part of the clinical examination, some limitations of this test include variability in force during the tapping procedure, subjectivity in qualifying the response, and the fact that different responses can be produced by exerting different amounts of force. Marshall and Little examined these limitations by measuring the amount of force needed to produce patellar DTR responses that were graded as hyporeflexic, normoreflexic, and hyperreflexic in persons without neural pathology and measured the amount of joint angle excursion in the latter two using an electrogoniometer.[206] The median peak tap force required to produce hyporeflexia was 12.8 Newtons (N), normoreflexia was 38.0 N, and hyperreflexia was 85.2 N. The authors suggest that the DTR response be quantified by dividing the quotient of knee excursion by peak tendon tap force and that this measure be known as briskness.[206]

Sensory Integrity. Testing of sensibility is an essential component of the examination of individuals with peripheral nerve injury and can help localize a nerve lesion, and facilitate diagnosis, prognosis, and selection of interventions including patients' educational needs. Sensory test selection should be based on the expected progression of sensory return:

Pain and temperature
↓
Sharp, pressure
↓
Moving 2-point discrimination
↓
Static 2-point discrimination

Sensory Testing. Sensory testing is most commonly performed with hand-held tools. Consequently, some variables cannot be fully controlled, including the amount of force used when applying the testing instrument, the amount of vibration because of shaking of the clinician's hand, the amount of time the device touches the client's skin, and the speed at which the device is applied to the skin.[207] Not all of these variables are significant for all types of sensory testing and thus will be discussed where pertinent to each tool.

For sensory testing, the examiner should ensure a mutually agreeable communication system, establish patient understanding of the testing procedure, and maximize patient comfort. Additionally, for all cutaneous sensory testing, vision should be occluded (Fig. 18-17, *A*), and after orientation to testing procedures, distracting noise and activities in the testing environment should be minimized. Comfort may improve accuracy as the client will be less likely to reposition, thus minimizing extrane-

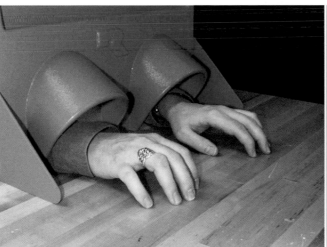 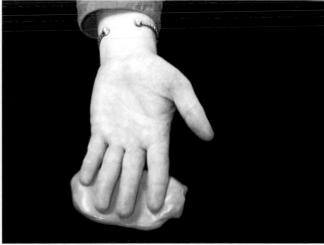

A   **B**

FIG. 18-17 Positioning for sensory testing. **A,** Vision occluded; **B,** resting hand in putty.

TABLE 18-12	Autonomous Sensory Zones for Terminal Nerves	
Nerve	Surface	Body Segment
Ulnar	Volar	Small finger, distal to DIP joint
Median	Volar	Distal to the DIP joint of index finger and IP joint of the thumb
Radial	Dorsal	First webspace, anatomical snuffbox (may be overlap of lateral antebrachial cutaneous nerve)
Superficial peroneal	Dorsal	Mid-dorsum of the foot
Deep peroneal	Dorsal	First dorsal webspace
Tibial	Plantar	Heel

DIP, Distal interphalangeal; *IP,* interphalangeal.

ous proprioceptive inputs. The body part to be tested should rest on a supportive surface to minimize extraneous movement and stretching of tissues (Fig. 18-17, *B*).[208]

Each nerve root and peripheral nerve receives sensory input from a specific area of the body. These areas are distinct but overlap to some degree because adjacent nerves can project into the same region. To localize a nerve injury, the clinician should examine areas where the probability of overlap is minimized (Table 18-12).

The ability to detect vibration is the first sensory function that is diminished with early peripheral nerve compression.[209-211] The ability to sense vibration may be tested with a hand-held tuning fork. This is done by first striking the tuning fork against a surface and then applying the single round end of the tuning fork over a bony prominence in the area of innervation and asking if the patient perceives the vibration. The sensitivity and specificity of this test are not known. Computer-controlled vibrometers, either with a fixed or variable frequency, are thought to more reliably quantify vibratory sensory loss. Force-defined vibrometers, which first measure skin compliance and then adjust the vibrometer for the force required to overcome skin compliance, have been shown to be reliable and highly sensitive for early detection of compressive neuropathy.[212]

Sensation of cutaneous pressure is best tested with nylon monofilaments (Fig. 18-18). These have been shown to have high sensitivity, as high as 91%,[213] but low specificity for perception of touch.[214] Of all hand-held manual devices, monofilaments appear to have the highest reliability.[215] Monofilaments are made of a single nylon thread attached to a plastic, hand-held rod. The end of the thread is pressed against the area being tested until it bends, and the subject is asked to note if they did or did not feel pressure from the thread.

Monofilaments of different thickness and stiffness are available, corresponding to the amount of force required to bend them, ranging from 0.008 gm to 279.4 gm. Semmes-Weinstein monofilament rods (one of the more common types of these monofilaments) are marked with a number (ranging from 1.65-6.65) that represents the $\log_{10}$ of the force in grams required to bend them. The monofilaments requiring the least force to bend can only be felt when sensation is normal, whereas some of the

monofilaments that require more force to bend may be felt even when sensation is impaired. The 1.65 to 2.83 monofilament represents the upper end of the normal range for most people without injury for most parts of the body and is recommended as the standard for normal sensation.[216-218] Exceptions are for the face, which is more sensitive and can usually feel a finer 2.44 monofilament, and the plantar surface of the foot, which is less sensitive and can usually only feel the 3.22 to 3.61 monofilament or thicker.[219]

When testing with monofilaments (Table 18-13), the clinician should begin with the "normal" monofilament for the area of the body being tested and progress to larger monofilaments until one is felt. A form can be used for recording monofilament testing findings. The monofilament is applied perpendicular to the skin and should generally be pressed until it bends. This is required for consistent application of force. The larger 4.56 and 6.65 monofilaments will not bend with manual pressure and should be pressed until they produce blanching of the patient's skin under the tip of the thread. Most monofilaments should be applied up to 3 times and held in place for up to approximately 1 second each time and then removed. An area may be retested after an approximate 1 second wait. To retest an area wait for at least another second before reapplying. The larger 4.56 and 6.65 monofilaments should only be applied once. For most clients, an uninvolved site should be used for comparison to establish a baseline.

In addition to testing for perception of vibration and light touch threshold, static 2-point discrimination (s2pd) and moving 2-point discrimination (m2pd) tests, known as density tests, can be used to quantify sensory perception in a given area. Static 2pd testing examines slow-adapting sensory nerve fibers, and m2pd testing examines fast-adapting sensory nerve fibers.[220] Both tests are reported to have high reliability.[221]

Two-point discrimination, whether static or moving, is also considered a functional test because s2pd and m2pd have been found to be predictive of a subject's ability to recognize objects by feeling them.[222] To carry out these tests in a standardized fashion, the clinician can choose between frequently used hand-held instruments, for example, the Disk-Criminator (Neuroregan, Bel Air, Md), Boley gauge (Research Designs, Inc, Houston, Tex), or other similar aesthesiometers. Use of a paper clip to determine s2pd and m2pd, while handy and economical, is not standardized. The Disk-Criminator (Fig. 18-19, *A*) has stationary sets of probes positioned around the perimeter of the disks, as well as one single probe. The Boley gauge has one stationary probe and another moving probe that can be positioned manually. With either device, the clinician applies one or two probes to the skin, without causing the body part to move (thus causing undesired stimulation of proprioceptive receptors) for 5 seconds. The patient is asked to identify whether he or she was touched with one or two of the probes. This is repeated, with 3-4 seconds rest between applications, until the patient can no longer distinguish between being touched with one or two probes. Interpretation for 2pd findings are listed in Table 18-14. Moving 2pd is determined as described previously,

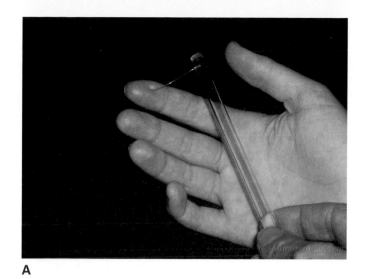

A

SEMMES-WEINSTEIN MONOFILAMENT
SENSORY TESTING RESULTS

Date: _____ Patient: _____

Comments	Filament	Interpretation	Force (gms)
	1.65 – 2.83 (green)	Normal	.008 – 0.08
	3.22 – 3.61 (blue)	Diminished light touch	.172 – 0.217
	3.84 – 4.31 (purple)	Diminished protective sensation	.445 – 2.35
	4.56 (red)	Loss of protective sensation	4.19
	6.65 (red)	Deep pressure sensation	279.4
	(red lined)	Tested with no response	

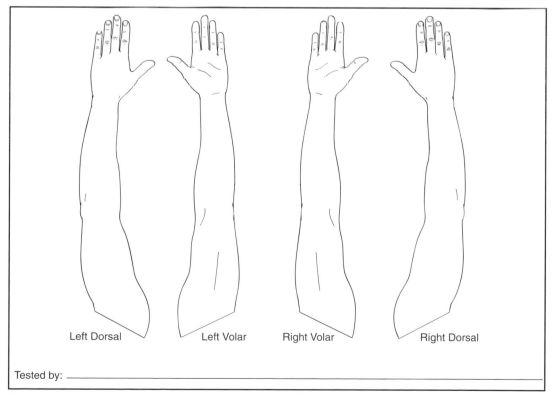

Left Dorsal   Left Volar   Right Volar   Right Dorsal

Tested by: _____

B

FIG. 18-18 **A,** Monofilament testing of tactile sensation. **B,** Sample recording sheet for monofilament testing. *B Courtesy North Coast Medical, Morgan Hill, Calif.*

TABLE 18-13	Interpretation of Monofilament Test Findings	
Filament	**Interpretation**	**Color**
1.65-2.83	Normal	Green
3.22-3.61	Diminished light touch	Blue
3.84-4.31	Diminished protective sensation	Purple
4.56-6.65	Loss of protective sensation	Red
over 6.65	Untestable	Red striped

TABLE 18-14	2-Point Discrimination in the Hand
Static 2 Point Discrimination	**Interpretation**
Less than 6 mm	Normal
6-10 mm	Fair
11-15 mm	Poor
One point perceived	Protective
No points perceived	Anesthetic

Data from American Society for Surgery of the Hand: *Examination and Diagnosis,* ed 2, Rosemont, Ill, 1983, The Society.

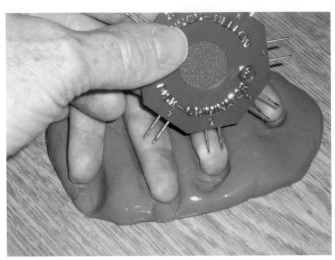

A

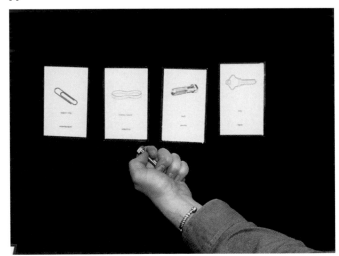

B

FIG. 18-19 A, Testing of 2-point discrimination with the Disk-Criminator. **B,** Items from the Moberg pick-up test for tactile gnosis.

except that the examiner moves the probes in a longitudinal, proximodistal manner.[223]

Variables that significantly affect the reliability of 2pd measures with any device include the amount and duration of force application and in the case of m2pd, the rate of motion. Although some authors recommend standardizing the force by applying sufficient pressure to cause blanching, it has been shown that blanching occurs with a wide range of forces, ranging from a mean of 19.16 gm to a mean of 36.49 gm with 1 point and from 2.38 gm to 14.91 gm when applying 2 points.[221]

Tactile Gnosis Testing. Patients with peripheral nerve injuries affecting sensation in the hand may have difficulty with tactile gnosis, which is the ability of the hand to perform complex functions by feel. A number of tests have been devised and evaluated for assessment and measurement of tactile gnosis. These include the Moberg pick-up test (Fig. 18-19, *B*) and the shape and texture identification (STI) test.

The pick-up test, as described by Ng et al, is performed first with vision available and then with vision occluded.[224] The client is asked to pick up 12 objects (coins [2 sizes], a key, a paper clip, screw, washer, safety pin, nail, wing nut, and metal nuts [3 sizes]) from a table, one at a time, and place them in a small container as quickly as possible. The time required is recorded. Then the test is repeated with the other hand. Finally, the client is asked to identify each object with vision and without vision. Dellon later modified the test to include standard metal objects.[225]

The STI test, introduced by Lundborg and Rosen, which involves the patient identifying the shape and texture of a variety of objects, has been found to have good sensitivity (95%), although poor specificity (40%) for identifying CTS, but good specificity (90%) and sensitivity (100%) for identifying patients with recent nerve laceration and repair.[226] This test has also been shown to be responsive to early but not later improvements after partial nerve lacerations, in contrast to 2pd testing, which is insensitive to early changes but responsive to later changes.[227] These findings suggest that the STI may be a good test for evaluating patients with severe sensory involvement, as occurs with total nerve lacerations and early in recovery, but is not specific enough to accurately differentiate higher levels of ability or less severe involvement.

Multifunction Computer-Controlled Devices for Sensory Testing. A number of computer-controlled tools are available for sensory testing. One of these, the Automated Tactile Tester (ATT) (Topical Testing, Inc, Salt Lake City, Utah) measures pressure sensitivity, as well as vibration, temperature, and pain sensation, while controlling for amplitude of application, rate of application, and length of time the stimulus is applied.[228] The ATT has been found to be more sensitive and reliable for testing light touch and vibration after surgical decompression for CTS than the usual manually applied devices, Semmes-Weinstein monofilaments and a tuning fork.[229]

Cardiovascular/Pulmonary. Peripheral nerve injury often occurs in conjunction with damage to other structures and for this reason, assessment of peripheral circulation is essential (see Chapter 29).

Function

Work, Community, and Leisure Integration. Compression neuropathy may be associated with activities that involve repetitive movements or vibration. However, since this is not a universal association and since the majority of people with CTS or ulnar entrapment do not perform jobs that involve repetition[230,231] and most people with repetitive strain injuries do not have compression neuropathy,[232] it should *not* be assumed that a patient's nerve injury is related to their occupation.

EVALUATION, DIAGNOSIS, AND PROGNOSIS

Most clients who fall into the *Guide for Physical Therapist Practice*[233] preferred practice pattern 5F: Impaired peripheral nerve integrity and muscle performance associated with peripheral nerve injury will have the following types of abnormal examination findings: Loss of or diminished strength, loss of or diminished ROM, impaired sensation, and hyporeactive stretch reflexes. In addition, integumentary integrity may be secondarily compromised. The following section describes rehabilitation interventions that have been shown to optimize outcomes for patients with peripheral nerve injury.

INTERVENTION

Clients with peripheral nerve injuries are referred for rehabilitation before and after surgical interventions and when surgery is not anticipated. After peripheral nerve injury, interventions should progress from those that focus on protection and immobilization to those that focus on restoring physical and functional abilities as the nerve recovers. These interventions should be modified according to findings on the examination, the level and mechanism of injury, and any associated injuries.

PATIENT EDUCATION

Clients with absent or impaired protective sensation should be instructed in measures to protect skin integrity. For patients with upper extremity involvement, this should include abstaining from holding cigarettes or cooking at a stovetop. For those with lower extremity involvement, this should include wearing shoes whenever walking. All patients with sensory impairment should be especially vigilant during activity involving use of sharp objects such as nail clippers, and patients who require splinting should regularly inspect under the splint for areas of pressure, rashes, and signs of maceration.

Personal and ergonomic factors may increase the risk for nerve compression or entrapment. Since smoking and obesity increase the risk for CTS, wellness programs that promote smoking cessation and weight reduction may reduce the incidence or severity of CTS.[234]

THERAPEUTIC EXERCISE

Strength Training. Although muscle strengthening exercises will not increase strength in patients with complete motor *denervation*, strengthening exercises can be effective with partial innervation and during reinnervation. Strengthening exercises may be started as soon as the patient can perform active muscle contraction (see Chapter 5). The use of electrical stimulation for strengthening denervated muscles is discussed in detail the section on Electrotherapeutic Modalities.

JOINT RANGE OF MOTION AND MUSCLE STRETCHING

Once immobilization for acute nerve injury is no longer necessary, joint ROM and muscle stretching may be needed to regain ROM and soft tissue length lost because of immobilization. After surgical nerve repair soft tissue lengthening should be performed with caution, particularly if the nerve was repaired under tension or with a graft. Muscle stretching is recommended when nerve compression or entrapment is caused by muscle shortening, as with cubital tunnel syndrome due to tightness of the flexor carpi ulnaris or piriformis syndrome due to tightness of the piriformis muscle compressing the sciatic nerve. Muscle stretching is also recommended when motor nerve injury causes weakness of one muscle and resultant shortening of its antagonist.

SENSORY RETRAINING

Sensory desensitization and reeducation programs are generally performed together or in sequence in patients with sensory nerve injuries that cause reduced sensation or pain. These interventions are intended to reduce hyperesthesia and promote reorganization of cortical representation of the involved limb.

Desensitization. Desensitization programs are described by several authors[235-237]; however, no published controlled studies evaluating the effectiveness of these interventions were found. Frykman and Waylett, who described a graded, self-introduced application of less to more irritating sensory stimuli, recommend 20-30 minute sessions, 2-3 times daily.[235] Barber later described a similar graded introduction of stimuli but recommended a specific progression from fixed textures, to loose materials in a container for limb immersion, to vibration, applied 3-4 times daily for 10 minutes each time.[236] Media commonly used for desensitization programs are shown in Fig. 18-20.

Sensory Reeducation. After nerve injury, even with optimal surgical repair, cell death and axonal misdirection can result in poor sensory localization and poor functional outcome.[131,238] The initial nerve injury, as well as axonal misdirection during regeneration, can alter sensory representation because of cortical reorganization.[239,240] The degree of cortical reorganization varies according to the nature of the injury. Crush injuries, where the basement membranes remain relatively intact, cause less axonal misdirection[131] and therefore little cortical reorganization after recovery.[241] In contrast, after complete nerve lacerations and repair, there is much distortion

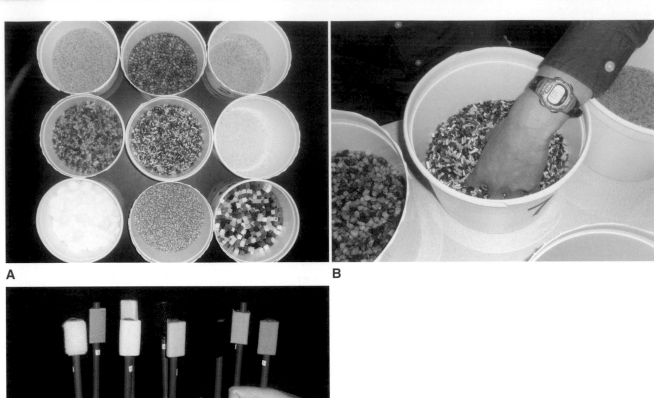

FIG. 18-20 Media for graded desensitization. **A** and **B,** Containers of loose materials; **C,** tactile sticks.

of somatosensory cortical maps causing previously well-defined areas to become diffuse[240] and adjacent areas to expand.[242]

Sensory reeducation may improve functional outcome after nerve injury by facilitating more appropriate cortical reorganization. Animal studies, with adult monkeys with peripheral nerve injuries, suggest that the following four components are necessary for sensory reeducation to be effective. First, stimulation must be spatially discrete rather than generalized to avoid "perceptual confusion." Second, areas of skin with normal sensation should be stimulated less than areas with abnormal sensation to avoid under representation of the areas with abnormal sensation. Third, stimulation must be actively pursued by the client and correct (versus incorrect) responses heavily and specifically rewarded, while praise for random attempts should be avoided. Fourth, training should be designed to improve both spatial and temporal discrimination.[243] There is some suggestion that training should also occur bilaterally[244] because tactile sensory inputs to

one side can activate the ipsilateral, as well as the contralateral, cerebral hemisphere.[245]

Various studies in human patients have found that sensory education can improve sensory outcome and function after peripheral nerve injury. Imai, Tajima, and Natsumai found that 24 patients who performed a 15-20 minute sensory reeducation program involving identification of the roughness of sandpaper and identification of the shapes of wooden forms and metal objects, once or twice a day after median nerve repair at the wrist performed better on object identification tests ($p < 0.05$) and had lower cutaneous pressure thresholds, although they did not perform better on tests of s2pd and m2pd than 22 patients who did not participate in this activity.[246,247] Similarly, a larger, prospective randomized controlled trial of 65 subjects with digital nerve injuries found that patients who received early tactile stimulation with a rotating or static stimulus several times a day had better sensory recovery than patients who did not receive sensory reeducation ($p < 0.02$).[248]

Based on these findings, it is recommended that sensory reeducation be included in the treatment of patients with sensory loss after peripheral nerve injury. Sensory reeducation programs generally include introduction and identification of increasingly complex tactile inputs with and without vision occluded. Stimulation should be focused on the area with reduced sensation and correct performance should be consistently and strongly reinforced.

MANUAL THERAPY TECHNIQUES

Nerve Mobilization. Nerve gliding techniques (Figs. 18-21 to 18-24) are commonly employed after nerve injury or repair with the goal of mobilizing nerves from sites of compression or entrapment after a period of immobilization.[249] Studies suggest that nerve gliding, when performed in conjunction with tendon gliding, may improve function in patients otherwise immobilized for nerve compression injury.

A prospective randomized trial with 28 subjects (36 hands) with CTS found that subjects who performed tendon and nerve gliding exercises for 4 weeks and who were provided with wrist splints had statistically significantly ($p < 0.03$) greater lateral pinch strength than subjects who were only provided with a wrist splint. However, symptom severity and functional status were not significantly different between the groups.[250] Similarly, a larger study involving 240 hands with CTS found that only 43% of those who performed tendon and nerve gliding exercises required surgical intervention as compared to 71.2% of those who did not perform these exercises.[251]

After surgical nerve repair, some recommend delaying all forms of mobilization to avoid disruption of the repair. Chao et al found in an in vitro study of 100 digital nerve transections in 10 human cadavers with 0-10 mm of nerve resected before suturing that when tendon gliding was performed in a splint there were no nerve disruptions when up to 5 mm of the nerve was transected, and when gliding was performed without a splint, there were no nerve disruptions when up to 2.5 mm of the nerve was transected.[252] A similar study with fewer subjects found that nerve repairs with up to 5 mm of resection were not disrupted by passive mobilization when limited by an extension blocking splint, and repairs with up to 2.5 mm of resection could withstand mobilization through full passive ROM.[253]

Although these results may lead the clinician to initiate early controlled passive mobilization after nerve injury and repair, it is important to keep in mind that nerve mobilization does pose risks to nerve regeneration. For example, application of continuous passive motion for 10 minutes, twice daily for 6 weeks after nerve repair in a canine model, beginning on postoperative day 1, was found to result in more scar formation and nerve hypovascularity than did immobilization.[254] Furthermore, surgical nerve repair techniques that minimize nerve tension were found in a study of sciatic nerve surgical repair in rats to optimize recovery as measured by nerve conduction velocity, muscle cross-sectional area, proprioceptive function, and motor function.[255] Given the conflicting evidence about the risks and benefits of nerve mobilization after nerve injury, further research is needed to clarify the optimal timing of nerve mobilization after different types of nerve injury.

PRESCRIPTION, APPLICATION, AND FABRICATION OF DEVICES AND EQUIPMENT

Splinting and Orthotics. Orthotics may be used to protect repaired nerves or insensate areas, rest limb segments to assist in resolving inflammation, promote function, or prevent deformity after nerve injury. For at least 3-4 weeks after nerve repair, orthotics are generally used for immobilization and to minimize tension on the nerve.[256] However, as noted previously, it is uncertain if such immobilization improves outcome.[257] Soft, nonrestrictive splints made of neoprene can also be used to protect nerves or areas with sensory loss as a result of nerve injury from thermal or mechanical trauma.

Body segments are often immobilized to reduce inflammation of musculoskeletal structures, and many authors recommend using splints to manage compressive neuropathies under the premise that this will help resolve an underlying inflammatory state. Despite the fact that histological studies suggest that edema and fibrosis rather than inflammation are more commonly associated with nerve compression,[258] studies indicate that splinting does help reduce symptoms from nerve compression. A systematic review of nonoperative treatment practices of CTS suggests that splinting does reduce symptoms but that surgery is more effective,[259] and elbow splinting alone or in conjunction with steroid injection were both found to be similarly effective treatments for cubital tunnel syndrome, with both decreasing symptoms and increasing NCV.[260]

Evidence indicates that full-time splint wear is more effective than just nighttime wear for reducing symptoms caused by nerve compression. Walker et al found that patients with CTS who wore a splint full-time had better symptom control and nerve conduction than those who only wore the splint at night ($p < 0.05$). A weakness of this study was that some subjects assigned to night-time wear only wore the splint more than instructed and some full-time wear subjects wore the splint less than instructed.[261]

Although functional splints (Fig. 18-25) can dynamically assist or substitute for muscle function after motor denervation, few studies are available to help clinicians and clients make more informed decisions regarding use of splints for these purposes. Functional orthotics for upper extremity nerve injuries have been found to be most useful for subjects with nerve injuries involving the dominant hand,[262] and ankle-foot orthoses (AFO) have been found to increase activity level while not decreasing muscle strength in patients with unilateral dorsiflexor paralysis.[263]

A single-subject study comparing three different splint designs (a static volar wrist cock-up splint, a dynamic tenodesis suspension splint, and a dorsal wrist cock-up splint with dynamic finger extension) and no splint after

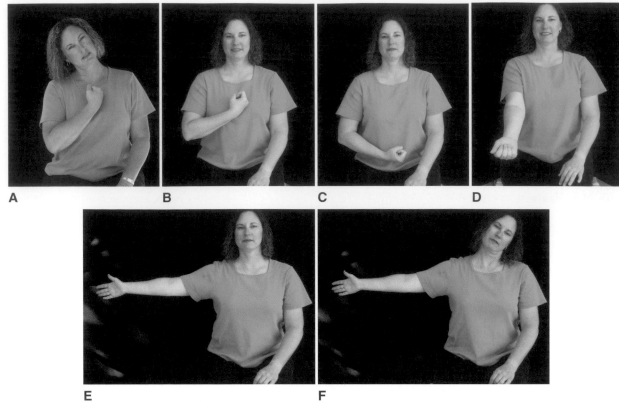

FIG. 18-21 Brachial plexus gilding exercise. **A,** The head is laterally flexed toward the affected side with the elbow, wrist, and fingers of the affected side in flexion. **B,** The head comes to the neutral position. **C,** The hand is moved across the chest and down to the hip level. **D,** The patient gradually extends the elbow and increasingly abducts the shoulder into the position in **E. F,** Lateral cervical flexion to the opposite side is the final component of this maneuver.

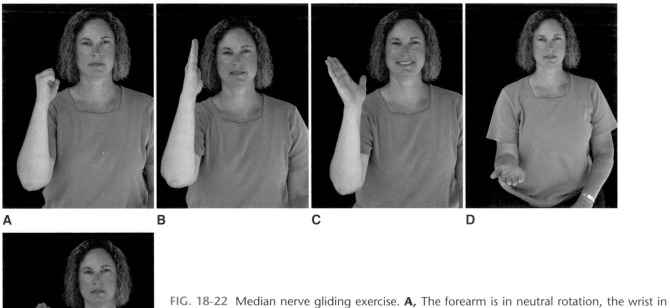

FIG. 18-22 Median nerve gliding exercise. **A,** The forearm is in neutral rotation, the wrist in neutral extension, and the fingers and thumb are flexed. **B,** The wrist remains in neutral, the fingers extend, and the thumb lies in neutral beside the index finger. **C,** While the thumb remains in the neutral position, the wrist is extended while finger extension is maintained. **D,** The wrist is returned to neutral extension, and with the fingers and thumb also in neutral extension, the forearm is supinated. **E,** With the forearm still in supination, a gentle stretch is applied to the thumb.

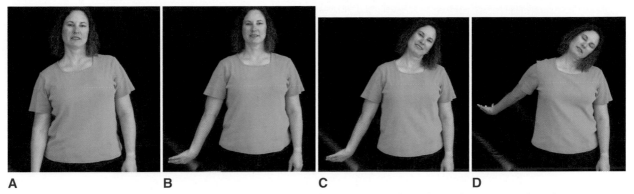

FIG. 18-23 Radial nerve gliding exercise. The patient stands with the body In a relaxed posture. **A,** The shoulder is depressed. **B,** The arm is internally rotated and the wrist is flexed. **C,** The neck is laterally flexed away from the affected side. **D,** The shoulder is extended while wrist flexion is maintained.

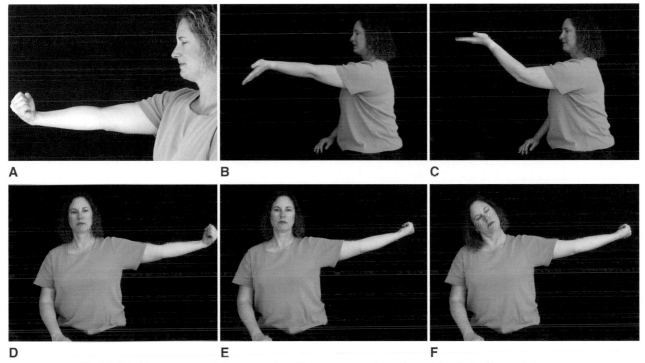

FIG. 18-24 Ulnar nerve gliding exercise. The sequence is performed only to the point where slight tension is produced. When this point is reached, the patient is asked to back off slightly. The first three positions emphasize the distal ulnar nerve and begin with a position of minimal stress. **A,** The head is in the midline and the shoulder is forward flexed and adducted. The elbow is extended and the wrist and fingers are flexed. **B,** The wrist and fingers are extended. **C,** The elbow is flexed. The final three positions in the sequence focus on the proximal ulnar nerve with the distal segment in a more neutral position. **D,** The shoulder is abducted, the elbow is extended and the wrist brought to neutral. **E,** External rotation of the shoulder is added. **F,** The neck is laterally flexed away from the affected side.

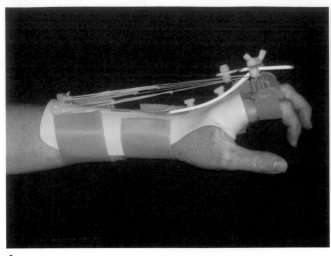

A

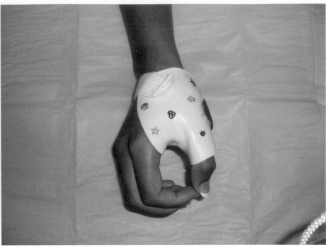

B

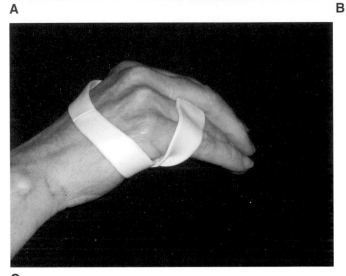

C

FIG. 18-25 Functional splints. **A,** A median nerve palsy splint designed to position the thumb to allow opposition. **B,** A radial nerve palsy splint designed to assist wrist and finger extension. **C,** An ulnar nerve palsy splint designed to prevent hyperextension of the MCP joints and allow the long finger extensors to extend the fingers when the intrinsic muscles are not able to contract. All of these splints are intended to be used during functional activities.

radial nerve injury found that the patient had significantly better function with the two dynamic splints but not with the static splint.[264] Despite this, the subject preferred wearing the static splint because it was supportive, easy to don, and had better cosmesis.

In general, the functional impact of a splint should always be carefully evaluated since this may differ among individuals. A small study with five subjects investigating the functional impact of knee immobilizers (made-to-fit Becker knee extension splint) for femoral nerve palsy found that two subjects reported falling less in the following year and that overall, after 5-7 days of using the orthosis, walking distance increased from a mean of 66 feet to a mean of 269 feet.[265]

Nerve injury often results in muscle weakness or imbalance. In this circumstance antideformity splints can be used to promote a more normal balance of forces or redirect forces. Table 18-15 describes some of the orthotics commonly used for upper and lower extremity nerve palsies (see also Chapter 34).

Assistive Devices. Patients with peripheral nerve injuries may need assistive devices for a short period of time while waiting for reinnervation or reconstructive surgery, such as a nerve or tendon transfer, or for the long-term, if motor reinnervation does not occur (see Chapter 33).

ELECTROTHERAPEUTIC MODALITIES

In patients with peripheral nerve injuries, electrical stimulation (ES) can be used to stimulate denervated muscle and facilitate muscle contraction in weakened reinnervated muscle and for pain management. The application of ES to promote peripheral nerve regeneration is also being investigated.

Electrical Stimulation. Some clinicians use ES to try to preserve muscle function and reduce the rate of atrophy and fibrosis in denervated muscle. Such stimulation is generally provided via surface electrodes using direct current stimulation. The research regarding the application of ES to denervated muscle has had mixed outcomes. This is most likely because of variations in treatment parameters, types of electrodes (transdermal versus implanted), timing of treatment, and the muscle being stimulated. Most studies examining the effects of ES on denervated muscle have used animal models and have explored two questions. First, does electrical stimulation retard or prevent

TABLE 18-15	Splints for Upper and Lower Extremity Peripheral Nerve Injuries		
Nerve Lesion	**Type of Splint***	**Indication**	**Rationale**
High median nerve	Elbow, wrist, and IF/MF extension restriction splint	Postsurgical	Decrease tension on repaired nerve.
Low median nerve	Wrist/hand flexion immobilization or restriction splint (dorsal blocking splint)	Postsurgical	Decrease tension on repaired nerve when tendons also injured.
	Thumb/opposition/abduction immobilization splint (opponens splint) (web spacer)	Functional and antideformity	Position the thumb in opposition to the index finger to promote pinching activities. Maintain web space.
High radial nerve	Elbow flexion/wrist extension immobilization splint	Postsurgical	Minimize tension on radial nerve.
	Wrist/MP/thumb extension mobilization splint	Functional	Utilizes tenodesis.
	Wrist/MP/thumb extension immobilization splint	Antideformity	Maintain length of extrinsic flexors and prevent overstretching of extensors.
	Wrist extension splint (cock-up splint)	Functional, antideformity	Prevent wrist drop.
	Wrist extension immobilization splint	Postsurgical	Decrease tension on repaired nerve.
Posterior interosseous nerve	MP extension mobilization splint	Functional	Maintain extension of MP joints, promote active flexion.
High ulnar nerve	Wrist flexion immobilization splint (dorsal blocking splint)	Postsurgical	Decrease tension on repaired nerve.
	Metacarpophalangeal extension restriction splint (figure-of-eight splint)	Functional, antideformity	Transmit EDC force distal to assist in interphalangeal extension, fourth and fifth digits if FDP innervated.
Cubital tunnel syndrome	Elbow flexion restriction splint	Symptom reduction or postsurgical	Limit stretch of the ulnar nerve. May restrict flexion of the elbow.
Low ulnar nerve	Metacarpophalangeal extension restriction splint	Functional, antideformity	Transmit EDC force distal to assist in interphalangeal extension (fourth and fifth digits).
Digital nerve	MP flexion, IP extension immobilization splint	Postsurgical	Protect repair. Hand-based or digital-based, volar or dorsal, depending on site of injury.
Femoral nerve	Long leg brace with spring-loaded knee	Functional	Assist in ambulation.
	AFO	Functional antideformity	Assist in ambulation.

*Common names of splints are provided in parentheses, splints are described using the American Society of Hand Therapists Splint Classification System.

IF, Index finger; *MF,* middle finger; *MP,* metaphalangeal; *IP,* interphalangeal; *AFO,* ankle-foot orthoses; *EDC,* extensor digitorum communis; *FDP,* flexor digitorum profundus; *AFO,* ankle foot orthosis.

muscle atrophy? Second, does electrical stimulation interfere with or promote reinnervation? Factors that should be considered when evaluating the research on the use of ES include that rates of atrophy in denervated muscle vary between muscle fiber type, within species and between species, and that rates of atrophy may vary, depending on the amount of passive stretch imposed on the denervated muscle.

Many authors suggest that electrical stimulation of denervated muscle in animals minimizes muscle atrophy and fibrosis while nerve regeneration takes place.[266-268] Others report that ES of denervated muscle does not produce this desired effect.[269-271] Overall, most studies that have found ES to be effective for this application have used implanted electrodes in animals, producing a high level of compliance and a regular schedule of intervention less likely to be found in a clinical situation. It is suggested that poorer outcomes in human studies may be a result of poor compliance, low frequency of treatments, the use of external electrodes, and inadequate stimulation levels for the depth of muscles requiring stimulation.[272] Furthermore, muscle fatigue and the potential for skin damage may have limited the effectiveness of ES for treatment of denervated muscle in humans.[273]

Overall, well-controlled animal studies using implanted electrodes have shown that ES with 0.4-7 ms pulse width, with 200 to 800 contractions per day, can reduce muscle atrophy in denervated muscle, when compared with unstimulated denervated controls, and can maintain muscle mass and maximum force generation capacity at the same level as in innervated controls.[274]

In humans, similar benefits have been found when implantable electrodes were used. Nicolaidis and Williams implanted electrodes in 15 human subjects with peripheral nerve transections and applied stimulation for 127-346 days. Other treatment parameters included a voltage between the minimum required to generate muscle twitch to a maximum of 10.5 V, a frequency of 130 Hz, a pulse width of 1.007 ms, and an on : off time ratio of 1.5/24 seconds. The outcomes of this treatment were compared to outcomes of others studies where ES was not provided, and the authors reported improved grip strength, pinch strength, and MMT outcomes for patients with ulnar and median nerve injuries and improved MMT outcomes for elbow, wrist, and digital extension for patients with radial nerve injuries.[275] These assessments were based on comparison with patients from other studies and were not evaluated statistically.

Although the evidence from animal studies seem to indicate that ES may help patients with denervated muscle maintain muscle strength and prevent atrophy until the muscle is reinnervated, there is evidence to suggest that this intervention may not accelerate nerve regeneration or may even retard nerve regneration.[276-278] Herbison et al's study comparing electrically stimulated soleus muscles (stimulated daily for 8 hours, with 4 mA, 4 ms pulse at 10 Hz) with nonstimulated soleus muscles in rats with bilaterally crushed sciatic nerves found that although the stimulation reduced atrophy, it did not improve nerve regeneration.[279] Furthermore, Love et al found that ES applied for 7 days with either trains of 0.2 ms pulses, at 20 pps for 10 seconds every 30 seconds or with 0.2 ms pulses, at 100 Hz for 600 ms every 60 seconds diminished axonal sprouting in partially denervated rat soleus muscles compared with unstimulated controls ($p < 0.02$).[280]

Electrical Stimulation for Neural Regeneration. Various investigators have studied whether ES can accelerate nerve recovery or improve the specificity of nerve regeneration. Although ES is not yet generally used clinically for these purposes, it may be adopted in the future if results continue to be positive. Some studies have shown positive results with the application of ES to injured nerves. For example, continuous ES with pulsed electrical current with a 0.2 ms pulse duration and frequency of 4 pps applied after nerve crush injuries in rabbits for 24 hours daily for 4 weeks was found to result in faster recovery of twitch force and tetanic tension than a control condition without stimulation.[281] Similarly, after transection and sutured repair of femoral nerves in rats, ES applied for 1 day to 2 weeks with 0.1-ms duration pulses of 3-volt amplitude delivered in a continuous 20 pps train, was found in one study to accelerate nerve recovery, with stimulated nerves taking 3 weeks to regenerate as compared to 8-10 weeks for unstimulated controls, and with stimulated nerves having more specific motor reinnervation.[282]

Electrical Stimulation for Transdermal Drug Delivery (Iontophoresis). Iontophoresis with a corticosteroid may help reduce symptoms in patients with nerve injuries with inflammation. Banta evaluated the effect of iontophoresis on CTS by initially treating a group of 23 patients with CTS with wrist splinting and nonsteroidal antiinflammatory drugs (NSAIDS) for 6 months. Four of these patients (17%) had symptomatic improvement. For the remaining 19 who failed this initial 6 months of wrist splinting and NSAIDs alone, iontophoresis with dexamethasone sodium phosphate was added. In this latter group, 58% of hands (11 of 19) showed improvement.[283] This suggests that iontophoresis with a corticosteroid may be effective for some patients with inflammatory nerve injuries. Since iontophoresis can cause skin burns where the electrodes are placed, these electrodes should not be placed on skin with reduced sensation.

PHYSICAL AND MECHANICAL MODALITIES

Heat. Heat is not commonly used for treatment of patients with nerve injury because it can increase inflammation during the acute recovery phase. However, heat may be used in the later rehabilitation of patients with peripheral nerve injury to facilitate stretching of muscles that have shortened as a result of weakness or denervation

of the antagonist and for pain management. A prospective, randomized controlled study investigating the effects of a low-level heat wrap (104° F) on wrist pain of various etiologies, including CTS, found that patients with CTS showed statistically significant improvement in pain ($p = 0.001$), joint stiffness ($p = 0.004$), grip strength ($p = 0.003$), and patient-rated wrist evaluation (PRWE) scores ($p = 0.0015$) compared to subjects taking oral placebos.[284]

Cold. Cryotherapy may occasionally be used to control inflammation and edema after trauma that includes damage to peripheral nerves, surgical nerve repair, or decompression,[285] or when soft tissue inflammation causes nerve compression. However, there has been little experimental investigation of the effectiveness of cryotherapy in these circumstances. In general, the role of cryotherapy in managing nerve lesions is limited because cold can delay nerve regeneration and nerves may be damaged if cooled excessively. There are reports of superficial nerve damage as a consequence of cryotherapy being applied for other reasons in an area over a superficial nerve[286,287] and of phrenic nerve injury as a consequence of cooling of the heart before cardiac surgery.[288,289]

Ultrasound. Pulsed ultrasound may promote recovery from nerve injury by nonthermal mechanisms. Furthermore, unlike continuous ultrasound, which increases tissue temperature and may adversely affect nerve latencies, pulsed ultrasound at intensities up to 1.0 W/cm^2 has been found to have little or no effect on nerve latencies.[290] A randomized, double-blind controlled study of 34 patients with electrodiagnostically confirmed bilateral CTS, where pulsed ultrasound (20%) at 1 MHz, 1.0 W/cm^2 was applied for 15 minutes for 20 treatments 2-5 times per week over the carpal tunnel of one wrist, while sham ultrasound was applied to the other wrist, found that those treated with ultrasound had less pain and better motor distal latency and sensory NCV than those who received the sham treatment ($p < 0.0001$).[291] This was true directly after completion of the intervention, 8 weeks after starting, and a 6-month follow-up.

Despite conflicting evidence, treatment with continuous ultrasound, which can heat tissues, is generally not recommended after nerve injuries because this intervention may exacerbate inflammation in an injured nerve or surrounding tissues. For example, in one study, continuous ultrasound at 3 MHz frequency, at either 1.5 or 0.8 W/cm^2 intensity was found to reduce NCV in patients with chronic CTS when sham ultrasound did not.[292] In contrast, a study of the effects of continuous ultrasound on acute experimentally-induced CTS in rabbits found that continuous ultrasound at 3 MHz frequency, 1.5 W/cm^2 intensity applied for 5 minutes resulted in greater recovery of compound muscle action potential (CMAP) amplitude than ultrasound at 0.2 W/cm^2 or sham ultrasound.[293]

Hydrotherapy. Despite a dearth of evidence, contrast baths, which involve immersing a limb segment in alternating cold and hot water, are often used clinically in patients with edema from any cause, including peripheral nerve injury.[294,295] It is proposed that the alternating cooling and heating will cause alternating vasoconstriction and vasodilation, respectively, to pump fluid out of an edematous area. However, there is very little published research on the effectiveness of this intervention for any application and none showing that this is an effective treatment for reducing edema.[296] Furthermore, it has been shown that contrast baths at temperatures commonly used clinically (15° C for the cold and 40° C for the hot) do not cause sufficient changes in soft tissue temperature to cause alternating vasoconstriction and vasodilation.[297]

Laser Light Therapy. Laser light therapy, also known as low level laser therapy (LLLT), is thought to reduce inflammation[298,299] and promote formation of new blood vessels[300] and proliferation of fibroblasts.[301] For nerves specifically, studies have produced conflicting results, showing that LLLT may result in decreased[302,303] or increased[304,305] distal latencies, reduced NCV,[306] and increased action potential amplitude. Furthermore, some have not found LLLT to have any significant effects on nerve conduction.[307-309] Some studies in animal models have also suggested that LLLT may promote nerve regeneration[310] or reduce nerve degeneration after injury.[311] Although the evidence is conflicting, LLLT is commonly used around the world to treat patients with peripheral nerve injuries, and since its initial Food and Drug Administration (FDA) clearance for treatment of pain associated with CTS in 2002, its use has rapidly increased for this and many other applications in the United States.

The clinically based evidence for the use of LLLT for patients with nerve injuries is also conflicting. Evidence in support of this intervention includes a small study of patients with CTS, with 10 treated subjects and 30 control subjects, that found that LLLT using a 830-nm wavelength GaAs laser, with a treatment dose of 1080 mJ applied 6 times, resulted in reduced symptom severity (pain, numbness, and tingling) and improvements in sensory nerve conduction 15 days after treatment only in the experimental group.[312] However, on reevaluation at 10 weeks and 54 weeks after treatment, both the experimental and the untreated controls had returned to their pretreatment states. Other uncontrolled[302] or poorly controlled studies[313] on the use of LLLT for CTS also suggest that this may be an effective intervention. Additionally, a small double-blind, placebo-controlled study with 16 experimental subjects and 14 controls on the effects of LLLT in patients with trigeminal neuralgia found that in the treatment group, 10 had complete resolution of symptoms, 2 had a reduction of pain and the remaining had little to no resolution of pain, whereas in the control group, 1 person had complete resolution of symptoms, 4 had some reduction of pain, and 9 had little or no effect.[314] In contrast to these findings, another small double-blind, randomized controlled trial with 15 subjects with electrodiagnostically-verified CTS found that the treated group, who received treatment 3 times per week for 5 weeks using a GaAlAs laser with a 860-nm wavelength with a 60-mW beam applied for 15 seconds to deliver at treatment dose of 6 J/cm^2, had similar findings on the Levine CTS Questionnaire, the Purdue Pegboard Test, and NCS, as the control group.[315]

SURGICAL INTERVENTION

Although rehabilitation clinicians do not perform surgery, they are often involved in the care of patients with nerve injuries that are surgically treated. Several factors determine the need for surgical interventions, including nature of the injury, whether the injury produces a closed or open wound, and the amount of time between injury and presentation. For severe nerve transections that present early, surgical nerve repair is generally indicated. If a nerve injury is associated with an open wound, the wound is generally surgically explored, whereas closed wounds are often observed for up to 3 months and only surgically explored if evidence of nerve regeneration is lacking. Surgery is also often indicated when pressure on a chronically compressed nerve produces symptoms.

The primary options for surgical nerve repair are end-to-end coaptation and nerve graft (autograft, allograft). End-to-end coaptation, after partial or complete nerve transection, involves suturing the epineurium of the separated nerve endings together (known as epineural repair) or suturing individual fascicles or groups of fascicle endings together (known as fascicular repair). Individual fascicle repair is uncommon because the many sutures required can cause excessive scaring.

If there is a gap between the nerve endings because the proximal and distal nerve segments have retracted or a portion of the nerve was so damaged it needed to excised, then a repair by end-to-end coaptation, which would require bringing the proximal and distal nerve stumps together, would place excessive tension on the nerve. In this circumstance, a nerve graft may be used. A conduit may also be placed around a nerve lesion or an area of nerve repair to reduce adhesion of the nerve to surrounding tissues and to direct nerve growth.

CASE STUDY 18-1

TRANSECTION OF THE ULNAR NERVE

Examination
Patient History

TR is a 31-year-old, left-handed construction worker who fell through glass and sustained a puncture wound to the left cubital tunnel, resulting in transection of the ulnar nerve. He underwent an ulnar nerve repair without anterior transposition on the day of injury and was placed in a long-arm, above elbow cast postoperatively. He presented to physical therapy 2 weeks after surgery. TR has no other medical issues. Since his injury, the patient has been on medical leave from work. Functional limitations include that the patient is completing 100% of bilateral tasks with his nondominant right hand. To manage mealtime activities, he purchases fast food or prepares ready-to-eat meals. Before his injury, the patient prepared his own meals four to five times per week. He has managed independent dressing by selecting clothing with few or no fasteners. The patient stated that he planned to return to work on modified duty in 1 week (3 weeks from date-of-injury) and full duty in 2 weeks.

Tests and Measures
Musculoskeletal

Posture TR's sitting and standing postures are within normal limits (WNL). His left shoulder is held in a position of slight elevation, perhaps to accommodate the weight of the cast.

Anthropometric Characteristics A hand volumeter was used to avoid submersing to the level of the surgical incision. Volumetric testing revealed moderate edema in the left hand with displacement of 37 cc more water than the right. The hands were warm to touch and of normal color. The 11-cm surgical incision was dry, red within 0.2 cm beyond the wound margins, and without odor, and the area surrounding the wound (along the medial and posterior elbow) was pink, tender, and edematous. Circumferential measures of the elbow taken in line with the elbow crease were 26 cm on the right and 32 cm on the left. Sutures were still in place.

Range of Motion and Muscle Length Initial measurements of passive and active motion were taken with care in order to not cause pain. Passive ROM (PROM) about the left shoulder and elbow were deferred in order to not place tension on the ulnar nerve. Active ROM (AROM) of the shoulder, elbow, and wrist joint were taken with the proximal and distal joint to each tested joint placed in such a position to not place tension on the ulnar nerve. Right upper extremity ROM was full but is provided as reference for those measures that are not full on the left. Results were as follows:

Joint motion	Right AROM	Left AROM	Left PROM
Shoulder flexion	0-180°	0-120°	NT
Shoulder hyperextension	0-60°	0-40°	NT
Shoulder abduction	0-180°	0-150°	NT
Elbow flexion	0-140°	15-60°	NT
Wrist extension	0-80°	0-20°	0-60°
Wrist flexion	0-75°	0-40°	0-75°
Wrist ulnar deviation	0-40°	0-25°	0-40°
Thumb CMC adduction	Full	Full†	NT
Thumb MCP flexion	0-50°	0-40°	NT
MCP abduction			
Index	0-25°	0-10°	0-25°
Middle (radial/ulnar)	0-15°, 0-15°	0-5°, 0°	0-15°, 0-15°
Ring	0-20°	0°	0-20°
Small	0-35°	20°‡	0-35°
MCP flexion*			
Index	0-90°	0-90°	0-90°
Middle	↓	0-90°	↓
Ring		−15°	
Small	▼	−20°	▼
PIP flexion*			
Index	0-100°	0-100°	0-100°
Middle	0-105°	0-105°	0-105°
Ring	0-110°	15-90°	0-110°
Small	0-110°	20-90°	0-110°
DIP flexion*			
Index	0-70°	0-70°	0-75°
Middle	0-70°	0-70°	0-75°
Ring	0-70°	0°	0-70°
Small	0-70°	0°	0-70°

*Composite metacarpophalangeal (MCP), proximal interphalangeal (PIP), and distal interphalangeal (DIP) passive flexion is full, indicating adequate length of the extensor digitorum communis.
†Thumb carpometacarpal (CMC) adduction carried out by the abductor pollicis brevis.
‡Small finger abduction because of contraction of the extensor digiti minimi.

Muscle Performance Manual muscle testing revealed weakness of the muscles innervated by the ulnar nerve, with flattening of the hypothenar eminence, as follows:

Muscle	Right	Left
Flexor carpi ulnaris	5/5	0/5
Flexor digitorum profundus (III and IV)	5/5	0/5
Abductor digiti minimi	5/5	0/5
Opponens digiti minimi	5/5	0/5
Flexor digiti minimi	5/5	0/5
Lumbricales (III and IV)	5/5	0/5
Dorsal interosseus	5/5	0/5
Palmar interosseous	5/5	0/5
Adductor pollicis	5/5	0/5

Pinch and grip strength was measured at the sixth postoperative week using a dynamometer and pinch meter. The dynamometer handle was set on the second level. Average measures (3 trials) were as follows:

Test	Right	Left
Grip	110 lb	48 pounds
2-point pinch	22 lb	19 pounds
3-point pinch	27 lb	18 pounds
Lateral pinch	30 lb	8 pounds

Left-hand grip strength measures were approximately 44% of the right (nondominant hand). Left 2-point pinch strength average was 86% of the right, left three-point pinch strength average 66% of the right, and left lateral pinch strength average was 27% of the right. On testing lateral pinch strength, Froment's sign was noted.

Neuromuscular

Pain TR reported pain about the elbow at a level of 5/10 with activity and 2/10 at rest.

Peripheral Nerve Integrity There was a positive Tinel's sign at the left inferior cubital tunnel with pain radiating proximally and distally.

Sensory Integrity With vision occluded, sensory testing using Semmes-Weinstein monofilaments showed absent sensation (using the 6.65+ monofilament) along the ulnar border of the volar and dorsal hand, along the volar small finger and ulnar half of the ring finger, along the dorsal surface of the small and ring finger metacarpals, and along the dorsal small finger and ulnar half of the ring finger. Given this finding, 2-point discrimination was not pursued initially.

Cardiovascular/Pulmonary: The Allen's test, performed over the radial and ulnar arteries at the wrist, was followed by timely flushing of the skin.

Evaluation, Diagnosis and Prognosis

Findings included presence of edema, timely wound healing, muscle paralysis in muscles innervated by the ulnar nerve, and absent sensation along the ulnar nerve distribution. These findings are consistent with ulnar nerve injury at the cubital tunnel. Consequently, TR is at risk for developing joint contractures and muscle shortening, as well as being susceptible to injury to the skin. Functionally, the patient's participation in activities of daily living (ADLs), work, and leisure activity is reduced. The patient is relatively young, which should facilitate a favorable outcome, but he has risk factors that could impede progress, including insufficient nutrient intake associated with dietary changes because of decreased independence in meal preparation and employment that includes forceful and repetitive activity. Full motor recovery may be expected in 1 year and good sensory recovery in 1-2 years.

Intervention
Skin Protection
TR was instructed in measures to protect skin integrity while participating in meal preparation and to visually monitor all activities involving sharp instruments. He was encouraged to use a protective glove when cooking. To minimize tissue damage because of skin dryness, the patient was instructed to use a moisturizing lotion several times per day. On his return to work, the patient was provided with recommendations to wear a protective glove with a rubberized fabric in the palm to both protect the skin and increase his ability to maintain objects in the hand by increasing friction (between the glove and an object) and to use cylindrical foam tubing around handles of tools.

Edema Management
The patient was provided with written materials instructing him to elevate the left arm while sleeping to minimize accumulation of fluids in the distal extremity. A light compressive garment was provided to minimize edema but to not be so restrictive as to compress the nerve.

Muscle Stretching and Range of Motion
Muscle stretching and passive joint ROM exercises were incorporated due to lack of expected progress to increase the length of the triceps and maintain length of the extensor digitorum communis muscle/tendons, the extrinsic digital flexors, and the volar PIP joint capsule of the ring and small finger. The triceps muscle may have become shortened because of postoperative immobilization and movement restriction to minimize tension on the ulnar nerve. The extensor digitorum communis muscle often becomes shortened as a result of the loss of the opposing flexor digitorum profundus. The digital flexors sometimes are shortened because of postoperative positioning. The volar PIP joint capsule often becomes short as a result of the inefficiency of the extensor digitorum communis to alone effectively extend the PIP joint. The patient was instructed how to avoid overstretching the ulnar nerve.

Strength Training
Active contraction of uninvolved muscles of the left upper extremity was initiated at the onset of rehabilitation to maintain ROM throughout the limb. A resistive exercise program was initiated at 6 weeks after surgery when innervation to the flexor carpi ulnaris was evident. This program of resistive exercise was progressively modified with sequential return of the ulnar nerve innervated muscles as expected in the following order: Flexor carpi ulnaris, flexor digitorum profundus (III and IV), abductor digiti minimi, opponens digiti minimi, flexor digiti minimi, lumbricales (III and IV), dorsal and palmar interossei, and adductor pollicis. Resisted exercise progressed in three phases as follows: Moving the limb segment through full AROM, place and hold exercises, moving the limb segment through full ROM and against gravity (for the flexor carpi ulnaris), and moving the limb segment against increasing resistance. The latter phase was implemented once each muscle reached a grade 3+/5. The amount of resistance required to engage the patient in this level of exercise was at 70% of his 1 repetition maximum. TR was instructed to complete 10 repetitions and engage in exercises 3 times per day each day.

Sensory Retraining
When TR began to perceive moving touch along the volar surface of the small and ring fingers, a sensory reeducation program was initiated. The program included object, shape, and material identification through tactile exploration for at least 15-20 minutes, once or twice a day. On attempting to identify the above inputs, the patient was to visually confirm whether his response was correct.

Toward the end of his rehabilitation, a desensitization program was initiated as part of a home program as a result of complaints of hypersensitivity along the ulnar digits. TR was informed of possible but unconfirmed benefits of desensitization protocols. He was instructed to obtain materials from his home that were nonirritating, potentially irritating, and definitely irritating and to apply these textures for 20-30 minute sessions, 2-3 times daily.

Nerve Mobilization
TR was provided with written instruction and demonstration in ulnar nerve gliding techniques by the fifth postoperative week with full flexion of the elbow avoided until the sixth postoperative week.

Splinting and Orthotics
At the time of the initial evaluation, a thermoplastic anterior elbow splint was fabricated to maintain the elbow in almost full extension. By the fourth week, wear of this splint decreased to night only and was discontinued by 5 weeks. At this time, a neoprene sleeve was applied at night to gently restrict flexion of the elbow while sleeping, without being compressive to the nerve. On reinnervation of the flexor digitorum profundus, a splint was fabricated to block the MCP joint of the ring and small finger in flexion, for the purposes of transmitting extensor digitorum communis force distally to the PIP joint.

Electrical Stimulation
On reinnervation of muscles supplied by the ulnar nerve, ES was used to enhance muscle contraction during exercises to increase strength and muscle hypertrophy. Initially, parameters were set to not cause excessive fatigue of newly innervated muscle.

Ultrasound
Pulsed ultrasound was used initially to reduce possible chronic inflammation, resulting in edema and pain about the elbow.

Outcome
Eighteen months after his initial injury, TR had full AROM and PROM in the left upper extremity. He had mild inter-

mittent "burning" sensations in the fifth digit. Grip measures increased on the left by 50%. Lateral pinch, 2-point pinch, and 3-point pinch increased by 30%, 32%, and 55%, respectively. The patient returned to work, with modifications, 2 months after his injury. During the course of treatment, he sustained one partial thickness burn injury to the tip of the ring finger from placing his hand on a hot stove.

Please see the CD that accompanies this book for a case study describing the examination, evaluation, and interventions for a patient with carpal tunnel syndrome.

CHAPTER SUMMARY

This chapter describes the examination, evaluation, and intervention for patients with peripheral nerve injury. Motor function, sensation, and sympathetic function is likely to be compromised, thus requiring examination of muscle strength, length, and balance and examination of quantitative and qualitative sensory functions, as well as examination of skin integrity. Intervention for patients with nerve injury may be brief, and the goals of treatment aimed toward relieving the causative factors, or long-term, while waiting for reinnervation of motor and sensory endorgans. In the latter case, treatment emphasis may shift to prevention of associated deformities and injury to skin, as well as facilitation of functional independence. Treatment may include patient education, edema management, muscle strengthening and lengthening, desensitization, sensory reeducation, electrical stimulation, ultrasound, splinting, and training with assistive devices.

ADDITIONAL RESOURCES

Useful Forms

Recording sheet for monofilament testing
British Medical Research Council (BMRC) Scale of Nerve Function

Books

Dyck PJ, Thomas PK: *Peripheral Neuropathy,* ed 4, Philadelphia, 2005, WB Saunders.
Senneff JA: *Numb Toes and Aching Soles: Coping with Peripheral Neuropathy,* San Antonio, 1999, Medpress.
Senneff JA: *Numb Toes and Other Woes: More on Peripheral Neuropathy,* San Antonio, 2001, Medpress.

Web Sites

The Neuropathy Association: www.neuropathy.org
Peripheral neuropathy: http://www.ninds.nih.gov/disorders/peripheralneuropathy/peripheralneuropathy.htm

GLOSSARY

Action potential: The change in electrical potential of a nerve when it is stimulated.
Afferent: Carrying impulses toward a center, as in nerves transmitting impulses toward the central nervous system.
Autonomic nervous system (ANS): Efferent pathways that include the sympathetic and parasympathetic divisions, which regulate smooth muscle, cardiac muscle, and glandular activity.
Axon: A projection or outgrowth of a nerve cell that conducts impulses away from the cell body.
Central nervous system (CNS): Nerves that are wholly contained within the brain and spinal cord.

Cranial nerves: Twelve pairs of nerves that have their origin in the brain.
Dendrite: Branching and tapering extensions of the axon that receive signals from other neurons.
Denervation: Loss of nerve supply.
Double-crush syndrome: Two or more lesions along the same nerve that produce a set of symptoms and that would be less observable if only one lesion existed.
Efferent pathways: Nerve cells carrying impulses away from the central nervous system.
Electromyogram (EMG): A graphic record of the electrical activity associated with contraction of a muscle.
Fascicle: A bundle of fibers, as in a nerve fiber tract.
Glia: Cells and fibers that form the supporting elements of the nervous system.
Infarction: Insufficiency or cessation of blood supply resulting in tissue necrosis.
Ischemia: Local deficiency of blood supply can be caused by mechanical obstruction of the circulation.
Mononeuropathy: An isolated nerve lesion.
Mononeuropathy multiplex: Asymmetrical lesions of multiple nerves.
Motor unit: A single alpha motor neuron and all the muscle fibers it innervates.
Myelin: Lipids and proteins that form a sheath around certain nerves.
Nerve conduction velocity (NCV): The speed at which electrical impulses can be propagated along the axon.
Neuroma: Abnormal growth of nerve cells.
Neurons: Nerve cells.
Neurotransmitter: A chemical agent released by a presynaptic cell that stimulates or inhibits the postsynaptic cell.
Nodes of Ranvier: A short interval in the myelin sheath of a nerve.
Peripheral nervous system (PNS): Nerves that may originate in the brain or spinal cord but end peripherally and include cranial and spinal nerves.
Plasmalemma: Plasma membrane.
Plexus: A network of nerves, or blood or lymphatic vessels.
Polyneuropathy: Symmetrical diffuse nerve dysfunction.
Schwann cells: Any of the cells that cover the nerve fibers in the peripheral nervous system and form the myelin sheath.
Synapse: The meeting point of the axon terminal of one neuron and a dendritic ending or cell body of another neuron or cell.
Wallerian degeneration: The degenerative changes of an axon and its myelin sheath distal to a focal lesion.

References

1. Nolte J: *The Human Brain,* ed 4, St. Louis, 1999, Mosby.
2. Flores AJ, Lavernia J, Owens PW: Anatomy and physiology of peripheral nerve injury and repair, *Am J Orthop* 29:167-173, 2000.
3. Rydevik B, Brown MD, Lundborg G: Pathoanatomy and pathophysiology of nerve root compression, *Spine* 9(1):7-15, 1984.
4. Breidenbach WB, Terzis JK: The blood supply of vascularized nerve grafts, *J Reconstr Microsurg* 3:43-58, 1986.
5. Lundborg G, Myers R, Powell H: Nerve compression injury and increased endoneurial fluid pressure: A "miniature compartment syndrome," *J Neurol Neurosurg Psychiatry* 46(12):1119-1124, 1983.
6. Olsson Y: Microenvironment of the peripheral nervous system under normal and pathological conditions, *Crit Rev Neurobiol* 5(3):265-311, 1990.
7. Deleted.
8. Lundborg G, Dahlin L: Pathophysiology of nerve trauma. In Omer GE, Spinner M, Van Beek AL (eds): *Management of Peripheral Nerves,* ed 2, Philadelphia, 1998, WB Saunders.
9. McLellan DL, Swash M: Longitudinal sliding of the median nerve during movement of the upper limb, *J Neurol Neurosurg Psychiatry* 39:566-570, 1976.
10. Byl C, Puttlitz C, Byl N, et al: Strain in the median and ulnar nerves during upper-extremity positioning, *J Hand Surg* 27A:1032-1040, 2002.
11. Wright TW, Glowczewskie F, Cowin D, et al: Ulnar nerve excursion and strain at the elbow and wrist associated with upper extremity motion, *J Hand Surg* 26A:655-662, 2001.
12. Gelberman RH, Yamaguchi K, Hollstien SB, et al: Changes in interstitial pressure and cross-sectional area of the cubital tunnel and of the ulnar nerve with flexion of the elbow. An experimental study in human cadavera, *J Bone Joint Surg Am* 80(4):492-501, 1998.

13. Borrelli J, Kantor J, Ungacta F, et al: Intraneural sciatic nerve pressure relative to the position of the hip and knee: A human cadaveric study, *J Orthop Trauma* 14:255-258, 2000.

14. Pechan J, Julis I: The pressure measurement in the ulnar nerve. A contribution to the pathophysiology of the cubital tunnel syndrome, *J Biomech* 8:75-79, 1975.

15. Lundbourg G, Rydevik B: Effects of stretching the tibial nerve of the rabbit. A preliminary study of the intraneural circulation of the barrier function of the perineurium, *J Bone Joint Surg* 78:54-65, 1973.

16. Clark WL, Trumble TE, Swiontkowski MF, et al: Nerve tension and blood flow in a rat model of immediate and delayed repairs, *J Hand Surg* 17A:677-687, 1992.

17. Fleming P, Lenehan B, O'Rourke S, et al: Strain on the human sciatic nerve in vivo during movement of the hip and knee, *J Bone Joint Surg Br* 85(3):363-365, 2003.

18. Wantanabe S, Yamaga M, Kato T, et al: The implication of repeated versus continuous strain on nerve function in a rat forelimb model, *J Hand Surg* 26A(4):663-669, 2001.

19. Nohuchia MP, Paley D, Bhave A, et al: Nerve lesions associated with limb-lengthening, *J Bone Joint Surg Am* 85:1502-1510, 2003.

20. Wall EJ, Massie JB, Kwan MK, et al: Experimental stretch neuropathy. Changes in nerve conduction under tension, *J Bone Joint Surg Br* 74(1):126-129, 1992.

21. Sunderland S, Bradley KC: Stress-strain phenomena in human peripheral nerves, *Brain* 84:102-119, 1961.

22. Liu CT, Benda CE, Lewey FH: Tensile strength of human nerves: Experimental physiological and histological study, *Arch Neurol Psychiatry* 59:322-336, 1948.

23. Brown R, Pedowitz R, Rydevik B, et al: Effects of acute graded strain on efferent conduction properties in the rabbit tibial nerve, *Clin Orthop* 296:288-294, 1993.

24. Rydevik BL, Kwan MK, Myers RR, et al: An in vitro mechanical and histological study of acute stretching on rabbit tibial nerve, *J Orthop Res* 8(5):694-701, 1990.

25. Sakurai M, Miyasaka Y: Neural fibrosis and the effect of neurolysis, *J Bone Joint Surg Br* 68(3):483-488, 1986.

26. Westkaemper JG, Varitimidid SE, Sotereanos DG: Posterior interosseous nerve palsy in a patient with rheumatoid synovitis of the elbow, *J Hand Surg* 24A:727-731, 1999.

27. Kornblauth ID, Freedman MK, Sher DO, et al: Femoral, saphenous palsy after tourniquet use: a case report, *Arch Phys Med Rehabil* 84.909-911, 2003.

28. Lin CC, Jawan B, de Villa MV, et al: Blood pressure cuff compression injury of the radial nerve, *J Clin Anesth* 13(4):306-308, 2001.

29. On AY, Ozdemir O, Aksit R: Tourniquet paralysis after primary nerve repair, *Am J Phys Med Rehabil* 79(3):298-300, 2000.

30. Koo JT, Szabo RM: Compression neuropathies of the median nerve, *J Am Soc Surg Hand* 4(3):156-175, 2004.

31. Gelberman RH, Hergenroeder PT, Hargens AR, et al: The carpal tunnel syndrome. A study of carpal canal pressures, *J Bone Joint Surg Am* 63(3):380 383, 1981.

32. Dahlin LB, Sjostrand J, McLean WG: Graded inhibition of retrograde axonal transport by compression of rabbit vagus nerve, *J Neurol Sci* 76(2-3):221-230, 1986.

33. Dahlin LB, McLean WG: Effects of graded experimental compression on slow and fast axonal transport in rabbit vagus nerve, *J Neurol Sci* 72(1):19-30, 1986.

34. Rydevik B, Lundborg G, Bagge U: Effects of graded compression on intraneural blood blow. An in vivo study on rabbit tibial nerve, *J Hand Surg* 6A:3-12, 1981.

35. Gelberman RH, Szabo RM, Hargens AR: Pressure effects on human peripheral nerve function. In Hargens AR (ed): *Tissue Nutrition and Viability*, New York, 1986, Springer-Verlag.

36. Mackinnon SE, Dellon AL, Hudson AR, et al: Chronic human nerve compression—a histological assessment, *Neuropathol Appl Neurobiol* 12(6):547-565, 1986.

37. Lundborg G: Structure and function of intraneural microvessels as related to trauma, edema formation and nerve function, *J Bone Joint Surg* 57A:938-948, 1975.

38. Szabo RM, Sharkey NA: Response of peripheral nerve to cyclic compression in a laboratory rat model, *J Orthop Res* 11(6):828-833, 1993.

39. Chang KY, Ho ST, Yu HS: Vibration induced neurophysiological and electron microscopical changes in rat peripheral nerves, *Occup Environ Med* 51(2):130-135, 1994.

40. Stromberg T, Dahlin LB, Brun A, et al: Structural nerve changes at wrist level in workers exposed to vibration, *Occup Environ Med* 54(5):307-311, 1997.

41. Lundborg G, Dahlin LB, Danielsen N, et al: Intraneural edema following exposure to vibration, *Scand J Work Environ Health* 13(4):326-329, 1987.

42. Dahlin LB, Lundborg G: Vibration-induced hand problems: role of the peripheral nerves in the pathophysiology, *Scand J Plast Reconstr Surg Hand Surg* 35(3):225-232, 2001.

43. Eguchi K, Majima M: Sciatic neuropathy caused by disorder of a nutrient artery: a case report of thromboembolism secondary to femoral artery aneurysm, *Arch Phys Med Rehabil* 82:253-255, 2001.

44. Wietholter H, Kruger J, Melville C, et al: Photochemically induced experimental ischemic neuropathy: A clinical, electrophysiological and immunohistochemical study, *J Neurol Sci* 117(1-2):68-73, 1993.

45. Korthals JK, Korthals MA, Wisniewski HM: Progression of regeneration after nerve infarction, *Brain Res* 552(1):41-46, 1991.

46. Delegal MK, Gorrie J: IV inserted to nerve results in radial nerve injury: $155,000 arbitration award, *Health Risk Manage* 23(1):1-2, 2001.

47. Chang WK, Mulford GJ: Iatrogenic trigeminal sensorimotor neuropathy resulting from local anesthesia: A case report, *Arch Phys Med Rehabil* 81:1591-1593, 2000.

48. Villarejo FJ, Pascual AM: Injection injury of the sciatic nerve (370 cases). *Childs Nerv Syst* 9:229, 1993.

49. Peuker E, Gronemeyer D: Rare but serious complications of acupuncture: Traumatic lesions, *Acupuncture Med* 19(2):103-108, 2001.

50. Khan R, Birch R: Iatrogenic injuries of peripheral nerves, *J Bone Joint Surg Br* 83:1145-1148, 2001.

51. Suneson A, Hansson HA, Seeman T: Peripheral high-energy missile hits cause pressure changes and damage to the nervous system: Experimental studies on pigs, *J Trauma* 27:782-789, 1987.

52. Kline DG: Civilian gunshot wounds to the brachial plexus, *J Neurosurg* 70:166-174, 1989.

53. Smith KL: Nerve response to injury and repair. In Mackin EJ, Callahan AD, Skirvin TM, et al (eds): *Rehabilitation of the Hand and Upper Extremity*, ed 5, St. Louis, 2002, Mosby.

54. Haveman J, Van Der Zee J, Wondergem J, et al: Effects of hyperthermia on the peripheral nervous system: a review, *Int J Hyperthermia* 20(4):371-391, 2004.

55. Pierre-Jerome C, Bekkelund SI: Magnetic resonance assessment of the double-crush phenomenon in patients with carpal tunnel syndrome: A bilateral quantitative study, *Scand J Plast Reconstr Surg Hand Surg* 37(1):46-53, 2003.

56. Nassif T, Steiger E: Post-traumatic distal nerve entrapment syndrome, *J Reconstr Microsurg* 15(3):159, 1999.

57. Golovchinsky V: Double crush syndrome in lower extremities, *Electromyogr Clin Neurophysiol* 38(2):115-120, 1998.

58. Wilbourn AJ, Gilliatt RW: Double-crush syndrome: A critical analysis, *Neurology* 49(1):21-29, 1997.

59. Chaudhry V, Clawson LL: Entrapment of motor nerves in motor neuron disease: Does double crush occur? *J Neurol Neurosurg Psychiatry* 62(1):71-76, 1997.

60. Morgan G, Wilbourn AJ: Cervical radiculopathy and coexisting distal entrapment neuropathies: Double-crush syndromes? *Neurology* 50(1):78-83, 1998.

61. Seddon HJ: Three types of nerve injury, *Brain* 66:238-288, 1943.

62. Sunderland S: Anatomy and physiology of nerve injury, *Muscle Nerve* 13(9):771-784, 1990.

63. Seddon HJ, Medawar PB, Smith H: Rate of regeneration of peripheral nerves in man, *J Physiol* 102:191, 1943.

64. Mackinnon SE: New directions in peripheral nerve surgery, *Ann Plast Surgery* 22:257-273, 1989.

65. Samii M: Diagnosis and management of intracranial nerve lesions. In Omer GE, Spinner M, Van Beek AL (eds): *Management of Peripheral Nerves*, ed 2, Philadelphia, 1998, WB Saunders.

66. Teerijoki-Oksa T, Jaaskelainen SK, Forssell K, et al: Recovery of nerve injury after mandibular sagittal split osteotomy. Diagnostic value of clinical and electrophysiologic tests in the follow-up, *Int J Oral Maxillofac Surg* 33(2):134-140, 2004.

67. Kraut RA, Chahal O: Management of patients with trigeminal nerve injuries after mandibular implant placement, *J Am Dent Assoc* 133(10):1351-1354, 2002.

68. Lydiatt DD: Litigation and the lingual nerve, *J Oral Maxillofac Surg* 61(2):197-200, 2003.

69. Ellis E, McFadden D, Simon P, et al: Surgical complications with open treatment of mandibular condylar process fractures, *J Oral Maxillofac Surg* 58(9):950-958, 2000.

70. Oliver P: Iatrogenic facial nerve palsies, *Surg Clin North Am* 60:629-635, 1980.

71. Singhi P, Jain V: Bell's palsy in children, *Semin Pediatr Neurol* 10(4):289-297, 2003.

72. Blankenship LD, Basford JR, Strommen JA, et al: Hypoglossal nerve palsy from cervical spine involvement in rheumatoid arthritis: 3 case reports, *Arch Phys Med Rehabil* 83:269-272, 2002.

73. Chang DJ, Paget SA: Neurological complications of rheumatoid arthritis, *Rheum Dis Clin North Am* 19:955-973, 1993.

74. van Wilgen CP, Dijkstra PU, van der Lann BF, et al: Shoulder complaints after neck dissection: is the spinal accessory nerve involved? *Br J Oral Maxillofac Surg* 41:7-11, 2003.

75. Chandawarker RY, Cervino AL, Pennington GA: Management of iatrogenic injury to the spinal accessory nerve, *Plast Reconstr Surg* 111(2):611-617, 2003.

76. Yavuzer G, Tuncer S: Accessory nerve injury as a complication of cervical lymph node biopsy, *Am J Phys Med Rehabil* 80:622-623, 2001.

77. Venkatesh B, Walker D: Hypoglossal neurapraxia following endotracheal intubation, *Anaesth Intensive Care* 25(6):699-700, 1997.

78. Rubio-Nazabal E, Marey-Lopez J, Lopez-Facal S, et al: Isolated bilateral paralysis of the hypoglossal nerve after transoral intubation for general anesthesia, *Anesthesiology* 96(1):245-247, 2002.

79. Dubuisson AG, Kline DG: Brachial plexus injury: a survey of 100 consecutive cases from a single service, *Neurosurg* 51(3):673-682, 2002.

80. Arslan E, Unai S, Bagis S, et al: Unilateral brachial plexus injury occurring after reduction mammaplasty, *Aesthetic Plast Surg* 26:372-374, 2002.

81. Ecker JL, Greebburg JA, Norwitz ER, et al: Birth weight as a predictor of brachial plexus injury, *Obstet Gynecol* 89:643-647, 1997.

82. Bar J, Dvir A, Hod M, et al: Brachial plexus injury and obstetrical risk factors, *Int J Gynaecol Obstet* 73:21-25, 2001.

83. Allen A, Sorab J, Gonick B: Risk factors for shoulder dystocia: An engineering study of clinician-applied forces, *Obstet Gynecol* 77:352-355, 1991.

84. Sandmire HF, DeMott RK: Erb's palsy causation: A historical perspective, *Birth* 29(1):52-54, 2002.

85. Hoeksma AF, Wolf H, Oei SL: Obstetrical brachial plexus injury: Incidence, natural course and shoulder contracture, *Clin Rehabil* 14(5):523-526, 2000.

86. Nehme A, Kany J, Sales-De-Gauzy J, et al: Obstetrical brachial plexus palsy. Prediction of outcome in upper root injuries, *J Hand Surg Br* 27(1):9-12, 2002.

87. Waters PM, Smith GR, Jaramillo D: Glenohumeral deformity secondary to brachial plexus birth palsy, *J Bone Joint Surg Am* 80(5):668-677, 1998.

88. Van der Sluijs JA, Van Ouwerkert WJR, de Gast A, et al: Deformities of the shoulder in infants younger than 12 months with an obstetric lesion of the brachial plexus, *J Bone Joint Surg Br* 83:551-555, 2001.

89. Wood VE, Frykman GK: Winging of the scapula as a complication of first rib resection: a report of six cases, *Clin Orthop* 149:160-163, 1980.

90. Ernst GP, Shippey D: Manual therapy rounds. Long thoracic neuropathy resulting from first rib palpation, *J Manual Manip Ther* 7(2):92-96, 1999.

91. Hester P, Caborn DN, Nyland J: Cause of long thoracic nerve palsy: A possible dynamic fascial sling cause, *J Shoulder Elbow Surg* 9(1):31-35, 2000.

92. Vastamaki M, Goransson H: Suprascapular nerve entrapment, *Clin Orthop* 297:135-143, 1993.

93. Kaspi A, Yanai J, Pick CG, et al: Entrapment of the distal suprascapular nerve. An anatomical study, *Int Orthop* 12(4):273-275, 1988.

94. Zehetgruber H, Noske H, Lang T, et al: Suprascapular nerve entrapment. A meta-analysis, *Int Orthop* 26(6):339-343, 2002.

95. Ide J, Maeda S, Takagi K: Does the inferior transverse scapular ligament cause distal suprascapular nerve entrapment? An anatomic and morphologic study, *J Shoulder Elbow Surg* 12(3):253-255, 2003.

96. Wong CA, Scavone BM, Dugan S, et al: Incidence of postpartum lumbosacral spine and lower extremity nerve injuries, *Obstet Gynecol* 101:279-288, 2003.

97. Cardosi RJ, Cox CS, Hoffman MS: Postoperative neuropathies after major pelvic surgery, *Obstet Gynecol* 100(2):240-244, 2002.

98. Natelson SE: Surgical correction of proximal femoral nerve entrapment, *Surg Neurol* 48(4):326-329, 1997.

99. Gruson KI, Moed BR: Injury of the femoral nerve associated with acetabular fracture, *J Bone Joint Surg Am* 85(3):428-431, 2003.

100. Simmons C Jr, Izant TH, Rothman RH, et al: Femoral neuropathy following total hip arthroplasty. Anatomic study, case reports, and literature review, *J Arthroplasty* 6:57-66, 1991.

101. DeHart MM, Riley LH Jr: Nerve injuries in total hip arthroplasty, *J Am Acad Orthop Surg* 7(2):101-111, 1999.

102. Mihalko WM, Phillips MJ, Krackow KA: Acute sciatic and femoral neuritis following total hip arthroplasty. A case report, *J Bone Joint Surg Am* 83(4):589-592, 2001.

103. Becker DA, Gustilo RB: Double-chevron subtrochanteric shortening derotational femoral osteotomy combined with total hip arthroplasty for the treatment of complete congenital dislocation of the hip in the adult. Preliminary report and description of a new surgical technique, *J Arthroplasty* 10(3):313-318, 1995.

104. Kim DH, Murovic JA, Tiel RL, et al: Intrapelvic and thigh-level femoral nerve lesions: management and outcomes in 119 surgically treated cases, *J Neurosurg* 100(6):989-996, 2004.

105. Hsieh LF, Liaw ES, Cheng HY, et al: Bilateral femoral neuropathy after vaginal hysterectomy, *Arch Phys Med Rehabil* 79(8):1018-1021, 1998.

106. Kvist-Poulsen H, Borel J: Iatrogenic femoral neuropathy subsequent to abdominal hysterectomy: Incidence and prevention, *Obstet Gynecol* 60(4):516-520, 1982.

107. Irvin W, Andersen W, Taylor P, et al: Minimizing the risk of neurologic injury in gynecologic surgery, *Obstet Gynecol* 103(2):374-382, 2004.

108. Pezina M: Contribution to the etiological explanation of the piriformis syndrome, Acta Anat 105:181, 1979.

109. Cai C, Kamath A, Nesathurai S: Traumatic sciatic nerve contusion, *J Back Musculoskel Rehabil* 15(2):89-92, 2000.

110. Barrack RL: Neurovascular injury: Avoiding catastrophe, *J Arthroplasty* 19(4):104-107, 2004.

111. Bradshaw C, McCrory P, Bell S, et al: Obturator nerve entrapment: a cause of groin pain in athletes, *Am J Sports Med* 25(3):402-408, 1997.

112. Hattori Y, Doi K, Saeki Y, et al: Obturator nerve injury associated with femur fracture fixation detected during gracilis muscle harvesting for functioning free muscle transfer, *J Reconstr Microsurg* 20(1):21-23, 2004.

113. Pecina M, Lucijanic I, Rosic D: Surgical treatment of obturator nerve palsy resulting from extrapelvic extrusion of cement during total hip arthroplasty, *J Arthroplasty* 16(4):515-517, 2001.

114. Dahlin LB: The biology of nerve injury and repair, *J Am Soc Surg Hand* 4(3):143-155, 2004.

115. Heumann R, Korsching S, Bandtlow C, et al: Changes of nerve growth factor synthesis in nonneuronal cells in response to sciatic nerve transaction, *J Cell Biol* 104:1623-1631, 1987.

116. Brushart TM: Motor axons preferentially reinnervate motor pathways, *J Neurosci* 13:2730-2738, 1993.

117. Liss AG, Wiberg M: Loss of nerve endings in the spinal dorsal horn after a peripheral nerve injury: An anatomical study in Macaca fascicularis monkeys, *Euro J Neuro* 9:2187-2192, 1997.

118. Frykman GK: The quest for better recovery from peripheral nerve injury: current status of nerve regeneration research, *J Hand Ther* 83-88, 1993.

119. Rosen B, Lundborg G, Dahlin LB, et al: Nerve repair: Correlation of restitution of functional sensibility with respect to cognitive capacities, *J Hand Surg* 19B:452-458, 1994.

120. Duteille F, Petry D, Poure L, et al: A comparative clinical and electromyographic study of median and ulnar nerve injuries at the wrist in children and adults, *J Hand Surg* 26B(1):58-60, 2001.

121. Polatkan S, Orhun E, Polatkan O, et al: Evaluation of the improvement of sensibility after primary median nerve repair at the wrist, *Microsurgery* 18:192-196, 1998.

122. Tajima T, Imai H: Results of median nerve repair in children, *Microsurgery* 10(2):145-146, 1989.

123. Barios C, Pablos J: Surgical management of nerve injuries of the upper extremity in children: a 15 years survey, *J Ped Orthop* 11:641-645, 1991.

124. Lundborg G, Rosen B: Sensory relearning after nerve repair, *Lancet* 358:809-810, 2001.

125. Bolitho DG, Boustred B, Hudson A, et al: Primary epineural repair of the ulnar nerve in children, *J Hand Surg* 24A:16-20, 1999.

126. Almquist E, Olofsson O: Sensory-nerve conduction velocity and two point discrimination in sutured nerves, *J Bone Joint Surg Am* 52:791-796, 1970.

127. Almquist E, Smith OA, Fry L: Nerve conduction velocity, microscopic, and electronic microscopy studies comparing repaired adult and baby monkey median nerves, *J Hand Surg* 8:406-410, 1983.

128. Todnem K, Lundemo G: Median nerve recovery in carpal tunnel syndrome, *Muscle Nerve* 23:1555-1560, 2000.

129. Porter P, Venkateswaran B, Stephenson H, et al: The influence of age on outcome after operation for the carpal tunnel syndrome: A prospective study, *J Bone Joint Surg Br* 84(5):688-691, 2002.

130. Friedenberg SM, Zimprich T, Harper CM: The natural history of long thoracic and spinal accessory neuropathies, *Muscle Nerve* 25(4):535-539, 2002.

131. Bontioni EN, Kanje M, Dahlin LB: Regeneration and functional recovery in the upper extremity of rats after various types of nerve injuries, *J Periph Nerv Sys* 8:159-168, 2003.

132. Ma J, Novikov LN, Kellerth JO: Early nerve repair after injury to postganglionic plexus: Experimental study of sensory and motor neuronal survival in rats, *Scan J Plat Reconstr Hand Surg* 37:1-9, 2003.

133. Lam N, Thurston A: Association of obesity, gender, age, and occupation with carpal tunnel syndrome, *Aust N Z J Surg* 68(3):190-193, 1998.

134. Richardson JK, Green DF, Jamieson SC, et al: Gender, body mass and age as risk factors for ulnar mononeuropathy at the elbow, *Muscle Nerve* 24(4):551-554, 2001.

135. Karatas GK, Gogus F: Suprascapular nerve entrapment in newsreel cameramen, *Am J Phys Med Rehabil* 82(3):192-196, 2003.

136. Nathan PA, Keniston RC, Myers LD, et al: Obesity as a risk factor for slowing of sensory conduction of the median nerve in industry. A cross-sectional and longitudinal study involving 429 workers, *J Occup Med* 34:379-383, 1992.

137. Ravindran M: Two cases of suprascapular neuropathy in a family, *Br J Sports Med* 37(6):539-541, 2003.

138. Grana W: Medial epicondylitis and cubital tunnel syndrome in the throwing athlete, *Clin Sports Med* 20(3):541-548, 2001.

139. Glousman RE: Ulnar nerve problems in the athlete's elbow, *Clin Sports Med* 9(2):365-377, 1990.

140. Szabo RM, Slater RR, Farver TB, et al: The value of diagnostic testing in carpal tunnel syndrome, *J Hand Surg* 24A:704-714, 1999.

141. Novak CB, MacKinnon SE: Repetitive use and static postures: a source of nerve compression and pain, *J Hand Ther* 10(2):151-159, 1997.

142. Waylett-Rendall J, Seibly DS: A study of the accuracy of a commercially available volumeter, *J Hand Ther* 4(1):10-13, 1994.

143. Dodds RL, Nielsen KA, Shirley AG, et al: Test-retest reliability of the commercial volumeter, *Work* 22(2):107-110, 2004.

144. Megens AM, Harris SR, Kim-Sing C, et al: Measurement of upper extremity volume in women after axillary dissection for breast cancer, *Arch Phys Med Rehabil* 82(12):1639-1644, 2001.

145. Mawdsley RH, Hoy DK, Erwin PM: Criterion-related validity of the figure-of-eight method of measuring ankle edema, *J Orthop Sports Phys Ther* 30(3):149-153, 2000.
146. Petersen EJ, Irish SM, Lyons CL, et al: Reliability of water volumetry and the figure of eight method on subjects with ankle joint swelling, *J Orthop Sports Phys Ther* 29(10):609-615, 1999.
147. Tatro-Adams D, McGann SF, Carbone W: Reliability of the figure-of-eight method of ankle measurement, *J Orthop Sports Phys Ther* 22(4):161-163, 1995.
148. Pellecchia GL: Figure-of-eight method of measuring hand size: reliability and concurrent validity, *J Hand Ther* 16(4):300-304, 2003.
149. Waylet J, Seibly D: A study to determine the average deviation accuracy of a commercially available volumeter, *J Hand Surg* 71:300, 1987.
150. van Velze CA, Kluever I, van der Merwe CA, et al: The difference in volume of dominant and nondominant hands, *J Hand Ther* 4(1):6-9. 1991
151. Matev B: Cubital tunnel syndrome, *Hand Surg* 8(1):127-131, 2003.
152. Cooper H, Dodds Wn, Adams ID, et al: Use and misuse of the tape measure as a means of assessing muscle strength and power, *Rheumatol Rehabil* 20(4):211-218, 1981.
153. Dellon A, Curtis R, Edgerton M: Reeducation of sensation in the hand after nerve injury and repair, *Plast Reconstr Surg* 53:297-305, 1974.
154. Gilbert A, Tassin JL: Obstetrical palsy: a clinical, pathologic, and surgical review. In Teriz JK (ed): Microreconstruction of nerve injuries, Philadelphia, 1987, WB Saunders.
155. Bae DS, Waters PM, Zurakowski D: Reliability of three classifications systems measuring active motion in brachial plexus birth palsy, *J Bone Joint Surg Am* 85(9):1733-1738, 2003.
156. Mallet J: Obstetrical paralysis of the brachial plexus. II. Therapeutics. Treatment of sequelae. Priority for the treatment of the shoulder. Method for the expression of results, *Rev Chir Orthop Reparatrice Appar Mot* 58(suppl 1):166-168, 1972.
157. Michelow BJ, Clarke HM, Curtis CG, et al: The natural history of obstetrical brachial plexus palsy, *Plast Reconstr Surg* 93(4):675-681, 1994.
158. Clarke HM, Curtis CG: An approach to obstetrical brachial plexus injuries, *Hand Clin* 11:563-581, 1995.
159. Curtis C, Stephens D, Clarke HM, et al: The Active Movement Scale: An evaluative tool for infants with obstetrical brachial plexus palsy, *J Hand Surg* 27A:470-478, 2002.
160. Manente G, Torrieri F, Pineto F, et al: A relief maneuver in carpal tunnel syndrome, *Muscle Nerve* 22(11):1587-1589, 1999.
161. Spindler HA, Dellon AL: Nerve conduction studies and sensibility testing in carpal tunnel syndrome, *J Hand Surg* 7A:260-263, 1982.
162. American Association of Electrodiagnostic Medicine, American Academy of Neurology, and American Academy of Physical Medicine and Rehabilitation: Practice parameters for electrodiagnostic studies in carpal tunnel syndrome: Report of the American Association of Electrodiagnostic Medicine, American Academy of Neurology, and American Academy of Physical Medicine and Rehabilitation, *Muscle Nerve* 25:918-922, 2002.
163. Witt JC, Hentz JG, Clarke Stevens J: Carpal tunnel syndrome with normal nerve conduction studies, *Muscle Nerve* 29:515-522, 2004.
164. Grundberg AB: Carpal tunnel decompression in spite of normal electromyography, *J Hand Surg* 8A(3):348-349, 1983.
165. Concannon MJ, Gainor B, Petroski GF, et al: The predictive value of electrodiagnostic studies in carpal tunnel syndrome, *Plast Reconstr Surg* 100:1452-1458, 1997.
166. Glowacki KA, Breen CJ, Sachar K, et al: Electrodiagnostic testing and carpal tunnel release outcome, *J Hand Surg* 21A:117-121, 1996.
167. Werner R, Gell N, Franzblau A, et al: Prolonged median sensory latency as a predictor of carpal tunnel syndrome, *Muscle Nerve* 24:1462-1467, 2002.
168. Nathan PA, Keniston RC, Myers LD, et al: Natural history of median nerve sensory conduction in industry: Relationship to symptoms and carpal tunnel syndrome in 558 hands over 11 years, *Muscle Nerve* 21:711-721, 1998.
169. Werner RA, Franzblau A, Albers JW, et al: Use of screening nerve conduction studies for predicting future carpal tunnel syndrome, *Occup Environ Med* 54:96-100, 1997.
170. Montagna P, Liguori R: The motor Tinel sign: A useful sign in entrapment neuropathy? *Muscle Nerve* 23(6):976-978, 2000.
171. Henderson WR: Clinical assessment of peripheral nerve injuries. Tinel's test, *Lancet* 2:801-804, 1948.
172. Khoo D, Carmichael SW, Spinner RJ: Ulnar nerve anatomy and compression, *Orthop Clin N Am* 27(2):317-337, 1996.
173. Seror P: Tinel's sign in the diagnosis of carpal tunnel syndrome, *J Hand Surg* 12B(3):364-365, 1987.
174. Monsivais JJ, Sun Y: Tinel's sign or percussion test? Developing a better method of evoking a Tinel's sign, *J South Orthop Assoc* 6(3):186-189, 1997.
175. Novack CB, Mackinnon SE, Brownlee R, et al: Provocative sensory testing in carpal tunnel syndrome, *J Hand Surg* 17B:204-208, 1992.
176. Spicher C, Kohut G, Miauton J: At which stage of sensory recovery can a tingling sign be expected? A review and proposal for standardization and grading, *J Hand Ther* 12(4):298-308, 1999.
177. Elvey R: Brachial plexus tension test and the pathoanatomical origin of arm pain. In Glascow E, Tavomey L (eds): *Aspects of Manipulative Therapy,* Melbourne, 1979, Lincoln Institute of Health Sciences.
178. Butler D: *Mobilization of the Nervous System,* Melbourne, 1991, Churchill Livingstone.
179. Hunter JM, Whitenack SH: Entrapment neuropathies of the brachial plexus and its terminal nerves: Hunter traction tests for differential diagnosis. In Macklin EJ, Callahan AD, Osterman AL (eds): *Rehabilitation of the Hand and Upper Extremity,* ed 5, St. Louis, 2002, Mosby.
180. Kleinrensink GJ, Stoeckart R, Vleeming A, et al: Mechanical tension in the median nerve. The effects of joint position, *Clin Biomech* 10:240-244, 1995.
181. Klienrensink GJ, Stoeckart R, Mulder PGH, et al: Upper limb tension tests as tools in the diagnosis of nerve and plexus lesions. Anatomical and biomechanical aspects, *Clin Biomech* 15:9-14, 2000.
182. Coppieters M, Stappaerts K, Janssens K, et al: Reliability of detecting "onset of pain" and "submaximal pain" during neural provocation testing of the upper quadrant, *Physiother Res Int* 7(3):146-156, 2002.
183. Coppieters MW, Stappaertos KH, Evaraert DG, et al: Addition of tests components during neurodynamic testing: Effect on range of motion and sensory responses, *J Orthop Sports Phys Ther* 31(5):226-237, 2001.
184. Buehler MJ, Thayer DT: The elbow flexion test. A clinical test for the cubital tunnel syndrome, *Clin Orthop* 233:213-216, 1988.
185. Novak CB, Lee GW, Mackinnon SE, et al: Provocative testing for cubital tunnel syndrome, *J Hand Surg* 19A(5):817-820, 1994.
186. Phalan GS: The carpal-tunnel syndrome: Seventeen years' experience in diagnosis and treatment of six hundred fifty-four hands, *J Bone Joint Surg Am* 48:211-228, 1996.
187. Seror P: Phalen's test in diagnosis of carpal tunnel syndrome, *J Hand Surg* 13(4):383-385, 1988.
188. Durkan JA: New diagnostic test for carpal tunnel syndrome, *J Bone Joint Surg Am* 73(4):535-538, 1991.
189. Williams TM, Mackinnon SE, Novak CB, et al: Verification of the pressure provocative test in carpal tunnel syndrome, *Ann Plast Surg* 29(1):8-11, 1992.
190. Tetro AM, Evanoff BA, Holstein SB: A new provocative test for carpal tunnel syndrome. Assessment of wrist flexion and nerve compression, *J Bone Joint Surg Br* 80(3):493-498, 1992.
191. Beatty RA: The piriformis muscle syndrome: A simple diagnostic maneuver, *Neurosurgery* 34(3):512-514, 1994.
192. Fishman LM, Dombi GW, Michaelsen C, et al: Piriformis syndrome: Diagnosis, treatment, and outcome—a 10-year study, *Arch Phys Med Rehabil* 83:295-301, 2002.
193. Kuschner SH, Ebramzadeh E, Johnson D, et al: Tinel's sign and Phalen's test in carpal tunnel syndrome, *Orthopedics* 15(11):1297-1302, 1992.
194. Williams TM, Mackinnon SE, Novak CB, et al: Verification of the pressure provocative test in carpal tunnel syndrome, *Ann Plast Surg* 29(1):8-11, 1992.
195. Gellman H, Gelberman RH, Tan AM, et al: Carpal tunnel syndrome: An evaluation of the provocative diagnostic tests, *J Bone Joint Surg Am* 68:735-737, 1986.
196. Priganc VW, Henry SM: The relationship among five common carpal tunnel syndrome tests and the severity of carpal tunnel syndrome, *J Hand Ther* 316:225-236, 2003.
197. Koris M, Gelberman RH, Duncan K, et al: Carpal tunnel syndrome. Evaluation of a quantitative provocational diagnostic test, *Clin Orthop* 251:157-161, 1990.
198. Szabo RM, Slater RR Jr, Farver TB, et al: The value of diagnostic testing in carpal tunnel syndrome, *J Hand Surg* 24A(4):704-714, 1999.
199. Massy-Westropp N, Grimmer K, et al: A systematic review of the clinical diagnostic tests for carpal tunnel syndrome, *J Hand Surg* 25A(1):120-127, 2000.
200. MacDermid JC, Wessel J: Clinical diagnosis of carpal tunnel syndrome: a systematic review, *J Hand Ther* 17(2):309-319, 2004.
201. O'Rianin S: New and simple test of nerve function in hand, *BMJ* 3:615-616, 1973.
202. Moberg E: Objective methods for determining the functional value of sensibility in the hand, *J Bone Joint Surg Br* 40(3):454-476, 1958.
203. Cales L, Weber RA: Effect of water temperature on skin wrinkling, *J Hand Surg* 22(4):747-749, 1997.
204. Phelps PE, Walker E: Comparison of the finger wrinkling test results to established sensory tests in peripheral nerve injury, *Am J Occup Ther* 31(9):565-572, 1977.
205. Stromberg WB, McFarlane RM, Bell JL, et al: Injury of the median and ulnar nerves: 150 cases with an evaluation of Moberg's ninhydrin test, *J Bone Joint Surg Am* 43:717-730, 1961.
206. Marshall GL, Little JW: Deep tendon reflexes: A study of quantitative methods, *J Spinal Cord Med* 25(2):94-99, 2002.
207. Bell-Krotoski JA, Buford WL: The force/time relationship of clinically used sensory testing instruments, *J Hand Ther* 76-85, 1988.
208. Brand PW, Hollister A: *Clinical Mechanics of the Hand,* ed 2, St. Louis, 1993, Mosby.
209. Gelberman RH, Szabo RM, Williamson RV, et al: Sensibility testing in peripheral-nerve compression syndromes: An experimental study in humans, *J Bone Joint Surg Am* 65:632-637, 1983.

210. Szabo RM, Gelberman RH, Dimick MP: Sensibility testing in patients with carpal tunnel syndrome, *J Bone Joint Surg Am* 66:60-64, 1984.
211. Szabo RM, Gelberman RH, Williamson RV, et al: Vibratory sensory testing in acute peripheral nerve compression, *J Hand Surg* 9A:104-109, 1984.
212. Hubbard MC, MacDermid JC, Kramer JF, et al: Quantitative vibration threshold testing in carpal tunnel syndrome: Analysis strategies for optimizing reliability, *J Hand Ther* 18:24-30, 2004.
213. Gellman H, Gelberman RH, Tan AM, et al: Carpal tunnel syndrome. An evaluation of the provocative diagnostic tests, *J Bone Joint Surg Am* 68:735-737, 1986.
214. MacDermid JC, Kramer JF, Roth JH: Decision making in detecting abnormal Semmes-Weinstein monofilament thresholds in carpal tunnel syndrome, *J Hand Ther* 7:158-162, 1994.
215. Bell-Krotoski J, Tomancik E: The repeatability of testing with Semmes-Weinstein monofilaments, *J Hand Surg* 12A:155-161, 1987.
216. Von Prince K, Butler B: Measuring sensory function of the hand in peripheral nerve injuries, *Am J Occup Ther* 21:385-396, 1967.
217. Bell-Krotoski JA, Fess EE, Figarola JH, et al: Threshold detection and Semmes-Weinstein monofilaments, *J Hand Ther* 8:155-162, 1995.
218. Werner Jl, Omer GE: Evaluating cutaneous pressure sensitivity of the hand, *Am J Occup Ther* 24:347-356, 1970.
219. Jeng C, Michelson J, Mizel M: Sensory thresholds of normal human feet, *Foot Ankle Int* 21:501-504, 2000.
220. Dellon AL: The moving two-point discrimination test: clinical evaluation of the quickly adapting fiber/receptor system, *J Hand Surg* 3:474-481, 1978.
221. Dellon AL, Mackinnon SE, Crosby PM: Reliability of two point discrimination measurements, *J Hand Surg* 12A:693-696, 1987.
222. Callahan AD: Sensibility assessment for nerve lesions-in-continuity and nerve lacerations. In Mackin EJ, Callahan AD, Osterman AL (eds): *Rehabilitation of the Hand and Upper Extremity,* ed 5, St. Louis, 2005, Mosby.
223. Novack CB: Evaluation of hand sensibility: A review, *J Hand Ther* 14:266-272, 2001.
224. Ng CL, Ho DD, Chow SP: The Moberg pickup test: results of testing with a standard protocol, *J Hand Ther* 12(4):309-312, 1999.
225. Dellon AL: *Evaluation of Sensibility and Reeducation of Sensation in the Hand,* Baltimore, 1981, Williams & Wilkins.
226. Rosen B, Lundborg G: A new tactile gnosis instrument in sensibility testing, *J Hand Ther* 11(4):251-257, 1998.
227. Rosen B, Jerosch-Herold C: Comparing the responsiveness over time of two tactile gnosis tests: Two-point discrimination and the STI test, *Br J Hand Ther* 5(4):114-119, 2000.
228. Horch K, Hardy M, Jimenez S, et al: An automated tactile tester for evaluation of cutaneous sensibility, *J Hand Surg* 17A:829-837, 1992.
229. Jiminez S, Hardy M, Horch K, et al: A study of sensory recovery following carpal tunnel release, *J Hand Ther* 6(2):124-129, 1993.
230. Dias JJ, Burke FD, Wildin CJ, et al: Carpal tunnel syndrome and work, *J Hand Surg* 29b(4):329-333, 2004.
231. Descatha A, Leclerc A, Chastang JF, et al: Incidence of ulnar nerve entrapment at the elbow in repetitive work, *Scand J Work Environ Health* 30(3):234-240, 2004.
232. Barthel HR, Miller LS, Deardorff WW, et al: Presentation and response of patients with upper extremity repetitive use syndrome to a multidisciplinary rehabilitation program: a retrospective review of 24 cases, *J Hand Ther* 11(3):191-199, 1998.
233. American Physical Therapy Association: *Guide to Physical Therapist Practice,* ed 2, Alexandria, Va, 2001, The Association.
234. Nathan PA, Meadows KD, Istvan JA: Predictors of carpal tunnel syndrome: an 11-year study of industrial workers, *J Hand Surg* 27A:644-651, 2002.
235. Frykman GK, Waylett J: Rehabilitation of peripheral nerve injuries, *Orthop Clin North Am* 12(2):361-379, 1981.
236. Barber LM: Desensitization of the traumatized hand. In Hunter JM (ed): *Rehabilitation of the Hand,* St. Louis, 1990, Mosby.
237. Anthony MS: Sensory Re-education. In Clark GL, Wilgis EFS, Aiello B, et al (eds): *Hand Rehabilitation: A Practical Guide,* New York, 1993, Churchill Livingstone.
238. Lundborg G: A 25-year perspective of peripheral nerve surgery: evolving neuroscientific concepts and clinical significance, *J Hand Surg* 25A:391-414, 2000.
239. Merzenich MM, Kaas JH, Wall JT, et al: Progression of change following median nerve section in the cortical representation of the hand in areas 3b and 1 in adult owl and squirrel monkeys, *Neuroscience* 10:639-665, 1983.
240. Wall JT, Kaas JH, Sur M, et al: Functional reorganization in somatosensory cortical areas 3b and 1 of adult monkeys after median nerve repair: possible relationships to sensory recovery in humans, *J Neurosci* 6:218-233, 1986.
241. Wall JT, Felleman DJ, Kaas JH: Recovery of normal topography in the somatosensory cortex of monkeys after nerve crush and regeneration, *Science* 221:771-773, 1983.
242. Silva AC, Rasey SK, Wu X, et al: Initial cortical reactions to injury of the median and radial nerves to the hands of adult primates, *J Comp Neurol* 366:700-716, 1996.

243. Merzenich MM, Jenkins WM: Reorganization of cortical representations of the hand following alterations of skin inputs induced by nerve injury, skin island transfers and experience, *J Hand Ther* 6(2):89-104, 1993.
244. Lunborg G: Nerve injury and repair—challenge to plastic brain, *J Peripher Nerv Sys* 8:209-226, 2003.
245. Oliveri M, Rossini PM, Pasqualetti P, et al: Interhemispheric asymmetries in the perception of unimanual and bimanual cutaneous stimuli. A study using transcranial magnetic stimulation, *Brain* 122:1721-1729, 1999.
246. Imai H, Tajima T, Natsumi Y: Successful reeducation of functional sensibility after median nerve repair at the wrist, *J Hand Surg* 16A(1):60-65, 1991.
247. Imai H, Tajima T, Natsuma Y: Interpretation of cutaneous pressure threshold, *Microsurgery* 10:142-144, 1989.
248. Cheng AS, Hung L, Wong JM, et al: A prospective study of early tactile stimulation after digital nerve repair, *Clin Orthop Relat Res* 384:169-175, 2001.
249. Trotten PA, Hunter JA: Therapeutic techniques to enhance nerve gliding in thoracic outlet syndrome and carpal tunnel syndrome, *Hand Clinics* 7(3):505-520, 1991.
250. Akalin E, El O, Peker O, et al: Treatment of carpal tunnel syndrome with nerve and tendon gliding exercises, *Am J Phys Med Rehabil* 81:108-113, 2002.
251. Rozmaryn LM, Dovell S, Rothman ER, et al: Nerve and tendon gliding exercises and the conservative management of carpal tunnel syndrome, *J Hand Ther* 11:171-179, 1998.
252. Chao RP, Braun SA, Ta KT, et al: Early passive mobilization after digital nerve repair and grafting, *Plast Reconstr Surg* 108(2):386-391, 2001.
253. Malczewski MC, Zamboni WA, Haws MJ, et al: Effect of motion on digital nerve repair in a fresh cadaver model, *Plast Reconstr Surg* 96:1672, 1995.
254. Lee A, Constantinescu M, Butler P: Effect of early mobilization on healing of nerve repair: histologic observations in a canine model, *Plast Reconstr Surg* 104(6):1718-1725, 1999.
255. Schmidhammer R, Zandieh S, Hopf R, et al: Alleviated tension at the repair site enhances functional regeneration: The effect of full range of motion mobilization on the regeneration of peripheral nerves–histologic, electrophysiologic, and functional results in a rat model, *J Trauma* 56(3):571-584, 2004.
256. Watchmaker GP, Mackinnon SE: Advances in peripheral nerve repair, *Clin Plast Surg* 24:63-73, 1997.
257. Cook AC, Szabo RM, Birkholz SW, et al: Early mobilization following carpal tunnel release. A prospective randomized study, *J Hand Surg* 20B(2):228-230, 1995.
258. Kerr CD, Sybert DR, Albarracin NS: An analysis of the flexor synovium in idiopathic carpal tunnel syndrome: Report of 625 cases, *J Hand Surg* 17A(6):1028-1030, 1992.
259. Muller M, Tsui D, Schnurr R, et al: Effectiveness of hand therapy interventions in primary management of carpal tunnel syndrome: A systematic review, *Hand* 17(2):210-228, 2004.
260. Hong CZ, Long HA, Kanakamedala RV, et al: Splinting and local steroid injection for the treatment of ulnar neuropathy at the elbow: Clinical and electrophysiological evaluation, *Arch Phys Med Rehabil* 77(6):573-577, 1996.
261. Walker WC, Metzler M, Cifu DX, et al: Neutral wrist splinting in carpal tunnel syndrome: a comparison of night-only versus full-time wear instructions, *Arch Phys Med Rehabil* 81(4):424-429, 2000.
262. Paternostros-Sluga T, Keilani M, Posch M, et al: Factors that influence the duration of splint wear in peripheral nerve lesions, *Am J Phys Med Rehabil* 82:86-95, 2003.
263. Geboers JF, Janssen-Potten JM, Seelen HAM, et al: Evaluation of effect of ankle-foot orthosis use on strength restoration of paretic dorsiflexors, *Arch Phys Med Rehabil* 82:856-860, 2001.
264. Hannah SD, Hudak PL: Splinting and radial nerve palsy: a single-subject experiment, *J Hand Ther* 14:195-201, 2001.
265. Jones VA, Stubblefield MD: The role of knee immobilizers in cancer patients with femoral neuropathy, *Arch Phys Med Rehabil* 85(2):303-307, 2004.
266. Kanaya F, Tajima T: Effect of electrostimulation on denervated muscle, *Clin Orthop* 283:296-301, 1992.
267. Mokrusch T, Engelhardt A, Eichhorn KF, et al: Effects of long-impulse electrical stimulation on atrophy and fibre type composition of chronically denervated fast rabbit muscle, *J Neurol* 237(1):29-34, 1990.
268. Dennis RG, Dow DE, Faulkner JA: An implantable device for stimulation of denervated muscles in rats, *Med Eng Phys* 25(3):239-253, 2003.
269. Nix WA: Effects of intermittent high frequency electrical stimulation on denervated EDL muscle of rabbits, *Muscle Nerve* 13:580-585, 1990.
270. Girlanda P, Dattola R, Vita G, et al: Effect of electrotherapy in denervated muscles in rabbits: an electrophysiological and morphological study, *Exp Neurol* 77:483-491, 1982.
271. Pachter BR, Eberstien A, Goodgold J: Electrical stimulation effect on denervated skeletal myofibers in rats: A light and electron microscope study microscope study, *Arch Phys Med Rehabil* 63:427-430, 1982.

272. Nicolaidis SC, Williams HB: Muscle preservation using an implantable electrical system after nerve injury and repair, *Microsurgery* 21(6):241-247, 2001.
273. Woodcock AH, Taylor PN, Ewins DJ: Long pulse biphasic electrical stimulation of denervated muscle, *Artif Organs* 23(5):457-459, 1999.
274. Dow DE, Cederna PS, Hassett CA, et al: Number of contractions to maintain mass and force of a denervated rat muscle, *Muscle Nerve* 30:77-86, 2004.
275. Nicolaidis SC, Williams HB: Muscle preservation using an implantable electrical system after nerve injury and repair, *Microsurgery* 21(6):241-247, 2001.
276. Merletti R, Pinelli P: A critical appraisal of neuromuscular stimulation and electrotherapy in neurorehabilitation, *Eur Neurol* 19(1):30-32, 1980.
277. Schimrigk K, McLaughjlin J, Gruninger W: The effect of electrical stimulation on the experimentally denervated rat muscle, *Scan J Rehabil Med* 9:55-60, 1997.
278. Tam SL, Archibald V, Jassar B, et al: Increased neuromuscular activity reduces sprouting in partially denervated muscles, *J Neurosci* 21;654-667, 2001.
279. Herbison GJ, Jaweed MM, Ditunno JF: Acetylcholine sensitivity and fibrillation potentials in electrically stimulated crush-denervated rat skeletal muscle, *Arch Phys Med Rehabil* 64:217-220, 1983.
280. Love FM, Son Y, Thompson WJ: Activity alters muscle reinnervation and terminal sprouting by reducing the number of Schwann cell pathways grow to link synaptic sites, *J Neurobiol* 54:566-576, 2003.
281. Nix WA, Hopf HC: Electrical stimulation of regenerating nerve and its effect on motor recovery, *Brain Res* 272:21-25, 1983.
282. Al-Majed AA, Neumann CM, Brushart TM, et al: Brief electrical stimulation promotes the speed and accuracy of motor axonal regeneration, *J Neurosci* 20(7):2602-2608, 2000.
283. Banta CA: A prospective, nonrandomized study of iontophoresis, wrist splinting, and antiinflammatory medication in the treatment of early-mild carpal tunnel syndrome, *J Occup Med* 36(2):166-168, 1994.
284. Michlovitz S, Hun L, Erasala GN, et al: Continuous low-level heat wrap therapy is effective for treating wrist pain, *Arch Phys Med Rehabil* 85(9):1409-1416, 2004.
285. Hochberg J: A randomized prospective study to assess the efficacy of two cold-therapy treatments following carpal tunnel release, *J Hand Ther* 14(3):208-215, 2000.
286. Moeller JL, Monroe J, McKeag DB: Cryotherapy-induced common peroneal nerve palsy, *Clin J Sport Med* 7(3):212-216, 1997.
287. Bassett FH 3rd, Kirkpatrick JS, Engelhardt DL, et al: Cryotherapy-induced nerve injury, *Am J Sports Med* 20(5):516-518, 1992.
288. Chandler KW, Rozas CJ, Kory RC, et al: Bilateral diaphragmatic paralysis complicating local cardiac hypothermia during open heart surgery, *Am J Med* 77(2):243-249, 1984.
289. Efthimiou J, Butler J, Woodham C, et al: Diaphragm paralysis following cardiac surgery: role of phrenic nerve cold injury, *Ann Thorac Surg* 52(4):1005-1008, 1991.
290. Moore JH, Gieck JH, Saliba EN, et al: The biophysical effects of ultrasound on median nerve distal latencies, *Electromyogr Clin Neurophysiol* 40(3):169-180, 2000.
291. Ebenbichler GR, Resch KL, Nicholakis P, et al: Ultrasound treatment for treating the carpal tunnel syndrome: randomized "sham" controlled trial, *BMJ* 7(316):731-735, 1998.
292. Oztas O, Turan B, Bora I, et al: Ultrasound therapy effect in carpal tunnel syndrome, *Arch Phys Med Rehabil* 79(12):1540-1544, 1998.
293. Paik NJ, Cho SH, Han TR: Ultrasound therapy facilitates the recovery of acute pressure-induced conduction block of the median nerve in rabbits, *Muscle Nerve* 26:356-361, 2002.
294. Breger Stanton D, Bear-Lehman J, et al: Contrasts baths: What do we know about their use? *J Hand Ther* 16(4):343-346, 2003.
295. Rivenburgh DW: Physical modalities in treatment of tendon injuries, *Clin Sports Med* 11:645-659, 1992.
296. Cote DJ, Prentice WE, Hooker DN, et al: Comparison of three treatment procedures for minimizing ankle sprain swelling, *Phys Ther* 68(7):1072-1076, 1988.
297. Higgins D, Kaminski TW: Contrast therapy does not cause fluctuations in human gastrocnemius intramuscular temperature, *J Athl Train* 33(4):336-340, 1998.
298. Mester E, Mester AF, Mester A: The biomedical effects of laser application, *Lasers Surg Med* 5(1):31-39, 1985.
299. Brosseau L, Welch V, Wells G, et al: Low level laser therapy for osteoarthritis and rheumatoid arthritis: A meta-analysis, *J Rheumatol* 27:1961-1969, 2000.
300. Garavello I, Baranauskas V, da Cruz Hofling MA: The effects of low laser irradiation on angiogenesis in injured rat tibiae, *Histol Histopathol* 19(1):43-48, 2004.
301. Lagan KM, McKenna T, Witherow A, et al: Low-intensity laser therapy/combined phototherapy in the management of chronic venous ulceration. A placebo-controlled study, *J Clin Laser Med Surg* 20:109-116, 2002.
302. Weintraub MI: Noninvasive laser neurolysis in carpal tunnel syndrome, *Muscle Nerve* 20(8):1029-1031, 1997.
303. Basford JR, Hallman HO, Matsumoto JY, et al: Effects of 830 nm continuous wave laser diode irradiation on median nerve function in normal subjects, *Lasers Surg Med* 13(6):597-604, 1993.
304. Greathouse DC, Currier DP, Gilmore RL: Effects of clinical infrared laser on superficial radial nerve conduction, *Phys Ther* 65:1184-1187, 1985.
305. Baxter GD, Walsh DM, Allen JM, et al: Effects of low intensity infrared laser irradiation upon conduction in the human median nerve in vivo, *Exp Physiol* 79(2):227-234, 1994.
306. Kasai S, Kono T, Sakamoto T, et al: Effects of low-power laser irradiation on multiple unit discharges induced by noxious stimuli in the anesthetized rabbit, *J Clin Laser Med Surg* 12(4):221-224, 1994.
307. Walsh DM, Baxter GD, Allen JM: Lack of effect of pulsed low-intensity infrared (820 nm) laser irradiation on nerve conduction in the human superficial radial nerve, *Lasers Surg Med* 26(5):485-490, 2000.
308. Comelekoglu U, Bagis S, Buyukakilli B, et al: Acute electrophysiological effect of pulsed gallium-arsenide low-energy laser irradiation on isolated frog sciatic nerve, *Lasers Med Sci* 17(1):62-67, 2002.
309. Bagis S, Comelekoglu U, Sahin G, et al: Acute electrophysiological effect of pulsed gallium-arsenide low energy laser irradiation on configuration of compound nerve action potential and nerve excitability, *Lasers Surg Med* 30:376-380, 2002.
310. Miloro M, Halkias LE, Mallery S, et al: Low-level laser effect on neural regeneration in Gore-Tex tubes. *Oral Surg Oral Med Oral Pathol Oral Radiol Endod* 93(1):27-34, 2002.
311. Rochkind S, Rousso M, Nissan M, et al: Systemic effects of low-power laser irradiation on the peripheral and central nervous system, cutaneous wounds, and burns, *Lasers Surg Med* 9:174-182, 1989.
312. Padua L, Padua R, Moretti C, et al: Clinical outcome and neurophysiological results of low-power laser irradiation in carpal tunnel syndrome, *Lasers Med Sci* 14:196-202, 1999.
313. Naeser MA, Hahn KK, Lieberman BE, et al: Carpal tunnel syndrome pain treated with low-level laser and microamperes transcutaneous electric nerve stimulation: A controlled study, *Arch Phys Med Rehabil* 83:978-988, 2002.
314. Eckerdal A, Lehmann B: Can low reactive-level-laser therapy be used in the treatment of neurogenic facial pain? A double-blind, placebo controlled investigation of patients with trigeminal neuralgia, *Laser Ther* 8:247-252, 1996.
315. Irvine J, Chong SL, Amirjani N et al: Double-blind randomized controlled trial of low level laser therapy in carpal tunnel syndrome, *Muscle Nerve* 30(2):182-187, 2004.

Chapter 19

Polyneuropathies

Mohamed Ibrahim

CHAPTER OUTLINE

OBJECTIVES

After reading this chapter, the reader will be able to:
1. Define different types of polyneuropathies.
2. Differentiate the motor and sensory dysfunctions commonly seen in patients with polyneuropathies.
3. Compare and contrast methods of examining patients with polyneuropathy.
4. Identify specialized equipment needs, assistive technology, and rehabilitation intervention considerations appropriate for patients with polyneuropathy.
5. Design effective rehabilitation intervention programs for patients with polyneuropathies.

Polyneuropathies are peripheral neuropathies affecting multiple nerves. *Polyneuropathy* affects approximately 2,400 individuals per 100,000 (2.4%), and this prevalence increases with age to a maximum of 8,000 per 100,000 (8%).[1,2] Annually, *peripheral neuropathy* is newly diagnosed in 118 people per 100,000.[3,4]

It is important to distinguish among different kinds of peripheral nervous system (PNS) dysfunctions. Polyneuropathy generally refers to a bilateral symmetric distur-bance of peripheral nerve function.[5] When the spinal nerve roots or the roots and the peripheral nerve trunks are involved these are termed polyradiculopathy and polyradiculoneuropathy, respectively. *Mononeuropathy* is a focal lesion of one peripheral nerve, and multiple mononeuropathy, or mononeuropathy mutiplex, is defined as multifocal isolated lesions of more than one peripheral nerve.[5] Neuropathies with different anatomical distribu-tions have characteristic causes, primary underlying pathology (*demyelination* or axonal degeneration), and tend to affect sensory, motor or a combination of both types of nerves. These associations are summarized in (Table 19-1). This chapter discusses pathology, examination, evaluation, and rehabilitation intervention for patients with impaired motor function and sensory integrity associated with acute and chronic polyneuropathies. The examination, evalua-tion, and rehabilitation intervention for patients with peripheral nerve injuries are covered in Chapter 18.

There are many types and causes of polyneuropathy. This chapter focuses on the types of polyneuropathy that occur most commonly in patients treated by rehabilitation clinicians in the developed Western world today.

PATHOLOGY

ACQUIRED DEMYELINATING POLYNEUROPATHIES

Guillain-Barré Syndrome. Guillain-Barré syndrome was first described by Landry in 1859 as an acute ascend-ing paralysis not caused by polio.[6,8] Later, in a series of case reports beginning in 1916, a group of French neurologists, Guillain, Barré, and Strohl, described key features of a syn-drome characterized by flaccid paralysis and areflexia.[7,8] The condition was initially named Landry-Guillain-Barré-Strohl syndrome* in recognition of their work but is now

---

*American and English literature uses the term Guillain-Barré syndrome in all recent publications. However, the terms acute inflammatory demyelinating polyneuropathy, acute infective polyneuritis, Guillain-Barré-Strohl syndrome, Landry-Guillain-Barré syndrome, idiopathic polyneuritis, postinfectious polyneuritis, acute toxic neuronitis, mononeuronitis, radiculoneuritis, polyradiculoneuritis, myeloradiculoneuritis, acute immune-mediated polyneuritis, and acute inflammatory polyneuropathy are all also used to describe this syndrome.

TABLE 19-1	Causes and Anatomical Distribution of Neuropathies					
Examples	Subtype	Predominantly Sensory	Mixed	Predominantly Motor	Axonal Degeneration	Demyelination
MONONEUROPATHY						
Entrapment neuropathies/ trauma	Neurapraxia	Yes		Yes		Yes
	Axonotmesis	Yes		Yes	Yes	
	Neurotmesis	Yes		Yes	Yes	
MULTIPLE MONONEUROPATHY						
Diabetic mononeuropathy		Yes	Yes	No		
Vasculitis		No	Yes	No		
AIDS		Yes		Yes	Yes (excluding acute)	No
Focal CIDP		Yes		Yes		
POLYNEUROPATHY						
Acquired demyelinating polyneuropathies	GBS (acute infective polyneuritis)	No	Yes	Yes	Yes	Yes
	CIDP					Yes
Neuropathies associated with systemic disorders	Diabetic neuropathies	Yes	Yes	No	Yes	Yes
	Nutritional deficiency (vitamins)	Yes	Yes		Yes	No
	Renal failure (uremia)		Yes		Yes	No
	Hepatic disorders	Yes	Yes		No	Yes (chronic)
	Critical illness neuropathy	No	Yes	Yes	Yes	No
Hereditary and idiopathic peripheral neuropathy	Hereditary motor and sensory neuropathies (CMT)	Yes		Yes	Yes	Yes
	Hereditary sensory and autonomic neuropathies	Yes	No	No		
Neuropathies associated with drugs, metals, and industrial agents	Neurotoxic drugs*	Yes	Yes	No	Yes (excluding acute)	No
	Alcoholic neuropathy	Yes		Yes	Yes	Yes
	Metal toxicity (lead)	Yes		Yes	Yes	Yes
Neuropathies associated with infection	HIV	Yes		Yes	Yes (excluding acute)	No

*For example, cisplatin, nitrofurantoin, and vincristine.

AIDS, Acquired immunodeficiency syndrome; *CIDP,* chronic inflammatory demyelinating polyneuropathy; *GBS,* Guillain-Barré syndrome; *CMT,* Charcot-Marie-Tooth disease; *HIV,* human immunodeficiency virus.

known as *Guillain-Barré syndrome (GBS)* or *acute inflammatory demyelinating polyneuropathy (AIDP).*[9]

GBS is an inflammatory disorder of the peripheral nerves, with a number of variants. In 1956, Charles Miller Fisher reported on a few patients who presented with ataxia, areflexia, and ophthalmoplegia with no weakness.[10] This variant of GBS, which affects 3% to 5% of patients with GBS, is now known as Miller Fisher syndrome.[11]

In most cases, clinical, electrophysiological, and pathological findings indicate that GBS is an autoimmune disease directed against myelin, hence the name, acute inflammatory demyelinating polyneuropathy. Recent publications describe variations in this process, including one where the immune process is directed against the axon itself, known as *acute motor sensory axonal neuropathy* (AMSAN).[12,13] Additionally, some reports from around the world describe a primary motor axonal form of GBS, known as *acute motor axonal neuropathy* (AMAN).[14-16] However, this latter form of GBS is not common in North America.[17] Characteristics of these and other variants of GBS are described in Table 19-2. The target area of these and other variants are shown in Fig. 19-1.

Incidence. GBS is the most common cause of acquired acute and subacute areflexic paralysis in humans, with an annual incidence of 1-2 per 100,000.[18-22] Although the mean age of occurrence is 40 years of age, GBS can affect people of any age from infants to the very old. Furthermore, GBS affects people of all races and nationality, with men affected slightly more often than women and whites slightly more often than blacks.[23-29]

Etiology and Pathogenesis. Although GBS often seems to be preceded by an acute bacterial or viral infection,[25,30-33] to date there is no evidence to indicate that GBS is

TABLE 19-2   Guillain-Barré Syndrome and Variants

Weakness Predominates			Weakness Does Not Predominate		
AIDP	AMAN	AMSAN	Miller Fisher Syndrome	Acute Panautonomic Neuropathy	PSN
CLINICAL PICTURE					
Paresthesia and pain followed by leg weakness	Affects children and young adults primarily in northern China and sporadically in the United States	Sudden weakness followed by quadriplegia and respiratory insufficiency	Diplopia, followed in 3-4 days by limb and gait ataxia; areflexia	Usual onset in 1-2 weeks but may be up to 8 weeks; dizziness, lightheadedness, nausea, vomiting, diarrhea, constipation	Large fiber, ataxia, areflexic, sensory neuropathy; No motor involvement
Disease progresses over days to 4 weeks	Preceded by diarrhea	Preceded by diarrhea	Sensory loss and mild muscle weakness	Orthostatic hypotension, heat intolerance, dry eyes	Tremor, autonomic features
80% recover in 6 months	Prognosis similar to AIDP	Longer recovery than AIDP	Excellent prognosis		
Mortality 3%-5%	Mortality <5%	Mortality 5%-10%			
CEREBRAL SPINAL FLUID					
Protein elevated in 90% of cases	Protein elevated after first week	Protein elevated without pleocytosis	Protein elevated after 7-10 days	Protein elevated without pleocytosis in most patients	
ELECTROMYOGRAPHY					
75% partial motor conduction block in proximal nerves	Reduced CMAP with normal conduction velocities	Marked CMAP reduction	Decreased amplitude of sensory nerve action potential	NCS usually normal	Involves sensory nerves more than motor nerves
30%-40% partial motor conduction block in routine studies	Sensory conduction velocities normal	Absent sensory nerve action potential	Motor conduction velocities normal	Autonomic reflex tests: Sinus arrhythmia lost to deep breathing	
Demyelination at week 3-4	Diffuse denervation by 2-3 weeks	Increased fibrillations at 2-3 weeks	Normal sensory conduction velocities	Reduced sudomotor function	

Modified from Kissel JT, Cornblath DR, Mendell JR: Guillain-Barré syndrome. In Mendell JR, Cornblath DR, Kissel JT (eds): *Diagnosis and Management of Peripheral Nerve Disorders,* Oxford, 2001, Oxford University Press.
AIDP, Acute inflammatory demyelinating polyneuropathy; *AMAN,* acute motor axonal neuropathy; *AMSAN* acute motor sensory axonal neuropathy; *CMAP,* compound action potential; *NCS,* nerve conduction studies; *PSN,* pure sensory neuropathy.

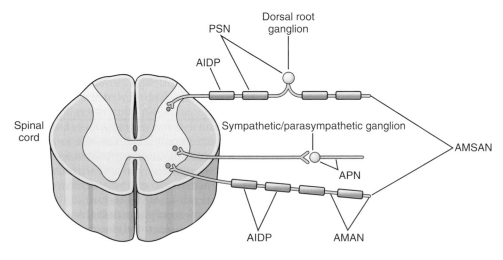

FIG. 19-1 Guillain-Barré syndrome target area anatomy and physiology. *AIDP,* Acute inflammatory demyelinating polyradiculoneuropathy; *AMAN,* acute motor axonal neuropathy; *AMSAN,* acute motor sensory axonal neuropathy; *APN,* acute panautonomic neuropathy; *PSN,* pure sensory neuropathy.

communicable nor are there specific genetic factors that increase vulnerability to GBS.[34] Approximately two-thirds of the cases are preceded by an acute, influenza-like illness (presumed viral infection), or diarrhea (presumed bacterial infection) from which the patient has recovered by the time the neuropathy becomes symptomatic.[35] Evidence suggests that GBS may be preceded by a variety of viral infections, including Epstein-Barr virus, cytomegalovirus, human immunodeficiency virus (HIV),[36] influenza virus,[37-39] coxsackie virus, herpes simplex virus, hepatitis A and C viruses, mumps,[40] and measles.[40] Bacterial infections from *Campylobacter jejunei*,[25,31-33] *Mycoplasma pneumoniae*,[29,41] *Borrelia burgdorferi* (Lyme disease),[34] and *Escherichia coli*,[29,41] may also precede GBS in some individuals.[37] Furthermore, a strong association is reported between GBS and a post-surgical state,[29,41,42] Hodgkin's disease,[29,41,43] pregnancy,[44] immunization,[37-40,45,46] and various drugs.[47] Breakdown of myelin, a characteristic of GBS, is thought to result from an autoimmune reaction toward nerve components.[48,49]

In AIDP, the classic form of GBS, deposition of complement components on the outer surface of the myelinated nerve fibers is thought to cause the myelin to degenerate. Once the entire myelin sheath is affected, macrophages attack Schwann cells that produce the myelin. This process penetrates through all the layers of myelin that surround a nerve until it finally reaches the basal lamina.[50] Recent work suggests that autoimmune reactivity may also be directed toward nonmyelin proteins involved in Schwann cell-axon interactions.[51]

In AMAN and AMSAN, myelin wrapped around the nerve is displaced, causing the nodes of Ranvier to lengthen and the axon below the node to swell[52] (Fig. 19-2). Macrophages move to this swollen area of the axon and separate the terminal loops of myelin from the axolemma. In AMSAN, this causes most of the axons within the nerve to degenerate,[16] whereas in AMAN, only a few of the axons degenerate.[14,15,52]

In Miller Fisher syndrome there is patchy demyelination,[29,30] and in the pure sensory neuropathy (PSN) form of GBS, inflammation of the dorsal roots and sensory ganglia have been demonstrated.[53]

Clinical Presentation. Despite the many variants of GBS, all present with the common features of acute or subacute peripheral nerve dysfunction, taking about 2-4 weeks to cause peak neurological deficits. All variants are commonly preceded by a trigger (upper respiratory tract infection, gastrointestinal infection, surgery, pregnancy, immunizations, etc), although this may be difficult to determine from the history. The neurological signs and symptoms partially or completely resolve over weeks to months, with the long-term prognosis depending on the site and extent of axonal injury. A good functional recovery is expected in most but not all cases, and this syndrome has a mortality of about 2% to 5%, generally from respiratory failure or infection.[50]

Clinically, GBS variants can be divided into those where weakness predominates and those where weakness does not predominate. AIDP, AMAN, and AMSAN fall into the first group. The second group includes Miller Fisher syndrome, acute panautonomic neuropathy, and PSN.[50]

Sensory loss is usually found in AIDP and AMSAN; however, in AMAN, there is no sensory involvement. Furthermore, Miller Fisher syndrome presents primarily with ataxia and ophthalmoplegia. Panautonomic neuropathies and PSN are the rarest forms of GBS. Table 19-2 provides further information about each variant's clinical presentation.

Chronic Inflammatory Demyelinating Polyradiculoneuropathy. *Chronic inflammatory demyelinating polyradiculoneuropathy* (CIDP) has a similar clinical presentation to GBS but with a slower onset and more chronic course. Patients with what appeared to be a chronic from of GBS have been described in the literature for many years and their disorders were given a variety of names, including polyneuritis idiopathica, nonfamilial

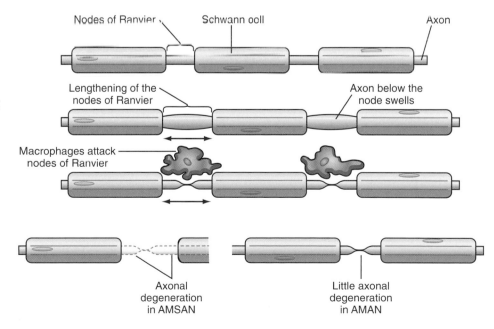

FIG. 19-2 Pathogenesis of acute motor axonal neuropathy *(AMAN)* and acute motor sensory axonal neuropathy *(AMSAN)* variants of Guillain-Barré syndrome. Note that in both variants, myelin wrapped around the nerve is displaced, causing the nodes of Ranvier to lengthen, and the axon below the node to swell. Macrophages move to this swollen area of the axon and separate the terminal loops of myelin from the axolemma. In AMSAN this causes most of the axons within the nerve to degenerate, whereas in AMAN, only a few of the axons degenerate.

hypertrophic neuritis, relapsing or recurrent neuritis, idiopathic neuritis, or chronic GBS.[54,55] As early as 1890, Eichhorst reported a case of recurrent neuritis.[56,57] Later, DeJong reported on twelve patients with recurrent symptoms of GBS, four of whom developed the full-blown syndrome more slowly than usual, over a 5-6 month period.[58] An ad hoc subcommittee of the American Academy of Neurology published proposed diagnostic criteria for CIDP in 1991 (Table 19-3).[59] These criteria are generally used today, although some recent publications suggest that they are too restrictive, causing many patients with CIDP to remain undiagnosed and untreated.[60,61]

Incidence. The prevalence of CIDP is generally reported to be one to 2 per 100,000.[62,63] However, since CIDP is often not recognized, and the diagnosis is rarely made outside of tertiary care referral centers, this estimate is probably low.[55] A recent study reported a prevalence of 7.7 per 100,000 in Vest-Agder, Norway.[64] CIDP can occur at any age[57] and has a mean age of onset of 47.6 years; however, the incidence does increase with age.[63] CIDP also occurs more often in males than in females (2 : 1 ratio).[63,65]

Etiology and Pathogenesis. Although the pathogenesis of CIDP is not proven, most authors consider it to be an autoimmune disease, caused by either humoral or cell-mediated immunity directed against myelin or Schwann cell antigens.[66] Multifocal demyelination of the peripheral nerves, mainly of the spinal roots, plexuses, and the proximal portions of the nerve trunks, as well as the distal peripheral nerves, has been reported in patients with CIDP. Nerve enlargement (onion bulb formation),

TABLE 19-3	Criteria for Diagnosis of Chronic Inflammatory Demyelinating Polyradiculoneuropathy (CIDP)	
Test	**Diagnostic Criteria**	**Finding**
Clinical	A. Mandatory	Progressive or relapsing muscle weakness for 2 months or longer.
		Symmetrical proximal and distal weakness in upper or lower extremities.
		Hyporeflexia or areflexia; usually involves all four limbs.
	B. Supportive	Large-fiber sensory loss predominates over small-fiber sensory loss.
	C. Exclusion	Mutilation of hands or feet, retinitis pigmentosa, ichthyosis, appropriate history of drug or toxic exposure know to cause a similar peripheral neuropathy, or family history of genetically based peripheral neuropathy.
		Sensory level.
		Unequivocal sphincter disturbance.
Electrodiagnostic (physiological)	A. Mandatory	NCS, including studies of proximal nerve segment in which the predominant process is demyelination.
		Must have three of the following four:
		1. Reduction in NCV in two or more motor nerves:
		• <80% of LLN, if amplitude >80% of LLN
		• <70% of LLN, if amplitude <80% of LLN
		2. Partial conduction block or abnormal temporal dispersion in one or more motor nerves (not at usual site of entrapment).
		3. Prolonged distal latencies in two or more nerves:
		• >125% of ULN, if amplitude >80% of LLN
		• >150% of ULN if amplitude <80% of LLN
		4. Absent F wave or prolonged minimum F-wave latencies in two or more motor nerves:
		• >120% of ULN, if amplitude >80% of LLN
		• >150% of ULN, if amplitude <80% of LLN
	B. Supportive	Reduction in sensory NCV to <80% of LLN.
		Absent H reflexes.
Pathological	A. Mandatory	Nerve biopsy showing unequivocal evidence of demyelination and remyelination:
	B. Supportive	1. Subperineurial or endoneurial edema.
		2. Mononuclear cell infiltration.
		3. Onion-bulb formation.
		4. Prominent variation in the degree of demyelination between fascicles.
	C. Exclusion	Vasculitis, neurofilamentous swollen axons, amyloid deposits, or intracytoplasmic inclusion in Schwann cells or macrophages, indicating adrenoleukodystrophy, metachromatic leukodystrophy, globoid cell leukodystrophy, or other evidence of specific pathology.
CSF	A. Mandatory	Cell count <10⁵/ml if HIV-seronegative or <50⁵/ml if HIV-seropositive.
		Negative VDRL.
	B. Supportive	Elevated protein.
Diagnostic categories	Definite	Clinical A and C, physiological A, pathological A and C, and CSF A.
	Probable	Clinical A and C, physiological A, and CSF A.
	Possible	Clinical A and C and physiological A.

From Ad Hoc Subcommittee of the American Academy of Neurology AIDS Task Force: *Neurology* 41:617-618, 1991.
NCS, Nerve conduction studies; *NCV,* nerve conduction velocity; *LLN,* lower limit of normal; *ULN,* upper limit of normal; *HIV,* human immunodeficiency virus; *CSF,* cerebrospinal fluid; *VDRL,* Venereal Disease Research Laboratory.

demyelination, and remyelination have also been found at autopsy.[67] Although scarce lymphocytic infiltration can be found in sural nerve biopsies, biopsies are frequently normal and do not show demyelination or inflammation, despite this syndrome being called "chronic inflammatory demyelinating polyradiculoneuropathy."[57,68,69] This may be because the sural nerve in patients with CIDP may not represent what is happening at the level of the nerve root[55] or because the damage is occurring to the axon itself.[70]

Clinical Presentation. CIDP generally presents with slowly progressive or relapsing motor and/or sensory symptoms in more than one limb, developing over at least 8 weeks.[54,57,59] There is symmetrical involvement of the proximal and distal muscles, with atrophy being less pronounced than the weakness. Although depressed or absent reflexes are found in all patients, these are generally confined to the ankles. Eighty percent of patients also have sensory disturbances (numbness).[54,65]

Some patients with CIDP present atypically, with symptoms similar to lumbar stenosis or cauda equina syndrome (see Chapter 8), caused by inflammation and recurrent demyelination and remyelination of the hypertrophied lumbar nerve roots.[71-73] Other patients present primarily or only with sensory symptoms.[74]

CIDP and GBS are differentiated clinically by the criterion of how long it takes for maximum deficits to develop (Table 19-4). CIDP develops over more than 8 weeks, whereas GBS symptoms peak in less than 4 weeks. Another difference is that CIDP responds to corticosteroids, whereas GBS does not, and respiratory muscles are often involved in GBS but are not affected in CIDP. Finally, although prognosis for recovery from GBS is usually good, CIDP has a poor prognosis and most patients do not fully recover.

Although children are rarely affected by CIDP,[75] when affected, their disease course is generally similar to that of adults.[76] Compared to the clinical presentation in adults, children often have weakness and loss of reflexes and sensation and rarely have pain or cranial nerve involvement. Children generally have an abrupt onset of symptoms and present with gait abnormalities and other significant neurological dysfunctions. The initial response of children with CIDP to immune modulating therapy is often excellent.[75,77]

NEUROPATHIES ASSOCIATED WITH SYSTEMIC DISORDERS

Diabetic Neuropathies. One of the most common complications of diabetes mellitus in the Western world is neuropathy. Virtually every type of peripheral nerve fiber can be affected, including sensory, autonomic, and motor nerve fibers.[78] Therefore diabetic neuropathy can have diverse presentations.[79] The term, *diabetic neuropathy,* includes all of these, and no single classification system identifies all subtypes.[80-82] Nonetheless, most diabetic neuropathies can be classified as focal or multifocal neuropathies, or as polyneuropathies, as shown in Table 19-5.[80-82]

Incidence. Because of underreporting and variations in diagnostic criteria, the exact prevalence of diabetic neuropathy is not known. However, it is clear that a very large number of people are affected by diabetic neuropathy.[83] Over 18 million Americans have diabetes, and this number increases by 5% each year.[84] Peripheral neuropathy is a common complication of diabetes, with 5% of patients already having diabetic neuropathy when their diabetes is diagnosed and up to 50% of patients with diabetes for over 25 years having symptoms of neuropathy.[85] In one study, clinical symptoms of diabetic neuropathy were present in 32% of subjects with diabetes and this number increased to 83.5% when quantitative neurological examination and nerve conduction studies (as described later) were used to make the diagnosis.[86] Another study reported evidence of neuropathy in 59% of patients with type I diabetes and in 66% of patients with

TABLE 19-4	Comparison of Guillain-Barré Syndrome (GBS) with Chronic Inflammatory Demyelinating Polyneuropathy (CIDP)	
	GBS	**CIDP**
Duration to develop full clinical picture	<4 weeks	>8 weeks
Responds to corticosteroids	No	Yes
Respiratory muscle	Usually affected	Generally not affected
Prognosis	Better	Worse
Recovery	>80% recover in 6-8 months	>80% fail to have spontaneous recovery

TABLE 19-5	Classification of Diabetic Neuropathies		
Focal	**Multifocal**	**Polyneuropathies**
Cranial neuropathies	Multiple mononeuropathies	Sensory polyneuropathies
Mononeuropathies	Diabetic thoracolumbar radiculoneuropathies*	Sensorimotor polyneuropathies
Compressive neuropathies	Diabetic lumbosacral radiculoplexopathies†	Autonomic neuropathy
		Treatment-induced neuropathy‡
		Acute painful diabetic neuropathy§

*Also called truncal radiculoneuropathy, thoracoabdominal neuropathy, truncal mononeuropathy, thoracic polyradiculoneuropathy.
†Also called proximal diabetic neuropathy, Bruns-Garland syndrome.
‡Also called insulin neuritis.
§Also called diabetic cachectic neuropathy, diabetic amyotrophy.[80-82]

type II diabetes,[87] and it is estimated that 30% of hospitalized patients with diabetes and 20% of patients in the community with diabetes have diabetic neuropathy.[88] Historically, the diagnosis of diabetic neuropathy depended primarily on signs and symptoms. Now, electrophysiological testing is used to diagnose cases where the presentation is unclear.[81]

Etiology and Pathogenesis. Over the past 20 years, research has helped to clarify the pathogenesis of diabetic neuropathy. However, the exact processes that cause this problem are still unclear, and it is difficult to combine the most popular theories into one consistent explanation. These theories include that nerve damage is caused by altered polyol metabolism, poor microvascular circulation, toxic glycosylation end-products, oxidative stress, low levels of neurotrophic factors, and/or by excess of products of essential fatty acid metabolism.[81,84,85]

It is proposed that altered polyol metabolism contributes to the development of diabetic neuropathy.[89] Polyol is a general term for sugar alcohols, which include glucose. Since the uptake of glucose by peripheral nerves is not insulin-dependent, when blood sugar levels are high, peripheral nerves take up a lot of glucose. This glucose is converted to sorbitol, and one theory is that the sorbitol exerts osmotic pressure, drawing fluid into the nerve, which causes swelling and damage.[81,82] However, recent research indicates that high concentrations of sorbitol in nerves do not cause nerve damage and it may be that it is the high metabolic flux of glucose through the polyol pathway that damages the peripheral nerves.[90,91]

Alternatively, diabetic neuropathy may be caused by microvascular ischemia. Diabetes is known to cause microvascular vasoconstriction and atherosclerosis, capillary basement membrane thickening, and endothelial cell hypertrophy.[78,92] This in turn results in decreased endoneurial blood flow and diminished oxygen tension and hypoxia, which may eventually lead to nerve damage and neuropathy.[93-96]

Reduced levels of nerve growth factor (NGF) in diabetes may also contribute to the development of diabetic neuropathy. NGF is a neurotrophic factor that is similar to insulin in molecular, structural, and physiological properties. Low serum levels of NGF in patients with diabetes have been found to correlate with their degree of peripheral neuropathy.[97,98] The formation of advanced glycosylation end products, oxidative stress, and protein kinase C (PKC) may also affect the development of diabetic neuropathy.[78,81,82]

Clinical Presentation. Diabetic neuropathy most commonly presents with distal symmetrical sensorimotor signs and symptoms. Typically, the distribution follows a length-dependent pattern, with the most distal extremities (the toes) being involved first, followed by the feet, and spreading up the legs in a stocking distribution.[80] The neuropathy may advance to involve the fingers, spreading up to the hands and forearms in a glove distribution.[83,99] Later still, the trunk may be affected in an anterior wedge-shaped pattern (Fig. 19-3).[80,100] There are usually sensory changes and mild weakness of the ankle dorsiflexor and toe extensor muscles, accompanied by electromyographic (EMG) evidence of denervation.[80,82] Distal muscle weak-

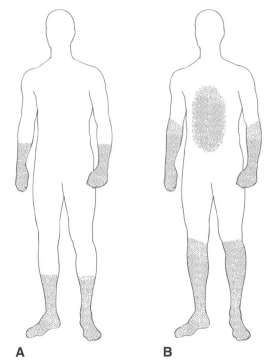

A   **B**

FIG. 19-3 Sensory loss in length dependent polyneuropathy. **A,** Stocking-glove distribution. **B,** Truncal sensory loss occurs in advanced cases, usually when the limbs are affected up to the knees and elbows.

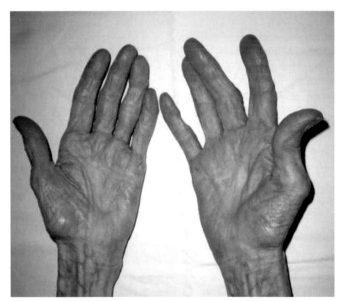

FIG. 19-4 Advanced case of diabetic neuropathy with thenar eminence muscle wasting bilaterally. *Courtesy Rehab R US Physical Therapy, Brooklyn, NY.*

ness and atrophy can be profound in advanced cases (Fig. 19-4). Positive symptoms, such as paresthesias, burning, tingling, aching, cold sensation, lancinating (sharp) pain, or pain produced by normal touch *(allodynia)* or by a change in temperature, are often reported.[99,101] When there is pain, it is often worse at night.[80] Negative signs and symptoms, such as sensory loss, depression or absence of ankle jerks, and loss of vibratory sensation, are often present and may not be reported by patients but should be sought out with a thorough examination.[99,101]

Charcot arthropathy, also known as neuropathic arthropathy, is a condition that affects some diabetic patients about 8-10 years after the onset of sensory loss from peripheral neuropathy. Charcot arthropathy is caused by lack of pain sensation and proprioception that result in unnoticed injuries to joints, generally in the foot. Repeated small injuries, such as strains and even fractures, tend to occur as the joint becomes more unstable until finally the joints are permanently destroyed and the foot becomes deformed. Sensory loss accompanied by vascular insufficiency is considered to be the primary cause of foot ulcers, which often result in amputations in patients with diabetes (see Chapter 30 for further information on neuropathic ulcers). Sensorimotor polyneuropathy is present in 85% of patients with diabetes who undergo amputation.[102]

The autonomic nerve involvement that commonly accompanies diabetic sensorimotor polyneuropathy may also cause postural hypotension, impotence (erectile dysfunction, initially with preserved ejaculation and orgasm), bladder atony, gastroparesis and nocturnal diarrhea, postprandial sweating, and diminished distal limb sweating.[82]

HEREDITARY MOTOR AND SENSORY NEUROPATHIES

Charcot-Marie-Tooth (CMT) Disease. *Charcot-Marie-Tooth* (CMT) *disease* (also called hereditary motor and sensory neuropathy) is a clinically and genetically heterogeneous group of inherited peripheral nerve disorders that can affect the sensory and/or motor nerves. It usually presents with distal weakness and sensory loss that starts in the patients' teens or twenties and progresses gradually over their lifetimes.

The first descriptions of this syndrome came from Jean-Martin Charcot and Pierre Marie of France, who in 1886 described a syndrome of progressive muscular atrophy of the feet and legs, followed by atrophy of the hand and forearm muscles, tightness of Achilles tendons, and pes cavus, with the lower extremities resembling an inverted champagne bottle (Fig. 19-5).[103,104] Shortly thereafter, Howard Henry Tooth of the United Kingdom described a group of his patients with an inherited progressive symmetrical atrophy of the distal (peroneal) muscles that began early in life and was caused by peripheral nerve dysfunction.[104,105] More recently, CMT has been divided into different classifications based on the type of nerve degeneration and the clinical presentation as well the mode of inheritance and other genetic information.[104,106,107] The classifications of CMT and related disorders are presented in Table 19-6.[108]

Incidence. In the United States, one in 2,500 people are affected CMT (about 100,000 Americans), which makes it the most common inherited neurological disorder.[109] The prevalence varies between geographical locations; the incidence is 28.2 per 100,000 in Spain,[110] 17.5 per 100,000 in Japan, and 10.8 per 100,000 in Italy.[111,112]

Etiology and Pathogenesis. CMT is caused by mutations in genes that produce proteins involved in the structure and function of either the peripheral nerve axons or the myelin sheath, thus causing an axonal or demyelinating neuropathy.[106,107] In CMT1A, a demyelinating neuropathy that accounts for 80% of CMT1 and 70% of all CMT,[113,114] chromosome 17 undergoes gene mutations (duplication) that alter proteins (PMP22) responsible for myelin production by Schwann cells in the peripheral nervous system.[108] PMP22 is overproduced, leading to defective axon myelination.[108] Histological examination reveals the presence of many thinly myelinated and remyelinated nerve fibers, with multiple onion bulbs (i.e., Schwann cell proliferation), more pronounced in the distal than proximal nerves.[115] Typically, the axon is present in the center of the onion bulb and the myelin sheath is thin or absent.

In axonal neuropathies, such as CMT2, there is typically loss of myelinated nerve fibers, axonal atrophy, and small clusters of thinly myelinated regenerating axons. Myelin wrinkling, Wallerian-like degeneration, and remyelination are also found.[115]

Clinical Presentation. CMT neuropathy affects both motor and sensory nerve fibers. Therefore patients with CMT typically present with distal muscle weakness or atrophy, structural foot abnormalities, soft tissue complications (e.g., calluses, ulcers), and EMG abnormalities. Furthermore, absent or diminished deep tendon reflexes and impaired sensation are also present to varying degrees in certain forms of CMT.[116] Findings are similar among affected family members.[104]

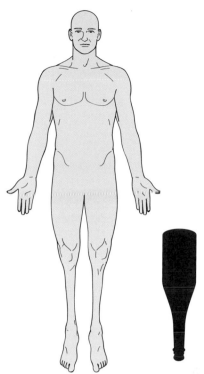

FIG. 19-5 Inverted champagne bottle appearance of lower extremities in Charcot-Marie-Tooth disease. *Redrawn from Feldman EL, Stevens MJ, et al: A practical two-step quantitative clinical and electrophysiological assessment for the diagnosis and staging of diabetic neuropathy,* Diabetes Care *17:1281-1289, 1994.*

TABLE 19-6	Classification of Charcot-Marie-Tooth Neuropathy and Related Disorders				
Type	**Disease**	**Inheritance**	**Process**	**Gene**	**Mechanism**
CMT type 1	CMT1A	AD	Demyelinating	PMP22	Duplication
	CMT1B	AD	Demyelinating	P$_o$	Point mutation
	CMT1C	AD	Demyelinating	LITAF	
	CMT1D	AD	Demyelinating	EDGR2	Point mutation
CMT type 2	CMT2A	AD	Axonal	KIF 1Bβ	
	CMT2B	AD	Axonal	RAB7	
	CMT2C	AD	Axonal		
	CMT2D	AD	Axonal		
DSD	DSD-A	AD or AR	Demyelinating	PMP22	Point mutation
	DSD-B	AD or AR	Demyelinating	P$_o$	Point mutation
	DSD-C	AD or AR	Demyelinating	EDGR2	Point mutation
CMT type 4	CMT4A	AR	Demyelinating	GDAP1	
	CMT4B	AR	Demyelinating	MTMR2	
	CMT4C	AR	Demyelinating		
	CMT4D	AR	Demyelinating	NDRG1	
X-linked dominant CMT	CMT1X	X-linked	Demyelinating	Cx32	Point mutation
	CMT2X	X-linked	Axonal		
HNPP	HNPPA	AD	Demyelinating	PMP22	Deletion
	HNPPB				
DI	DI-CMT	DI			

Data from Berciano J, Combarros O: *Curr Opin Neurol* 16:613-622, 2003.
CMT, Charcot-Marie-Tooth disease; *DSD,* Dejerine-Sottas disease; *AD,* autosomal dominant; *AR,* autosomal recessive; *HNPP,* hereditary neuropathy with pressure palsies; *DI,* Dominant-intermediate.

Generally, distal muscle weakness (dorsiflexors and evertors) results in foot drop and a steppage gait with frequent tripping or falls. Pes cavus and hammertoes, which are also common, are caused by weakness in the intrinsic foot muscles and the unequal action of the long toe flexors and extensors.[104] Typically, few patients seek help, suggesting that they experience few symptoms, that they are accustomed to their symptoms and manage well functionally, or that they believe that no help is available.[104]

CMT symptoms usually present in the second or third decade of life, ranging from infancy to mid-adulthood, depending on the CMT subtype.[115,118] Symptoms usually progress gradually and vary in severity. Some may have such mild symptoms that they do not notice, while others with a severe form of the disorder may be severely compromised because of respiratory muscle involvement.[115,118] CMT is rarely fatal, and most people who have the disease have a normal life expectancy.[109,115]

The different genetic subtypes of CMT have similar presentations, making them difficult to distinguish by clinical presentation alone. In CMT1A, most patients seek medical care for pes cavus, hammertoes, and painful calluses, and most patients do not present with the classic "inverted champagne bottle" shaped lower extremities.[115] Upper limb weakness has been reported in about two-thirds of patients with CMT1A[107,115]; more than 50% have an absent muscle stretch reflex, and one-third of patients have a postural or essential tremor.[115] Finally, nerve enlargement (e.g., of the greater auricular, ulnar, peroneal nerves) can be palpated in up to 50% of patients with CMT1.[107,115]

CMT type 2 has 4 subtypes. It has autosomal-dominant inheritance and causes an axonal neuropathy. CMT2A presents clinically very much like CMT1 but without slowing of nerve conduction velocity (NCV).[115,118] In CMT1, NCV is less than 38 meters per second (m/sec) because of the demyelination, whereas in CMT2 the NCV is above 38 m/sec because there is axonal degeneration but no demyelination.[108,117]

Patients with CMT2B generally have poorly healing foot ulcers that can result in lower extremity amputations.[115,118] CMT2C is characterized by vocal cord paralysis, leading to a hoarse voice; diaphragmatic and intercostals muscle weakness, leading to impaired respiratory function; and proximal muscle weakness, leading to difficulty in arising from a chair.[115] Patients with CMT2D have hand weakness before the distal lower limbs are involved.[118]

Dejerine-Sottas disease (DSD) is a demyelinating subtype of CMT characterized by onset at birth, hypotonia, generalized limb and trunk weakness, ataxia, enlarged palpable peripheral nerves, and absent muscle stretch reflexes.[115,119] DSD can have an autosomal-dominant or a recessive mode of inheritance.[115] Table 19-7 includes a summary and further details of the clinical presentation of CMT.

TOXIC NEUROPATHIES

Alcoholic Neuropathy. Neuropathy as a complication of excessive alcohol consumption was first reported over 200 years ago.[120,121] Controversy still exists as to whether *alcoholic neuropathy* is a direct toxic effect of alcohol or is caused by secondary nutritional deficiencies common in alcoholics.[121-124] This debate persists in part because the clinical presentation of alcoholic neuropathy is similar to that of neuropathy caused by certain nutritional deficiencies such as thiamine deficiency.[123] In addition, because alcohol provides so many calories, many alcoholics have little other nutritional intake and are

TABLE 19-7   Clinical Presentation of Charcot-Marie-Tooth Neuropathy

	CMT Type 1A, 1B, 1C	CMT Type 2A, 2B, 2D	CMT Type 2C	DSD	CMT Type 4A	CMT Type 4B	CMT Type 4C	X-linked (CMTX)	HNPP
Onset	First decade	First or second decade	Infancy	Infancy	Before 2 years of age	Before 2-3 years of age	Before 10 years of age	First or second decade	Second or third decade
Muscle weakness	Distal	Distal	Vocal cord and respiratory muscles	Generalized limb and trunk	Severe distal, progresses to proximal	Proximal and distal, progresses to hands	Distal, progresses to hands	Distal	Presents as multiple compression neuropathy
Reflexes	Majority areflexic	Minority areflexic	Loss or diminished TDR	Areflexia	Areflexia	Areflexia	Areflexia	Diminished distally	Loss of distal stretch reflex
Sensory	Loss	Loss	Loss (minimal)	Loss (severe)	Loss (mild)	Loss (mild)	Loss (mild)	Loss	Mononeuropathy pattern loss
Postural tremor	33% of cases	Less than CMT1		Ataxia					
Palpable nerve	In 50% of cases	No	No	Common				Not common	
Pes cavus and hammertoe	Common	Common	May be present	Common and scoliosis	Common and scoliosis	Common and scoliosis	Common or pes cavus or planus	Common	May be present
NCV UE	<40 m/sec		<20 m/sec	≈20-30 m/sec	≈14-17 m/sec	≈20-30 m/sec			
NCV LE	<30 m/sec		<10 m/sec	≈20-30 m/sec	≈14-17 m/sec	≈20-30 m/sec			

Data from Mendell JR, Sahenk Z. Hereditary motor and sensory neuropathies and giant axonal neuropathy. In Mendell JR, Cornblath DR, Kissel JT (eds): *Diagnosis and Management of Peripheral Nerve Disorders*, Oxford, 2001, Oxford University Press.
CMT, Charcot-Marie-Tooth disease; *DSD*, Dejerine-Sottas disease; *HNPP*, hereditary neuropathy with pressure palsies; *LE*, lower extremities; *NCV*, nerve conduction studies; *UE*, upper extremities.

therefore often relatively malnourished.[122] Furthermore, alcohol may interfere with gastrointestinal absorption of nutrients, exaggerating malnutrition.[122]

Current evidence, however, gives greatest support to the hypothesis that alcoholic neuropathy is primarily a result of the toxic effects of alcohol. This is supported by the finding that neuropathy develops in alcoholics who are not malnourished and that nutritional supplementation alone does not alter the course of neuropathy in these patients.[123,125,126] Alcoholic neuropathy presents with a gradual decrease in sensory and motor peripheral nerve function in patients who chronically consume excessive amounts of alcohol.

Incidence. The exact incidence of alcoholic neuropathy is not known. However, some reports suggest that about 10% to 15% of chronic alcoholics develop clinically apparent neuropathy.[126,127] This increases to approximately 30% when detailed electrophysiological assessment is used for diagnosis.[125,128] Furthermore, up to three-fourths of alcoholics show some degree of sensory dysfunction on detailed sensory testing with a vibrometer, tuning fork, or thermal threshold tests.[129-131] Alcoholic neuropathy is more common in men than in women, and the incidence increases with age and rate of consumption.[121,129]

Etiology and Pathogenesis. Although the precise pathogenesis and pathophysiology of alcoholic neuropathy remain unclear, it is known that alcoholic neuropathy causes axonal involvement of both myelinated and unmyelinated peripheral nerve fibers and can cause segmental demyelination.[123,124,132]

Clinical Presentation. Taking a good history is key to detecting long-standing alcohol abuse. Ethanol alcohol consumption of 100 gm per day for 3 years has been suggested as the minimum amount likely to cause alcoholic neuropathy.[121,122] Generally, alcoholic neuropathy presents initially with distal sensory or sensorimotor findings, including symmetrical distal loss of all sensory modalities (light touch, pin prick, vibration, and temperature), foot and calf pain, and diminished ankle reflexes.[129-131] The sensory loss is in a stocking-glove distribution (see Fig. 19-3). Almost 50% of patients with alcoholic neuropathy have muscle weakness, progressing to foot drop, gait disturbances, and wrist drop, depending on the severity of the disease.[122] Generally, weakness is more pronounced in the lower extremities than in the upper extremities.[122,123]

Alcoholic neuropathy is usually associated with a number of other medical conditions, including liver cirrhosis, gastrointestinal bleeding, Wernicke-Korsakoff syndrome (a brain disorder caused by thiamine deficiency), alcoholic cerebellar degeneration, and alcoholic dementia. However, many patients seek medical assistance for pain from neuropathy rather than for symptoms associated with these conditions.

EXAMINATION

A thorough examination is required to establish a diagnosis and prognosis (including plan of care) and select interventions for patients with suspected polyneuropathy.[133]

PATIENT HISTORY

Patients with polyneuropathy generally present with complaints of motor or sensory disturbance, or both. When there are motor disturbances the patient may report muscle incoordination, distal weakness (causing frequent tripping and difficult walking on uneven surfaces), or proximal weakness (causing difficulty with getting out of a chair and with going up and down stairs). Sensory presentations include feelings of tingling, burning, stabbing, throbbing, clumsiness, cold, hot, wooden, and/or dead.

The progression of symptoms may indicate their likely cause. However, some patients with polyneuropathy present with an unclear history, particularly if the symptoms developed very gradually, as in many inherited neuropathies.[134] Such patients may have had subtle symptoms since childhood that presented as poor performance in sports, frequent falls, or frequent ankle sprains and only now have developed severe enough symptoms to seek out medical advice or intervention. In contrast, other causes of polyneuropathy, such as GBS, produce symptoms that develop rapidly, over a few days to up to 4 weeks;[135] whereas, symptoms of CIDP develop over more than 8 weeks, and alcoholic or diabetic neuropathy symptoms generally develop over years.[136]

The family history can help distinguish different types of polyneuropathy because some types, particularly CMT, are inherited. The clinician should ask about similar symptoms in immediate and more distant family members, including children, parents, siblings, aunts, uncles, cousins, and grandparents. Questions about family members should also include information about the use of assistive devices, functional limitations, and any complaints similar to those of the patient.

A social and occupational history can help identify risk factors for certain types of polyneuropathies. Welders, printers, and manufacturers of batteries are often exposed to lead and are therefore at risk for neuropathy from lead toxicity.[137,138] Patients with a history of drug or alcohol abuse are at increased risk for alcoholic neuropathy,[121,124] and HIV-related neuropathies are more common among intravenous drug users and men who have sex with men.[36]

The patient's past medical history can also be revealing and should focus on surgeries, illnesses, and medications. Recent surgeries or illness, as explained earlier, can precipitate GBS. Side effects of medication can lead to toxic neuropathy. A history of multiple nerve entrapment is usually associated with hereditary neuropathies.

SYSTEMS REVIEW

The systems review is used to target areas requiring further examination and to define areas that may cause complications or indicate a need for precautions during the examination and intervention processes. See Chapter 1 for details of the systems review.

TESTS AND MEASURES

Clinicians should have the proper tools for performing tests and measures on patients with suspected polyneuropathy. These tools include a goniometer, a tape measure, a hand-held dynamometer, a pinch gauge, a reflex hammer, a tool that allows measurement of 2-point discrimination and sensation (safety pins and brush), a tuning fork (to test vibratory sensation), and monofilaments to measure touch sensitivity.[139,142]

A standard paper and pencil screening tool may also be used to screen patients for early signs and symptoms of polyneuropathy. The Michigan Neuropathy Screening Instrument can help identify patients with polyneuropathy.[79,140]

Musculoskeletal

Anthropometric Characteristics. Certain skeletal deformities, masses, and atrophy are associated with certain polyneuropathies (see Table 19-11). Pes cavus, with or without hammer toes, is common in CMT neuropathies. Children with DSD usually present with scoliosis or kyphoscoliosis.

Muscle Performance. Muscle strength should be tested in all patients with polyneuropathy. Manual muscle testing (MMT) is a reliable and valid method for testing the strength of major muscle groups (see Chapter 5).[141-143] However, for more objective and quantitative data, measurement with a hand-held dynamometer is recommended.[114,145] The Vigorimeter is a hand-held dynamometer with established interobserver and intraobserver reliability (analysis of variance [ANOVA] $r = 0.95$-0.97) and criterion validity (when compared to the arm scale $p \leq 0.0005$) for measurement of grip strength in patients with polyneuropathy (83 with GBS and 22 with CIDP).[146]

Polyneuropathies have characteristic presentations, distributions, and courses of muscle weakness. For most polyneuropathies, weakness progresses from distal to proximal, starting with the intrinsic foot muscles; followed by the extensor digitorum brevis, anterior tibialis, posterior tibialis; and finally the lower parts of the thigh muscles (Fig. 19-6). This sequence causes a steppage gait early on, secondary to bilateral foot drop, and later as atrophy develops, a physical appearance resembling an inverted champagne bottle (see Fig. 19-5).[147]

Neuromuscular

Cranial Nerve Integrity. Cranial nerve (CN) function distinguishes among different types of polyneuropathy and is therefore important for evaluation, diagnosis, and prognosis. Patients with diabetic neuropathy commonly loose their sense of smell (CN I) and develop optic neuritis (CN II).[148] Patients with CMT[104] and inflammatory demyelinating neuropathy[148] also often have optic nerve atrophy. Facial muscle weakness is not uncommon in GBS and CIDP.[149,152] Vocal cord paralysis can occur in CMT type 2C, leading to hoarseness of voice.[150]

Reflex Integrity. The distribution of changes in muscle stretch reflexes can often distinguish polyneuropathy, which usually causes bilateral and symmetrical loss, from mononeuropathy or multiple mononeuropathy, which causes unilateral decreases or loss. Furthermore, length-dependent polyneuropathy presents with changes in distal reflexes, whereas inflammatory demyelinating polyradiculoneuropathies frequently have a diffuse presentation.

Sensory Integrity. Abnormal or absent sensation is common in patients with polyneuropathies. It is impor-

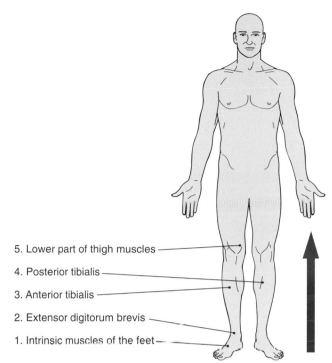

5. Lower part of thigh muscles
4. Posterior tibialis
3. Anterior tibialis
2. Extensor digitorum brevis
1. Intrinsic muscles of the feet

FIG. 19-6 Progression of most polyneuropathies from distal to proximal, starting with weakness of the intrinsic foot muscles, followed by the extensor digitorum brevis, anterior tibialis, posterior tibialis, and finally the lower parts of the thigh muscles. *Redrawn from Feldman EL, Stevens MJ, et al: A practical two-step quantitative clinical and electrophysiological assessment for the diagnosis and staging of diabetic neuropathy,* Diabetes Care *17:1281-1289, 1994.*

tant to test for different modalities of sensation because pain and temperature are carried by small nerve fibers, vibration and proprioception by large nerve fibers, and light touch by both small and large fibers (Table 19-8).[151,152] Testing should be performed on both sides, proximally and distally, and on the upper and lower extremities for comparison. Sensory testing of the trunk is also important to evaluate for certain conditions such as diabetic truncal radiculoneuropathy (see Fig. 19-3).

Cardiovascular/Pulmonary

Aerobic Capacity and Endurance. Breathing may be impaired in any polyneuropathy that affects the motor nerves to the diaphragm or trunk muscles. This is of particular concern in GBS where involvement of the trunk or diaphragm may be severe and comes on rapidly, necessitating intubation and ventilator-assisted breathing in some patients.[147]

Integumentary

Integumentary Integrity. Clinicians should inspect the skin for trophic changes, skin discoloration, sweat pattern abnormalities, and ulceration, particularly on the feet. Foot ulcers are common in patients with diabetic polyneuropathies, as well as in those with other sensory and *autonomic neuropathies*[149] (see Chapter 30).

Trophic changes, such as hair loss in the lower leg, occur in length-dependent polyneuropathies, such as

TABLE 19-8	Sensory Testing for Patients with Polyneuropathy Affecting Different Types of Nerves			
Nerve Type	Myelination	Sensation	Clinical Testing Tool	QST
Small fiber	Unmyelinated	Pain	Safety pin	HPDT
	Myelinated	Temperature	Hot/cold water tube	WDT
				CDT
Small/large fiber		Light touch	Cotton swab	No test available
Large fiber	Myelinated	Vibration	Tuning fork	VDT
	Myelinated	Proprioception	Passive movement by examiner	No test available

QST, Quantitative Sensory Testing; HPDT, heat pain nociception detection thresholds; WDT, warm detection thresholds; CDT, cool detection thresholds; VDT, vibratory detection thresholds.

TABLE 19-9	Normal Values for Distal Latency, Compound Muscle Action Potential Amplitude, and Nerve Conduction Velocities				
	Nerve	Site of Stimulation	Distal Latency (ms)	CMAP	NCV (m/sec)
Motor	Median	Elbow	3.49 ± 0.34	7.0 ± 2.7	63.5 ± 6.2
	Ulnar	Above elbow	2.59 ± 0.39	5.5 ± 1.9	61.0 ± 5.5
	Tibial	Knee	3.96 ± 1.00	5.1 ± 2.2	48.5 ± 3.6
	Peroneal	Ankle	3.77 ± 0.86	5.1 ± 2.3	52.0 ± 6.2
Sensory	Median	Wrist	2.84 ± 0.34	38.5 ± 15.6	56.2 ± 5.8
	Ulnar	Wrist	2.54 ± 5.3	35.0 ± 14.7	54.8 ± 5.3
			Latency to Recording Site		
F wave	Median	Elbow	22.8 ± 1.9		
	Ulnar	Above elbow	23.1 ± 1.7		
	Tibial	Above knee	39.9 ± 3.2		
	Peroneal	Knee	39.6 ± 4.4		

Modified from Kimura J: *Electrodiagnosis in Diseases of Nerve and Muscle: Principles and Practice,* New York, 2001, Oxford University Press. *CMAP,* Compound muscle action potential; *NCV,* nerve conduction velocities.

alcoholic or other toxic neuropathies, secondary to denervation of hair follicles. Furthermore, autonomic denervation of sweat glands can cause the skin to become thin and dry (see Table 19-11).[149]

Electrodiagnostic Testing. EMG and nerve conduction studies (NCS) are among the most informative, widely available, and reliable tests for examination of patients with peripheral neuropathy.[153-155] Electrodiagnostic testing is generally performed by a physician (usually a neurologist or a physiatrist) but may be performed by suitably trained and qualified physical therapists. These studies help identify the type of fibers involved (motor, sensory, or both), the underlying pathophysiology (axonal damage versus demyelination), and the pattern of involvement (symmetrical, asymmetrical, or multifocal).[153,155] NCS can identify 80% of patients with diabetic neuropathy and 80% to 100% of patients with GBS.[156,157]

Motor NCS record a number of parameters, including NCV, distal latency, compound action potential (CMAP) amplitude, and duration. Normal values for these parameters are presented in Table 19-9. Demyelination causes slowed conduction velocity, prolonged distal latencies, temporal dispersion, and conduction block (Fig. 19-7).[151] Axonal damage causes decreased CMAP amplitude, without changes in distal motor latency or NCV.[1,151] Since decreased limb temperature and increased age can cause decreased NCVs, the limb temperature should be kept above 32° C throughout the study, and age-appropriate normative data should be used for comparison.[152,158]

Sensory NCS and H-reflex studies can determine if the dorsal root ganglia and large myelinated axons are affected.[158] Since sensory fibers are usually affected first in length-dependent neuropathy, sensory NCS are often used to diagnose large fiber polyneuropathy.[158] Special techniques that measure responses from small myelinated and unmyelinated sensory axons can be used to determine whether the nerve root and anterior horn cell are intact.[152]

Quantitative Sensory Testing. Quantitative sensory testing (QST) is a systematic, precise procedure for testing large and small sensory nerve fibers (myelinated and unmyelinated) that cannot be tested by conventional NCS.[159-161] QST involves stimulating the patient with quantified sensory stimuli and determining thresholds for sensory perception, based on the patient's response.[159,161] Perception thresholds for light touch pressure, vibration, thermal sensations (cold and warm), and heat and cold pain thresholds can be measured noninvasively using QST. These procedures can be used to assess the function of A-delta (small diameter myelinated) and C (unmyelinated) sensory nerve fibers.[160,162]

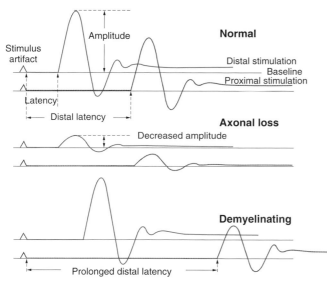

FIG. 19-7 Changes in compound muscle action potential (CMAP) with axonal and demyelinating lesions.

A computer-assisted device for QST, known as computer-assisted sensory examination (CASE), has been developed. This device determines vibratory detection thresholds (VDT), warm detection thresholds (WDT), cool detection thresholds (CDT), heat-pain detection thresholds (HPDT), and sensations using a number of different algorithms for presenting various sensory stimuli (see Table 19-8).[163] Although QST has an established role in diagnosing small-fiber neuropathy, it does have a number of shortcomings.[163-165] Patients may deliberately perform

poorly on the test, and mental fatigue, boredom, confusion, and drowsiness may affect the test results.[163]

Semmes-Weinstein Aesthesiometer for Sensory Assessment. In the late 1950s, Josephine Semmes and Sidney Weinstein developed nylon monofilaments for quantitative examination of cutaneous sensory perception. These monofilaments distinguish between normal, diminished light touch, diminished protective sensation, and loss of protective sensation (Table 19-10). These monofilaments have well-established reliability (*kappa* = 0.92).[166-168]

The Semmes-Weinstein monofilament complete set includes 20 monofilaments of different lengths and diameters. When the tip of the fiber is pressed against the skin at right angles, the force of application increases as the operator advances the probe until the fiber bends. After the fiber bends, continued advancement bends the fiber more but does not increase the force on the skin. This allows one to apply a reproducible force using a hand-held probe. Testing with these monofilaments has certain shortcomings, including lack of specificity (sometimes producing pain, as well as force sensations), and fragility (leaving most sets without one or more filaments). (See Chapter 18 for further details of how to use Semmes-Weinstein monofilaments.) Later, Weinstein develop the Weinstein Enhanced Sensory Test (WEST) (Fig. 19-8), which provides greater sensitivity and accuracy.

EVALUATION, DIAGNOSIS, AND PROGNOSIS

Most patients who fall into the *Guide to Physical Therapy Practice*[136] preferred practice pattern 5G: Impaired motor function and sensory integrity associated with acute or chronic polyneuropathy will typically have the following abnormal examination findings: Muscle weakness in one or more extremities, diminished or lost deep tendon reflexes, and abnormal tone, strength, and sensation. They may also have various other abnormal examination findings, as summarized in Table 19-11.

TABLE 19-10	Monofilament Sensory Testing Interpretation		
Plantar Thresholds	Hand and Dorsal Foot Thresholds	Monofilament Label	Force (gm)
Normal	Normal	1.65	0.008
		2.36	0.02
		2.44	0.04
		2.83	0.07
	Diminished light touch	3.22	0.16
		3.61	0.4
Diminished light touch	Diminished protective sensation	3.84	0.6
		4.08	1
		4.17	1.4
		4.31	2
Diminished protective sensation	Loss of protective sensation	4.56	4
		4.74	6
		4.93	8
Loss of protective sensation		5.07	10
		5.18	15
		5.46	26
		5.88	60
		6.10	100
		6.45	180
		6.65	300

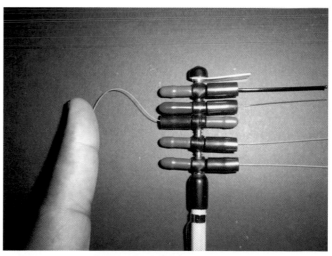

FIG. 19-8 The Weinstein Enhanced Sensory Test (WEST).

TABLE 19-11	Examination Findings and Likely Diagnosis in Patients with Polyneuropathy	
Impairments	**Functional Limitations**	**Pathology/Medical Diagnosis**
LOWER LIMB		
Distal muscle weakness	Frequent tripping/difficulty walking	Distal denervation
Foot drop	High-steppage gait	GBS
Proximal muscle weakness	Difficulty getting up from deep chair/stairs and rising from squatting position	CMT (hereditary)
Pes cavus and hammertoes	Difficulty walking	Distal denervation
Loss of hair extending up to the midcalf	None	Length-dependent neuropathies
Thin and dry skin	None	Length-dependent neuropathies
Ulceration	None	Hereditary sensory neuropathy or diabetic neuropathy
UPPER LIMB		
Proximal muscle weakness	Difficulty reaching overhead, shaving, combing hair	CMT disease (hereditary)
Distal muscle weakness	Difficulty opening doors, buttoning, and manipulating small objects, etc	Distal denervation
Repeated trauma to joint, pathological fracture, and osteomyelitis	Loss of pain sensation	Neuropathic joint, Charcot joint
TRUNK		
Scoliosis–kyphoscoliosis	Difficulty breathing	Denervation of paraspinal muscle

GBS, Guillain-Barré syndrome; *CMT,* Charcot-Marie-Tooth disease.

INTERVENTION

This section includes discussion of evidence-based interventions for patients with polyneuropathies. These include patient education and exercise, physical modalities, electrical stimulation (ES), and the use of orthoses and other durable medical equipment. Sackett et al defined evidence-based medicine as "the integration of best research evidence with clinical expertise and patient values."[169] The research used for deriving the recommendations below are primarily randomized controlled trials (RCT) or quasi-RCT. Other kinds of research are included in some cases but are not used as a primary source for clinical recommendations.

Publications were sought from the following electronic databases: MEDLINE (from 1966 to January 2005), CINAHL (from January 1982 to January 2005), and Cochrane Reviews. The following search terms: Neuropathy, polyneuropathy, Guillain-Barré, CIDP, polyradiculoneuritis, polyneuritis, as well as terms specific to the interventions, were used.

PATIENT AND FAMILY EDUCATION

Patient and family education regarding the progression and course of recovery, and the need for compliance with instructions, can impact the success of rehabilitation.[170] Compliance with instruction and recommendations for home activities including exercise can be influenced by variables related to the patient, the disease, the interventions, and interactions between the patient and the practitioner.[171,172]

The factors that specifically influence the compliance of patients with polyneuropathy with instructions and recommendations have not been evaluated. However, patient compliance with exercise programs has been studied in other patient populations.[173-175] Lack of positive feedback, degree of helplessness, and barriers that patients perceive or encounter were among the main factors for noncompliance.[174]

The effects of patient education on clinical and functional outcomes in patients with polyneuropathy have been evaluated in a few studies. A systematic review of the effect of patient education in diabetic foot care, based on eight RCTs, found that the evidence suggests that patient education may have positive but short-lived effects on patient knowledge and behavior and may reduce foot ulceration and amputations, especially in high-risk patients.[176] In addition, failure to comply with educational recommendations is associated with poor outcomes, including recurrent foot ulceration in patients with diabetes.[170]

EXERCISE

Evidence for the effect of exercise for patients with polyneuropathy is very limited in both quantity and quality. There are only a few RCTs, and these have only a few subjects each (Table 19-12).[177-182] Therefore current recommendations are based on these few trials and the outcomes of uncontrolled and nonrandomized trials and observational studies.

Studies indicate that various types of exercise, including progressive strengthening, balance, moderate resistance and higher resistance dynamic, exercise resulted in improvements in impairments and functional abilities, including muscle strength, six- and nine-minute walk tests, tandem stance, unipedal stance, SF-36 scores, and maximal isokinetic and isometric strength in patients with polyneuropathies.

In a prospective randomized controlled single blind trial, Lindeman et al found improvements in isokinetic knee extensor torque and 6-meter walk test performance, without increases in creatine phosphokinase (CPK) levels (an indicator of muscle breakdown), in 29 patients with

TABLE 19-12	Trials on the Effects of Exercise in Patients with Peripheral Neuropathy				
Condition	**Research Method (No. of Patients)**	**Exercise Type**	**Outcome Measure**	**Beneficial**	**Reference**
CMT (type I or II)	RCT (29)	Progressive strengthening exercise	Muscle strength* 6MWT* Questionnaire on functional performance	Yes	Lindeman[177]
Peripheral neuropathy associated with diabetes mellitus	Quasi-RCT (20)	Progressive strengthening and balance exercise	Tandem stance time* Functional reach Unipedal stance* ABC scale score	Yes	Richardson[178]
Chronic peripheral neuropathy	Quasi-RCT (28)	Home exercise program	Average muscle score Handgrip force 9MWT SF-36*	Yes	Ruhland[179]
Limited joint mobility and peripheral neuropathy	Not RCT (11)	Passive mobilization	Mobility of the ankle and foot joints	No	Dijs[180]
HMSN, MD, and other neuromuscular conditions	Not RCT (27)	Home exercise program, moderate resistance dynamic exercise	Maximal isokinetic and isometric strength*	Yes	Aitkens[181]
HMSN, MD, and LGD	Not RCT (10)	Home exercise program, higher resistance dynamic exercise	Maximal isometric and isokinetic strength of the elbow flexors* and knee extensors	Yes	Kilmer[182]

*Refers to improvements in outcome.
CMT, Charcot-Marie-Tooth disease; *RCT,* randomized controlled trial; *6MWT,* 6-minute walk test; *9MWT,* 9-minute walk test; *HMSN,* hereditary motor sensory neuropathy; *MD,* muscular dystrophy; *LGD,* limb girdle dystrophy.

CMT disease who exercised as compared to a control group who did not exercise.[177] The exercise consisted of weight lifting, with weights adjusted to patient performance, performed 3 times a week for 24 weeks.[177]

A study of twenty patients with peripheral neuropathy associated with diabetes mellitus showed improvements in functional reach, unipedal and tandem stance times, as well as higher scores on the activities-specific balance confidence (ABC) scale (see Chapter 13), in patients who participated in a 3-week exercise program consisting of upright unipedal and bipedal toe raises, heel raises, and resisted foot inversion and eversion, as compared with a group who did not exercise.[178]

A prospective quasi-RCT evaluated the effects of a home exercise program consisting of general muscle stretches, strengthening using resistance from elastic bands and bicycling or walking at an intensity to produce a heart rate of 60% to 70% of estimated maximum, in 28 patients with chronic peripheral neuropathy. The subjects were instructed to exercise daily for 6 weeks. At the end of this period the subjects had increased muscle strength but no improvements in pulmonary function test performance, walking velocity, or SF-36 scores. There were no reports of adverse effects of exercise.[179]

There are concerns, based on studies on animals that have found reduced reinnervation in response to short-term intense exercise, that too much exercise may adversely impact patients with partial denervation or those in the process of reinnervation.[183] Some studies also suggest that high levels of neuromuscular activity produced by ES or excessive exercise can be detrimental par-

ticularly in muscles that are extensively denervated. Furthermore, excessive exercise may reduce axonal sprouting and increase motor unit loss, as compared to conditions that produce normal physiological levels of muscle activation.[184] Concerns of overwork weakness from animal studies have led to avoidance of exercise in patients with polyneuropathies such as GBS and CIDP. However, studies (see Table 19-12) have found that moderate exercise produces improvements in various strength measures, including isokinetic knee extensor torque and 6-meter walk test, without adverse effects as measured by CPK or questionnaire, in patients with peripheral nerve diseases.[177] Similarly, in patients with post-polio syndrome, moderate intensity exercise increased muscle strength without reducing the number of motor units.[185]

To avoid overwork, exercise should be adjusted so that it does not produce delayed onset muscle soreness or post-exercise soreness that worsens rather than improves over time.[186,187] It has also been suggested that eccentric exercise be avoided, since this type of activity causes more muscle damage and postexercise soreness than isometric and concentric contractions in healthy persons.[188-190]

The Borg rating of perceived exertion (RPE) may also be used to guide the cardiovascular intensity of exercise in patients with polyneuropathies (see Chapter 23).[186,191,192] It is suggested that to increase their cardiovascular endurance patients with neuromuscular diseases, including those with polyneuropathy, start their exercise at very light intensity and gradually increase to the level of somewhat difficult.[186] Further guidelines and recommendations for exercise in patients with peripheral nerve

TABLE 19-13 Published Exercise Guidelines for Patients with Peripheral Neuropathy

Conditions	Recommendations	Source
Neuromuscular diseases	Adopt an active lifestyle. Moderate-intensity (defined by frequency, load, and duration) resistive strengthening exercise programs. Moderate aerobic exercise training program may be recommended without concern about any deleterious effect. Reduce fatigue by using brief work-rest-interval training programs.	Fowler[194]
Neuromuscular diseases	Resistance exercise with a relatively slow rate of progression may be beneficial if the degree of weakness is not severe. High-intensity resistance exercise has no advantage over more moderate program.	Kilmer[193]
Neuromuscular diseases	Aerobic conditioning is encouraged. Avoid eccentric exercise. Brace the joints with inadequate muscle support. Start exercise at a low level and progress gradually. Begin strength training with 20% of the maximum weight the patient can lift. Do 8-15 repetitions of each resisted exercise. Patients with severely affected muscles, with less than 10% of the normal strength, are unlikely to benefit from exercising these muscles. Patients with rapidly progressive disease will not benefit from strength or endurance exercise.	Forrest[186]
Guillain-Barré syndrome	Assess overwork weakness. Submaximal strength training. Aerobic training using Borg scale of perceived exertion. Recruit/train fast-twitch muscle fibers. Intense eccentric contractions should be avoided. Practice functional activities.	Bassile[191]

and neuromuscular diseases are summarized in Table 19-13.[186,191,193,194]

PHYSICAL MODALITIES

Although heat and cold are of limited benefit in patients with polyneuropathy,[195] if patients have other indications for such interventions, it is essential that their ability to sense temperature be carefully examined because the absence of such sensation increases the risk for burns. The application of deep or superficial heating agents is contraindicated in patients with impaired or absent temperature sensation. The patient should be able to distinguish between very cold, cold, room temperature, warm, and hot for the application of heat to be safe.[196]

Recently, a device that emits monochromatic infrared (890-nm wavelength) light from an array of light-emitting diodes (LEDs) has been cleared by the Food and Drug Administration (FDA) for the treatment of diabetic peripheral neuropathy.[197] This device has an array of 60 LEDs attached to a control unit that pulses the light at 292 times per second. This device is thought to increase circulation by promoting the release of nitric oxide to cause arterial and venous dilation. A recent double-blind, randomized, placebo-controlled study by Leonard et al reported significant improvements in foot sensation, balance, and pain in 27 subjects treated with this device who had diabetic peripheral neuropathy with loss of protective plantar sensation.[198] All subjects received an active or placebo treatment three times per week for 40 minutes each, and then both groups received active treatments for an additional 2 weeks. Other studies have shown that treatment

with this device can improve sensation and balance and reduce the frequency of falls in patients with peripheral neuropathy (Table 19-14).[197-200] Further studies are needed to establish and confirm the effectiveness of this intervention in patients with different types of polyneuropathy.

The role of low level laser therapy (LLLT) in the management of peripheral neuropathy has also been evaluated and debated in the literature. Early results were promising.[201,202] However, other trials have not shown such clear benefit.[200]

ELECTRICAL STIMULATION

ES has been evaluated and used as an intervention for patients with various types of polyneuropathy. It has been used to produce contractions in denervated muscles and at a sensory or motor level to control pain.

Denervated Muscle. Motor denervation is common in patients with polyneuropathy, and the appropriateness of ES to retard atrophy in denervated muscle has been debated in the literature for over 70 years. Studies of the effects of ES in animals with muscle denervation have produced conflicting results with some showing prevention or retardation of the effects of muscle denervation, including muscle atrophy,[203-205] and other studies finding this intervention to be ineffective or even detrimental.[206-208] These differences may be a result of differences in the ES interventions. In human patients electric stimulation has not been shown to enhance reinnervation of totally denervated muscles with peripheral neuropathies.[209] There are also concerns about applying ES to patients with dener-

TABLE 19-14 | Trials on the Effects of Light Therapy on Patients with Peripheral Neuropathy

Condition (No. of Patients)	Research Method	Modalities Type	Beneficial	Reference
Diabetic peripheral neuropathy (27)	Quasi-RCT	Infrared light from LEDs	Yes	Leonard[198]
Peripheral neuropathy due to diabetes and alcohol (38)	Non-RCT	Infrared light from LEDs	Yes	Kochman[199]
Diabetic peripheral neuropathy (49)	Non-RCT	Infrared light from LEDs	Yes	Kochman[197]
Diabetic sensorimotor polyneuropathy (50)	RCT	Low intensity infrared laser	No	Zinman[200]

RCT, Randomized controlled trials.

TABLE 19-15 | Trials on the Effects of Electrical Stimulation on Pain in Patients with Peripheral Neuropathy

Condition (No. of Patients)	Research Method	Mode of Application	Beneficial	Reference
Peripheral neuropathy (24)	RCT	TENS using carbon rubber electrodes	Yes	Thorsteinsson[218]
Diabetic peripheral neuropathy (10)	Quasi-RCT	Implanted spinal electrodes	Yes	Tesfaye[219]
Diabetic peripheral neuropathy (31)	RCT	TENS using carbon rubber electrodes	Yes	Kumar[220]
Diabetic peripheral neuropathy (8)	Non-RCT pilot study	TENS using stocking electrodes	Yes	Armstrong[221]
Diabetic peripheral neuropathy (50)	Quasi-RCT	Percutaneous stimulation	Yes	Hamza[222]
Diabetic peripheral neuropathy (30)*	Quasi-RCT	TENS using stocking electrodes	No	Oyibo[223]

*Only 14 completed.
RCT, Randomized controlled trials; *TENS*, transcutaneous electrical nerve stimulation.

vation because in animals axonal sprouting, a naturally occurring phenomenon, has been found to be inhibited by ES of denervated muscle fibers.[210-212]

Pain Management. Nerve damage that results from demyelination or axonal damage of sensory and/or motor nerves in patients with polyneuropathy can result in neuropathic pain.[213,214] This pain may be improved by the use of transcutaneous electrical nerve stimulation (TENS).[215-217] The evidence on the effectiveness of TENS for pain associated with diabetic peripheral neuropathy is contradictory. Although a number of studies have found TENS to reduce pain in this population, one RCT found that this intervention was no more effective than placebo (Table 19-15).[218-223] It would be expected that if TENS parameters preferentially stimulate the A-beta myelinated fibers while avoiding stimulation of C and A-delta fibers, transient pain relief would be provided during the stimulation.[224] In addition, one study found that using TENS for up to 1 week also resulted in reduction of pain for a number of weeks after the treatment was stopped.[225]

ORTHOSES

An orthosis is an externally applied device intended to correct and/or prevent deformity and improve function[226] (see Chapter 34). When using orthoses in patients with polyneuropathy and impaired sensation, particular attention should be paid to distributing pressure evenly over a large area and frequently inspecting the skin for early signs of breakdown.[195] The most commonly used lower extremity orthosis in patients with polyneuropathy is the total contact cast used in patients with neuropathic ulcers[227] (see Chapter 30). This device is designed to redistribute pressure on the foot, minimize shearing force, and protect wounds from contamination and infection.[170,228,229] In addition, ankle-foot orthoses (AFOs) may also be used to prevent plantar flexion contractures and assist with gait in patients with polyneuropathies that cause ankle dorsiflexor weakness.

CASE STUDY 19-1

GUILLAIN-BARRÉ SYNDROME

Examination
Patient History
PR is a 41-year-old woman who was admitted to the hospital with lower extremity weakness (inability to walk), facial tenderness, and numbness and tingling of the limbs. The lower extremity weakness was symmetrical and affected both proximal and distal muscles. Seven days before hospitalization, PR had flu-like symptoms. NCS results were consistent with a sensory-motor peripheral demyelinating neuropathy, and the patient was diagnosed with GBS. Two days after admission, PR developed labored breathing, was unable to move her lower extremities, and developed weakness of the upper limbs and trunk. PR was placed on a ventilator in the intensive care unit.

Systems Review
Heart rate 62 bpm, blood pressure 114/72 mm Hg, and respiratory rate is 12 breaths per minute.

Test and Measures
One Week after Admission to the Hospital
Range of Motion Functional passive ROM of all joints was within normal limits.

Muscle Performance Strength was graded by MMT as 2+/5 in the upper extremities and 1/5 in the lower extremities.

Function PR was completely dependent in bed mobility (rolling, sit to supine, supine to sit), and transfers (sit to stand, bed to chair, bed to commode).

Evaluation, Diagnosis, and Prognosis

PR had impaired bed mobility, transfers, and balance. The preferred practice pattern is 5G: Impaired motor function and sensory integrity associated with acute or chronic polyneuropathies.

Intervention

During the 8 weeks after her initial hospitalization, PR received physical therapy once or twice each day. Interventions included lower extremity stretching, strengthening exercises, endurance training, bed mobility training, standing balance training, gait training, and patient and family education. AFOs were initially applied to both feet to prevent ankle plantar flexion contractures and were later used during ambulation to optimize gait.

Outcome

Two Weeks after Admission to the Acute Care Hospital

Function PR was transferred to a skilled nursing facility for further rehabilitation.

Four Weeks after Initial Admission to the Hospital

Range of Motion Functional active ROM of all joints was within normal limits.

Muscle Performance Strength was graded by MMT as 3+/5 in the upper extremities and 3/5 in the lower extremities.

Function PR required minimal assistance for bed mobility (rolling, sit to supine, supine to sit), and moderate assistance for transfers (sit to stand, bed to chair, bed to commode).

Eight Weeks after Initial Admission to the Hospital

Range of Motion Functional active ROM of all joints was within normal limits.

Muscle Performance Strength was graded by MMT as 4+/5 in the upper extremities and 4/5 in the lower extremities.

Function PR was independent in bed mobility (rolling, sit to supine, supine to sit), and required contact guard assistance or verbal cueing for transfers (sit to stand, bed to chair, bed to commode).

Gait: By the eighth week, PR could walk 200 feet with a front-wheeled walker and close supervision. She stopped 2-3 times during this walk because of fatigue and left lower extremity pain. She also had the following gait deviations: Bilateral foot drop, poor heel contact, slow cadence, and diminished step length bilaterally. Fatigue affected all gait parameters negatively.

Overall, PR made excellent progress during this 8-week time period. At discharge from the skilled nursing facility, she could ambulate with a wheeled walker with only distant supervision, and she had almost full return of her lower extremity strength. Continued daily strengthening exercises were recommended to maximize her functional recovery, which is likely to be complete.

Please see the CD that accompanies this book for a case study describing the examination, evaluation, and interventions for a patient with diabetic polyneuropathy.

CHAPTER SUMMARY

Polyneuropathies are conditions that affect the function of multiple peripheral nerves. Polyneuropathies can have a wide range of etiologies and presentations that may impact their affect on patient function and selection of the ideal plan of care and interventions. Most polyneuropathies are associated with reduced sensation and strength, particularly in the distal extremities. There is some evidence that rehabilitation intervention, including patient and family education, exercise, physical modalities, ES, and orthotics, may reduce impairments and functional limitations in patients with polyneuropathies. However, more well-designed trials are needed to ascertain the effectiveness of these and other interventions in this patient population.

ADDITIONAL RESOURCES

Useful Forms

Michigan Neuropathy Screening Instrument
Activities-Specific Balance Confidence (ABC) Scale
Berg Balance Scale

Books

Ahroni JH: *101 Foot Care Tips for People with Diabetes,* Alexandria, 2000, American Diabetes Association.

Brown WF, Bolton CF, Aminoff MJ: *Neuromuscular Function and Disease: Basic, Clinical, and Electrodiagnostic Aspects,* Philadelphia, 2002, WB Saunders.

Dyck PJ: *Peripheral Neuropathy,* Philadelphia, 1993, WB Saunders.

Ouvrier RA, McLeod JG, Pollard JD: *Peripheral Neuropathy in Childhood,* New York, 1990, Raven Press.

Senneff JA: *Numb Toes and Aching Soles: Coping with Peripheral Neuropathy,* San Antonio, 1999, MedPress.

Staal A, Van Gijn J, Spaans F: *Mononeuropathies: Examination, Diagnosis and Treatment,* Philadelphia, 1999, WB Saunders.

Weiner WJ, Goetz CG: *Neurology for the Non-Neurologist,* Philadelphia, 1999, Lippincott Williams & Wilkins.

Web Sites

Alcoholic polyneuropathy: www.nlm.nih.gov/medlineplus/ency/article/000714.htm

Charcot-Marie-Tooth Disease Fact Sheet: www.ninds.nih.gov/disorders/charcot_marie_tooth/detail_charcot_marie_tooth.htm

Diabetic Neuropathies: www.diabetes.niddk.nih.gov/dm/pubs/neuropathies/index.htm

Neuromuscular Disease Center: www.neuro.wustl.edu/neuromuscular/index.html

GBS/CIDP Syndrome Foundation International: www.gbsfi.com/index.html

Chronic Inflammatory Demyelinating Polyneuropathy (CIDP): www.ninds.nih.gov/disorders/cidp/cidp.htm

Guillain-Barré Syndrome Information: www.ninds.nih.gov/disorders/gbs/gbs.htm

CIDP International Organization: www.cidpusa.org

The Neuropathy Association: www.neuropathy.org

National Diabetes Fact Sheet: www.diabetes.org/diabetes-statistics/national-diabetes-fact-sheet.jspl

GLOSSARY

Acute inflammatory demyelinating polyneuropathy (AIDP): Most common variant of GBS. An autoimmune disease directed against myelin.

Acute motor axonal neuropathy (AMAN): A variant of GBS that primarily affects the motor nerve axons.

Acute motor sensory axonal neuropathy (AMSAN): A variant of GBS that primarily affects the motor and sensory nerve axons.

Alcoholic neuropathy: Decreased nerve functioning caused by damage from excessive drinking of alcohol.

Allodynia: The sensation of pain in response to sensory stimulation that is usually not painful.

Autonomic neuropathy: Damage to nerves that regulate autonomic functions, including blood pressure, heart rate, bowel and bladder emptying, and digestion.

Charcot-Marie-Tooth (CMT) disease: A group of inherited, slowly progressive disorders that result from progressive damage to nerves. Symptoms include numbness and muscle atrophy that first occur in the feet and legs and then in the hands and arms.

Chronic inflammatory demyelinating polyradiculoneuropathy (CIDP): An autoimmune disease directed against myelin or Schwann cell antigens that causes slowly progressive or relapsing motor and/or sensory symptoms in more than one limb, developing over at least 8 weeks.

Demyelination: Loss of myelin.

Diabetic neuropathy: A common complication of diabetes mellitus in which nerves are damaged as a result of hyperglycemia (high blood sugar levels).

Guillain-Barré syndrome (GBS): An autoimmune disease directed against myelin that causes progressive muscle weakness or paralysis over a few days, which often starts a few days after resolution of an infectious illness.

Mononeuropathy: Dysfunction of a single nerve or nerve group.

Peripheral neuropathy: Dysfunction of the peripheral nerves.

Polyneuropathy: Generally, a bilateral symmetrical disturbance of peripheral nerve function.

References

1. Hughes RA: Peripheral neuropathy, *BMJ* 324:466-469, 2002.
2. Martyn CN, Hughes RA: Epidemiology of peripheral neuropathy, *J Neurol Neurosurg Psychiatry* 62:310-318, 1997.
3. Hughes RA: Diagnosis of chronic peripheral neuropathy, *J Neurol Neurosurg Psychiatry* 71:147-148, 2001.
4. Hughes RA: Management of chronic peripheral neuropathy, *Proc Roy Coll Phys (Edinburgh)* 30:321-327, 2000.
5. Thomas PK, Ochoa J: Clinical features and differential diagnosis. In Dyck PJ (ed): *Peripheral Neuropathy*, Philadelphia, 1993, WB Saunders.
6. Landry O: Note sur la paralysie ascendante aigue, *Gaz Hebd Med Chir* 6:472-474, 1859.
7. Guillain G, Barré JA, Strohl A: Sur un syndrome de radiculo-nevrite avec hyperalbuminose du liguide cephalo-rachidien sans reaction cellulaire: Remarques sur les caracters clinques des reflexes tendineux, *Bull Mem Soc Med Hop Paris* 40:1462-1470, 1916.
8. Guillain G, Barré JA, Strohl A: Radiculoneuritis syndrome with hyperalbuminosis of cerebrospinal fluid without cellular reaction. Notes on clinical features and graphs of tendon reflexes. 1916], *Ann Med Interne (Paris)* 150:24-32, 1999.
9. Arnason BG, Soliven B: Acute inflammatory demyelinating polyradiculoneuropathy. In Dyck PJ (ed): *Peripheral Neuropathy*, Philadelphia, 1993, WB Saunders.
10. Fisher CM: An unusual variant of idiopathic polyneuritis (syndrome of ophthalmoplegia, ataxia, and areflexia), *N Engl J Med* 57-65, 1956.
11. Phillips MS, Stewart S, Anderson JR: Neuropathological findings in Miller Fisher syndrome, *J Neurol Neurosurg Psychiatry* 47:492-495, 1984.
12. Feasby TE, Gilbert JJ, Brown WF, et al: An acute axonal form of Guillain-Barré polyneuropathy, *Brain* 109 (Pt 6):1115-1126, 1986.
13. Feasby TE, Hahn AF, Brown WF, et al: Severe axonal degeneration in acute Guillain-Barré syndrome: evidence of two different mechanisms? *J Neurol Sci* 116:185-192, 1993.
14. Griffin JW, Li CY, Ho TW, et al: Pathology of the motor-sensory axonal Guillain-Barré syndrome, *Ann Neurol* 39:17-28, 1996.
15. Hafer-Macko C, Hsieh ST, Li CY, et al: Acute motor axonal neuropathy: An antibody-mediated attack on axolemma, *Ann Neurol* 40:635-644, 1996.
16. McKhann GM, Cornblath DR, Griffin JW, et al: Acute motor axonal neuropathy: a frequent cause of acute flaccid paralysis in China, *Ann Neurol* 33:333-342, 1993.
17. Gupta SK, Taly AB, Suresh TG, et al: Acute idiopathic axonal neuropathy (AIAN): A clinical and electrophysiological observation, *Acta Neurol Scand* 89:220-224, 1994.
18. Hankey GJ: Guillain-Barré syndrome in Western Australia, 1980-1985, *Med J Aust* 146:130-133, 1987.
19. Radhakrishnan K, el Mangoush MA, Gerryo SE: Descriptive epidemiology of selected neuromuscular disorders in Benghazi, Libya, *Acta Neurol Scand* 75:95-100, 1987.
20. Halls J, Bredkjaer C, Friis ML: Guillain-Barré syndrome: diagnostic criteria, epidemiology, clinical course and prognosis, *Acta Neurol Scand* 78:118-122, 1988.
21. Kinnunen E, Farkkila M, Hovi T, et al: Incidence of Guillain-Barré syndrome during a nationwide oral poliovirus vaccine campaign, *Neurology* 39:1034-1036, 1989.
22. Ballesteros M, Lasky T, Nash D, et al: Guillain-Barré syndrome incidence based on hospital discharge data, *J Infect Dis* 178:1228, 1998.
23. Ho TW, Li CY, Cornblath DR, et al: Patterns of recovery in the Guillain-Barré syndromes, *Neurology* 48:695-700, 1997.
24. A prospective study on the incidence and prognosis of Guillain-Barré syndrome in Emilia-Romagna region, Italy (1992-1993). Emilia-Romagna Study Group on Clinical and Epidemiological Problems in Neurology, *Neurology* 48:214-221, 1997.
25. Feasby TE, Hughes RA: Campylobacter jejuni, antiganglioside antibodies, and Guillain-Barré syndrome, *Neurology* 51:340-342, 1998.
26. Jiang GX, Pedro-Cuesta J, Fredrikson S, et al: Guillain-Barré syndrome in south-west Stockholm, 1973-1991, 2. Clinical epidemiology, *Ital J Neurol Sci* 18:49-53, 1997.
27. Jiang GX, Cheng Q, Ehrnst A, et al: Guillain-Barré syndrome in Stockholm County, 1973-1991, *Eur J Epidemiol* 13:25-32, 1997.
28. Jiang GX, Cheng Q, Link H, et al: Epidemiological features of Guillain-Barré syndrome in Sweden, 1978-93, *J Neurol Neurosurg Psychiatry* 62:447-453, 1997.
29. Ropper AH: The Guillain-Barré syndrome, *N Engl J Med* 326:1130-1136, 1992.
30. Hahn AF: Guillain-Barré syndrome, *Lancet* 352:635-641, 1998.
31. Allos BM: Campylobacter jejuni infection as a cause of the Guillain-Barré syndrome, *Infect Dis Clin North Am* 12:173-184, 1998.
32. Hao Q, Saida T, Kuroki S, et al: Antibodies to gangliosides and galactocerebroside in patients with Guillain-Barré syndrome with preceding Campylobacter jejuni and other identified infections, *J Neuroimmunol* 81:116-126, 1998.
33. Yuki N, Miyatake T: Guillain-Barré syndrome and Fisher's syndrome following Campylobacter jejuni infection, *Ann N Y Acad Sci* 845:330-340, 1998.
34. Gorson KC, Ropper AH: Guillain-Barré syndrome. In Cros D (ed): *Peripheral Neuropathy: A Practical Approach to Diagnosis and Management*, Philadelphia, 2001, Lippincott Williams & Wilkins.
35. Pentland B, Donald SM: Pain in the Guillain-Barré syndrome, *Pain* 59:159-164, 1994.
36. Cornblath DR, McArthur JC, Kennedy PG, et al: Inflammatory demyelinating peripheral neuropathies associated with human T-cell lymphotropic virus type III infection, *Ann Neurol* 21:32-40, 1987.
37. Hurwitz ES, Schonberger LB, Nelson DB, et al: Guillain-Barré syndrome and the 1978-1979 influenza vaccine, *N Engl J Med* 304:1557-1561, 1981.
38. Schonberger LB, Hurwitz ES, Katona P, et al: Guillain-Barré syndrome: Its epidemiology and associations with influenza vaccination, *Ann Neurol* 9(suppl):31-38, 1981.
39. Lasky T, Terracciano GJ, Magder L, et al: The Guillain-Barré syndrome and the 1992-1993 and 1993-1994 influenza vaccines, *N Engl J Med* 339:1797-1802, 1998.
40. Rees J, Hughes R: Guillain-Barré syndrome after measles, mumps, and rubella vaccine, *Lancet* 343:733, 1994.
41. Ropper AH, Wijdicks EFM, Truax BT: *Guillain-Barré Syndrome*, Philadelphia, 1991, FA Davis.
42. Arnason BG, Asbury AK: Idiopathic polyneuritis after surgery, *Arch Neurol* 18:500-507, 1968.
43. Case records of the MGH Weekly clinicopathological exercises: Case 8-1990. A 45-year-old woman with Hodgkin's disease and a neurologic disorder, *N Engl J Med* 322:531-543, 1990.
44. Jiang GX, Pedro-Cuesta J, Strigard K, et al: Pregnancy and Guillain-Barré syndrome: a nationwide register cohort study, *Neuroepidemiology* 15:192-200, 1996.

45. Ropper AH, Victor M: Influenza vaccination and the Guillain-Barré syndrome, *N Engl J Med* 339:1845-1846, 1998.
46. Salisbury DM: Association between oral polio vaccine and Guillain-Barré syndrome? *Lancet* 351:79-80, 1998.
47. Awong IE, Dandurand KR, Keeys CA, et al: Drug-associated Guillain-Barré syndrome: A literature review, *Ann Pharmacother* 30:173-180, 1996.
48. Ho TW, McKhann GM, Griffin JW: Human autoimmune neuropathies, *Annu Rev Neurosci* 21:187-226, 1998.
49. Steck AJ, Schaeren-Wiemers N, Hartung HP: Demyelinating inflammatory neuropathies, including Guillain-Barré syndrome, *Curr Opin Neurol* 11:311-318, 1998.
50. Kissel JT, Cornblath DR, Mendell JR: Guillain-Barré syndrome. In Mendell JR, Cornblath DR, Kissel JT (eds): *Diagnosis and Management of Peripheral Nerve Disorders,* Oxford, 2001, Oxford University Press.
51. Kwa MS, van Schaik IN, de Jonge RR, et al: Autoimmunoreactivity to Schwann cells in patients with inflammatory neuropathies, *Brain* 126:361-375, 2003.
52. Griffin JW, Li CY, Macko C, et al: Early nodal changes in the acute motor axonal neuropathy pattern of the Guillain-Barré syndrome, *J Neurocytol* 25:33-51, 1996.
53. Gibbels E, Giebisch U: Natural course of acute and chronic monophasic inflammatory demyelinating polyneuropathies (IDP). A retrospective analysis of 266 cases, *Acta Neurol Scand* 85:282-291, 1992.
54. Barohn RJ, Kissel JT, Warmolts JR, et al: Chronic inflammatory demyelinating polyradiculoneuropathy. Clinical characteristics, course, and recommendations for diagnostic criteria, *Arch Neurol* 46:878-884, 1989.
55. Kissel JT, Mendell JR: Chronic inflammatory demyelinating polyradiculoneuropathy. In Mendell JR, Cornblath DR, Kissel JT (eds): *Diagnosis and Management of Peripheral Nerve Disorders,* Oxford, 2001, Oxford University Press.
56. Nattrass FJ: Recurrent hypertrophic neuritis, *J Neurol Psychopathol* 2:159, 1921.
57. Dyck PJ, Prineas J, Pollard J: Chronic inflammatory demyelinating polyradiculoneuropathy. In Dyck PJ (ed): *Peripheral Neuropathy,* Philadelphia, 1993, WB Saunders.
58. DeJong RN: The Guillain-Barré syndrome. Polyradiculoneuritis with albuminocytologic dissociation, *Arch Neurol Psychiatry* 44:1044-1050, 1940.
59. Report from an Ad Hoc Subcommittee of the American Academy of Neurology AIDS Task Force: Research criteria for diagnosis of chronic inflammatory demyelinating polyneuropathy (CIDP), *Neurology* 41:617-618, 1991.
60. Sander HW, Latov N: Research criteria for defining patients with CIDP, *Neurology* 60:S8-S15, 2003.
61. Berger AR, Bradley WG, Brannagan TH, et al: Guidelines for the diagnosis and treatment of chronic inflammatory demyelinating polyneuropathy, *J Peripher Nerv Syst* 8:282-284, 2003.
62. Lunn MP, Manji H, Choudhary PP, et al: Chronic inflammatory demyelinating polyradiculoneuropathy: a prevalence study in south east England, *J Neurol Neurosurg Psychiatry* 66:677-680, 1999.
63. McLeod JG, Pollard JD, MaCaskill P, et al: Prevalence of chronic inflammatory demyelinating polyneuropathy in New South Wales, Australia, *Ann Neurol* 46:910-913, 1999.
64. Mygland A, Monstad P: Chronic polyneuropathies in Vest-Agder, Norway, *Eur J Neurol* 8:157-165, 2001.
65. Dyck PJ, Lais AC, Ohta M, et al: Chronic inflammatory polyradiculoneuropathy, *Mayo Clin Proc* 50:621-637, 1975.
66. van der Meche FG, van Doorn PA: Guillain-Barré syndrome and chronic inflammatory demyelinating polyneuropathy: Immune mechanisms and update, *Ann Neurol* 37(suppl 1):S14-S31, 1995.
67. Reid VA, Black KR, Menkes DL, et al: Chronic inflammatory demyelinating polyradiculoneuropathy: Diagnosis and management. In Cros D (ed): *Peripheral Neuropathy: A Practical Approach to Diagnosis and Management,* Philadelphia, 2001, Lippincott Williams & Wilkins.
68. Molenaar DS, Vermeulen M, de Haan R: Diagnostic value of sural nerve biopsy in chronic inflammatory demyelinating polyneuropathy, *J Neurol Neurosurg Psychiatry* 64:84-89, 1998.
69. Matsumuro K, Izumo S, Umehara F, et al: Chronic inflammatory demyelinating polyneuropathy: Histological and immunopathological studies on biopsied sural nerves, *J Neurol Sci* 127:170-178, 1994.
70. Notermans NC, Wokke JH, Van den Berg LH, et al: Chronic idiopathic axonal polyneuropathy. Comparison of patients with and without monoclonal gammopathy, *Brain* 119(Pt 2):421-427, 1996.
71. Goldstein JM, Parks BJ, Mayer PL, et al: Nerve root hypertrophy as the cause of lumbar stenosis in chronic inflammatory demyelinating polyradiculoneuropathy, *Muscle Nerve* 19:892-896, 1996.
72. Ginsberg L, Platts AD, Thomas PK: Chronic inflammatory demyelinating polyneuropathy mimicking a lumbar spinal stenosis syndrome, *J Neurol Neurosurg Psychiatry* 59:189-191, 1995.
73. De Silva RN, Willison HJ, Doyle D, et al: Nerve root hypertrophy in chronic inflammatory demyelinating polyneuropathy, *Muscle Nerve* 17:168-170, 1994.
74. Oh SJ, Joy JL, Kuruoglu R: "Chronic sensory demyelinating neuropathy:" chronic inflammatory demyelinating polyneuropathy presenting as a pure sensory neuropathy, *J Neurol Neurosurg Psychiatry* 55:677-680, 1992.
75. Simmons Z, Wald JJ, Albers JW: Chronic inflammatory demyelinating polyradiculoneuropathy in children. I. Presentation, electrodiagnostic studies, and initial clinical course, with comparison to adults, *Muscle Nerve* 20:1008-1015, 1997.
76. Hattori N, Ichimura M, Aoki S, et al: Clinicopathological features of chronic inflammatory demyelinating polyradiculoneuropathy in childhood, *J Neurol Sci* 154:66-71, 1998.
77. Simmons Z, Wald JJ, Albers JW: Chronic inflammatory demyelinating polyradiculoneuropathy in children: II. Long-term follow-up, with comparison to adults, *Muscle Nerve* 20:1569-1575, 1997.
78. Duby JJ, Campbell RK, Setter SM, et al: Diabetic neuropathy: an intensive review, *Am J Health Syst Pharm* 61:160-173, 2004.
79. Simmons Z, Feldman EL. Update on diabetic neuropathy. *Curr Opin Neurol* 15:595-603, 2002.
80. Thomas PK, Tomlinson DR: Diabetic and hypoglycemic neuropathy. In Dyck PJ (ed): *Peripheral Neuropathy,* Philadelphia, 1993, WB Saunders.
81. Gominak S, Parry GJ: Neuropathies and Diabetes. In Cros D (ed): *Peripheral Neuropathy: A Practical Approach to Diagnosis and Management,* Philadelphia, 2001, Lippincott Williams & Wilkins.
82. Mendell JR: Diabetic neuropathies. In Mendell JR, Cornblath DR, Kissel JT (eds): *Diagnosis and Management of Peripheral Nerve Disorders,* Oxford, 2001, Oxford University Press.
83. Vinik AI, Holland MT, Le Beau JM, et al: Diabetic neuropathies, *Diabetes Care* 15:1926-1975, 1992.
84. US Department of Health and Human Services, CDC: *National diabetes fact sheet,* Available at: www.cdc.gov/diabetes/pubs/factsheet.htm. 2003.
85. Pirart J: Diabetes mellitus and its degenerative complications: a prospective study of 4,400 patients observed between 1947 and 1973, *Diabetes Care* 1:168-188, 1978.
86. Fedele D, Comi G, Coscelli C, et al: A multicenter study on the prevalence of diabetic neuropathy in Italy. Italian Diabetic Neuropathy Committee, *Diabetes Care* 20:836-843, 1997.
87. Dyck PJ, Kratz KM, Karnes JL, et al: The prevalence by staged severity of various types of diabetic neuropathy, retinopathy, and nephropathy in a population-based cohort: the Rochester Diabetic Neuropathy Study, *Neurology* 43:817-824, 1993.
88. Shaw JE, Zimmet PZ: The epidemiology of diabetic neuropathies, *Diabetes Rev* 7:245-252, 1999.
89. Tomlinson DR: Polyols and myo-inositol in diabetic neuropathy—of mice and men, *Mayo Clin Proc* 64:1030-1033, 1989.
90. Sheetz MJ, King GL: Molecular understanding of hyperglycemia's adverse effects for diabetic complications, *JAMA* 288:2579-2588, 2002.
91. Oates PJ: Polyol pathway and diabetic peripheral neuropathy, *Int Rev Neurobiol* 50:325-392, 2002.
92. Giannini C, Dyck PJ: Basement membrane reduplication and pericyte degeneration precede development of diabetic polyneuropathy and are associated with its severity, *Ann Neurol* 37:498-504, 1995.
93. Low PA, Lagerlund TD, McManis PG: Nerve blood flow and oxygen delivery in normal, diabetic, and ischemic neuropathy, *Int Rev Neurobiol* 31:355-438, 1989.
94. Malik RA, Masson EA, Sharma AK, et al: Hypoxic neuropathy: relevance to diabetic neuropathy, *Diabetologia* 33:311-331, 1990.
95. Sladky JT, Tschoepe RL, Greenberg JH, et al: Peripheral neuropathy after chronic endoneurial ischemia, *Ann Neurol* 29:272-278, 1991.
96. Cameron NE, Cotter MA: The relationship of vascular changes to metabolic factors in diabetes mellitus and their role in development of peripheral nerve complications, *Diabetes Metab Rev* 10:189-224, 1994.
97. Faradji V, Sotelo J: Low serum levels of nerve growth factor in diabetic neuropathy, *Acta Neurol Scand* 81:402-406, 1990.
98. Apfel SC, Arezzo JC, Brownlee M, et al: Nerve growth factor administration protects against experimental diabetic sensory neuropathy, *Brain Res* 634:7-12, 1994.
99. Vinik AI, Park TS, Stansberry KB, et al: Diabetic neuropathies, *Diabetologia* 43:957-973, 2000.
100. Waxman SG, Sabin TD: Diabetic truncal polyneuropathy, *Arch Neurol* 38:46-47, 1981.
101. Calissi PT, Jaber LA: Peripheral diabetic neuropathy: current concepts in treatment, *Ann Pharmacother* 29:769-777, 1995.
102. Pinzur MS: The diabetic foot, *Compr Ther* 28:232-237, 2002.
103. Charcot JM, Marie P: Sur une forme particulière d'atrophie musculaire progressive souvent familial débutant par les pieds et les jambs et atteignant plus tard les mains, *Rev Méd (Paris)* 86, 1886.
104. Dyck PJ, Chance P, Lebo R, Carney A: Hereditary motor and sensory neuropathies. In Dyck PJ (ed): *Peripheral Neuropathy,* Philadelphia, 1993, WB Saunders.
105. Tooth HH: *The Peroneal Type of Progressive Muscular Atrophy,* London, 1886, HK Lewis & Co.

106. Reilly MM: Classification of hereditary motor and sensory neuropathies, *Curr Opin Neurol* 13:561-564, 2000.
107. Harding AE, Thomas PK: The clinical features of hereditary motor and sensory neuropathy types I and II, *Brain* 103:259-280, 1980.
108. Berciano J, Combarros O: Hereditary neuropathies, *Curr Opin Neurol* 16:613-622, 2003.
109. National Institute of Neurological Disorders and Stroke: Charcot-Marie-Tooth Disease Fact Sheet. Available at: www.ninds.nih.gov/health_and_medical/pubs/CMT.htm. 2004.
110. Combarros O, Calleja J, Polo JM, et al: Prevalence of hereditary motor and sensory neuropathy in Cantabria, *Acta Neurol Scand* 75:9-12, 1987.
111. Morocutti C, Colazza GB, Soldati G, D'Alessio C, et al: Charcot-Marie-Tooth disease in Molise, a central-southern region of Italy: An epidemiological study, *Neuroepidemiology* 21:241-245, 2002.
112. Kurihara S, Adachi Y, Wada K, et al: An epidemiological genetic study of Charcot-Marie-Tooth disease in Western Japan, *Neuroepidemiology* 21:246-250, 2002.
113. Lupski JR, Oca-Luna RM, Slaugenhaupt S, et al: DNA duplication associated with Charcot-Marie-Tooth disease type 1A, *Cell* 66:219 232, 1991.
114. Raeymaekers P, Timmerman V, Nelis E, et al: Duplication in chromosome 17p11.2 in Charcot-Marie-Tooth neuropathy type 1a (CMT 1a). The HMSN Collaborative Research Group, *Neuromuscul Disord* 1:93-97, 1991.
115. Mendell JR, Sahenk Z: Hereditary motor and sensory neuropathies and giant axonal neuropathy. In Mendell JR, Cornblath DR, Kissel JT (eds): Diagnosis and Management of Peripheral Nerve Disorders, Oxford, 2001, Oxford University Press.
116. Chance PF: Genetic studies in polyneuropathy. In Cros D (ed): *Peripheral Neuropathy: A Practical Approach to Diagnosis and Management,* Philadelphia, 2001, Lippincott Williams & Wilkins.
117. Zhou L, Griffin JW: Demyelinating neuropathies, *Curr Opin Neurol* 16:307-313, 2003.
118. De Jonghe P, Timmerman V, FitzPatrick D, et al: Mutilating neuropathic ulcerations in a chromosome 3q13-q22 linked Charcot-Marie-Tooth disease type 2B family, *J Neurol Neurosurg Psychiatry* 62:570-573, 1997.
119. Guzzetta F, Ferriere G, Lyon G: Congenital hypomyelination polyneuropathy. Pathological findings compared with polyneuropathies starting later in life, *Brain* 105:395-416, 1982.
120. Jackson J: A peculiar disease resulting form the use of ardent spirits, *N Engl J Med Surg* 11:351, 1822.
121. Windebank A: Polyneuropathy due to nutritional deficiency and alcoholism. In Dyck PJ (ed): *Peripheral Neuropathy,* Philadelphia, 1993, WB Saunders.
122. So Y: Nutritional and alcoholic neuropathies. In Cros D (ed): *Peripheral Neuropathy: A Practical Approach to Diagnosis and Management,* Philadelphia, 2001, Lippincott Williams & Wilkins.
123. Erdem S, Kissel JT, Mendell JR: Toxic neuropathies: Drugs, metals, and alcohol. In Mendell JR, Cornblath DR, Kissel JT (eds): *Diagnosis and Management of Peripheral Nerve Disorders,* Oxford, 2001, Oxford University Press.
124. D'Amour ML, Butterworth RF: Pathogenesis of alcoholic peripheral neuropathy: direct effect of ethanol or nutritional deficit? *Metab Brain Dis* 9:133-142, 1994.
125. Monforte R, Estruch R, Valls-Sole J, et al: Autonomic and peripheral neuropathies in patients with chronic alcoholism. A dose-related toxic effect of alcohol, *Arch Neurol* 52:45-51, 1995.
126. Estruch R, Nicolas JM, Villegas E, et al: Relationship between ethanol-related diseases and nutritional status in chronically alcoholic men, *Alcohol Alcohol* 28:543-550, 1993.
127. Boyd DH, MacLaren DS, Stoddard ME: The nutritional status of patients with an alcohol problem, *Acta Vitaminol Enzymol* 3:75-82, 1981.
128. Scholz E, Diener HC, Dichgans J, et al: Incidence of peripheral neuropathy and cerebellar ataxia in chronic alcoholics, *J Neurol* 233:212-217, 1986.
129. Sosenko JM, Soto R, Aronson J, et al: The prevalence and extent of vibration sensitivity impairment in men with chronic ethanol abuse, *J Stud Alcohol* 52:374-376, 1991.
130. Hilz MJ, Zimmermann P, Rosl G, et al: Vibrometer testing facilitates the diagnosis of uremic and alcoholic polyneuropathy, *Acta Neurol Scand* 92:486-490, 1995.
131. Hilz MJ, Zimmermann P, Claus D, et al: Thermal threshold determination in alcoholic polyneuropathy: An improvement of diagnosis, *Acta Neurol Scand* 91:389-393, 1995.
132. Tredici G, Minazzi M: Alcoholic neuropathy. An electron-microscopic study, *J Neurol Sci* 25:333-346, 1975.
133. American Physical Therapy Association: Guide to physical therapist practice, second edition, *Phys Ther* 81:9-746, 2001.
134. Barohn RJ: Approach to peripheral neuropathy and neuronopathy, *Semin Neurol* 18:7-18, 1998.
135. Kissel JT, Cornblath DR, Mendell JR: Guillain-Barré syndrome. In Mendell JR, Cornblath DR, Kissel JT (eds): *Diagnosis and Management of Peripheral Nerve Disorders,* Oxford, 2001, Oxford University Press.
136. Pollard JD: Chronic inflammatory demyelinating polyradiculoneuropathy, *Curr Opin Neurol* 15:279-283, 2002.
137. Rubens O, Logina I, Kravale I, et al: Peripheral neuropathy in chronic occupational inorganic lead exposure: a clinical and electrophysiological study, *J Neurol Neurosurg Psychiatry* 71:200-204, 2001.
138. Yeh JH, Chang YC, Wang JD: Combined electroneurographic and electromyographic studies in lead workers, *Occup Environ Med* 52:415-419, 1995.
139. Mueller MJ: Identifying patients with diabetes mellitus who are at risk for lower-extremity complications: Use of Semmes-Weinstein monofilaments, *Phys Ther* 76:68-71, 1996.
140. Feldman EL, Stevens MJ, Thomas PK, et al: A practical two-step quantitative clinical and electrophysiological assessment for the diagnosis and staging of diabetic neuropathy, *Diabetes Care* 17:1281-1289, 1994.
141. Kendall FP, McCreary EK, Provance PG: *Muscles, Testing and Function,* Baltimore, 1993, Williams & Wilkins.
142. Silver M, McElroy A, Morrow L, et al: Further standardization of manual muscle test for clinical study: applied in chronic renal disease, *Phys Ther* 50:1456-1466, 1970.
143. Frese E, Brown M, Norton BJ: Clinical reliability of manual muscle testing. Middle trapezius and gluteus medius muscles, *Phys Ther* 67:1072-1076, 1987.
144. Piao C, Yoshimoto N, Shitama H, et al: Validity and reliability of the measurement of the quadriceps femoris muscle strength with a hand-held dynamometer on the affected side in hemiplegic patients, *J UOEH* 26:1-11, 2004.
145. Mathiowetz V: Comparison of Rolyan and Jamar dynamometers for measuring grip strength, *Occup Ther Int* 9:201-209, 2002.
146. Merkies IS, Schmitz PI, Samijn JP, et al: Assessing grip strength in healthy individuals and patients with immune-mediated polyneuropathies, *Muscle Nerve* 23:1393-1401, 2000.
147. Sabin T: Generalized peripheral neuropathy: Symptoms, signs, and syndromes. In Cros D (ed): *Peripheral Neuropathy: A Practical Approach to Diagnosis and Management,* Philadelphia, 2001, Lippincott Williams & Wilkins.
148. Mendell JR, Kolkin S, Kissel JT, et al: Evidence for central nervous system demyelination in chronic inflammatory demyelinating polyradiculoneuropathy, *Neurology* 37:1291-1294, 1987.
149. Mendell JR, Kissel JT, Cornblath DR: Clues to diagnosis of peripheral neuropathy: History and examination of the patient. In Mendell JR, Cornblath DR, Kissel JT (eds): *Diagnosis and Management of Peripheral Nerve Disorders,* Oxford, 2001, Oxford University Press.
150. Dyck PJ, Litchy WJ, Minnerath S, et al: Hereditary motor and sensory neuropathy with diaphragm and vocal cord paresis, *Ann Neurol* 35:608-615, 1994.
151. Poncelet AN: An algorithm for the evaluation of peripheral neuropathy, *Am Fam Phys* 57:755-764, 1998.
152. Olney RK: Clinical trials for polyneuropathy: the role of nerve conduction studies, quantitative sensory testing, and autonomic function testing, *J Clin Neurophysiol* 15:129-137, 1998.
153. Donofrio PD, Albers JW: AAEM mini monograph #34—Polyneuropathy: Classification by nerve conduction studies and electromyography, *Muscle Nerve* 13:889-903, 1990.
154. Thrush D: Investigation of peripheral neuropathy, *Br J Hosp Med* 48:13-22, 1992.
155. McLeod JG: Investigation of peripheral neuropathy, *J Neurol Neurosurg Psychiatry* 58:274-283, 1995.
156. Oh SJ: *Clinical Electromyography Nerve Conduction Studies,* Baltimore, 1993, Williams & Wilkins.
157. Oh SJ: *Principles of Clinical Electromyography: Case Studies,* Baltimore, 1998, Williams & Wilkins.
158. Cornblath DR, Chaudhry V: Electrodiagnostic evaluation of the peripheral neuropathy patient. In Mendell JR, Cornblath DR, Kissel JT (eds): *Diagnosis and Management of Peripheral Nerve Disorders,* Oxford, 2001, Oxford University Press.
159. Dyck PJ, Zimmerman IR, O'Brien PC, et al: Introduction of automated systems to evaluate touch-pressure, vibration, and thermal cutaneous sensation in man, *Ann Neurol* 4:502-510, 1978.
160. Mendell JR, Cornblath DR: Evaluation of the peripheral neuropathy patient using Quantitative Sensory Testing. In Mendell JR, Cornblath DR, Kissel JT (eds): *Diagnosis and Management of Peripheral Nerve Disorders,* Oxford, 2001, Oxford University Press.
161. Stewart J, Freeman R: Quantitative Sensory Testing. In Brown WF, Bolton CF, Aminoff MJ (eds): *Neuromuscular Function and Disease: Basic, Clinical, and Electrodiagnostic Aspects,* Philadelphia, 2002, WB Saunders.
162. Dyck PJ, O'Brien PC: Quantitative sensation testing in small-diameter sensory fiber neuropathy, *Muscle Nerve* 26:595-596, 2002.
163. Siao P, Cros DP: Quantitative sensory testing, *Phys Med Rehabil Clin N Am* 14:261-286, 2003.
164. Gruener G, Dyck PJ: Quantitative sensory testing: methodology, applications, and future directions, *J Clin Neurophysiol* 11:568-583, 1994.

165. Dyck PJ, O'Brien PC: Quantitative sensation testing in epidemiological and therapeutic studies of peripheral neuropathy, *Muscle Nerve* 22:659-662, 1999.
166. Anderson AM, Croft RP: Reliability of Semmes Weinstein monofilament and ballpoint sensory testing, and voluntary muscle testing in Bangladesh, *Lepr Rev* 70:305-313, 1999.
167. Bell-Krotoski J, Tomancik E: The repeatability of testing with Semmes-Weinstein monofilaments. *J Hand Surg* 12A:155-161, 1987.
168. van Brakel WH, Khawas IB, Gurung KS, et al: Intra- and inter-tester reliability of sensibility testing in leprosy, *Int J Lepr Other Mycobact Dis* 64:287-298, 1996.
169. Sackett DL: Evidence-Based Medicine: How to Practice and Teach EBM, Edinburgh, 2000, Churchill Livingstone.
170. Helm PA, Walker SC, Pullium GF: Recurrence of neuropathic ulceration following healing in a total contact cast, *Arch Phys Med Rehabil* 72:967-970, 1991.
171. Meichenbaum D, Turk DC: *Facilitating Treatment Adherence: A Practitioner's Guidebook*, New York, 1987, Plenum Press.
172. Jensen GM, Lorish C, Shepard K: Understanding patient receptivity to change: teaching for treatment adherence. In Shepard K, Jensen GM (eds): *Handbook of Teaching for Physical Therapists*, Boston, 1997, Butterworth-Heinemann.
173. Chen CY, Neufeld PS, Feely CA, et al: Factors influencing compliance with home exercise programs among patients with upper-extremity impairment, *Am J Occup Ther* 53:171-180, 1999.
174. Sluijs EM, Kok GJ, van der ZJ: Correlates of exercise compliance in physical therapy, *Phys Ther* 73:771-782, 1993.
175. Jensen GM, Lorish CD: Promoting patient cooperation with exercise programs: Linking research, theory, and practice, *Arthritis Care Res* 7:181-189, 1994.
176. Valk GD, Kriegsman DM, Assendelft WJ: Patient education for preventing diabetic foot ulceration. A systematic review, *Endocrinol Metab Clin North Am* 31:633-658, 2002.
177. Lindeman E, Leffers P, Spaans F, et al: Strength training in patients with myotonic dystrophy and hereditary motor and sensory neuropathy: A randomized clinical trial, *Arch Phys Med Rehabil* 76:612-620, 1995.
178. Richardson JK, Sandman D, Vela S: A focused exercise regimen improves clinical measures of balance in patients with peripheral neuropathy, *Arch Phys Med Rehabil* 82:205-209, 2001.
179. Ruhland JL, Shields RK: The effects of a home exercise program on impairment and health-related quality of life in persons with chronic peripheral neuropathies, *Phys Ther* 77:1026-1039, 1997.
180. Dijs HM, Roofthooft JM, Driessens MF, et al: Effect of physical therapy on limited joint mobility in the diabetic foot. A pilot study, *J Am Podiatr Med Assoc* 90:126-132, 2000.
181. Aitkens SG, McCrory MA, Kilmer DD, et al: Moderate resistance exercise program: its effect in slowly progressive neuromuscular disease, *Arch Phys Med Rehabil* 74:711-715, 1993.
182. Kilmer DD, McCrory MA, Wright NC: The effect of a high resistance exercise program in slowly progressive neuromuscular disease, *Arch Phys Med Rehabil* 75:560-563, 1994.
183. Okajima Y, Maloney FP: Overwork weakness in rats with acrylamide neuropathy, *Am J Phys Med Rehabil* 68:66-69, 1989.
184. Tam SL, Archibald V, Jassar B, et al: Increased neuromuscular activity reduces sprouting in partially denervated muscles, *J Neurosci* 21:654-667, 2001.
185. Chan KM, Amirjani N, Sumrain M, et al: Randomized controlled trial of strength training in post-polio patients, *Muscle Nerve* 27:332-338, 2003.
186. Forrest G, Qian X: Exercise in neuromuscular disease, *NeuroRehabilitation* 13:135-139, 1999.
187. Clarkson PM, Nosaka K, Braun B: Muscle function after exercise-induced muscle damage and rapid adaptation, *Med Sci Sports Exerc* 24:512-520, 1992.
188. Newham DJ, McPhail G, Mills KR, et al: Ultrastructural changes after concentric and eccentric contractions of human muscle, *J Neurol Sci* 61:109-122, 1983.
189. Newham DJ, Mills KR, Quigley BM, et al: Pain and fatigue after concentric and eccentric muscle contractions, *Clin Sci (Lond)* 64:55-62, 1983.
190. McCully KK, Faulkner JA: Injury to skeletal muscle fibers of mice following lengthening contractions, *J Appl Physiol* 59:119-126, 1985.
191. Bassile C: Guillain-Barré syndrome and exercise guidelines, Neurol Rep 20:31-36, 1996.
192. Borg GA: Psychophysical bases of perceived exertion, *Med Sci Sports Exerc* 14:377-381, 1982.
193. Kilmer DD: Response to resistive strengthening exercise training in humans with neuromuscular disease, *Am J Phys Med Rehabil* 81:S121-S126, 2002.
194. Fowler WM Jr: Role of physical activity and exercise training in neuromuscular diseases, *Am J Phys Med Rehabil* 81:S187-S195, 2002.
195. Stillwell K, Thorsteinsson G: Rehabilitation procedures. In Dyck PJ (ed): *Peripheral Neuropathy*, Philadelphia, 1993, WB Saunders.
196. Bélanger A: *Evidence-Based Guide to Therapeutic Physical Agents*, Philadelphia, 2002, Lippincott Williams & Wilkins.
197. Kochman AB, Carnegie DH, Burke TJ: Symptomatic reversal of peripheral neuropathy in patients with diabetes, *J Am Podiatr Med Assoc* 92:125-130, 2002.
198. Leonard DR, Farooqi MH, Myers S: Restoration of sensation, reduced pain, and improved balance in subjects with diabetic peripheral neuropathy: A double-blind, randomized, placebo-controlled study with monochromatic near-infrared treatment, *Diabetes Care* 27:168-172, 2004.
199. Kochman A: Monochromatic infrared photo energy and physical therapy for peripheral neuropathy: Influence on sensation, balance, and falls, *J Geriat Phys Ther* 27:18-21, 2004.
200. Zinman LH, Ngo M, Ng ET, et al: Low-intensity laser therapy for painful symptoms of diabetic sensorimotor polyneuropathy: a controlled trial, *Diabetes Care* 27:921-924, 2004.
201. Basford JR: Low-energy laser therapy: Controversies and new research. *Lasers Surg Med* 9:1-5, 1989.
202. Kalinina OV, Alekseeva NV, Burtsev EM: Infrared laser therapy in distal diabetic polyneuropathy, *Zh Nevrol Psikhiatr Im S S Korsakova* 98:23-25, 1998.
203. Valencic V, Vodovnik L, Stefancic M, et al: Improved motor response due to chronic electrical stimulation of denervated tibialis anterior muscle in humans, *Muscle Nerve* 9:612-617, 1986.
204. Carraro U, Catani C, Saggin L, et al: Isomyosin changes after functional electrostimulation of denervated sheep muscle, *Muscle Nerve* 11:1016-1028, 1988.
205. Yanai A, Harii K, Okabe K: Preventing denervation atrophy of a grafted muscle, *J Reconstr Microsurg* 7:85-92, 1991.
206. Girlanda P, Dattola R, Vita G, et al: Effect of electrotherapy on denervated muscles in rabbits: An electrophysiological and morphological study, *Exp Neurol* 77:483-491, 1982.
207. Nix WA, Dahm M: The effect of isometric short-term electrical stimulation on denervated muscle, *Muscle Nerve* 10:136-143, 1987.
208. Nix WA: Effects of intermittent high frequency electrical stimulation on denervated EDL muscle of rabbit, *Muscle Nerve* 13:580-585, 1990.
209. Herbison GJ, Jaweed MM, Ditunno JF Jr: Exercise therapies in peripheral neuropathies *Arch Phys Med Rehabil* 64:201-205, 1983.
210. Brown MC, Holland RL: A central role for denervated tissues in causing nerve sprouting, *Nature* 282:724-726, 1979.
211. Schimrigk K, McLaughlin J, Gruninger W: The effect of electrical stimulation on the experimentally denervated rat muscle, *Scand J Rehabil Med* 9:55-60, 1977.
212. Eberstein A, Eberstein S: Electrical stimulation of denervated muscle: is it worthwhile? *Med Sci Sports Exerc* 28:1463-1469, 1996.
213. Backonja MM: Defining neuropathic pain, *Anesth Analg* 97:785-790, 2003.
214. Dworkin RH, Backonja M, Rowbotham MC, et al: Advances in neuropathic pain: Diagnosis, mechanisms, and treatment recommendations, *Arch Neurol* 60:1524-1534, 2003.
215. Melzack R, Wall PD: Pain mechanisms: A new theory, *Science* 150:971-979, 1965.
216. Shealy CN, Mortimer JT, Reswick JB: Electrical inhibition of pain by stimulation of the dorsal columns: Preliminary clinical report, *Anesth Analg* 46:489-491, 1967.
217. Shealy CN: Six years' electrical stimulation for control of pain, *Adv Neurol* 4:775-782, 1974.
218. Thorsteinsson G, Stonnington HH, Stillwell GK, et al: Transcutaneous electrical stimulation: a double-blind trial of its efficacy for pain, *Arch Phys Med Rehabil* 58:8-13, 1977.
219. Tesfaye S, Watt J, Benbow SJ, et al: Electrical spinal-cord stimulation for painful diabetic peripheral neuropathy, *Lancet* 348:1698-1701, 1996.
220. Kumar D, Marshall HJ: Diabetic peripheral neuropathy: amelioration of pain with transcutaneous electrostimulation, *Diabetes Care* 20:1702-1705, 1997.
221. Armstrong DG, Lavery LA, Fleischli JG, et al: Is electrical stimulation effective in reducing neuropathic pain in patients with diabetes? *J Foot Ankle Surg* 36:260-263, 1997.
222. Hamza MA, White PF, Craig WF, et al: Percutaneous electrical nerve stimulation: A novel analgesic therapy for diabetic neuropathic pain, *Diabetes Care* 23:365-370, 2000.
223. Oyibo SO, Breislin K, Boulton AJ: Electrical stimulation therapy through stocking electrodes for painful diabetic neuropathy: A double blind, controlled crossover study, *Diabet Med* 21:940-944, 2004.
224. Wittink H, Allan J, Hoskins Michel T, et al: Management of selected syndromes. In Wittink H, Hoskins Michel T (eds): *Chronic Pain Management for Physical Therapists*, Boston, 1997, Butterworth-Heinemann.
225. Marchand S, Charest J, Li J, et al: Is TENS purely a placebo effect? A controlled study on chronic low back pain, *Pain* 54:99-106, 1993.

226. Kott K: Orthoses for patients with neurological disorders. In Seymour R (ed): *Prosthetics and Orthotics Lower Limb and Spinal,* Philadelphia, 2002, Lippincott Williams & Wilkins.

227. Helm PA, Walker SC, Pullium G: Total contact casting in diabetic patients with neuropathic foot ulcerations, *Arch Phys Med Rehabil* 65:691-693, 1984.

228. Harrelson JM: Management of the diabetic foot, *Orthop Clin North Am* 20:605-619, 1989.

229. Rajbhandari SM, Jenkins RC, Davies C, et al: Charcot neuroarthropathy in diabetes mellitus, *Diabetologia* 45:1085-1096, 2002.

Chapter 20

Nonprogressive Spinal Cord Disorders

Lynda L. Spangler

CHAPTER OUTLINE

OBJECTIVES

After reading this chapter, the reader will be able to:
1. Describe the most common types of spinal cord injuries and their primary sequelae.
2. Choose and perform appropriate tests and measures for an individual with spinal cord injuries based on information gathered from the history and systems review.
3. Propose a diagnosis and prognosis for functional recovery of an individual with spinal cord injuries based on evaluation of examination results.
4. Develop a plan of care for the physical therapy management of an individual with spinal cord injuries.
5. Execute the plan of care, including chosen interventions, and periodic reevaluation and modification of the plan as indicated, with moderate guidance.
6. Recognize the impact of spinal cord injuries on physical, emotional, social, and psychological health.
7. Participate in the decision-making process for equipment recommendation and home program establishment for an individual with spinal cord injuries.

Injuries and illnesses that affect the spinal cord are devastating for the individual involved and for those who surround them. A fleeting moment can mark the difference between being independently mobile and being dependent on personal determination, mechanical equipment, and other people for all daily activities. The occurrence of *spinal cord injury* (SCI) is statistically low compared to many other diagnoses, but the personal and financial expense is high.

There are approximately 247,000 people in the United States (US) today living with SCI, and approximately 11,000 people in the US, equivalent to 40 per million, are newly diagnosed with SCI each year.[1,2] This group includes people of all age groups and ethnicities. Trauma is the most common cause of SCI, although most of the information applies similarly to SCIs of nontraumatic origin.

Data concerning the traumatic spinal cord–injured population in the US is gathered by the National Spinal Cord Injury Database (NSCID) and processed at the Nation Spinal Cord Injury Statistical Center (NSCISC). The following data is based on figures from current and past reports of the NSCID and NSCISC.[1,2]

Motor vehicle accidents (MVAs) account for the largest percentage of SCIs (about half). Other causes of SCI include falls, violent acts (stab and gun shot wounds), and sports injuries. The proportion of injuries represented by each of these groups is shown in Fig. 20-1. Although the incidence of SCI because of these primary causes has remained fairly constant over the last 30 years, there are some noteworthy changes in overall distribution. The proportion of injuries as a result of sports has decreased, presumably because of better training techniques and emergency care and improvements in protective equipment. With the aging of the US population in general, the percentage of SCI attributed to falls has increased. Below the age of 45, the leading cause of SCI is MVAs, but after age 45, falls become the leading mechanism of injury. Acts of violence have declined from a peak of 21% in 1990-1992 but remain disproportionately higher among African-Americans and Hispanics compared to other racial groups.

PATHOLOGY

The neurological deficits associated with SCI occur when sufficient force is exerted on the spinal cord to cause nerve damage. The forces may be direct, as when an object like a bullet or a bone fragment directly enters the spinal canal and severs some or all of the nerves of the spinal cord. More often forces are indirect, with the spinal cord remaining physically contiguous, but the neural components being adversely affected by secondary damage that impacts the site of injury and the surrounding tissues.

The mechanism of injury dictates the initial type of mechanical damage to the spine, the spinal cord, and surrounding structures. Flexion (or hyperflexion) injuries (Fig. 20-2, *A*) occur when forces cause anterior movement of one segment of the spine on another (e.g., forward contact of a lower part of the body with an immovable object, causing extreme flexion in higher segments) and can result in posterior ligament disruption, posterior intervertebral disk herniation or tear, and vertebral body fracture and/or dislocation.[3-5] Extension (or hyperextension) injuries (Fig. 20-2, *D*) occur when forces are directed toward the posterior surface of the body (e.g., backward contact of the lower part of the body with an immovable object) and may result in tearing of the anterior longitudinal ligament, tear or anterior herniation of the intervertebral disk, and fractures of the posterior spine elements with compression and/or subluxation. Flexion

and extension injuries are most likely to occur where the spine is the most flexible and has the greatest bending moment. In the cervical spine the greatest flexion moment occurs at C5-6 and the greatest extension moment occurs at C4-5, making these the segments most vulnerable to flexion and extension injuries, respectively.[5]

Axial loading (vertebral compression) with sufficient vertical force, from the cranial or caudal end or both, can cause one or more vertebral bodies to burst.[4,6] A burst fracture produces bone fragments that scatter and cause damage to surrounding tissues, often including the spinal cord (Fig. 20-2, *C*). Rotational injury occurs when one segment of the body is forcefully twisted longitudinally on another segment that is either stable or moving in the opposite direction.[3] The opposing movements create a rotational force that can have a variety of results, including stretching and tearing of neural tissue, ligament tears, and vertebral fractures (Fig. 20-2, *D*).

The primary damage to the spinal cord is classified as a concussion if there is injury as a result of violent movement or a blunt blow that results in temporary loss of function.[4] In contrast, a contusion is when the surface of the spinal cord and its coverings remain intact, but there is loss of neural tissue (grey and/or white matter) in the central portion of the cord. The injury is considered a laceration or maceration if the glia is disrupted and there is possible direct disruption of the spinal cord tissue.

Secondary damage to the spinal cord is damage that occurs after the primary structural damage and that extends beyond the area of initial trauma.[6,7] Secondary damage occurs at the site of the primary lesion and over time may spread as far as four spinal segments above and/or below the initial lesion.[4,5,7] Initially, there is necrotic destruction of axons where they were damaged by the trauma. This is followed by a progression of tissue injury that is only partially understood but is most likely related in part to vascular and immune system responses.

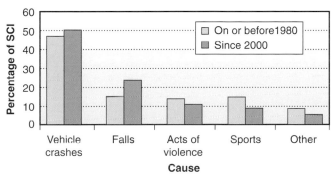

ETIOLOGY OF SPINAL CORD INJURY

FIG. 20-1 Causes of spinal cord injury *(SCI). Data from the National Spinal Cord Injury Database.*

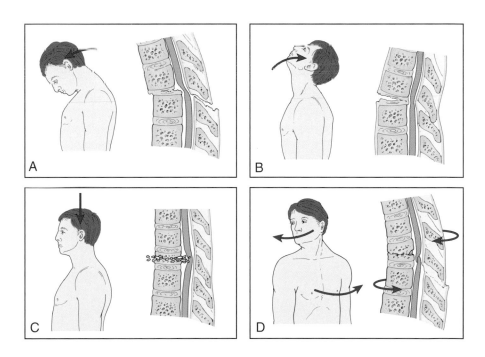

FIG. 20-2 Mechanisms of SCI. **A,** Flexion; **B,** extension; **C,** axial loading; **D,** rotation.

Changes in blood flow because of ischemia and/or hemorrhage contribute to local nerve cell destruction. At the site of injury, intraparenchymal hemorrhage contributes to early tissue damage because of sheer stress on vessels located centrally in the grey matter and in a margin of the surrounding white matter.[7] The vessels in the periphery of the spinal cord are relatively spared from this early damage, owing to the greater compliance (and thus reduced sheering force) of the white matter. The microvascular damage to the grey matter results in diminished blood flow to the spinal cord and impairment of autoregulation. Ischemic damage in this region can also occur as a result of vasogenic edema (secondary to breakdown of the blood-spinal cord barrier), by direct compression by surrounding tissues, or as the result of local vasospasm.

It appears that immune cells trigger posttraumatic inflammatory responses that contribute to the acute and chronic secondary pathogenesis of SCI.[4,7-10] Hemorrhage and disruption of the blood-spinal cord barrier allows inflammatory cells to infiltrate the injured area of the spinal cord, beginning at the first hour after injury and continuing over a period of weeks. These cells are associated with neuronal death and demyelination and other changes in the white matter, including Wallerian degeneration. Further detrimental effects can also be attributed to changes in ion levels and free radical production in the spinal cord.

Some aspects of the immune response may promote recovery from SCI.[4,7] Beneficial immune responses may include scavenging of cellular debris and release of nerve growth factors. These and other actions can have a neuroprotective function and may enhance neural regeneration.

Despite the predominance of destructive forces, some nerve tissue in the spinal cord may be spared, particularly in the peripheral regions. The amount of the nerve preservation, combined with appropriate early medical intervention to minimize primary and secondary damage, will dictate the degree of motor and sensory function preserved at and below the level of injury.

Since traumatic physical impact is the primary cause of SCI, it is not surprising that many other injuries can be associated with SCI. For all persons enrolled in the NSCID between 1985 and 1995, 29% had fractures and 29% had loss of consciousness. Traumatic pneumothorax or hemothorax occurred in 18% of cases. Traumatic brain injury severe enough to impair cognitive or emotional functioning was also reported in 11.5% of the SCI population.

Although trauma is the cause of most SCIs, there are other pathologies that can cause spinal cord damage. Nontraumatic causes include any injury or disease process that results in damage to the neural components of the spinal cord, such as transverse myelitis and multiple sclerosis.[11] The cord may also be damaged by compressive forces from tumors, spinal degeneration, or intervertebral disk distension. Vascular events can also cause ischemia or hemorrhage in the spinal cord or spinal column. Congenital malformation of the spine or spinal canal, such as spina bifida (see Chapter 15) or severe scoliosis (see Chapter 4), may also result in spinal cord damage.

Spinal cord injury is described according to the pattern and degree of preserved motor and sensory function after injury. The International Standards for Neurological Classification of Spinal Cord Injury is a set of descriptors that attempts to standardize discussion and classification of SCI internationally.[12] According to this system, the *skeletal level* refers to the spinal level at which the greatest vertebral damage is found. The *neurological level* of injury is defined as the most caudal segment of the spinal cord with normal sensory and motor function on both sides of the body. If the segment at which normal function occurs differs greatly between sides of the body or between sensory and motor function, then this classification can be subdivided to better describe the function. The neurological level might thus be described as R-sensory, L-sensory or R-motor, L-motor, with accompanying spinal levels noted for each. When the term *sensory level* is used, it refers to the most caudal segment of the spinal cord with normal sensory function on both sides of the body, and the *motor level* is similarly defined for motor function. The motor level is sometimes divided into upper extremity motor scores (UEMS) and lower extremity motor scores (LEMS), with similar processes also used to divide upper and lower extremity sensory function.

An incomplete SCI is one with partial preservation of sensory and/or motor function below the neurological level that also includes some function of the lowest sacral segment. A complete injury is defined as one that causes absence of all sensory and motor function below the neurological level, including the lowest sacral segment. *Zone of partial preservation* (ZPP) is a term associated with complete injuries and refers to those dermatomes and myotomes caudal to the neurological level where some modalities of function remain. It is important to note that although these definitions are recognized for research and documented classification, in the clinical setting an individual with any sparing of function below the neurological level of injury is frequently considered to have an incomplete SCI, whereas an individual without detectable sparing is often considered to have a complete SCI, regardless of sacral segment function.

A SCI is termed *tetraplegia* (or *quadriplegia*) if the impairment or loss of motor and/or sensory function is a result of damage of the neural elements in the cervical segments of the spinal cord. Tetraplegia results in impairments involving the UEs, as well as more caudal functions. *Paraplegia* is loss of function in the thoracic, lumbar, or sacral segments, resulting in sparing of UE function but possible impairments in the trunk, pelvis, and LEs (depending on the level of the lesion).

An injury to the spinal cord above the cauda equina (approximately the L1-2 intervertebral space in adults) will preserve the sacral reflex arc, but damage upper motor neurons (UMNs) and lower motor neurons (LMNs).[5,13] This type of injury is characterized by motor weakness or paralysis, hypertonia, cocontraction, and hyperreflexia below the level of the lesion. SCI to regions caudal to the beginning of the cauda equina will damage only LMNs, resulting in destruction of the sacral reflex arc and loss of reflexes, muscle atrophy, flaccid paralysis, and fibrillations below the injury level.

SPINAL SHOCK

A major contributing factor to complications during the acute phase of SCI is a phenomenon called *spinal shock* (also known as areflexia). Spinal shock is characterized by a total loss of sensory, motor, and autonomic control below the level of the lesion. It occurs immediately at the time of injury and can last for days to weeks after the injury.[4,5] During this period, there is flaccid paralysis of all musculature below the level of the lesion, including the smooth muscles of the visceral systems.

Where upper motor neurons are affected, resolution of spinal shock is signified by the return of deep tendon reflexes and the onset of *spasticity* in skeletal and visceral muscles. Where only lower motor neurons are affected, skeletal muscle and visceral muscles remain flaccid after the resolution of spinal shock.

Because of spinal shock, many individuals with SCI have low tone and good flexibility below their injury level early on, during the acute management phase, but may develop potentially limiting hypertonicity, spasticity, and contractures as their rehabilitation progresses and the spinal shock resolves (see later discussion of spasticity).

AUTONOMIC DYSREFLEXIA

Autonomic dysreflexia (AD; also known as autonomic hyperreflexia) is a serious, life-threatening emergency caused by uncontrolled episodes of hypertension that can occur in individuals with SCI at or above the T6 level. AD occurs after the period of spinal shock, as reflexes and autonomic responses return. A survey of the model SCI systems (1996-1998) found that 7.9% of patients experienced AD during rehabilitation.[14] In patients with complete tetraplegia, the incidence was as high as 29%. Because of the frequency and the danger of AD, it is extremely important for therapists dealing with individuals with SCI to be able to recognize the symptoms of AD and to respond appropriately when AD occurs.

AD is the result of an uncontrolled autonomic response to a noxious stimulus from either an external or internal (visceral) source. The most common causes for AD are bladder or bowel distention, although there are other causes, such as a blocked catheter, bowel impaction, or urinary tract infection.[4,15] A noxious stimulus normally causes a sympathetic response that results in vasoconstriction and an increase in blood pressure (BP). In an individual without SCI, the body compensates for this phenomenon with inhibitory impulses that cause vasodilation and a normalization of BP. Spinal cord injury prevents activation of the body's normal compensation mechanism below the level of injury, and results in steadily escalating blood pressure. If not treated immediately, the rising BP may cause damage to the brain, kidneys, eyes or heart due to subarachnoid hemorrhage, seizure, renal or retinal hemorrhage, or myocardial infarction respectively.[16,17]

Symptoms of AD reflect the pathological sympathetic response and high BP (elevation of systolic BP by 20-40 mm or more above the patient's baseline): Initial flushing of the skin above the injury level and sweating followed by the fairly rapid onset of a severe, pounding headache; possible blurred vision; and worsened sweating with chills or goose bumps (in the absence of fever).[16,17] There may be a period of cardiac arrhythmias and bradycardia as the body attempts to compensate for the elevated BP. The individual may also experience an unexplained feeling of apprehension or anxiety. All members of the treatment team (especially the individual with SCI and their family) must be taught to recognize these symptoms and to respond to AD as a medical emergency.

Interventions by therapists and other medical personnel should include an immediate check for obvious sources of noxious stimuli (kinked urinary catheter, distended bladder, tight or twisted clothing, positioning resulting in abdominal compression, etc) and removal of the stimulus if possible.[17] If the person is prone or supine, they should be brought into a sitting position to reduce intracranial pressure. BP and heart rate should be monitored immediately and frequently. Caregivers should also notify the individual's nurse and/or physician and prepare to activate the emergency medical system if removing the most obvious stimuli does not result in immediate resolution of signs and symptoms. It may be necessary to administer BP-reducing medications until the noxious stimulus can be identified and resolved. After an episode of AD, symptoms and BP should be monitored for at least 2 hours to check for and prevent recurrence.

PRESSURE ULCERS

Pressure ulcers (also known as decubitus ulcers or pressure sores) are one of the most frequent problems after SCI and are a major cause of hospital readmission. Pressure ulcers are characterized by ischemic ulceration of soft tissue as a result of unrelieved pressure and shearing forces. (See Chapter 28 for more information on pressure ulcer etiology, examination, evaluation and interventions.)

Sixty percent to 80% of individuals with SCI will develop a pressure ulcer at some time during their lifetime, and 30% will have more than one ulcer.[18,19] Many individuals (approximately 30%) will develop their first pressure ulcer during their initial hospital stay after injury, and the trend continues over a lifetime, with surveys of SCI populations showing that in a given postinjury year, approximately 20% or more individuals have a pressure ulcer.[20] In the US alone, the Centers for Disease Control and Prevention (CDC) estimates the annual cost of treating SCI-related pressure ulcers at 1.2 billion dollars.[21] These direct medical costs are compounded by the economic, vocational, social, and psychological costs to the individual who requires an extended period of wound care.

Risk factors for pressure ulcer development include sensory loss, prolonged pressure, immobility, shearing forces, skin maceration, and inadequate nutrition. These factors may be compounded by substance abuse, obesity, smoking, poor hygiene, psychosocial stressors, and noncompliance with preventive behaviors (e.g., proper bed positioning).[5,20,21] Although any area of bony prominence is at risk for ulcer development, during acute care, the sacrum, heels, and scapulae are particularly susceptible because of prolonged supine positioning. As an individual

TABLE 20-1	Pressure Ulcer Prevention
Prevention Technique	**Suggested Strategies**
Proper positioning in bed and in wheelchair	1. Good postures and positions with bony prominences protected and pressure distributed equally over large surface areas. 2. Use of pressure distribution equipment such as wheelchair cushions, custom mattresses, and alternating pressure mattress pads.
Frequent changes in position	1. Every 2 hours when in bed. 2. Every 15-20 minutes when seated.
Keep skin clean and dry	1. Good bowel and bladder care with immediate cleansing after episodes of incontinence. 2. Thorough cleansing and drying of skin at least once daily. 3. Inspect skin for areas of redness in AM and PM. 4. Use of recommended commercial skin care products.
Nutrition	1. Diet with adequate calories, protein, vitamins, and minerals. 2. Sufficient water intake. 3. Limit alcohol.
Clothing	1. Avoid clothes that are either too tight or too loose fitting. 2. Avoid clothes with thick seams, buttons, or zippers in areas of pressure.
Activity	1. Regular cardiovascular exercise. 2. Gradual build-up of skin tolerance for new activities, equipment, and positions. 3. Avoid movements that rub, drag, or scratch the skin.

begins to spend more time out of bed in a wheelchair, the ischia become at greater risk.

Prevention of pressure ulcers involves multiple members of the health care team. Table 20-1 includes some of the steps that should be taken to reduce pressure ulcer risk. If a pressure ulcer develops, immediate intervention includes getting and keeping the area clean and avoiding as much as possible any position that puts pressure on the affected area.[19] Additional physical therapy wound care interventions may be utilized during the recovery process. Physical therapy may also play a role in helping to modify mobility and positioning to help protect the skin during a period of wound healing.

EXAMINATION

PATIENT HISTORY

Patient history obtained from the medical record and the patient interview is used to help guide the testing and measurement portion of the examination.[22] For the SCI population, records should be reviewed for background information, including but not limited to patient demographics (age, sex, etc), previous medical conditions and interventions, developmental history, and family history.

Specifics related to the current injury should include medical conditions directly and indirectly related to the SCI, medications, and clinical laboratory and other diagnostic tests. It is essential to review the medical and surgical history related to the SCI (mechanism of injury, fractures, stabilization surgeries, etc.) because this will indicate likely primary and secondary impairments requiring further examination, and will also warn of precautions that may need to be observed.

The patient and family interview gathers information that allows the therapist to develop an idea of the patient's lifestyle before the SCI. Information obtained during the interview should include living environment, prior functional level, educational level, school and/or employment situation, social habits, previous health habits, recreational/hobby interests, general personality characteristics, and life goals.[22] This information will guide evaluation, interventions, and discharge planning. Patients should also be assessed for understanding of their current condition and the associated medical prognoses. The final piece of the patient interview is discussion of the patient's goals and expected outcomes for their rehabilitation and the role that they expect therapy to play in their recovery.[11] The therapist should be clear about what the patient can expect from therapy, what therapy expects from the patient, and how the interdisciplinary rehabilitation team functions.

SYSTEMS REVIEW

The systems review is used to target areas requiring further examination and to define areas that may cause complications or indicate a need for precautions during the examination and intervention processes. See Chapter 1 for details of the systems review.

Physical therapists (PTs) can make better clinical decisions regarding patient care if they understand the global influence of SCI on multiple body functions. During the systems review, it is important to recognize how changes in system functions may affect the individual's participation in the rehabilitation process. The following describes the impact the SCI can have on multiple body systems.

Gastrointestinal System. At the time of SCI, gastrointestinal (GI) complications are less common and less severe than many other deficits, but those that occur can be dangerous and deserve careful consideration. Ileus (profoundly decreased bowel motility) can occur during the period of spinal shock, with loss of bowel sounds for 24-72 hours after injury.[4,5] GI hemorrhage occurs in 3% to 5% of patients with SCI. The use of corticosteroids to reduce acute inflammation and resulting secondary injury at the site of SCI may increase the risk of GI bleeding. Prophylactic medications are often used to reduce the incidence of GI bleeds.[5] Chronic GI complications associated with SCI include an elevated incidence of gallstone disease, esophageal disease, abdominal pain, abdominal distention, autonomic dysreflexia associated with the GI tract, gastric dilation (with or without the presence of ileus), and superior mesenteric artery syndrome.

SCI can also disrupt the normal motility and evacuation of the colon. Patients with alterations in bowel function secondary to SCI are described as having a neurogenic bowel.[23,24] The effect of SCI on colon and anorectal function depends on the level of the injury. There are two general patterns of dysfunction. Complete SCI above the sacral spinal cord segments results in an UMN or reflexic bowel where the external anal sphincter cannot voluntarily relax. With this condition, intact nerve connections in the colon wall (from higher spinal regions) do allow for reflex coordination of stool propulsion. This combination of intact propulsion without sphincter relaxation results in stool retention and can contribute to some of the other GI conditions described. Complete SCI at the sacral segments (or the cauda equina) results in a LMN or areflexive bowel. With this condition, peristalsis is reduced and the denervated sphincter has low tone. This combination results in poor stool movement and an increased risk for fecal incontinence secondary to the hypotonic sphincter.

The primary intervention used to control neurogenic bowel dysfunction is a regular bowel program that is initiated during acute hospitalization.[24] The program always includes diet and fluid management and regularly scheduled bowel elimination. Elimination may be assisted or controlled with chemical or mechanical stimulation, positioning, medications, or elimination devices. The goal of the bowel program is to prevent impaction or unplanned bowel movements. The bowel program must be continued throughout the individual's life or until neurological recovery improves volitional bowel function.[5]

Bladder Management. Establishing a consistent and effective method of emptying the bladder is one of the first routines that needs to be developed after SCI. Failure to regularly and completely drain the bladder can result in urinary tract infection (the most common complication among SCI survivors), kidney dysfunction, renal calculi, and other genitourinary problems.

The pathology associated with bladder function follows similar patterns to the bowel function as noted. SCI lesions above the conus medullaris (UMN injuries) will result in a reflexive neurogenic bladder, with possible spasticity, voiding difficulties, detrusor muscle hypertrophy, and urethral reflux.[1,5] Lesions below the conus medullaris (LMN injuries) result in a nonreflexive bladder characterized by flaccidity with decreased sphincter muscle tone and an inability to empty spontaneously.

Examination of bladder function after SCI includes multiple tests, generally ordered or performed by a urologist, to determine the pattern and extent of bladder control problems. These tests include ultrasound renal scans, urinalysis, intravenous pyelograms (IVPs), urodynamic testing, and various bladder scans (e.g., cystourethrograms and cystoscopy).[4,5] After bladder function is evaluated, a bladder management program with goals of emptying the bladder effectively, minimizing the risk of infection, and preventing incontinence between voids is instituted.

The primary intervention for bladder management in the acute stages of SCI (during the period of spinal shock) is catheterization (either indwelling or intermittent).[5,11] During the rehabilitation phase of SCI, interventions for a reflexive (UMN) bladder may include timed voiding with manual stimulation (tapping on the suprapubic area, etc), timing of reflexive voids, and intermittent catheterization

at gradually increasing intervals. In some instances, a long-term indwelling catheter may be used. A nonreflexive (LMN) bladder may be managed with intermittent catheterization and/or with techniques like the Valsalva maneuver (creating an increase in intraabdominal pressure) and the Credé method (unidirectional massage over the bladder area) to assist with emptying. For both UMN and LMN lesions, medications may be used to help control bladder or sphincter tone and assist with bladder training.

Changes in Bone Density and Bone Formation. Major changes in bone metabolism that start within a few days after SCI result in steady decreases in bone mineral density (BMD). This bone loss leads to osteoporosis, with resulting increased risk of fractures. The exact mechanism of this phenomenon is unknown, but it may be related to neurological, circulatory system, and/or hormonal changes, combined with the effects of immobility following injury.[4,25,26] What is known is that there is significant (20% to 50%+) loss of BMD in multiple body areas below the level of SCI with greater losses in trabecular than cortical bone. Results of one comprehensive study confirmed that BMD in the LEs was reduced by 22% at 3 months after complete SCI and by approximately 32% at 14 months postinjury.[27] Garland et al examined the BMD of a population of patients with SCI who had suffered fractures at the knee (the most common site of fracture in chronic SCI) and found that these individuals had a BMD of only 49% of that of an analogous able-bodied control group.[28]

Research related to preventing this bone loss in patients with SCI has produced mixed results. Some studies have reported a decrease in the rate of bone loss with activities like standing, assisted gait, or electrical stimulation–induced cycling.[29,30] Other attempts to reproduce these results have not found significant changes in BMD.[25] Newer technologies allowing more effective and less invasive BMD measurement should assist with continuing efforts to find techniques to minimize bone loss after injury.[26]

Neurogenic *heterotopic ossification* (HO) is defined as abnormal bone growth within the extraarticular soft tissues. Progressive HO can result in severe restriction of muscle and joint movement. Although the exact pathophysiology of HO is not well understood, it is generally accepted that microtrauma and mechanical stress to the musculotendinous apparatus induces ossification directly by releasing osteoblast-stimulating factors or indirectly by instituting a local inflammatory response.[31,32]

HO is common in joints distal to the level of SCI and most often occurs at the hips and knees. In severe cases, HO causes restrictions severe enough to limit mobility, complicate hygiene, and predispose the individual to pressure ulcers. HO has been reported to occur in 16% to 53% of individuals with new SCI. Individuals with complete SCI, with severe spasticity, and those with existing pressure ulcers are at greater risk for developing HO. HO usually develops within the first 6 months postinjury and stabilizes within 18-24 months after onset.[11]

Interventions for HO involve prophylactic medications and gentle mobilization of muscles and joints.[11] Cautious passive range of motion (ROM) and joint mobilization exercises to prevent tissue shortening should be initiated as soon as the patient is stable and should be performed consistently during rehabilitation.[31,32] Delaying the onset of ROM activities increases the risk that tissue shortened by periods of immobility will be traumatized by later ROM activities and that aggressive ROM exercises begun at this later point may actually contribute to microtrauma and the formation of HO. In severe cases of HO, surgery may be indicated to remove the excess bone and try to regain joint movement required for functional mobility.

Respiratory Considerations. Individuals with spinal cord compromise are at risk for developing respiratory complications. Pneumonia is the leading cause of death for all persons with SCI, and pulmonary embolism is the second leading cause of death within the first year after injury.[33] Within the first year after injury, an individual with SCI is more than 80 times more likely to die of pneumonia or influenza than others in the general population. The risks remain elevated compared to the general population for the remainder of the lifespan for individuals requiring ventilator support. After completion of rehabilitation, if stable, unassisted respiration is achieved, mortality rates related to respiratory disease approach population norms. The incidence of pulmonary complications is also found to be directly correlated to age (higher with older age) and with the level and completeness of SCI (greater with higher level of injury and with complete injuries).

For individuals with tetraplegia, the work of breathing is increased because of a number of factors, including inspiratory muscle paresis or paralysis, decreased chest wall mobility, expiratory muscle paresis or paralysis, altered position of the diaphragm, postural changes, and decreased functional mobility.[34] Depending on the level of injury, there may also be complete or partial loss of primary and secondary muscles of respiration (Table 20-2).

Complete spinal cord lesions at or above C3 result in complete paralysis of the diaphragm and require immediate resuscitation and life-long mechanical ventilator support to sustain life. Mechanical ventilation may also be required on a temporary or long-term basis for individuals with acute ascending edema in a lower cervical SCI, for patients with preexisting pulmonary disease, or for patients with direct trauma to the lungs or abdomen.

TABLE 20-2	Respiratory Muscle Innervation
Muscles	**Innervation Level**
INSPIRATION	
Diaphragm	C3, C4, C5 (via phrenic nerve)
External intercostals	T1-12
Sternocleidomastoids	Cranial nerve XI (spinal accessory nerve)
Scalenes	C1, C2
Additional accessory muscles: Trapezii, pectoralis minor, serratus anterior	
EXPIRATION	
Internal intercostals	T1-12
Abdominals	T7-L1

For individuals with lower cervical or high thoracic SCI, injury may result in complete or partial paralysis of the diaphragm, intercostal, and abdominal muscles. This can decrease inspiratory and expiratory flow, tidal volume, and vital capacity. Weakness of the inspiratory muscles results in alveolar hypoventilation, hypoxemia, and hypercapnia, making the individual prone to atelectasis and pulmonary infections.[33,34] With reduced abdominal muscle function, there is loss of support for the visceral contents, which in turn reduces support of the diaphragm and causes the resting position of the diaphragm to be lower, resulting in decreased excursion and marked reduction in inspiratory capacity. This alters breathing dynamics, resulting in *paradoxical breathing*, where the abdomen rises and the chest is pulled in on inspiration and the abdomen falls and the chest expands on expiration.[5] This altered breathing pattern results in flattening of the upper chest wall, expansion of the abdominal wall, and ultimately musculoskeletal changes in the trunk.[4] Passive expiratory volume is decreased for these individuals because of the loss of elastic recoil of the low tone abdominal wall, and forced expiration is limited by loss of intercostal and abdominal muscle function. There may be a paralyzed or weak cough, with reduced ability to clear secretions and increased risk of pulmonary infections.

Within several months after injury, as strength and mobility increase, vital capacity should improve for patients with an intact diaphragm. Vital capacity may also be helped by providing support for the abdominal wall with an external devices (e.g., an abdominal binder), or by the development of mild trunk spasticity.[34] However, severe thoracic spasticity may decrease chest wall compliance and increase the work of breathing (see Chapter 26).

Cardiovascular. Three major acute cardiovascular conditions are associated with SCI. Autonomic dysreflexia and pulmonary embolism (PE) have been mentioned previously. Deep vein thrombosis (DVT) is the third complication that is of particular concern, especially during early postinjury management.

Factors contributing to DVT in the SCI population include decreased or absent muscle function, prolonged periods of decreased functional mobility, and loss of sympathetic innervation. These combine to cause vasodilation and pooling of blood in the venous system.[5,35] Failure to recognize and treat DVT can result in PE and death. Green et al reviewed the rehabilitation records of 243 patients with SCI and found that thromboembolism is more likely to develop in patients who are older, obese, and have flaccid paralysis or cancer.[36] Clinical signs of DVT may include swelling, localized warmth or redness of the affected extremity, pain in the calf with muscle stretch (if sensation is present), and fever.[3] Because clinical signs have poor sensitivity and specificity for DVT, medical screening tests may be indicated for patients with SCI.[5] Active DVT is managed with anticoagulation medications and occasionally with surgical placement of a vascular filter.[37] DVT and PE are of greatest concern during acute SCI management (within 7-10 days postinjury) and have very low incidence (less than 1% per year beyond 2 years postinjury) in chronic SCI populations.[37]

There is conflicting evidence about the effects of SCI on the risk for cardiovascular diseases such as hypercholesterolemia, hypertension, and coronary artery disease. Questions remain about how much of observed cardiovascular changes are directly related to metabolic and systemic alterations resulting from SCI and/or how much they are attributable to lifestyle and activity level changes after injury. For example, in individuals with paraplegia, total cholesterol, LDL, and triglycerides, as well as adiposity, have all been found to be higher among persons who were depressed.[38] Further research is needed to identify the relationship between SCI and cardiovascular risk factors and to develop guidelines for minimizing these risks.

Sexual Function. Questions about sexual function will likely arise for both male and female SCI patients during the rehabilitation process. Because sexuality is a sensitive issue, patients may approach the subject with any member of the treatment team with whom they feel a level of confidence and trust, including their primary PT. For this reason, it is important for therapists to have at least a basic knowledge of how SCI affects sexual function and available referral and reference information to direct questions beyond the therapist's knowledge. All patients should be encouraged to seek medical and counseling advice to deal constructively with concerns about sexuality and sexual function.

Male Sexual Function. Male sexual function after SCI is altered based on the level of injury. Sensory function is often absent or impaired after injury, resulting in absent or changed responses to tactile stimuli below the injury level. Erectile function may be altered at two levels. Psychogenic erections (erections resulting from sensory input that produce erotic emotions) are mediated at the T10-T12 spinal levels. SCI at or above this level will result in loss of psychogenic erection, whereas injury below this level or incomplete injury may result in preservation of this function. Reflex erections (erections that occur involuntarily and do not require input from the brain) occur via activation of sensory nerves at S2-S4. Most men with SCI are able to have reflex erections if there is not direct damage to these spinal segments.

While some erectile ability is often preserved, the quality and duration of the erection may or may not be sufficient for intercourse. For individuals with erectile dysfunction secondary to SCI, there are multiple intervention options for improving sexual function, including oral medications, medications injected or inserted into the penis, penile implants, and vacuum devices with tension rings. A physiatrist and a urologist familiar with SCI should discuss the advantages and risks of these options with each individual before using any erectile aids.

Even with erection sufficient for sexual activity, as many as 90% of men with SCI are not able to ejaculate during intercourse.[39] Problems with the synergy of the pathways from the brain for triggering response to sensory input, from T10-T12 for emission and S2-S4 for ejaculation, can result in disrupted ejaculatory function. Some men may also experience retrograde ejaculation, in which alterations in sphincter control of the genitourinary system results in semen being ejaculated into the bladder rather than out through the urethra. Even if ejaculation is possible, the motility rate of sperm for men with SCI is 20% compared to 70% in able-bodied men.[40]

Poor ejaculatory function combined with poor sperm motility and concentration results in very low fertility rates for men with SCI.[41,42] Because of this, a number of interventions have been developed to assist men with SCI to father children. Some of these techniques include penile vibratory stimulation, rectal probe ejaculation, and medical harvesting of semen. These techniques are combined with intrauterine insemination or in vitro fertilization to attempt pregnancy. Although these techniques greatly enhance the chances of successful pregnancy, they are very expensive and require significant time and emotional stress for both partners.

Female Sexual Function. The impact on sexual function for women with SCI is significantly less than for their male counterparts. For 60% or more of women, there is a period of amenorrhea for approximately 5 months after injury.[24] Although beyond that initial period there are no major physiological changes that alter reproductive function, other changes are worth noting.

SCI may result in a lessening or absence of vaginal lubrication secondary to the inability of sexual response input from the brain to reach the sacral region (similar to the effects on the psychogenic erection response in the male). Lubricants can help to compensate for this problem. Depending on the level and completeness of the SCI, there may be a loss of muscular control in the genital region and decreased muscle function may result in less friction during intercourse. Changes in sexual position may help to minimize this effect.[43]

Sensory loss may alter the experience of orgasm after SCI. In a study of patients in the SCI Model System, 54% of sexually active women reported experiencing orgasm.[44] Shifts in erogenous zones (often to areas above the injury level) have also been reported.

Pregnancy is possible for women with any level of spinal injury. Because of this, women with SCI need to consider the same issues related to contraception as women without SCI. If a woman with SCI chooses to become pregnant, there are several factors that put her in a higher risk pregnancy category: Pressure of the fetus, complicating bowel and bladder programs; weight gain, affecting mobility skills and increasing pressure ulcer risk; increased risk for urinary tract infections; changes in patterns of spasticity; decreased respiratory capacity from pressure of the fetus on the diaphragm; cardiovascular changes; and alterations in normal feeling of and response to contractions during labor.[45,46] AD also occurs more often during all stages of pregnancy, particularly during labor. Despite these complicating factors (most of which are to a lesser extent issues for able-bodied women during pregnancy), women with SCI can safely give birth to children with the guidance of a physiatrist and obstetrician who are familiar with the special needs of women with SCI.

TESTS AND MEASURES

The patient history and systems review should guide the clinician's selection of specific tests and measures for each individual. The purpose of this component of the examination is to allow for more detailed identification of impairments, functional limitations, and disabilities. In turn, the identified areas of limitation will be used for the formulation of functional outcome goals, intervention plans, and other aspects of the plan of care. This section summarizes the tests and measures most frequently used with the spinal cord–injured population. This list is intended as a general guide and is not a comprehensive list of every test a therapist may decide is applicable for a given patient.

Musculoskeletal

Posture. Observation of sitting posture should focus on the ability to remain upright against gravity, symmetry, scapula position, use of UEs to assist with and maintain posture, and position of lower trunk and pelvis. Lack of symmetry may indicate a difference in preservation of motor function between the right and left sides. Asymmetry may also indicate unequal weight distribution, increasing the risk of skin breakdown. Scapular position is an early indicator of muscle balance and control in the scapular region. The use of UE support and/or extremes of pelvic anterior or posterior tilt to maintain trunk control are compensations that often indicate poor active trunk control. (See Chapter 4 for detailed information on the examination of posture.)

Anthropometric Characteristics. General body composition and proportion are noted. Relationship of limb length to trunk length is important, since longer limbs will provide the advantage of a longer lever arm for closed chain UE activities but will also necessitate increased control for management of flaccid or spastic LEs. Obesity will increase the demand on extremities during mobility and may prevent achievement of the ROM at the pelvis and hips required for many mobility skills. An individual who is very thin or who has lost a large amount of weight during acute care may have more prominent bony prominences, with increased susceptibility to pressure ulcers.

Range of Motion. Complete evaluation of all motions available at all joints is important in examination of patients with SCI, because extremes of ROM often play important roles in compensating for strength deficits. Standard goniometric testing is indicated but may be complicated by medical precautions, presence of spinal stabilization devices or orthoses, or by the patient's inability to tolerate some standard testing positions. Any variation from a standard testing position or procedure should be noted.

Muscle Performance. Manual muscle testing (MMT) is performed for all muscle groups[5,22] (see Chapter 5). The American Spinal Injury Association (ASIA) and the International Medical Society of Paraplegia developed an SCI examination system known as the International Standard for Neurological Classification of Spinal Cord Injury (Fig. 20-3).[47] ASIA recommends testing the strength of a designated key muscle group on each side in each of the 10 paired myotomes, using a rostral to caudal sequence. The strength of the muscle is recorded using the traditional 0-5 MMT scale. These motor scores are added together to determine a total motor score. The physician also tests for the presence of muscle strength in the external anal sphincter and records the presence (yes) or absence (no)

of contraction on the examination form. These scores are combined with sensory scores (see neuromuscular examination section) and other information to aid in the determination of diagnosis and prognosis for the individual with SCI.

Because people with specific muscle weakness will use other muscles to accomplish a movement where possible (known as substitution), palpation is critical when muscle testing individuals with SCI.[5] Common substitutions are noted in Box 20-1. Since proximal joints and body segment stabilization is often impaired because of neurological deficits, external stabilization of proximal regions may be needed during testing to accurately assess distal strength. For example, a tetraplegic patient may not be able to provide strong resistance for biceps muscle testing unless external trunk support is provided to prevent the patient from falling forward during the test. As with ROM measurement, complications may prevent the use of standard testing positions. Use of alternative positions at the time of examination should be noted and kept consistent for subsequent reexamination.

Joint Integrity and Mobility. Joint integrity and mobility are frequently assessed during the ROM examination, using palpation and observation during active, active assistive. and passive movement. Because of the increased demand for UE weight bearing during mobility for SCI patients, the integrity of the scapulothoracic, shoulder, elbow, and wrist joints are of particular concern in this population.

Neuromuscular

Cognition. A basic cognitive screen, such as the Mini-Mental State Examination (MMSE), is often administered to determine the patient's potential for participation in rehabilitation.[48] Because the NSCID reports loss of consciousness in 28.2% of SCI patients and head injury sufficient to affect cognitive or emotional function in 11.5% of cases, it is important to recognize signs of traumatic brain injury and the possible need for further neuropsychological testing. (See Chapter 16 for further information on examination of patients with traumatic brain injury.)

Pain. The incidence of pain after SCI varies greatly, but pain can significantly impact the rehabilitation process, functional mobility, quality of life, and the psychological well being of many people with SCI. In a large study of patients with SCI attending regular health assessments, Budh et al found that 63.7% of patients reported pain, with 32.3% reporting that the pain was severe enough to have a negative impact on their quality of life.[49] A survey of patients during rehabilitation had similar results (79% and 37.9%, respectively).[50] Pain usually starts soon after the injury but may also start much later.

Quantifying and qualifying pain after SCI is complicated because methods used for studying pain in patients with SCI vary and because there is no single, widely accepted or validated method of classifying post-SCI pain.[51,52] The McMaster University Evidence-Based Practice Center conducted an extensive literature search on SCI–related neuropathic pain[52] and found 132 studies that met their search criteria; only 6 of 132 were randomized controlled trials (RCTs), and many had deficiencies in

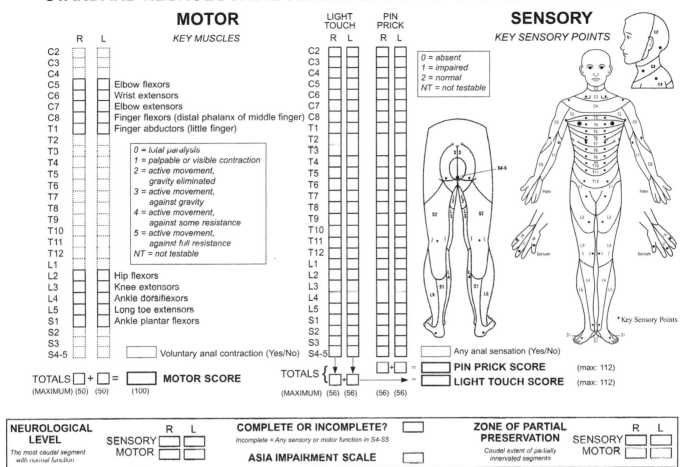

FIG. 20-3 American Spinal Injury Association (ASIA) Examination Form. *Courtesy American Spinal Injury Association, Atlanta, Ga.*

reporting that limited the assessment of their validity, relevance, precision, and therefore their clinical application. There were no studies that evaluated the role of treatment algorithms or multidisciplinary approaches to pain management. No conclusions could be drawn about effective pain management for individuals with SCI.

Pain after SCI can generally be categorized as nociceptive pain or neuropathic pain. Nociceptive pain occurs when intact peripheral nociceptors in partially or fully innervated parts of the body are activated by local irritation or damage to nonneural tissues. This category includes musculoskeletal and visceral pain. Neuropathic pain occurs as a result of direct damage to neural tissue within the peripheral and/or central nervous system. This includes pain patterns like central pain, radicular pain, and complex regional pain syndrome. Pain in SCI can be further divided by its location above, at, or below the level of injury.

The presence, intensity, and location of pain is noted at the time of examination and is periodically reexamined. Pain may be measured with a variety of standard pain

scales, indices, and questionnaires as described in Chapter 22.

Reflex Integrity. Reflexes are tested using a tap of a reflex hammer on the tendon of a relaxed muscle. Biceps, triceps, quadriceps, and triceps surae tendons are some of the most commonly tested.[13] In the acute period, spinal shock may result in areflexia. Periodic reexamination of reflex activity is therefore indicated to determine the end of the spinal shock period, as well as to aid in diagnosis.

Sensory Integrity. Testing of light touch, pain (sharp/dull), discriminative touch, temperature sensation, proprioception, and kinesthesia are performed for the entire body. For light touch, pain discrimination, temperature, and 2-point discriminative testing the appropriate stimulus is applied to a single point on the body and the patient is asked to provide a verbal response about whether they are aware of the stimulus and/or what they feel at the point of application.[53] For SCI patients, stimuli are tested according to dermatome patterns to aid in the ultimate evaluation of the neurological level of the SCI.

BOX 20-1   Common Substitutions in Manual Muscle Testing

Upper Extremities and Scapula

Upper Trapezius
- Levator scapula can substitute; it produces scapular elevation and adduction of the medial border of the scapula.

Middle Trapezius
- Rhomboids can substitute; they produce scapular adduction and medial rotation of the inferior angle of scapula.
- Levator scapula can possibly substitute; it produces scapular elevation and adduction of the medial border of the scapula.

Rhomboids
- Middle trapezius can substitute, it produces pure adduction of the medial border of the scapula.
- Patient can lift hand off buttock using the shoulder extensors (posterior deltoid, teres major, latissimus dorsi, and long head triceps).
- Patient can also lift hand off buttock by tipping the scapula anteriorly using the pectorals, especially pectoralis minor with coracobrachialis.

Serratus Anterior
- Pectoralis minor and coracobrachialis can substitute.
- Scapula should not wing off the chest/thoracic wall in the prone-on-elbows position.

Biceps
- Brachioradialis can substitute where elbow flexion occurs in the midposition of pronation and supination; but the patient will not be able to flex the elbow in full supination.

Pectoralis Major
- The patient can substitute for the adduction/internal rotation component of this muscle with the long head of biceps, coracobrachialis, and anterior deltoid, possibly latissimus dorsi.
- Remember the segmental innervation for the clavicular components of pectoralis major is C5-6, while the segmental innervation of the sternal components of pectoralis major is C7-8 to T1 (possibly a small amount of C6).

Triceps
- The patient can use the external rotators of the shoulder (supraspinatus, infraspinatus, teres minor) to place the arm in a positions where gravity will extend the elbow.
- When weight bearing on the upper extremity, the patient can use some external rotation of the shoulder coupled with gravity; however, some of the final locking of the elbow in extension is done by the pectoralis major, the long head of biceps, and the coracobrachialis.

Deltoid
- Paralysis of the middle fibers of the deltoid is compensated for by the long head of biceps, long head of triceps, clavicular pectoralis, major external rotators of the shoulder, and serratus anterior.

Shoulder External Rotators
- Patient can substitute by depressing the shoulder so that gravity can rotate the shoulder.
- Patient can substitute with the supinators of the forearm and the extensors of the wrist to help rotate wrist and arm with gravity.

Supinator
- Patient can substitute with biceps, shoulder external rotators, brachioradialis, and wrist extensors.

Shoulder Internal Rotators
- Pectoralis minor and coracobrachialis can substitute by protracting the shoulder so gravity can rotate the shoulder internally.
- Patient can also substitute with pronators, wrist flexors, and brachioradialis.

Pronators
- Patient can substitute with shoulder internal rotators and brachioradialis.

Wrist Extensors
- Patient can substitute by externally rotating the shoulder so that gravity can extend the wrist.
- Patient can substitute by supinating the forearm so that gravity can extend the wrist.
- Patient can substitute with any of the long finger extensors.

Wrist Flexors
- Patient can substitute by internally rotating the shoulder so that gravity can flex the wrist.
- Patient can substitute by pronating the forearm so that gravity can flex the wrist.

Latissimus Dorsi
- Patient can substitute with teres major, posterior deltoid, lower trapezius, and possible long head of triceps.

Long Finger Flexors
- The patient can substitute by utilizing the tenodesis effect, whereby wrist extension produces passive tension on the long finger flexors; some finger flexion, especially at the interphalangeal joints, can occur.

BOX 20-1 | **Common Substitutions in Manual Muscle Testing—cont'd**

Long Finger Extensors
- Patient can substitute by utilizing the tenodesis effect, whereby wrist flexion produces passive tension on the long finger extensors; some finger extension especially at the interphalangeal joints can occur.

Trunk
Abdominals (Upper)
- Patient can substitute with head and neck flexors, pectoralis major and minor, and serratus anterior.

Obliques
- Patient can substitute with latissimus dorsi if the upper extremities are fixed.

Quadratus Lumborum
- Patient can substitute with latissimus dorsi or obliques.

Lower Extremities
Hip Flexors
- Patient can substitute with the lower abdominals, which tilt the pelvis posteriorly and cause the lower extremity to swing forward with momentum.
- Patient can substitute with lower obliques, which rotate the pelvis anteriorly, causing the lower extremity to swing forward.
- Hip adductors can flex hip.
- Latissimus dorsi can cause some flexion and abduction of the hip as the patient unilaterally elevates the pelvis.

Hip Extensors
- Patient can substitute with the lumbar extensor muscles, which tilt the pelvis anteriorly and cause the lower extremity to swing posteriorly with momentum.
- It may seem like you palpate some hip extensors as the patient maximally contracts the hip flexors then relaxes because the lower extremity will move posteriorly on rebound or recoil.
- Patient can substitute with the longitudinal fibers of adductor magnus.
- Patient can substitute with quadratus lumborum.

Hip Abductors
- Patient can substitute for gluteus medius and minimus using either latissimus dorsi or the obliques to elevate or "hike" the pelvis.
- Patient can substitute with sartorius, which will also flex the hip.
- Patient can abduct the hip with tensor fascia lata.

Hip Adductors
- Patient can substitute with some of the hip flexors.
- Patient can substitute using lower abdominals to rotate the pelvis forward, allowing gravity to adduct the lower extremity.

Hip Internal Rotators
- Patient can substitute using lower abdominal muscles to rotate the pelvis forward so gravity internally rotates the lower extremity.

Hip Extensor Rotators
- Patient can substitute using lower back extensors to rotate the pelvis backward so gravity externally rotates the lower extremity.

Knee Flexors
- Patient can substitute for semimembranosus and semitendinosus using sartorius and gracilis.
- Patient can substitute with the rebound phenomenon from the quadriceps.

Quadriceps
- Patient can substitute in sitting position simply by leaning the truck backward, thus initiating a swinging motion of the legs upward.
- Patient can substitute in supine or side lying positions by using adductor magnus to extend the hip and knee.

Foot Inversion
- Patient can substitute by rotating the hips internally and by using the medial gastrocnemius.

Foot Eversion
- Patient can substitute by rotating the hip externally and by using the lateral gastrocnemius.

Adapted from Nixon V: *Spinal Cord Injury: A Guide to Functional Outcomes in Physical Therapy Management.*

The ASIA classification system uses examination of light touch (cotton) and pin prick (safety pin) tested at specific points in each of the 28 dermatomes on both sides of the body[47] (see Fig. 20-3). Test results are scored on a 3-point scale: 0 = absent, 1= impaired, 2 = normal (with NT = not testable). The scores are then summed across dermatomes and sides of the body to generate two sensory scores: A Pin Prick score and a Light Touch score.

Motor Function—Control and Learning. Motor control varies, depending on the type of injury and the resulting loss or preservation of motor function. Complete SCI causes total loss of voluntary movement below the level of injury but spasticity, which produces an involuntary increase in muscle tone, can still occur and may interfere, or be used to assist, with motor control and mobility skills. In incomplete injuries, there will be some overlap of voluntary control and spasticity across spinal levels making the resultant motor function more difficult to predict.

The pathological synergy patterns and spasticity frequently associated with other nonprogressive UMN central nervous system disorders, such as stroke[13,53,54] (as described in Chapter 16), differ somewhat from the abnormal movement patterns commonly seen in SCI. Spasticity in SCI is caused by changes in neural control and in the muscles themsleves.[13,55,56] Inhibitory interneuron responses to Ia afferent activity are diminished, resulting in hyperreflexia. Nonreciprocal inhibition is reduced, resulting in muscle hypertonia. Transmission from cutaneous afferents to motor neurons is facilitated, resulting in exaggerated reflex responses to normally innocuous stimuli (e.g., withdrawal reflex of the entire LE in response to light touching of the thigh). And the mechanical properties of the muscles change as a result of muscle fiber atrophy, fibrosis, and alterations in contractile properties from phasic toward tonic. This combination of changes can result in weakness, impaired coordination, changes in posture, and involuntary movements.[5,57]

The incidence of spasticity in SCI is difficult to ascertain because there is no universally agreed on way to measure spasticity in this population. Thirty-two percent of the persons in the NSCID were reported to have spasticity before discharge from rehabilitation and 42.7% reported spasticity by 1 year after their injury. For this database, spasticity was defined as "spasticity severe enough to have warranted a trial of medication or surgical treatment." A study of SCI patients admitted to the University of Michigan Model Spinal Cord Injury Care System between 1985 and 1988 showed that spasticity was present in 67% of patients when spasticity was defined as "patient showed increase deep tendon reflexes, increased muscle tone during passive movements or involuntary muscle spasms."[58] In this same study, 37% of patients with spasticity required antispasticity medications. This is fairly consistent with the previously noted NSCID statistics. Higher incidences of spasticity have been noted with tetraplegia (versus paraplegia), and with incomplete injuries at any level (especially in acute phases of recovery) as compared with complete injuries.[58]

In addition to the motor control issues previously discussed, if spasticity is severe and uncontrolled, it may contribute to muscle and joint contractures, interfere with activities of daily living (ADLs) and mobility skills, prevent proper positioning, impair hygiene, increase the risk for pressure ulcers, interfere with sleep, create pain, and cause other disruptions to quality of life.[5,11,59-62] The presence and severity of spasticity is also influenced by the individual's physiological state[60] and may be increased by physiological stressors,[5,61] such as urinary tract infection, fever, menstruation, bowel or bladder distention, mechanical shortening/contractures of muscles, changes in environmental temperature, presence of pressure ulcers, tight clothing, and emotional stress.

Several authors[11,59,60] note that mild spasticity may improve ADL function by increasing muscle tone, by helping to support circulation, or by the individual intentionally using various stimuli to trigger reflexive responses at desired times (e.g., to manipulate LEs during mobility or to empty the bladder). Although this claim is consistent with this author's experience, literature searches did not produce any published evidence to validate, quantify, or refute these statements.

Spasticity in SCI is often measured by noting how much or how often spastic movements interfere with functional activities. Frequently recorded items may include the following (1) frequency of spasticity preventing or interfering with performance of ADLs (transfers, bed mobility, stable sitting, driving), (2) frequency with which spasticity-related pain prevents or interferes with these activities, (3) whether or how often spasticity interferes with sleep, and (4) whether resistance to passive stretch is present and whether it prevents full passive ROM. Scales designed to measure muscle tone, like the Modified Ashworth Scale,[59,63] may also be utilized, but these scales generally reflect only the baseline hypertonia associated with SCI and may not be valid to describe all of the other aspects of SCI spasticity as noted previously. A search of the literature failed to reveal any evidence to determine the reliability or validity of these or other tests of muscle tone in the SCI population.

Cardiovascular/Pulmonary

Circulation. Persons with high level SCI are particularly prone to orthostatic hypotension because of decreased venous return, decreased cardiac output, and pooling of blood in dependent body parts,[5] so careful initial measurement and ongoing observation of blood pressure is required in this population. As noted previously, AD is a dangerous consequence of SCI that results in circulatory changes and requires frequent BP monitoring. (See Chapter 22 for further information on blood pressure measurement and AD.)

Ventilation and Respiration/Gas Exchange. Examination of respiratory function may include measurement of oxygen saturation, respiratory muscle strength (diaphragm, abdominals, pectorals, serratus, scalenes, sternocleidomastoid, latissimus), respiratory capacities, respiratory rate, and chest expansion.[5,15] Oxygen saturation may be measured with a pulse oximeter. Vital capacity and inspiratory and expiratory reserve volumes may be measured using a spirometer.[5,64] Kelley et al found that 92.4% of 278 individuals with SCI tested were able to produce acceptable and reproducible spirometry testing efforts with minor modifications to the American Thoracic Society testing standards.[65]

Respiratory pattern (especially the presence of paradoxical breathing), chest shape and symmetry, ability to cough, and duration of phonation (length of vocalization and syllables per breath) are noted and recorded. Auscultation may be performed to determine the types and location of breath sounds. The use of respiratory assistive devices like ventilators or positive pressure ventilatory support should also be noted, along with the settings and critical values that have been determined for the patient.[5,66]

Aerobic Capacity and Endurance. Examination of endurance and aerobic capacity in individuals with SCI must be performed by using tests that do not require the ability to ambulate (the skill most often used to judge cardiovascular fitness in able-bodied individuals). One of the most frequently used alternatives for research and training is performance on arm ergometry tests.[67-69] Heart rate, power output, and oxygen uptake ($\dot{V}O_2$) may all be measured with continuous or interval arm ergometry. For individuals without a normal heart rate response to exercise because of sympathetic system alterations, ratings of perceived exertion (e.g., the Borg Ratings of Perceived Exertion [RPE] scale[70]) may be used to determine exercise intensity[67] (see Chapter 23).

Function

Basic Mobility and Self-Care. A review of functional mobility skills is completed. The examination should include the following functions: Rolling in bed to both sides, rolling from supine to prone and returning to supine, moving supine to/from long sitting, transitioning from supine to/from sitting at edge of bed, and transferring from bed or mat to/from a wheelchair. Additional ADL and instrumental ADL (IADL) skills may be examined based on the patient's level of function.

The ability to perform mobility skills may be recorded using any of a number of functional mobility scales. Hadley performed an extensive review of the applicability, validity, and reliability of functional outcome measures for the acute SCI population.[71] The review concluded that there was insufficient evidence to support any standard for functional outcome measurement. It was recommended that the Functional Independence Measure (FIM) be utilized by clinicians working with SCI patients. The FIM is a 7-level scale that designates major gradations in behavior from dependence to independence on 18 different self-care items (transfers, eating, bowel and bladder management, social cognition, etc).[72] It has been shown to be reliable and valid with variety of rehabilitation populations.[73]

In addition to FIM, a variety of other general rehabilitation scales have been used with persons with SCI. The Modified Barthel Index (MBI) is an example. Additional scales have been created for more specific use with SCI, including the Quadriplegic Index of Function (QIF) and the Spinal Cord Independence Measure (SCIM).[71]

Locomotion and Gait. For most acute patients with SCI the primary means of locomotion is by wheelchair. Initial examination of wheelchair mobility includes observing the individual's ability to manage wheelchair parts (wheel locks, foot rests, etc) and to propel the chair on level surfaces. For higher level tetraplegic patients, the skills required for managing the control mechanism of a power wheelchair may need to be tested. The patient should be tested on his or her ability to perform an effective pressure-relief technique when seated in the wheelchair.

More extensive tests have been developed to measure additional dimensions of wheelchair propulsion such as endurance, speed, and exertion. The Wheelchair Circuit is a test that was specifically developed to assess manual wheelchair mobility in persons with SCI. The tests consists of 8 wheelchair skills (Box 20-2) and results in 3 test scores: Ability (whether an item can be performed), performance time (measured on the figure-of-eight course and a 15-m sprint), and physical strain (primarily measured by heart rate). A longitudinal study of 74 patients, comparing performance on the Wheelchair Circuit test at the beginning and completion of inpatient rehabilitation, found that this test is a valid and responsive instrument for evaluation of wheelchair mobility in subjects with a variety of SCIs. The ability and time scores on the Wheelchair Circuit test positively correlated with performance on the FIM mobility performance measures (transfers to bed/chair/wheelchair, transfer to toilet, transfer to tub, and walk/wheelchair propulsion).[74]

Standard gait assessment tools (see Chapter 32) and functional measures, such as the FIM and MBI, may be used to assist with gait examination and determination of level of independence with gait skills in individuals with SCI who can ambulate. Two scales have recently been developed to assist with the standardized description of gait in patients with SCI. The Spinal Cord Injury Functional Ambulation Inventory (SCI-FAI) is an observational gait assessment instrument with three domains: Gait parameters, assistive device use, and a walking mobility score (based on typical walking practices and timed test).[75] A study with 22 subjects reviewed both live and on videotape by 4 raters found that this test had moderate-good interrater reliability and good intrarater reliability.[75] An additional group of 19 subjects with SCI showed a 44.7% increase in score after an intensive walking training program, indicating that this test is also a valid and sensitive measure of functional gait change in this population.

The Walking Index for Spinal Cord Injury (WISCI)[76,77] is a 20-point hierarchical scale that incorporates gradations of functional limitation (based on physical assistance and assistive devices required) for walking after SCI. A 10-m walk is used to score the examination. Interrater reliability for the WISCI was found to be excellent (100%) for trained users performing observations of 40 video cases.[76] Significant positive correlations have been shown between the WISCI and other commonly used mobility scales (MBI, FIM, SCIM, and Rivermead Mobility Index).[78] There is also a strong positive correlation ($p < 0.0001$) between the WISCI and the ASIA LEMS.

EVALUATION, DIAGNOSIS, AND PROGNOSIS

The information gathered during the examination process is used to formulate a physical therapy diagnosis. Most patients with spinal cord injuries fall into the preferred practice pattern 5H: Impaired motor function, peripheral nerve integrity, and sensory integrity associated with nonprogressive disorders of the spinal cord, as described in the *Guide to Physical Therapist Practice* (the *Guide*).[22] According to the *Guide,* 80% of patients classified in this pattern can be expected to achieve optimal motor function, peripheral nerve integrity, sensory integrity, and functional mobility in the course of 9 months of physical therapy, with 4 to 150 visits. Multiple factors (e.g., cognitive status,

BOX 20-2   The Wheelchair Circuit Test

Item 1: Figure-of-8 Shape

Three markers are placed on the floor in a straight line and 1.50 m apart. The subject sits in the wheelchair with front casters behind the first marker and turned backward. At the starting signal, the subject propels the wheelchair as fast as possible in a shape of an 8 around the other 2 markers. Time is recorded from the moment the subject starts until the front casters pass the first marker again.

Ability score 0: The subject cannot perform this item within 60 seconds (sec).
Ability score 1: The subject performs this item correctly within 60 sec.
Performance time: Time needed to perform this item.

Item 2: Crossing a Doorstep

A wooden doorstep (height: 0.04 m) is placed in an otherwise level doorway. One meter in front and behind the doorstep a marker is placed on the floor. The subject sits in the wheelchair with front casters behind the first marker and turned backward. At the starting signal, the subject propels the wheelchair forward, negotiates the doorstep, and propels further forward onto the second marker. Time is recorded from the moment the subject starts until the front casters pass the second marker.

Ability score 0: The subject cannot perform this item within 120 sec.
Ability score 0.5: The subject is able to cross the doorstep with the front casters (within 120 sec) but cannot pass the doorstep with the rear wheels.
Ability score 1: The subject performs this item correctly within 120 sec.

Item 3: Mounting a Platform

A wooden platform (height: 0.1 m) is placed on the floor, one side against the wall. Two meters in front of the platform, a marker is placed on the floor. The subject sits in the wheelchair with front casters behind the first marker and turned backward. At the starting signal, the subject propels the wheelchair forward and mounts the platform. Time is recorded from the moment the subject starts until all four wheels are on the platform.

   Note: This item is only performed if the subject was able to cross the doorstep in Item 2 (Ability score: 1).
Ability score 0: The subject cannot perform this item within 120 sec.
Ability score 0.5: The subject is able to mount the platform with the front casters (within 120 sec) but cannot pass the doorstep with the rear wheels.
Ability score 1: The subject performs this item correctly within 120 sec.

Item 4: 15 m Sprint

Two markers are placed on the floor, 15 m apart. The subject sits in the wheelchair, with the front casters behind the first marker and turned backward. At the starting signal, the subject propels the wheelchair toward the second marker as fast as possible. Time is recorded from the moment he/she starts until the front casters pass the second marker.

Ability score 0: The subject cannot perform this item within 60 sec.
Ability score 1: The subject performs this item correctly within 60 sec.
Performance time: Time needed to perform this item.

Item 5: 3% Slope

This item is carried out with the subject propelling their wheelchair on a wheelchair-adjusted treadmill. At the starting signal, the velocity of the belt is set at 0.56 m/s. Ten seconds later the slope is raised 3% (which takes 12 sec), and when this inclination is reached, the subject keeps propelling the wheelchair for another 10 sec before the inclination is returned to 0% (which again takes 12 sec). The test ends when the treadmill has returned to horizontal position.

Ability score 0: The subject cannot perform this item.
Ability score 1: The subject performs this item correctly.
Strain: The maximum heart rate reached during the performance of the item.

Item 6: 6% Slope

This item is exactly the same as the 3% slope item, except for the inclination of the slope, which is increased to 6%. Both the increasing and decreasing of the slope take 23 sec.

   Note: This item is only performed if the subject was able to perform Item 5 (Ability score: 1).
Ability score 0: The subject cannot perform this item.
Ability score 1: The subject performs this item correctly for 180 sec.

Item 7: Wheelchair Propulsion

This item is carried out with the subject propelling the wheelchair on a wheelchair-adjusted treadmill. At the starting signal, the velocity of the belt is set at 0.56, 0.83, or 1.1 m/sec, depending on the subject's ability. The subject propels the wheelchair for 180 sec.

Ability score 0: The subject cannot perform this item.
Ability score 1: The subject performs this item correctly for 180 sec.

BOX 20-2   **The Wheelchair Circuit Test—cont'd**

Item 8: Transfer

A line is placed on the floor 1 m from a treatment table and parallel to it. The table is set at the same height as the top of the seat cushion in the wheelchair. The subject sits in the wheelchair with the front casters behind the line and turned backward. At the starting signal, the subject performs a transfer from the wheelchair to the table. First the subject drives up to the table and puts the wheelchair in position, then makes a transfer, with his or her legs hanging over the edge of the table, and finally places his or her legs on the table, while remaining seated. The subject is allowed to use the assistive device(s) he or she normally uses to perform a transfer. Time is recorded from the moment the subject starts until the subject sits on the table with both legs lying on the table.

Note: This item is not carried out if the subject has a score less than 3 on the FIM transfer item bed/chair/wheelchair. The research assistant is not allowed to lift any part of the subject's body to help in performing the item.

Ability score 0: The subject cannot perform this item within 300 sec.

Ability score 0.5: The subject is able to perform a transfer (within 300 sec) but cannot do this in the manner described above.

Ability score 1: The subject performs this item correctly within 300 sec.

Kilkens OJ, Post MW, van der Woude LH, Dallmeijer AJ, van den Heuvel WJ: *Arch Phys Med Rehabil* 83(12):1783–1788, 2002.

---

living environment, and psychological and socioeconomic factors) may modify the frequency of visits or the total duration of the plan of care. Findings like pressure ulcer, fracture, and ventilator dependency may require classification in other patterns in addition to practice pattern 5H. Individuals with SCI may require multiple episodes of care over the lifetime to ensure safety and to adapt to changes in physical condition, environment, caregiver status, or task demands.

Evaluation of SCI usually includes grading the degree of impairment using the ASIA Impairment Scale[47] (Fig. 20-4). The Impairment Scale is based on the results of the ASIA motor and sensory scores (see section on Examination) and has been shown to characterize sensory, motor and functional impairment.[71,79-81] For some comparisons (e.g., LEMS as a predictor of gait[82] and UEMS as a correlate to motor FIM scores[83]), a better prediction of functional abilities may be obtained by using the separate UEMS and LEMS to describe different dimensions of the effect of impairment on function, rather than using the total motor score. The ASIA Impairment Scale is scored from A, which is more impaired, to E, which is normal sensory and motor function. Note that for an individual to receive a grade of C or above, he or she must not have a complete SCI because this score requires the presence of sensory or motor function in the sacral segments S4-S5. In addition, the individual must have either voluntary anal sphincter contraction or sparing of motor function more than three levels below the motor level.

A number of clinical syndromes associated with incomplete SCI result in typical patterns of impairment (Table 20-3).[3,5,13,47] Recognizing these syndromes can help predict functional limitations and can assist with treatment planning.

Prognosis for functional recovery after SCI is complicated by the infinite variety of patterns of neurological loss and preservation possible with spinal cord damage. Incomplete injury recovery can be partially predicted by examination results and diagnostic categorization. For complete injuries (without other complicating medical factors), Table 20-4 summarizes the functional outcomes that may be expected by the end of the initial episode of care.

ASIA IMPAIRMENT SCALE

☐ **A = Complete:** No motor or sensory function is preserved in sacral segments S4–S5.

☐ **B = Incomplete:** Sensory but not motor function is preserved below the neurological level, including sacral segments S4–S5.

☐ **C = Incomplete:** Motor function is preserved below the neurological level, and more than half the key muscles below the neurological level have muscle grade less than 3.

☐ **D = Incomplete:** Motor function is preserved below the neurological level, and at least half the key muscles below the neurological level have muscle grade of 3 or more.

☐ **E = Normal:** Motor and sensory function are normal.

CLINICAL SYNDROMES

☐ Central cord
☐ Brown-Séquard
☐ Anterior cord
☐ Conus medullaris
☐ Cauda equina

FIG. 20-4 The ASIA Impairment Scale. *Courtesy American Spinal Injury Association, Atlanta, Ga.*

TABLE 20-3	Spinal Cord Injury Syndromes	
Name of Syndrome	**Pattern of Neurological Injury**	**Associated Impairments**
Central cord syndrome	Injury to the central portion of the cord, with sparing of peripheral areas. Occurs almost exclusively in the cervical region.	Sparing of sacral sensation. Weakness more severe in the UEs with lesser impairment or preservation of function in the LEs.
Brown-Séquard syndrome	Anterior to posterior hemisection of the spinal cord or other injury resulting in unilateral cord damage.	Ipsilateral proprioceptive and motor loss, and contralateral loss of sensitivity to light touch, pressure, pain, and temperature.
Anterior cord syndrome	Destruction of the anterior portions of the white and gray matter of the cord, with preservation of posterior components.	Complete loss of motor function and some loss of light touch and temperature sensation. Sparing of proprioception and discriminative touch.
Posterior cord syndrome	Destruction of the posterior portions of the cord, with relative preservation of anterior components.	Severe impairment of proprioception, discrimination, and vibration. Motor function minimally affected or preserved.
Cauda equina syndrome	Damage to the lumbar or sacral nerve roots caudal to the level of spinal cord termination.	Sensory loss and flaccid paralysis of LE muscles, bladder, and bowels.

UEs, Upper extremities; *LE,* Lower extremities.

TABLE 20-4	Functional Outcomes after Spinal Cord Injury					
C4	**C5**	**C6**	**C7-C8**	**T1-T8**	**T9-T12**	**L1-L3**
RESPIRATION						
VC 30%-50% of normal Independently directs TA required for bronchial hygiene	VC up to 60% of normal Directs assistance with some portions of bronchial hygiene Performs SA coughing techniques	VC 60%+ of normal Independent with bronchial hygiene, including SA coughing	VC 60%-80% or normal Independent with bronchial hygiene, including SA coughing	VC 80% or more of normal Independent with bronchial hygiene	VC 80% or more of normal Independent with bronchial hygiene	Independent with bronchial hygiene
PRESSURE RELIEF						
Modified independent in sitting with appropriately equipped power WC Independent to direct total assistance required for positioning in bed	Modified independent with appropriately equipped power WC Modified assistance in sitting in manual WC Moderate assistance with bed rails for positioning in bed	Modified independent with pressure relief in sitting in manual WC Minimal assistance to modified independent with positioning in bed with bed rails	Independent pressure relief in sitting in manual WC and in unsupported sitting Modified independent to independent with bed positioning	Independent with pressure relief in sitting and with bed positioning	Independent with pressure relief in sitting and with bed positioning	Independent with pressure relief in sitting and with bed positioning
ROLLING						
TA Independently directs assistant	Moderate assistance with bed rails	Minimal assistance to modified independent with bed rails	Modified independent to independent	Independent	Independent	Independent
SIT TO SUPINE						
TA Independently directs assistant	Moderate-to-maximal assistance Independently directs assistant	Minimal assistance to modified independent with adaptive devices	Modified independent to independent	Independent	Independent	Independent

TABLE 20-4	Functional Outcomes after Spinal Cord Injury—cont'd					
C4	**C5**	**C6**	**C7-C8**	**T1-T8**	**T9-T12**	**L1-L3**
SEATED SCOOTING						
TA Independently directs assistant	Maximal assistance Independently directs assistant	Minimal assistance Independently directs assistant	Independent on level surfaces	Independent on level surfaces and uneven surfaces/inclines	Independent on level surfaces and uneven surfaces/ inclines	Independent on level surfaces and uneven surfaces/inclines
LEVEL SURFACE TRANSFERS						
TA, using mechanical or manual lift techniques Independently directs assistant	Moderate-to-maximal assistance with sliding board or similar assistive device Independently directs assistant	Minimal assistance with adaptive equipment (sliding board)	Modified independent to independent	Independent	Independent	Independent
UNEVEN SURFACE TRANSFERS (CAR, TOILET, ETC)						
TA, using mechanical or manual lift techniques Independently directs assistant	Total-to-maximal assistance with sliding board or similar assistive device Independently directs assistant	Maximal-to-moderate assist with device Independently directs assistant	Minimal assistance to modified independent	Modified independent to independent	Independent	Independent
FLOOR TRANSFER						
TA Independently directs assistant	TA Independently directs assistant	TA Independently directs assistant	Maximal-to-moderate assistance	Variable-to-moderate assistance to modified independence	Minimal assistance to independence	Modified independent to independent
Modified independent with appropriately equipped power WC	Modified independent with power WC Modified independent on smooth level surfaces with manual WC with modified hand rims and appropriate seating Maximal assist with uneven/rough surfaces Dependent with curbs but independent to direct assistance	Modified independent with power WC Modified independent on smooth level surfaces with manual WC with adaptations (plastic-coated rims, gloves) Moderate-to-minimal assist with uneven/rough surfaces Dependent with curbs but independent to direct assistance	Modified independent level surface with manual WC Modified independent on uneven/rough surfaces with modified push rims and/or WC gloves/cuffs Minimal assist with curbs to modified independent with curbs	Modified independent level surfaces Modified independent on rough/uneven surfaces Minimal assist to modified independent curbs Stairs maximal-to-minimal assistance	Modified independent with level and uneven surfaces Modified independent curbs Stairs moderate assist to modified independence	Modified independent level and uneven surfaces Modified independent curbs Stairs moderate assist to modified independence
NA	NA	NA	NA	Maximal-to-minimal assistance with standing and limited level surface ambulation with KAFOs and assistive device	Modified independent on level surfaces with KAFOs and assistive device	Modified independent with appropriate orthotics and with assistive device on level and uneven surfaces

*With orthotics and appropriate assistive device (not including body weight–supported or electronically assisted ambulation).
VC, Vital capacity; *TA*, total assistance; *SA*, self-assisted; *WC*, wheelchair; *NA*, not applicable; *KAFOs*, knee-ankle-foot orthoses.

INTERVENTION

Because of the global effects of SCI, case management needs to be team-based and include interventions for multiple musculoskeletal and neuromuscular systems. The rehabilitation team may include nursing, medicine (specifically physicians with specialization in physical medicine and rehabilitation), occupational therapy, physical therapy, speech and language therapy, psychology, social work, and recreation therapy. Other medical specialists and allied health practitioners may be involved, depending on the exact nature of the patient's needs. The remainder of this chapter addresses basic intervention options in the acute and rehabilitation phases of recovery from SCI. Because of the infinite combinations of motor and sensory loss and preservation after injury, no single intervention plan can be applied to the majority of patients with SCI. The following suggestions will need to be modified according to the results of a thorough examination and evaluation process.

THE ACUTE PHASE

Early intervention in the acute stage of recovery from SCI focuses on prevention of secondary complications from immobility and beginning the transition to upright postures. Emphasis is placed on passive and active assistive exercise, positioning to prevent skin breakdown and preserve ROM, and on maintaining or restoring as much respiratory function as possible.

Patient-Related Instruction. Education of the patient and any identified caregivers must begin at the time of onset of therapy services. The patient must learn to direct the assistance he or she needs to control their physical care, their comfort, and their psychosocial needs. In particular, physical therapy instruction in the acute setting will include instruction in bed positioning, skin inspection and pressure ulcer risk factors, respiratory exercises, and assisted ROM exercises. Instructions should be provided and learning assessed for accuracy, since an error in understanding could lead to submaximal care and possible complications in recovery. Once the patient is stable he or she should also begin to be educated about the long-term rehabilitation process.

Therapeutic Exercise. Passive ROM (PROM) exercises are used to minimize shortening of muscles and articular structures. Traditional ROM exercises are provided to all limbs, trunk, and cervical region as allowed by immobilization devices and by medical restrictions to movement. ROM exercises are begun as soon as the patient is medically stable and cleared for activity. Because of the possible risk of increased incidence of HO development associated with delayed onset of ROM, early intervention is stressed. A standard ROM protocol usually includes twice daily exercises of all joints through full available ROM for 5-10 repetitions.[5,11] This ROM frequency is arbitrary, with no evidence found to support the efficacy of this or any other protocol in the SCI population. There is some evidence that frequent shorter periods of stretch may have little effect on muscle extensibility[84,85] and that longer periods of stretching may be required to maintain muscle length after SCI. The need for more prolonged stretching is partially met with appropriate bed positioning as described later in this section. Despite the lack of evidence to support ROM exercises, it is recommended that until more research is done to better define stretching parameters, ROM exercises be used for their possible contributions to flexibility, circulatory function, prevention of pressure ulcers, and as a means to reintroduce the patient to the concept of movement in preparation for active mobility.

Some extra precautions must be taken when performing ROM exercise with an individual with SCI because of the future ROM required for mobility and the hypotonicity present during early recovery:

1. Extreme or forceful ROM is avoided because of the risk of soft tissue trauma and possible predisposition to HO.
2. Straight leg raises and combined hip and knee flexion may be limited in acute phases, particularly after lower thoracic or lumbar surgery, because of the possible stretch on dural tissue and lumbar structures.
3. Combined movements of the wrist and fingers are rarely applied in the same directions (e.g., wrist flexion combined with finger flexion or wrist extension with finger extension) to avoid overstretching the long finger flexor or extensor tendons. The natural passive movement of the fingers into flexion with wrist extension will be utilized by many patients to perform grasp functions (called *tenodesis grip*), so preservation of some tightness in the long finger flexors in combination with wrist extension must be preserved. Concomitantly, extensor length must be preserved to allow the passive opening of the tenodesis grip when the wrist is flexed. The exception to this rule occurs if the patient is developing severe spasticity, at which time, prolonged stretching or splinting may be required to prevent contractures of the involved muscle groups.
4. Because of the need for strength and mobility in the shoulder and scapula for all future mobility skills, these areas must be addressed along with distal extremity motions.
5. During the areflexive period of spinal shock, care should be taken to fully support the limbs during ROM to prevent trauma to intermediate joints.

While ROM is initially a passive activity performed by the therapist or trained caregiver, as patient progress allows, these exercises are advanced to active assistive or active exercise, and the patient is instructed in how to perform self-ROM exercises for maintaining flexibility.

Positioning. Because of the prolonged period of time most acute SCI patients spend in bed, it is very important that correct positioning be used to reduce the risk of pressure ulcers, maintain postural and skeletal alignment, and reduce the secondary effects of spasticity. A pressure-relief bed, mattress, or mattress overlay should always be used in addition to constant monitoring of positioning and skin condition. Turning between positions is generally performed every 2 hours.

When the patient is supine, the following posture is recommended:

Body Area	Anatomical Point	Position
LEs	Hips	In extension and slightly abducted, with neutral rotation
	Knees	In extension, but supported and not hyper-extended
	Ankles	In dorsiflexion, generally with the use of an orthotic device
	Toes	Extended
UEs (for patients with tetraplegia)	Shoulders	In adduction, slight flexion, neutral rotation
	Elbows	In extension, especially in the presence of biceps function without opposing triceps function. Air splints or other orthotic devices may be used to maintain elbow extension in the case of biceps spasticity
	Wrists	In extension of approximately 30-45 degrees. A schedule of intermittent splinting may be used to facilitate proper wrist position
	Fingers	In slight flexion

Patients are rarely positioned in direct sidelying because of the pressure this places on the bony prominences at the shoulder and hip. Instead, they are positioned slightly away from sidelying in the supine direction. In this position, the hips and knees are slightly flexed and the upper leg is slightly posterior to the lower, with padding provided between the limbs (especially at the knees and ankles). The lower side shoulder is flexed to about 90 degrees and is slightly protracted, the elbow extended, and the forearm supinated and supported on a pillow. The upper arm is supported on a pillow in shoulder flexion and elbow extension.

Prone positioning is an excellent option for prolonged stretching of hip and knee flexors and is an especially good position for patients with a good prognosis for recovery of ambulation. The presence of medical devices (e.g., tracheotomy or feeding tube) may complicate but does not preclude the use of the prone position in early intervention. The presence of a Halo brace is not necessarily a contraindication for prone-lying, but many patients with a Halo have to be slowly introduced to time spent prone secondary to the initial helpless feeling of lying face down and because the feeling of compression on the chest may create a perceived change in respiratory function. In fact, prone positioning improves oxygenation and may increase circulation to dependent lung regions.[86] Even if a patient with a Halo does not tolerate prolonged prone positioning, he or she should still be turned to prone for a few minutes daily to allow skin inspection and cleaning under the posterior portion of the Halo vest and to help with respiratory secretion mobilization.

As the patient's condition stabilizes, he or she may be progressed to upright sitting. An abdominal binder and LE ace wrapping are used for vascular support, and the individual is gradually raised into a sitting position in bed or in a reclining wheelchair with elevating leg rests, while BP and heart rate are monitored and the patient is observed for signs of light-headedness or dizziness. When the patient can tolerated sitting in this position for extended periods (15-30 minutes), the patient can be progressed to sitting with the LEs in a dependent position.

Airway Clearance. Many individuals with SCI, especially at the cervical level, require mechanical ventilation during their acute management. Patients with complete injuries above C4 will require life-long full or partial ventilatory support. Physical therapy interventions during acute patient management will include techniques for improving respiratory muscle strength and endurance and improving airway clearance and for minimizing the respiratory complications of prolonged immobilization. Treatment should be closely coordinated with other members of the treatment team, including nursing, respiratory therapy, speech therapy, and occupational therapy.

Interventions chosen are based on the results of the pulmonary examination and evaluation. If airway secretions are present or suspected, interventions may include positioning for postural drainage, percussion, and vibration (see Chapter 24). These interventions are applied to lung areas involved (as noted on radiograph or with auscultation), and the treatment time is determined by the changes in airway clearance. Treatments may take 20-30 minutes and are continued as long as there are productive secretions (with induced cough or suctioning) and breath sounds are improving.[66] A change in breath sounds from diminished or absent before treatment to crackles, rhonchi, or vesicular during and after treatment indicates effective secretion mobilization. Periodic suctioning and/or assisted coughing may be used to clear the mobilized secretions. A pneumatic vest that supplies mechanical vibration to the entire chest wall may also be used to mobilize secretions. Once a patient is more active and can mobilize secretion with coughing, passive airway clearance techniques may be discontinued.

An abdominal binder to support breathing may be used once the patient is performing some spontaneous breathing. The binder is applied in the area 2-3 inches below the xiphoid process and extending slightly below the anterior superior iliac spine (ASIS).[66] Binders placed too high may impair inspiration, and binders that extend too low may cause skin breakdown. Although the use of abdominal binders to support respiration is controversial, there is evidence that binders can help some individuals.[87,88] Vital capacity, respiratory rate, breathing pattern, and oxygen saturation may be monitored in supine and in sitting with and without the binder to determine if the binder is helping a specific individual.

To support weaning from mechanical ventilation, respiratory muscle training may be performed with inspiratory muscle training devices and/or with abdominal weight training.[5,66] Manual cues and facilitation may be used to target specific muscles and excursions during exercise. The duration and resistance of training is progressed slowly to prevent respiratory muscle fatigue. As respiratory endurance improves interventions for mobility may be added during the periods when the patient is off of the ventilator. During the weaning process continuous positive airway pressure may be used to assist breathing when the patient is off of mechanical ventilation.

Patients with higher cervical SCI may be taught a technique called glossopharyngeal breathing (GPB), which uses the upper accessory muscles (innervated by the cranial nerves) to expand the oral cavity to draw air into the mouth and create a negative inspiratory pressure to facilitate inspiration. The air is then "pushed" into the lungs by pulling the chin and tongue back toward the neck, creating a positive pressure in the mouth. This air "gulping" or "stroke" is repeated multiple (≈3-12) times per breath.[89] Some patients who would otherwise be ventilator-dependent can use GPB to allow extended time off of the ventilator. For others, it serves an emergency procedure to sustain breathing for short periods in the case of temporary failure of mechanical ventilatory support.

Pain Management. Interventions for pain management vary with the type of pain. Although any structure above or below the injury level may be affected, nociceptive pain is often musculoskeletal in nature and frequently occurs above the level of injury secondary to the increased stresses of weight bearing and mobility placed on the UEs.[90] The shoulder is the most common site of pain above the level of injury. Nociceptive pain symptoms are addressed with similar regimens to those used for able-bodied populations, including the use of analgesic and antiinflammatory medications, rest, lifestyle modifications, therapeutic modalities, and exercise.[90,91] Additional interventions for people with SCI may involve ergonomic assessment and modification of wheelchair seating and propulsion technique.[92,93] No controlled study evidence was found for SCI patients related to the efficacy of various interventions for nociceptive pain. In a self-report study of pain management in 120 individuals with SCI, 40 had tried physical therapy and 50% of them rated it as making pain "considerably better" or "disappear."[52]

Neuropathic pain is more difficult to classify and treat, particularly if it occurs below the injury level. Treatment options for this type of pain are similar to those used in other patients with chronic pain and may include medication (e.g., opioids, antidepressants, anticonvulsants, and antispasticity agents), psychosocial support, cognitive-behavioral therapy, and surgical intervention.[52,91,93] Spinal cord stimulation and drug infusions are additional possibilities.[94] Few clinical studies have been done to evaluate the effectiveness of any given treatment, and none of these interventions is consistently effective. Further

research is required to develop effective methods for management of neuropathic pain after SCI.[52,91,93-95]

THE REHABILITATION PHASE

During the rehabilitation phase of recovery, interventions focus on training mobility skills and providing education in self-care to the individual with SCI. This phase will at a minimum include training in pressure relief techniques, bed mobility skills, transfer training, wheelchair mobility skills, respiratory care, and gait training (when appropriate). Training for each of these tasks may be accompanied by specific exercises to increase the strength, flexibility, or control components necessary to increase task performance and efficiency. Information in this section of the chapter is categorized according to task and includes descriptions of techniques that may be used for achieving and improving task performance.

Patient-Related Instruction

Pressure Relief in Sitting. Patients with SCI are at an increased risk for developing pressure ulcers during their initial episode of care after injury. It is therefore imperative that pressure relief techniques are taught as soon as possible after injury and frequently reinforced throughout the rehabilitation process. The patient must understand the importance of these skills, and all team members must cue and reinforce their performance.

When seated, tissue around the ischial tuberosities is at greatest risk for breakdown. If the patient has a kyphotic posture with a posterior pelvic tilt, the area over the sacrum is also at increased risk.[96,97] Recommendations about how long and often pressure should be relieved over the bony prominences to reduce ulcer risk vary greatly.[11,18,19] Most sources agree that pressure relief should initially be performed for 15 seconds or more, at least every 15-30 minutes. However, recent evidence suggests that this may not be sufficient for reoxygenation of compressed tissue. Based on monitoring of transcutaneous oxygen levels during pressure relief, studies have concluded that most subjects tested required 1.5-2 minutes of pressure relief to restore oxygen equivalent to baseline unloaded levels.[98,99]

For patients with tetraplegia at or above the C4 level, pressure relief is performed by an assistant or a powered system tilting or reclining the wheelchair (Fig. 20-5). An assistant can tilt the wheelchair by sitting behind the wheelchair, grasping its push handles, and tilting the chair back onto its rear wheels until the chair is tilted at least 65 degrees (the back of the chair may be resting on the assistant's knees).[100] Some wheelchairs have a mechanism that allows the back of the wheelchair to be reclined separately from the seating surface. With this type of mechanism the chair back should be reclined as far back as comfortably possible (120-150 degrees)[101] and the legs elevated. Further weight shifting can be accomplished by partially rolling the individual to each side once in the supine position. A disadvantage of reclining the patient is that this involves changing the patient's position relative to the chair. The patient then needs to be repositioned when the chair is returned to the upright position after the pressure relief, and this can trigger spasticity. It is also important to realize that some angles of recline that reduce ischial pressure can increase surface shear force and thus risk of tissue breakdown.[101]

For patients with SCI at the C5-6 level with good head and neck control and some UE function (not including triceps), several techniques may be used to assist with pressure relief in a manual wheelchair. The individual may lean forward with the chest moving toward the thighs (Fig. 20-6, *A*). Henderson et al found this technique to be more effective in reducing pressure over the ischial tuberosities than tilting the chair back by 35 or 65 degrees.[100] The most difficult part of this technique is learning to recover from the forward position without triceps function. Patients can be taught to use their anterior shoulder muscles to push up to sitting, or to throw

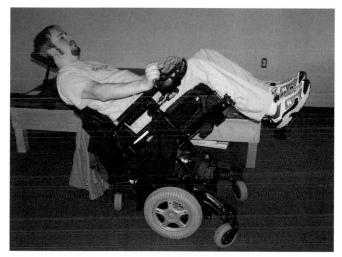

FIG. 20-5 Passive pressure relief using a tilt-in-space wheelchair.

one arm back and "hook" the back of the chair or push handle to pull themselves back to an upright position. Another technique is to lean sideways in the wheelchair as far as possible, using the opposite arm (i.e., left arm for right lean) to hook the wheelchair back or push handle (with the forearm for individuals with C5 function and with wrist extension for individuals with C6 function) to control the lean and to recover from the lean (Fig. 20-6, *B*). This technique must be then repeated to the opposite side for bilateral pressure relief.

For individuals with functional use of the triceps, pressure relief may be performed using the push-up technique (Fig. 20-6, *C*). This involves placing the hands on the wheelchair tires or arm rests and lifting the body off of the seat with a push-up motion. Some individuals without triceps function may be able to perform a version of this skill, if their seating configuration allows them to position the UEs in way that passively locks the elbow into extension while the shoulders depressors are used to create the lifting force. The disadvantage of the push-up technique is that it contributes further to the over use of the shoulders and wrist already inherent in wheelchair mobility.[102] It is also extremely difficult for someone to maintain the push-up position long enough to allow sufficient tissue perfusion (1.5-2 minutes).

In addition to regular pressure relief techniques, it is essential that every individual with SCI use a seat cushion designed to distribute pressure when sitting in the wheelchair or on any surface for an extended period of time. Wheelchair cushions are available in four basic types, each with advantages and disadvantages. Cushions that use air for support consistently reduce pressure over bony prominences[103,104] and are generally lightweight, but they require regular maintenance and provide a less stable surface for performing mobility skills. Gel cushions require minimal maintenance and are generally easier to

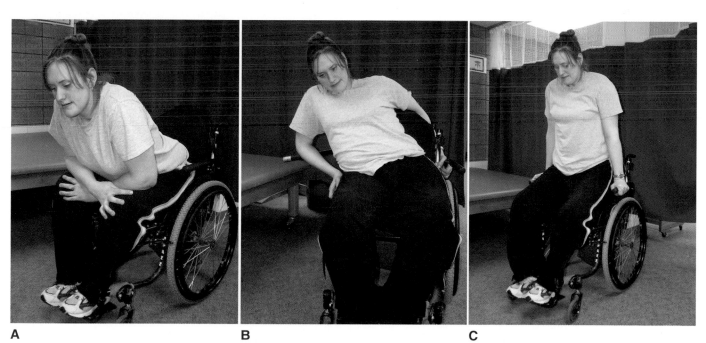

A   B   C

FIG. 20-6 Active pressure relief techniques. **A,** Forward lean; **B,** side lean; **C,** push-up.

move on and off of but can be heavy and trap moisture. Foam cushions come in a large variety of shapes and various combinations of foam density and material. The effectiveness of the pressure relief and the longevity of the material vary greatly between types of foam, and careful assessment is needed to match the fit, the mobility needs, and the pressure distribution requirements of the individual to the characteristics of the cushion. Other cushions are made from any of a number of synthetic materials in a variety of configurations (e.g., honeycomb construction), with variable attributes related to pressure distribution, positioning, and mobility skills.

Gait and Locomotion Training

Wheelchair Mobility. Training individuals with any level of SCI to use a wheelchair is essential for independent daily mobility. After an initial period of skill and endurance training, an individual should be able to propel his or her wheelchair throughout an average day at the community level without creating muscle soreness or fatigue. The level of SCI will dictate the skills required and the type of wheelchair needed to meet this goal.

Individuals with SCI at C4 or above will use a power wheelchair for mobility. Power chairs may be controlled by any of a number of control mechanisms that are matched to the patient's mobility. Small movements of the head, chin, lips, breath, or shoulders can be used to control the chair and to control power pressure relief options. A variety of hand and arm mounting systems enable individuals to drive a wheelchair with limited UE motion. Portable ventilators can be mounted on power wheelchairs to allow ventilator-dependent individuals to be mobile at the household and community levels. Initial practice with powered mobility should be done in an open area with the wheelchair controls adjusted to a slow speed. As the individual's skills progress, he or she should be instructed in using the chair on uneven terrain, around obstacles, in public places, and on elevators. The power chair user must be able to direct the management and maintenance of all parts of his or her wheelchair, including the mechanism that disengages the drive mechanism and allows the wheelchair to be pushed by an assistant in case of mechanical failure.

SCI at the midcervical level (C5-6) results in motor control that allows limited manual wheelchair propulsion. Specially designed push rims on the wheelchair give patients projections or tacky surfaces that can be used to "grip" the rim in the absence of finger function. For these individuals, the wheelchair push stroke involves planting the hands on the rims behind the hips and pulling with the biceps to start the propelling motion, following through with a squeeze motion of the anterior shoulder and chest muscles to complete the push stroke. The wheelchair should be adjusted to allow maximum maneuverability, while at the same time having stable seat and back support sufficient to allow maximum push stroke efficiency without compensatory postural changes.[105,106] While most individuals with this level of SCI can be independent on smooth level surfaces with manual wheelchair propulsion, community level mobility often requires the use of a power-assist manual wheelchair or a power wheelchair.

Most individuals with complete SCI at or below C7 will use a manual wheelchair for mobility. The push stroke for these individuals involves grasping the push rim behind the hips (with modifications to the rim as needed with cervical injuries), pushing forward on the rims, allowing the hands to drop down and then extending the shoulders during the recovery phase, and then gripping the rims again. In this way the push stroke becomes a circular motion rather than a back and forth "sawing" type of motion. A small but interesting study by Boninger et al found that individuals who propel with a greater percentage of force directed radially toward the wheelchair axle instead of parallel to the axle were at an increased risk for progression of MRI findings consistent with shoulder injury.[92] This at-risk group consisted primarily of women. Although the number of subject in this study (n = 14, 8 men and 6 women) does not allow for definitive conclusions about the relationship of push stroke to shoulder injury, it does highlight the need for providing teaching interventions and equipment that maximize propulsion while minimizing risks for future injury and impairment.

After mastering the basic push stroke required for propulsion on a level surface, manual wheelchair users should be instructed in a variety of additional skills that they can then adapt to their daily needs. The ability to open and close doors, operate an elevator, and perform ADL tasks from the seated position should all be taught during the patient's rehabilitation. The "wheelie" skill should also be introduced (Fig. 20-7) to allow for balance during steep descents, to unload the front of the wheel-

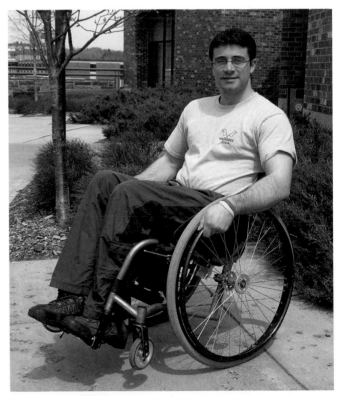

FIG. 20-7 Patient with complete T10 paraplegia balancing in the wheelie position.

chair to improve mobility over rough surfaces, and as a component of the skill of ascending curbs. The wheelie position is achieved by giving a firm forward push on the hand rims from a position just behind the hips, while at the same time leaning the head and shoulders back. This results in the front castors of the chair coming off the floor and all of the weight being transferred to the rear wheels. With practice most individuals can learn to maintain the chair in a balanced position with weight on the rear wheels only. When training a patient in this skill, the therapist must maintain a firm grip on the wheelchair push handles or on a safety strap looped around the rear of the wheelchair frame. This allows the therapist to help the patient get tilted far enough back to find the balanced position, while also preventing the patient from losing their balance backward.

Patients should be taught to protect themselves in the case of a fall. If falling backward, the individual should lean forward with their head turned (to avoid having their legs fall directly into their face) and try to grasp the front of the wheelchair frame. At no time should they try to reach back and catch themselves to prevent a fall; this puts the UE at high risk for shoulder injury or dislocation.

Ascending and descending curbs are skills that require repeated practice to master. A low curb can be ascended using a wheelie to lift the front wheels up over the curb, pushing the chair forward until the rear wheels are against the curb, leaning the trunk as far forward as possible, and then pulling up and pushing forward on the hand rims. This technique requires good UE and grip strength. A low curb may be descended by backing down the curb with the rear wheels while leaning as far forward as possible over the front of the chair. Once the back of the chair is on the lower surfaces, the front end is moved off the curb by turning to the side or by using a wheelie to lift the front end and pulling back away from the curb. A more efficient technique for ascending curbs is to have the chair rolling forward throughout the ascent so that the forward momentum of the moving chair provides most of the force needed to get up the curb (Fig. 20-8). This involves approaching the curb with the chair rolling at a steady, moderate speed; just as the footplate is about to reach the curb the front end is lifted with a wheelie, and as soon as the front of the chair clears the curb, the upper body is thrown forward (lean or fall, depending on trunk control) while the arms continue the push stroke. Descending the curb is performed similarly by approaching the curb rolling and performing a small wheelie at the edge of the curb to hold up the front end of the chair as the rear wheels descend the curb, thus allowing the rear wheels to land on the lower surface either slightly before or at the same time as the front castors. Note that both of these skills require a good sense of timing, motor coordination, and a fair command of the wheelie skill. Patients should be assisted to allow success during early practice and should be closely guarded to prevent injury as they progress with their training.

In addition to learning wheelchair mobility skills, the individual must also be comfortable with the mechanics of the wheelchair: Managing leg rests and arm rests (required for transfers), using the wheel locks, making the chair compact for travel (this may involve folding the chair and/or removing the wheels), making mechanical adjustments to alter the performance of the chair (camber, seat to back angle, etc), and performing basic maintenance.

Gait. Traditionally, gait training for individuals with SCI focused on using orthotics and assistive devices to allow individuals to bear weight on their LEs and achieve upright positioning and a limited measure of functional mobility in standing. While this approach maintains some utility and is discussed later in this section, more recent investigation has led to a shift in intervention paradigm that seeks to better exploit the spinal neural circuitry. Treatment programs consistent with this paradigm include various forms of "locomotor training," which are

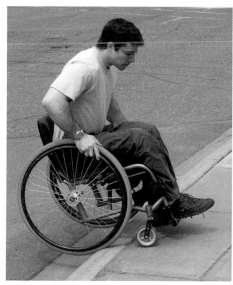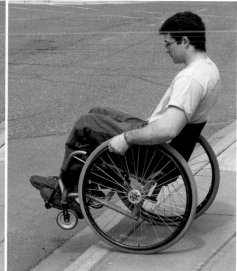

FIG. 20-8 Patient with complete T10 paraplegia ascending and descending a curb.

A   B

sometimes combined with additional modalities (e.g., functional electrical stimulation [FES], drug therapies) and other traditional therapy interventions.

Locomotor Training. Locomotor training takes advantage of neural networks in the spinal cord called *central pattern generators* (CPGs) that can produce rhythmic neural activity without supraspinal and proprioceptive input. CPGs may provide basic motor patterns, with the higher centers and sensory inputs initiating and modifying these patterns. The presence of CPGs contributing to a variety of movements is well established in a number of vertebrates other than humans, and evidence from these animals suggests that repetitive motor training may provide sufficient input to modify or enhance CPG motor output.[107-111] While the presence and exact function of CPGs in humans is more controversial, studies have shown that individuals with complete and incomplete SCI can produce locomotor-type movements and EMG patterns when LE stepping movements are assisted externally to provide appropriate sensory cues to the spinal cord.[112-114]

The evidence supporting the existence of human CPGs has led to the development of a number of interventions aimed at using these neural pathways to produce locomotor movement in patients with SCI. This is generally done by suspending the individual above a treadmill with a harness connected to a device that allows a portion of the person's body weight to be lifted off of their feet. As the treadmill starts to move the LEs are passively moved or electrically stimulated to produce a stepping pattern that is as kinematically correct as possible. Over time, the repetitive stepping practice results in greater spontaneous stepping and the amount of body weight suspended and the amount of assistance provided are decreased as tolerated. The goal of this intervention is to maximize the use-dependent plasticity of the spinal neural networks to increase the effectiveness of ambulation.

Many variations of this basic approach have been used with varying results. A review of research with locomotor training on a treadmill with FES found that benefits included decreased physiological cost of walking (reduced by a factor of 2) and an increase in maximal walking speed (mean increase of 0.50 meters per second [m/sec]).[115] In a single case study, Carhart et al combined epidural spinal cord stimulation with partial weight-bearing treadmill therapy (locomotor training) and noted a decrease in the effort of walking (from 8/10 to 3/10 on the Borg Scale) and a 100% increase in walking speed for this individual.[116] Stewart et al studied nine subjects with chronic SCI (mean time since injury: 8.1 years) who were trained with body weight–supported treadmill training (BWST) with manual assistance provided as need by therapists.[117] After 6 months of progressive BWST, these investigators noted increased walking velocity (on the treadmill) of 135% and a 55% increase in the time walking per session on the treadmill. Four of the nine subjects also showed measurable improvement in functional overground walking as rated on the Wernig Walking Scale. Interestingly, these patients also had significant reductions in total cholesterol and changes in muscle fiber properties that included increases in the size of type I and IIa fibers. Field-Fote and Tepavac applied BWST combined with FES to the peroneal

nerve of 14 subjects with chronic, incomplete SCI. After 36 sessions of training over 12 weeks, mean overground walking speed increased by 84% and treadmill walking speed increased by 158%.[118] Nine of the 14 subjects also had increased intralimb consistency and coordination. In addition to physical and functional benefits, locomotor training has also been associated with psychological gains, including increased confidence, self-esteem, hope, and quality of life in patients with SCI.[119-121]

Although the results of these studies are very promising, many had very small numbers of subjects and varied intervention strategies and there were many possible confounding factors such as spontaneous recovery and other simultaneous therapy interventions. Locomotor training is a promising treatment option for patients with SCI; however, it has yet to be definitively shown that any one type of locomotor training is effective for a broad range of individuals with SCI or if locomotor training is more effective than traditional gait training techniques for this population.

Recent developments in locomotor training techniques include using mechanical robotic devices to provide the assistance needed during gait (to decrease strain on the therapist and increase the time the patient spends in training during a given session),[122] using implanted electrical stimulators (known as neuroprostheses) to produce contractions of muscles needed for standing and mobility, and combining locomotor training with drug therapies that may enhance CPG activity and/or plasticity in preserved pathways.

Therapists wishing to use locomotor training interventions will find a huge variation in protocols used for training in various research trials. A number of researchers involved in locomotor training have developed a standardized BWST protocol to be used in a current multicenter study of the efficacy of locomotor training after SCI.[123] This protocol includes 1 hour of step training with BWST 5 days per week, with the goal of 20 minutes of continuous stepping within that time period. Percentage of body-weight support at the initiation of training ranges from 20% to 50%. Treadmill speeds vary by patient ability but are aimed at reaching speeds of at least 2 to 2.5 miles per hour, as soon as possible. Assistance with stepping is provided manually as needed to the LEs, trunk, and pelvis. This protocol is fairly representative of many of the other articles noted, with the possible exception of 5 days per week of training as compared with 3 days used in a number of other studies. Locomotor training is very much task specific, and it is therefore essential to incorporate the skills practiced in BWST into a program of overground ambulation to make the skill as functional as possible.

Lessons learned from animal and human locomotor gait training studies have shown that there are several gait parameters therapists should try to achieve during BWST in order to maximize the effectiveness of the neural input.[107,124,125] The maximum weight-loading (i.e., with the least amount of body-weight support) that can be tolerated without deterioration of the gait pattern should be used. Treadmill speeds should be as close as possible to the patient's normal gait speed (before injury); for most people this is at least 2.0 m/sec. At the end of stance phase, full hip extension ROM should be facilitated and synchronized with loading of the opposite limb to trigger an ipsilateral flexion response and contralateral loading response. Kinematics at the knee and ankle should also be as normal as possible. UE weight bearing should be avoided, and reciprocal arm swing encouraged. Sensory stimulation that conflicts with sensory information associated with locomotion should be minimized (e.g., stimulation of extensor afferents during swing phase).

Gait Training with Bilateral KAFOs. In patients with complete SCI or incomplete SCI without functional ambulation skill, interventions may include bracing accompanied by instruction in alternative gait patterns. The most commonly taught pattern is a 2-point swing-through pattern with the use of forearm crutches and bilateral knee-ankle-foot orthoses (KAFOs) with the knee joints locked in extension and the ankles locked in slight dorsiflexion. To utilize this technique effectively, individuals must have normal UE function with excellent strength and endurance and preferably some preservation of active trunk control (T8 and below). They must also have full passive hip extension, ankle dorsiflexion, and lumbar extension ROM.

The most efficient KAFO gait sequence is as follows (Fig. 20-9):

1. Momentary balance is achieved by extending the hips and trunk with weight shifted forward over the ball of the foot and arms extended with the crutch tips behind the position of the feet. In this position the locked ankle of the brace is providing the forward stability.
2. Both crutches are lifted and extended forward simultaneously, and weight is transferred to the crutches in a forward falling motion.

3. Full weight is then born on the UEs while both legs are lifted and simultaneously swung through to a point in front of the crutch tips.
4. A forceful push on the crutches is used at the same time the trunk is extended to push the hips forward into extension and achieve the balance position noted in item 1.

Repetition of this momentary balance followed by forward "fall" creates the gait sequence. Although this sequence can be mastered by some individuals, the energy demand is so high, the burden on the UE joints so great, and the risk of loss of balance so significant that most people choose to use a wheelchair as their primary means of locomotion. Mobility with the KAFOs is then reserved for spaces that are too small to accommodate a wheelchair (e.g., bus or plane aisles), for short distance mobility, or for doing ADLs that require short periods of standing (reaching objects from overhead cabinets, etc).

Functional Training in Self-Care and Home Management

Mobility Skills. The limited use of multiple muscle groups after SCI requires that the patient use alternative methods for performing mobility skills. Unlike many other physical therapy applications where the patient is trying to return to a previously known movement pattern, many SCI patients will need to learn new and different ways of performing everyday movements. For many individuals with SCI the rehabilitation process will involve the slow and difficult process of learning to use the UEs to compensate for absent or weak LE movement. The PT performs a key role in helping the individual to discover the most effective and efficient means of mobility according to their particular pattern of movement preservation.

What follows is a description of several functional postures that are key to mobility and ADLs, with training techniques that can be used to increase control within the postures and techniques that can be taught to help with transitions between these functional postures. Refer to the outcomes chart in the prognosis section of this chapter for guidelines related to the amount of assistance that may be needed for these techniques for patients with different levels of SCI.

Basic Postures

Prone on Elbows. The prone-on-elbows posture is useful for bed positioning, rolling, and progressing to sitting positions. This position also relieves pressure from posterior structures after periods of sitting or lying supine and stretches anterior hip muscles at the hips and trunk that can easily become shortened with prolonged sitting. The prone-on-elbows position is a very stable position with a large base of support that is used extensively during the rehabilitation process to improve all levels of motor control (mobility, stability, controlled mobility, and skill) in partial weight bearing at the shoulder in preparation for full UE weight-bearing activities like transfers. One precaution to consider for this position is whether the individual has sufficient lordosis to comfortably achieve the position. This position should be avoided in individuals with extremely unstable shoulder joints that may be traumatized by even partial weight bearing.

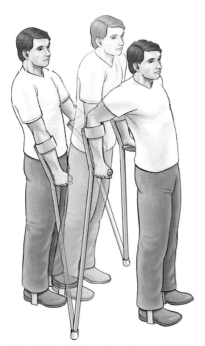

FIG. 20-9 Gait with bilateral KAFOs.

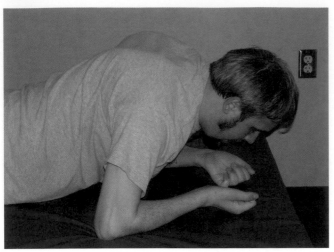

FIG. 20-10 Individual with complete C5 tetraplegia in the prone-on-elbows position. Note the scapular winging indicating poor innervation of the serratus anterior muscles and the wide base of support used for lateral stability.

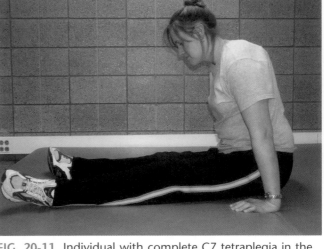

FIG. 20-11 Individual with complete C7 tetraplegia in the long-sitting position with head forward for balance.

Push-ups in the prone-on-elbows position (Fig. 20-10) emphasize strengthening of the serratus anterior and anterior shoulder muscles and eccentric control of scapular musculature. These are vital points of control for progressing independence with functional mobility. Individuals with weak or absent (above C6 level) serratus anterior function will have marked winging of the scapulae during prone-on-elbows push-ups.

Progression through the stages of motor control in the prone-on-elbows position may be facilitated with combinations of various activities including:

1. Mobility—Assuming the prone-on-elbows position from sidelying or prone, push-ups.
2. Stability—Weight bearing in the position, manually applied joint approximation, alternating isometrics in multiple directions, and rhythmic stabilization.
3. Controlled mobility—Controlled anterior-posterior and side to side weight shifts, push-ups (on elbows or onto hands), unilaterally supporting on one arm while unweighting and/or reaching with the other (static dynamic movement).
4. Skill—"Walking" on the elbows side to side and forward and back (commando type movements).

Supine on Elbows. The supine-on-elbows position is primarily used to increase flexibility and mobility at the shoulder and in preparation for moving from supine to long sitting. Similar to the prone-on-elbows position to enhance motor control, activities like weight shifting, stability activities, and side-to-side movements may be practiced in this position. The process of assuming the supine-on-elbows position is described in the section on transitioning from supine to long sit.

Quadruped and Tall Kneeling. The quadruped and tall-kneeling positions function as progressions from the positions noted previously. They require more muscular and motor control because of the decreased base of support and longer lever arms for movement. In most cases patients in the tall-kneeling position will use UE support on a table or bolster to assist in maintaining upright trunk posture.

For individuals with tetraplegia and high paraplegia, these positions are useful for practicing motor control in partial weight bearing through the entire UE with the elbow maintained in extension. Individuals without triceps control will need the therapist's assistance to keep the elbows extended when in the quadruped or tall-kneeling position. A therapy ball or large bolster may also be placed under the trunk to give support during quadruped activities. Tall kneeling is used most often with individuals who have partial preservation of trunk function, where the UEs can be used to control movement through a support surface.

Individuals with complete lower paraplegia or with incomplete injuries at any level may be put in these postures to challenge trunk, pelvic, and LE control in preparation for activities requiring upright balance and control in sitting and standing. The quadruped position may be assumed from prone on elbows or from side sitting; both provide a significant challenge at the mobility level of motor control. The kneeling position is assumed from quadruped, generally using UEs for assist. Once in kneeling the individual is encouraged to find a balance position with hips and trunk extended and weight bearing on arms minimized. Once either of these positions is achieved, isometric and dynamic activities can be added to challenge the individual's skills at progressive levels of motor control.

Long Sitting. Long sitting is the primary position used during dressing and other ADLs, especially for individuals without trunk or full UE control (Fig. 20-11). Long sitting is also a stable position for practicing and progressing associated skills. Stability is provided by the large base of support and by the taut hamstring muscles holding the pelvis in a stable midway position. It is important that hamstring length is not too short, which would pull the pelvis into a posterior pelvic tilt, nor too long, which would allow the pelvis to fall into an anterior tilt. Either of these would be less stable than a midway position.

Ideally, hamstring length should allow approximately 100 degrees of passive straight leg raise.

Activities in long sitting would be similar to those practiced in the prone-on-elbows position. Push-ups in this position help with strength and allow practice in preparation for mastering transfer skills. This position also allows practice of static and dynamic balance activities with bilateral or unilateral UE support, or without arm support. The patient should learn to transition from a supported position with the hands in front of the hips, to a position with the hands behind the hips with the upper body supported on the extended arms. This transition requires the ability to maintain balance briefly without UE support. For individuals with trunk muscle innervation, long sitting is a good position to begin trunk strengthening and practice of static and dynamic control.

Short Sitting. The ability to maintain balance and move in the short-sit position is crucial for independence with transfers, mat or bed mobility, and some ADLs and to have the arms free for functional activities. Most patients with SCI at or below the C5 level can find a position in short sitting where they can maintain static balance without UE support and have some degree of dynamic balance in this position with UE weight bearing. It is important during sitting activities that the feet are supported with hips and knees near 90-degree angles to allow partial weight to be borne on the feet to stabilize the lower body. It is also essential for patients with cervical injuries that the hands are positioned with fingers flexed when weight bearing on the UEs in sitting to avoid overstretching the long finger flexors and weakening the possible tenodesis grip.

The amount of preservation of active movement will determine what postures and compensatory balance strategies must be used to function in the short-sitting position. Patients with low thoracic injury levels should be able to achieve a fairly upright static posture with little or no posterior pelvic tilt. Dynamic movements will be possible in a small "cone of stability," with movements of the head, shoulder, and arms used to create and control weight shifting. Moving much beyond the base of support will require support on at least one UE. Patients with high thoracic or lower cervical injuries will most often maintain static balance with a combination of posterior pelvic tilt, trunk flexion, and forward head position. In this position, they may be able to unload one or both UEs for brief periods of time with compensatory movements of head and UEs (Fig. 20-12), but their stability remains poor and almost any dynamic movement in the seated position will require use of one or both UEs for weight bearing to increase the base of support.

As with long sitting, patients should learn to transition from a forward-propped position (hands in front of hips), to a backward-lean position (hands and shoulders behind hips) in short sitting. In order to maintain elbow extension in these weight-bearing positions, individuals without triceps function will need to mechanically lock the elbows by positioning the extremity in shoulder external rotation with the hand in a fixed position distally. This posture moves the elbow joint in front of the line of force through the UE and passively maintains the elbow in

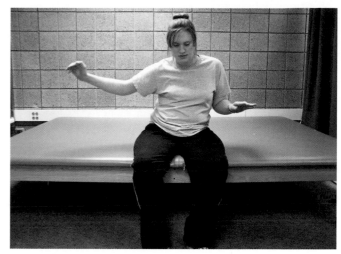

FIG. 20-12 Individual with a C7 incomplete SCI using her head and arms to compensate for limited balance during static short-sitting without upper extremity support. Note the scoliotic collapse of her trunk.

extension. During a forward lean with hands fixed, the anterior deltoid and the clavicular head of the pectoralis major can also be used to draw the humerus into adduction, thus creating a push-up motion that moves the extremity toward extension at the elbow.

The same sequence of activities used in the prone-on-elbows position to move through the stages of motor control may be used in the short-sitting position. It is particularly important that the patient master a push-up from the short-sitting position sufficient to clear the buttocks from the seating surface as this is required for scooting and transfer activities. This skill is performed by locking the elbows in extension, using the fixed shoulders and scapula as a fulcrum, then leaning the head forward and lifting the trunk and pelvis, using scapular depressors (lower trapezius muscles among others) and any available trunk musculature. The mechanics of this motion are contrary to the "normal" use of the scapular depressors where the pelvis and trunk are fixed and concentric contraction draws the scapulae down relative to the trunk. In this case, the scapulae are fixed and concentric contraction of the depressors draws the trunk and pelvis upward relative to the scapulae.[126] Mastery of this skill requires much practice as it requires high levels of strength, endurance, and motor control.

Transitioning Between Positions

Rolling. Rolling is taught early in rehabilitation because it is essential for many ADLs (e.g., dressing), for independence in bed mobility and bed positioning and is a building block for other mobility skills (e.g., moving from supine to sitting). Initial training for rolling is performed on a treatment mat, but the patient must be able to perform this skill on a bed for it to be functional. Whenever possible, rolling is taught without the use of assistive devices such as bed rails, webbing loops, or an over-bed trapeze. However, some individuals with complete cervical injuries may need assistive devices to perform this skill independently.

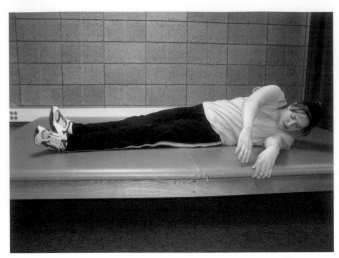

FIG. 20-13 Individual with a C7 incomplete SCI rolling from supine to sidelying using her head and upper extremity reach to turn her upper body.

Moving from supine to sidelying requires a coordinated sequence of movements. Most people will use slight variations of the following (Fig. 20-13):

1. The arms are extended over the chest as far as possible. For individuals without triceps, the hands may be pressed together or the arms lowered slightly toward the hips to allow gravity to help maintain as much elbow extension as possible.
2. Both arms are rocked from side to side in a symmetrical pattern to generate momentum.
3. Flexion and rotation of the head are combined with the arm motion to help move the upper body in the desired direction.
4. Once momentum is gained with the rocking motions of the arm and head, a single forceful rock is used to start the turn, followed by reaching as far as possible with the upper arm, protracting the shoulder, elongating the trunk, and turning the head to rotate the upper body toward prone.
5. The lower body passively follows the upper body into the rotated position.
6. The patient returns to supine by reaching back with the upper arm and turning the head in the desired direction of movement, thus rotating the upper trunk toward supine. Horizontal abduction of the lower shoulder can assist this motion. Once the upper body has rolled past midline, the lower body will follow because of gravity. If needed, the UEs and head can be rocked or forcefully "thrown" in the direction of movement to further turn the upper body to help complete the lower body roll.

During early training, rolling can be made easier in several ways. The roll may be started from a partially turned position rather than from full supine. The LEs may be crossed passively before starting the roll to partially tilt the pelvis and help move the lower body. For individuals without triceps function, air splints may be used to maintain elbow extension and increase the lever arm of the UE rocking motion. With elbows extended, weights may be

added at the wrist to increase the momentum of the rocking motion. The entire mat table may be propped up on one side to tilt the table in the desired direction to allow gravity to further assist with the roll. The therapist may also provide help with the reaching motion in step 4 or help the pelvis to turn to complete the roll. These same techniques may be reversed to further challenge the skill after it has been mastered: Tilting the mat table so the roll is performed up hill, partially flexing the UEs to shorten the lever arm of the rocking motion, providing some manual resistance to the roll at the shoulders or pelvis.

Suggested exercises that may be used to practice components of this activity include bilateral symmetrical UE proprioceptive neuromuscular facilitation (PNF) patterns, incorporating inspiration and expiration with the rhythmic rocking and reaching motions, and strengthening exercise for the serratus anterior and pectoral muscles to facilitate the reach and trunk elongation required to complete the roll.

Supine to Long Sitting Transition. Being able to come to a sitting position from supine assists with ADLs, bed mobility, and preparation for transfers. Several techniques may be used to achieve this skill, depending on the functional muscle groups available. The selected techniques will depend most on whether the triceps muscles and the abdominal muscles are functioning.

Individuals without good triceps or abdominal muscle function will generally use their biceps and assistive devices to move from supine to sitting. Bed rails of various heights and sizes can be used to provide leverage for maneuvering. Some individuals may use a series of webbing loops attached to the foot of the bed (a webbing "ladder") to pull up into a sitting position. The patient puts one forearm through a loop of the ladder, contracts the biceps to partially raise the body, then puts the other arm through the next loop, and pulls further forward. This is repeated, using successive loops, until the body is in the upright long-sitting position.

A technique commonly used for moving from supine to long sitting consists of rolling to the side and then "walking" the upper trunk around on the elbows until the sitting position is achieved. Again, each individual will vary the technique slightly, but the primary steps are the following (Fig. 20-14):

1. Roll toward prone as described (Fig. 20-14, *A*).
2. Move from sidelying or three-quarters–prone to partial-prone lying on elbows. This is a difficult maneuver that usually combines shoulder abduction and depression of the lower arm with horizontal adduction of the upper arm to lever into the on-elbows position (Fig. 20-14, *B*). Functional use of triceps enables a push-up motion onto elbows or directly onto the hands with the elbows extended.
3. The upper body is "walked" on elbows toward the legs. As the legs are approached, it may be possible to use the upper arm to pull on the hips or legs to bring the upper body further toward the legs (Fig. 20-14, *C*).
4. Transition from on-elbows position to on-hands position. Without triceps this involves a push-up motion using pectoral muscles proximally with

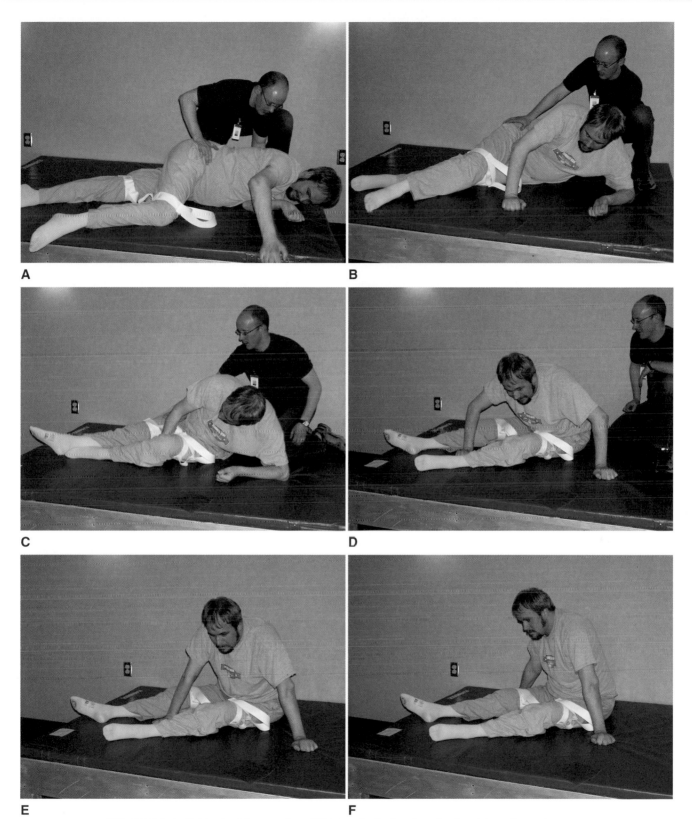

FIG. 20-14 Individual with complete C5 tetraplegia (no functioning triceps) moving from supine to long sitting using the sidelying "walk around" technique.

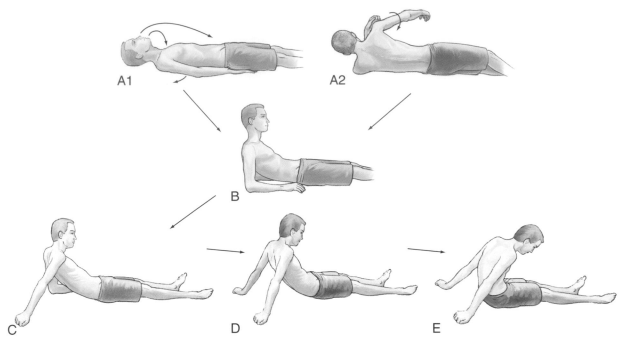

FIG. 20-15 Moving from supine to long sitting using a supine on elbows technique; for individuals with paraplegia or lower cervical tetraplegia.

hands fixed distally (Fig. 20-14, *D*), or "hooking" the legs with the upper arm, pulling with biceps sufficiently to unload the lower arm, which is then quickly repositioned in the extended position. With triceps, this maneuver can be achieved with a traditional push-up maneuver.

5. The upper body is then walked around alternately weight bearing on extended UEs until a balanced long-sitting position is achieved (Fig. 20-14, *E* and *F*).

For individuals with paraplegia or lower cervical tetraplegia, alternative techniques for coming to long sitting are also possible. One possible sequence is as follows (Fig. 20-15):

1. In supine, the hands are caught under the hips and elbow flexion and neck flexion are used to pull up into a position of supine on elbows (Fig. 20-15, *A1*). Alternately, the move is begun from sidelying, with the upper arm rapidly extended at the shoulder with the elbow flexed as the body rolls toward supine to "catch" the weight on that elbow (Fig. 20-15, *A2*). Head lean and rocking of the shoulders are then used to shift the weight onto one elbow while the other shoulder is extended and the flexed elbow is positioned for weight bearing (Fig. 20-15, *B*).

2. Body weight is shifted to one elbow with head and upper body lean while the other arm is fully extended at the shoulder (with the momentum of the shoulder movement used to create elbow extension in the absence of strong triceps), and the hand is then planted on the mat with elbow extended.

This requires good strength and flexibility of the shoulder girdle (Fig. 20-15, *C*).

3. Weight is then shifted onto the arm in extension with a combined rocking and leaning motion until the original support arm is unweighted and can also be reached back into the extended position (Fig. 20-15, *D*)

4. From the position of supporting on extended arms, the upper body is moved forward by leaning the head forward, alternate side shifting, and slow forward movements of the hands until a balanced long-sitting position is achieved (Fig. 20-15, *E*).

This technique may also be used by some higher level tetraplegics with exceptional balance and proximal UE control.

For patients with at least partial control of the abdominal muscles, a head and trunk curl motion can be used to initiate coming to sitting and then augmented as needed by pushing up with the UEs. With fully intact abdominal muscles, patients with lower paraplegia may be able to perform a traditional sit-up, although they may need to use their UEs for assistance because the LE muscles will not be able to stabilize the pelvis.

Exercises that may be used to practice components of this activity include PNF mobility and controlled mobility techniques while in supine on elbows, partially prone on elbows, or in long sitting with weight on extended arms; static and dynamic balance activities in long sitting; biceps curls in the supine position; and push-ups and partial push-ups in prone, long sitting, or short sitting.

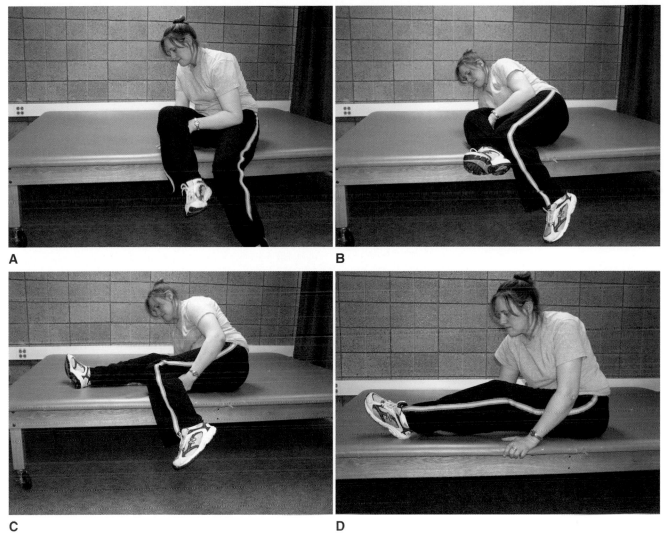

FIG. 20-16 Individual with incomplete C7 tetraplegia moving from short-sitting to long-sitting.

Transitioning from Short Sitting to Long Sitting to Supine. When transferring from a wheelchair to lying down, the individual generally goes from sitting in the wheelchair to short sitting on another surface, then getting the legs on to the new surface and ultimately moving into a supine position. These transitions require good balance and coordination, as well as sufficient hamstring length. LE and/or trunk spasticity can interfere with these transitions.

Individuals with midcervical tetraplegia can use the following steps to bring their legs up onto the bed, moving from short sitting to long sitting. In this example the individual is turned to his or her right (Fig. 20-16):

1. In the short-sitting position, scoot as far back as possible on the seating surface (at least until the popliteal fossa contacts the edge) and partially turn the upper body toward the end of the bed where the feet will ultimately be positioned.

2. Support on the lead (right) arm while using the trailing (left) arm to begin lifting the right leg onto the mat (Fig. 20-16, *A*). For individuals without grasp function, the wrist or the forearm is hooked under the leg to lift it, or the leg is lifted with a webbing leg loop secured around the distal thigh. At this point, it may be necessary to drop onto the elbow of the lead arm to gain enough stability and leverage to lift the weight of the leg (Fig. 20-16, *B*).

3. Once the lead leg is securely on the mat, the body may be scooted sideways, further onto the mat, using a partial long-sit push-up technique or, if propped on elbow in step 2, by pulling the body on the elbows in commando fashion.

4. The second leg is then lifted onto the mat using a similar technique as the first, the legs are then straightened into extension, and balance achieved in long sitting (Fig. 20-16, *C* and *D*).

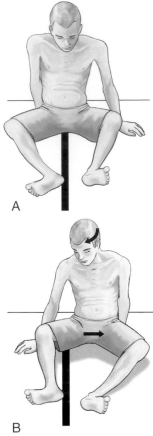

FIG. 20-17 Seated scooting. Note the use of the head-hips relationship.

5. Any of the supine to long sitting techniques described earlier can be reversed to complete the transition to supine (lean to side and "walk" around on elbows, extend arms behind body, and flex elbows into supine-on-elbows position).

Seated Scooting. The ability to move from side to side in the seated position improves functional capabilities in transfers and bed mobility. Scooting can be performed with similar techniques in the long-sitting and the short-sitting position (Fig. 20-17):

1. Weight is supported on extended UEs with one arm positioned next to the body, and the arm on the lead side (desired direction of movement) abducted to place the hand a small distance from the hip.
2. A push-up is performed with the head lowered and leaned forward as described in the short sitting section above (Fig. 20-17, *A*).
3. Once the hips are off the mat the head is rotated to the side away from the desired direction of movement, and the hips are twisted in the desired direction (Fig. 20-17, *B*).
4. The hips are then lowered to the mat and the arms repositioned to attain a balanced position.
5. Weight bearing is shifted to the lead arm, and the following arm is used to pull the legs toward the lead arm and back into alignment with the pelvis.

Patients without good grip may use webbing leg loops to help control the LEs.

During these actions the head is always moving in the opposite direction from the hips around a pivot point at the shoulders; the head is lowered and brought forward to raise the hips, and the head is moved to the side to move the hips in the opposite direction. This principle is known as the *head-hips relationship* and is frequently used during mobility skills involving UE weight bearing.

Transfers. Transitioning from one surface to another (e.g., from a wheelchair to bed) requires combinations of the mobility, balance, and motor control developed in the postures and movement sequences described previously. The basic sequence of the transfer is similar in most circumstances, although the individual's pattern of motor preservation, body proportions, endurance, and personal preferences will determine the exact technique used for various transfer situations. In all situations, the following general guidelines should be observed during transfers:

1. The buttocks should be lifted and not dragged between surfaces. If the individual cannot do this alone, manual assistance should be provided and/or a sliding board or similar device should be used to minimize shear forces during scooting.
2. The environment should be arranged before transferring to allow the most level, controlled transfer possible.
3. Use of momentum for movement should be minimized, with emphasis placed on slow, controlled movements.
4. Early in transfer training, just enough assistance and instruction should be provided to allow for successful performance of the skill. It is important that the individual accomplish the task as independently as possible so that they gain a sense of independence and control.

The transfer is generally begun by positioning the transfer surfaces. When transferring from the wheelchair, the chair is generally positioned at a 30- to 45-degree angle to the mat table (or other surface). This allows the patient to stay in front of the wheelchair wheel during the transfer. The feet are then positioned in preparation for the transfer; with rigid frame chairs, one or both feet may be left on the foot plate and turned slightly in the direction of the transfer, with folding frame chairs, the footrests are usually removed and the feet placed flat on the floor, and for individuals with poor balance control the feet may be lifted onto the mat to put the individual in a more stable long-sit position before beginning the scooting portion of the transfer. The pelvis is then moved forward slightly in the chair to bring the hips closer to the transfer surface, to move the hips anterior to the wheelchair wheel, and to put some weight through the LEs (Fig. 20-18, *A*). Tetraplegic patients often achieve this forward scooting by twisting the head and upper body with one arm hooked around the push handle of the wheelchair, and then repeating this technique on the other side.

If a sliding board is required (generally for individuals with midcervical SCI without triceps or during initial training for patients with lower level injuries) the board is

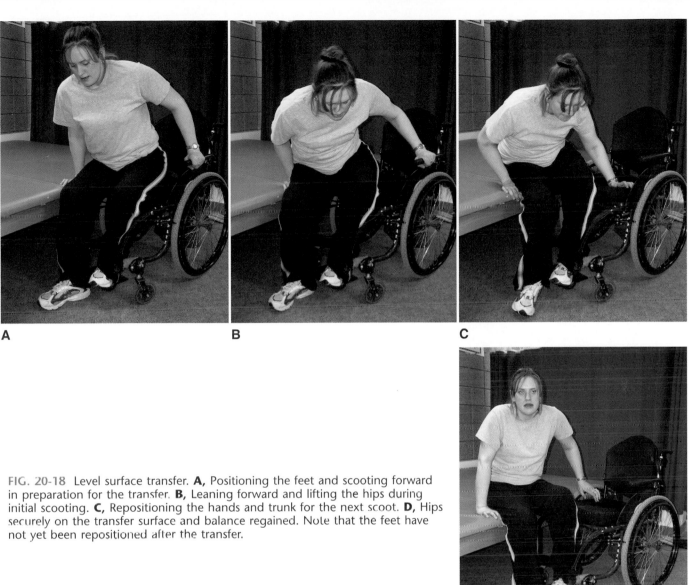

FIG. 20-18 Level surface transfer. **A,** Positioning the feet and scooting forward in preparation for the transfer. **B,** Leaning forward and lifting the hips during initial scooting. **C,** Repositioning the hands and trunk for the next scoot. **D,** Hips securely on the transfer surface and balance regained. Note that the feet have not yet been repositioned after the transfer.

placed under the midthigh of the lead leg and angled toward the ischial tuberosity on the opposite side. The individual then leans the head forward, performs a push-up, lifts the hips, and pivots the head away from the transfer surface—thus using the head-hips relationship to swing the hips toward the transfer surface (Fig. 20-18, *B*). The hips are lowered, balance is regained and hands repositioned (see Fig. 20-18, *C*), and then the sequence is repeated until the hips are securely positioned on the transfer surface (Fig. 20-18, *D*). The legs may be repositioned after each scoot, if needed for balance, or they may be left to trail the body and repositioned after the final sitting position is achieved. Variations on this basic technique are used for transfers to a bathtub bench, toilet, car, or any other relatively level surface.

Patients with high cervical level injuries will be physically dependent for transfers but should become independent in directing the required assistance before they are discharged from rehabilitation. A mechanical lift can be used to transfer a patient in the hospital or the modified home setting. A mechanical lift, although cumbersome at times, reduces the long-term strain on caregivers who have to repeatedly lift and move an individual. In situations where a mechanical lift is impractical, a pivot transfer with a sliding board and assistance by one or two people is generally used. Note that it is still important that the person being transferred has their feet on the floor, if possible, to allow partial weight bearing through the legs (which are braced by the assistant's legs) and reduce the lift required during the transfer. The head-hips relationship should also be employed; the individual being transferred has his or her head and upper trunk turning away from the transfer surface and hips moving toward the transfer surface. In this case, the weight-bearing pivot point for the head-hips relationship is the feet of the individual being transferred. Care must be taken to avoid pulling on the UEs during assisted transfers to avoid straining unstable shoulder joints.

Transferring from the floor into the wheelchair is an advanced skill that is mastered only after the individual has mastered level surface transfers and developed considerable strength, flexibility, and coordination. Variations on a few basic techniques are used to accomplish this skill. The first technique begins with the individual positioned next to and approximately parallel to the front edge of the wheelchair. The lead hand is placed on the wheelchair seat, and the other hand is placed next to the hip (Fig. 20-19, *A*). The legs may be flexed up and held in place by leaning into them with the head and shoulders, or they may be left straight during the transfer. The individual then leans the head as far forward as possible and pushes with the arms to raise their hips to the edge of the wheelchair seat (Fig. 20-19, *B* and *C*). Once the lead hip is securely on the seat a series of small lifts and scoots may be used to bring both hips firmly onto the

seating surface. The trunk is brought into the upright position by pushing up with the arms on the front of the wheelchair frame or seat (Fig. 20-19, *D*). This skill can be made easier by removing the wheelchair cushion from the chair (effectively reducing the height required with the lift) and using it under the hips on the floor (effectively raising the floor surface and further reducing the lift required). The skill may also be trained or simplified by using intermediate height surfaces to break-up the task.

Another technique for moving from the floor to a chair is to use a front push-up from an intermediate quadruped position. The knees are positioned by the front of the wheelchair and the individual pulls himself or herself up on the chair until his or her weight is distributed on the knees on the floor and on the chest resting on the seat of the chair. A push-up is then performed with the hands on the wheelchair seat until the hips clear the edge of the chair. The individual then twists and pivots the trunk to move the lead hip onto the seating surface. The hands are then repositioned, and additional push-ups are performed to bring the hips fully into the seated position. Because of the large twisting motion required by this technique, it is most effectively used by an individual with some degree of active trunk control.

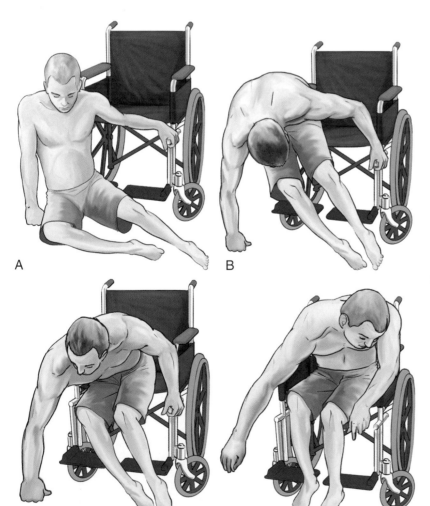

A

B

C

D

FIG. 20-19 Floor to chair transfer using "one hand up, one hand down" technique.

Another option is to use a back push-up (Fig. 20-20). The individual begins in sitting with his or her back to the chair seat and reaches back and up with both arms until the hands are on the top of the wheelchair frame or the front edge of the seat. A push-up is then performed to lift the body into the chair. This technique requires a lot of strength in a mechanically disadvantageous position of extreme shoulder extension and elevation.

Although some individuals with SCI will master independent floor transfers, all patients with SCI should be independent in directing others to safely and effectively move them from the floor to a chair. This should be practiced in the rehabilitation setting so that when the individual either intentionally or accidentally finds

themselves on the floor or ground they are not intimidated by the circumstances and can be in control of safely returning to the wheelchair.

Functional Training in Leisure Integration or Reintegration. Advances in wheelchair and other adaptive device technology have made many leisure and recreational opportunities open to individuals with SCI. Sports like tennis, basketball, and quad rugby draw many participants and have competitions at every level from local to international. Recreational activities like snow skiing and water skiing may also be enjoyed by individuals with all levels of mobility (Fig. 20-21). Specific competitions and team events have been developed for individuals using power wheelchair mobility. Therapists can assist in prepa-

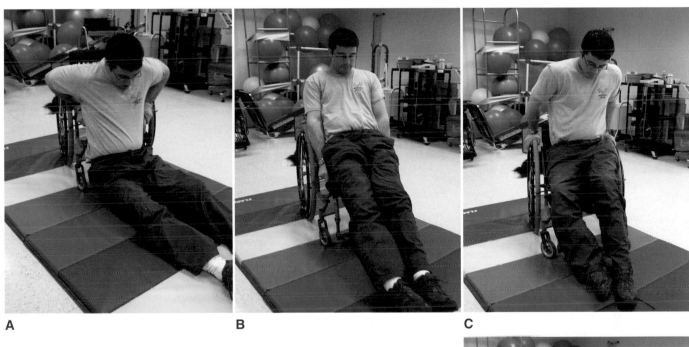

A   **B**   **C**

FIG. 20-20 Individual with complete T10 paraplegia performing floor-to-chair transfer using the back push-up technique. Note spasticity producing extension of the trunk and lower extremities in **B.**

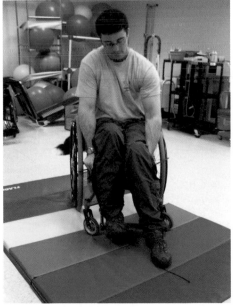

D

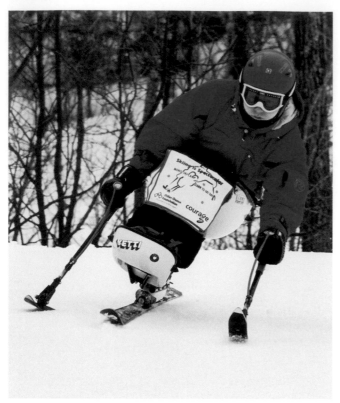

FIG. 20-21 Individual with paraplegia participating in a snow skiing event.

ration for these activities by providing assessment for adaptive devices, training in activity-specific mobility skills, strength building and conditioning, and education about injury prevention and management. Referral should also be made to school, community, state, and national programs that can provide information and assistance that will allow individuals to pursue areas of interest.

Airway Clearance Techniques. As the patient becomes more medically stable and physically active during rehabilitation, a number of respiratory interventions may be added to those begun during the acute phase. Initial emphasis is on improving active mobilization and expectoration of secretions. Expectoration is addressed by techniques designed to improve the ability to cough. Intervention may involve manual assistive cough techniques, including but not limited to "quad cough" (forceful expiration assist provided via a Heimlich-type or abdominal thrust maneuver), costophrenic assist, anterior chest compressions, or trunk counter-rotation.[5,11,89] Patients may learn to do self-assisted versions of the quad cough by using techniques like positioning their hands under the rib cage and using biceps to pull up and in, or by timing a forward trunk lean with the expulsion phase of coughing. Individuals with sufficient balance and inspiratory lung volume may also learn to utilize an independent airway clearance strategy called active cycle of breathing (ACB) followed by a forced expiratory technique (FET)[89,127] (see Chapter 24).

Once the individual is upright, obtaining proper postural alignment will assist with facilitation of respiratory muscles. Alignment should include slight shoulder retraction (opening of the anterior chest wall), shoulder neutral or external rotation, thoracic spine extension, and pelvic positioning that avoids excessive posterior tilt. This alignment facilitates recruitment of primary and accessory breathing muscles and prevents the development of secondary postures (e.g., kyphosis) that may impair respiratory capacity.[5,89]

Pairing respiratory efforts with complimentary movements and cues can help to maximize both the breathing effort and the mobility skills.[5,89] If a task involves trunk extension (over head reaching, UE PNF flexion patterns, rolling sidelying to supine, etc), it may be paired with inspiration (expansion of thoracic cage). Conversely, movements involving thoracic flexion and compression (forward lean or reach, rolling supine to sidelying with head and upper trunk flexion pattern, PNF extension patterns) should be paired with expiratory efforts. Concentric trunk and extremity movements can be paired with concentric respiratory movements and eccentric with eccentric. Manual cues and verbal cues can also be used to facilitate the appropriate combination of movements, with strong cues associated with concentric (inspiratory or expiratory) breathing efforts and slower, softer cues associated with eccentric (expiratory) breathing efforts. By combining the appropriate cues and movements, the efficiency of both mobility and breathing are increased and the benefits of interventions for training mobility skills are compounded.

The endurance and power of the respiratory system can be augmented with training of the respiratory musculature. The length and control of expiratory efforts can be practiced with common activities like singing, humming, or blowing through a straw or blow toy, etc. Incentive spirometers with target ranges can be used for repetitive breathing exercise. Utilizing ventilatory muscle training devices (VMTs) strengthens breathing by adding resistance to respiratory muscle contractions. Most VMT training programs are used during the rehabilitation phase for 15-20 minutes, 2 times per day, 5-7 days per week for approximately 6 weeks. Studies have shown improvement in inspiratory muscle strength and endurance, and subjective reports of decreased breathing effort with the use of VMT training.[128,129]

CASE STUDY 20-1

COMPLETE SPINAL CORD INJURY AT T10

Examination
Patient History
JD is a 20-year-old student who was involved in a MVA 22 days ago. He was admitted to the trauma center with a fracture and complete SCI at the level of T10. He sustained fractures of his ninth, tenth, and eleventh ribs on the right. He was initially immobilized in a thoracolumbosacral orthosis (TLSO) of a plastic body-jacket style. He underwent spinal stabilization surgery. His stay was complicated by pneumonia with decreased secretion clear-

ance. Acute therapies involved ROM, positioning in bed and transitioning to sitting, patient and family education, and active breathing exercises. JD was unable to tolerate assisted coughing or manual facilitation for respiration because of pain from soft tissue bruising and rib fractures. JD used the TLSO at all times when out of bed and no brace when in bed per his physician's instructions. After 3 weeks in the hospital, the pneumonia was resolving and JD was considered medically stable and appropriate for further rehabilitation in an inpatient rehabilitation center.

Past medical history was significant only for a right knee meniscectomy 3 years ago with good functional recovery. JD's medications at time of admission to inpatient rehabilitation included heparin (prophylaxis for DVT), meperidine (Demerol) for pain, and docusate sodium (Colace) as a stool softener. His resolving pneumonia was also being treated with antibiotics.

Systems Review

The patient is 5 foot 11 inches tall and weighs 183 lb. Heart rate was 80 bpm and BP was 110/68 mm Hg at rest in supine and remained unchanged on coming to sit in bed. Respiratory rate was 14 breaths per minute with a diaphragmatic breathing pattern.

Tests and Measures

Musculoskeletal

Range of Motion Active ROM in both UEs was grossly within normal limits. LE PROM was within normal limits except dorsiflexion was not measured in the end range of hip flexion and straight leg raise was not tested because of JD's recent spine surgery.

Muscle Performance Strength throughout both UEs was greater than or equal to 4/5 on manual muscle testing. JD had no active movement or visible contractions in either LE and strength was therefore graded as 0/5. Lower extremities are hypotonic throughout. Trunk strength was not tested formally with resisted motion through ROM because of pain and postsurgical restrictions. However, JD could isometrically contract his upper abdominal muscles sufficiently to produce a visible and palpable contraction. He is able to breathe with a normal breathing pattern when cued but prefers a shallow, diaphragmatic breathing pattern with little anteroposterior chest expansion at rest because it is less painful.

Neuromuscular

Arousal, Attention, Cognition JD is alert and oriented, and his cognition is grossly intact.

Pain JD reported some back pain around the surgical site. Rib pain was present at all times (rated 2/10 at rest) and increased with deep breathing, moving, and donning the TLSO (8/10 at worst). Oral medications were being used for pain, with pain remaining less than or equal to 3/10 during mobility with the medications.

Sensory Integrity JD had intact sensation in all modalities (light touch, sharp, vibration, kinesthesia, proprioception, and pain) above the umbilicus and absent sensation in all modalities below the umbilicus.

Motor Function—Control and Learning Coordination was grossly within normal limits (WNL) in both UEs.

LE coordination could not be tested secondary to the absence of active movement.

Cardiovascular/Pulmonary: JD was noted to be short of breath during wheelchair propulsion and practice of mobility skills. JD's vital capacity was measured to be 40% lower than normal for a person of his age and height.

Integumentary

Integumentary Integrity JD's skin was intact throughout the extremities, sacrum, and ischia with no areas of redness. Surgical incisions covered with dressings were present at the thoracic spine and over the bone graft donor site at the pelvis. These sites were not directly observed because occlusive dressings were in place, but nursing reported that the wounds were healing gradually without evidence of infection.

Function

Gait, Locomotion, and Balance JD could propel his wheelchair independently on a smooth, level surfaces for 50 feet. Sitting at the edge of a treatment mat, JD could maintain his balance statically with bilateral UE support with stand-by assistance. He was unable to maintain sitting balance without using his UEs, and he had poor dynamic balance.

Assistive and Adaptive Devices JD used a manual wheelchair with swing-away leg rests. A pressure relief cushion was used at all times in the wheelchair. He had been using an over-head trapeze for mobility in bed but was trying to wean off of this device. The bed JD was using had a pressure relieving over-lay. He used a long-handled reacher and a leg loop for ADL skills and an incentive spirometer to encourage deep breathing.

Self-Care and Home Management JD required maximal assistance from one person and a sliding board to transfer between level surfaces. He required moderate assistance from one person for all bed mobility. JD was dependent for all ADLs except that he could feed himself independently after he, his food, and utensils had been set-up. JD was incontinent of bowel and bladder. His indwelling catheter had been removed, and he was started on an intermittent catheterization program that he was learning to perform himself. He was on an every other day bowel elimination program.

Evaluation, Diagnosis, and Prognosis

JD presented with impairments of loss of muscle function and sensation below T10 and diminished respiratory capacity. His injury was classified as ASIA A, complete paraplegia. FIM scores were 2 for transfers and 2 for locomotion.

Functional limitations included limited ability with transfers, ADLs, IADLs, decreased endurance, and decreased functional mobility at either the wheelchair or ambulatory level. He was at high risk for complications of the respiratory, GI, and integumentary systems and for depression. He was also unable at the time of evaluation to perform in his roles as student, employee, and recreational athlete.

JD's findings were consistent with preferred practice pattern 5H: Impaired motor function, peripheral nerve integrity, and sensory integrity associated with nonprogressive disorders of the spinal cord.

Goals

1. JD and his identified caregivers will be independent with the skills required to prevent, recognize, and provide initial treatment for potential secondary complications of SCI.
2. JD will be independent with all bed mobility without adaptive devices.
3. JD will be independent with all approximately level transfers required for performance of ADLs.
4. JD will be modified independent with wheelchair mobility for at least 500 feet on indoor surfaces and community surfaces that meet accessibility codes.
5. JD will require moderate assistance or less with advanced transfers and advanced wheelchair mobility skills.
6. JD and his caregivers will be independent with home exercise programs for flexibility, strengthening, and endurance training.
7. JD will have respiratory capacity and endurance equal to approximately 80% of normal for his age and height.

Prognosis

JD's prognosis is good because of his supportive social structure, his intact cognitive skills, and his normal UE function. Factors that may have limited or slowed his progress were the restrictions in movement imposed by the TLSO and the pain present with activities that stress the rib fracture and thoracic surgery areas.

Plan of Care

Approximately 50 visits over a 4-week period.

Intervention

Patient-Related Instruction

Education: Because JD is at high risk for skin breakdown and because this complication could impede progress in all other areas of mobility training, providing education and training in skin care was vital for JD. Skin care training included education for JD and his caregivers about pressure relief techniques, bed and wheelchair positioning, and skin protection during mobility skills. JD was encouraged to turn every 2 hours in bed and to perform a pressure relief technique (he preferred a forward lean because push-ups increased his rib and back pain) for 2 minutes out of every 15 minutes of sitting. Physical therapy also reinforced education related to skin care from other rehabilitation team members including diet (especially hydration), hygiene, bowel, and bladder programs.

Procedural Interventions

Respiratory Training: Because of his history of pneumonia and his altered preferred breathing pattern, improving respiratory function was a priority for early care for JD. Mobilizations and other manual techniques that otherwise may have been applicable to respiratory care were not aggressively performed because rib fractures and pain prevented these procedures. Therefore respiratory training consisted of incentive spirometry, ventilatory muscle training twice a day for 3 weeks until active effort improved, breathing techniques education and practice, cardiovascular conditioning, and positioning for postural drainage.

Mobility Skills Training: Mobility skills training was the focus of JD's physical therapy. Mobility skills included training in the use of his wheelchair, mobility in bed, training in sitting balance, and transfer training. JD was trained to use his wheelchair on level and uneven surfaces and on ramps and stairs (with assistance as needed), and was trained in how to manage doorways, elevators and escalators. Bed mobility skills training included training in rolling and moving from supine to sitting, and from sitting to supine. JD was also trained to maintain balance when long sitting and short sitting and to transfer on level surfaces, up and down uneven surfaces, in and out of a vehicle, up and down from the floor, on and off of a commode, and into and out of a bathtub.

Training in ADLs and IADLs: Training in ADLs and IADLs were coordinated with other rehabilitation team members to teach and reinforce skills required for dressing, bathing, toileting, utilizing adapted equipment, and performing household and community level tasks.

Therapeutic Exercise: Therapeutic exercises included flexibility exercises and training in self range of motion activities for the LEs. In addition, muscle strength and endurance training was performed with an emphasis on the shoulder and scapular muscles utilized during mobility skills.

Modalities: The use of FES and biofeedback were considered for muscle reeducation but were not introduced during the initial treatment sessions.

Gait Training: Gait training was initiated with standing in a standing frame for building tolerance to being in an upright position and to maintain ROM. In addition, JD participated in body weight–supported locomotor training. At the time of initial training, JD required maximal assistance for stepping during gait training. It was planned that his standing and gait training programs would be progressed, depending on the level and degree of return of LE strength.

Integration: JD was introduced to wheelchair level sport and recreation activities as part of his functional training. An opportunity was arranged for him to meet with a peer counselor. JD was referred to a community organization that provides sport and recreational opportunities for individuals with disabilities.

Please see the CD that accompanies this book for a case study describing the examination, evaluation, and intervention for a patient with anterior cord syndrome.

CHAPTER SUMMARY

SCI alters the function of multiple body systems, including the GI, skeletal, respiratory, cardiovascular, genitourinary, integumentary, musculoskeletal, and neuromuscular systems. Many of these changes require ongoing medical management and changes in an individual's activities of daily living. Some of the possible systemic effects of SCI, such as pressure ulcers or AD, are potentially life-threatening. A careful plan of care developed and administered by a diverse team of rehabilitation professionals is necessary to manage the acute needs of the SCI patient and provide a rehabilitation process that will prepare the individual to lead a healthy and fulfilling life after injury.

ADDITIONAL RESOURCES

Useful Forms

ASIA Standard Neurological Classification of Spinal Cord Injury Form
The Wheelchair Circuit Test
Walking Index for Spinal Cord Injury (WISCI)

Web Sites

Paralyzed Veterans of America: www.pva.org
Spinal Cord Injury Information Network: www.spinalcord.uab.edu
The National SCI Statistical Center: www.NSCISC@uab.edu
The American Spinal Injury Association (ASIA): www.asia-spinalinjury.org
The Miami Project to Cure Paralysis: www.miamiproject.miami.edu
Wheelchair Sports, USA: www.wsusa.org

GLOSSARY

Anterior cord syndrome: Destruction of the anterior portion of the spinal cord that results in a pattern of impairments characterized by complete loss of motor function and some loss of light touch and temperature sensation, with sparing of proprioception and discriminative touch.

Autonomic dysreflexia (AD): A serious, life-threatening emergency condition that is the result of an uncontrolled autonomic response to a noxious stimulus from either an external or an internal (visceral) source.

Brown-Séquard syndrome: Damage to one-half of the spinal cord, resulting in a pattern of impairments characterized by ipsilateral proprioceptive and motor loss and contralateral loss of pain and temperature sensation.

Cauda equina syndrome: Damage to the lumbar or sacral nerve roots, resulting in sensory loss and flaccid paralysis below the injury level.

Central cord syndrome: Injury to the central portion of the spinal cord, resulting in a pattern of impairments characterized by weakness more severe in UEs than in LEs, with sparing of sacral sensation.

Central pattern generators: Neural circuits within the spinal cord that are able to produce.

Head-hips relationship: Descriptive term describing a mechanical principle used during mobility skills, with UE weight bearing the shoulders act as a fulcrum; the head and hips move in opposite directions around this point.

Heterotopic ossification (HO): Abnormal bone growth within the extraarticular soft tissues that can result in severe restriction of muscle and joint movement.

Motor level: The most caudal segment of the spinal cord with normal motor function on both sides of the body.

Neurological level: The most caudal segment of the spinal cord with normal sensory and motor function on both sides of the body.

Paradoxical breathing: An abnormal breathing pattern common in tetraplegia and occurring occasionally in high paraplegia, in which the abdomen rises and the chest is pulled in on inspiration and the abdomen falls and the chest expands on expiration.

Paraplegia: Loss of function in the thoracic, lumbar, or sacral segments of the spinal cord, resulting in sparing of UE function but possible impairments in the trunk, pelvis, and LEs, depending on the segment of the lesion.

Pressure ulcer: A common complication of SCI characterized by ischemic ulceration of soft tissue as a result of unrelieved pressure and shearing forces.

Quadriplegia: SCI affecting all four extremities; synonym for tetraplegia.

Sensory level: The most caudal segment of the spinal cord with normal sensory function on both sides of the body.

Skeletal level: The spinal level at which the greatest vertebral damage is found after spinal injury.

Spasticity: A disorder that can occur below the level of SCI characterized by velocity-dependent hypertonia, resulting from a combination of multiple changes in neural control and muscle properties.

Spinal cord injury (SCI): Damage to the neurological components of the spinal cord as the result of primary or secondary effects of disease or trauma.

Spinal shock: A temporary condition that occurs after acute SCI, characterized by a total loss of sensory, motor, and autonomic control below the level of the lesion.

Tenodesis grip: Use of the passive properties of the long finger flexors to perform grasp functions. With the finger flexors slightly tight, the motion of wrist extension is used to pull the fingers toward the palm in a grasping motion.

Tetraplegia: Loss of function because of damage of the neural elements in the cervical segments of the spinal cord, resulting in impairment or loss of motor and/or sensory function involving the upper extremities, as well as more caudal functions.

Zone of partial preservation (ZPP): Those dermatomes and myotomes caudal to the neurological level that remain partially innervated (in the absence of sacral function) in complete SCI.

References

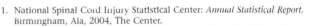

1. National Spinal Cord Injury Statistical Center: *Annual Statistical Report,* Birmingham, Ala, 2004, The Center.
2. National Spinal Cord Injury Statistical Center: *Spinal Cord Injury Facts and Figures at a Glance,* Birmingham, Ala, 2004, The Center.
3. Senelick R, Dougherty K: *The Spinal Cord Injury Handbook,* Birmingham, Ala, 1998, HealthSouth Press.
4. Fuller KS: Traumatic spinal cord injury. In Goodman CC, Fuller KS, Boissonnault WG (eds): *Pathology: Implications for the Physical Therapist,* ed 2, Philadelphia, 2003, WB Saunders.
5. Buchanan LE, Nawoczenski DA (eds): *Spinal Cord Injury: Concepts and Management Approaches,* Baltimore, 1987, Williams & Wilkins.
6. Basso DM: Neuroanatomical substrates of functional recovery after experimental spinal cord injury: Implications of basic science research for human spinal cord injury, *Phys Ther* 80(8):808-817, 2000.
7. Mautes A, Weinzierl M, Donovan F, et al: Vascular events after spinal cord injury: contribution to secondary pathogenesis, *Phys Ther* 80:673-687, 2000.
8. Dusart I, Schwab ME: Secondary cell data and the inflammatory reaction after dorsal hemisection of the rat spinal cord, *Eur J Neurosci* 6:712-724, 1994.
9. Beattie MS, Bresnahan JC: Cell death, repair, and recovery of function after spinal cord contusion injuries in rats. In Kalb RG, Strettmatter SM (eds): *Neurobiology of Spinal Cord Injury,* Totowa, NJ, 2000, Human Press.
10. Bregman BS: Transplants and neurotrophins modify the response of developing and mature CNS neurons to spinal cord injury. In Kalb RG, Strettmatter SM (eds): *Neurobiology of Spinal Cord Injury,* Totowa, NJ, 2000, Human Press.
11. Bromley I: *Tetraplegia and Paraplegia: A Guide for Physiotherapists,* ed 3, Edinburgh, 1998, Churchill Livingstone.
12. Marino RJ (ed): *International Standards for Neurological Classification of Spinal Cord Injury,* ed 5, Chicago, Ill, 2000, American Spinal Injury Association.
13. Lundy-Ekman L: *Neuroscience: Fundamentals for Rehabilitation,* Philadelphia, 1998, WB Saunders.
14. Chen D, Apple DF, Hudson LM, et al: Medical complications during acute rehabilitation following spinal cord injury—current experience of the model systems, *Arch Phys Med Rehabil* 80:1397-1401, 1999.
15. Carter P, Edwards S: General principles of treatment. In Edwards S (ed): *Neurological Physiotherapy,* ed 2, Edinburgh, 2002, Churchill Livingstone.
16. Blackmer J: Rehabilitation medicine: Autonomic dysreflexia, *Can Med Assoc J* 169(9):931-935, 2003.
17. Consortium for Spinal Cord Medicine Clinical Practice Guidelines: *Acute Management of Autonomic Dysreflexia: Individuals with Spinal Cord Injury Presenting to Health-Care Facilities,* Washington, DC, 2001, Paralyzed Veterans of America.
18. Spinal Cord Injury InfoSheet No. 13: *Prevention of Pressure Sores through Skin Care,* Birmingham, Ala, 2000, Medical RRTC on Secondary Conditions of SCI.
19. Consortium for Spinal Cord Medicine Clinical Practice Guidelines: *Pressure Ulcer Prevention and Treatment Following Spinal Cord Injury,* Washington, DC, 2000, Paralyzed Veterans of America.
20. Krause JS: Skin sores after spinal cord injury: Relationship to life adjustment, *Spinal Cord* 36:51-56, 1998.

21. Centers for Disease Control and Prevention/National Center for Injury Prevention and Control: *Injury Fact Book 2001-2002,* Available at http://www.cdc.gov/ncipc/fact_book/25_Spinal_Cord_Injury.htm. Accessed September 9, 2004.
22. American Physical Therapy Association: *Guide to Physical Therapist Practice,* ed 2, Alexandria, Va, 2001, The Association.
23. Steins SA, Bergman SB, Goetz LL: Neurogenic bowel dysfunction after spinal cord injury: clinical evaluation and rehabilitative management, *Arch Phys Med Rehabil* 78:S86-S102, 1997.
24. Consortium for Spinal Cord Medicine Clinical Practice Guidelines: *Neurogenic Bowel Management in Adults with Spinal Cord Injury,* Washington, DC, 1998, Paralyzed Veterans of America.
25. Eser P, deBruin ED, Telley I, et al: Effect of electrical stimulation-induced cycling on bone mineral density in spinal cord-injured patients, *Eur J Clin Invest* 33(5):412-419, 2003.
26. Szollar SM, Martin EME, Sartoris DJ, et al: Bone mineral density and indexes of bone metabolism in spinal cord injury, *Am J Phys Med Rehabil* 77:28-35, 1998.
27. Garland DE, Stewart CA, Adkins RH, et al: Osteoporosis after spinal cord injury, *J Orthop Res* 10:371-378, 1992.
28. Garlamd DE, Maric Z, Adkins RH, et al: Bone mineral density about the knee in spinal cord injured patients with pathological fractures, *Contemp Orthop* 26:375-379, 1993.
29. Hangartner TN, Rodgers MM, Glaser RM, et al: Tibial bone density loss in spinal cord injured patients. Effects of RES exercise, *J Rehabil Res Dev* 31:50-61, 1994.
30. Bloomfield SA, Mysiw WJ, Jackson RD: Bone mass and endocrine adaptations to training in spinal cord injured individuals, *Bone* 19:61-68, 1996.
31. Silver J: Letter to the editor, *Spinal Cord* 41:421-422, 2003.
32. Van Kuijk A, Geurts A, van Kuppevelt H: Letter to the editor, *Spinal Cord* 41:423-424, 2003.
33. Spinal Cord Injury InfoSheet No. 19: *Understanding and Managing Respiratory Complications after SCI,* Birmingham, Ala, 2001, Office of Research Services.
34. Clough P: Restrictive lung dysfunction. In Hillegass E, Sadowsky HS (eds): *Essentials of Cardiopulmonary Physical Therapy,* ed 2, Philadelphia, 2001, WB Saunders.
35. Chiou-Tan FY, Garza H, Chan KT, et al: Comparison of Dalteparin and Enoxaparin for deep venous thrombosis prophylaxis in patients with spinal cord injury, *Am J Phys Med Rehabil* 82(9):678-685, 2003.
36. Green D, Hartwig D, Chen D, et al: Spinal cord injury risk assessment for thromboembolism, *Am J Phys Med Rehabil* 82(12):950-956, 2003.
37. Chiou-Tan FY, Garza H, Chan KT, et al: Comparison of Dalteparin and Enoxaparin for deep venous thrombosis prophylaxis in patients with spinal cord injury, *Am J Phys Med Rehabil* 82(9):678-685, 2003.
38. Kemp B, Spungen E, Adkins R, et al: The relationship among serum lipid levels, adiposity, and depressive symptomology in persons aging with spinal cord injury, *J Spinal Cord Med* 23:216-220, 2000.
39. Spinal Cord Injury InfoSheet No 3: *Sexual Function for Men with SCI,* Birmingham, Ala, 2000, Office of Research Services.
40. Amador M, Lynne C, Brackett N: *A Guide and Resource Directory to Male Fertility Following Spinal Cord Injury/Dysfunction,* Miami, Fla, 2000, Miami Project to Cure Paralysis.
41. Amble J, Lannoye-Amble R: The winding road of infertility: the successful path to parenthood with an SCI, *SCI Nurs* 19(3):113-116, 2002.
42. Cardenas D, Farrell-Roberts L, Sipski M, et al: In Stover S, DeLisa J, Whiteneck G, eds. *Spinal Cord Injury: Clinical Outcomes from the Model Systems,* Gaithersburg, Md, 1995, Aspen Publishers.
43. Spinal Cord Injury InfoSheet No. 21: *Sexuality for Women with Spinal Cord Injury,* Birmingham, Ala, 2002, Office of Research Services.
44. Jackson A, Wadley V: A multicenter study of women's self-reported reproductive health after spinal cord injury, *Arch Phys Med Rehab* 80(11):1420-1428, 1999.
45. Spinal Cord Injury InfoSheet No. 14: *Pregnancy for Women with Spinal Cord Injury,* Birmingham, Ala, 2003, Office of Research Services.
46. Bake E, Cardenas D, Benedetti T: Risks associated with pregnancy in spinal cord injured women, *Obstet Gynecol* 80:425-428, 1992.
47. Marino RJ (ed): *International Standards for Neurological Classification of Spinal Cord Injury,* ed 5, Chicago, Ill, 2000, American Spinal Injury Association.
48. Folstein MF, Folstein SE, McHugh PR: Mini-mental state: a practical method for grading the cognitive state of patients for the clinician, *J Psychiatr Res* 12:189-198, 1975.
49. Budh C, Lund I, Ertzgaard P, et al: Pain in a Swedish spinal cord injury population, *Clin Rehabil* 17:685-690, 2003.
50. McDonald H, Fish W: Pain during spinal cord injury rehabilitation: Client perspectives and staff attitudes, *SCI Nurs* 19:125-131, 2003.
51. Bryce T, Kristjan R: Epidemiology and classification of pain after spinal cord injury, *Top Spinal Cord Inj Rehabil* 7(2):1-17, 2001.
52. Widerstrom-Noga EG, Turk DC: Types and effectiveness of treatments used by people with chronic pain associated with spinal cord injuries: Influence of pain and psychosocial characteristics, *Spinal Cord* 41(11):600-609, 2003.
53. Schmitz TJ. In O'Sullivan SB, Schmitz TJ: *Physical Rehabilitation: Assessment and Treatment,* ed 4, Philadelphia, 2001, FA Davis.
54. Dietz V, Trippel M, Berger W: Reflex activity and muscle tone during elbow movement in patients with spastic paresis, *Ann Neurol* 30:767-779, 1991.
55. Segal RL, Wolf SL: Operant conditioning of spinal stretch reflexes in patients with spinal cord injuries, *Exp Neurol* 130:202-213, 1994.
56. Sedgwick EM, Benfield J: Spasticity II: Physiological measurements. In Illis LS (ed): *Spinal Cord Dysfunction,* Oxford, 1992, Oxford University Press.
57. Coffey RJ, Cahill D, Steers W, et al: Intrathecal baclofen for intractable spasticity of spinal origin: Results of a long-term multicenter study, *J Neurosurg* 78:226-232, 1993.
58. Maynard FM, Karunas RS, Waring WP: Epidemiology of spasticity following traumatic spinal cord injury, *Arch Phys Med Rehabil* 71:566-569, 1990.
59. Beck T: Current spasticity management in children with spinal cord injury, *SCI Nurs* 19:28-31, 2002.
60. Satkunam L: Rehabilitation Medicine: Management of adult spasticity, *Can Med Assoc J* 169(11):1173-1179, 2003.
61. Illis LS: Spasticity I: Clinical aspects. In Illis L (ed): *Spinal Cord Dysfunction: Intervention and Treatment,* Oxford, 1992, Oxford University Press.
62. Thompson A: Drug treatment or neurological disability. In Edwards S (ed): *Neurological Physiotherapy,* Edinburgh, 2002, Churchill Livingstone.
63. Bohannon RW, Smith MB: Interrater reliability of a Modified Ashworth Scale of muscle spasticity, *Phys Ther* 67:206-207, 1987.
64. Watchie J: *Cardiopulmonary Physical Therapy,* Philadelphia, 1995, WB Saunders.
65. Kelley A, Garshick E, Gross ER, et al: Spirometry testing standard in spinal cord injury, *Chest* 123(3):725-730, 2003.
66. Ciesla, ND: Physical therapy associated with respiratory failure. In Deturk WE, Cahalin LP (eds): *Cardiovascular and Pulmonary Physical Therapy: An Evidence-Based Approach,* New York, 2004, McGraw Hill.
67. Hick AL, Martin KA, Ditor DS, et al: Long-term exercise training in persons with spinal cord injury: effects on strength, arm ergometry performance and psychological well-being, *Spinal Cord* 41:34-43, 2003.
68. Groot PCE, Hjeltnes N, Heijboer AC, et al: Effect of training intensity on physical capacity, lipid profile and insulin sensitivity in early rehabilitation of spinal cord injured individuals, *Spinal Cord* 41:673-679, 2003.
69. Davis GM: Exercise capacity of individual with paraplegia, *Med Sci Sports Exerc* 25:423-432, 1993.
70. Borg GAV: Psychophysical bases of perceived exertion, *Med Sci Sport Exerc* 14:377-381, 1970.
71. Hadley MN: Clinical assessment after acute cervical spinal cord injury, *Neurosurgery* 50(3):S21-S29, 2002.
72. Guide for the Uniform Data Set for Medical Rehabilitation, version 5.0, section III: *Functional Independence Measure,* Buffalo, NY, 1996, UB Foundation Activities.
73. Dodds TA, Martin DP, Stolov WC, et al: A validation of the functional independence measurement and its performance among rehabilitation inpatients, *Arch Phys Med Rehab* 74:531-536, 1993.
74. Kilkens OJ, Kallmeijer AJ, de Whitte LP, vander Woude LH, Post MW: The wheelchair circuit: construct validity and responsiveness of a test to assess manual wheelchair mobility in persons with spinal cord injury, *Arch Phys Med Rehab* 85(3):424-431, 2004.
75. Field-Fote EC, Fluet GG, Schafer SD, et al: The spinal cord injury functional ambulation inventory (SCI-FAI), *J Rehabil Med* 33:177-181, 2001.
76. Ditunno JF, Ditunno PL, Graziani V, et al: Walking index for spinal cord injury (WISCI): an international multicenter validity and reliability study, *Spinal Cord* 38:234-243, 2000.
77. DitunnoPL, Dituno JF: Walking index for spinal cord injury (WISCI II): scale revision, *Spinal Cord* 39:654-656, 2001.
78. Marganti B, Scivoletto G, Ditunno P, Ditunno JF, Molinari M: Walking index for spinal cord injury (WISCI): criterion validation, *Spinal Cord* 43:27-33, 2005.
79. Bode RK, Heinemann AW, Chen D: Measuring the impairment consequences of spinal cord injury, *Am J Phys Med Rehabil* 78(6):582-594, 1999.
80. Kirschblum SC, Memmo P, Kim N, Campagnolo D, Millis S: Comparison of the revised 2000 American Spinal Injury Association classification standards with the 1996 guidelines, *Am J Phys Med Rehabil* 81:502-505, 2002.
81. Curt A, Dietz V: Ambulatory capacity in spinal cord injury: significance of somatosensory evoked potentials and ASIA protocol in predicting outcome, *Arch Phys Med Rehab* 78(1):39-43, 1997.
82. Waters RL, Adkins R, Yakura J, Vigil D: Predication of ambulatory performance based on motor scores derived from standards of the American spinal injury association, *Arch Phys Med Rehab* 75(7):756-760, 1994.
83. Marino RJ, Graves DE: Metric properties of the ASIA motor score: subscales with functional activities, *Arch Phys Med Rehab* 85(11):1804-1810, 2004.

84. Harvey L, Byak A, Ostrovskaya M, et al: Randomised trial of the effects of four weeks of daily stretch on extensibility of hamstring muscles in people with spinal cord injuries, *Austral J Physiother* 49:176-181, 2003.

85. Harvey LA, Herbert RD: Muscle stretching for treatment and prevention of contracture in people with spinal cord injury, *Spinal Cord* 40:1-9, 2002.

86. Dellinger R: Inhaled nitric oxide versus prone positioning in acute respiratory distress syndrome, *Crit Care Med* 28:572-574, 2000.

87. Bonaventura CD, Gastaldi AC: Effect of abdominal binder on the efficacy of respiratory muscles in seated and supine tetraplegic patients, *Physiotherapy* 89(5):290-295, 2003.

88. Goldman JM, Rose LS, Williams SJ, Silver JR, Denison DM: Effects of abdominal binders on breathing in tetraplegic patients, *Thorax* 41(12):940-945, 1986.

89. Massery M, Cahalin L: Physical therapy associated with ventilatory pump dysfunction and failure. In Deturk WE, Cahalin LP (eds): *Cardiovascular and Pulmonary Physical Therapy: An Evidence-Based Approach,* New York, 2004, McGraw Hill.

90. Apple D: Pain above the injury level, *Top Spinal Cord Inj Rehabil* 7(2):18-29, 2001.

91. Wegener ST, Haythornthwaite JA: Psychological and behavioral issues in the treatment of pain after spinal cord injury, *Top Spinal Cord Inj Rehabil* 7(2):73-83. 2001.

92. Boninger M, Dicianno B, Cooper R, et al: Shoulder magnetic resonance imaging abnormalities, wheelchair propulsion, and gender, *Arch Phys Med Rehabil* 84(11):1615-1620, 2003.

93. Kezar LB, Ness TJ: Systemic medications, *Top Spinal Cord Inj Rehabil* 7(2):57-72, 2001.

94. Penn R: Treatment of pain in persons with spinal cord injury: spinal cord stimulation and intrathecal drugs, *Top Spinal Cord Inj Rehabil* 7(2):51-56, 2001.

95. Agency for Healthcare Research and Quality, Public Health Service, US Department of Health and Human Services: Management of chronic central neuropathic pain following traumatic spinal cord injury: Executive summary of evidence report/technology assessment: No. 45, *J Pain Palliat Care Pharmacother* 17(2):99-109, 2003.

96. Minkel JL: Seating and mobility considerations for people with spinal cord injury, *Phys Ther* 80(7):701-709, 2000.

97. Defloor T, Grypdonck MH: Sitting posture and prevention of pressure ulcers, *Appl Nurs Res* 12(3):136-142, 1999.

98. Bogie KM, Nuseibeh I, Bader DL: Early progressive changes in tissue viability in the seated spinal cord injured subject, *Paraplegia* 33(3):141-147, 1995.

99. Coggrave MJ, Rose LS: A specialist seating assessment clinic: Changing pressure relief practice, *Spinal Cord* 41(12):692-695, 2003.

100. Henderson JL, Price SH, Brandstater ME, et al: Efficacy of three measures to relieve pressure in seated persons with spinal cord injury, *Arch Phys Med Rehabil* 75(5):535-539, 1994.

101. Hobson DA: Comparative effects of posture on pressure and shear at the body-seat interface, *J Rehabil Res Dev* 29(4):21-31, 1992.

102. Nawoczenski DA, Clobes SM, Gore SL, et al: Three-dimensional shoulder kinematics during a pressure relief technique and wheelchair transfer, *Arch Phys Med Rehabil* 84(9):1293-1300, 2003.

103. Defloor T, Grypdonck MH: Do pressure relief cushions really relieve pressure? *West J Nurs Res* 22(3):335-350, 2000.

104. Yuen HK, Garrett D: Comparison of three wheelchair cushions for effectiveness of pressure relief, *Am J Occup Ther* 55(4):470-475, 2001.

105. Tomlinson JD: Managing maneuverability and rear stability of adjustable manual wheelchair: An update, *Phys Ther* 80:904-911, 2000.

106. Minkel JL: Seating and mobility considerations for people with spinal cord injury, *Phys Ther* 80:701-709, 2000.

107. Dietz V, Harkema SJ: Locomotor activity in spinal cord-injured persons, *J Appl Physiol* 96:1954-1960, 2004.

108. MacKay-Lyons M: Central pattern generation of locomotion: A review of the evidence, *Phys Ther* 82:69-79, 2002.

109. Field-Fote EC: Spinal cord control of movement: Implications for locomotor rehabilitation following spinal cord injury, *Phys Ther* 80:477-484, 2000.

110. Basso DM: Neuroanatomical substrates of functional recovery after experimental spinal cord injury: Implications of basic science research for human spinal cord injury, *Phys Ther* 80:808-817, 2000.

111. de Leon RD, Roy R, Edgerton VR: Is the recovery of stepping following spinal cord injury mediated by modifying existing neural pathways or by generating new pathways? A perspective, *Phys Ther* 81:1904-1911, 2001.

112. Harkema SJ, Hurley SL, Patel UK, et al: Human lumbosacral spinal cord interprets loading during stepping, *J Neurophysiol* 77:797-811, 1997.

113. Beres-Jones JA, Harkema SJ: The human spinal cord interprets velocity-dependent afferent input during stepping, *Brain* 127:2232-2246, 2004.

114. Wernig A, Muller S, Nanassy A, et al: Laufband therapy based on "rules of spinal locomotion" is effective in spinal cord injured persons, *Eur J Neurosci* 7:823-829, 1997.

115. Barbeau H, Fung J, Leroux A, et al: A review of the adaptability and recovery of locomotion after spinal cord injury. In McKerracher L, Doucet G, Rossignol S (eds): *Progress in Brain Research,* vol 137, Boston, 2002, Elsevier Science.

116. Carhart MR, Jiping H, Herman R, et al: Epidural spinal-cord stimulation facilitates recover of functional walking following incomplete spinal cord injury, *IEEE Trans Neur Sys Rehabil Engin* 12(1):32-41, 2004.

117. Stewart B, Tarnoplsky M, Hicks A, et al: Treadmill training-induced adaptations in muscle phenotype in person with incomplete spinal cord injury, *Muscle Nerve* 204:61-68, 2004.

118. Field-Fote EC, Tepavac D: Improved intralimb coordination in people with incomplete spinal cord injury following training with body weight support and electrical stimulation, *Phys Ther* 82(7):707-715, 2002.

119. Lawless AR, Davis S, Bowden M, et al: Locomotor training, progression and outcomes after incomplete spinal cord injury: A case study. Poster presented at Combined Sections Meeting of The American Physical Therapy Association, New Orleans, February, 2005.

120. Hannold E, Young M, Rittman M, et al: Locomotor training experiences: Cognitive-emotional reactions and training benefits identified by persons with incomplete spinal cord injury. Poster presented at Combined Sections Meeting of The American Physical Therapy Association, New Orleans, February, 2005.

121. Agarwal S, Triolo R, Kobetic R, et al: Long-term user perceptions of an implanted neuroprosthesis for exercise, standing, and transfers after spinal cord injury, *J Rehabil Res Dev* 40(3):241-252, 2003.

122. Colombo G, Matthias J, Schreier R, et al: Treadmill training of paraplegic patients using a robotic orthosis, *J Rehabil Res Dev* 37(6):693-700, 2000.

123. Dobkin B, Apple D, Barbeau H, et al: Methods for a randomized trial of weight-supported treadmill training versus conventional training for walking during inpatient rehabilitation after incomplete traumatic spinal cord injury, *Neurorehab Neural Repair* 17(3):153-167, 2003.

124. Behrman AL, Harkema SJ: Locomotor training after human spinal cord injury: A series of case studies, *Phys Ther* 80:688-700, 2000.

125. Field-Fote EC: The injured spinal cord: Pathology and potential. Presented at American Physical Therapy Association Combined Sections Meeting, Tampa, February, 2003.

126. Bernard PL, Codine P, Minier J: Isokinetic shoulder rotator muscles in wheelchair athletes, *Spinal Cord* 42:222-229, 2004.

127. Down AM: Physiological basis for airway clearance techniques and clinical applications of airway clearance techniques. In Frownfelter DL, Dean E (eds): *Principles and Practice of Cardiopulmonary Physical Therapy,* ed 3, St. Louis, 1996, Mosby.

128. Rutchik A, Weissman AR, Almenoff PL, et al: Resistive inspiratory muscle training in subjects with chronic cervical spinal cord injury, *Arch Phys Med Rehabil* 79(3):293-297, 1998.

129. Liaw M, Lin M, Cheng P, Wong MA, et al: Resistive inspiratory muscle training: Its effectiveness in patients with acute complete cervical cord injury, *Arch Phys Med Rehabil* 81:752-756, 2000.

Chapter 21

Disorders of Consciousness: Coma, Vegetative State, and Minimally Conscious State

Susan Grieve

CHAPTER OUTLINE

OBJECTIVES

After reading this chapter, the reader will be able to:
1. Define and understand the uses of the terms coma, vegetative state, and minimally conscious state.
2. Identify and distinguish between the clinical criteria and characteristics of coma, vegetative state, and minimally conscious state.
3. Understand the pathology causing altered or impaired consciousness.
4. Understand the prognostic indicators for coma, vegetative state, and minimally conscious state and how to tailor rehabilitation interventions and recommendations accordingly.

Over the past two decades, advances in medical technology have reduced mortality from severe medical disease and brain injuries significantly, allowing many people to survive despite being in severely impaired states of *consciousness*. It is predicted that 30% to 40% of survivors of brain injury and approximately 80% of survivors of cardiac arrest will remain in a state of impaired consciousness after medical stabilization.[1,2] Although some of these people regain some degree of consciousness, many have severely limited neurological function and continue to have disorders of consciousness for prolonged periods and often for the rest of their lives. These patients are often admitted to rehabilitation facilities for management by a multidisciplinary rehabilitation team.

The role of rehabilitation for patients with disorders of consciousness includes prevention of deterioration and maintenance of the sensory-motor system and other vital body functions to avoid medical complications and maximize functional outcomes.[3] Through careful and ongoing examination and appropriate intervention, clinicians may also clarify the patient's diagnosis and prognosis and optimize clinical outcomes. All rehabilitation professionals must understand the definitions, clinical features, research evidence, and prognostic indicators of the different disorders of consciousness to help with resource allocation and to provide patients and their families with the most effective interventions. This chapter discusses current rehabilitation examination, evaluation, and intervention for patients with disorders of consciousness. For rehabilitation specialists, these disorders most commonly include *coma, vegetative state,* and *minimally conscious state,* resulting from trauma, tumor, stroke, cerebral anoxia, and/or metabolic dysfunction. Coma, vegetative state, and minimally conscious state may be permanent conditions or transient states from which patients may evolve or regress.

The *Guide to Physical Therapist Practice* (the *Guide*) classifies these patients under preferred practice pattern 5I: Impaired arousal, range of motion, and motor control associated with coma, near coma, or vegetative state.[4] The terminology used in this chapter is slightly different from that used in the *Guide* to be more consistent with most of the current literature on states of impaired consciousness. In this chapter, the terms "minimally conscious," as well as "coma" and "vegetative state," are used, whereas the term "near coma" is not. The definitions and diagnostic criteria sections further discuss the use of these terms.

PATHOLOGY

Understanding the pathology of impaired consciousness first requires knowledge of intact or normal consciousness. Consciousness is studied by various disciplines, including neurophysiology, philosophy, psychology, and psychiatry. All agree that the essential components of normal or intact consciousness are arousal and awareness of self and the environment.[5] Arousal, the more primitive element of consciousness, is clinically intact if a person opens his or her eyes either spontaneously or in response to an external stimulus. Arousal requires a functioning ascending *reticular activating system* (ARAS). The ARAS is a diffuse network of nerves located in the upper two thirds of the brainstem that connects to the thalamus and the cerebral cortex (Fig. 21-1). The ARAS may be activated by somatosensory stimuli, such as touch and sound, or by basic needs, such as hunger or thirst.

Awareness, the more complex component of consciousness, involves not only awareness of self but also awareness of the relationship of self to the environment. The combination of self-awareness and the awareness of one's relationship to the environment requires cerebral functioning and leads to conscious cognitive behavior. Awareness requires cerebral hemisphere function, whereas arousal does not. Arousal requires only a functioning upper brainstem. Arousal can occur without awareness, but awareness is not possible without arousal.

It may be helpful to think of arousal as the light switch and awareness as the light bulb (Fig. 21-2). For consciousness to be normal, a person must have a functioning ARAS in the brainstem (the light switch), functioning cerebral hemispheres (the light bulb), and functioning connections through the thalamus (wiring) to send information between the two. Injuries or medical conditions that affect any of these areas in the central nervous system (CNS) can impair or alter consciousness.

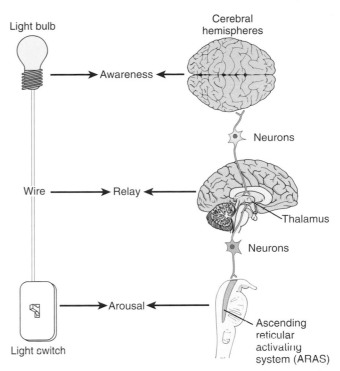

FIG. 21-2 Light bulb and light switch analogy for arousal as it relates to awareness.

There are three mechanisms by which the cerebral hemispheres, thalamus, and/or the brainstem may be affected to alter consciousness. The first is a structural lesion caused by conditions such as stroke, tumor, abscess, or trauma. The second results from toxic or metabolic abnormalities, and the third results from diffuse brain insults such as anoxia.[6]

A structural lesion above the tentorium is classified as *supratentorial*, and one involving structures below the tentorium is classified as *subtentorial* (Fig. 21-3). Supratentorial lesions that affect consciousness involve either the cerebral hemispheres or the thalamus, whereas consciousness-impairing subtentorial lesions are in the brainstem. Clinically, a supratentorial structural lesion may initially cause localizing hemispheric signs, including contralateral motor and/or sensory impairments, as is typical after a middle cerebral artery stroke (see Chapter 16). If the

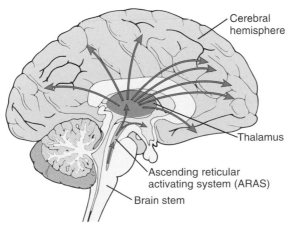

FIG. 21-1 Areas of the brain responsible for consciousness: The ARAS in the brainstem and the cerebral hemispheres.

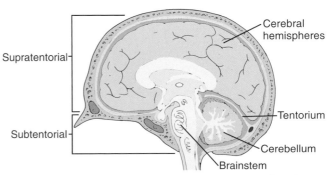

FIG. 21-3 Division of the brain into supratentorial and subtentorial structures by the tentorium.

damage from a stroke progresses, by extension or by causing swelling, to cause bihemispheric compromise or brain herniation, or there is some type of lesion affecting both hemispheres, then consciousness may become impaired. A structural lesion in the ARAS of the brainstem, a subtentorial area, will usually present clinically with initial rapid changes in or loss of consciousness with or without hemispheric or cranial nerve signs. Subdural hematoma is the most common nontraumatic supratentorial lesion to cause impairment of consciousness, accounting for 80% of cases, whereas brainstem infarct accounts for 71% of subtentorial lesions causing alteration of consciousness.[6]

Alterations of consciousness from toxic causes may be a result of excessive intake of substances, such as alcohol or other psychoactive drugs, or a result of poor elimination or toxin production because of kidney or liver dysfunction. In addition, hypoglycemia or severe hyperglycemia may also impair consciousness. Toxic and metabolic abnormalities are the most common nontraumatic causes of impaired consciousness, accounting for 47% of emergency room presentations for "coma of unknown origin."[6] Of these, 55% are caused by alcohol or other drugs. When consciousness is impaired by toxic or metabolic causes, patients typically present clinically with somnolence or *delirium* preceding the state of coma. They generally do not have focal neurological signs such as localized motor or sensory abnormalities.

Consciousness may also be impaired by diffuse brain damage as the result of subarachnoid hemorrhage, infection, cerebral anoxia secondary to cardiac arrest, or diffuse axonal injury secondary to trauma. Diffuse brain damage is the least common cause of impaired consciousness, accounting for only 4.5% of patients presenting with nontraumatic causes of coma. Table 21-1 lists the more common nontraumatic causes of impaired consciousness.

After trauma, the two leading causes of coma are toxic/metabolic insults, primarily from drug overdose, and cardiac arrest causing diffuse global ischemia. Some believe that with increased access to automated defibrillators in public places and a greater public interest in learning basic life support, more people may survive cardiac arrest after prolonged impairment of circulation to all areas, including the brain. This will consequently increase the incidence of "cardiac arrest coma."[2]

Many medical conditions can also cause impaired consciousness and unresponsiveness. Coma can be thought of as the final common pathway in many untreated disease states. The underlying cause of impaired consciousness may give an indication of patient prognosis and be used to guide rehabilitation interventions and family education.

CLINICAL DEFINITIONS AND CRITERIA FOR DIAGNOSIS OF DISORDERS OF CONSCIOUSNESS

One of the problems facing clinicians who care for patients with impaired consciousness is the lack of consistent nomenclature for defining disorders of consciousness.[7] Several studies have shown that between 18% and 43% of patients with a diagnosis of coma or vegetative

TABLE 21-1	Nontraumatic Causes of Impaired Consciousness*	
Diagnosis		**Percentage**
METABOLIC/TOXIC		
1. Exogenous toxins (e.g., drug abuse, EtOH intoxication)		34
2. Endogenous toxins (e.g., liver, renal failure)		27
TOTAL		61
DIFFUSE BRAIN INJURY		
1. Anoxia/ischemia		17
2. Infection		4
3. Subarachnoid hemorrhage		3
4. Concussion		3
TOTAL		34
SUPRATENTORIAL LESION		
1. Intracerebral hematoma		11
2. Subdural hematoma		7
3. Cerebral infarct		2
4. Brain tumor		2
5. Brain abscess		1
6. Epidural hematoma		0.5
TOTAL		23.5
SUBTENTORIAL LESION		
1. Brainstem infarct		13
2. Brainstem hemorrhage		2
3. Cerebellar hemorrhage		1
4. Brainstem tumor		0.5
5. Cerebellar abscess		0.5
TOTAL		17

*From a sample of 292 patients with initial diagnosis "coma of unknown etiology" (nontraumatic), with some patients having more than one cause.
Adapted from Kandel ER, Schwartz JH, Jessell TM (eds): *Principles of Neuroscience,* ed 3, New York, 1991, Elsevier.
EtOH, Ethyl alcohol.

state residing in nursing homes or admitted to inpatient rehabilitation centers were diagnosed incorrectly.[8-10] A clinically correct medical diagnosis is not only paramount in determining the neurological and functional prognosis of patients with impaired consciousness but is also one of the primary factors influencing rehabilitation decisions regarding the type, intensity, and duration of specific interventions. Understanding the criteria for each disorder and the differences among them allows allied health professionals involved in the rehabilitation of patients with impaired consciousness to most accurately determine an individual's expected functional outcome and amount of time needed to achieve that outcome. An appropriate plan of care that identifies specific interventions, frequency of treatment, duration of treatment, anticipated goals, and expected outcomes can then be developed by all members of the rehabilitation team. Rehabilitation professionals should also understand the criteria for each disorder and the differences among them so that changes in patient behavior and movement can be accurately monitored and those responsible for making a medical diagnosis of a specific disorder can be alerted if there is a change in the patient's level of consciousness.

The American Congress of Rehabilitation Medicine,[11] The Multi-Society Task Force on Persistent Vegetative

State,[12,13] and The Aspen Neurobehavioral Conference[14] have attempted to standardize the criteria and nomenclature used to identify disorders of consciousness. Their recommendations are summarized here.

COMA

Coma is the neurobehavioral diagnostic term for a patient in a state of "unarousable unawareness." This description was first used by Plum and Posner in their widely referenced text *The Diagnosis of Stupor and Coma*, first published in 1966. The latest edition (third) published in 1982 expands the description of coma to "the total absence of awareness of self and environment even when the subject is externally stimulated."[6] Using this definition as a basis, the Aspen Neurobehavioral Conference defined coma as "complete failure of the arousal system with no spontaneous eye opening and inability to awaken by the application of vigorous sensory stimuli."[14] The Multi-Society Task Force on Persistent Vegetative State referenced Plum and Posner[6] in their definition of coma as "sustained pathologic unconsciousness that results from dysfunction of the RAS in the brainstem or of both cerebral hemispheres. The eyes remain closed and the patient cannot be aroused."[12,13] The American Congress of Rehabilitation Medicine again referenced Plum and Posner[6] in their description of coma as a "diagnostic term that denotes unarousability and loss of the capacity for environmental interaction. A patient in a coma cannot be aroused to a wakeful state by any means."[11]

Criteria for diagnosis of coma

The patient's eyes do not open either spontaneously or to external stimulation.
The patient does not follow any commands.
The patient does not mouth or utter recognizable words.
The patient does not demonstrate intentional movement (may show reflexive movement such as posturing, withdrawal from pain, or involuntary smiling).
The patient cannot sustain visual pursuit movements of the eyes through a 45-degree arc in any direction when the eyes are held open manually.
The above criteria are not secondary to use of paralytic agents.[1]

VEGETATIVE STATE

Jennett and Plum first used the term "persistent vegetative state" in 1972 to label the population of patients who demonstrated "arousal in the absence of awareness."[15] Patients in the vegetative state have some activity in the ARAS but lack relay (thalamic) or cerebral function. Over the past 10 years, there has been a great deal of discussion and controversy in the medical community regarding the use of the term "persistent" in labeling patients in a vegetative state.[11,14,16] Many believe that use of the term "persistent" implies that a patient in this state cannot make any improvements. This may cause payers to withdraw or

withhold payment for rehabilitation services for these patients. Several groups and authors recommend discontinuing the use of the modifier "persistent," arguing that its use adds nothing to the meaning of the diagnosis or prognosis of vegetative state.[11,14,16] The Multi-Society Task Force on PVS introduced the term "permanent" vegetative state to indicate the low probability of meaningful recovery if the vegetative state extends beyond 12 months after brain damage because of trauma and beyond 3 months after brain damage from any other cause.[13] It is generally agreed that only the terms "vegetative state" and "permanent vegetative state" be used in describing patients who demonstrate arousal in the absence of awareness after brain injury.

"The vegetative state is a clinical condition of complete unawareness to the self and the environment accompanied by sleep-wake cycles with either complete or partial preservation of hypothalamic and brainstem autonomic functions."[12]

Criteria for diagnosis of vegetative state

The patient has no awareness of self or environment; inability to interact with others.
The patient shows no evidence of sustained, reproducible, purposeful, or voluntary behavioral responses to visual, auditory, tactile, or noxious stimuli.
The patient shows no evidence of language comprehension or expression.
The patient does have periods of intermittent wakefulness and sleep-wake cycles.
The patient does have sufficiently preserved hypothalamic and autonomic functions to survive with medical care.
The patient is bowel and bladder incontinent.
The patient has variably preserved cranial nerve reflexes (pupillary, oculocephalic, corneal, vestibulo-ocular, gag) and spinal reflexes.

MINIMALLY CONSCIOUS STATE

The term "minimally conscious state" does not appear in the *Guide*[4] but is found in the literature concerning patients in low-level neurological states that cause impaired consciousness. The American Congress of Rehabilitation Medicine first used the term "minimally responsive state" in 1995 to describe patients who were no longer in a coma or vegetative state but who remained severely disabled. This diagnostic term was recently changed to "minimally conscious state" because patients in a vegetative state have reflex responses, so the term "minimally responsive" fails to clearly distinguish between vegetative state and minimally responsive state. The distinguishing feature between these states is the presence of some cognitive function in the latter state, which is therefore most clearly termed the "minimally conscious state."[17]

The Aspen Neurobehavioral Conference Workgroup in 2002 developed a position paper that defined and established diagnostic criteria for the minimally conscious state.[14] Through a review of the literature on disorders of consciousness, members of the work group determined that there were insufficient data to establish evidence-based guidelines for diagnosis, prognosis, and management of the minimally conscious state. The group therefore developed a consensus-based definition for minimally conscious state based on the behavioral diagnostic criteria used in current practice.

"The minimally conscious state is a condition of severely altered consciousness in which minimal but definite behavioral evidence of self or environmental awareness is demonstrated."[14]

Criteria for diagnosis of minimally conscious state

The patient follows simple commands.

The patient can gesture or verbally express yes/no responses (regardless of accuracy).

The patient is capable of intelligible verbalization.

The patient demonstrates purposeful behavior not due to reflexive activity.

Unlike the criteria for coma or vegetative state in which a patient must meet all of the criteria for a diagnosis, an individual is determined to be in a minimally conscious state if only one or more of the above criteria are met.

NEAR COMA

The preferred practice pattern 5I: Impaired arousal, range of motion, and motor control associated with coma, near coma and vegetative state, included in the *Guide*,[4] includes the term "near coma." This term appears in the Coma/Near Coma scale, as described later, but is not used elsewhere in current literature. The definition of near coma according to the Coma/Near Coma scale is "consistently responsive to stimuli presented to two sensory modalities and/or inconsistently or partially responsive to simple commands."[18] Since the publication of this scale and of the *Guide*, the term "near coma" has fallen out of favor. It appears that the diagnostic category "minimally conscious state" is now used to describe patients who were previously described as in near coma. Patients in a minimally conscious state are unconscious but occasionally show signs of consciousness such as tracking with their eyes, reaching for an object when asked, or grabbing for someone's hand. Since the term "near coma" is no longer in current usage in other literature, it is not used in this chapter and where relevant, has been replaced with the term "minimally conscious state."

Other terms used in the medical community to describe decreased levels of alertness but that have not been defined as diagnostic categories are *stupor, somnolent, obtunded,* and delirium.

DIFFERENTIAL DIAGNOSIS OF DISORDERS OF CONSCIOUSNESS

Correct diagnosis of a disorder of consciousness requires not only an understanding of the specific clinical features and behavioral characteristics of each but also an under-

standing of conditions which can mimic these states. One such condition is *locked-in syndrome*. This syndrome often results from a stroke at the base of the pons in the brainstem. Patients with this condition have a functioning ARAS, as well as normal thalamic and cortical connections, and therefore have intact normal consciousness; however, all motor pathways to the face, trunk, and limbs are lost. Thus these patients are awake and fully aware of their condition and environment but cannot move. Often the ability to blink and move the eyes vertically are spared and become the patient's only means of communicating. Patients with locked-in syndrome are frequently misdiagnosed as being in a persistent vegetative state.[10,19]

Brain death is another term sometimes confused with coma and vegetative state. For a patient to be brain dead they must meet three neurological criteria: coma, absent brainstem reflexes and apnea.[20] The concept of brain death was developed in the late 1950s and 1960s, with the advent of intensive care units (ICUs) and sophisticated ventilators that made it possible to maintain respiration in patients with severe irreversible brain injuries. The principal aim of the concept was to facilitate organ transplantation by providing justification for the removal of organs from individuals who were not dead by cardiopulmonary criteria.[21] Before the development of effective ventilators, these patients usually died within minutes because of the irreversible stoppage of respiration and heartbeat. Brain death is considered legally equivalent to death, and although cardiopulmonary function may occasionally be supported for prolonged periods, most patients lose cardiopulmonary function within a few days despite maximal support[22] and there are no documented cases of recovery of any degree of consciousness in patients who meet the criteria for brain death. Given their poor prognosis, patients who are brain dead are not candidates for rehabilitation. Table 21-2 summarizes the major clinical criteria for coma, vegetative state, minimally conscious state, locked-in-syndrome and brain death.

EXAMINATION

PATIENT HISTORY

A rehabilitation examination should begin with a thorough patient history. For the patient with a disorder of consciousness most of this information will be found in the medical chart. The chart review should focus on four areas. First, the etiology of the disorder should be determined because this information can provide insight into the prognosis for recovery. Second, the findings of all neurological examinations before the current examination should be reviewed. These findings can illustrate any trend in the patient's neurological condition, whether improving or deteriorating, and over what time frame. This will help determine prognosis for recovery and give a baseline for comparison with findings from the current examination. Third, nursing notes may provide valuable information about the patient's current activity level, vital sign stability, and areas of skin breakdown. Fourth, the patient's medications should be reviewed, looking particularly for those that may cause sedation or other side effects that

TABLE 21-2	Clinical Criteria for Coma, Vegetative State, Minimally Conscious State, Locked-In Syndrome, and Brain Death			
Coma	**Vegetative State**	**Minimally Conscious State**	**Locked-In Syndrome**	**Brain Death**
Eyes do not open spontaneously or to external stimuli. Does not follow commands. Does not mouth or utter meaningful words. Does not demonstrate intentional movement. Cannot sustain visual pursuit. Not under the influence of any paralytic agent.	Eyes open spontaneously. Sleep-wake cycles present. No evidence of awareness of self or environment. Inability to interact with others. No language comprehension or expression. No purposeful movement. No visual pursuit. Bowel/bladder incontinence. Variably preserved cranial nerve reflexes.	Follows simple commands. Gestures or verbal yes/no responses. Intelligible verbalization. Purposeful behavior not a result of reflex activity. Minimally conscious state if one or more criteria are met.	Eyes open spontaneously or in response to external stimulation. Unable to follow motor commands except eye blink or some vertical eye movement. Caused by total paralysis below the level of the oculomotor nuclei in the brainstem. Full awareness of self and the environment. Able to communicate through eye movement.	Coma. Absent brainstem reflexes (pupillary response, corneal, oculocephalic, oculovestibular, and gag). Apnea. Completely unresponsive to external visual, auditory, and tactile stimuli. Incapable of communication in any manner.

may confound the examination (tremors, weakness, hypotension, tachycardia, nystagmus, respiratory depression).[23] Together, these four elements of the patient history will influence the frequency, intensity, and types of rehabilitation interventions best suited for the patient.

SYSTEMS REVIEW

The systems review is used to target areas requiring further examination and to define areas that may cause complications or indicate a need for precautions during the examination and intervention processes. See Chapter 1 for details of the systems review.

Patients with a disorder of consciousness typically undergo a period of bed rest, and it is therefore important for clinicians to understand the physiological effects of bed rest on body systems when performing the systems review.

Cardiovascular/Pulmonary. Bed rest significantly affects the cardiovascular and pulmonary system. Signs of orthostatic intolerance begin within 3-4 days of complete bed rest.[24] Both the central and peripheral components of the system are affected. Centrally, as the heart muscle atrophies, stroke volume decreases and heart rate (HR) increases to maintain cardiac output. This substantially decreases an individual's capacity to respond to increases in physical demand, including changes in position from supine to sitting or standing, as well as exercise. Peripherally, within 3-4 weeks of bed rest, blood volume shifts to the thorax. Any change in position from supine causes the volume of blood in the thorax to decrease, decreasing venous return to the heart and reducing cardiac output. This reduction in cardiac output is counteracted by a surge in HR, sometimes by more than 35 beats per minute (bpm), when moving a patient from supine to standing.[25]

Initial examination of the cardiovascular/pulmonary system involves systematic observation to determine how much ventilatory support a patient is receiving (see Chapter 26). Respiratory therapists are an invaluable source of information regarding the respiratory status of these patients and in most cases are part of the rehabilitation team. If the patient is not using a ventilator, his or her spontaneous respiratory rate (RR) and pattern should be recorded. The brainstem controls RR and pattern, and if these are abnormal, brainstem dysfunction may be present.

Integumentary. The initial examination of the integumentary system also involves systematic observation. The patient should be visually examined from head to toe for any areas of skin breakdown or potential skin breakdown (see Chapter 28), and these findings should be recorded on a body chart and reported to the patient's nurse or physician. The location of dressings should also be recorded on a body chart because these may affect patient positioning. Also, note any changes in skin color, such as bruising or redness.

Musculoskeletal. The effects of bed rest on the musculoskeletal system are many. Strength loss is greatest during the first week of immobilization with skeletal muscle strength decreasing by 1% to 1.5% per day with strict bed rest and by 1.3% to 5.5% with cast immobilization.[26] With bed rest, tendons and ligaments also lose strength internally and in their connections to muscle and bone. Bone loss occurs, with the ratio of bone formation to bone resorption decreasing because there is less stress placed on the bones in the gravity-eliminated position. As bed rest continues, bones become less dense and more prone to fracture. Trabecular bone, as found in the neck of the femur, is more susceptible to resorption than cortical bone. Joints also remodel in response to bed rest, with cartilage degenerating, synovium atrophying, and fibrofatty tissue infiltrates appearing.[26]

When examining the musculoskeletal system of patients in low-level neurological states, the rehabilitation specialist must know if the patient's condition is caused by trauma. In this case, clinicians should note on a body chart any fracture sites and any physician ordered precautions to movement. Fracture sites may involve any area, but special attention should be given to the cranium and vertebral column because any movement of unstable fractures in these areas can further damage neurological structures. Gross range of motion (ROM), possible contracture formation, and signs of increased contracture risk (such as foot drop or increased tone in the upper/lower extremities) should also be noted. The patient's height and weight should be recorded as these may influence selection of patient movement and transfer approaches.

Neuromuscular. The neuromuscular system should be carefully examined in this patient group. Patients should be observed for abnormal spontaneous or reflexive movement patterns that are common in patients with severe brain damage. Table 21-3 lists and describes the more common motor patterns observed in patients with disorders of consciousness and possible causes of each. As a rule, crossing of the legs, normal shifts in posture, yawning, and sneezing indicate less severe impairments of consciousness.[5] Turning toward a noxious stimulus is a reflexive response, but turning away from a noxious response may be purposeful.[5] Gross whole body flexion, extension, and adduction in response to tactile stimuli are reflex responses indicating deep bicerebral or brainstem dysfunction.[5] A response that consists of upper extremity flexion together with lower extremity extension is known as a decorticate response. A response consisting of exten-sion of both the upper and lower extremities is known as a decerebrate response and indicates more advanced motor dysfunction, generally caused by deep bilateral cerebral hemispheric lesions or compression of the brainstem. Fig. 21-4 illustrates *decorticate* and *decerebrate posturing*. A grasp reflex in response to tactile stimulation of the palm is sometimes present as is trismus or biting down spontaneously or in response to something placed in the mouth. These reflexes may be mistaken for purposeful movement, particularly by family and friends of the patient who may perceive them as a sign of "waking up" or conscious attempts at hand holding or eating.

Spontaneous ocular movements are also common in patients with disorders of consciousness, specifically roving eye movements from side to side or up and down and blinking at rest or in response to light, sound, or threat. These eye movements do not indicate that the patient is moving toward a higher state of arousal or awareness. Rehabilitation clinicians should be aware that nystagmus is uncommon in patients who are in a coma or vegetative state.[6] Nystagmus is produced by the attempt to bring the eyes back to midline and is seen clinically as quick horizontal eye movements. This requires interaction of the brainstem with the cerebral cortex and this interaction is lacking in patients who are in a coma or vegetative state. Consistent visual tracking is one of the first

TABLE 21-3	Motor Patterns Commonly Seen in Patients with Disorders of Consciousness	
Observation	**Description**	**Likely Cause**
Grasp reflex	Patient's fingers flex around examiner's when palm is stroked.	Cerebral dysfunction.
Decorticate posture	Upper extremity flexion, lower extremity extension.	Cerebral dysfunction.
Decerebrate posture	Upper extremity and lower extremity extension.	More advanced motor system dysfunction than decorticate posture. Deep bilateral cerebral lesions or brainstem dysfunction. Can also be seen with advanced metabolic dysfunction.
Gross body flexion, extension, or adduction		Reflex response, deep bicerebral or brainstem dysfunction.
Yawning, sneezing, and/or crossing legs; normal shifts in posture		Less severe disorders of consciousness. Seen as a positive prognostic indicator.
Trismus	Biting down spontaneously or on something placed in the mouth.	Dysfunction above the midpons.
Turning toward a noxious stimulus		Always a reflexive response (abnormal).
Turning away from a noxious stimulus		May be purposeful.

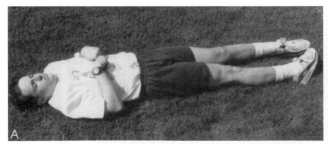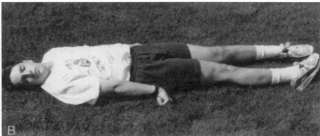

FIG. 21-4 **A,** Decorticate posture; **B,** decerebrate posture. *From Magee D:* Orthopedic Physical Assessment, *ed 4, Philadelphia, 2005, Saunders.*

indicators that a patient is no longer in a vegetative state and has achieved some level of awareness.[12]

TESTS AND MEASURES

The final step in the examination of a patient with a disorder of consciousness is performance of specific tests and measures. Tests and measures should be administered on initial patient contact and should be readministered at regular intervals to check for signs of changes in neurological status such as development of new purposeful movement. Initial examination by rehabilitation professionals of patients in a coma, vegetative state, or minimally conscious state commonly takes place in the ICU, where multiple monitoring lines, sedating drugs, and mechanical ventilatory support machines may complicate the examination. In this setting, rehabilitation professionals are most often asked to initiate interventions that assist in maintaining full extremity ROM and reduce the risk of contractures and pressure ulcers. As patients move from the ICU to step-down units and general medical floors, rehabilitation clinicians can examine patients more accurately and completely and adjust interventions accordingly.

Musculoskeletal

Range of Motion. Active ROM (AROM) and passive ROM (PROM) are measured with a goniometer. It is beyond the scope of this chapter to review the goniometric measurement technique and normal ranges for each joint. These can be found in other texts.[27] Two studies have shown that PROM measured by goniometry demonstrates poor reliability and suggest the poor results may be due to the type of underlying disease or injury and type of instrument used.[28,29]

Posture. Recently, a group of investigators looked at the effects of postural change on levels of arousal and awareness.[30] In a pilot study, 12 patients, 5 in a vegetative state and 7 in a minimally conscious state, were assessed both lying in bed and in a standing position using a tilt table. Patients' behaviors were recorded in each position and assigned a score based on the Wessex Head Injury Matrix (WHIM), a 62-point scale ranking behaviors in patients with disorders of consciousness.[31] Low scores are given to behaviors suggestive of low levels of arousal and

awareness and high scores assigned to behaviors suggesting the opposite. Eight of the 12 patients (three in a vegetative state and five in a minimally conscious state) showed improvements in the number and type of behaviors observed while in the standing position. The implications of this finding for rehabilitation remain unclear, but it is suggested that neurological assessment to classify patients as being in a vegetative or minimally conscious state take place with the patient in a standing position if possible.[30]

An older study suggests that assisting patients who are in a vegetative state to a correct sitting position can inhibit abnormal reflexes and movements caused by neurological damage.[32] In this study, changes in reflexes were assessed by clinical observation and not by standardized tests, but these results do suggest that patients should be neurologically assessed in positions other than supine.

Neuromuscular

Arousal, Attention, and Cognition. Coma scales and cognitive function scales have been developed with the aim of achieving standardization in determining level of consciousness for clinical research, as well as for monitoring changes during acute illness, and serving as prognostic indicators.[33] Most coma and cognitive function scales are composite scales that include measures of motor function, level of disability, and levels of arousal, attention, and cognition.

The Glasgow Coma Scale (GCS), developed in 1974, is the scale most widely used in emergency departments, community hospitals, and research literature worldwide[34] (Table 21-4). Originally developed for use with patients after traumatic brain injury, this scale has also proven to be a reliable predictor of outcome for patients in coma with brain damage from nontraumatic causes.[35] The GCS shows high interrater and intrarater reliability when used by paramedics, physicians and nurses.[36,37]

The GCS consists of three categories: Eye opening, best motor response, and best verbal response. Each category has a numerical scale assigned to specific responses. Scores for eye opening range from 1-4, for best motor response from 1-6, and for best verbal response 1-5. The totals for all categories are summed to give the final score. Total scores range from 3-15, with a score of 8 or less defining

TABLE 21-4		The Glasgow Coma Scale (GCS)			
Eye Opening		**Best Motor Response**		**Best Verbal Response**	
Spontaneous	4	To verbal command	6	Oriented and converses	5
To speech	3	To painful stimulus	5	Disoriented and converses	4
To pain	2	Flexion withdrawal	4	Inappropriate words	3
No response	1	Flexion abnormal	3	Incomprehensible sounds	2
		Extension	2	No response	1
		No response	1		
E score		M score		V score	

Total Score = E score + M score + V score.
Interpretation: ≤8 = Coma; ≥9 = Not in a coma; 9-11 = Moderate severity; ≥12 = Minor injury.

coma. A score of 9-11 indicates moderately severe brain injury, and a score of greater than or equal to 12 indicates minor injury. Overall criticisms of the GCS are its failure to include brainstem reflexes, its bias toward best motor response, and its inability to obtain a verbal score from intubated patients.[38]

The Glasgow Outcome Scale (GOS) was developed in 1975 with the goal of developing a standardized language for clinical research to describe the outcomes of groups of patients with severe brain damage[39] (Table 21-5). The original scale, which is still generally used today, has 5 categories: Dead, persistent vegetative state, severe disability, moderate disability, and good recovery. In 1985 an expanded version of the GOS was developed with 8 categories to more accurately describe outcomes in the research literature by capturing subtle improvements in higher levels of functional performance.[40] The GOS is not intended to provide a detailed individual assessment of impairment and disability.[39,41] The interrater reliability of the scale is quite poor, in some instances only 50%.[42,43] Several studies show improved interrater reliability of 85% and test-retest reliability of 98% when a specific structured interview is used to determine GOS category.[41,44-46] A detailed description of the expanded version of the GOS, as well as administration and scoring guidelines, can be found in other sources.[47]

The Disability Rating Scale (DRS) was developed in 1982 to quantitatively assess disability in patients with severe brain injury.[48] This scale may be used to assess patients from the state of coma to full recovery. The scale is primarily used for patients with traumatic brain injury, although a few studies have used it as an outcome measure for patients with nontraumatic causes of severe brain injury.[49-51] The DRS is more sensitive to small changes in progress over time than the GOS.[48] The DRS was devel-

oped to specifically quantify the more subtle changes in individual patients that may occur when recovering from severe brain injury. The scale has a range from 0-30 with scores correlating with 10 levels of disability from death (30) to no disability (0). The scale is frequently used in rehabilitation centers to document progress and as a research tool in the literature quantifying outcomes from brain injury.[51] Five studies have shown the DRS to have a high interrater and test-retest reliability of up to 98% and high concurrent and predictive validity of up to 67%.[48,52-55] The DRS form and scoring guidelines can be found, along with directions and tips for administering the scale, at the Center for Outcome Measurement in Brain Injury (COMBI) web site (see Additional Resources).

The Rancho Los Amigos Levels of Cognitive Function Scale (LCFS) was developed in 1972 as a descriptive scale outlining the sequence of behavioral and cognitive recovery that typically takes place in patients after traumatic brain injury[56] (Table 21-6). The scale is frequently initially administered on admission to a trauma center and is re-administered as the patient moves through acute, sub-acute, and inpatient rehabilitation. The scale does not require cooperation from the patient because a level is assigned

TABLE 21-6	Level of Cognitive Functioning Scale (LCFS)

Level I: No Response.
Patient does not respond to external stimuli and appears asleep.
Level II: Generalized Response.
Patient reacts to external stimuli in nonspecific, inconsistent, and nonpurposeful manner with stereotypic and limited responses.
Level III: Localized Response.
Patient responds specifically and inconsistently with delays to stimuli but may follow simple commands for motor action.
Level IV: Confused, Agitated Response.
Patient exhibits bizarre, nonpurposeful, incoherent, or inappropriate behaviors, has no short-term recall, and attention is short and nonselective.
Level V: Confused, Inappropriate, Nonagitated Response.
Patient gives random, fragmented, and nonpurposeful responses to complex or unstructured stimuli. Simple commands are followed consistently, memory and selective attention are impaired, and new information is not retained.
Level VI: Confused, Appropriate Response.
Patient gives context appropriate, goal-directed responses, dependent on external input for direction. There is carry-over for relearned but not for new tasks and recent memory problems persist.
Level VII: Automatic, Appropriate Response.
Patient behaves appropriately in familiar settings, performs daily routines automatically, and shows carry-over for new learning at lower than normal rates. Patient initiates social interactions, but judgment remains impaired.
Level VIII: Purposeful, Appropriate Response.
Patient oriented and responds to the environment but abstract reasoning abilities are decreased relative to premorbid levels.

TABLE 21-5	Glasgow Outcome Scale	
Score/Category	**Definition**	
1: Dead	A. As a direct result of brain trauma.	
	B. Regained consciousness, died from secondary complications.	
2: Persistent vegetative state	Remains unresponsive and speechless for an extended period of time.	
	May open eyes and show sleep-wake cycles but an absence of function in the cerebral cortex.	
3: Severe disability (conscious but disabled)	Dependent for daily support secondary to mental and/or physical disability.	
4: Moderate disability (disabled but independent)	Can travel by public transport and work in a sheltered environment; can be independent as far as daily life is concerned.	
	Disabilities include varying degrees of dysphasia, hemiparesis, or ataxia, as well as intellectual and memory deficits and personality change.	
5: Good recovery	Resumption of normal life, even though there may be minor neurological and pathological deficits	

based on observations of the patient's responses to external stimuli. The scale is recorded in roman numerals and consists of 8 levels ranging from I: No response to VIII: Purposeful appropriate response. Patients can plateau at any level of the scale, which may indicate a temporary or permanent leveling off in the recovery process. The LCFS is not intended as a prognostic tool for patients with brain injury. The scale is intended for patients with traumatic causes of brain injury only and is primarily a means of standardizing communication between rehabilitation clinicians and between clinicians and patients' family members. The level assigned to a patient is determined by how closely the patient's behavioral responses fit the descriptors associated with each level of the scale. The LCFS has been shown to have interrater reliability of 89%, test-retest reliability of 82%, and a concurrent and predictive validity of between 59% and 79%.[7,54]

Patients in a coma are assigned LCFS level I or II, patients in a vegetative state or minimally conscious state are typically assigned level II or III. Levels III through VIII describe a patient exhibiting some degree of awareness or conscious behavior.

The Coma/Near Coma (CNC) scale was developed in 1992 to measure small clinical changes in patients with severe brain injuries who function at the very low levels characteristic of the vegetative state.[57] The scale is used with patients with injury resulting from either traumatic or nontraumatic causes. The CNC scale has five levels from "no coma" to "extreme coma." A level is assigned based on 11 items that are scored to indicate the severity of sensory, perceptual, and primitive response deficits. The CNC scale is useful for recognizing patients in low-level neurological states most likely to respond to further rehabilitation.[57,58] Interrater reliability of the CNC is reported to be between 95% and 97%.[57] Validity of the scale was established by significant correlations between scores on the CNC and the DRS.[57] The CNC scale, as well as directions and tips for administering the scale, can be found the COMBI web site (see Additional Resources). The CNC scale does not appear often in the literature concerning outcomes or treatment of patients with disorders of consciousness, and as discussed previously, the language of the scale used to label scoring levels does not correlate with the current language used in describing patients with disorders of consciousness.

WHIM is a 62-point scale ranking behaviors in patients with disorders of consciousness. Low scores are given to behaviors suggestive of low levels of arousal and awareness and high scores assigned to behaviors suggesting the opposite. The scale was developed in 2000 in England and has undergone only preliminary testing of validity and reliability.[59]

Cranial Nerve Integrity. Rehabilitation clinicians do not usually test cranial nerve function or reflexes in this population, but an understanding of these tests and their results gives information regarding brainstem integrity and overall prognosis. As mentioned previously, the ARAS is located in the upper two thirds of the brainstem, specifically the upper pons and midbrain, and is responsible for the arousal component of consciousness. Awareness and cognitive functioning are not possible without arousal,

and this requires a functioning ARAS. The nuclei of the cranial nerves (CNs) are located throughout the brainstem, so by testing certain CN reflexes that have nuclei surrounding the ARAS, inferences about brainstem integrity can be made. It is generally thought that if cranial nerve reflexes are present, brainstem function is intact, but if the reflexes are absent, one cannot be sure that brainstem function is absent. Various illicit drugs, antibiotics, neuromuscular-blocking agents, and vestibular diseases can block CN reflexes.[6] Fig. 21-5 illustrates the location of the ARAS in the brainstem and the surrounding CNs and nuclei.

The CN reflexes commonly tested in this population are the pupillary light reflex (CN II and III), corneal reflex (CN V and VII), and/or the oculocephalic and oculovestibular reflexes (CN III, IV, VI, and VIII). Shining a bright light into each eye and looking for direct and consensual constriction of the pupil tests the pupillary reflex (Fig. 21-6). The corneal reflex is tested by touching each cornea with a cotton swab, looking for the eyelids to shut (and/or upward deviation of the eyes, an ocular movement known as Bell's phenomenon) (Fig. 21-7). The oculocephalic reflex test, also known as the doll's eye phenomenon, is tested by rapidly moving the patient's head from one side to the other, then up and down, briefly

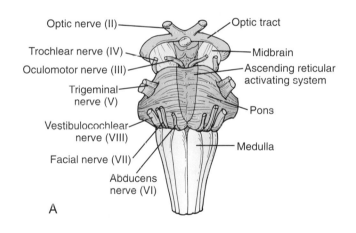

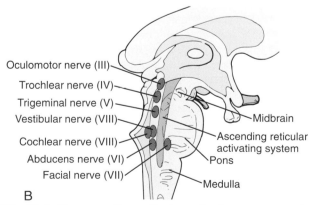

FIG. 21-5 The ascending reticular activating system and the surrounding cranial nerves and nuclei. **A,** Anterior view; **B,** midsagittal view.

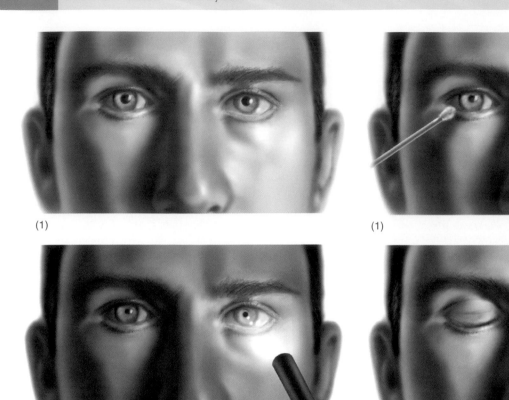

(1)

(2)

FIG. 21-6 Cranial nerve reflexes: The pupillary light reflex test (CN II and III).

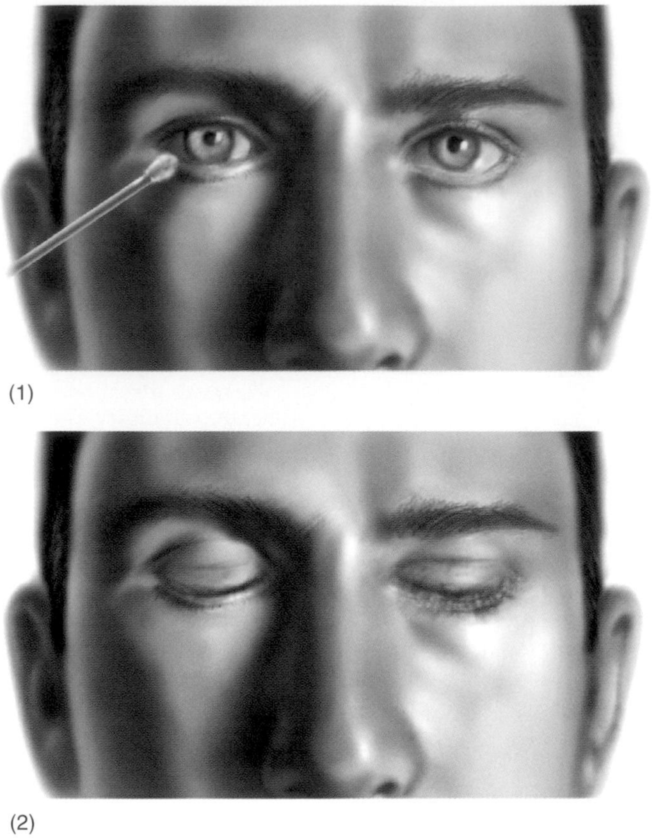

(1)

(2)

FIG. 21-7 Cranial nerve reflexes: The corneal reflex test (CN V and VII).

holding the endpoints (Fig. 21-8). The patient's eyes are watched for movement in the opposite direction to the movement of the head, indicating a positive test or intact reflex. The oculocephalic reflex test is not used if there is concern that the patient may have an unstable cervical spine so that rapid movement of the head from side to side or up and down is contraindicated. The oculovestibular reflex test is often referred to as caloric stimulation and elicits the same but stronger response than the oculocephalic reflex. The integrity of the patient's tympanic membranes must be assessed before caloric stimulation is done, since the test involves introducing cold and warm water into the ears (Fig. 21-9). To test the reflex, the patient's head is elevated 30 degrees from horizontal and a small amount of ice water is first used to irrigate each ear canal separately. The eyes of an unconscious patient should deviate toward the side of irrigation. Then, both ear canals are irrigated simultaneously with ice water, producing an upward deviation of both eyes and then with warm water to produce a downward deviation of the eyes. Fig. 21-6 illustrates the normal results of these four CN reflex tests. Very scant evidence exists regarding the reliability of these tests. One study found the interobserver reliability of cranial reflex tests to be 69%.[60]

Reflex Integrity. Abnormal deep tendon reflexes and tone abnormalities (see Chapters 16 and 17) are common in patients in coma, vegetative state, or minimally conscious state. The terms hypertonia, hypotonia, *spasticity*, and *clonus* are commonly used to describe these findings.

Cardiovascular/Pulmonary

Ventilation and Respiration/Gas Exchange. It is not uncommon for patients in vegetative state and minimally conscious state to have a fever, elevated systolic blood pressure (BP), and high HR during the acute phase of recovery.[61-63] Tests and measures for RR, BP, temperature, HR, and oxygen saturation of patients in vegetative and minimally conscious states can be found in Chapter 22.

Integumentary. Patients with disorders of consciousness are at increased risk for pressure ulcers because of their impaired mobility, as well as impaired nutritional and respiratory status (see Chapter 28).

EVALUATION, DIAGNOSIS, AND PROGNOSIS

Prognosis for recovery from conditions causing disorders of consciousness vary greatly with age, underlying etiology of the low-level state, depth of unresponsiveness, length of unresponsiveness, and response to brainstem reflex testing. The state of complete unarousal and unresponsiveness characteristic of patients in a coma rarely continues beyond 14 days, with patients usually dying or becoming vegetative within that time frame.[7,64,65]

COMA FROM TRAUMATIC CAUSES

The prognosis for traumatic coma differs from that for nontraumatic coma. In general, patients with coma resulting from trauma achieve better outcomes than patients in

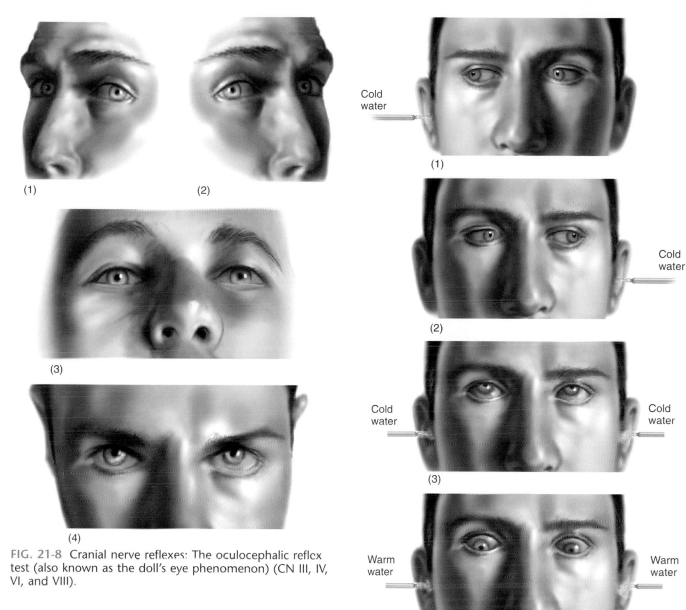

FIG. 21-8 Cranial nerve reflexes: The oculocephalic reflex test (also known as the doll's eye phenomenon) (CN III, IV, VI, and VIII).

FIG. 21-9 Cranial nerve reflexes: The oculovestibular reflex tests (also known as caloric reflexes) (CN III, IV, VI, and VII).

coma from nontraumatic causes.[66] Younger age and higher GCS score 1 week after injury are the most reliable predictors of functional recovery at 6 months in patients with coma from trauma. Outcome data from the Coma Data Bank shows that the mortality rate for patients admitted to a hospital with coma resulting from trauma is 36%. Of the remaining 64% who do not die, 27% have a good recovery and return to their former activity level, 16% are independent but not at their former level of activity, 16% are severely disabled, and 5% remain in a vegetative state.

COMA FROM NONTRAUMATIC CAUSES

Two studies identified four clinical features that appear to impact prognosis after nontraumatic coma. These features are coma etiology, depth of coma, duration of coma, and clinical signs.[67,68]

Metabolic/toxic etiologies, specifically coma induced by drug overdose, have the best prognosis. Patients with coma caused by drug overdose often present as deeply comatose with depressed brainstem reflexes because of the

effects of the drugs on the brainstem. These patients show high levels of motor activity, and all have the potential for a good prognosis. The probability of waking from coma within 2 weeks is 8 times better for drug-induced coma than for coma from other nontraumatic causes. Coma resulting from hypoxic/global ischemic etiologies has the next most favorable prognosis followed by ischemic stroke. Patients with hemorrhagic etiologies of coma have the worst prognosis for functional recovery.[65]

Depth of coma as measured by the GCS is also predictive of outcome in nontraumatic coma. Patients with higher scores 6 hours after the onset of coma have better outcomes. The 2-week outcome for patients with an initial GCS score of 3-5 is 14.8% awake and 85.2% dead or vegetative; the 2-week outcome for patients with an initial score of 6-8 is 53.1% awake and 46.9% dead or vegetative.[64] Patients with an initial GCS of 6-8 were 7 times more likely to awaken by 2 weeks than those with initial scores of 3-5.[64]

Patients in a coma of nontraumatic etiology whose eyes open within 6 hours of onset of coma have a 1 in 5 chance for a good recovery, whereas those whose eyes do not open within 6 hours have a 1 in 10 chance for a good recovery. No motor response within 6 hours leaves only a 3% chance for good recovery, whereas patients who show flexion withdrawal to noxious stimuli have a greater than 15% chance for a good recovery. Patients have only an 8% chance for a good recovery if they make no noise within 6 hours, whereas those who groan within 6 hours have a 30% chance of achieving good recovery.[65] The longer a patient remains in a coma the worse his or her chance of a good outcome. If a comatose state lasts 3 days or longer, the chance for a good recovery is only 7% and drops to 2% by day 14.[65]

Other clinical signs identifying patients likely to have a poor outcome are the absence of CN reflexes (corneal, pupillary light, oculocephalic, and oculovestibular) at 24 hours after onset of coma.[65] Patients in coma because of cardiac arrest who lack pupillary and corneal reflexes at 24 hours after onset of coma and who have no motor response at 72 hours after onset of coma have a very small chance of meaningful neurological recovery.[2,69]

VEGETATIVE STATE

In 1994 the Multi-Society Task Force on Persistent Vegetative State completed a literature review of studies involving 754 vegetative patients to determine guidelines for prognosis for recovery.[13] The group distinguished between awareness and recovery of function. Awareness was present if patients achieved consistent voluntary behavioral responses to visual and auditory stimuli and some type of consistent interaction with others. Recovery of function was measured using the "good recovery," "moderate disability," and "severe disability" categories of the GOS. The good recovery and moderate disability categories specify independent function, whereas the severe disability category indicates dependence with activities of daily living. The Multi-Society Task Force categorized their findings by age (adult: ≥16 years old versus child: <16 years old) and cause of vegetative state (traumatic versus nontraumatic). The Task Force's conclusions and numerical tables regarding prognosis 1 year after injury for those in a vegetative state at 1 month, 3 months, and 6 months postinjury are widely accepted by the medical and legal professions. For numerical tables, the reader is referred to the Multi-Society Task Force consensus statement, part 2.[13] Table 21-7 summarizes these findings.

In general, recovery of awareness 1 year after brain injury that resulted in vegetative state is unlikely in adults and children who are in this state because of traumatic injury. The prognosis for recovery of awareness after traumatic injury is slightly better for children than for adults up to 1 year after injury. However, recovery of function after traumatic injury is similar in children and adults, with both having a slightly better prognosis for functional recovery if awareness returns by 6 months after injury. Recovery of awareness after 3 months is rare in adults and children with vegetative state resulting from nontraumatic injury. Prognosis for recovery of function is poor for adults and only slightly better for children, 3 months after nontraumatic injury. The Multi-Society Task Force found no cases of functional recovery that exceeded "severe disability" if vegetative state continued 1 year after injury.

MINIMALLY CONSCIOUS STATE

Because the term "minimally conscious state" is relatively new, there is limited information on the prognosis for patients in this state.[14] The Aspen Neurobehavioral Conference formally defined the term in 1997 and stated "there is as yet inadequate information in the research literature to corroborate the natural history and prognosis for patients in minimally conscious state."[14] The group suggested that "recovery from MCS should depend upon type and severity of neuropathology" and that the relative worse prognosis for nontraumatic injury versus traumatic injury for patients in vegetative state holds true for recovery of patients in minimally conscious state.[14] The only definite conclusion put forth by the conference regarding the prognosis for patients in minimally conscious state is

TABLE 21-7	Prognosis and Recovery Indicators for Patients Who Remain in a Vegetative State 1 Month after Injury from Traumatic or Nontraumatic Causes			
Traumatic Cause			**Nontraumatic Cause**	
Recovery of Awareness	**Recovery of Function**		**Recovery of Awareness after 3 Months Vegetative**	**Recovery of Function after 3 Months Vegetative**
CHILDREN				
Unlikely after 1 year. Better prognosis for children than adults up to 1 year after injury.	If aware by 6 months after injury, better functional recovery.		Rare	Only slightly better than for adults.
ADULTS <40 YEARS OF AGE				
Unlikely but slightly better prognosis than older adults.	If aware by 6 months after injury, better functional recovery.		Rare	Poor
ADULTS >40 YEARS OF AGE				
Poor chance of recovery of awareness after 3 months after injury.	Poor chance of recovery of function after injury.			

that "patients in minimally conscious state at 12 months after injury of any cause are likely to remain, at best, severely disabled according to the Glasgow Outcome Scale."[14] The Aspen Neurobehavioral Conference group strongly suggests further research is needed to develop guidelines for recovery and prognosis in this population.

Research suggests that patients in a minimally conscious state may show more continuous improvement and attain slightly more favorable outcomes, as measured by the DRS, by 1-year postinjury than patients diagnosed with vegetative state.[70] One study followed 104 patients with a diagnosis of vegetative state or minimally conscious state admitted to a rehabilitation-based coma intervention program. The study did not mention the types of rehabilitation interventions provided to the patients. Results showed that functional outcomes at 3, 6, and 12 months postinjury were significantly more favorable for patients initially in minimally conscious state than for patients initially in vegetative state. Higher levels of motor agitation and visual tracking were recorded in the minimally conscious state group, suggesting that this may differentiate between these two populations. The authors of this study strongly suggest that more research in this area is needed.

INTERVENTION

There are no evidence-based guidelines regarding the care and rehabilitation of patients with disorders of consciousness.[71,72] A standard treatment approach is lacking for patients in this practice pattern, and little has been discovered to advance rehabilitation techniques.[30] Despite this, it is widely recommended that active rehabilitation begin early.[58,65] Several reports have highlighted the generic benefits of early rehabilitation,[14,58,62,73] and most rehabilitation centers follow consensus-based guidelines for the care and treatment of these patients.

The Aspen Neurobehavioral Conference recommends that treatment interventions focus on four areas: Augmenting communication, promoting meaningful behavioral responsiveness, preventing complications, and facilitating nursing care.[14] It has been suggested that for patients who lack awareness (coma and vegetative state), treatment should be focused on "maintaining or attaining physical health so that there is a useful body for the brain to control should recovery of awareness occur."[61]

The Aspen Neurobehavioral Conference proposes that treatment interventions be classified into two categories: Basic interventions, consisting of treatments that are vital to maintaining physical health, such as ROM, positioning protocols, and tone normalizing methods; and optional interventions or those considered to be nonessential but appropriate on a case by case basis. Sensory stimulation programs and pharmacological trials are given as examples of optional interventions.[14] Casting of limbs with goals of improving ROM and decreasing hypertonia is also considered to be an optional intervention.

BASIC INTERVENTIONS

Range of Motion Exercises. It has been a long-held belief in the rehabilitation community that daily ROM exercises in bed-bound patients assist with maintaining joint ROM, preventing contractures, and reducing the risk

of developing *heterotopic ossification*, all common outcomes in patients with severe neurological injury. However, this belief is not substantiated by the research literature. The incidence of heterotopic ossification in patients with severe brain injuries is 76%. The hips and shoulders are most commonly affected.[61] There are no studies evaluating the effect of PROM on the incidence of heterotopic ossification.

The incidence of contractures in brain-injured patients has been shown to be 84%; the joints most commonly affected are the hips, followed by the shoulders, ankles, and elbows.[74] A statistically significant increase in the number of contractures with increased duration of low-level neurological state and immobility due to neurological injury has also been shown.[74,75] Contractures can result from central and/or peripheral factors. Centrally, hypertonia or resistance to passive movement often results from CNS pathology. There is no evidence that PROM reduces centrally mediated contractures. Peripheral factors contributing to contracture formation are the structural changes that occur in soft tissues with prolonged immobilization. These include the shortening of ligaments, tendons, joint capsules, and muscle fibers; fibrofatty tissue proliferation in joints; and intraarticular adhesions.[76] There are no studies evaluating the effect of PROM in reducing the effects of peripheral factors in contracture formation.

As stated earlier, maintaining functional PROM in certain joints is key in assisting with the long-term care of these generally bed-bound patients because reduced ROM can cause difficulty with turning and positioning. Stretching increases the extensibility of soft tissues and is used widely as an intervention to increase joint mobility. A systematic review of the literature examining the effects of stretching on joint ROM in healthy subjects without contractures was completed in 2002.[77] This review indicates that stretching does produce increases in joint ROM that is evident 1 day or more after stopping the intervention in people without contractures or without risk for contractures. It is cautioned that the studies reviewed were not of high quality and that at the time no studies existed that determined the effects of stretching on patients with contractures or at risk for contracture formation.

A second systematic review completed in 2002 looked at the effects of passive muscle stretching on spasticity and joint ROM in children in vegetative state and minimally conscious state.[78] This review concluded that there is limited evidence supporting the use of passive muscle stretching to improve ROM and reduce spasticity in this patient population. However, the study's authors recommend that these findings be interpreted with caution because of the poor quality and limited number of studies available for review.

Despite the lack of evidence supporting the use of passive stretching to minimize contracture and spasticity in patients, most agree that stretching should be used as an intervention until the results of further studies emerge.[77-79] It has been suggested that to maximize the probability of attaining a clinical effect, soft tissues should be stretched for at least 20 minutes a day or maybe for as long as 12 hours a day.[80]

Positioning Protocols. Positioning protocols should be developed in conjunction with the nursing staff whose primary concerns are to avoid the development of pressure ulcers secondary to prolonged bed rest, to mobilize static lung secretions, and to prevent aspiration to reduce the risk of pneumonia. Aspiration pneumonia is common in patients with disorders of consciousness.[62,63] Evidence indicates that positioning patients in a semirecumbent position by elevating the head of the bed reduces the risk of aspiration pneumonia in patients confined to bed.[81,82] This presents difficulty because it is in direct conflict with goals of controlling pressure, friction, and shear to reduce the risk of pressure ulcer formation. From a rehabilitation perspective, correct positioning in a wheelchair (see the section on Normalizing Tone) has been shown to temporarily reduce abnormal tone and reflexes,[33] and standing a patient with the aid of a tilt table can sometimes facilitate higher level behavioral responses.[31] These techniques may be included in the positioning schedule for patients with disorders of consciousness.

Normalizing Tone. Tone abnormalities are common in patients in with disorders of consciousness. High tone can lead to posturing, which can result in contracture formation and positioning difficulties.[63] A number of physical interventions are thought to decrease tone in hypertonic muscles. These include electrical stimulation, vibration, altering body position, and prolonged muscle stretch (including splinting).[83] However, there is no evidence that physical interventions permanently normalize tone in hypertonic muscles. Several authors advocate the use of sitting programs with patients in vegetative state because clinical observation seems to suggest that proper sitting position can temporarily normalize tone.[33,74] This has not been evaluated by research.

OPTIONAL INTERVENTIONS

Sensory Stimulation. Sensory stimulation is the application of environmental stimuli by an external agent for the purpose of promoting arousal and behavioral responsiveness.[84] Formalized sensory stimulation programs as a treatment for patients in a coma or vegetative state became popular in the 1980s despite a lack of scientific evidence proving or disproving their effectiveness. The programs varied in intensity and frequency of intervention, as well as targeted senses. At a minimum, most programs included stimulation of visual, auditory, olfactory, kinesthetic, and tactile senses.

Proponents of such programs contended that patients with disorders of consciousness suffered from environmental deprivation and that this "deprivation could lead to widespread impairments of intellectual and perceptual processes accompanied by changes in cerebral electrical activity."[85] Controversy concerning the benefits of such programs continued throughout the 1990s, prompting the Cochrane Collaboration in 1999 to formally assess the effectiveness of sensory stimulation programs through a systematic review of the literature. Including only randomized controlled trials that compared sensory stimulation with standard rehabilitation programs, the Cochrane group found "no reliable evidence to support or rule out the effectiveness of multi-sensory programs in patients in

coma or vegetative state."[86] There is no literature on the effectiveness of sensory stimulation programs in patients in minimally conscious state. Clinicians need to understand the high degree of uncertainty of outcomes with these programs and take into account other prognostic factors for outcome before initiating or recommending sensory stimulation intervention.

Casting. The use of casts in management of tone in adults with impaired consciousness is controversial. Three goals are suggested for casting in these patients: Improved ROM, decreased spasticity, and improved function. A systematic review of the literature published in 2003 revealed that improved PROM is the only outcome supported by the current evidence. There is insufficient evidence to support the theory that casting decreases spasticity or improves function in brain-injured adults.[87]

CASE STUDY 21-1

CLOSED HEAD INJURY

Examination
Patient History

BT was admitted to a trauma center with a diagnosis of closed head injury and loss of consciousness secondary to assault. BT was brought to the trauma center by ambulance. His history was obtained from chart notes. No family was present. Per the ambulance report, BT was found unconscious on a street corner. The duration of his unconscious state could not be verified. He was intubated at the scene. His admission radiographs showed he had temporal and occipital skull fractures, multiple rib fractures, and a right forearm fracture. CT scans showed evidence of two large subdural hematomas. His GCS score on admission was recorded as 10 and dropped to 7 on day 2 of his hospitalization. He remained in the ICU for treatment to control suspected cerebral edema and was closely monitored for further neurological decline or recovery. On hospital day 5, his GCS score was recorded as 8 and a physical therapy consult was ordered and initiated. A chart review revealed that BT was approximately in his middle twenties and had intact pupillary light, corneal, and oculovestibular reflexes on admission. The oculocephalic reflex was not tested because of the contraindication to rapid head movements with suspected cervical spine trauma. BT remained on a ventilator and was to begin a weaning trial the following morning. Medications included narcotics to lessen pain suspected with BT's multiple fractures.

Systems Review

BT required a ventilator to support his breathing, and his vital signs were stable. Respiratory therapy was to begin ventilator weaning trials the following morning. There were no areas of skin breakdown. CN nerve reflexes were intact. Initial admission GCS score of 10 was recorded as eyes opening (E) to speech = 3, best motor response (M) localizes pain = 5, and best verbal response (V) incomprehensible sounds = 2. He was not in a coma at this time. BT's decline in neurological status was indicated by his second GCS score of 7; E = 1 no response, M = 4 flexion withdrawal, and V = 2 incomprehensible sounds. At this time, BT was in a coma as defined by a GCS of below or equal to 8. The GCS recorded on the morning of BT's physical therapy examination was 8: E = 1 no response, M = 5 localizes to pain, and V = 2 incomprehensible sounds. An LCFS level of II (generalized response) was recorded on the morning of his physical therapy examination.

Tests and Measures

Musculoskeletal

Range of Motion BT's PROM was tested in the lower extremities and left upper extremity. Right upper extremity ROM testing was deferred because of the unstable right forearm fracture and pending orthopedic evaluation. There were no limits in PROM in the joints tested, however, a mild increase in resistance to movement was felt throughout.

Muscle Performance/Strength Formal strength testing was not performed because BT was not alert and could not follow commands, but when testing ROM, he did spontaneously move his left arm and legs. These observations were recorded.

Neuromuscular

Arousal, Attention, and Cognition During his physical therapy examination, BT opened his eyes spontaneously. He did not follow commands. His eyes appeared to be roving from side to side and not tracking. These observations were recorded, and the physician notified. Spontaneous eye opening would change his overall GCS score to 11 (if no other areas changed), indicating he was no longer in a coma but had an injury of moderate severity according to the scale. His LCFS level remained at II.

Reflex Integrity Clonus and Babinski's sign testing were normal, and muscle stretch reflexes were equal but hyperresponsive bilaterally.

Evaluation, Diagnosis, and Prognosis

BT's initial physical therapy examination was limited by continued ventilatory support, pending orthopedic consultation to determine the stability and plan for his rib and forearm fractures, and lack of medical clearance to begin mobilizing BT to the edge of the bed. Despite this, it was determined that his GCS score and therefore his neurological status were continuing to improve. BT's ability to spontaneously open his eyes indicated that he was now alert and no longer in a coma. However, he showed no signs of awareness. He was determined to now be in a vegetative state. Evidence shows that the prognosis for recovery from coma or vegetative state as a result of trauma is far better than the prognosis for recovery from coma or vegetative state from other causes; 40% of patients in coma from trauma return to full independence although 16% not to their former activity level. It was recommended that BT be transferred to an acute rehabilitation center, once medically stabilized, to maximize his chances for full functional recovery.

Intervention

BT was seen daily for physical therapy intervention, including ROM and assisting nursing with positioning.

His neurological status was closely monitored. On hospital day 7, BT was extubated, and his right forearm fracture stabilized with a splint. Clearance was given to assist BT to the edge of the bed, which was done on hospital day 8 with nursing assistance. BT was dependent in transferring from supine to sitting at the edge of the bed and for maintaining balance in the sitting position. His vital signs remained stable in the sitting position, but he showed no increase in awareness to the environment. It was recommended that BT be assisted to a lift chair daily with the help of physical therapy, nursing, and/or the hospital lifting team. On hospital day 10, after positioning BT in a sitting position, it was noticed that he followed the clinician around the room with his eyes and that he inconsistently assisted with ROM exercises. His LCFS level was recorded as III (localized response). This information was reported to the physician, who, after examination, determined BT to now be in a minimally conscious state with a GCS of 11. The patient was transferred on hospital day 11 to a traumatic brain injury unit of an acute inpatient rehabilitation center where his care and monitoring continued.

Outcome

While in the acute care hospital, BT did not loose any PROM of his extremities and developed no skin breakdown. His tolerance for upright activity improved, and his neurological status showed steady improvements with improving GCS scores and LCFS levels.

Please see the CD that accompanies this book for a case study describing the examination, evaluation, and interventions for a patient with metabolic coma.

CHAPTER SUMMARY

The past two decades have provided advances in medical technology that have caused the mortality from severe brain injuries to decrease significantly. Patients who previously would have died are living in a vegetative or minimally conscious state and are being evaluated for admission to rehabilitation facilities with greater frequency. Rehabilitation professionals working together as a multidisciplinary team must understand the prognostic indicators for this population to make the most appropriate and informed recommendations for rehabilitation.

The role of rehabilitation in the early stages of injury is to help prevent deterioration of the sensory-motor system and to maintain physical health to reduce the risk of complications associated with prolonged bed rest. Clinicians also have the responsibility of monitoring changes in the behavior and function of these patients and understanding what these changes might indicate. It is imperative that all rehabilitation professionals understand the differences between specific definitions, clinical features, and prognostic indicators for this group of patients so appropriate decisions regarding care can be made.

There is a lack of evidenced-based data concerning behavior measurement, rehabilitation interventions, and outcomes for patients in preferred practice pattern 5I. Quality research is needed in this area to develop rehabilitation programs consisting of interventions that have the potential to optimize recovery of awareness and function in these patients.

ADDITIONAL RESOURCES

Useful Forms

Activities-Specific Balance Confidence (ABC) Scale
Disability Rating Scale (DRS)
Glasgow Coma Scale (GCS)
Glasgow Outcome Scale (GOS)
Rancho Los Amigos Levels of Cognitive Function Scale (LCFS)

Books

Jennett B: *The Vegetative State: Medical Facts, Ethical and Legal Dilemmas,* London, 2002, Cambridge University Press.
Plum F, Posner JB: *The Diagnosis of Stupor and Coma,* ed 3, Philadelphia, 1982, FA Davis.
Young B, Ropper A, Bolton C: *Coma and Impaired Consciousness,* New York, 1998, McGraw Hill.

Web Sites

Brain Injury Association: www.biausa.org
Center for Outcome Measurement in Brain Injury (COMBI): www.tbims.org/combi
Coma Recovery Association: www.comarecovery.org
National Institute of Neurological Disorders and Stroke: www.ninds.nih.gov/index.htm
National Rehabilitation Information Center (NARIC): www.naric.com

GLOSSARY

Clonus: Spasmodic alternation of muscular contraction and relaxation believed to result from alteration of the normal pattern of motoneuron discharge.

Coma: A neurobehavioral diagnosis indicating the patient is unarousable and without sleep-wake cycles. The patient has no ability to interact with the environment. Eyes do not open spontaneously or to external stimulation and the patient does not follow any commands.

Consciousness: The totality in psychology of sensations, perceptions, ideas, attitudes, and feelings of which an individual or a group is aware at any given time or within a given time span; waking life (as that to which one returns after sleep, trance, or fever) in which one's normal mental powers are present; the upper part of mental life of which the person is aware as contrasted with unconscious processes.

Decerebrate posturing: Extension of the elbow, internal rotation of the shoulders, and extension of the lower extremities. Usually occurs with lesions affecting the midbrain portion of the brainstem.

Decorticate posturing: Flexion of the upper extremities and extension of the lower extremities. Usually occurs with lesions affecting the corticospinal tracts. Usually more favorable than decerebrate posturing.

Delirium: An abnormal mental state characterized by disorientation, irritability, fear, visual hallucinations, and misperception of sensory stimuli. Delirium is characterized by rapid onset and rarely persists longer than 7 days. Delirium is common with toxic and metabolic disorders of the nervous system.

Heterotopic ossification: The appearance of ectopic bone in soft tissue usually in periarticular locations. Can present clinically with erythema, warmth, and edema and decreased ROM.

Locked-in-syndrome: A neurobehavioral diagnosis referring to patients who are alert, aware of the environment, and able to interact with it but who cannot move or speak. Communication is usually through limited eye movements (blinking or vertical movements). The syndrome is the result of a brainstem lesion usually involving the pons.

Minimally conscious state: A neurobehavioral diagnosis indicating severely altered consciousness in which minimal but definite behavioral evidence of self- or environmental awareness is demonstrated. The patient's eyes open spontaneously or

in response to stimulation; the patient follows commands inconsistently.

Obtunded: A decreased alertness and interest in the environment, slow response to stimuli and increased sleep time with drowsiness characterizing awake time.

Reticular activating system: A part of the reticular formation that extends from the brainstem to the midbrain and thalamus with connections distributed throughout the cerebral cortex and that controls the degree of activity of the central nervous system (as in maintaining sleep and wakefulness and in making transitions between the two states).

Somnolent: Inclined to or heavy with sleep.

Spasticity: Velocity-dependent resistance to passive movement.

Stupor: A state of deep sleep from which a patient can be awoken with vigorous and repeated stimuli. Once the stimulation is stopped, the patient falls back into a state of unresponsiveness.

Subtentorial (infratentorial): Occurring or made below the tentorium cerebelli.

Supratentorial: Relating to, occurring in, affecting, or being the tissues overlying the tentorium cerebelli.

Vegetative state: A neurobehavioral diagnosis indicating complete loss of ability to interact with the environment but with intact sleep-wake cycles. The patient's eyes open spontaneously or in response to stimulation; the patient does not follow any commands.

References

1. Marshall LF, Becker DD, Bowers SA, et al: The national traumatic coma data bank, *J Neuro Surg* 59:276-284, 1983.
2. Booth CM, Boone RH, Tomlinson G, et al: Is the patient dead, vegetative or severely neurologically impaired? *JAMA* 291:870-879, 2004.
3. Pilon M, Sullivan SJ: Motor profile of patients in minimally responsive and persistent vegetative states, *Brain Inj* 10:421-437, 1996.
4. American Physical Therapy Association: *Guide to Physical Therapist Practice,* ed 2, Alexandria, Va, 2001, The Association.
5. Young B, Ropper A, Bolton C: *Coma and Impaired Consciousness,* New York, 1998, McGraw Hill.
6. Plum F, Posner JB: *The Diagnosis of Stupor and Coma,* ed 3, Philadelphia, 1982, FA Davis.
7. Giacino JT, Zasler ND: Outcome after severe traumatic brain injury: Coma, the vegetative state and the minimally responsive state, *J Head Trauma Rehabil* 10:40-56, 1995.
8. Childs NL, Mercer WN, Childs HW: Accuracy of diagnosis of persistent vegetative state, *Neurology* 43:1465-1467, 1993.
9. Tresch DD, Farrol HS, Duthie EH, et al: Clinical characteristics of patients in persistent vegetative state, *Arch Internal Med* 151:930-932, 1991.
10. Andrews K, Murphy L, Munday R, et al: Misdiagnosis of the vegetative state: Retrospective study in a rehabilitation unit, *BMJ* 313:13-16, 1996.
11. American Congress of Rehabilitation Medicine: Recommendations for the use of uniform nomenclature pertinent to patients with severe alterations in consciousness, *Arch Phys Med Rehabil* 76:205-209, 1995.
12. Multi-Society Task Force on PVS: Medical aspects of the persistent vegetative state (1), *N Engl J Med* 330:1499-1508, 1994.
13. Multi-Society Task Force on PVS: Medical aspects of the persistent vegetative state (2), *N Engl J Med* 330:1572-1578, 1994.
14. Giacino JT, Zasler ND, Katz DI, et al: Development of practice guidelines for the assessment and management of the vegetative and minimally conscious states, Aspen Neurobehavioral Conference, *J Head Trauma Rehabil* 12:79-89, 1997.
15. Jennett B, Plum F: Persistent vegetative state after brain injury: A syndrome in search of a name, *Lancet* 1:734-737, 1972.
16. Jennett B: *The Vegetative State: Medical Facts, Ethical and Legal Dilemmas,* London, 2002, Cambridge University Press.
17. Giacino J, Ashwal S: The minimally conscious state: Definition and diagnostic criteria, *Neurology* 58:349-353, 2002.
18. Rappaport M, Dougherty AM, Kelting DL: Evaluation of coma and vegetative states, *Arch Phys Med Rehabil* 73:628-634, 1992.
19. Childs NL, Mercer WN, Childs HW: Accuracy of diagnosis of persistent vegetative state, *Neurology* 43:1465-1467, 1993.
20. Wijdicks EF: The diagnosis of brain death, *N Engl J Med* 344:1215-1221, 2001.
21. Kerridge IH, Saul P, Lowe M, et al: Death, dying and donation: Organ transplantation and the diagnosis of death, *J Med Ethics* 28:89-94, 2002.
22. Shewmon DA: Chronic "brain death:" Meta-analysis and conceptual consequences, *Neurology* 51:1538-1545, 1998.
23. Ciccone CD: *Pharmacology in Rehabilitation,* ed 3, Philadelphia, 2002, FA Davis.
24. Convertino V, Hung J, Goldwater D, et al: Cardiovascular responses to exercise in middle-aged men after 10 days of bed rest, *Circulation* 65:134-140, 1982.

25. Balocchi R, DiGarbo A, Michelassi C, et al: Heart rate and blood pressure response to short-term head-down bed rest: A nonlinear approach, *Methods Inf Med* 39:157-159, 2000.

26. Bloomfield SA: Changes in musculoskeletal structure and function with prolonged bed rest, *Med Sci Sports Exerc* 29:197-206, 1997.

27. Young GB, Ropper AH, Bolton CF: *Coma and Impaired Consciousness*, New York, 1998, McGraw-Hill.

27. Norkin CC, White DJ: *Measurement of Joint Motion: A Guide to Goniometry*, ed 3, Philadelphia, 2003, FA Davis.

28. Gajdosik RL, Florence JM, King WM, et al: Clinical measurement of range of motion: Review of goniometry emphasizing reliability and validity, *Phys Ther* 67:1867-1872, 1987.

29. Elveru RA, Rothstein JM, Lamb RL: Goniometric reliability in a clinical setting: Subtalar and ankle joint measurements, *Phys Ther* 68:672-677, 1988.

30. Elliott L, Coleman M, Shiel A, et al: Effect of posture on levels of arousal and awareness in vegetative and minimally conscious state patients: A preliminary investigation, *J Neuro Neurosurg Psych* 76:298-299, 2005.

31. Shiel A, Horn SA, Wilson BA, et al: The Wessex Head Injury Matrix (WHIM) main scale: A preliminary report on a scale to assess and monitor patient recovery after severe head injury, *Clin Rehabil* 14:408-416, 2000.

32. Shaw R: Persistent vegetative state: Principles and techniques for seating and positioning, *Head Trauma Rehabil* 1:31-37, 1986.

33. Wisner DH: History and current scoring systems for critical care, *Arch Surg* 127:352, 1992.

34. Teasdale G, Jennett B: Assessment of coma and impaired consciousness: A practical scale, *Lancet* 2:81-84, 1974.

35. Sacco RL, Van Gool R, Mohr JP, et al: Nontraumatic coma, Glasgow coma score and coma etiology as predictors of 2-week outcome, *Arch Neurol* 47:1181-1184, 1990.

36. Menegazzi JJ, Davis EA, Sucov AN, et al: Reliability of the Glasgow coma scale when used by emergency physicians and paramedics, *J Trauma* 34:46-48, 1993.

37. Heron R, Davie A, Gillies R, et al: Interrater reliability of the Glasgow coma scale scoring among nurses in sub-specialties of critical care, *Aust Crit Care* 14:100-105, 2001.

38. Sternbach GL: The Glasgow coma scale, *J Emerg Med* 19:67-71, 2000.

39. Jennett B, Bond M: Assessment of outcome after severe brain damage: A practical scale, *Lancet* 1:480-484, 1975.

40. Hall K, Cope DN, Rappaport M: Glasgow outcome scale and disability rating scale: comparative usefulness in following recovery in traumatic head injury, *Arch Phys Med Rehabil* 66:35-37, 1985.

41. Wilson JT, Pettigew LE, Teasdale GM: Emotional and cognitive consequences of head injury in relation to the Glasgow outcome scale, *J Neurol Neurosurg Psychiatry* 69:204-209, 2000.

42. Anderson SI, Housley AM, Jones PA, et al: Glasgow outcome scale: an inter-rater reliability study, *Brain Inj* 7:309-317, 1993.

43. Maas AI, Braakman R, Schouten HJ, et al: Agreement between physicians on assessment of outcome following severe head injury, *J Neurosurg* 58:321-325, 1983.

44. Pettigrew LE, Wilson JT, Teasdale GM: Assessing disability after head injury: Improved use of the Glasgow outcome scale, *J Neurosurg* 89:939-943, 1998.

45. Wilson JT, Edwards P, Fiddes H, et al: Reliability of postal questionnaires for the Glasgow outcome scale, *J Neurotrauma* 19:999-1005, 2002.

46. Pettigrew LE, Wilson JT, Teasdale GM: Reliability of ratings on the Glasgow outcome scale from in-person and telephone structured interviews, *J Head Trauma Rehabil* 18:252-258, 2003.

47. Wilson JTL, Pettigrew LEL, Teasdale GM: Structured interviews for the Glasgow Outcome Scale and the Extended Glasgow Outcome Scale: Guidelines for their use, *J Neurotrauma* 15:573-585, 1998.

48. Rappaport M, Hall K, Hopkins K, et al: Disability rating scale for severe head trauma: Coma to community, *Arch Phys Med Rehabil* 63:118-123, 1982.

49. Huang ME, Wartella JE, Kreutzer JS: Functional outcomes and quality of life in patients with brain tumors: a preliminary report, *Arch Phys Med Rehabil* 82(11):1540-1546, 2001.

50. Gray DS, Burnham RS: Preliminary outcome analysis of a long-term rehabilitation program for severe acquired brain injury, *Arch Phys Med Rehabil* 81(11):1447-1456, 2000.

51. Williams GR, Jiang JG: Development of an ischemic stroke survival score, *Stroke* 31(10):2414-2420, 2000.

52. Hall K, Cope DN, Rappaport M: Glasgow outcome scale and disability rating scale: Comparative usefulness in following recovery in traumatic head injury, *Arch Phys Med Rehabil* 66:35-37, 1985.

53. Eliason MR, Topp BW: Predictive validity of Rappaport's disability rating scale in subjects with acute brain dysfunction, *Phys Ther* 64:1357-1360, 1984.

54. Gouvier WD, Blanton PD, LaPorte KK, et al: Reliability and validity of the disability rating scale and the levels of cognitive functioning scale in monitoring recovery from severe head injury, *Arch Phys Med Rehabil* 68:94-97, 1987.

55. Fleming JM, Maas F: Prognosis of rehabilitation outcome in head injury using the Disability Rating Scale, *Arch Phys Med Rehabil* 75:156-163, 1994.

56. Hagen C, Malkmus D, Durham P: *Rancho Los Amigos Levels of Cognitive Functioning Scale*, Downey, Calif, 1972, Rancho Los Amigos Hospital.

57. Rappaport M, Dougherty AM, Kelting DL: Evaluation of coma and vegetative states, *Arch Phys Med Rehabil* 73:628-634, 1992.

58. Talbot LR, Whitaker HA: Brain-injured persons in an altered state of consciousness: Measures and intervention strategies, *Brain Inj* 8:689-699, 1994.

59. Shiel A, Horn SA, Wilson BA, et al: The Wessex Head Injury Matrix (WHIM) main scale: A preliminary report on a scale to assess and monitor patient recovery after severe head injury, *Clin Rehabil* 14:408-416, 2000.

60. Born JD, Hans P, Albert A, et al: Interobserver agreement in assessment of motor response and brain stem reflexes, *Neurosurgery* 4:513-517, 1987.

61. Whyte J, Laborde A, DiPasquale MC: Assessment and treatment of the vegetative and minimally conscious patient. In Rosenthal M, Griffith ER, Kreutzer J, et al (eds): *Rehabilitation of the Adult and Child with Traumatic Brain Injury*, ed 3, Philadelphia, 1999, FA Davis.

62. Sandel ME: Medical management of the comatose, vegetative, or minimally responsive patient, *NeuroRehabilitation* 6:9-17, 1996.

63. Whyte J, Glenn MB: The care and rehabilitation of the patient in a persistent vegetative state, *Head Trauma Rehabil* 1:39-53, 1996.

64. Sacco RL, Van Gool R, Mohr JP, et al: Nontraumatic coma, Glasgow coma score and coma etiology as predictors of 2-week outcome, *Arch Neurol* 47:1181-1184, 1990.

65. Bates D. The prognosis of medical coma, *J Neurol Neurosurg Psychiatry* 71:20-23, 2001.

66. Marshall LF, Gautille T, Klauber MR, et al: The outcome of severe closed head injury, *J Neurosurg* 75:28-33, 1991.

67. Jorgensen EO, Malchow-Moller A: A natural history of global and critical brain ischemia, *Resuscitation* 9:133-191, 1981.

68. Levy DE, Bates D, Caronna JA, et al: Prognosis in non-traumatic coma, *Ann Intern Med* 94:293-301, 1981.

69. Levy DE, Caronna JJ, Singer BH, et al: Predicting outcome from hypoxic-ischemic coma, *JAMA* 253:1420-1426, 1985.

70. Giacino J, Kalmar K: The vegetative and minimally conscious states: A comparison of clinical features and functional outcome, *J Head Trauma Rehabil* 12:36-51, 1997.

71. Giacino JT, Zasler ND, Katz DI, et al: Development of practice guidelines for assessment and management of the vegetative and minimally conscious states, *J Head Trauma Rehabil* 12(4):79-89, 1997.

72. Pape T, Senno R, Guernon A, et al: A measure of neurobehavioral functioning after coma. Part II: Clinical and scientific implementation, *J Rehabil Res Dev* 42:19-28, 2005.

73. Andrews K: Managing the persistent vegetative state. Early skilled care offers the best hope for optimal recovery, *BMJ* 305:486-487, 1992.

74. Yarkony GM, Sahgal V: Contractures. A major complication of craniocerebral trauma, *Clin Orthop* 219:93-96, 1987.

75. Yarkony GM, Bass LM, Keenan V, et al: Contractures complicating spinal cord injury: incidence and comparison between spinal cord center and general hospital acute care, *Paraplegia* 23:265-271, 1985.

76. Binkley J: Overview of ligament and tendon structure and mechanics: Implications for clinical practice, *Physiother Canada* 41:24-29, 1989.

77. Harvey L, Herbert R, Crosbie J: Does stretching induce lasting increases in joint ROM? A systematic review, *Physio Ther Res Intern* 7:1-13, 2002.

78. Leong B: Critical review of passive muscle stretch: implications for the treatment of children in vegetative and minimally conscious states, *Brain Inj* 16:169-183, 2002.

79. Harvey L, Batty J, Crosbie J, et al: A randomized trial assessing the effects of 4 weeks of daily stretching on ankle mobility in patients with spinal cord injury, *Arch Phys Med Rehabil* 81:1340-1347, 2000.

80. Harvey L, Herbert RD: Muscle stretching for treatment and prevention of contracture in people with spinal cord injury, *Spinal Cord* 40:1-9, 2002.

81. Hixson S, Sole M, King T: Nursing strategies to prevent ventilator-associated pneumonia, *AACN Clin Issues* 1:76-90, 1998.

82. Reignier J, Thenoz-Jost N, Fiancette M, et al: Early enteral nutrition in mechanically ventilated patients in the prone position, *Crit Care Med* 1:94-99, 2002.

83. Whyte J, Glenn MB: The care and rehabilitation of the patient in a persistent vegetative state, *Head Trauma Rehabil* 1:39-53, 1996.

84. Giacino J: Sensory stimulation: theoretical perspectives and the evidence for effectiveness, *NeuroRehabilitation* 6:69-78, 1996.

85. Le Winn EB, Dimancescu MD: Environmental deprivation and enrichment in coma, *Lancet* 2:156-157, 1978.

86. Lombardi F, Taricco M, DeTanti A, et al: Sensory stimulation for brain injured individuals in coma or vegetative state, *Cochrane Database Syst Rev* (2):CD001427, 2002.

87. Mortenson PA, Eng J: The use of casts in the management of joint mobility and hypertonia following brain injury in adults: A systematic review, *Phys Ther* 83:648-658, 2003.

Chapter 22

Vital Signs

Brian K. Peterson

CHAPTER OUTLINE

OBJECTIVES

After reading this chapter, the reader will be able to:
1. Identify the vital signs.
2. Discuss the importance and physiological implications of each vital sign.
3. Describe and perform appropriate procedures to measure the vital signs, including pulse, respiratory rate, blood pressure, pain level, and oxygen saturation.
4. Identify normal ranges for the vital signs.
5. Know when to monitor vital signs during rehabilitation.

Vital signs are critical indicators of a person's health and current medical status. The body's cells and organs require a relatively constant internal environment to function and the vital signs reflect whether specific body systems (circulatory, pulmonary, neurological, and endocrine) are functioning appropriately.[1] Vital signs often provide the first indication of harmful physiological changes or disturbances in the body and may also be the first indication of a return to a more stable condition.[2]

There are four traditional vital signs (also known as cardinal signs): Temperature, *pulse*, respiratory rate, and blood pressure (BP). Two additional measures, pain level and oxygen saturation, were more recently added to these. Pain level was added because many patients have pain, and pain is often why patients seek medical help. Thus pain can be an indicator of patient progress, status, and comfort.[1] Additionally, the level of oxygen saturation, as measured by pulse oximetry, provides information about the amount of oxygen a patient is carrying in their blood and can indicate changes in cardiac, circulatory, and pulmonary status.

Recording baseline measurements of vital signs during the initial patient contact is important for comparison with future measurements. Regular recording and documentation of vital signs may reveal sudden or gradually progressive changes that might not otherwise be observed. Accurate reliable measurements of the vital signs are needed to detect such changes. Knowledge of normal ranges of vital signs is also important for patient evaluation and direction of interventions.

This chapter provides information about the vital signs of temperature, pulse, BP, respiratory rate, pain level, and oxygen saturation. Included is information about the implications of the vital sign, measurement methods, evidence regarding the reliability and validity of different measurement approaches, normal ranges for each vital sign, and suggestions for when each should be measured during the management of patients involved in rehabilitation.

TEMPERATURE

IMPLICATIONS OF TEMPERATURE

Heat is produced by virtually every chemical reaction within the body, and core body temperature represents the balance between heat production and heat loss. Body temperature is tightly regulated within a narrow physiological range but may increase significantly in response to infection or increased physical activity. Many other factors, such as *ambient temperature,* circadian rhythm, neurological function, clothing, age, gender, menstrual cycle, pregnancy, emotion, and injury, influence core body temperature. Body temperature is regulated primarily by the hypothalamus, which acts like a thermostat, keeping core body temperature near a set point of approximately 37° C (98.6° F). The hypothalamus continuously monitors body temperature and directs the heat producing and heat loss mechanisms to keep the temperature near the set point.

Infection may alter the set point of the hypothalamus, shifting the balance toward heat production and away from heat loss so that the core body temperature increases. Increased temperature may stimulate defense responses to quell the infection. Once the stress of the infection has been eliminated, the set point resets to the individual's normal baseline, allowing heat-reducing mechanisms to restore the normal temperature.

There are both external and internal thermoregulatory mechanisms. Heat may be transferred by conduction, convection, conversion, radiation, and evaporation. Conduction is the transfer of heat to a substance or object through direct contact. Convection is the transfer of heat by mass flow of a liquid or gas past a surface. Air or fluids generally cool or heat the body by convection. Air next to the body becomes warmed by conduction, and since warmer air is less dense than cooler air, it rises to produce a convection current. The warm air is replaced by cool air, and the process continues. The greater the temperature difference between the body surface and the environment, the more rapidly the air exchange takes place and the more quickly heat is lost. Circulating blood in the body transfers heat by convection. The body adjusts its rate of heat transfer by *vasodilation* (an increase in the diameter of the blood vessels) and *vasoconstriction* (a decrease in the size of the blood vessels) in response to information processed in the hypothalamus regarding increasing or decreasing temperature. Temperature increases promote peripheral vasodilation and increased blood flow to the skin to help eliminate heat from the body and reduce the core temperature. Conversely, temperature decreases promote peripheral vasoconstriction to shunt blood to the core and preserve body heat. Conversion is the production of heat by conversion from another form of energy. Both metabolism and ultrasound produce heat in the body by conversion. Radiation is the transfer or emission of heat in the form of electromagnetic waves between objects that are not in contact with one another. For example, the sun warms us by radiation. Evaporation describes the process by which thermal energy (heat) is conducted away from a surface as liquid becomes a vapor. Evaporation is reduced when there is already moisture in the air. Therefore the higher the relative humidity the less effectively evaporation can cool the body.

If temperature regulation cannot keep up with environmental changes, core body temperature may shift excessively downward, resulting in *hypothermia* (too low a temperature) or upward resulting in hyperthermia (too high a temperature). Hypothermia is defined as body temperature of 35° C (95° F) or lower. If unchecked, hypothermia causes a sequence of symptoms beginning with a sense of cold, progressing to shivering, vasoconstriction, muscle rigidity, decreased BP, confusion, loss of reflexes, loss of spontaneous movement, coma, and death, usually by cardiac *arrhythmia,* when core temperature falls to 21.2°-29.4° C (70°-85° F).

METHODS FOR MEASURING TEMPERATURE

Body temperature may be measured with various types of thermometers and at various sites. Thermometer types include mercury-in-glass thermometers, electronic thermometers, *tympanic membrane* thermometers, and disposable/single-use thermometers. Sites for temperature measurement include oral, axillary, tympanic membrane, and rectal. The procedure for rectal temperature measurement is not described because rehabilitation clinicians are unlikely to perform this procedure.

The gold standard measurement of body temperature is the pulmonary artery catheter,[3] which provides continuous precise monitoring of temperature but requires an invasive medical procedure for placement. Pulmonary artery catheter temperature measurement is not discussed further in this text but is used for comparison with the noninvasive measures described.

Types of Thermometers

Mercury-in-Glass Thermometer. Mercury-in-glass thermometers are discussed because they have been used extensively in the past both institutionally and in research. However, there is a growing trend nationally and internationally to phase out or ban the use of mercury thermometers and other equipment containing mercury, such as *sphygmomanometers,* because of the toxicity of mercury to the individual and the environment. There are currently at least 10 states in the United States that have banned the sale of mercury thermometers. Local city and county ordinances banning mercury thermometers are also in effect in certain areas. In practice, electronic,

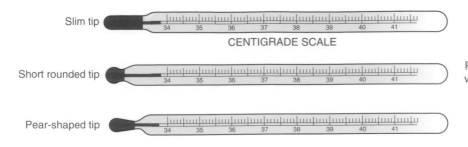

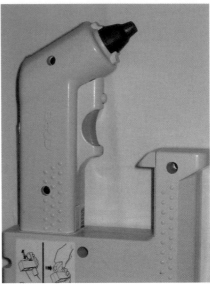

FIG. 22-1 Mercury-in-glass thermometers with three different types of tips.

tympanic membrane, and single-use thermometers will be encountered much more commonly than the mercury-in-glass thermometer.

Mercury-in-glass thermometers consist of a sealed glass tube calibrated in degrees Centigrade and/or degrees Fahrenheit, with a mercury-filled reservoir at one end. The mercury in the reservoir expands with increased temperature, climbing higher up the thermometer, and it contracts and recedes as the temperature falls. Mercury-in-glass thermometers generally have one of three different tips: Slim (oral or axillary) tip, the short-rounded tip (also known as stubby), and the pear-shaped (rectal) tip[1] (Fig. 22-1).

Tympanic Membrane Thermometers. Tympanic membrane thermometers use an *otoscope*-like probe that is inserted into the external auditory canal to detect and measure thermal infrared energy emitted from the tympanic membrane (Fig. 22-2). A scan button is pressed to start the measurement, and an audible signal indicates that the temperature is ready to be recorded from the digital display.

Tympanic thermometers are minimally invasive, record temperatures in approximately 3 seconds, register temperatures in the range of 25°-43° C, have no direct contact with mucous membranes, and work only if the disposable probe cover is in place.[4] The probe lens, however, can be easily damaged if not handled carefully. It is important to check the lens before each use and to replace its protective cover when not in use.[4] Operator handedness, patient position, and ear (right or left) have been shown not to produce clinically significant variability,[5] although mean tympanic measurements from a single ear were found to agree less than the mean of both ears when compared to temperature measurement by pulmonary artery catheter.[6] Obstruction of the tympanic membrane by cerumen may lower tympanic measurements.[7]

Tympanic thermometers have been found to be accurate, easily usable clinically,[8] and satisfactory for routine intermittent temperature measurement.[9] They are as accurate as indwelling rectal probes and are suitable for estimating core temperature when a pulmonary artery catheter is not in place or is contraindicated.[10] Tympanic membrane thermometers are the most sensitive noninvasive devices for measuring body temperature greater than 37.5° C and are better for detecting temperature shifts after acetaminophen than single-use or mercury-in glass-thermometers.[11] Some authors find tympanic and oral electronic thermometer measurements equally acceptable if

FIG. 22-2 A tympanic membrane thermometer resting in its storage base.

pulmonary artery catheter and rectal temperatures are not available or contraindicated.[12]

Significant variations in temperature measurement have been found among different types and makes of tympanic thermometers,[10,13,14] which may be attributed at least in part to different people using the devices.[5] Even though the tympanic thermometer produces more variable results, the mean readings are not significantly different from those taken with a mercury-in-glass thermometer.[15] Inaccuracies are more likely in children if the thermometer is calibrated for an adult, the incorrect size probe is used, or if the child is less than 1 year old where even the smallest tip available is likely to fit poorly.[14,16] Additionally, inaccuracies may occur with incorrect positioning,[10] leading some researchers to recommend that an electronic oral measurement be taken before a tympanic measurement to first check if they correlate.[17]

Electronic Thermometers. Electronic thermometers detect temperature changes using a thermoresistive device in which the electrical resistance changes in response to changes in temperature (Fig. 22-3). This device may be a thermistor or a thermocouple and is incorporated into the tip of a probe. Thermistors are very small and therefore respond rapidly to changes in temperature.[18] The current flow from a thermistor is translated into a temperature reading that is displayed on a digital readout. Electronic thermometers display either a predicted equilibrium temperature based on measurements taken over 15-30 seconds (in predictive mode) or an actual equilibrium temperature that is generally achieved in a minute or less (in continuous mode).[4]

Electronic thermometers are relatively easy to use and measure temperatures from 31.6°-42.2° C in predictive mode and from 26.7°-42.2° C in continuous mode.[18] The low range available in continuous mode makes this device useful for measuring temperature in hypothermic patients. Electronic thermometers are portable and can be

used to measure oral, axillary, and rectal temperatures. Axillary temperature is measured in the same way as with a mercury-in-glass thermometer but using the electronic probe and waiting for the signal to indicate that the temperature is ready on the digital display. There are separate color-coded probes for oral and rectal measurements, and the disposable probe cover needs to be in place to operate, which helps reduce the risk of cross-contamination.[1,18] An audible signal indicates when the temperature on the digital display is ready to be recorded.

Giuliano et al found that oral measurements using an electronic thermometer produced more accurate and reproducible measurements than tympanic thermometers and therefore recommend these be used when pulmonary artery catheter placement is not indicated.[17] Pugh-Davies et al found that although the average accuracy of oral temperature measures taken with mercury-in-glass and electronic thermometers were not significantly different, the electronic thermometers produced greater fluctuation of readings with up to 23% of electronic measurements differing by 0.5° C or more when only 6% of mercury-in-glass thermometer readings varied this much.[19]

Disposable/Single Use Thermometers. Single-use thermometers usually consist of a plastic strip with a matrix of dots arranged to correspond with temperature registered in degrees Centigrade and/or Fahrenheit (Fig. 22-4). The dots contain two heat-sensitive chemicals that change color in response to temperature. This type of thermometer is usually calibrated to measure temperatures between 35.5°-40.5° C (96.0° F-104° F) and takes 1 minute to measure an oral temperature, and 3 minutes to measure an axillary or rectal temperature.[4,20]

Single-use thermometers have the advantages of being sterile when opened; unbreakable; easy to use; suitable for oral, axillary, and rectal temperature measurement; and possibly decreasing the risk of cross infection.[4,20] The main disadvantages are that the chemicals within the dots may degenerate if stored above 35° C, cost may increase if repeated measurements are required, and as mentioned previously, they can only measure temperatures between 35.5°-40.5° C.[4,20]

Single-use thermometers have been shown to produce accurate, precise, and clinically valid temperature readings in children with and without fever when compared to electronic, tympanic membrane, and mercury-in-glass thermometers.[11,21,22] They are often recommended for clinical use because of their accuracy and efficiency.[11,22] They

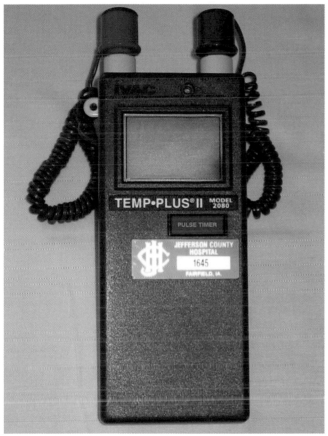

FIG. 22-3　An electronic thermometer.

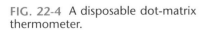

FIG. 22-4　A disposable dot-matrix thermometer.

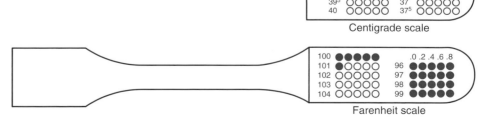

Centigrade scale

Farenheit scale

are also an appropriate choice when treating patients under isolation or with communicable diseases.

Oral and axillary procedure and placement for using disposable thermometers is essentially the same as the mercury-in-glass thermometer. Remember to turn the dots inward when measuring at the axillary site.

Whatever type of thermometer used, correct and consistent procedure must be followed to ensure accuracy and reliability, and the same site and instrument should be used for repeated measurements to accurately reflect changes in body temperature over time.[4,21]

Site of Temperature Measurement.
Core body temperature may be estimated by measurement at oral, axillary, tympanic membrane, or rectal sites using the various types of thermometers as described. Site and instrument selection is determined partly by the patient's age, medical condition, comfort, ease of access to site, and instrument availability.

Pontious et al compared measurement at different sites using disposable, tympanic and mercury-in-glass thermometers on children aged 5 and under in the emergency department and found the most accurate sites in descending order to be oral, axillary, tympanic membrane, and rectal.[11] Regarding precision, the sites in descending order were oral, tympanic membrane, rectal, and axillary. Age, behavior, febrile status, and tympanic bulge did not significantly change accuracy.[11] Schmitz et al measured temperatures in rapid sequence in febrile adult patients in the intensive care unit using a tympanic thermometer and an electronic thermometer at oral, axillary, and rectal sites and a pulmonary artery catheter for reference.[12] They found that rectal temperatures most closely agreed with the pulmonary artery catheter, followed by the oral, tympanic, and axillary sites. The rectal site was recommended as the site of choice, but if rectal temperature measurement is contraindicated, both oral and tympanic temperatures are acceptable substitutes.

Romano et al compared axillary and rectal temperature measurements taken with an electronic digital thermometer, with measurements taken with two different tympanic thermometers, and with a pulmonary artery catheter in pediatric patients in an intensive care unit. The rectal and tympanic measures correlated best with the pulmonary artery catheter.[10]

Although evidence from the studies cited previously and others indicate that axillary temperature measurements are the least sensitive, some authors have found that axillary placement using a mercury-in-glass thermometer can be accurate enough for clinical use.[3,23]

When taking a temperature orally, placing the thermometer in the *sublingual pocket* (Fig. 22-5) gives the most accurate estimate of core body temperature because this area, which is on both sides of the *frenulum* under the tongue, is closest to the sublingual arteries.[13,21,24] The sublingual pocket is an acceptable and convenient site for most hospital patients but may be difficult to reach in confused or unconscious patients, young children, and those with oral inflammation or trauma.[18]

Most of the problems with accuracy of oral temperature measurement result from environmental influences on the buccal cavity.[18] *Tachypnea* (rapid breathing) may

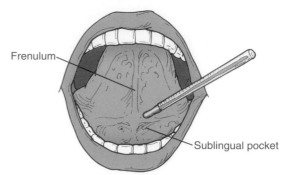

FIG. 22-5 The sublingual pocket area on either side of the frenulum underneath the tongue gives the most accurate estimate of core body temperature measured orally.

significantly reduce sublingual temperature.[25] Drinking ice water has been shown to decrease oral temperatures by up to 3° C for up to 15 minutes, and hot drinks may increase oral temperatures by about 1° C.[26,27] Smoking before temperature measurement has little effect; however, smoking during measurement may increase oral temperature by up to 2° C.[28] Based on these observations, oral temperatures should not be taken for at least 15 minutes after the intake of cold drinks or even hot foods, and the patient should not smoke while having their oral temperature measured.

Procedure.
The recommended procedures for measuring body temperature vary slightly from one source to another, but the procedures presented here reflect accepted practice for obtaining oral, axillary, and tympanic temperature readings.[1,29,30]

Oral measurement with mercury-in-glass thermometer

1. The patient should be resting comfortably allowing easy access to the measurement site.
2. Don disposable gloves.
3. Grasp and hold the tip of the thermometer away from the reservoir. If color coded, the tip will be blue.
4. Read the level of mercury at eye level by rotating the thermometer until the scale is visible.
   A. If the temperature is above 35.5° C (96° F), shake the mercury below that level with a few quick flicks of the wrist.
   B. Be sure to stand clear of any objects you may hit with the thermometer and be sure to hold onto it securely.
5. Cover the end of the thermometer with a plastic sleeve if available.
6. Place the thermometer gently under the patient's tongue into the sublingual pocket (see Fig. 22-5).
7. Have the patient gently hold the thermometer with their lips. Instruct them to keep the thermometer still and in place and to not bite down.
8. The thermometer remains in place for 3 minutes.

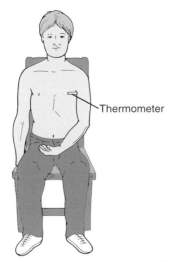

FIG. 22-6 Thermometer positioning for axillary temperature measurement of a person seated with forearm resting across abdomen. Mercury-in-glass, electronic, or disposable thermometers may be used in this manner.

9. Remove the thermometer gently, discard the plastic sleeve, and wipe away any remaining secretions with a clean tissue.
10. Read the thermometer at eye level and record the temperature.

Axillary measurement with mercury-in-glass thermometer

1. Prepare the thermometer as you would for steps 1-4 for measuring oral temperature.
2. Have the patient lie down supine if possible. Otherwise, they should sit comfortably.
3. Make sure the axilla is dry. Abduct the arm to expose the axilla. Place the thermometer tip at the center of the axilla then reposition the arm to the side of the patient with the forearm across the abdomen to hold the thermometer in place (Fig. 22-6).
4. The thermometer remains in place for at least 3 minutes, but it may need to be left in place 6-9 minutes to reach a stable temperature.
5. Remove and discard the plastic cover and wipe off any remaining secretions with a clean tissue.
6. Read the thermometer at eye level and record the temperature.

Tympanic Membrane Thermometer. The tympanic membrane thermometer measures temperature via an infrared sensor tip inserted into the patient's ear (Fig. 22-7). The procedure for using this device is as follows:

1. The patient should be in a comfortable position either lying or sitting with the head turned away from the examiner.
2. Make a note if there is excess ear wax in the auditory canal.

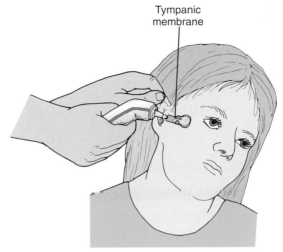

FIG. 22-7 Position of tympanic membrane thermometer. One hand pulls pinna of the ear up, out, and back to help position the tip of the thermometer forward.

3. Cover the sensor tip of the thermometer with the protective plastic sheath, making sure it locks in place.
4. Insert the tip into the auditory canal according to the manufacturers positioning directions. These may include:
   A. Pulling the *pinna* of the ear up, out, and back for an adult.
   B. Moving the tip in a figure-of-eight pattern to situate the tip of the probe.
   C. Make sure the probe fits snugly and does not move.
   D. Point the tip toward the nose.
5. Once the probe is properly placed, press the scan button and wait for an audible signal indicating that the temperature is ready to be read on the display.
6. Remove the tip from the ear and discard the plastic cover.
7. Record the temperature.

Electronic Thermometer
1. Don disposable gloves.
2. Make sure the oral/blue probe is attached and slide one of the plastic probe covers onto the probe until it locks.
3. Gently place the probe in the sublingual pocket (see Fig. 22-5) under the patient's tongue.
4. Instruct the patient to hold the probe in place with the lips closed until the signal is heard.
5. Read and record the temperature on the display.
6. Remove the probe and push the eject button to discard the plastic probe cover.

Measurement Time. Electronic and tympanic membrane thermometers make a sound to indicate when they have completed measuring the temperature. Most electronic thermometers register a temperature in less than a minute[18] in either the predictive or continuous mode, and tympanic membrane thermometers register temperature in about 3 seconds.[4] Disposable thermometers have measurement times of 1 minute for oral measurement and 3

TABLE 22-1	Body Temperature Ranges		
Measurement Site	Adult Normal Ranges (° C)	Men (° C)	Women (° C)
Oral	33.2-38.2	35.7-37.7	33.2-38.1
Rectal	34.4-37.8	36.7-37.5	36.8-37.1
Tympanic	35.4-37.8	35.5-37.5	35.7-37.5
Axillary	35.5-37.0		

minutes for axillary and rectal measurements.[20] Recommendations for how long to insert a mercury-in-glass thermometer varies from 3-10 minutes, with 3 minutes generally recommended for oral measurements and 5 minutes for axillary.[3,20,22,31]

NORMAL TEMPERATURE RANGES

Even though the normal adult core temperature range of 36°-38° C (96.8°-100.4° F)[1,2,32] is well accepted, there is evidence suggesting that the lower end of this range may need to be lowered further and that there are differences between men and women. Table 22-1 provides temperature ranges at different sites for men and women based on a review of studies in which the researchers' evidence was considered to be strong to fairly strong.[33]

Average normal temperatures are reported as 37° C (98.6° F) measured orally, 37.6° C (99.6° F) measured rectally, and 36.4° C (97.6° F) measured at the axilla.[3] It has also been traditionally accepted that axillary temperature is 0.6° C (1° F) lower than oral temperature and 1.2° C (2° F) lower than rectal temperature.[3] The implication that axillary temperatures are not an accurate estimation of core temperature because of the presumed 1.2° C (2° F) temperature difference has been found true only 5% of the time, lending support to the argument that axillary temperatures accurately reflect core temperature.[3]

RELEVANCE OF TEMPERATURE MEASUREMENT TO REHABILITATION

Most outpatients will likely have a normal temperature, but occasionally a patient may not look well or may complain of fever or chills, at which time measuring their temperature would be indicated. If the patient has recently had surgery, check the incision site for heat, redness, swelling, drainage, and tenderness to evaluate for local infection. If the patient's temperature is abnormal, contact their physician and consider canceling the therapy session.

Inpatients are often admitted with an infection-related diagnosis. Review their temperature in the vital signs section of the chart to determine if it is nearing acceptable values. Patients with abnormal temperatures are likely to have reduced activity tolerance that will be more severe the greater the abnormality.

PULSE

IMPLICATIONS OF PULSE MEASUREMENTS

A patient's peripheral pulse rate approximates their heart rate. The quality and regularity of the peripheral pulse may also give other information about cardiovascular function. The simplest and most common way of taking a pulse is by counting the number of pulse waves felt in a specified amount of time at a location where a superficial artery can be palpated.

Under normal conditions, the cardiac electrical and mechanical cycle is initiated at the sinoatrial (SA) node located within the posterior wall of the right atrium. The SA node spontaneously depolarizes and repolarizes, initiating each cycle of contraction and relaxation and setting the normal heart rate. SA node depolarization first initiates atrial contraction. The depolarization then travels through the heart to the atrioventricular (AV) node where it is delayed briefly to allow for complete emptying of the atria. The signal then spreads throughout the ventricles initiating their contraction and subsequent ejection of blood out into the arterial system.[34]

Blood ejected from the heart distends the arterial walls and rapidly travels in a pulsatile wave from the aorta to the arteries in the extremities. The wave produced by blood moving through the arteries with each heartbeat produces the palpable pulse. Palpating an artery that lies close to the surface of the body allows this wave to be felt. The number of times the pulse wave is counted in 1 minute is the pulse rate. An estimation of the pulse rate can be calculated if the pulse is counted for 15 seconds and then multiplied by 4 to derive the heart rate in beats per minute (bpm).

Pulse has characteristics of rhythm and strength, in addition to rate. Rhythm reflects the regularity of the heartbeat and strength reflects the volume of blood ejected. Documentation should include the heart rate, strength, and rhythm. For example, a pulse may be reported as 60 bpm, strong and regular, or as 70 bpm, weak and irregular.

The heart rhythm is generally noted as being regular when the beats occur at evenly spaced intervals, or irregular when the beats are unevenly spaced. Even though irregular heartbeats may be *benign,* they may indicate potentially life-threatening cardiac dysfunction and should be reported to the physician to determine if more sophisticated monitoring or intervention is needed.

The pulse strength is generally noted as strong, bounding/full, or weak. A strong pulse is normal. It can be palpated easily with mild pressure of the fingers and is not easily obliterated. A bounding or full pulse is even more pronounced and not easily obliterated with firm palpation. A weak pulse is one that is difficult to palpate and is easily obliterated with mild or light palpation. Weak pulses are also known as feeble or thready and may indicate a decreased stroke volume. Pulse strength may also be numerically graded as in Table 22-2.

In addition to measuring the pulse to assess cardiac function, the quality of the pulse at peripheral sites can be used to assess local arterial perfusion. For example, a weak or absent femoral pulse can indicate that the lower extremity is not getting enough blood and a weak or absent pedal pulse can indicate that the foot is not getting enough blood. The ankle brachial index (ABI) is a simple and reliable measure of peripheral blood flow to assist identification of peripheral arterial disease (PAD) in the

TABLE 22-2		Identifying Pulse Strength
Number System	**Description**	**Definition**
0	Absent	No pulsation is felt despite best efforts at palpation.
1+	Thready	Pulse is not easily felt; slight pressure will obliterate it.
2+	Weak/feeble	Slightly stronger than a thready pulse and light pressure will still obliterate it.
3+	Normal	Pulse is easily felt, but it takes moderate pressure to obliterate it.
4+	Bounding	Pulse is strong and is not obliterated with moderate pressure.

Adapted from Timby BK: *Fundamental Skills and Concepts in Patient Care,* ed 7, Philadelphia, 2003, Lippincott, Williams and Wilkins.

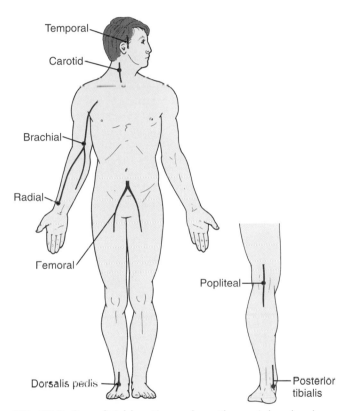

FIG. 22-8 Superficial locations where the peripheral pulses may be assessed.

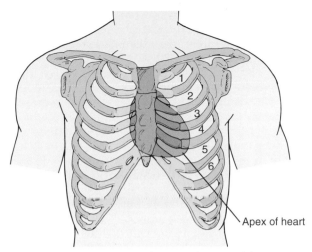

FIG. 22-9 Site to locate and assess the apical heart rate.

legs. The ABI is the ratio of the systolic BP at the ankle and the arm. The stated normal range varies between 0.95-1.2, depending on the source. An ABI below 0.95 or one that drops after exercise is a cause for concern and may indicate the presence of PAD (see Chapter 29).

METHODS FOR ASSESSING PULSE

The pulse may be assessed peripherally at sites where an artery is close to the skin (Fig. 22-8) or apically, on the chest over the heart (Fig. 22-9). The peripheral pulse most commonly assessed is the radial artery at the distal radial portion of the wrist because this site is easily accessible and the pulse is generally readily palpated here. Other sites that are easily palpated include the carotid artery at the neck, the brachial artery at the antecubital fossa or inner portion of the upper arm between the biceps and the triceps, the temporal artery on the head, and the dorsalis pedis, posterior tibial, femoral, and popliteal arteries on the lower extremities. These sites may be used if the radial pulse site is not accessible or if assessment of circulation in another part of the body is required. Additionally, the *apical* rate may be compared with the radial rate to check that all cardiac contractions are producing a peripheral pulse.

Procedure. The recommended procedures for measuring the pulse vary slightly from one source to another, but the procedures presented here reflect accepted practice for measuring the radial pulse at the wrist.[1,2,29,30] Similar procedures should be used for measuring the pulse at the other peripheral sites.

Equipment: watch or clock that indicates seconds

1. The patient should rest for at least 5 minutes before the pulse is taken.
2. Explain to the patient what you are doing and why and how they can cooperate to get better results.
3. Position the patient comfortably, either sitting or supine, with the forearm supported and wrist slightly extended. If the patient is in bed, raise it to a height that allows easy access to the site chosen for measurement.
4. Press the flat part of the fingertips of your index, middle, and/or ring fingers in the shallow trough just medial to the radial border of the wrist and feel for a recurring pulsation. Do not use your thumb because it has its own pulse that may be mistaken for the patient's.
5. Observe your watch or clock and count the number of pulsations that occur in 15 or 30 seconds and multiply by 4 or 2, respectively. If this is the first measurement or if the pulse is irregular, count for a full minute.

6. Record the pulse rate, rhythm, strength, and peripheral site used.
7. Report any anomalies to the physician.

If the pulse is too weak to be palpable at a peripheral site, if there is significant irregularity, or when measuring the heart rate in an infant, the apical heart rate may be measured by direct palpation or auscultation with a stethoscope over the apex of the heart. The heart's apex or point of maximal impulse (PMI) is generally located in the fifth intercostal space, slightly below the nipple in adults, in line with or just medial to the middle of the left clavicle (midclavicular line, MCL) (see Fig. 22-9). In infants and children the apex of the heart is slightly higher than in adults, generally in the third or fourth intercostal space in infants and in the fourth intercostal space in children under the age of 7 years.[29]

Additionally, weak peripheral pulses that are difficult to palpate by hand may be detected and counted using a Doppler ultrasound (DUS) device. This device detects movement of blood and converts the movement information to a sound. Transmission gel is applied to the site to be assessed or to the plastic case housing the probe's transducer. The probe is maneuvered over the artery until a pulsing sound is heard, either through headphones or with a speaker (Fig. 22-10). Arterial sounds must be distinguished from venous sounds, since both may be heard simultaneously. Arteries produce a distinct pulsation with a pumping quality, whereas veins produce sounds that are intermittent and vary with respiration. If the arterial sounds are not clearly heard, reposition the probe to improve clarity. Once the arterial pulse can be heard clearly, hold the probe in place and count the number of arterial pulses for 1 minute. After completing the measurement, wipe off the gel from the probe and the skin and clean the probe with any recommended cleaning solution.

Occasionally, if the peripheral pulse is irregular, skips, or is otherwise difficult to count, the apical and radial pulses are compared. The rates at both sites should be within two beats of each other.[1] A greater difference is known as a pulse deficit. A peripheral pulse rate may be

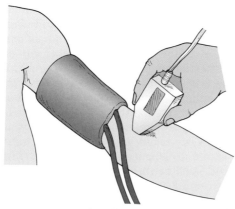

FIG. 22-10 Using Doppler ultrasound at the brachial artery to measure blood pressure.

lower if the heart's contractions are not strong enough to produce a pulse peripherally with every beat.

In addition to methods using palpation, auscultation, or DUS, there are a number of devices that monitor heart rate electronically. Some of these devices are available to the public for monitoring heart rate at rest and during activity at home, and some devices are intended for medical professionals to use in hospitals or clinics. The professional devices generally combine measurement of heart rate with measurement of other vital signs or cardiac performance parameters.

NORMAL RANGES

Normal resting pulse rate in adults ranges from 60-100 bpm.[30] *Tachycardia* or rapid pulse rate is defined as a pulse rate greater than 100 bpm at rest. Rapid and sustained tachycardia overworks the heart and can prevent adequate peripheral oxygenation by reducing cardiac output. When the heart rate increases, the heart has less time to fill with blood between contractions, resulting in less blood being ejected with each contraction.[30] *Bradycardia* or a slow pulse rate is defined as a heart rate of less than 60 bpm at rest.[2] Although bradycardia may be pathological, physical training with exercise commonly produces low resting heart rates in highly trained athletes that are not pathological.[35-37] The resting heart rate can be lower than 40 bpm in professional cyclists[38] and other endurance athletes. Although the exact mechanism of this training–induced resting bradycardia is not understood, it is likely due to both an increase in parasympathetic influence and a decrease in sympathetic influence.[39]

Although there is a normal range for the resting pulse rate, a number of factors, including age, time of day, gender, body build, activity, stress, body temperature, blood volume, and anemia, as well as various medications, may alter this rate. The heart rate is typically lower in the morning than in the evening.[30] After puberty, the pulse is generally about 7-8 beats slower in males than females.[2,29,30] Tall slender people usually have a slower heart rate than shorter heavier people.[2,30] Exercise increases heart rate acutely, during, and shortly after the activity. However, regular aerobic exercise reduces the resting heart rate and causes it to rise more slowly with exertion. This causes both resting and exercise pulse to be lower than average in trained athletes.[29,30,35-37] In addition, physiological changes, such as sympathetic stimulation as a result of fear, anger, excitement, or pain, as well as increases in body temperature, dehydration, excessive blood loss, and anemia, will produce increases in the heart rate.[1,2,29,30] Furthermore, many drugs may increase or decrease the resting heart rate. For example, digitalis preparations and sedatives slow heart rate, whereas caffeine, nicotine, cocaine, thyroid replacement hormones, and epinephrine will all increase heart rate.[1,2,29,30]

Age consistently affects the resting heart rate, with the rate gradually decreasing from birth to adulthood to finally reach the average adult range of 60-100 bpm by adolescence[1,2,29,30] (Table 22-3).

RELEVANCE OF PULSE TO REHABILITATION

Pulse rate is often used as a measure of cardiac work when setting exercise intensity and goals in deconditioned

TABLE 22-3	Normal Pulse Rates at Various Ages	
Age	Approximate Range (bpm)	Approximate Average (bpm)
Newborn	100-180	140
1-12 months	80-140	120
1-2 years	70-130	110
3-6 years	75-120	100
7-12 years	75-110	95
Adolescence	60-100	80
Adulthood	60-100	80

Data from Perry AG, Potter PA: *Clinical Nursing Skills and Techniques,* ed 5, St. Louis, 2002, Mosby; DeWit SC: *Rambo's Nursing Skills for Clinical Practice,* ed 4, Philadelphia, 1994, WB Saunders.
bpm, Beats per minute.

patients and those undergoing cardiac rehabilitation (see Chapters 23 and 25). Slower heart rates indicate less cardiac work, and slower heart rates at the same overall workload indicate improvement in cardiac conditioning, as long as medications that influence heart rate have not been changed. In general, conditioning exercise is prescribed based on a target heart rate that is related to the individual's resting heart rate and predicted maximum heart rate. Therapy should be stopped immediately and the physician contacted if a patient has an abnormal pulse along with symptoms of shortness of breath or light-headedness because these may indicate life-threatening cardiac or pulmonary pathology.

RESPIRATORY RATE

IMPLICATIONS OF RESPIRATORY RATE MEASUREMENT

Breathing, which includes respiration and ventilation, is the multistep physiological process that delivers oxygen to and removes carbon dioxide from the human body (see Chapter 26). Respiration is the process of exchanging gases between the alveoli and the blood, and ventilation is the movement of air into and out of the lungs.

Ventilation is made up of two phases. Inspiration (inhalation or breathing in) fills the lungs with air. Expiration (exhalation or breathing out) expels air from the lungs. The primary inspiratory muscles are the diaphragm and the external intercostals. Smaller accessory muscles, the scalenes, sternocleidomastoids, and pectorals, also aid inspiration during exertion or under certain pathological conditions.[40] Expiration is largely passive while at rest and during light activity and results from the relaxation of the inspiratory muscles and the recoil of the lungs through their natural elasticity. The chest cavity decreases in size and air is expelled from the lungs. Moderate to heavy exercise enlists the internal intercostals and abdominal muscles to pull the ribs back down and pull in the abdominal cavity to forcefully expel more air from the lungs.[34]

Automatic control of respiration resides in the medulla and is influenced by peripheral and central chemoreceptors monitoring arterial partial pressure of oxygen (PaO_2), partial pressure of carbon dioxide ($PaCO_2$), and pH. Respiration can also be controlled to some extent voluntarily.

Respiratory rate is the number of breaths or the number of times a cycle of inspiration and expiration is completed in 1 minute.

METHODS FOR ASSESSING RESPIRATORY RATE

The clinician should try to assess the rate and regularity of breathing as well as the depth of breathing to determine if an adequate volume of air is being exchanged. Unusual sounds produced with respiration are noted because they may indicate additional pathology (see Chapters 24 and 26).

Procedure

1. The patient should be inactive for 5 minutes before testing.
2. Make sure the patient is comfortable in supine or a more upright sitting position and that the chest can be observed. If necessary, move blankets or bed linen for better viewing.
3. Since patients often voluntarily alter their breathing if they are aware that you are counting the respiratory rate, it is best to count when the patient is unaware that you are counting. It may be helpful to count respiratory rate while appearing to count pulse or while the patient is holding a thermometer in the mouth to measure temperature.
4. Count the number of times the chest rises and falls for a full minute if there appears to be anything unusual. Count for 30 seconds if breathing is noiseless and effortless then multiply by two. If unable to observe the chest clearly, place a hand on the patient's upper abdomen to feel the inspiration and expiration cycle and count the number of times it rises and falls.
5. Record the respiratory rate, rhythm, and depth and any abnormalities that may be observed.

NORMAL RANGES

The normal range of respiratory rate varies with age and gender. In general, respiratory rate is higher in the newborn than in the adult and slightly higher in adult women than men. Typical ranges are 30-60 breaths per minute (breaths/min) in the newborn, 20-40 breaths/min in early childhood, 15-28 breaths/min in late childhood, 18-22 breaths/min in adolescence, 14-18 breaths/min in adult males, and 16-20 breaths/min in adults females.[2,30]

Respiratory rates that lie outside accepted norms may need follow-up by the physician. A rapid respiratory rate, faster than 20 breaths/min in an adult, is known as tachypnea, and a slow respiratory rate, slower than 10 breaths/min is known as bradypnea. Tachypnea commonly occurs during fever with the rate increasing by about 4 breaths/min for each 0.5° C (1° F) increase in temperature.[2] Hyperventilation is when the rate and depth of breathing increase enough to lower blood levels of carbon dioxide. This may occur during periods of high anxiety, following severe exertion, or with fever and diabetic acidosis.[2] Bradypnea may be a result of sedating drugs such as morphine,[30] head injury, or increased intracranial pressure affecting the respiratory center.[2] If an adult's respiratory rate falls below 10 respirations per minute and the depth is shallow they may become apprehensive, restless, confused, dizzy, or less conscious because of inadequate delivery of oxygen to the brain.[2] Apnea is the absence of breathing and may occur for short periods or for periods that are long enough to be life-threatening. If prolonged, apnea can cause brain damage or lead to serious abnormal cardiac rhythms.[30]

BLOOD PRESSURE

BP is the pressure exerted by the blood on the arterial walls. It is determined by the contractile force exerted by the left ventricle of the heart, the amount of blood ejected with each heartbeat (i.e., the stroke volume), and the resistance of the blood vessels to flow. BP reflects the effectiveness of the heart's contraction, the adequacy of blood volume, and the presence of obstruction or interference to blood flow through the vessels.[2] Arterial BP changes cyclically with the heartbeat. The maximum arterial BP is known as the systolic BP and the minimum arterial BP is known as the diastolic BP.

Systolic BP represents the peak ventricular contractile force pushing the blood through the vascular system, whereas diastolic pressure represents the minimum pressure in the arteries between heartbeats while the ventricles are refilling. BP is recorded as systolic/diastolic in millimeters of mercury (mm Hg), for example, 120/80 mm Hg. The standard unit of mm Hg describes the height to which a column of mercury can be sustained by the pressure exerted within the arteries.

METHODS FOR MEASURING BLOOD PRESSURE

BP is generally measured noninvasively using a sphygmomanometer and a stethoscope. A sphygmomanometer is a device that measures the pressure (the manometer) and an occlusive cuff. The manometer uses a glass column of mercury, a calibrated aneroid dial, or an electronic device to measure and display the pressure (Figs. 22-11 to 22-13). The occlusive cuff has an inflatable bladder that wraps around the limb to occlude the artery and a bulb to inflate the cuff. When using a mercury or aneroid manometer, a stethoscope must be used to listen for the heart sounds (Fig. 22-14). When using an electronic manometer, no stethoscope is needed. A sphygmomanometer with an aneroid dial and a stethoscope are the most popular devices for measuring BP today because these devices are economical, simple to use, and easy to handle and provide accurate results quickly while avoiding the hazards associated with mercury.

A mercury manometer is a calibrated transparent tube with a reservoir containing mercury. They have the advantages of consistently providing accurate readings, being easy to maintain, and not losing calibration.[41] The level of the top of the convex *meniscus* at the top of the column of mercury is used for readings. One must read the meniscus at about eye level or have it positioned in a direct line

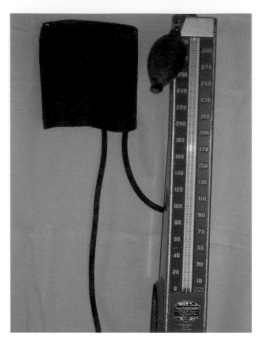

FIG. 22-11 Mercury sphygmomanometer with arm cuff, inflation bulb, and manometer.

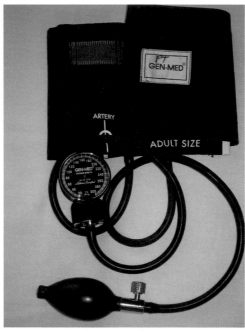

FIG. 22-12 Aneroid sphygmomanometer with arm cuff, inflation bulb, and manometer.

with the eye to avoid visual distortion that may skew the readings.

The aneroid manometer is made of a sealed canister with thin metal walls. One of the walls is flexible and moves with changes in pressure. This movement causes a needle on the calibrated dial to shift, indicating the pressure in mm Hg. Aneroid manometers are generally accurate, but their readings will vary with changes in outside temperature and they may be less accurate than mercury

Electric sphygmomanometers use aneroid manometer technology and an electronic device to measure the maximum and minimum pressure after inflation of the cuff. This type of device displays diastolic and systolic BP on a digital display. These devices also require regular maintenance and accuracy checks.

BP cuffs range in size to fit different size limbs from the arm of a newborn, infant, child, small adult, adult, or large adult to the thigh. Small children require a narrower cuff with a shorter bladder, whereas muscular, large, or obese patients need a wider cuff with a longer bladder.[2] The bladder should be long enough to encircle at least 80% of the limb in the adult and the entire limb in the child.[41,43] Regular adult cuffs are generally 12-13 cm (4.8-5.2 inches) wide and 22-23 cm (8.5-9 inches) long.[1] The appropriately-sized cuff must be used to assure valid measurement. If the cuff is too small, too narrow, or too short, it will overestimate the BP, and if it is too large, it will to a lesser degree underestimate the BP.[41,44] Therefore clinicians should have several cuff sizes available to suit the typical patient population that they encounter.

All equipment should be maintained and regularly calibrated according to manufacturer recommendation or facility policy. If the device does not meet standards, it should be replaced. Knight et al found in a study evaluating the accuracy and safety of a wide range of medical instruments in medical clinics that 69.1% of mercury manometers and 95.7% of aneroid sphygmomanometers examined had no service records. Of those that did have service records, only 8.1% of the mercury and 0.9% of the aneroid instruments had a record of a service check in the last 12 months. None of the instruments met all quality standards, and 3.9% of the mercury and 6.1% of the aneroid instruments met less than half of the quality standards. Only two thirds of mercury and 38.8% of aneroid devices were accurate at all pressure levels tested. The researchers concluded that the level of defects noted could have an impact on diagnosis and monitoring of BP abnormalities, particularly hypertension (high BP).[45] Two additional studies also report significant enough variances in sphygmomanometer accuracy to affect decisions in patient follow-up and care.[46,47]

Procedure. The procedures described here for measuring BP reflect commonly accepted practice.[41,43] Positioning of the patient and therapist is critical to obtaining accurate results. The clinician must be in a good position to view the manometer, and the patient must be positioned so that the results are not adversely affected by discomfort or undue exertion.

The upper arm is most commonly used to obtain BP, although other sites can be used and are discussed briefly after this general description. The initial measurement should be taken in both arms.

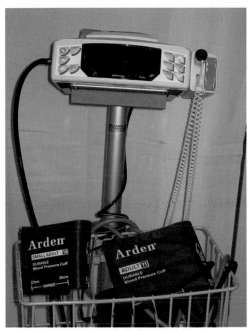

FIG. 22-13 Combination unit with electronic BP device, thermometer, and pulse oximeter.

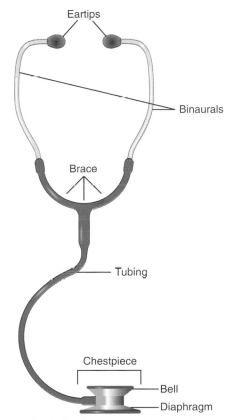

FIG. 22-14 Stethoscope and its various parts.

manometers if not calibrated regularly and handled gently.[42] Aneroid manometers should be recalibrated every 6-12 months or if their readings differ by more than 2-4 mm Hg from those taken with a mercury sphygmomanometer.[41] They tend to underread pressure when decalibrated.[41,42]

1. The patient should be seated comfortably for at least 5 minutes in a chair with their feet on the floor before measuring their BP. The patient should refrain from smoking, exercising, or ingesting caffeine for 30 minutes before the measurement is taken. The patient may be supine

or standing if necessary. The surroundings should be quiet if possible.

2. The arm is supported at the level of the heart whether the patient is seated, supine, or standing. BP measures increase when the arm is below heart level and decrease when the arm is above heart level.[48-50] If measuring BP in a position other than sitting, note this position for consistency. The patient should not have to hold their arm at heart level actively or the isometric contraction involved may artificially increase the BP measurement. Crossing the legs should also be avoided as this has been found to elevate both systolic and diastolic pressures.[51]

3. Select the appropriately-sized cuff and position the manometer gauge so that the view is unobstructed, in line with the eyes, and the gauge indicates zero mm Hg while the cuff is deflated. The air bladder should be long enough to encircle at least 80% of the limb.

4. Expose the upper arm and apply the cuff directly on the skin. Clothing may prevent correct placement of the cuff and interfere with readings. Wrap the deflated cuff evenly around the upper arm so the center of the bladder is directly over the brachial artery in the antecubital fossa. Arrows on the cuff generally mark the area that should be over the brachial artery. The elbow should be slightly bent, and the lower border of the cuff should be placed approximately 1 inch above the antecubital fossa in adults (Fig. 22-15).

5. If this is the initial examination, perform a preliminary palpatory determination of systolic pressure as follows. This gives the approximate systolic pressure and serves as a benchmark to ensure that enough pressure is used to exceed systolic pressure to occlude the artery while avoiding unnecessarily over inflating the cuff. Palpate the radial or brachial artery with the fingertips. Close the valve on the bulb. Pump the cuff 30 mm Hg past the point where the pulse is no longer felt. Slowly release the cuff pressure by about 2 mm Hg per second and note the point where the pulse reappears. Mentally make a note of both of these numbers. The latter is the

approximate systolic BP, whereas the former will be used in the procedure for precise measurement as described in the next steps. Wait at least 2 minutes to make any further measurements. This time allows the blood trapped in the veins to be released and prevents false high systolic readings.

6. Place the earpieces of the stethoscope in your ears. The earpieces of the stethoscope should be pointing slightly forward in the direction of the ear canal to more clearly hear sounds. Make sure that the stethoscope tubing is hanging freely without rubbing or bumping anything that may interfere with the sounds to be auscultated. Place the diaphragm of the stethoscope over the brachial artery in the antecubital fossa firmly enough that all surface edges of the diaphragm are in contact with the skin. Rapidly inflate the cuff about 30 mm Hg above the point where the pulse was previously noted to disappear.

7. Gradually deflate the cuff at about 2 mm Hg per second while listening for the pulse with the stethoscope. The systolic BP is the number at which the pulse is first heard. The diastolic BP is the number at which the sound of the pulse is no longer heard. Once the diastolic BP is reached, the cuff can be deflated quickly all the way to zero. If readings are difficult to obtain, do not stop midway and try to reinflate to repeat the reading as this will produce unreliable results. Wait at least 2 minutes before repeating any measurement to confirm accuracy. If sounds are heard all the way down to zero, use the point where muffling of sound begins (fourth phase/fourth Korotkoff sound) (Table 22-4 and Fig. 22-16) and record that number as the diastolic reading.

8. If this is the initial examination, repeat the procedure on the other arm. There should be no more than 10 mm Hg difference between arms. The arm with the higher reading should be the one used for subsequent measurements.

9. Remove the cuff.

10. Record your findings and note from which arm the measurement was taken.

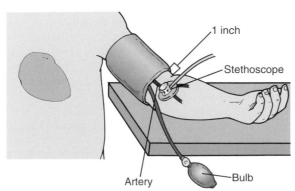

FIG. 22-15 Position of the arm with the cuff and stethoscope to measure blood pressure.

TABLE 22-4	Korotkoff Sounds and Phases
Korotkoff Sound (Phase)	**Characteristics**
1	Resembles a faint clear tapping that gradually grows louder to a sharp thump.
2	A swishing, blowing sound that increases as the cuff is deflated.
3	A softer knocking, thumping sound than phase 1.
4	A muffling or softening of the prior tapping and knocking sounds that generally fades.
5	Disappearance of sound all together.

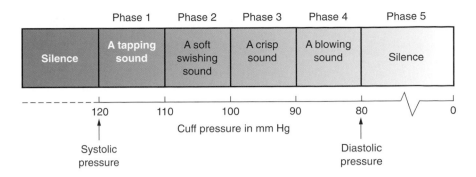

	Phase 1	Phase 2	Phase 3	Phase 4	Phase 5
Silence	A tapping sound	A soft swishing sound	A crisp sound	A blowing sound	Silence

FIG. 22-16 Korotkoff sounds corresponding to phases 1-5 during auscultation of blood pressure.

Cuff pressure in mm Hg: 120 — Systolic pressure, 110, 100, 90, 80 — Diastolic pressure, 0

Although differences between BP readings in the two arms may indicate pathology, differences are not uncommon, even in the absence of pathology.[52,53] One author found diastolic BP differences of up to 10 mm Hg in 40% of subjects and systolic BP differences of up to 20 mm Hg in 23% of subjects without known disease.[52] Another researcher reported significant differences in mean inter-arm systolic BP and mean absolute systolic BP and diastolic BP.[53] Therefore BP should be routinely measured in both arms, at least during the initial examination, and the same arm should be used consistently for all comparisons or follow-up measures.[52,53] Some researchers recommend using the right arm consistently for all measurements because the BP in the right arm has been found to generally be higher,[52] whereas others recommend using the arm with the higher initial measure for that individual.[53]

KOROTKOFF SOUNDS

Measuring BP by auscultation involves listening for sounds over an artery as the cuff is deflated. These sounds change through the cardiac cycle and are known as the five Korotkoff sounds or phases (see Table 22-4 and Fig. 22-16).

The first Korotkoff sound (phase 1) is the first sound heard as the cuff is deflated from its maximum pressure. The first Korotkoff sound is a faint clear tapping that gradually gets louder. The pressure when this sound is first heard is the systolic BP. Phase 4 is when the sound becomes abruptly muffled, and phase 5 is when the sound becomes inaudible. The pressure at which phase 5 starts is generally recorded as the diastolic pressure. However, if the sound never becomes inaudible or becomes inaudible at an extremely low pressure, then the pressure at the beginning of phase 4 is considered the diastolic pressure. For complete accuracy, the BP from both the fourth and fifth phases may be recorded. For example, 125/82/0 would indicate that 125 systolic pressure would be the fourth Korotkoff sound and zero would indicate that the muffled fourth Korotkoff sounds were heard all the way to a zero reading on the manometer.[41,82] The fourth Korotkoff sound is typically used to denote diastolic pressure in children under the age of 13 years, pregnant women, patients with other high cardiac output states, and those with peripheral vasodilation because heart sounds often do not become silent in these populations.[41]

ALTERNATIVE BLOOD PRESSURE SITES

Although BP is generally measured in the upper arm, thigh measurement of BP using the popliteal artery is indicated in certain circumstances, including when BP cannot be measured on either arm because of burns, trauma, or bilateral mastectomy; when BP in one thigh is to be compared with BP in the other thigh; or when the BP cuff available is too large for the upper extremity.[29]

The procedure for measuring BP at the thigh is similar to that used for the arm except that the patient must be lying down, ideally prone to expose the popliteal fossa, or if necessary, supine, with the knee slightly bent. The popliteal pulse is auscultated in the popliteal fossa, similar to the brachial pulse in the antecubital fossa of the arm, to listen for the Korotkoff sounds.

Many wrist-cuff devices are available to measure BP in the forearm. They are appealing because of their convenience and portability, and a few studies report that they are comparable to standard upper arm auscultatory and electronic sphygmomanometers.[54,55] However, the majority of evidence has not found wrist-cuff sphygmomanometers to be accurate or reliable enough for practical use, and these are therefore not recommended.[11,56-59]

AGE-RELATED CONSIDERATIONS FOR BLOOD PRESSURE MEASUREMENT PROCEDURE

In infants, a pediatric stethoscope with a smaller diaphragm should be used for auscultation and the lower edge of the cuff can be placed closer to the antecubital fossa than in the adult because infants' arms are so much smaller. Arm and thigh pressure are essentially equivalent in children under 1 year of age, and therefore BP may be measured at the thigh if this is more convenient.[29]

In children, it is best to explain the steps and what it will feel like first and then demonstrate on a doll or stuffed animal if available. The bladder should be wide enough to cover about 40% of the arm and long enough to wrap around 80% to 100% of the arm's circumference. Ideally, BP measurements should be taken before uncomfortable procedures so that the measure is not artificially elevated. In children over 1 year of age, the thigh BP is about 10 mm Hg higher than the arm BP.

In the elderly the cuff pressure should not remain high for any longer than necessary to minimize the risk of damaging fragile skin. Also, if the patient is taking any antihypertensive medication, one should note which one and when the last dose was taken.[6]

CONTRAINDICATIONS TO MEASURING BLOOD PRESSURE

BP should not be measured on the patient's arm when the patient has had breast or axilla surgery, the patient has an intravenous line or has had a recent blood transfusion on that limb, or if the patient has an arteriovenous fistula (for renal dialysis) in that limb. The thigh should not be used if there has been a recent surgery on that hip or lower extremity.

NORMAL RANGES

Normal BP in adults is less than 120/80 mm Hg. Hypertension is defined as a BP with either the systolic or the diastolic BP being at or above the cut-off of 140/90 mm Hg[43,60] (Table 22-5).

The prevalence of hypertension, particularly systolic hypertension, increases with advancing age to the point where approximately 50% of people aged 60-69 years, approximately 75% of those over age 70, and approximately 90% of those aged 80-85 years meet hypertensive criteria[61-63] (Table 22-6). Although greater emphasis used to be placed on controlling diastolic BP rather than systolic BP, it has been found that diastolic BP is more important for individuals under the age of 50 and that after the age of 50, which is when most people develop hypertension, systolic BP has a greater impact than diastolic BP on cardiovascular disease risk.[61-66]

Isolated systolic hypertension (ISH) is not uncommon in the elderly and poses a serious public health concern.[67-69] Adequate control of ISH reduces total mortality, cardiovascular morbidity, and the incidence of stroke and heart failure.[70-72] However, studies have shown that diastolic BP is generally more readily and effectively controlled than systolic BP.[73-76]

Increased BP (systolic or diastolic) is an independent risk factor for all forms of cardiovascular disease, including heart attack, stroke, heart failure, peripheral vascular disease, and kidney failure.[41,43] The risk increases progressively as BP gets higher. The risk for death as a result of ischemic heart disease and stroke increases progressively and linearly as systolic BP increases above 115 mm Hg and diastolic BP increases above 75 mm Hg. For every 20 mm Hg rise in systolic BP and for every 5 mm Hg rise in diastolic BP, the mortality from ischemic heart disease and stroke doubles.[77]

TABLE 22-5	JNCVII Blood Pressure Classification
Category	**BP (mm Hg)**
Normal	<120/80
Prehypertension	120-139/80-89
Hypertension	≥140/90
Stage I	140-159/90-99
Stage II	≥180/110

From Chobanian AV, Bakris GL, Black HR, et al: *Hypertension*, 42:1206-1252, 2003.
JNCVII, Seventh Report of the Joint National Committee on Prevention, Detection, Evaluation, and Treatment of High Blood Pressure; *BP*, blood pressure.

The Seventh Report of the Joint National Committee on Prevention, Detection, Evaluation, and Treatment of High Blood Pressure (JNCVII) includes a designation of prehypertension (120-139/80-89 mm Hg). This is not a disease category but a standard to identify individuals at increased risk of developing hypertension in the hopes that early intervention and education to promote a healthier lifestyle may decrease BP, slow the progression to hypertension, or prevent it entirely.[43]

Cardiovascular disease risk is determined in part by BP but also by associated risk factors, including smoking, dyslipidemia, diabetes mellitus, age, gender, obesity, and family history. Prevention through risk factor modifica-

TABLE 22-6	Factors Affecting Blood Pressure
Factor	**Impact**
Age	Systolic BP gradually increases through life. Diastolic BP increases until 50-60 years of age. Newborn mean systolic BP is 73 mm Hg. Ages 10-19 BP ranges from 124-136/77-84 mm Hg for boys and 124-127/63-74 mm Hg for girls. Geriatric adult BP commonly ranges from 140-160/90 mm Hg.
Gender	Women typically have lower BP than men until after menopause.
Exercise	Physical exertion increases BP acutely and decreases resting BP over time.
Position	BP can fall after a change of position from lying to sitting or sitting to standing (see section on Orthostatic Hypotension).
Medications/drugs	Many medications may increase or decrease BP. Antihypertensives, diuretics, beta-blockers, calcium channel blockers, vasodilators, ACE inhibitors, and narcotic medications all decrease BP. Stimulants, such as caffeine, generally increase BP.
Sympathetic nervous system stimulation	Stress, anxiety, fear, and pain increase BP.
Obesity	Obesity predisposes people to hypertension.
Diurnal variations	BP is usually lowest in the morning when metabolic rate is the lowest, rises throughout the day, and peaks in late afternoon when the person is mentally awake and physically active.
Fever/heat/cold	Increased metabolic rate associated with fever may elevate BP. External heat associated with vasodilation may decrease BP. Cold associated with vasoconstriction may increase BP.
Smoking	Smoking causes vasoconstriction, which increases peripheral resistant resulting in elevated BP. BP may remain elevated acutely for up to 15 minutes after smoking.[43]
Race/ethnicity	Typically, African-American men over 35 years of age have higher BP than European men of the same age.

BP, Blood pressure; *ACE*, angiotensin-converting enzymes.

tion is considered better than treatment. This mainly involves lifestyle changes such as decreasing caloric intake to decrease body weight, moderating alcohol consumption, increasing exercise, stopping smoking, decreasing fat intake, and decreasing stress. If and when these measures fail, then the physician may decide to prescribe medications.

WHITE COAT HYPERTENSION

White coat hypertension (WCH), also known as the white coat effect or isolated office hypertension, is the presence of higher BP when measured in the physician's office than at other times.[6] It has been found that some people do have higher BPs when measured by a physician than they typically do at home or when their BP is measured by a technician. One study found that 33% of patients had WCH (defined in this study as an increase in systolic BP by 10 mm Hg or in diastolic BP by 5 mm Hg) when measured by a general practitioner as compared with measurements taken by a nurse or by the patient themselves. Interestingly, 10% of patients in this study had a markedly lower BP when measured by the general practitioner than when measured by the nurse or with self-measurement, indicating a possible reverse WCH effect in at least some patients. Self-measurement of BP or ambulatory BP measurement can be used to differentiate WCH from true elevated BP.[43,60]

Whether WCH is a benign phenomenon or carries increased cardiovascular risk is still not known. WCH should not be taken lightly since it presents the possibility of misdiagnosing a patient as hypertensive and subjecting them to unnecessary medications and their side effects. However, failing to treat true hypertension can also have severe long-term consequences. If WCH is suspected, JNCVII advocates self-monitoring of BP at home and at work to check for differences compared to the doctor's office so that those with self-measured values of less than 130/80 mm Hg, despite elevated measures in the office, may generally avoid more aggressive medical intervention.[13]

SALT AND HYPERTENSION

There is a general consensus that dietary sodium affects BP. Salt is implicated in the pathogenesis of coronary artery disease and strokes. This may be due to its effects on BP and/or other independent mechanisms. Dietary sodium may harm the cardiovascular system in ways that aggravate the effects of hypertension such as increasing left ventricular mass and thickening and stiffening the conduit arteries. It appears that a modest reduction in salt intake for 4 weeks or more reduces BP significantly in both hypertensive and normotensive people, supporting recommendations for modestly reducing salt intake to decrease BP and cardiovascular mortality risk. However, studies have found that abruptly reducing salt intake to very low levels after acute salt loading does not provide benefit.

HYPOTENSION

Hypotension is generally defined as a systolic BP of 90 mm Hg or lower, although in some adults such a low BP may be normal.[1] Signs and symptoms of clinically significant hypotension include tachycardia, dizziness, mental confusion, restlessness, cool, clammy, pale or *cyanotic* skin, and *syncope*.[29] Low BP in conjunction with symptoms of shock or circulatory collapse indicates a dangerous condition that can rapidly progress to death unless treated.[2] Shock may be caused by a reduction in BP as a result of a wide range of causes, including hemorrhage, vomiting, diarrhea, burns, myocardial infarction, and overwhelming infection. Signs and symptoms of shock include hypotension, tachycardia, cold clammy skin, dizziness, blurred vision, and apprehension. The presence of low BP and any of these symptoms may indicate onset of shock or circulatory collapse and should be taken seriously, including ensuring immediate medical attention.

ORTHOSTATIC HYPOTENSION

Orthostatic hypotension, also known as postural hypotension, is a transient decrease in BP, occurring in response to a change in position, generally when moving from lying down to an upright position. It is typically defined by a decline of 20 mm Hg or more in systolic BP or a decline of 10 mm Hg or more in diastolic BP.[87,88] Orthostatic hypotension is common in patients when they first try to get up after a protracted period of bed rest.[89] When the patient stands, blood pools in the legs and trunk and causes venous return to transiently fall. This in turn decreases cardiac output and subsequently BP and cerebral perfusion.[88] Normally, autonomic reflexes quickly restore BP by causing vasoconstriction and a transient increase in heart rate to prevent dizziness or lightheadedness. However, if pooling is severe or if the autonomic response is delayed or inadequate, the patient will feel lightheaded and may faint.[88] Certain medications, including diuretics and beta-blockers, may promote or aggravate orthostatic hypotension.[87]

RELEVANCE OF BLOOD PRESSURE TO REHABILITATION

Physical therapists (PTs) can participate in improving public health by providing education about exercise and other lifestyle-related interventions that help to reduce resting BP and thus the community burden of hypertension and its sequelae. BP measures are used to indicate a patient's baseline hemodynamic status during rehabilitation and to guide the safety and vigor of activities during rehabilitation. Patients frequently perform exercises, such as treadmill walking, running, upper body ergometer pedaling, or cycling on a stationary bicycle, as a component of their physical therapy interventions. Although these exercises can be beneficial, they all place demands on the cardiovascular system and should be tailored to the individual needs and limitations of the patient.

Typically, systolic BP rises rapidly and diastolic pressure rises slightly during the first few minutes of aerobic exercise and then both level off.[34] With resistance training, systolic BP rises more dramatically. High-level resistance training can cause rises in systolic BP that can be harmful for individuals with preexisting hypertension or heart disease and therefore loads should be kept lower in such patients. Aerobic exercise performed with the arms produces a greater rise in systolic and diastolic BP than lower extremity exercise performed at the same intensity (as measured by percent of maximal oxygen uptake).[34] Therefore upper body ergometry should be avoided or used with caution and should generally be replaced with lower extremity exercise in those with increased cardio-vascular risk. Although exercise causes an acute increase in BP, regular submaximal aerobic and resistance training do not cause long-term increases in resting BP but rather result in lowered BP for 2-3 hours after exercise, lowered resting BP, and blunting of the BP response to this form of exercise.[34]

AUTONOMIC DYSREFLEXIA

The interruption of autonomic pathways by spinal cord injury (SCI) can cause dysfunction of the autonomic nervous system (see Chapter 20). SCI cranial to the sympathetic outflow may be complicated by a phenomenon known as autonomic dysreflexia (AD). Although AD is generally associated with injuries at or above the T6 level, there have been cases reported with SCI as low as the T8 and T10 level. AD occurs in between 19% and 70% of patients with SCI.

AD is an acute syndrome manifested by cardiovascular symptoms and characterized by a sudden increase in BP.[91] Along with paroxysmal hypertension, AD generally causes a throbbing headache, profuse sweating above the level of the spinal lesion, facial flushing, bradycardia, or tachy-cardia.[90,92,99-101] Headache is one of the most common symptoms of AD, occurring in approximately 50% of patients.[102] Less commonly, AD causes nasal congestion, piloerection, paresthesias, shivering, desire to void, anxiety, malaise, nausea, dullness in the head, or blurred vision.[90,99-101] Untreated, AD can cause seizures, strokes, cardiac arrhythmias, and death.[91,100-105]

The main objective sign of AD is a dramatic increase in systolic BP and diastolic BP,[90] which can reach as high as 250-300 mm Hg and 200-220 mm Hg, respectively.[102,106] Most authors consider a rise in systolic BP of 30-40 mm Hg or 20% of the baseline value to be diagnostic of AD when it occurs in conjunction with at least one of the following: Headache, flushing, piloerection, sweating, and chills.[90] Even though bradycardia is considered to be a sign of AD, a study found that this only occurred in only 10% of the cases surveyed,[102] whereas tachycardia has been reported to occur in up to 38% of cases.[107]

The onset of AD is rapid and often dramatic,[90] and prac-tically any cutaneous or visceral stimulus below the level of the spinal cord lesion can precipitate the AD reaction.[99] Common triggers for AD are distention or contraction of the hollow organs or activation of pain receptors. More than one stimulus occurring simultaneously may make the reaction more severe and easier to bring on.[90] Bowel and bladder distention are perhaps the most common causes of AD.[90] However, catheterization and manipula-tion of an indwelling catheter are also well-known pre-cipitating factors.[108] Additional precipitating factors, although less common, are gastric ulcers,[109] gastro-esophageal reflux,[110] skeletal fractures below the level of the spinal cord lesion,[111,112] pregnancy,[113,114] labor,[115] sexual activity,[90] surgery,[116] and numerous others.[117]

REHABILITATION AND AUTONOMIC DYSREFLEXIA

Because of its life-threatening potential, clinicians working with patients with SCIs must be familiar with and understand the signs and triggers for AD. Patients with SCI should be positioned carefully to avoid pain and undue pressure on the bladder or abdomen. One should keep in mind that aggressive stretching or range of motion (ROM) activities that stimulate nociceptors can trigger an AD reaction. In addition, urinary catheters should be checked for blockage, twisting of the tubing, or overfilling of the bag.

An AD reaction should be treated as a medical emer-gency, and institutional policies for such situations should be followed. In addition, the patient should be kept as upright as possible and inspected for any possible trigger-ing mechanism. Keep in mind that the trigger may be something as simple as tight clothing or sitting on a wrinkle in clothing. All potential triggers should be resolved as quickly as possible. For example, tight cloth-ing should be loosened or removed and catheter tubing should be unkinked. The therapy session should be discontinued so that the patient is able to recover and stabilize.

PAIN*

IMPLICATIONS OF PAIN

Pain is an unpleasant sensory and emotional experience associated with actual or potential tissue damage or described in terms of such damage.[118] It is the most common symptom that brings patients to their health care practitioner, and patients' goals in rehabilitation fre-quently involve relieving pain. Measurement of pain helps evaluate the cause and source of symptoms, selection of interventions, and outcome assessment of the rehabilita-tion management.

The case to consider pain as the fifth vital sign stems from attempts to overcome barriers to relieving pain,[119] goals to improve patient/practitioner communication,[120] and attempts to improve the overall quality of patient care.[121] Pain should be taken seriously and addressed even if the patient does not want to complain about it or if pain is an expected part of the patients' condition.[122]

Pain is not just the result of nociceptive signals reach-ing the brain but also encompasses an individual's expe-rience of the sensation interwoven within their past and present experiences and emotions. Therefore, to be suc-cessful, pain management may need to address these issues, as well as the nociceptive aspect of pain.[123]

Pain measurement may include information about the nature, location, severity, and duration of the patient's experience of pain, as well as the degree to which the pain results in functional limitation or disability. Various methods and assessment tools have been developed to quantify and qualify both experimentally induced and

---

*The information on measurement of pain in this chapter is adapted from Cameron MH: *Physical Agents in Rehabilitation,* ed 2, Philadelphia, 2003, WB Saunders.

clinical pain. These methods are based on patients rating their pain on visual analog or numeric scales; comparing their present pain with that experienced in response to a predefined, quantifiable pain stimulus; or selecting words from a list to describe their present experience of pain. Different tools provide different amounts and types of information and require differing amounts of time and cognitive ability to complete.

VISUAL ANALOG AND NUMERIC SCALES

Visual analog and numeric scales assess pain severity by asking the patient to indicate the present level of pain on a drawn line or to rate the pain numerically on a scale of 1 10 or 1 100.[124] With the visual analog scale (VAS), the patient marks a position on a horizontal or vertical line, where one end of the line represents no pain and the other end represents the most severe pain possible or the most severe pain the patient can imagine (Fig. 22-17). With the numeric rating scale (NRS), 0 is no pain and 10 or 100, depending on the scale used, is the most severe pain possible or the most severe pain the patient can imagine. The horizontal VAS has been validated and shown to be reliable.[125]

Scales similar to the visual analog or numeric scales have been developed for use with individuals who have difficulty using these scales. For example, children who understand pictures but are too young to understand numeric representations of pain can use a scale with faces with different expressions to represent different experiences of pain (Fig. 22-18). The faces pain scale (FPS) is often used for children (3-12 years old) or individuals who are unable to communicate verbally.[126,127] This type of scale can also be used to assess pain in patients with limited comprehension because of language barriers or cognitive deficits. Pain scales are also available for rating pain in very young children and infants. These are based on describing the child's behavior, from inconsolable, constant crying to smiling.

These simple scales are frequently used to assess the severity of a patient's clinical pain because they are quick and easy to administer, are easily understood, and provide readily quantifiable data.[124] Herr et al compared the psy-chometric properties and usability of five common pain scales used in younger adults (25-55 years of age) to see if could be used with older adults (65-94 years of age). All pain scales tested (VAS, verbal rating scale [VRS], verbal descriptor scale [VDS; see semantic differential scales later], FPS, and 21-point NRS) were determined to be valid and reliable with either age group even if mild-to-moderate cognitive deficits were present. The NRS was preferred for both groups when reporting their pain intensity, whereas the VDS demonstrated the best psychometric properties.[128]

VAS and NRS provide only a single measure of the patient's pain complaint and do not provide information about the patient's affective response to pain or the effect of the pain on his or her functional activity level. Despite the findings of Herr at al[128] the reliability of visual analog and numeric rating may still vary among individuals and within the patient group examined, although the two scales have a high degree of agreement between them.[129] These types of measures are most useful in the clinical setting when a quick estimate of a patient's perceived progress or response to different activities or treatment interventions is desired.

COMPARISON WITH A PREDEFINED STIMULUS

Pain quantification methods that involve comparison with a predefined painful stimulus are intended to provide a greater degree of intersubject reliability than visual analog and numeric scales. For this type of assessment, the individual compares the severity of his or her symptoms with a predefined stimulus, resulting in more similar ratings among individuals. These measures are not used clinically but are used in some research as they are readily standardized.[130,131]

SEMANTIC DIFFERENTIAL SCALES

Semantic differential scales consist of word lists and categories that represent various aspects of the patient's pain experience. The patient is asked to select words from these lists that best describe his or her present experience of pain. These types of scales are designed to collect a broad

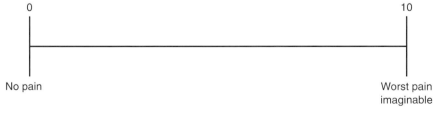

FIG. 22-17 Visual analog scale (VAS) for pain.

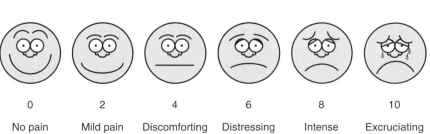

FIG. 22-18 Pain scale using graphic representations to assist small children or those with a language barrier. *Adapted from Wong DL, Perry SE, Hockenberry MJ: Maternal Child Nursing Care, ed 2, St. Louis, 2002, Mosby.*

range of information about the patient's pain experience and to provide quantifiable data for intrasubject and intersubject comparisons. The semantic differential scale included in the McGill Pain Questionnaire, or variations of this scale, are commonly used to assess pain[132-134] (Fig. 22-19). This scale includes descriptors of sensory, affective, and evaluative aspects of the patient's pain and groups the words into various categories within each of these aspects. The categories include temporal, spatial, pressure, and thermal to describe the sensory aspects of the pain; fear, anxiety, and tension to describe the affective aspects of the pain; and the cognitive experience of the pain based on past experience and learned behaviors to describe the eval-

uative aspects of the pain. The patient circles the one word in each of the applicable categories that best describes the present pain.[132,134]

Semantic differential scales have a number of advantages and disadvantages compared with other types of pain measures. They allow assessment and quantification of various aspects of the pain's scope, quality, and intensity. Counting the total number of words chosen provides a quick gauge of the pain severity. A more sensitive assessment of pain severity can be obtained by adding the rank sums of all the words chosen to produce a pain-rating index. For greater specificity with regard to the most problematic area, an index for the three major categories of the

---

What does your pain feel like?

Some of the words below describe your *present* pain. Indicate which words describe it best. Leave out any word group that is not suitable. Use only a single word in each appropriate group—the one that applies *best*.

1	2	3	4
1 Flickering	1 Jumping	1 Pricking	1 Sharp
2 Quivering	2 Flashing	2 Boring	2 Cutting
3 Pulsing	3 Shooting	3 Drilling	3 Lacerating
4 Throbbing		4 Stabbling	
5 Beating		5 Lancinating	
6 Pounding			

5	6	7	8
1 Pinching	1 Tugging	1 Hot	1 Tingling
2 Pressing	2 Pulling	2 Burning	2 Itchy
3 Gnawing	3 Wrenching	3 Scalding	3 Smarting
4 Cramping		4 Searing	4 Stinging
5 Crushing			

9	10	11	12
1 Dull	1 Tender	1 Tiring	1 Sickening
2 Sore	2 Taut	2 Exhausting	2 Suffocating
3 Hurting	3 Rasping		
4 Aching	4 Splitting		
5 Heavy			

13	14	15	16
1 Fearful	1 Punishing	1 Wretched	1 Annoying
2 Frightful	2 Gruelling	2 Blinding	2 Troublesome
3 Terrifying	3 Cruel		3 Miserable
	4 Vicious		4 Intense
	5 Killing		5 Unbearable

17	18	19	20
1 Spreading	1 Tight	1 Cool	1 Nagging
2 Radiating	2 Numb	2 Cold	2 Nauseating
3 Penetrating	3 Drawing	3 Freezing	3 Agonizing
4 Piercing	4 Squeezing		4 Dreadful
	5 Tearing		5 Torturing

FIG. 22-19 Semantic differential scale from the McGill Pain Questionnaire. *From Melzack R: The McGill Pain Questionnaire: major properties and scoring methods,* Pain *1:277-299, 1975.*

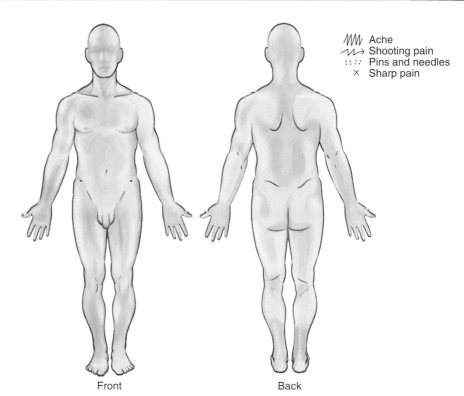

FIG. 22-20 Body diagram to record pain symptoms.

Ache
Shooting pain
Pins and needles
× Sharp pain

Front   Back

questionnaire can also be calculated.[134] The primary disadvantages of this scale are that it is time consuming to administer, and it requires the patient to have an intact cognitive state and a high level of literacy. Given these advantages and limitations, the most appropriate use for this type of scale is when detailed information about a patient's pain is needed such as in a chronic pain treatment program or in clinical research.

OTHER MEASURES

Other measures or indicators of pain that may provide additional useful information about the individual's pain complaint and clinical condition include daily activity/pain logs indicating which activities ease or aggravate the pain, body diagrams on which the patient can indicate the location and nature of the pain (Fig. 22-20), and open-ended, structured interviews.[135] Physical examination that includes observation of posture and assessment of strength, mobility, sensation, endurance, response to functional activity testing, and soft tissue tone and quality can also add valuable information to the evaluation of the severity and cause(s) of a patient's pain complaint.

In addition to the severity and nature of pain, pain can be described according to its presentation over time as constant or intermittent. Constant pain is pain that is present at all times. The person is never pain free, although the severity of the pain may vary over time. Intermittent pain is pain that is not always present. The pain comes and goes, and the patient has some pain-free periods, although these may be brief. Chemically-induced pain associated with an inflammatory process is often constant. Mechanical pain, which is generally associated with positioning, malalignment, or pressure, is usually intermittent.

In selecting the measures for assessing pain, one should consider the duration of the symptoms, the cognitive abilities of the patient, and the amount of time appropriate to assess this aspect of the patient's complaint. In many situations, a simple VAS may be sufficient to provide information regarding a progressive decrease in pain as the patient recovers from an acute injury. However, in more complex or prolonged cases, more detailed measures, such as semantic differential scales or a combination of several measures, are more appropriate.

ARTERIAL OXYGEN SATURATION

IMPLICATIONS OF ARTERIAL OXYGEN SATURATION

As early as 1988, it was suggested that arterial oxygen saturation be considered a vital sign.[136] Arterial oxyhemoglobin saturation, more commonly known as arterial oxygen saturation (SaO_2), is the degree to which hemoglobin in the blood is bound to oxygen. Each hemoglobin molecule has four oxygen binding sites and is considered to be 100% saturated when all four sites are bound to oxygen. Oxygen saturation is generally measured by percentage saturation and may be as high as 100%. Values of 95% to 100% are considered normal, and pulse oximetry generally provides reliable measures of oxygen saturation in the range of 70% to 100%.[137]

SaO_2 may be measured by pulse oximetry or through an arterial blood gas (ABG) analysis from a sample of arterial blood. Pulse oximetry *(SpO_2)* is generally preferred because it is simple, painless, accurate, noninvasive, and provides instantaneous, continuous measures of oxygen saturation.[137] Pulse oximetry is used to monitor hypoxia in patients with moderate-to-severe pulmonary disease and also the effectiveness of oxygen supplementation in many patients.[136]

Although many factors influence SaO₂, the most important influence is the partial pressure of oxygen (PaO₂). Under normal circumstances, this is around 100 mm Hg at sea level. The greater the PaO₂ the higher the SaO₂ will be and vice versa. However, this relationship is not linear (Fig. 22-21). Oxygen-hemoglobin binding increases very rapidly as the partial pressure of oxygen increases from 10-60 mm Hg, and then rises much more slowly as PaO₂ increases from 70-100 mm Hg. Thus, at a PaO₂ of 60 mm Hg, approximately 90% of the hemoglobin is saturated with oxygen, and beyond this point further increases in PaO₂ will only saturate the remaining 10% of unbound hemoglobin. This relationship protects the body from large variations in oxygen saturation in response to typical PaO₂ fluctuations that may occur with respiratory diseases and with commonly encountered PaO₂ changes that result from flying or changes in elevation.

Oxygen-hemoglobin binding is also affected by blood pH, body temperature, and the PaCO₂.[137] The dissociation curve shifts to the right in response to lowered pH, increased PaCO₂, or increased body temperature. Each of these may act singly or in combination with the others. As the dissociation curve shifts to the right, the hemoglobin loses its affinity for oxygen, facilitating the breaking of bonds holding oxygen to hemoglobin so that for any given PaO₂, more oxygen is freed from the hemoglobin molecule. The reverse is true if pH is increased, PaCO₂ is lowered, or body temperature is lowered.

HOW PULSE OXIMETRY WORKS

A pulse oximeter consists of a sensor connected to a microprocessor (Fig. 22-22). Most sensors resemble a small clothespin or a flat patch. The clothespin type sensor is typically secured to a fingertip, and the patch sensor may be taped to the skin, wrapped around a digit, or wrapped about the foot of an infant or small child. The sensor has a light-emitting diode (LED) light source and a light detector or photodetector positioned directly opposite the LED. The LED produces alternating bursts of red and infrared light. Unoxygenated hemoglobin absorbs more of the red light and oxygenated hemoglobin absorbs more of the infrared light. The photodetector measures how much of each type of light passes through the tissue and transmits this information to a microprocessor that calculates the SpO₂ from this data. Pulse oximeters only monitor light absorption that varies in a pulsatile manner and will therefore only work if applied to an area with good arterial flow.[137] The device generally displays both arterial oxygen saturation and the pulse rate.

Pulse oximetry is generally accurate to ±2% of the displayed number.[138] A meta-analysis of published works investigating the accuracy of oxygen saturation measured by pulse oximetry in healthy individuals compared to oxygen saturation measured by ABG analysis found pulse oximetry to be valid and accurate (weighted mean correlation coefficient = 0.893).[139] This indicates that in healthy individuals measures of oxygen saturation by pulse oximetry correlate well with the accepted gold standard of ABG measurement. In contrast, a more recent study found that the correlation between pulse oximetry and ABG analysis was not good enough to replace ABGs in patients presenting to the emergency department with chronic obstructive pulmonary disease.[140] However, most authors and researchers continue to recommend the use of pulse oximeters for continuous monitoring of oxygen saturation in the emergency department, critical care,

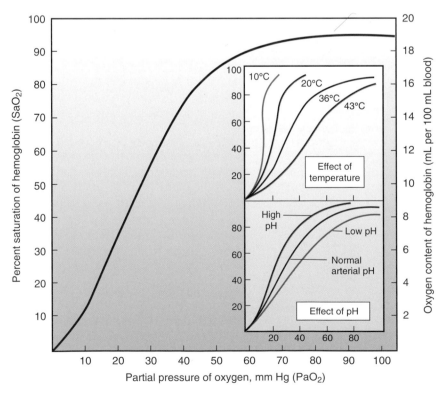

FIG. 22-21 Oxygen-hemoglobin dissociation curve. Normal saturation is easily maintained at PaO₂ values ranging from 80-100 mm Hg. PaO₂ below 60 mm Hg, which results in approximately 90% saturation (SaO₂), will cause a rapid decline in SaO₂. Therefore 90% SaO₂ is generally considered the lowest acceptable safe level of oxygen saturation. The curve is shifted to the left by a lower temperature or by an increase in pH. The curve is shifted to the right by a higher temperature, or by a decrease in pH. *Redrawn from McArdle WD, Katch FI, Katch VL:* Essentials of Exercise Physiology, *Philadelphia, 1994, Lea & Febiger.*

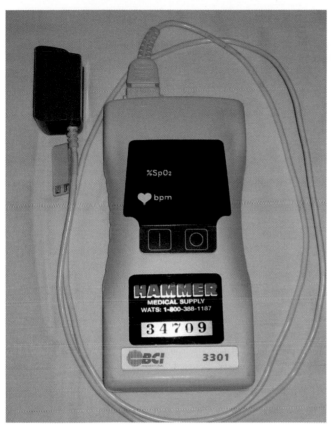

FIG. 22-22 A pulse oximeter with a fingertip sensor.

operating room, and respiratory ward settings where the trend of readings can be as informative as the absolute value.[140]

METHOD FOR MEASURING ARTERIAL OXYGEN SATURATION

Descriptions of the procedure for measuring SpO_2 vary slightly from one source to another. The procedure here reflects common accepted practice.[1,137] Before measuring an individual's arterial oxygen saturation you should, if possible, be aware of their hemoglobin level, previous baseline arterial oxygen saturation and temperature. Additionally, check to see if the patient has a current or has past history of using oxygen therapy.

Procedure

1. Explain what you are going to do, why, and how the patient can cooperate.
2. Wash your hands.
3. Provide for patient privacy, position patient comfortably, and try to ensure that the patient is breathing regularly.
4. Choose the site for application of the sensor. The sensor should be applied to an area of high vascularity such as the finger-tip, toe, earlobe, pinna of the ear, or the bridge of the nose. It should have adequate perfusion, be as motionless as possible, and free of any substance that may interfere with the light transmission through the tissue.

5. Choose the appropriate sensor for the selected location. In infants, if finger or toe sensors of the appropriate size are not available, then an adhesive type sensor may be used.
6. If using the finger, have the forearm supported and choose a finger without nail polish or artificial nails. If necessary, remove the polish or artificial nail. If that is not possible, use a toe or place the sensor sideways on the finger rather than over the nail bed.
7. Place the sensor on the patient. Let the patient know that it will not hurt and that they will feel only a little pressure. Make sure it is aligned correctly. If pulse oximetry is to be continuous, be sure to move sensors secured by spring tension every 2 hours as a safety precaution.
8. Turn on the oximeter, and observe the pulse intensity display and listen for an audible beeping sound. Correlate the oximeter pulse with a palpated pulse for accuracy.
9. Have the patient remain still, and inform them that an alarm will sound if the sensor falls off or if the patient displaces the sensor. If necessary, cover the sensor with a towel or washcloth to prevent bright ambient light from shining on the sensor, which may distort readings.
10. Leave the sensor in place until the oximeter reaches a stable value and the pulse display reaches full strength during each cardiac cycle. Read the SpO_2. If the SpO_2 is less than 95%, retake it or find an alternate site to retake the measurement unless the patient is known to have habitually low readings.
11. Document the SpO_2, pulse rate, sensor site, activity level, patient position, date, time, and, if the patient is on supplemental oxygen, the delivery rate and method of delivery. Discuss the findings with the physician as needed.

FACTORS AFFECTING RELEVANCE AND ACCURACY OF PULSE OXIMETRY READINGS

A number of factors may affect the clinical relevance and accuracy of SpO_2 measurements taken using pulse oximetry. These include patient factors, such as hemoglobin level, carbon monoxide inhalation, and the type of hemoglobin, as well as factors during the test such as motion, ambient light, wearing nail polish, and mechanical problems with the device.

Hemoglobin Level. Arterial oxygen hemoglobin saturation must be interpreted in the context of the patient's complete clinical picture, particularly their hemoglobin level. Even though a patient may have a high level of saturation, oxygen delivery to the tissues will be poor if the hemoglobin level is low.[137] Normal hemoglobin levels typically range from about 12-16 g/dL for women and 13-18 g/dL for men. Each gram of hemoglobin can carry about 1.34 ml of oxygen when fully saturated.[137] To determine overall oxygen-carrying capacity of the blood, multiply 1.34 ml/g by the patient's hemoglobin level in g/dL and by SpO_2. The normal range for oxygen-carrying capacity is 19-20 ml/dL.[137] For example, a woman with a hemoglobin level of 15 g/dL and an SpO_2 of 97% will have an oxygen-carrying capacity of 1.34 ml/g × 15 g/dL × 0.97 = 19.50 ml/dL, which is within the normal range. In contrast, a patient with a low hemoglobin level of 12 g/dL with a 97% SpO_2 would have a oxygen-carrying capacity of 1.34 ml/g × 12 g/dL × 0.97 = 15.6 ml/dL, which is well below the normal range of 19-20 ml/dL. A reduction in oxygen-carrying capacity causes a reduction in the amount of oxygen delivered to the tissues and will produce the same symptoms as low SpO_2.

Carbon Monoxide Inhalation. *Carboxyhemoglobin* absorbs light similarly to oxyhemoglobin, and pulse oximeters cannot differentiate between hemoglobin saturated with carbon monoxide or oxygen. Therefore patients who have inhaled a significant amount of carbon monoxide may have pulse oximeter readings that give the false impression of being normal. If carbon monoxide poisoning is suspected, only an ABG test should be used to determine oxygen saturation.[137]

Type of Hemoglobin. Pulse oximetry can be used in patients with sickle cell anemia because even though SpO_2 is underestimated, the difference is not clinically significant.[141] Pulse oximetry can also be used in infants and neonates, who have fetal hemoglobin (HbF), because it provides accurate, reliable, and clinically acceptable estimates of arterial hemoglobin in this population.[142-144]

Low Perfusion States. Low perfusion states that weaken or eliminate peripheral pulses will decrease the precision of the pulse oximeter readings because the device must detect pulsatile flow to function.[137] Patients at risk for low perfusion are those with hypotension, peripheral vascular disease, peripheral vasoconstriction, peripheral edema, and hypothermia and those who are hypovolemic or in cardiac arrest.[1,137] These conditions can easily lead to unreliable readings. In patients who are cold but not hypothermic, it is recommended that more central sites, such as the forehead or earlobes, be used or peripheral sites be warmed, to avoid inaccuracies caused by distal peripheral vasoconstriction.[137]

Motion During the Test. A variety of errors can be produced by patient movement during the measurement of arterial blood saturation by pulse oximetry. These include reduced accuracy, loss of signal, false desaturation alarms, and missed hypoxic events.[145] Erratic movement, especially in small children and neonates, may partially dislodge the sensor, which in turn disrupts the light transmission through the tissue. Up to 71% of pulse oximeter alarms involving pediatric critical care patients have been found to be false alarms.[146] Furthermore, rhythmic movements may make it difficult for the sensor to distinguish pulsatile flow, and other movements, such as shivering, exercise, and vibration, during transport may dislodge the sensor.[137] Therefore the patient should be as still as possible when measuring oxygen saturation. Newer devices, with different hardware and software designed to tolerate or compensate for movement, have been found to produce more reliable and accurate results than older units when patients are moving.[145-149]

Ambient Light. Ambient light can alter pulse oximeter readings if there is enough light of similar wavelengths to those produced by the sensor's LED.[150] This has been documented to occur with bright fluorescent lighting and can be rectified by simply covering the sensor with an opaque towel.[150]

Fingernail Polish. Fingernail polish, particularly dark polish, may interfere with pulse oximetry readings at the fingers or toes. Therefore, if the patient is wearing dark nail polish, either remove the polish from a finger or toe and use this digit or measure oxygen saturation at an alternate site. If necessary, the sensor may be placed sideways on the finger or toe.[137]

Mechanical Problems. Pulse oximeters like any other mechanical device need to be maintained and calibrated regularly. If inconsistencies are suspected in a unit, have it checked immediately and continue with a unit that is known to be in good working order.

NORMAL VALUES

Oxygen saturation values of 95% to 100% are generally considered normal. Values under 90% could quickly lead to a serious deterioration in status, and values under 70% are life-threatening.[29] Patients may deteriorate considerably before there is a dramatic change in oxygen saturation because, as discussed previously, the PaO_2 may fall from 100 mm Hg to 60 or 70 mm Hg before the oxygen saturation drops to 90%. Signs of deterioration include low BP, increased respiratory rate, and increased pulse rate.[137] Other signs of altered oxygen saturation that would indicate checking SpO_2 are altered respiratory rate; depth or rhythm; unusual breath sounds; cyanotic appearance of nail beds, lips, or mucous membranes; dusky skin; confusion; decreased level of consciousness; and dyspnea.[1,29]

CLINICAL APPLICATION

Pulse oximetry is a valuable tool to evaluate patients' exercise tolerance or progress in a rehabilitation program. Additionally, documentation of SpO_2 values with therapeutic intervention can lend support to the need for supplemental home oxygen therapy.

CHAPTER SUMMARY

Vital signs are indicators of a patients' general health. A history of recorded vital signs provides a view of a patient's health status over time and current measurements are valuable indicators of acute changes. The rehabilitation provider should be able to differentiate between normal and abnormal findings and have the proper skills and tools to gather and document vital sign measures (Fig. 22-23). Accurate and reliable measures contribute to and aid in goal setting and treatment planning and are needed for safe and effective patient management during therapeutic interventions.

GLOSSARY

Ambient temperature: The temperature in one's immediate location.
Apical: Of, at, or forming the apex of a structure.

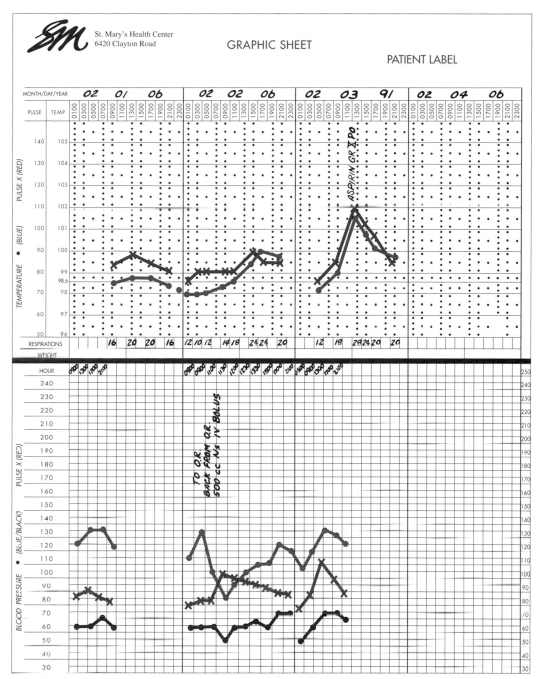

FIG. 22-23 Example of a vital signs documentation sheet. *Courtesy St. Mary's Health Center, St. Louis, MO.*

Arrhythmia: Irregularity or loss of rhythm, especially of the heartbeat. Also known as dysrhythmia.

Benign: Not recurrent or progressive. The opposite of malignant.

Bradycardia: A slow heart rate usually less than 60 beats per minute.

Carboxyhemoglobin: Compound of hemoglobin and carbon monoxide formed in poisoning by carbon monoxide.

Cyanotic: Pertaining to the bluish, grayish or dark purple discoloration of the skin, resulting from abnormal amounts of reduced hemoglobin in the blood.

Frenulum: Fold of mucous membrane that extends from the floor of the mouth to the inferior surface of the tongue along its midline.

Hypothermia: Having a body temperature below normal, usually considered 35° C (95° F) and below.

Meniscus: The curved upper surface of a liquid in a container. The surface is convex if the liquid does not wet the container and concave if it does.

Otoscope: A device for examination of the ear.

Pinna: The auricle or projected part of the exterior ear that collects and directs sound waves into the ear.

Pulse: The regular expansion felt over an artery as the wave of blood passes through the vessel in time with the heartbeat.

Sphygmomanometer: The instrument used to determine BP through the use of an arm cuff and an aneroid dial or a calibrated column of mercury.

Spo₂: Estimation of arterial blood saturation by pulse oximetry.

Sublingual pocket: The area to the back and underneath the tongue on either side of the frenulum.

Syncope: A transient loss of consciousness from inadequate blood flow to the brain. Also known as fainting or swooning.

Tachycardia: Abnormally rapid heart rate, usually considered over 100 bpm in adults at rest.

Tachypnea: Abnormally rapid respiration or rate of breathing.

Tympanic membrane: Eardrum. The membrane serving as the lateral wall of the tympanic cavity and separating it from the external acoustic meatus.

Vasoconstriction: Decrease in the caliber of a blood vessel.

Vasodilation: Increase in the caliber of a blood vessel.

Vital signs: The critical indicators of a person's health and current medical status (i.e., pulse, body temperature, respiration, BP, oxygen saturation, and perceived pain).

References

1. Perry AG, Potter PA: *Clinical Nursing Skills and Techniques*, ed 5, St. Louis, 2002, Mosby.
2. DeWit SC: *Rambo's Nursing Skills for Clinical Practice*, ed 4, Philadelphia, 1994, WB Saunders.
3. Guiffre M, Heidenreich T, Carney-Gersten P, et al: The relationship between axillary and core body temperature measurements, *Appl Nurs Res* 3(2):52-55, 1990.
4. O'Toole S: Alternatives to mercury thermometers, *Prof Nurs* 12(11):783-786, 1997.
5. Weiss ME, Sitzer V, Clarke M, et al: A comparison of temperature measurements using three ear thermometers, *Appl Nurs Res* 11(4):158-166, 1998.
6. Stavem K, Saxholm H, Smith-Erichsen N: Accuracy of infrared ear thermometry in adult patients, *Intensive Care Med* 23:100-105, 1997.
7. Doezema D, Lunt M, Tandberg D: Cerumen occlusion lowers infrared tympanic membrane temperature measurement, *Acad Emerg Med* 2:17-19, 1995.
8. Shinozaki T, Deane R, Perkins FM: Infrared tympanic thermometer: evaluation of a new clinical thermometer, *Crit Care Med* 16(2):148-150, 1988.
9. Erickson RS, Yount ST: Comparison of tympanic and oral temperatures in surgical patients, *Nurs Res* 40(2):90-93, 1991.
10. Romano MJ, Fortenberry JD, Autrey E, et al: Infrared tympanic thermometry in the pediatric intensive care unit, *Crit Care Med* 21(8):1181-1185, 1993.
11. Pontious SL, Kennedy A, Chung KL, et al: Accuracy and reliability of temperature measurement in the emergency department by instrument and site in children, *Pediatr Nurs* 20(1):58-63, 1994.
12. Schmitz T, Bair N, Falk M, et al: A comparison of five methods of temperature measurement in febrile intensive care patients, *Am J Crit Care* 4(4):286-292, 1995.
13. Erickson R: Oral temperature differences in relation to thermometer and technique, *Nurs Res* 29(3):157-164, 1980.
14. Gayle F, Brown M: Comparing three methods of temperature taking: oral mercury-in-glass, oral Diatek and tympanic First Temp, *Nurs Res* 44(22):120-122, 1995.
15. Dowding D, Freeman S, Nimmo S, et al: An investigation into the accuracy of different types of thermometers, *Prof Nurs* 18(3):166-168, 2002.
16. Wilshaw R, Beckstrand R, Waid D, et al: A comparison of the use of tympanic, axillary and rectal thermometers in infants, *Pediatr Nurs* 14(2):88-93, 1999.
17. Giuliano KK, Scott SS, Elliot S, et al: Temperature measurement in critically ill orally intubated adults: a comparison of pulmonary artery core, tympanic and oral methods, *Crit Care Med* 27(10):2188-2193, 1999.
18. Closs J: Oral temperature measurement, *Nurs Times* 83(1):36-39, 1987.
19. Pugh-Davies S, Kassab JY, Thrush AJ, et al: A comparison of mercury and digital clinical thermometers, *J Adv Nurs* 11:535-543, 1985.
20. Buswell C: Comparing mercury and disposable thermometers, *Prof Nurs* 12(5):359-362, 1997.
21. Pontius S, Kennedy AH, Shelley S, et al: Accuracy and reliability of temperature measurements by instrument and site, *Pediatr Nurs* 9(2):114-123, 1994.
22. Board M: Comparison of disposable and glass mercury thermometers, *Nurs Times* 91(33):36-37, 1995.
23. Eoff MJ, Joyce B: Temperature measurement in children, *Am J Nurs* 81(5):1010-1011, 1981.
24. Blainey CG: Site selection in taking body temperature, *Am J Nurs* 74:1859-1861, 1974.
25. Tandberg D, Sklar D: Effect of tachypnea on the estimation of body temperature by an oral thermometer, *N Engl J Med* 308:945-946, 1983.
26. Woodman EA, McConnell PS, Simms L: Sources of unreliability in oral temperatures, *Nurs Res* 16(3):276-279, 1967.
27. Forster B, Adler DC, Davis M: Duration of effects of drinking iced water on oral temperature, *Nurs Res* 19(2):169-170, 1970.
28. Lee RE, Atkins E: Spurious fever, *Am J Nurs* 72(6):1094-1095, 1972.
29. Kozier B, Erb G, Berman A, et al: *Techniques in Clinical Nursing: Basic to Intermediate Skills*, ed 5, New Jersey, 2004, Pearson Prentice Hall.
30. Timby BK: *Fundamental Skills and Concepts in Patient Care*, ed 7, Philadelphia, 2003, Lippincott, Williams & Wilkins.
31. Baker N, Bidwell-Cerone S, Gaze N, et al: The effect of type of thermometer and length of time inserted on oral temperature measurements of afebrile subjects, *Nurs Res* 33(2):109-111, 1984.
32. Severine JE, Mckenzie NE: Advances in temperature monitoring: a far cry from shake and take, *Nursing* 27(5):1-16, 1997.
33. Sund-Levander M, Forsberg C, Wahren LK: Normal oral, rectal, tympanic and axillary body temperature in adult men and women: a systematic literature review, *Scand J Car Sci* 16:122-128, 2002.
34. McArdle WD, Katch FI, Katch VL: *Essentials of Exercise Physiology*, Philadelphia, 1994, Lea & Febiger.
35. Maciel BC, Gallo L, Marin Neto JA, et al: Parasympathetic contribution to bradycardia induced by endurance training in man, *Cardiovasc Res* 19:642-648, 1985.
36. Ekblom B, Kilbom ASA, Soltysiak J: Physical training, bradycardia, and autonomic nervous system, *Scand J Clin Lab Invest* 32:251-256, 1973.
37. Roeske WR, O'Roarke RA, Klein A, et al: Noninvasive evaluation of ventricular hypertrophy in professional athletes, *Circulation* 53:286-292, 1976.
38. Wilcockson J, Von Neupauer KS: Brother Klodi: Is Ullrich's understudy ready for the big time? *VeloNews* 34 (1):40-41, 2005.
39. Scheuer J, Tipton CM: Cardiovascular adaptations to physical training, *Ann Rev Physiol* 39:221-251, 1977.
40. Marieb EN: *Human Anatomy and Physiology*, ed 2, Redwood City, 1992, Benjamin/Cummings.
41. Perloff D, Grim C, Flack J, et al: Human blood pressure determined by sphygmomanometry, *Circulation* 88(5):2460-2470, 1993.
42. Yarows SA, Quin K: Accuracy of aneroid sphygmomanometers in clinical usage: University of Michigan experience, *Blood Press Monit* 6(2):101-106, 2001.
43. Chobanian AV, Bakris GL, Black HR, et al: National High Blood Pressure Education Program Coordinating Committee: Seventh report of the joint national committee on prevention, detection, evaluation, and treatment of high blood pressure, *Hypertension* 42:1206-1252, 2003.
44. Rastam L, Prineas RJ, Gomez-Marin O: Ratio of cuff width/arm circumference as a determinant of arterial blood pressure measurements in adults, *J Intern Med* 227, 225-232, 1990.
45. Knight T, Leech F, Jones A, et al: Sphygmomanometers in use in general practice: an overlooked aspect of quality in patient care, *J Hum Hypertens* 15, 681-684, 2001.
46. Markandu N, Whitcher F, Arnold A, et al: The mercury sphygmomanometer should be abandoned before it is proscribed, *J Hum Hypertens* 14, 31-36, 2000.
47. Beevers M, Morgan H: An audit of blood pressure measurement in two teaching hospitals, *J Hum Hypertens* 7, 98, 1997.
48. Hemingway T, Guss D, Abdelnur D: Arm position and blood pressure measurement, *Ann Intern Med* 140(1):74-75, 2004.
49. Mourad A, Carney S: Arm position and blood pressure: An audit, *Intern Med J* 34(5):290-291, 2004.
50. Mourad A, Carney S, Gillies A, et al: Arm position and blood pressure: a risk factor for hypertension? *J Hum Hypertens* 17(6):389-395, 2003.
51. Foster-Fitzpatrick L, Ortiz A, Sibilano H, et al: The effect of crossed leg on blood pressure measurement, *Nurs Res* 48,105-108, 1999.
52. Cassidy P, Jones K: A study of inter-arm blood pressure differences in primary care, *J Hum Hypertens* 15, 519-522, 2001.
53. Lane D, Beevers M, Barnes N, et al: Inter-arm differences in blood pressure: When are they clinically significant? *J Hypertens* 20, 1089-1095, 2002.
54. Mourad A, Gillies A, Carney S: Inaccuracy of wrist-cuff oscillometric blood pressure devices: An arm position artefact? *Blood Press Monit* 10(2):67-71, 2005.
55. Yarrows SA: Comparison of the Omron HEM-637 wrist monitor to the auscultation method with the wrist position sensor on or disabled, *Am J Hypertens* 17(1):54-58, 2004.
56. Kikyua M, Chonan K, Imai Y, et al: Accuracy and reliability of wrist-cuff devices for self-measurement of blood pressure, *J Hypertens* 20:629-638, 2002.
57. Zweiker R, Schumacher M, Fruhwald FM, et al: Comparison of wrist blood pressure measurement with conventional sphygmomanometry at a cardiology outpatient clinic, *J Hypertens* 18(8):1013-1018, 2000.
58. Rogers P, Burke V, Stroud P, et al: Comparison of oscillometric blood pressure measurements at the wrist with an upper-arm auscultatory mercury sphygmomanometer, *Clin Exp Pharma Physiol* 26(5-6):477-481, 1999.
59. Palatini P, Longo D, Toffanin G, et al: Wrist blood pressure overestimates blood pressure measured at the upper arm, *Blood Press Monit* 9(2):77-81, 2004.

60. Guidelines Subcommittee: World Health Organization International Society of Hypertension Guidelines for the management of hypertension., *J Hypertens* 17(2):151-183, 1999.
61. Burt VL, Whelton P, Roccella EJ, et al: Prevalence of hypertension in the U.S. adult population. Results from the Third National Health and Nutrition Examination Survey, 1988-1991, *Hypertension* 25(3):305-313, 1995.
62. Vasan RS, Beiser A, Seshadri S, et al: Residual lifetime risk for developing hypertension in middle-aged women and men: The Framingham Heart Study, *JAMA* 287(8):1003-1010, 2002.
63. Franklin SS, Gustin W, Wong ND, et al: Hemodynamic patterns of age-related changes in blood pressure. The Framingham Heart Study, *Circulation* 96(1):308-315, 1997.
64. Banegas J, de la Cruz J, Rodriguez-Artalejo F, et al: Systolic vs diastolic blood pressure: community burden and impact and impact on blood pressure staging, *J Hum Hypertens* 16(3):163-167, 2002.
65. Tin L, Beevers D, Lip G: Systolic vs. diastolic blood pressure and the burden of hypertension, *J Hum Hypertens* 16:147-150, 2002.
66. Franklin SS, Larson MG, Khan SA, et al: Does the relation of blood pressure to coronary heart disease risk change with aging? The Framingham Heart Study, *Circulation* 103(9):1245-1249, 2001.
67. Sulbaran T, Silva E, Maestre G: Isolated systolic hypertension: a new challenge in medicine, *J Hum Hypertens* 16(suppl 1):S44-S47, 2002.
68. Leonetti G, Cuspidi C, Facchini M, et al: Is systolic pressure a better target for antihypertensive treatment than diastolic pressure? *J Hypertens* 18(suppl 3):S13-S20, 2000.
69. Perry HM Jr, Miller JP, Baty JD, et al: Pretreatment blood pressure as a predictor of 21 year mortality, *Am J Hypertens* 13(6):724-733, 2000.
70. Kostis JB, Davis BR, Cutler J, et al: Prevention of heart failure by antihypertensive drug treatment in older persons with isolated systolic hypertension. SHEP Cooperative Research Group, *JAMA* 278(3):212-216, 1997.
71. SHEP Cooperative Research Group: Prevention of stroke by antihypertensive drug treatment in older persons with isolated systolic hypertension. Final results of the Systolic Hypertension in the Elderly Program (SHEP), *JAMA* 265(24):3255-3264, 1991.
72. Staessen JA, Thijs L, Fagard R, et al: Predicting cardiovascular risk using conventional vs ambulatory blood pressure in older patients with systolic hypertension: Systolic Hypertension in Europe Trial Investigators, *JAMA* 282(6):539-546, 1999.
73. Hyman DJ, Pavlik VN: Characteristics of patients with uncontrolled hypertension in the United States, *N Engl J Med* 345:479-486, 2001.
74. Loyd-Jones DM, Evans JC, Larson MG, et al: Differential control of systolic and diastolic blood pressure: factors associated with lack of blood pressure control in the community, *Hypertension* 36:594-599, 2000.
75. Cushman WC, Ford CE, Cutler JA, et al: Success and predictors of blood pressure control in diverse North American settings: The Antihypertensive and Lipid-Lowering Treatment to Prevent Heart Attack Trial (ALLHAT), *J Clin Hypertens* 4(6):393-404, 2002.
76. Black HR, Elliott WJ, Neaton JD, et al: Baseline characteristics and early blood pressure control in the CONVINCE trial, *Hypertension* 37(1):12-18, 2001.
77. Lewington S, Clarke R, Qizilbash N, et al: Age-specific relevance of usual blood pressure to vascular mortality: A meta-analysis of individual data for one million adults in 61 prospective studies. Prospective Studies Collaboration., *Lancet* 360:1903-1913, 2002.
78. Pickering T, James G, Boddie G, et al: How common is white coat hypertension? *JAMA* 259(2):225-228, 1988.
79. Kumpusalo E, Teho A, Laitila R, et al: Janus Faces of the White Coat Effect: Blood pressure not only rises, it may also fall, *J Hum Hypertens* 16:725-728, 2002.
80. Mancia G, Parati G, Pomidossi G, et al: Alerting reaction and rise in blood pressure during measurement by physician and nurse, *Hypertension* 31:1185-1189, 1987.
81. Celis H, Fagard RH: White-coat hypertension: A clinical review, *Eur J Intern Med* 15(6):348-357, 2004.
82. Beevers D: Salt and cardiovascular disease: not just hypertension, *J Hum Hypertens* 15:749-750, 2001.
83. De Wardener H, MacGregor G: Harmful effects of dietary salt in addition to hypertension, *J Hum Hypertens* 16:213-223, 2002.
84. He F, MacGregor G: Effect of modest salt reduction on blood pressure: a meta-analysis of randomized trials. Implications for public health, *J Hum Hypertens* 16:761-770, 2002.
85. Midgley J, Matthew A, Greenwood C, et al: Effect of reduced dietary sodium on blood pressure: a meta-analysis of randomized controlled trials, *JAMA* 275:1590-1597, 1996.
86. Grandal N, Galloe A, Garred P: Effect of sodium restriction on blood pressure, rennin, aldosterone, catecholamines, cholesterols and triglycerides: A meta-analysis, *JAMA* 279:1383-1391, 1998.
87. Poon IO, Braun U: High prevalence of orthostatic hypotension and its correlation with potentially causative medications among elderly veterans, *J Clin Pharm Therapeut* 30(2):173-178, 2005.
88. Bradley JG, Davis KA: Orthostatic Hypotension, *Am Fam Phys* 68(12):2393-2398, 2003.
89. Sclater A, Alagiakrishnan K: Orthostatic hypotension. A primary care primer for assessment and treatment, *Geriatrics* 59(8):22-27, 2004.
90. Karlsson AK: Autonomic dysreflexia, *Spinal Cord* 37:383-391, 1999.
91. Naftchi NE, Richardson JS: Autonomic dysreflexia: Pharmacological management of hypertensive crises in spinal cord injured patients, *J Spinal Cord Med* 20(3):355-360, 1997.
92. Vaidyanathan S, Soni BM, Watt JWH, et al: Pathophysiology of autonomic dysreflexia: long term treatment with terazosin in adult and pediatric spinal cord injury patients manifesting recurrent dysreflexic episodes, *Spinal Cord* 36:761-770, 1998.
93. Gimovski ML, Ojeda A, Ozaki R, et al: Management of autonomic hyperreflexia associated with low thoracic spinal cord lesion, *Am J Obstet Gynecol* 153:223-224, 1985.
94. Kiker JD, Woodstide JR, Jelinek GE: Neurogenic pulmonary edema associated with autonomic dysreflexia, *J Urology* 128:1038-1039, 1982.
95. Moeller BA Jr, Scheinberg D: Autonomic dysreflexia in injuries below the sixth thoracic segment, *JAMA* 224:1295, 1973.
96. Braddom RL, Rocco JF: Autonomic dysreflexia. A survey of current treatment, *Am J Phys Med Rehabil* 70:234-241, 1991.
97. Snow JC, et al: Autonomic hyperreflexia during cystoscopy in patients with high spinal cord injuries, *Paraplegia* 15:327-332, 1978.
98. Lindan R, Joiner E, Freehafer AA, et al: Incidence and clinical features of autonomic dysreflexia in patients with spinal cord injury, *Paraplegia* 18:285-292, 1980.
99. Erickson RP: Autonomic hyperreflexia: pathophysiology and medical management, *Arch Phys Med Rehabil* 61:431-440, 1980.
100. Eltorai I, Kim R, Vulpe M, et al: Fatal cerebral hemorrhage due to autonomic dysreflexia in a tetraplegic patient: Case report and review, *Paraplegia* 30:355-360, 1992.
101. Lee BY, Karmaker MG, Herz BL, et al: Autonomic dysreflexia revisited, *J Spinal Cord Med* 18:75-87, 1995.
102. Kewalramani LS: Autonomic dysreflexia in traumatic myelopathy, *Am J Phys Med* 59:1-21, 1980.
103. Yarkony GM, Katz RT, Yeong-Chi W: Seizures secondary to autonomic dysreflexia, *Arch Phys Med Rehabil* 67:834-835, 1986.
104. Pine ZM, Miller SD, Alonso JA: Atrial fibrillation associated with autonomic dysreflexia, *Am J Phys Med Rehabil* 70:271-273, 1991.
105. Kursh ED, Freehafer A, Persky L: Complications of autonomic dysreflexia, *J Urology* 118:70-72, 1977.
106. Kurnick N: Autonomic hyperreflexia and its control in patients with spinal cord lesions, *Ann Intern Med* 44:678-685, 1956.
107. Scott MB, Morrow JW: Phenoxybenzamine in neurogenic bladder dysfunction after spinal cord injury. II. Autonomic dysreflexia, *J Urology* 119:483-484, 1978.
108. Perkash I: Autonomic dysreflexia and detrusor-sphincter dyssynergia in spinal cord injury patients, *J Spinal Cord Med* 20:365-370, 1997.
109. Finestone HM, Teasell RW: Autonomic dysreflexia after brainstem resection. A case report, *Am J Phys Med Rehabil* 72:395-397, 1993.
110. Donald IP, Gear MW, Wilkinson SP: A life threatening respiratory complication of gastro-esophageal reflux in a patient with tetraplegia, *Postgrad Med J* 63:397-399, 1987.
111. Beard JP, Wade WH, Barber DB: Sacral insufficiency stress fracture as etiology of positional autonomic dysreflexia: case report, *Paraplegia* 34:173-175, 1996.
112. Givre S, Freed HA: Autonomic dysreflexia: a potentially fatal complication of somatic stress in quadriplegics, *J Emerg Med* 7:461-463, 1989.
113. Craig DI: The adaptation to pregnancy of spinal cord injured women, *Rehabil Nurse* 15:6-9, 1990.
114. Craig DI: Spinal cord injury and pregnancy: the stories of two women, *SCI Nurse* 11:100-104, 1994.
115. McGregor JA, Mecuwsen J: Autonomic hyperreflexia: a mortal danger for spinal cord damaged women in labor, *Am J Obstet Gynecol* 151:330-333, 1985.
116. Eltorai IM, Wong DH, Lacerna M, et al: Surgical aspects of autonomic dysreflexia, *J Spinal Cord Med* 20(3):361-364, 1997.
117. Teasell RW, Arnold JMO, Krassioukov A, et al: Cardiovascular consequences of loss of supraspinal control of the sympathetic nervous system after spinal cord injury, *Arch Phys Med Rehabil* 81:506-516, 2000.
118. Mersky H: The definition of pain, *Eur J Psychiatry* 6:153-159, 1991.
119. Lynch M: Pain as the fifth vital sign, *J Intraven Nurs* 24(2):85-94, 2001.
120. Davis MP, Walsh D: Cancer pain: how to measure the fifth vital sign, *Cleve Clin J Med* 71(8):625-632, 2004.
121. Chanvej L, Petpichetchian W, Kovitwanawong N, et al: A chart audit of postoperative pain assessment and documentation: the first step to implement pain assessment as the fifth vital sign in a university hospital in Thailand, *J Med Assoc Thai* 87(12):1447-1453, 2004.
122. Schaffer I: Postoperative pain as the fifth vital parameter, *Medicinski Pregled* 54(5-6):283-287, 2001.
123. Mckenzie R, May S: *The Human Extremities: Mechanical Diagnosis and Therapy*, Wellington, 2000, Spinal Publications.
124. Downie W, Leatham PA, Rhind VM, et al: Studies with pain rating scales, *Ann Rheum Dis* 37(4):378-381, 1978.

125. Maio RF, Garrison HG, Spaite DW, et al: Emergency Medical Services Outcomes Project (EMSOP) IV: Pain measurement in out-of-hospital outcomes research, *Ann Emerg Med* 40:172-179, 2002.

126. Luffy R, Grove SK: Examining the validity, reliability, and preference of three pediatric patient measurement tools in African-American children, *Pediatr Nurs* 29:54-59, 2003.

127. Tyler DC, Tu A, Douthit J, et al: Toward validation of pain measurement tools for children: a pilot study, *Pain* 52:301-309, 1993.

128. Herr KA, Spratt K, Mobily PR, et al: Pain intensity assessment in older adults: use of experimental pain to compare psychometric properties and usability of selected pain scales with younger adults, *Clin J Pain* 20:207-219, 2004.

129. Grossman SA, Sheidler VR, McGuire DB, et al: A comparison of the Hopkins Pain Rating Instrument with standard visual analogue and verbal description scales in patients with cancer pain, *J Pain Symptom Manage* 7(4):196-203, 1992.

130. Posner J: A modified submaximal effort tourniquet test for evaluation of analgesics in healthy volunteers, *Pain* 19:143-151, 1984.

131. Kast EC: An understanding of pain and its measurement, *Med Times* 94:1501-1503, 1966.

132. Melzack R: The McGill Pain Questionnaire: major properties and scoring methods, *Pain* 1:277-299, 1975.

133. Byrne M, Troy A, Bradley LA, et al: Cross-validation of the factor structure of the McGill Pain Questionnaire, *Pain* 13(2):193-201, 1982.

134. Prieto EJ, Hopson L, Bradley LA, et al: The language of low back pain: factor structure of the McGill Pain Questionnaire, *Pain* 8(1):11-19, 1980.

135. Ransford AO, Cairns D, Mooney V: The pain drawing as an aid to the psychological evaluation of patients with low back pain, *Spine* 1(2):127-134, 1976.

136. Neff TA: Routine oximetry: A fifth vital sign? (editorial), *Chest* 94(2):227, 1988.

137. Carroll P: Pulse oximetry at your fingertips, *RN* 60(2):22-27, 1997.

138. Carroll P: Using pulse oximetry in the home, *Home Healthc Nurse* 15(2):89-95, 1997.

139. Jensen LA, Onyskiw JE, Prasad NGN: Meta-analysis of arterial oxygen saturation monitoring by pulse oximetry in adults, *Heart Lung* 27:387-408, 1998.

140. Kelly AM, McAlpine R, Kyle E: How accurate are pulse oximeters in patients with acute exacerbations of chronic obstructive airway disease? *Respir Med* 95(5):336-340, 2001.

141. Fitzgerald R, Johnson A: Pulse oximetry in sickle cell anemia, *Crit Care Med* 29(9):1803-1806, 2001.

142. Brouillette RT, Waxman DH: Evaluation of the newborn's blood gas status. National Academy of Clinical Biochemistry, *Clin Chem* 43(1):215-221, 1997.

143. Rajadurai VS, Walker AM, Yu VY, et al: Effect of fetal haemoglobin on the accuracy of pulse oximetry in preterm infants, *J Pediatr Child Health* 28(1):43-46, 1992.

144. Denjean A, Bridey F, Praud JP, et al: Accuracy of measurements of HbF with OSM3 in neonates and infants, *Eur Respir J* 5(1):105-107, 1992.

145. Barker SJ: Motion-resistant pulse oximetry: A comparison of new and old models, *Anesth Analg* 95(4):967-972, 2002.

146. Lawless ST: Crying wolf: False alarms in a pediatric intensive care unit, *Crit Care Med* 22:981-985, 1994.

147. Bohnhorst B, Peter CS, Poets CF: Pulse oximeters' reliability in detecting hypoxemia and bradycardia: A comparison between a conventional and two new generation oximeters, *Crit Care Med* 28:1565-1568, 2000.

148. Hay WW, Rodden DJ, Collins SM, et al: Reliability of conventional and new pulse oximetry in neonatal patients, *J Perinatol* 22(5):360-366, 2002.

149. Torres A, Skender K, Wohrley J, et al: Pulse oximetry in children with congenital heart disease; effects of cardiopulmonary bypass and cyanosis, *Intensive Care Med* 19(4):229-234, 2004.

150. Amar D, Neidzwiski J, Wald A, et al: Fluorescent light interferes with pulse oximetry, *J Clin Monit* 5(2):135-136, 1989.

Chapter 23

Deconditioning

Ahmed Samir Elokda, Kevin Helgeson

OBJECTIVES

After reading this chapter, the reader will be able to:
1. Discuss the risk factors for pathologies associated with the consequences of deconditioning.
2. Apply the best methods and tools for examining a patient with deconditioning.
3. Understand how the disablement model and the *Guide to Physical Therapist Practice* are used to evaluate and diagnose a patient with deconditioning.
4. Use evidence-based interventions for patients with deconditioning.

$\mathcal{D}$econditioning is the decline of normal anatomical and physiological function caused by disease, aging, or inactivity.[1] *Deconditioning* can affect multiple body systems, and a decline in the function of any one system may affect the other systems. The cardiopulmonary system is most affected by deconditioning, and this secondarily has the greatest effect on the musculoskeletal system. Deconditioning of the cardiopulmonary system impairs the transport of blood and oxygen to the body's tissues, including the skeletal muscles that provide for mobility of the body. Musculoskeletal deconditioning leads to changes in muscle cellular metabolism, decreased capillarization, and decreased ability to work for long periods.[1]

Deconditioning can occur in many patients seen by a physical therapist (PT), ranging from high-level athletes who cannot perform sports-specific physical training because of injury to patients in the intensive care unit and less active elderly individuals. Patients with a high level of physical fitness will have a more rapid decline in physiological function with periods of extended immobility than patients with low levels of fitness.[2] Periods of immobility or decreased activity quickly result in a decline in maximal oxygen consumption rate, total blood volume, and stroke volume. These changes can be measured after as little as 2 weeks of inactivity.[1,2] Measures of pulmonary function, heart rate, and muscle metabolism decline more slowly, with measurable changes occurring after at least 30 days of inactivity.[1]

A deconditioned patient needs to be examined for impairments, functional limitations, and disabilities to develop a plan of care. A patient with deconditioning will present with *endurance impairments* that can be measured by whole body activities or with repeated movements of an extremity, as described in the section on Tests and Measures. The rehabilitation clinician should consider the patient's primary pathological conditions, co-morbidities, and psychosocial factors that may have contributed to deconditioning, as well as his or her current level of activity when evaluating the patient and developing a plan of care. The disablement model is used to describe how patients with deconditioning are examined, evaluated, and diagnosed.

PATHOLOGY

The *Guide to Physical Therapist Practice* (the *Guide*) includes the preferred practice pattern 6B: Impaired aerobic capacity/endurance associated with deconditioning.[3] This practice pattern describes physical therapy management for patients with deconditioning who develop the impairments of decreased aerobic capacity and/or endurance. To fully implement the disablement model for a patient in this practice pattern, the PT must consider the relationships between the patient's endurance impairment and functional limitations. The functional limitations related to the endurance impairment will be activities or tasks the patient cannot perform for long enough or with enough repetitions to be efficient or carry out in a typically expected or competent manner. For the patient classified in this preferred practice pattern, the endurance impairment is considered their chief impairment because it is most closely related to their functional limitations.

A patient who is primarily categorized as having conditions that best fit other practice patterns in the musculoskeletal, neuromuscular, or integumentary sections of the *Guide* may also have deconditioning and endurance impairments.[3] Therefore the information presented in this chapter may serve as a useful reference for patients primarily categorized in other preferred practice patterns who develop problems related to deconditioning. The musculoskeletal preferred practice pattern 4C: Impaired muscle performance (see Chapter 5) is closely related to deconditioning, since the loss of muscle endurance, the inability to perform repetitive work tasks, and decreased functional work capacity described in the inclusion criteria of this pattern may also be found in a patient fitting the deconditioning pattern. The impaired muscle performance pattern should be used for problems that primarily affect the musculoskeletal system in a specific region of the body, whereas the deconditioning pattern would be used for problems of a more global nature, affecting multiple systems.

PROCESSES THAT RESULT IN DECONDITIONING

The effects of detraining in athletic subjects and of bed rest in subjects without pathologies have been well studied.[1,2,4] The effects on the cardiopulmonary, musculoskeletal, and endocrine systems in these subjects serve as the basis for our understanding of the effects of deconditioning on patients with conditions that result in endurance impairments.

Maximum oxygen uptake ($\dot{V}O_{2max}$) rate is considered the best indicator of cardiopulmonary fitness.[5,6] $\dot{V}O_{2max}$ is the maximum amount of oxygen in milliliters (ml) that one can use in 1 minute (min) per kilogram (kg) of body weight. $\dot{V}O_{2max}$ is determined by measuring the amount of oxygen the body consumes during an activity such as walking, running, or bicycling with maximal effort. $\dot{V}O_{2max}$ in a healthy adult is usually in the range of 24-50 ml of oxygen/kg of body weight/min.[6] $\dot{V}O_{2max}$ has been shown to decline with inactivity, with the decline being fastest during the first month of inactivity but ongoing, albeit at a slower rate, for at least the next 2 months.[1,2] Changes in stroke volume, blood volume, heart rate, and ventilatory capacity all contribute to the decline in $\dot{V}O_{2max}$.

The oxygen consumption rate at rest is about 3.5 ml/kg/min. Activities of daily living (ADLs), such as grooming, preparing a meal, and slow walking, require an oxygen consumption rate of 7 to 10 ml/kg/min. The inability to tolerate activities that require an oxygen consumption rate higher than 18 ml/kg/min has been used as a criterion for disability.[5] Activities, such as prolonged standing, walking at 3 miles per hour (mph), and climbing stairs, are examples of activities that could not be sustained by a person with a maximum oxygen consumption rate of 18 ml/kg/min.[7]

Inactivity. Cardiac stroke volume has been shown to decline, by approximately 12%, during the first 30 days of inactivity or bed rest.[2] This decrease is primarily a result of decreased filling of the left ventricle during diastole.[8] When the left ventricle is less full at the end of diastole, it has less blood available to pump out with each stroke and is able to exert less force because the ventricle is not optimally stretched. Associated with this decrease in stroke volume is a decline in blood volume and increase in heart rate at submaximal levels of activity.[1,9] The maximum ventilatory capacity of the lungs also declines, showing a 10% to 15% decline after 4 weeks of inactivity.[2]

Inactivity also affects the mitochondrial enzymes necessary for aerobic metabolism in muscles. Levels of these enzymes decline significantly within 1 month of inactivity, making the mitochondria rely more on anaerobic metabolism for energy production.[10] The quantity of capillaries within the muscles also decline with inactivity.[11] Muscle capillarization affects the amount of oxygen that can diffuse to muscle tissues and the rate of removal of metabolic waste products. The rates of decline in muscle mitochondrial metabolism and in capillarization are affected by the activity level of the individual, as well as genetic influences.[2]

Inactivity causes muscle mass to decline because of atrophy. With atrophy, the amount of actin and myosin in muscle and the overall muscle cross-sectional area decrease.[12] Inactivity generally causes the most atrophy in the muscles responsible for weight bearing and mobility, especially the lower extremity extensor muscles (see Chapter 5 for further information on the effects of inactivity on muscle performance).[11]

Inactivity and bed rest also affect anaerobic metabolism and neuroendocrine responses to exercise. Studies show that 3 days of bed rest result in a decrease in insulin-mediated glucose uptake and diminished levels of cortisol and growth hormone.[13,14] Inactivity can also decrease leukocyte (white blood cell) counts, affecting the body's immune response and ability to fight infection.[15]

Aging. Aging is a gradual process that influences a person's function and endurance levels. Physical effects of aging include loss of bone mineralization, loss of muscle mass, reduction in mitochondrial enzymes, reduced pulmonary function, and vascular insufficiency.[16-18] All of these changes contribute to deconditioning of the aging adult. Each individual ages at a different rate as a result of the interaction of genetic predisposition, behaviors, ongoing and new disease processes, psychosocial factors, physical activity levels, and living environment. For healthy older adults, the rate of decline in physiological functional capacity is largely determined by the volume and intensity of exercise they maintain as they age.[19]

The effects of aging on endurance and functional activities have been extensively studied and reviewed.[16,17,19] Aging of the cardiovascular and musculoskeletal systems have the greatest influence on deconditioning. Aging is associated with reduced cardiac output during periods of exercise and decreased maximal cardiac output.[18] Maximal cardiac output declines at a rate of 1% per year during adulthood.[20] Declining cardiac muscle function reduces both contraction force and conduction through the myocardium, resulting in a decreased stroke volume and heart rate response to exercise.[21] Changes in the responses of the myocardium and peripheral vessels to beta-adrenergic stimulation and decreased arterial wall compliance are also responsible for decreased cardiovascular responses during exercise.[22]

Skeletal muscle atrophies with aging as a result of a decrease in the number of muscle fibers accompanied by an increase in connective and fatty tissues within the muscle.[23] The size of type II muscle fibers decreases with age, resulting in a greater percentage of type I fiber mass, particularly in the lower extremity muscles. These changes can cause muscle strength to decrease by up to 40% by the age of 80.[24] This decrease in strength can limit the amount of activity the aging adult can perform. Decreased lower extremity strength and decreased weight-bearing activities are also associated with loss of bone mineral density and osteoporosis (see Chapter 3).[17]

Obesity. Obesity can also contribute to deconditioning. A sedentary lifestyle and voluntary inactivity have been associated with rising obesity rates in the United States.[25-27] Obesity contributes to deconditioning by accelerating the progression of atherosclerosis, increasing the risk of type II diabetes and its pathological consequences, and reducing tolerance of activities that maintain physical fitness. Obesity has also contributed to a rise in type II diabetes and heart disease in younger populations.[28] Multiple physical and psychosocial factors influence the progression of obesity. Many of these factors also limit the performance of physical activities and thus the individual's ability to reverse obesity and deconditioning.

A patient with deconditioning may have multiple pathological conditions that contribute to their endurance impairment. The therapist should have an understanding of these conditions and the interventions that are already being used to address them when planning their examination and plan of care. The examination of the patient with deconditioning emphasizes the patient's tolerance of endurance activities and the factors that could motivate the patient to increase their activity level.

EXAMINATION

PATIENT HISTORY

When examining a patient with deconditioning the therapist should gather data from the patient and other sources, such as the medical chart and/or family members, about the patient's medical history and current health status. The therapist should use the patient history to help organize the rest of the examination and begin evaluating for the presence of pathologies, impairments, functional limitations, and disabilities and their relationships. The history should include information about the patient's general health (physical, psychological, and social functions), current level of activity, and any related symptoms, such as fatigue, dyspnea, or angina, during activities. In particular, the patient history should include information about the patient's general health that may guide the systems review to look for conditions that would preclude the patient's participation in a rehabilitation program that includes conditioning exercises.

Motivation. To improve their functional abilities, most patients with deconditioning will need to begin and maintain an exercise program. A patient's history of exercise participation and activities and possibly history of participation in recreational or competitive sporting activities will help the therapist select the types of interventions that will most likely result in the patient beginning and maintaining an exercise program. The patient's social history and habits, living environment, employment, and exercise habits and history may all influence exercise participation and continuation.

An exercise program is a voluntary behavior that requires a certain level of physical exertion and period of time to complete and maintain.[6] *Patient motivation* has been shown to be the single most important factor for continuing an exercise program.[29-31] The therapist needs to determine if the patient is ready to change his or her behavior to start and maintain an exercise program. The assessment and facilitation of motivation should be specific to the patient's background, current needs, and developmental status.[32]

There are many theories on how to best affect a patient's motivation to change behavior, and three of these theories, the behavior modification theory, the social cognitive theory, and the stages of change theory, are briefly reviewed here.

The *behavior modification theory* is frequently applied in rehabilitation and health promotion. According to this theory, reward and feedback about the performance of a behavior are the greatest determinants of maintaining that behavior.[33] This theory advocates patient involvement with planning their exercise program and setting goals for behavior, receiving feedback on their success, and revising the plan as needed.

The *social cognitive theory* proposes that a person's self-efficacy is the primary factor influencing behavior change. Self-efficacy is the belief in one's abilities to organize and execute actions required to manage situations.[34] A person's self-efficacy about exercise is mediated and improved through their cognition. Therefore the therapist should first assess the patient's beliefs about exercise and the patient's confidence that he or she can and will maintain an exercise program. Discussing beliefs about exercise can also help patients who have repeatedly lapsed in maintaining exercise programs to develop effective strategies for continuing their program.[6,35]

The *stages of change theory* is part of a transtheoretical model of motivation and behavior change.[36-38] According to this theory, there are five stages to a person's emotional and intellectual preparation for and actualization of change. The therapist can determine which stage a patient is in and thus his or her readiness for change from many of the questions included in the general patient history or by asking a series of specific questions about the patient's activity level and intentions to participate in physical activities (Box 23-1).[6,39]

From Reed GR, Velicer WF, Prochaska JO, et al: *Am J Health Promot* 12(1):57-66, 1997.

BOX 23-1 | Questionnaire to Determine Stage of Change for Exercise

Please read all of the following statements first, and after reading them, place an X by the one statement that represents your present exercise status.

Regular exercise is defined as exercising 3 times per week at 20 minutes per time or more at moderate intensity or higher (at least some light sweating, for example, fast walking, swimming, cycling, running, soccer, and aerobics; not included are activities like bowling, fishing, or horseshoes).

Please mark only ONE of the five statements.

1. ____I currently do not engage in exercise, and I am not thinking about starting.
2. ____I currently do not engage in exercise, but I am thinking about starting.
3. ____I currently do engage in some exercise but not on a regular basis.
4. ____I currently do engage in regular exercise, but I have only begun in the past 6 months.
5. ____I currently do engage in regular exercise, and I have done so for longer than 6 months.

Stages of Change

The patient's chosen statement will approximately match the following stages.

1. Precontemplation is the stage at which there is no intention to starting an exercise program in the foreseeable future. Many individuals in this stage are unaware or under aware of their problems.
2. Contemplation is the stage in which people are aware that problems exist and are seriously thinking about starting exercise but have not yet made a commitment to take action.
3. Preparation is a stage that combines intention and behavioral criteria. Individuals in this stage are intending to start exercise in the next month or have started but not at an adequate level to improve their physical fitness.
4. Action is the stage in which individuals modify their behavior and environment in order to start and maintain an exercise program at a level to improve their physical fitness.
5. Maintenance is the stage in which people work to prevent relapse and have maintained their exercise program for longer than 6 months.

SYSTEMS REVIEW

The systems review is used to target areas requiring further examination and to define areas that may cause complications or indicate a need for precautions during the examination and intervention processes. See Chapter 1 for details of the systems review.

Because many of the tests of endurance require ambulation, the patient's gait should be briefly examined before beginning these tests. The patient's overall stability and safety with walking activities should be evaluated, and any significant gait deviations should be noted (see Chapter 32). The effect of fatigue on gait stability and safety should be monitored during the endurance tests.

TESTS AND MEASURES

Patients with deconditioning may have a range of other problems requiring measurement of musculoskeletal, neuromuscular, cardiorespiratory, and/or integumentary function. However, since deconditioning is primarily a condition of altered cardiorespiratory function, tests and measures should focus on this area. Cardiorespiratory conditioning depends on the interdependent functioning of the cardiovascular, pulmonary, musculoskeletal, and neurological systems.[40] The therapist should choose valid and reliable measures for assessing a patient's conditioning, taking into consideration the patient's history and safety, as well as the available clinical resources and skills. The tests and measures described cover areas of greatest importance for deconditioned patients.

Musculoskeletal. The patient with deconditioning should be generally examined with tests and measures of posture, range of motion (ROM), and muscle performance.

Anthropometric Characteristics. Body composition should be measured in the deconditioned patient because this can affect his or her tolerance of certain types of exercise programs. A patient who is obese has an increased risk for developing overuse injuries during an exercise program.[41] *Body mass index* (BMI) is the most commonly used general indicator of body composition (Fig. 23-1). BMI is equal to a person's weight in kilograms (kg) divided by their height in meters (m) squared (kg/m^2).[42] Although BMI is often substituted for information from specific tests of body composition, one should keep in mind that it does not differentiate musculoskeletal weight from fat.[43] BMI may be used to screen for risk factors associated with obesity.[44] Patients with BMI greater than 30 should be referred for nutrition counseling, and patients with BMI greater than 35 need regular medical follow-up.[45]

More accurate but more cumbersome measures of body composition and body fat percentage are achieved through underwater weighing, skinfold measurements, or through bioelectrical impedance analysis (BIA).[42] Underwater weighing is the gold standard indirect method for assessing body composition and involves comparing the patient's weight in air to their weight when fully submerged in water after a complete exhalation. The time and equipment needed to perform this procedure precludes its use in most clinical settings. Skinfold measurements can also be used to estimate body fat. With an accurate caliper and an experienced tester, this approach produces reliable and valid results in most patients. BIA estimates the percentage of body fat by using a low level current to measure body impedance. This is an easier, less invasive, and less technically-demanding method than skinfold measurements, but measurements in patients with excessive water retention or tissue edema may be inaccurate and yield inaccurate estimations of body composition. Using body fat percentage, obesity is generally regarded as greater than 30% for adult men and greater than 40% for adult women. Minimal or essential body fat percentages are 5% for men and 10% for women.[42]

Neuromuscular

Arousal, Attention, and Cognition (Fatigue). A report of fatigue during the patient history may be an indication of deconditioning, and fatigue that is not the result of

To determine BMI, locate the height of interest in the left-most column and read across the row for that height to the weight of interest. Follow the column of the weight up to the top row that lists the BMI. A BMI of 18.5 to 24.9 is the healthy-weight range, BMI of 25 to 29.9 is the overweight range, and BMI of 30 and above is in the obese range.

BMI	19	20	21	22	23	24	25	26	27	28	29	30	31	32	33	34	35
Height							**Weight in Pounds**										
4'10"	91	96	100	105	110	115	119	124	129	134	138	143	148	153	158	162	167
4'11"	94	99	104	109	114	119	124	128	133	138	143	148	153	158	163	168	173
5'	97	102	107	112	118	123	128	133	138	143	148	153	158	163	158	174	179
5'1"	100	106	111	116	122	127	132	137	143	148	153	158	164	169	174	180	185
5'2"	104	109	115	120	126	131	136	142	147	153	158	164	169	175	180	186	191
5'3"	107	113	118	124	130	135	141	146	152	158	163	169	175	180	186	191	197
5'4"	110	116	122	128	134	140	145	151	157	163	169	174	180	186	192	197	204
5'5"	114	120	126	132	138	144	150	156	162	168	174	180	186	192	198	204	210
5'6"	118	124	130	136	142	148	155	161	167	173	179	186	192	198	204	210	216
5'7"	121	127	134	140	146	153	159	166	172	178	185	191	198	204	211	217	223
5'8"	125	131	138	144	151	158	164	171	177	184	190	197	203	210	216	223	230
5'9"	128	135	142	149	155	162	169	176	182	189	196	203	209	216	223	230	236
5'10"	132	139	146	153	160	167	174	181	188	195	202	209	216	222	229	236	243
5'11"	136	143	150	157	165	172	179	186	193	200	208	215	222	229	236	243	250
6'	140	147	154	162	169	177	184	191	199	206	213	221	228	235	242	250	258
6'1"	144	151	159	166	174	182	189	197	204	212	219	227	235	242	250	257	265
6'2"	148	155	163	171	179	186	194	202	210	218	225	233	241	249	256	264	272
6'3"	152	160	168	176	184	192	200	208	216	224	232	240	248	256	264	272	279
	Healthy Weight						**Overweight**					**Obese**					

From U.S. Department of Health and Human Services, U.S. Department of Agriculture: *Dietary guidelines for Americans 2005*, ed 6, Washington, DC, 2005, Authors. Accessible at *www.healthierus.gov/dietaryguidelines*.

Source: National Institutes of Health, National Heart, Lung, and Blood Institute: *Evidence report of clinical guidelines on the identification, evaluation, and treatment of overweight and obesity in adults*, Bethesda, Md, 1998, Author.

FIG. 23-1 Body mass index is body weight in kilograms divided by height in meters squared (kg/m^2).

deconditioning may also severely limit activity participation by a deconditioned patient. Fatigue can be measured with tools such as the Visual Analog Scale for Fatigue or the Fatigue Severity Scale (Fig. 23-2).[46,47] Patients with more severe limitations may benefit from assessment of multiple dimensions of function using the Multidimensional Assessment of Fatigue[47,48] or the Chronic Fatigue Syndrome–Activities and Participation Questionnaire, which have been validated for use with patients undergoing rehabilitation.[49]

Pain. A patient with deconditioning may have episodic or chronic pain that should be assessed and monitored. Measurement of pain intensity by a pain scale, words, or pictures can be performed during an exercise program (see Chapter 22).

Cardiovascular/Pulmonary. Examination of a patient with deconditioning should focus on assessment of cardiopulmonary function. Measurements of the vital signs of heart rate, blood pressure (BP), and respiratory rate (see Chapter 22) provide basic information about the patient's cardiopulmonary function and readiness for active exercise and serve as a baseline for responses to exercise.[50] Findings of an abnormal heart rate or BP will affect the intensity of exercise chosen for the patient and may require a referral of the patient to another health care provider.

During the past week, I have found that:

	Strongly Disagree 1	Moderately Disagree 2	Mildly Disagree 3	Neither Agree or Disagree 4	Mildly Agree 5	Moderately Agree 6	Strongly Agree 7
My motivation is lower when I am fatigued.							
Exercise brings on my fatigue.							
I am easily fatigued.							
Fatigue interferes with my physical functioning.							
Fatigue causes frequent problems for me.							
My fatigue prevents sustained physical functioning.							
Fatigue interferes with carrying out certain duties and responsibilities.							
Fatigue is among my three most disabling symptoms.							
Fatigue interferes with my work, family or social life.							
Total							

FIG. 23-2 Fatigue Severity Scale. *From Krupp LB, LaRocca NG, Muir-Nash J, et al:* Arch Neurol *46(10):1121-1123, 1989.*

A fatigue score is calculated by adding the score for each answer and dividing it by nine.

For a patient with a history of cardiac and pulmonary disease, auscultation of heart and breath sounds and observation of heart rhythm on an electrocardiogram can help determine the current status of their pathology and be used to monitor for changes in myocardial function during exercise.[6,51]

Ventilation and Respiration/Gas Exchange. Patients who report discomfort with breathing during activities should rate their dyspnea before and during exercise and may also need pulmonary function testing.[52,53] Fig. 23-3 is a dyspnea scale that can be used to subjectively rate discomfort with breathing.

Aerobic Capacity and Endurance. As noted previously, the measure that most accurately reflects an individual's cardiorespiratory functional fitness is their maximal oxygen uptake $\dot{V}O_{2max}$.[6,54] A patient with a $\dot{V}O_{2max}$ of less than 60% of the average $\dot{V}O_{2max}$ for individuals of the same age and gender is considered to have impaired aerobic capacity or endurance.[55]

0 = No dyspnea
1 = Mild, not noticeable to an observer
2 = Mild, noticeable to an observer
3 = Moderate difficulty, patient can continue with activities
4 = Severe difficulty, patient cannot continue with activities

FIG. 23-3 Dyspnea scale. *From Williams MA (ed):* Guidelines for Cardiac Rehabilitation and Secondary Prevention Programs, *ed 4, Champaign, Ill, 2004, Human Kinetics.*

Although maximal aerobic testing is the gold standard for assessing maximum aerobic capacity, this type of testing requires the patient to reach a state of maximal oxygen uptake that may put the patient at risk, cause excessive fatigue, or not be achievable because of fatigue

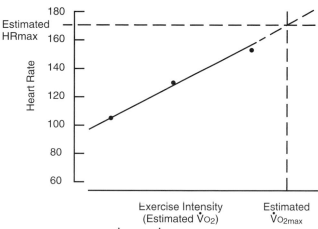

FIG. 23-4 Estimated $\dot{V}O_{2max}$. $\dot{V}O_{2max}$ estimated from a 50-year-old patient's submaximal modified Bruce protocol test. Maximum heart rate is 170 (220-50). A straight line of best fit from measures of heart rate and $\dot{V}O_2$ taken during three stages of the protocol is extrapolated to the estimated maximum heart rate. This patient's estimated $\dot{V}O_{2max}$ is 42 ml/kg/min. *From Guiccione A: Geriatric Physical Therapy, ed 2, St. Louis, 2005, Mosby.*

TABLE 23-1	Modified Bruce Protocol*		
Stage	Speed/Grade (mph/Percent)	Oxygen Cost (ml/kg/min)	METs
1	1.7/0	7.0	2
2	1.7/5	12.3	3.5
3	1.7/10	17.5	5
4	2.5/12	24.5	7
5	3.4/14	33.3	9.5
6	4.2/16	45.5	13
7	5.0/18	42.0	16

*After a short warm-up, the treadmill is set at 1.7 mph at 0% grade and the grade is increased every 3 minutes.
Data from Franklin DA (ed). *ACSM's Guidelines for Exercise Testing and Prescription*, ed 6, Baltimore, 2000, Lippincott Williams & Wilkins.
METs, Metabolic equivalents.

or limitations from other impairments. Clinicians assessing the aerobic capacity of patients with deconditioning therefore generally use submaximal aerobic testing to estimate the patient's $\dot{V}O_{2max}$.[6,40,56] Tests for estimating $\dot{V}O_{2max}$ primarily use changes in the patient's heart rate with increasing workloads to determine the cardiorespiratory response to aerobic demand. Because heart rate has a linear relationship with oxygen uptake, heart rate can be used to estimate a person's oxygen uptake during the test and to estimate $\dot{V}O_{2max}$. When submaximal testing is used, the $\dot{V}O_{2max}$ is estimated by extrapolating from the heart rate at different levels of work achieved during the test to the patient's predicted maximum heart rate as shown in Fig. 23-4.[6,57]

Stationary bicycling and treadmill walking are the most common activities used to provide a workload when estimating $\dot{V}O_{2max}$.[54,56] The benefits of using a stationary bicycle include patient safety, the portability and relatively low price of stationary bicycles, and the ability to accurately measure vital signs during the test. However, patients who are not familiar with bicycling may have difficulty maintaining a consistent workload during the test because they cannot maintain a consistent cadence.[56] Exercise tests using stationary bicycles have been found to have prediction errors of less than 10% for estimating $\dot{V}O_{2max}$.[57] Treadmill walking may be appropriate for a patient familiar with using a treadmill for exercise. Because of the variability of a patient's familiarity with walking on a treadmill, tests using a treadmill have a greater prediction error of up to 17% for estimating $\dot{V}O_{2max}$.[58] Walking tests for distances or time may also be used when a stationary bicycle and treadmill are not available or appropriate. These tests usually assess heart rate at the end of a period of walking and have a prediction error of less than 10%.[59,60]

The *modified Bruce protocol* is a protocol of exercise progression commonly used in clinical settings for estimating $\dot{V}O_{2max}$ in patients with low functional capacity[40,54] (Table 23-1). This protocol correlates highly with direct measurements of $\dot{V}O_{2max}$.[61] The modified Bruce protocol uses a treadmill that starts at a slow walking speed (1.7 mph) with a 0 degree grade of ramping, compared to the standard Bruce protocol that starts at 1.7 mph with a 10% grade. The workload at the beginning of the modified Bruce protocol requires approximately a $\dot{V}O_{2max}$ of 7.0 ml/kg/min, which is twice the aerobic power used at rest. The grade of the ramp and/or the speed of the treadmill are then gradually increased in a standardized manner at 3-minute intervals.[62]

The Astrand/Rhyming and YMCA protocols are alternative reliable methods for estimating $\dot{V}O_{2max}$ using a bicycle ergometer rather than a treadmill. These protocols allow accurate estimation of aerobic power while the patient is seated and pedaling with their lower extremities.[6,54,56] The Astrand/Rhyming protocol is preferred for patients with low functional capacity because it is a single-stage test that uses one workload. This test is performed having the patient pedal at a rate of 50 revolutions per minute at a set workload (50 or 100 Watts for men, 50 or 75 Watts for women) for 6 minutes. The average heart rate measured at the fifth and sixth minute is used to estimate $\dot{V}O_{2max}$ using a nomogram. The estimated $\dot{V}O_{2max}$ is then adjusted by an age-correction factor.[6]

Patients with higher levels of fitness can use the YMCA protocol, which is a multistage test where the work load is increased every 3 minutes. The first stage of the test involves cycling for 3 minutes at a low workload, and based on the patient's heart rate at the end of 3 minutes, the workload is increased to higher levels. Depending on the patient's response during this second stage the workload can be increased for a third and fourth stage. The patient's heart rate at each workload during the test is then extrapolated to their age-predicted maximum heart rate to estimate $\dot{V}O_{2max}$ (see Fig. 23-4).[6,58]

The patient's heart rate, BP, and lung sounds are monitored before, during, and after the exercise test. Heart rate is measured by palpation of the pulse or with a cardiac monitor. The test is usually terminated when the patient reports exhaustion or when the heart rate reaches 85% of the person's age-predicted maximum. Criteria for stopping the test before these events include the onset of angina symptoms, a drop of 20 mm Hg or more in systolic BP, systolic BP rising to greater than 260 mm Hg, diastolic BP rising to greater than 115 mm Hg, or development of any other signs of poor perfusion such as confusion, cyanosis, or nausea (Box 23-2).[6,33]

A self-paced walking test for a set distance can also be used as a baseline measurement of conditioning for patients who cannot maintain a consistent walking speed on a treadmill or pedaling speed on a stationary bicycle. The distance walked in a 2- or 6-minute test can be used for indoor settings with a measured walking course.[63] These tests have been found to be reliable in patients with pulmonary diseases and in other patient populations.[64] The self-paced walking tests do not require the patient to maintain a steady workload during the test and should not be used to estimate $\dot{V}O_{2max}$.[58]

Function

Self-Care and Home Management. Patients with deconditioning are often limited in their self-care and home management abilities. The patient's ability to perform ADLs and work can be assessed by interview or by use of a number of functional abilities tools (Table 23-2). These tools can be used to determine functional limitations at baseline, when the patient is first seen, and to set goals for improving functional status.

The Barthel Index is a performance-based tool based on assessing performance of ten ADLs (Fig. 23-5). It is suitable for patients with low functional abilities. It is widely used in rehabilitation settings because of its high intratester reliability and content validity.[65-67]

The Lower Extremity Functional Scale (LEFS) is suitable for patients with higher functional abilities (Fig. 23-6). It is based on a self-report of the individual's functional status using a five-point scale to measure their ability to perform twenty activities ranging from self-care and transfers to standing, walking, and running. The LEFS has good reliability and construct validity when compared to other instruments that measure functional status.[68]

The Functional Independence Measure (FIM) was developed for patients in rehabilitation settings, using a seven point scale to measure a patient's independence with activities such as dressing, bathing, and transfers. The FIM scales have high content validity and reliability.[69] The FIM scale for independence with locomotion can be used to set rehabilitation goals and assess outcome. The FIM locomotion scale has been found to correlate positively with scores on the LEFS.[70]

EVALUATION, DIAGNOSIS, AND PROGNOSIS

Evaluation is a dynamic process in which the therapist makes clinical judgments about the data collected in the examination.[3] During the examination of a patient with deconditioning, the therapist will interpret findings for their relevance to the patient's problems and to help plan interventions. Employing the disablement model helps the clinician prioritize the patient's functional limitations and determine their relationship to the patient's chief impairment, endurance impairment, and other impairments. The relationship between the endurance impairment and functional limitations will determine the most appropriate interventions for improving endurance and functional abilities. Most patients with deconditioning fall into the preferred practice pattern 6B: Impaired aerobic capacity/endurance associated with deconditioning.[3]

The plan of treatment for a patient with deconditioning should be individualized according to the goals and abilities of the patient. Patients in this preferred practice pattern generally achieve optimal aerobic capacity and endurance and the highest level of functioning in home, work, community, and leisure environments over the course of 6-12 weeks of therapy with a range of 6-30 visits per episode of care.[3] The prognosis within this range for each individual depends primarily on the patient's level of fitness and functional abilities on presentation, their baseline level of fitness, co-morbidities, and their willingness to participate in a program that will improve their fitness level. Exercise activities may be just one component of an overall plan to improve the patient's endurance and fitness. The prognosis for returning to previous levels

---

BOX 23-2	**Criteria for Stopping an Exercise Test**

Preferred criteria:
1. Patient requests stopping because of fatigue.
2. Heart rate reaches 85% of age-predicted maximum.

Criteria to stop for safety reasons:
1. Onset of angina.
2. Systolic BP drops 20 mm Hg or more.
3. Systolic BP >260 mm Hg.
4. Diastolic BP >115 mm Hg.
5. Signs of poor perfusion such as confusion, cyanosis, or nausea.

From Franklin BA (ed): *ACSM's Guidelines for Exercise Testing and Prescription,* ed 6, Baltimore, 2000, Lippincott, Williams & Wilkins. *BP,* Blood pressure.

TABLE 23-2	Recommended Functional Assessment Tools for Deconditioned Patients		
Tool	**Scale Content**	**Recommended Population**	**Advantages**
Barthel Index	10 ADLs	Acute and rehabilitation settings	Sensitive to small changes in function
Lower Extremity Functional Scale	20 Functional activities	Musculoskeletal conditions	Measures moderate to higher levels of function
Functional Independence Measure	ADLs and functional activities, including locomotion	Rehabilitation settings	Appropriate for multidisciplinary use

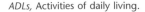

ADLs, Activities of daily living.

BARTHEL INDEX

Activity	Score
Feeding 0 = unable 5 = needs help cutting, spreading butter, etc., or requires modified diet 10 = independent	0 5 10
Bathing 0 = dependent 5 = independent (or in shower)	0 5
Grooming 0 = needs help with personal care 5 = independent face/hair/teeth/shaving (implements provided)	0 5
Dressing 0 = dependent 5 = needs help but can do about half unaided 10 = independent (including buttons, zippers, laces, etc.)	0 5 10
Bowels 0 = incontinent (or needs to be given enemas) 5 = occasional accident 10 = continent	0 5 10
Bladder 0 = incontinent or catheterized and unable to manage alone 5 = occasional accident 10 = continent	0 5 10
Toilet Use 0 = dependent 5 = needs some help, but can do some things alone 10 = independent (on and off, dressing, wiping)	0 5 10
Transfers (bed to chair and back) 0 = unable, no sitting balance 5 = major help (one or two people, physical), can sit 10 = minor help (verbal or physical) 15 = independent	0 5 10 15
Mobility (on level surfaces) 0 = immobile or < 50 yards 5 = wheelchair independent, including corners, >50 yards 10 = walks with help of one person (verbal or physical) >50 yards 15 = independent (but may use any aid; for example, stick) >50 yards	0 5 10 15
Stairs 0 = unable 5 = needs help (verbal, physical, carrying aid) 10 = independent	0 5 10
Total (0-100)	

The Barthel ADL Index: Guidelines

1. The index should be used as a record of what a patient does, not as a record of what a patient could do.

2. The main aim is to establish a degree of independence from any help, physical or verbal, however minor and for whatever reason.

3. The need for supervision renders the patient not independent.

4. A patient's performance should be established using the best available evidence. Asking the patient, friends/relatives, and nurses are the usual sources, but direct observation and common sense are also important. However direct testing is not needed.

5. Usually the patient's performance over the preceding 24-48 hours is important, but occasionally longer periods will be relevant.

6. Middle categories imply that the patient supplies over 50 percent of the effort.

7. Use of assistive devices to be independent is allowed.

FIG. 23-5 Barthel Index. *From Maboney FI, Barthel D: Functional evaluation: the Barthel Index,* Maryland State Med J 14:61-65, 1965.

We are interested in knowing whether you are having any difficulty at all with the activities listed below because of your lower limb problem for which you are currently seeking attention. Please provide an answer for each activity.

Today, do you or would you have any difficulty at all with (circle one number on each line).

FIG. 23-6 Lower Extremity Functional Scale.

Activities	Extreme Difficulty or Unable to Perform Activity	Quite a Bit of Difficulty	Moderate Difficulty	A Little Bit of Difficulty	No Difficulty
a) Any of your usual work, housework, or school activities	0	1	2	3	4
b) Your usual hobbies, recreational, or sporting activities	0	1	2	3	4
c) Getting into or out of the bath	0	1	2	3	4
d) Walking between rooms	0	1	2	3	4
e) Putting on your shoes or socks	0	1	2	3	4
f) Squatting	0	1	2	3	4
g) Lifting an object, like a bag of groceries from the floor	0	1	2	3	4
h) Performing light activities around your home	0	1	2	3	4
i) Performing heavy activities around your home	0	1	2	3	4
j) Getting into or out of a car	0	1	2	3	4
k) Walking 2 blocks	0	1	2	3	4
l) Walking a mile	0	1	2	3	4
m) Going up or down 10 stairs (about 1 flight of stairs)	0	1	2	3	4
n) Standing for 1 hour	0	1	2	3	4
o) Sitting for 1 hour	0	1	2	3	4
p) Running on even ground	0	1	2	3	4
q) Running on uneven ground	0	1	2	3	4
r) Making sharp turns while running fast	0	1	2	3	4
s) Hopping	0	1	2	3	4
t) Rolling over in bed	0	1	2	3	4
Column Totals:					

Score: _____ /80

of fitness and improving quality of life should be discussed and clarified with the patient before initiating interventions.

INTERVENTION

Interventions for a patient with deconditioning should focus on improving functional abilities, especially those related to ADLs and activities of independent living. Aerobic exercise and weight training programs have been shown to most effectively improve aerobic capacity,[33,71,72] and thus directly enhance the deconditioned patient's ability to use aerobic metabolism at rest and during activity. In addition to aerobic exercise, interventions for deconditioning should include communication, education, and coordination with the individual's other medical treatments.

COMMUNICATION

For a patient with severe deconditioning in an acute or long-term care setting, communication of which and how much activity a patient can perform safely can guide other health care providers and patient's family members to avoid encouraging the patient to over or under exert. Activities should not be unnecessarily limited nor should too much assistance be given. Activities should also be paced to allow optimal function through the course of the day. It is also important to communicate the nature of a patient's signs of fatigue to avoid over exertion. Coordination of the patient's medical treatment and rehabilitation sessions should limit their overall fatigue and improve their performance during therapeutic and functional activities.[33]

In an outpatient setting, communication with the patient, the patient's family, and caregivers should convey expectations of the patient's activities during rehabilitation sessions and during their daily activities. The patient and family should see their daily activities as part of the rehabilitation program. The family will need to learn to assist at an appropriate level so that the patient can increase their independence. This should be explicitly discussed with the patient and family so that the treatment plan is constructed with their input and progression of functional abilities is accurately assessed.

EDUCATION

The patient and family should receive education about the benefits of increased physical activity. Understanding the physiological and psychological benefits of exercise will help reinforce the patient's goals for treatment and assist the patient in adhering to the exercise program. The patient should also be educated to differentiate signs of normal physiological responses to exercise, such as increased respiratory and heart rate, from signs of fatigue that require rest.

The patient should understand that periods of rest during the day are important for pacing their activities and limiting fatigue. The patient should also use rest periods to prepare for potentially fatiguing activities, such as family functions or visits to medical professionals.[33] The patient and family should also be educated regarding safety issues. The patient and family should have a list of phone numbers to call, including their Emergency Medical System (911), in case problems or an emergency situation arise.

MOTIVATION

Because a patient's motivation has been shown to be the most important determinant of maintaining an exercise program,[29-31] the therapist should employ interventions to improve the patient's motivation and confidence to optimize the likelihood that they will maintain an exercise program. The therapist should discuss with the patient his or her beliefs about exercise and address issues about how the patient will maintain his or her exercise program. The discussion should include the patient's history of exercise and physical activities to help the therapist understand the types of activities and programs that have been successful and to avoid activities that the patient does not believe will be effective.[6,35]

Using the five stages from the stages of change theory (see Box 23-1) allows the therapist to employ behavioral and cognitive interventions that are appropriate for the patient's emotional and intellectual preparedness for starting and maintaining an exercise program (Table 23-3). An example is a patient in the Preparation stage who has begun some independent exercise but not at the recommended frequency each week. Appropriate strategies for this stage include helping the patient identify barriers to increasing the frequency of exercise, changing activities or behaviors that take up the time that could be used for exercise, and identifying family or friends who will support increasing exercise frequency. The patient could also document barriers overcome for each exercise session and the factors that contributed to not

TABLE 23-3	Interventions Appropriate for Different Stages of Change
Stage of Change	**Appropriate Intervention**
Precontemplation	Provide information about beginning an exercise program. Do not attempt to force a person into the contemplation stage.
Contemplation	Ask questions regarding what they can do to begin preparations for an exercise program. Have person consider their psychological and environmental barriers to beginning an exercise program.
Preparation	Problem solve with the patient as to what they need to do to start and become consistent with an exercise program.
Action	Help patient to anticipate problems and changes in environment or social support and to make alternative plans for maintaining their exercise program.
Maintenance	Congratulate patient on maintaining their exercise program, offer assistance if problems do arise.

exercising on designated days to better understand the factors that contribute to adherence to an exercise plan.[37,73]

AEROBIC EXERCISE

The foundation of therapeutic exercise programs for patients with deconditioning is aerobic activity.[74-76] The physiological effects of aerobic exercise on the cardiopulmonary system in healthy populations are well established.[75-77] The therapist should design the therapeutic exercise program to also directly or indirectly affect the functional limitations and disabilities of patients with deconditioning.

Recent studies with different patient populations have measured the effects of aerobic exercise on functional limitations. A study of 34 patients with osteoarthritis of the knee found that a 12-week walking program improved performance in tests of walking function.[78] A study of patients after total hip replacement found that those patients who completed a program of lower extremity exercise and walked for 30 minutes at least 3 times per week for 12 weeks demonstrated improvements in walking speed and performance.[79] Two studies that included 45 patients with stroke found that a home or community-based 8-week program of aerobic exercise improved lower extremity functions related to walking and mobility.[80,81] Studies of patients on hemodialysis who participate in endurance training programs have also been shown to have improved physical performance and less skeletal muscle wasting.[82,83]

Aerobic activities should be prescribed with a specified level of intensity, duration, and frequency. The therapist should base this prescription on the information gathered during the examination and modify the exercise program based on the response of the patient. The patient may initially be limited in the mode or type of aerobic activities he or she can perform, but as the patient progresses, the mode of exercise should be based on the patient's goals and individual preference.

Acute Care Inpatient Setting. For a patient in the acute care inpatient setting, the primary goal of an exercise program is to improve the patient's functional abilities to prepare for discharge home or to another health care facility. The exercise program will have other benefits, but because of the short duration of most inpatient hospital stays, the primary goal is to decrease fatigue with functional activities. The inpatient exercise program can also be the first stage of a more comprehensive, long-term exercise program that changes physiological function, improves endurance, and prepares the patient to return to his or her societal roles.[72]

For the patient with severe deconditioning, periods of sitting upright in bed or in a chair may be the first step of the conditioning exercise program. The patient may then be progressed to periods of standing and walking for short distances (less than 50 feet). Walking distance may be limited by fatigue or by monitoring or treatment equipment in a hospital room. Upper extremity active ROM exercises in a sitting or standing position can also be used to increase cardiovascular demand and thus improve function and endurance.[33,72]

The ambulatory patient may initially use walking as the primary mode of exercise, with walking distance and speed used to progress exercise intensity and monitor exercise tolerance. Patients who report fatigue with walking may be able to walk further if they take short rest periods, either in standing or sitting, between walking bouts. A walking exercise program can be progressed by increasing the total walking time, speed, or distance and/or by reducing the frequency and duration of rest periods. The patient's heart rate, respiratory rate, dyspnea rating, and *rating of perceived exertion* (RPE) (see Box 23-3 and the section on Exercise Intensity) should be monitored during the exercise session to determine the intensity of walking activities.[72] The patient's BP, heart rhythm, and oxygen saturation levels (see Chapter 22) should be monitored before, during, and after these periods of walking to assess the patient's cardiorespiratory tolerance of the exercise session.

General guidelines for stopping an exercise session

Heart rate: A drop below the resting rate or an increase of more than 20-30 beats per minute (bpm) above the resting rate.
Systolic blood pressure: A drop of more than 10 mm Hg below the resting rate.
Oxygen saturation level: Below 90%.[84]
Symptoms: Angina, significantly increased dyspnea.[6,33]

Depending on their length of stay, prior level of conditioning, and level of deconditioning at the initiation of exercise, a patient in an inpatient setting may progress to tolerate longer periods of exercise and other modes and forms of exercise. A stationary bicycle or arm ergometer can be transported to the patient's room or floor for more prolonged endurance exercises. The patient's pedaling speed or work level can then be used to progress and monitor the intensity of this exercise. Patients may also be able to use the long corridor and stairs of a hospital or rehabilitation center to increase their walking endurance. Upper extremity ROM exercises using light resistance with sets of 12-15 repetitions are also recommended.[5,33]

Outpatient Setting. A patient in the outpatient setting will generally have time for and tolerate a more comprehensive and long-term exercise program than the patient in the inpatient setting. The therapist and patient should set goals for the exercise program based on the patient's functional, vocational, and recreational activities. The exercise program can be designed to improve performance of these activities, maintain and improve overall fitness, and often reduce the risk of recurrence of their disease processes.[33,76] Exercise appropriate at this stage should also improve physiological parameters.

The exercise prescription should be based on objective measures of physiological function, on what is attainable for the patient based on their general health and medical history, and on evidence of the effectiveness of exercise. To reduce deconditioning, an exercise prescription should primarily involve activities to improve aerobic function, but some patients will also need activities to improve their strength and flexibility.

In the outpatient setting, whether in a clinic or health club, the patient will likely have a range of exercise modes and equipment available for their aerobic exercise program. The therapist should select equipment that is safe for the patient and that the patient feels comfortable using. The treadmill is the most common mode for endurance exercise because it has controls to easily change the speed and slope of incline. The patient should use a speed and incline that allows safe walking with good balance and efficient lower and upper extremity movement. Other equipment that allows movements similar to walking are the elliptical trainer and cross-country gliders, although these may require more balance and coordination, so the patient should be closely monitored as they learn to use this equipment.

The prescription of an exercise program for a patient with deconditioning needs to be individualized, based on the patient's current medical condition and fitness level and available equipment or exercise settings. Although the exercise prescription for the patient should be based on scientific evidence, the design and progression of the program should be continually evaluated and modified according to the patient's response. The exercise prescription is usually defined by the parameters of exercise intensity, duration, and frequency.

The exercise session should include warm-up and cool-down periods, during which the activity level is slowly increased to and then later decreased from the prescribed levels. The warm-up period is intended to reduce the risk of cardiac arrhythmias and ischemia and improve muscle performance.[71,85,86] The warm-up period may include static stretching of large muscle groups and should also involve moving these muscle groups to prepare them and the cardiovascular system for the exercise session. The patient should be closely monitored during the cool-down period because adverse cardiac events are thought to occur most often during this period.[6] The cool-down period should be long enough to allow the heart rate and BP to return toward resting levels.

Exercise Intensity. The intensity of exercise after the warm-up period should be determined primarily by the physiological response of the patient. The American College of Sports Medicine (ACSM) recommends beginning the exercise program for unfit individuals at 55% to 65% of the estimated maximum heart rate or at 40% to 50% of the *heart rate reserve* (HRR).[73,76] Measures of exercise intensity based on the patient's heart rate rather than oxygen consumption are generally used because heart rate can easily be monitored during an exercise session.

When using a percentage of the maximum heart rate to prescribe exercise intensity, maximum heart rate is generally estimated to be 220 minus the patient's age.[76] Thus a patient's initial exercise goal would be between 0.55 × (220 – patient's age) and 0.65 × (220 – patient's age). This method may be inaccurate in deconditioned patients because their maximum heart rate may actually be lower than the estimated 220 – age.[71]

The HRR method (also known as the *Karvonen method*) is therefore the preferred method for exercise prescription for deconditioned patients.[76] HRR is equal to the maximum heart rate minus the resting heart rate. To calculate the target heart rate using the Karvonen method, use the following formula:

([maximum heart rate – resting heart rate] × goal percentage of HRR) + resting heart rate

For this method, maximum heart rate is ideally the symptom-limited maximum heart rate as determined by a graded exercise test, although when this is not available, 220 minus the patient's age may be used as an estimate. For example, for a 50-year-old patient with a resting heart rate of 80 bpm whose target heart rate is 50% of HRR, the target heart rate would be: ([220 – 50 – 80] × 0.50) + 80 = 125 bpm.[76] This compares with a target heart rate of 94 to 111 based on 55% to 65% of the age-predicted maximum heart rate alone.

Using either method for estimating target heart rate, the clinician should keep in mind that this is only an estimate of the appropriate work level for the patient. During each exercise session the intensity of the exercise should be slowly progressed toward this level while monitoring the patient's tolerance of the activity by his or her respiratory effort and rate and fatigue level. A patient who cannot tolerate exercise at the calculated level should have the target level decreased or the mode of the exercise changed to better match their current fitness level.[33,71] As the patient progresses with their exercise program the intensity level can be gradually increased toward the maximal recommended levels of 90% of maximum heart rate or 85% of HRR.[71]

Another common method for monitoring exercise intensity during exercise uses the patient's own perception of their level of exertion. The RPE scale, as proposed by Borg, rates a patient's exertion using words such as "light" or "hard" with corresponding numbers 6-20 to describe the patient's workload (Box 23-3).[86,87] The RPE scale correlates well with other physiological measures of exertion and can be used reliably by patients, with instruction.[88] The RPE scale can be used along with heart rate to monitor exercise intensity. A RPE level of 10-12 would be appropriate for deconditioned patients beginning an exercise program.[71] A patient's perceived exertion will change with different modes of exercise, and the prescribed level of exertion would need to be adjusted for each mode of exercise.[33,71] When patients are ready to perform an independent exercise program, they may use the RPE scale to maintain a specified level of intensity.[71]

A *metabolic equivalent* (MET) is a another commonly used and convenient measure of activity intensity that can be used for exercise monitoring and prescription. One MET is equivalent to the energy used at rest, which is equivalent to approximately 3.5 ml of oxygen/kg/min.[6] The ACSM's Guidelines for Exercise Testing and Prescription includes tables of MET ranges for ADLs and recreational activities (Table 23-4).[6] These tables can help the therapist direct the deconditioned patient to an appropriate level of activity.

BOX 23-3 Borg RPE Scale

Instructions to the Borg-RPE-Scale®

6	No exertion at all
7	
8	Extremely light
9	Very light
10	
11	Light
12	
13	Somewhat hard
14	
15	Hard (heavy)
16	
17	Very hard
18	
19	Extremely hard
20	Maximal exertion

Borg-RPE-Scale®
© Gunnar Borg 1970, 1985, 1998

During the work we want you to rate your perception of exertion, i.e. how heavy and strenuous the exercise feels to you and how tired you are. The perception of exertion is mainly felt as strain and fatigue in your muscles and as breathlessness or aches in the chest.

Use this scale from 6 to 20, where **6** means "No exertion at all" and **20** means "Maximal exertion."

9 Very light. As for a healthy person taking a short walk at his or her own pace.

13 Somewhat hard. It still feels OK to continue.

15 It is hard and tiring, but continuing is not terribly difficult.

17 Very hard. It is very strenuous. You can still go on, but you really have to push yourself and you are very tired.

19 An extremely strenuous level. For most people this is the most strenuous exercise they have ever experienced.

Try to appraise your feeling of exertion and fatigue as spontaneously and as honestly as possible, without thinking about what the actual physical load is. Try not to underestimate, nor to overestimate. It is your own feeling of effort and exertion that is important, not how it compares to other people's. Look at the scale and the expressions and then give a number. You can equally well use even as odd numbers.

Any questions?

"Borg's RPE Scale," Borg G, 1994.

Exercise Duration and Frequency. The total volume of training depends on the exercise intensity and duration.[76,89] To maximize the benefits of an exercise program the exercise intensity should be progressed toward a target level, as previously described, and the duration of activities should be adjusted to the patient's tolerance. The optimal intensity and duration of exercise to improve and maintain aerobic fitness is controversial. Initially, a patient may tolerate only 5-minute or shorter bouts of exercise with rest periods in between. The patient can then be progressed by increasing the duration of the bouts and decreasing the duration of rest periods by a few

TABLE 23-4 Metabolic Equivalent (MET) Ranges for Various Activities

Activity	METs
Bowling	2-4
Billiards	2.5
Shuffleboard	2-3
Music playing	2-3
Fishing: Standing from a bank	2-4
Canoeing: Two person	3-5
Golf: Power cart	2-3
Golf: Walking with pull cart	5
Dancing	3-8
Table tennis	3-5
Bicycling at 10 mph	7

From Franklin BA (ed): *ACSM's Guidelines for Exercise Testing and Prescription,* ed 6, Baltimore, 2000, Lippincott Williams & Wilkins.

minutes each session.[71,74] A deconditioned patient should ideally maintain a low-to-moderate intensity of exercise for 20-60 minutes to gain physiological benefits of aerobic training.[76] As the duration of the exercise is increased, the intensity may need to be temporarily decreased, based on the patient's tolerance for the longer duration. These parameters may also affect adherence to the exercise program.[76,90]

The ACSM recommends two to five exercise sessions per week for improving aerobic capacity in deconditioned patients.[76] However, patients with severe deconditioning may initially do better with brief, daily sessions of exercise and functional activities.[56,72] As patients increase their tolerance for longer durations and intensity of exercise and activities, the frequency of exercise sessions can be adjusted to maximize performance and allow for longer durations of recovery, as demonstrated in the case study at the end of this chapter.[71,76]

WEIGHT TRAINING

Patients with deconditioning may also benefit from an exercise program that includes resistive weight training. A resistive weight training program will improve muscle strength impairments and may improve associated functional limitations.[31] Some patients prefer resistive weight training to aerobic exercise because of their perceived need to improve strength-related activities.[91]

There are a number of published studies examining the effects of combining resistive exercises with aerobic exercises in patients with coronary artery disease (CAD). A study of 18 men with CAD found that the combined exercise method increased both lower extremity strength and aerobic performance more than aerobic exercise alone.[92] However, another study of 36 patients with CAD found that combined resistive and aerobic training had more effect on strength but a similar effect on aerobic capacity as an aerobic training program alone.[93] A study of 40 men with CAD compared the effects of a combined aerobic and resistive exercise training program to a combined aerobic exercise and volleyball program. The group participating in aerobic and resistive exercise had greater gains in strength and endurance and greater confidence to participate in common physical tasks than the other group.[94] Improvements in overall strength in deconditioned patients may also improve emotional well-being and adherence to an exercise program.[91]

CIRCUIT WEIGHT TRAINING

Patients with deconditioning may also benefit from weight training using a *circuit weight training* (CWT) program.[71,72,76] CWT is defined as the performance of 10-15 repetitions using 40% to 60% of one repetition maximum (1RM) in a continuous fashion and moving from one exercise station or machine to another with short rest periods between stations. The circuit should contain 5-15 different exercise stations, each used 2-3 times per session, and sessions should be done 3-5 times per week.[95] The continuous activity of performing moderate resistance exercise and moving quickly from station to station is proposed to engage aerobic metabolism.[96] However, although CWT in healthy, untrained males has shown to increase strength by 20% to 40% after 8-20 weeks of training,[95-97] it has been found to improve aerobic capacity only by 5% to 10%.[95,98]

CASE STUDY 23-1

CHRONIC OBSTRUCTIVE PULMONARY DISEASE WITH EMPHYSEMA

Examination
Patient History

TD is a 76-year-old man with a history of chronic obstructive pulmonary disease (COPD) with emphysema. He uses oxygen therapy primarily at night and a nebulized bronchodilator twice per day. He was referred to physical therapy by his pulmonologist because of decreased endurance and decreased ability to perform basic ADLs, especially preparing meals and cleaning his kitchen. He lives alone, and his activities have decreased over the past 3 months primarily because of his son moving out of town and the colder winter weather. His son had been able to visit twice a week to assist him with his home cleaning and was taking him out to community activities. TD appears to be emotionally distressed as he discusses how he relies on his son for assistance and support. He relates that he knows he should be exercising more and reports that his dyspnea has been limiting his food intake. TD is concerned that he will be unable to maintain his independent living status.

A consultation with the referring pulmonologist reveals that this patient's pulmonary function only decreased slightly in the past 3 months. The pulmonologist suggested a referral to a pulmonary rehabilitation program that was refused by the patient, but the patient did request help in getting started with an independent exercise program. He reports no significant musculoskeletal problems, other than occasional mid-back discomfort from certain sitting positions. He denies problems with coordinating movements with upper or lower extremities.

Systems Review

TD has a cachetic appearance, with a barrel chest and hypertrophy of the accessory respiratory muscles. He is 5 foot 9 inches tall and weighs 132 lb (BMI = 19.5). He has a resting BP of 128/86, heart rate is 82 bpm, and respiratory rate is 18 breaths/minute. His oxygen saturation was measured at 92%, with a dyspnea rating at rest of 4/10. Auscultation of the lungs finds reduced breath sounds in the middle and lower lobes.

Fatigue Severity Scale average score = 6.1.

Tests and Measures
Musculoskeletal

Range of Motion Normal active ROM of the upper and lower extremities except for limited hip extension bilaterally due to limited extensibility of the hip flexor muscles. He experienced orthopnea when positioned in supine.

Muscle Performance A test of upper extremity endurance was performed by having the patient stand holding a dowel with his arms elevated to 90 degrees. After 80 seconds, he reported more shortness of breath and requested to stop the test. Dyspnea rating at the end of the test was 7/10.

Cardiovascular/Pulmonary

Aerobic Capacity and Endurance TD completed a 6-minute self-paced walk test without the use of oxygen.[99] He walked 210 m with two short standing rest periods. At the end of the test, his oxygen saturation was 88% with a dyspnea rating of 8/10. He used pursed lip breathing during the last 4 minutes of the test. His heart rate at the end of the test was 112 bpm, with a BP of 140/104 mm Hg. His vital signs and dyspnea rating returned to resting levels within 10 minutes of sitting rest.

Evaluation, Diagnosis, and Prognosis

TD appears to have deconditioning because of emphysema that has resulted in decreased overall home and community activities. He has decreased endurance as demonstrated by decreased standing and walking tolerance activities. He is motivated to begin an endurance exercise program but indicates he would like to perform the program at home.

Due to his problems related to housekeeping, meal preparation, and eating, he may benefit from a referral to occupational therapy for an evaluation of his home environment and instruction in energy conservation methods and a referral to a dietician to improve his caloric intake. His decreased social interactions are also a concern. A discussion with TD about resuming some of his usual community activities will be addressed at a later visit.

Goals

1. Increase self-paced 6-minute walk to 300 m within 3 months.
2. Increase arm elevation tolerance to 3 minutes with moderate dyspnea.
3. Patient will improve endurance and learn energy conservation methods.
4. Patient will self-initiate participation in community activities.

Prognosis

The improvements should be attainable with a consistent home exercise program (HEP). If TD is not able to improve his functional abilities, a referral to a pulmonary rehabilitation program will be suggested.

Intervention

HEPs with minimal supervision have been shown to improve exercise tolerance and activities for patients with obstructive respiratory diseases.[100,101] TD started with a daily home walking program and with upper extremity exercises. He was instructed to use a 10-point dyspnea scale to monitor and set the intensity of these activities.

Initially, he was instructed to walk twice per day for a 4-minute period with a sitting rest between the periods. The rest should last until his dyspnea returned to 4/10 level. Additionally, he should stop walking if his dyspnea reached or exceeded a level of 8/10. He was instructed to walk on the sidewalk by his house or in his garage if the weather does not allow outside walking. The walking periods will be increased by 1 minute per period per week.

Upper extremity exercises were also recommended as these can decrease dyspnea and improve upper extremity function.[102,103] Initially, TD was given only one upper extremity exercise, which involved raising a dowel above his head while in a standing position. He was to start with 3 sets of 10 repetitions, with an approximate 1-minute rest period between sets. The arm raising exercises are to stop if he reaches a dyspnea rating of 8/10.

Please see the CD that accompanies this book for case studies describing the examination, evaluation, and interventions for a patient with fatigue and weight gain and a patient with deconditioning after surgery.

CHAPTER SUMMARY

Deconditioning is the decline of normal anatomical and physiological function caused by disease, aging, or inactivity. Deconditioning primarily affects the cardiopulmonary system and its ability to supply the musculoskeletal system with oxygen for aerobic metabolism. This can result in impaired endurance and reduced ability to perform normal activities long enough or with enough repetitions to complete desired activities or tasks. The interaction of disease, aging, and decreased activities can result in deconditioning and impaired endurance and functional limitations.

Interventions for a patient with deconditioning should focus on improving their functional abilities, especially those related to ADLs and activities of independent living. Interventions to reverse the effects of deconditioning and improve endurance and functional abilities primarily involve aerobic exercise. Because exercise programs for a patient with deconditioning need to be consistently followed for multiple weeks and months, an individualized exercise prescription should be fashioned for each patient to optimize the physiological effects of the exercise and to enhance the patient's motivation to continue with the exercise program. An individualized exercise program will include the type of activity, the intensity level and how the intensity will be monitored, the duration of the activity, and how often the activity will be performed daily or on a weekly basis. The exercise program should be reevaluated on a consistent basis to assess for progression towards the treatment goals and to adjust the exercise parameters.

ADDITIONAL RESOURCES

Useful Forms

Fatigue Severity Scale
Dyspnea scale
Barthel Index
Lower Extremity Functional Scale

Books

Franklin BA (ed): *ACSM's Guidelines for Exercise Testing and Prescription,* ed 6, Baltimore, 2000, Lippincott, Williams & Wilkins.

Noonan V, Dean E: Submaximal exercise testing: Clinical application and interpretation, *Phys Ther* 80(8):782-807, 2000.

Franklin BA: Abnormal cardiorespiratory responses to acute aerobic exercise. In *ACSM's Resource Manual for Guidelines for Exercise Testing and Prescription,* ed 4, Baltimore, 2001, American College of Sports Medicine.

Williams MA (ed): *Guidelines for Cardiac Rehabilitation and Secondary Prevention Programs,* ed 4, Champaign, Ill, 2004, Human Kinetics.

Web Sites

American Heart Association: www.justmove.org/
America on the Move: www.americaonthemove.org/
American Association of Cardiovascular and Pulmonary Rehabilitation: www.aacvpr.org/
American College of Sports Medicine: www.acsm.org/health%2Bfitness/index.htm

GLOSSARY

Behavior modification theory: A theory for patient motivation and behavior change frequently used in rehabilitation and health promotion. According to this theory, reward and feedback about performance of a behavior are the greatest determinants of maintaining that behavior.

Body mass index (BMI): A general indicator of body composition calculated as weight in kilograms divided by height in meters squared (kg/m^2).

Circuit weight training (CWT): The performance of exercises with 10-15 repetitions using 40% to 60% of 1 RM in a continuous fashion, moving from one exercise station or machine to another with short rest periods between stations.

Deconditioning: The decline of normal anatomical and physiological function caused by disease, aging or inactivity.

Endurance impairment: The primary impairment for individuals with deconditioning that can be measured by whole body activities or with repeated movements of an extremity.

Heart rate reserve (HRR): Estimated maximum heart rate minus the resting heart rate. This can be used to determine aerobic exercise intensity.

Karvonen method: Formula for determining target heart rate using the heart rate reserve: ([HRR − resting heart rate] × goal percent of HRR) + resting heart rate.

Maximum oxygen uptake ($\dot{V}O_{2max}$): The maximum amount of oxygen consumption of the body during activity. This is the best indicator of cardiopulmonary fitness.

Metabolic equivalent (MET): One MET is the rate of energy consumption at rest, which is approximately 3.5 ml of oxygen /kg/min. The MET is a convenient measure of intensity for prescribing activity levels.

Modified Bruce protocol: A protocol for exercise testing commonly used in clinical settings for estimating $\dot{V}O_{2max}$ in patients with low functional capacity.

Patient motivation: A patient's internal state that activates their behavior and gives it direction. Motivation is the single most important factor for determining if a patient will maintain an exercise program.

Rating of perceived exertion (RPE): A common method for monitoring exercise intensity during exercise, using the patient's own perception of his or her level of exertion.

Social cognitive theory: A theory of patient motivation for behavior change that proposes that a person's self-efficacy is the primary factor influencing behavior change.

Stages of change theory: Part of the transtheoretical model of motivation and behavior change. This theory describes a person's emotional and intellectual preparedness for change in terms of five stages.

References

1. Mujika I, Padilla S: Cardiorespiratory and metabolic characteristics of detraining in humans, *Med Sci Sports Exerc* 33(3):413-421, 2001.
2. Coyle EF: Detraining and retention of adaptation induced by endurance training. In *ACSM's Resource Manual for Guidelines for Exercise Testing and Prescription,* ed 4, Baltimore, 2001, American College of Sports Medicine.
3. American Physical Therapy Association: Guide to Physical Therapist Practice, second edition, *Phys Ther* 81:9-744, 2001.
4. Dudley GA, Ploutz-Synder LL: Deconditioning and bed rest: Musculoskeletal response. In *ACSM's Resource Manual for Guidelines for Exercise Testing and Prescription,* ed 4, Baltimore, 2001, American College of Sports Medicine.
5. Fletcher GF, Balady GJ, Amsterdam EA, et al: Exercise standards for testing and training: a statement for healthcare professionals from the American Heart Association, *Circulation* 104(14):1694-1740, 2001.
6. Franklin BA: *ACSM's Guidelines for Exercise Testing and Prescription,* ed 6, Baltimore, 2000, Lippincott Williams & Wilkins.
7. Ainsworth BE, Haskell WL, Whitt MC, et al: Compendium of physical activities: An update of activity codes and MET intensities, *Med Sci Sports Exerc* 32(suppl 9):S498-504, 2000.
8. Coyle EF, Martin WH, Dinacore DR, et al: Time course of loss adaptations after stopping prolonged intense endurance training, *J Appl Physiol* 57:1857-1864, 1984.
9. Thompson PD, Cullinane EM, Eshleman R, et al: The effects of caloric restriction or exercise cessation on the serum lipid and lipoprotein concentrations of endurance athletes, *Metabolism* 33(10):943-950, 1984.
10. Coyle EF, Martin WH, Bloomfield SA: Effects of detraining on responses to submaximal exercise, *J Appl Physiol* 59:853-859, 1985.
11. Klausen K, Andersen LB, Pelle I: Adaptive changes in work capacity, skeletal muscle capillarization and enzyme levels during training and detraining, *Acta Physiol Scand* 113:9-16, 1981.
12. Manfredi TG, Fielding RA, O'Reilly KP, et al: Plasma creatine kinase activity and exercise-induced muscle damage in older men, *Med Sci Sports Exerc* 23(9):1028-1034, 1991.
13. Oshida Y, Yamanouchi K, Hayamizu S, et al: Effects of training and training cessation on insulin action, *Int J Sports Med* 12(5):484-486, 1991.
14. Smorawinski J, Nazar K, Kaciuba-Uscilko H, et al: Effects of 3-day bed rest on physiological responses to graded exercise in athletes and sedentary men, *J Appl Physiol* 91(1):249-257, 2001.
15. Murdaca G, Setti M, Brenci S, et al: Modifications of immunological and neuro-endocrine parameters induced by anti-orthostatic bed rest in human healthy volunteers, *Minerva Med* 94(6):363-378, 2003.
16. Lewis CB, Bottomley JM: *Geriatric Rehabilitation: A Clinical Approach,* ed 2, Upper Saddle River, NJ, 2003, Prentice Hall.
17. Guiccone AA: *Geriatric Physical Therapy,* ed 2, St. Louis, 2000, Mosby.
18. Cheitlin MD: Cardiovascular physiology changes with aging, *Am J Geriatr Cardiol* 12(1):9-13, 2003.
19. Tanaka H, Seals DR: Dynamic exercise performance in Masters athletes: Insight into the effects of primary human aging on physiological functional capacity, *J Appl Physiol* 95(5):2152-62, 2003.
20. Dehn MM, Bruce A: Longitudinal variations in maximal oxygen uptake with age and activity, *J Appl Physiol* 33:805-807, 1972.
21. Rodeheffer FJ: Exercise cardiac output is maintained with advancing age in health human subjects, *Circulation* 69:203-213, 1984.
22. Shimada K, Kitazumi T, Sadakne N: Age related changes of baroreflex function, plasma norepinephrine, and blood pressure, *Hypertension* 7:113-117, 1985.
23. Overend TJ, Cunningham DA, Paterson DH, et al: Thigh composition in young and elderly men determined by computed tomography, *Clin Physiol* 12:629-640, 1992.
24. Lexell J, Taylor CC, Sjostorm M: Total number, size and proportion of different fiber types studied in whole vastus lateralis muscle from 15 to 83 years old men, *J Neurol Sci* 84:275-294, 1988.
25. Hill JO, Melanson EL: Overview of the determinants of overweight and obesity: Current evidence and research issues, *Med Sci Sports Exerc* 31(suppl 11):S515-521, 1999.
26. Jebb SA, Moore MS: Contribution of a sedentary lifestyle and inactivity to the etiology of overweight and obesity: Current evidence and research issues, *Med Sci Sports Exerc* 31(suppl 11):S534-541, 1999.
27. Patrick K, Norman GJ, Calfas KJ, et al: Diet, physical activity, and sedentary behaviors as risk factors for overweight in adolescence, *Arch Pediatr Adolesc Med* 158(4):385-390, 2004.
28. Goldberg RB: Prevention of type II diabetes, *Med Clin North Am* 82:805-821, 1998.
29. Damrosch S: General strategies for motivating people to change their behavior, *Health Promot* 26:833-843, 1991.
30. Dishman RK, Ickes W, Morgan WP: Self-motivation and adherence to habitual physical activity, *J Appl Soc Psych* 10:115-132, 1980.
31. Lee RE, Nigg CR, DiClemente CC, et al: Validating motivational readiness for exercise behavior with adolescents, *Res Q Exerc Sport* 72:401-410, 2001.
32. Jitamontree N: Evidence-based protocol: Exercise promotion, *J Gerontol Nurs* 27:7-18, 2001.
33. Williams MA (ed): *Guidelines for Cardiac Rehabilitation and Secondary Prevention Programs,* ed 4, Champaign, Ill, 2004, Human Kinetics.
34. Bandura A: Self-efficacy: Toward a unifying theory of behavior change, *Psychological Rev* 84:191-215, 1977.
35. Plonczynski DJ: Measurement of motivation for exercise, *Health Educ Res* 15:695-705, 2000.
36. Prochaska JO, Velicer WF: The transtheoretical model of health behavior change, *Am J Health Promot* 12(1):38-48, 1997.
37. Marshall SJ, Biddle SJ: The transtheoretical model of behavior change: A meta-analysis of applications to physical activity and exercise, *Ann Behav Med* 23(4):229-246, 2001.
38. Reed GR, Velicer WF, Prochaska JO, et al: What makes a good staging algorithm: examples from regular exercise, *Am J Health Promot* 12(1):57-66, 1997.
39. Marttila J, Nupponen R: Assessing stage of change for physical activity: How congruent are parallel methods? *Health Educ Res* 18:419-428, 2003.
40. Noonan V, Dean E: Submaximal exercise testing: clinical application and interpretation, *Phys Ther* 80(8):782-807, 2000.
41. Suni JH, Oja P, Miilunpalo SI, et al: Health-related fitness test battery for adults: Associations with perceived health, mobility, and back function and symptoms, *Arch Phys Med Rehabil* 79:559-569, 1998.
42. Going S, Davis R: Body composition. In *ACSM's Resource Manual for Guidelines for Exercise Testing and Prescription,* ed 4, Baltimore, 2001, American College of Sports Medicine.
43. Ravaglia G, Forti P, Maioli F: Measurement of body fat in healthy elderly men: A comparison of methods, *J Gerontol A Biol Sci Med Sci* 54:M70-76, 1999.
44. Deurenberg P, Weststrate JA, Seidell JC: Body mass index as a measure of body fatness: age and sex-specific prediction formulas, *Br J Nutr* 65:105-114, 1991.
45. Riley R: Nutrition and weight management. In *ACSM's Resource Manual for Guidelines for Exercise Testing and Prescription,* ed 4, Baltimore, 2001, American College of Sports Medicine.
46. Krupp LB, LaRocca NG, Muir-Nash J, et al: The fatigue severity scale, *Arch Neurol* 46(10):1121-1123, 1989.
47. Winstead-Fry P: Psychometric assessment of four fatigue scales with a sample of rural cancer patients, *J Nurs Meas* 6(2):111-122, 1998.
48. Aaronson LS, Teel CS, Cassmeyer V, et al: Defining and measuring fatigue, *Image J Nurs Sch* 31:45-51, 1999.
49. Nijs J, Vaes P, McGregor N, Van Hoof E: Psychometric properties of the Dutch Chronic Fatigue Syndrome–Activities and Participation Questionnaire, *Phys Ther* 83:444-454, 2003.
50. Eason JM: Cardiopulmonary assessment, *Cardiopulm Phys Ther* 10:135-142, 1999.
51. Sansoy V, Watson DD, Beller GA: Significance of slow upsloping ST-segment depression on exercise stress testing, *Am J Cardiol* 15:709-712, 1997.
52. Mahler DA, Wells CK: Evaluation of clinical methods for rating dyspnea, *Chest* 93:580-586, 1988.
53. Weaver TE, Narsavage GL, Guilfoyle MJ: The development and psychometric evaluation of the pulmonary functional status scale: An instrument to assess functional status in pulmonary disease, *J Cardiopulm Rehabil* 18:105-111, 1998.
54. American Thoracic Society, American College of Chest Physicians statement on cardiopulmonary exercise testing, *Am J Respir Crit Care Med* 167:211-277, 2003.
55. Bruce RA, Kusumi F, Hosmer D: Maximal oxygen intake and nomographic assessment of functional aerobic impairment in cardiovascular disease, *Am Heart J* 85(4):546-562, 1973.
56. McConnell TR: Cardiorespiratory assessment of apparently healthy populations. In *ACSM's Resource Manual for Guidelines for Exercise Testing*

and Prescription, ed 4, Baltimore, 2001, American College of Sports Medicine.

57. Macsween A: The reliability and validity of the Astrand nomogram and linear extrapolation for deriving VO_{2max} from submaximal exercise data, *J Sports Med Phys Fitness* 41(3):312-317, 2001.

58. Ragg KE, Murray TF, Karbonitt LM, et al: Errors in predicting functional capacity form a treadmill exercise stress test, *Am Heart J* 100:581-583, 1980.

59. Cahalin L, Pappagianopoulos P, Prevost S, et al: The relationship of the 6-min walk test to maximal oxygen consumption in transplant candidates with end-stage lung disease, *Chest* 108:452-459, 1995.

60. Solway S, Brooks D, Lacasse Y, et al: A qualitative systematic overview of the measurement properties of functional walk tests used in the cardiorespiratory domain, *Chest* 119:256-270, 2001.

61. Foster C, Jackson AS, Pollock ML, et al: Generalized equations for predicting functional capacity from treadmill performance, *Am Heart J* 107(6):1229-1234, 1984.

62. Kaminsky LA, Whaley MH: Evaluation of a new standardized ramp protocol. the BSU/Bruce Ramp protocol, *J Cardiopulm Rehabil* 18.438-444, 1998.

63. Butland RJ, Pang J, Gross ER, et al: Two-, six-, and 12-minute walking tests in respiratory disease, *BMJ* 284:1607-1608, 1982.

64. Eiser N, Willsher D, Dore CJ: Reliability, repeatability and sensitivity to change of externally and self-paced walking tests in COPD patients, *Respir Med* 97(4):407-414, 2003.

65. Mahoney FI, Barthel DW: Functional evaluation: The Barthel Index, *Md State Med J* 14:61-65, 1965.

66. Wolfe CD, Taub NA, Woodrow EF, et al: Assessment of scales of disability and handicap for stroke patients, *Stroke* 22:1242-1244, 1991.

67. Gresham GE, Phillips TF, Labi ML: ADL status in stroke: Relative merits of three standard indexes, *Arch Phys Med Rehabil* 61:355-358, 1982.

68. Binkley JM, Stratford PW, Lott SA, et al: The lower extremity functional scale (LEFS): Scale development, measurement properties and clinical application, *Phys Ther* 79:371-383, 1999.

69. Kidd D, Stewart G, Baldry J, et al: The Functional Independence Measure: A comparative validity and reliability study, *Disabil Rehabil* 17:10-14, 1995.

70. Stratford PW, Binkley JM, Watson J, et al: Validation of the LEFS on patients with total joint arthroplasty, *Physiother Can* 52:97-105, 2000.

71. Holly RG, Shaffrath JD: Cardiorespiratory endurance. In *ACSM's Resource Manual for Guidelines for Exercise Testing and Prescription,* ed 4, Baltimore, 2001, American College of Sports Medicine.

72. Hillegass EA, Sadowsky HS: *Cardiopulmonary Physical Therapy,* ed 2, Philadelphia, 2001, WB Saunders.

73. Rosen CS: Is the sequencing of change processes by stage consistent across health problems? A meta-analysis, *Health Psychol* 19(6):593-604, 2000.

74. Lemura LM, von Duvillard SP, Mookerjee S: The effects of physical training of functional capacity in adults ages 46 to 90: A meta-analysis, *J Sports Med Phys Fitness* 40(1):1 10, 2000.

75. Fleg JL, Piña IL, Balady G: Assessment of functional capacity in clinical and research applications. An advisory from the Committee on Exercise, Rehabilitation, and Prevention, Council on Clinical Cardiology, American Heart Association, *Circulation* 102:1591-1597, 2000.

76. American College of Sports Medicine Position Stand: The recommended quantity and quality of exercise for developing and maintaining cardiorespiratory and muscular fitness and flexibility in healthy adults, *Med Sci Sports Exerc* 30(6):975-991, 1998.

77. Wilmore JH, Stanforth PR, Gagnon J, et al: Cardiac output and stroke volume changes with endurance training: the HERITAGE Family Study, *Med Sci Sports Exerc* 33(1):99-106, 2001.

78. Talbot LA, Gaines JM, Huynh TN, et al: A home-based pedometer-driven walking program to increase physical activity in older adults with osteoarthritis of the knee: a preliminary study, *J Am Geriatr Soc* 51(3):387-392, 2003.

79. Jan MH, Hung JY, Lin JC, et al: Effects of a home program on strength, walking speed, and function after total hip replacement, *Arch Phys Med Rehabil* 85(12):1943-1951, 2004.

80. Eng JJ, Chu KS, Kim CM, et al: A community-based group exercise program for persons with chronic stroke, *Med Sci Sports Exerc* 35(8):1271-1278, 2003.

81. Duncan P, Richards L, Wallace D, et al: A randomized, controlled pilot study of a home-based exercise program for individuals with mild and moderate stroke, *Stroke* 29(10):2055-2060, 1998.

82. Deligiannis A: Exercise rehabilitation and skeletal muscle benefits in hemodialysis patients, *Clin Nephrol* 61(suppl 1):S46-50, 2004.

83. Kopple JD, Storer T, Casburi R: Impaired exercise capacity and exercise training in maintenance hemodialysis patients, *J Ren Nutr* 15(1):44-48, 2005.

84. American Thoracic Society: Standards for the diagnosis and care of patients with chronic obstructive pulmonary disease, *Am J Respir Crit Care Med* 136:225-244, 1995.

85. Foster C, Dymond DS, Carpenter J, et al: Effect of warm-up on left ventricular response to sudden strenuous exercise, *J Appl Physiol* 53(2):380-383, 1982.

86. Franklin BA (ed): Abnormal cardiorespiratory responses to acute aerobic exercise. In *ACSM's Guidelines for Exercise Testing and Prescription,* ed 6, Baltimore, 2000, Lippincott, Williams & Wilkins.

87. Borg GA: Psychophysical basis of perceived exertion, *Med Sci Sports Exerc* 14.377-381, 1982.

88. Williams JG, Eston RG: Determination of the intensity dimension in vigorous exercise programmes with particular reference to the use of the rating of perceived exertion, *Sports Med* 8(3):177-189, 1989.

89. Pollock ML, Ward A, Ayres JJ: Cardiorespiratory fitness: response to differing intensities and durations of training, *Arch Phys Med Rehabil* 58(11):467-473, 1977.

90. Sallis JF, Hovell MF, Hofstetter CR: Predictors of adoption and maintenance of vigorous physical activity in men and women, *Prev Med* 21(2).237-251, 1992.

91. Ewart CK: Psychological effects of resistive weight training: Implications for cardiac patients, *Med Sci Sports Exerc* 21(6):683-688, 1989.

92. McCartney N, McKelvie RS, Haslam DR, et al: Usefulness of weightlifting training in improving strength and maximal power output in coronary artery disease, *Am J Cardiol* 67(11):939-945, 1991.

93. Pierson LM, Herbert WG, Norton HJ, et al: Effects of combined aerobic and resistance training versus aerobic training alone in cardiac rehabilitation. *J Cardiopulm Rehabil* 21(2):101-110, 2001.

94. Ewart CK, Stewart KJ, Gillilan RE, et al: Self-efficacy mediates strength gains during circuit weight training in men with coronary artery disease, *Med Sci Sports Exerc* 18(5):531-540, 1986.

95. Gettman LR, Pollock ML: Circuit weight training: A critical review of its physiological benefits, *Phys Sportsmed* 9(1):44 66, 1981.

96. Gettman LR, Ayres JJ, Pollock ML, et al: The effect of circuit weight training on strength, cardiorespiratory function, and body composition of adult men, *Med Sci Sports Exerc* 10(3):171-176, 1978.

97. Harber MP, Fry AC, Rubin MR, et al: Skeletal muscle and hormonal adaptations to circuit weight training in untrained men, *Scand J Med Sci Sports* 14(3):176-185, 2004.

98. Wilmore JH, Parr RB, Girandola RN, Ward P, et al: Physiological alterations consequent to circuit weight training, *Med Sci Sports Exerc* 10(2):79-84, 1978.

99. ATS Committee on Proficiency Standards for Clinical Pulmonary Function Laboratories: ATS statement: Guidelines for the six-minute walk test, *Am J Respir Crit Care Med* 166(1):111-117, 2002.

100. Ferrari M. Vangelista A, Vedovi F, et al: Minimally supervised home rehabilitation improves exercise capacity and health status in patients with COPD, *Am J Phys Med Rehabil* 83(5):337-343, 2004.

101. Wijkstra PJ, Ten Vergert EM, van Altena R, et al: Long term benefits of rehabilitation at home on quality of life and exercise tolerance in patients with chronic obstructive pulmonary disease, *Thorax* 50(8).824-828, 1995.

102. Couser JI Jr, Martinez FJ, Celli BR: Pulmonary rehabilitation that includes arm exercise reduces metabolic and ventilatory requirements for simple arm elevation, *Chest* 103(1):37-41, 1993.

103. Martinez FJ, Vogel PD, Dupont DN, et al: Supported arm exercise vs unsupported arm exercise in the rehabilitation of patients with severe chronic airflow obstruction, *Chest* 103(5):1397-1402, 1993.

104. Larsson P, Olofsson P, Jakobsson E, et al: Physiological predictors of performance in cross-country skiing from treadmill tests in male and female subjects, *Scand J Med Sci Sports* 12(6):347-353, 2002.

105. Ng AV, Demment RB, Bassett DR, et al: Characteristics and performance of male citizen cross-country ski racers, *Int J Sports Med* 205-209, 1988.

Chapter 24

Airway Clearance Dysfunction

Jan Stephen Tecklin

CHAPTER OUTLINE

OBJECTIVES

After reading this chapter, the reader will be able to:
1. Identify four common causes of airway clearance dysfunction.
2. Describe associations between specific pathological findings and airway clearance techniques.
3. Apply valid and reliable tests to determine whether airway clearance techniques are appropriate for a particular patient.
4. Design and execute safe and effective interventions for improving airway clearance.
5. Document and communicate the examination findings, prognosis, plan of care, and reexamination findings for any patient with airway clearance dysfunction.
6. Identify when airway clearance techniques should be taught to a patient's family members.

$\mathcal{A}$irway clearance dysfunction is a problem common to individuals with a wide variety of medical and surgical diagnoses. Airway clearance dysfunction implies an inability to adequately clear the airways of obstructing material such as mucus, secretions, fluid, cellular debris, inflammatory exudate, or other items such as aspirated foreign objects. Many immediate and potentially adverse outcomes may result from an inability to clear the airways,

including airway obstruction, inflammation, infection, *atelectasis,* abnormal ventilation/perfusion relationships, and deterioration of arterial blood gas (ABG) values. Airway obstruction occurs in many groups of individuals and is a defining feature of chronic obstructive pulmonary disease (COPD) in adults and of cystic fibrosis (CF) in children, adolescents, and adults.

PATHOLOGY

Airway clearance dysfunction occurs in many diseases and conditions. In reviewing the codes from the *International Classification of Diseases—Ninth revision* (ICD9)[1] that are listed in the *Guide to Physical Therapist Practice*[2] for preferred practice pattern 6C: Impaired ventilation, respiration/gas exchange, and *aerobic capacity*/endurance associated with airway clearance dysfunction, it appears that patients in three large diagnostic groups are at risk for airway clearance dysfunction. One group includes patients with disorders caused by chronic inhalation of particulate matter, including organic (generally tobacco smoke) and inorganic dusts; another group of patients have infectious disorders; and the third large group is associated with operative procedures, including cardiovascular and orthopedic procedures and solid organ transplantation. In addition, the nature of the pathological process in CF, which leads to tenacious and voluminous bronchial secretions, inevitably produces airway clearance problems.

EXAMINATION

PATIENT HISTORY

The patient history should include questions about the following areas:

Employment/work Does the patient's current employment contribute to the airway dysfunction? Is there exposure to fumes, dusts, gases or other particulate matter? Such exposure often causes and/or exacerbates lung disease.[3,4] Does the physical disability limit the ability to perform work-related tasks?

Living environment Does the home or other discharge destination provide space and resources (including adequate electrical outlets) for necessary respiratory support items such as oxygen, a ventilator, and suction devices?

General health status Is the patient mobile at home? Is the patient depressed? Depression is common in individuals with COPD.[5] Has there been a change in community, leisure, and social function because of the illness?

Social/health habits Is the patient a smoker and has there been an attempt to stop smoking? It is clear that smoking cessation, even on an intermittent basis, can reduce the long-term decline in pulmonary function associated with smoking.[6] Can and does the patient participate in fitness activities? Long-term exercise for individuals with chronic lung disease may reduce self-reported disability and improve functional status.[7]

Medical/surgical history Were there recent hospitalizations or illnesses? Are there co-morbidities that may affect rehabilitation participation and effort?

Current condition/chief complaint What current concern has led to the request for rehabilitation intervention and is this a recurrence? What are the current therapeutic interventions? Has the patient been performing any type of airway clearance or exercise regimen? What are the patient's and family's expectations for this episode of care?

Functional status/activity level Was the patient previously independent at home and with activities of daily living (ADLs)? What is the current and recent status regarding work and community activities?

Medications What medications is the patient taking and can these be expected to impact the physical therapy regimen? Patients with airway clearance dysfunction often use aerosolized *bronchodilator* and *mucolytic* medications. Taking these before airway clearance and exercise interventions can optimize benefits from such treatments.[8]

Clinical Tests. Available records should be reviewed. Pulmonary function test results and ABG values can help guide the appropriate intensity of interventions and the need for rest during interventions.

SYSTEMS REVIEW

The systems review is used to target areas requiring further examination and to define areas that may cause complications or indicate a need for precautions during the examination and intervention processes. See Chapter 1 for details of the systems review.

TESTS AND MEASURES
Musculoskeletal

Posture. Posture is commonly altered by chronic lung disease, particularly when hyperinflation is present for a long period of time.[9] An examination of postural align-

ment should therefore be performed on any patient with chronic lung disease (see Chapter 4).[10] Patients with long-term hyperinflation have several typical findings, including tight pectoral, sternocleidomastoid, scalene, and scapular muscles and an increased anterior-posterior (AP) diameter of the thorax. The normal ratio of the AP diameter to the transverse diameter of the thorax in the absence of hyperinflation is approximately $1:2$. This ratio is termed the *thoracic index*. In the presence of hyperinflation, the thoracic index increases and is often $\geq 2:1$. This is termed a barrel chest.[11] The muscle shortening and increase in thoracic index associated with hyperinflation are generally accompanied by an increase in thoracic kyphosis. Overall, the rigidity of the continually enlarged thoracic cage reduces both thoracic excursion and spinal flexibility. Measurement of chest circumference with a tape measure at the level of the xiphoid process can be used to determine thoracic expansion. Chest calipers, also called pelvimeters, may also be used to determine the thoracic index and changes in thoracic index with active efforts at chest expansion and with hyperinflation.

Range of Motion. Because of the degree of chronic inactivity and lack of mobility in many individuals with chronic lung disease, it is important to test range of motion (ROM) at all major joints in this group of patients. Shoulder girdle and thoracic spine ROM are of particular importance to assure that chest expansion is not impeded by soft tissue tightness or lack of joint mobility. In addition, people with chronic lung disease, who commonly are not able to be very active, tend to spend a great deal of time seated or supine, which often reduces ROM in the lower extremities. Examination of ROM using classical goniometric techniques, inclinometry, and observation of functional ROM are all appropriate in this population.

Muscle Performance. Individuals with COPD often have muscle weakness in their extremities, shoulder girdle, neck, and chest that limits physical activity.[12] There is increasing evidence that peripheral muscle dysfunction exists independent of ventilation limitations in individuals with COPD and CF.[12] Studies indicate that chronic lung disease results in muscle weakness and that oxidative stress reduces muscle endurance in individuals with COPD.[13] Regardless of the cause, it is clear that the peripheral muscle strength deficits in this population lead to exercise limitation and intolerance.[14-16]

With airway clearance dysfunction, the patient benefits from an effective cough. The power behind a cough is achieved by a sudden and forceful contraction of the abdominal muscles and expiratory muscles of the thorax. Expiratory muscle function is reflected by maximal static expiratory pressure and peak expiratory flow (see Chapter 26).[17,18] These can be measured easily and inexpensively with an analog "bugle" dynamometer or a digital device.[19]

Neuromuscular

Pain. Assessment of pain—both its source and perceived level—is an important part of the examination of the patient with airway clearance difficulties. Chest wall pain resulting from musculoskeletal problems is common. This pain is usually nonsegmental, localized to the anterior chest, and aggravated by deep breathing and has a palpable source. Chest wall pain is also usually unrelated to exercise. In contrast, chest pain caused by cardiac ischemia (angina pectoris) is typically a viselike, crushing midline pain that radiates to the jaw and arm and is aggravated by exercise. Thoracic nerve root inflammation can also cause chest pain, but this will follow a dermatomal distribution.

If the patient has chest wall pain, a pain scale (see Chapter 22) should be used to determine the level of pain. A pain diary may be helpful to determine the effects of pain on daily activity and to evaluate the effects of interventions on this symptom.

Cardiovascular/Pulmonary

Ventilation and Respiration/Gas Exchange. Two important indicators of potential problems with respiration include the rate of perceived exertion (RPE) and the level of *dyspnea,* commonly quantified with the revised 10-point Borg Scale[20] and with dyspnea scales, respectively. The Borg Scale of perceived exertion was originally a scale with a range of scores from 6 to 20 (see Box 23-3). A score of 6 indicated no exertion at all and 20 indicated very, very hard exertion. The scale was later revised to a 10-point scale from 0-10 with 0 equating to no exertion at all and 10 indicating very, very strong exertion (Box 24-1). This revision has been shown to be both valid and reliable in more than 400 consecutive patients with dyspnea in an emergency department.[21] It has also been shown to be reproducible over long time periods.[22]

There are numerous dyspnea scales that range from simple and unidimensional to more complex and multidimensional (see Fig. 23-3). In addition, dyspnea measures often appear within more wide-ranging questionnaires about respiratory diseases and their effects on the quality of life. A visual analog scale (VAS) similar to the visual analog scale used to quantify pain severity (see Chapter 22) can also be used to quantify dyspnea. A 10-cm horizontal line is presented with end points of "not breathless at all" to "worst breathlessness I can imagine." The patient indicates his or her level of breathlessness on the line. Scoring of breathlessness on the VAS has strong concurrent validity with the Borg Scale[23] and is reproducible at varying levels of exercise.[24]

Two very commonly employed valid and reliable disease-specific instruments that include dyspnea are the Chronic Respiratory Questionnaire (CRQ)[25] and the St. George's Respiratory Questionnaire (SGRQ).[26] Both instruments are self-report questionnaires that examine the impact of respiratory problems on daily life. Both have been used extensively in research and allow for ready comparison of results from different studies.[27] (See Additional Resources for information on obtaining copies of these instruments.)

Many of the findings associated with impaired ventilation and gas exchange have a direct bearing on procedural intervention selection. These findings are best gathered through the tools of a traditional chest examination, which include inspection, *auscultation,* palpation, and percussion.

Inspection. The inspection phase of the chest examination involves looking at the patient, specifically seeking

signs of problems with breathing. Inspection should first focus on the patient's general appearance. The therapist evaluates body type as normal, obese, or cachectic and then examines posture, taking particular note of any spinal misalignment or unusual postures as noted previously. The therapist should look for and document the presence of kyphosis, scoliosis, and forward bend, or professorial posture (Fig. 24-1).

During inspection of the extremities the therapist should look for nicotine stains on the fingers, digital clubbing, painful swollen joints, tremor, and edema. Nicotine stains suggest a history of heavy smoking and are important in the evaluation of the unconscious patient. Clubbing of the fingers or toes is associated with cardiopulmonary and small bowel disease.[28] Painful swollen joints in certain patients with lung disease may indicate pseudohypertrophic pulmonary osteoarthropathy rather than the osteoarthritis or rheumatoid arthritis more familiar to physical therapists (PTs).[29] Bilateral pedal edema may indicate cor pulmonale or right-sided heart failure in those with long-standing chronic lung disease.

The therapist should also note all equipment used in managing the patient. For example, the use of a cardiac monitor, a Swan-Ganz catheter, or a left ventricular assist device suggests potential or actual cardiac rhythm disturbances or hemodynamic or cardiac output problems, respectively.

When inspecting the head and neck, the therapist should check the face for signs of respiratory distress and oxygen desaturation. Signs commonly seen in individuals with significant respiratory distress include flaring of the alae nasi and cyanosis of the mucous membranes.[30]

Inspection of the unmoving chest should include looking for congenital defects such as pectus carinatum (pigeon breast) and pectus excavatum (funnel chest or hollow chest). The therapist should next inspect the rib angles and intercostal spaces. Normally, the rib angles are less than 90 degrees, and the ribs attach to the vertebrae at an angle of about 45 degrees. The spaces between the ribs are broader posteriorly than anteriorly. Widening of the rib angles and broadening of the anterior intercostal spaces suggests hyperinflation of the lungs. Inspection of the musculature around the chest often reveals bilateral trapezius and sternocleidomastoid muscle hypertrophy as a result of overuse of these accessory muscles of ventilation associated with acute respiratory distress and chronic dyspnea. However, a prominent appearance of these muscles is most often caused by an increase in thoracic kyphosis and a forward-head position rather than actual muscle hypertrophy.[31] The two hemithoraces should be compared for asymmetry such as unilateral chest wall retraction.

Inspection of the moving chest begins with assessment of the respiratory rate, which normally ranges from 12-20 breaths per minute (breaths/min) in adults. This normal, or eupneic, pattern of breathing supplies one breath for every four heartbeats. Tachypnea refers to a ventilatory rate faster than 20 breaths/min. Bradypnea refers to a ventilatory rate slower than 10 breaths/min. Fever affects ventilatory rate which increases by 3-4 breaths/min for every

BOX 24-1 **Borg CR10 Scale**

Instruction. Use this rating scale to report how strong your perception is. It can be exertion, pain, or something else. Ten (10) or "Extremely strong"—"Maximal" is a very important intensity level. It serves as a reference point on the scale. This is the most intense perception or feeling (e.g., of exertion) you have ever had. It is, however, possible to experience or imagine something even more intense. That is why we've placed "Absolute maximum" outside and further down on the scale without any corresponding number, just a dot "•". If your experience is stronger than "10," you can use a larger number.

First look at the verbal expressions. Start with them and then the numbers. If your experience or feeling is "Very weak," you should say "1," if it is "Moderate," say "3." Note that "Moderate" is "3" and thus weaker than "Medium," "Mean," or "Middle." If the experience is "Strong" or "Heavy" (it feels "Difficult") say "5." Note that "Strong" is about 50 percent, or about half, of "Maximal." If your perception is "Very strong" ("Very intense") choose a number from 6 to 8, depending upon how intense it is. Feel free to use half-numbers like "1.5" or "3.5," or decimals like "0.3," "0.8," or "2.3." It is very important that you report what you actually experience or feel, not what you think you should report. Be as spontaneous and honest as possible and try to avoid under- or over-estimating. Look at the verbal descriptors and then choose a number.

When rating *perceived exertion* give a number that corresponds to your feeling of exertion, that is, how hard and strenuous you perceive the work to be and how tired you are. The perception of exertion is mainly felt as strain and fatigue in your muscles and as breathlessness or aches in the chest. It is important that you only think about what you feel, and not about what the actual load is.

1   Very light. As for a healthy person taking a short walk at his or her own pace.
3   Moderate is somewhat but not especially hard. It feels good and not difficult to go on.
5   The work is hard and tiring, but continuing isn't terribly difficult. The effort and exertion are about half as intense as "Maximal."
7   Quite strenuous. You can still go on, but you really have to push yourself you are very tired.
10 An extremely strenuous level. For most people this is the most strenuous exertion they have ever experienced.
•   Is "Absolute maximum ," for example "12" or even more.
Any questions?

0   **Nothing at all**
0.3
0.5   **Extremely weak**   **Just noticeable**
0.7
1   **Very weak**
1.5
2   **Weak**   **Light**
2.5
3   **Moderate**
4
5   **Strong**   **Heavy**
6
7   **Very strong**
8
9
10   **Extremely strong**   **"Maximal"**
11
✦
•   **Absolute maximum**   **Highest possible**

Borg CR10 Scale
© Gunnar Borg 1982, 1998

"The Borg CR-10 Scale," Borg G, 2003.

degree Fahrenheit of fever, and by even more in young children[32] (see Chapter 22 for further details of how to measure respiratory rate). Next, the therapist inspects the ratio of inspiratory and expiratory time (the I : E ratio). Normally, expiration lasts twice as long as inspiration, giving an I : E ratio of 1 : 2. In obstructive lung disease, expiration is prolonged, commonly producing I : E ratios of 1 : 4 or 1 : 5.

When examining the moving chest, one also examines the sounds associated with breathing. Detection of *stridor*, a crowing sound during inspiration, suggests upper airway obstruction and may indicate laryngospasm.[33] *Stertor*, a snoring noise created when the tongue falls back into the lower palate, may be heard in patients with depressed consciousness. Expiratory grunting, commonly heard in infants with respiratory distress, may be a physiological attempt to prevent premature airway collapse. Gurgling sounds heard during inspiration and expiration may indicate copious secretions in the larger airways. The therapist next determines the pattern of breathing to identify the rate, depth and regularity of the ventilatory cycle. Some commonly encountered breathing patterns appear in Table 24-1.

After inspecting the pattern and sounds of breathing, the therapist determines the symmetry and synchrony of breathing. The timing and relative motion of one hemithorax to the other and to the abdomen are compared during both normal tidal breathing and deep breathing. Individuals with respiratory muscle dysfunction because of neuromuscular disease often have asymmetrical or paradoxical thoracic motion. Paradoxical motion occurs when the diaphragm or rib cage muscula-

ture are impaired preferentially. Paradoxical motion involves chest wall motion contradictory to the expected inspiratory motion.[34] The chronically hyperinflated thorax and flattened diaphragm, often seen with severe COPD, can result in a simultaneous in-drawing of the lower ribs and expansion of the upper ribs during inspiration.[35] Gross observation of the respiratory muscles facilitates detection of accessory inspiratory or expiratory muscle activity. Moreover, careful observation of the intercostal spaces may reveal inspiratory retraction associated with decreased pulmonary compliance or expiratory bulging associated with expiratory obstruction.[36]

Inspection of the chest continues with evaluation of speech, breath, cough, and sputum. Speech patterns associated with breathing difficulties or specific breath problems can often be recognized during casual conversation, particularly shortness of breath that causes frequent interruptions in speech known as "dyspnea of phonation." This may be quantified by the number of words that can be spoken between sequential breaths and called, for example, "three word dyspnea" or "four word dyspnea." Malodorous breath detected during conversation may indicate anaerobic infection of the mouth or respiratory tract.[37]

If a patient has complaints of coughing, the clinician next identifies characteristics of the cough, including whether it is persistent, paroxysmal, or occasional; dry or productive; and the circumstances associated with the onset or cessation of coughing. Examination of voluntary coughing can also assist in patient evaluation because certain cough characteristics are associated with different pathologies. For example, patients with COPD often cough with poor inspiratory effort and negligible abdominal muscle compression, making the cough ineffective for airway clearance. Patients with COPD also often have

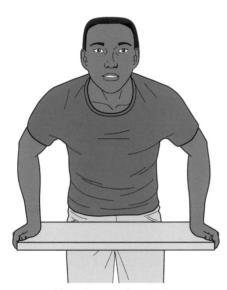

FIG. 24-1 Forward-bend or professorial posture.

TABLE 24-1	Breathing Patterns Commonly Found in the Examination of Patients with Airway Clearance Problems
Pattern of Breathing	**Description**
Apnea	Absence of ventilation
Fish-mouth	Apnea with concomitant mouth opening and closing; associated with neck extension and bradypnea
Eupnea	Normal rate, normal depth, regular rhythm
Bradypnea	Slow rate, shallow or normal depth, regular rhythm; associated with drug overdose
Tachypnea	Fast rate, shallow depth, regular rhythm; associated with restrictive lung disease
Hyperpnea	Normal rate, increased depth, regular rhythm
Cheyne-Stokes respiration (periodic)	Increasing then decreasing depth, periods of apnea interspersed with somewhat regular rhythm; associated with critically ill patients
Biot's respiration (cluster)	Slow rate, shallow depth, apneic periods, irregular rhythm; associated with CNS disorders such as meningitis
Apneustic	Slow rate, deep inspiration followed by apnea, irregular rhythm; associated with brainstem disorders
Prolonged expiration	Fast inspiration, slow and prolonged expiration yet normal rate, depth, regular rhythm; associated with obstructive lung disease
Orthopnea	Difficulty breathing in postures other than erect
Hyperventilation	Fast rate, increased depth, regular rhythm; results in decreased arterial carbon dioxide, tension; called "Kussmaul breathing" in metabolic acidosis; also associated with CNS disorders such as encephalitis
Psychogenic dyspnea	Normal rate, regular intervals of sighing; associated with anxiety
Dyspnea	Rapid rate, shallow depth, regular rhythm; associated with accessory muscle activity
Doorstop	Normal rate and rhythm; characterized by abrupt cessation of inspiration when restriction is encountered; associated with pleurisy

From Irwin S, Tecklin JS: *Cardiopulmonary Physical Therapy: A Guide to Practice*, ed 4, Philadelphia, 2004, Elsevier Science.
CNS, Central nervous system.

much paroxysmal coughing that can be very fatiguing because it is so frequent and ineffective.

Sputum inspection attempts to estimate or measure the quantity of expectorate raised per day. In addition to quantity, the color and consistency of any sputum raised should be evaluated.

The inspection phase of the chest examination closes with a brief examination of the abdomen to detect anything that may affect diaphragmatic function. Findings affecting diaphragm function may include morbid obesity; previous and recent abdominal surgeries, including colostomy; or insertion of a feeding tube. Findings from the inspection phase of the examination may be further elucidated and validated by the auscultation phase of the chest examination,.

Auscultation. Auscultation provides information about which parts of the lungs are being ventilated during breathing and about the location and presence of secretions in the lungs. Poor ventilation of an area may be addressed by breathing retraining or positional change, whereas accumulation of secretions may be addressed by specific airway clearance activities. During chest auscultation the patient should breathe in and out deeply with the mouth open.

A wide range of terminology is used to describe breath sounds.[38] Breath sounds are generated by the vibration and turbulence of airflow into and out of the airways and lung tissue during inspiration and expiration. Normal breath sounds can be divided into four specific types: Tracheal, bronchial, bronchovesicular, and vesicular. Each of these is considered normal when heard over a specific region of the thorax. However, when heard in a different region, these sounds are considered abnormal. Tracheal breath sounds are high-pitched, loud noises that sound like wind blowing through a pipe. There is a distinct absence of sound during the transition from inspiration to expiration. These sounds are considered normal when heard over the trachea. Bronchial breath sounds, which are similar to but quieter than tracheal sounds, are normal when heard next to the sternum near the major airways. When heard in any other area of the lungs, bronchial sounds usually indicate lung tissue that is consolidated, compressed, filled with fluid, or airless because of atelectasis. Vesicular breath sounds are low-pitched muffled sounds that have been described as a rustling sound similar to a gentle breeze blowing through the leaves of a tree.[39] Vesicular sounds are louder, longer, and higher in pitch during inspiration than expiration and are considered normal over all areas of the lung except where tracheal or bronchial sounds are expected. Vesicular breath sounds are abnormal if they are diminished or absent. Diminished or absent vesicular breath sounds can occur when underlying lung tissue is poorly ventilated, or when extensive hyperaeration reduces the transmission of vesicular sounds from the lung tissue. Bronchovesicular sounds, as one might expect, combine characteristics of bronchial and vesicular sounds. Inspiration and expiration are heard for similar times, at the same pitch, and with a slight break between the two phases. These sounds are normal when heard next to the sternum at the costosternal border at the sternal

angle and between the scapulae from about T3 through T6.[40]

Adventitious breath sounds are breath sounds that are always abnormal. These sounds are commonly placed into two categories (although more exist): *Crackles,* previously called rales, and *wheezes,* previously called rhonchi. Crackles are nonmusical sounds that may be mimicked by rolling several strands of hair near your ear or by listening to a bowl of cereal that crackles when the milk is added. Crackles may be heard throughout inspiration or only at its termination. Inspiratory crackles are common at the bases of the lungs in an erect subject. Inspiratory crackles may represent the sudden opening of airways previously closed by gravity and therefore may be a sign of abnormal lung deflation.[41,42] Expiratory crackles may be rhythmical or nonrhythmical. Rhythmical crackles may indicate the reopening of previously closed airways. Nonrhythmical crackles are generally low pitched and occur throughout the ventilatory cycle. They may indicate the presence of fluid in the large airways.

Wheezes are continuous and musical sounds that sound like whistling or growling. Wheezes are probably produced by air flowing at high velocities through narrowed airways. Their pitch varies with the velocity of airflow and the diameter of the airway. Wheezes may be monophonic (single tone) or polyphonic (multiple tones) and may be heard during inspiration or expiration. Inspiratory wheezes may be caused by airway stenosis and other types of intrinsic or extrinsic obstruction such as bronchospasm or foreign-body aspiration. Expiratory wheezes are more common than inspiratory wheezes.[39] They tend to be low pitched and polyphonic and may reflect unstable airways that have collapsed. Expiratory wheezes are associated with diffuse airway obstruction as may occur in patients with extensive secretions in their airways as associated with chronic bronchitis or cystic fibrosis. Monophonic expiratory wheezes occur when only one airway reaches the point of collapse.

Other adventitious sounds that may be detected during auscultation of the lungs include rubs and crunches. Rubs are coarse, grating leathery sounds. Pleural rubs are heard concurrently with the ventilatory cycle, whereas pericardial rubs are heard during the cardiac cycle. Rubs generally indicate inflammation.[39] Crunches are crackling sounds heard over the pericardium during systole and suggest the presence of air in the mediastinum, called mediastinal emphysema.

With these definitions and descriptions in mind, the therapist compares the quality, intensity, pitch, and distribution of the breath and voice sounds of homologous bronchopulmonary segments of the anterior, lateral, and posterior aspects of the chest. Fig. 24-2 presents one method for auscultating the chest.

On completing auscultation, the therapist must record and interpret the findings in a nomenclature acceptable to the institution. Normal breath and voice sounds in all bronchopulmonary segments suggest a normal examination. If inspection was also normal and the patient denied all pulmonary symptoms, one considers this portion of the chest examination normal and further examination is deferred. If breath sounds are abnormal or if adventitious

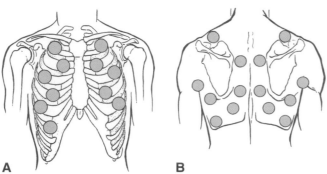

FIG. 24-2 A suggested method for chest auscultation. **A,** Anteriorly; **B,** posteriorly. *From Buckingham EB: A Primer of Clinical Diagnosis, ed 2, New York, 1979, Harper & Row. In Irwin S, Tecklin JS:* Cardiopulmonary Physical Therapy: A Guide to Practice, *ed 4, St. Louis, 1995, Mosby.*

sounds are present, the examination findings are abnormal but at this point inconclusive. Generally, decreased or absent breath sounds or inspiratory crackles suggest reduced ventilation. Crackles during both ventilatory cycles suggest impaired secretion clearance. Monophonic, biphasic wheezing suggests stenosis or bronchial smooth–muscle spasm. Polyphonic wheezing suggests diffuse airway obstruction. The absence of crackles and wheezes does not, however, ensure the absence of acute disease because patients with chronic obstructive lung disease may have hyperinflation so severe that adventitious sounds cannot be heard through the excessive air in the lungs. In summary, auscultation either confirms the findings of inspection or identifies areas of impaired ventilation or impaired secretion clearance.

Palpation. In general, palpation refines the information obtained previously. It further identifies any thoracoabdominal asymmetry or asynchrony detected during inspection by further examining the position of the mediastinum and motion of the thorax. Palpation of accessory muscles of inspiration permits specific examination of muscle activity identified grossly during inspection. The sternocleidomastoid and scalene muscle groups are the primary accessory muscles of inspiration.[43] Normally, accessory muscles are inactive during quiet breathing. Palpation of increased accessory muscle activity during inspiration indicates that the work of breathing is increased. Their use during stressful situations, such as physical exertion or acute illness, may be appropriate, but accessory muscle use during rest may add unnecessarily to the work of breathing. Patients with airway clearance dysfunction who have chronic lung disease often habitually and unnecessarily use their accessory muscles. Intervention may be directed at reducing accessory muscle use to conserve energy.

Steps for palpating the activity of accessory muscles of breathing
1. Position the patient with his or her back toward you.
2. Place your thumbs over the spinous processes so that your fingers reach around to the anterolateral aspect of the neck.

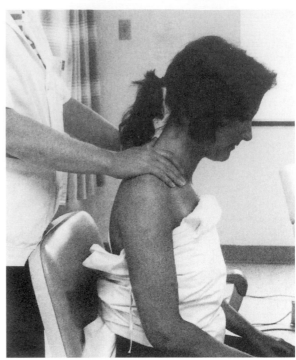

FIG. 24-3 Palpation of scalene muscle activity. *From Irwin S, Tecklin JS:* Cardiopulmonary Physical Therapy: A Guide to Practice, *ed 4, St. Louis, 1995, Mosby.*

3. Feel for activity and movement of scalenes and sternocleidomastoid muscles (Fig. 24-3).
4. Examine the area through at least two respiratory cycles.

The position of the mediastinum is generally determined by palpating the position of the trachea, which is normally in the midline. A lateral shift in the mediastinum, as determined by a shift of the trachea, occurs when intrathoracic pressure or lung volume differs between the two hemithoraces. The mediastinum shifts toward the affected side when lung volume is unilaterally decreased. The mediastinum shifts toward the unaffected side or contralaterally when pressure or volume is unilaterally increased.

Palpation can also be used to compare expansion of the upper, middle, and lower lobes of the lungs during quiet and deep breathing. In each case the therapist places the hands on the appropriate portion of the thorax and asks the patient to take in a normal or deep breath. The therapist compares the timing and extent of movement of each hand as the chest expands. Lobar motion, as reflected by thoracic motion, is considered normal when both hands move the same amount at the same time. This phase of palpation allows the therapist to localize any disproportionate expansion observed during inspection. For example, if inspection reveals asymmetrical chest expansion, palpation may not only localize the problem to the right upper lobe but may also identify a shift of the mediastinum to the right of midline. Together these signs suggest that the problem is either a loss of volume in the right upper lobe or an increase of volume in the left upper lobe.

Vocal fremitus is the vibration produced by the voice and transmitted to the chest wall, where it can be detected by the hand as a tactile vibration called *fremitus*. The therapist evaluates fremitus by comparing the intensity of the vibrations detected by each hand during quiet breathing and speech. It is normal for the vibrations to be equal and moderate during speech. Fremitus is abnormal when it is increased or decreased. Increased fremitus suggests a loss or decrease in ventilation in the underlying lung because sound is transmitted more strongly through non–air-filled lung tissue.[44] Decreased fremitus suggests increased air within the underlying lung because sound is transmitted more poorly through hyperinflated lung tissue.[37]

Rhonchal fremitus describes vibrations detected during quiet breathing caused by turbulent airflow through or around retained secretions in the airways. Rhonchal fremitus is therefore always abnormal. Identification of rhonchal fremitus permits the therapist to locate secretions or to better identify reasons for decreased breath sounds found during auscultation.

Palpation may also be used to identify and localize some types of chest pain to help determine the safety of continuing further examination and intervention. Palpation facilitates identification of characteristics and descriptors associated with the pain for more complete and effective communication with the patient's physician and may provide information about the source of chest pain, which may include musculoskeletal problems, coronary artery disease, malignancy, cervical disk or nerve root disease, thoracic outlet syndrome, herpes zoster, or pulmonary embolism. Identifying the probable anatomical source of chest pain requires associating the type of pain and its stimulus (Table 24-2). Matching the sensory distribution of the pain to the appropriate anatomical structure may also help the therapist identify the anatomical source of the pain. Table 24-3 presents the segmental innervation of the structures of the chest and abdomen. Fig. 24-4 illustrates the distribution of the cervical and thoracic dermatomes.

When chest pain is identified, the therapist should also ask about the onset, character, duration, and severity of this pain. Chest pain associated with cardiac disease is important to identify because of its serious potential consequences. Such pain is often described as heaviness or crushing pain that radiates toward the neck, jaw, left

TABLE 24-3	Segmental Innervation of the Chest and Abdomen
Cord Segments	**Structure**
T1-4	Mediastinal contents: Heart, aorta, pulmonary vessels
T3-8	Descending aorta
T4-8	Esophagus
T3-5	Trachea and bronchi
T7-9	Upper abdominal viscera
C5-T1	Chest wall; apical parietal pleura
T2-8	Remainder parietal; upper pericardial pleura
T6-8	Peripheral diaphragm
C3-5	Central diaphragm; lower pericardial pleura
T2-10	Intercostal muscles; ribs
C5-T1	Pectoral muscles
C3-4	Skin overlying shoulders
T1-2	Upper arms, inner surface
T3-8	Skin on chest wall

Adapted from Edmeads J, Billings RF: Neurological and psychological aspects of chest pain. In Levene DL (ed): *Chest Pain: An Integrated Diagnostic Approach,* Philadelphia, 1977, Lea and Febiger.

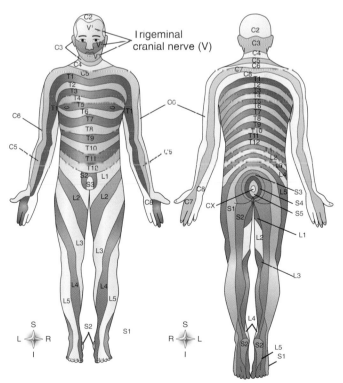

FIG. 24-4 Dermatome distribution of the spinal nerves. *From Thibodeau GA, Patton KT:* Anatomy and Physiology, *ed 6, St. Louis, 2006, Mosby.*

TABLE 24-2	Guideline for Identifying the Probable Source of Chest Pain	
Symptom Characteristics	**Effective Stimulus**	**Anatomical Source**
Sharp	Fine touch	Skin
Superficial	Pinprick	
Burning	Heat	
Precisely localize	Cold	
Dull or sharp	Movement	Chest wall
Intermediate depth	Deep pressure	
Aching		
Generally located		
Dull	Ischemia	Thoracic viscera
Deep	Distention	
Aching	Muscle spasm	
Diffuse, vaguely localized		

Adapted from Edmeads J, Billings RF: Neurological and psychological aspects of chest pain. In Levene DL (ed): *Chest Pain: An Integrated Diagnostic Approach,* Philadelphia, 1977, Lea and Febiger.

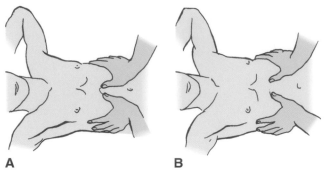

A   **B**

FIG. 24-5 Palpation of diaphragmatic motion. **A,** At rest. **B,** At the end of a normal inspiration. *From Cherniack RM, Cherniack L, Naimark A:* Respiration in Health and Disease, *ed 2, Philadelphia, 1972, WB Saunders. In Irwin S, Tecklin JS:* Cardiopulmonary Physical Therapy: A Guide to Practice, *ed 4, St. Louis, 1995, Mosby.*

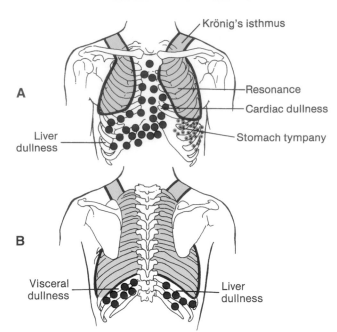

FIG. 24-6 Normal resonance pattern of the chest with percussion. **A,** Anteriorly; **B,** posteriorly. *Adapted from Irwin S, Tecklin JS:* Cardiopulmonary Physical Therapy: A Guide to Practice, *ed 4, St. Louis, 1995, Mosby.*

upper extremity, and midscapular region and generally is not affected by palpation.[45]

During the last phase of palpation, movement of the diaphragm is identified as normal or abnormal. Fig. 24-5 presents one method of examining diaphragmatic motion. Normal motion of the diaphragm produces equal upward motion of the costal margins. Inward motion of the costal margins during inspiration is associated with a flattened diaphragm that commonly occurs in individuals with chronic airway clearance dysfunction and COPD.[46] Flattening of the diaphragm caused by severe hyperinflation may reduce the ability of the diaphragm to contract because it alters the length-tension relationship of the muscle fibers.[46]

Percussion. Percussion (mediate percussion) is the fourth and final part of the chest examination. It enables the clinician to associate any symptoms and signs previously uncovered that suggest changes in lung density, and it allows one to establish the borders of abnormally dense lung areas and normally occurring organs. Finally, percussion allows examination of the extent of diaphragmatic motion. Percussion is performed by tapping the finger of one hand against the middle finger of the other hand placed on the chest wall. The middle finger should be placed at rib interspaces. The sound produced by the tapping will be affected by the density of the underlying tissue, with denser tissue (poorly inflated lung or other solid tissue) sounding flat or dull and less dense tissue (hyperinflated lung) sounding hyperresonant or tympanic. When examining lung density by percussion, the therapist may identify one of three sounds or notes: Normal, dull, or tympanic. (It should be noted that physicians identify five notes: Tympanic, hyperresonant, resonant, dull, and flat, but three serve the purpose for PTs.) A normal note is produced when percussion is performed over the thorax adjacent to resonant lung of normal density. A dull note is soft, brief, high-pitched, and thud-like and is heard over the thorax with lung of increased density because it is less air-filled. A dull note can be simulated by percussion over the liver or the thigh. A tympanic note is loud, lengthy, low pitched, and hollow and is heard over the thorax in areas of excessive air such as

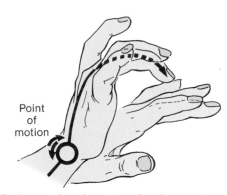

FIG. 24-7 Correct hand position for diagnostic percussion. *Adapted from Buckingham EB:* A Primer of Clinical Diagnosis, *ed 2, New York, 1979, Harper & Row.*

hyperinflated lung. A tympanic note can be simulated by percussion over the empty stomach.

Normally dense, resonant lung can be found from the clavicle to the sixth rib anteriorly, the eighth rib laterally, and the tenth rib posteriorly (Fig. 24-6). The correct hand position for percussion is presented in Fig. 24-7.

In a normal examination, the resonance is similar across homologous lung segments (i.e., in lung segments in similar positions within each hemithorax). Moreover, to be normal, the resonance must extend throughout the anatomical limits of the lungs. Abscesses, tumors, cysts, pneumonia, and areas of atelectasis can produce changes in lung density and result in abnormal percussive notes. Lung borders are affected by volume changes in either the abdomen or lungs. Abnormally high lung bases are associated with increased abdominal volume as seen in pregnancy. Abnormally low lung bases are associated with increased lung volumes because of hyperinflation as is typical in chronic obstructive lung disease. These and other variations in lung borders can be identified by mediate percussion.[47]

Aerobic Capacity and Endurance. Among the many reasons for testing for aerobic capacity and endurance are the following: (1) identifying through standardized protocols the baseline ability of the patient, (2) determining the capacity of the patient to perform functional activities, (3) predicting the response of the patient to physiological demands during periods of increased or stressful physical activity, and (4) recognizing symptoms that may limit the patient's ability to respond to an increased workload. The many modes of testing range from noting symptomatic responses to a standard exercise challenge to instrumented technically sophisticated invasive aerobic testing in an exercise laboratory. Exercise testing to determine aerobic capacity typically involves progressive or incremental increases in exercise intensity while walking on a treadmill or riding a bicycle ergometer, as described in detail in Chapter 23.

Function

Orthotic, Protective, and Supportive Devices. Individuals with respiratory difficulty leading to airway clearance dysfunction often use supplemental oxygen devices, including metal oxygen cylinders of various sizes, liquid oxygen systems, oxygen concentration devices, and oxygen from wall-mounted oxygen sources in hospitals and nursing homes (as described in detail in Chapter 26). Oxygen may be delivered from these sources by nasal cannula or mask. The PT must determine the level of oxygen being used and portability of the oxygen device if gait training and ambulation activities are employed.

EVALUATION, DIAGNOSIS, AND PROGNOSIS

Outcomes from therapy for the patient with airway clearance dysfunction can include significant reduction in a pathological process such as atelectasis. Most commonly, impairments that improve will include ABG levels, pulmonary function test performance, breathing pattern and rate, and dyspnea scores. Rating of perceived exertion during activities will also commonly improve, as well as participation in functional abilities such as transfers, ambulation and other modes of mobility. Safety, health, wellness, and patient satisfaction can also be affected by instruction of the patient and family in home use of airway clearance techniques.

INTERVENTION

COORDINATION, COMMUNICATION, AND DOCUMENTATION

Coordination, communication, and documentation are interventions used for all patients and are particularly important for this preferred practice pattern because patients with impaired airway clearance generally have needs for intervention by many different types of health care professionals. Patients may need various types of equipment, help at home, or placement in some type of

assisted living situation and often require ongoing case management. In addition, collaboration with various agencies, such as home care practitioners, equipment providers, and third party payers, is often necessary to ensure continuation of care across varied settings. Complex cases often include an interdisciplinary effort that requires communication across and between disciplines, with occasional referral to other professionals not involved with the team.

PATIENT/CLIENT-RELATED INSTRUCTION

Education and training about the lung disease underlying the airway clearance dysfunction is critically important for self efficacy in patients in this preferred practice pattern.[18] The American Thoracic Society cites education as one of the four major components of any pulmonary rehabilitation program and includes the items in the following list as important parts of the educational component:[49]

1. Structure and function of the lung
2. Information regarding their specific disease
3. Instruction and participation in correct inhaler technique
4. Airway clearance techniques
5. Breathing, relaxation, and panic control techniques
6. Respiratory muscle training
7. Exercise principles
8. ADLs and instrumental ADLs (IADLs)
9. Nutrition interventions and considerations
10. Medications—their effects and side effects
11. Psychosocial interventions and means of coping with stress, anxiety, and depression
12. Avoidance of environmental irritants
13. Smoking cessation
14. Oxygen rationale and proper use of oxygen-delivery devices
15. Travel and leisure activities
16. Sexuality
17. End-of-life issues and planning for those with progressive diseases

Individualized teaching or a series of short, interactive lectures are commonly employed. Videotapes, digital video disks (DVDs), and CD ROMs are available regarding specific topics as are various Internet web sites. If the patient seems overwhelmed by the amount of information presented, it may be helpful to provide them with a well-organized notebook to refer to as needed. The ultimate goal for patient-related instruction in individuals with airway clearance dysfunction is to provide basic knowledge about their disease, its medical management, and daily techniques and activities to enhance their quality of life while recognizing the limitations imposed by the disease process.

AIRWAY CLEARANCE TECHNIQUES

Airway clearance techniques include a range of therapeutic interventions intended to clear the airways of secretions and other debris in individuals with pulmonary disease or respiratory impairment or those who are at risk for developing those conditions. The interventions include various physical maneuvers, manual procedures, breathing techniques, use of equipment, and instruction.

A PT, a respiratory therapist, a nurse or other health care worker, a family member, or the patient may apply airway clearance techniques to maintain patent airways and thereby reduce or eliminate airway obstruction, enhance ventilation, and reduce the likelihood of new or continuing infection of the respiratory tract.

The medical profession recognizes that providing airway clearance intervention is important despite its high costs in terms of treatment time and financial resources. Several major "state-of-the-art" reviews on airway clearance interventions have appeared in the literature over the past quarter century.[50-52] At least two professions, physical therapy and respiratory therapy, have promulgated standards of practice regarding some of the skills employed in airway clearance.[2,53] Interdisciplinary educational efforts that incorporate the professions involved in airway clearance have received federal funding in past decades. Furthermore, more than "... two generations of physicians have been taught that retention of excessive secretions in the respiratory tract is not only bad for pulmonary function but can also be lethal to the patient."[54]

Airway clearance, in one of its many forms, is a universally employed intervention for patients with virtually all types of pediatric and adult lung diseases. There are many approaches, specific techniques, and traditions for removal of secretions and other debris from the patient's airway. However, there is a dearth of well-designed, methodologically sound, properly carried out, statistically adequately analyzed studies to support one particular technique over another. The choice of airway clearance approach should therefore be based on patient needs, therapist skill, and personal choices regarding the effectiveness of these techniques. This section presents the major approaches and techniques for airway clearance.

Breathing Strategies for Airway Clearance

Forced Expiratory Technique. The forced expiratory technique (FET) employs a forced expiration or huff after a medium-sized breath.[55] The patient is instructed to take a medium breath (to midlung volume) then tighten the abdominal muscles firmly while huffing (expiring forcibly but with an opened glottis), without contracting the throat muscles. The "huff" should be maintained long enough to mobilize and remove distal bronchial secretions without stimulating a spasmodic cough. The important part of FET is the period (15-30 seconds) of relaxation with gentle diaphragmatic breathing following 1 or 2 huffs. This helps relax the airways as secretions continue to be mobilized during the deep breathing. Once secretions are felt in the larger, uppermost airways, a huff or double cough should remove them.

Active Cycle of Breathing Technique. Because of alleged misinterpretation of the technique by other practitioners, the FET was reconfigured into the active cycle of breathing technique (ACBT). ACBT uses several individual breathing strategies in sequential combination to accomplish the goals of mobilization and evacuation of bronchial secretions. As with FET, self-treatment without the need for an assistant or caregiver is the major advantage to ACBT. A suggested sequence for ACBT is as follows:

- Breath control, another name for diaphragmatic breathing, is performed for 15-30 seconds in a quiet, relaxed manner.
- Several attempts at thoracic expansion are performed. (There is divergence of opinion regarding the necessity of having the patient assume one of the many postural drainage positions during this phase. Some might also suggest using the manual techniques of percussion or vibration during the expiratory phase of breathing.)
- Breath control is repeated for 15-30 seconds.
- Thoracic expansion is repeated.

This alternating cycle of breath control and thoracic expansion may continue until the patient feels ready to expectorate the built-up secretions. FET and huffing or coughing, as described, is performed next to help evacuate the accumulated secretions. The repeated sequence of breath control and expansion is begun again.

Autogenic Drainage. Autogenic drainage (AD) is another airway clearance technique that permits self-treatment.[56] AD is performed in a sitting position and requires that patients determine (through proprioceptive, sensory, and auditory signals) when bronchial secretions are present in the smaller, medium, or larger airways. The patient then learns to breathe at low, medium, and high lung volumes to mobilize secretions in those airways.

Sequence of autogenic drainage

1. The patient sits upright with a minimum of distractions in the room.
2. After a brief period of diaphragmatic breathing, the patient exhales to a low lung volume and breathes at a normal *tidal volume* at that low lung volume. This is the "unsticking phase" of AD.
3. As the patient becomes aware of secretions in those smaller airways, breathing becomes a bit deeper and moves into midlung volume. This is the "collecting phase" in which secretions are mobilized proximally into the midsized airways.
4. At this point, breathing becomes deeper at normal to high lung volumes. The patient is asked to suppress coughing until it cannot be avoided. This "evacuation phase" enables secretions to accumulate in central airways and be evacuated by huffing or a cough, using minimal effort.

Proponents of AD believe it can be applied in all types of obstructive lung disease and for postoperative treatment and can be taught to children as young as 5-6 years of age. Intensive training in the technique is necessary before it can be used effectively. Recent research on AD found that ACBT and AD were comparable in improving ventilation, removing secretions, and enhancing pulmonary function.[57] AD in subjects with CF was less likely to cause oxygen desaturation during treatment than traditional postural drainage with percussion (as described in the section on Manual and Mechanical Technique).[58] Another study examined the effects of either AD or ACBT randomized as a treatment to 30 males with COPD over a

20-day period. The two techniques were comparable in that each improved performance on standard pulmonary functions tests and perception of dyspnea. However, AD resulted in better improvement in both oxygen saturation and *hypercapnia.*[59]

Coughing and Huffing. Coughing and huffing is an effective means of removing secretions and is critically important for the individual with airway clearance dysfunction. Coughing may be reflexive or voluntary. A reflexive cough has four phases: Irritation, inspiration, compression, and expulsion, whereas a voluntary cough has only the latter three phases. To be effective for airway clearance, either type of cough must generate enough force to clear secretions from the larger airways and move secretions from as far down as the twelfth generation of bronchial branching.[60]

Huffing is a popular airway clearance technique consisting of a single large inspiration followed by short expiratory efforts interrupted by pauses. The glottis remains open during huffing to reduce the potential for side effects that may occur from cough (bronchoconstriction, spasms of coughing, and marked swings in thoracic pressure or cerebral blood flow). Huffing has been recommended in lieu of coughing because it is thought to reduce the physical work of the activity. However, research has not shown huffing to be any more energy efficient than coughing.[61]

Some studies have shown that coughing alone can be as effective at airway clearance as traditional bronchial drainage with percussion in certain patient populations, particularly those with intact strength such as patients with CF.[62,63] If these techniques fail to clear the airway, endotracheal suctioning may be necessary, but where possible, coughing or huffing are preferred because suctioning can injure the tracheal epithelium and may cause sudden *hypoxemia* or vagal stimulation, which may lead to cardiac dysrhythmias.[64,65]

Proper cough technique, which facilitates airway clearance, requires that the patient sequentially (1) inspires to or near a maximal inspiration; (2) closes the glottis; (3) "bears down" by tightening the abdominal, perineal, gluteal, and shoulder depressor muscles to increase intrathoracic and intraabdominal pressures; and (4) suddenly opens the glottis to enable the pressurized inspired air to suddenly escape to provide the expulsive force. The patient should cough no more than two times during each expulsive, expiratory phase—a "double cough." To continue beyond this "double cough" usually produces little added benefit. Proper cough technique after surgery may also require incisional splinting. Splinting an abdominal or thoracic incision is commonly performed by having the patient hold a small pillow firmly against the incision while attempting to cough or using the hands to approximate the edges of the incision while attempting to cough. There is no scientific evidence that this type of splinting improves cough, but there is a great deal of anecdotal commentary on the usefulness of the techniques. Following are techniques that can be used to improve cough:

1. Positioning—sitting in the forward leaning posture with the neck flexed, the arms supported, and the feet firmly planted on the floor—promotes effective coughing (Fig. 24-8).

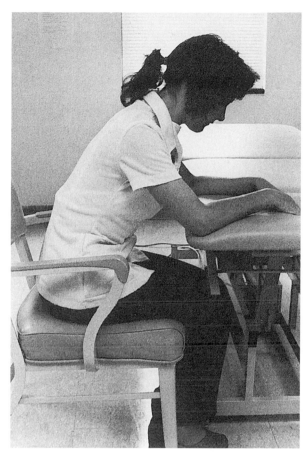

FIG. 24-8 Recommended position for effective coughing. *From Irwin S, Tecklin JS:* Cardiopulmonary Physical Therapy: A Guide to Practice, *ed 4, St. Louis, 1995, Mosby.*

2. Tracheal stimulation—pressure or vibration applied to the extrathoracic trachea—may elicit a reflex cough.
3. Pressure applied to the midrectus abdominis area after inspiration—may improve cough effectiveness if the pressure is suddenly released.
4. Pressure applied along the lower costal borders during exhalation—may improve the effectiveness of an impaired cough.

Manual and Mechanical Techniques

Postural Drainage with Chest Percussion, Vibration, and Shaking. This group of techniques is often referred to as "chest physiotherapy," "chest PT," "postural drainage," "bronchial drainage," or simply "physio" and represents the classic and traditional approach to airway clearance that has been used for many decades. Although the evidence for superiority of this technique over other more modern approaches is lacking, a number of studies have found it to be as effective as some of the newer equipment-intensive approaches to airway clearance described, including high-frequency chest compression,[66] intrapulmonary percussive ventilation (IPV),[67] and treatment with Flutter devices.[68] Furthermore, the experience of several generations of committed physicians, PTs, respiratory therapists and nurses has borne out the ongoing utility of

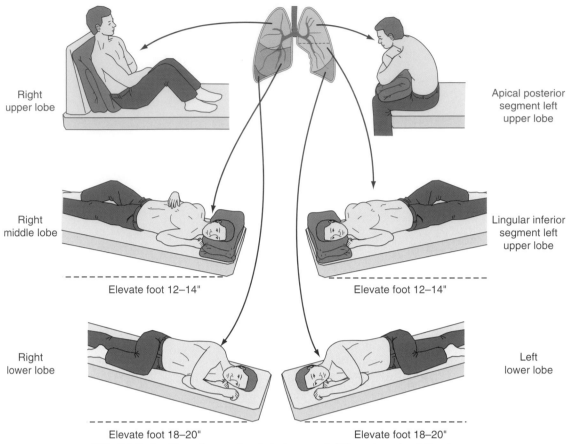

Right
upper lobe

Apical posterior
segment left
upper lobe

Right
middle lobe

Lingular inferior
segment left
upper lobe

Elevate foot 12–14"   Elevate foot 12–14"

Right
lower lobe

Left
lower lobe

Elevate foot 18–20"   Elevate foot 18–20"

FIG. 24-9 Positions for postural drainage of different parts of the lungs.

this approach to airway clearance. In addition, the face validity of airway clearance for properly selected patients is undeniable. As a result, most patients with chronic and acute respiratory problems that produce voluminous secretions are currently treated with some airway clearance technique, whether it be manual or mechanical.

Positioning. Before manual or mechanical approaches are used to loosen and mobilize secretions, it is generally recommended that the patient be positioned to optimally drain a particular lung segment or lobe. This requires that the area to be drained is uppermost, with the bronchus from the area in as close to a vertical position as possible or reasonable. Some refer to this notion as the "ketchup bottle theory." To get ketchup from the bottle, it must be turned upside down (and shaken).[69] Fig. 24-9 shows positions for postural drainage of different parts of the lungs.

These positions may need to be modified under certain conditions, including increased intracranial pressure, decreased arterial oxygen tension, decreased cardiac output, decreased forced expiratory volume in 1 second (FEV_1), decreased specific airway conductance, pulmonary hemorrhage (hemoptysis), gastroesophageal reflux (particularly common in infants and children), and severe dyspnea. Typically, the modification consists of reducing the angle for head-down positions for the middle lobe, lingula, and lower lobes. With severe dyspnea or gastroesophageal reflux and with increased intracranial pressure, all positions for the middle lobe, lingula, and lower lobes

should be performed with the patient flat with no decline. Recent research indicates that in infants with CF, the head–down tipped position should be avoided for the first year of life because this position stimulates gastroesophageal reflux that can adversely affect lung tissue.[70]

Percussion and Vibration. Often referred to as "manual techniques" of airway clearance, percussion and vibration of the thorax are performed to loosen accumulated secretions. These techniques are intended to enhance movement of secretions to the more proximal airways during positioning for gravity-assisted postural drainage. Some clinicians also advocate "chest shaking," a more vigorous type of vibration. Percussion and vibration are usually performed in an area of the thorax corresponding to the lung segment being drained while the patient is positioned specifically to allow gravity to assist in secretion drainage.

Percussion, a massage stroke originally called "tapotement," involves rhythmically clapping with a cupped hand for 2-5 minutes over the appropriate area of thorax being drained by gravity (Fig. 24-10). Percussion may feel uncomfortable but should not be painful; a layer of clothing or towel may be employed to reduce any discomfort.

Vibration often follows percussion, although some advocate its use in lieu of percussion, particularly in postoperative treatment and in those for whom percussion should be done with caution (see Table 24-4). Vibration involves placing one's hands on the area previously per-

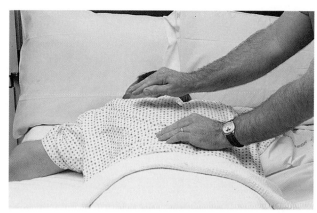

FIG. 24-10 Correct hand position for therapeutic chest percussion. *From Potter PA, Perry AG:* Fundamentals of Nursing, *ed 6, St. Louis, 2005, Mosby.*

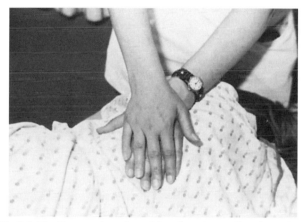

FIG. 24-11 Correct hand position for chest vibration. *From Frownfelter D, Dean E:* Cardiovascular and Pulmonary Physical Therapy: Evidence and Practice, *ed 4, St. Louis, 2006, Mosby.*

TABLE 24-4	Conditions in Which Caution in the Application of Therapeutic Percussion Is Recommended
Type of Condition	**Characteristics**
Cardiovascular	Chest wall pain
	Unstable angina
	Hemodynamic lability
	Low platelet count
	Anticoagulation therapy
	Unstable or potentially lethal dysrhythmias
Musculoskeletal	Osteoporosis
	Prolonged steroid therapy
	Costochondritis
	Osteomyelitis
	Osteogenesis imperfecta
	Spinal fusion
	Rib fracture or flail chest
Pulmonary	Bronchospasm
	Hemoptysis
	Severe dyspnea
	Untreated lung abscess
	Pneumothorax
	Immediately after chest tube removal
	Pneumonia or other infectious process
	Pulmonary embolus
Oncological	Cancer metastasis to the ribs or spine
	Carcinoma in the bronchus
	Resectable tumor
	Osteoporosis secondary to chemotherapeutic agents
Miscellaneous	Recent skin grafts
	Burns
	Open thoracic wounds
	Skin infection in the thoracic region
	Subcutaneous emphysema in the head or back regions
	Immediately after cataract surgery

cussed (Fig. 24-11) and having the patient perform several deep breaths using sustained maximal inspiration as in the ACBT maneuver. During the expiratory phase, the therapist performs a fine, tremulous vibration to the chest wall. This may be repeated several times, although in individuals with copious secretions, the first vibratory effort often stimulates coughing and evacuation of secretions and debris.

As with positioning, there are pathological conditions that may be contraindications to manual techniques or that may require that such techniques be applied cautiously (Table 24-4). The basis for the recommendations in Table 24-4 is not always clear.

Mechanical Devices for Airway Clearance

High-Frequency Chest Wall Oscillation. High-frequency chest wall oscillation (HFCWO) is provided by a device that uses an air compressor and a garment (a vest) that has inflatable bladders attached to the compressor by large, flexible tubing (Fig. 24-12). The compressor pumps bursts of air at varying frequencies (1-20 Hz) and varying pressures into the bladders within the vest. The bursts

of air entering the vest bladder transmit oscillations or vibrations to the chest wall. Studies on HFCWO in dogs suggest that the bursts of air produce a shearing force on secretions within the airways and increase airflow into and out of the airways.[70] Clinical studies have shown that HFCWO is as effective in the short term as manual bronchial drainage techniques.[66,71] Warwick and Hansen followed 16 patients with CF using HFCWO for a period of 22 months. They determined that regression slopes for pulmonary function were slightly improved when compared to the period of time before instituting HFCWO.[72] HFCWO produced changes in 50 patients with CF hospitalized for acute pulmonary exacerbation equivalent to the improvements typically produced by traditional postural drainage with percussion and vibration.[66] Tecklin and colleagues found that HFCWO applied to 102 children with CF produced similar outcomes in terms of various pulmonary function tests, clinical radiology scores, and days hospitalized across 1 year, as did bronchial drainage techniques applied to 55 other children with CF.[72] HFCWO, which is typically used twice each day at several different frequencies for a total of 30 minutes per treat-

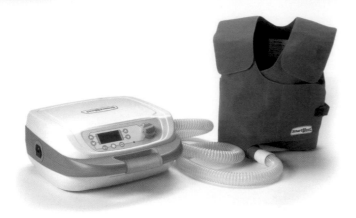

FIG. 24-12 High-frequency chest wall oscillation (HFCWO) device. *Courtesy Electromed, Inc., New Prague, Minn.*

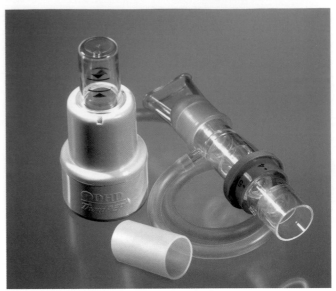

FIG. 24-13 A positive expiratory pressure (PEP) device. *Courtesy Smiths Medical, Rockland, Mass.*

ment, can be used concurrently with nebulized bronchodilators and mucolytics, whose deposition may increased by the enhanced airflow generated by HFCWO.[73] Originally used for young adults with CF, HFCWO is now also used in other people with long-term need for airway clearance such as those who have undergone heart/lung transplantation and those with respiratory pump dysfunction secondary to chronic neuromuscular disorders.

Intrapulmonary Percussive Ventilation. Intrapulmonary percussive ventilation (IPV) is a type of airway clearance administered via a pneumatic device called a high-frequency intrapulmonary percussive device. The patient breathes through a mouthpiece that delivers a preset driving pressure and frequency of intra-airway oscillations from a nebulizer-like apparatus. The device automatically activates during exhalation to provide intrapulmonary percussion at 11-30 Hz. The device simultaneously delivers positive expiratory pressure at 2-8 cm H_2O and an aerosol inhalation of normal saline at 1 ml/min, with particle size distribution of 2-4 μm. During the percussive bursts of air and saline into the lungs, the inspiratory flow opens airways and enhances secretion mobilization. Although it is not used as frequently in the United States as other modes of airway clearance, some data support the efficacy of IPV. Newhouse and colleagues found no significant differences among IPV, traditional chest physical therapy, and Flutter in the ability to produce sputum in subjects with CF.[74] Varekojis et al found that dry sputum weights were not different among IPV, HFCWO, and vigorous chest physical therapy delivered for 2 days each in 24 subjects with CF.[67] IPV appears to be a reasonable alternative for airway clearance, although it has not been a particularly popular approach in the United States.

Positive Expiratory Pressure. Positive expiratory pressure (PEP) breathing employs another mechanical device for airway clearance dysfunction (Fig. 24-13). This device tries to maintain airway patency by applying positive pressure during expiration with the goal of dislodging and moving secretions proximally in the respiratory tract. PEP was originally provided via an anesthesia face mask, but a mouthpiece can also be used to deliver this treatment. As the patient exhales, the valve of the PEP device provides a positive pressure of 10-20 cm H_2O within the airways. This positive pressure stabilizes the small airways and prevents their collapse, which would otherwise trap the secretions distal to the point of collapse and interfere with evacuation of secretions by huffing or coughing. In addition to assisting in secretion removal, PEP may help reduce air trapping by stabilizing the small airways and thus enhancing collateral ventilation through pores of Kohn and canals of Lambert (interconnections between adjacent alveolar sacs and respiratory bronchioles, respectively). When using PEP, patients should take a large breath in and then breathe out slowly. While breathing out, the patient will experience positive pressure from the PEP device. Many PEP devices have an indicator that shows how much pressure is being exerted. Pressure of 10-20 cm H_2O should be maintained throughout the full expiration. This procedure is repeated for 10-20 breaths and is followed by huffing or coughing to expel accumulated secretions. Some recommend performing the PEP maneuver while the patient is in bronchial drainage positions.

PEP has been shown to be more effective than bronchial drainage and vibratory positive expiratory pressure in patients with cystic fibrosis.[75,76] PEP is an effective, inexpensive, well-researched, and universally employed airway clearance device. It can be used effectively by people who can understand and follow the instructions. It is not particularly useful, however, for patients with significant neuromuscular weakness or dyscoordination who may not be able to achieve adequate flows to receive the benefits.

Use of a PEP device
Therapist washes hands and assembles the PEP device.

Patient sits upright with elbows resting on a table.
Patient completes a diaphragmatic breath with a larger than normal volume.
Patient holds the inspiratory breath for 2-3 seconds.
Patient exhales fully but not forced to functional residual capacity (FRC) through the device.
The pressure manometer should read 10-20 cm H_2O pressure during exhalation.
Therapist adjusts the orifice to result in an inspiratory-to-expiratory time ratio of 1 : 3.
Patient performs 10-20 breaths.
Follow with huffing or coughing.
Repeat the cycle of 10-20 breaths at least 3-4 times.

Vibratory Positive Expiratory Pressure. Two vibratory positive expiratory pressure devices, the Flutter (Axcan-Pharma, Birmingham, Ala) (Fig. 24-14) and the Acapella (Smiths Medical, Rockland, Mass) (Fig. 24-15), are commonly employed. Each adds oscillation during the expi-ratory cycle of PEP breathing. The Flutter employs a pipelike device with a metal ball that is dislodged and reseated in its reservoir during expiratory effort. The dislodgment and reseating of the ball opens and closes the expiratory port, which in turn oscillates the expiratory airflow. The Acapella oscillates airflow using a magnet and a rocker with a metal pin. The variable distance between the pin and the magnet should be matched and set to the patient's needs to create the appropriate resistance and desired length of expiration.

The Flutter is more technique-dependent than the Acapella because the Flutter must be positioned correctly for the ball to be properly dislodged against gravity. The Flutter was shown to have similar clinical efficacy to manual airway clearance techniques in a well-designed and controlled 2-week study in hospitalized patients in which patients with CF were randomized to a Flutter group or a chest physical therapy group. After the 2-week period, there were no differences between the groups in pulmonary function changes and exercise tolerance.[77]

A recent paper by Volsko et al shows that performance characteristics of the Acapella are similar to the Flutter.[78] Additionally, the Acapella can be used at very low expiratory flows and can generate PEP at any angle because it is not gravity dependent.[78]

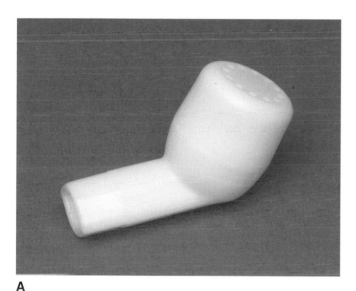

A

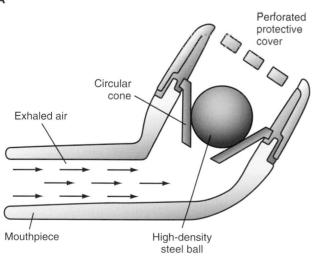

Perforated protective cover

Circular cone

Exhaled air

Mouthpiece

High-density steel ball

B

FIG. 24-14 The Flutter device. *Courtesy Axcan Pharma, Birmingham, Ala.*

Suggested sequence for use of the Flutter and the Acapella
Therapist washes hands and makes sure device is ready for use.
Patient is seated with back and head erect.
Patient places device in mouth and inhales more deeply than normal but not fully.
Patient holds the inspiratory breath for 2-3 seconds.
Patient now exhales fully but not forced through the device.
Patient must hold cheeks firmly (not puffed out) to direct oscillation into the airways.
Patient repeats each inspiratory/expiratory cycle 5-10 times and suppresses cough.
Patient next takes 2 deep breaths in and out through the device.
Patient attempts to remove sputum via huffing or coughing.
Patient repeats the entire process 2-3 times

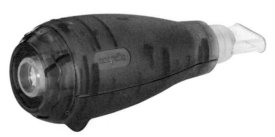

FIG. 24-15 The Acapella airway clearance device. *Courtesy Smiths Medical, Rockland, Mass.*

Assistive Devices. Percussors and vibrators have been used to assist with manual techniques of airway clearance for many years. These devices have been shown to produce similar changes in patients with CF in both pulmonary function and secretion production as unassisted manual airway clearance techniques alone but with less effort.[79] These devices may be powered by compressed gas or electricity. Because an electrical motor could generate a spark that could cause an explosion around high concentrations of oxygen, the use of electrically powered devices is contraindicated around patients receiving supplemental oxygen.

THERAPEUTIC EXERCISE

Aerobic Capacity/Endurance Conditioning or Reconditioning. Patients with pulmonary disease with associated inability to clear their airway often experience dyspnea on exertion that leads to abstaining from any activity that precipitates this unpleasant sensation. This continued avoidance of activity further decreases exercise tolerance and in turn lowers the patient's dyspnea threshold, thereby resulting in dyspnea with even minimal physical exertion such as produced by performing ADLs. Exercise is the most common and useful intervention to break this vicious cycle of deterioration. A cautionary note is that the work of breathing during physical activity in patients with airway clearance dysfunction and COPD may constitute a major portion of their oxygen consumption, which may reduce their ability to achieve the workload one might expect. Therefore the therapist must administer the exercise program judiciously and with close monitoring for signs of early fatigue that may include cyanosis and abnormal vital signs.

Rehabilitation interventions to improve aerobic capacity and exercise tolerance vary widely. They may be formal, based on a strictly derived exercise prescription, or informal, started from an arbitrary point and progressed according to a patient's symptoms and tolerance. They may require equipment like treadmills or bicycle ergometers or merely require enough space to permit obstacle-free walking. Participants may have either subacute pulmonary disease or chronic pulmonary disease of varying severity, and the exercise regimen may begin in any setting from intensive care to home. Exercise may be administered while the patient breathes room air or supplemental oxygen. Completion of the programs may require several days, several months, or longer. Some indications for oxygen-supplemented exercise include right heart failure, cor pulmonale, resting partial pressure of arterial oxygen (PaO$_2$) of 50 mm Hg or less on room air, inability to tolerate exercise while breathing room air,[80] and oxygen saturation below 80% during physical exertion and while performing ADLs when breathing room air.[81]

Preparation for any aerobic exercise program requires determining the degree and type of monitoring needed to preserve the patient's safety. No formal guidelines that establish the monitoring requirements for informal exercise programs have been published; this determination must be made according to individual circumstances. Final preparation for any exercise program requires that the therapist and patient identify a mutually acceptable goal for the program and develop a plan for periodically evaluating progress toward that goal, often with the advice of a physician.

There are clear instances in which an exercise session should be terminated. Some of these reasons for termination are physiological, and others are symptom related. The exercise session should be terminated in the presence of the following:

- Premature ventricular contractions in pairs, runs, or increasing frequency
- New onset atrial dysrhythmias: Tachycardia, fibrillation or flutter
- Heart block, second or third degree
- Angina
- ST-segment changes of greater than or equal to 2 mm in either direction
- Persistent HR or BP decline
- Elevation of diastolic pressure by more than 20 mm Hg above resting or to more than 100 mm Hg
- Dyspnea, nausea, fatigue, dizziness, headache, blurred vision
- Intolerable musculoskeletal pain
- Heart rate greater than target rate
- Patient pallor or diaphoresis

Aerobic exercise training for patients with airway clearance dysfunction has been shown to produce benefits that include improved exercise tolerance, reduced dyspnea, and enhanced quality of life.[82-85] Troosters et al randomly assigned 100 individuals with COPD to either a 6-month outpatient rehabilitation program that involved aerobic exercise training or to regular medical therapy.[85] Among patients who completed the 6-month rehabilitation program, significant and clinically important changes were demonstrated in 6-minute walking distance, maximal exercise performance, peripheral and respiratory muscle strength, and quality of life. Although the formal rehabilitation ended after 6 months, many of the benefits were still evident at an 18-month follow-up session.[61]

Body Mechanics and Postural Stabilization Training. Body mechanics and postural stabilization training have two potential benefits for the patient with airway clearance dysfunction and COPD. One benefit—reducing general body work—is discussed more fully in the section on Functional Training in Self-Care and Home Management. The second benefit is to use postural stabilization and proper body positioning to reduce the work of breathing and diminish the effects of dyspnea. Many anecdotal examples of dyspnea relief in the forward-flexed posture have precipitated research into proper positions for the patient with COPD. It is clear that the seated, forward-leaning posture is the preferred position to reduce dyspnea in patients with severe and moderate limitations of maximal inspiratory pressure associated with COPD. The forward-leaning posture produces a significant increase in maximum inspiratory pressures, thereby relieving the sensation of dyspnea.[86] In addition, this position may increase FRC in those with airflow limitations because the thorax approaches a similar position to prone in which FRC is increased.[87] In patients who are unable to tolerate functional walking because of either musculoskeletal stress or dyspnea, a high walker may be adapted

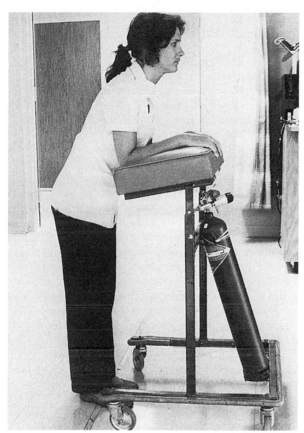

FIG. 24-16 A high walker to permit assumption of a forward-leaning posture in standing. *From Irwin S, Tecklin JS: Cardiopulmonary Physical Therapy: A Guide to Practice, ed 4, St. Louis, 1995, Mosby.*

to permit forward leaning, thereby reducing the work of breathing and the perception of dyspnea to permit the desired activity (Fig. 24-16).

Flexibility Exercises. Exercise to improve flexibility for the patient with airway clearance dysfunction and COPD may include stretching exercises to promote muscle lengthening, exercises to improve ROM, and mobilization exercises to improve joint function. There is little or no experimental evidence to support the use of flexibility exercises in this patient population. However, it seems intuitive that maintaining or improving thoracic and shoulder girdle flexibility would enhance respiratory effort by increasing thoracic compliance. A more flexible chest wall should require less muscular work to inflate the thorax. A similar benefit of increased thoracic compliance and reduced work of breathing may be implied for improving motion of a tight shoulder girdle in the patient with pulmonary disease. Many individuals with COPD have an increased AP thoracic diameter and a hyperinflated and often fixed thoracic cage, particularly during periods of dyspnea.[88] One suspects that using exercise to prevent or treat the fixed thoracic cage should be beneficial despite the dearth of evidence.

A series of flexibility exercises has been recommended as part of a traditional "warm-up" for a pulmonary rehabilitation session (Table 24-5). Although this program has not been formally evaluated from a scientific perspective, it serves as a model for a major long-established pulmonary rehabilitation program.[89] These exercises may be used as a regular exercise routine to improve or maintain good thoracic and shoulder girdle motion.

Breathing Exercises. To increase *alveolar ventilation,* therapists teach breathing exercises that are intended to influence the rate, depth, or distribution of ventilation or muscular activity associated with breathing. The breathing strategies commonly recommended to improve ventilation and oxygenation include diaphragmatic breathing, also referred to as breathing control, pursed-lip breathing, segmental breathing, low-frequency breathing, and sustained maximal inspiration breathing exercises. ACBT and AD are also breathing strategies, but they are used primarily with airway clearance and were discussed earlier in this chapter.

Diaphragmatic Breathing Exercises. The diaphragm is the principal muscle of inspiration. Historically, when muscles other than the diaphragm assumed a role in inspiration, therapeutic efforts were directed toward restoring a more normal, diaphragmatic pattern of breathing. The return to diaphragmatic breathing was thought to relieve dyspnea.

Diaphragmatic breathing exercises are intended to enhance diaphragmatic descent during inspiration and diaphragmatic ascent during expiration. Diaphragmatic descent is assisted by directing the patient to protract the abdomen gradually during inhalation. One assists diaphragmatic ascent by directing the patient to allow the abdomen to retract gradually during exhalation or by directing the patient to contract the abdominal muscles actively during exhalation. Although the exact techniques used to teach diaphragmatic breathing vary, in principle they are similar. They all recommend that the patient assume a comfortable position, usually one-half to three-quarters upright sitting, before beginning, and that the patient's hips and knees be flexed to relax the abdominal and hamstring muscles respectively. Diaphragmatic breathing exercises are then taught as follows:

Diaphragmatic breathing exercises

1. Place the patient's dominant hand over the midrectus abdominis area.
2. Place the patient's nondominant hand on the midsternal area.
3. Direct the patient to inhale slowly through the nose.
4. Instruct the patient to watch the dominant hand as inspiration continues.
5. Encourage the patient to direct the air so that the dominant hand gradually rises as inspiration continues.
6. Caution the patient to avoid excessive movement under the nondominant hand.
7. Apply firm counterpressure over the patient's dominant hand just before directing the patient to inhale.
8. Instruct the patient to inhale as you lessen your counterpressure as inspiration continues.

TABLE 24-5	"Warm-up" Flexibility Exercises for Pulmonary Rehabilitation
Body Area	**Exercise**
Cervical	Look up/down (nod "yes").
	Look left/right (shake "no").
	Move left ear to left shoulder.
	Move right ear to right shoulder.
Shoulder and upper extremity	Shoulder circles forward and backward.
	Shoulder shrugs (up/relax).
	Shoulder blade squeeze: Rest your hands on your shoulders, touch your elbows together in front of your body, pull them apart, try to push them backward. Squeeze your shoulder blades together as you push back. Breathe IN as you push your elbows backward, and breathe OUT as you bring your elbows together in front.
	Front arm raises (shoulder flexion): Lift your arms overhead, lower them in front of you slowly, as if pushing against resistance. Breathe IN when lifting, and breathe OUT when lowering.
	Side-arm raises (abduction): Lift your arms out to the side and up overhead, lower them back to your sides slowly, as if pushing against resistance. Breathe IN as you lift, and breathe OUT as you lower.
	Arm circles forward: With your arms fully extended and raised to shoulder level, slowly make small circles with your arms, then reverse. (If the patient is extremely short of breath, he or she may lower the arms.)
Trunk	Trunk rotation (side to side twists): Start with your arms extended in front of you and slowly twist to the right and then to the left. Try not to move your hips.
	Side-bending (right and left): Reach one arm up over your head and lean to the opposite side, then reverse. Blow OUT as you bend, and breathe IN as you straighten.
Lower extremity	Wall slide: Stand with your hips and buttocks pressed as flat as you can against a wall. Shoulders should be relaxed. Slowly lower your body as if you were going to sit in a chair. Keep your hips above the level of your knees. Hold this position. Try to increase the holding time to at least 2 minutes.
	Hip flexion: Marching in place.
	Toe tapping.
	Gastrocnemius/soleus stretch: Stand facing a wall about a foot away and put your hands on the wall in front of you at about shoulder height. With knees extended, lean your body into the wall to put a stretch on your large calf muscles.
General instructions	Begin with 3-5 repetitions of each exercise and then increase gradually to 7-10 repetitions. Once 10 repetitions of each can be done, a 1-lb weight may be added to the arm exercises.
	Perform pursed-lip breathing throughout your activity. Remember to have patients breathe "IN" through the nose and "OUT" through pursed lips. Remind them to not hold their breath.

9. Practice the exercise until the patient no longer requires manual assistance of the therapist to perform the exercise correctly.
10. Progress the level of difficulty by sequentially removing auditory, visual, and tactile cues. Thereafter, progress the exercise by practicing it in varied positions including seated, standing, and walking.

Diaphragmatic breathing exercises have also been administered concurrently with relaxation training with the goal of eliminating unnecessary muscle activity, particularly excessive use of the accessory inspiratory muscles. In the past, increased diaphragmatic strength was assumed when increased resistance to abdominal protraction was tolerated, as with weights placed over the abdomen, but this notion has not held up to objective scrutiny.[90]

Evaluation of the effectiveness of diaphragmatic breathing exercises has been the objective of much research over the past several decades. A recent and excellent review by Cahalin et al concluded that "there was great inconsistency among the many published studies regarding the operational definitions and techniques employed for teaching or demonstrating diaphragmatic breathing."[91] The outcomes examined in the many studies in this review included ventilation, severity of COPD symptoms, thoracic motion, and various tests of pulmonary function. Many normal subjects, as well as patients with COPD, who were able to increase tidal volume during diaphragmatic breathing exercises and who had good chest wall biomechanics, were able to direct greater ventilation toward the lower lobes during the exercise session, albeit with some paradoxical chest wall motion.[92-95] However, in individuals with more advanced COPD, diaphragmatic breathing resulted in reduced chest wall coordination, increased dyspnea, and less mechanically efficient breathing, making the use of these techniques questionable in those with more advanced disease.[96,97] The effects of diaphragmatic breathing on pulmonary function, respiratory rate and ABG measurements are more encouraging. Sergysels et al examined diaphragmatic breathing with low frequency and high tidal volumes in patients with moderate COPD while at rest and during bicycle exercise and found that PaO_2, peak oxygen consumption, vital capacity and total lung capacity, and diffusion capacity all increased when diaphragmatic breathing was employed at rest and with exercise.[98] In Vitacca et al's study, diaphragmatic breathing training, although associated with impaired chest wall function and increased dyspnea, resulted in a significant increase in blood oxygenation along with a decrease in carbon dioxide levels.[97] Diaphragmatic breathing exercises will continue to be used clinically as research more clearly defines the optimal methods for this intervention and the expected outcomes. The objectives and potential outcomes of diaphragmatic breathing are summarized in Table 24-6.

Pursed-Lip Breathing Exercises. Pursed-lip breathing is another method, often associated with relaxation activities, suggested for improving ventilation and oxygenation and relieving respiratory symptoms in individuals with airway clearance dysfunction.[99] One method of pursed-lip breathing advocates passive expiration,[100] whereas the other recommends abdominal muscle contraction to prolong expiration.[101] Current use of the technique usually encourages passive rather than forced expiration. Pursed-lip breathing with passive expiration is performed as follows:

Pursed-lip breathing
1. Position the patient comfortably.
2. Place your hand over the midrectus abdominis area to detect activity during expiration.
3. Direct the patient to inhale slowly.
4. Instruct the patient to purse the lips before exhalation.
5. Instruct the patient to relax the air out through the pursed lips and refrain from abdominal muscle contraction.
6. Direct the patient to stop exhaling when abdominal muscle activity is detected.
7. Progress the intensity of the exercise by substituting the patient's hand for yours, removing tactile cues, and having the patient perform the exercise while standing and exercising.

Thoman and colleagues found that pursed-lip breathing significantly decreased respiratory rate, increased tidal volume, improved alveolar ventilation as measured by partial pressure of arterial carbon dioxide ($PaCO_2$), and enhanced the ventilation of previously underventilated areas of the lungs in patients with COPD.[102] Mueller and colleagues also found that pursed-lip breathing improved ventilation and oxygenation in individuals with COPD, at

TABLE 24-6	Objectives and Potential Outcomes of Diaphragmatic Breathing Exercises
Therapeutic objectives	Alleviate dyspnea
	Reduce the work of breathing
	Reduce the incidence of postoperative pulmonary complication
Physiological objectives	Improve ventilation
	Improve oxygenation
Potential outcomes	Eliminate accessory muscle action
	Decrease respiratory rate
	Increase tidal ventilation
	Improve distribution of ventilation
	Decrease need for postoperative therapy

rest and during exercise.[100] Several studies have found that this approach improves symptoms, as well as improving objective measures of ventilation and enhancing exercise tolerance and efficiency in patients with COPD.[103-105]

One study on the effects of providing external expiratory resistance to intubated patients with COPD found that this intervention did not improve gas exchange or breathing pattern in this group of subjects in ways it has been shown to improve in nonintubated patients with COPD.[106]

Research has failed to fully explain the symptomatic benefits some patients ascribe to pursed-lips breathing. One theory is that pursed-lip breathing is effective because the slight resistance to expiration increases positive pressure within the airways and helps to keep open the small bronchioles that otherwise collapse because of loss of support associated with lung tissue destruction. Alternatively, or additionally, pursed-lip breathing could be effective because it slows the respiratory rate. At the very least, pursed-lip breathing appears to reduce respiratory rate and increase tidal volume, thereby not compromising minute ventilation. It is recommended that clinicians continue to teach pursed-lip breathing exercises to patients complaining of dyspnea.

Segmental Breathing Exercises. Segmental breathing, also referred to as localized expansion breathing, is another type of exercise used to improve ventilation and oxygenation in individuals with airway clearance dysfunction. This exercise presumes that inspired air can be actively directed to a specific area of lung by emphasizing and increasing movement of the thorax overlying that lung area. This intervention has been recommended to prevent the accumulation of pleural fluid, to reduce the probability of atelectasis, to prevent the accumulation of tracheobronchial secretions, to decrease *paradoxical breathing*, to prevent the panic associated with uncontrolled breathing, and to improve chest wall mobility.[107] The attempt to preferentially enhance localized lung expansion uses manual counterpressure against the thorax to encourage the expansion of that specific area of thorax in the hopes of improving ventilation to a specific part of the lung.

Segmental breathing exercises

1. Identify the surface landmarks demarcating the affected area.
2. Place your hand or hands on the chest wall overlying the bronchopulmonary segment or segments requiring treatment (i.e., the areas of lung you hope to expand).
3. Apply firm pressure to that area at the end of the patient's expiratory maneuver. (Pressure should be equal and bilateral across a median sternotomy incision.)
4. Instruct the patient to inspire deeply through his or her mouth, attempting to direct the inspired air toward your hand, saying, "Breathe into my hand, or make my hand move as you breathe in."
5. Reduce hand pressure as patient inspires. (At end inspiration, the instructor's hand should be applying no pressure on the chest.)
6. Instruct the patient to hold his or her breath for 2-3 seconds at the completion of inspiration.
7. Instruct the patient to exhale.
8. Repeat sequence until patient can execute the breathing maneuver correctly.
9. Progress the exercises by instructing the patient to use his or her own hands or a belt to execute the program independently.

Evaluation of the effectiveness of segmental breathing begins with validation of its underlying premise that ventilation can be directed to a predetermined area. One study on lateral basal expansion exercises concluded that this type of segmental breathing exercise failed to improve local ventilation in patients with emphysema.[108] Another study also failed to find any change in the distribution of ventilation when subjects with lung restriction breathed segmentally but showed clearly that when subjects were placed in sidelying, both ventilation and blood flow in the dependent lung improved.[109] There is a lack of persuasive evidence linking segmental breathing with other therapeutic effects. However, it is quite clear and demonstrable that improving local chest wall motion can improve breathing by converting intercostal muscle shortening into lung volume expansion.[110]

Sustained Maximal Breathing Exercises. Breathing exercises during which a maximal inspiration is sustained for about 3 seconds have also been associated with improved oxygenation.[111] Currently, sustained maximal inspiration is more commonly employed as part of the ACBT and is used in association with airway clearance techniques as described previously.

Relaxation Exercise Techniques. Relaxation exercise and training are currently used as adjunctive therapy for many different diseases, including such divergent entities as gastroesophageal reflux, nausea after chemotherapy, behavioral aspects of autism, and mild hypertension. However, despite many anecdotal reports, particularly regarding care of the patient with asthma, there is little data to demonstrate discrete pulmonary benefits of relaxation.[112] Relaxation techniques coupled with breathing strategies and hypnosis have recently been shown to result in some symptomatic improvement in children with dyspnea.[113] Relaxation techniques are often administered to decrease unnecessary muscle contraction throughout the body and thereby reduce general body work. The traditional method or approach involves muscle contraction followed by relaxation, whereas a newer technique employs visual imagery to achieve the desired effects.

Strength, Power, and Endurance Training. Endurance training that focuses primarily on aerobic benefits has been used for decades in pulmonary rehabilitation programs. The issue of muscle strength and resistance exercise to improve strength and reduce related symptoms has only recently come to the fore as a means of improving physical functioning in patients with chronic airway clearance dysfunction. Recent work indicates that people with COPD have peripheral muscle weakness that is likely multifactorial in origin.[114] Among those factors are disuse atrophy, inadequate nutrition, long-term hypercapnia and hypoxemia, reduced anabolic steroid levels, and myopathy from continuous or periodic corticosteroid use. Muscle strength, particularly lower extremity strength, is reduced in individuals with COPD when compared to age-matched controls.[95] Although there is great patient-to-patient variability in this muscular dysfunction, research has demonstrated a 20% to 30% deficit in quadriceps strength in those with moderate-to-severe COPD. Muscle endurance is similarly decreased in this population. These deficits may limit exercise capacity and function in those with COPD.[12,115,116]

There is a growing body of evidence that strength training is beneficial and should become part of a comprehensive physical therapy program for patients with airway clearance dysfunction and COPD. The primary benefits of strength training in this population are improved muscle strength, endurance, function, and exercise tolerance and reduced dyspnea.[117-120] Although these benefits are reasonably well accepted, recent studies call into question the benefit of such exercises on patients' quality of life.[121,122] Since the preponderance of evidence indicates that strength training can improve impairments associated with quality of life, a comprehensive intervention plan for the patient with airway clearance dysfunction should include resistance training, as well as endurance training. Features of a resistance exercise program for patients with airway clearance dysfunction are described in Table 24-7.[123]

Functional Training in Self-Care and Home Management, Work, Community, and Leisure Integration/Reintegration. There is little direct evidence regarding functionally specific training programs and improvement in ADLs in patients with airway clearance dysfunction. However, it appears from recent data that whether the physical rehabilitation program focuses on endurance training using treadmill or bicycle ergometry or employs more traditional calisthenics, the intervention produces significant improvement in functional performance and overall health.[124]

Several studies have attempted to develop and validate ADL profiles for the patient with chronic airway clearance dysfunction. These profiles include the Manchester Respi-

TABLE 24-7	Features of a Resistance Exercise Program for Patients with Airway Clearance Dysfunction
Frequency	Each major muscle group to be trained should be exercised 2-3× per week.
	Specific suggestions will depend on where the program is carried out: At home, outpatient, inpatient, and other sites.
Intensity	Muscle load is typically and reasonably safely initiated with 50%-60% of the 1 repetition maximum (1RM) established during the examination.
	Repetitions are typically 10 per muscle group at outset of program. One set of repetitions is a good starting point. A degree of success should be built in to the prescription for the psychological benefits and to increase a likelihood of adherence. A rest period should provide time between the sets for recovery.
Mode	Various types of resistance devices may be employed—exercise tables, benches, pulleys, free weights, etc. Exercise should focus on the large muscle groups of the lower and upper extremities, as well as trunk musculature such as latissimus dorsi. To ensure continued interest and to vary the training stimulus, it is important to vary the types of exercise and consider including eccentric, concentric, isometric, isotonic, and isokinetic exercises.
Duration	ACSM recommends a 10-12 week duration followed by a period of active recovery using alternative forms of exercise.
Progression	Begin with lighter loads and increase number of repetitions and sets as the patient begins to demonstrate tolerance at each particular level of activity.

ACSM, American College of Sports Medicine.

ratory Activities of Daily Living questionnaire and the London Chest Activity of Daily Living scale.[125,126] One study demonstrated improvement in physical function, as measured by the Chronic Respiratory Questionnaire (CRQ) and the Medical Outcomes Study 36-Item Short Form Health Survey (SF-36), after pulmonary rehabilitation.[127] Unlike patients with neuromuscular or musculoskeletal deficits who may need to learn new strategies and adapted tasks to regain functional independence, it appears that those with COPD need to gain control over their dyspnea and disease to use existing functional skills. These self-care skills have not been lost but have gone unused because of the physical and emotional impact of the severe dyspnea and resultant physical deconditioning that has accrued over months and years of disabling lung disease. Among the various functional tasks that may need to be relearned or adapted are the following:

- Bed mobility and transfers—use of transfer boards and overhead trapeze bars
- Self-care such as bathing, grooming, dressing—raised toilet seat, long-handled brush, shower seat
- Household activities and related chores such as yard work—long-handled tools, rolling bench
- Activity adaptation to conserve energy break complex or difficult tasks into component parts, motorized mobility device
- Injury prevention—use of grab-bars, walking aids

DEVICES AND EQUIPMENT

There are various oxygen sources and delivery devices available for use in the home, at work, or in the community. Oxygen may be supplied in gas cylinders of varying sizes. These cylinders must be replaced or refilled periodically to replenish the oxygen supply and most are large, bulky, and heavy. However, recent technology has made much smaller devices, such as liquid oxygen containers and oxygen concentrators, available (Fig. 24-17). These devices can supply oxygen for up to several hours of oxygen, depending on patient usage. Liquid oxygen systems have been available for use at home for many years. There is usually a large reservoir in the home from which a small, portable knapsack–size container may be

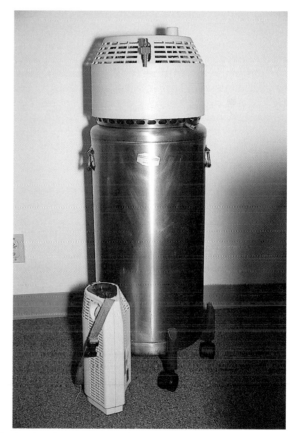

FIG. 24-17 Stationary and portable liquid oxygen units. *From Potter PA, Perry AG: Fundamentals of Nursing, ed 6, St. Louis, 2005, Mosby.*

filled for outside use. Oxygen concentrators, which have also been available for several years, are electrically powered and use a molecular sieve to separate oxygen from the ambient air and concentrate and store the oxygen. These devices are economical for use in the home and for activities immediately around the house, such as gardening, but are too large to take out into the community.

Oxygen must be delivered from its source to the patient via a device. Oxygen catheters may be inserted into the nasal passage or via a small surgical incision directly into the trachea, with a transtracheal device. Oxygen masks placed over the nose and mouth may also be used. These sometimes have a reservoir that enables high concentrations of oxygen to be provided. The most commonly used device is a nasal cannula that provides a small prong into each nostril for oxygen delivery (Fig. 24-18).

Mechanical ventilators are commonly used for patients with airway clearance disorders when acute or chronic respiratory failure occurs such as after acute disease processes, trauma, or surgery (see Chapter 26). Basic modes of mechanical ventilation are briefly identified in Table 24-8. When the patient with airway clearance dysfunction is receiving mechanical ventilation, it is important to note the parameters of ventilation, particularly when breathing strategies and retraining are to be employed. Certain modes and limitations of mechanical ventilation may or may not allow certain breathing strategies.

Assistive devices, such as canes and walkers, are often indicated to assist with ambulation and enhance stability and safety.[2] When recommending such assistive devices for the patient with airway clearance dysfunction, the therapist must be aware that crutches, walkers, and similar devices tend to increase the oxygen requirement when compared to unassisted ambulation.[128] A cost-benefit decision about such devices must be made.[129] A wheeled walker can, however, be very helpful for individuals with chronic airway clearance dysfunction. The walker not only offers support and stabilization but with a basket or small platform can be used to carry a small oxygen delivery system during community activities. Motorized scooters are useful for community mobility outside the home for shopping, work, and recreational activities in individuals with significant airway clearance dysfunction. There are lift systems for automobile storage of the scooters to facilitate patient use. Motorized scooters and the appropriate lift devices are expensive but often make the difference between being housebound or active in the community.

CASE STUDY 24-1

CHRONIC BRONCHITIS

Examination
Patient History

NT is a 66-year-old woman with a long-established history of chronic bronchitis. She was admitted to the hospital in acute respiratory distress and was diagnosed with bacterial pneumonia. Because NT previously participated in a pulmonary rehabilitation program, a physical therapy consultation was requested. She reported a 110 pack per year history of cigarette smoking. NT reported that it now exhausts her to prepare her meals and perform other IADLs. She has no significant medical or surgical history other than her lung disease and recent osteoporosis of the vertebrae, which she reports is secondary to her medications. She is currently taking antibiotics for her infection, oral and inhaled bronchodilators, and oral and inhaled corticosteroids. Her ABG values on admission were pH: 7.33, $PaCO_2$: 45, bicarbonate (HCO_3): 20, and base excess (BE): −4. These values revealed the need for oxygen via nasal cannula at 2 L/min. Pulmonary function testing was deferred because of respiratory distress, but recent values indicated a severe obstructive deficit with moderate increases in residual volume consistent with COPD and hyperinflation.

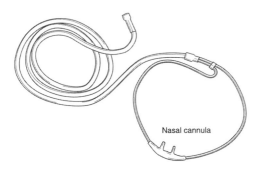

Nasal cannula

FIG. 24-18 Nasal cannula for oxygen delivery. *From Hillegass EA, Sadowsky HS:* Essentials of Cardiopulmonary Physical Therapy, *ed 2, Philadelphia, 2001, Saunders.*

TABLE 24-8	Basic Modes of Mechanical Ventilation
Mode	**Description**
Control	The patient is guaranteed a predetermined number of mechanical breaths and is unable or not permitted to initiate a mechanical breath or breathe spontaneously.
Assist	The patient is permitted to initiate a mechanical breath but is not guaranteed a predetermined number of mechanical breaths.
Assist-control	The patient is guaranteed a predetermined number of mechanical breaths and is permitted to initiate additional mechanical breaths.
Intermittent mandatory ventilation (IMV)	The patient is guaranteed a predetermined number of mechanical breaths but is permitted to initiate spontaneous breaths through the ventilator.

Systems Review

Heart rate is 100 beats per minute (bpm), RR is 24 breaths/min with clear distress, BP is 130/85 mm Hg.

Tests and Measures

Musculoskeletal

Posture NT has forward head and shoulders and a significant thoracic kyphosis.

Range of Motion Grossly symmetrical and full functional ROM.

Muscle Performance Mild loss of strength in the lower extremities.

Cardiovascular/Pulmonary

Circulation NT has minimal pedal edema.

Chest Examination

Inspection NT is in acute respiratory distress with tachypnea, flaring of the nares, use of accessory muscles of inspiration, and prolonged expiration with an I : E ratio of 1 : 4. Perioral cyanosis, digital clubbing, and cough produced thick, yellowish sputum without evidence of blood. Her thorax appeared symmetrical.

Palpation NT has minimal thoracic excursion with a very limited right hemithorax. No shift in the mediastinum was seen. Vocal fremitus was increased in the lower right posterior and lateral thorax. Some rhonchal fremitus was palpated in that same area. Dullness to mediate percussion was noted in the lower right posterior and lateral thorax in generally the same area in which increased vocal fremitus was felt.

Auscultation Distant breath sounds throughout the lungs, except for bronchial and bronchovesicular sounds in the lower right posterior and lateral thorax. Coarse crackles and low-pitched wheezing were noted in that area on the right, along with some scattering of these sounds throughout the lung fields. These findings were consistent with hyperinflation throughout the lungs and consolidation and increased mucus secretion in the right lower lobe.

Aerobic Capacity and Endurance Testing NT's recent worsening of fatigue during community activities and her decreasing ability to participate in ADLs are indications for additional tests. NT was asked to perform a 6-minute walk test. She was not able to complete this test. She could walk 100 feet in 2 minutes but could not continue because of severe fatigue. She reported dyspnea that was consistent with a rating of 4 on the American Thoracic Society Breathlessness Scale. She also reported a rating of 9/10 on the revised Borg RPE scale at the end of the 6-minute walk test.

Integumentary: Cyanosis around the lips and nail beds, along with some moderate clubbing of the fingers.

Evaluation, Diagnosis, and Prognosis

This case represents an acute exacerbation of a chronic disability whose basic pathological changes are largely irreversible. Nonetheless, through reduction of the many impairments noted in the examination, one may expect to see notable improvement in NT's functional abilities.

Findings gathered during the examination lead to a choice of diagnostic patterns between preferred practice pattern 6C: Impaired ventilation, respiration/gas exchange, and aerobic capacity/endurance associated with airway clearance dysfunction, or pattern 6F: Impaired ventilation and respiration/gas exchange associated with respiratory failure. Because the medical criteria for respiratory failure includes a $PaCO_2$ of ≥ 50 mm Hg, this patient should be classified as pattern 6C.

Goals

1. NT should be able to perform ADLs and IADLs in an independent manner.
2. NT is expected to resume some of her community-based activities without risk of physical deterioration.
3. With continued adherence to her home program as identified during the outpatient portion of her plan of care, NT should have a reduced risk of recurrence, as well as an improved ability to manage her disease.
4. NT's overall health status is expected to improve with concomitant reduction in health care costs.
5. NT's sense of self-confidence and her quality of life are expected to improve.

Intervention

Airway Clearance Techniques

NT was treated with bronchial drainage, percussion, and vibration during her hospital admission. Because NT lives alone, she requires an airway clearance technique that she can perform independently. She was instructed in proper use of AD. She was able to demonstrate the technique, and it was reviewed with her on a weekly basis for 3 consecutive weeks as an outpatient to ensure that she was using it correctly.

Therapeutic Exercise

Aerobic exercise training using bedside cycle ergometry was performed until NT could travel to the physical therapy department, after which she began endurance walking on a motorized treadmill. She used supplemental oxygen during her exercise until the point of hospital discharge. She continued with outpatient rehabilitation that included both treadmill exercise and free walking while at home. Strengthening exercises were performed every other day in an effort to improve muscle power throughout her weakened lower extremities.

Flexibility exercises were used on alternate days to the strengthening exercises. These exercises were aimed at improving thoracic mobility in an effort to enhance motion of the thorax and the thoracic spine and reduce the degree of kyphosis. Relaxation exercises were integrated with a program of instruction in diaphragmatic breathing. These exercises were intended to reduce the muscular effort associated with overly active accessory muscles and to offer a means of dealing with the anxiety associated with breathlessness and dyspnea.

Please see the CD that accompanies this book for a case study describing the examination, evaluation, and interventions for a newborn patient with meconium aspiration.

CHAPTER SUMMARY

This chapter focuses on individuals with airway clearance dysfunction, particularly patients with COPD and CF. The principles and skills described are applicable to any patient with airway clearance dysfunction, including infants in the neonatal intensive care unit and young adults with neurological trauma that has resulted in inability to cough and clear secretions. Basic chest examination techniques—inspection, palpation, mediate percussion, and auscultation—are described and are appropriate for any patient with respiratory or pulmonary disease. Interventions described include specific approaches to airway clearance and therapeutic exercise for strength, aerobic fitness, and breathing retraining.

ADDITIONAL RESOURCES

Useful Forms

Dyspnea Scale

Chronic Respiratory Disease Questionnaire (CRQ): www.atsqol.org/sections/instruments/ae/pages/crq.html

St. George's Respiratory Questionnaire: www.atsqol.org/sections/instruments/pt/pages/george.html

Books

Irwin S, Tecklin JS (eds): *Cardiopulmonary Physical Therapy: A Guide to Practice,* ed 4, Philadelphia, 2004, Elsevier.

Burton GG, Hodgkin JE, Ward JJ (eds): *Respiratory Care: A Guide to Practice,* ed 4, St. Louis, 1997, Mosby-Yearbook.

Wilkins RL, Stoller JK: *Egan's Fundamentals of Respiratory Care,* ed 7, Philadelphia, 2004, Elsevier.

Web Sites

American Thoracic Society: www.thoracic.org/

American College of Chest Physicians: www.chestnet.org/

American Lung Association: www.lungusa.org/

Pulmonary Breath Sounds: http://jan.ucc.nau.edu/~daa/heartlung/breathsounds/contents.html

GLOSSARY

Aerobic capacity: Another term for maximal oxygen uptake ($\dot{V}O_{2max}$). The highest amount of oxygen consumed during maximal exercise.

Alveolar ventilation: The volume of gas expired from the alveoli to the outside of the body per minute.

Atelectasis: Alveolar collapse because of poor lung expansion or complete obstruction of an airway.

Auscultation: Listening with a stethoscope.

Bronchodilator: Medication that reduces bronchial smooth muscle spasm and thereby causes an increase in caliber of a bronchial tube.

Crackles: Nonmusical sounds (previously called rales) that may be mimicked by rolling several strands of hair near your ear or by listening to a bowl of cereal that crackles when milk is added. Crackles may represent the sudden opening of previously closed airways. Expiratory crackles may indicate the presence of fluid in the large airways.

Dyspnea: Shortness of breath. A subjective difficulty or distress in breathing.

Fremitus: Vibrations within the thorax that can be palpated.

Hypercapnia: Increased carbon dioxide level in the arterial blood.

Hypoxemia: Low or insufficient oxygen in the arterial blood.

Mucolytic: A medication capable of dissolving or decreasing the viscosity of mucus.

Paradoxical breathing: Moving the belly in during inspiration and out during expiration.

Stertor: A snoring noise created when the tongue falls back into the lower palate.

Stridor: A crowing sound during inspiration.

Thoracic index: Ratio of the anteroposterior diameter to the transverse diameter of the thorax.

Tidal volume: The volume of air inspired or expired in a single breath during regular breathing.

Wheezes: Whistling sounds probably produced by air flowing at high velocities through narrowed airways.

References

1. American Medical Association: *International Classification of Diseases: Clinical Modification,* ninth revision, Chicago, 2000, AMA.
2. American Physical Therapy Association: Guide to Physical Therapist Practice, second edition, *Phys Ther* 81(1):S114-S1115, 2001.
3. Chan-Yeung M, Enarson DA, Kennedy SM: Impact of grain dust on respiratory health, *Am Rev Respir Dis* 145:476-487, 1992.
4. Sydbom A, Blomberg A, Parnia S, et al: Health effects of diesel exhaust emissions, *Eur Respir J* 17(4):733-746, 2001.
5. de Godoy DV, de Godoy RF: A randomized controlled trial of the effect of psychotherapy on anxiety and depression in chronic obstructive pulmonary disease, *Arch Phys Med Rehabil* 84(8):1154-1157, 2003.
6. Pelkonen M, Notkola IL, Tuikainen H, et al: Smoking cessation, decline in pulmonary function and total mortality: A 30 year follow up study among the Finnish cohorts of the Seven Countries Study, *Thorax* 56(9):703-707, 2001.
7. Berry MJ, Rejeski WJ, Adair NE, et al: A randomized, controlled trial comparing long-term and short-term exercise in patients with chronic obstructive pulmonary disease, *J Cardiopulm Rehabil* 23(1):60-68, 2003.
8. Tecklin JS, Holsclaw DS: Bronchial drainage with aerosol medications in cystic fibrosis, *Phys Ther* 56(9):999-1003, 1976.
9. Cassart M, Gevenois PA, Estenne M: Rib cage dimensions in hyperinflated patients with severe chronic obstructive pulmonary disease, *Am J Respir Crit Care Med* 154:800-805, 1996.
10. Posture: Alignment and Muscle Balance. In Kendall FP, McCreary EK, Provance PG (eds): *Muscles, Testing and Function,* ed 4; Philadelphia, 1993, Lippincott, Williams & Wilkins.
11. Malasanos L, Barkauskas V, Stoltenberg-Allen K: *Health Assessment,* ed 4, St. Louis, 1990, Mosby.
12. Gosselink R, Troosters T, Decramer M: Peripheral muscle weakness contributes to exercise limitation in COPD, *Am J Respir Crit Care Med* 153(3):976-980, 1996.
13. Koechlin C, Couillard A, Simar D, et al: Does oxidative stress alter quadriceps endurance in chronic obstructive pulmonary disease? *Am J Respir Crit Care Med* 169:1022-1027, 2004.
14. Storer TW: Exercise in chronic pulmonary disease: Resistance exercise prescription, *Med Sci Sports Exerc* 33(7 suppl):S680-692, 2001.
15. Moser C, Tirakitsoontorn P, Nussbaum E, et al: Peripheral muscle weakness and exercise capacity in children with cystic fibrosis, *Am J Respir Crit Care Med* 159:748-754, 2000.
16. Bernard S, LeBlanc P, Whitton F, et al: Peripheral muscle weakness in patients with chronic obstructive pulmonary disease, *Am J Respir Crit Care Med* 158:629-634, 1998.
17. Black LF, Hyatt RE: Maximal respiratory pressures: normal values and relationship to age and sex, *Am Rev Respir Dis* 99:696-702, 1969.
18. Wang AY, Jaeger RJ, Yarkony GM, et al: Cough in spinal cord injured patients: the relationship between motor level and peak expiratory flow, *Spinal Cord* 35:299-302, 1997.
19. Sobush DC, Dunning M 3rd: Assessing maximal static ventilatory muscle pressures using the "bugle" dynamometer. Suggestion from the field, *Phys Ther* 64:1689-1690, 1984.
20. Borg G: Psychophysical bases of perceived exertion, *Med Sci Sports Exerc* 14(5):377-381, 1982.
21. Kendrick KR, Baxi SC, Smith RM: Usefulness of the modified 0-10 Borg scale in assessing the degree of dyspnea in patients with COPD and asthma, *J Emerg Nurs* 26(3):216-222, 2000.
22. Wilson RC, Jones PW: Long-term reproducibility of Borg scale estimates of breathlessness during exercise, *Clin Sci* (London) 80:309-312, 1991.
23. Wilson RC, Jones PW: A comparison of the visual analog scale and the modified Borg scale for the measurement of dyspnea during exercise, *Clin Sci* 76:277-282, 1989.
24. Muza SR, Silverman MT, Gilmore GC, et al: Comparison of scales used to quantitate the sense of effort to breathe in patients with chronic obstructive pulmonary disease, *Am Rev Respir Dis* 141:909-913, 1990.
25. Guyatt GH, Berman LB, Townsend M, et al: A measure of quality of life for clinical trials in chronic lung disease, *Thorax* 42(10):773-778, 1987.
26. Jones PW, Quirk FH, Baveystock CM, et al: A self-complete measure of health status for chronic airflow limitation. The St George's Respiratory Questionnaire, *Am Rev Respir Dis* 145(6):1321-1327, 1992.
27. Carrieri-Kohlman V, Stulbarg MS: Dyspnea: Assessment and management. In Hodgkin JE, Celli BR, Connors GL: *Pulmonary Rehabilitation,* ed 3, Philadelphia, 2000, Lippincott Williams & Wilkins.

28. Myers KA, Farquhar DR: The rational clinical examination. Does this patient have clubbing? *JAMA* 286(3):341-347, 2001.

29. May T, Rabaud C, Amiel C, et al: Hypertrophic pulmonary osteoarthropathy associated with granulomatous *Pneumocystis carinii* pneumonia in AIDS, *Scand J Infect Dis* 25(6):771-773, 1993.

30. Tecklin JS: The patient with airway clearance dysfunction. In Irwin S, Tecklin JS (eds): *Cardiopulmonary Physical Therapy: A Guide to Practice*, ed 4, St. Louis, 2004, Mosby.

31. Peche R, Estenne M, Gevenois PA, et al: Sternomastoid muscle size and strength in patients with severe chronic obstructive pulmonary disease, *Am J Respir Crit Care Med* 153(1):422-425, 1996.

32. Gadomski AM, Permutt T, Stanton B: Correcting respiratory rate for the presence of fever, *J Clin Epidemiol* 47(9):1043-1049, 1994.

33. Hassan WU, Henderson AF: Cough and stridor: Who should investigate the patient? *J Laryngol Otol* 107(7):639, 1993.

34. Estenne M, De Troyer A: Relationship between respiratory muscle electromyogram and rib cage motion in tetraplegia, *Am Rev Respir Dis* 132:53-59, 1985.

35. Gilmartin JJ, Gibson GJ: Mechanisms of paradoxical rib cage motion in patients with obstructive pulmonary disease, *Am Rev Respir Dis* 134:683-687, 1986.

36. Burnside JW: *Adam's Physical Diagnosis*, ed 15, Baltimore, 1974, Williams & Wilkins.

37. Turck M: Foul breath and a productive cough, *Hosp Pract* 20(5A):50, 1985.

38. Pulmonary terms and symbols. A report of the ACCP-STS Joint Committee on Pulmonary Nomenclature, *Chest* 67(5):583-593, 1975.

39. Lehrer S: *Understanding Lung Sounds*, Philadelphia, 1984, WB Saunders.

40. Murray JF: Physical examination. In Murray JF, Nadel JA: *Textbook of Respiratory Medicine*, ed 3, Philadelphia, 2000, WB Saunders.

41. Forgacs P: Lung sounds, *Br J Dis Chest* 63:1, 1969.

42. Nath AR, Capel LH: Inspiratory crackles and mechanical events of breathing, *Thorax* 29:695, 1974.

43. Campbell EJM: Accessory muscles. In Campbell EJM, Agostini E, Davis JN (eds): *The Respiratory Muscles*, ed 2, Philadelphia, 1970, WB Saunders.

44. Seidel HM, Ball JW, Dains JE, et al: *Mosby's Guide to Physical Examination*, ed 2, St. Louis, 1991, Mosby-Yearbook.

45. Irwin S: Cardiac disease and pathophysiology. In Irwin S, Tecklin JS (eds): *Cardiopulmonary Physical Therapy: A Guide to Practice*, ed 4, St. Louis, 2004, Mosby.

46. Laghi F, Tobin MJ: Disorders of the respiratory muscles, *Am J Respir Crit Care Med* 168(1):10-48, 2003.

47. Yernault JC, Bohanda AB: Chest percussion, *Eur Respir J* 8:1756-1760, 1995.

48. Lorig KL, Sobel DS, Stewart AL, et al: Evidence suggesting that a chronic disease self-management program can improve health status while reducing hospitalization: A randomized trial, *Med Care* 37:5-14, 1999.

49. Pulmonary rehabilitation—1999. American Thoracic Society, *Am J Respir Crit Care Med* 159:1666-1682, 1999.

50. Proceedings of the Conference on the Scientific Basis of Respiratory Therapy, *Am Rev Respir Dis* 110:1-204, 1974.

51. Williams MT: Chest physiotherapy and cystic fibrosis. Why is the most effective form of treatment still unclear? *Chest* 106:1872-1882, 1994.

52. Thomas J, Cook DJ, Brooks D: Chest physical therapy management of patients with cystic fibrosis. A meta-analysis, *Am J Respir Crit Care Med* 151:846-850, 1995.

53. AARC Clinical Practice Guidelines: Postural drainage therapy, *Respir Care* 12:1418-1426, 1991.

54. Murray JF: The ketchup-bottle method, *N Engl J Med* 300:1155-1157, 1979.

55. Pryor JA, Webber BA, Hodson ME, et al: Evaluation of the forced expiratory technique as an adjunct to postural drainage in treatment of cystic fibrosis, *BMJ* 2(6187):417-418, 1979.

56. Dab I, Alexander F: The mechanism of autogenic drainage studied with flow volume curves, *Monogr Paediatr* 10:50-53, 1979.

57. Miller S, Hall DO, Clayton CB, et al: Chest physiotherapy in cystic fibrosis: a comparative study of autogenic drainage and the active cycle of breathing techniques with postural drainage, *Thorax* 50(2):165-169, 1995.

58. Giles DR, Wagener JS, Accurso FJ, et al: Short-term effects of postural drainage with clapping vs autogenic drainage on oxygen saturation and sputum recovery in patients with cystic fibrosis, *Chest* 108(4):952-954, 1995.

59. Savci S, Ince DI, Arikan H: A comparison of autogenic drainage and the active cycle of breathing techniques in patients with chronic obstructive pulmonary diseases, *J Cardiopulm Rehabil* 20(1):37-43, 2000.

60. Scherer PW: Mucus transport by cough, *Chest* 80(6 suppl):830-833, 1981.

61. Pontifex E, Williams MT, Lunn R, et al: The effect of huffing and directed coughing on energy expenditure in young asymptomatic subjects, *Aust J Physiother* 48(3):209-213, 2002.

62. de Boeck C, Zinman R: Cough versus chest physiotherapy. A comparison of the acute effects on pulmonary function in patients with cystic fibrosis, *Am Rev Respir Dis* 129(1):182-184, 1984.

63. Rossman CM, Waldes R, Sampson D, et al: Effect of chest physiotherapy on the removal of mucus in patients with cystic fibrosis, *Am Rev Respir Dis* 126(1):131-135, 1982.

64. Chulay M: Arterial blood gas changes with a hyperinflation and hyperoxygenation suctioning intervention in critically ill patients, *Heart Lung* 17:654-661, 1988.

65. Mathias CJ: Bradycardia and cardiac arrest during tracheal suction–mechanisms in tetraplegic patients, *Eur J Intensive Care Med* 2(4):147-156, 1976.

66. Arens R, Gozal D, Omlin KJ, et al: Comparison of high frequency chest compression and conventional chest physiotherapy in hospitalized patients with cystic fibrosis, *Am J Respir Crit Care Med* 150:1154, 1994.

67. Varekojis SM, Douce FH, Flucke RL, et al: A comparison of the therapeutic effectiveness of and preference for postural drainage and percussion, intrapulmonary percussive ventilation, and high-frequency chest wall compression in hospitalized cystic fibrosis patients, *Respir Care* 48(1):24-28, 2003.

68. Homnick DM, Anderson K, Marks JH: Comparison of the flutter device to standard chest physiotherapy in hospitalized patients with cystic fibrosis: A pilot study, *Chest* 114(4):993-997, 1998.

69. Murray JF: The ketchup-bottle method, *N Engl J Med* 300(20):1155-1157, 1979.

70. King M, Zidulka A, Phillips JM, et al: Tracheal mucus clearance in high-frequency oscillation: Effect of peak flow bias, *Eur Respir J* 3:6-13, 1990.

71. Warwick WJ, Hansen LG: The long-term effect of high-frequency chest compression therapy on pulmonary complications of cystic fibrosis, *Pediatr Pulmonol* 11:265, 1991.

72. Tecklin JS, Clayton R, Scanlin T: High frequency chest wall oscillation vs. traditional chest physical therapy in cystic fibrosis—a large one-year, controlled study, 14th Annual North American Cystic Fibrosis Conference, November 11, 2000, Baltimore, Md.

73. Chambers C, Klous D, Nantel N, et al: Does high-frequency chest compression (HFCC) during aerosol therapy affect lung deposition? *Am J Respir Crit Care Med* 157(suppl 3):A131, 1998.

74. Newhouse PA, White F, Marks JH, et al: The intrapulmonary percussive ventilator and flutter device compared to standard chest physiotherapy in patients with cystic fibrosis, *Clin Pediatr* 37:427-432, 1998.

75. McIlwaine PM, Wong LT, Peacock D, et al: Long-term comparative trial of conventional postural drainage and percussion versus positive expiratory pressure physiotherapy in the treatment of cystic fibrosis, *J Pediatr* 131:570-574, 1997.

76. McIlwaine PM, Wong LT, Peacock D, et al: Long term comparative trial of positive expiratory pressure versus oscillating positive expiratory pressure (flutter) physiotherapy in the treatment of cystic fibrosis, *J Pediatr* 138:845-850, 2001.

77. Gondor M, Nixon PA, Mutich R, et al: Comparison of Flutter device and chest physical therapy in the treatment of cystic fibrosis pulmonary exacerbation, *Pediatr Pulmonol* 28:255-260, 1999.

78. Volsko TA, DiFiore J, Chatburn RL: Performance comparison of two oscillating positive expiratory pressure devices: Acapella versus flutter, *Respir Care* 48(2):124-130, 2003.

79. Maxwell M, Redmond A: Comparative trial of manual and mechanical percussion technique with gravity-assisted bronchial drainage in patients with cystic fibrosis, *Arch Dis Child* 54(7):542-544, 1979.

80. Garrod R, Paul EA, Wedzicha JA: Supplemental oxygen during pulmonary rehabilitation in patients with COPD with exercise hypoxemia, *Thorax* 55:539-543, 2000.

81. Soguel Schenkel N, Burdet L, de Muralt B, et al: Oxygen saturation during daily activities in chronic obstructive pulmonary disease, *Eur Respir J* 9:2584-2589, 1996.

82. Foglio K, Bianchi L, Bruletti G, et al: Long-term effectiveness of pulmonary rehabilitation in patients with chronic airway obstruction, *Eur Respir J* 131:125-132, 1999.

83. Goldstein RS, Gort EH, Stubbing D, et al: Randomised controlled trial of respiratory rehabilitation, *Lancet* 344:1394-1397, 1994.

84. Berry MJ, Rejeski WJ, Adair NE, et al: Exercise rehabilitation and chronic obstructive pulmonary disease stage, *Am J Respir Crit Care Med* 160:1248-1253, 1999.

85. Troosters T, Gosselink R, Decramer M: Short- and long-term effects of outpatient rehabilitation in patients with chronic obstructive pulmonary disease: A randomized trial, *Am J Med* 109(3):207-212, 2000.

86. O'Neill S, McCarthy DS: Postural relief of dyspnea in severe chronic airflow limitation: Relationship to respiratory muscle strength, *Thorax* 38:595-600, 1983.

87. Numa AH, Hammer J, Newth CJ: Effect of prone and supine positions on functional residual capacity, oxygenation, and respiratory mechanics in ventilated infants and children, *Am J Respir Crit Care Med* 156:1185-1189, 1999.

88. Filippelli M, Duranti R, Gigliotti F, et al: Overall contribution of chest wall hyperinflation to breathlessness in asthma, *Chest* 124(6):2164-2170, 2003.

89. Hilling L, Smith J: Pulmonary rehabilitation. In Irwin S, Tecklin JS (eds): *Cardiopulmonary Physical Therapy*, ed 3, St. Louis, 1995, Mosby.

90. Merrick J, Axen K: Inspiratory muscle function following abdominal weight exercises in healthy subjects, *Phys Ther* 61(5):651-656, 1981.

91. Cahalin LP, Braga M, Matsuo Y, et al: Efficacy of diaphragmatic breathing in person with chronic obstructive pulmonary disease: A review of the literature, *J Cardiopulm Rehabil* 22:7-21, 2002.

92. Sackner MA, Silva G, Banks JM, et al: Distribution of ventilation during diaphragmatic breathing in obstructive lung disease, *Am Rev Respir Dis* 109:331-337, 1974.

93. Brach BB, Chao RP, Sgroi ML, et al: 133Xenon washout patterns during diaphragmatic breathing. Studies in normal subjects and patients with chronic obstructive pulmonary disease, *Chest* 71:735-739, 1977.

94. Sackner MA, Gonzalez HF, Jenouri G, et al: Effects of abdominal and thoracic breathing on breathing pattern components in normal subjects and in patients with chronic obstructive pulmonary disease, *Am Rev Respir Dis* 130(4):584-587, 1984.

95. Sackner MA, Gonzalez HF, Rodriguez M, et al: Assessment of asynchronous and paradoxic motion between rib cage and abdomen in normal subjects and in patients with chronic obstructive pulmonary disease, *Am Rev Respir Dis* 130:588-593, 1984.

96. Gosselink RA, Wagenaar RC, Rijswijk H, et al: Diaphragmatic breathing reduces efficiency of breathing in patients with chronic obstructive pulmonary disease, *Am J Respir Crit Care Med* 151:1136-1142, 1995.

97. Vitacca M, Clini E, Bianchi L, et al: Acute effects of deep diaphragmatic breathing in COPD patients with chronic respiratory insufficiency, *Eur Respir J* 11:408-415, 1998.

98. Sergysels R, DeCoster A, Degre S, et al: Functional evaluation of a physical rehabilitation program including breathing exercises and bicycle training in chronic obstructive lung disease, *Respiration* 38:105-111, 1979.

99. Schutz K: Muscular exercise in the treatment of bronchial asthma, *NY J Med* 55:635, 1935.

100. Mueller RE, Petty TL, Filley GF: Ventilation and arterial blood gas changes induced by pursed lips breathing, *J Appl Physiol* 28:784, 1970.

101. Westreich N, Paguyo N, Cohen S, et al: Breathing retraining: Mount Sinai Hospital emphysema-chronic bronchitis clinic, *Minn Med* 53:621-622, 1970.

102. Thoman RL, Stoker GL, Ross JC: The efficacy of pursed lips breathing in patients with chronic obstructive pulmonary disease, *Am Rev Respir Dis* 93:100-106, 1966.

103. Casciari RJ, Fairshter RD, Harrison A: Effects of breathing retraining in patients with chronic obstructive pulmonary disease, *Chest* 79:393-398, 1981.

104. Bianchi R, Gigliotti F, Romagnoli I, et al: Chest wall kinematics and breathlessness during pursed-lip breathing in patients with COPD. *Chest* 125(2):459-465. 2004.

105. Dechman G, Wilson CR: Evidence underlying breathing retraining in people with stable chronic obstructive pulmonary disease, *Phys Ther* 84(12):1189-1197, 2004.

106. Lourens MS, van den Berg B, Hoogsteden HC, et al: Effect of expiratory resistance on gas-exchange and breathing pattern in chronic obstructive pulmonary disease (COPD) patients being weaned from the ventilator, *Acta Anaesthesiol Scand* 45:1155-1161, 2001.

107. Watts N: Improvement of breathing patterns, *Phys Ther* 48(6):563-576, 1968.

108. Campbell EJM, Friend J: Action of breathing exercise in pulmonary emphysema, *Lancet* 19:325, 1955.

109. Martin DJ, Ripley H, Reynolds J, et al: Chest physiotherapy and the distribution of ventilation, *Chest* 69:174-178, 1976.

110. Cappello M, De Troyer A: On the respiratory function of the ribs, *J Appl Physiol* 92(4):1642-1646, 2002.

111. Ward RJ, Danziger F, Bonica JJ, et al: An evaluation of postoperative respiratory maneuvers, *Surg Gynecol Obstet* 123:51-54, 1976.

112. Erskine-Milliss J, Schonell M: Relaxation therapy in asthma: A critical review, *Psychosom Med* 43:365-372, 1981.

113. Anbar RD: Self-hypnosis for management of chronic dyspnea in pediatric patients, *Pediatrics* 107(2):E21, 2001.

114. Bernard S, LeBlanc P, Whittom F, et al: Peripheral muscle weakness in patients with chronic obstructive pulmonary disease, *Am J Respir Crit Care Med* 158:629-634, 1998.

115. Hamilton AL, Killian KJ, Summers E, et al: Muscle strength, symptom intensity, and exercise capacity in patients with cardiorespiratory disorders, *Am J Respir Crit Care Med* 152:2021-2031, 1995.

116. Mador MJ, Bozkanat E: Skeletal muscle dysfunction in chronic obstructive pulmonary disease, *Respir Res* 2(4):216-224, 2001.

117. O'Donnell DE, McGuire M, Samis L, et al: General exercise training improves ventilatory and peripheral muscle strength and endurance in chronic airflow limitation, *Am J Respir Crit Care Med* 157:1489-1497, 1997.

118. Mador MJ, Kufel TJ, Pineda LA, et al: Effect of pulmonary rehabilitation on quadriceps fatigability during exercise, *Am J Respir Crit Care Med* 163(4):930-935, 2001.

119. Spruit MA, Gosselink R, Troosters T, et al: Resistance versus endurance training in patients with COPD and peripheral muscle weakness, *Eur Respir J* 19(6):1072-1078, 2002.

120. Casaburi R, Bhasin S, Cosentino L, et al: Effects of testosterone and resistance training in men with chronic obstructive pulmonary disease, *Am J Respir Crit Care Med* 15:870-878, 2004.

121. Bernard S, Whittom F, Leblanc P, et al: Aerobic and strength training in patients with chronic obstructive pulmonary disease, *Am J Respir Crit Care Med* 159:896-901, 1999.

122. Mador MJ, Bozkanat E, Aggarwal A, et al: Endurance and strength training in patients with COPD, *Chest* 125(6):2036-2045, 2004.

123. Storer TW: Pulmonary rehabilitation: Resistance exercise prescription, *Med Sci Sports Exerc* 33(7 suppl):S690-692, 2001.

124. Normandin EA, McCusker C, Connors M: An evaluation of two approaches to exercise conditioning in pulmonary rehabilitation, *Chest* 12:1085-1091, 2002.

125. Yohannes AM, Roomi J, Winn S, et al: The Manchester Respiratory Activities of Daily Living questionnaire: Development, reliability, validity, and responsiveness to pulmonary rehabilitation, *J Am Geriatr Soc* 48:1496-1500, 2000.

126. Garrod R, Bestall JC, Paul EA, et al: Development and validation of a standardized measure of activity of daily living in patients with severe COPD: The London Chest Activity of Daily Living scale (LCADL), *Respir Med* 94:589-596, 2000.

127. Camp PG, Appleton J, Reid WD: Quality of life after pulmonary rehabilitation: assessing change using quantitative and qualitative methods, *Phys Ther* 80:986-995, 2000.

128. Bhambhani YN, Clarkson HM, Gomes PS: Axillary crutch walking: effects of three training programs, *Arch Phys Med Rehabil* 71(7):484-489, 1990.

129. Holder CG, Haskvitz EM, Weltman A: The effects of assistive devices on the oxygen cost, cardiovascular stress, and perception of non-weight-bearing ambulation, *JOSPT* 18:537-542, 1993.

Chapter 25

Congestive Heart Failure

Jennifer Dekerlegand

CHAPTER OUTLINE

OBJECTIVES

After reading this chapter, the reader will be able to:
1. Define congestive heart failure and identify implications for rehabilitation interventions.
2. Understand the etiology and pathology of heart failure.
3. Describe classification systems for heart failure.
4. Identify the examination procedures used to diagnose heart failure.
5. Perform a comprehensive rehabilitation examination and evaluation for a patient with heart failure.
6. Provide effective rehabilitation interventions for patients with heart failure.
7. Evaluate and modify as needed an exercise prescription based on a patient with heart failure's response to the program.
8. Examine methods to measure outcomes of treatment of patients with heart failure, including exercise testing and self-report measures.

Heart failure affects 5 million people in the United States, with approximately 550,000 new cases being diagnosed each year.[1] According to the Centers for Medicare and Medicaid, heart failure is the most frequent Medicare diagnosis at hospital admission, and 250,000 deaths each year are caused by heart failure.[1] Whether a clinician works in an acute care hospital, an acute rehabilitation facility, an outpatient clinic, a long-term care facility, or in the home setting, they will certainly encounter patients with heart failure. Hallmarks of heart failure include decreased activity tolerance, decreased function, and edema. Patients with heart failure can benefit from the expertise of therapists to improve these deficits.

Heart failure is a progressive disease that results from the heart's gradual inability to pump enough blood to meet the body's demands. In the past, the term congestive heart failure was used to describe patients who presented with heart failure and the classic signs and symptoms of volume overload. However, we now realize that many patients with heart failure have reduced activity tolerance without evidence of fluid retention. Therefore, since the 1990s, *heart failure* has become the preferred term because it causes less confusion about the presenting signs and symptoms in these patients.

Until recently, heart failure research focused on interventions aimed at reducing mortality and decreasing signs and symptoms in patients diagnosed with heart failure. There were also a few studies on interventions intended to prevent or reduce the risk of heart failure. The New York Heart Association, the American College of Cardiology (ACC), and the American Heart Association (AHA) developed guidelines for classifying heart failure into one of four stages (see Table 25-5), with recommended interventions for each of these stages.[2] This chapter presents and analyzes the evidence on the rehabilitation examination, evaluation, and interventions for patients in all stages of heart failure.

PATHOLOGY

Heart failure is a clinical syndrome resulting from a reduction in the heart's ability to fill with blood or eject blood to the rest of the body. There are many disease processes that can progress to heart failure. Structural causes of heart failure include disorders of the *myocardium*, pericardium, endocardium, or great vessels. Heart failure can also be caused by valvular disease, coronary artery disease (CAD), hypertension, *cardiomyopathy,* alcohol or drug abuse, and myocarditis.[2]

Hypertension causes heart failure because it leads to high peripheral arterial pressure and resistance, which increases the afterload on the heart, making it more difficult for the heart to eject blood. Cardiomyopathy of any type, restrictive, hypertrophic, or dilated, can also lead to heart failure. In *restrictive cardiomyopathy* the walls of the ventricle become stiff because of abnormal infiltration of the heart muscle. This stiffness prevents the heart from filling or ejecting blood adequately. Causes of restrictive cardiomyopathy include *amyloidosis, sarcoidosis,* and hemochromatosis. *Hypertrophic cardiomyopathy* is characterized by thickening of the walls of the heart as a result of abnormal growth and abnormal arrangement of cardiac muscle cells. The thickening reduces the size of the heart chambers and can also restrict the heart's ability to fill, both of which limit the heart's ability to pump blood. *Dilated cardiomyopathy* is characterized by stretching and thinning of the heart muscle with consequent cardiac enlargement and increased filling but reduced ejection of blood. The various types of cardiomyopathy are depicted in Fig. 25-1.

CLASSIFICATION OF HEART FAILURE

Heart failure may be classified according to a variety of classification schemes. It is generally classified by whether

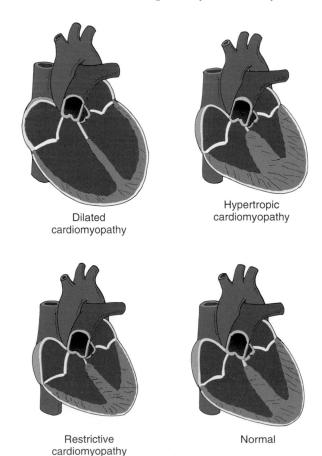

Dilated cardiomyopathy

Hypertropic cardiomyopathy

Restrictive cardiomyopathy

Normal

FIG. 25-1 Types of cardiomyopathies and the normal heart.

it most affects systolic (ejection of blood from the heart) or diastolic (filling of the heart with blood) heart function. Systolic failure can be further divided according to its etiology as ischemic or nonischemic. Although the signs and symptoms of all types of heart failure may be similar, appropriate management can vary, depending on classification.[3]

Heart function is quantified either by *echocardiography* or by nuclear multiple-gated acquisition (MUGA) scanning, with the primary index generally being left ventricular *ejection fraction* (EF).[4] The left ventricular EF is the percentage of the *end-diastolic volume* (i.e., the amount of blood in the left ventricle when it is full, at the end of *diastole*) pumped from the left ventricle with each heartbeat. A normal EF is between 55% and 65%. *Systolic dysfunction* is defined as an EF below 40%. In contrast, *diastolic dysfunction* is characterized by a normal EF with reduced filling.[4] Systolic dysfunction is easier to detect than diastolic dysfunction because the reduced EF can be readily detected by echocardiography. Both systolic and diastolic heart failure can present with similar symptoms, including fatigue, *dyspnea,* and decreased exercise tolerance.

As noted, systolic dysfunction can be further categorized as ischemic or nonischemic. *Ischemic heart failure* is the breakdown of the heart muscle because of lack of blood flow to the coronary vessels and may occur with or without myocardial infarction. Approximately 50% to 70% of patients diagnosed with heart failure have ischemic systolic dysfunction.[5] Nonischemic heart failure is systolic heart failure that results from any process other than CAD. It can have many causes, including hypertension, alcohol abuse, valvular disease, and viral or other infectious diseases. Nonischemic systolic heart failure is also associated with pregnancy and certain medications or may be idiopathic. The prognosis for patients with ischemic heart failure is worse than for those with nonischemic failure, probably because more of these patients have other co-morbidities such as diabetes mellitus.[6]

From 20% to 70% of patients with heart failure have diastolic dysfunction, characterized by a normal left ventricular EF.[7-9] Patients with diastolic dysfunction are more often female, older, and obese and more likely to have high blood pressure (BP) and less likely to have CAD than patients with systolic heart failure.[9] With diastolic dysfunction, there is impaired filling of the left ventricle because of thickening, stiffening, and/or impaired relaxation of the walls of the heart. With aging, the heart's elasticity decreases, leading to increased myocardial stiffness.[10,11] Diastolic heart failure is usually detected after exclusion of other possible reasons for heart failure symptoms.

CHARACTERISTICS OF HEART FAILURE CONTRIBUTING TO EXERCISE INTOLERANCE

Regardless of etiology or classification, heart failure is characterized by the inability of the heart to meet the demands of the body. This results in the hallmark symptom of heart failure: Decreased exercise tolerance. A normal exercise response requires the coordination of multiple systems, including the cardiac, pulmonary, vascular, and musculoskeletal. During exercise, *cardiac output,* which is the product of heart rate (HR) multiplied by *stroke volume,* should be able to increase to four to six times its resting level. Patients with heart failure can often only achieve half this normal increase in cardiac output during exercise.[12]

Central hemodynamic characteristics of heart failure contribute to exercise intolerance. These include abnormal pressures within the heart, reduced left ventricular EF, reduced cardiac output, and increased pulmonary capillary wedge pressure. Although a low EF is diagnostic of systolic heart failure, exercise tolerance correlates poorly with EF.[13] Patients with a similar EF can present with very different severities of functional impairment and exercise intolerance. Furthermore, although medications may rapidly improve central hemodynamics, including stroke volume and EF, exercise tolerance may not improve until weeks to months later. The fact that central factors alone cannot account for exercise intolerance in patients with heart failure has led researchers to search for other mechanisms that may contribute to the decreased exercise tolerance observed in these patients. New evidence suggests that a number of peripheral factors, including alterations in sympathetic and other neurohormonal control mechanisms, as well as changes in skeletal muscle, pulmonary, and vascular function, may contribute to the reduced activity tolerance seen in this population.

The low BP typical of heart failure activates the sympathetic nervous system, which leads to tachycardia at rest, decreased HR variability, and decreased peripheral vasodilation. Increased blood levels of norepinephrine observed in patients with heart failure support the notion that heart failure is associated with increased sympathetic nervous system activation.[14,15] This sympathetic activation helps to compensate for the low output that occurs with heart failure by increasing HR, thereby increasing cardiac output and by stimulating vasoconstriction, which increases systemic BP. However, prolonged sympathetic activation may worsen heart failure by increasing the resistance to the outflow of blood from the heart.

The renin-angiotensin-aldosterone system is also activated in heart failure. This causes increased production of angiotensin II, which increases HR, impairs cardiac filling, and increases coronary vasoconstriction and peripheral vascular resistance.

Vasodilation may also be impaired in patients with heart failure because of increased vascular stiffness that results from increased sodium and fluid in the vascular tissue, chronic vascular deconditioning, and endothelial dysfunction in peripheral and coronary vessels.

Early reports attributed skeletal muscle abnormalities in heart failure patients to poor perfusion of the muscles as a result of the reduction in cardiac output. However, medications that augment cardiac output and muscle perfusion have not been found to improve muscle performance in these patients.[16,17] Studies show that a combination of skeletal muscle abnormalities that include altered metabolism, muscle atrophy, decreased blood flow to the muscles, and the conversion of muscle fiber type from slow twitch to fast twitch contribute to exercise intolerance in patients with heart failure.[18-20]

Pulmonary system abnormalities can also contribute to exercise intolerance in patients with heart failure. Patients with heart failure have abnormalities in pulmonary function testing, and one of the most common complaints of patients with heart failure is shortness of breath with exertion.[21] These signs and symptoms normalize after cardiac transplantation. The mechanisms underlying these changes are unclear. There is some contribution from changes in the muscles of respiration, including atrophy, increased lactic acid production, and muscle hypoxia, that are similar to the changes that occur in the peripheral muscles. Furthermore, there is evidence of increased use of accessory muscles during breathing.[22] Some have also attributed respiratory changes to abnormal increases in heart chamber pressures; however, elevated pressures have not been found to correlate with exercise testing results in this population.[23] After a group of patients completed a program of aerobic training, heart pressures were unchanged, despite a 23% increase in maximal oxygen uptake ($\dot{V}O_{2max}$) and a reduction in dyspnea.[23]

EXAMINATION

Examination of the patient with heart failure consists of a comprehensive patient history and a systems review, followed by the appropriate tests and measures. As with other rehabilitation diagnoses, the examination will be tailored to meet the specific needs of the individual patient. Factors that will vary the selection of procedures used in examination of the patient with heart failure may include age, social history, diagnosis of chronic or acute heart failure, time since onset of initial heart failure diagnosis, other current medical conditions, and patient goals.

PATIENT HISTORY

The examination must include a comprehensive patient history that can be gathered from the patient's inpatient or outpatient chart, as well as through direct interview with the patient or family members. In addition to general demographics, such as age, gender, and race, it is important to assess the family and caregiver support for the patient. Heart failure is a progressive disease, often characterized by exacerbations that can be kept to a minimum with the support of family and friends reinforcing compliance with the medical regimen.

Employment history should include information about job responsibilities and activities, such as the frequency of stair climbing, heavy lifting, pushing, pulling, or extreme temperature work environments, as these can affect job performance and the clinical status of the patient with heart failure. Home environment and structure should be documented along with any equipment the patient is using or has available for future use. Equipment that may be useful to the patient with heart failure includes motorized wheelchairs, oxygen delivery devices, stair glides, exercise equipment, adaptive bathroom equipment, and home monitoring equipment such as scales, BP units, and HR monitors. The history should also document the health and social habits of the patient, including compliance with medications, diet, exercise routine, medical follow-up, as well as assessment of smoking, drug, and alcohol use.

The history should continue with documentation of the medical and surgical history, current medications, and clinical tests. Commonly used medications in this population and their indications and potential side effects are included in Table 25-1. Clinical tests commonly include echocardiograms, cardiac catheterizations, exercise testing, laboratory tests, electrocardiograms, and radiographic imaging. Additionally, the clinician should determine if the patient has a pacemaker or implanted cardiac defibrillator (ICD) and the settings of these devices, as these may affect the initiation and termination of rehabilitation interventions. Likewise, the history should document any recent arrhythmias with the associated patient symptoms.

Finally, the patient's current functional status, complaints, and symptoms should be thoroughly discussed and documented. The therapist should determine if the patient has symptoms typical for heart failure, including fatigue, shortness of breath, reduced exercise and activity tolerance and peripheral edema; what kind and duration of activity brings on each of these symptoms; how long they last; and what relieves these symptoms. Common signs and symptoms seen in the patient with heart failure are included in Box 25-1.

SYSTEMS REVIEW

The systems review is used to target areas requiring further examination and to define areas that may cause complications or indicate a need for precautions during the examination and intervention processes. See Chapter 1 for details of the systems review.

TESTS AND MEASURES

Musculoskeletal. Musculoskeletal tests and measures may include quantification of range of motion (ROM), flexibility, postural alignment, joint integrity and mobility (see Chapter 4). Anthropometric characteristics relative to heart failure may include determination of body

TABLE 25-1	Medications Used in the Treatment of Heart Failure			
Drug Class	**Examples**	**Therapeutic Effects**	**Adverse Effects**	**Exercise Implications**
ACE inhibitors	Benazepril (Lotensin) Enalapril (Vasotec) Lisinopril (Zestril) Quinapril (Accupril)	Promote vasodilation and lower BP.	Persistent cough, orthostasis, skin rash, change in sense of taste, renal dysfunction, elevated potassium levels	Watch for episodes of hypotension and arrhythmias.
ARBs	Candesartan (Atacand) Irbesartan (Avapro) Losartan (Cozaar) Valsartan (Diovan)	Promote vasodilation and lower BP.	Orthostasis, rash, facial swelling, renal dysfunction, elevated potassium levels	Watch for episodes of hypotension and arrhythmias.
Antiarrhythmics	Amiodarone (Cordarone, Pacerone) Sotalol (Betapace)	Prevent arrhythmias, including atrial fibrillation and flutter.	Thyroid dysfunction, GI upset, pulmonary fibrosis, ataxia, liver dysfunction	Prolonged use can lead to pulmonary dysfunction, reduced coordination and tremor.
Anticoagulants	Warfarin (Coumadin) Enoxaparin (Lovenox)	Prevent formation of blood clots.	Nosebleeds, bleeding of the gums, bruising	Monitor INR for risk of increased bleeding.
Beta-blockers	Carvedilol (Coreg) Metoprolol (Lopressor, Toprol XL)	Decrease myocardial demand.	Fatigue, weakness, orthostasis, decreased sexual ability, wheezing, and bradycardia	Will demonstrate blunted heart rate response to exercise, monitor for bradycardia.
Digitalis preparations	Digoxin (Digitek, Lanoxin)	Increase force of the heart's contractions.	Suppressed appetite, nausea/vomiting, headache, visual deficits, and irregular rhythms	Monitor for arrhythmias.
Potassium	Potassium chloride (K-Dur, Klor-Con)	Used in conjunction with some diuretics to prevent low potassium levels.	Nausea, diarrhea, and rarely, abnormal heart-beats	Monitor for arrhythmias.
Vasodilators	Isosorbide dinitrate (Isordil) Isosorbide mononitrate (Imdur ISMO) Nitroglycerin	Increase vasodilation to decrease workload on the heart.	Orthostasis, headaches, flushing, heart palpitations, nasal congestion, joint pain, and/or rash	Monitor for hypotension.
Inotrope	Milrinone (Primacor)	Decrease myocardial workload.	Ventricular arrhythmias, hypotension, decreased potassium	Monitor for hypotension and arrhythmias.
Diuretics	Bumetanide (Bumex) Furosemide (Lasix) Spironolactone (Aldactone) Hydrochlorothiazide	Decrease fluid accumulation in periphery/lungs.	Orthostasis, frequent urination, renal dysfunction, altered potassium levels	Monitor for hypotension and arrhythmias from changes in potassium.

ACE, Angiotensin-converting enzyme; *BP,* blood pressure; *INR,* international normalized ratio; *GI,* gastrointestinal; *ARBs,* angiotensin-receptor blockers.

BOX 25-1	Common Signs and Symptoms in Patients with Heart Failure

- Dyspnea
- Fatigue
- Paroxysmal nocturnal dyspnea
- Peripheral edema
- JVD
- Rales
- Abnormal heart sounds (S3, S4)
- Ascites/liver congestion/hepatomegaly
- Decreased functional exercise capacity
- Angina
- Renal insufficiency/failure
- Hypotension
- Orthopnea
- Tachycardia

JVD, Jugular venous distention.

TABLE 25-2	Calculation and Classification of Body Mass Index (BMI)

BMI = Body Weight in Kilograms/ (Height in Meters)^2

Classification	BMI (kg/m^2)
Underweight	<18.5
Normal	18.5-24.9
Overweight	25-29.9
Class of Obesity	
I	30-34.9
II	35-39.9
III	>40

Adapted from *Arch Intern Med* 158:1855-1867, 1998.

mass index (BMI). BMI is based on the patient's weight and height. The formula for calculating BMI and the interpretation of its values are given in Table 25-2.

Neuromuscular. Tests and measures for neuromuscular examination generally include examination of reflex and sensory integrity, as well as motor function. These tests are usually not required in the patient with heart failure. However, aspects of the neuromuscular examination that are important in patients with heart failure are measures of arousal, attention, and cognition and of pain.

Arousal, Attention, and Cognition. Recent research suggests that some degree of cognitive dysfunction is commonly associated with heart failure. An initial study using neuropsychological testing in 68 patients with heart failure found that 30% had four or more cognitive deficits and only 9% of the sample had normal results.[24] Another study compared neuropsychological test results in three groups of elderly patients, including a group with heart failure, a group with other types of cardiovascular disease, and a group that was disease-free. The investigators found greater cognitive deficits in the heart failure group in four of the seven parts of the testing.[25] These parts of the testing focused on verbal learning and attention. Another investigation of cognitive impairment in patients with

heart failure found the greatest deficits in memory, attention, problem solving, and motor response.[26] This study found that EF was not related to the level of cognitive impairment.[26] Cognitive deficits in patients with heart failure are thought to be caused by cerebral infarction and/or cerebral hypoperfusion. The challenge is how to reliably measure and document these cognitive deficits. Although there is not sufficient evidence to recommend specific tools to measure cognitive dysfunction in patients with heart failure,[27] it is important for clinicians to recognize the potential presence of these deficits and to adjust their interventions accordingly.

Pain. A global pain assessment should include the use of a visual analog scale and a pain drawing to measure pain intensity and location at rest and during activity (see Chapter 22). More specifically, in patients with heart failure, symptoms of angina and dyspnea that may limit performance of functional tasks should be measured. Angina is typically rated on a 1 to 4 scale (Table 25-3). For patients with ischemic heart disease, exercise should not precipitate symptoms exceeding a rating of 2. Dyspnea can also be rated on the Dyspnea Index, which is rated on a 0 to 4 scale (Table 25-4). The Dyspnea Index score is the number of breaths required while the patient counts out loud from 1 to 15. Patients should not exceed a score of 2 at any time during rehabilitation interventions.

Cardiovascular/Pulmonary. Most of the tests and measures performed in the examination of patients with heart failure should focus on assessing circulation and aerobic capacity. As discussed previously, the clinical

TABLE 25-3	Angina Scale

Stage	Description
1	Onset of angina; mild but recognized as the usual angina-of-effort pain or discomfort with which the subject is familiar.
2	Some pain, moderately severe and definitely uncomfortable but still tolerable.
3	Severe anginal pain at a level that the subject will wish to stop exercising.
4	Unbearable chest pain; the most severe pain the subject has felt.

From Allred EN, Bleecker ER, Chaitman BR, et al: *Environ Health Perspect* 91:89-132, 1991; Allred EN, Bleecker ER, Chaitman BR, et al: *N Engl J Med* 321:1426-1432, 1989.

TABLE 25-4	Dyspnea Index

Level	Description
0	Able to count aloud to 15 without taking a breath
1	Must take one breath in order to complete counting aloud to 15
2	Must take two breaths in order to complete counting aloud to 15
3	Must take three breaths in order to complete counting aloud to 15

From Watchie J: *Cardiopulmonary Physical Therapy: A Clinical Manual,* Philadelphia, 1995, WB Saunders.

presentation of heart failure results from vascular, musculoskeletal, pulmonary, cardiac, and hematological abnormalities and can cause peripheral and *pulmonary edema,* dyspnea, *orthopnea* (shortness of breath with lying supine), *jugular venous distention* (JVD), abnormal heart sounds, and exercise intolerance. The examination should therefore include tests and measures of fluid accumulation, jugular venous distention, HR and BP, and lung and heart sounds to provide a baseline for comparison with later reexamination and an objective indication of a patient's response to treatment interventions.[28]

Circulation

Fluid Accumulation. When the heart cannot pump fluid through the vasculature adequately, fluid may accumulate in the periphery, centrally, and/or in the lungs. Therefore fluid status can be used to assess the severity of disease and the effectiveness of some treatment interventions in heart failure. Fluid status can be assessed by monitoring body weight, detecting JVD, and evaluating for the presence and degree of pulmonary and peripheral edema. Since short-term volume changes can readily be detected by measuring body weight with a scale, heart failure management guidelines recommend daily weight monitoring for patients with heart failure. Clinicians should pay particular attention to a patient's weight as a weight gain of 3 or more pounds in 3 days can be a sign of decompensation.

Jugular Venous Pressure. Jugular venous pressure (JVP) is the pressure of blood in the jugular veins. JVP will be elevated in patients with heart failure when they cannot pump blood out of the heart adequately, causing blood to accumulate in the venous system. JVP is examined by observing the height and characteristics of the pulse of the internal and external jugular veins with the patient lying at a 45-degree angle, with the head turned slightly to avoid compression of the vein by the sternocleidomastoid muscle[29] (Fig. 25-2). The height of the pulsation above the sternal angle can be used to estimate mean *right atrial pressure*.[29,30] A height of 3-4 cm is normal, and a height of more than 4-5 cm from the sternal angle is consistent with JVD, elevated right atrial pressure, and fluid retention.

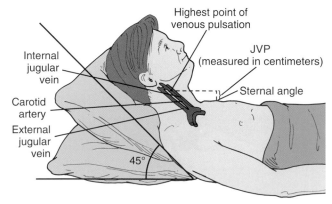

FIG. 25-2 Measurement of jugular venous pressure (JVP). *Redrawn from Seidel HM:* Mosby's Guide to Physical Examination, *ed 5, St. Louis, 2003, Mosby. In Frownfelter D, Dean E:* Cardiovascular and Pulmonary Physical Therapy: Evidence and Practice, *ed 4, St. Louis, 2006, Mosby.*

In a study of 50 patients with heart failure, assessment of jugular venous pressure was found to have a high specificity (90%) but low sensitivity (30%) for impaired left ventricular function.[28] Furthermore, a study that included 2,569 patients with heart failure found that patients with elevated JVP had significantly more hospitalizations for heart failure and more deaths from heart failure than those without elevated JVP.[30] These findings demonstrate the importance of JVP for monitoring change and determining prognosis for patients with heart failure.

Heart Rate and Rhythm. Although HR should be assessed during the systems review for many patients, particular attention should be paid to specific examination of HR and rhythm in the patient with heart failure as these are often indicators of the patient's physiological status and prognosis and may predict the patient's tolerance for activity-based interventions (see Chapter 22 for detailed descriptions of methods of measuring HR and rhythm). Tachycardia, which is a HR greater than 100 beats per minute (bpm) at rest, is a common compensatory attempt to maintain cardiac output in patients with heart failure. Resting tachycardia in the absence of other causes can be attributed to a heightened sympathetic drive from poor ventricular performance.

Abnormal heart rhythms are called arrhythmias (or dysrhythmias). Arrhythmias can provide prognostic information in the heart failure population.[31] According to the Framingham study, the rate of sudden death (i.e., death caused by arrhythmia) is increased by 9 times in heart failure. Approximately 50% of deaths in patients with heart failure are caused by arrhythmias, most commonly fast ventricular arrhythmias. Atrial arrhythmias, including atrial fibrillation and flutter, occur in 10% to 30% of patients with heart failure, and the incidence is proportional to the degree of heart failure.[32] Therefore it is important for therapists to monitor heart rhythm, on telemetry if available, at baseline, as well as during and after interventions.

Because of the risk of arrhythmias and sudden death, many patients with heart failure have pacemakers and/or ICDs. ICDs can recognize and terminate rapid heart rhythms. Clinicians should determine the settings of any device therapy and modify interventions as necessary. Patients are at risk for inappropriate firing of the ICD during exercise if the HR exceeds the programmed threshold. At a minimum, therapists should determine the threshold for ICD firing from the medical history to prevent such inappropriate discharges from occurring during the interventions.

Blood Pressure. BP is used to assess systemic perfusion (see Chapter 22 for detailed descriptions of methods of measuring BP). BP must be measured at least at baseline and after each intervention and if there are any signs or symptoms of decompensation. Both the underlying pathology of heart failure and the medications used to treat it can cause hypotension (low BP). BP goals for these patients may be lower than normal and will vary on an individual basis, depending on the patient's tolerance. It is not uncommon for a patient with dilated cardiomyopathy to tolerate a systolic BP as low as 80-90 mm Hg without symptoms. However, the clinician should monitor each patient for signs and symptoms of hypotension intolerance, including cool, clammy extremities; complaints of dizziness, particularly when rising from supine or sitting; fatigue; and/or blurred vision.

Heart Sounds. Heart sounds can be heard by auscultation of the heart through the chest wall with a stethoscope. Heart sounds generally reflect the closing of the heart valves and include normal and abnormal sounds. The first heart sound *(S1)* is the sound heard with the closing of the mitral and tricuspid valves and is best heard with placement of the diaphragm of the stethoscope at the apex of the heart. The second heart sound *(S2)* represents aortic and pulmonic valve closures and is best auscultated with the diaphragm of the stethoscope at the second intercostal space. S1 precedes S2, and together these compose the "lub-dub" sounds.

The third heart sound *(S3)* may be normal (physiological) or abnormal (pathological). A physiological S3 is sometimes heard in children and young adults, but an S3 in a person over 30 years of age is generally pathological and is commonly present in older patients with heart failure. The pathological S3 is often an early sign of heart failure. If present, the S3 heart sound occurs immediately after the S2, coinciding with the period of rapid ventricular filling, and is a soft and low frequency sound that is best heard with the bell of the stethoscope lightly rested over the chest wall.[29] Despite findings that interrater agreement on the presence of an S3 heart sound is low to moderate, and that its sensitivity and specificity for the presence of heart failure are also only fair to good (sensitivity 51%, specificity 90% for patients with heart failure),[33] the presence of abnormal heart sounds along with JVD is associated with increased heart failure hospitalization, heart failure deaths, and death from all causes in patients with heart failure.[30]

The fourth heart sound *(S4)* is an abnormal heart sound that can be heard immediately before S1 and indicates increased resistance to ventricular filling due to high atrial pressure or increased ventricular thickness. The presence of an S4 may indicate myocardial infarction or shock.

Aerobic Capacity and Endurance

Lung Sounds. Lung sounds can be assessed by chest auscultation (see Chapter 24). *Crackles* are adventitious or abnormal breath sounds that sound like bubbling or popping and can reflect fluid overload in the lungs because of an acute exacerbation of or onset of heart failure. If crackles that were not present at baseline start during an intervention, the session should be terminated and the health care team notified. However, crackles are neither sensitive nor specific signs of heart failure. With optimal medical management, many patients with severe heart failure may not present with crackles, since they will not accumulate excessive fluid in the lungs. Crackles may be a sign of other pulmonary problems, most commonly atelectasis. Therefore the presence of crackles on auscultation of the lungs should be used in conjunction with other test findings, such as peripheral edema and body weight measurements, to assess fluid status in heart failure.

A variety of measures of aerobic capacity and endurance are used to monitor and document the severity and progression of heart failure. These include the *New York Heart Association* (NYHA) *Classification system,* clinical exercise testing, and the 6-Minute Walk Test (6MWT).

New York Heart Association Classification System. The NYHA Classification system is a simple and widely used tool that classifies patients with heart failure into one of four classes according to their degree of symptoms at rest and with activity. In the early stages of heart failure, the heart may function adequately both at rest and with activity. With progression of the disease, the heart will first not be able to meet the demands of the body with activity, and patients will begin to demonstrate clinical signs and symptoms with activity. With further progression of the disease, patients will demonstrate signs and symptoms of heart failure even at rest. The NYHA Classification system is the system most commonly used by physicians to prognosticate and monitor the effectiveness of treatment interventions in heart failure.[34] The classes used in this system, I to IV with I indicating less severity and higher numbers indicating greater severity, are described in Table 25-5. Classification is based on the patient's self-report of signs and symptoms. Patients can move between classes, either up or down, depending on the severity of their disease at the time.

The NYHA Classification system has been examined for its ability to predict mortality. With optimal treatment, there is a 1-year mortality of 10% to 15% for stable patients classified in NYHA class I and II, 15% to 20% for patients classified in class III, and 20% to 50% for patients classified in class IV.[35]

The NYHA Classification system is often criticized because it only documents self-reported signs and symptoms and does not provide guidance for treatment interventions. Therefore a new approach for heart failure classification was developed that emphasizes the appropriate treatment interventions, depending on the stage of the disease.[2] This system classifies patients into one of four stages, A to D, that can be used for selection of medical treatment interventions (Fig. 25-3). Stage A includes patients with a high risk for developing left ventricular dysfunction, with the emphasis on risk factor modification as the treatment intervention. Stage B includes patients with left ventricular dysfunction without any symptoms, with treatment interventions also focused on prevention. Stage C includes patients with left ventricular dysfunction and presenting symptoms. At stage C, medical and pharmacological interventions are

TABLE 25-5	New York Heart Association Classification of Heart Failure
NYHA class	**Description**
I	No symptoms with ordinary exertion
II	Symptoms with ordinary exertion
III	Symptoms with less than ordinary exertion
IV	Symptoms at rest

Data from The Criteria Committee of the New York Heart Association: *Nomenclature and Criteria for the Diagnosis of the Heart and Great Vessels,* ed 6, Boston, 1964, Little Brown.

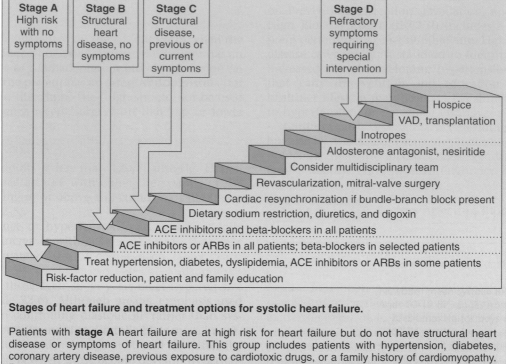

| Stage A High risk with no symptoms | Stage B Structural heart disease, no symptoms | Stage C Structural disease, previous or current symptoms | Stage D Refractory symptoms requiring special intervention |

Hospice
VAD, transplantation
Inotropes
Aldosterone antagonist, nesiritide
Consider multidisciplinary team
Revascularization, mitral-valve surgery
Cardiac resynchronization if bundle-branch block present
Dietary sodium restriction, diuretics, and digoxin
ACE inhibitors and beta-blockers in all patients
ACE inhibitors or ARBs in all patients; beta-blockers in selected patients
Treat hypertension, diabetes, dyslipidemia, ACE inhibitors or ARBs in some patients
Risk-factor reduction, patient and family education

Stages of heart failure and treatment options for systolic heart failure.

Patients with **stage A** heart failure are at high risk for heart failure but do not have structural heart disease or symptoms of heart failure. This group includes patients with hypertension, diabetes, coronary artery disease, previous exposure to cardiotoxic drugs, or a family history of cardiomyopathy. Patients with **stage B** heart failure have structural heart disease but have no symptoms of heart failure. This group includes patients with left ventricular hypertrophy, previous myocardial infarction, left ventricular systolic dysfunction, or valvular heart disease, all of whom would be considered to have New York Heart Association (NYHA) class I symptoms. Patients with **stage C** heart failure have known structural heart disease and current or previous symptoms of heart failure. Their symptoms may be classified as NYHA class I, II, III, or IV. Patients with **stage D** heart failure have refractory symptoms of heart failure at rest despite maximal medical therapy, are hospitalized, and require specialized interventions or hospice care. All such patients would be considered to have NYHA class IV symptoms.

FIG. 25-3 Stages and treatment options for patients with heart failure. *VAD,* Ventricular assist device; *ACE,* angiotensin-converting enzymes; *ARBs,* angiotensin-receptor blockers. *Redrawn from Jessup M, Brozena S:* N Engl J Med *348(20):2007-2018, 2003.*

recommended to alleviate symptoms and slow disease progression. Stage D is for those patients with advanced stage refractory heart failure. At stage D, specialized pharmacological and surgical treatment interventions are recommended. With this staging system, once patients reach stage C or D and have symptoms, they cannot revert to stage A or B, indicating that although symptoms may be controlled with medications the disease is continuing to progress.

Exercise Testing. The standard clinical method for assessing functional aerobic capacity and endurance is exercise testing. Exercise testing uses a bicycle or a treadmill and gradually and progressively increases the workload until a maximal, symptom-limited, or submaximal level is reached. During the test, the patient's heart rhythm and rate, BP, and signs and symptoms are closely monitored. The test is terminated using specific guidelines as outlined in Box 25-2[36] (see also Chapter 23). Information obtained from exercise testing can be used to classify patients into functional classes and can be used to guide exercise prescription using the work level the patients

attained according to *metabolic equivalents* (METs), maximal HR, or $\dot{V}O_{2max}$.

One measure of functional capacity obtained by exercise testing is a MET level. One MET is equivalent to 3.5 ml oxygen/kg/min, which is the typical *oxygen consumption rate* ($\dot{V}O_2$) of a healthy adult at rest. MET levels are independent of body weight and can be used for exercise prescription or to estimate energy requirements for specific activities. Energy expenditure in MET levels for various activities are well documented in published tables.[37,38] Sample MET levels for common activities of daily living (ADLs) are included in Table 25-6. Activities that require a greater MET level require more consumption of oxygen and energy. The information from Table 25-6 can be used to educate patients about activities that they can perform safely at home or at work. Patients with a maximum activity tolerance of less than 5 METs, as determined by exercise testing, have a worse prognosis than those who achieve more than 5 MET level of exercise.[37,38] Most ADLs require a MET level of less than 5.

TABLE 25-7	Weber's Functional Classification of Patients with Heart Failure According to Aerobic Capacity

Class	$\dot{V}o_2$ (ml/kg/min)	Deterioration in Functional Capacity
A	>20	Mild or absent
B	16-20	Mild to moderate
C	10-15	Moderate to severe
D	<10	Severe

Data from Weber KT, Kinasewitz GT, Janicki JS, et al: *Circulation* 65:1213-1223, 1982.
$\dot{V}o_2$, Maximal oxygen uptake.

Ventilatory gas exchange can also be measured during exercise testing to provide additional information about functional capacity. Measures of gas exchange, including peak oxygen consumption rate ($\dot{V}o_2$), *anaerobic threshold* (AT), and other ventilatory parameters, can be used to guide exercise prescription, prognosis, and treatment interventions. Peak $\dot{V}o_2$ is the highest oxygen consumption rate attained during an exercise test. Peak $\dot{V}o_2$ is a strong predictor of morbidity and mortality in patients with heart failure.[39-41] $\dot{V}o_2$ has been recommended as an objective measure (in contrast to the subjective criteria used for the NYHA classification system) for classifying patients with heart failure into functional classes as shown in Table 25-7.[42] Peak $\dot{V}o_2$ and AT are also used to time the referral of a patient for heart transplant evaluation.[41,43] Oxygen consumption measurements are reliable and reproducible, provide an accurate assessment of functional capacity, and can help distinguish between pulmonary and cardiac causes of a patient's symptoms.[11-13] However, this type of testing may not be available at all facilities because it requires expensive equipment, personnel training, and time.

Six-Minute Walk Test. The Six-Minute Walk Test (6MWT) is a simple clinical tool that can be used by clinicians to assess submaximal exercise capacity. This tool is a useful measure for documenting baseline function and the effectiveness of therapy interventions, including exercise training. The 6MWT can be used more frequently than other types of exercise testing because it is quick and easy, requires minimal equipment, and is well tolerated by patients. For the 6MWT the patient is instructed to walk along a hallway as far as they can in 6 minutes. The American Thoracic Society has published guidelines for this procedure that can serve as a reference for clinicians on the indications, protocol, safety measures, and guidelines for interpreting the 6MWT.[44] The test has been found most useful in patients with moderate-to-severe heart failure and in elderly patients and those with neurological or orthopedic limitations, which can compromise the safety of other types of exercise testing.

The usefulness of the 6MWT was first determined by comparing it to exercise testing. The 6MWT distance has been found to correlate moderately with peak $\dot{V}o_2$ on exercise testing in patients with heart failure.[45-47] The 6MWT distance has also been found to be an independent predictor of hospitalization rate and mortality.[48,49] In a group of 541 stable outpatients with heart failure, a 6MWT distance of less than 200 m was associated with the greatest risk of mortality and death because of worsening heart failure after a median follow-up time of 32 months.[50] In a study of 45 patients with advanced heart failure (mean EF 20% ± 6%) walking less than 300 m on the 6MWT was found to predict death, the need for inotropic support, or placement of a mechanical device within 6 months.[45] The 6MWT is easy to administer and well-tolerated and demonstrates good reproducibility in patients with heart failure.[51] However, it does not distinguish patients in NYHA class II and III as well as a graded exercise test, and it is less sensitive to changes than clinical exercise testing.[52]

Medical Tests for Patients with Heart Failure. Several medical tests can provide useful information about cardiac function in patients with heart failure. These are described here briefly to give the rehabilitation clinician an idea of their utility and interpretation.

TABLE 25-6	Metabolic Equivalent Levels for Activities of Daily Living

Activity	MET Level Range
Sitting	1-2
Eating	1-2
Dressing	2-3
Toileting	2-3
Bathing/showering	2-4
Walking on level surfaces 2 mph	2-3
Walking on level surfaces 3 mph	3-4
Walking up a flight of stairs	4-7
Sexual intercourse	3-5
Shoveling snow	6-7
Vacuuming	3-4
Washing dishes	2-3
Gardening	2-4
Washing a car	6-7

Adapted from Ainsworth BE, Haskell WL, Leon AS, et al: *Med Sci Sports Exerc* 25:71-80, 1993.
MET, Metabolic equivalent.

Echocardiography uses ultrasound to image the heart in real time. It can provide information about the size of the heart chambers, the thickness of the heart walls, valve form and function, EF, relative pressures within the heart chambers, and wall motion. EF is most readily determined by echocardiography, and therefore echocardiography is often used to track the progression of systolic heart failure. Remember that patients with diastolic dysfunction have a normal EF. As systolic heart failure progresses, producing severe symptoms and an EF of less than 30%, other parameters, such as ventricular dimensions, severity of right ventricular dysfunction, and mitral and tricuspid valve regurgitation, may be more useful indicators of disease progression.[4]

Catheters can be used to measure pressures at various sites in the heart and blood vessels. Right and left *heart catheterization* can provide important information about cardiac function and hemodynamics, including pulmonary artery pressure and pulmonary capillary wedge pressure, which have been shown to be predictors of outcome in patients with heart failure.[53] A pulmonary artery catheter may be left in place while the patient is in the intensive care unit, to allow close hemodynamic monitoring while medications are given and to guide selection of treatment interventions for patients with heart failure. Right atrial pressure, an indicator of right ventricular filling volume, is normally between 2 and 8 mm Hg. Pulmonary artery pressure, an indicator of pulmonary vascular resistance, is normally 15-30/4-12 mm Hg.

Function

Self-Care and Home Management. Quality of life (QOL) measures are often used to determine a patient's sense of the effects of a disease process on his or her life. Two disease-specific measures have been developed to assess QOL in patients with heart failure: Minnesota Living with Heart Failure Questionnaire (LHFQ) and the Kansas City Cardiomyopathy Questionnaire (KCCQ). The LHFQ was developed to assess patient perceptions of the effects of heart failure and its treatment on daily life.[54] This questionnaire uses a 0- ("no") to 5-point ("very much") Likert scale to assess 21 limitations commonly reported by patients with heart failure. Scores are determined by summing the 21 responses for a maximum total score of 105. A physical domain score can be calculated by summing 8 questions found to be related to dyspnea and fatigue as determined by factor analysis.[55] An emotional dimension score can be determined from the sum from 5 other questions. This questionnaire was found to be valid and reliable (test-retest reliability = 0.93) in a study evaluating the effects of enalapril (an angiotensin-converting enzyme [ACE] inhibitor) compared to placebo on QOL in patients with heart failure.[55] However, the LHFQ has been criticized for its poor discriminative ability in patients with moderate to severe heart failure (NYHA class II and III).[56,57]

Because of the limitations of the LHFQ, a second disease-specific QOL measure, the KCCQ, was developed.[58] This tool has 23 items within 8 domains: Physical status, symptoms, symptom stability, social limitations, self-efficacy, QOL, functional status, and clinical summary. A

study of 129 NYHA patients with class I-IV heart failure, found that this tool was more responsive than the LHFQ and more sensitive to a patient's change in status.[58] Therefore this scale is recommended for detection of self-reported changes in QOL after interventions in patients with heart failure. A copy of the KCCQ can be found on the CD that accompanies this book.

EVALUATION, DIAGNOSIS, AND PROGNOSIS

Most patients classified into the preferred practice pattern 6D: Impaired aerobic capacity/endurance associated with cardiovascular pump dysfunction or failure have abnormal examination findings in the categories of cardiopulmonary tests and measures. According to the *Guide,*[59] it is anticipated that 80% of patients classified into this pattern with cardiovascular pump dysfunction will achieve optimal aerobic capacity and endurance and the highest level of functioning in home, work, community, and leisure environments over the course of 6-12 weeks, with a range of 3-30 visits during a single continuous episode of care.[59] For the patient with cardiovascular pump failure, achievement of these goals will take 8-16 weeks with a range of 14-44 visits.[59]

INTERVENTION

The mainstays of medical interventions for patients with heart failure are medications that optimize fluid balance and cardiac preload, afterload, and contractility. More recently, surgery, including heart transplantation and placement of left ventricular assist devices (VADs), has been successful in some patients with severe heart failure. Rehabilitation interventions for patients with heart failure focus primarily on different types exercise. Appropriate exercise, in combination with optimal medical care, can improve function, symptoms, and QOL in patients with chronic heart failure.[60-62] Exercise training provides benefit primarily by altering the peripheral factors that contribute to exercise intolerance rather than by changing left ventricular function. Functional and symptomatic improvements have been reported when training is performed consistently 3 times per week for 3 or more weeks for 20-40 minutes per session at an intensity of 40% to 70% of $\dot{V}O_{2max}$, as determined by a graded exercise test.[12,63]

In the past, patients with heart failure were instructed not to exercise for fear that this additional stress on an already failing heart would exacerbate their condition. In addition, bedrest was recommended because it was theorized that the supine position would promote diuresis by increasing renal blood flow and reduce systemic vascular resistance and thus decrease stress on the heart.[64] However, the many risks of inactivity, including deep vein thrombosis, pulmonary embolism, skin breakdown, muscle atrophy, and deconditioning, as well as advancements in drug therapy, prompted reconsideration of these restrictions. Furthermore, recent research has demonstrated that exercise can provide many benefits to this population.

During exercise, the heart maintains cardiac output by increasing HR and stroke volume. In people with good cardiac function, during the early phase of exercise, cardiac output is increased by rapidly increasing stroke volume and gradually increasing HR.[65] With continued exercise, stroke volume plateaus and any further need for a rise in cardiac output is met by increasing HR. In patients with heart failure, exercise is limited by an inadequate cardiac output response because of a reduction in both stroke volume and HR. These patients have a reduced stroke volume at rest as a result of a decreased EF and have a blunted stroke volume response to exercise. Patients with heart failure also often have a high resting HR to compensate for their reduced stroke volume but are not able to further increase this rate in response to maximal workloads. The higher resting HR and lower peak exercise HR limit the HR reserve (HRR) substantially. The combination of limited responses in stroke volume and HR contribute to a decreased peak exercise response to exercise in patients with heart failure.[66] Table 25-8 summarizes the differences in exercise responses between people with and without heart failure.

Alterations in gas exchange also limit exercise tolerance in this patient population. Fluid accumulation in the lungs results in abnormal gas exchange and can cause shortness of breath. Patients with heart failure also have more vasoconstriction at rest because of elevated sympathetic tone, which further limits the delivery of oxygenated blood to the muscles. Reduced oxygen extraction combined with reduced cardiac output limits the delivery of oxygen to the working skeletal muscles. In addition, skeletal muscle changes in patients with heart failure, including reduction in the size of muscle fibers and change of muscle fiber types, can further contribute to early fatigue during exercise.[67]

Various pharmacological interventions are used to improve exercise tolerance in patients with heart failure, but these have met with limited success.[15,68-70] Therefore investigators have sought out alternative means, such as exercise therapy, to improve exercise and activity tolerance in the population with heart failure. Much of the research in this area focuses on trying to identify the optimal exercise regimen for patients with heart failure.

AEROBIC EXERCISE

Aerobic exercise is any continuous activity that involves rhythmic contraction of large muscle groups and increases the rate of aerobic metabolism. Since aerobic exercise was the primary type of exercise used in cardiac rehabilitation for patients after myocardial infarction, aerobic exercise was the first to undergo investigation for optimizing function in patients with heart failure. Potential benefits of aerobic exercise include improvements in central hemodynamics, such as increases in cardiac output, HR, and stroke volume during exercise, and decreases in cardiac demand at rest. Potential peripheral improvements include improved delivery of oxygen to the working muscles, improved oxygen extraction by the muscles, and improved skeletal muscle fiber function.[71]

Exercise prescription in heart failure can be challenging because many factors can limit exercise tolerance. Initially, exercise studies focused on patients with heart failure who were less debilitated (NYHA class I and II) because of concerns that exercise could have adverse effects in patients with more advanced disease.[63] More recently, studies have also demonstrated that exercise benefits patients with severely reduced left ventricular function (NYHA class III and IV).[12]

One of the first randomized trials using exercise training in patients with heart failure was published in 1996.[60] Forty men with heart failure were randomly assigned to usual care or usual care plus exercise and were followed for 6 months. The exercise consisted of a 43-minute session, 3 times per week for 24 weeks. Each session consisted of a 5-minute warm-up, followed by 11 minutes each on a treadmill, upper body ergometer, and stationary bicycle and then another 5 minute cool-down period. Patients exercised at an intensity of 60% of HRR in the first 2 weeks and then 80% of HRR in subsequent sessions (see Chapter 23 for a discussion of HRR). Despite an almost a 30% drop-out rate, the exercise group had significantly higher peak $\dot{V}O_2$, exercise duration tolerance and peak power output than the usual care group.[60] This study provided preliminary support for the safety and effectiveness of moderate intensity exercise in patients with heart failure.

A number of later studies support these initial findings, demonstrate additional benefits to exercise, and delineate factors that may optimize exercise in patients with heart failure. For example, a European study of 134 patients

TABLE 25-8	**Responses to Exercise in People with and without Heart Failure**	

Measure	Response in People without Heart Failure	Response in People with Heart Failure
Cardiac output	Increased to 4-6 times resting level with maximal exercise.	Less than 50% of the increase seen in people without heart failure.
Heart rate	Linear increase in heart rate with a twofold to fourfold increase with maximal exercise.	The heart rate does not linearly increase to meet the demands of exercise, resulting in a blunted heart rate response.
Stroke volume	Increases by 20%-50%, at least 100 ml in response to maximal exercise.	Decreased stroke volume at rest. Peak stroke volume increase of 50-65 ml with exercise.
Cardiac contractility	Increased force of contraction.	No change in force of contraction.
$\dot{V}O_2$	Peak $\dot{V}O_2$ averages 30-40 ml/kg/min.	Peak $\dot{V}O_2$ averages 10-20 ml/kg/min.
Blood pressure	Systolic BP increases, diastolic BP changes minimally from baseline.	Both systolic and diastolic BP change minimally from baseline.
Peripheral vascular dilation	Vasodilation leads to decreased peripheral resistance.	No vasodilation.

Adapted from Pina IL, Apstein CS, Balady GJ, et al: *Circulation* 107(8):1210-1225, 2003.
$\dot{V}O_2$, Maximal oxygen uptake; *BP,* blood pressure.

with chronic heart failure evaluated the effects of different types and duration of exercise. They divided the patients into two groups. One group performed cycle ergometry for 20 minutes, and the second group performed calisthenic exercise and stationary running in addition to 20 minutes of cycle ergometry.[72] Both groups exercised 4-5 days per week for an average of 8 weeks (range 6-16 weeks). All subjects demonstrated a significant training effect, with an average 13% improvement in peak $\dot{V}O_2$ and 17% improvement in exercise duration. However, those who participated in the exercise for more weeks and those in the group who performed more exercise per session showed greater improvements, demonstrating that at least to some degree, more exercise is better in this population.

Another randomized trial examined the effects of short bouts of exercise in patients with heart failure. The subjects for this study were seventy males with heart failure. For the first 2 weeks of the study, they performed 10 minutes of supervised stationary cycling 4-6 times per week. After 2 weeks, they performed 20 minutes of stationary cycling per day independently at home at 70% of peak $\dot{V}O_2$. The subjects demonstrated significant improvements in NYHA classification, exercise time, and exercise capacity, and their left ventricular EF increased significantly from a mean of 30% to 35%.[73] This study suggests that short bouts of exercise can improve outcomes in patients who cannot tolerate longer 30-40 minute exercise sessions.

The significant, although small, effect on EF noted in the study cited in the previous paragraph was not found in a study with 49 patients with mild-to-moderate heart failure who performed interval training using cycle ergometry at a ratio of 90 seconds of exercise, followed by a 30-second rest at an intensity of 80% of $\dot{V}O_{2max}$, progressing from 15 minutes twice a week to 45 minutes 3 times a week over a 4-month period. In this study, although there were no adverse events and exercise capacity improved significantly, left ventricular function and EF did not change significantly from baseline (although it did increase from 37% to 42%).[74]

A number of trials have attempted to evaluate the effect of exercise on factors related to QOL, as well as exercise performance and physiological characteristics. Belardinelli and colleagues randomized 99 patients to either a moderate exercise group or a no exercise group.[62] The exercise group performed cycle ergometry for 40 minutes three times per week at 60% of peak $\dot{V}O_2$ for 8 weeks and thereafter for 1 hour twice a week. No adverse cardiac events occurred during the study, and those in the experimental group had a better QOL, lower mortality, and fewer hospital readmissions, as well as higher peak $\dot{V}O_2$ than those who did not exercise. This was one of the first controlled studies to demonstrate long-term benefits from exercise training in patients with heart failure.

Improvements in QOL and depression in response to exercise have also been documented in patients with heart failure.[74-76] Afzal and colleagues found improvements in self-care activities, depression and anxiety, shortness of breath, and well-being after a group of patients completed a cardiac rehabilitation program consisting primarily of aerobic exercises.[75] Another study found 51 patients with chronic heart failure who participated in a 12-week exercise program had better disease-specific QOL and physical performance after completing the program.[76]

Since many patients do not have access to supervised exercise programs or exercise equipment, a number of studies have evaluated the effects of exercise without use of these resources. One such study randomized 79 patients with a mean EF of 27% ± 8.8% to usual care or a 12-week home walking program. Peak $\dot{V}O_2$ and self-reported measures of function did not change from baseline at 3 months; however, 6MWT distance did increase significantly.[77] A second study randomized 40 patients to either a usual care group or a usual care plus home walking and resistive exercise group to evaluate the effects of home exercise on exercise capacity and QOL.[78] These investigators also found no significant differences in peak $\dot{V}O_2$ but found that self-reported fatigue, emotional function, and mastery were better in the group that exercised.[78] Although these studies had small sample sizes and produced limited gains, they do provide preliminary evidence that a home walking program is safe and well tolerated in this population.[77,78]

How aerobic exercise improves function and peak $\dot{V}O_2$ in patients with heart failure remains unclear. Some studies suggest that this increase is explained by an increase in peak HR, with reports that increased peak HR accounts for up to 46% of the increase in peak $\dot{V}O_2$ in the training groups.[60] Other studies indicate that $\dot{V}O_2$ is improved by an increase in stroke volume accompanied by an increase in peak lower extremity blood flow.[79] Still others hypothesize that the increases produced by exercise are caused by a decrease in systemic vascular resistance.[80-83] Although the mechanisms for the benefits of exercise in patients with heart failure need further elucidation, the present evidence does support the use of aerobic exercise in patients with stable heart failure to improve exercise and activity tolerance, as well as QOL.

RESISTIVE TRAINING

Despite the benefits of aerobic exercise in patients with heart failure, there are still concerns that certain types of exercise, particularly resistance training, may increase the size of the ventricles. This concern is based on the fact that BP increases can increase afterload on the heart, which could then promote left ventricular dilatation. Since resistive training can produce high peak BPs, the concern is greatest with this type of exercise. Although the benefits of resistive exercise that have been demonstrated in other populations, including increasing strength and power and improving balance, all of which may contribute to improved performance of functional activities, most agree that isometric resistance exercise should be avoided in patients with heart failure because it increases afterload on the heart to such a degree. However, mild-to-moderate resistive training may be used in patients with heart failure with close monitoring for signs or symptoms of worsening heart failure, such as increased fatigue and dyspnea.[84]

A number of studies have evaluated the effects of resistance training in patients with heart failure. Delagardelle and colleagues compared the effects of 40 minutes of aerobic exercise or aerobic exercise combined with resistive training in 20 male patients with heart failure.[85] The aerobic exercise group used a cycle ergometer for the entire time, and the combined exercise group cycled for 20 minutes and performed resistance exercise consisting of 3 sets of 30 repetitions at 60% of a one repetition maximum (1RM) of leg extensions, leg curls, seated arm press, pull downs, rowing, and lateral arm abductions for the other 20 minutes. Both groups demonstrated improvements in strength, which were not significantly different between groups, and left ventricular EF was also not significantly different between groups at the end of the study (26.7% at baseline to 31.6% at 3 months in the combined group and 30.7% at baseline to 27.2% at 3 months in the aerobic training only group).[85] Another similar study found that there were significant short-term gains in left ventricular function in patients with heart failure who performed a program that combined moderate upper body resistive training and bicycle ergometry.[86]

Although these studies suggest that moderate resistive training in combination with aerobic exercise may be safe in this population, firm recommendations on the use of resistive training in heart failure cannot be made until further studies assess the long-term effects of this type of intervention on cardiac function.

INTERVAL TRAINING

Interval training consists of short bouts of exercise followed by periods of rest applied in a repeated sequence. Interval training allows the muscles to work harder than they could with steady-state exercise without excessively stressing the cardiovascular system. Interval training with 30 seconds of exercise followed by 60 seconds of rest at an intensity of 75% of peak $\dot{V}O_2$ produced a lower *rate-pressure product*, lower *rate of perceived exertion* (RPE), and lower increases in plasma *catecholamine* levels than steady-state exercise at the same intensity.[87] The safety of this type of exercise makes it appealing for patients with heart failure.

Interval training may be performed using a stationary bicycle or a treadmill, and a variety of exercise-to-rest ratios may be used, including 15 seconds/60 seconds, 10 seconds/60 seconds, or 30 seconds/60 seconds for a total of 15-30 minutes.[88,89] Interval training may be gradually progressed in intensity by lengthening the exercise period or shortening the rest periods.

Meyer and colleagues demonstrated that interval training could safely improve peak $\dot{V}O_2$ in patients with heart failure.[90] They had 18 patients with severe heart failure (mean EF = $21 \pm 1\%$) perform stationary cycling for 15 minutes and treadmill walking for 10 minutes 5 times per week for 3 weeks. With both types of exercise, the intervals were 30 seconds of work followed by 60 seconds of rest and exercise intensity was 50% of a maximum work rate determined by a steep-ramp test (a submaximal exercise test that constantly and continuously increases workload to provide an accurate estimate of oxygen uptake[91]). The authors found that the exercise program was well tolerated and that peak $\dot{V}O_2$ increased from 12.2 ± 0.7 to 14.6 ± 0.7 ml/kg/min ($p < 0.001$) without any adverse events.[90] This study suggests that a work-to-rest ratio of 30 seconds

to 60 seconds is safe and can allow patients with heart failure to improve their exercise capacity with minimal cardiac stress.

EXERCISE SAFETY IN HEART FAILURE

Despite the fact that evidence indicates that exercise can help patients with heart failure, there are still concerns about the safety of exercise training in this population. In standard outpatient cardiac rehabilitation programs, observational studies estimate the incidence of cardiovascular complications from exercise in patients with heart failure to be 1 for every 60,000 participant-hours.[92] In a review of the literature on exercise training in patients with heart failure, which included 20 studies with a combined sample of 467 patients, the AHA found only 19 reported adverse cardiac events, which included heart failure exacerbations, ventricular tachycardia, atrial fibrillation, hypotension, and exhaustion but no reported deaths.[93] They found that the three most important factors affecting the risk of exercise in patients with heart failure were the patient's age, the intensity of the exercise, and the presence of ischemic heart disease.

Based on this review, the AHA developed standards for exercise testing and training in patients with heart failure.[93] In their most recent recommendations, they encourage aerobic activity to improve activity and exercise tolerance, except during periods of decompensation, but advise patients with heart failure to avoid heavy labor or exhaustive sports.[94] However, neither the AHA nor any other group provides specific recommendations for exercise in this population, although the AHA's risk stratification system does provide some helpful guidelines for adjusting exercise intensity in patients with NYHA class I to III heart failure.[93-95]

EXERCISE PRESCRIPTION FOR PATIENTS WITH HEART FAILURE

To safely prescribe exercise for a patient with heart failure, one must first determine if the patient can safely perform any exercise at all. Patients with decompensated heart failure should not exercise. Signs of decompensated heart failure that should exclude patients from participating in exercise include the acute onset of crackles, signs of worsening pulmonary edema, ventricular arrhythmias, uncontrolled atrial fibrillation, bradycardia, symptomatic hypotension, and dyspnea and fatigue at rest. Further contraindications and relative contraindications to exercise in the heart failure population are listed in Box 25-3.

Because of the complexity of heart failure, there is no specific consensus for exercise prescription. The AHA guidelines recommend clinicians individualize exercise prescription in patients with heart failure, considering baseline functional status, findings from a thorough physical assessment, and a comprehensive review of the literature. When prescribing exercise for patients with heart failure, the exercise mode, intensity, duration, and frequency should be specified. The following sections review the evidence on these different components of exercise prescription for patients with heart failure.

Exercise Mode. The mode of exercise refers to the type of activity performed. At a minimum, the exercise

BOX 25-3	Relative and Absolute Contraindications for Exercise for a Patient with Heart Failure

- Systolic BP >240 mm Hg or diastolic BP >110 mm Hg
- Decrease in systolic BP by more than 10 mm Hg from baseline
- Angina > level 2 on the Angina Scale
- Dyspnea ≥ level 2 on the Dyspnea Index
- Symptoms of worsening failure such as pallor, excessive fatigue, or mental confusion
- ECG abnormalities such as second or third degree heart block, ventricular arrhythmias, acute ST changes, onset of left or right bundle-branch block, uncontrolled atrial fibrillation
- Resting systolic BP <80 mm Hg
- Decreased HR response to exercise
- HR elevation close to ICD firing threshold
- New onset of pulmonary rales
- New onset of S3 heart sound
- Borg RPE Scale rating of >13 on the 6-20 scale

Adapted from American College of Sports Medicine: *ACSM's Guidelines for Exercise Testing and Prescription,* Baltimore, 2000, Williams & Wilkins.
BP, Blood pressure; *ECG,* electrocardiogram; *HR,* heart rate; *ICD,* implanted cardiac defibrillator; *RPE,* rate of perceived exertion.

prescription should include some form of aerobic exercise. The exercise should include activities that are predominately aerobic in nature such as walking and/or stationary cycling. Cycle ergometry has the advantages of easy reproducibility, allowing exercise at a very low workload, and being safe for patients with deficits in dynamic balance. Because of fluctuations in the environment, outdoor cycling is recommended only for clinically stable NYHA class I and II patients and not for patients in class III or IV.[63] Cycling in a recumbent or semirecumbent position is generally discouraged, as it may limit exercise tolerance by increasing venous return and thereby pulmonary edema and by decreasing diaphragmatic excursion, although there is no strong evidence to support this recommendation.[96]

Walking can be performed by a wide range of patients with heart failure because its speed can easily be varied. Patients with a documented peak $\dot{V}O_2$ of at least 13 ml/kg/min can generally tolerate treadmill speeds as high as 3.7 mph, with less fit patients (peak $\dot{V}O_2$ of 8 ml/kg/min) generally tolerating speeds of 1.9 mph or less.[97] Quell and colleagues found that brisk walking could elicit an adequate training effect in patients with heart failure.[98] Jogging is generally not advised because even a slow jogging speed of 3 mph is only tolerated in patients with a $\dot{V}O_2$ of 20 ml/kg/min or greater.[63]

Exercise Frequency and Duration. In most studies of exercise in patients with heart failure the subjects have exercised 3-5 times per week for 10-60 minutes per session. In all patients with heart failure the clinician must monitor patients closely for any signs or symptoms of intolerance during or following exercise and should adjust exercise frequency and duration accordingly. Severely compromised patients may require a longer rest interval

between exercise sessions, with a gradual progression to a frequency of 3-5 times per week, and/or shorter sessions initially with a gradual progression of duration over time.

Exercise frequency and duration should be individualized to the patient according to their baseline functional level and level of impairment. The American College of Sports Medicine (ACSM) recommends that patients with a functional capacity of less than 3 METs will generally tolerate multiple daily bouts of exercise lasting 5-10 minutes. Patients functioning at a 3-5 MET level will tolerate and benefit from 1-2 daily sessions daily of 15 minutes each and those with a functional capacity of greater than 5 METs are recommended to exercise 3-5 times per week for 20-30 minutes each session, with close monitoring for any signs or symptoms of intolerance.[36] Interval training may also be used in patients who do not tolerate sustained exercise throughout the exercise period.

Exercise prescription in all patients, and particularly those with cardiac conditions, should always include adequate warm-up and cool-down periods. The warm-up period should include 5-10 minutes of intermittent or continuous low-intensity aerobic activity at approximately 25% to 50% of the patient's functional capacity. This phase can also include gentle stretching to reduce the risk of musculoskeletal injuries, especially in a deconditioned population.[99,100] In patients with heart disease, adequate warm-up is thought to reduce the risk of myocardial ischemia by promoting opening of collateral vessels and preventing vascular spasm and redistribution of blood from areas at risk. After the warm-up, exercise can be progressed to the goal intensity level. The cool-down should be similar to the warm-up. This will allow the HR and BP to gradually return to preexercise levels. This will enhance venous return and decrease the risk of postexercise hypotension.[101] Patients with heart failure who do not adequately cool down are also thought to be at increased risk of arrhythmias because of myocardial irritability from the large volume of blood returned to the heart when exercise stops suddenly.

Exercise Intensity. As with other populations, the intensity of aerobic exercise in a patient with heart failure can be prescribed as a percentage of peak $\dot{V}O_2$, a percentage of peak HR or according to the Borg RPE Scale (see Box 23-3). Generally, patients with heart failure can tolerate an initial intensity ranging from 40% to 70% of peak $\dot{V}O_2$, or an intensity corresponding to ten beats per minute below the level where symptoms such as shortness of breath or angina occur. Because of the abnormal HR response to exercise and the frequent use of beta-blocker therapy in patients with heart failure, determining exercise intensity using HR can be difficult. Therefore the Borg RPE Scale is often recommended for setting exercise intensity in patients with heart failure. The Borg RPE Scale ranges from 6-20 and has a linear relationship to the HR response with increasing intensity of exercise.[102] Exercising at a Borg RPE rating of 11-14 ("light" to "somewhat hard") on this scale corresponds to a HR response between 40% to 70% of peak $\dot{V}O_2$ and is generally appropriate for patients with heart failure.[102]

Although many studies of exercise in patients with heart failure set exercise intensity according to percentage of peak $\dot{V}O_2$ or HRR as determined by an exercise test, clinicians often do not have access to the results of an exercise test. In these circumstances the Borg RPE Scale, in conjunction with individual clinical judgment, may be used to set the most appropriate exercise intensity.

Exercise Progression. Progression of exercise will depend on the patient's baseline functional status, activity tolerance, vital sign response, and subjective complaints. Patients with a low initial exercise capacity will generally make faster initial progress than those who start at a high functional capacity. Training can be considered as occurring in three stages: The initial stage, the improvement stage, and the maintenance stage.[36] Progression from one stage to another is based on the patient attaining specific intensity and duration goals. These three stages are outlined further in Table 25-9. Exercise should be progressed sequentially with adjustments first made to duration, then frequency, and finally the intensity of the program.

HEART TRANSPLANTATION

Heart transplantation may be indicated in patients with end-stage heart failure that is refractory to optimal pharmacological support. Indications for transplant include NYHA class III or IV heart failure, cardiac index of less than 2.0 L/min/m², exercise capacity less than 14 ml/min/kg, age less than 70 years, and adequate psychosocial support. Contraindications include active sepsis, renal insufficiency, ongoing substance abuse, severe pulmonary disease, severe peripheral vascular disease or cerebrovascular disease, malignancy, human immunodeficiency virus (HIV) infection, morbid obesity, fixed *pulmonary hypertension,* and uncontrolled diabetes.[103]

Heart transplantation is the last resort for patients with heart failure because although it can produce good outcomes, it is fraught with complications and the availability of hearts for transplantation is far less than the demand. According to the Organ Procurement and Transplantation Network (OPTN), in 2003 there were 4,200 patients waiting for a heart transplant, with 2,500 transplants performed each year. It is estimated that 30% of patients waiting for a heart transplant will die before receiving one because of the shortage of organs. One-year

survival after heart failure is now 86% with 75% of patients surviving for 5 years or more. Patients are listed and receive an organ for transplantation using a system established by the United Network for Organ Sharing (UNOS) that prioritizes patients according to disease severity and listing time. Once a patient reaches the top of the list, potential organs must be matched to the recipient's body size and blood type.

The transplant procedure is performed using a *median sternotomy* approach with anastomosis at the vena cava, aorta, and pulmonary arteries. The immediate postoperative care is similar to that provided after other open-heart procedures and generally includes observation of sternal precautions for 6-8 weeks after the procedure (Box 25-4). However, cardiac vagal denervation and side effects of antirejection medications can limit function and exercise tolerance. Cardiac output after heart transplant is approximately 25% to 30% lower than in the normal population. BP is typically elevated at rest, with a greater systolic BP response to exercise. Peak $\dot{V}O_2$ is also lower than in age matched controls (usually 70% to 80% of age-matched controls).[104]

Exercise training is recommended as part of a comprehensive posttransplant management plan that includes proper nutrition, drug therapy, and frequent medical and surgical follow-up. When prescribing exercise for patients after heart transplant, one must keep in mind that they will respond differently because their heart is denervated. The loss of vagal input makes heart transplant recipients have an elevated HR at rest. Their HR will rise little if at all when exercise is started. With continued exertion, their HR will rise gradually and slightly to a lower peak during maximal exercise than in age-matched healthy people without heart transplants (Fig. 25-4). Because of this abnormal HR response, HR should not be used as a target for exercise prescription in patients with heart transplants. In this population, a target Borg RPE Scale rating of 12-14 can serve as a guide for exercise intensity.

Since some of the immunosuppressive agents used after organ transplantation increase the risk for bone density loss and osteoporosis, weight-bearing exercise, as well as resistive training, are recommended in this population (see Chapter 3). Outpatient cardiac rehabilitation, which is generally initiated 6-8 weeks after surgery once the sternum has healed, has been shown to improve exercise tolerance and QOL in patients after heart transplant.[71,105]

TABLE 25-9	Exercise Progression for the Patient with Heart Failure*	
Stage	Intensity	Duration**
Initial	Low level 40%-50% of peak $\dot{V}O_2$	10-15 minutes
Improvement	Primary goal to increase intensity 50%-70% of peak $\dot{V}O_2$	15-30 minutes
Maintenance	Primary goal to maintain intensity 70% of peak $\dot{V}O_2$	30-35 minutes

Data from American College of Sports Medicine: *ACSM's Guidelines for exercise testing and prescription,* Baltimore, 2000, Williams & Wilkins.
*First progress exercise duration, then frequency, then intensity.
**Not including warm-up and cool-down.
$\dot{V}O_2$, Maximal oxygen uptake.

BOX 25-4	Sternal Precautions*

- No lifting >10 lb.
- No lifting of both hands above the head at the same time.
- No placing of both hands behind the back at the same time.
- No driving for 6-8 weeks or until surgeon provides clearance.
- No pushing or pulling anything >5-10 lb.
- Encourage splinted coughing techniques.

*Sternal precautions are facility dependent, and the reader is referred to the policies of the specific institution for further details.

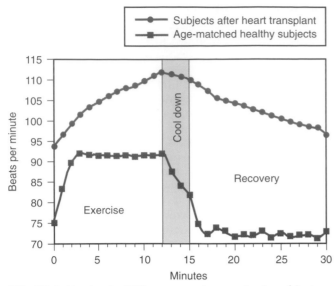

FIG. 25-4 Heart rate (HR) response to exercise in subjects after heart transplant and age-matched healthy subjects.

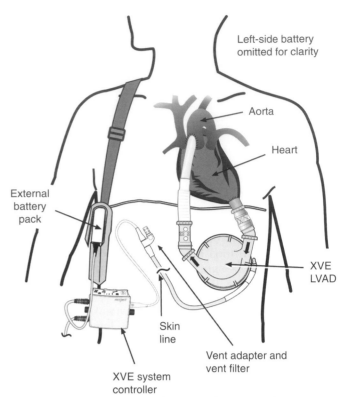

FIG. 25-5 Ventricular assist device (VAD).

MECHANICAL ASSIST DEVICES

Mechanical assist devices are devices that can be used to provide either temporary or permanent support for a failing heart. These devices include intraaortic balloon pumps (IABPs), ventricular assist devices (VADs), and cardiopulmonary bypass machines (CPBs). VADs can provide support to either the right or the left ventricle or both (Fig. 25-5). Indications for mechanical assist devices include recovery after cardiac surgery or acute myocardial infarction, as a bridge to heart transplantation or as destination therapy. Mechanical assist devices are implanted when cardiac output is insufficient to perfuse the vital organs despite maximal pharmacological support. The Food and Drug Administration (FDA) recently approved the Heart-Mate VAD for use as destination therapy, so that patients can have the device implanted permanently. Previously, VADs were only approved as a "bridge" for patients until a heart was available for transplant. Therapists may see patients with these devices in a variety of settings beyond the acute care hospital.

VADs are implanted using a medial sternotomy as with other types of cardiac surgery. Although many facilities follow sternal precautions for 6-8 weeks after medial sternotomy (see Box 25-4), early progressive mobilization has been shown to improve outcomes in patients with left VADs (LVADs).[106] LVADs have also been shown to improve functional exercise tolerance in patients with heart failure. A study comparing submaximal exercise tolerance in patients with heart failure and patients with LVADs found that those with the LVAD could walk further than those without the LVAD.[107] Similarly, a study comparing exercise testing in patients with moderate-to-severe heart failure to a group with an LVAD found peak $\dot{V}O_2$ to be significantly higher in the LVAD group than in the heart failure group and hemodynamic measurements at rest to be better in the LVAD group.[108]

CASE STUDY 25-1

NYHA CLASS III HEART FAILURE

Examination
Patient History
AT, a 58-year-old man, presents to the hospital with complaints of dyspnea and weight gain of 6 lb over the past 2 days. His history is significant for idiopathic dilated cardiomyopathy, diabetes, hypertension, and hypercholesterolemia, and he had an ICD placed 2 years ago. AT was admitted from the emergency room to the coronary intensive care unit for diuresis, right heart catheterization, and possible initiation of new medications. A physical therapy consultation was requested. AT is on disability because of his cardiac condition but was independent in all ADLs before this hospital admission. He reports frequent shortness of breath. His ICD threshold is set at 185 bpm, and the ICD has fired one time; he had blurred vision prior to the firing. Medications include Lanoxin (digoxin), Lasix (furosemide), Coumadin (warfarin), NovoLog (insulin), Cordarone (amiodarone), Zestril (lisinopril), Klonopin (clonazepam), Aldactone (spironolactone), and Coreg (carvedilol).

Medical Test Results
Echocardiogram: Left ventricular EF of 15% with moderate-to-severe mitral regurgitation and moderate-to-severe tricuspid regurgitation.

Right Heart Catheterization: Right atrial pressure 20 mm Hg, right ventricular pressure 52/20 mm Hg, pulmonary artery pressure 54/28 mm Hg, pulmonary capillary wedge pressure 20 mm Hg, cardiac output 4.63 L/min, cardiac index 2.18.

Systems Review

HR was 100 bpm, RR was 28 breaths per minute (breaths/min), and BP was 90/50 mm Hg.

Tests and Measures

Musculoskeletal: Upper and lower extremity strength and ROM grossly within functional limits.

Anthropometric Characteristics BMI was 28.

Neuromuscular: Static and dynamic balance grossly normal. Light touch sensation intact throughout.

Pain Pain level 0/10. The patient has no complaints of angina, therefore this scale was not assessed.

Cardiovascular/Pulmonary

Circulation JVP distended to approximately 4 cm above the sternal angle.

HR was 100 bpm, rhythm irregularly irregular (atrial fibrillation). 2+ pitting edema in both ankles. Heart auscultation revealed a soft S4 with a normal S1 and S2. No S3 was appreciated. Oxygen saturation was 99% on room air.

Ventilation and Respiration/Gas Exchange Lungs were clear to auscultation. Dyspnea at rest graded as 1.

Aerobic Capacity and Endurance 6MWT: Distance walked 850 feet, with 1 minute rest during the 6-minute time frame, HR ranged from 100-130 bpm, BP ranged from 92/50 mm Hg to 110/55 mm Hg during the test.

Borg RPE Scale: Score ranged from 8 at rest to 13/20 with activity.

Function

Self-Care and Home Management Independent in bed mobility and transfers, required supervision without a device for walking 200 feet to the gym. QOL score on the Minnesota LHFQ was 20.

Evaluation, Diagnosis, and Prognosis

AT was determined to be in NYHA class III heart failure and stage C of the AHA system. He is overweight. He had a low EF consistent with systolic heart failure, abnormal right heart catheterization values, as well as signs and symptoms consistent with heart failure. AT had impairments in aerobic capacity, symptoms in response to activity consistent with heart failure, abnormal responses to incremental increases in exercise demand, and decreased tolerance of ADLs.

AT was diagnosed with preferred practice pattern 6D: Impaired aerobic capacity associated with cardiopulmonary pump dysfunction. The plan of care included progressive aerobic exercise, resistive training, and patient education with goals of safely improving his aerobic capacity and functional activity level during a range of 6-12 sessions, contingent on his length of stay.

Goals

1. Patient will be independent in self-monitoring during exercise.
2. Patient will be able to perform 20 minutes of aerobic exercise with appropriate vital sign response, per the ACSM guidelines for safe exercise training.
3. Patient will be independent in home exercise program.
4. Patient will be able to complete all ADLs with a Borg RPE Scale rating of less than 13 on the 6-20 scale.

Intervention

Session 1 (Day 3 of Hospital Stay)

Ambulation 200 feet with monitoring of vital signs, RPE, and dyspnea index.

Initial measures: HR was 100 bpm, irregularly irregular. BP was 90/50 mm Hg, Borg RPE Scale: 6, Dyspnea Index 1.

Measures directly after ambulation: HR was 115 bpm, irregularly irregular. BP was 78/30 mm Hg, Borg RPE Scale: 8, Dyspnea Index 2. Patient complained of dizziness.

Measures 5 minutes after ambulation completed were unchanged from those taken directly after ambulation.

AT was returned to his room, and the session was terminated because of an abnormal response to exercise as demonstrated by the decreased systolic and diastolic BP. The nurse and medical team were informed of this response, and it was hypothesized AT was hypovolemic because of over diuresis. His medications were adjusted accordingly.

Session 2 (Day 4 of Hospital Stay)

Ambulation 200 meters with monitoring of vital signs, Borg RPE, and Dyspnea Index.

Initial measures: HR was 100 bpm, irregularly irregular. BP was 90/50 mm Hg, Borg RPE Scale: 6, Dyspnea Index 1.

Measures directly after ambulation: HR was 110 bpm, irregularly irregular. BP was 95/50 mm Hg, Borg RPE Scale: 8, Dyspnea Index 1.

Given AT's good tolerance of ambulation, as demonstrated by his vital sign response, he was instructed in light warm-up exercises while seated in a chair that consisted of ankle pumps, knee extension and hip flexion for 30 repetitions with a 3-lb cuff weight for all the exercises. He also performed biceps curls and shoulder presses for 30 repetitions with a 1-lb dumbbell. Measures after completing warm-up exercises: HR was 105 bpm, BP was 88/50 mm Hg, Borg RPE Scale: 8, Dyspnea Index 1.

Given AT's good tolerance of the warm-up walk to the gym and the warm-up exercises, these activities were followed by ambulation on a treadmill. The treadmill speed was set at 1.2 mph for the first 5 minutes, then progressed to a speed of 1.5 mph for 5 minutes, and then reduced back to a speed of 1.2 mph for a 5-minute cool-down period. His maximum RPE during this activity was 13 at the end of the 5 minutes at 1.5 mph.

Measures after completing treadmill walking: HR was 110 bpm, BP was 90/50 mm Hg, Dyspnea Index 2.

Sessions 3 to Discharge from Hospital

Therapy was continued at a frequency of 3 times per week until discharge. AT was progressed on the treadmill, first increasing the time and followed by increasing the speed, all while maintaining the RPE rating of less than 13. While performing his exercise program, AT continued to receive education on proper use of the Borg RPE Scale and Dyspnea Index, which were to be performed with his home exercise program on discharge.

Please see the CD that accompanies this book for a case study describing the examination, evaluation, and interventions for a patient after heart transplantation.

CHAPTER SUMMARY

Heart failure is a progressive disease that results from the heart's inability to pump blood to meet the demands of the body. Patients with heart failure commonly present with intolerance of ADLs and exercise. Heart failure is globally classified as either systolic or diastolic dysfunction, with both types presenting with similar symptoms of fatigue, dyspnea, and decreased exercise tolerance. The NYHA Classification system and the ACC and AHA heart failure guidelines can be used to classify the severity of heart failure and its resultant functional limitations and to guide medical treatment interventions. Diagnostic tests, such as echocardiography and right and left heart catheterization, can provide further information on the prognosis of patients with heart failure. Rehabilitation clinicians should perform a comprehensive examination of patients with heart failure that includes measurement of peripheral edema and JVP; auscultation of the heart and lungs; measurement of vital signs at baseline, during activity, and after all interventions; and some form of assessment of exercise tolerance. Exercise tolerance can easily be assessed using the 6MWT, which can be performed in any clinical setting and can provide reliable and prognostic information for this population. Self-reported function can also be quantified using two disease-specific quality of life tools, the Minnesota LHFQ or the KCCQ.

Despite the many factors that can limit exercise tolerance, exercise training is safe and effective in patients with heart failure. These patients require individualized exercise programs that can include aerobic, resistive, and interval training. Aerobic exercise is the most researched mode of exercise for patients with heart failure. Its documented benefits include improved exercise capacity, improved QOL, and reduced fatigue and dyspnea. Research is now being conducted to study the effects of exercise on mortality in patients with heart failure, as this is not yet known.

When pharmacological support is no longer able to maintain an adequate cardiac output, patients may be referred for cardiac transplantation or placement of a VAD. Clinicians should be able to recognize the signs and symptoms of rejection and be familiar with the mechanics of the assist devices when treating patients who have undergone these procedures.

ADDITIONAL RESOURCES

Useful Forms

6-Minute Walk Test (6MWT)
Kansas City Cardiomyopathy Questionnaire (KCCQ)
Living with Heart Failure (LHFQ): www.mlhfq.org/_dnld/mlhfq_
    questionnaire.org

Books

American College of Sports Medicine: *ACSM's Guidelines for Exercise Testing and Prescription,* Baltimore, 2000, Williams & Wilkins.
Jessup MLL, Loh E (eds): *Heart Failure: A Clinicians' Guide to Ambulatory Diagnosis and Treatment (Contemporary Cardiology),* Totowa, NJ, 2003, Humana Press.

Web Sites

Heart Failure Society of America: www.hfsa.org
American Heart Association: www.americanheart.org

GLOSSARY

Aerobic exercise: Continuous, rhythmic exercise that involves large muscles and increases the rate of aerobic metabolism.

Amyloidosis: A disease characterized by deposits of amyloid in the tissues and organs.

Anaerobic threshold (AT): An indirect measure of endurance obtained from an exercise stress test. The point at which the blood is unable to buffer lactic acid during exercise.

Cardiac output: Amount of blood ejected from the heart, expressed in liters per minute. Cardiac output is equal to the product of heart rate multiplied by stroke volume.

Cardiomyopathy: A disease of the heart muscle that can result in heart failure.

Catecholamine: Chemicals released from the medulla of the adrenal gland that include norepinephrine and epinephrine.

Crackles: Adventitious or abnormal breath sounds that can reflect acute fluid accumulation in the distal airways of the lungs.

Diastole: Period of the heart's pumping cycle where the heart muscle relaxes to allow the heart to fill with blood.

Diastolic dysfunction: Decreased ability of the heart to accept blood.

Dilated cardiomyopathy: Disease of the cardiac muscle with dilation of the ventricles.

Dyspnea: Shortness of breath.

Echocardiography: Diagnostic test that uses ultrasound to assess structures and function of the heart.

Ejection fraction (EF): The percentage of end-diastolic volume ejected from the left ventricle with each heartbeat.

End-diastolic volume: The volume of blood in the left ventricle at the end of diastole.

Heart catheterization: Procedure performed under fluoroscopy where a catheter is inserted into the left side or right side of the heart to measure pressures and/or assess the coronary arteries and heart valves.

Heart failure: Previously called congestive heart failure. Inability of the heart to pump enough blood to meet the demands of the organs.

Hypertrophic cardiomyopathy: Disease of the heart muscle that results in excessive thickening of the left ventricle.

Ischemic heart failure: Heart failure that is caused by an inadequate supply of blood to the heart muscle.

Jugular venous distention (JVD): Distention or stretching of the jugular veins because of fluid overload.

Median sternotomy: Surgical incision using a midline cut through the sternum.

Metabolic equivalent (MET): Energy requirement while resting, which is the energy used to burn 3.5 ml of oxygen per kilogram of body weight per minute.

Myocardium: Heart muscle.

New York Heart Association (NYHA) Classification system: System used to classify patients with heart failure according to subjective limitations in functional activities.

Orthopnea: Shortness of breath with lying supine.

Oxygen consumption rate ($\dot{V}O_2$): Amount of oxygen consumed while performing an activity, measured by exercise testing.

Pulmonary edema: Excessive fluid accumulation in the lungs.

Pulmonary hypertension: Abnormal elevation of the pulmonary artery pressure.

Rate of perceived exertion (RPE): Subjective rating of exercise intensity.

Rate-pressure product: Heart rate multiplied by systolic blood pressure. An index of myocardial oxygen requirement.

Restrictive cardiomyopathy: Disease of the heart muscle that is characterized by fibrosis of the ventricles and leads to diastolic dysfunction.

Right atrial pressure: Pressure of the blood in the right atrium.

S1: The first heart sound, which is produced by closing of the atrioventricular valves.

S2: The second heart sound, which is produced by the closing of the aortic and pulmonic valves of the heart.

S3: The third heart sound, which is produced by vibrations in the ventricle walls with the sudden rush of blood from the atria. This sound may be normal in younger patients and may be a sign of heart failure in older patients.

S4: An abnormal heart sound that can be heard in patients with heart failure and that reflects poor ventricular compliance.

Sarcoidosis: Disease characterized by nodules in the organs and tissues.

Stroke volume: The volume of blood ejected from the left ventricle with each heart beat.

Systolic dysfunction: Inability of the heart to eject blood.

References

1. American Heart Association: *Heart Disease and Stroke Statistics-2003 Update,* Dallas, 2002, The Association.
2. Hunt SA, Baker DW, Chin MH, et al: ACC/AHA Guidelines for the Evaluation and Management of Chronic Heart Failure in the Adult: Endorsed by the Heart Failure Society of America, *Circulation* 104(24):2996-3007, 2001.
3. Connolly K: New directions in heart failure management, *Nurse Pract* 25(7):23, 27-28, 31-34, 42-43, 2000.
4. Echeverria HH, Bilsker MS, Myerburg RJ, et al: Congestive heart failure: Echocardiographic insights, *Am J Med* 75(5):750-755, 1983.
5. Gheorghiade M, Bonow RO: Chronic heart failure in the United States: A manifestation of coronary artery disease, *Circulation* 27 97(3):282-289, 1998.
6. Dries DL, Sweitzer NK, Drazner MH, et al: Prognostic impact of diabetes mellitus in patients with heart failure according to the etiology of left ventricular systolic dysfunction, *J Am Coll Cardiol* 38(2):421-428, 2001.
7. Tecce MA, Pennington JA, Segal BL, Jessup ML: Heart failure: Clinical implications of systolic and diastolic dysfunction, *Geriatrics* 54(8):24-33, 1999.
8. Kessler KM: Heart failure with normal systolic function. Update of prevalence, differential diagnosis, prognosis, and therapy, *Arch Intern Med* 148(10):2109-2111, 1988.
9. Hogg K, Swedberg K, McMurray J: Heart failure with preserved left ventricular systolic function; epidemiology, clinical characteristics, and prognosis, *J Am Coll Cardiol* 43(3):317-327, 2004.
10. Mendes LA, Davidoff R, Cupples LA, et al: Congestive heart failure in patients with coronary artery disease: the gender paradox, *Am Heart J* 134:207-212, 1997.
11. Davie AP, Francis CM, Caruana L, et al: The prevalence of left ventricular diastolic filling abnormalities in patients with suspected heart failure, *Eur Heart J* 18(6):981-984, 1997.
12. Pina IL, Apstein CS, Balady GJ, et al: Exercise and heart failure: A statement from the American Heart Association Committee on exercise, rehabilitation, and prevention, *Circulation* 107(8):1210-1225, 2003.
13. Mancini DM, Eisen H, Kussmaul W, et al: Value of peak exercise oxygen consumption for optimal timing of cardiac transplantation in ambulatory patients with heart failure, *Circulation* 83(3):778 786, 1991.
14. Leclerc KM, Levy WC: The role of norepinephrine in exercise impairment in congestive heart failure, *Congest Heart Fail* 9(1):25-28, 2003.
15. Mancini DM, LeJemtel TH, Factor S, et al: Central and peripheral components of cardiac failure, *Am J Med* 28 80(2B):2-13, 1986.
16. Kataoka T, Keteyian SJ, Marks CR, et al: Exercise training in a patient with congestive heart failure on continuous dobutamine, *Med Sci Sports Exerc* 26(6):678-681, 1994.
17. Mancini DM, Schwartz M, Ferraro N, et al: Effect of dobutamine on skeletal muscle metabolism in patients with congestive heart failure, *Am J Cardiol* 65(16):1121-1126, 1990.
18. Clark A, Volterrani M, Swan JW, et al: Leg blood flow, metabolism and exercise capacity in chronic stable heart failure, *Int J Cardiol* 55(2):127-135, 1996.
19. Clark AL, Poole-Wilson PA, Coats AJ: Exercise limitation in chronic heart failure: central role of the periphery, *J Am Coll Cardiol* 28(5):1092-1102, 1996.
20. Okita K, Yonezawa K, Nishijima H, et al: Skeletal muscle metabolism limits exercise capacity in patients with chronic heart failure, *Circulation* 98(18):1886-1891, 1998.
21. Braith RW, Limacher MC, Staples ED, et al: Blood gas dynamics at the onset of exercise in heart transplant recipients, *Chest* 03(6):1692-1698, 1993.
22. Mancini DM, Henson D, LaManca J, et al: Respiratory muscle function and dyspnea in patients with chronic congestive heart failure, *Circulation* 86(3):909-918, 1992.
23. Sullivan MJ, Higginbotham MB, Cobb FR: Exercise training in chronic heart failure delays ventilatory anaerobic threshold and improves submaximal exercise performance, *Circulation* 79(2):324-329, 1989.
24. Callegari S, Majani G, Giardini A, et al: Relationship between cognitive impairment and clinical status in chronic heart failure patients, *Monaldi Arch Chest Dis* 58(1):19-25, 2002.
25. Trojano L, Antonelli Incalzi R, Acanfora D, et al: Cognitive impairment: a key feature of congestive heart failure in the elderly, *J Neurol* 250(12):1456-1463, 2003.
26. Bennett SJ, Sauve MJ: Cognitive deficits in patients with heart failure: a review of the literature, *J Cardiovasc Nurs* 18(3):219-242, 2003.
27. Riegel B, Bennett JA, Davis A, et al: Cognitive impairment in heart failure: Issues of measurement and etiology, *Am J Crit Care* 11(6):520-528, 2002.
28. Stevenson LW, Perloff JK: The limited reliability of physical signs for estimating hemodynamics in chronic heart failure, *JAMA* 261(6):884-888, 1989.
29. Perloff JK: The jugular venous pulse and third heart sound in patients with heart failure, *N Engl J Med* 345(8):612-614, 2001.
30. Drazner MH, Rame JE, Stevenson LW: Prognostic importance of elevated jugular venous pressure and a third heart sound in patients with heart failure, *N Engl J Med* 345(8):574-581, 2001.
31. Stevenson WG, Stevenson LW, Middlekauff HR, et al: Improving survival for patients with atrial fibrillation and advanced heart failure, *J Am Coll Cardiol* 28(6):1458-1463, 1996.
32. Maisel WH, Stevenson LW: Atrial fibrillation in heart failure: Epidemiology, pathophysiology, and rationale for therapy, *Am J Cardiol* 91(6A):2D-8D, 2003.
33. Patel R, Bushnell DL, Sobotka PA: Implications of an audible third heart sound in evaluating cardiac function, *West J Med* 158(6):606-609, 1993.
34. The Criteria Committee of the New York Heart Association: *Nomenclature and Criteria for the Diagnosis of the Heart and Great Vessels,* ed 6, Boston, 1964, Little, Brown.
35. Uretsky BF, Sheahan RG: Primary prevention of sudden cardiac death in heart failure: will the solution be shocking? *J Am Coll Cardiol* 30(7):1589-1597, 1997.
36. American College of Sports Medicine: *ACSM's Guidelines for Exercise Testing and prescription,* Baltimore, 2000, Williams & Wilkins.
37. Ainsworth BE, Haskell WL, Leon AS, et al: Compendium of physical activities: classification of energy costs of human physical activities, *Med Sci Sports Exerc* 25(1):71-80, 1993.
38. Ainsworth BE, Haskell WL, Whitt MC, et al: Compendium of physical activities: an update of activity codes and MET intensities, *Med Sci Sports Exerc* 32(9 suppl):S498-504, 2000.
39. Arena R, Humphrey R: Comparison of ventilatory expired gas parameters used to predict hospitalization in patients with heart failure, *Am Heart J* Mar 143(3):427-432, 2002.
40. Arena R, Myers J, Aslam SS, et al: Peak VO$_2$ and VE/VCO$_2$ slope in patients with heart failure: a prognostic comparison, *Am Heart J* 147(2):354-360, 2004.
41. Osada N, Chaitman BR, Miller LW, et al: Cardiopulmonary exercise testing identifies low risk patients with heart failure and severely impaired exercise capacity considered for heart transplantation, *J Am Coll Cardiol* 31(3):577-582, 1998.
42. Weber KT, Kinasewitz GT, Janicki JS, et al: Oxygen utilization and ventilation during exercise in patients with chronic cardiac failure, *Circulation* 65(6):1213-1223, 1982.
43. Myers J, Gullestad L, Vagelos R, et al: Cardiopulmonary exercise testing and prognosis in severe heart failure: 14 mL/kg/min revisited, *Am Heart J* 139:78-84, 2000.
44. ATS statement. Guidelines for the six-minute walk test, *Am J Respir Crit Care Med* 166(1):111-117, 2002.
45. Cahalin LP, Mathier MA, Semigran MJ, et al: The six-minute walk test predicts peak oxygen uptake and survival in patients with advanced heart failure, *Chest* 110(2):325-332, 1996.
46. Peeters P, Mets T: The 6-minute walk as an appropriate exercise test in elderly patients with chronic heart failure, *J Gerontol A Biol Sci Med Sci* 51(4):M147-151, 1996.
47. Faggiano P, D'Aloia A, Gualeni A, et al: Assessment of oxygen uptake during the 6-minute walking test in patients with heart failure: Preliminary experience with a portable device, *Am Heart J* 134(2 Pt 1):203-206, 1997.
48. Bittner V, Weiner DH, Yusuf S, et al: Prediction of mortality and morbidity with a 6-minute walk test in patients with left ventricular dysfunction. SOLVD Investigators, *JAMA* 270(14):1702-1707, 1993.
49. Shah MR, Hasselblad V, Gheorghiade M, et al: Prognostic usefulness of the six-minute walk in patients with advanced congestive heart failure secondary to ischemic or nonischemic cardiomyopathy, *Am J Cardiol* 88(9):987-993, 2001.
50. Curtis JP, Rathore SS, Wang Y, et al: The association of 6-minute walk performance and outcomes in stable outpatients with heart failure, *J Card Fail* 10(1):9-14, 2004.
51. Riley M, McParland J, Stanford CF, et al: Oxygen consumption during corridor walk testing in chronic cardiac failure, *Eur Heart J* 13(6):789-793, 1992.
52. Lucas C, Stevenson LW, Johnson W, et al: The 6-min walk and peak oxygen consumption in advanced heart failure: Aerobic capacity and survival, *Am Heart J* 138:618-624, 1999.

53. Jessup MLL, Loh E (eds): *Heart Failure: A Clinicians' Guide to Ambulatory Diagnosis and Treatment (Contemporary Cardiology)*, Totowa, NJ, 2003, Humana Press.

54. Rector TS, Cohn JN: Assessment of patient outcome with the Minnesota Living with Heart Failure questionnaire: Reliability and validity during a randomized, double-blind, placebo-controlled trial of pimobendan. Pimobendan Multicenter Research Group, *Am Heart J* 124(4):1017-1025, 1992.

55. Rector TS, Kubo SH, Cohn JN: Validity of the Minnesota Living with Heart Failure questionnaire as a measure of therapeutic response to enalapril or placebo, *Am J Cardiol* 71(12):1106-1107, 1993.

56. Packer M, Colucci WS, Sackner-Bernstein JD, et al: Double-blind, placebo-controlled study of the effects of carvedilol in patients with moderate to severe heart failure. The PRECISE Trial. Prospective Randomized Evaluation of Carvedilol on Symptoms and Exercise, *Circulation* 94(11):2793-2799, 1996.

57. Colucci WS, Packer M, Bristow MR, et al: Carvedilol inhibits clinical progression in patients with mild symptoms of heart failure. US Carvedilol Heart Failure Study Group, *Circulation* 94(11):2800-2806, 1996.

58. Green CP, Porter CB, Bresnahan DR, et al: Development and evaluation of the Kansas City Cardiomyopathy Questionnaire: A new health status measure for heart failure, *J Am Coll Cardiol* 35(5):1245-1255, 2000.

59. American Physical Therapy Association: *Guide to Physical Therapist Practice*, ed 2, Alexandria, Va, 2001, American Physical Therapy Association.

60. Keteyian SJ, Levine AB, Brawner CA, et al: Exercise training in patients with heart failure. A randomized, controlled trial, *Ann Intern Med* 124(12):1051-1057, 1996.

61. Hambrecht R, Niebauer J, Fiehn E, et al: Physical training in stable chronic heart failure: effects on cardiorespiratory fitness and ultrastructural abnormalities of leg muscles, *J Am Coll Cardiol* 25(6):1239-1249, 1995.

62. Belardinelli R, Georgiou D, Cianci G, et al: Randomized, controlled trial of long-term moderate exercise training in chronic heart failure: Effects on functional capacity, quality of life, and clinical outcome, *Circulation* 99(9):1173-1182, 1999.

63. Meyer K: Exercise training in heart failure: Recommendations based on current research, *Med Sci Sports Exerc* 33(4):525-531, 2001.

64. Pashkow FJD, Dafoe WA (ed): *Clinical Cardiac Rehabilitation: A Cardiologist's Guide*, ed 2, Baltimore, 1999, Williams & Wilkins.

65. Sullivan MJ, Knight JD, Higginbotham MB, et al: Relation between central and peripheral hemodynamics during exercise in patients with chronic heart failure. Muscle blood flow is reduced with maintenance of arterial perfusion pressure, *Circulation* 80(4):769-781, 1989.

66. White M, Yanowitz F, Gilbert EM, et al: Role of beta-adrenergic receptor downregulation in the peak exercise response in patients with heart failure due to idiopathic dilated cardiomyopathy, *Am J Cardiol* 76(17):1271-1276, 1995.

67. Mancini DM, Walter G, Reichek N, et al: Contribution of skeletal muscle atrophy to exercise intolerance and altered muscle metabolism in heart failure, *Circulation* 85(4):1364-1373, 1992.

68. Davies SW, Lipkin DP: Exercise physiology and the role of the periphery in cardiac failure, *Curr Opin Cardiol* 7(3):389-396, 1992.

69. Coats AJ: Exercise and heart failure, *Cardiol Clin* 19(3):517-524, 2001.

70. Cohen-Solal A, Logeart D, Guiti C, et al: Cardiac and peripheral responses to exercise in patients with chronic heart failure, *Eur Heart J* 20(13):931-945, 1999.

71. Stewart KJ, Badenhop D, Brubaker PH, et al: Cardiac rehabilitation following percutaneous revascularization, heart transplant, heart valve surgery, and chronic heart failure, *Chest* 123(6):2104-2111, 2003.

72. Experience from controlled trials of physical training in chronic heart failure. Protocol and patient factors in effectiveness in the improvement in exercise tolerance. European Heart Failure Training Group, *Eur Heart J* 19(3):466-475, 1998.

73. Hambrecht R, Gielen S, Linke A, et al: Effects of exercise training on left ventricular function and peripheral resistance in patients with chronic heart failure: A randomized trial, *JAMA* 283(23):3095-3101, 2000.

74. Willenheimer R, Erhardt L, Cline C, et al: Exercise training in heart failure improves quality of life and exercise capacity, *Eur Heart J* 19(5):774-781, 1998.

75. Afzal A, Brawner CA, Keteyian SJ: Exercise training in heart failure, *Prog Cardiovasc Dis* 41(3):175-190, 1998.

76. Meyer K, Laederach-Hofmann K: Effects of a comprehensive rehabilitation program on quality of life in patients with chronic heart failure, *Prog Cardiovasc Nurs* 18(4):169-176, 2003.

77. Oka RK, De Marco T, Haskell WL, et al: Impact of a home-based walking and resistance training program on quality of life in patients with heart failure, *Am J Cardiol* 85(3):365-369, 2000.

78. Corvera-Tindel T, Doering LV, Woo MA, et al: Effects of a home walking exercise program on functional status and symptoms in heart failure, *Am Heart J* 147(2):339-346, 2004.

79. Sullivan MJ, Higginbotham MB, Cobb FR: Exercise training in patients with severe left ventricular dysfunction: Hemodynamic and metabolic effects, *Circulation* 78(3):506-515, 1988.

80. Gielen S, Erbs S, Schuler G, et al: Exercise training and endothelial dysfunction in coronary artery disease and chronic heart failure. From molecular biology to clinical benefits, *Minerva Cardioangiol* 50(2):95-106, 2002.

81. Johnson W, Lucas C, Stevenson LW, et al: Effect of intensive therapy for heart failure on the vasodilator response to exercise, *J Am Coll Cardiol* 33(3):743-749, 1999.

82. Linke A, Schoene N, Gielen S, et al: Endothelial dysfunction in patients with chronic heart failure: Systemic effects of lower-limb exercise training, *J Am Coll Cardiol* 37(2):392-397, 2001.

83. Wilson JR, Frey MJ, Mancini DM, et al: Sympathetic vasoconstriction during exercise in ambulatory patients with left ventricular failure, *Circulation* 79(5):1021-1027, 1989.

84. Effron MB: Effects of resistive training on left ventricular function, *Med Sci Sports Exerc* 21(6):694-697, 1989.

85. Delagardelle C, Feiereisen P, Autier P, et al: Strength/endurance training versus endurance training in congestive heart failure, *Med Sci Sports Exerc* 34(12):1868-1872, 2002.

86. Karlsdottir AE, Foster C, Porcari JP, et al: Hemodynamic responses during aerobic and resistance exercise, *J Cardiopulm Rehabil* 22(3):170-177, 2002.

87. Meyer K, Samek L, Schwaibold M, et al: Physical responses to different modes of interval exercise in patients with chronic heart failure-application to exercise training, *Eur Heart J* 17(7):1040-1047, 1996.

88. Meyer K, Samek L, Schwaibold M, et al: Interval training in patients with severe chronic heart failure: analysis and recommendations for exercise procedures, *Med Sci Sports Exerc* 29(3):306-312, 1997.

89. Braith RW, Welsch MA, Feigenbaum MS, et al: Neuroendocrine activation in heart failure is modified by endurance exercise training, *J Am Coll Cardiol* 34(4):1170-1175, 1999.

90. Meyer K, Foster C, Georgakopoulos N, et al: Comparison of left ventricular function during interval versus steady-state exercise training in patients with chronic congestive heart failure, *Am J Cardiol* 82(11):1382-1387, 1998.

91. Myers J, Buchanan N, Walsh D, et al: Comparison of the ramp versus standard exercise protocols, *J Am Coll Cardiol* 17(6):1334-1342, 1991.

92. Pollock ML, Franklin BA, Balady GJ, et al: AHA Science Advisory. Resistance exercise in individuals with and without cardiovascular disease: benefits, rationale, safety, and prescription, *Circulation* 101(7):828-833, 2000.

93. Fletcher GF, Balady GJ, Amsterdam EA, et al: Exercise standards for testing and training: a statement for healthcare professionals from the American Heart Association, *Circulation* 104(14):1694-1740, 2001.

94. Consensus recommendations for the management of chronic heart failure. On behalf of the membership of the advisory council to improve outcomes nationwide in heart failure, *Am J Cardiol* 83(2A):1A-38A, 1999.

95. Moser DKR: *Improving Outcomes in Heart Failure*, Rockville, Md, 2001, Aspen.

96. Humphrey R, Bartels MN: Exercise, cardiovascular disease, and chronic heart failure, *Arch Phys Med Rehabil* 82(suppl 1):S76-81, 2001.

97. Franklin BA, Pamatmat A, Johnson S, et al: Metabolic cost of extremely slow walking in cardiac patients: implications for exercise testing and training, *Arch Phys Med Rehabil* 64(11):564-565, 1983.

98. Quell KJ, Porcari JP, Franklin BA, et al: Is brisk walking an adequate aerobic training stimulus for cardiac patients? *Chest* 122(5):1852-1856, 2002.

99. Thacker SB, Gilchrist J, Stroup DF, et al: The impact of stretching on sports injury risk: a systematic review of the literature, *Med Sci Sports Exerc* 36(3):371-378, 2004.

100. Hart LE: Effects of stretching on muscle soreness and risk of injury: A meta-analysis, *Clin J Sport Med* 13(5):321-322, 2003.

101. Dimsdale JE, Hartley LH, Guiney T, et al: Postexercise peril. Plasma catecholamines and exercise, *JAMA* 251(5):630-632, 1984.

102. Borg GA: Psychophysical bases of perceived exertion, *Med Sci Sports Exerc* 14(5):377-381, 1982.

103. Spann JC, Van Meter C: Cardiac transplantation, *Surg Clin North Am* 78(5):679-690, 1998.

104. Marzo KP, Wilson JR, Mancini DM: Effects of cardiac transplantation on ventilatory response to exercise, *Am J Cardiol* 69(5):547-553, 1992.

105. Kavanagh T: Physical training in heart transplant recipients, *J Cardiovasc Risk* 3(2):154-159, 1996.

106. Morrone TM, Buck LA, Catanese KA, et al: Early progressive mobilization of left ventricular assist devices is safe and optimizes recovery before heart transplantation, *J Heart Lung Transplant* 15(4):423-429, 1996.

107. Foray A, Williams D, Reemtsma K, et al: Assessment of submaximal exercise capacity in patients with left ventricular assist devices, *Circulation* 94(9 suppl):II222-226, 1996.

108. Mancini D, Goldsmith R, Levin H, et al: Comparison of exercise performance in patients with chronic severe heart failure versus left ventricular assist devices, *Circulation* 98(12):1178-1183, 1998.

Chapter **26**

Respiratory Failure

Robert L. Dekerlegand, Lawrence P. Cahalin, Christiane Perme

CHAPTER OUTLINE

OBJECTIVES

After reading this chapter, the reader will be able to:
1. Describe the prevalence and incidence of respiratory failure and its economic impact on society.
2. Describe normal physiological processes associated with ventilation and respiration.
3. Describe pathophysiological processes leading to respiratory insufficiency and failure.
4. Classify types of respiratory failure.
5. Identify common diseases and diagnoses associated with respiratory failure.
6. Identify potential complications of respiratory failure and discuss their impact on rehabilitation and functional capacity.
7. Be familiar with evidence for and be able to apply commonly used, reliable, and valid rehabilitation tests and measures for individuals with respiratory failure.
8. Describe and apply rehabilitation interventions for individuals with respiratory failure and demonstrate understanding of their proposed mechanisms of action.

Respiratory failure is caused by impairment of gas exchange between ambient air and circulating blood because of reduced intrapulmonary gas exchange or reduced movement of gases in and out of the lungs.[1] Breathing is a multistep physiological process with the vital purposes of delivering oxygen to and removing carbon dioxide from the human body. Efficient maintenance of appropriate blood gases is vital to survival and provides the energy needed for daily activities. By breathing, the lungs allow gases to be exchanged between the environment and the blood through the terminal airways known as the *alveoli*. Breathing involves two linked processes, *respiration* and *ventilation*. Respiration is the process of gas exchange between the alveolar air spaces and the blood, and ventilation is the movement of air in and out of the lungs. These processes interact and both need to function efficiently to balance oxygen (O_2) supply and demand and to eliminate metabolic waste products such as carbon dioxide (CO_2). The body relies on the cardiovascular system's ability to transport O_2 and CO_2 and on the tissue's ability to extract and utilize O_2 while producing and eliminating CO_2. Together, the respiratory and cardiovascular systems and the tissues' ability to extract and utilize O_2 make up the O_2 transport system (Fig. 26-1). Respiratory insufficiency and subsequent failure occur when the pulmonary system cannot maintain a steady state of gas exchange in response to the metabolic demands of the body, resulting in inadequate delivery of O_2 and/or inadequate elimination of CO_2.

Respiratory failure is a common and severe health problem. Acute respiratory failure has been shown to be associated with a 58% overall mortality in children.[2] In adults, respiratory failure is generally due to either acute respiratory distress syndrome (ARDS) or chronic obstructive pulmonary disease (COPD). The incidence of ARDS is 1.5 to 17.9 cases per 100,000 and approximately 24 million adults in the United States have evidence of COPD, as demonstrated by impaired lung function.[3] COPD is currently the fourth leading cause of death in the United States and predicted to be the third leading cause of death by the year 2020. COPD is also anticipated to be the fifth leading cause of disability in the world by 2020.[4] As respiratory failure becomes more common, rehabilitation professionals will play a growing role in providing preventive education and procedural interventions that help restore lost functional capacity and improve quality of life while containing costs associated with complications of respiratory failure.

Respiratory failure is a state or condition that may result from a disease, condition, or process. In general,

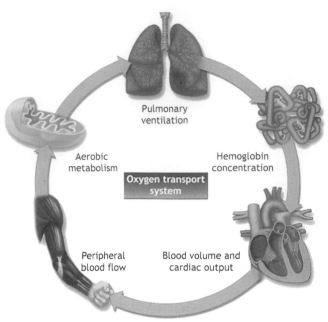

FIG. 26-1 The oxygen transport system. This system mobilizes oxygen into the body and eliminates carbon dioxide. *From McArdle WD, Katch FI, Katch VL: Exercise Physiology: Energy, Nutrition, and Human Performance, ed 5, Philadelphia, 2001, Lippincott, Williams & Wilkins.*

BOX 26-1	Diagnoses Associated with Respiratory Failure (ICD-9 Codes)

Poliomyelitis (045)	Emphysema (492)
Cystic fibrosis (277.0)	Asthma (493)
Parkinson's disease (332)	Bronchiectasis (494)
Huntington's chorea (333.4)	Pneumothorax (512)
Spinocerebellar disease (334)	Pulmonary edema (514)
Amyotrophic lateral sclerosis (335.20)	Lung involvement in conditions classified elsewhere (517)
Multiple sclerosis (340)	Inflammatory pulmonary fibrosis (515)
Quadriplegia (344.00)	
Guillain-Barré syndrome (357.00)	Other disorder of the lung (518)
Muscular dystrophy (359.1)	Acute respiratory failure (518.81)
Viral pneumonia (480)	
Bacterial pneumonia (482)	Disorders of the diaphragm (519.4)
Chronic bronchitis (491)	Curvature of the spine (737)
	Burns (941-949)

ICD-9, International Classification of Diseases, ninth revision.

respiratory failure can be caused by disorders of the airways, the lung tissue, or the skeletal, muscular, and neural components of the respiratory system. Regardless of the underlying pathology, the rehabilitation professional should assess the degree of resulting functional limitation to select the most appropriate interventions to progress the patient toward realistic goals. Box 26-1 lists diagnoses commonly associated with respiratory failure.[5]

The preferred practice patterns addressed in this chapter are 6E: Impaired ventilation and respiration/gas exchange associated with ventilatory pump dysfunction or failure and 6F: Impaired ventilation, respiration/gas exchange associated with respiratory failure. Preferred practice pattern 6G: Impaired ventilation, respiration/gas exchange, and aerobic capacity/endurance associated with respiratory failure in the neonate is not specifically covered because this is not a common area of practice for the entry level practitioner. However, much of the information that applies to adults can also be applied to this population.

PATHOLOGY

For the O_2 transport system to function effectively and efficiently, each component, as shown in Fig. 26-1, must work optimally. Although small deficiencies in one component may be compensated for by other systems, when deficiencies increase or are prolonged or demands increase, compensation generally fails and respiratory failure ensues. Since activity increases demands on the O_2 transport system, the rehabilitation professional may be able to compensate for reduced O_2 transport by curtailing the patient's activity level or intensity.

RESPIRATORY ANATOMY

The respiratory system can be divided into four components: The skeletal components, the muscular components, the lungs and airways, and the neural control centers.

Skeletal Components of the Respiratory System. The skeletal components of the respiratory system are the thoracic vertebrae, the sternum, and the ribs, which together make up the thorax (Fig. 26-2). The thorax contains and protects the heart, lungs, and the major vessels. It provides a stable base for attachment of the muscles of respiration and allows for lung expansion. The upper portion of the rib cage is much less mobile than the lower portion. For optimal ventilation, the lungs and thus the thorax must be able to expand in all dimensions: Anterior-posterior, superior-inferior, and medial-lateral. This requires appropriate rib mobility. Limitations or restrictions in the ability of either the lungs or ribs to expand will increase the workload (O_2 demand) of the respiratory system, limit how much air can move into the airways, and may indirectly contribute to respiratory muscle fatigue and failure.

Muscular Components of the Respiratory System. The muscular components of the respiratory system consist of the primary breathing muscle, the diaphragm, and the accessory muscles of ventilation (Fig. 26-3). These muscles together affect the volume of air in the lungs and the flow of air through the airways. Contraction of the respiratory muscles creates negative pressure to "pull" air into the airways. If at any time the diaphragm cannot sustain ventilation, the accessory muscles will assist. Any muscle that attaches directly to the thorax can act as an accessory muscle of ventilation.

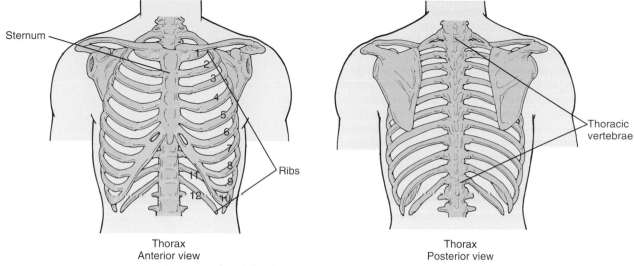

FIG. 26-2 The skeletal components of the respiratory system.

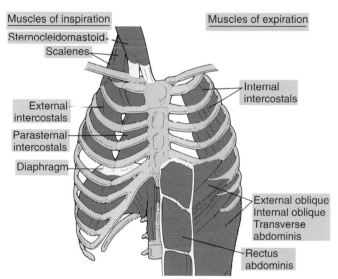

FIG. 26-3 The muscular components of the respiratory system.

The accessory muscles are best understood by dividing them into muscles of inspiration and muscles of expiration as shown in Table 26-1 and Fig. 26-3.

The diaphragm is innervated by the phrenic nerve, which is composed of nerve roots from C3, C4, and C5. (Remember: "C3, 4, 5 keeps the phrenic nerve alive!") The diaphragm originates from the upper three lumbar vertebrae, the lower border of the rib cage, and the xiphoid process of the sternum. The fibers converge to form and insert on the common central tendon. The diaphragm is the only muscle that works in three dimensions and that has a bony origin but does not have a bony insertion. At rest the diaphragm is elevated in a domed-shaped position that optimizes the length-tension relationship of the fibers and thus the efficiency of its contraction. In some disease processes, such as emphysema, the resting position of the diaphragm may change creating a mechanical disadvantage that impairs muscle contraction force generation.[6]

The position of the diaphragm also varies among normal individuals and is affected by age, weight, and thoracic dimensions.[7] As the diaphragm contracts, it flattens and lowers (Fig. 26-4), increasing thoracic volume and producing most (if not all) of the negative inspiratory pressure required to inhale air at rest. The diaphragm is primarily composed of slow-twitch oxidative muscle fibers (type I fibers) that are resistant to fatigue but it also contains fast-twitch glycolytic muscle fibers (type II fibers) that are designed for strength.[8] This combination of fibers not only enables the diaphragm to sustain breathing day in and day out but also allows it to generate increased force when needed.

When the diaphragm initially contracts, it begins to flatten and descend, drawing air into the lungs and producing an observable rise of the abdomen.[9] As contraction progresses, the diaphragm continues to descend until it touches the abdominal contents. At this point, the central tendon becomes "fixed" or stationary. When the diaphragm contracts further, it pulls up on the ribs causing an observable expansion of the lower border of the rib cage. To achieve maximal lung expansion the accessory muscles of ventilation must expand the upper chest. The sequential abdominal rise, lateral costal expansion, and upper chest rise overlap to some degree but all contribute to achieving optimal lung capacity during inhalation.[9] The rate of inhalation and control of breathing can also affect the penetration of air into the lungs. Controlled slow breathing may allow inhaled air to reach deeper within the airways.[10,11]

Lungs and Airways. The organs of respiration, the lungs, are located within the thorax. The two lungs, the left and the right, are each subdivided into lobes and segments (Fig. 26-5). Air enters the lungs via the trachea that branches into the left and right mainstem bronchi at the level of the sternal angle anteriorly and the spinous process of T3 posteriorly. The airways then continue to branch into the smaller lobar bronchi, followed by the segmental bronchi, and then into the bronchioles to finally reach the alveoli where gas exchange takes place

TABLE 26-1	Muscles of Breathing		
	Origin	Insertion	Innervation
MUSCLES OF INSPIRATION			
Diaphragm	Xiphoid process Lower 6 costal cartilages Anterior surfaces of the lumbar vertebrae	Central tendon	Phrenic nerve (C3-C5)
External intercostals	Inferior border of the superior rib Fibers run inferomedially	Superior border of the inferior rib	T1-T12
Upper trapezius	Medial aspect of the superior nuchal line	Distal one third of the scapula	Spinal accessory nerve (CN XI)
Sternocleidomastoid	Manubrium and medial third of the clavicle	Mastoid process	Spinal accessory nerve (CN XI)
Scalenes	Transverse processes of C3-C7	First and second ribs	C4-C8
Serratus anterior	Upper 8 ribs	Medial border of the scapula	Long thoracic nerve (C5-7)
Pectoralis major	Clavicle and sternum	Lateral lip of the intertubercular groove of the humerus	Medial and lateral pectoral nerve (C5-T1)
Pectoralis minor	Ribs 2-4 or 3-5	Coracoid process of the scapula	Medial and lateral pectoral nerve (C5, T1)
Abdominals			T5-L1
Latissimus dorsi	Spinous processes of T6-T12, L1-L5, upper sacral vertebrae, and the iliac crest	Intertubercular groove of the humerus	Thoracodorsal nerve, C6-C8
MUSCLES OF EXPIRATION			
Abdominals			T5-L1
Internal intercostals	Inferior border of the superior rib Fibers run inferolaterally	Superior border of the inferior rib	T1-12

Data from Clarkson H: *Musculoskeletal Assessment: Joint ROM and Manual Muscle Strength*, ed 2, Philadelphia, 2000, Lippincott Williams & Wilkins.
CN, Cranial nerve.

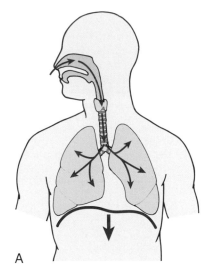
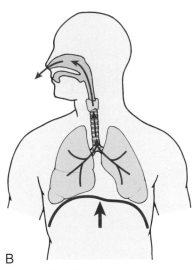

A
The diaphragm descends
with muscle contraction (inspiration).

B
The diaphragm rises
with muscle relaxation (expiration).

FIG. 26-4 The diaphragm is the primary muscle of respiration. **A,** The diaphragm descends with muscle contraction (inspiration); **B,** the diaphragm rises with muscle relaxation (expiration).

(Fig. 26-6). There may be 23 to 25 levels of airway branching. The airways from the trachea down to approximately the seventeenth level of branching only conduct air to the *respiratory airways*. No gas exchange occurs in these *conducting airways*. The respiratory airways, where gas exchange takes place, begin after approximately the seventeenth branching. These airways are characterized by the appearance of alveoli, with the number of alveoli increasing with further branching of the airways. The airways are protected primarily by the epiglottis and a functional cough. They are kept clear of mucus and foreign material by the "mucociliary escalator"[12] (see Chapter 24).

RESPIRATORY PHYSIOLOGY

Neural Control of Breathing. Breathing is designed to facilitate *alveolar ventilation* and is under both voluntary and involuntary control. The neural respiratory control center is located within the pons and medulla of the brainstem. It is here that information from the motor cortex, chemoreceptors in the periphery, and mechanoreceptors in the skeletal muscle and the lung tissues is integrated to produce efferent impulses that control the respiratory muscles to alter the rate and depth of breathing in response to the metabolic demands of the body.[13]

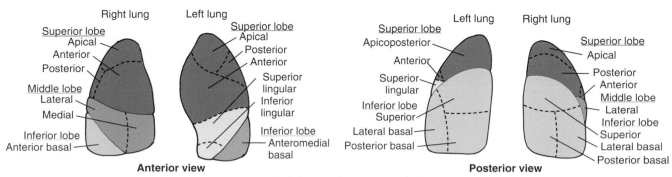

FIG. 26-5 The lobes and segments of the lungs.

Most breathing is under involuntary control and responds to input from mechanoreceptors and chemoreceptors. Under normal resting conditions, breathing is primarily under chemical control.[13] Central and peripheral chemoreceptors sense levels of CO_2 and O_2, respectively, and determine respiratory drive. The central chemoreceptors in the brainstem respond to blood levels of CO_2 to provide the primary drive for breathing. As CO_2 levels rise, they stimulate increased ventilation to blow off the extra CO_2. This mechanism is often referred to as the hypercapnic drive for breathing. The peripheral chemoreceptors in the aortic arch and the common carotid arteries respond to blood O_2 levels. If O_2 levels fall below normal, these receptors stimulate increased ventilation. This serves as a back-up for the hypercapnic drive, and this response is often referred to as the hypoxic drive or the secondary drive for breathing.

In addition to the strategically located chemoreceptors, mechanoreceptors in the lungs and the peripheral skeletal muscles respond to stretch or movement to regulate the overall breathing pattern. As the lungs near full inspiratory volume, mechanoreceptors inhibit inhalation and facilitate exhalation so that the lungs do not become overstretched. Mechanoreceptors in the skeletal muscles are also thought to play a role in stimulating breathing at the initial stages of exercise.

The airways and the pulmonary vessels are under a degree of autonomic control. Sympathetic activation causes airway dilation and suppression of secretion production, whereas parasympathetic activation has the opposite effect. The pulmonary vessels are primarily affected by their O_2 level and constrict in response to low O_2 levels. This phenomenon is known as hypoxic vasoconstriction.[14]

In addition to these involuntary breathing control mechanisms, breathing can also be voluntarily controlled via the motor cortex. This type of control is used to perform volitional activities such as blowing out birthday candles, singing, taking a deep breath before submerging in water, and to some extent during exercise.

Pulmonary Function Tests and Lung Volumes.
The ventilatory pump system controls the volume of air moving in and out of the airways and the rate at which the air moves. Normal values for lung volumes, capacities, and flow rates are listed and defined in Table 26-2, and volumes and capacities are shown graphically in Fig. 26-7. A lung capacity is the sum of two or more volumes.

Conducting zone	Trachea	0
	Primary bronchus	1
	Bronchus	2
		3
		4
	Bronchi	5-10
	Bronchioles	11-16
Respiratory zone	Respiratory bronchioles	17
		18
		19
	Alveolar ducts	20
		21
		22
	Alveolar sacs	23

FIG. 26-6 Airway branching. The trachea to the seventeenth level of branching is the conducting zone. Gas exchange takes place after the seventeenth level in the respiratory zone. *From McArdle WD, Katch FI, Katch VL: Exercise Physiology: Energy, Nutrition, and Human Performance, ed 5, Philadelphia, 2001, Lippincott Williams & Wilkins.*

Lung volumes and capacities vary in the normal individual based on body size, gender, height, and weight and can be compromised by pathology. Compromised lung volumes and capacities are often associated with restrictive lung diseases.

Measures commonly used to evaluate airway function are forced vital capacity (FVC), forced expiratory volume in 1 second (FEV_1) and forced midexpiratory flow ($FEF_{25\%-75\%}$). FVC is the volume of air moved from maximal inhalation to maximal exhalation. To measure FVC the patient is asked to inhale maximally and then forcefully blow out into a measuring device or spirometer until their

TABLE 26-2	Lung Volumes Associated with Ventilation	

Volumes	Definition	Adult Normal Values
Tidal volume (TV)	Volume of air inspired or expired per breath	600-500 ml
Inspiratory reserve volume (IRV)	Volume of air from end of tidal inspiration to maximal inspiration	3000-1900 ml
Expiratory reserve volume (ERV)	Volume of air from end tidal expiration to maximal expiration	1200-800 ml
Total lung capacity (TLC)	Volume of air in the lungs at the end of maximal inspiration	6000-4200 ml
Residual volume (RV)	Volume of air in the lungs after maximal expiration	1200-1000 ml (20%-25% TLC)
Vital capacity (VC)	Volume of air from maximal inspiration to maximal expiration	4800-3200 ml
Inspiratory capacity (IC)	Volume of air from tidal expiration to maximal inhalation	3600-2400 ml
Functional residual capacity (FRC)	Volume of air in the lungs after a tidal expiration	2400-1800 ml (40%-50% TLC)
Forced vital capacity (FVC)	Volume of air forcefully exhaled from maximal inspiration to maximal expiration	4800-3200 ml

Flows	Definition	Adult Normal Values
Forced expiratory volume in 1 second (FEV$_1$)	Volume of air moved in the first second of an FVC maneuver	75%-80% FVC
FEV$_1$/FVC ratio		0.75-0.80
Peak expiratory flow (PEF)	Peak flow reached during an FVC maneuver	9-10 L/sec

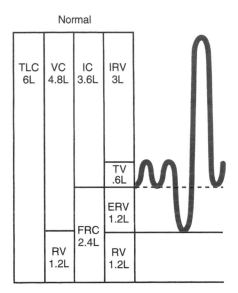

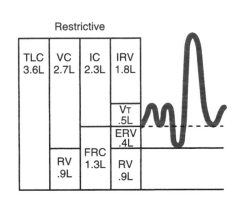

FIG. 26-7 Lung volumes and capacities. *TLC,* Total lung capacity; *VC,* vital capacity; *RV,* reserve volume; *IC,* inspiratory capacity; *FRC,* functional residual capacity; *IRV,* inspiratory reserve volume; *TV,* tidal volume; *ERV,* expiratory reserve volume. *From Hillegass E, Sadowsky HS:* Essentials of Cardiopulmonary Physical Therapy, *ed 2, Philadelphia, 2001, Saunders.*

lungs feel completely empty. The total volume moved during this forced maneuver is the FVC. FEV$_1$ is the volume of air moved during the first second of the FVC maneuver and represents air movement through the larger airways. FEF$_{25\%-75\%}$ is the flow rate during the middle portion of the FVC maneuver and is affected by the integrity of the small airways. Compromised flow rates are often associated with obstructive pulmonary diseases.

Arterial–Alveolar Oxygen Difference. The difference in O$_2$ concentration between the arterial blood and the air within the alveoli is known as the *arterial–alveolar oxygen difference,* or gradient, and is abbreviated as PAO$_2$–PaO$_2$. This value reflects the adequacy of gas exchange within the lung. PAO$_2$–PaO$_2$ will widen if diffusion between the alveoli and the pulmonary circulation is impaired and less O$_2$ reaches the bloodstream from the alveoli. PAO$_2$–PaO$_2$ is normally less than 20 mm Hg but may be as low as 10 mm Hg in children and as high as 30 mm Hg in the elderly.[15]

Ventilation and Perfusion. Ventilation (V̇) refers to the movement of a volume of air from the atmosphere in

and out of the airways and is highly dependent on the ability of the respiratory muscles to generate force to bring air into the lungs. *Minute ventilation* (MV) is the volume of air moved in 1 minute and is usually measured liters per minute (L/min). MV is equal to the tidal volume multiplied by the respiratory rate:

$$MV = TV \times RR$$

where:
MV = minute ventilation
TV = tidal volume
RR = respiratory rate in breaths per minute (breaths/min)

Maximal voluntary ventilation (MVV) is an individual's maximal MV and contributes to their overall functional aerobic capacity, which is also affected by all the entire O$_2$ transport system. MVV can be measured with pulmonary function tests. MVV is rarely reached at maximal aerobic capacity and is not a limiting factor in individuals without pulmonary dysfunction. However, those with pulmonary disease may approach their MVV with certain activities or exercise.[16] When an individual's MV reaches about 50% of their MVV, they will feel short of breath.[17] At 70% of MVV the respiratory muscles will begin to fatigue, and 90% MVV is only sustainable for a short period of time.[18] Ventilatory reserve (MVV − MV) is associated with outcome (progression to respiratory failure) in individuals experiencing COPD exacerbations.[19] Although rehabilitation professionals may not always have exact objective measurements of these values, these concepts should be considered when working with patients with respiratory compromise and when selecting exercise intensities.

Perfusion ($\dot{Q}$) of the lungs refers to the amount of blood flowing through the lungs. *Alveolar perfusion* has the greatest effect on respiration because only the blood that reaches the alveoli participates in gas exchange. The pulmonary circulation is primarily determined by the status and integrity of the cardiovascular system. Conditions, such as congestive heart failure, pulmonary embolism, and hypertension, may reduce pulmonary perfusion and thus interfere with respiration.

Ventilation and perfusion are not distributed equally through the lungs.[20-23] When an individual is upright, gravity causes more perfusion in the inferior portions and more ventilation in the superior portions of the lungs.[24] Therefore, because the dependent portions are less inflated, they have the greatest potential for expansion (i.e., they have the greatest amount of reserve volume). Thus if ventilation is increased beyond normal levels, the extra ventilation will likely occur inferiorly.

Ventilation and Perfusion Matching. Ventilation and perfusion must match for adequate gas exchange and respiration to occur. Normally, the $\dot{V}:\dot{Q}$ ratio ranges from 0.6 to 3.0, with the lesser value representing the dependent portions of the lung where there is more perfusion ($\dot{Q}$) and less ventilation ($\dot{V}$), and the higher value representing the upper portions of the lung where there is more ventilation ($\dot{V}$) and less perfusion ($\dot{Q}$).[25] Optimal gas exchange occurs where $\dot{V}$ and $\dot{Q}$ are equal and the $\dot{V}:\dot{Q}$ ratio = 1. In the upright position, this occurs in the middle lung zones. The overall distribution of ventilation and perfusion within the lungs creates an aggregate $\dot{V}:\dot{Q}$ match that allows for optimal gas exchange within the lungs under normal conditions. $\dot{V}:\dot{Q}$ mismatch reduces gas exchange and limits respiratory function and may occur if either ventilation or perfusion are impaired.

Dead space refers to areas within the lungs in which the air is not participating in respiration and thus breathing is impaired. Dead space can be anatomical (normal) or physiological (abnormal or pathological). Anatomical dead space consists of areas that normally have a high $\dot{V}:\dot{Q}$ ratio such as the conducting airways (i.e., the trachea through approximately generation 17 of the bronchi). It is normal for the air in these locations not to participate in gas exchange. Physiological, or pathological, dead space describes areas where air that should be participating in respiration does not do so due to a disease process or abnormal condition that limits perfusion but not ventilation. For example, physiological dead space may occur when a pulmonary embolism occludes blood flow (perfusion) to a given area of the lungs, limiting alveolar perfusion.

With *pulmonary shunt,* perfusion is greater than ventilation ($\dot{Q} > \dot{V}$). This may occur normally in the dependent portions of the lungs but can also be pathological. The classic example of pulmonary shunt is in areas of *atelectasis* (collapse of the airways) or consolidation (filling of alveoli with secretions). These conditions reduce ventilation but not perfusion.

Respiration. Respiration is the process of exchange of gases between the atmosphere and the tissues. This process involves the acquisition of O_2 and the elimination of CO_2 and occurs through diffusion in the alveoli. Four primary factors affect diffusion in the lungs: Partial pressures of gases, surface area available for gas exchange, thickness of the membrane, and time. The partial pressures of O_2 and CO_2 are the "driving" forces of gas exchange and diffusion (Fig. 26-8). Gases will diffuse from an area with higher partial pressure to an area with lower partial pressure to move toward equilibrium. Partial pressures are discussed in greater detail in the section on arterial blood gases.

The relevant surface area is the area of alveolar membrane in contact with air and blood. As an aggregate, the alveoli have the largest surface area of all the airways, being on average 118 m^2 in adult males and 91 m^2 in adult females, equivalent to approximately $\frac{1}{4}$ of a professional basketball court.[26,27] The total alveolar surface area involved with respiration depends on the number and size of the alveoli and can be affected by various disease states and by the amount of ventilation. The alveolar membrane is made up of a single layer of endothelial cells, creating a very thin membrane through which gas exchange can occur. Certain diseases and/or the presence of mucus may increase airway thickness or limit the number of alveoli participating in respiration. Infiltrates from pneumonia may reduce the number of alveoli available for ventilation, and emphysema will reduce alveolar surface area by destroying the alveolar walls. Both will ultimately limit alveolar gas exchange and impair respiratory function.

The final component that affects diffusion is the amount of time the gas is in contact with the alveoli. Alterations in gas partial pressures, alveolar surface area, or alveolar membrane thickness may potentially be

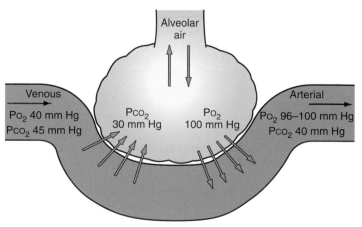

FIG. 26-8 Gas exchange occurs through diffusion in the alveoli.

TABLE 26-3　Normal Arterial Blood Gas Values and Common Simplified Abnormalities*

	pH	$Paco_2$ (mm Hg)	Pao_2 (mm Hg)	HCO_3 (mEq/L)
Normal	7.35-7.45	35-45	>80	22-26
Respiratory acidosis	<7.35	>45	>80	22-26
Respiratory alkalosis	>7.45	<45	>80	22-26
Metabolic acidosis	<7.35	35-45	>80	>26
Metabolic alkalosis	>7.45	35-45	>80	<22

*These represent pure uncompensated states of either respiratory or metabolic acidosis/alkalosis and may or may not be associated with varying degrees of hypoxemia depending on the severity of illness.

compensated for by increasing the contact time for diffusion.

Arterial Blood Gases. Arterial blood gases (ABGs) are measures of the partial pressure of O_2 (Pao_2), partial pressure of CO_2 ($Paco_2$), levels of bicarbonate (HCO_3), and the pH of arterial blood and are primary indicators of the respiratory and ventilatory status and overall physiological state of the body. Under normal circumstances, respiration balances O_2 supply and demand, as well as CO_2 production and elimination. The normal ranges for the components of the ABGs, along with common acid-base disorders, are summarized in Table 26-3. For an ABG to be considered normal, all values must be within normal limits.

Breathing primarily affects $Paco_2$, pH, and Pao_2. Inadequate ventilation (hypoventilation) causes $Paco_2$ to increase and Pao_2 to decrease by limiting respiration. The increase in $Paco_2$ will cause pH to fall and make the blood more acidic. An increase in ventilation (hyperventilation) will cause $Paco_2$ to decrease. The decrease in $Paco_2$ will cause pH to rise and make the blood more alkaline. Hyperventilation generally does not significantly affect Pao_2 because this value is close to its maximum under normal conditions and cannot increase further.

Work of Breathing. *Work of breathing* (WOB) is the amount of energy or O_2 consumption needed by the respiratory muscles to produce enough ventilation and respiration to meet the metabolic demands of the body. Under normal resting circumstances, the WOB is about 5% of $\dot{V}O_{2max}$.[28] In individuals with pulmonary problems, WOB may exceed 50% of $\dot{V}O_2$ max, reducing their energy reserve and exercise capacity and stressing other systems to compensate.[29,30]

WOB is affected by various factors. The first factor is the metabolic needs of the body. As the body demands more energy, WOB needs to increase to provide adequate ventilation. WOB is also affected by how much force the respiratory muscles must exert to overcome the resistance to airflow to move air in and out of the airways and maintain adequate lung volumes. The final determinant of WOB is the rate at which the muscles need to generate force, which is represented by the respiratory rate. WOB is determined by how hard and how fast the respiratory muscles must contract. $\dot{V}:\dot{Q}$ mismatching and impaired diffusion from various disease processes can also make the respiratory system inefficient, increasing ventilatory demands and the WOB.[29-31]

Airway Resistance. Airway resistance is the force opposing air flow in the airways. Airway resistance depends on the radius and length of the airway, according to Poiseuille's law as expressed in the following equation:

$$R = 8\ell n/\pi r^4$$

where:
R = resistance
ℓ = length of the airway
n = gas viscosity
r = radius of the airway

Since resistance is inversely proportional to the radius to the fourth power, anything that changes the radius or diameter of the airway will tremendously affect resistance to airflow. For example, if bronchoconstriction as a result of asthma or airway obstruction as a result of mucus causes the airway radius to decrease by a factor of two, the resistance will increase by a factor of 2^4 (i.e., 16). In this case, the respiratory muscles will need to generate much more pressure to overcome this resistance and produce adequate airflow. Generating more pressure will require increased WOB and energy expenditure.

Elasticity. *Elasticity* refers to the ability of the lungs and chest wall to recoil or deflate passively during exhalation. Since exhalation is normally passive at rest, it consumes no energy and therefore does not contribute to the overall work of breathing. The elastic recoil of the lungs and chest wall is similar to a balloon deflating without any external pressure when you let go of it after it is inflated. It deflates as a result of the elasticity, or passive recoil, of the balloon. Conditions that decrease the elasticity of the lungs may prevent passive exhalation. In this scenario, the accessory muscles of exhalation may need to contract and expend additional energy to maintain adequate ventilation and prevent hyperinflation of the lungs. The net result will be an increased WOB, which may eventually result in respiratory muscle fatigue or the inability to maintain adequate respiration.

If airway resistance increases, as with bronchoconstriction from asthma, passive elastic recoil may not generate enough force to overcome this resistance and empty the lungs. In this scenario, the body will need to use the accessory muscles of breathing to complete exhalation. This increase in muscle activity increases the WOB. This problem is exacerbated by the fact that when air is unable to get out, the trapped air functions as dead space and does not participate in respiration, making even less O_2 available to the body to produce energy.

Compliance. Lung *compliance* refers to the change in lung volume per unit of pressure change, and the standard

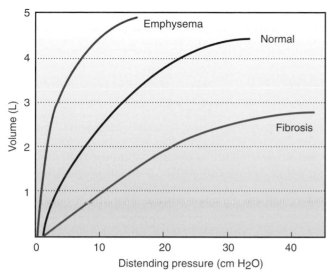

FIG. 26-9 Lung compliance is the change in lung volume per unit of pressure change. *From http://oac.med/jhmi.edu/ res_phys/Encyclopedia/Compliance/Compliance.html. Copyright 1995 Johns Hopkins University.*

compliance curve is shown in Fig. 26-9. Lung compliance affects the ability of the lungs to expand during inspiration. The less compliant the tissue, the more "stiff" or resistant to expansion it will be. Anyone who has attempted to blow up a balloon has experienced this concept. The initially low compliance of the balloon makes it very difficult to inflate. Thus high pressures and much energy are required to inflate the balloon. Efficient ventilation requires that both the lungs and the chest wall be compliant. The respiratory muscles will need to exert more inspiratory force if either lungs and or chest wall compliance are decreased, thereby increasing the WOB.

A number of musculoskeletal, neurological, and pulmonary conditions can also affect lung or chest wall expansion. For example, severe scoliosis can significantly restrict thoracic expansion and thus limit lung expansion. Neurological conditions, such as cerebrovascular accidents, may increase muscle tone in the trunk restricting chest wall expansion.[31,32] Chest expansion may also be limited by neurologic conditions that paralyze the respiratory muscles.[33] For example, individuals with mid- or high-cervical spinal cord injury may have paralyzed respiratory muscles that cannot generate force to draw air into the lungs and therefore limit chest wall and lung expansion.[34]

Surface Tension. The term surface tension refers to the cohesive state that occurs at a liquid-gas interface or liquid-liquid interface.[35] Within the lungs, this occurs at the interface between the alveolar membrane and the airway. Increased surface tension increases cohesion within the alveoli, pulling the alveoli closed. The alveolar cells produce a specialized liquid, *surfactant,* that decreases the surface tension in the airways reducing the amount of energy required to expand the lungs.[36] When surface tension increases, more force is needed to expand the lungs, increasing the WOB. This occurs in respiratory distress syndrome in premature newborns because until around 36 weeks of gestation the fetus produces immature surfactant that inadequately reduces surface tension.[36] The resulting increased WOB causes most of these infants to initially need ventilatory assistance.

PATHOPHYSIOLOGY OF RESPIRATORY FAILURE

Respiratory failure refers to the inability of the body to maintain adequate gas exchange to meet its metabolic demands. Many factors affect gas exchange, but ventilation, diffusion, and perfusion are the primary contributors. Ventilation requires the respiratory muscles to produce sufficient force to sustain ventilation at all times and in response to a range of demands. If the WOB exceeds the capacity of the individual, fatigue and eventually respiratory failure will occur. Even if the muscles can generate enough force, diseases of the lung and airways may make this effort futile. Respiratory failure can be classified as being due to hypoventilation, $\dot{V}:\dot{Q}$ mismatch, abnormal diffusion, or a combination of these factors.[37-39]

Hypoventilation. Hypoventilation refers to a state of decreased or inadequate ventilation. Many factors can contribute to hypoventilation. However, the primary causes of hypoventilation are central nervous system depression, neurological disease, or disorders of the respiratory muscles.[33,37]

Under normal circumstances, ventilation maintains a steady state between O_2 supply and demand and between CO_2 production and elimination. Tidal volumes exceed the volume of dead space in the conducting airways so that air reaches the alveoli for gas exchange to take place. Hypoventilation, which causes low tidal volumes, will decrease alveolar ventilation that in turn will decrease the potential for gas exchange. When gas exchange fails to keep the circulating concentrations of O_2 and CO_2 within the normal range, this indicates respiratory insufficiency and potential failure.

Ventilation-Perfusion Mismatch. Mismatching of ventilation and perfusion ($\dot{V}:\dot{Q}$ mismatch) is one of the more frequent causes of respiratory failure or inadequate gas exchange. As explained previously, ventilation-perfusion matching is determined by the distribution of air and blood flow in the lungs. Many factors, including diseases and body position, can affect the $\dot{V}:\dot{Q}$ ratio and lead to excessive dead space or areas of shunt.[20,22,37,40] In either case the result of the $\dot{V}:\dot{Q}$ mismatch is impaired gas exchange in the affected areas of lungs and a decreased ability to maintain a steady state of O_2 and CO_2 concentrations.

In some instances, where $\dot{V}:\dot{Q}$ mismatching only occurs in part of the lungs, the body may be able to compensate by redistributing perfusion or increasing ventilation within the lungs to maintain appropriate $\dot{V}:\dot{Q}$ matching overall. Hypoxic vasoconstriction is a physiological reflex aimed at minimizing $\dot{V}:\dot{Q}$ mismatch to preserve respiration.[14] In response to low ventilation ($\dot{V}<\dot{Q}$) of an area, the body also decreases the perfusion ($\dot{Q}$) to this area through vasoconstriction to try to keep ventilation and perfusion matched and thus maintain gas exchange. This is an example of the cardiovascular components of the O_2 transport system attempting to compensate for pulmonary impairments at the expense of increased workload. This compensation may effectively keep circulating CO_2 and O_2 levels within normal limits. If it fails, CO_2 levels will rise stimulating an increase in respiratory rate. This will increase the WOB and may eventually lead to respiratory fatigue or failure.

Diffusion Abnormalities. Gas exchange occurs at the alveolar level by diffusion and depends on alveolar surface area, partial pressures of O_2 and CO_2, the thickness of the alveolar wall, and time. Isolated abnormalities of diffusion are less common contributors to respiratory failure than $\dot{V}:\dot{Q}$ mismatching; however, impaired diffusion may result in $\dot{V}:\dot{Q}$ mismatching.[37] Inadequate diffusion increases the overall WOB by interfering with gas exchange. In the presence of other abnormal conditions, such as respiratory muscle weakness, the body may not be able to sustain the additional WOB and respiratory fatigue or failure may result.

Classification of Respiratory Failure. With inadequate respiration, O_2 levels decrease *(hypoxia)* and CO_2 levels increase *(hypercapnia)*. The increase in CO_2 produces a decrease in blood pH. Respiratory failure can alter all aspects of the ABGs. The ABG criteria for respiratory failure are a PaO_2 of less than 60 mm Hg, a $PaCO_2$ greater than 50 mm Hg, or a pH of less than 7.3.[37,38]

Respiratory failure can be classified as primarily hypoxic (know as type I) or as primarily hypercapnic (known as type II). Hypoxic respiratory failure is primarily characterized by abnormally low PaO_2 and a normal or close to normal $PaCO_2$, whereas hypercapnic respiratory failure is primarily characterized by an abnormally elevated $PaCO_2$ that may or may not be associated with hypoxia.[38]

Respiratory failure can also be classified as acute or chronic depending on its time course. Acute respiratory failure occurs over a short period of time (minutes to hours), whereas chronic respiratory failure develops over a longer period of time (days to months). The patient history can help determine the acuity of respiratory failure, and ABGs can help distinguish between acute and chronic hypercapnic respiratory failure. With acute hypercapnic respiratory failure, CO_2 levels rise, causing a fall in arterial pH. Over time, the kidneys can compensate for this change by retaining bicarbonate (HCO_3) to bring the pH back toward normal. Thus, with acute hypercapnic respiratory failure, $PaCO_2$ is elevated and pH is low, whereas with chronic hypercapnic respiratory failure, $PaCO_2$ is elevated, but pH is almost normal. The acuity of hypoxemic respiratory failure cannot be determined from ABG values since PaO_2 does not influence pH. Acute hypoxemia can be differentiated from chronic hypoxemia by the history and the presence or absence of clinical indicators of long-standing hypoxemia such as polycythemia (an increase in the number of red blood cells).

It is important to distinguish between acute and chronic respiratory failure because individuals in the acute stages of respiratory failure should limit their activity since increasing the O_2 demand may worsen their condition. However, early mobilization, positioning, and breathing exercises can help these patients by improving ventilation, enhancing $\dot{V}:\dot{Q}$ matching, and stimulating respiratory drive. For individuals with chronic respiratory failure or

those at risk of developing failure, rehabilitation interventions should focus on improving breathing efficiency and improving overall conditioning through strength and aerobic training (see Chapter 23).

EXAMINATION

PATIENT HISTORY

The patient history may be obtained directly from the patient if they are not intubated or unconscious. Otherwise the history may be obtained from the patient's chart, other health care providers and the patient's family members. One should try to ascertain the primary and secondary reasons for respiratory failure; the patient's prior level of respiratory function, including activity tolerance and need for supplemental O_2; and the course of his or her respiratory decline. One should also consider if any medications are contributing to the current respiratory failure, if the patient has a history of depression or anxiety, and whether the patient has a history of diabetes or neurological disorders.

SYSTEMS REVIEW

The systems review is used to target areas requiring further examination and to define areas that may cause complications or indicate a need for precautions during the examination and intervention processes. See Chapter 1 for further details of the systems review.

For the patient with respiratory failure the systems review should include examination of the level of consciousness and the ability to follow commands. The chart should also be reviewed for vital signs, ABG values, and results of cardiovascular tests such as cardiac catheterization, echocardiography, electrocardiogram (ECG), and cardiac enzymes.

TESTS AND MEASURES

Musculoskeletal. The primary musculoskeletal tests and measures for persons with respiratory failure are measurements of upper and lower extremity range of motion (ROM), strength and endurance, and joint integrity and mobility in preparation for upright activities and progression of functional and exercise training.

Neuromuscular. The primary neuromuscular tests and measures for persons with respiratory failure are measurements of cognition (e.g., attention and arousal), reflexes, sensation, coordination, motor function (e.g., control and learning), balance, and pain. Many of the tests and measures used by physical therapists (PTs) to examine the neuromuscular function of patients without respiratory failure can be used or adapted for use in patients with respiratory failure.

Integumentary. The integumentary system should be examined frequently in patients with respiratory failure who are bed bound (see Chapter 28).

Cardiovascular/Pulmonary

Ventilator Settings and Oxygen Requirements. For the patient on a ventilator, the ventilator settings and O_2 requirements should be checked before other tests and measures are performed. Fig. 26-10 provides an overview

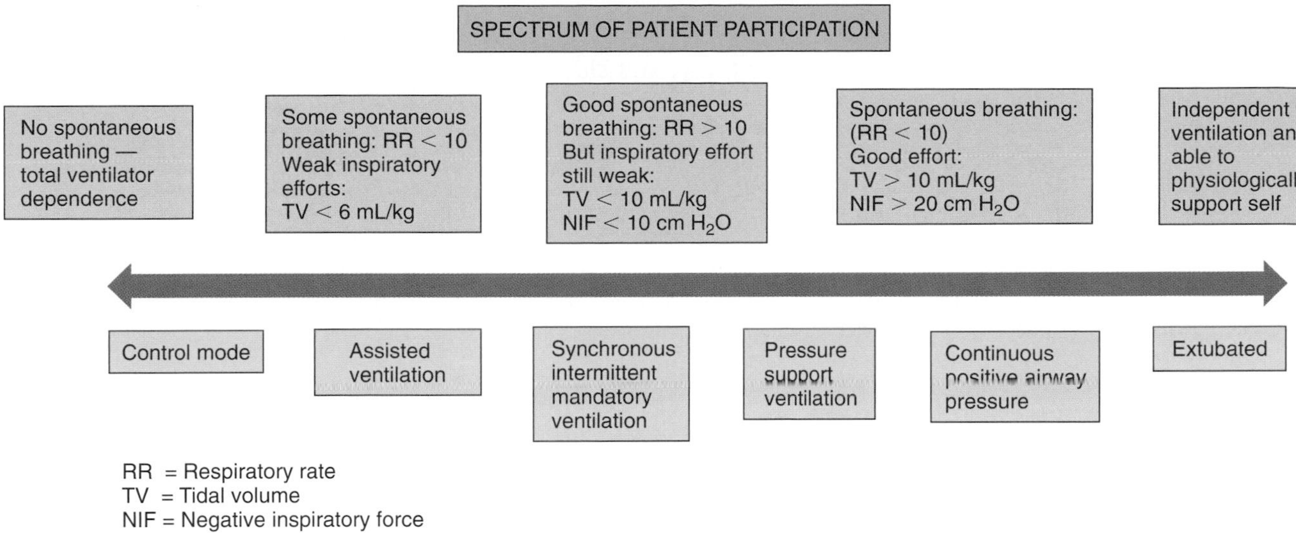

SPECTRUM OF PATIENT PARTICIPATION

FIG. 26-10 Overview of ventilator settings.

of typical ventilator settings. Moving from the right to the left of this figure illustrates the increasing need for ventilatory support and decreasing respiratory performance. Similarly, patients receiving more O_2 are likely to have poorer O_2 transport and a greater dependency on supplemental O_2. Supplemental O_2 can be provided with mechanical ventilation and is often described in terms of percentage of inspired O_2. Patients receiving a greater percentage of inspired O_2 have poorer O_2 transport and are in greater need of additional O_2.

Arterial Blood Gases, Oxygen Saturation, and Noninvasive Carbon Dioxide Measures. As discussed previously, ABG measures can be used to examine O_2 transport and respiratory performance.[11-13] Table 26-3 presents common blood gas abnormalities. When interpreting ABGs, one should first determine if the pH is greater (alkalosis) or less than 7 (acidosis).[40] With a primary respiratory acidosis because of hypoventilation, which often occurs with respiratory failure, the pH will be low and the $PaCO_2$ will be high.

Measures of O_2 saturation, as discussed in detail in Chapter 22, also provide information about respiratory performance and O_2 transport. O_2 saturation is the amount of O_2 saturating the hemoglobin molecule. Normal O_2 saturation is 95% or greater, mild hypoxemia is an O_2 saturation level between 90% and 95% and moderate and severe hypoxemia are O_2 saturation levels between 80% and 90% and less than 75% and 80%, respectively.[42-44] O_2 saturation may be measured intermittently as a component of the ABG and continuously or intermittently with a pulse oximeter worn on the finger, earlobe, or other body part (see Chapter 22)

CO_2 levels provide specific information about alveolar ventilation. CO_2 levels are obtained with the ABGs and may also be measured transcutaneously, although this is thought to be less accurate, particularly in infants or children.[44,45]

Auscultation of the Heart and Lungs. Auscultation of the heart and lungs should be performed in persons with respiratory failure. Chest auscultation and many other aspects of the chest examination are covered in detail in Chapter 24. Although the accuracy and reliability of this examination is only modest, it is a standard measurement technique used by almost all health care providers. Auscultation of the chest may detect the presence of certain cardiac or pulmonary disorders, the presence or absence of retained pulmonary secretions, and if secretion removal techniques are needed and successful.

Cardiovascular Tests and Measures. The heart rate and blood pressure of a person with respiratory failure should be examined while the patient is resting, in various body positions, and during exercise or functional activities (see Chapter 22). In patients receiving mechanical ventilation, one should be aware that intrathoracic pressure may be increased by the positive pressure ventilation, which may reduce venous return, causing a decrease in blood pressure. Therefore one should always examine for signs or symptoms of hypotension in persons receiving mechanical ventilation. Other common cardiovascular findings in persons with respiratory failure include faster resting and exercise heart rates, as well as more easily produced anginal symptoms because of more rapid heart rate with activity and poorer O_2 transport.

Chest Wall and Abdominal Motion. Chest wall and abdominal motion should be examined in patients with respiratory failure. This examination may be performed using observation, palpation, and measurement of chest expansion.

Observation. Observation of the breathing pattern should include comparison of the magnitude of upper chest movement (superior to the xiphoid process) and lower chest wall movement (abdominal area around the umbilicus) and determination of the synchrony of these motions.

Palpation. Movements of the upper and lower chest during inspiration and expiration should also be evaluated by palpation. The therapist should place one hand on the patient's lower chest (abdominal area) and one hand on the patient's upper chest (midsternal area) to evaluate for areas of hypermobility or hypomobility and timing and coordination of the breathing pattern. Posterior palpation over the bases of the lungs, between the scapulae, and on the shoulders (on the superior and posterior aspect of the trapezius) may also be used to examine and evaluate chest wall motion. Although palpation can give general information about the presence and severity of chest wall motion abnormalities, more reliable and precise methods for measuring chest wall excursion in patients with respiratory failure are available.

Measurement of Chest Expansion. A tape measure can be used to quantify chest wall excursion in different areas of the thorax. Measurement of chest wall excursion at the levels of the sternal angle (where the second rib meets the sternum), the xiphoid process, and a midpoint between the xiphoid process and the umbilicus can give information about upper, middle, and lower chest wall motion, respectively. The bucket-handle motion of the ribs most affects expansion at the level of the midpoint between the xiphoid process and the umbilicus, whereas the pump-handle motion of the ribs most affects expansion at the levels of the sternal angle and the xiphoid process.

To optimize reliability the anatomical landmark can be identified with a marker (especially the site midpoint between the xiphoid and the umbilicus) and the tape measure should be level and pulled taut but not so tight that it prevents inspiration at the site being measured. A spring-loaded metal phalange at the end of the tape measure can decrease measurement error. Once the tape is in place the subject is asked to exhale and then inhale normally (not maximally). The tape measure should move horizontally as the subject inhales and the distance from pre-inspiration to end of normal inspiration is measured.

The amount (distance) of chest wall motion during normal breathing (which can be referred to as tidal volume breathing) should be recorded in centimeters or inches. Chest wall motion during a maximal inspiration can also be measured in a similar manner.

Respiratory inductive plethysmography is considered by some to be the "gold standard" for evaluating chest wall excursion and the relationship between upper and lower chest wall excursion.[46] Inductive plethysmography is performed by placing two elastic straps around the thorax, one at the level of the nipples and the other at the level of the umbilicus. These straps have electrical wires sewn into them, allowing them to detect and measure changes in length and thus chest wall motion at the two sites. Inductive plethysmography has been found to be an accurate and reliable method for monitoring synchrony of breathing, as well as episodes of sleep apnea, and is therefore commonly used in the intensive care unit (ICU) and sleep laboratories.

Respiratory Muscle Strength and Endurance. Respiratory muscle weakness can affect the severity and prognosis of respiratory failure, contribute to abnormal breathing patterns and guide selection of interventions. A number of different techniques can be used to measure breathing muscle strength including manual muscle testing, measurements of maximal inspiratory pressure (MIP) and maximum expiratory pressure (MEP), and tests of breathing muscle strength via weighted breathing (weights added to the abdominal area of a supine patient).

Manual muscle testing of the respiratory muscles is difficult since it is virtually impossible to perform a manual muscle test of the diaphragm, and it is very difficult to quantify the combined strengths of the accessory muscles of breathing and their contribution to breathing. However, several of the methods used to examine diaphragmatic motion previously described can be adapted so that manual resistance applied during inspiration indirectly gauges inspiratory muscle strength. Attempting to resist the (1) pushing away of the fingertips from under the lower ribs bilaterally, (2) bucket-handle motion of the lower ribs bilaterally, or (3) outward movement of the abdomen during inspiration may all provide indirect manual measurements of diaphragmatic muscle strength. However, there is no published research evaluating the reliability, validity, sensitivity, or specificity of this method of examination despite the fact that such techniques are commonly employed.

Measurement of MIP and MEP has become more common in recent years, and several different devices using hand-held manometers or electronic pressure transducers are available for measuring MIP and MEP. Most of these devices provide accurate and reliable measures, although the electronic devices have been found to be better. Additionally, in mechanically ventilated patients, the ventilator can often produce a measure of MIP and MEP. All of these devices work similarly, measuring the amount of negative pressure developed during a maximal inspiration (i.e., MIP) and the amount of positive pressure developed during a maximal expiration (i.e., MEP). This pressure is generally expressed in units of centimeters of water (cm H_2O).

MIP and MEP are measured by asking the patient to inhale as quickly and forcefully as possible after a maximal expiration (near residual volume) and then exhale as quickly and forcefully as possible after a maximal inspiration (total lung capacity). If the patient is on a mechanical ventilator, a hand-held device can be attached to an endotracheal tube (ETT) or *tracheostomy* or the respiratory pressure measurement mode on the ventilator can be used if available. Ideally, the patient should be seated in a chair with the hips perpendicular to the back, but this may be difficult for patients receiving mechanical ventilation. Encouragement to breathe forcefully during the measurement of both MIP and MEP and ensuring a good seal at the mouth piece or ETT/tracheostomy site are important to optimize measurement accuracy and reliability.

Respiratory muscle endurance can be estimated by placement of progressively greater weights on the abdominal area of a patient with respiratory failure, through use of the mechanical ventilator or a variety of other methods. The most commonly used method is testing how long a person can sustain a breathing load of 70% to 85% of MVV. Inspiratory muscle endurance may also be measured by starting with a low load of 20% to 30% of MIP and progressively increasing the load every 2 minutes by 20% increments until the person can no longer sustain the load for 2 minutes.[47] Similar results may be obtained by starting breathing at a load of 90% MIP and gradually decreasing this load in 5% decrements until the load can be sustained for greater than 10 minutes. With this type of testing, end-tidal CO_2 and O_2 saturation levels, inspiratory muscle use, and level of dyspnea are often monitored, and testing is terminated if the CO_2 level becomes abnormal, if a paradoxical breathing pattern occurs, or if a patient reports severe dyspnea (Borg modified rating of perceived exertion [RPE] $\geq 7/10$). Measurement of ventilatory muscle endurance using this method has been found to be safe, reproducible, and representative of other measurements often accepted as a measure of ventilatory muscle endurance, but very little literature has examined such tests in persons receiving mechanical ventilation.

Function. The primary functional tests and measures for the person with respiratory failure include measurements of bed mobility, transfer ability, sitting ability, standing ability, walking ability, and activities of daily living (ADLs). A variety of methods to examine each of these areas exist and although patients with respiratory failure are frequently intubated or receiving noninvasive positive pressure ventilation (NIPPV), the same tests and measures used for other patients receiving physical therapy are applicable. It is important to frequently reassess each of these tests and measures so that a patient's rehabilitation program can be progressed optimally.

EVALUATION, DIAGNOSIS, AND PROGNOSIS

The information obtained during the examination provides an indication of the patient's baseline functional status and can be used to monitor outcomes and direct patient evaluation, diagnosis, prognosis, and interventions. The initial physical therapy goals are generally directed toward preventing secondary complications of bed rest, whereas the ultimate goals of physical therapy for patients requiring prolonged mechanical ventilation are to minimize loss of mobility, maximize independence, and facilitate weaning.

The outcomes for patients with respiratory failure who receive rehabilitation management and mechanical ventilation are listed in Box 26-2. They include both favorable and unfavorable outcomes.[48-61] Performing serial examinations and evaluations and monitoring patients should improve prognosis.[49-61] Of utmost importance is the greater likelihood of favorable outcomes when exercise training is performed.[49-71] Since intubation for mechanical ventilation can cause complications that increase the WOB, such patients should be reevaluated after extubation.[72,73]

INTERVENTION

MEDICAL MANAGEMENT OF RESPIRATORY FAILURE

Medical interventions for patients with respiratory failure either treat the disease causing the failure or provide support to maintain ventilation and respiration when the cause cannot be eliminated. Interventions aimed at treating diseases that cause respiratory failure are described in depth in a range of medical texts and are not discussed further here. Supportive measures, mechanical ventilation, and supplemental O_2 are discussed in the following section.

Supplemental Oxygen. Supplemental O_2 is indicated when the patient can sustain sufficient WOB to maintain ventilation independently but cannot maintain adequate levels of oxygenation. Supplemental O_2 can be delivered by a wide range of devices varying in complexity and the amount of O_2 they can deliver.

Oxygen Delivery Sources. All O_2 delivery systems consist of a supply source and a delivery device. O_2 may be supplied from a portable reservoir in the form of an O_2 gas tank or a liquid O_2 system. In hospitals, patients may receive O_2 from a fixed main hospital supply through a wall hook-up. To avoid confusion with other medical gases, all O_2 tanks and ports are colored green.

The amount of time a portable O_2 gas tank will last depends on its size, how full it is (measured as the

---

BOX 26-2	**Possible Outcomes for Patients Receiving Mechanical Ventilation**
Adverse Outcomes	**Favorable Outcomes***
1. Infection	1. Improved survival by resolving respiratory failure
2. Deconditioning and muscle weakness	2. Improved pulmonary, cardiovascular, and multisystem function
3. Altered cardiovascular and pulmonary function	3. Rapid wean from mechanical ventilation
4. Greater dependency on anaerobic metabolism	4. Ability to exercise and increase functional activities
5. Poor nutritional status	5. Improved psychological function
6. Hypertension/hypotension	6. Exercise training adaptations
7. Anxiety/psychosis	a. Improved skeletal and cardiac muscle function
8. Depression	b. Lower resting heart rate and blood pressure
9. Osteoporosis	c. Lower rate pressure product
10. Psychological dysfunction	d. Increased peak O_2 consumption
11. Physiological dysfunction after endotracheal intubation or tracheostomy	e. Increased lean muscle mass
12. Ventilator dependency	f. Decreased body weight and body fat
	g. Greater heart rate responsiveness during exercise
	h. Improved lipid and blood sugar profiles
	i. Decreased rate of bone mineral loss

*Many of the favorable outcomes can only be achieved with exercise training.

pressure of the gas in pounds per square inch [psi]), and the flow rate. O_2 tank sizes are letter coded. The most common tanks are small E-cylinders, with a volume of approximately 700 L, and large H-cylinders, with a volume of approximately 7,000 L. Standard O_2 tanks are filled to a pressure of 2,200 psi of gaseous O_2 when full.[29] The amount of time a tank will last can be calculated using the following equation:[28]

$$T = [P \times k]/\text{flow rate}$$

where:
T = time left in minutes
P = pressure in psi
k = 0.28 for an E-cylinder and 3.14 for an H-cylinder
flow rate = L/min

With liquid systems, the amount of O_2 available is measured by weight rather than pressure. This weight can be converted to a volume of gas; 1 L of liquid O_2 weighs 2.5 lb and makes 860 L of O_2 gas. The amount of time a liquid system will last can be calculated by the following steps:[28]
1. Determine the weight of liquid O_2 left in the system:

Weight (lb) of liquid O_2 = current weight of container (lb) – weight of empty container (lb)

2. Calculate the volume of gas in the given weight:

$$\text{Gas volume remaining (L)} = \frac{\text{weight (lb) of } O_2 \text{ liquid} \times 860}{2.5 \text{ (lb/L)}}$$

3. Calculate the time left:

$$\text{Time left (min)} = \frac{\text{gas volume remaining (L)}}{\text{flow rate (L/min)}}$$

Oxygen Delivery Devices. O_2 is usually delivered from the supply to the patient by a nasal canula or a face mask. The nasal canula is used most often. The amount of O_2 delivered to a patient by this device is affected by the concentration and rate of delivery as well as the patient's respiratory rate, depth, and pattern of breathing. This device can deliver between 24 and 44% O_2 at a flow rate of 1/16 to 6 L/min. It consists of nasal prongs that sit in the patient's nasal passageway on one end and a connector that attaches to the O_2 source on the other end. It is recommended that at flow rates of more than 3 L/min a humidifier be used with this device to minimize drying of the nasal mucosa.

If adequate O_2 saturation cannot be maintained by the nasal canula or if flow rates greater than 6 L/min are required, a face mask should be considered. Face masks vary in complexity and in the concentration of O_2 they can deliver for a given flow rate. The most commonly used masks are the simple mask, the venturi mask, the rebreather mask, and the nonrebreather mask. These masks and their estimated O_2 concentration delivery and corresponding flow rates are listed in Table 26-4.

Oxygen Dosage. Dosage or the amount of O_2 delivered can be expressed in terms of flow rate, generally in L/min, or in terms of concentration. O_2 concentration is expressed as the percentage of O_2 inspired (FiO$_2$). FiO$_2$ may range from 21% (the concentration of O_2 in room air) to 100% depending on the device. When O_2 is delivered by nasal canula the dosage is given in L/min, whereas when

TABLE 26-4	Oxygen Provided by Common Delivery Devices	
Device	Flow (L/min)	FiO$_2$ (%)
Nasal canula	1-6	24-44
Simple face mask	5-10	35-55
Venturi mask	Set, depending on FiO$_2$ desired	24-55
Rebreather mask	Set, depending on FiO$_2$ desired	60-90
Nonrebreather mask	6-10	60-100

a face mask is used, the dose may be given in either form. When using a nasal canula, the estimated FiO$_2$ can be calculated using the following equation:

$$\text{FiO}_2 = (\text{Flow rate in L/min} \times 4) + 20$$

This can be used to maintain a comparable dosage when switching from a nasal canula to a face mask or other delivery device.

Oxygen Is a Medication. O_2 is classified by the Food and Drug Administration (FDA) as a medication. Therefore only a physician may prescribe the O_2 dosage and how it should be delivered, except in an emergency. In nonemergency situations, rehabilitation professionals should modify O_2 demand by altering patient activity or exercise intensity or adjust the O_2 supply if the physician orders titration of delivery to demand or within a given range. For example, a physician may request that O_2 be titrated up to 6 L/min via nasal canula to keep O_2 saturation above 90%.

Mechanical Ventilation. Patients with respiratory insufficiency or failure who cannot sustain the necessary WOB independently can have their breathing supported by mechanical ventilation. Indications for mechanical ventilation include acute respiratory failure, impending respiratory failure, need for protection of the airway, secretion management, upper airway obstruction, and to allow for paralysis or sedation.[38] Mechanical ventilators are used most often in the intensive care or critical care setting. However, patients who are expected to need support from a mechanical ventilator for a prolonged period may be seen in a variety of settings, including inpatient rehabilitation facilities and at home.

A mechanical ventilator substitutes for or assists the patient's ventilatory pump to allow breathing to occur. Supplemental O_2 is usually administered in conjunction with the mechanical assistance to maintain oxygenation. Ventilator design has progressed over time to better mimic normal physiological ventilation, with one major exception, mechanical ventilators support ventilation by applying positive pressure to the airways, "pushing" air with varying O_2 concentrations into the lungs, whereas normal physiological breathing is driven by negative pressure that essentially "pulls" air into the airways. This difference can cause complications.

When examining a patient who is using a ventilator, the rehabilitation professional should note the route of intubation, mode of ventilation, rate setting, tidal volume (TV), amount of positive end-expiratory pressure (PEEP), pressure support (PS), and the FiO$_2$. This information may be gathered directly from the ventilator and indicates the amount of support being provided by the ventilator.

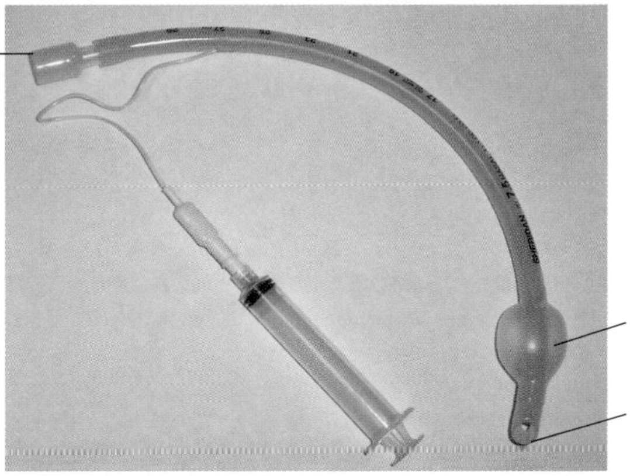

Proximal
end of ETT,
connects to
ventilation
system

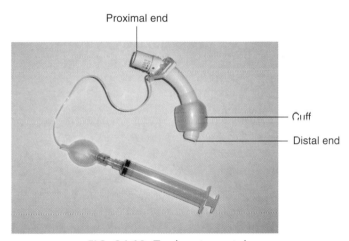

Cuff

Distal end
of ETT
(sits at the
carina)

FIG. 26-11 Endotracheal tube (ETT).

Proximal end

Cuff

Distal end

FIG. 26-12 Tracheostomy tube.

Route of Intubation. The route of intubation is the way the patient is connected to the ventilator. There are four basic routes of intubation: Via a nasopharyngeal airway, an oropharyngeal airway, an ETT, or a tracheostomy. The first two are generally seen in emergent situations and occasionally in the ICU for short-term airway management but are generally not seen in the rehabilitation field. The latter two airways are more commonly seen in patients requiring prolonged mechanical ventilation.

In general, ET intubation, with an ETT (Fig. 26-11) is used for short-term intubation. A standard ETT is a long, flexible tube that is inserted through the mouth into the trachea. The distal end of the tube sits just above the level of the carina, just before the trachea bifurcates into the left and right mainstem bronchi. The cuff, which is at the distal end of the ETT, is inflated to hold the tube in place and maintain a seal to ensure that the breath enters the lungs and does not escape out through the upper airways. The proximal end exits the patient's mouth and is connected to the ventilator through a series of tubing. This tubing and all its connections are termed the ventilator circuit. ETTs come in various sizes based on the patient's size and age.

When an ETT is present, the rehabilitation professional must ensure that it does not dislodge or advance within the airways during activities because this may disconnect the patient from the ventilator or render the ventilator nonfunctional. The tube has numbered markings on the outside to indicate its placement. The clinician should note which marking lines up with the patient's teeth or other fixed landmark before starting treatment, during treatment, and at the end of treatment. If the therapist suspects that the ETT has moved, they should immediately alert the physician, nurse, or respiratory therapist to ensure appropriate tube placement.

Tracheostomy is indicated when long-term use of the ventilator is expected and consists of surgical placement of a tube in the trachea through an opening made at the level of the jugular notch, below the glottis and vocal cords. Tracheostomy tubes come in various sizes and types (Fig. 26-12). The tube prevents the patient from speaking or performing a functional cough unless it is fenestrated with an opening that allows air to flow out the upper airways and over the vocal cords. The distal end of the tube may or may not have a cuff as in the ETT, and the proximal end is attached to the ventilator circuit.

Some patients may be able to speak when off the mechanical ventilator by occluding the tracheostomy with a finger or a speaking valve. The rehabilitation professional should consult with the physician and the speech therapist to determine who may tolerate this. However, whenever occluding the tracheostomy to facilitate speech, the cuff *must be deflated*.

Modes of Ventilation. The mode of ventilation determines whether the ventilator or the patient initiates breathing and which performs most of the work of breathing (see Fig. 26-10). Current ventilators allow for selection of various modes of mechanical ventilation.

Controlled Ventilation, Assisted Ventilation, and Assist Control. With controlled ventilation (CV) the mechanical ventilator controls all aspects of ventilation, including FiO_2, respiratory rate, and volume and pressure of each delivered breath, and the patient does not need to actively breathe at all. The patient may be completely paralyzed or sedated as the ventilator is doing all the WOB. With assisted ventilation (AV) the patient controls the rate and rhythm of breathing. When the ventilator senses negative pressure as the patient initiates a breath it delivers a breath at a preset volume, pressure, or flow rate. With AV the respiratory muscles are active and initiate the breath, but the ventilator is doing most of the work. If the patient does not initiate the breath, the ventilator will not be triggered. With the assist control (AC) mode, which combines CV and AV, the ventilator delivers the breath along with the patient's inspiratory effort at a preset volume and/or pressure as in the AV mode, thereby allowing the patient to control the rate and rhythm if able. However, if the patient does not initiate a breath within a predetermined period, the ventilator will still deliver the breath. This allows the patient to initiate breaths but provides the safety of delivering a breath if the patient fails to initiate breathing. With all of these modes, most if not all of the WOB is performed by the ventilator.

Synchronized Intermittent Mandatory Ventilation. Synchronized intermittent mandatory ventilation (SIMV) mode delivers a breath at a set volume and pressure and at a rate that coordinates with the patient's respiratory cycle. Although this mode has a set rate, it will not deliver a breath if the patient is exhaling and it will only deliver "mandatory" breaths if the patient-initiated breaths do not meet the minimum ventilator settings. In SIMV mode, the patient and the ventilator contribute to the WOB to varying degrees, depending on the set rate, pressure, and volume. The higher the minimum settings (i.e., rate, pressure support, TVs) on the ventilator the less likely the patient will achieve them and thus the ventilator will perform more work. Similarly, the lower the minimum settings the more WOB will be performed by the patient.

Continuous Positive Airway Pressure. With continuous positive airway pressure (CPAP) mode the patient controls the respiratory rate, rhythm, and volume, and the ventilator maintains positive pressure throughout inspiration and expiration to decrease the overall WOB. The amount of assistance given by the ventilator is directly related to the pressure setting on the ventilator. CPAP mode is frequently used when weaning a patient from a ventilator, as it allows the patient to breathe independently but provides enough assistance to overcome the resistance of breathing through a long narrow tube.

Other Ventilator Settings. In addition to the modes, various settings can be manipulated on a ventilator to optimize the assistance given and mimic normal ventilation and respiration. Additional settings include the rate and TV, PS, PEEP, and the FiO_2.

Rate and TV can be set in various combinations to maximize ventilation based on the patient's physiological needs much the same way the normal individual manipulates rate and TV to maintain adequate MV. The rate and TV are based on the patient's needs and how much work they can contribute to the breathing process.

PS represents the amount of positive pressure "pushing" the breath into the airways. The amount of PS depends on the needs and physiological constraints of the patient. In general, pressure is set as low as possible to avoid damaging the lungs. Damage from excessive pressure is known as barotrauma.

PEEP is the pressure in the airways at the end of expiration and is approximately 5 cm H_2O under normal physiological conditions. This pressure is needed to maintain functional residual capacity (FRC) and prevent airway collapse. It is usually set at 5 cm H_2O on a ventilator, although it may be set higher in some circumstances to aid in ventilation and oxygenation.

The amount of O_2 in the inspired air can be manipulated by setting the FiO_2 between 21%, which represents room air, and 100%, or pure O_2.

Complications of Mechanical Ventilation. Most of the complications associated with mechanical ventilation occur during intubation or as a result of the positive pressure ventilation. During insertion of an ETT, there may be tracheolaryngeal injury. This may only become apparent after extubation when the patient has a hoarse voice, cough, persistent sputum production, or *hemoptysis*. A small percentage of the population (2%) have a tracheoinnominate artery that may rupture with trauma from an artificial airway and cause life-threatening bleeding.[74]

The positive pressure can cause barotrauma because of overdistention of the alveoli. This will cause fluid to infiltrate the airways and lung tissue. The incidence of barotrauma ranges from 4% to 48%, with the highest incidence occurring in ARDS, where high positive pressures are needed to maintain oxygenation.[75] Barotrauma can cause long-term fibrosis of the lungs that permanently limits ventilatory capacity.

Positive pressure can also cause a *pneumothorax* as a result of alveolar rupture. When an alveolus ruptures, air may escape from the lungs and become trapped in the pleural space. This trapped air will restrict lung expansion and in severe cases can cause the lung to collapse.

With prolonged use, the cuff at the distal end of an ETT or tracheotomy tube can cause tracheal necrosis. The presence of the artificial airway also increases the risk for pneumonia and promotes secretion production, which can worsen respiratory failure.[76]

Complications of mechanical ventilation are not confined to the pulmonary system. Cardiovascular complications of mechanical ventilation include pulmonary hypertension, decreased cardiac output, hypotension, and cardiac dysrhythmias. Pressure ulcers are also common in ventilated patients because of immobility, loss of muscle mass, decreases in range of motion, difficulty maintaining hygiene, and malnutrition.

One of the greatest challenges of prolonged mechanical ventilation may be the overall effect on the ventilatory muscles themselves. The mechanical ventilator is often used to assist the muscles of ventilation. However, assisting these muscles promotes disuse atrophy and when the artificial ventilation is removed, the respiratory muscles may not have the strength and endurance to sustain ventilation. In this circumstance, mechanical ventilation may need to be "weaned" gradually over time to allow the muscles to regain strength.[75,77,78]

Weaning from Mechanical Ventilation. Weaning from mechanical ventilation is the process of gradually decreasing ventilatory support until the individual can sustain spontaneous breathing. Weaning may be needed to allow the strength and endurance of the respiratory muscles to improve or to allow the underlying cause of the respiratory failure to resolve. When weaning, the energy demand of breathing at rest may compromise the ability to exercise. Under normal circumstances, only about 5% of the maximum energy available at rest is used to breathe, and the remaining 95% is potentially available to perform exercise or ADLs. When weaning from mechanical ventilation, more energy will be needed for breathing, leaving less of a reserve for other activities. If pushed too hard, the patient may fail the weaning process. However, if not pushed at all, the patient will probably get weaker. The rehabilitation professional must carefully select and monitor the level of activity for the optimal outcome.

The process of weaning from mechanical ventilation varies among patients, physicians, and facilities. Many hospitals have "weaning protocols" or pathways to help guide this process. There are also evidence-based guidelines for weaning in the literature.[78] Weaning is generally initiated when the patient shows signs of being able to breathe adequately without support by meeting "weaning criteria." Examples of weaning criteria are: O_2 saturation maintained at greater than 92%, FiO_2 requirements less than 40% to 50%, respiratory rate less than 35, respiratory rate to TV ratio less than 100 breaths/min/L, and no signs of distress.[38] When these criteria are met, trials of breathing without support are attempted. If the patient is intubated for a prolonged period, these trials may be gradually increased in duration until the patient can breathe independently for 24 hours, at which time they are extubated. If the patient cannot be extubated after 3 months of weaning trials, the patient is generally considered ventilator dependent.

Noninvasive Mechanical Ventilation. Noninvasive mechanical ventilation is any form of assisted ventilation where an ETT is not used. This type of assisted ventilation is usually provided via a face mask. Evidence suggests that the use of noninvasive mechanical ventilation in patients in the ICU may reduce the need for intubation or reintubation and that outpatients with COPD who receive noninvasive mechanical ventilation are able to exercise more than similar patients who do not receive this intervention.[62-69] A meta-analysis on the acute effects of noninvasive mechanical ventilation in patients with COPD (in which 15 studies were found and 7 met inclusion criteria) found that this intervention significantly reduced dyspnea during exercise and increased exercise duration.[65] The authors hypothesized that these acute effects would facilitate training adaptation in persons with COPD over time.[65] A study on the long-term effects of noninvasive mechanical ventilation in 14 patients with COPD, 7 of whom used noninvasive mechanical ventilation during exercise (experimental group) and 7 of whom exercised with supplemental O_2, found that the experimental group had a significantly greater increase in peak VO_2 with a significantly lower ventilatory requirement.[66] Another study of 39 patients with severe COPD found that noninvasive mechanical ventilation improved exercise duration and peak workload.[68]

REHABILITATION INTERVENTIONS

New technologies in the areas of mechanical ventilation and critical care medicine have allowed many critically ill patients to survive and have led to a dramatic increase in the number of patients who are ventilator-dependent. Patients who require mechanical ventilation have limited mobility because of multiple medical problems, equipment, and weakness. The prolonged bed rest associated with a stay in the ICU can also lead to a significant loss of functional abilities. Patients requiring prolonged mechanical ventilation experience high morbidity, high costs of care, and poor functional outcomes. Rehabilita-tion programs for patients with respiratory failure are generally initiated in the ICU and focus on early mobilization and ambulation. Before returning home, these patients will continue to benefit from a rehabilitation program and often spend extended periods of time in acute care or rehabilitation units.

Positioning and Adjunctive Techniques for Clearance of Secretions. The use of different body positions to achieve optimal outcomes has been considered one of several critical adjunctive interventions for patients in respiratory failure receiving mechanical ventilation. The primary goals of proper positioning include the reduction of pulmonary complications and skin breakdown and promotion of optimal cardiovascular and pulmonary function. Different body positions achieve these outcomes by improving lung volumes, $\dot{V}:\dot{Q}$ matching, work of breathing, cardiovascular function (heart rate and blood pressure), redistribution of edema, and mucociliary transport and clearance.[48-51,53] A number of positions are typically used to achieve these key outcomes (Table 26-5).

The prone position has been found to most significantly improve $\dot{V}:\dot{Q}$ matching and FRC as well as redistribute edema in patients with ARDS receiving mechanical ventilation.[48-51,53] The upright body position, which replicates normal cardiovascular and pulmonary function during most functional activities, has also be found to significantly improve lung volumes and decrease the work of breathing in patients receiving mechanical ventilation.[48-51,53] However, not all patients receiving mechanical ventilation are able to attain a prone or upright position and therefore other positions are often

TABLE 26-5	**Positions Used for Optimal Outcomes with Mechanical Ventilation***
Position	**Potential Outcome**
Supine	Important position in SCI because of gravity effects
Quarter-supine	Facilitates a change in CVSC and PUL function
Sidelying	Facilitates a greater change in CVSC and PUL function
Quarter-prone	Facilitates a change in CVSC and PUL function
Prone	Facilitates a greater change in CVSC and PUL function
Trendelenburg	Extreme change in CVSC and PUL function
Reverse Trendelenburg	Extreme change in CVSC and PUL function
Semi-Fowler's position	Achieving more normal CVSC and PUL function
Fowler's position	Achieving more normal, functional CVSC and PUL function
Continuous rotation	Facilitates continuous change in CVSC and PUL function
Upright	Desired position for optimal CVSC and PUL function

*Moving patients in and out of these positions will help achieve outcomes as well as maintain optimal integumentary status.
SCI, Spinal cord injury; *CVSC,* cardiovascular; *PUL,* pulmonary.

TABLE 26-6	Traditional Secretion Clearance Techniques
Technique	**Method**
Deep breathing	Patient instructed to breathe deeply or is provided with increased TV breaths via mechanical ventilation or Ambu bag.
Percussion	Cupped hands gently percuss the chest in areas of retained secretions with a resulting "pop" being heard during percussion to unstick, loosen, and mobilize retained secretions in a manner similar to ketchup being mobilized to move forward by percussing the bottom of a ketchup bottle. Percussion is done continuously during inspiration and expiration for 3-5 minutes.
Vibrations	Vibration of the thorax over areas of retained secretions during exhalation.
Shaking	Moderately vigorous shaking of the thorax over areas of retained secretions during exhalation.
Coughing*	A variety of methods can be used to stimulate or facilitate a cough to mobilize retained secretions.
Huffing	Mobilization of retained secretions without closure of the glottis. Patient instructed to inhale maximally followed by a controlled expulsion of air making the sound of a "huff" during the exhalation.
Suctioning	Sterile techniques are employed as a catheter is introduced into the ETT or tracheostomy after which gentle pressure on the carina will facilitate a cough and secretions can be suctioned. Hyperoxygenation is often performed before and after suctioning.

*A cough is differentiated from a huff by an expulsion of air with a closed glottis. Other methods to stimulate or facilitate a cough include (1) increasing the tidal volume and inspiratory capacity, (2) gentle tactile stimulation to the trachea ("tracheal tickle"), abdominals, or other expiratory muscles during exhalation, or (3) assistive cough techniques (e.g., Heimlich maneuver) in persons unable to cough independently because of neuromuscular disorders.
TV, Tidal volume; *ETT*, endotracheal tube.

used. Alternating right and left sidelying is commonly used to improve $\dot{V} : \dot{Q}$ matching and clearance of airway secretions in the uppermost lung. Positioning together with specific postural drainage positions may also improve cardiovascular and pulmonary function.[48-51,53]

Patients with respiratory failure receiving mechanical ventilation who also have neurological and/or musculoskeletal disorders may benefit from a positioning program to prevent the development of contractures and pressure ulcers (especially in the sacral and heel areas). An optimal positioning program should include training of patients, nurses, and family members in utilization of positions that are most effective for individual patients. Information sheets describing positions with schematics of body positions to be used may facilitate optimal outcomes for persons receiving mechanical ventilation in the hospital, home, or rehabilitation unit.[49,53]

Traditional secretion clearance techniques, as described in detail in Chapter 24, can also be used in patients with retained secretions who cannot mobilize them through the use of different body positions or active movement alone. Table 26-6 describes several of the traditional secretion clearance techniques. Perhaps the most important of these techniques is deep breathing exercises followed by coughing or huffing. Facilitating coughs through education in coughing, assisted cough techniques, or huffing may improve mucociliary transport and subsequently improve O_2 transport.[52,54,55]

Breathing in mechanically ventilated patients may also be improved through the use of breathing assist techniques (BATs). This approach uses gentle manual thoracic mobilization in specific positions (Table 26-7). There is limited research on the effectiveness of BATs. BATs were designed to improve ventilation via neuroreflexive mechanisms based on neural communication between respiratory muscle spindle and proprioceptive activity and the command centers for breathing.[56]

Functional and Exercise Training. There is limited research on the effects of functional and exercise training in people with respiratory failure receiving mechanical ventilation.[48-51,53] Therefore most of the support for this type of intervention is based on expert opinion and inferred from changes known to accompany exercise in healthy and diseased individuals (Box 26-3).

A recent comprehensive overview on the effects of exercise and mobilization on acutely ill patients (including patients receiving mechanical ventilation) presented specific guidelines regarding safety and progression of exercise for patients in the ICU.[61] The primary examination areas for patients in the ICU included the medical background, cardiovascular considerations, and respiratory considerations for each patient. Further examination and management techniques were addressed under each of these three primary areas.[61] The examination and management techniques addressed under respiratory considerations and most relevant to patients receiving mechanical ventilation included oxygenation, hypercapnia, breathing pattern, and characteristics of mechanical ventilation. Patients receiving mechanical ventilation were considered appropriate for mobilization when (1) oxygenation, hypercapnia, and the breathing pattern were relatively normal or within acceptable limits, (2) they were able to tolerate more supportive ventilatory modes (pressure control ventilation or SIMV with high mandatory rates) during exercise, (3) they were alert and able to follow commands, and (4) the level of weaning from mechanical ventilation was such that mobilization did not induce excessive demand on the respiratory or cardiovascular systems.[61]

The acceptable limits of oxygenation, hypercapnia, and breathing pattern may be patient specific and should be considered a relative indication/contraindication for exercise training. Despite the important role and need of more supportive ventilatory modes during exercise, patients requiring high levels of ventilatory support at rest are often quite ill (with more and worse co-morbidities) and likely to have significantly limited respiratory reserve. Therefore mobility training should be postponed or minimized until lower levels of ventilatory support at rest are required (Box 26-4).[61]

Only one study has examined the effects of exercise training in patients with respiratory failure receiving

TABLE 26-7	Breathing Assist Techniques (BATs)	
Components	**Purpose**	**Method**
Facilitation of exhalation by assisting the motion of the rib cage	1. Assist exhalation by improving expiratory flow and volume. 2. Decrease dynamic hyperinflation. 3. Increase thoracic mobility.	Hands are placed on the thorax,* providing a gentle diagonal compressive pressure (force = weight of the hands) mimicking the downward and inward motion of the ribcage (opposite the upward and outward "bucket-handle" motion of inspiration) throughout exhalation. Should be done slowly.
Facilitation of inspiration by utilizing the elasticity of the costal cartilage	1. Assist inspiration by decreasing intrathoracic pressure. 2. Improve inspiratory and expiratory flows and volumes. 3. Increase ventilation to the entire lung (distal to proximal) either bilaterally or unilaterally. 4. Decrease dynamic hyperinflation. 5. Loosen secretions. 6. Stimulate a cough.	Hands are placed on the thorax,* providing gentle but firm diagonal compressive pressure at end expiration or early inspiration, after which the hands are quickly removed. Rapid removal of hands from the thorax after a gentle but firm compressive pressure at end of thoracic ROM is to utilize the elastic recoil of the chest wall and promote bucket-handle motion and other wanted thoracic movements during inspiration. Rapid removal of hands is analogous to pulling the hands away after touching a hot surface like a stove and is critical in facilitating successful inspiration.
Elevation of the rib cage via quick stretch to the costal muscles	1. Assist inspiration by decreasing intrathoracic pressure. 2. Increase inspiratory flow and volume. 3. Increase ventilation to the distal lung region.	Hands are placed on the thorax* (often in an area of decreased chest wall excursion or decreased breath sounds†) and provide gentle diagonal pulsatile pressure up the ribs during inspiration.
Assisting the motion of the rib cage	1. Assist inspiration by decreasing intrathoracic pressure. 2. Increase inspiratory flow and volume. 3. Increase thoracic mobility.	Hands are placed on the thorax* with the fingertips positioned in one or more intercostals spaces with which the ribs are gently and slowly pulled outward during inspiration.
Extension of the trunk to elevate the rib cage	1. Assist inspiration by decreasing intrathoracic pressure. 2. Increase inspiratory flow and volume. 3. Increase ventilation to the underlying lung region.	With the patient in supine, the hands (or a towel) are placed in the thoracic or lumbar region and gently pulled upward, extending the trunk during inspiration, which should be combined with a gentle pulsatile lift throughout inspiration.
Shaking and kneading	1. Assist inspiration or exhalation by altering the intrathoracic pressure. 2. Improve inspiratory and expiratory flows and volumes. 3. Increase ventilation to the underlying lung region. 4. Decrease dynamic hyperinflation. 5. Loosen secretions. 6. Stimulate a cough. 7. Patient relaxation.	The hands are placed on the thorax* (often in an area of decreased chest wall excursion or decreased breath sounds†) and provide (1) a gentle superficial stroking on a horizontal plane of the thorax during inspiration (using part of or the whole hand) mimicking a shake and (2) massaging the thorax in a circular motion mimicking the kneading of bread.
Other techniques such as cough assist or diaphragmatic stretch	1. Assist cough. 2. Elicit a stronger diaphragmatic contraction to produce many of the effects listed above.	To assist coughing, hands are placed on the thorax* (often in an area of decreased chest wall excursion or decreased breath sounds†) and provide support or gentle compressive pressure to assist coughing. To stretch the diaphragm, gentle compression applied to the abdominal area at the end of exhalation (providing an inward and upward pressure) may elicit an improved diaphragmatic contraction.

*The location of the hands on the thorax depends on the individual and observed patient needs.
†BATs are provided, based on auscultation, palpation, and visual observation examination results. Abnormal breath sounds and palpated or visualized abnormalities in the biomechanics of breathing are absolute indications for the provision of BATs—often directly to the area of the abnormality.
From Bethune D: *Physiother Canada* 27(5):241-245, 1975.
ROM, Range of motion.

mechanical ventilation.[70] This study involved 80 patients with COPD and acute respiratory failure, 61 receiving invasive mechanical ventilation and 19 receiving noninvasive mechanical ventilation. The patients were randomized to stepwise pulmonary rehabilitation (n = 60), which included passive mobilization, respiratory and lower extremity muscle training, and for some patients, treadmill ambulation, or to standard medical therapy (n = 20). Only the stepwise pulmonary rehabilitation group had significantly increased MIP and performance on the 6-minute walk test, although both groups had comparable and significant improvements in symptoms.[70]

Overall, the evidence indicates that exercise may accelerate weaning, decrease hospital length of stay, and improve the sense of well-being in patients with respiratory failure receiving mechanical ventilation.

BOX 26-3	Functional and Exercise Training Methods and Results

Methods	Anticipated Results*
Passive ROM/stretching	Maintain/improve joint ROM
Active-assisted ROM	Maintain/improve joint ROM/strength
Active ROM†	Maintain/improve joint ROM/strength
Resistive exercise	Maintain/improve muscle strength/endurance
Bed mobility training‡	Improve physiological and functional activity
Transfer training	Improve physiological and functional activity
Sitting	Improve physiological and functional activity
Self-care	Improve functional activity
Standing	Improve physiological and functional activity
Balance and coordination	Improve trunk stability and functional activity
Walking	Maintain/improve physiological function

ROM, Range of motion.

*All functional and exercise training has the potential to decrease the risk of thromboembolism. Sitting exercises are performed before standing exercises so that patients can better accommodate to orthostasis and be less likely to experience orthostatic hypotension. Active ROM exercise in sitting or standing may improve or possibly even prevent orthostatic hypotension.

†Active ROM accompanied by electrical stimulation (35-Hz pulse width 350 μsec for 25 minutes, 2 × day, 5 days/week for 4 weeks) in COPD patients with peripheral muscle hypotonia and atrophy receiving mechanical ventilation produced significant improvements in peripheral muscle strength and decreased number of days needed to transfer from bed to chair.[11]

‡Bed mobility and transfers can be performed safely under most circumstances in the ICU but require that the following measures: (1) all mechanical ventilation tubing and intravenous lines recognized and positioned so that they do not hinder mobility and do not become disconnected, (2) use of appropriate mobility and transfer equipment (e.g., pillows, sheets, sliding board, walkers, reclining chairs), and (3) ICU staff assistance during mobilization and transfer efforts.

BOX 26-4	Criteria for Postponing Functional and Exercise Training

1. Hypotension associated with fainting, dizziness, and/or diaphoresis
2. Severe intolerable dyspnea
3. Saturation less than 90% on supplemental O_2
4. Significant chest pain or discomfort
5. Extreme fatigue
6. Patient wishes to stop

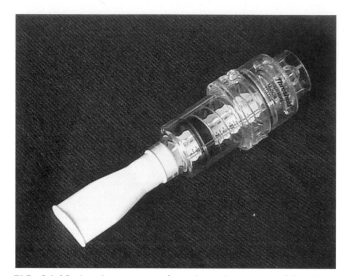

FIG. 26-13 Inspiratory muscle trainer. *From Frownfelter D, Dean E: Cardiovascular and Pulmonary Physical Therapy: Evidence and Practice, ed 4, St. Louis, 2006, Mosby.*

Inspiratory Muscle Training. Inspiratory muscle training (IMT) is a type of exercise that involves using a device that provides resistance to inspiration[79-87] (Fig. 26-13). If not using mechanical ventilation, the patient places their mouth around a mouth piece and then breathes in and out of the device. If using mechanical ventilation, the IMT device can be used via the ventilator tubing.[86] This type of training is intended to increase inspiratory muscle strength and endurance by applying the same principles as those governing exercise intended to improve performance of other muscles (see Chapter 5). Increasing inspiratory muscle strength and endurance may then increase function in patients with respiratory failure and assist in weaning from mechanical ventilation.[84,85]

A number of studies have evaluated the effectiveness of IMT (Table 26-8).[79-87] Overall, these studies demonstrate that IMT can improve pulmonary function, increase MIP, and decrease wean time from mechanical ventilation.[79-87] However, there is one report of severe but nonfatal bradycardia with syncope occurring in one patient after IMT and another report of hypoxia occurring during IMT.[82,83] Therefore, although IMT appears to be a beneficial adjunct for patients receiving mechanical ventilation, heart rate and O_2 saturation should be monitored during treatment sessions. Since the studies on IMT all used different treatment protocols and generally different devices, the ideal protocol or device for IMT is not known. In some studies, IMT was used alone, whereas in others it was combined with other interventions, including other types of exercise, positioning and bronchodilator medications. In addition, the rate of IMT progression varied. Thus, in clinical practice, protocols for IMT vary. A suggested protocol for performing IMT with a patient using a typical IMT device is provided in Box 26-5.

Behavioral Interventions. Behavioral, emotional, and psychological issues affect many patients with respiratory failure receiving mechanical ventilation. Individuals constrained to a bed with very little movement or stimulation who depend on a mechanical device for every breath often find this experience psychologically stressful, resulting in emotions and behaviors that range from fear and complacency to anger and hostility.[88] A recent study

TABLE 26-8	Studies of Inspiratory Muscle Training in Patients Receiving Mechanical Ventilation		
Author/Study Type/No.	**Diagnosis/Experimental Intervention/ Length of Training (Days)**	**Study Measurements**	**Outcomes**
Belman[79]/PE/2	COPD with respiratory failure: Isocapnic hyperpnea breathing for 15 minutes (if possible), 3-6 × day using bypass mode of a Bear I Ventilator and 100% CO_2 rebreathing through the inspiratory line of the ventilator (3 and 5).	VE, end-tidal CO_2, MSVC	Both patients weaned successfully without complication after 3-5 days of isocapnic hyperpnea breathing showing a progressive increase in VE during training and increases in MSVC after extubation.
Aldrich and Karpel[80]/PE/4	CHF, COPD, pneumonia, and breast cancer: IMT via P-flex at 15%-20% of MIP for 5-15 minutes and duration was increased by 5-10 minutes until 30 minutes of IMT was performed, after which resistance was increased (based on symptoms and RR) and duration was decreased to 15 minutes. Also, weaning trails were attempted 2 × week (10-24).	MIP, VC, RR, ABGs	3 of the 4 patients were weaned successfully and were found to increase mean MIP from 38-54 cm H_2O and have greater IME. The patient not successfully weaned had the lowest body weight and showed no increase in MIP, VC, or tolerance to T-piece trial.
Abelson and Brewer[81]/PE/4	One patient with COPD and 3 patients with cervical SCI: IMT via P-flex and Calculair with 1 of 6 resistive settings for 15 minutes at a "previously determined TV," 2 × day progressively increasing the IMT program to the next resistance setting (with a smaller orifice through which one inspires) once 15 minutes of IMT at a specific resistance setting was completed (21-71).	IMT resistance level, VC, MIP, and motivation/ general outlook	4 patients receiving MV increased their IMT resistance, VC, MIP, and apparently underwent successful weaning from MV with improved motivation/general outlook.
Aldrich, Karpel, Uhrlass, et al[82]/ PE/27	SCI, idiopathic neuropathy, Guillain-Barré syndrome, and COPD: RIMT through an adjustable nonlinear resistor, the P-flex IMT, with gradual increases in the duration of resistance. When initial T-piece tolerance was <2 hours, 2-10 breaths of MV were given during IRT session; MV was provided between sessions for all subjects (10-46).	RR, VC, MIP, and T-piece tolerance duration	12 patients weaned successfully, 5 weaned to nocturnal ventilation, and 10 remained unweanable. Neuromuscular diseases showed greater results than those with primary lung diseases; 6/10 patients who could not be weaned showed signs of improvement during IRT; 8/10 died, mostly from pneumonia. One of the successfully weaned and one of patients weaned to nocturnal ventilation died.
Bruton[83]/PE/27	Postsurgical, acute-on-chronic COPD, acute respiratory failure, acute renal failure, and posttrauma: Supine with torso elevated to 45 degrees, patient continued with mode of MV until moment of measurement, by the TIRE device. Subjects exhaled to residual volume and then encouraged to make a single maximal inspiratory effort for as long as possible. Before measurement, all inspired 100% oxygen for 1-2 minutes to reduce likelihood of hypoxia (NR).	SMIP and peak MIP	SMIP can be used as an indicator of extubation success. SMIP and peak MIP measurements resulted in significant differences between extubation success and failure groups and between success and not tried groups but not between failure groups and not tested groups. There was no relationship between extubation outcome and original reason for ventilation.
Martin, Davenport, Franceschi, et al[84]/PE/10	COPD, MI, and post-CABG, tetraplegia, CHF, pneumonia, polyneuropathy, pancreatitis, and Wegener granulomatosis: PEP IMT (by inhaling through the exhalation orifice) for IMT ranges of 4-20 cm H_2O and Threshold IMT for IMT at ranges >20 cm H_2O attached to	IMT resistance and duration of spontaneous breathing periods	9/10 patients were successfully weaned and the one patient who was not successfully weaned was one of the oldest subjects suffering from aspiration pneumonia and who was unable to tolerate spontaneous breathing periods. Mean IMT resistance increased from 7 cm H_2O

Continued

TABLE 26-8	Studies of Inspiratory Muscle Training in Patients Receiving Mechanical Ventilation—cont'd		
Author/Study Type/No.	**Diagnosis/Experimental Intervention/ Length of Training (Days)**	**Study Measurements**	**Outcomes**
	tracheostomy tubes with 15-mm and 22-mm adapters performed 3-5 sets of 6 reps for a total of 18-30 training breaths/day, 5-7 days/week with patients in approximately 30° head-up tilt. Training was progressed via Borg RPE 0-10 so that if RPE was <6/10 the IMT resistance was increased, and if the RPE was >8/10, the resistance was decreased (however, the amount of resistance change was not reported). Spontaneous breathing periods were gradually increased as tolerated (10-144).		to 18 cm H_2O and changes in the spontaneous breathing durations over the mean IMT period of 44 days culminating in the successful wean were not reported.
Gutierrez, Harrow, Haines[85]/PE/7	Cervical SCI caused by trauma: C2 (high tetraplegia), C4-7 (low tetraplegia): Included pretraining optimization through Trendelenburg positioning, tracheal suctioning, bronchodilator aerosolization, transient hyperinflation of the lungs, and removal of tracheal tube inner cannula; inspiratory and expiratory resistance muscle training with the Resistex PEP therapy trainer, on ventilator and off ventilator endurance muscle training. (High tetraplegia: 30-60; low tetraplegia: 365-455)	PImax, PEmax, VC, on ventilator endurance duration, and off ventilator breathing time	For the low tetraplegia patients, PImax increased 75%, PEmax increased 71%, VC increased 59%, on ventilator endurance increased 91.6%, and off ventilator breathing time increased 76.7%; 4/5 (one died) low tetraplegics were successfully weaned. High tetraplegic patients improved their ability to spontaneously ventilate; both groups increased inspiratory and expiratory muscle strength, VC, on and off ventilator endurance.
Sprague and Hopkins[86]/PE/6	Postsurgical and cancer of the cervical spine with x-ray therapy and chemotherapy: Used the Threshold IMT, which provided a specific, measurable resistance that was constant through each breath and was independent of flow rate; resistance was increased as patient progressed followed by UBTs (9-28).	MIP, RR, oxygen saturation, Borg RPE scale, training pressures in cm/H_2O	All 6 patients who were previously diagnosed "failure to wean," were successfully weaned with increases in both their training pressures and MIP. However, it was not determined why the patients benefited from IST. Some possibilities: (1) inspiratory muscle pump failure was addressed, (2) standardization of breathing techniques, (3) routine UBTs following the IST, (4) nonspecific training effects.
Liaw, Lin, Cheng, et al[87]/TE/20	Acute complete cervical cord injury Experimental group received training with a Diemolding Healthcare Division inspiratory muscle trainer for 15-20 minutes per session, 2 × day, 7 days a week for 6 weeks (42).	Spirometry, lung volume test, MIP, MEP, and modified Borg scale measurements	Both the control group and the experimental group demonstrated improvements in their pulmonary parameters, however, the RIMT group showed greater improvements: TLC, TLC % predicted, VC, minute ventilation, FEV_1 % predicted, and resting Borg scale were significantly greater in those who were in the RIMT group.

PE, Pre-experimental; *COPD,* chronic obstructive pulmonary disease; *VE,* ventilator extubation; *MSVC,* maximal sustained ventilatory capacity; *CHF,* congestive heart failure; *IMT,* inspiratory muscle training; *MIP,* maximum inspiratory pressure; *RR,* respiratory rate; *VC,* vital capacity; *ABG,* arterial blood gases; *IME,* inspiratory muscle endurance; *TV,* tidal volume; *MV,* mechanical ventilation; *RIMT,* resistive inspiratory muscle training; *IRT,* inspiratory resistance training; *SMIP,* sustained maximal inspiratory pressure; *TIRE,* test of incremental respiratory endurance; *NR,* not reported; *MI,* myocardial infarction; *CABG,* coronary artery bypass graft; *PEP,* positive expiratory pressure; *RPE,* rating of perceived exertion; *SCI,* spinal cord injury; *PImax,* maximal inspiratory pressure; *PEmax,* maximal expiratory pressure; *UBT,* unassisted breathing trials; *IST,* inspiratory strength training; *TE,* true experimental; *MEP,* maximum expiratory pressure; *TLC,* total lung capacity; *TLC %,* TLC predicted percentage; FEV_1 *% predicted,* forced expiratory volume in 1 second predicted percentage.

BOX 26-5   A Typical Method for Performing Inspiratory Muscle Training

1. Obtain baseline pulmonary function tests including MIP, MEP, FEV_1, FVC, and TV with ventilated patients and MIP alone in nonventilated patients.
2. Position the patient supine or sitting. If the patient is supine, elevate the head of the bed at least 45 degrees. Have the patient's legs and arms in a relaxed position.
3. Set the IMT at 50% of the participant's baseline MIP measurement.
4. If necessary, give a gentle quick stretch in an inward and upward direction to the participant's abdomen (level of umbilicus and upper chest) at the end of exhalation to facilitate inhalation.
5. Verbally encourage inhalation to help the patient overcome the resistance felt during inspiration, and exhale along with the patient to ensure as much air as possible is expelled from the lungs.
6. Instruct the patient to breathe in and out as normally as possible despite feeling some resistance when breathing in. They should increase their effort to overcome this resistance and then breathe out with usual force.
7. The patient should perform 4-6 sets of 8 repetitions, or stop sooner if fatigued.
8. Between each set the patient may rest and be put back on mechanical ventilation if necessary until the training begins again.
9. The RPE scale should be used to evaluate the amount of effort the patient experiences. 0 represents no effort required with breathing, 1 represents the least amount of effort needed to breathe and 10 represents the most amount of effort needed to breathe with the trainer. After each set, the patient should grade his or her effort on the RPE scale. If the patient's RPE is between 1 and 5, increase the resistance by 1-2 cm H_2O. If their rating is 6-8, do not change the amount of resistance. If their rating is 9-10, reduce the resistance by 1-2 cm H_2O.

MIP, Maximum inspiratory pressure; *MEP*, maximum expiratory pressure; FEV_1, forced expiratory volume in 1 second; *FVC*, forced vital capacity; *TV*, tidal volume; *IMT*, inspiratory muscle training, *RPE*, rating of perceived exertion.

---

of patients' recollections of their ICU experience during prolonged mechanical ventilation found that most patients remembered the majority of their ICU stay and most notably remembered the ETT.[89] Most recollections were of moderately to extremely bothersome experiences, including pain, fear, anxiety, lack of sleep, feeling tense, inability to speak or communicate, lack of control, nightmares, and loneliness.

Several studies suggest that relaxation biofeedback therapy can decrease weaning times in patients receiving mechanical ventilation.[90-93] This effect is likely due to reductions in respiratory rate and occlusion pressure at 1 second from the onset of inspiration and thus a decrease in neural respiratory drive. Two studies using IMT included targeted feedback of information about resistive breathing efforts with IMT.[79,83] This feedback was also thought to shorten weaning times. In addition, the functional and exercise training methods discussed previously may also improve patients' sense of psychological well-being by providing proprioceptive, visual, and general sensory stimulation.[48-71] Accelerated weaning from mechanical ventilation may improve the ICU experience for patients and their families, as well as the rest of the health care team.

Fig. 26-14 shows a psychological and behavioral hypothesis-oriented algorithm that may be useful for patients with respiratory failure receiving mechanical ventilation. This algorithm is based on an extensive review of the literature regarding psychosocial and behavioral issues of patients in the ICU requiring mechanical ventilation.[94-98] Identification of one or more of the primary characteristics listed at the top of this algorithm identifies the potential for a psychosocial or behavioral issue. Appropriate referral to the health care providers listed along the right arm of the decision tree is likely to improve the patient's psychosocial and behavioral impairments. However, such problems may not be identified initially and may only become apparent during exercise sessions, as shown in the left arm of the decision tree. This highlights the importance of physical therapy in identifying psychosocial and behavioral issues during serial exercise training sessions.

CASE STUDY 26-1

BRONCHIOLITIS OBLITERANS ORGANIZING PNEUMONIA

Examination
Patient History

DN, a 42-year-old woman, was admitted to the hospital with end-stage bronchiolitis obliterans organizing pneumonia (BOOP). On the same day, she underwent bilateral lung transplantation. In the immediate postoperative period, DN developed hypoxemic respiratory failure as a result of pneumonia and required mechanical ventilation. The patient has had BOOP for several years and has been experiencing progressively greater difficulty breathing and performing functional tasks. She has been hospitalized 10 times over the past year with the last 2 hospitalizations lasting approximately 3 weeks each. Her past medical history is also significant for hypertension, Cushing's syndrome because of chronic steroid use, osteoporosis, and osteopenic fractures of her thoracic vertebrae. DN was referred to physical therapy on the fifth day after her lung transplantation surgery. Since the patient was not able to talk, most of the patient history was obtained from her medical chart. The patient's medical condition was also discussed with the attending physician, as well as the patient's nurse. The patient's medications included Solu-Medrol, CellCept, Prograf, Vancomycin, Bactrim, Zithromax, Levaquin, Metoprolol, Hydralazine, Epivir, Acyclovir,

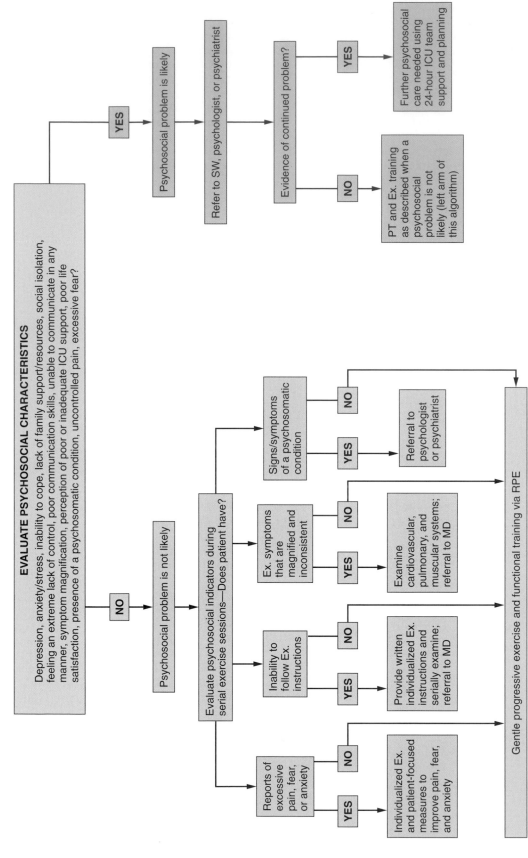

EVALUATE PSYCHOSOCIAL CHARACTERISTICS

Depression, anxiety/stress, inability to cope, lack of family support/resources, social isolation, feeling an extreme lack of control, poor communication skills, unable to communicate in any manner, symptom magnification, perception of poor or inadequate ICU support, poor life satisfaction, presence of a psychosomatic condition, uncontrolled pain, excessive fear?

YES → Psychosocial problem is likely → Refer to SW, psychologist, or psychiatrist → Evidence of continued problem?

Evidence of continued problem?
- YES → Further psychosocial care needed using 24-hour ICU team support and planning
- NO → PT and Ex. training as described when a psychosocial problem is not likely (left arm of this algorithm)

NO → Psychosocial problem is not likely → Evaluate psychosocial indicators during serial exercise sessions—Does patient have?

Reports of excessive pain, fear, or anxiety
- YES → Individualized Ex. and patient-focused measures to improve pain, fear, and anxiety
- NO

Inability to follow Ex. instructions
- YES → Provide written individualized Ex. instructions and serially examine; referral to MD
- NO

Ex. symptoms that are magnified and inconsistent
- YES → Examine cardiovascular, pulmonary, and muscular systems; referral to MD
- NO

Signs/symptoms of a psychosomatic condition
- YES → Referral to psychologist or psychiatrist
- NO

Gentle progressive exercise and functional training via RPE

FIG. 26-14 Psychosocial and behavioral algorithm for patients receiving mechanical ventilation. *Ex,* Exercise; *MD,* medical doctor; *RPE,* rating of perceived exertion; *SW,* social worker.

Prevacid, and Ambien. The patient also received the following medications as needed: Fentanyl for pain, Benadryl for itching, Lorazepam for anxiety, and Reglan and Zofran for nausea.

Systems Review

HR is 93 bpm, RR is 23 breaths/min, BP is 146/97 mm Hg, and O_2 saturation is 92%.

Ventilator Settings
SIMV: 8 breaths/min
TV: 450 ml
PS: 15 cm H_2O
FiO_2: 0.6
PEEP: 8 cm H_2O

Arterial Blood Gases: pH: 7.45, PCO_2: 40 mm Hg, PO_2: 65 mm Hg, O_2 saturation: 93%, Base excess: 4 mEq/L, HCO_3: 27.9

Chest X-Ray: Bibasilar pulmonary parenchymal infiltrates.

Tests and Measures

Musculoskeletal

Range of Motion Active-assisted ROM is within normal limits throughout all major joints.

Muscle Strength: Muscle strength is at least 3/5 in all four extremities, except both hips are 2/5. Manual resistance for extremity strength testing was deferred due to the recent surgical procedure. Maximal inspiratory and expiratory muscle strength was not initially assessed.

Neuromuscular

Sensation Grossly intact to light touch and deep pressure on all four extremities.

Function

Functional Mobility Supine to sit with maximal assistance; turning side to side with maximal assistance; unable to stand; bed to chair with maximal assistance.

Activities of Daily Living Patient is dependent for all ADLs.

Evaluation, Diagnosis, and Prognosis

DN presents with the following impairments:
- Impaired ventilation
- Impaired gas exchange
- Impaired muscle performance
- Impaired aerobic capacity

Her functional limitations are:
- Inability to perform bed mobility and transfer activities independently
- Inability to ambulate
- Inability to perform self-care or any instrumental ADLs

The physical therapy diagnosis is preferred practice pattern 6F: Impaired ventilation, respiration, aerobic capacity and endurance associated with respiratory failure.

DN has severe functional limitations as a result of recent lung transplant and need for mechanical ventilation. She was sedentary for an extended period before the surgery because of the severity of her lung disease. Given her current medical condition and co-morbidities associated with mechanical ventilation, it is likely that DN will require comprehensive inpatient rehabilitation to achieve her highest level of function. It is expected that DN will be independent in ADLs and ambulate without an assistive device as her medical condition improves.

Goals

DN was unable to talk because of ET intubation and could not extensively participate in decision making regarding her physical therapy goals and plan of care. Physical therapy goals and treatment plans will be updated every 2-3 weeks as part of the reexaminations and reevaluations. Short-term goals to be achieved in 2 weeks:
1. Move from supine to sitting with moderate assistance.
2. Move from sitting to standing with maximal assistance.
3. Ambulate 20-30 feet with a walker and moderate assistance.

The rehabilitation criteria for her discharge from ICU were:
1. Independent bed mobility and transfers.
2. Independent ambulation with appropriate assistive device.
3. Ability to ambulate more than 500 feet.
4. Independent with basic ADLs.

The plan of care for physical therapy included:
1. Positioning and adjunctive techniques.
2. Functional and exercise training.
3. Inspiratory muscle training.
4. Behavioral feedback.
5. Strengthening exercises with emphasis on lower extremities.
6. Bed mobility activities.
7. Transfer training.
8. Progression to standing with walker and gait training as appropriate.
9. Weaning from mechanical ventilation.

Initially, the frequency of treatments was daily. The frequency was planned to increase to two times per day when tolerated.

Intervention

Before each physical therapy session, the ventilator settings and vital signs were noted and the patient's status discussed with nursing staff. Vital signs that were continuously monitored included O_2 saturation, heart rate, respiratory rate, and blood pressure and these were used to determine tolerance of the physical therapy session. As prescribed by the physician, O_2 saturation equal to or greater than 90% on supplemental O_2 was required throughout all physical therapy sessions. Regular discussions with the pulmonary physician and respiratory therapists optimized coordination of the weaning process and physical therapy treatments. Weight bearing, upright position, getting out of bed, and gait training were emphasized in each of the physical therapy treatments. Furthermore, after physical therapy sessions, DN was placed in positions to modify her WOB and to optimize cardiovascular function and drainage of retained pulmonary secretions.

Leg strengthening exercises using resistance from elastic bands were initiated immediately after the initial physical therapy evaluation. DN was initially able to perform 3 sets of 10 repetitions, and gradually increased to 50 repetitions. Mobility training included progression of activity from supine to sitting on the edge of the bed. DN was encouraged to sit on the edge of the bed for at least 10 minutes and perform one or a combination of the following activities: Leg exercises, trunk control, unsupported sitting, and ADLs (e.g., brushing teeth, combing hair, washing face). Standing with a walker and assistance was attempted as part of the initial evaluation and on a daily basis. DN could not stand during her first 3 sessions, despite use of a walker and the assistance of two people. Once DN was able to stand, pre-gait activities were initiated, including weight shifting and steps in place and sideways with a walker. On postoperative day 14, DN underwent tracheotomy because of failure to wean and need for prolonged mechanical ventilation. Some of the factors that were limiting her ability to start ambulation were high respiratory rate, O_2 desaturation, and extreme fatigue with standing activities.

On discussion with the physician, it was decided that DN would benefit from increased ventilatory support and supplemental O_2 to tolerate increased levels of activity. An order was written for DN to be placed on the following ventilator settings during PT sessions: Pressure support of 15 cm H_2O, FiO_2 60%, and PEEP of 5 cm H_2O. It was also decided that the patient would begin gentle IMT.

On postoperative day 16, DN began IMT at 7 cm H_2O for 30 seconds, after which her RPE score was 9/10. IMT was therefore stopped, and DN was placed on pressure support of 15 cm H_2O, FiO_2 60%, and PEEP of 5 cm H_2O. The patient's high RPE score appeared to be partly a result of anxiety. Therefore biofeedback training was provided during the next IMT session later the same day. A mirror was placed in front of the patient before IMT, and she was instructed to observe her chest and abdominal area move during inspiration and expiration. She appeared excited to be in control of her breathing and observed her chest and abdominal motion during IMT, which enabled her to complete 2 minutes of IMT before she complained of fatigue with an RPE score of 6/10.

On postoperative 17, DN was reassessed and none of the goals set for her had been achieved. This was attributed to her multiple medical problems, including respiratory failure, transient myocardial dysfunction leading to congestive heart failure, renal insufficiency, and weakness arising from prolonged bed rest. The plan was to continue to work toward her physical therapy goals set on initial evaluation. At this time, DN's IMT was progressed and continued to be performed with "mirror" behavioral biofeedback training. The IMT threshold was increased to 10 cm H_2O for 2 minutes after which the patient's RPE score was 4/10 and IMT was continued for 2 additional minutes with a 4-minute RPE score of 6/10. The IMT program was progressed in this manner until the patient could comfortably perform 10 minutes at an intensity that elicited an RPE score of 6/10. During IMT the patient was allowed to observe her breathing in a mirror and was instructed to focus on breathing from her abdomen and expanding the area during inspiration.

On postoperative day 18, gait training using a portable ventilator was initiated. Gait distance increased from 30 feet on day 18 to 80 feet on day 22. After several gait sessions with the portable ventilator, the physician was very optimistic about DN's functional progress and decided to start trials of spontaneous breathing off the ventilator with intermittent IMT followed by ventilatory support. DN was now showing improvement in overall strength and endurance, and a decision was made to assess her ability to tolerate gait activities without ventilatory support. On postoperative day 23, she was able to ambulate 90 feet without ventilator support. At this point, since DN required less assistance and showed great improvement in gait pattern, the focus of the physical therapy sessions was to gradually increase gait distance to improve endurance. DN no longer required behavior biofeedback via the mirror during IMT sessions, which had progressed to several times per day at 12-16 cm H_2O for 5-10 minutes with less ventilatory support after the IMT sessions.

DN was reassessed on postoperative day 33 and her therapy goals were achieved. Her new goals are the rehabilitation criteria, set at the initial assessment, for discharge from ICU. On day 35, DN demonstrated interest in improving her upper extremity strength. Overhead pulleys with 2-lb weights were installed on the bed, and after instruction, DN initiated arm exercises independently. On day 37, DN was transferred to the telemetry floor after remaining off the ventilator for 48 hours continuously. On postoperative days 40 and 41, DN requested twice daily treatments, which she emphatically stated needed to consist of walking activities. Her tracheostomy was removed on postoperative day 43, and DN was placed on O_2 by nasal cannula since supplemental O_2 was still needed. On postoperative day 48, DN was discharged directly home with a referral for outpatient physical therapy.

Outcomes
At the time of hospital discharge, DN was independent with all bed mobility, transfers, and ADLs and could ambulate 550 feet with a front-wheeled walker.

CHAPTER SUMMARY

The primary function of the respiratory system is to bring O_2 into the body and release CO_2. The respiratory system can be divided into the musculoskeletal pump system, the gas exchange unit, and its neural control centers. Respiratory failure is a state or condition in which the respiratory system fails to meet the body's needs for gas exchange. When respiratory failure occurs, arterial CO_2 concentration will increase and O_2 concentration will decrease. Many pathological conditions can cause respiratory failure, but the physiological mechanisms causing failure include: (1) diffusion abnormalities, (2) hypoventilation, and (3) $\dot{V}:\dot{Q}$ mismatching.[37]

Respiratory failure can be classified as either type I (hypoxic) or type II (hypercapnic), depending on the primary blood gas abnormality. Individuals may live in chronic states of respiratory failure or may experience sudden acute bouts of failure. Medical management is generally supportive in nature (i.e., mechanical ventilation and/or supplemental O_2). This chapter focuses on rehabilitation intervention for patients receiving mechanical ventilation also includes approaches that can be applied to other individuals with respiratory failure.

Rehabilitation of the individual with respiratory failure requiring mechanical ventilation is an area in need of further investigation. A limited number of studies have examined the rehabilitation of such patients. The most evidence-based areas of rehabilitation for such patients, with clinically applicable results, are in the areas of IMT and behavioral feedback as adjunctive methods for weaning patients from mechanical ventilation. Patients weaning from mechanical ventilation who perform IMT appear to have improved breathing muscle strength and endurance, some measures of pulmonary function, and most importantly, are able to wean from mechanical ventilation when previously they had failed. Behavioral feedback and biofeedback mechanisms also improve several measures of respiratory function and hasten weaning from mechanical ventilation. Other rehabilitation efforts discussed in this chapter that are performed by PTs with a limited evidence base but strong physiological rationale include positioning and adjunctive techniques, as well as functional and exercise training.

ADDITIONAL RESOURCES

Books

DeTurk W, Cahalin L: *Cardiovascular and Pulmonary Physical Therapy: An Evidence-based Approach*, 2004, McGraw-Hill.

Irwin S, Tecklin JS (eds): *Cardiopulmonary Physical Therapy: A Guide to Practice*, ed 4, Philadelphia, 2004, Elsevier.

Web Sites

American Association for Respiratory Care: www.aarc.org
Cardiovascular and Pulmonary Section of the American Physical Therapy Association: www.cardiopt.org
American Thoracic Society: www.thoracic.org

GLOSSARY

Alveolar perfusion: The amount of blood flow that comes in contact with the alveoli and participates in respiration.

Alveolar ventilation: The amount of air flow that comes in contact with the alveoli and participates in respiration.

Alveoli: The distal terminal air sacs in the lungs where gas exchange occurs.

Arterial–alveolar oxygen difference (PAO_2–PaO_2): The difference between the partial pressure of O_2 in the alveoli and the partial pressure of O_2 in the arterial blood.

Atelectasis: A collapsed airway or section of the lung in which air cannot move through the airways and participate in gas exchange.

Compliance: A measure of the ease of expansion of the lungs and chest wall.

Conducting airways: Airways within the lungs that serve as a conduit for air to travel down to the alveoli. Because of the absence of alveoli, gas exchange does not occur in these airways. These are found in the upper airways from generation 0-16.

Dead space: Air within the lungs that does not participate in respiration.

Elasticity: The ability of an object to return to its original state after being deformed.

Hemoptysis: Expectoration of blood.

Hypercapnia: An increased level of CO_2 in the circulating blood.

Hypoxia: A decreased level of O_2 in the circulating blood.

Maximal voluntary ventilation: The most amount of air an individual can move in and out of the airways over 1 minute. It is determined by the maximal respiratory rate and vital capacity.

Minute ventilation: The amount of air moved into or out of the lungs over 1 minute.

Pneumothorax: Air in the pleural cavity.

Pulmonary shunt: Blood flow moving through the lungs that does not participate in respiration.

Respiration: The process of gas exchange between the atmospheric air and the pulmonary capillary bed.

Respiratory airways: The airways in the tracheobronchial tree where gas exchange may occur due to the presence of alveoli. These airways generally begin at generation 17.

Surfactant: Substance produced by the alveolar cells that reduces surface tension in the airways.

Tracheostomy: A surgical incision in the trachea through which an artificial airway may be placed.

Ventilation: Air flow through the airways.

Work of breathing (WOB): The energy cost of breathing.

References

1. Beers MH, Berknow R (ed): *The Merck Manual of Diagnosis and Therapy*, ed 17, New York, 1999, John S. Wiley.
2. Karande S, Murkey R, Ahuja S, et al: Clinical profile and outcome of acute respiratory failure, *Ind J Pediatr* 70:865-869, 2003.
3. Atabai K, Matthay MA: The pulmonary physician in critical care. 5: Acute lung injury and the acute respiratory distress syndrome: Definitions and epidemiology, *Thorax* 57(5):452-458, 2002.
4. Roche N, Huchon G: Epidemiology of chronic obstructive disease, *Rev Prat* 54(13):1408-1413, 2004.
5. American Physical Therapy Association: Guide to Physical Therapist Practice, second edition, *Phys Ther* 81(1):9-746, 2001.
6. Ruel M, Deslauriers J, Maltais F: The diaphragm in emphysema, *Chest Surg Clin N Am* 8:381-399, 1998.
7. Suwatanapongched T, Gierada DS, Slone RM, et al: Variation in diaphragm position and shape in adults with normal pulmonary function, *Chest* 123(6):2019-2027, 2003.
8. Polla B, D'Antona G, Bottinelli R, et al: Respiratory muscle fibers: Specialization and plasticity, *Thorax* 59(9):808-817, 2004.
9. Poole DC, Sexton WL, Farkas GA, et al: Diaphragm structure and function in health and disease, *Med Sci Sports Exerc* 29(6):738-754, 1997.
10. Laube BL, Jashnani R, Dalby RN, et al: Targeting aerosol deposition in patients with cystic fibrosis: Effects of alterations in particle size and inspiratory flow rate, *Chest* 118(4):1069-1076, 2000.
11. Brand P, Friemel I, Meyer T, et al: Total deposition of therapeutic particles during spontaneous and controlled inhalations, *J Pharm Sci* 89(6):724-731, 2000.
12. Houtmeyers E, Gosselink R, Gayan-Ramirez G, et al: Regulation of mucociliary clearance in health and disease, *Eur Respir J* 13(5):1177-1188, 1999.
13. McArdle WD, Katch FI, Katch VL: *Exercise Physiology: Energy, Nutrition, and Human Performance*, ed 5, Philadelphia, 2001, Lippincott Williams & Wilkins.
14. Moudgil R, Michelakis ED, Archer SL: Hypoxic pulmonary vasoconstriction, *J Appl Physiol* 98(1):390-403, 2005.
15. Dean E: Preferred practice patterns in cardiopulmonary physical therapy: A guide to physiologic measures, *Cardiopulm Phys Ther* 10(4):124-134, 1999.
16. Blackie SP, McElvaney NG, Wilcox PG, et al: Normal values and ranges for ventilation and breathing pattern at maximal exercise, *Chest* 100(1):136-142, 1991.
17. Rampulla C, Baiocchi S, Dacosta E, et al: Dyspnea on exercise. Pathophysiologic mechanisms, *Chest* 101:248S-252S, 1992.
18. Hamnegard CH, Wragg S, Kyroussis D, et al: Diaphragm fatigue following maximal ventilation in man, *Eur Respir J* 9:241-247, 1996.
19. Beachey WD, Olson DE: Quantifying ventilatory reserve to predict respiratory failure in exacerbations of COPD, *Chest* 97(5):1086-1091, 1990.
20. Moriya E, Kawakami K, Sudoh M, et al: The effect of body position on ventilation and perfusion in the lung, *Physiologist* 30(1 suppl):S60-61, 1987.
21. Dean E: Effect of body position on pulmonary function, *Phys Ther* 65(5):613-618, 1985.
22. Kim MJ, Hwang HJ, Song HH: A randomized trial on the effects of body positions on lung function with acute respiratory failure patients, *Int J Nurs Stud* 39(5):549-555, 2002.
23. Ross J, Dean E, Abboud RT: The effect of postural drainage positioning on ventilation homogeneity in healthy subjects, *Phys Ther* 72(11):794-799, 1992.
24. Norton LC, Conforti CG: The effects of body position on oxygenation, *Heart Lung* 14(1):45-52, 1985.

25. Wagner PD, Laravuso RB, Uhl PR, et al: Continuous distributions of ventilation-perfusion ratios in normal subjects breathing air and 100 percent O$_2$, *J Clin Invest* 54(1):54-68, 1974.

26. Colebatch HJ, Ng CK: Estimating alveolar surface area during life, *Respir Physiol* 88(1-2):163-170, 1992.

27. Hansen JE, Ampaya EP: Human air space shapes, sizes, areas, and volumes, *J Appl Physiol* 38:990-995, 1975.

28. Hillegass E, Sadowsky HS (ed): *Essentials of Cardiopulmonary Physical Therapy,* ed 2, Philadelphia. 2001, WB Saunders.

29. Aliverti A, Macklem PT: How and why exercise is impaired in COPD, *Respiration* 68(3):229-239, 2001.

30. Bell SC, Saunders MJ, Elborn JS, et al: Resting energy expenditure and oxygen cost of breathing in patients with cystic fibrosis, *Thorax* 51(2):126-131, 1996.

31. Haas A, Rusk HA, Pelosof H, et al: Respiratory function in hemiplegic patients, *Arch Phys Med Rehabil* 48(4):174-179, 1967.

32. Narain S, Puckree T: Pulmonary function in hemiplegia, *Int J Rehabil Res* 25(1):57-59, 2002.

33. Laghi F, Tobin MJ: Disorders of the respiratory muscles, *Am J Respir Crit Care Med* 168(1):10-48, 2003.

34. Winslow C, Rozovsky J: Effect of spinal cord injury on the respiratory system, *Am J Phys Med Rehabil* 82(10):803-814, 2003.

35. *Taber's Cyclopedic Medical Dictionary,* ed 17, Philadelphia, 2005, FA Davis.

36. Scanlan C, Spearman CB, Sheldon RL (eds): *Egan's Fundamentals of Respiratory Care,* ed 5, Philadelphia, 1990, Mosby.

37. Greene KE, Peters JI: Pathophysiology of acute respiratory failure, *Clin Chest Med* 15(1):1-12, 1994.

38. Markou NK, Myrianthefs PM, Baltopoulos GJ: Respiratory failure: An overview, *Crit Care Nurs Q* 27(4):353-379, 2004.

39. Raju P, Manthous CA: The pathogenesis of respiratory failure: An overview, *Respir Care Clin N Am* 6(2):195-212, 2000.

40. Wagner PD, et al: Ventilation-perfusion inequality in chronic obstructive pulmonary disease, *J Clin Invest* 59(2):203-216, 1977.

41. Shapiro B, Peruzzi W, Kozelowski-Templin R: *Clinical Application of Blood Gases,* ed 5, St. Louis, 1994, Mosby-Year Book.

42. Williams AJ: ABC of oxygen: assessing and interpreting arterial blood gases and acid-base balance, *BMJ* 317(7167):1213-1216, 1998.

43. Andrews JL Jr, Copeland BE, Salah RM, et al: Arterial blood gas standards for healthy young nonsmoking subjects, *Am J Clin Pathol* 75(6):773-780, 1981.

44. McBride DS Jr, Johnson JO, Tobias JD: Noninvasive carbon dioxide monitoring during neurosurgical procedures in adults: End-tidal versus transcutaneous techniques, *South Med J* 95(8):870-874, 2002.

45. Stock MC: Noninvasive carbon dioxide monitoring, *Crit Care Clin* 4(3):511-526, 1988.

46. Cohn MA, Rao S, Broudy M, et al: The respiratory inductive plethysmograph: A new non-invasive monitor of respiration, *Bull Eur Physiopathol Respir* 18(4):643-658, 1982.

47. Martyn JB, Moreno RH, Pare PD, et al: Measurement of inspiratory muscle performance with incremental threshold loading, *Am Rev Respir Dis* 135(4):919-923, 1987.

48. Dean E, Ross J: Discordance between cardiopulmonary physiology and physical therapy. Toward a rational basis for practice [see comment], *Chest* 101(6):1694-1698, 1992.

49. Ciesla ND: Chest physical therapy for patients in the intensive care unit, *Phys Ther* 76(6):609-625, 1996.

50. Paratz J: Haemodynamic stability of the ventilated intensive care patient: A review, *Aust J Physiother* 38:167-172, 1992.

51. Dean E: Oxygen transport: A physiologically-based conceptual framework for the practice of cardiopulmonary physiotherapy, *Physiotherapy* 80(6):347-355, 1994.

52. Jaeger RJ, Turba RM, Yarkony GM, et al: Cough in spinal cord injured patients: Comparison of three methods to produce cough [see comment], *Arch Phys Med Rehabil* 74(12):1358-1361, 1993.

53. Stiller K: Physiotherapy in intensive care: Towards an evidence-based practice, *Chest* 118(6):1801-1813, 2000.

54. Braun SR, Giovannoni R, O'Connor M: Improving the cough in patients with spinal cord injury, *Am J Phys Med* 63(1):1-10, 1984.

55. Bach JR: Mechanical insufflation-exsufflation. Comparison of peak expiratory flows with manually assisted and unassisted coughing techniques, *Chest* 104(5):1553-1562, 1993.

56. Puckree T, Cerny F, Bishop B: Does intercostal stretch alter breathing pattern and respiratory muscle activity in conscious adults? *Physiotherapy* 88(2):89-97, 2002.

57. Vianello A, Corrado A, Arcaro G, et al: Mechanical insufflation-exsufflation improves outcomes for neuromuscular disease patients with respiratory tract infections, *Am J Phys Med Rehabil* 84(2):83-88; 89-91, 2005.

58. Winck JC, Goncalves MR, Lourenco C, et al: Effects of mechanical insufflation-exsufflation on respiratory parameters for patients with chronic airway secretion encumbrance, *Chest* 126(3):774-780, 2004.

59. Sancho J, Servera E, Diaz J, et al: Efficacy of mechanical insufflation-exsufflation in medically stable patients with amyotrophic lateral sclerosis, *Chest* 125(4):1400-1405, 2004.

60. Sancho J, Servera E, Vergara P, et al: Mechanical insufflation-exsufflation vs. tracheal suctioning via tracheostomy tubes for patients with amyotrophic lateral sclerosis, *Am J Phys Med Rehabil* 82(10):750-753, 2003.

61. Stiller K, Phillips A: Safety aspects of mobilizing acutely ill patients, *Physiother Theory Pract* 19: 239-257, 2003.

62. Ceriana P, Delmastro M, Rampulla C, et al: Demographics and clinical outcomes of patients admitted to a respiratory intensive care unit located in a rehabilitation center [see comment], *Respir Care* 48(7):670-676, 2003.

63. Nava S, Confalonieri M, Rampulla C: Intermediate respiratory intensive care units in Europe: A European perspective [see comment], *Thorax* 53(9):798-802, 1998.

64. Nava S, Evangelisti I, Rampulla C, et al: Human and financial costs of noninvasive mechanical ventilation in patients affected by COPD and acute respiratory failure, *Chest* 111(6):1631-1638, 1997.

65. van't Hul A, Kwakkel G, Gosselink R: The acute effects of noninvasive ventilatory support during exercise on exercise endurance and dyspnea in patients with chronic obstructive pulmonary disease: A systematic review, *J Cardiopulm Rehabil* 22(4):290-297, 2002.

66. Costes F, Agresti A, Court-Fortune I, et al: Noninvasive ventilation during exercise training improves exercise tolerance in patients with chronic obstructive pulmonary disease, *J Cardiopulm Rehabil* 23(4):307-313, 2003.

67. Bianchi L, Foglio K, Pagani M, et al: Effects of proportional assist ventilation on exercise tolerance in COPD patients with chronic hypercapnia, *Eur Respir J* 11(2):422-427, 1998.

68. Johnson JE, Gavin DJ, Adams-Dramiga S: Effects of training with heliox and noninvasive positive pressure ventilation on exercise ability in patients with severe COPD, *Chest* 122(2):464-472, 2002.

69. Soo Hoo GW: Nonpharmacologic adjuncts to training during pulmonary rehabilitation: the role of supplemental oxygen and noninvasive ventilation, *J Rehabil Res Devel* 40:81-97, 2003.

70. Nava S: Rehabilitation of patients admitted to a respiratory ICU, *Arch Phys Med Rehab* 79(7):849-854, 1998.

71. Zanotti E, Felicetti G, Maini M, et al: Peripheral muscle strength training in bed-bound patients with COPD receiving mechanical ventilation: Effect of electrical stimulation [see comment], *Chest* 124(1):292-296, 2003.

72. Ishaaya AM, Nathan SD, Belman MJ: Work of breathing after extubation, *Chest* 107(1):204-209, 1995.

73. Kaplan J, Schuster D: Physiological consequences of tracheal intubation, *Clin Chest Med* 12:425-432, 1991.

74. Pingleton SK: Complications of acute respiratory failure, *Am Rev Respir Dis,* 137(6):1463-1493, 1988.

75. Hussain SN, Vassilakopoulos T: Ventilator-induced cachexia, *Am J Respir Crit Care Med* 166:1307-1308, 2002.

76. Sassoon CS: Ventilator-associated diaphragmatic dysfunction, *Am J Respir Crit Care Med* 166:1017-1018, 2002.

77. Hendra K, Celli B: Physiologic responses to long-term ventilation, *Respir Care Clin N Am* 8(3): 447-462, 2002.

78. MacIntyre NR, Cook DJ, Ely EW Jr, et al: Evidence-based guidelines for weaning and discontinuing ventilatory support: A collective task force facilitated by the American College of Chest Physicians, the American Association for Respiratory Care, and the American College of Critical Care Medicine, *Chest* 120(6 Suppl):375S-395S, 2001.

79. Belman MJ: Respiratory failure treated by ventilatory muscle training (VMT). A report of two cases, *Eur J Respir Dis* 62(6):391-395, 1981.

80. Aldrich TK, Karpel JP: Inspiratory muscle resistive training in respiratory failure, *Am Rev Respir Dis* 131(3):461-462, 1985.

81. Abelson H, Brewer K: Inspiratory muscle training in the mechanically ventilated patient, *Physiother Canada* 39(5):305-307, 1987.

82. Aldrich TK, Karpel JP, Uhrlass RM, et al: Weaning from mechanical ventilation: Adjunctive use of inspiratory muscle resistive training, *Crit Care Med* 17(2):143-147, 1989.

83. Bruton A: A pilot study to investigate any relationship between sustained maximal inspiratory pressure and extubation outcome, *Heart Lung* 31(2):141-149, 2002.

84. Martin AD, Davenport PD, Franceschi AC, et al: Use of inspiratory muscle strength training to facilitate ventilator weaning: a series of 10 consecutive patients, *Chest* 122(1):192-196, 2002.

85. Gutierrez CJ, Harrow J, Haines F: Using an evidence-based protocol to guide rehabilitation and weaning of ventilator-dependent cervical spinal cord injury patients, *J Rehabil Res Devel* 40(5):99-110, 2003.

86. Sprague SS, Hopkins PD: Use of inspiratory strength training to wean six patients who were ventilator-dependent, *Phys Ther* 83(2):171-181, 2003.

87. Liaw M, Lin MC, Cheng PT, et al: Resistive inspiratory muscle training: its effectiveness in patients with acute complete cervical cord injury, *Arch Phys Med Rehabil* 81(6):752-756, 2000.

88. Gale J, O'Shannick G: Psychiatric aspects of respiratory treatment and pulmonary intensive care unit, *Adv Psychosom Med* 14:93-108, 1985.

89. Rotondi AJ, Chelluri L, Sirio C, et al: Patients' recollections of stressful experiences while receiving prolonged mechanical ventilation in an intensive care unit [see comment], *Crit Care Med* 30(4):746-752, 2002.

90. Holliday JE, Hyers TM: The reduction of weaning time from mechanical ventilation using tidal volume and relaxation biofeedback, *Am Rev Resp Dis* 141(5 Pt 1):1214-1220, 1990.

91. Yarnal JR, Herrell DW, Sivak ED: Routine use of biofeedback in weaning patients from mechanical ventilation, *Chest* 79(1):127, 1981.

92. Corson JA, Grant JL, Moulton DP, et al: Use of biofeedback in weaning paralyzed patients from respirators, *Chest* 76:543-545, 1979.

93. Holliday J, Shapiro M, Durham R: Optimization of P100 for reducing ventilator weaning time using tidal volume and relaxation feedback, *Am Rev Respir Dis* 143:A684, 1991.

94. Green T, Gidron Y, Friger M, et al: Relative-assessed psychological factors predict sedation requirement in critically ill patients, *Psychosom Med* 67(2):295-300, 2005.

95. Douglas SL, Daly BJ: Caregiving and long-term mechanical ventilation [comment], *Chest* 126(4):1387-1388, 2004.

96. Johnson P: Reclaiming the everyday world: How long-term ventilated patients in critical care seek to gain aspects of power and control over their environment, *Intensive Crit Care Nurs* 20:190-199, 2004.

97. Hewitt-Taylor J: Children who require long-term ventilation: Staff education and training, *Intensive Crit Care Nurs* 20(2):93-102, 2004.

98. Chlan LL: Description of anxiety levels by individual differences and clinical factors in patients receiving mechanical ventilatory support, *Heart Lung* 32(4):275-282, 2003.

Chapter 27

Lymphatic System Disorders

Ahmed Samir Elokda

OBJECTIVES

After reading this chapter, the reader will be able to:
1. Understand the anatomy and the physiology of the lymphatic system.
2. Discuss the risk factors for pathologies associated with the consequences of lymphedema.
3. Apply the best methods and tools for examining a patient with lymphedema.
4. Understand how the disablement model and the *Guide to Physical Therapist Practice* are used to evaluate and diagnose a patient with lymphedema.
5. Use evidence-based interventions for patients with lymphedema.

*R*ehabilitation clinicians treat patients with a variety of systemic disorders, including disorders of the *lymphatic system*. This chapter discusses the rehabilitation of patients with lymphatic disorders who fall into the *Guide to Physical Therapist Practice* (the *Guide*)[1] preferred practice pattern 6H: Impaired circulation and anthropometric dimensions associated with lymphatic system disorders. Through discussion of anatomy and physiology of the lymphatic system, common classifications of lymphatic system disorders, and the examination, evaluation, and interventions for patients with lymphatic system disorders, this chapter will help practitioners understand and differentiate among lymphatic system disorders and provide them with the tools to effectively evaluate and treat patients presenting with disorders of the lymphatic system. Although the lymphatic system includes an immune function, *lymphedema* (which is caused by dysfunction of the lymphatic circulatory system) is the major focus of this chapter.

It is estimated that 250 million persons worldwide have lymphedema.[2] *Filariasis*, a disease involving infestation of the lymphatics with filarial worms, is the most common cause of lymphedema worldwide. The World Health Organization (WHO) estimates that 120 million people, including 40 million in Africa and 700,000 in the Americas, have lymphatic filariasis.[3] In the United States, however, lymphedema is usually iatrogenic and results from radiation and/or surgery used to treat breast cancer.[2] Among this population, 10% to 40% develop some degree of ipsilateral upper extremity lymphedema.[2]

Although lymphedema rarely impacts life expectancy, except when it affects the small intestine, if untreated or uncontrolled, it can impair quality of life by reducing mobility and activity and by predisposing the individual to infection.[4] Lymphedema can affect a person's quality of life, including activities of daily living, recreation, and work, and it is estimated that 30% of people with lymphedema in the upper extremities have reduced shoulder and/or arm function.[5-8]

THE LYMPHATIC CIRCULATORY SYSTEM

The lymphatic system has two main functions. It transports *lymph* from the periphery to the venous system to maintain fluid balance, and it serves an immune function, helping to protect the body from infection. The lymphatic system is made up of lymph (i.e., lymphatic fluid), *lymphatic vessels, lymph nodes,* and the lymphatic organs: The spleen, thymus, and tonsils (Fig. 27-1).[9]

Lymph is a fluid that originates from the blood plasma and enters the capillaries from the arteries. When blood enters the capillaries, some of the intercellular fluid diffuses out of the blood circulation. Approximately 90% of this fluid is reabsorbed by the venous system in the venous leg of the capillary loop. The remaining approximately 10% contains macromolecular proteins that cannot be reabsorbed by the venous system. This fluid and the proteins are returned to the circulation by the lymphatic system in the form of lymph.[9]

Lymph primarily contains proteins, immune cells, fat (which is present in intestinal lymph also known as *chyle*), and waste products. Lymph protects the body from foreign organisms and other materials by removing them from the interstitial fluid. Lymph tissue (the nodes and

organs) contains macrophages, B- and T-lymphocytes, plasma cells, and reticular cells. Substances typically removed via lymph and the lymphatic system include excess interstitial fluid and normal by-products of cellular processes.[9,10]

Although the lymphatic system transports fluid around the body it differs from the blood circulatory system in a number of ways as shown in Table 27-1.[10,11]

Lymph flows through lymph-specific capillaries that run through both superficial and deep tissues. Protein-rich lymph collects at lymph nodes that filter and produce components of lymph. The nodes produce lymphocytes, particularly when an immune reaction is required, and they regulate the protein content of lymph. The average person has about 650 lymph nodes located in clusters or chains around the lymphatic vessels (see Fig. 27-1). The size of lymph nodes can vary widely, from a few millimeters to 1-2 cm in diameter in their normal state and up to 8 cm in diameter, or more, when activated or diseased.[9]

A lymph node has a fibrous capsule on the outside, with a cortex surrounding the medulla on the inside (Fig. 27-2). The cortex is more densely structured than the medulla and is divided into two levels. The outer cortex contains B-lymphocytes, dendritic reticular cells, and macrophages, and the inner cortex, also known as the paracortex, contains T-lymphocytes and interdigitating reticular cells. All areas of the node are active in the immune response, engulfing and destroying invading bacteria, viruses, and other cellular debris.[9,11]

Lymph moves through the body powered by intrinsic and extrinsic pumping mechanisms. Intrinsic pumping is provided by spontaneous contraction of lymphatic vessels. If this intrinsic pump fails, lymphatic circulation depends on extrinsic pumping by skeletal muscles to compress the lymphatic vessels. Arterial pulsations, respiration, and massage may also contribute in a small way to lymph propulsion.[10] The lymphatic circulation is a one-way transport mechanism that moves fluid from the interstitium to the blood circulatory system.[11]

The spleen and thymus have supportive immune functions. The spleen produces some lymphocytes and also destroys defective red blood cells and blood-borne pathogens. The thymus is classified as one of the primary central lymphatic organs because it produces genetically imprinted T-lymphocytes prenatally until early adulthood. These T-lymphocytes participate in the humoral immune response and trigger development of other lymphatic organs. There are collectors at the base of the tonsils that collect lymphatic fluid from the area of the head and neck.[9,12]

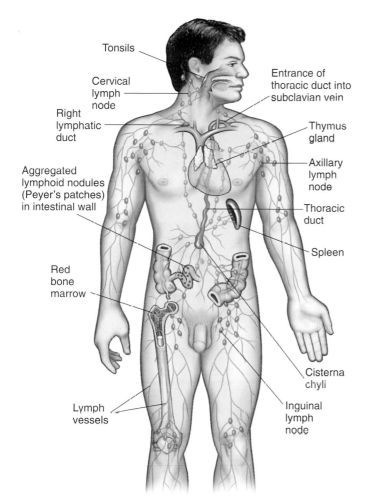

FIG. 27-1 The lymphatic system. *From Thibodeau GA, Patton KT:* Anatomy and Physiology, *ed 6, St. Louis, 2006, Mosby.*

TABLE 27-1	Differences Between Lymphatic and Blood Circulation	
	Lymph	**Blood**
Direction	One way	Circular
Flow	1-2 L/day	≈5 L/min
Pumping mechanism	Intrinsic contractions of lymph trunks	Separate pump (heart), calf muscle (second heart)
Continuity	No continuous column of fluid	Continuous column of fluid
Effect of dependency on pressure	None	Increases venous pressure
Effect of obstruction	Accumulation of high protein fluid (>1.5 g/dl)	Accumulation of low protein fluid (<1.0 g/dl)

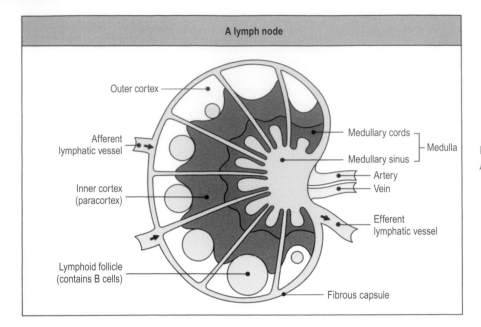

FIG. 27-2 A lymph node. *From Janeway C:* Immunobiology, *ed 5, New York, 2001, Garland Science.*

ANATOMY OF THE LYMPHATIC CIRCULATORY SYSTEM

The lymphatic circulatory system is made up of the lymphatic vessels and the lymph nodes. The vessels are organized into a superficial system (also known as subcutaneous or epifascial) and a deep system. The superficial system drains the cutis and subcutis, and the deep system drains lymph from the extremities, muscles, bones, joints, and viscera. Perforating vessels connect the two systems and can conduct lymph from the deep system to the superficial system.[9,13,14]

The superficial lymphatic circulatory system begins distally with very narrow vessels, the lymphatic capillaries. These are single-layered vessels made of endothelial cells, and they have no valves. All the lymphatic vessels beyond the capillaries have valves to prevent fluid backflow. The capillaries empty into precollectors, which originate in the interstitium just under the epidermis. The precollectors are medium-sized vessels made up of an inner endothelial layer surrounded by two layers of smooth muscle controlled by the autonomic nervous system. The precollectors flow into larger diameter vessels known as collectors, which divide into several branches and transport lymph to regional lymph nodes. From the nodes, the lymph enters larger diameter vessels, the lymphatic trunks.[9]

Capillaries → Precollectors → Collectors →
Lymph nodes → Lymphatic trunks =
Superficial lymphatic circulatory system

The deep lymphatic vessels run deep to the fascia, parallel to the major arteries and accompanying veins, and drain the muscles, bones, joints, and viscera of the entire body, except for the upper right quadrant and face. These vessels drain into deep lymph collectors that are similar to but wider than the superficial collectors, and the collectors then drain to lymph nodes and join with fluid from the superficial system to drain into the lymphatic trunks.[9,13,14] If the vessels or nodes of the deeper circulation are removed, all of the fluid may be forced to travel in the superficial circulation. This can lead to congestion, fluid extravasation, and edema.[9]

The lymph from the lower portion of the body collects in a dilated vessel in the lumbar region of the abdominal cavity, the cisterna chyli. The cisterna chyli extends for about 6 cm just to the right of the abdominal aorta and at the level of the twelfth thoracic vertebra it narrows to become the thoracic duct. Lymph from the rest of the body, except for the upper right quadrant, drains into the thoracic duct more cranially. The thoracic duct empties into the base of the left subclavian vein to be mixed with blood. Lymph from the lymphatic vessels in the upper right quadrant of the body empties into the right *lymphatic duct* and then into the base of the right subclavian vein (Fig. 27-3).

PHYSIOLOGY OF LYMPH TRANSPORT

The primary task of the lymphatic system is to transport interstitial fluid and its components from the interstitium back to the venous system. The balance of hydrostatic and colloidal osmotic pressure in the capillaries and interstitium allows this process to occur.[15]

The endothelial cells that make up the lymphatic capillaries overlap to form "swinging flaps" (Fig. 27-4). When the interstitial hydrostatic pressure exceeds the hydrostatic pressure inside the vessels the flaps open and fluid moves into the lymphatic capillaries. This is known as the filling phase.[16] When the pressure in the capillaries equals the interstitial pressure, the swinging flaps close and the lymphatic capillaries open to the precollectors, allowing lymph to flow into them. This is known as the emptying phase.[16] Once the protein-rich lymph is in the precollectors, the intrinsic and extrinsic pumps propel the lymph fluid to its final destination, the venous circulatory system.

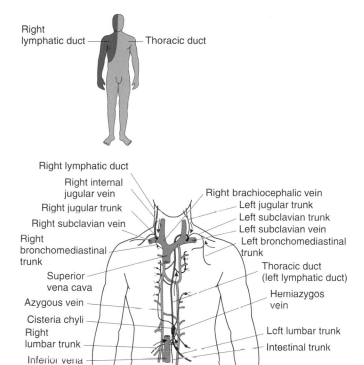

FIG. 27-3 Lymph drainage through the thoracic duct and the right lymphatic duct. *From Casley-Smith JR, Casley-Smith JR:* Modern Treatment for Lymphoedema, *ed 5, Adelaide, Australia, 1997, Lymphoedema Association of Australia. Inset from Goodman CC, Boissonnault WG, Fuller KS:* Pathology: Implications for the Physical Therapist, *2e, Philadelphia, 2003, Saunders.*

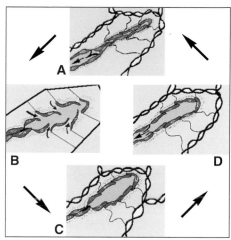

FIG. 27-4 Lymph formation. **A,** The initial lymph vessel is empty and collapsed. **B,** Filling phase. **C,** The initial lymph vessel is filled with lymph. **D,** The pressure inside the initial lymph vessels opens the valve to the precollector and thus the lymph flows toward the precollector. *Földi/Földi/Kubik: Lehrbuch der Lymphologie, 6th edition © Elsevier GmbH, Urban & Fischer Verlag München.*

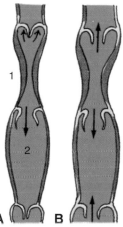

FIG. 27-5 Structure and function of the valve segments. **A,** Normal function. **B,** Dilated lymph vessel with valvular insufficiency and reflux. 1, Contracted segment (emptying phase). 2, Relaxed segment (filling phase). *Földi/Földi/Kubik: Lehrbuch der Lymphologie, 6th edition © Elsevier GmbH, Urban & Fischer Verlag München.*

PATHOLOGY

When functioning properly, anatomically and physiologically, the lymphatic circulatory system can accommodate a certain degree of variability in the amount interstitial fluids and large molecular weight substances it needs to transport from the periphery to the central venous system. It can increase its transport capacity by developing more collateral vessels as well as more lymphovenous anastomoses and lympholymphatic anastomoses, and it can accommodate more plasma proteins by producing more macrophages. If the lymphatic system becomes overloaded, due to an excessive increase in load or, more commonly, due to damage that limits its ability to accommodate, fluids and other substances may accumulate in the interstitium causing swelling known as lymphedema. As proteins in the accumulated fluid degrade, chronic inflammation and cell proliferation may then occur.

LYMPHEDEMA

Lymphedema is a symptom of lymphatic transport malfunction that occurs when the lymphatic load exceeds the transport capacity of the lymphatic circulatory system. Lymphedema presents clinically with swelling of the soft tissues because of accumulation of protein-rich fluid.

Once it occurs, lymphedema often progresses because the initial buildup of macromolecules in the interstitium causes an increase in interstitial oncotic pressure that "pulls" yet more fluid out of the vessels into the interstitium. The prolonged presence of swelling and proteins leads to inflammation and fibrosis and provides a suitable medium for repeated local infection of the lymph vessels *(lymphangitis)* and the surrounding soft tissues *(cellulitis).* Persistent dilatation of the lymphatics, in addition to incompetent valves, leads to further stagnation (Fig. 27-5). Lymphedema most commonly occurs in the extremities but can also occur in the face, neck, abdomen, and genitalia.

Lymphedema may be classified according to its etiology as primary (also known as idiopathic) or secondary.[4]

Primary Lymphedema. Primary lymphedema is a benign condition that is generally caused by malformation of the lymph vessels and/or lymph nodes. There may be aplasia (lack of development), hypoplasia (too few or too small), or hyperplasia (too many or too large) of any of the lymph vessels or nodes.[4] Primary lymphedema may be congenital (present at birth), or may be classified as lymphedema praecox if the onset is after birth but before the age of 35 years or as lymphedema tardum if the onset is after the age of 35. Lymphedema tardum is a primary benign condition that may develop when local inflammation from a musculoskeletal injury, local infection, or insect bite causes an increase in fluid load in a person with a congenital anatomical predisposition. However, lymphedema that develops in adulthood is more frequently secondary lymphedema associated with a malignancy.[4]

Secondary Lymphedema. Secondary lymphedema is lymphedema that occurs in the absence of any anatomical malformation. Secondary lymphedema may develop at any age and may be caused by a malignant tumor obstructing lymph flow, a traumatic injury such as a fracture or injury to tissue surrounding a normal lymphatic flow, or by filariasis (filarial worm infestation that damages the lymph nodes or lymphatic vessels). Iatrogenic lymphedema may also occur as the result of medical interventions such as radiation therapy or lymph node removal for treatment of cancer, particularly breast cancer.[4] Congenital secondary lymphedema can be caused by an anomalous hair floating in the amniotic fluid, wrapping around a limb, and constricting lymphatic flow from the fingers, toes, or genitalia.[4]

Other less common causes of secondary lymphedema include artificial lymphedema, which is self-inflicted by the patient applying a tourniquet to the extremity, causing venous and lymphatic congestion. In some cases, this has been combined with forceful bludgeoning of the extremity to induce an inflammatory response, thus increasing the rate of congestion.

Stages of Lymphedema. If lymphedema is not treated, it progresses through the following stages.

Stage 0. Stage 0 (latency/subclinical stage) lymphedema is characterized by reduction of the normal lymph transport capacity. During this stage, there is approximately 30% more fluid in the interstitium than normal and the patient may feel discomfort, heaviness, and aching in the affected limb, but there will be no measurable increase in volume.

Stage I. Stage I lymphedema (reversible lymphedema) is characterized by the presence of protein-rich edema and is associated with a measurable increase in volume. Stage I lymphedema causes the tissue to feel soft and doughy, and pitting edema, in which the skin remains indented for a few minutes after removal of firm finger pressure, is present. At this stage the edema is reversible. The edema may be visible and palpable at the end of a day, but it reduces or completely disappears with rest overnight or with elevation. Activity, heat, and humidity may cause or increase stage I lymphedema. Stemmer's sign, defined as the inability to lift the thickened cutaneous folds at the dorsum of the toes or fingers, is negative or borderline positive in stage I lymphedema (Fig. 27-6).[17]

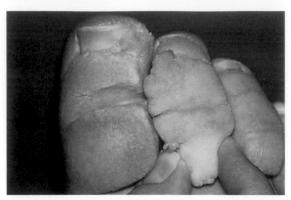

FIG. 27-6 Stemmer's sign. *From Browse N, Burnand K, Mortimer P:* Diseases of the Lymphatics, *London, 2003, Arnold.*

Stage II. Stage II lymphedema (spontaneously irreversible lymphedema) presents with increased volume, replacement of some of the protein-rich lymphatic fluid with tissue fibrosis, and a positive Stemmer's sign. The skin may thicken or break down, and there is a greater risk of recurrent infection because the lymph does not move. Pitting is also much more difficult to induce than with the stage I lymphedema because the tissue is stiffer and filled with more lymph fluid and interstitial fibrosis.[17]

Stage III. Stage III lymphedema (lymphostatic elephantiasis) is characterized by *subcutaneous fibrosclerosis* (hardening of the soft tissues under the skin) and severe skin alterations, including *hyperkeratosis* (a thickening of the outer layer of the skin) and papillomatosis (the development of numerous papillomas). In most but not all cases, there is more swelling in stage III lymphedema than in stage II.[17,18] Since grading is based on pathological and anatomical factors, a large volume does not necessarily imply a higher stage of lymphedema.

The stages of lymphedema are sequential, but their duration can vary and lymphedema may not progress through all the stages. Typically, tissue changes seen as lymphedema progresses or becomes more chronic include proliferation of connective tissue, increased production of collagen fibers, an increase in fatty deposits in the affected limb, and fibrotic changes.[16] Secondary skin changes can also occur in both primary and secondary lymphedema and may include development of cellulitis, hyperkeratosis, and fungal infections (Fig. 27-7).

EXAMINATION

PATIENT HISTORY

The history for any patient with lymphedema should cover patient demographics, including age, sex, and country or countries of residence, as these can influence the likelihood and underlying etiology of lymphedema, as well as its prognosis. In addition, one should obtain a complete medical history, asking specifically about any history of cancer. Since edema may have causes other than lymphatic dysfunction, if the cause of edema is unknown, the patient should also be asked about

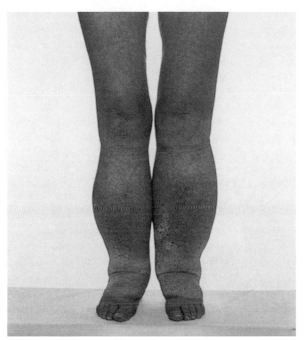

FIG. 27-7 Edema of both lower legs with early skin thickening and hyperkeratosis. *From Browse N, Burnand K, Mortimer P:* Diseases of the Lymphatics, *London, 2003, Arnold.*

any history of peripheral vascular, thyroid, renal, or cardiac disease, as well as any history of local surgery or trauma.

The progression, nature, and severity of the patient's edema should also be covered. This includes when the patient first noticed problems with the affected limb, including any sense of heaviness or swelling, how signs and symptoms have progressed, and the nature of the current signs and symptoms. One should determine if the patient has swelling, how severe it is, if it reverses with rest or overnight, and if there is pain, skin changes, or infection or any other associated problems.

Finally, the patient history should also cover the nature and degree of functional limitations caused by the lymphedema, as well as the nature and effectiveness of any compensation or intervention the patient has tried in order to reduce symptoms and optimize function.

SYSTEMS REVIEW

The systems review is used to target areas requiring further examination and to define areas that may cause complications or indicate a need for precautions during the examination and intervention processes. See Chapter 1 for details of the systems review.

TESTS AND MEASURES
Musculoskeletal

Anthropometric Characteristics. Edema is the most characteristic sign of lymphedema. Edema is generally measured by water displacement using a volumeter (see Fig. 18-10) or through circumferential measures with a flexible tape measure.[19] Results of these tests should be compared with the uninvolved limb and over time.

When using a volumeter, the same level surface should be used for all measurements in the same client, and extraneous movement should be minimized. The volumeter is filled with water until it overflows. The client should remove jewelry before immersing the limb in the volumeter. For the upper extremity, the hand is immersed until it rests lightly between the middle and ring fingers on the dowel inside the volumeter. For the lower extremity, the foot is positioned so that the medial border and heel of the immersed foot touch the sides of the volumeter. Chapter 18 contains information on the reliability and validity of this approach for measuring edema and limb volume.

Girth measurements taken with a flexible tape measure can also be used for documentation and comparison of edema. Girth measurements should be taken at consistent locations relative to anatomical landmarks for valid comparison between limbs and over time.

Both volumetric measurements and girth measurements have been shown to be reliable,[20,21] but the two methods cannot reliably be interchanged.[22] Thus clinicians should not substitute one measure or method for the other when calculating volume but should maintain the same measurement method for each measurement obtained.

Lymphedema may also be staged as stage 0 to stage III according to the descriptions provided earlier in this chapter.

Range of Motion. Range of motion (ROM) should be checked in all major joints in the affected and contralateral limb.

Muscle Performance. Since lymphedema can lead to disuse and thus generalized reduced strength in an affected limb, strength for movements in the primary planes of motion in the affected and contralateral limb should be estimated using manual muscle tests. More specific testing with isokinetic dynamometry or other tools is generally not indicated.

Neuromuscular

Pain. If the patient reports the presence of pain, one should determine its severity, nature, and location, as well as easing and aggravating factors (see Chapter 22 for pain measurement tools).

Sensory Integrity. Should the patient report sensory changes, including numbness or tingling, or if they have a secondary medical diagnosis associated with sensory changes, such as diabetes or peripheral vascular disease, sensory testing should be performed.

Cardiovascular/Pulmonary

Circulation. Physicians may use a number of methods to examine the anatomy and patency of the lymphatic circulation. These include *lymphangiography*, lymphoscintigraphy, computed tomography (CT) scan, magnetic resonance imaging (MRI), and Doppler ultrasound.

Lymphangiography is a radiographic method for examining the lymphatic vessels and nodes in which an oily contrast medium is injected into a lymphatic vessel in the foot or hand. This method formerly was the criterion standard for examining the anatomy and patency of the lymphatic system. However, because the contrast medium used for this technique can cause lymphatic endothelial inflammation, leading to scarring, atrophy, and even luminal obliteration, it has been replaced by other safer and less invasive techniques and is generally no longer used.

Lymphoscintigraphy, which involves the injection of a water-based radionuclide contrast material that does not damage the lymphatic tissues, has now largely replaced lymphangiography for imaging the lymphatic vessels. The radionuclide material is injected near a finger or toe of the affected limb and creates images of the lymph flow that define lymphatic anatomy and patency. This technique can also evaluate flow dynamics and direction and determine the severity of any obstructions.

CT and MRI are also occasionally recommended for delineating lymph node architecture. However, since these approaches are much more expensive than lymphoscintigraphy and provide little additional information about lymph circulation, they are reserved for cases where there is suspicion of malignancy and imaging of surrounding tissue is also needed.

Doppler ultrasound, which is used to evaluate blood flow in the veins, is sometimes used to evaluate flow in the lymphatics and is commonly used to evaluate for deep vein thrombosis when the cause of lower extremity edema is in question.

Integumentary

Integumentary Integrity. The skin in the affected area should be visually inspected and palpated. During the early stages of lymphedema the skin may thicken, obscuring milder swelling. With progression of lymphedema the skin will develop creases, horny scale, and hyperkeratosis and later, papillomas and then fibrosis.

Function

Gait, Locomotion, and Balance. When lymphedema affecting the lower extremity alters ROM and strength, gait and balance may also be affected and should therefore be examined (see Chapters 13 and 32) (Fig. 27-8).

EVALUATION, DIAGNOSIS, AND PROGNOSIS

Information from all aspects of the examination, including the patient history, systems review, and tests and measures, are interpreted together by the clinician to derive a treatment diagnosis. Patients falling into the preferred practice pattern 6H: Impaired circulation and anthropometric dimensions associated with lymphatic systems disorders, as described in the *Guide,*[1] typically have edema, impaired skin integrity, pain, and some limitation in their ability to perform functional tasks such as dressing. According to the *Guide,* 80% of patients in this preferred practice pattern can be expected to demonstrate optimal circulation and anthropometric dimensions and the highest level of functioning in home, work, community, and leisure environments over the course of 1-8 weeks of physical therapy intervention with 5-24 visits. A number of factors, including accessibility and availability

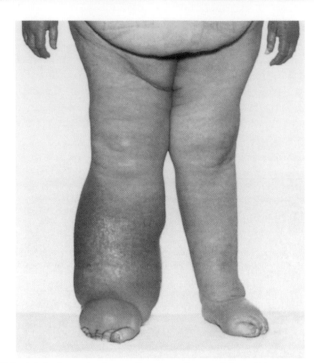

FIG. 27-8 Lymphedema that interferes with walking. *From Browse N, Burnand K, Mortimer P:* Diseases of the Lymphatics, *London, 2003, Arnold.*

of resources, adherence to interventions, age, chronicity and severity of the condition, comorbidities, level of impairment, decline in functional independence, living environment, overall health status, psychological and socioeconomic factors, and the amount of social support, may modify the frequency of visits or the duration of an episode of care. Patients may require multiple episodes of care for lymphedema management over their lifetime.

INTERVENTION

Interventions for patients with lymphedema focus on education and procedures to facilitate proximal flow of lymphatic fluid. Recommended procedural interventions include a variety of manual techniques, compression approaches, and exercise. Since all lymph fluid that returns from the interstitium ultimately enters the cardiovascular circulatory system, before initiating any lymphedema treatment the therapist should consider the potential consequences to the cardiopulmonary system if lymphatic drainage is successful. Patients with known or suspected cardiac involvement are at greatest risk for adverse effects of treatment because any lymphatic fluid that may be successfully removed from an edematous limb or body part will initially increase cardiac load. Furthermore, since the kidneys help to remove excess fluid from the circulatory system, in patients with reduced renal function, the additional circulatory load may overload the kidneys. If therapy is to be initiated, the patient's condition must be monitored for any untoward side effects that may suggest cardiac or renal overload. Should any new symptoms, particularly shortness of breath, chest pain, or diaphoresis, or changes in laboratory values (increased blood urea nitrogen or creatinine) indicating worsening kidney function, occur during treatment, the therapy should be immediately discontinued and the patient's physician contacted. Further interventions should be postponed until the patient is evaluated and cleared by the physician for further treatment.

Several other medical conditions are contraindications to certain components of lymphedema therapy. Patients with an infection, a blood clot, or malignancy in the involved limb should not receive compression or manual techniques because these may spread the problem through the circulatory system to other areas, most notably the heart and lungs.

EDUCATION

Patients with lymphedema are at risk for a worsening of their condition and for a number of complications, particularly infection. Therefore patients with lymphedema should be instructed to observe the following precautions.[23] Since lymphedema in most patients results from an irreversible anatomical change, these precautions will generally need to be observed for the patient's lifetime.

- No blood pressure measurements on the involved extremity.
- No needle sticks or blood draws on the involved extremity.
- All wounds on the affected limb, no matter how small (e.g., insect bites, paper cuts, hangnail, etc), should be treated immediately.
- Protect the hands and feet of the involved extremities from mechanical trauma and burns at all times.
- Avoid constricting jewelry and clothing.
- Avoid overheating local body parts or rise in core body temperature.
- Avoid lifting heavy objects; no heavy handbags with over-the-shoulder straps.

Education may be provided verbally or in the form of written materials, including pamphlets or brochures.

PROCEDURES

The treatment of lymphedema can be difficult, costly, and time consuming and is generally best performed by a multidisciplinary team.[21-28] Procedures for the management of lymphedema include surgical and pharmacological interventions, as well as manual procedures typically performed by a physical or occupational therapist.

Surgical Interventions. There are two general types of surgery for lymphedema, debulking (reduction surgery), which involves removing excess fluid and tissues, and physiological procedures that attempt to improve lymphatic circulation. Evidence indicates that debulking procedures are associated with significant adverse effects, including infection and poor wound healing, and these are therefore rarely performed.[29,30] Although physiological procedures are not associated with such adverse effects, their effectiveness is also limited.

Pharmacological Interventions. A number of pharmacological interventions have been suggested as adjunctive measures for the management of lymphedema. Coumarin (1,2-benzopyrone or 5,6-benzo-[alpha]-pyrone) (not related to the anticoagulant Coumadin) gained some popularity in the 1980s when some studies suggested that

it helped to reduce lymphedema by stimulating proteolysis by macrophages and by increasing the number of macrophages within the affected site.[31] Use of this medication has since fallen out of favor because it was only found to be effective in a few studies[32,33] and there were reports of abnormal liver function tests in up to 6% of treated patients.[34] The long-term effects of coumarin treatment are not known. Antibiotics are often used to treat acute and chronic infections associated with lymphedema, including cellulitis and lymphangitis. Some have suggested that diuretics be used to treat the fluid retention associated with lymphedema; however, since the fluid is not within the vessels, this is generally not effective.[35]

Manual Interventions. Although a number of manual therapy approaches have been recommended for the treatment of lymphedema, the approach with the greatest support at this time is complete decongestive physical therapy (CDPT). This approach is divided into two phases.

The first phase, also known as the intensive phase, involves meticulous skin care, manual lymph drainage (MLD), bandaging, and exercises with the bandage on. Ideally, during this phase, treatment should be provided twice a day for 4-6 weeks. At the end of the phase, when the edema is under control, the patient should be fitted with a compression garment.

During the second phase, also known as the self-management phase, the patient performs his or her own skin care and MLD and applies a custom-sized compression garment during the day and wears a bandage at night. During this phase, the patient may perform exercises wearing the bandage or the compression garment.

Meticulous skin care is the cornerstone of both phases of CDPT. This involves careful cleansing and the application of low-pH lotions and emollients to keep the skin supple.[36-38] Careful drying, particularly in areas of creases, is also essential to avoid topical fungal and bacterial overgrowth and infection.[39-43]

MLD is a generic term for the massage used to reduce lymphedema. MLD techniques gained popularity in the United States in the 1990s as reports of their effectiveness emerged.[44] Vodder, a massage therapist by training, is credited as being the first to directly massage the chronically enlarged lymph node in an attempt to decrease its size.[45] Michael and Ethel Földi followed up on this work in their clinic, where they successfully reduced lymphedema and maintained its reduction using MLD techniques.[46-48]

MLD massage is intended to increase the movement of lymph and interstitial fluid. The basic hand positions used for MLD are based on the anatomy and function of the lymphatic system. The approach involves combining a number of strokes, described as stationary circles, pumping, scooping, and rotary strokes. Each stroke consists of a working (stretching) and resting phase, where the pressure smoothly increases and decreases, respectively. Each stroke lasts at least 1 second and is repeated 5-7 times, and all strokes are applied in the direction of lymph flow. When there is congestion or obstruction caused by surgery, trauma, or radiation, strokes are applied toward the intact lymphatic pathways. The most proximal areas, which are those closest to the venous angle where the lymphatics enter the venous system, should be treated first to clear the way for drainage from more distal areas. Thus, when treating lymphedema in the extremities, treatment begins proximally and continues distally. In general, each session lasts 40-90 minutes. MLD should not be performed in patients with acute kidney infections or renal failure, those with edema caused by heart failure, deep venous thrombosis (DVT), or pregnant women.

Most of the studies evaluating the effectiveness of MLD have been carried out on patients with secondary lymphedema caused by breast cancer treatment (Table 27-2). Overall, these studies have found that MLD significantly reduces excess limb volume, as well as pain, discomfort, heaviness, fullness, and hardness of the affected limb. MLD is most effective when used in conjunction with compression bandaging and garments, exercise, and skin care. Unfortunately, most of the research on MLD is of low quality (rated level III or lower). Additional higher quality studies are needed to provide strong evidence-based recommendations for treatment.

Compression

Pneumatic Compression Pumping. Compression is applied by surrounding a limb with a device that can apply inwardly-directed pressure. A variety of pneumatic devices may be used to apply compression for the treatment of extremity lymphedema.[53] A number of studies have shown that pneumatic compression pumping can produce positive clinical outcomes, including reduced girth and discomfort and improved function.[54-61] However, the use of pneumatic compression for the treatment of lymphedema is controversial, with some authors claiming that it is ineffective and that it worsens or accelerates the fibrosis associated with lymphedema.[62-64] Segers and colleagues contend that there is disagreement about the effect of compressive therapies because different amounts of pressure have different positive and adverse effects and because the pressure meters on pneumatic compression devices are often inaccurate.[65]

Some pneumatic compression devices use single-chamber sleeves, whereas others have multichambered, sequentially-inflating sleeves that allow pumping to

TABLE 27-2	Studies Evaluating Effectiveness of Manual Lymphatic Drainage			
Study Design	Level of Evidence	Subjects (Sample Size)	Outcome/Intervention	Summary of Results (Conclusions and Implications)
Qualitative design[49]	III	Persons with cancer-related lymphedema who had completed a 3-week course of MLD treatment (6).	Interviews were conducted and transcribed. Common themes were identified.	Themes identified included response to MLD treatment, experience of relaxation during MLD, and resources involved in the provision of MLD treatment.
Cross-sectional study[7]	III	Breast cancer survivors treated in Vermont (148).	Respondents were asked if they felt increased swelling, numbness, pain, or decreased function. Pain and shoulder function were rated on a 10-point scale.	63% of respondents had numbness. 35% had swelling. 40% had pain. 30% had decreased shoulder/arm function.
Cross-sectional study[50]	III	40 women with lymphedema and 10 physicians that treat lymphedema (50).	This study identified knowledge about and treatment received for lymphedema in breast cancer survivors.	60% of women received pamphlets from their health care providers. Most women receiving treatment reported using multiple therapies.
Randomized controlled trial[51]	I	Participants were drawn from a lymphedema treatment center in a large cancer hospital (31).	Group A received 3 weeks of daily MLD followed by 6 weeks without treatment, then 3 weeks of SLD. Group B received 3 weeks of SLD followed by 6 weeks without treatment and then 3 weeks of MLD.	MLD reduced limb volume and dermal thickness. SLD produced a nonsignificant reduction in limb volume. MLD improved emotional function, pain, and heaviness in affected extremities.
Single subject study[52]	III	60-year-old woman with postmastectomy lymphedema of the left upper extremity (1).	The subject was seen 3 × week for 8 weeks. The first 4 weeks the subject received CDPT with MLD and the second 4 weeks the subject received CDPT without MLD.	The results showed a greater decrease in edema when MLD was used with CDPT. There was also a greater increase in function when MLD was used.

MLD, Manual lymphatic drainage; *SLD,* simple lymphatic drainage; *CDPT,* complete decongestive physical therapy.

progress from distal to proximal.[66] Multichambered sleeves are thought to be more effective because they can pump fluid progressively more proximally. Although no studies have directly compared these different types of sleeves, there is a report of a multichambered sleeve being effective in a patient with lymphedema who previously failed to respond to treatment with a single-chamber sleeve.[55]

The recommended treatment parameters for pneumatic compression are 30 seconds of compression followed by a 5-second rest period for the upper extremity or a 10-second rest period for the lower extremity, with pressure of 45 mm Hg for the upper extremity, 60 mm Hg for the lower extremity during compression, and at or near 0 mm Hg during the rest period to allow the vessels to refill.[66] Treatment sessions should initially last 20 minutes, and patients should be closely monitored for any adverse reactions, particularly numbness or tingling because of compression of sensory nerves or systemic side effects because of fluid overload. If no complications arise, treatment duration may be increased by 10 minutes per day up to a maximum of 1 hour.[66] A second session may be added if patient improvement continues.[66]

There are a number of precautions and contraindications for pneumatic compression pumping. Precautions to treatment are the following:

- Decreased sensation in the proposed treatment area.
- Pain, redness, numbness, or tingling in the extremity after treatment.
- Lymphatic vessel dilation or becoming visible during or after treatment.
- Increase in swelling proximal to the sleeve.
- Changes in skin texture at the base of the limb.

If any of these occur during treatment, the treatment should be modified or discontinued.

Contraindications to pneumatic compression therapy are the following:[63,68,69]

- Brachial plexus lesions.
- Radical breast surgery with radiation.
- Bilateral mastectomy.
- After pelvic surgery, if proximal portions of lower extremities have begun to swell.
- Primary lymphedema.
- Swelling present in abdomen or genitalia.
- Lymphatic vessel dilated or visible before treatment.
- Lower extremity ankle brachial index (ABI) of <0.8 (see Chapter 29).
- Suspected DVT in the limb.
- Infection in the limb.
- Malignancy in the limb or proximal to the limb to be treated.
- Ongoing radiation therapy for active cancer in the limb or surrounding area.
- Renal or cardiac insufficiency.
- Uncontrolled hypertension.

Compressive Bandaging. Compressive bandaging should be applied using short-stretch bandage materials that generate low resting pressures and high working pressures. Resting pressure is the constant pressure exerted by a bandage when the individual is at rest and not moving. The more elastic a bandage is, and the more initial tension applied to it, the more resting pressure it will exert. Working pressure is the pressure that is exerted when muscles inside a compressive bandage attempt to expand as a result of active contraction. This active muscle contraction increases the pressure in the tissue if the tissue is wrapped by a bandage. The more rigid (less compliant) the bandage material is, the more working pressure will develop in response to an active muscle contraction.

The amount of pressure exerted by a compression bandage is generally expressed in millimeters of mercury (mm Hg). Compression bandages should be applied so that they create a pressure gradient, with more compression distally than proximally. An appropriate pressure gradient will generally be produced by wrapping a bandage with equal tension all the way up. This gradient occurs because, according to Laplace's law (Pressure = Tension/Radius), if tension is kept constant when a bandage is applied to a limb that increases in radius, as happens when going from the foot to the ankle and then up the calf, less pressure will be exerted proximally than distally. This will facilitate movement of fluid from the distal foot and ankle complex in a proximal direction. A bandage should be applied concentrically, with equal tension, and overlapping and slipping bandages should be avoided.

Clinically, one type of bandage or multiple layers of different types of bandages may be used. Multilayer bandaging allows one to take advantage of different properties of different types of bandages, with some exerting more resting pressure and others exerting more working pressure (Fig. 27-9). Several layers of nonextensible bandages will generate higher working pressures while maintaining lower resting pressures.[69] Multilayer bandaging has claimed to reverse skin changes, stop lymphorrhea (the light amber-colored fluid that drains from open skin areas), and soften underlying fibrosis; however, its clinical efficacy has not been demonstrated in randomized controlled trials.[69]

Compression Garments. Compression garments may also be used for compression therapy and have been shown to effectively reduce lymphedema.[68,71] Garments are available for various body parts, including the legs, arms, and trunk, and are available in different sizes and amounts of compression. Compression garments may be ready-made or custom-fit. The therapist must follow manufacturer recommendations for measuring patients for custom-fit garments to ensure proper fit and effective treatment.

The lightest compression garment is the surgical antiembolism stocking. This garment provides up to 17 mm Hg of compression and is only suitable for prevention of thromboses or emboli in immobile patients and not for the treatment of lymphedema.[70] Compression stockings suitable for the treatment of edema are available in four classes of compression and can be used in combination to exert even more pressure. Although recommendations vary, in general, 30 mm Hg of compression is appropriate for the upper extremity and 80 mm Hg is appropriate for the lower extremity.[24,62,67,71-73] The compression class, degree of compression, pressure provided, and indications

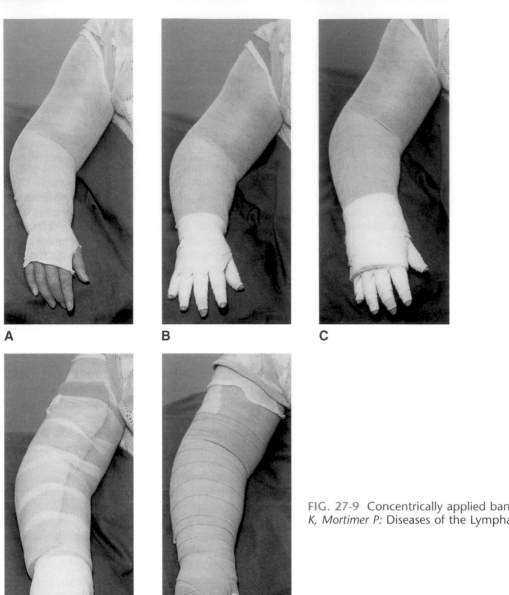

A   **B**   **C**

D   **E**

FIG. 27-9 Concentrically applied bandage. *From Browse N, Burnand K, Mortimer P:* Diseases of the Lymphatics, *London, 2003, Arnold.*

for use for different compression garments are described in Table 27-3.

EXERCISE

Exercise is another essential component of CDPT. Exercise is thought to reduce lymphedema because skeletal muscle contraction increases pressure around the lymphatics, helping to push fluid proximally.[74] Exercise may also increase lymph vessel contraction, improve lymph circulation, enhance fluid transport by the thoracic duct by increasing deep breathing, and help to normalize intersti-

tial hydrostatic pressure.[37,75-79] Furthermore, exercise may help reduce ROM restrictions and weakness caused by disuse of the involved extremity.[74] Exercises of the involved extremity should initially be performed while wearing compressive bandaging.[80] As the lymphedema begins to subside, the exercises should be continued while wearing compressive garments. It is suggested that limitations to mobility and muscular weakness be treated along with the lymphedema so the entire muscle chain and all associated joints can recover and be incorporated into the regimen of decongestive exercise therapy. Exercise for

TABLE 27-3	Compression Garments	
Compression Class	Degree of Compression	Pressure Provided
Antiembolism	Very light	Up to 17 mm Hg
1	Light	18-21 mm Hg
2	Medium	23-32 mm Hg
3	Strong	34-46 mm Hg
4	Very strong	>49 mm Hg

Földi/Földi/Kubik: *Lehrbuch der Lymphologie,* 6th edition © Elsevier GmbH, Urban & Fischer Verlag München.

the patient with lymphedema should include a warm-up of stretching followed by strengthening, endurance, and coordination activities, as well as breathing exercises.[28,69,78,81,82]

CASE STUDY 27-1

EARLY STAGE I SECONDARY LYMPHEDEMA

Examination
Patient History
JS is a 65-year-old obese man who was referred to outpatient cardiac rehabilitation 3 weeks after a 3-vessel coronary artery bypass graft (CABG). His other medical problems include peripheral vascular disease, insulin-dependent diabetes mellitus, hypercholesterolemia, hyperlipidemia, and hypertension. His surgical history includes a femoral-popliteal bypass of the right lower extremity 4 months ago. The patient reported that he recently developed swelling of the lower extremities, abdomen, and scrotum. The lower extremity edema reduced slightly with elevation but returned rapidly after the legs were lowered. JS also has a nonhealing wound on the medial aspect of his left lower leg that has been present for more than 3 years and that did not improve with conventional wound care. Since JS does not have heart failure, his physician suspected that his swelling was caused by secondary lymphedema, as a result of removal of his saphenous vein and thus lymphatic overload, and referred him to a therapist for conservative management. The patient's medications are insulin, metoprolol (a beta-blocker), and lisinopril (an angiotensin-converting enzyme [ACE] inhibitor).

Systems Review
Heart rate is 68 bpm and blood pressure is 160/90 mm Hg. JS is 5 feet 9 inches tall and weighs 260 lb.

Tests and Measures
Musculoskeletal
Anthropometric Measures Edema was present in both legs. Girth was 15 inches around both ankles and 25 inches around both knees. Stemmer's sign was positive bilaterally.

Range of Motion JS has fair trunk and hip ROM but limited active and passive ROM at the knees and ankles.

Muscle Performance Strength was grossly 4–/5 in the upper extremities and 4/5 in the lower extremities.

Neuromuscular
Pain JS reported pain at level of 5/10 in his low back and lower extremities that reduced with rest and elevation of the lower extremities.

Cardiovascular/Pulmonary
Circulation Capillary refill at the nail beds of the toes and pedal pulses were minimally reduced.

Integumentary
Integumentary Integrity Pitting was easy to induce at the distal lower extremities. The skin on both legs appeared tight and shiny. Apart from the wound on the medial aspect of the left lower leg, JS has no skin infections in the large skin folds or nail fungus. The chest and leg incisions were clean with mild serosanguineous fluid draining from the leg incision.

Function
Gait, Locomotion, and Balance JS has fair dynamic and static sitting and standing balance. He walks with a slightly waddling gait because of his obesity and lower extremity swelling and weakness.

Self-Care and Home Management JS's abdominal, scrotal, and lower extremity edema causes difficulty with donning clothes, toileting, and sitting. He requires assistance for transfers because of the additional energy demand.

Assistive and Adaptive Devices JS uses a straight cane when walking.

Evaluation, Diagnosis, and Prognosis
JS's edema, impaired skin integrity, pain, and limitations in his ability to perform functional tasks are consistent with the preferred practice pattern 6H: Impaired circulation and anthropometric dimensions associated with lymphatic systems disorders. He is anxious to begin his treatment and understands the effort he will need to exert to achieve an optimal outcome.

Goals
JS wants to decrease his lower extremity and back pain, increase his mobility into and out of the tub and shower, be able to fit into normal clothing without making alterations, and decrease the size of his legs.

Prognosis
JS is likely to achieve good edema resolution and functional recovery with 8 weeks of intensive CDPT.

Plan of Care
Compression, MLD, and cardiovascular conditioning exercise.

Intervention
JS received treatment, including meticulous skin care, MLD, compression bandaging and exercise, 3 times per week for

8 weeks (a total of 24 sessions). Between therapy sessions, JS bandaged himself independently and performed a home exercise program. At the end of the 8 weeks, when his girth measurements plateaued, JS was measured for a full pantyhose compression garment with open toes to wear during the day and was instructed to bandage at night.

ADDITIONAL RESOURCES

Lymphedema Therapist Training Programs

- *Academy of Lymphatic Studies*
Web site: www.acols.com
Home office: Sebastian, FL
Telephone: 772-589-3355
Fax: 772-589-0306

- *Boris-Lasinski School*
Home office: Woodbury, Long Island, NY
Telephone: 516-364-2200
Fax: 516-364-1844

- *Casley-Smith Courses in the United States*
Home office: Decatur, GA
Telephone: 404-377-9883 ext 2
Fax: 404-377-9336
E-mail: CLTcourses@cs.com

- *Dr. Vodder School–North America*
Web site: www.vodderschool.com
Home Office: Victoria, British Columbia, Canada
Telephone: 250-598-9862 or 800-522-9862
Fax: 250-598-9841

- *Klose Training & Consulting, LLC*
Web site: www.klosetraining.com
Home office: Red Bank, NJ
Telephone: 732-530-7888 or 866-621-7888
Fax: 732-530-2802

- *The Lymphedema Consultants*
Home office: Pittsburgh, PA
Telephone: 412-364-3720
Fax: 412-364-3119
E-mail: tlc.consultants@verizon.net

- *The Norton School of Lymphatic Therapy*
Web site: www.nortonschool.com
Home office: Red Bank, NJ
Telephone: 732-842-4414 or 866-445-9674 (44LYMPH)
Fax: 732-842-5299

- *The Upledger Institute*
Web site: www.upledger.com
Home office: Palm Beach Gardens, FL
Telephone: 561-622-4334
Fax: 561-622-4771

Lymphedema-Related Links

Lymphology Association of North America (LANA): www.clt-lana.org/
International Society of Lymphology: www.u.arizona.edu/~witte/ISL.htm
Updated ISL Consensus Document: www.u.arizona.edu/~witte/2003consensus.pdf
Lymphedema Association of Quebec: www3.sympatico.ca/rachelp
Lymphovenous Canada: www.lymphovenous-canada.com
The Lymphatic Research Foundation: www.lymphaticresearch.org
Nederlands Lymfoedeem Netwerk: www.lymfoedeem.nl
Dutch Lymphedema Physiotherapist Association: www.nvfl.nl
Lymphoedema Association of Australia: www.lymphoedema.org.au
British Lymphology Society: www.lymphoedema.org

Lymphedema Organization of Sweden: http://user.tninet.se/~kwn630i/index.html

Breast Cancer–Related Links

The Susan G. Komen Breast Cancer Foundation: www.komen.org
National Breast Cancer Coalition: www.natlbcc.org
NABCO: www.nabco.org
Y-Me: www.y-me.org
The Breast Cancer Alliance: www.breastcanceralliance.org
Community Breast Health Project: www-med.stanford.edu/CBHP
Breast Cancer Answers: www.canceranswers.org

Primary Lymphedema–Related Links

National Association for Rare Disorders (NORD): www.rarediseases.org
University of Pittsburgh, Department of Human Genetics: www.pitt.edu/AFShome/g/e/genetics/public/html/lymph/

GLOSSARY

Cellulitis: Diffuse acute inflammation of the skin and subcutaneous tissue.

Chyle: The cloudy liquid product of digestion taken up by the small intestine, consisting mostly of emulsified fat. Chyle passes from the small intestine to the lymphatic system for transport to the venous circulation.

Filariasis: Disease caused by the presence of parasitic worms that occlude the lymphatic channels.

Hyperkeratosis: A condition marked by thickening of the outer layer of the skin that can result from normal use, chronic inflammation or genetic disorders.

Lymph: The fluid that is collected from tissue throughout the body and that moves through the lymphatic vessels. Most of the cells in lymph are lymphocytes.

Lymph nodes: Small bean-shaped bodies located along the course of lymphatic vessels. Lymph nodes produce lymphocytes and monocytes. They act as filters keeping particulate matter, such as bacteria, from gaining entrance into the bloodstream.

Lymphangiography (lymphography): The x-ray examination of lymph glands and lymphatic vessels after an injection of contrast medium.

Lymphangitis: Inflammation of one or more lymphatic vessels.

Lymphatic ducts: Terminal lymph vessels that convey lymph to the bloodstream.

Lymphatic system: The tissues and organs (including the bone marrow, spleen, thymus, and lymph nodes) that produce and store cells that fight infection and the network of vessels that carry lymph.

Lymphatic vessels: A body-wide network of channels that transports lymph to the immune organs and into the bloodstream.

Lymphedema: A disorder characterized by swelling caused by accumulation of lymph in soft tissues.

Subcutaneous fibrosclerosis: Hardening below the skin caused by abnormal formation of fibrous tissue.

References

1. American Physical Therapy Association: Guide to Physical Therapist Practice, second edition, *Phys Ther* 81:9-744, 2001.
2. Humble CA: Lymphedema: Incidence, pathophysiology, management, and nursing care, *Oncol Nurs Forum* 22(10):1503-1509, 1995.
3. World Health Organization: Sixth meeting of the Technical Advisory Group on the global elimination of lymphatic filariasis, Geneva, Switzerland, 20-23 September 2005, *Weekly Epidemiol Rec* 80(46):401-408, 2005.
4. Földi M, Földi E: Lymphostatic diseases. In Földi M, Földi E, Kubik S: *Textbook of Lymphology for Physicians and Lymphedema Therapists,* Munich, 2003, Urban & Fischer.
5. Andersen L, Hojris I, Erlandsen M, et al: Treatment of breast-cancer-related lymphedema with or without manual lymphatic drainage, *Acta Oncologica* 39(3):399-405, 2000.

6. Johansson K, Albersson M, Ingvar C, et al: Effects of compression bandaging with or without manual lymph drainage treatment in patients with postoperative arm lymphedema, *Lymphology* 32:103-110, 1999.

7. Bosompra K, Ashikaga T, O'Brien P, et al: Swelling, numbness, pain, and their relationship to arm function among breast cancer survivors: A disablement process model perspective, *Breast J* 8(6):338-348, 2002.

8. Velanovich V, Szymanski W: Quality of life of breast cancer patients with lymphedema, *Am J Surg* 177:184-188, 1999.

9. Kubik S: Anatomy of the lymphatic system. In Földi M, Földi E, Kubik S: *Textbook of Lymphology for Physicians and Lymphedema Therapists*, Munich, 2003, Urban & Fischer.

10. Levick JR, McHale N: The physiology of lymph production and propulsion. In Browse N, Burnand K, Mortimer P: *Diseases of the Lymphatics*, London, 2003, Arnold.

11. Guyton AC, Hall JE: *Textbook of Medical Physiology*, ed 11, Philadelphia, 2005, WB Saunders.

12. Kaiserling E: Lymphatic tissue and its vessel systems. In Földi M, Földi E, Kubik S: *Textbook of Lymphology for Physicians and Lymphedema Therapists*, Munich, 2003, Urban & Fischer.

13. Weissleder H, Schuchhardt C: Anatomy fundamentals. In Weissleder H, Schuchhardt C: *Lymphedema Diagnosis and Therapy*, ed 3, Köln, 2001, Viavital Verlag.

14. Kelly DG: *A Primer on Lymphedema*, Upper Saddle River, NJ, 2002, Prentice Hall.

15. Weissleder H, Schuchhardt C: Physiology fundamentals. In Weissleder H, Schuchhardt C: *Lymphedema Diagnosis and Therapy*, ed 3, Köln, 2001, Viavital Verlag.

16. Földi M, Földi E: Physiology and pathophysiology of the lymphatic system. In Földi M, Földi E, Kubik S: *Textbook of Lymphology for Physicians and Lymphedema Therapists*, Munich, 2003, Urban & Fischer.

17. Weissleder H: Examination methods. In Weissleder H, Schuchhardt C: *Lymphedema Diagnosis and Therapy*, ed 3, Köln, 2001, Viavital Verlag.

18. Weissleder H, Schuchhardt C: Pathophysiology fundamentals. In Weissleder H, Schuchhardt C: *Lymphedema Diagnosis and Therapy*, ed 3, Köln, 2001, Viavital Verlag.

19. DeVore GL, Hamilton GF: Volume measure of the severely injured hand, *Am J Occup Ther* 22:16-18, 1968.

20. Waylett-Rendell J, Seibly DS: A study of the accuracy of a commercially available volumeter, *J Hand Ther* 4:10-13, 1991.

21. Whitnet SL, Mattocks L, Irrgang JJ, et al: Reliability of lower extremity girth measurements and right- and left-side differences, *J Sports Rehabil* 4:108-115, 1995.

22. Karges JR, Mark BE, Stikeleather SJ, et al: Concurrent validity of upper extremity volume estimates: Comparison of calculated volume derived from girth measurements and water displacement volume, *Phys Ther* 83:134-145, 2003.

23. Goodman CC: The cardiovascular system. In Goodman CC, Boissonnault WG: *Pathology: Implications for the Physical Therapist*, Philadelphia, 1998, WB Saunders.

24. Grabois M: Breast cancer. Postmastectomy lymphedema. State of the art review, *Phys Med Rehabil Rev* 8:267-277, 1994.

25. Brennan MJ: Lymphedema following the surgical treatment of breast cancer: A review of pathophysiology and treatment, *J Pain Symp Manage* 7(2):110-116, 1992.

26. Levinson SF: Rehabilitation of the patient with cancer or human immunodeficiency virus. In Dellisa JA (ed): *Rehabilitation Medicine Principles and Practice*, ed 2, Philadelphia, 1993, JB Lippincott.

27. Nelson PA: Rehabilitation of patients with lymphedema. In Kottke FJ, Lehmann JF (eds): *Krusen's Handbook of Physical Medicine and Rehabilitation*, ed 4, Philadelphia, 1990, WB Saunders.

28. Brennan MJ, Depomopolo RW, Garden FH: Focused review: Postmastectomy lymphedema, *Arch Phys Med Rehabil* 77:S74-80, 1996.

29. Savage RC: The surgical management of lymphedema (review), *Surg Gynecol Obstet* 160(3):283-290, 1985.

30. Savage RC: The surgical management of lymphedema (review), *Surg Gynecol Obstet* 159(5):501-508, 1984.

31. Pillar NV, Morgan RG, Casley-Smith JR: A double-blind, cross-over trial of 0-(beta-hydroxy-ethyl)-rutoside (benzopyrene) in the treatment of the arms and legs, *Br J Plast Surg* 41(1):20-27, 1988.

32. Casley-Smith JR, Morgan RG, Piller NB: Treatment of lymphedema of the arms and legs with 5,6-benzo-[alpha]-pyrone, *N Engl J Med* 329(16):1158-1163, 1993.

33. Loprinzi CL, Sloan J, Kugler J: Lack of effect of coumarin in women with lymphedema after treatment for breast cancer, *N Engl J Med* 340:346-350, 1999.

34. Loprinzi CL, Sloan J, Kugler J: Coumarin-induced hepatotoxicity, *J Clin Oncol* 15(9):3167-3168, 1997.

35. Garden FH, Gillis TA: Principles of cancer rehabilitation. In Braddon RL (ed): *Physical Medicine and Rehabilitation*, Philadelphia, 1996, WB Saunders.

36. Földi E, Földi M, Weissleder H: Conservative treatment of lymphedema of the limbs, *Angiology* 36(3):171-180, 1985.

37. Mallon EC, Ryan TJ: Lymphedema and wound healing, *Clin Dermatol* 12:89-93, 1994.

38. Ko D, Lerner R, Klose G, et al: Effective treatment of lymphedema of the extremities, *Arch Surg* 133:452-458, 1998.

39. Ohkuma M: Cellulitis seen in lymphedema. In Nishi M, Uchino S, Yabuki S (eds): *Progress in Lymphology XII*, Amsterdam, 1990, Elsevier.

40. Ohkuma M: Mycotic infection in lymphedema. In Cluzan RV, Pecking AP, Lokiec FM (eds): *Progress in Lymphology XIII*, Amsterdam, 1992, Elsevier.

41. Thiadens SRJ: A study of infection in 353 lymphedema patients and antibiotic therapy. In Cluzan RV, Pecking AP, Lokiec FM (eds): *Progress in Lymphology XIII*, Amsterdam, 1992, Elsevier.

42. Olszewski WL, Jamal S, Dworczynski A, et al: Bacteriological studies of skin, tissue and fluid and lymph in filial lymphedema, *Lymphology* 27(suppl):345-348, 1994.

43. Bedna K, Svestkova S: Incidence rate of recurrent erysipelas in our lymphoedema patients, *Lymphology* 27(suppl):519-522, 1994.

44. Boris M, Weindorf S, Lasinkski S, et al: Persistence of lymphedema reduction after noninvasive complex lymphedema therapy, *Oncology* 11:99, 1997.

45. Wittlinger H: *Textbook of Dr. Vodder's Manual Lymph Drainage*, vol 1, ed 4, Brussels, 1992, Haug International.

46. Földi E: Comprehensive lymphedema treatment center, *Lymphology* 27:505-507, 1994.

47. Anonymous: The diagnosis and treatment of peripheral lymphedema, *Lymphology* 28:113-117, 1995.

48. Földi M: Treatment of lymphedema, *Lymphology* 27:1-5, 1994.

49. Woods M: The experience of manual lymph drainage as an aspect of treatment for lymphoedema, *Int J Palliat Nurs* 9(8):336-342, 2003.

50. Paskett ED, Stark N: Lymphedema: Knowledge, treatment, and impact among breast cancer survivors, *Breast J* 6(6):373-378, 2000.

51. Williams AF, Vadgama A, Franks PJ, et al: A randomized controlled crossover study of manual lymphatic drainage therapy in women with breast cancer related lymphoedema, *Eur J Cancer Care* 11:254-261, 2002.

52. Aldridge R, Clifft J: Effect of manual lymphatic drainage on edema and function in a patient with postmastectomy lymphedema, *J Sec Women's Health* 26(1):25-33, 2002.

53. Swedborg I: Effects of treatment with an elastic sleeve and intermittent pneumatic compression in postmastectomy patients with lymphedema of the arm, *Scand J Rehab Med* 9:131, 1984.

54. Bunce IH, Mirolo BR, Hennessey JM, et al: Post-mastectomy lymphedema treatment and measurement, *Med J Aust* 161(2):125-128, 1994.

55. Klein MJ, Alexander MA, Wright JM, et al: Treatment of adult lower extremity lymphedema with the Wright linear pump: Statistical analysis of a clinical trial, *Arch Phys Med Rehabil* 69:202-206, 1988.

56. Kim-Sing C, Basco VE: Postmastectomy lymphedema treated with the Wright linear pump, *Can J Surg* 5:368-370, 1987.

57. Pappas CJ, O'Donnell TF Jr: Long-term results of compression treatment for lymphedema, *J Vasc Surg* 16(4):555-562, 1992.

58. Richmand DM, O'Donnell TR Jr, Zelikovski A: Sequential pneumatic compression for lymphedema: A controlled trial, *Arch Surg* 120(10):11116-11119, 1995.

59. Zanolla R, Monzeglio C, Balzarini A, et al: Evaluation of the results of three different methods of postmastectomy lymphedema treatment, *J Surg Oncol* 26(3):210-213, 1984.

60. Brorson H, Svensson H: Liposuction combined with controlled compression therapy reduces arm lymphedema more effectively than controlled compression therapy alone, *Plast Recon Surg* 102:1058-1067, 1998.

61. Szuba A, Achalu R, Rockson SG: Decongestive lymphatic therapy for patients with breast carcinoma-associated lymphedema: A randomized, prospective study of a role for adjunctive intermittent pneumatic compression, *Cancer* 95:2260-2267, 2002.

62. Földi E, Földi M, Clodius L: The lymphedema chaos: A lancet, *Ann Plast Surg* 22:505-515, 1989.

63. American College of Sports Medicine: *Guidelines for Exercise Testing and Prescription*, Philadelphia, 1991, Lea and Febiger.

64. Boris M, Weindorf S, Lasinski B, et al: Lymphedema reduction by noninvasive complex lymphedema therapy, *Oncology* 9:95-106, 1994.

65. Segers P, Belgrado JP, Leduc A, et al: Excessive pressure in multichambered cuffs used for sequential compression therapy, *Phys Ther* (82):1000-1008, 2002.

66. Kelly DG: Other intervention options. In Kelly DG (ed): *A Primer on Lymphedema*, Upper Saddle River, NJ, 2002, Prentice Hall.

67. Casley-Smith JR, Casley-Smith JR: Modern treatment of lymphedema I complex physical therapy: The first 200 Australian limbs, *Aust J Dermatol* 33(2):61-68, 1992.

68. Bertelli G, Venturini M, Forno G, et al: An analysis of prognostic factors in response to conservative treatment of postmastectomy lymphedema, *Surg Gynecol Obstet* 455-460, 1992.

69. Badger CMA, Peacock JL, Mortimer PS: A randomized controlled, parallel-group clinical trial comparing multi-layer bandaging followed by hosiery versus hosiery alone in the treatment of lymphedema of the limb, *Cancer* 88:2832-2837, 2000.

70. Asmussen PD, Strössenreuther RHK: Compression therapy. In Földi M, Földi E, Kubik S: *Textbook of Lymphology for Physicians and Lymphedema Therapists*, Munich, 2003, Urban & Fischer.

71. Johnson G, Kupper C, Farrar DJ, et al: Graded compression stockings, *Arch Surg* 117:69-72, 1982.
72. Casley-Smith JR: Modern treatment of lymphedema, *Mod Med Aust* 70-83, 1992.
73. Ohkuma M: Lymphedema treated by microwave and elastic dressing, *Int J Dermatol* 31(9):660-663, 1992.
74. Strössenreuther RHK: Decongestive kinesiotherapy, respiratory therapy, physiotherapy and other physical therapy techniques. In Földi M, Földi E, Kubik S: *Textbook of Lymphology for Physicians and Lymphedema Therapists*, Munich, 2003, Urban & Fischer.
75. Casley-Smith JR: Varying total tissue pressures and the concentration of initial lymphatic lymph, *Microvasc Res* 25:369-379, 1983.
76. Leduc O, Peeters A, Borgeois P, et al: Scintigraphic demonstration of its efficacy on colloidal protein reabsorption during muscle activity, *Progress in Lymphology XII*, Amsterdam, 1990, Elsevier.
77. Weissleder H, Schuchhaardt C: *Lymphedema Diagnosis and Therapy*, ed 2, Bonn, 1997, Kagerer.
78. Lerner R: What's new in lymphedema therapy in America? *Int J Angiol* 7:191-196, 1998.
79. Wittlinger H: *Textbook of Dr. Vodder's Manual Lymphatic Drainage II*, Heidelberg, Germany, 1989, Karl R. Hang Publishers.
80. Kelly DG: Complete decongestive therapy: A five part intervention on lymphedema. In Kelly DG (ed): *A Primer on Lymphedema*, Upper Saddle River, NJ, 2002, Prentice Hall.
81. Hutzschenreuter P, Brummer H: Lymphangiomotoricity and tissue pressure, *Z Lymphol* 10(2):55-57, 1986 (article in German).
82. Földi M: Are there enigmas concerning the pathophysiology of lymphedema after breast cancer treatment? *NLN Newsletter* 10(4):1-4, 1998.

Chapter 28

Tissue Healing and Pressure Ulcers

Rose Little Hamm

CHAPTER OUTLINE

OBJECTIVES

After studying this chapter, the reader will be able to:
1. Discuss causative factors and risk factors for pressure ulcers.
2. Analyze the tissue and cellular changes that occur in pressure ulcers.
3. Identify patients at risk for developing pressure ulcers and establish an appropriate preventive plan of care.
4. Effectively use risk assessment and wound evaluation scales.
5. Examine and evaluate patients with pressure ulcers.
6. Diagnose a pressure ulcer according to stage and/or tissue involvement.
7. Plan and implement effective interventions for prevention and treatment of pressure ulcers.

Impaired integumentary integrity resulting in acute and chronic pressure ulcers (PUs) is a concern for patients of all ages. A PU is "any lesion caused by unrelieved pressure resulting in damage of underlying tissue."[1] Rehabili-tation professionals can help resolve and prevent PUs through patient mobilization, positioning, and family and caregiver education.

This chapter discusses the general management of chronic wounds, with a focus on PUs. This chapter provides information that applies to wounds in general and to pressure ulcers in particular, and Chapters 29 to 31 refer to this chapter for general wound management.

EPIDEMIOLOGY

The *prevalence* and *incidence* of PUs depend on the patient population and the medical setting, ranging from as low as 0.29% in children to as high as 44% in adults who sustain spinal cord injuries during childhood (Table 28-1).[2-11]

The financial implications of PUs for the medical system are staggering and worsening as the median age of the population increases. One study found that when hospitalized patients developed partial- or full-thickness PUs, their average hospital length of stay increased from 12.8 days to 30.4 days, and their mean unadjusted hospital costs increased from $13,924 to $37,288.[12] The reported average cost of caring for a full-thickness PU in the home health care setting using traditional methods is more than $20,000.[13] The hospital cost for treating patients with PUs can range from $20,000 to $70,000, depending on the severity of the wound and the required interventions.[14] In addition to the high financial cost of PU care, PUs can also have detrimental psychological and social effects for both patients and their families. Pain, change in body image, patient and family stress, loss of work days, loss of functional mobility, and reduced ability to provide self-care can all be caused by PUs.[15-17]

NATIONAL ORGANIZATIONS

The two major organizations in the United States advocating for research on, prevention of, treatment for, and education about PUs are the National Pressure Ulcer Advisory Panel (NPUAP) and the Agency for Health Care Policy Research (AHCPR), now known as the Agency for

TABLE 28-1 Prevalence and Incidence of Pressure Ulcers in Various Populations

Population Surveyed	Prevalence(P) or Incidence(I)	Reference
Four pediatric-specific health care databases	P: 0.47%	Baldwin[2]
	I: 0.29%	
Pediatric ICU patients	I: 27%	Curley[3]
Patients two days after surgery	I: 21.2%	Schoonhoven[4]
Elderly patients with hip fractures	I: 8.8%	Baumgarten[5]
Adult SCI patients injured during childhood	P: 44%	Vogel[6]
Patients admitted to long-term care from hospitals	P: 11.9%	Baumgarten[7]
Patients admitted to long-term care from other sources	P: 4.7%	
Tertiary care facilities	I: 8.5%	Bergstrom[8]
VA medical centers	I: 7.4%	
Skilled nursing homes	I: 23.9%	
43,000 patients in 356 acute care facilities	P: 14.8% (overall)	Amlung[9]
	P: 7.1% (nosocomial)	
Community-based older adults receiving home health care	I: 3.2%	Bergquist[10]
Elderly patients (>65 years) in general medical practice	P: 0.31%-0.70%	Margolis[11]
	I: 0.18%-3.36% (varied with age)	

ICU, Intensive care unit; *SCI,* spinal cord injury.

Healthcare Research and Quality (AHRQ). The NPUAP, established in 1987, is an independent nonprofit professional organization composed of a panel of experts whose mission is to "improve patient outcomes in PU prevention and management through education, public policy, and research."[18] The NPUAP was instrumental in amending the Omnibus Budget Reconciliation Act (OBRA) of 1987 for quality of care for patients in long-term care facilities and in drafting the Healthy People 2010 Pressure Ulcer Prevention Objective that was formulated by the National Academy of Science. In 1989, OBRA established the AHCPR as the primary Federal Agency "to enhance the quality, appropriateness, and effectiveness of health care services."[1] As part of the United States Department of Health and Human Services, the AHCPR supports research for improving the quality of health care, reducing medical costs, and broadening access to essential services.[19] In 1994, with seven NPUAP members contributing to the effort, the AHCPR published guidelines for the prevention and treatment of PUs.[1,20] These publications established the standards for PU wound description, evaluation, prevention, and medical treatment and also rated the strength of the evidence for the effectiveness of different wound care interventions, including management of tissue loads in reclining and sitting positions, *debridement* and cleansing techniques, dressings, adjunctive therapies (e.g., electrical stimulation, ultraviolet, ultrasound, infrared), management of bacterial colonization and infection, surgical repair, education, and quality improvement.[1] The recommendations made in these guidelines are the basis for the interventions discussed in this chapter.

PATHOLOGY

Pressure ulcers usually occur over bony prominences (e.g., the sacrum, ischial tuberosities, greater trochanters, heels, malleoli, medial femoral condyles, elbows, scapular spine, vertebral spine, and occiput) where the weight of the body is distributed over a small area, thereby producing high local pressure. This pressure reduces blood flow to the tissues, reducing oxygen and nutrient delivery to the skin and subcutaneous tissue, causing the tissue to die. The body responds to this tissue *necrosis* by a sequence of events that can heal the wound. If the pressure is not relieved and the tissue damage exceeds the body's capacity for repair, a PU forms and over a period of time becomes visible as a chronic wound.

WOUND HEALING

Acute wounds, in which the tissue damage is recent and the healing environment is ideal, heal by a predictable and timely sequence of events that occur in a continuum traditionally characterized by five healing phases: Hemostasis, inflammation, proliferation, epithelialization, and remodeling.[21-23]

The first phase of healing, hemostasis, begins as soon as tissue destruction occurs (Fig. 28-1). Platelets rapidly aggregate and adhere to the exposed collagen in the injured tissue, thereby slowing or stopping bleeding. Platelet aggregation also activates *Hageman factor* (clotting factor XII) to initiate clotting by converting prothrombin into thrombin, which then triggers the conversion of fibrinogen into fibrin. Fibrin forms the coagulum or soft

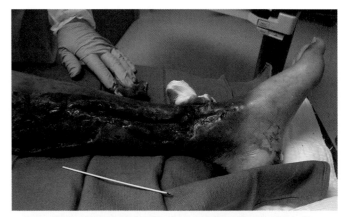

FIG. 28-1　A wound in the hemostasis phase of healing.

plug of a wound. Excessive clotting is prevented by *prostacyclin,* a substance released by the negatively charged endothelial cells, and that inhibits platelet aggregation. The hemostatic process, also referred to as the coagulation cascade, lasts for approximately 30 minutes after the initial injury and prevents excessive bleeding, edema, and further tissue damage. During hemostasis, various cells, proteins, chemicals, and enzymes are also released or attracted to the wound site to initiate the inflammatory response.

The second phase of healing, inflammation, is a complex sequence of events involving numerous cells and chemicals (Figs. 28-2 and 28-3). This phase lasts 3-7 days and begins with neutrophils invading the injured area to lyse and clear away the nonviable cellular components, a process termed *phagocytosis.* During the early phase of inflammation, platelets and neutrophils release growth factors needed for the next steps of tissue repair. Eosinophils are also involved in phagocytosis of dead cells. Mast cells and basophils release histamine to increase vascular permeability and release chemotactic factors to attract the next group of cells to the injured area. The next group of cells includes monocytes (which become macrophages when they leave the capillaries and enter the

interstitial space) and lymphocytes (which regulate the body's immune response to microbes that enter the wounded area). The macrophages continue phagocytosis by producing enzymes, including *collagenases* and *proteases,* which promote autolytic debridement. During this phase, platelets, macrophages, fibroblasts, and keratinocytes also release growth factors that facilitate the synthesis of collagen to form new capillary walls, extracellular matrix, basement membrane, and epidermis. Macrophages, the regulatory cells of the inflammatory phase, are also necessary for the transition from the inflammatory phase to the proliferative phase.

Detectable signs of inflammation (redness, warmth, swelling, and pain) are caused by inflammatory factors released into the tissue during the inflammatory phase of healing. These factors include *prostaglandins, kinins* (e.g., bradykinin), and *anaphylatoxins.* Inflammation can reduce function in the area of the wound and in the patient overall. Patients with more severe wounds may also develop systemic fever during this phase. In the inflammatory phase, healthy systemic processes provide the cellular and chemical components necessary for healing. However, if the natural debridement or lysis process is not completed, the wound may become chronically inflamed, with persistent edema, erythema, and drainage. If chronic inflammation occurs, bacteria, necrotic tissue, and drainage must be managed effectively so that the wound can progress to the next phase of healing, proliferation.

The visible hallmark of the proliferative phase of healing is the new capillary bed, termed *granulation tissue* (Fig. 28-4). Fibroblasts, the most prevalent cells during proliferation, produce the collagen that forms the connective tissue that gives granulation tissue structure. Lymphocytes produce antibodies to prevent wound infection and endothelial cells produce the new capillaries of the granulation tissue. During this phase, macrophages continue to phagocytose devitalized tissue and bacteria. If the granulation tissue grows without the development of a basement membrane, hypergranulation will occur and epithelial cells will not be able to migrate over the excessive granulation tissue. Myofibroblasts, which contain actin (also responsible for muscle fiber contraction), are also prevalent in granulation tissue and can contract to bring the edges of the wound toward each other and

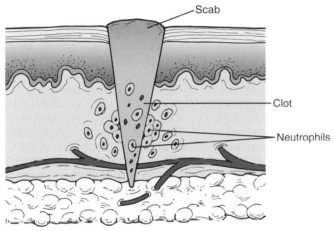

FIG. 28-2 Cellular and noncellular components of the inflammatory phase of healing. *Redrawn from Cameron MH: Physical Agents in Rehabilitation: From Research to Practice, ed 2, Philadelphia, 2003, Saunders.*

Labels: Scab, Clot, Neutrophils

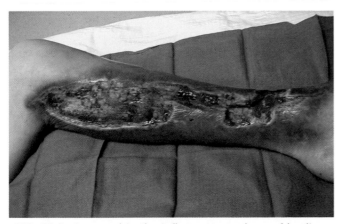

FIG. 28-3 A wound in the inflammatory phase of healing.

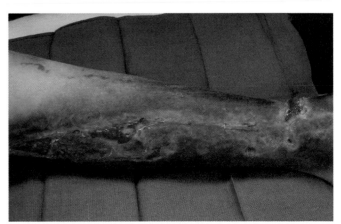

FIG. 28-4 A wound in the proliferative phase of healing.

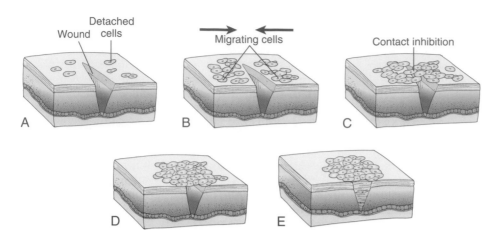

FIG. 28-5 Schematic diagram of epithelialization. *Redrawn from Cameron MH:* Physical Agents in Rehabilitation: From Research to Practice, *ed 2, Philadelphia, 2003, Saunders.*

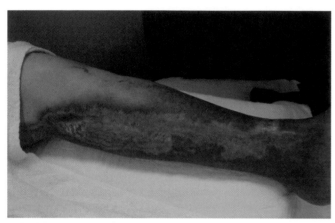

FIG. 28-6 A wound in the epithelialization phase of healing.

reduce the wound size. This process is called wound contraction. A combination of growth factors (e.g., platelet-derived growth factors, epithelial growth factors, transforming growth factors), fibronectin, and *glycosaminoglycans* (GAGs) regulate the proliferative process in preparation for wound closure.

As with proliferation, the fourth phase of healing, epithelialization, involves tissue regeneration (Figs. 28-5 and 28-6). During this phase, beginning from the wound edges or from intact hair follicles and sweat ducts, epithelial cells migrate across the wound bed and produce a single-cell thick layer to cover the granulation tissue. This layer lies over the basement membrane, which is produced by basal cells that advance just a few cells ahead of the epithelial cells. Adhesive *glycoproteins,* such as fibronectin and laminin, adhere the new epithelial cells to the underlying lamina.

Remodeling, the fifth and final phase of wound healing, lasts from several weeks to 2 years after the initial tissue injury. During this phase, collagen in the dermal layer is reorganized to optimize tissue strength, maximize tissue mobility, and minimize scarring. Fibroblasts lay down new collagen fibers in some areas, while collagenase lyses excess collagen in other areas. When this deposition and lysis are balanced, they produce sufficient collagen fibers, with appropriate alignment, to withstand the forces

applied to the tissue, and the collagen transitions from predominantly type III to the preinjury type I collagen. During remodeling, the skin also returns to its genetically determined color and the subcutaneous tissue returns to its normal vascularity, marking the end of the wound healing process. Scar formation is a superficial sign of inner remodeling.

The entire area of a small wound may be in the same healing phase at any one time; however, in most wounds, especially PUs, different areas are often in different phases of healing. The phase of wound healing should be identified to allow for optimal clinical management.

The complete sequence of tissue healing just described occurs in response to acute wounds with full-thickness skin loss. Superficial wounds, where only the epidermis is involved, do not require new collagen formation to close; therefore, after hemostasis and inflammation, they move directly to the epithelialization phase.

Clean full-thickness wounds with little or no tissue loss generally heal with minimal collagen deposition and thus minimal scarring, provided that the edges are kept approximated and secured during healing. This is termed healing by primary intention. In contrast, full thickness wounds with significant contamination or tissue loss may be left open to prevent accumulation of drainage. These wounds generally heal over a longer period with sufficient collagen production to result in a large scar. This is known as healing by secondary intention (Fig. 28-7). If a wound cannot heal in the normal sequence in a timely manner, it is referred to as a chronic wound.

CHRONIC WOUNDS

Any of the phases of healing can be delayed or arrested, causing an acute wound to become chronic. In these circumstances, interventions are required to reinitiate or facilitate healing. Chronic wounds are defined as those that "fail to progress through a normal, orderly, and timely sequence of repair or wounds that pass through the repair process without restoring anatomic and functional results."[24] Without adequate treatment of the wound etiology and comorbidities, the wound fluid will also develop properties that inhibit healing, such as increased *matrix metalloproteinases* (MMPs) and extracellular matrix and decreased tissue protease inhibitors.[25] The primary factors that predispose wounds to chronicity are the following:[21]

- Moderate-to-large amounts of necrotic tissue.
- High burden of microorganisms, with or without clinical infection.
- Chronic inflammation with persistently high numbers of neutrophils and macrophages.
- Impaired hemodynamics (e.g., hypoxia, ischemia, or edema).
- Senescent fibroblasts and keratinocytes that are unresponsive to growth factors; visible signs may include rolled edges or red, nongranulated tissue in the wound base.
- Abnormally high levels of growth-inhibiting proteases, especially metalloproteinases, that cause collagen degradation and can prevent development of a healthy extracellular matrix.
- Overgrowth of epithelium because of insufficient underlying connective tissue.

Because PUs develop insidiously rather than as the result of an isolated incident, they usually have many characteristics of chronic wounds by the time they reach the attention of the health care team and are evaluated. The exception would be the early stage I ulcer that is treated early by effective removal of the causative factors. If there are no other impediments to healing, a stage I PU will heal quickly. However, with chronic PUs, changes in the interstitial fluid composition and the periwound fiber structure delay healing and weaken the periwound tissue.[26]

CAUSES OF PRESSURE ULCERS

There are four primary causes of PUs—shear, friction, pressure, and moisture (Fig. 28-8). Many other risk factors also predispose patients to PU formation. Determination and elimination of the causative factors, as well as evaluation and modification of risk factors, are integral to effective PU prevention and treatment.

Shear. When skin is in contact with a support surface and the underlying tissue moves parallel to the support surface and the skin, shear forces develop in the subcutaneous fascia, muscle, and adipose tissue. For example, shear forces are exerted on the subcutaneous tissue at the spine and sacrum when a patient is in bed with the head

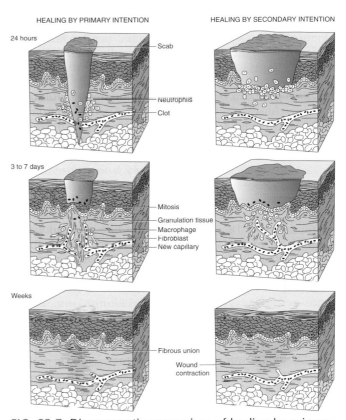

FIG. 28-7 Diagrammatic comparison of healing by primary intention *(left)* and secondary intention *(right)*. *Adapted from Cameron MH: Physical Agents in Rehabilitation: From Research to Practice, ed 2, Philadelphia, 2003, Saunders.*

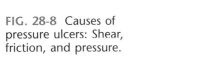

FIG. 28-8 Causes of pressure ulcers: Shear, friction, and pressure.

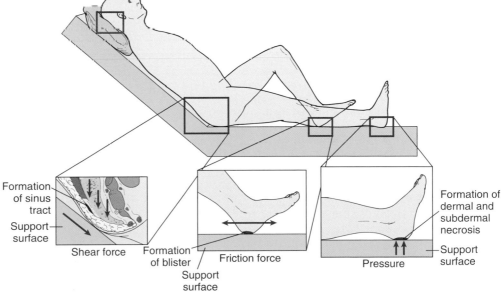

elevated by as little as 10 degrees from horizontal or when the patient's cervical and upper thoracic spine is flexed.[27] A wheelchair-bound patient who slides forward and downward is also subject to destructive shear forces on the soft tissues overlying the sacrum. Shear forces compress, distort, or tear cutaneous and subcutaneous capillaries, resulting in tissue ischemia, initially in the deeper tissues and subsequently in the skin.[28] The resulting tissue destruction can cause deep tracts of necrosis along fascial planes called sinus tracts, and these frequently become sites of infection. This type of damage may exist for quite some time before skin changes are visible. In addition to sinus tracts, PUs caused by shear forces have cratered walls and are round or oval shaped. Shear forces can be minimized by positioning the patient horizontally and by distributing forces on the support surface uniformly to reduce sliding movements that cause shear forces.[27,29,30]

Pressure. Pressure is the amount of force per unit area (see Fig. 28-8). When the external pressure applied to tissue exceeds the capillary closing pressure in that tissue, the capillaries become occluded, preventing blood flow and causing tissue hypoxia or anoxia and eventual cell death. Capillary closing pressure, defined as the pressure that occludes the smallest vessels, ranges from approximately 20 to 40 mm Hg. For example, the average capillary closing pressure in the forefinger of a healthy adult male is 32 mm Hg at the arterial end of the capillary.[31] When a person lies in a standard hospital bed without a pressure-reducing surface, the pressure exerted on the greater trochanters and the heels is 50-95 mm Hg; when a person sits in a chair, the pressure exerted on the ischial tuberosities can be as high as 300-500 mm Hg.[32] If this much pressure is applied for a short period of time, the tissue can reperfuse when the pressure is relieved, preventing tissue damage; however, if this much pressure is exerted over a prolonged period, PUs may develop. The duration and amount of pressure that can be tolerated without cell death varies among patients and tissue type.[33] Therefore individual risk assessment, frequent skin inspection, and personalized turning schedules are recommended to reduce the risk of tissue damage.[11]

Friction. Friction occurs where two surfaces rub against each other (e.g., skin of the heels or elbows sliding on bed linens; see Fig. 28-8). Friction can destroy the superficial layers of the skin, including the epidermis and upper dermis, resulting in blisters, abrasions, or skin tears. A subsequent inflammatory reaction causes extrusion of watery transudate from the damaged area, further adding to skin destruction by causing maceration. These processes can eventually cause PUs. Unlike shear forces that cause ulcers to begin in deep tissue, wounds caused by friction begin with surface skin damage that then exposes subcutaneous tissue, making it more vulnerable to shear or pressure forces and bacterial contamination.[34] Wounds caused by friction tend to be painful because the nerve endings are exposed. Friction can be eliminated by lifting the patient slightly before repositioning; by protecting vulnerable areas with pillows, foam protectors, or rigid positioners; and by placing protective dressings over at-risk or damaged skin.

Moisture. Prolonged exposure of the skin to excessive moisture macerates the epidermis and increases the susceptibility of tissue to destruction from shear and friction, facilitates bacterial access to the subcutaneous tissue, and delays healing of an existing wound. Normal skin is slightly acidic to protect it from bacterial penetration and infection.[35] If skin is exposed to moisture from urinary or fecal incontinence, complications are more likely because this increases surface pH and bacterial exposure.[36] Excessive skin moisture can be prevented by use of moisture barrier creams; management of incontinence with catheters, fecal pouches, and use of bowel and bladder training programs (especially for spinal cord injured patients); and placement of appropriate absorbent padding on the support surface.

Risk Factors for Pressure Ulcer Formation. Risk factors are circumstances that predispose patients to PU formation or to impaired healing when the skin and subcutaneous tissue are subjected to the causative factors just discussed. The National Pressure Ulcer Long-Term Study found that 53% of the residents in 109 surveyed long-term care facilities were at risk of developing a PU, based on criteria from the Braden Scale (see section on Risk Assessment Scales).[37] Risk factors for all populations may include immobility, joint contractures, decreased sensation, increased age, poor nutrition, incontinence (fecal and urinary), comorbidities, altered mental status, and psychosocial factors.[20] Additional risk factors have been identified in studies of specific patient populations (Table 28-2).[3,5,37-46] PU risk factors may be classified as extrinsic or intrinsic. Extrinsic risk factors include physical factors, such as equipment, orthoses, clothing, foreign objects, or medical apparatus, that can exert damaging pressure on patient skin and underlying tissue; intrinsic factors include patient comorbidities or physical attributes, as well as medications that increase tissue vulnerability to PU formation (Box 28-1 and Table 28-3).[47] Effective treatment of PUs includes identifying and managing the risk factors while eliminating or reducing the causative factors.

Risk Assessment Scales. Several risk assessment scales have been developed to screen patients and determine their vulnerability to PU formation. Selection of a risk assessment tool involves consideration of the facility setting, the patient population, the raters using the tool, and the scale's validity and reliability within a given setting.[36] The Norton Scale,[20,48,49] the Braden Scale,[20,50-52] the Minimum Data Set (MDS),[53,54] the Outcomes and Assessment Information Set (OASIS),[55-58] and the Spinal Cord Injury Pressure Ulcer Scale (SCIPUS)[59,60] are the most commonly used PU risk assessment scales that have been tested for reliability and validity in various settings (Table 28-4). Copies of many of these scales, including examination forms and scoring details, can be found on the CD that accompanies this book.

The Norton Scale and the Braden Scale. The Norton Scale and the Braden Scale (the Braden Scale for Predicting Pressure Sore Risk) are the PU risk assessment tools recommended in the AHRQ *Guidelines* because they have been extensively evaluated.[1,20] When using the Norton or Braden Scales, patients should be assessed at the time of admission and at frequent intervals thereafter because

TABLE 28-2	Pressure Ulcer Risk Factors for Specific Patient Populations	
Patient Population	**Risk Factors**	**Reference**
Elderly hip fracture patients	Longer wait before surgery Intensive care unit stay Longer surgical procedure General anesthesia	Baumgarten[5]
Pediatric ICU patients	Use of mechanical ventilation Mean arterial pressures ≤50 mm Hg Lower Braden Q scores	Curley[3]
Patients with severe closed head injury	Use of semirigid cervical collars	Chendrasekhar[38]
Patients in a neurological ICU or intermediate unit	Braden score ≤13 Low BMI	Fife[39]
Patients in a burn center	Concurrent injuries Infection Surgical procedures Older age	Fritsch[40]
Patients in long-term care facilities	Involuntary weight loss Dehydration Severity of illness Incontinence and catheter use History of PUs Diabetes Male gender Dependency in ADLs	Horn[37]
Nonambulatory SCI patients	Low BMI Medications for pain and/or spasticity History of smoking, alcohol, and drug use Poor family support	Krause[41]
Patients in ICU	Surgical procedures Fecal incontinence Hypoalbuminemia (preoperative) Altered sensation Moisture of the skin Impaired circulation Use of inotropic drugs Diabetes mellitus Immobility High APACHE II score	Keller[42]
Elderly hospitalized patients	Use of sedatives before admission	Lindquist[43]
Elderly bedridden patients	Increased platelet aggregation	Matsuyama[44]
Mobility-impaired, hospitalized patients	Hypoalbuminemia Confusion Malnourished Use of a catheter	Reed[45]
Pediatric patients seen in a hospital wound clinic	Diagnosis of myelodysplasia Paralysis Impaired sensation High activity level Immobility	Samaniego[46]

ICU, Intensive care unit; *SCI,* spinal cord injury; *BMI,* body mass index; *PUs,* pressure ulcers; *ADLs,* activities of daily living.

their condition may change over time. Preventive interventions are selected according to the noted impairments. When an ulcer occurs, it is recommended that the patient be reassessed more frequently to monitor for risk of ulceration at other anatomical sites.[36]

The Minimum Data Set (MDS). All Medicare- and Medicaid-certified long-term care facilities are mandated to perform periodic comprehensive assessments of each of their residents, including assessment of PU risk. The MDS, a component of the Resident Assessment Instrument (RAI), includes a tool for basic assessment of patients' clinical and functional impairments. Patients are assessed within 14 days of admission, quarterly, and upon any change in medical status. Skin condition is one of 16 assessed aspects of patient well-being. The criteria for skin assessment can be used to establish an effective PU prevention program, and the entire data set is helpful for developing a comprehensive wound care plan.

A chart review study of 555 residents of 8 nursing homes found the MDS and the Braden Scale to be valid

BOX 28-1	Extrinsic and Intrinsic Risk Factors for Pressure Ulcer Formation

Extrinsic	Intrinsic
• Older age • Poor family support • Psychosocial factors • Use of braces, orthoses, or other semirigid support devices • Poorly fitting beds and wheelchairs • External devices such as catheters and tubes • Shear, pressure, and friction forces • Moisture against the skin	• Low body mass • Atrophy • Medications, especially sedatives • Immobility • Joint contractures • Paralysis • Impaired sensation • Impaired circulation • Comorbidities • Confusion • Hypoalbuminemia • Urinary/fecal incontinence • Chemotherapy or radiation therapy • Malnutrition • Low diastolic blood pressure • Fever

TABLE 28-3	Medications that Affect Wound Healing

Medication (Class: Examples)	Function	Affect on Wound Healing
Fluoroquinolones: Ciprofloxacin, lomefloxacin, norfloxacin, ofloxacin	Antibiotic; inhibits bacterial DNA replication; effective against wide range of gram-positive and gram-negative bacteria, including *S. aureus*	Decreases bacterial load; may cause diarrhea, a contributing factor for pressure ulcers; may cause skin rash or itching
Cephalosporins: Cefazolin, cephalexin, cefotaxime	Antibiotic; inhibits bacterial cell membrane synthesis	Decreases bacterial load; may cause diarrhea or hypersensitivity reactions
Aminoglycosides: Streptomycin, gentamicin, neomycin	Antibacterial; interrupts protein synthesis, thereby leading to bacterial cell death; effective against aerobic gram-negative bacteria	Decreases bacterial load; may cause frequent urination
Penicillins: Penicillin, oxacillin, amoxicillin, methicillin, vancomycin	Antibiotic; inhibits bacteria cell wall function	Decreases bacterial load; may cause diarrhea or hypersensitivity reactions; may lead to resistant strains that require isolation
Aspirin	Antiinflammatory and antiplatelet	Inhibits platelet-induced thrombus formation, may delay inflammatory response to injury; may cause gastrointestinal bleeding
NSAIDs: Ibuprofen, naproxen sodium	Antiinflammatory	May delay inflammatory response to healing
Corticosteroids: Cortisone, dexamethasone, hydrocortisone, prednisolone, prednisone	Antiinflammatory; decreases synthesis of prostaglandins and leukotrienes; immunosuppressive	Inhibit migration of monocytes and neutrophils toward site of injury; delay inflammatory response to healing; aggravate diabetes mellitus, thereby increasing blood sugars and impeding delivery of oxygen to wound; increase risk of infection; catabolic effect on collagenous tissue
Acetic acid	Topical antiseptic; effective against *Pseudomonas*	Toxic to human fibroblasts and keratinocytes; lowers wound pH and inhibits formation of granulation tissue
Dakin's solution (low concentration bleach)	Topical antiseptic; helps dissolve necrotic tissue	Acts as a chemical debrider; cytotoxic to healthy granulation tissue; damages fibroblasts and endothelial cells
Hibiclens	Topical antiseptic and antimicrobial; safe to use on intact skin	Not intended for full-thickness wounds
Hydrogen peroxide	Topical antimicrobial	Toxic to fibroblasts; may cause oxygen gas emboli
Povidone-iodine	Topical antiseptic	Toxic to fibroblasts and polymorphonucleocytes; may cause stinging and burning of tissue

NSAIDs, Nonsteroidal antiinflammatory drugs.

TABLE 28-4	Pressure Ulcer Risk Assessment Scales			
Scale (Year Published)	**Recommended Population/Setting**	**Risk Categories Assessed**	**Scale Interpretation**	**References**
Norton Scale (1962)	Elderly in acute hospital setting	Physical condition Mental condition Activity Mobility Incontinence	Scale of 1-4; 1 highest Score range: 5-20 ≤16 = at risk <12 = at high risk	Bergstrom[20] Barton[48] Norton[49]
Braden Scale (1988)	Acute care Intensive care Nursing home Any patient regardless of skin color Older population	Sensory perception Moisture Activity Mobility Nutrition Friction and shear	Scale of 1-4; 1 highest Score range: 6-23 <12 high risk 12-14 moderate risk 15-16 mild risk 17-18 low risk	Bergstrom[20] Ayello[50] Bergstrom[51] Bergstrom[52]
Minimum Data Set (MDS; 1987)	Long-term care facilities	Ulcers Type of ulcer History of resolved ulcers Other skin problems or lesions present Skin treatments Foot problems and care	Scale/score not provided for risk evaluation; used to determine payment category	Vap[53] Hawes[54]
Outcomes and Assessment Information Set (OASIS; 1999 with ongoing revisions)	Home health care setting	Psychosocial support Sensory status Integumentary status Elimination status Cognitive function Toileting Transferring Ambulation	Scale/score not provided for risk evaluation; used to determine payment category	Hittle[55] Madigan[56] Madigan[57] Madigan[58]
Spinal Cord Injury Pressure Ulcer Scale (SCIPUS; 1996)	SCI patients in acute and long-term care settings	Extent of paralysis Level of activity Mobility Urinary incontinency Moisture Pulmonary disease Serum creatinine Albumin	Score 0-25 0-12 low risk 13-18 moderate risk 19-20 high risk 21-25 very high risk	Salzberg[59] Salzberg[60]

SCI, Spinal cord injury.

for identifying risk factors for PU formation.[53] The MDS was more sensitive than the Braden Scale for the prediction of PU incidence in long-term care facilities. They recommend that the Braden Scale be used immediately upon resident admission to assess for risk factors and the MDS be used to predict ulcer formation.[53] A study testing the reliability of the MDS in 13 nursing homes in 5 states found intraclass correlation of 0.7 or higher for key areas of functional status (e.g., cognition, activities of daily living [ADLs], continence, and diagnosis); 0.6 or higher for 63% of the items, and 0.4 or higher for 89% of the items.[54] If the MDS is the only assessment tool used for residents admitted to long-term care facilities, delaying administration by up to 14 days from admission may be detrimental to those at high risk for ulcer formation; therefore assessment at the time of admission is recommended.

Outcomes and Assessment Information Set (OASIS). The OASIS is an extensive and comprehensive assessment form developed by the Health Care Financing Administration (HCFA) for use in the home health care setting.

OASIS includes items specific to wounds, including the presence of PUs, tissue involvement, and the healing phase of existing ulcers. Although used primarily to establish reimbursement, the other areas, such as psychosocial support, sensory status, integumentary status, elimination status, cognitive functioning, toileting, transferring, and ambulation, included in this tool can assist the evaluator by identifying patients at risk for PUs and providing preventive information to patients and caregivers.

Spinal Cord Injury Pressure Ulcer Scale (SCIPUS). The SCIPUS was developed for assessing pressure ulcer risk in patients with spinal cord injuries. A follow-up study of SCI patients in the acute phase (within 30 days of admission) compared the reliability and sensitivity of various PU risk assessment scales not intended for use with SCI patients (Norton, Braden, Gosnell, Abruzzese scales) with the SCIPUS, which was not intended for risk assessment during acute hospitalization.[60] Although the Braden Scale was found to be the most accurate of the general purpose scales, it was a poor overall predictor of PU formation in this patient population. Of the 226 patients studied,

97.3% had a Braden score of 18 or less. A cutoff score of ≤10 provided the highest balance of sensitivity (74.7%) and specificity (56.6%) for the Braden Scale. The authors concluded that if the Braden Scale is used for SCI patients, a score of ≤10 is most appropriate for identifying those at risk for PU formation.[60] As a result of this study, the original SCIPUS was modified for use with the SCI patient during acute hospitalization. The authors recommend that the SCIPUS be used daily to assess all SCI patients in the acute care setting.

EXAMINATION

PATIENT HISTORY

Examination of a patient with a PU begins with a thorough history focused on the causes of wound formation. Pertinent questions to ask patients about onset, medical history, and functional status include but are not limited to the following:

- When and how did the wound begin?
- Can any event be associated with the onset (e.g., a recent illness, a new pair of shoes, a change of equipment)?
- What other signs or symptoms are present (e.g., fever, itching, pain, burning)?
- What alleviates or aggravates the pain (e.g., prolonged sitting, rolling, scooting)?
- Is the wound improving or regressing?
- What other disease processes are present?
- What medications (with dosages) are being taken, including prescription, herbal, and over-the-counter medicines?
- Are there any allergies that may alter the type of dressing used (e.g., silver, sulfa, adhesives)?
- What are the patient's alcohol, tobacco, and drug use habits?
- What is the patient's physical activity level?
- What kind of assistive device is required for functional activities?
- What are the goals of the patient and the caregiver?[61]

For hospitalized patients, long-term care residents, and especially cognitively impaired patients, much of this information can be obtained from the medical chart or during the functional assessment. Whenever possible, however, information regarding onset, pain, and aggravating and alleviating factors should be obtained directly from the patient. Components of the history that are usually obtained from the medical chart or from the referring physician include the medical and surgical history, medications, nutritional status, clinical tests, and detrimental environmental conditions.

Nutritional Status. The need for adequate nutrition to prevent and treat PUs is well documented. According to the National Pressure Ulcer Long-Term Study of 2,490 residents in 109 long-term care facilities, the two nutrition-related factors that most affect PU risk are involuntary weight loss of more than 10% of the total body weight (increased risk 74%) and dehydration (increased risk 42%).[37,62,63] In addition to adequate calories, wound healing requires sufficient protein intake. The caloric needs of wound and periwound tissue increases to 50%

above baseline and the protein requirement increases to 2-2.5 times above baseline.[64] Clinical tests used to assess nutritional status and to measure the effectiveness of nutritional supplements are serum albumin and prealbumin levels. Albumin levels of less than 3.5 g/dl and prealbumin levels of less than 20 g/dl are considered indicators of poor nutritional status.[65] Albumin levels indicate nutrition over the prior 1-3 months and prealbumin indicates nutritional status over the prior 2-3 days. Other nutritional components necessary for optimal wound healing include fats, fatty acids, and carbohydrates (a major source of energy for healing). In addition, vitamins A, B complex, C, and E and the trace elements zinc, copper, and iron influence PU formation and healing.[65,66]

Psychosocial Issues. Psychosocial assessment of a patient with a PU may identify issues that may benefit or interfere with healing potential. The patient's ability, willingness, and motivation to alter lifestyle habits should be factored into treatment planning and goal setting. The support of family, friends, and caregivers may also be necessary for successful treatment in the home setting. Stress has been found to delay healing of acute and chronic wounds,[67,68] most likely through downregulation of the cellular immune response.[69,70] Depression and/or polypharmacy may also influence healing by reducing appetite and motivation for activity.[71] Drug and alcohol abuse (both of which may cause *protein-energy malnutrition*) and any form of tobacco use (which causes tissue hypoxia) can also affect healing potential.[72]

SYSTEMS REVIEW

The systems review is used to target areas requiring further examination and to define areas that may cause complications or indicate a need for precautions during the examination and intervention processes. See Chapter 1 for details of the systems review.

TESTS AND MEASURES

The wound examination should begin with observation to describe the wound tissue and drainage, skin color, edema, wound edges, and odor.

Tissue Description. Tissue description helps identify the depth of the PU and phase(s) of healing in the wound bed. When *eschar* is present, the tissue should be described before and after debridement, and the wound should be diagnosed or staged only after debridement. Estimating the amount of each tissue type as a percentage of the total wound area can also provide data for assessing change. Tissue types include the following:

- **Eschar** is black, brown, yellow, or grey tissue that may be dry and hard, or in the presence of an underlying infection, soft and "mushy." In PUs, the eschar may also have a rubbery texture. Eschar is composed of dead cells and should therefore be removed from most wounds to determine depth of tissue involvement, to facilitate healing, and to decrease risk of infection.
- **Yellow slough,** often visible under the eschar during the inflammatory phase of healing, is the softer and lighter necrotic debris that collects as the by-product of *autolysis.*

- **Granulation tissue** is the red, "beefy-looking" tissue that results from angiogenesis and deposition of type III collagen. The color can vary from an anemic salmon-color to a healthy, bright red, indicating that the wound is ready for surgical closure or that epithelialization can be supported. Granulation tissue is required for closure for any wound healing by secondary intention. It serves to fill in full-thickness wound cavities and matures into scar tissue during the remodeling phase of healing.
- **Devitalized fascia** is dull, fibrous connective tissue that can be tan or grey.
- **Healthy muscle** is striated, reddish, and sensate when pinched with forceps; devitalized muscle is brownish-grey and insensate.
- **Healthy tendons** are shiny, stringy, and covered with a fibrous sheath of connective tissue containing synovial or fatty fluid, termed paratenon.
- **Healthy bone** is light tan with intact periosteum that gives it a moist appearance. Bone without periosteum is light to dark tan and very dry; necrotic bone is dark brown and requires surgical debridement.
- **Fat,** when healthy, appears as shiny globules. Fat has a poor vascular supply and therefore when exposed, usually dies rapidly and shrivels.

Most wounds contain various tissue types that can be identified and quantified during the initial evaluation and periodic reassessment. Once the types of tissue present in a wound have been identified, all necrotic tissue should be removed while the healthy, vital tissue that provides the resources for new tissue to develop and for healing to progress should be protected.

Drainage. Drainage, a by-product of wound metabolism, is evaluated for quality and quantity (e.g., scant, minimal, moderate, or copious). Serous drainage is a clear, watery fluid that flows from blood vessels, collects in the extracellular spaces, and results in edema if the skin remains intact. If the skin is not intact, serous drainage appears as clear fluid seeping from the opening. If the fluid has a low protein concentration (specific gravity <1.015) it is termed transudate.[73] Sanguineous drainage is bloody drainage. Red sanguineous drainage occurs with recent bleeding, before hemostasis occurs, whereas brownish drainage is from old blood. Serosanguineous drainage is serous fluid with a slight bloody tinge. *Exudate* is pale yellow viscous drainage composed of serum, blood cells, plasma proteins, and lysed debris. Exudate, which has a specific gravity more than 1.015 because of the high protein concentration,[73] is frequently present in the acute inflammatory stage of mild injuries.

Seropurulent drainage is slightly thicker and yellower than exudate, and indicates colonization of the wound by bacteria but not necessarily active infection. In contrast, *purulence,* a thick necrotic drainage frequently accompanied by a foul odor, is a sign of infection. Odor can vary in type and severity. For example, green or greenish-blue drainage accompanied by a distinctive sweet odor is typical of *Pseudomonas* infection. A putrid foul odor is indicative of deep, chronic infection with anaerobic bacteria. Extensive necrotic tissue may have an odor that can only be described as that of nonviable tissue. Certain dressings can have a strong odor; therefore odor is assessed after removal of the dressing and thorough wound cleansing.

Periwound Skin Color. Periwound skin color can provide information about the type of wound and the status of the surrounding tissue. Any change in skin color and the extent of the change should be documented because reduction or increase in the degree and size of color changes are indicators of improvement or decline in wound status. Skin color is presented here as it relates to PUs.

Erythema is redness of the skin that may result from an inflammatory response (reactive hyperemia), from underlying infection, or from unrelieved pressure. In darker-skinned patients, erythema may be more difficult to see; however, accompanying changes in warmth or texture may be detected. Erythema may be blanchable or unblanchable, meaning it does or does not pale with pressure. Normal skin will pale when the blood is pushed out of the capillaries (refer to capillary refill time). Unblanchable erythema in the periwound area is a sign of the inflammatory response to healing or a sign of infection. Unblanchable redness or prolonged refill time in the foot indicates microvascular or small vessel disease. Dark-red discoloration, a result of repeated shear forces, may also be referred to as pre-ulcer or a purple ulcer. Blanched, white periwound skin is typical of maceration that occurs when moisture is inadequately managed. Darker skin tones around the periphery of an open PU are often an indication of extensive undermining.

Edema. Edema, caused by excess fluid in the interstitial tissue, can be multifactorial in origin and can occur with any type of wound. Edema in the area of a PU usually indicates infection or inflammation.

Wound Edges. The appearance of the wound edges can indicate the type of wound and the healing processes occurring within the wound site.

- Even edges are typical of arterial ulcers or surgically induced wounds.
- Irregular edges are typically seen in venous ulcers or PUs with undermining.
- Closed or rolled edges, signs of halted healing, appear curled or raised with epithelial cell migration stopping at the granulation edge. The cells at the edge are senescent, meaning they are unable to reproduce. Rolled edges are sometimes referred to as epibole and may require debridement to facilitate epithelialization.
- *Hyperkeratosis,* also termed callus, is overdevelopment of the horny cell layer of skin as a result of continuous tissue stress. The appearance is dry, thick, adhered epidermal tissue.
- Epithelialization is the migration of epithelial cells over granulation tissue. The percentage of the edges that are epithelializing should be determined.

Wound Size. The initial examination should also include a measure of wound size. In addition to dimensions, usually reported in centimeters, the measurement method and patient position should be documented to ensure valid and reliable assessment of progress. When using the perpendicular method, length (L) is the longest

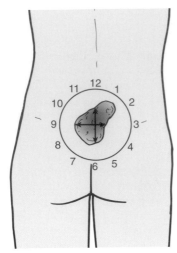

FIG. 28-9 Clockwise method of measuring pressure ulcer size.

Tracing, which provides an exact wound outline, may also be included in the documentation for later comparisons. A study comparing the reliability and validity of acetate tracings with that of computerized planimetry on 45 human and 38 animal wounds found that tracing had excellent concurrent validity on human wounds; however, it was poor for small animal wounds.[77]

Technique for Tracing Wound Outline

- Place a clear film over the wound.
- Place a piece of clear acetate film with a measuring guide over the first layer of film.
- Trace the wound edges with an indelible pen on the top film layer.
- Note orientation, undermining, tunneling, bony prominences, or erythema.
- Label the tracing with the patient's name and the measurement date.
- Discard the film that was next to the wound.

---

measurement of the wound regardless of orientation and width (W) is the longest distance perpendicular to the length. Measurements are documented as L × W, with length first. The perpendicular method can yield an approximate surface area for superficial wounds or wound openings but may be incomplete for complex wounds.

When using the clockwise method, length is the longest dimension along a 12:00-6:00 plane in an anatomical orientation (12:00 is cephalic and 6:00 is caudal) and width is the longest dimension on a 3:00-9:00 plane perpendicular to 12:00-6:00. Fig. 28-9 illustrates clockwise orientation. The clockwise method is useful for sacral ulcers that tend to be irregularly shaped. Sacral ulcers should be observed with the patient lying on both sides because undermining and tunneling may be obscured in some positions.

A study conducted in an outpatient wound care clinic evaluated accuracy of wound measurements by 16 clinicians, comparing the clinician's usual method with the perpendicular and clockwise methods.[74] Using the standard error of measurement as an index of the relative amount of error for each method, the perpendicular method was determined to be the most accurate of the three when compared with measurements using computer-assisted planimetry. The intraclass correlation coefficient (ICC) for the perpendicular method was 0.962 and for the clockwise method was 0.682.[75]

Volumetric measurements, useful for small or cavity wounds, are estimated by multiplying the wound length by width by depth. The depth is measured by placing a sterile swab perpendicular to the wound bed, marking the distance from the wound bed to the surface on the swab shaft, and measuring the distance with a graduated guide. The volume of larger wounds can also be estimated by using a large syringe to fill the wound with either sterile saline or amorphous gel. If spillage is a problem because of the wound shape or location, the volume can be measured by stretching an adhesive transparent film over the wound cavity and by injecting the liquid through the film and into the wound space.[76]

Photographs provide a visual description of the wound and complement documentation. Polaroid cameras provide immediate documentation, and digital cameras may be convenient and cost-effective because no film is required, unsatisfactory photographs can be deleted, and the details of the wound bed are more discernible because of the increased resolution. If the photographs and measuring guides are gridded, surface area can be calculated by counting the number of x/y intersections visible within the wound bed. This area does not, however, account for depth or provide any measure of volume. Care must be taken with photographing wounds to obtain consistent indicators of color and size.

Suggestions for Optimal Wound Photographs

- Position the patient with the wound easily visualized in the view box.
- Adjust the lighting for equal illumination throughout without shadows.
- Use blue or green towels around the wound to eliminate conflicting background and to absorb light, thereby minimizing glare.
- Close curtains or shades so that only fluorescent light exists in the room.
- Hold the camera at a 90-degree angle to the wound to avoid distortion of the shape.
- Take more than one photograph at different settings.
- Label photographs with the patient's name, medical record number, examination date, patient position, and wound location.

Subcutaneous wound extensions require probing and cleansing because they can conceal bacteria and facilitate infection. The size of wound extensions, as well as the size of the exposed wound, are indicators of wound severity and may be a measure of intervention efficacy. The four types of wound extensions are undermining, sinus tract, tunneling, and fistulas. Undermining, defined as a fan-shaped destruction of connective tissue between the dermis and subcutaneous tissue, may be indicated by red or brawny discoloration that extends beyond the wound edges. A sinus tract is a long, narrow opening along a fascial plane that may connect to an underlying, deeper abscess. Palpation of a hard, indurated area adjacent to an open wound may indicate the presence of an abscess. Tunneling is a tract that connects two open wounds. A fistula is tunneling that connects with a body cavity or organ (e.g., the small or large intestine). Undermining and sinus tracts are the types of subcutaneous wound extensions most frequently associated with PUs and occur most commonly in the areas of the sacrum and trochanters.

Undermining and tunneling are measured by slowly inserting a moistened sterile alginate or cotton-tipped applicator into the wound extensions and probing to the deepest parts for sinuses or abscesses. (Alginate-tipped applicators are preferable to cotton ones because alginate fibers that adhere to the wound are absorbed, whereas cotton fibers can become irritants and provide a nidus for infection if left in the wound bed.) Because the area being probed may not be visualized, probing should stop immediately when resistance is felt in order to avoid damaging tissue. The depth of the extension is marked on the applicator, measured with a graduated guide, and documented, along with the presence of any drainage, purulence, or blood on the applicator tip. The location of the extension is usually indicated according to the clockwise method of measuring or in relation to an anatomical landmark.[76]

Clinical Tests. In addition to the clinical tests that help determine a patient's wound healing potential based on nutritional status (serum albumin, prealbumin, and *body mass index* [BMI]), several other clinical tests are recommended in specific conditions (Table 28-5).

Ankle-Brachial Index. Determination of *ankle-brachial index* (ABI), a measure of lower extremity arterial blood flow, is recommended for patients with diabetes or peripheral vascular disease who develop heel PUs. The values are used to determine healing potential, the safety of debridement, and the need for revascularization (see Chapter 30 for details of how to measure ABI).

Blood Glucose Levels. Blood glucose levels should be checked in a patient with a chronic wound because approximately one third of those who are diabetic are unaware that they have the disease.[78] Diabetes impedes wound healing by impairing blood flow through the small vessels at the wound surface, reducing red blood cell permeability, and reducing the amount of oxygen and nutrients that are delivered to the injured tissue.[79] In addition, immune function is impaired if blood glucose levels are persistently elevated above 200 mg/dl. Abnormally elevated glucose levels may indicate the presence of undiagnosed infection requiring antibiotics and optimization of glucose control (see Chapter 30 for further information on chronic wounds associated with diabetes).

Cultures. Cultures are reserved for wounds with clinical signs of infection, which for PUs has been expanded beyond the classical signs of warmth, pain, erythema, and

TABLE 28-5	Clinical Tests for Patients with Pressure Ulcers	
Clinical Test	**Normal Values**	**Interpretation of Abnormal Values**
Serum albumin	3.2-4.5 gm/dl	<3.5 gm/dl: Poor nutritional status
		3.0-3.5: Mild
		2.5-3.0: Moderate
		<2.5: Severe
Prealbumin	15-35 mg/dl	<5 mg/dl: Poor prognosis
		5-10.9 mg/dl: Significant risk; aggressive nutritional support indicated
		11-15 mg/dl: Increased risk; monitor status biweekly
BMI	20-25	<16: Severely underweight
		16-19: Underweight
		26-30: Mild obesity
		31-40: Moderate obesity
		>40: Severe obesity
ABI	1.0	>1.2: Not reliable in diabetics because of arterial calcification
		0.8-1.0: Mild PAOD
		0.5-0.8: Moderate PAOD
		<0.5: Severe PAOD
Fasting plasma glucose	<110 mg/dl	110-126: Prediabetes
		>126: Diagnosis of diabetes
		>200: Impaired healing

BMI, Body mass index; *ABI,* ankle-brachial index; *PAOD,* peripheral arterial occlusive disease.

edema to also include purulent drainage, delayed healing, discoloration of granulation tissues, pocketing at the base of the wound, foul odor, and breakdown of recently formed new tissue.[80] All wounds have some bacteria present, and most chronic wounds are colonized with bacteria, meaning that organisms are present on the wound bed. In most cases, the host's immune system can manage the bacterial load without interfering with healing. In these situations, cultures are unnecessary and are not cost-effective.[81] If the organisms penetrate the wound tissue, infection occurs and the healing process is interrupted. Exactly when healing is affected depends on the type and amount of bacteria, as well as host immunity.

The AHRQ *Guidelines* recommended culturing fluid obtained by needle aspiration or biopsy of ulcer tissue[1]; however, recent studies indicate that a swab culture from the properly prepared wound bed (i.e., after debridement of necrotic tissue and cleansing with normal saline) correlates adequately with a tissue biopsy.[82-84] In addition, a swab culture is not traumatic to a poorly healing wound site and is less expensive than a biopsy.[81] The quantitative definition of infection is >10[5] organisms/gram tissue[85]; however, qualitative clinical infection depends on the host immune system and the strain of bacteria.

Proper Technique for Taking Cultures
- Prepare the wound bed: Cleanse the wound bed with normal saline and debride as much necrotic

tissue as possible so that the culture is from deeper wound tissue.

- Swab the wound bed: Roll the tip of a sterile swab for a full rotation over the area of the wound that appears to be infected. Placing pressure on the tissue as the swab is rolled helps extrude more of the tissue fluid. Avoid contact of the swab with adjacent skin to minimize contamination.
- Use needle aspiration for wound extensions: Purulent drainage from wound extensions (sinuses, undermining, tunnels) is best collected by aspiration with a sterile needle syringe with care to avoid touching the periwound tissue.
- Protect the culture: Immediately place the swab in the transport medium.
- Label the culture: Label the transport container with the patient's name, medical record number, collection date, and location of the wound.
- Deliver to the laboratory: Deliver the culture to the laboratory as soon as possible.

Pain. Pain assessment can indicate the cause and extent of a wound and the appropriate pain management approaches. The nature, onset, duration, and exacerbating and relieving factors, as well as pain severity, are aspects of pain to be considered in making the diagnosis. Pain caused by hypoxia or ischemia, which is usually deep and cramping in quality, and pain that results from neuropathy, which is usually burning, lancinating, or electric-like,[86] are discussed in Chapters 29 and 30, respectively. Throbbing, localized pain, termed nociceptive, is often experienced with infection. Deep pain that increases with pressure may indicate the presence of osteomyelitis.[87] Superficial tenderness or burning can occur with exposed nerve endings, may be accompanied by sharp shooting pains, and can make sharp debridement difficult for the patient to tolerate. Pain when red striated tissue is pinched with forceps indicates the tissue is viable muscle and should not be debrided. Pain severity can be assessed using a variety of scales as described in Chapter 22.

A study of patients with PUs found that 100% of the patients reported pain related to the ulcer with a mean intensity of 5.80/10 (±2.93). The verbal descriptors (from the McGill Pain Questionnaire) used most frequently to describe the pain were throbbing, sharp, burning, aching, and tugging.[88]

Although the best pain assessment tool for patients with chronic wounds has yet to be identified, the literature consistently supports the need for measuring pain and using this information to guide the treatment of patients with acute and chronic wounds.

Sensory Integrity. Testing for sensation is especially important in patients with chronic wounds and diabetic or peripheral neuropathies, SCI, or prolonged immobility. Sensation of light touch, pressure, temperature, vibration, and proprioception should all be tested. For patients at risk for PU formation, assessment of vulnerable areas (feet, sacrum, trochanters, shoulders) will assist in selecting appropriate protective equipment. For SCI patients, one should determine the spinal level where sensation stops and teach off-loading strategies to prevent wounds in insensate areas (see Chapter 20).

EVALUATION, DIAGNOSIS, AND PROGNOSIS

Any soft tissue wound may be classified according to the depth and type of tissue involved.[89] According to the classification scheme used by the *Guide to Physical Therapist Practice* (the *Guide*),[89] wounds can be classified according to depth into one of five preferred practice patterns. These patterns are: 7A: Primary prevention/risk reduction for integumentary disorders; 7B: Impaired integumentary integrity associated with superficial skin involvement; 7C: Impaired integumentary integrity associated with partial-thickness skin involvement and scar formation; 7D: Impaired integumentary integrity associated with full-thickness skin involvement and scar formation, and 7E: Impaired integumentary integrity associated with skin involvement extending into fascia, muscle, or bone and scar formation. Partial thickness is defined as involving the epidermis and dermis; full thickness is defined as the complete destruction of the dermal layers and extending into the subcutaneous tissue.

The NPUAP published a staging system specifically for PUs in 1989 and revised this system in 1998. This system was adopted by the AHCPR and is universally used in the medical community to describe PUs. The staging system, intended for use with PUs only, is based on the deepest layer of tissue involvement at the time of the initial evaluation.[36] The characteristics of the stages as revised in 1998 and the *Guide*'s preferred practice patterns related to the integumentary system are shown in Table 28-6. Fig. 28-10 shows examples of the four NPUAP PU stages.

Necrotic PUs are not staged until debridement is completed because staging depends on identifying the type of tissue at the ulcer base. After debridement of necrotic tissue, the wound depth and amount of tissue involvement can be determined. Also, wounds are not staged in reverse when healing occurs. In other words, a stage III does not become a stage II as the wound granulates, and a stage II does not become a stage I as it reepithelializes. The correct nomenclature would be a stage III PU in the proliferative phase or a stage II in the epithelialization or remodeling phase. Each wound is described according to the deepest layer of tissue involvement and the healing phase at the time of assessment. If a wound deteriorates during the period of intervention, at reassessment the stage can be advanced to reflect deeper tissue involvement.

Several instruments have been developed to monitor wound healing, including the Pressure Ulcer Scale for Healing, the Sussman Wound Healing Tool, the Sessing Scale, and the Pressure Sore Status Tool.

In 1997 the Pressure Ulcer Scale for Healing (PUSH) tool was developed as an alternative to reverse staging of PUs.[90] The PUSH tool categorizes ulcers according to severity in 4 elements: Length, width, amount of exudate, and tissue type, with lower grades being smaller, clean wounds and higher grades correlating with larger wounds with heavier exudate and more nonviable tissue (necrosis and slough).

TABLE 28-6	National Pressure Ulcer Advisory Panel (NPUAP) Pressure Ulcer Stages Compared to the *Guide*'s Integumentary System Preferred Practice Patterns

NPUAP Stage	Preferred Practice Pattern
No comparable stage	7A: Primary prevention/risk reduction for integumentary disorders
Stage I: Observable pressure-related alteration of intact skin whose indicators, as compared to adjacent or opposite area on the body, may include changes in skin color (red, blue, and purple tones), skin temperature (warmth or coolness), skin stiffness (hardness, edema), and/or sensation (pain).	7B: Impaired integumentary integrity associated with superficial skin involvement
Stage II: Partial-thickness skin loss involving epidermis and/or dermis. The ulcer is superficial and presents clinically as an abrasion, a blister, or a shallow crater.	7C: Impaired integumentary integrity associated with partial-thickness skin involvement and scar formation
Stage III: Full-thickness skin loss involving damage or necrosis of subcutaneous tissue that may extend down to, but not through, underlying fascia. The ulcer presents clinically as a deep crater with or without undermining of adjacent tissue.	7D: Impaired integumentary integrity associated with full-thickness skin involvement and scar formation
Stage IV: Full-thickness skin loss with extensive destruction, tissue necrosis, or damage to muscle, bone, or supporting structures (e.g., tendon, joint capsule).	7E: Impaired integumentary integrity associated with skin involvement extending into fascia, muscle, or bone and scar formation

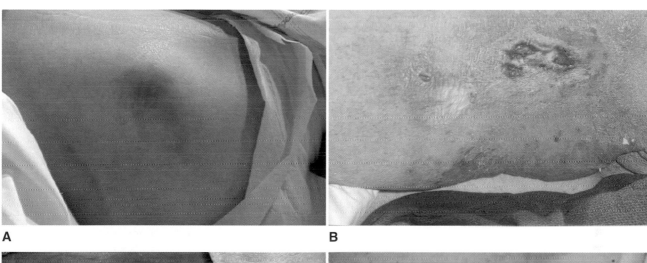

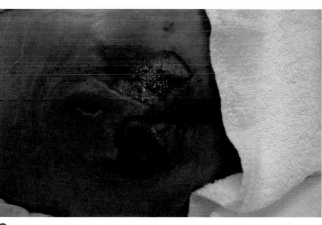

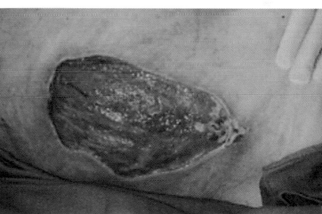

A

B

C

D

FIG. 28-10 Pressure ulcers in NPUAP stages. **A,** Stage I; **B,** stage II; **C,** stage III; **D,** stage IV.

Specific definitions for scoring interpretation are provided for each element, and the total score can range from 0-17. If the total score decreases, the wound is healing; if it increases, the wound is regressing. Advantages of the PUSH tool are that it contains very basic information, making each ulcer easy to score; the data is sensitive to progression; and the scores can be used to calculate a wound healing rate by the following equation:

Wound healing rate = (Admission score −
    Discharge score)/Number days in hospital or care

Wound healing rates can be used to monitor facility performance, to determine the effectiveness of wound care programs, and to track trends of patients with wounds within a facility.[91] Disadvantages of the PUSH tool are that only one wound is scored on each assessment form, making it burdensome if a patient has several PUs, and wound progress or lack of it can be easily identified without use of the assessment tool.[92] Two studies of 372 subjects reported that the PUSH tool accounted for 58% to 74% of the wound healing variance over 10 weeks in Study 1 and 40% to 57% over 12 weeks in Study 2. Sensitivity of the model to total healing was measured with regressive analysis. The PUSH accounted for 39% of the variance over 6 weeks and 31% of the variance over 12 weeks ($p < 0.001$; Studies 1 and 2, respectively).[93]

The Sussman Wound Healing Tool (SWHT) was developed as a physical therapy diagnostic tool to monitor and track the effectiveness of physical interventions on wound healing.[94] This tool includes 10 wound tissue attributes (associated with changes in healing phases) that are scaled as present (1) or absent (0). Five of the attributes are considered "not good for healing," and five are considered "good for healing." A decrease in the "not good" score and an increase in the "good" score would indicate that the wound is progressing through the healing phases and improving. In addition, there are nine descriptions of depth and undermining that are used as parameters for wound healing, and there is a key for indicating wound location and healing phase. Advantages of the SWHT are its adaptability to a computerized database, its ability to target wounds that are not progressing, and its relative simplicity.[95] Disadvantages are that it has not been evaluated for reliability and validity and it was based on the acute healing model although it is intended for use with chronic wounds.[92]

The Pressure Sore Status Tool (PSST) includes information on wound location and shape and 13 other wound descriptors.[96] Each descriptor is graded on a scale of 0-5 (minimal to severe) and a total score, between 0 and 65, is calculated. A score of 0 represents tissue health; 13, tissue regeneration; and 65, wound degeneration. As a wound improves, its score will decrease. Advantages of the PSST are that it can be used to monitor overall healing or groups of characteristics (e.g., necrotic tissue or exudate), it can be used to assist in setting goals, and it can be used to assess the effectiveness of interventions.[96] The PSST has been evaluated for content validity (average index for tool = 0.91), interrater reliability ($r = 0.91$; $p < 0.001$), and intrarater reliability ($r = 0.99$; $p < 0.001$).[96] The main disadvantage of the PSST is that it is complex, requiring training of the evaluator and taking approximately 15 minutes to complete.[97] It is therefore considered better suited for research than for clinical use.[92]

In summary, no one tool is ideal for assessing wound status or healing in all circumstances and settings. The PSST has undergone more validation than the PUSH but the PUSH tool is thought to use the best methodology[91] and therefore is most likely to become a universal assessment tool.

INTERVENTION

PREVENTION BASED ON RISK FACTORS

Although labor intensive and costly, comprehensive PU prevention programs have been shown to decrease the incidence of PUs and are cost-effective in both acute and long-term care facilities. Implementation of a prevention program in 2 long-term care facilities (patient populations 150 and 110) resulted in an 87% and 76% decrease respectively in the PU incidence after 5 months. Prevention included risk assessment with the Braden Scale, implementation of the AHRQ *Guidelines* for skin care and early treatment,[20] nutritional supplementation, and use of pressure-relieving devices, in addition to nursing staff education.[98] The same study reported an average additional monthly cost for this program for a high-risk patient of $519[73] and an initial per patient expense of $277 for pressure-relieving devices (mattress and cushion).

Guidelines for Pressure Ulcer Prevention Based on Risk Assessment[20]

For bed-bound individuals
- Reposition at least every 2 hours.
- Use pillows or foam wedges to keep bony prominences from direct contact.
- Use devices that totally relieve pressure on the heels.
- Avoid positioning directly on the trochanter.
- Elevate the head of the bed as little and for as short a time as possible.
- Use lifting devices to move rather than drag individuals during transfers and position changes.
- Place at-risk individuals on a pressure-reducing mattress. Do not use doughnut-type devices.

For chair-bound patients
- Reposition at least every hour.
- Have patient shift weight every 15 minutes if able.
- Use pressure-reducing devices for seating surfaces. Do not use doughnut-type devices.
- Consider postural alignment, distribution of weight, balance and stability, and pressure relief when positioning individuals in chairs or wheelchairs.
- Use a written plan.

Skin care
- Inspect skin at least once a day.
- Individualize bathing schedule. Avoid hot water. Use a mild cleansing agent.

- Minimize aggravating environmental factors such as low humidity and cold air. Use moisturizers for dry skin.
- Avoid massage over bony prominences.
- Use proper positioning, transferring, and turning techniques.
- Use lubricants to reduce friction injuries.

Moisture/incontinence
- Cleanse skin at time of soiling.
- Minimize skin exposure to moisture. Assess and treat urinary incontinence. When moisture cannot be controlled, use underpads or briefs that are absorbent and present a quick-drying surface to the skin.

Nutritional deficit
- Investigate factors that compromise an apparently well-nourished individual's dietary intake (especially protein or calories) and offer support with eating.
- Plan and implement a nutritional support and/or supplementation program for nutritionally compromised individuals.

Education
- Etiology and risk factors for PUs.
- Risk assessment tools and their application.
- Skin assessment.
- Selection and/or use of support surfaces.
- Development and implementation of an individualized program of skin care.
- Demonstration of positioning to decrease risk of tissue breakdown.
- Instruction on accurate documentation of pertinent data.

A 6-month study of 63 patients found that the incidence of PUs decreased from 23% to 5% after implementation of an intensive PU prevention protocol.[99] The mean cost for prevention and treatment of PUs were not significantly different before and after the program (before: $113 ± $345; after: $100 ± $157; $t = 0.27$, $p = 0.79$). However, the mean number of days to ulcer development increased significantly from 146 ± 61 days before the program to 158 ± 53 days after the program was initiated (log rank = 8.63, $p = 0.003$).

Another study of 63 nursing home patients looked at the clinical outcomes and costs of implementing a protocol for incontinence and PU prevention.[100] This study found that 60% of the 34 incontinent patients became dry and the number of patients who developed PU decreased from 16 before protocol implementation to 3 after implementation. The cost of this program for all 63 patients was $86,436 for 6 months ($9.09 ± $10.52/person per day), including $36,755 for toileting.

A comparison of two studies reporting the total expenditures for patient care, one to prevent PUs and one to treat PUs, revealed that in both cases the greatest expense is labor; however, for prevention, 46% of the total expenditures are labor,[100] whereas for treatment, labor accounts for 80% of costs.[101]

Some of the risk factors for PU (e.g., older age, history of chemotherapy, history of radiation treatment) are not modifiable. Other risk factors (e.g., confusion, poor family support, and psychosocial issues) necessitate referral to other professionals, including medical social workers, psychologists, psychiatrists, or other adult services. Fever, low diastolic blood pressure, medications, impaired circulation, and comorbidities may require medical attention in addition to preventive measures. Some of the risk factors that can be addressed by rehabilitation interventions are impaired circulation (see Chapter 30), impaired sensation as it relates to the diabetic foot (see Chapter 31), and poorly fitting wheelchairs (see Chapter 33).

Most PU risk factors can be addressed by five specific interventions identified as effective in preventing PUs or in facilitating wound healing. These interventions are: Caregiver education, use of support surfaces, positioning, moisture control, and adequate nutrition. Of these five, education received strength of evidence ratings of A and B.[1] The AHRQ *Guideline* further states that the education should be structured, organized, and comprehensive; should be directed at all levels of health care providers, patients, family, and caregivers; and should include information about the other four interventions.[1]

Support Surfaces. Support surfaces (including wheelchair cushions, bed overlays, and specialty mattresses) distribute pressure to decrease the amount of pressure over a body part at risk for PU formation. Support surfaces are divided into two categories: Pressure reducing, defined as a surface that inconsistently reduces the pressure below the capillary closing pressures in all positions, on all body locations (25-32 mm Hg), and pressure relieving, defined as a surface that consistently reduces the pressure below capillary closing pressures, in any position and in most body locations. Table 28-7 provides indications, advantages, disadvantages, and examples of different bed support surfaces.

Because it is universally accepted and federally mandated that support surfaces be used for patients at risk for or with existing PUs, recent research has been directed at determining the most cost-effective, efficacious support surface for different patient conditions. Study summaries about the effects of various bed and wheelchair support surfaces on wound incidence and healing rates are listed in Table 28-8.[102-116]

Interface pressure, defined as the pressure between a surface and the skin over a bony prominence, can be measured by a number of devices, ranging from hand-held sensors to large pressure-mapping devices. The ideal interface pressure would be lower than the patient's arterial capillary closing pressure, defined as the pressure that occludes the smallest vessels. The average capillary closing pressure in a healthy adult male forefinger is 32 mm Hg[31]; however, the values can vary, depending on body build, skeletal structure, amount of body fat, and the amount of soft tissue covering the bony prominences. Therefore the totality of patient risk factors must be considered when selecting equipment for prevention or treatment of PUs. If pressure sensors are not available, the support surface can be checked for adequate off-loading by placing the hand between the support surface (mattress or cushion)

and the base of the bed or wheelchair. If the bony prominence is palpable, the surface is said to have "bottomed out" and is not sufficiently reducing the interface pressure.

The low-air-loss (LAL) bed is intended to remove or reduce perspiration, provide localized cooling of the skin to prevent heat accumulation and thereby control the skin microclimate, and distribute the torso load (Fig. 28-11).[117] Lateral rotation beds that provide continuous side-to-side rotation have been shown to increase the oxygenation index (the ratio of arterial partial pressure of oxygen to fraction of inspired oxygen) and to decrease the incidence of ventilator-associated pneumonia.[118] The side-to-side rotation is not, however, sufficient off-loading to prevent PUs, as noted by a study of patients with pulmonary conditions using lateral rotation beds in an acute care hospital. An increased incidence of PUs of the sacrum, occiput, and heels was noted after 6 months of use, and reinstitution of repositioning, off-loading the heels, and turning the patient's head every 2 hours resulted in a 52% decrease in PU incidence.[119] Research for the optimal bed to prevent and treat PUs is ongoing, with new products continually being developed.

Wheelchair cushions, like beds, can be static or dynamic; nonpowered or powered; air, gel, or foam, and vary in size and shape. Unlike beds that distribute the weight over the entire body, cushions primarily protect the major weight-bearing surface in sitting (the ischial tuberosities) and transfer the weight to the area that is at least risk for PUs (the femurs). Some cushions are contoured to distribute the weight equally throughout the buttocks and posterior thighs; some are designed to eliminate pressure on the ischial tuberosities by providing a U-shaped pocket in which they are suspended (Isch-Dish, Span-America, Greenville, SC). Criteria for cushion selection are multifactorial and specific to each patient.

Criteria for Wheelchair Cushion Selection
Patient factors
- History or presence of ulceration
- Amount of skin moisture and incontinence
- Weight and height
- Sensation and ability to detect peak pressures
- The length of time the patient will be sitting each day

Functional factors
- Ability to off-load by shifting weight or performing push-ups
- Anticipated length of time the cushion will be used (short-term vs long-term)
- Amount of stability the patient needs from the cushion
- The type of chair the patient uses
- Cost and insurance reimbursement

Although no specific studies were found relating pressure reduction with doughnut-shaped cushions, it is generally accepted that these cushions are not effective in redistributing pressure on as much body surface area as possible, and they may contribute to ischemia in the tissue positioned inside the doughnut hole.

Clinicians have historically taught wheelchair-bound patients to do push-ups and weight shifts to allow reperfusion of the ischial and gluteal areas and thereby help prevent PU formation. A study of transcutaneous oxygen tension ($TcPO_2$) in the sitting (loaded) position and during pressure relief (unloaded) in SCI patients suggested that doing pressure lifts for 15-30 seconds is not sufficient to raise oxygenation to unloaded values.[120] The mean duration of pressure relief required to raise $TcPO_2$ to unloaded values was 1 minute 51 seconds. Therefore the authors recommend alternative methods of pressure relief.

Two specialty products designed for wheelchair pressure relief are the total contact seat (TCS) and the thoracic suspension orthosis (TSO). The TCS uses a prosthetic fitting technique to distribute sitting pressure and reduce resting pressure under the ischial tuberosities to below capillary pressure, presumed to be 1 pound per square inch *(psi)*. A comparison of the TCS with three standard cushions showed significantly lower pressures at all times using the TCS with sustained pressures below the postulated threshold for tissue damage.[116] The TSO consists of a custom-molded thoracolumbosacral orthosis suspended from the wheelchair frame (also referred to as the bucket design) so that the body weight is supported primarily by the thorax, thereby off-loading the lower body pressure areas.[121,122] The TSO is recommended for patients with chronic PUs, chronic pain with sitting, severe scoliosis, or bilateral lower extremity amputation (Fig. 28-12). A retrospective study of six patients with severe chronic PUs indicated they were able to either resume modified sitting or sit for longer periods of time when using the TSO.[123] A quantitative study of seating pressure in 10 subjects using a TSO found a 59.8% mean decrease in seating pressures during a 90-120 minute period of being suspended.[124]

Three meta-analyses of randomized controlled trials assessing the effectiveness of pressure relieving beds, mattresses, and cushions in the prevention and treatment of PUs summarized the high quality data in this area and reached the following conclusions:[125-127]

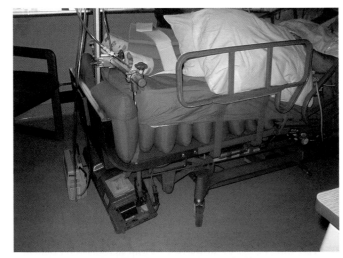

FIG. 28-11 Low-air-loss bed.

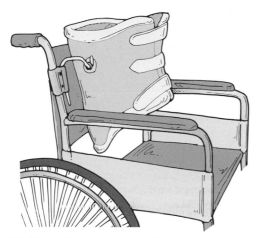

FIG. 28-12 Thoracic suspension orthosis is recommended for patients with chronic pressure ulcers, chronic pain with sitting, or bilateral lower extremity amputation. *Courtesy Fillauer, Inc, Chattanooga, Tenn.*

- Foam mattresses are more effective than standard hospital mattresses in moderate- to high-risk patients.
- Pressure relieving overlays in the operating room reduced the incidence of postoperative PUs.
- Air-fluidized beds and LAL beds improve the rate of wound healing.
- Seat cushions and constant low-pressure devices have not been adequately evaluated.

Positioners/Protectors. Positioners are support devices used to off-load bony prominences and to maintain optimal position of a body part, thereby reducing the risk of ulceration or promoting healing of an existing ulcer (Fig. 28-13). A positioner may also help prevent foot drop, maintain neutral hip position, keep the heels off the bed, or prevent ankles and knees from rubbing against each other. Positioners are constructed of rigid or semirigid frames with air, gel, foam, or lambs wool padding. Semirigid frames are recommended if the patient does not have the range of motion (ROM) needed for equal weight distribution throughout the device. For example, the ankle should achieve 0 degrees dorsiflexion if a rigid boot

is used, so that high pressures do not develop on the forefoot and Achilles tendon (Fig. 28-14). Other considerations in selecting a foot positioner are gait status (some styles have an ambulating surface, some do not), risk factors (e.g., fragile skin, insensate feet), and cost.

Protectors are soft devices that use foam, gel, air, fiber, or dimethicone to protect bony prominences (primarily on the heels and elbows) from shear and friction; however, protectors do not reduce pressure. Protectors are most useful when the patient has fragile skin and tends to slide against the linens or chair arms. The Rooke boot, an example of a substantial protector, is useful for the ischemic foot before surgery because it off-loads the heel, protects the toes, and maintains warmth. When a positioner or a protector is used on the heel, the lower leg should be elevated on a pillow to further reduce peak pressure where the heel touches the bed.

Positioning. Although appropriate support surfaces can help prevent PUs and facilitate wound healing, they are only an adjunct to proper positioning and frequent turning. After identification of risk factors and inspection of the skin, a turning schedule should be instituted when indicated. Although most turning schedules are based on a 2-hour sequence,[36,128] patients at high risk may need to be repositioned more frequently or areas that are at high risk or with existing ulcers may require continuous off-loading, thereby eliminating a position from the sequence.[1] For example, if a patient has a stage III PU on the right greater trochanter, right sidelying would be eliminated or minimized, depending on the tissue integrity of the sacrum and left side. Having a written schedule posted in the patient's room facilitates involving all disciplines in the turning program and can improve compliance.

The ideal sitting position is one that distributes the body weight to nonbony areas (e.g., the posterior thighs) and that off-loads the bony prominences. The "90/90/90" position, with the hips, knees, and ankles flexed approximately 90 degrees, is often recommended (Fig. 28-15). In this position, the femurs are parallel to the floor with all but the distal $1\frac{1}{2}$-2 inches supported on the sitting surface, the feet are supported on the floor or foot rests, the face is in a vertical position perpendicular to the floor, and the gaze is directed straight ahead. The weight is equally

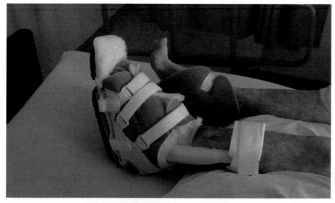

FIG. 28-13 Foot positioner and protector. Both require placement of a pillow under the calves for optimal off-loading of the heels.

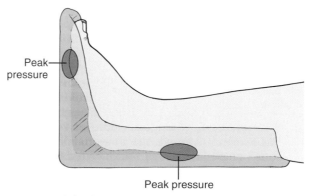

FIG. 28-14 If the foot cannot be dorsiflexed to 0 degrees, the Achilles tendon and plantar metatarsal heads are at risk for increased soft tissue pressure and ulcer formation.

distributed on both sides, and the natural spinal curves are supported by the chair back or by cushions. The "90/90/90" position distributes body weight most equally through the trunk and extremities and reduces the risk of high peak pressures leading to ulceration. Additional off-loading in sitting can be provided by armrests of sufficient height to support the upper body weight without causing excessive shoulder elevation.[27]

An alternative sitting position is with the wheelchair back semireclined, with the legs elevated on leg rests (Fig. 28-16).[129,130] After the ideal sitting position for a patient is

determined, the evaluator can isolate the physical limitation and seating deficits that prevent the position from being assumed and maintained. Chapter 34 provides more detail on evaluation, selection, and adaptation of wheelchairs. Table 28-9 outlines common errant sitting patterns and positions and recommended remedies.

The ideal position for a supine patient is with the weight distributed as evenly as possible throughout the entire body. This is best achieved with the bed as flat as possible. However, this position is not always comfortable, especially for the elderly patient (e.g., if the patient has back pain as a result of spinal stenosis), nor is it ideal for some pathological conditions (e.g., patients on mechani-

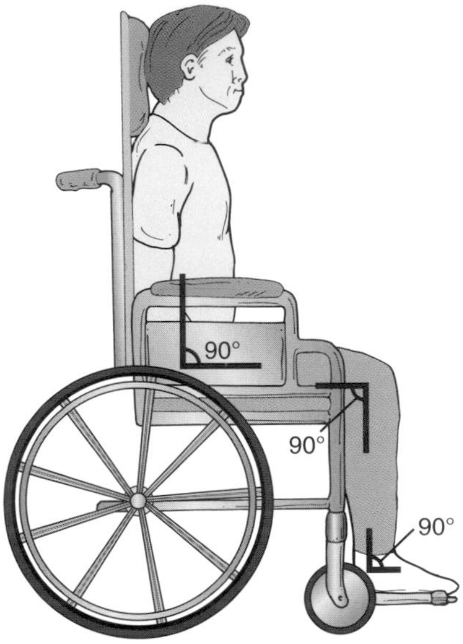

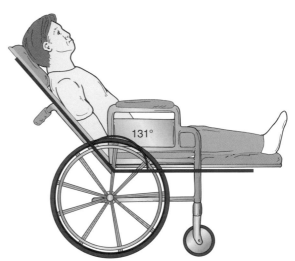

FIG. 28-15 The "90/90/90" sitting position in a wheelchair distributes body weight on the well-padded posterior thighs, off-loading the ischial tuberosities.

FIG. 28-16 Semi-reclining wheelchair position with the legs elevated on leg rests off-loads sacrum and prevents shear forces that occur with slumping positions.

TABLE 28-9 Causes and Solutions for Problematic Sitting Patterns

Problematic Position	Causes	Solutions
Buttocks sliding forward in seat, face looking toward ceiling	<90° hip flexion	Recline the chair till face is vertical
	Seat depth too short or too long	Modify to extend to within 1.5 inches of popliteal fossa
	Seat too high, feet do not touch the floor	Place cushion behind back
		Use a drop-seat or foot rests
		Minimize contact of the ball of the foot with foot rest
	Increased trunk extensor tone	Use a lap belt or pommel cushion to hold hips back in the chair
		Use a lower back rest
		Change seat or back angle
Forward trunk flexion, face looking at floor	Kyphosis	Use a wedge cushion
	>90° hip flexion contractures	
	Seat height too low	Add a seat cushion
	Foot rests too high	Lower foot rests or add a cushion
Weight unequally distributed side to side	Low trunk tone	Add trunk supports
	Chair too wide	Use narrower chair
	Structural deformity or post-surgical deformity	Use thicker cushion on the side with less weight or with lower pelvis
	Poor femoral position	Use contoured cushion to support femurs
		Use foam or towel roll between the chair and the lateral femur to maintain neutral hip

Adapted from Hamm R, Behringer B: *The Give and Take of Wound Management: A Guide to Making Clinical Decisions,* Irvine, Calif, 2004, ConceptMedia, Inc.
References: Rappl L: Management of pressure by therapeutic positioning. In Sussman C, Bates-Jensen BM (eds): *Wound Care: A Collaborative Practice Manual for Physical Therapists and Nurses,* Gaithersburg, Md, 1998, Aspen.

cal ventilation for whom a semirecumbent position of 45 degrees is recommended to prevent ventilator-associated aspiration pneumonia).[131,132] Box 28-2 lists some strategies to consider when adjusting the patient away from the ideal position, and Table 28-10 lists common problems for recumbent positions, associated risks, and recommended solutions.

Two alternative positions for the bed-bound patient are 30- and 150-degrees sidelying. Both positions off-load the sacrum without increasing pressure to the greater trochanter, and both can be comfortable for the patient (Fig. 28-17). To maintain 30-degrees sidelying, a foam wedge or pillow roll is placed under one side of the shoulders and hips to form a 30-degree angle between the pelvis and the support surface. A pillow under the upper leg and between the knees prevents pressure on the inside of the knees and ankles. A pillow under the uppermost extremity will also improve patient comfort. The 150-degrees sidelying position is maintained by placing a pillow or wedge under the chest, a pillow under the upper leg to prevent excessive hip internal rotation, and a small pillow or towel roll under the ankle of the lower leg (Fig. 28-18). Foam wedges with at least a 30-degree angle are excellent support devices and are available from commercial vendors.

The occiput is at risk for ulceration in the younger pediatric population,[3] especially if the head is larger than normal,[46] because at this age the occiput is proportionately the largest and heaviest bony prominence.[133] At around adolescence, pressure shifts from the occiput to areas typical for adults.[3,134] High occipital pressure was found to be consistently reduced with a 4-inch foam overlay.[134] However, a study of interface pressures on LAL beds using

---

BOX 28-2 | Strategies for Tissue Protection in the Supine Position

- Test interface pressure between skin over bony prominences and support surface with commercial pressure sensor or by placing hand between mattress and overlay. If point of concern (e.g., sacrum, heel, greater trochanter) can be palpated or if there is less than 1 inch of support between the hand and bony prominences, support surface has "bottomed out" and is not effective.
- Use pillows or foam protective devices to protect bony prominences from rubbing against each other or against mechanical devices.
- Maintain head of bed lower than 30° except during meals. Increasing head elevation increases risk for shear forces over the sacrum. For patients who have NG feeding tube or have COPD, both requiring that head of bed be higher than 30°, maintaining it below 45° is advised.
- Off-load heels with pillows under calves, knees, and thighs (not under heels) or with heel protectors. After patient is positioned, check heel by placing hand underneath to ensure nothing is pressing on any side. Convoluted foam heel protectors require caution and frequent skin checks, especially if the foot and lower leg are edematous and skin is fragile. Raised points of foam on the inner surface of these devices can cause pressure points that lead to skin breakdown.
- Maintain <25° of knee flexion by supporting the knees with a pillow or by gatching the bed.

NG, Nasogastric; *COPD*, chronic obstructive pulmonary disease.

TABLE 28-10 | Risks and Solutions for Problematic Recumbent Positions

Problem	Areas at Risk	Solution
Exaggerated trunk extension	Occiput and heels	Support head with pillow and flex knees and hips to reduce tone
Abnormal reflexes (e.g., tonic labyrinthine, asymmetrical tonic neck reflex)	Any bony prominence	Use firm support devices to reduce tone; avoid soft pillows that facilitate tone; use side-lying positions
Risk of aspiration; cardiopulmonary deficits; need HOB elevated >30°	Sacrum and heels	Off-load heels with pillows or protectors; limit time HOB is elevated >45°; keep below 30° if safe; sit in chair for meals if possible
Kyphosis, prominent spinous processes	Spinous processes; sacrum; coccyx	Elevate HOB slightly and support head and neck with pillows; in severe cases, place small towel roll along each side of the spine
Hip and knee flexion contractures (usually patient rolls to one side more than the other)	Inner knees, heels, greater trochanter, ischium, sacrum	Support the lower extremities in position of maximum extension; place a pillow between knees and ankles, turn side to side frequently
Postsurgical incisions or scars	Ischemia around incision; dehiscence; ulcer recurrence	Position off the affected area; use support surface
Foot drop	Heels	Use protective device; place a pillow under calf, knee, and thigh; use foam or pillows to support foot in neutral position

Adapted from Hamm R, Behringer B: *The Give and Take of Wound Management: A Guide to Making Clinical Decisions,* Irvine, Calif, 2004, ConceptMedia, Inc.
References: Rappl L: Management of pressure by therapeutic positioning. In Sussman C, Bates-Jensen BM (eds): *Wound Care: A Collaborative Practice Manual for Physical Therapists and Nurses,* Gaithersburg, Md, 1998, Aspen; Rappl L, Hagler D: Prevention and treatment of pressure ulcers. In Kloth L, McCullough JM (eds): *Wound Healing: Alternatives in Management,* ed 3, Philadelphia, 2002, FA Davis.
HOB, Head of bed.

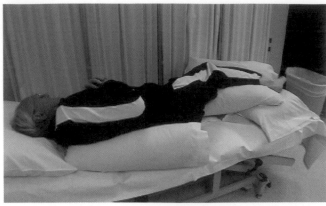

FIG. 28-17 Patient in 30-degree side-lying position to off-load the sacrum.

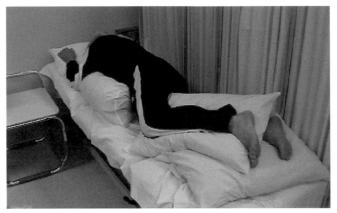

FIG. 28-18 Patient in 150-degree side-lying position to off-load the sacrum, greater trochanters, and scapulae.

10 healthy subjects found that occipital and heel pressures exceeded the accepted capillary closing pressure, suggesting that additional measures are needed to off-load the occiput and heels to prevent PU formation.[135] There is little literature on effective methods to off-load the occiput; however, suggestions from caregivers include the use of a gel or air-cell pad or a rolled towel under the area just proximal to the occiput. Turning the head from side to side every 2 hours is also recommended.[119] The use of doughnuts is discouraged because they contribute to venous congestion and edema inside the ring[1] and may contribute to the formation of PUs.[136]

Patients who wear rigid cervical collars are also at risk for occipital PUs.[137] Risk factors associated with the collars are pressure, accumulation of moisture, and increased skin temperature.[138] As with any rigid orthotic, the skin under the collar should be checked frequently, and the device should be adjusted for proper fit if any skin impairments are observed.

The amount of off-loading needed is different for every patient, depending on the impairments and the vulnerable areas of concern. After a thorough patient examination and evaluation, support surfaces and devices can be used creatively to establish an effective positioning and turning schedule specific for the patient. Through dili-

gence and cooperation, members of the health care team can ensure that the care plan is adhered to by all therapies and the goals are shared by all disciplines.

Moisture Management. Although moisture management is traditionally considered a function of nursing care, understanding the following principles and strategies for the incontinent patient is helpful for all rehabilitation caregivers:

- Bladder training or prompted voiding.[139]
- Cleanse after each incontinent episode with no-rinse cleaner.
- Apply a moisture barrier ointment or cream after every cleansing.
- Use absorbent underpads or briefs.
- Avoid thin plastic-backed underpads that hold moisture and heat against the skin.
- Use a catheter for urinary incontinence and a fecal pouch or rectal tube for fecal incontinence.
- Place absorbent material in skinfolds where perspiration may accumulate and cause skin impairment.
- Wash wheelchair cushions after every incontinent episode and allow the cushion to fully dry before using it again.

The National Pressure Ulcer Long-Term Care Study of 1524 subjects in 95 long-term care facilities reported that patients were significantly less likely to develop PUs if they wore disposable briefs.[37] However, if the patient is in a specialty bed designed to reduce skin moisture and temperature, pads or briefs that have plastic backing are contraindicated. These beds are especially beneficial for patients at risk for skin maceration from excessive perspiration. If the patient has a sacral or trochanteric PU, fishnet surgical panties are recommended to hold dressings in place and allow free flow of air on the surrounding skin.

Lewis-Byers evaluated two incontinence skin care protocols for 31 patients in a long-term care facility.[140] The protocols were (1) cleansing with soap and water followed by application of a moisturizing lotion, and (2) cleansing with a no-rinse pH-balanced liquid cleanser followed by application of a moisture barrier cream after the first incontinent episode each day. There was a trend toward maintained or improved skin integrity and lower pain scores in group 2; however, the study sample was too small to determine statistical significance.[140] A retrospective study of 34 skilled nursing facility (SNF) residents with incontinence compared the incidence of PUs with 3 months of standard care or with 3 months of standard care plus the use of a disposable perineal washcloth containing a skin protectant.[141] Five of the 34 incontinent residents (14.7%) developed PUs during the first 3 months with standard care; none developed PUs during the 3 months with standard care plus the use of a perineal washcloth with skin protectant ($p = 0.15$).[141] The authors concluded that the use of a skin protectant is effective in reducing the incidence of nosocomial sacral and buttock PUs, as is recommended by the AHRQ *Guidelines*.[20]

Nutrition. The goals of any nutrition intervention for patients with PUs are to provide sufficient calories, protein, fluid, vitamins, and trace elements to facilitate wound healing and closure.[64,65] For patients with nutritional deficits at risk for or with existing wounds, nutritional supplementation should be given orally if the patient can eat. If the gastrointestinal system is functioning, but the patient cannot swallow enough food to meet their nutritional needs, feeding of liquid may be provided temporarily by a nasogastric tube or by a gastrojejunostomy tube permanently inserted by a percutaneous endoscopic gastrostomy (PEG) procedure. If the gastrointestinal system is not functioning, nutrition may be provided intravenously by total parenteral nutrition (TPN). All nonoral alternative feeding methods have associated risks and are not as effective at meeting nutritional needs as oral feeding. Nutritional interventions are ordered by the physician, generally in consultation with a registered dietitian.

INTERVENTIONS BASED ON WOUND STAGE

After a PU has been debrided of necrotic tissue and staged (based on the amount of tissue loss as described), effective local interventions can be implemented (Table 28-11). The process of improving the wound to facilitate healing, termed wound-bed preparation, involves multiple interventions with the following goals: To remove devitalized tissue from the wound, including necrotic eschar and fibrinous tissue; to facilitate angiogenesis and thereby increase the amount of granulation tissue; to reduce the number of senescent cells (cells incapable of mitotic activity) in the wound bed and at the edges and thereby facilitate both angiogenesis and epithelialization; to decrease exudate and edema, both of which retard the healing process; and to decrease the bacterial burden.[142,143]

Wound-bed preparation begins with removal of the devitalized tissue (debridement), which may be accomplished by one or more techniques (Table 28-12). With debridement, much of the bacterial burden is removed; however, if clinical signs of infection (redness, drainage, edema, pain, odor, warmth) are present, a culture is indicated, followed by appropriate systemic or topical antibiotics. The removal of bacteria, exudate, and edema can be facilitated by a variety of techniques, including advanced dressings and physical modalities. After the necrotic tissue, exudate, and bacterial load have been removed, dressings that will effectively manage drainage and maintain a warm, moist wound environment are applied.

Wound Dressings. Wound dressings are identified as primary or secondary. Primary dressings are applied directly to the wound bed and secondary dressings are used to anchor or contain the primary dressings. The

TABLE 28-11	Intervention Based on Pressure Ulcer Stage
Stage	**Intervention**
Stage I	Determine the causative factors.
	Adapt seating and bed surfaces to reduce pressure, friction, or shear forces at the areas of concern.
	Protect macerated skin with a moisture barrier cream or ointment.
	Protect areas exposed to friction forces with a transparent film dressing.
	Encourage frequent changes of position.
Stage II	Consistently position the patient to reduce pressure at the areas of concern.
	Cleanse the wound and periwound tissue with normal saline or a wound cleanser.
	Remove any loose devitalized tissue.
	Cover with a transparent film dressing if there is no drainage or a hydrocolloid dressing if there is minimal to moderate drainage. Both dressings are semipermeable to prevent bacteria from entering the wound.
	Evaluate the need for an indwelling urinary catheter or absorbent pads to prevent skin exposure to excess moisture.
	Protect the periwound skin from maceration or friction.
Stage III and Stage IV	Consistently position the patient to relieve pressure at the areas of concern.
	Use a pressure-relieving support surface.
	Debride the wound of all necrotic tissue.
	Culture for infection (if signs of infection are observed) and treat with appropriate antibiotics and local antimicrobial dressings.
	Irrigate the wound daily with pulsed lavage with suction to remove slough, to decrease the bacteria load, and to help manage drainage.
	Assess for negative pressure therapy after more than 70% of the wound is free of necrotic tissue.
	Use a dressing appropriate for the bacterial load and drainage (e.g., alginates, foam fillers, hydrocolloids, collagen matrix dressings, or non-toxic topical ointments).
	Assess nutritional status and supplement diet as needed.
	Evaluate the need for surgical closure.
Post-Surgery	Maintain bed rest in a low–air loss mattress or air-fluidized bed for two to four weeks.
	Manage incontinence to keep flap dry and free of contaminants.
	Observe flap for changes that may indicate hematoma formation (dark red appearance), flap necrosis (black tissue), dehiscence (separation at suture site), seroma (pocket of clear fluid), or infection (white appearance under the skin).
Post-Healing	Assess for proper support surfaces to off-load the flap or graft.
	Monitor support surfaces for "bottoming out" phenomenon for at least two years.
	Monitor the skin of the flap or graft for at least two years.
	Rehabilitate the patient to maximum functional level.
	Educate the patient on the necessity to stop smoking in order to maintain tissue viability.
	Encourage continued good nutrition.

TABLE 28-12	Methods of Debridement

Type	Methods
Surgical	Performed in the operating room by a licensed physician, podiatrist, or physician's assistant.
	Not tissue-specific; removes all necrotic tissue down to and often including some viable tissue.
	Required in the following conditions:
	• The wound is life-threatening.
	• There is more necrotic tissue than can be removed at bedside.
	• The risk of bleeding is high and sutures or cauterization may be required.
	• Infected or necrotic bone is being removed.
	• Pain cannot be controlled by standard medications or topical anesthetics.
Sharp	Selective removal of necrotic, infected, or foreign tissue with sterile instruments (scalpels, scissors, tweezers, and forceps).
	Performed bedside or in an outpatient clinic.
	Requires a physician's referral when performed by allied health personnel.
Mechanical	Nonselective removal of devitalized tissue from the wound and periwound areas using friction or pressure.
	May be painful.
	Used for loose debris and exudate.
	Includes moist-to-damp dressings, abrasion, syringe irrigation, PLWS, and whirlpool.
Autolytic	Phagocytosis of necrotic tissue by white blood cells in natural body fluids.
	Facilitated by moisture-retentive dressings (e.g., transparent films, hydrocolloids, calcium alginates).
	Selective and pain-free.
	Effective for adhered superficial eschar; is inefficient for large amounts of eschar.
Enzymatic	Is the application of enzymes in a topical petrolatum based ointment to facilitate the liquefaction and digestion of nonviable wound tissue.
	Selective and pain-free.
	Helpful adjunct to sharp and autolytic debridement.
	Currently limited to two preparations:
	• Papain-urea based combinations.
	• Collagenase.

PLWS, Pulsed lavage with suction.

function and selection of the primary dressing is based on the wound characteristics (e.g., tissue type, healing phase, bacterial count). The function and selection of the secondary dressing is based on the purpose and consistency of the primary dressing and on the patient's functional status. The appropriate wound dressing will likely change as the needs of the wound change and may vary among different areas of a wound that are in different healing phases. Custom dressings consisting of two or more primary dressings and one secondary dressing may be indicated in a single wound, provided the primary dressings do not inactivate each other. The informed clinician, being resourceful with the available supplies, matches the primary dressing to the wound needs and the secondary dressing to the patient needs (Table 28-13).

Selecting the optimal dressing for a PU can appear to be a daunting task given the myriad of products available. A few basic principles, however, can make the decision quite simple. The advantages of a moist wound environment over dry or wet-to-dry methods are well documented,[144] therefore any dressing selected should keep the wound bed moist while keeping the periwound skin dry to protect it from maceration. If the wound bed tends to be dry, dressings that add moisture are advised. If there is drainage, the dressing should manage any excessive moisture. Periwound skin should also be protected with moisture barrier creams, protective films, or hydrocolloid dressings. When dressing a PU with a cavity, the cavity should be lightly filled with the dressing material so that there is no dead space to collect exudate and increase the risk of infection or abscess formation. Self-adhesive dress-

ings are recommended to avoid applying tape to the periwound skin because removing tape can cause skin tears. Many of the advanced dressings can remain in place for 24-72 hours or longer, reducing caregiver time and facilitating wound healing by limiting wound bed disturbance, and as a result, thereby decreasing the overall cost of treatment.

Although wound dressings that facilitate wound healing by creating a moist wound environment are currently accepted as standard of care in the medical community, some of the newer advanced biological topical medications and dressings are more controversial. Becaplermin gel (Regranex) is a platelet-derived growth factor that has been studied extensively for the treatment of diabetic ulcers.[145-148] One study reported that becaplermin gel is also effective in the treatment of PUs. In a randomized controlled trial of 124 adults with PUs, topical treatment with becaplermin gel was compared with a placebo gel until healing was achieved or for a maximum of 16 weeks. Becaplermin significantly increased the incidence of complete or >90% healing and significantly reduced the ulcer volume at end-point.[149] In addition, a meta-analysis of four phase II and III trials strongly supports the efficacy of becaplermin gel for facilitation of wound healing.[150] Although becaplermin gel is currently the only topical growth factor commercially available, topical formulations of transforming growth factor-beta 3[151] and nerve growth factors[152-154] are being investigated specifically for use with PUs with promising results.

Silver, in the forms of dilute silver nitrate liquid and silver sulfadiazine cream, has been used as a topical

TABLE 28-13	Dressing Categories			
Dressing Category	**Composition**	**Uses**	**Advantages**	**Disadvantages**
Wound cleansers				
• Normal saline	0.9% saline, sterile water	Cleansing wound Moist to damp dressing	Inexpensive	Contains no preservatives, should be discarded 24 hours after opening
• Cleansing solutions	Surfactants in assorted bases	Cleansing wound Mechanical debridement	Helps disrupt bond between necrotic tissue and wound bed Neutral pH	Reduces frictional force of sterile gauze
Gauze	100% cotton or synthetic fabric	Cleansing wound Filling cavity and sinus wounds Anchoring primary dressings	Available in a variety of sizes and shapes Inexpensive Conforms to wound shape Absorbs exudate	Dries easily Destroys healthy tissue if allowed to dry Needs to be changed twice per day Does not contain exudate
Transparent film	Polymer sheet with adhesive layer on one side	Autolytic debridement Reduce friction over bony prominences Superficial wounds with minimal drainage Secondary dressing over foam or gauze	Conforms easily to any shape Impermeable to bacteria Reduces friction between wound bed and contact surfaces Waterproof Adheres well to dry skin Can stay in place 3-7 days Cost effective	Nonabsorbent May cause periwound maceration May tear fragile skin if removed improperly Will not stick to moist areas
Hydrogel sheets	Hydrophilic polymers entrap water to form solid sheet	Thermal burns and painful wounds	Promotes epithelialization Soothes inflamed tissue Protects granulation tissue	Slippery Requires a secondary dressing
Amorphous	Polymers and water in a gel form	Dry eschar wounds Clean granulating wounds Exposed tendon and bone	Maintain moist wound environment Assume shape of cavity wounds Promotes autolysis Non-cytotoxic to granulation tissue Cost effective	Requires a secondary dressing May contribute to periwound maceration if applied too heavily
Hydrocolloids	Combination of adhesive layer, absorbent hydrocolloid layer, and semipermeable layer	Shallow full thickness wounds with minimal to moderate exudate Stage II or III pressure ulcers Macerated tissue	Absorbent Promotes granulation and epithelialization Promotes autolysis Protects skin from friction May not require second dressing Can stay in place 3-4 days Available in variety of sizes and shapes and in combination with other dressings	May roll at the edges Moderately expensive May create an odor as it absorbs exudate May tear fragile skin if removed improperly
Foams	Polyurethane	Wounds with minimal to copious exudates Cavity wounds (chips and pillows)	Available in a variety of sizes and shapes Highly absorbent Do not adhere to the wound bed Painless to remove	Expensive May require secondary dressing May be bulky Difficult to conform to some areas
Calcium alginates				
• Ropes or layers	Calcium salts of alginic acid which have been spun into fibers	Wounds with moderate to copious drainage	Highly absorbent Conforms to wound shape May be bacteriostatic and mildly hemostatic Decreases odor	Requires secondary dressing Not advised over bone or tendon because of dessication Difficult to remove if allowed to dry in wound bed
Collagen matrix	Collagen derived from bovine material with all cells extracted, freeze-dried, and shaped into sheets, particles, or gels	Any recalcitrant wound to facilitate collagen migration	Conforms to wound bed Promotes granulation and epithelialization	Expensive Requires secondary dressing

Continued

TABLE 28-13	Dressing Categories—cont'd			
Dressing Category	**Composition**	**Uses**	**Advantages**	**Disadvantages**
Topical dressings	Water or petrolatum-based gels and ointments containing active ingredients; used as primary dressing on wound bed (antimicrobials, growth factors, silver, enzymes)	Wounds requiring topical medications / Painful wounds (topical anesthetics)	Allows local application of antimicrobials without use of systemic antibiotics / Maintains moist wound environment while delivering active ingredient to wound bed	Usually requires prescription depending on active ingredient / Requires a secondary dressing / Risk of allergic reaction to active ingredient / Some may not be used simultaneously (e.g., enzymatic and silver sulfadiazine)
Small intestine submucosa (SIS) dressings	Collagen tissue extracted from porcine submucosa, processed to remove cells, and shaped into sheets	Full or partial thickness wounds of any etiology / Autograft donor sites / Second degree burns	Promote cell migration / Present no risk of rejection / Minimizes scarring / Reduces frequency of dressing changes (in place 5-7 days) / Has long shelf life	Expensive
Living skin equivalents	Human fibroblasts embedded in a bovine collagen matrix and bioabsorbable scaffold	Full or partial thickness flat wounds	Promote epithelialization / Noninvasive and painless / May help avoid skin grafting / Decreases scarring	Requires fully granulated, infection-free wound bed / Expensive / Short shelf-life (5 days)

antimicrobial medication for wound management for many years, especially with burn related wounds.[155] Silver sulfadiazine cream has also been used for treatment of PUs because of its ability to keep the wound bed moist and decrease bacterial load. Because the silver in silver nitrate liquid and silver sulfadiazine cream is released and absorbed quickly, these preparations must be applied twice daily, and an absorbent secondary dressing may be needed to manage exudates in moderate to heavily draining wounds. A new topical silver preparation, *nanocrystalline silver*, has recently become popular for wound management because the silver in it is absorbed only by the local tissue not systemically, making it safe for use on patients with end-stage renal disease. The nanocrystalline silver can also be incorporated into an absorbent dressing (e.g., hydrofiber or foam) and thus remain in place for 2-4 days. A laboratory study of a nanocrystalline silver-coated dressing demonstrated that the concentration of silver released over a 24-hour period was 70 mg/ml and inhibition of microbes (*P. aeruginosa* and *Staphylococcus aureus*) lasted for a minimum of 9 days with one application. In addition, the silver was "very rapidly" bactericidal.[156] In another study, the rat burn model was used to compare the effectiveness of nanocrystalline silver dressings with liquid silver nitrate. The mean percentage survival rate of the control group was 5%, the silver nitrate group was 0%, and the nanocrystalline silver group was 85%, suggesting that the slow-release silver is more effective than traditional methods in controlling sepsis that result from burn wound infections. Additionally, the authors state that because nanocrystalline silver acts rapidly against bacteria, the risk of bacterial resistance to the dressing is minimized.[155] An uncontrolled, prospective study of 29 patients with chronic ulcers, including 2 with pressure ulcers, showed marked clinical improvement of the wounds treated with nanocrystalline silver dressings, including decreased exudate, decreased purulence, and a decrease in wound surface bacterial load measured by semiquantitative swabs.[157] An additional positive effect of nanocrystalline silver was demonstrated in a pilot study of eight patients with chronic wounds in which the matrix metalloproteinases (MMPs) in chronic wound fluid was measured before and after treatment. A marked decrease in MMPs was noted in the first 2-3 days of treatment and was sustained with continued use of the nanocrystalline dressing.[158] (MMPs have been shown to degrade extracellular matrix and inhibit wound healing.) Antimicrobial activity of four silver-containing dressings against three microorganisms: A gram-positive bacterium, *S. aureus*, a gram-negative organism, and *Escherichia coli* was studied.[159] Acticoat (Smith & Nephew, Largo, Fla) produced the most rapid antimicrobial effect in vitro, which was ascribed to the rapid release of relatively large concentrations of highly active silver ions. Contreet-H (Coloplast, Marietta, Ga), a foam-based dressing, had a broad antimicrobial activity similar to Acticoat but with a slower onset of action. Actisorb Silver 220 (Johnson & Johnson, New Brunswick, NJ), a gel-based dressing, was less effective in the wound itself but was capable of removing bacteria from exudate. Avance (SSL International, UK) was minimally effective.

A study of nanocrystalline silver in a sodium carboxymethylcellulose fiber dressing (Aquacel Ag, ConvaTec, Princeton, NJ) has implications for the treatment of

PUs because of the dressing's absorbent qualities and its ability to be used to fill cavity wounds. A pilot study of 18 participants with chronic leg ulcers, all of whom were treated for 28 days with nanocrystalline silver in sodium carboxymethylcellulose fiber dressings, yielded the following findings: The overall mean wear time was 3.59 days, no leakage was observed in 69.8% of the dressing changes, pain scores were significantly reduced from baseline including with dressing changes, 39% of the wounds showed marked improvement and 56% showed mild improvement, and 2 of the 11 wounds infected at baseline resolved without the use of systemic antibiotics.[160] These studies indicate that nanocrystalline silver, particularly when used in conjunction with an absorbent dressing, may decrease the bacterial load of PUs, promote wound healing, and be cost-effective because fewer dressing changes are required during the treatment period.

Topical Antibiotics. The use of topical antibiotics is not recommended for wounds that are responding to conservative treatment with risk factor management and dressings. However, when a clean PU is not healing or a wound has persistent exudate after 2-4 weeks of standard care, the AHRQ *Guidelines* recommend a 2-week trial of topical antibiotics.[1] The antibiotic should be effective against gram-negative, gram-positive, and anaerobic organisms. This approach has sufficient strength of evidence to be rated A.[1]

Debridement. Debridement, the removal of nonviable tissue and foreign bodies from the wound bed, is an important part of wound-bed preparation. For stage IV wounds involving muscle, tendon, or bone, surgical debridement under anesthesia may be advised to avoid pain during the procedure and to allow for ready control of bleeding should this occur. For stage II and III PUs, selective sharp debridement at the bedside is usually feasible, in which case, local or systemic pain medications may be used to control pain if necessary. Selective sharp debridement is performed using a range of sterile surgical tools (e.g., scissors, scalpel, forceps, and curette) and either sterile or clean technique. The wound is first cleansed with a wound cleanser or normal saline. The necrotic tissue is removed by lifting and cutting with the forceps and scissors; by curettage in which the slough and soft exudate is scooped with the curette; or scoring, a technique of cross-hatching dry eschar to allow penetration of topical dressings that can soften the underlying connective tissue. Caution is required if the patient is on anticoagulants; if the $TcPO_2$ is less than 30 mm Hg, indicating compromised healing potential; or if the eschar is attached to vital tissue such as tendons or bone. In addition, if hard, dry eschar on a heel shows no signs of infection and is not interfering with function, it is recommended that the wound be treated conservatively, without debridement, until adequate circulation for healing has been confirmed.[161]

Debridement is continued in serial sessions after the initial debridement because wound healing is a dynamic process with changing tissue composition. During each treatment, the wound is observed closely for changes, and dressings are altered according to the needs of the tissue. Debridement should be terminated if any of the following conditions occur: Exposure of bones, tendons, nerves, or blood vessels or exposure of an unexpected sinus, tunnel, abscess, or fascial plane; all devitalized tissue has been removed; excessive bleeding; or the clinician is for any reason uncertain about continuing with tissue removal.

Debridement with tools may be augmented by use of topical enzymatic chemical debriders. Although these cannot substitute for surgical or sharp debridement when there is a large amount of necrotic tissue, they are effective for maintenance debridement or for removing adhered fibrous tissue that is difficult to debride with instruments.[162] The two active ingredient combinations currently used for enzymatic debridement are collagenase and a papain-urea combination. Collagenase ointment (Santyl) contains a partially purified preparation of collagenase enzyme derived from bacteria. The enzyme degrades nonviable collagen and converts it to gelatin, thereby facilitating the removal of the devitalized tissue.[163] The enzyme is selective for nonviable tissue and does not cause pain when applied. Papain-urea ointments (Panafil, Accuzyme) contain urea which denatures protein and disrupts its hydrogen bonds, and exposes the papain activators. This allows the papain enzymes to proteolyse the devitalized tissue. The papain-urea combination breaks down both viable and nonviable protein and may cause an inflammatory response and pain.[163] Therefore this type of preparation is recommended only for bulk debridement of necrotic tissue.

A laboratory study comparing the proteolytic activities of papain-urea and collagenase on different substrates indicated that papain-urea solubilizes matrices and extracellular matrix components, including casein, fibrin, native and heat-denatured collagen, and skin; however, it did not lyse elastin. Collagenase digested collagen, both native and heat denatured, as well as elastin and skin, but it did not digest fibrin. Clinically, this suggests that papain-urea would be effective for debridement of eschar, dried fibrinous exudate usually found in chronic venous ulcers, and burn eschar. Collagenase would be effective for burn eschar, heat-denatured collagen, and dermal ulcers.[164]

The effectiveness of collagenase and papain-urea preparations was evaluated in 26 long-term care patients with pressure ulcers in a randomized, prospective study.[165] Adequate off-loading was also provided with support surfaces and turning schedules. There was a significantly greater reduction in the area of nonviable tissue and increase in the area of granulation tissue for the wounds treated with papain-urea than for those treated with collagenase; however, there was no difference in wound size or amount of epithelialization between the two groups. In summary, enzymatic debridement may be a useful adjunct for removing devitalized tissue; however, interventions for off-loading tissue, reducing bacterial load, and managing exudate are still essential for effective treatment of any PU.

Adjunctive Therapies. Physical modalities, including electrical, light, sound, and mechanical energy to effect tissue changes at the cellular level, are used by physical therapists (PTs) to promote soft tissue healing in a variety of conditions.

Physical agents are a "broad group of procedures using various forms of energy that are applied to tissues in a systematic manner and that are intended to increase connective tissue extensibility; increase the healing rate of open wounds and soft tissue; modulate pain; reduce or eliminate soft tissue swelling, inflammation, or restriction associated with musculoskeletal injury or circulatory dysfunction; remodel scar tissue; or treat skin conditions."[23] Electrotherapeutic modalities, as they relate to wound healing, are a broad group of agents that use electricity to increase the rate of healing of open wounds, modulate or decrease pain, reduce bacterial load, and reduce or eliminate soft tissue swelling or inflammation. Negative pressure wound therapy (including pulsed lavage with suction and vacuum-assisted closure), electrical stimulation, ultraviolet C, and ultrasound are modalities that may be used for treatment of PUs; however, it is important to remember that they are adjunct therapies and not substitutes for standard care (i.e., tissue off-loading, debridement, and provision of a moist wound environment).

Pulsed Lavage with Suction. Given the fact that removal of bacteria, devitalized tissue, foreign bodies, and exudates facilitate wound closure, the clinician is faced with selecting the most effective method of removing these impediments. Pulsed lavage with suction (PLWS) combines low or high-pressure irrigation of normal saline at a controlled pressure (measured in pounds per square inch [psi]) and suction at a controlled subatmospheric pressure (measured in mm Hg) to remove debris, bacteria, and exudate from the wound bed (Fig. 28-19). A pressure range of 4-15 psi will safely mechanically debride a wound, remove bacteria, and stimulate angiogenesis.[166]

Recommended Pressure Ranges (in psi) for Pulsed Lavage with Suction

4-6: For sensitive areas, sinus tracts, tunneling, and painful wounds.
8-15: To decrease bacterial load in infected wounds.
9-15: To remove necrotic tissue.
15 and above: Use only with physician present.

The PLWS unit may be mains or battery-powered and includes a hand piece with a trigger to control the pressure, a tip to deliver the water into the wound bed and suction away the contaminated fluid, and two tubes—one connected to the bag of sterile normal saline and one connected to a suction pump (Fig. 28-20). Four systems, each with specific recommendations for providing patient care, are currently available. The Pulsavac System (Zimmer, Inc, Dover, OH) consists of a portable pump that can be transported to any patient care location and detachable, disposable handgun and tips. The Simpulse VariCare System (Davol, Inc, Cranston, RI) consists of a battery-operated hand piece that can be cleaned and stored for multiple treatments with the same patient when used with a special diverter tip that prevents the contaminated saline from traveling through the handpiece. The Davol Simpulse Plus System (Davol, Inc) is powered by medical air or nitrogen. The InterPulse System (Stryker, Inc, Kalamazoo, Mich) has a battery-powered hand piece with trigger-controlled pressure and disposable diverter tips.

Although much of the evidence on high-pressure irrigation (>8 psi) has been reported in the orofacial surgery and orthopedic literature, several studies have evaluated the effects of PLWS on acute and chronic wounds. Rodeheaver evaluated the effectiveness of high pressure irrigation for removing bacterial contamination in an animal model. Wounds on 4 groups of rats were contaminated with *S. aureus* and irrigated with saline delivered at 1, 5, 10, or 15 psi. Contaminant removal was 48.6%, 50.3%, 75.7%, and 84.8%, respectively.[167] Another study of postoperative appendectomy patients compared the infection rate of complicated surgical wounds treated with antibiotics (n = 40) or with antibiotics plus syringe irrigation of the wound with normal saline (n = 55).[168] In the group treated only with antibiotics, 72.5% of the patients developed wound infections; in the group treated with irrigation and antibiotics, 16.3% developed infections,

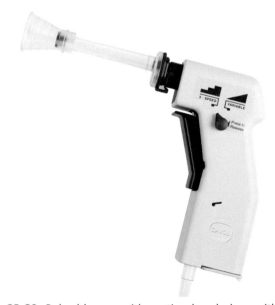

FIG. 28-20 Pulsed lavage with suction hand-piece with tip used to deliver water to the wound bed and suction contaminated fluid.

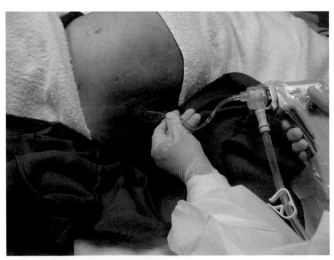

FIG. 28-19 Pulsed lavage with suction is used to remove debris, bacteria, and exudates from wound bed.

suggesting that irrigation of surgical wounds decreased postoperative infection rates. Bhandari studied the time-dependent effectiveness of high- and low-pressure lavage in removing aerobic bacteria from experimentally induced traumatic wounds with exposed bone in animals and found that high pressure (70 psi) removed bacteria more effectively than low pressure (1-2 psi) at all time points.[169] However, a study comparing the effectiveness of a 50-ml plastic syringe, a manual pump, and jet lavage for reducing bacterial load on nonbiological and biological surfaces found that although all techniques were effective, the manual pump was most effective.[170]

Based on the criteria in the AHRQ *Guidelines* for strength of evidence, PLWS is rated C.[1] More research is needed to determine the effects of PLWS on wound healing in patients. However, because of its advantages over other methods of wound cleansing, including whirlpool, PLWS is generally accepted as the treatment of choice for cleansing infected, necrotic, and draining wounds but is not generally recommended for healthy granulation tissue.

Advantages and Disadvantages. PLWS provides a higher pressure than syringe irrigation and delivers a larger amount of irrigating solution to the wound in a shorter length of time than bulb irrigation. PLWS can be used to treat bedridden and medically unstable patients (e.g., those in intensive care and cardiac care units) who cannot be transported to hydrotherapy for whirlpool treatment. It also enables treatment of isolated patients without risking exposure of other patients. Cross-contamination of multiple wounds on the same patient is reduced, and exposure to bacteria from other body parts, as may occur in full body submersion in a large whirlpool, is eliminated. The variable and controlled pressure and suction of PLWS allows adjustment to minimize pain. Treatment of foot ulcers with PLWS avoids the dependent position required for whirlpool treatment. In addition, PLWS is more time efficient than transporting patients to hydrotherapy and cleaning whirlpools. Specifically related to patients with PUs, PLWS enables patients to be treated in off-loaded positions and avoids transporting and treating patients with sacral ulcers in supine positions on hard surfaces.[171]

Indications and Contraindications. Indications for PLWS include stage III and IV PUs, especially those that are infected, draining, or necrotic. Irrigation performed before debridement will facilitate sharp debridement by loosening slough and softening eschar. Long flexible tips are available to treat areas of tunneling or undermining, where bacteria can colonize and exudate can collect. These tips deliver lower pressure and are safe to use in sinuses where the base of the wound is not visible.

Special Precautions. Special precautions are recommended for some unusual or complex wounds, such as tunneling wounds that cannot be observed or probed to the base, facial and groin wounds, wounds that expose major vessels, and wounds with excessive bleeding. Patients on anticoagulants, patients who are insensate, and patients who have pain not controlled by pain medications can also benefit from precautions. Precautionary measures include using lower pressure or different tips, lowering the suction to 60-80 mm Hg, or using a Yankauer suction tip rather than suctioning through the irrigation tip.

Method of Application. Depending on the size of the wound, 500-3,000 ml of sterile normal saline solution in intravenous-type bags is used for each treatment. A randomized single-blind cross-over trial comparing warmed saline and room temperature saline on laceration wounds in 38 patients concluded that warmed saline was better tolerated than room temperature saline.[172] Therefore the bag of saline should be warmed in a fluid warmer or microwave to body temperature before use.

Suction pressure is adjusted to 60-100 mm Hg. In wounds that are sensitive, close to major vessels, or have soft tissue that is easily pulled into the tip shield, lower suction is advised. In wounds with fragile tissue, crevices, or undermining that is difficult to suction, a Yankauer suction tube can be connected to the wall canister and used in conjunction with any irrigation tip. The pressure is selected according to the treatment goals, exposed tissue, and patient pain levels.

Infection control with the use of PLWS is important because of the aerosol nature of treatment and the possible spread of microbes in the wound.[173] The Centers for Disease Control has recently supported recommendations developed by Loehne,[174] including the wearing of personal protective equipment by all staff in the room at the time of treatment, providing treatment only in private patient or treatment rooms, strict disposal of contaminated waste in appropriate biohazard bags, and disinfection of horizontal surfaces after each treatment. Guidelines for disposal of body fluids in a biohazard bag state to include fluid in the suction canister and any dressing containing >20 cc drainage. To minimize contamination between treatments, reusable components of the PLWS system are stored between treatments, wrapped in sterile towels, sealed in a plastic bag, and labeled with the patient name, room number, and date of first use.

Outcomes. Expected outcomes of PLWS intervention include elimination of odor and exudate in 3-7 days, full debridement after 1-2 weeks, and advancement from the chronic to inflammatory phase in 1 week and to the proliferative phase in 2 weeks.[174] Treatment is discontinued after 1 week if no improvement is noted. Frequency of treatment initially is daily and may be decreased to 2-3 days per week to maintain a clean wound bed if surgical closure is expected. In stage III or IV PUs, once the wound bed is clean and more than 70% granulated, either advanced dressings that can be changed less frequently or vacuum-assisted closure is recommended.

Vacuum-Assisted Closure. The application of topical negative or subatmospheric pressure to open wounds was first reported in Europe in the early 1990s[175-177] and was introduced in the United States in 1997.[178] Early application involved the use of wall suction apparatus or surgical vacuum bottles; however, these systems lacked control and maintenance of required pressure levels.[179] Since that time, a purpose-designed vacuum-assisted closure (VAC) device (VAC, Kinetic Concepts, Inc, San Antonio, Tex) that uses a microprocessor-controlled pump has become widely accepted as an adjunctive therapy for wounds of all etiologies. VAC application consists of filling or covering the wound with sterile polyurethane foam with pores ranging from 400-600 µm in size, inserting a suction tube into the foam, and connecting the tube to the pump that contains a collection canister. The foam, part of the tubing, and periwound tissue are then sealed with an occlusive sterile drape (Figs. 28-21 and 28-22). Continuous or intermittent suction, ranging from 50-200 mm Hg, creates a vacuum that reduces edema, exudate, and bacteria. In addition, the closed wound environment is kept moist, thereby promoting healing and preventing contamination.

The first article on VAC therapy reported that negative pressure increased local blood flow by up to 4 times baseline and increased the rate of granulation by 63% to 103%.[180] Based on these results, a protocol of using continuous pressure for the first 48 hours of treatment to decrease edema and using intermittent pressure thereafter to optimize granulation tissue formation was developed.[181] A prospective, randomized controlled trial of VAC versus hydrogel dressings on 35 full-thickness PUs for a 6-week treatment period found that wound volume decreased by 42.1% with the hydrogel and by 51.8% with VAC ($p = 0.46$).[182] The mean number of polymorphonuclear (PMN)

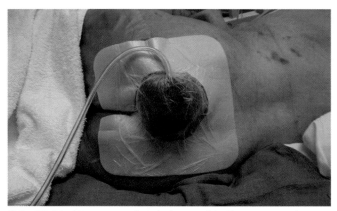

FIG. 28-21 Vacuum-assisted closure (VAC) on a sacral pressure ulcer.

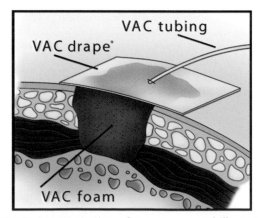

FIG. 28-22 A cross-section of a cavity wound illustrates the position of the foam and tubing.

cells and lymphocytes decreased in the VAC group ($p = 0.13$) and increased in hydrogel group ($p = 0.41$). Of the 15 ulcers with underlying osteomyelitis (confirmed by biopsy), 3 improved with the VAC and none improved with the hydrogel dressing. Given the clinical improvements noted in the VAC group, the authors concluded that VAC accelerates wound healing and promotes favorable histological changes, although the results were not statistically significant.[182] Another prospective, randomized controlled trial of VAC versus a control group with standard wound care with moist gauze and an occlusive dressing only was completed with 24 patients with 36 wounds (28 PUs), 18 randomized to each group. The wounds were evaluated at initiation of treatment, after 3 weeks, and after 6 weeks. At 6 weeks the wounds treated with the VAC were 78% smaller (by volume) as compared to a 30% reduction in the control group ($p = 0.038$). The most significant change in dimensions was for depth—66% for VAC and 20% for control ($p < 0.00001$).[183] This change in depth may not only result in faster wound closure but for larger wounds may allow for closure by skin grafting rather than by surgical flap.

Philbeck et al published a retrospective review of 1,032 home health patients with 1,170 wounds that failed to heal by conventional methods and that were subsequently treated with negative pressure.[13] Healing rates and closure times for stage III and IV PUs treated with VAC were compared to those reported by Ferrell in 1993 for PUs treated with LAL mattresses and normal saline dressings.[105] Closure rate with the VAC was 0.23 cm²/day. Based on this, the average wound in this study (22.2 cm²) would heal in 97 days and incur a cost of $14,546. The same wound using Ferrell's predicted healing rate would heal in 247 days and incur a cost of $23,465. These findings suggest that treatment with the VAC is a cost-effective intervention for chronic wounds.

Many case studies and retrospective reviews of the use of the VAC for treatment of wounds of various etiologies have been published; however, there are few randomized controlled trials of this intervention in human subjects. Therefore, based on the AHRQ *Guideline* criteria, VAC would have an evidence-based rating of B for treatment of PUs. This is supported by a Cochrane Review meta-analysis on the use of VAC for treatment of chronic wounds that states that there is weak evidence suggesting that topical negative pressure is superior to saline gauze dressings in healing chronic human wounds. They further state that the small samples of the existing trials and methodological limitations affect the interpretation of findings and suggest that cost, quality of life, pain, and comfort issues would also affect interpretation of efficacy.[184]

Advantages and Disadvantages. Advantages of VAC are the decrease in the number of dressings changes from 1-2 times per day to every 2-3 days and the ability of the occlusive drape to keep moisture (e.g., urinary and fecal incontinence, perspiration, and leaking exudates) away from the wound and periwound skin. The primary disadvantage is the expense with current estimates for pump rental of $75-$125 per day, in addition to the supplies (packaged to include foam, drape, and tubing for each dressing change), which cost approximately $20-$30 per application. Given the cost of one hospital day, however, cost savings are likely if use of this device shortens hospital stays.

Indications and Contraindications. VAC therapy is indicated for any cavity wound, dehisced or acute surgical wounds, skin grafts and flaps, traumatic wounds, and neuropathic stage III PUs or stage IV PUs, after adequate debridement has been achieved. It is contraindicated for wounds with more than 30% devitalized tissue, untreated osteomyelitis, wounds with cancerous or malignant tissue, and exposed blood vessels. Precautionary measures are recommended for wounds that have not achieved hemostasis or wounds that bleed easily because the patient is on anticoagulants. Precautionary measures include lowering the pressure or delaying initiation of therapy until active bleeding ceases. Wounds adjacent to major vessels or bypass grafts may be lined with nonadherent mesh under the polyurethane foam or dressed with denser, saline soaked foam available from the manufacturer. Wounds containing fistulas may require customized application of dressings and suction to adequately manage drainage.

Treatment Guidelines. The use of sterile technique and supplies are recommended for VAC application, although it is known that chronic wounds are generally not sterile. The entire cavity is filled with foam (including undermining and sinus tracks) to prevent accumulation of fluid in dead spaces—a condition that provides an environment for bacterial growth. Nonadherent mesh can be placed between the wound surface and the provided black foam to prevent granulation tissue from penetrating the foam, thereby decreasing destruction of new tissue and patient discomfort when removing the dressing. The foam should be cut and positioned so that some part of every piece touches another piece of foam. The occlusive drape needs to extend 3-5 cm beyond the wound edge to obtain a good seal and prevent leakage, and the suction tube needs to be embedded in the foam so that the drainage holes at the end of the tube are covered. Directions for starting therapy and changing the canister are included with every unit and are therefore not included here. The suction pressure should be set at between 50 and 125 mm Hg, according to patient comfort.

VAC dressings are changed as follows: Infected wounds, every 12 hours; heavily draining wounds, every 24 hours; clean wounds, every 48 hours; and meshed graft wounds, after 4-5 days. Full canisters can be changed without complete dressing changes. The wound is inspected daily, and the dressing is changed immediately if any of the following conditions are observed:

- Odor comes from the wound or canister, possibly a result of accumulation of blood in the foam.
- If hemostasis is not maintained in the wound bed and bleeding occurs, the negative pressure will suction blood and an alternative dressing is recommended.
- Foam is no longer tightly wrinkled, indicating the seal is lost and suction is insufficient.
- Suction is off for more than 2 hours. Accumulated drainage under the foam is an ideal environment for bacterial growth that may cause infection.

- Pain or discomfort under the foam is unrelieved by decreasing the pressure.
- Drainage accumulates under the adhesive drape. This may cause skin maceration.

Treatment with the VAC is usually discontinued when full granulation is achieved. Then another dressing that facilitates epithelialization or surgical closure should be considered. In summary, VAC is a versatile, effective adjunctive therapy for removal of edema, bacteria, and loose debris from wounds; for stimulating cell proliferation; and for providing protection from external contaminants.

Electrical Stimulation. Electrical stimulation (ES), with various treatment parameters, has been used for many years to facilitate tissue healing. The proposed rationales for applying electricity to facilitate tissue healing include the presence of an electrical charge in healing tissue, attraction of specific cell types by an applied electrical current (termed *galvanotaxis*), the stimulatory effect of electricity on cells to promote biosynthesis and replication, possible bactericidal effects of electricity, and effects of electricity on circulation and myofibroblast contraction. The strength of evidence for each of these mechanisms varies and is discussed briefly. A number of animal-based and clinical studies with patients support the effectiveness of electrical currents in accelerating closure of chronic wounds of various etiologies.

The surface of intact human skin has a negative charge of approximately -23mV, while the inner layers of the epidermis have a positive charge. This charge difference is a result of the sodium pump that pumps positively-charged sodium ions (Na+) into the inner layers of the epidermis, leaving negatively charged chloride ions (Cl−) on the surface. The difference between these charges is termed transepithelial potential (TEP). When a dermal wound occurs, a Na+ ion flows from the deeper wound bed to the surface, attracting the cells required for tissue repair (Fig. 28-23). The wound must stay moist for this current of injury to flow. This is one proposed rationale for the effectiveness of moist wound healing.[105] The current of injury continues through all phases of healing until a wound closes. Once a wound is closed, there is no further current flow.

The current of injury is thought to cause charged cells to move toward the area of opposite charge. Applied electrical currents with a fixed polarity (i.e., monophasic

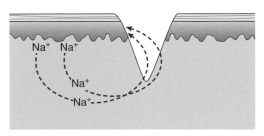

FIG. 28-23 The current of injury flows from the deeper wound bed to the surface when a wound occurs, attracting the cells required for tissue repair. Moist wound dressings maintain the current of injury and electrical stimulation facilitates the ionic flow.

currents) can also promote galvanotaxis, as has been demonstrated in vitro by Cho.[186]

An electrical current can be applied to a wound by placing electrodes on or near the wound bed (Fig. 28-24). The polarity of the electrode at the wound site is selected, depending on the type of cells required to facilitate or advance a particular healing phase. For example, during the inflammatory phase, platelets, macrophages, neutrophils, lymphocytes, and mast cells are required for phagocytosis, vasodilation, and release of growth factors; during the proliferative phase, fibroblasts are required for collagen synthesis and wound contraction; and during the epithelialization phase, epidermal cells are required for skin closure. The charge of each of the cell types involved in wound healing processes and the electrode to which they are attracted are listed in Table 28-14. Based on this information, the clinician can select the appropriate polarity for the active electrode according to the presence or absence of infection and the healing phase of the wound.[185]

In addition to attracting appropriate cells to an area, pulsed electrical currents have been shown to trigger calcium channels in fibroblast and lymphocyte cell membranes to open, increasing the level of intracellular calcium. Increased intracellular calcium induces exposure of additional insulin receptors on the cell surface and, if insulin is available, fibroblasts will increase their synthesis of proteins, including collagen and DNA. This effect is voltage dependent, with greatest effect occurring with

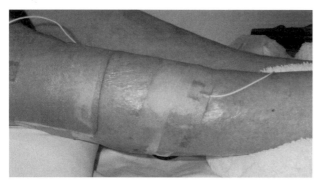

FIG. 28-24 Applying electrical stimulation to promote wound healing. *From Cameron MH: Physical Agents in Rehabilitation: From Research to Practice, ed 2, Philadelphia, 2003, Saunders.*

peak voltages of 60-90 volts, using high volt–pulsed current waveform.[187]

Although some have proposed that ES has direct bactericidal effects in wounds, this is controversial. In vitro studies have shown inhibition of bacterial growth with ES; however, the current amplitude and treatment durations used were greater than used in clinical studies.[188,189] It is not known if this effect is specific to pathogens or if such high levels of electricity may also damage healthy regenerating cells in the wound. Additionally, it is proposed that ES facilitates wound healing by improving blood flow to the area. However, this is probably not the primary mechanism underlying the effectiveness of this intervention since effective treatment protocols do not involve producing a muscle contraction, and circulation is most enhanced by ES when contractions are produced.[190]

Clinical Evidence. A number of studies have reported the beneficial effects of ES on diabetic wounds[191,192] and on animal models.[193-197] Several studies have evaluated the effects of ES on pressure ulcers. For example, in a study by Kloth and Feedar, patients with stage IV PUs were randomly assigned to a treatment group that received daily high-voltage pulsed current (HVPC), a monophasic pulsed electrical current.[198] A control group received a sham treatment with electrodes but no stimulation. The ES protocol included 45 minutes of HVPC at 105 pps at submotor intensity. The anode (+ pole) was placed over the wound for all patients initially, and the polarity was changed daily with four patients who had no measurable progress. Standard care was provided 24 hours per day for both groups. The treatment group wounds healed at the rate of 44.8% per week and healed 100% over a mean period of 7.4 weeks. The control group wounds increased in area an average of 11.6% per week and increased 28.9% over a mean period of 7.4 weeks.

Another study by Feedar and Kloth compared the effects of pulsed cathodal (–pole) current and sham treatment applied for 4 weeks to 47 patients with 50 stage II, III, and IV PUs.[199] Initially, twice daily treatment involved 30 minutes of ES with 128 pulses per second (pps) and a peak amplitude of 29.2 mA if the wound contained necrotic tissue or exudate. Three days after the wound was debrided or produced no exudate, the polarity was changed every 3 days until the wound was epithelializing. Thereafter, the pulse frequency was then reduced to 64 pps, and the active electrode polarity was changed daily

TABLE 28-14	Cell Charge and Attracting Electrode		
Cell Type	**Healing Phase**	**Charge**	**Electrode that Attracts the Cell**
Platelets	Hemostasis and inflammatory	Positive	Negative
Macrophages	Inflammatory	Negative	Positive
Neutrophils	Inflammatory	Negative (with infection)	Negative
		Positive (without infection)	Positive
Mast cells	Inflammatory	Negative	Positive
Fibroblasts	Proliferative	Positive	Negative
Epidermal cells	Epithelialization	Negative	Positive

From Sussman C, Byl N: Electrical stimulation for wound healing. In Sussman C, Bates-Jensen BM (eds): *Wound Care: A Collaborative Practice Manual for Physical Therapists and Nurses,* Gaithersburg, Md, 1998, Aspen; Hamm R, Behringer B: *The Give and Take of Wound Management: A Guide to Making Clinical Decisions,* Irvine, Calif, 2004, ConceptMedia, Inc.

until the wound was closed. After 4 weeks of treatment, the treatment group wounds were 44% of initial size and the control group wounds were 67% of initial size. The healing rates per week were 14% for the treatment group and 8.25% for the control group.

A more recent study on the effects of ES on chronic lower extremity ulcers of various etiologies involved 27 patients with 42 wounds. The subjects were randomly assigned to receive HVPC (100 μsec, 150 V, 100 Hz, cathodal) or a sham intervention. Treatments were given for 45 minutes 3 times per week for 4 weeks. Over the 4-weeks the size of the wounds in the active treatment group decreased by 44.3% (±8.8%) and the size of the wounds in the control group decreased by 16% (±8.9%).[200]

A meta-analysis of 15 studies found that on average the rate of wound healing with ES was 22% per week and with standard care provided to control groups was 9%. This is a net difference of 13% per week or an increase of 144% over the control rate. The authors of this analysis concluded that ES is effective for promoting healing of chronic wounds but that further research is needed to identify which currents are most effective and which wound etiologies respond best to this intervention.[201] According to the AHCPR *Guidelines,* the use of ES to promote PU healing gets an A rating based on strength of evidence.[1]

Indications and Contraindications. The effects of ES on wound and periwound tissue are related to the phase of wound healing rather than the wound etiology. Therefore, except for the listed contraindications, ES is considered safe for all types of wounds. Contraindications for ES include the presence of any neoplasm in or around the wound, untreated or nonresolving osteomyelitis in underlying bony structures, metal ions (e.g., silver from topical medications), any electronic implant that would be affected by the ES, and close proximity to any reflex center (carotid sinus, phrenic nerve, heart, or laryngeal muscles) that would be sensitive to ES. Therefore ES is not recommended on the chest or anterior neck.[185]

Treatment Guidelines. When using ES to treat wounds, the clinician selects the polarity of the active electrode (defined as the electrode on or in proximity to the wound), the type of electrodes and the conducting medium, the electrode placement, waveform, frequency, and the current amplitude. The polarity of the cells one wants to attract to the wound bed generally determines the polarity of the active electrode placed at the wound site. Kloth summarizes the selection as the following: Positive for epithelialization (galvanotaxis of negatively charged epithelial cells), positive for autolysis and reactivation of inflammatory phase (galvanotaxis of neutrophils and macrophages), and negative for granulation (galvanotaxis of fibroblasts).[185] Sussman recommends using the negative electrode for edema and inflammation, alternating polarity every 3 days for proliferation, and alternating daily for epithelialization and remodeling.[202] Both of these protocols are used with a HVPC waveform, a frequency of 30-120 pps, a sensory level current amplitude (75-150 V peak voltage), and daily treatments of 45-60 minutes duration.

The type of electrode depends on availability, wound size, wound location, and patient isolation. Because air transmits electricity poorly, the space between the wound bed and the electrode needs to be filled with a conducting medium to ensure transmission of the electric current. Unless a topical dressing, such as an enzymatic debrider, is being used, the conducting medium can remain on the wound after the ES treatment is completed and can thus be the primary dressing. Using the conducting gel as the primary dressing protects the wound bed, keeps the wound moist, maintains heat that accumulates during treatment, and conserves supplies. Saline-soaked gauze, amorphous hydrogel, and hydrogel sheets are excellent conducting media for the active electrode. For cavity wounds, the gauze is moistened with saline solution, fluffed, lightly packed into the wound cavity, covered with an aluminum foil electrode, and anchored with tape. A pre-gelled, self-adhesive electrode can be used for the dispersive electrode. After the ES treatment, an appropriate secondary dressing is applied over the gauze or hydrogel, or a new dressing is applied.

The active electrode may be placed directly over or just proximal to the wound, or two electrodes of the same polarity, each half the size of the wound area, may be placed on intact skin at either side of the wound (termed the straddling technique).[185] A dispersive electrode approximately the same size as the wound area is placed 15-30 cm proximal to the wound site. If the wound is deep, the dispersive electrode should be farther from the wound so the current will flow more deeply.

The current amplitude is adjusted to a level that causes the patient to feel a slight tingling without any motor activity. For the insensate patient, the amplitude is adjusted to a submotor level, i.e., it is increased until a contraction is seen and then decreased by approximately 10%. Additional recommendations for the application of electrical stimulation for the treatment of chronic wounds include the following:

- Remove all topical dressing residue that may contain petrolatum or heavy metal ions (for example, iodine or zinc).
- Cleanse the skin that will be under the electrodes with normal saline or soap and water to remove oils or debris that can impede good current flow.
- Perform sharp debridement before application of ES. The conducting medium can then remain in the wound as a primary dressing, thereby reducing the amount of time the wound is exposed to air.
- If the patient complains of tingling or burning under the dispersive electrode, check for dryness or poor skin contact. If either condition exists, interrupt treatment to moisten the electrode and reapply with good contact.
- After each treatment, inspect the skin under both active and dispersive electrodes for any signs of irritation.

Ultraviolet C. Ultraviolet (UV) radiation is electromagnetic radiation with a frequency range of $7.5 \times 10^{14}\text{-}10^{16}$ Hz and with wavelengths of 400-100 nm. UV radiation is divided into three spectral bands, UVA, UVB, and UVC, with UVA being the longest and UVC being the shortest at 290-100 nm. Only UVC is used to facilitate wound healing. UVC may facilitate healing in chronic wounds by stimulating fibroblasts to produce collagen, by killing bacteria and viruses, by causing vasodilation and thereby increasing capillary permeability and oxygen delivery to the affected tissue, by destroying senescent epithelial cells at the wound edge to enhance reepithelialization, by increasing production of growth factors, and by causing sloughing of necrotic tissue.[203] Wound contraction may also be facilitated by increased production of fibronectin in epithelial fibroblasts.[204]

Clinical Evidence. A series of in vitro studies evaluated the effects of UVC on the survival of methicillin-resistant *S. aureus* (MRSA), vancomycin-resistant *Enterococcus faecalis* (VRE), group A streptococcus (GAS), and select prokaryotic (*P. aeruginosa, Mycobacterium abscessus*) and eukaryotic (*Candida albicans, Aspergillus fumigatus*) organisms.[205-207] UVC (254 nm, 15.54 mW/cm^2 output) killed 99.9% of all of these organisms with an application of 5 seconds or longer.

Thai and colleagues reported on three patients with chronic ulcers infected with MRSA that were treated with UVC (250 nm, 180 seconds).[208] The treatment was applied 7 times over 14 days and then weekly for 1 month. Two of the wounds improved from heavy growth of MRSA to light growth, and one wound improved from light growth to occasional or scant growth.

These studies indicate that UVC can kill some of the pathogens that commonly infect wounds and may decrease the bacterial load of infected wounds. Because the effects of UVC on the skin have not been studied in controlled experiments, it is recommended that it only be used on clinically infected wounds and that its use be discontinued when the surface contamination is eliminated.[209]

Because of the limited number of reported studies on UVC in the treatment of PUs and the fact that most of the controlled trials have been animal studies, the strength of evidence rating for UVC issued by the AHCPR *Guidelines* is C.[1] There are no published systematic reviews on the effects of ultraviolet for wound healing.

Indications and Contraindications. UVC may be used for treatment of infected wounds, independent of etiology; however, there are a number of patients for whom any type of UV radiation is contraindicated:[209]

Contraindications for the Use of Ultraviolet C
- Acute onset of psoriasis, herpes simplex, or eczema in periwound skin
- Malignant wounds or cancer in periwound tissue
- Fever*
- Skin grafts
- Local erythema
- Acquired immunodeficiency syndrome (AIDS)/human immunodeficiency virus (HIV) infection
- Pulmonary tuberculosis*
- Cardiac, renal, or liver disease*
- Severe diabetes*
- Systemic lupus erythematosus
- Hyperthyroidism*

- Deep x-ray therapy
- Eye

---

*UVC is contraindicated if used in conjunction with UVA or UVB to large body surface areas.

Precautions are advised for patients with poor tolerance to sun exposure. Photosensitivity may also be increased by certain medications, including the antibiotics tetracyclines, sulfonamides, and quinolones; the phenothiazine antipsychotics; psoralens used for treatment of acute psoriasis; gold therapy used historically as an antiinflammatory agent in patients with rheumatoid arthritis; and the cardiac antiarrhythmic drugs, amiodarone hydrochloride and quinidine. Also, any recently irradiated tissue that is more susceptible to developing cancer should be treated with extreme caution,[181] although there have been no published reports of increased incidence of skin cancer with the use of UVC.[209]

Treatment Guidelines. Derma-wand (National Biological Corporation, Twinsburg, OH) is the only UVC device currently on the market in the United States. It is a relatively inexpensive, hand-held unit that is convenient to use for treatment of infected wounds (Fig. 28-25). Treatment with UVC should be preceded by a complete wound evaluation, sharp debridement of necrotic tissue, and removal of any residual dressing with normal saline. Both the patient and the therapist should avoid exposure of the eyes to UV radiation by wearing UV-blocking goggles. UV radiation therapy should be discontinued as soon as clinical signs of infections have resolved.

Procedure for Ultraviolet C Treatment of Infected Wounds
- Position the patient so the UV wand can be placed parallel to the wound bed and the rays can be

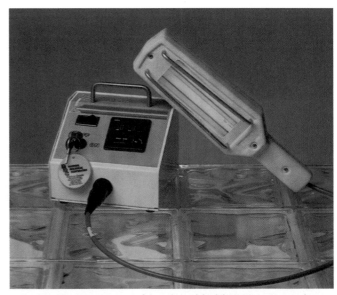

FIG. 28-25 Derma-wand is a hand-held UVC unit used to treat infected wounds. *Courtesy National Biological Corp, Twinsburg, OH.*

transmitted perpendicular to the tissue to maximize energy delivery to the wound.

- Apply a UV-blocking agent with an SPF of 30, a thick layer of petrolatum, or a cotton drape over the periwound skin for protection.
- Position the UVC lamp 2.5 cm from the wound.
- Expose the wound to UVC according to the following guidelines:
  - GAS infection: 4 seconds, twice per day
  - GAS plus *S. aureus*: 120 seconds, twice per day
  - MRSA: 90 seconds, daily
  - VRE: 45 seconds, daily
  - Antibiotic-susceptible bacteria: 30 seconds, daily
- Apply the appropriate dressing to the wound as soon as possible to prevent drying and cooling of the wound tissue.
- Clean the equipment with an antiseptic solution after each use.

Ultrasound. Ultrasound (US) is sound waves with a frequency of greater than 20 kHz (20,000 cycles per second). Therapeutic US is generally in the 1-3 MHz (1-3 million cycles per second) frequency range. When ultrasound waves are absorbed by tissue they cause a range of effects. Continuous US of sufficient intensity can cause a rise in tissue temperature that will cause vasodilation and an increase in local blood supply. This heating may be therapeutic; however, in areas with poor circulation (common in chronic wounds) the temperature rise may be excessive and burn the tissue. Lower intensities of pulsed US do not cause measurable increases in tissue temperature; however, pulsed US may promote tissue repair by nonthermal mechanisms. Nonthermal effects of US include cavitation, microstreaming, and acoustic streaming.

Cavitation is the production of small, gas-filled bubbles within conducting mediums and tissue fluids that absorb US. The intensities of US that can be produced by therapeutic US devices cause these bubbles to oscillate in size, becoming bigger and smaller. This is stable cavitation. Stable cavitation is thought to increase cell membrane permeability and diffusional properties. Much higher intensities of ultrasound can cause the bubbles to burst. This unstable cavitation can cause tissue damage but does not occur at the US intensities used in therapy.[210]

Microstreaming refers to microscopic fluid movements. US causes microstreaming next to cell membranes and around the bubbles produced by cavitation. Microstreaming is thought to enhance transport of ions and molecules involved in tissue healing. Acoustic streaming is a larger scale flow of fluids produced in the ultrasound field. This flow is also thought to enhance the flow of ions and molecules involved in wound healing. Stable cavitation, microstreaming and acoustic streaming are thought to underlie the following physiological changes associated with wound healing that have been observed with the application of US:

- Mast cell degranulation, resulting in a release of histamine and chemotactic factors into the periwound tissue and an initiation of the inflammatory healing phase.
- Increased vascular permeability, resulting in an increased flow of platelets, macrophages, leukocytes, and mast cells, all of which are active during the inflammatory phase of healing.
- Increased phagocytosis of hematoma material by macrophages and neutrophils.
- Stimulation of fibroblast activity, resulting in increased collagen synthesis, and in turn producing two positive healing effects—accelerated wound closure and stronger scar tissue.
- Stimulation of endothelial cell activity, resulting in accelerated dermal repair.[185]

Clinical Evidence. Laboratory studies of in vitro cells have provided some evidence that US can affect healing processes at the cellular level.[211] Selkowitz et al performed a double blind, single-case, baseline-AB study of the effect of pulsed low-intensity US on a 75-year-old patient with a stage III sacral PU. Healing rates were determined for a baseline period (50.8 mm^2/day), 2 weeks after application of pulsed low-intensity US with a total of 10 treatments (34 mm^2/day), and after 2 weeks of placebo US treatment (12.6 mm^2/day). Standard wound care was provided throughout the study period. The healing rate was significantly faster with the US as compared to the placebo, however, it was not significantly different from the baseline healing rate. The authors concluded that the effect of US was not appreciably different from that of standard care alone.

Lowe et al compared the effects of no treatment, treatment with 0.5W/cm^2, 3MHz, pulsed US applied for 5 minutes 3 times per week, and placebo treatment on wounds made on x-ray irradiated tissue in animals.[212] They found no difference in healing rates between groups, suggesting that US does not stimulate healing of radiation-impaired tissue.

In contrast, however, a study evaluating the effects of 0.5 W/cm^2 and 1.0 W/cm^2 US and placebo US on the healing rates of lower extremity venous wounds in humans found that the wounds in both active treatment groups healed significantly faster than those in the placebo group, with a tendency for those in the lower dose US group to heal fastest.[213] Johnson reported US to be useful for the management of chronic venous wounds through case studies, indicating that improvements were noted in healing rates, pain, pigmentation, and odor reduction.[214]

A randomized study of the effects of US on PUs on 88 subjects used 3.28 MHz, 0.1 W/cm^2, 3$\frac{3}{4}$-7$\frac{1}{2}$ minute treatment time, depending on the size of the wound, for a period of 12 weeks. At the end of the study, 40% of the wounds treated with US were healed and 44% of the wounds treated with sham US were healed. The researchers noted a tendency for US to be more effective on small wounds than on larger wounds.[215]

A discussion of the use of US in wound healing by Sussman suggests that delivery of US to recently injured tissue during the inflammatory phase (e.g., ecchymosis with bruising or erythema with stage I PU) will stimulate the release of growth factors from platelets, mast cells, and macrophages and thereby facilitate faster transition from the inflammatory to proliferative healing phase.[216]

A systematic review by Flemming and Cullum to assess the effectiveness of the use of US in the treatment of PUs led to the conclusion that there was no evidence of a benefit of US therapy in the treatment of PUs.[217] They further stated that the methodological limitations and small numbers of participants were a factor in the conclusions and beneficial effects could not be ruled out. As a result of the lack of control trials in human studies, US received a strength of evidence rating of C for treatment of PUs. Because of the effects noted in laboratory studies and the positive results in some studies, US is a modality that could be considered for recalcitrant wounds if standard care has not effected positive changes and if other modalities with more positive evidence are not available.

Indications and Contraindications. The indications for use of US in wound healing are acute wounds in the inflammatory healing phase (preferably within a few hours of onset), hematomas, bruises, and recalcitrant wounds. Contraindications are irradiated tissue; tumors or malignancies; pregnant uterus; deep vein thrombosis (DVT), emboli, or thrombophlebitis; ischemic or insensate tissue; pacemakers or implanted defibrillators; reproductive organs, eyes, stellate ganglion, central nervous system tissue; joint cement or plastic joint components. Precautions include use in hemophiliacs who are not receiving factor replacement, acute wound inflammation (avoid high-dose continuous US), bony prominences, and fractures (use lower intensity to avoid heating the periosteum or causing pain). US therapy should be discontinued if precautionary methods fail to eliminate pain.

Treatment Guidelines. The adjustable variables of US include frequency, duty cycle, intensity, coupling medium, size of the treatment area, and treatment duration. Control of each variable is determined by the intended effect and expected treatment outcome. As previously stated, the higher frequency of 3 MHz (which penetrates 1-2 cm) is used for shallow tissue, whereas 1 MHz (which penetrates up to 5 cm) is used for deeper tissue (Fig. 28-26). Although US can be applied in a continuous or pulsed mode, only pulsed mode, which optimizes nonthermal effects and minimizes thermal effects, is recommended for treatment of open wounds (Fig. 28-27). A 20% pulsed duty cycle is generally recommended because it is the duty cycle used in pulsed US studies. In general, the recommended ultrasound intensity for wound healing is 0.5-1.0 W/cm^2.

A coupling medium is used between the sound head and the treatment tissue to eliminate air spaces that deflect the sound waves. Water, transmitting gels, hydrogel sheets, and transparent films are effective coupling mediums. When using a transmitting gel from a nonsterile container, a sterile transparent film between the wound bed and the gel reduces the risk of contamination. When using a transparent film, all air bubbles should be pressed out before applying a thin layer of gel over the film. Hydrogel sheets used as a coupling medium can remain in place after US treatment and be used as a primary dressing. The coupling medium should extend several centimeters beyond the wound edge to enable treatment of periwound tissue. After treatment with ultrasound is complete, the hydrogel sheet should be trimmed to the size of the wound to avoid maceration of periwound skin. Water is used on distal areas over bony prominences and curved areas where maintaining full contact between the sound head and the treatment area (such as ankles, heels, elbows) is difficult. When water is the coupling medium, clean the container with antiseptic solution between treatments, use a container large enough to submerge the treatment area and the sound head, and fill the container with water several minutes before treatment so that air bubbles can

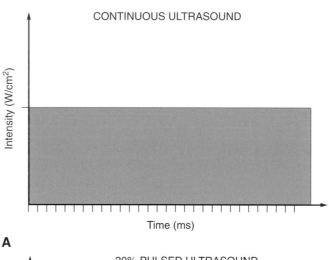

A

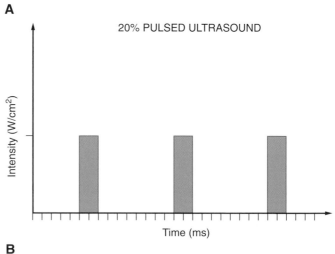

B

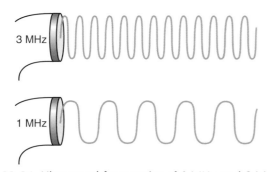

FIG. 28-26 Ultrasound frequencies of 1 MHz and 3 MHz. *Adapted from Cameron MH: Physical Agents in Rehabilitation: From Research to Practice, ed 2, Philadelphia, 2003, Saunders.*

FIG. 28-27 Continuous and 20% pulsed ultrasound. *Adapted from Cameron MH: Physical Agents in Rehabilitation: From Research to Practice, ed 2, Philadelphia, 2003, Saunders.*

dissipate. There are two guidelines for treatment times reported in the literature—1 min/cm² of treatment area or 5 minutes for each area that is 2 times the size of the sound head, with a recommended maximum time of 15 minutes.[216]

When applying US to a chronic wound using gel as the transmission medium, cleanse the sound head with an antiseptic agent before and after each treatment to prevent wound contamination, and warm the gel to approximately body temperature before putting it on the patient.

CASE STUDY 28-1

STAGE IV SACRAL PRESSURE ULCER

Examination
Patient History
LM is a 44-year-old woman admitted to an acute care hospital with complaints of severe abdominal pain, diminished appetite with nausea, and diarrhea for 4 days. Past medical history includes end-stage liver disease secondary to amyloidosis, resulting in a liver transplant 4 years ago, end-stage renal disease with hemodialysis 2 times per week, hypertension, and a DVT with onset 4 months ago. LM has also had a sacral ulcer for 4 months.

Medications include sirolimus (Rapamune), warfarin (Coumadin), prednisone; sevelamer HCl (Renagel), midodrine HCl (ProAmatine), and folic acid, calcium, and iron supplements.

Her nutritional status is compromised because of her abdominal symptoms and liver disease, and her albumin level is 2.7. Other clinical test results include creatinine of 4.5, BUN of 56, INR of 3.0, PTT of 40.8, and negative blood cultures.

Tests and Measures
Musculoskeletal
Posture The supine position most frequently observed was with the head of bed elevated >60 degrees; sitting tended to be in a bedside chair in a semireclining position.

Range of Motion Functional ROM of all joints, except the ankles, which were limited due to 3+ pedal edema.

Muscle Performance 2+/5 gross lower extremity strength, and 3–/5 gross upper extremity strength.

Integumentary
Integumentary Integrity LM has impaired integumentary integrity and several risk factors, including diminished BMI, medications, impaired mobility, numerous comorbidities, and poor nutritional status. Wound size: 3.7 × 3.4 cm with 2-3 cm of undermining from 10:00 to 2:00)

Tissue type: 85% yellow rubbery eschar, 15% red granulation of poor quality

Drainage: Minimal serosanguineous drainage on the old dressing

Periwound skin color: Brawny discoloration of the periwound skin, proximal > distal

Edema: Minimal

Odor: None

Sensation: Impaired to light touch

Pain level: 0/10 on the visual analog scale

Braden Scale score: 9

Function
Self Care LM has been wheelchair bound for more than 2 years.

Moderate to maximal assistance was required for all bed mobility and transfers.

Evaluation, Diagnosis, and Prognosis
LM's low score on the Braden Scale put her at high risk for developing additional PUs.

The preferred practice pattern is 7E: Impaired integumentary integrity associated with skin involvement extending into fascia, muscle, or bone and scar formation, also classified as a stage IV sacral PU (staged after debridement of all eschar).

Intervention
Planning appropriate interventions began with addressing each aspect of care recommended by the AHCPR *Guidelines*. In addition, LM was started on TPN to meet the caloric and protein needs for wound healing.

Managing Tissue Loads
LM was placed on a LAL bed and a turning schedule was posted for all disciplines to follow. A chair-sized air-cell cushion, to allow proper sitting position, was also provided.

Ulcer Care
Sharp debridement of the eschar was performed at the bedside with sterile sharp instruments, followed by daily serial debridement of underlying devitalized tissue and slough. An absorbent dressing was chosen each day, depending on the needs of the wound. Initially, hydrogel and an occlusive secondary dressing were used to facilitate autolysis of remaining necrotic tissue. When bleeding was an issue, calcium alginates were used; however, once the distal sacrum and coccyx were exposed, alginates were discontinued and hydrogel, sterile gauze, and transparent film were applied on a daily basis. The periwound skin was covered with hydrocolloid strips to prevent application of an adhesive covering on the fragile skin.

Managing Bacterial Colonization and Infection
There were no clinical signs of infection, therefore cultures were not indicated. At each treatment session, the wound was irrigated with PLWS using 1,000 ml of warmed normal saline, 6-12 psi pressure, and 80 mm Hg suction (because of a tendency to bleed). This helped to soften and release necrotic tissue, remove coagulum from bleeding, and keep the bacterial load low. Sterile technique was used with each treatment to reduce the risk of nosocomial infections.

Operative Repair of the Ulcer
Consultation by a plastic surgeon was obtained to evaluate LM for surgical closure of her wound but surgical closure was not recommended because it was thought that LM would be at high risk for failure given her

immobility, poor nutritional status, and multiple co-morbidities. A conservative approach for facilitating closure by secondary intention was agreed on by all disciplines.

Education

LM and her family were educated about the factors contributing to the ulcer formation, the optimal sidelying and sitting positions to off-load the sacrum, and the importance of keeping the head of the bed below 30 degrees.

Outcomes

At the time LM was discharged home, 10 days after her admission, the wound was debrided of all eschar and more than 60% of the exposed tissue was red but not granulating. The remainder of the wound bed was bone and devitalized adhered connective tissue. Because LM's insurance would not cover VAC and she refused to transfer to a SNF for continued care, she was discharged home with a specialty bed and daily home health care for dressing changes. Approximately 2 weeks later, she was readmitted to the hospital because of a general decline in her health and bleeding from the ulcer. The wound was 7 × 5 cm with 5 cm of undermining from 10:00 to 2:00. There was no granulation tissue, the sacrum was exposed and necrotic, and the soft tissue was dark red. Attempts to debride resulted in moderate bleeding that required prolonged pressure and silver nitrate to abate. INR was again high and warfarin dosages were adjusted. As the INR decreased to between 2 and 2.5, debridement of necrotic tissue was completed with PLWS and sharp technique. After 5 days, VAC therapy was initiated. Nonadherent mesh was placed over the exposed bone and black foam was used to fill the wound. Suction was initially set at 125 mm Hg in the continuous mode and was maintained at continuous for several days due to the amount of sanguineous drainage. Dressings were changed every other day, and PLWS and serial debridement were performed with each dressing change. Pressure relief measures were the same as during the first admission.

After 2 weeks, the tissue began to granulate, and after 3 weeks, the wound was contracting and the undermining was filling in. LM continued to refuse to transfer to a SNF, therefore, after 3½ weeks, she was transferred home with the specialty bed and home health providing daily wound care. At the time of discharge, the wound was 5 × 4 cm with 2-2.5 cm of undermining at 11:00 to 2:00. The tissue was more than 80% granulated, with less than 20% exposed bone and adherent connective tissue.

Please see the CD that accompanies this book for a case study describing the examination, evaluation, and interventions for a patient with a stage III and a stage IV pressure ulcer.

CHAPTER SUMMARY

Pressure ulcers are wounds that occur as a result of sustained pressure, shear, or friction in an area over a bony prominence. In addition, prolonged exposure to moisture can cause skin maceration, thereby contributing to PU formation. PUs occur in a wide range of patients, particularly those with limited mobility, poor nutrition, and multiple comorbidities. The first step to PU prevention is to identify risk factors and alter the patient's intrinsic and extrinsic environments to eliminate the circumstances that increase the risk for ulceration. Preventive strategies include pressure relief through modification of support surfaces and positioning, increasing mobility, optimizing nutrition, treating systemic disease processes, managing urinary and fecal incontinence, and educating patient and family members. Once a PU has developed, assessment of the patient's medical status and evaluation of the wound are used to determine appropriate interventions. Standard care consists of off-loading the affected area, frequent repositioning, debridement of devitalized tissue, and maintenance of a clean moist wound environment with appropriate dressings. Adjunctive modalities that may help facilitate wound healing include pulsed lavage with suction, negative pressure wound therapy, electrical stimulation, ultraviolet, and ultrasound.

ADDITIONAL RESOURCES

Useful Forms

Norton Scale
Braden Scale for Predicting Pressure Sore Risk
The Minimum Data Set (MDS): www.cms.hhs.gov/medicaid/mds20/
Outcomes and Assessment Information Set (OASIS): www.cms.hhs.gov/oasis
Spinal Cord Injury Pressure Ulcer Scale (SCIPUS)
Push Tool 3.0

Web Sites

Pressure Ulcer Scale for Healing, the Sussman Wound Healing Tool, the Sessing Scale, and the Pressure Sore Status Tool and other assessment tools: www.medal.org/ch21.html
National Pressure Ulcer Advisory Panel: www.npuap.org
National Institutes of Health information on pressure ulcers: www.nlm.nih.gov/medlineplus/pressuresores.html
Guidelines on pressure ulcer risk assessment and prevention from the UK National Health Service: www.nice.org.uk/guidance/CGB

GLOSSARY

Anaphylatoxins: Substances that induce the degranulation of mast cells, causing the release of histamine and increased vascular permeability.
Angiogenesis: New capillary formation.
Ankle-brachial index (ABI): The ratio of the systolic blood pressure at the ankle to the systolic brachial blood pressure. This number is used to assess the degree of peripheral vascular occlusion in the lower extremities.
Autolysis: The breakdown of necrotic tissue by the body's own white blood cells.
Body mass index (BMI): Weight in kilograms (kg)/height in meters squared (m^2).
Collagenase: An enzyme that catalyses the hydrolysis of collagen.
Debridement: The removal of necrotic or nonviable tissue from a wound with sharp instruments, mechanical force, enzymes, or autolysis.
Eschar: Black, grey, brown, or yellow nonviable tissue, usually dry or rubbery, within a wound.
Exudate: Pale yellow fluid drainage composed of blood cells, serum, and lysed debris.
Galvanotaxis: The attraction of living cells to an electrical charge.
Glycoproteins: Carbohydrate-protein complexes that regulate collagen interactions that lead to fibril formation.
Glycosaminoglycans (GAGs): Polysaccharide chains that form an inflexible gel which fills extracellular spaces. GAGs provide

mechanical support to tissues while allowing diffusion of water-soluble molecules and migration of cells.

Granulation tissue: The matrix of collagen, hyaluronic acid, and fibronectin that contains new capillary growth during the proliferative phase of healing.

Hageman factor (clotting factor XII): The enzyme in blood that initiates clotting by converting fibrinogen into fibrin.

Hyperkeratosis: Overdevelopment of the horny cell layer of skin.

Incidence: The number of individuals who develop a disease or disorder during a specified time.

Interface pressure: The pressure between a support surface and the skin covering a bony prominence.

Kinins: Substances produced by plasma during the early phases of inflammation that cause an increase in the microvascular permeability.

Matrix metalloproteinases (MMPs): Enzymes that degrade proteins in the extracellular matrix.

Nanocrystalline silver: Slow-release silver ions used in antimicrobial dressings, referred to as nanocrystalline because their size is measured in nanometers (10^{-9} meter).

Necrosis: Tissue death.

Phagocytosis: The process by which macrophages and neutrophils lyse and carry away nonviable cellular and noncellular components during the process of wound healing.

Prevalence: The number of individuals who have a disease or disorder at a defined time.

Prostacyclin: A substance released by the negatively charged endothelial cells that inhibits platelet aggregation, thereby preventing excessive clotting after tissue injury.

Prostaglandins: Unsaturated fatty acids produced by all cells in the body and released in response to injury to increase vascular permeability, facilitate neutrophil chemotaxis, and induce pain.

Protease: A protein-splitting or protcolytic enzyme.

Protein-energy malnutrition: Chronic, long-term deprivation of protein in the diet; results in poor healing potential.

psi: Pounds per square inch; the unit of measurement for the pressure exerted by water on tissue during the irrigation process.

Purulence: Thick necrotic drainage frequently accompanied by a foul odor; may have a high bacterial count if associated with infection.

Slough: Nonviable tissue within a wound that is the result of autolysis of dead cells.

References

1. Bergstrom N, Bennett MA, Carlson CE, et al: *Treatment of Pressure Ulcers,* Clinical Practice Guideline No. 15, Rockville, Md, 1994, USDHHS Public Health Service, AHCPR Publication No. 95-0652.
2. Baldwin KM: Incidence and prevalence of pressure ulcers in children, *Adv Skin Wound Care* 15(3):121-124, 2002.
3. Curley MA, Quigley SM, Lin M: Pressure ulcers in pediatric intensive care: incidence and associated factors, *Pediatr Crit Care Med* 4(3):284-290, 2003.
4. Schoonhoven L, Defloor T, Grypdonck MH: Incidence of pressure ulcers due to surgery. *J Clin Nurs* 11(4):479-487, 2002.
5. Baumgarten M, Margolis D, Berlin JA, et al: Risk factors for pressure ulcers among elderly hip fracture patients, *Wound Repair Regen* 11(2):96-103, 2003.
6. Vogel LC, Krajci KA, Anderson CJ: Adults with pediatric-onset spinal cord injury: Prevalence of medical complications, *J Spinal Cord Med* 25(2):106-116, 2002.
7. Baumgarten M, Margolis D, Gruber-Baldini AL, et al: Pressure ulcers and the transition to long-term care, *Adv Skin Wound Care* 16(6):299-304, 2003.
8. Bergstrom N, Braden B, Kemp M, et al: Multi-site study of incidence of pressure ulcers and the relationship between risk level, demographic characteristics, diagnoses, and prescription of preventive interventions, *J Am Geriatr Soc* 44(1):22-30, 1996.
9. Amlung SR, Miller WL, Bosley LM: The 1999 National Pressure Ulcer Prevalence Survey: a benchmarking approach, *Adv Skin Wound Care* 14(6):297-301, 2001.
10. Bergquist S, Frantz R: Pressure ulcers in community-based older adults receiving home health care. Prevalence, incidence, and associated risk factors, *Adv Wound Care* 12(7):339-351, 1999.
11. Margolis DJ, Bilker W, Santanna J, et al: Venous leg ulcer: Incidence and prevalence in the elderly, *J Am Acad Dermatol* 46(3):381-386, 2002.
12. Allman RM, Goode PS, Burst N, et al: Pressure ulcers, hospital complications, and disease severity: impact on hospital costs and length of stay, *Adv Wound Care* 12(1):22-30, 1999.
13. Philbeck TE, Whittington KT, Millsap MH, et al: The clinical cost effectiveness of externally applied negative pressure wound therapy in the treatment of wounds in home healthcare Medicare patients, *Ostomy Wound Manage* 45(11):41-50, 1999.
14. Ducker A: Pressure ulcers: Assessment, prevention, and compliance, *Case Manager* 13(4):61-64, 2002.
15. Franks PJ, Winterberg H, Moffatt CJ: Health-related quality of life and pressure ulceration assessment in patients treated in the community. *Wound Repair Regen* 10(3):133-140, 2002.
16. Langemo DK, Melland H, Hanson D, et al: The lived experience of having a pressure ulcer: a qualitative analysis, *Adv Skin Wound Care* 13(5):225-235, 2000.
17. Pittman J: The chronic wound and the family, *Ostomy Wound Manage* 49(2):38-46, 2003.
18. An introduction to the NPUAP. Available at http://www.npuap.org/his-intro.htm. Accessed 1/5/2004.
19. Agency for Healthcare Research and Quality (AHRQ). Available at http://www.ahcpr.gov.
20. Bergstrom N, Bennett MA, Carlson CE, et al: *Pressure Ulcers in Adults: Prediction and Prevention,* Clinical Practice Guideline No. 3, Rockville, Md, 1992, USDHHS Public Health Service, AHCPR Publication No. 92-0047.
21. Enoch S, Harding K: Wound bed preparation: the science behind the removal of barriers to healing, *Wounds* 15(7):213-229, 2003.
22. Kirsner RS, Bogensberger G: The normal process of healing. In Kloth L, McCullough JM (eds): *Wound Healing: Alternatives in Management,* ed 3, Philadelphia, 2002, FA Davis.
23. Ennis WJ: The microenvironment, *Wounds* Suppl B:1S-12S, 2004.
24. Lazarus GS, Cooper DM, Knighton DR, et al: Definitions and guidelines for assessment of wounds and evaluation of healing, *Arch Dermatol* 130:489-493, 1994.
25. Smith APS: Etiology of the problem wound. In Sheffield PJ, Smith APS, Fife CE (eds): *Wound Care Practice,* Flagstaff, Ariz, 2004, Best Publishing Company.
26. Edsberg LE, Cutway R, Anain S, et al: Microstructural and mechanical characterization of human tissue at and adjacent to pressure ulcers, *J Rehab Res Dev* 37(4):463-471, 2000.
27. Rappl L, Hagler D: Prevention and treatment of pressure ulcers. In Kloth L, McCullough JM (eds): *Wound Healing: Alternatives in Management,* ed 3, Philadelphia, 2002, FA Davis.
28. Wong RA: Chronic dermal wounds in older adults. In Guccione AA (ed): *Geriatric Physical Therapy,* ed 2, St. Louis, 2000, Mosby.
29. Edlich RF, Winters KL, Woodard CR, et al: Pressure ulcer prevention, *J Long Term Eff Med Implants* 14(4):285-304, 2004.
30. Jastremski CA: Pressure relief bedding to prevent pressure ulcer development in critical care, *J Crit Care* 17(2):122-125, 2002.
31. Landis EM: Micro-injection studies of capillary blood pressure in human skin, *Heart* 15:209, 1930.
32. Allman RM: Pressure ulcer. In Hazzard WR, Blass JP, Ettinger WH Jr, et al (eds): *Principles of Geriatric Medicine and Gerontology,* ed 4, New York, 1999, McGraw-Hill.
33. Kosiak M: Etiology and pathology of ischemic ulcers, *Arch Phys Med Rehab* 40:62-69, 1959.
34. Dinsdale SM: Decubitus ulcers: role of pressure and friction in causation, *Arch Phys Med Rehab* 55:147-152, 1974.
35. Rippke F, Schreiner V, Schwanitz HJ: The acidic milieu of the horny layer: new findings on the physiology and pathophysiology of skin pH, *Am J Clin Dermatol* 3(4):261-272, 2002.
36. Bates-Jensen BM: Pressure ulcers: Pathophysiology and prevention. In Sussman C, Bates-Jensen BM (eds): *Wound Care: A Collaborative Practice Manual for Physical Therapists and Nurses,* Gaithersburg, Md, 1998, Aspen.
37. Horn SD, Bender SA, Bergstrom N, et al: Description of the National Pressure Ulcer Long-Term Care Study, *J Am Geriatr Soc* 50(11):1816-1825, 2002.
38. Chendrasekhar A, Moorman DW, Timberlake GA: An evaluation of the effects of semirigid cervical collars in patients with severe closed head injury, *Am Surg* 64(7):604-606, 1998.
39. Fife C, Otto G, Capsuto EG, Brandt K, et al: Incidence of pressure ulcers in a neurologic intensive care unit, *Crit Care Med* 29(2):283-290, 2001.
40. Fritsch DE, Coffee TL, Yowler CJ: Characteristics of burn patients developing pressure ulcers, *J Burn Care Rehabil* 22(4):293-299, 2001.
41. Krause JS, Vines CL, Farley T, Sniezek J, et al: An exploratory study of pressure ulcers after spinal cord injury: Relationship to protective and risk behaviors, *Arch Phys Med Rehabil* 82:107-113, 2001.
42. Keller BP, Wille J, van Ramshorst B, et al: Pressure ulcers in intensive care patients: a review of risks and prevention, *Intensive Care Med* 28(10):1379-1388, 2002.
43. Lindquist LA, Feinglass J, Martin GJ: How sedative medication in older people affects patient risk factors for developing pressure ulcers, *J Wound Care* 12(7):272-275, 2003.

44. Matsuyama N, Takano K, Mashiko T, et al: The possibility of acute inflammatory reaction affects the development of pressure ulcers in bedridden elderly patients (article in Japanese), *Rinsho Byori* 47(11):1039-1045, 1999.

45. Reed RL: Low serum albumin levels, confusion, and fecal incontinence: Are these risk factors for pressure ulcers in mobility-impaired hospitalized adults? *Gerontology* 49:255-259, 2003.

46. Samaniego IA: A sore spot in pediatrics: risk factors for pressure ulcers, *Pediatr Nurs* 29(4):278-282, 2003.

47. Margolis DJ, Knauss J, Bilker W, et al: Medical conditions as risk factors for pressure ulcers in an outpatient setting, *Age Ageing* 32(3):259-264, 2003.

48. Barton A: Pressure ulcer described—1981, *J Tissue Validity* 15(2):8-9, 2005.

49. Norton D: Calculating the risk: Reflections on the Norton Scale, *Decubitus* 2(3):24-31, 1989.

50. Ayello EA: Predicting pressure ulcer sore risk, *Medsurg Nurs* 12(2):130-131, 2003.

51. Bergstrom N, Braden B: A prospective study of pressure sore risk among institutionalized elderly, *J Am Geriatr Soc* 40(8):747-758, 1992.

52. Bergstrom N, Braden B, Boynton P, et al: Using a research-based assessment scale in clinical practice, *Nurs Clin North Am* 30(3):539-551, 1995.

53. Vap PW, Dunaye T: Pressure ulcer risk assessment in long-term care nursing, *J Geront Nurs* 26(6):37-45, 2000.

54. Hawes C, Morris JN, Phillips CD, et al: Reliability estimates for the Minimum Data Set for nursing home resident assessment and care screening (MDS), *Gerontologist* 35(2):172-178, 1995.

55. Hittle DF, Shaughnessy PW, Crisler KS, et al: A study of reliability and burden of home health assessment using OASIS, *Home Health Care Serv Q* 22(4):43-63, 2003.

56. Madigan EA, Fortinsky RH: Additional psychometric evaluation of the Outcomes and Assessment Information Set (OASIS), *Home Health Care Serv Q* 18(4):49-62, 2000.

57. Madigan EA, Tullai-McGuinness S, Fortinsky RH: Accuracy in the Outcomes and Assessment Information Set (OASIS), *Res Nurs Health* 26(4):273-283, 2003.

58. Madigan EA, Fortinsky RH: Interrater reliability of the Outcomes and Assessment Information Set: Results from the field, *Gerontologist* 44(5):689-692, 2004.

59. Salzberg CA, Byrne DW, Cayten CG, et al: A new pressure ulcer risk assessment scale for individuals with spinal cord injury, *Am J Phys Med Rehabil* 75(2):96-104, 1996.

60. Salzberg CA, Byrne DW, Kabir R, et al: Predicting pressure ulcers during initial hospitalization for the acute spinal cord injury, *Wounds* 11(2):45-57, 1999.

61. Hamm R, Behringer B: *The Give and Take of Wound Management: A Guide to Making Clinical Decisions*, Irvine, Calif, 2004, ConceptMedia, Inc.

62. Demling RH, DeSanti L: Involuntary weight loss and the nonhealing wound: the role of anabolic agents, *Adv Wound Care* 12(1):1-14, 1999.

63. Demling RH, DeSanti L: Closure of the "non-healing wound" corresponds with correction of weight loss using the anabolic agent oxandrolone, *Ostomy Wound Manage* 44:58-68, 1998.

64. James JJ: Optimal wound healing: A comprehensive approach through metabolic, anabolic, and nutritional interventions. Involuntary optimal wound healing: A comprehensive approach through metabolic, anabolic, and nutritional interventions, *Wounds* 14(9):4-8, 2002.

65. Lewis B: Nutrition and wound healing. In Kloth L, McCullough JM (eds): *Wound Healing: Alternatives in Management*, ed 3, Philadelphia, 2002, FA Davis.

66. Moussavi RM: Serum levels of vitamins A, C, and E in persons with chronic spinal cord injury living in the community, *Arch Phys Med Rehabil* 84(7):1061-1067, 2003.

67. Whitney JD, Heitkemper MM: Modifying perfusion, nutrition, and stress to promote wound healing in patients with acute wounds, *Heart Lung* 28(2):123-133, 1999.

68. Norman D: The effects of stress on wound healing and leg ulceration, *Br J Nurs* 12(21):1256-1263, 2003.

69. Glaser R: Stress-related changes in proinflammatory cytokine production in wounds, *Arch Gen Psychiatry* 56(5):450-456, 1999.

70. Rozlog LA: Stress and immunity: implications for viral disease and wound healing, *J Periodontol* 70(7):786-792, 1999.

71. Rothstein JM: Pharmacology and physical therapy, *Phys Ther* 75(5):341, 1995.

72. Barclay L, Vega C: Smoking increases risk of wound infections even for simple wounds, Medscape Medical News. Available at http://www.medscape.com/viewarticle/458282_print. Accessed 4/4/2004.

73. Fantone JC, Ward PA: Inflammation. In Rubin E, Farber JL (eds): *Essential Pathology*, Philadelphia, 1995, JB Lippincott.

74. Richard J: Of mice and wounds: reproducibility and accuracy of a novel planimetry program for measuring wound area, *Wounds* 12(6):148-154, 2000.

75. Bryant JL, Brooks TL, Schmidt B, et al: Reliability of wound measuring techniques in an outpatient wound center, *Ostomy Wound Manage* 47(4):44-51, 2001.

76. Lampe KE: Methods of wound evaluation. In Kloth L, McCullough JM (eds): *Wound Healing: Alternatives in Management*, ed 3, Philadelphia, 2002, FA Davis.

77. Thawer HA: A comparison of computer-assisted and manual wound size measurement, *Ostomy Wound Manage* 48(10):46-53, 2002.

78. All About Diabetes. Available at http://www.diabetes.org/about-diabetes.jsp. Accessed July 4, 2002.

79. Collins N: Diabetes, nutrition, and wound healing, *Adv Skin Wound Care* 16(6):291-294, 2003.

80. Lindholm C: Pressure ulcers and infection—understanding clinical features, *Ostomy Wound Manage* 49(5A suppl):4-7, 2003.

81. Dow G: Bacterial swabs and the chronic wound: When, how, and what do they mean? *Ostomy Wound Manage* 49:8-13, 2003.

82. Bill TJ: Quantitative swab culture versus tissue biopsy: A comparison in chronic wounds, *Ostomy Wound Manage* 47(1):34-37, 2001.

83. Ratliff CR, Rodeheaver GT: Correlation of semi-quantitative swab cultures to quantitative swab cultures from chronic wounds, *Wounds* 14(9):329-333, 2002.

84. Sullivan PK: Assessment of wound bioburden development in a rat acute wound model: quantitative swab versus tissue biopsy, *Wounds* 16(4):115-123, 2004.

85. Robson MC: Infection in the surgical patient: an imbalance in the normal equilibrium, *Clin Plast Surg* 6:493, 1979.

86. Reddy M: Practical treatment of wound pain and trauma: A patient-centered approach. An overview, *Ostomy Wound Manage* 49(4A suppl):2-15, 2003.

87. Reddy M: Pain in pressure ulcers, *Ostomy Wound Manage* 49(4A suppl):30-35, 2003.

88. Quirino J: Pain in pressure ulcers, *Wounds* 15(12):381-389, 2003.

89. American Physical Therapy Association: *Guide to Physical Therapist Practice*, ed 2, Alexandria, Va, 1998, The Association.

90. Pressure Ulcer Scale for Healing. Available at http://www.npuap.org/push3-0.htm. Accessed 1/24/2004.

91. Pompeo M: Implementing the PUSH tool in clinical practice: Revisions and results, *Ostomy Wound Manage* 49(8):32-46, 2003.

92. Houghton PE, Woodbury MG: Assessment of wound appearance of chronic pressure ulcers. In Krasner DL, Rodeheaver GT, Sibbald RG (eds): *Chronic Wound Care: A Clinical Source Book for Healthcare Professionals*, ed 3, Wayne, Penn, 2001, HMP Communications.

93. Stotts NA: An instrument to measure healing in pressure ulcers: Development and validation of the Pressure Ulcer Scale for Healing (PUSH), *J Gerontol A Biol Sci Med Sci* 56(12):M795-799, 2001.

94. Sussman C, Swanson G: The utility of Sussman Wound Healing Tool in predicting wound healing outcomes in physical therapy, *Adv Wound Care* 10(5):74-77, 1997.

95. Sussman C, Bates-Jensen BM: Tools to measure wound healing. In Sussman C, Bates-Jensen BM (eds): *Wound Care: A Collaborative Practice Manual for Physical Therapists and Nurses*, Gaithersburg, Md, 1998, Aspen.

96. Bates-Jensen BM, Vredevoe DL, Brecht ML: Validity and reliability of the Pressure Sore Status Tool, *Decubitus* 5(6):20-28, 1992.

97. Woodbury MG: Pressure ulcer assessment instruments: A critical appraisal, *Ostomy Wound Manage* 45(5):42-45, 48-50, 53-55, 1999.

98. Lyder CH: A comprehensive program to prevent pressure ulcers in long-term care: exploring costs and outcomes, *Ostomy Wound Manage* 48(4):52-62, 2002.

99. Xakellis GC: Cost-effectiveness of an intensive pressure ulcer prevention protocol in long-term care, *Adv Wound Care* 11(1):22-29, 1998.

100. Frantz RA, Xakellis GC Jr, Harvey PC, et al: Implementing an incontinence management protocol in long-term care. Clinical outcomes and costs, *J Gerontol Nurs* 29(8):46-53, 2003.

101. Frantz RA, Gardner S, Specht JK, et al: Integration of pressure ulcer treatment protocol into practice: clinical outcomes and care environment attributes, *Outcomes Manag Nurs Pract* 5(3):112-120, 2001.

102. Jolley DJ, Wright R, McGowan S, et al: Preventing pressure ulcers with the Australian Medical Sheepskin: An open-label randomized controlled trial, *Med J Aust* 180(7):324-327, 2004.

103. Sanada H, Sugama J, Matsui Y: Randomised controlled trial to evaluate a new double-layer air-cell overlay for elderly patients requiring head elevation, *J Tissue Viability* 13(3):112-118, 2003.

104. Schultz A, Bien M, Dumond K, et al: Etiology and incidence of pressure ulcers in surgical patients, *AORN J* 70(3):434-439, 1999.

105. Ferrell BA, Osterweil D, Christenson P: A randomized trail of low-air-loss beds for treatment of pressure ulcers, *JAMA* 269(4):494-497, 1993.

106. Branom R, Rappl LM: "Constant force technology" versus low-air-loss therapy in the treatment of pressure ulcers, *Ostomy Wound Manage* 47(9):38-46, 2001.

107. Hardin JB, Cronin SN, Cahill K: Comparison of the effectiveness of two pressure-relieving surfaces: low-air-loss versus static fluid, *Ostomy Wound Manage* 46(9):50-56, 2000.

108. Goetz LL, Brown GS, Priebe MM: Interface pressure characteristics of alternating air cell mattresses in persons with spinal cord injury, *J Spinal Cord Med* 25(3):167-173, 2002.

109. McLane KM: Comparison of interface pressures in the pediatric population among various support surfaces, *J Wound Ostomy Continence Nurs* 29(5):242-251, 2002.

110. Rosenthal MJ, Felton RM, Nastasi AE, et al: Healing of advanced pressure ulcers by a generic total contact seat: 2 randomized comparisons with low air loss bed treatments, *Arch Phys Med Rehab* 84(12):1733-1742, 2003.

111. Economides NG: Evaluation of the effectiveness of two support surfaces following myocutaneous flap surgery, *Adv Wound Care* 8(1):49-53, 1995.

112. Conine TA: Pressure ulcer prophylaxis in elderly patients using polyurethane foam or Jay wheelchair cushions, *Int J Rehabil Res* 17(2):123-137, 1994.

113. Ragan R: Seat-interface pressures on various thicknesses of foam wheelchair cushions: A finite modeling approach, *Arch Phys Med Rehabil* 83(6):872-875, 2002.

114. Geyer MJ: A randomized control trial to evaluate pressure-reducing seat cushions for elderly wheelchair users, *Adv Skin Wound Care* 14(3):120-129, 2001.

115. Yuen HK, Garrett D. Comparison of three wheelchair cushions for effectiveness of pressure relief, *Am J Occup Ther* 55(4):470-475, 2001.

116. Rosenthal MJ, Felton RM, Hileman DL, et al: A wheelchair cushion designed to redistribute sites of sitting pressure, *Arch Phys Med Rehabil* 77(3):278-282, 1996.

117. Figliola RS: A proposed method for quantifying low-air-loss mattress performance by moisture transport, *Ostomy Wound Manage* 49(1):32-42, 2003.

118. Wang JY: Continuous lateral rotational therapy in the medical intensive care unit, *J Formos Med Assoc* 102(11):788-792, 2003.

119. Russell T, Logsdon A: Pressure ulcers and lateral rotation beds: A case study, *J Wound Ostomy Continence Nurs* 30(3):143-145, 2003.

120. Coggrave MJ, Rose LS: A specialist seating assessment clinic: Changing pressure relief practice, *Spinal Cord* 41(12):692-695, 2003.

121. Fillauer CE, Pritham CH: The thoracic suspension jacket—review of principles and fabrication, *Orthot Prosthet* 38(1):36-44, 1984.

122. Carlson JM, Wood SL: A flexible, air-permeable socket prosthesis for bilateral hip disarticulation and hemicorporectomy amputees, *J Pros Ortho* 10(4):110-115, 1998.

123. Rindflesch AB, Miller NE: The thoracic suspension orthosis—a seating option for patients with pressure ulcers, *J Spinal Cord Med* 25(4):306-309, 2002.

124. Harris GF, Coad JE, Pudlowski R, et al: Thoracic suspension: quantitative effects upon seating pressure and posture, *Paraplegia* 25:446-453, 1987.

125. Cullum N: Pressure ulcer prevention and treatment. A synopsis of the current evidence from research, *Crit Care Nurs Clin North Am* 13(4):547-554, 2001.

126. Cullum N: Beds, mattresses and cushions for pressure sore prevention and treatment, *Cochrane Rev Abstracts*. Posted 4/01/2003. Retrieved from http://www.medscape.com/viewarticle/454504 on 4/21/2004.

127. Cullum N, Nelson EA, Flemming K, et al: Systematic reviews of wound care management: (5) beds; (6) compression; (7) laser therapy, therapeutic ultrasound, electrotherapy and electromagnetic therapy, *Health Technol Assess* 5(9):1-221, 2001.

128. Braden BJ: Risk assessment in pressure ulcer prevention. In Krasner DL, Rodeheaver GT, Sibbald RG (eds): *Chronic Wound Care: A Clinical Source Book for Healthcare Professionals,* ed 3, Wayne, Penn, 2001, HMP Communications.

129. Defloor T, Grypdonck MH: Sitting posture and prevention of pressure ulcers, *Appl Nurs Res* 12(3):136-142, 1999.

130. Stinson MD, Porter-Armstrong A, Eakin P: Seat-interface pressure: a pilot study of the relationship to gender, body mass index, and seating position, *Arch Phys Med Rehabil* 84(3):405-409, 2003.

131. Cook DJ, Meade MO, Hand LE, et al: Toward understanding evidence uptake: Semi-recumbency for pneumonia prevention, *Crit Care Med* 30(7):1472-1477, 2002.

132. Helman DL: Effect of standardized orders and provider education on head-of-bed positioning in mechanically ventilated patients, *Crit Care Med* 31(9):2285-2290, 2003.

133. Jones I, Tweed C, Marron M: Pressure area care in infants and children: Nimbus Paediatric System, *Br J Nurs* 10(12):789-795, 2001.

134. Solis I, Krouskop T, Trainer N, et al: Supine interface pressure in children, *Arch Phys Med Rehabil* 69(7):524-526, 1988.

135. Ryan DW, Allen V, Murray A: An investigation of interface pressures in low air loss beds, *Int J Clin Pract* 51(5):296-298, 1997.

136. Crewe RA: Problems of rubber ring nursing cushions and a clinical survey of alternative cushions for ill patients, *Care Sci Pract* 5(2):9-11, 1987.

137. Blaylock B: Solving the problem of pressure ulcers resulting from cervical collars, *Ostomy Wound Manage* 42(4):26-33, 1996.

138. Black CA, Buderer NM, Blaylock B, et al: Comparative study of risk factors for skin breakdown with cervical orthotic devices: Philadelphia and Aspen, *J Trauma Nurs* 5(3):62-66, 1998.

139. Weir D: Pressure ulcers: Assessment, classification and management. In Krasner DL, Rodeheaver GT, Sibbald RG (eds): *Chronic Wound Care: A Clinical Source Book for Healthcare Professionals,* ed 3, Wayne, Penn, 2001, HMP Communications.

140. Lewis-Byers K, Thayer D, Kahl A: Evaluation of two incontinence skin care protocols in a long-term care setting, *Ostomy Wound Manage* 48(12):44-51, 2002.

141. Clever K, Smith G, Bowser C, et al: Evaluating the efficacy of a uniquely delivered skin protectant and its effect on the formation of sacral/buttock pressure ulcers, *Ostomy Wound Manage* 48(12):60-67, 2002.

142. Falanga V: Classifications for wound bed preparation and stimulation of chronic wounds, *Wound Repair Regen* 8:347-352, 2000.

143. Kirsner R: Wound bed preparation, *Ostomy Wound Manage* February:2-3, 2003.

144. Jones V, Harding K: Moist wound healing. In Krasner DL, Rodeheaver GT, Sibbald RG (eds): *Chronic Wound Care: A Clinical Source Book for Healthcare Professionals,* ed 3, Wayne, Penn, 2001, HMP Communications.

145. Cohen MA, Eaglestein WH: Recombinant human platelet-derived growth factor gel speeds healing of acute full-thickness punch biopsy wounds, *J Am Acad Dermatol* 45(6):857-862, 2001.

146. Embil JM: Recombinant human platelet-derived growth factor-BB (becaplermin) for healing chronic lower extremity diabetic ulcers: an open-label clinical evaluation of efficacy, *Wound Repair Regen* 8(3):162-168, 2000.

147. Guzman-Gaardearzabal E, Leyva-Bohorquez G, Salas-Colin S, et al: Treatment of chronic ulcers in the lower extremities with topical becaplermin gel .01%: A multicenter open-label study, *Adv Ther* 17(4):184-189, 2000.

148. Smiell JM, Wieman TJ, Steed DL, et al: Efficacy and safety of becaplermin (recombinant human platelet-derived growth factor-BB) in patients with non-healing lower extremity diabetic ulcers: a combined analysis of four randomized studies, *Wound Repair Regen* 7(5):335-346, 1999.

149. Rees RS, Robson MC, Smiell JM, et al: Becaplermin gel in the treatment of pressure ulcers: a phase II randomized, double-blind, placebo-controlled study, *Wound Repair Regen* 7(3):141-147, 1999.

150. Perry BH, Sampson AR, Schwab BH, et al: A meta-analytic approach to an integrated summary of efficacy: a case study of becaplermin gel, *Control Clin Trials* 23(4):389-408, 2002.

151. Hirshberg J, Coleman J, Marchant B, et al: TGF-beta3 in the treatment of pressure ulcers: a preliminary report, *Adv Skin Wound Care* 14(2):91-95, 2001.

152. Kohyama T, Liu X, Wen FQ, et al: Nerve growth factor stimulates fibronectin-induced fibroblast migration, *J Lab Clin Med* 140(5):329-335, 2002.

153. Landi F, et al: Topical treatment of pressure ulcers with nerve growth factor: a randomized clinical trial, *Ann Intern Med* 139(8):635-641, 2003.

154. Bernabei R, Landi F, Bonini S, et al: Effect of topical application of nerve-growth factor on pressure ulcers, *Lancet* 354(9175):307, 1999.

155. Burrell RE: Efficacy of silver-coated dressings as bacterial barriers in a rodent burn sepsis model, *Wounds* 11(4):64-71, 1999.

156. Wright JB: The comparative efficacy of two antimicrobial barrier dressings. In vitro examination of two controlled release of silver dressings, *Wounds* 10(6):179-188, 1998.

157. Sibbald RG, Browne AC, Coutts P, et al: Screening evaluation of an ionized nanocrystalline silver dressing in chronic wound care, *Ostomy Wound Manage* 47(10):38-43, 2001.

158. Kirsner RS, Orstead H, Wright JB: Matrix metalloproteinases in normal and impaired wound healing: a potential role of nanocrystalline silver, *Wounds* 13(3):4-12, 2001.

159. Thomas S, McCubbin P: A comparison of the antimicrobial effects of four silver containing dressings on three organisms, *J Wound Care* 12(3):101-107, 2003.

160. Vanscheidt W, Lazareth I, Routkovsky-Norval C: Safety evaluation of a new ionic silver dressing in the management of chronic ulcers, *Wounds* 15(11):371-378, 2003.

161. Tikva SJ, Kerstein MD: Is there a difference in outcome of heel ulcers in diabetic and non-diabetic patients, *Wounds* 12(4):96-101, 2000.

162. Falanga V: Wound bed preparation and the role of enzymes: A case for multiple actions of therapeutic agents, *Wounds* 14(2):47-57, 2002.

163. Zacur H, Kirsner RS: Debridement: Rationale and therapeutic options, *Wounds* 14(suppl E):2E-7E, 2002.

164. Hebda PA, Chia-Yee L: The effects of active ingredients of standard debriding agents—papain and collagenase—on digestion of native and denatured collagenous substrates, fibrin, and elastin, *Wounds* 13(5):190-194, 2001.

165. Alvarez OM: A prospective, randomized, comparative study of collagenase and papain-urea for pressure ulcer debridement, *Wounds* 14(8):293-301, 2002.

166. Luedtke-Hoffmann KA, Schafer DS: Pulsed lavage in wound cleansing, *Phys Ther* 80:292-300, 2000.

167. Rodeheaver GT, Pettry D, Thacker JG, et al: Wound cleansing by high pressure irrigation, *Surg Gynecol Obstet* 141(3):357-362, 1975.

168. Cervantes-Sanchez CR, Gutierrez-Vega R, Vazquez-Carpizo JA, et al: Syringe pressure irrigation of subdermic tissue after appendectomy can decrease the incidence of postoperative wound infection, *World J Surg* 24(1):38-41, 2000.

169. Bhandari M, Thompson K, Adili A, et al: High and low pressure irrigation in contaminated wounds with exposed bone, *Int J Surg Investig* 2(3):179-182, 2000.

170. Bahrs C, Schnabel M, Frank T, et al: Lavage of contaminated surfaces: An in vitro evaluation of the effectiveness of different systems, *J Surg Res* 112(1):26-30, 2003.

171. Scott RG, Loehne HB: Five questions and answers about pulsed lavage, *Adv Skin Wound Care* 13(1):133-134, 2000.

172. Ernst AA, Gershoff L, Miller P, et al: Warmed versus room temperature saline for laceration irrigation: a randomized clinical trial, *South Med J* 96(5):436-439, 2003.

173. Streed S: Aerolization of microorganisms during pulsatile lavage. Presented at the 1999 APIC Annual Educational Conference and International Meeting, June 1999, Baltimore, Md.

174. Loehne HB: Wound debridement and irrigation. In Kloth L, McCullough JM (eds): *Wound Healing: Alternatives in Management,* ed 3, Philadelphia, 2002, FA Davis.

175. Fleischmann W, Lang E, Kinzl L, et al: Vacuum assisted wound closure after dermatofasciotomy of the lower extremity, *Unfallchirurg* 99(4):283-287, 1996.

176. Kovacs L: Vacuum sealing: A new and promising regimen in the therapy of radiation ulcers, *Br J Surgery* 85:70, 1998.

177. Muller G: Vacuum dressing in septic wound treatment, *Langenbecks Arch Chir Suppl Kongressbd* 114:537-541, 1997.

178. Morykwas MJ, Argenta LC, Shelton-Brown EI, et al: Vacuum-assisted closure: A new method for wound control and treatment: Animal studies and basic foundation. *Ann Plast Surg* 38(6):553-562, 1997.

179. Banwell P, Withey S, Holten I: The use of negative pressure to promote healing, *Br J Plast Surg* 51(1):79, 1998.

180. Morykwas MJ, Argenta LC, Shelton-Brown EI, et al: Vacuum-assisted closure: a new method for wound control and treatment: animal studies and basic foundation, *Ann Plast Surg* 38(6):553-562, 1997.

181. Kloth LC: Adjunctive interventions for wound healing. In Kloth L, McCullough JM (eds): *Wound Healing: Alternatives in Management,* ed 3, Philadelphia, 2002, FA Davis.

182. Ford CN, Reinhard ER, Yeh D, et al: Interim analysis of a prospective, randomized trial of vacuum-assisted closure versus the health point system in the management of pressure ulcers, *Ann Plast Surg* 49(1):55-61, 2002.

183. Emmanuella J: A prospective, randomized trial of vacuum-assisted closure versus standard therapy of chronic non-healing wounds, *Wounds* 12(3):60-67, 2000.

184. Evans D: Topical negative pressure for treating chronic wounds, *Cochrane Rev Abstracts.* Retrieved from http://www.medscape.com/viewarticle/435423 on 1/25/2003.

185. Kloth LC: Electrical stimulation for wound healing. In Kloth L, McCullough JM (eds): *Wound Healing: Alternatives in Management,* ed 3, Philadelphia, 2002, FA Davis.

186. Cho MR, Thatte HS, Lee RC, et al: Integrin-dependent human macrophage migration induced by oscillatory electrical stimulation, *Ann Biomed Eng* 28(3):234-243, 2000.

187. Bourguignon GJ, Wenche JY, Bourguignon LYW: Electric stimulation of human fibroblasts causes an increase in Ca 2+ influx and the exposure of additional insulin receptors, *J Cell Physiol* 140:379-385, 1989.

188. Kincaid CB, Lavoie KH: Inhibition of bacterial growth in vitro following stimulation with high voltage, monophasic pulsed current, *Phys Ther* 69(8):651-655, 1989.

189. Szuminsky NJ, Albers AC, Unger P, et al: Effect of narrow, pulsed high voltages on bacterial viability, *Phys Ther* 74(7):660-667, 1994.

190. Mohr T, Akers TK, Wessman HC: Effect of high voltage stimulation on blood flow in the rat hind limb, *Phys Ther* 67(4):526-533, 1987.

191. Baker LL, Chambers R, DeMuth SK, et al: Effects of electrical stimulation on wound healing in patients with diabetic ulcers, *Diabetes Care* 20(3):405-412, 1997.

192. Lundeberg TCM, Eriksson SV, Malm M: Electrical nerve stimulation improves healing of diabetic ulcers, *Ann Plast Surg* 29:328-331, 1992.

193. Alvarez OM, Mertz PM, Smerbeck RV, et al: The healing of superficial skin wounds is stimulated by external electrical current, *J Invest Dermatol* 81:144-148, 1983.

194. Brown M, Gogia PP, Sinacore DR, et al: High voltage galvanic stimulation on wound healing in guinea pigs: longer term effects, *Arch Phys Med Rehabil* 76:1134-1137, 1995.

195. Smith J, Romansky N, Vomero J, et al: The effect of electrical stimulation on wound healing in diabetic mice, *J Am Podiatry Assoc* 74(2):71-75, 1984.

196. Taskan I, Ozyazgan I, Tercan M, et al: A comparative study of the effect of ultrasound and electrostimulation on wound healing in rats, *Plast Reconstr Surg* 100(4):966-972, 1997.

197. Thawer HA, Houghton PE: Effects of electrical stimulation on the histological properties of wounds in diabetic mice, *Wound Repair Regen* 9(2):107-115, 2001.

198. Kloth LC, Feedar JA: Acceleration of wound healing with high voltage, monophasic, pulsed current, *Phys Ther* 69(8):503-508, 1989.

199. Feedar JA, Kloth LC, Gentzkow GD: Chronic dermal ulcer healing enhanced with monophasic pulsed electrical stimulation, *Phys Ther* 71(9):639-649, 1991.

200. Houghton PE, Kincaid CB, Lovell M, et al: Effect of electrical stimulation on chronic leg ulcer size and appearance, *Phys Ther* 83(1):17-28, 2003.

201. Gardner SE, Frantz RA, Schmidt FL: Effect of electrical stimulation on chronic wound healing: A meta-analysis, *Wound Repair Regen* 7(6):495-503, 1999.

202. Sussman C, Byl N: Electrical stimulation for wound healing. In Sussman C, Bates-Jensen BM (eds): *Wound Care: A Collaborative Practice Manual for Physical Therapists and Nurses,* Gaithersburg, Md, 1998, Aspen.

203. Kloth LC: Physical modalities in wound management: UVC, therapeutic heating and electrical stimulation, *Ostomy Wound Manage* 41(5):18-25, 1995.

204. Morykwas MJ, Mark MW: Effects of ultraviolet light on fibroblast fibronectin production and lattice contraction, *Wounds* 10(4):111-117, 1998.

205. Conner-Kerr TA, Sullivan PK, Gaillard J, et al: The effects of ultraviolet radiation on antibiotic-resistant bacteria in vitro, *Ostomy Wound Manage* 44(10):50-56, 1998.

206. Sullivan PK, Conner-Kerr TA, Smith ST: The effects of UVC irradiation on group A streptococcus in vitro, *Ostomy Wound Manage* 45(10):50-54, 56-58, 1999.

207. Sullivan PK, Conner-Kerr TA: A comparative study of the effects of UVC irradiation on select prokaryotic and eucaryotic wound pathogens, *Ostomy Wound Manage* 46(10):28-34, 2000.

208. Thai TP, Houghton PE, Campbell KE, et al: Ultraviolet light C in the treatment of chronic wounds with MRSA: A case study, *Ostomy Wound Manage* 48(11):52-60, 2002.

209. Houghton PE, Campbell KE: Therapeutic modalities in the treatment of chronic recalcitrant wounds. I: Krasner DL, Rodeheaver GT, Sibbald RG (eds): *Chronic Wound Care: A Clinical Source Book for Healthcare Professionals,* ed 3, Wayne, Penn, 2001, HMP Communications.

210. Cameron MH: Ultrasound. In Cameron MH (ed): *Physical Agents in Rehabilitation,* ed 2, St. Louis, 2003, WB Saunders.

211. Selkowitz DM, Cameron MH, Mainzer A, et al: Efficacy of pulsed low-intensity ultrasound in wound healing: A single-case design, *Ostomy Wound Manage* 48(4):40-44, 46-50, 2002.

212. Lowe AS, Walker MD, Cowan R, et al: Therapeutic ultrasound and wound closure: lack of healing effect on x-ray irradiated wounds in murine skin, *Arch Phys Med Rehabil* 82(11):1507-1511, 2001.

213. Swist-Chmielewsak D: Experimental selection of best physical and application parameters of ultrasound in the treatment of venous crural ulceration (abstract only), *Pol Merkuriusz Lek* 12(72):500-505, 2002.

214. Johnson S: Low-frequency ultrasound to manage chronic venous leg ulcers, *Br J Nurs* 12:S14-24, 2003.

215. ter Riet G, Kessels AG, Knipschild P, et al: A randomized clinical trial of ultrasound in the treatment of pressure ulcers, *Phys Ther* 76(12):1301-1312, 1996.

216. Sussman C, Dyson M: Therapeutic and diagnostic ultrasound. In Sussman C, Bates-Jensen BM (eds): *Wound Care: A Collaborative Practice Manual for Physical Therapists and Nurses,* Gaithersburg, Md, 1998, Aspen.

217. Flemming K, Cullum N: Therapeutic ultrasound for pressure sores, *Cochrane Rev Abstracts.* Retrieved from http://www.medscape.com/viewarticle/435169 on 12/5/2002.

Vascular Ulcers

Bonnie J. Sparks-DeFriese

OBJECTIVES

After reading this chapter, the reader will be able to:
1. Describe the anatomy and function of the vascular system in the lower extremities.
2. Understand the etiology of different vascular ulcers.
3. Differentiate arterial from venous ulcers based on physical examination.
4. Design a plan of care for vascular ulcer management.
5. Apply information learned regarding vascular ulcer management to presented case studies.

*P*eripheral vascular insufficiency, a dysfunction of blood flow, often leads to soft tissue *ischemia* and ulceration. Although peripheral vascular insufficiency may occur anywhere in the body, it is most common in the distal lower extremities where the vessels are the longest. Insufficiency of the venous system, the arterial system, or both, can result in skin and soft tissue ulceration. Such vascular ulcers are complex, requiring treatment of not only the area of soft tissue damage but also the underlying pathology, as well as consideration of the likely life-long lifestyle changes needed to heal the wound and minimize the risk of recurrence.

Lower extremity vascular disease (LEVD) may cause pain, tissue loss, and changes in appearance and function. Venous ulcers are the most common of the vascular ulcers and generally have the best prognosis. In contrast, arterial ulcers are less common and have a much poorer prognosis; these ulcers often result in amputation. In some patients, both venous and arterial vessels are involved, presenting an even greater clinical challenge.

Differences in interventions and expected outcomes make it imperative that clinicians know the type of ulcer they are managing. A review of common tests, both noninvasive and invasive, is included in this chapter to guide the reader in accurately determining the etiology of a lower extremity ulcer and the status of the lower extremity blood vessels.

EPIDEMIOLOGY

Vascular ulcers can place great psychological, financial and physical strain on patients and their families and thus adversely impact their quality of life.[1] Leg ulcers affect approximately 2.5 million people in the United States.[2] The Wound, Ostomy and Continence Nurses Society (WOCN) reported that two million workdays are lost annually because of lower extremity vascular ulcers.[2] The average direct costs (for one patient with vascular ulcers) over a lifetime exceeds $40,000.[3]

Lower extremity ulcers may be caused by *arterial insufficiency, venous insufficiency,* or mixed vascular disease. Approximately 20% to 25% are caused by arterial or mixed disease, and the remainder are caused by venous disease.[4-9]

It is estimated that approximately 30% of people over the age of 66 have lower extremity arterial disease (LEAD).[2] In 1999 the Centers for Disease Control and Prevention (CDC) reported that 15.5 million people had *atherosclerosis* (hardening of the arteries). Before the age of 70, *peripheral arterial disease* (PAD) is more common in men, but thereafter there is no gender difference in prevalence.[10] Intermittent *claudication* (IC) is the most common symptom of PAD and is experienced by 2% to 3% of men and 1% to 2% of women aged 60 years and older.[11,12]

The American Venous Forum estimates that, at any given time, one person in every 1,000 in the United States has an unhealed venous ulcer.[8] The WOCN Guideline (2004) reported that LEVD is more common among the elderly and that 62% of patients with LEVD are female.[9]

PATHOLOGY

VASCULAR ANATOMY

The lower extremity vasculature is comprised of arterial, venous, and lymphatic vessels. Figs. 29-1 and 29-4 show the major vessels of the lower extremity arterial and venous systems. The anatomy of arteries and veins is briefly described in the following section (see Chapter 27 for more information on lymphatic circulation).

Arterial System. Arteries are elastic, strong, muscular contractile vessels that convey blood from the heart to the periphery. The major arteries in the lower extremities are the iliac, femoral, popliteal, and tibial arteries (Fig. 29-1).

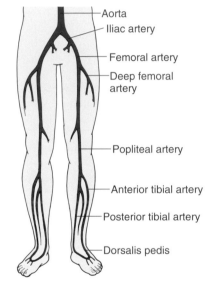

FIG. 29-1 The major arteries of the lower extremity.

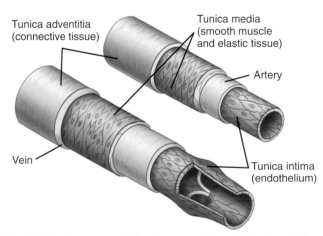

FIG. 29-2 Structure of blood vessels. *From Thibodeau GA, Patton KT:* Anatomy and Physiology, *ed 5, St. Louis, 1999, Mosby.*

All arteries have three layers, the tunica intima, tunica media, and tunica adventitia (Fig. 29-2). The tunica intima, the innermost layer, is composed of endothelium. The tunica media is made of smooth muscle and elastic connective tissue. The outermost layer, the tunica adventitia, is made of collagen fibers. The smooth muscle in the tunica media allows the artery to constrict or dilate. If the muscle in the tunica media is damaged, the vessel loses contractility and the rate of blood flow becomes fixed, preventing any increase in arterial blood supply in response to increased metabolic demand. Stenosis (narrowing) of the artery can also reduce blood flow. Downstream blood flow is reduced when there is 30% or greater stenosis of a peripheral artery and can reach a critical level when the arterial diameter is reduced by 50% or more.[13] Decreased flow can cause tissue ischemia, pain at rest, nonhealing wounds, and *gangrene*.[2]

Venous System. Veins, which convey blood from the periphery back to the heart, are made up of three layers that are similar to the arteries; however, the layers of the vein wall are thinner than in the arteries. The layers of the vein walls can be thin because the blood pressure in the veins is low.[14] The inner layer of smooth endothelium in the veins is folded at intervals to form unidirectional valves that prevent backflow of blood (Fig. 29-3). There are more valves in the leg veins than elsewhere because the blood often has to move against gravity to return to the heart.

There are deep and superficial venous systems in the lower extremities (Fig. 29-4). The primary superficial vein of the lower extremity is the saphenous vein. The saphenous system is connected to the deep system by numerous perforator veins. The main deep veins are the external iliac, femoral, popliteal, and tibial veins. Distal to the tibial veins there are many smaller veins with numerous crosslinking branches.

The deep veins of the legs are surrounded by skeletal muscles that contract and relax during ambulation and other activities. When these muscles contract, they compress the veins, pushing blood back toward the heart (Fig. 29-5). This muscular pump is required for good return of venous blood to the heart. The deep veins (femoral, popliteal, and tibial) lie within the muscle compartment of the leg and are "milked" by muscle contractions. Venous insufficiency can occur if the vein walls, the valves, or the muscles do not function normally.

In the upright position, the blood pressure in the veins in the lower extremities is about 100 mm Hg. If this pressure is unopposed, it will cause significant venous hypertension and peripheral *edema*. Contraction of the gastrocnemius muscle compresses and empties the deep veins, which promotes venous return and reduces the ambulatory pressure within the venous and capillary systems to less than 20 mm Hg. Thus normal venous function is characterized by high "standing" pressures or "resting" pressures and low "walking" pressures.[1]

VASCULAR ULCERS

Arterial Ulcers. Arterial insufficiency occurs when the blood flow in the arteries is not sufficient to meet the

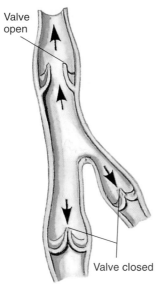

FIG. 29-3 Unidirectional valves in the veins prevent backflow of blood. *From Thibodeau GA, Patton KT: Anatomy and Physiology, ed 5, St. Louis, 1999, Mosby.*

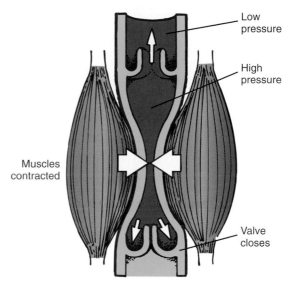

FIG. 29-5 Muscle contractions compress the veins, pushing blood back toward the heart. *From McCance K, Heuther S: Pathophysiology, ed 4, St. Louis, 2002, Mosby.*

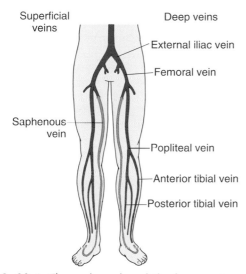

FIG. 29-4 The major veins of the lower extremity.

needs of the skin, muscles, and nerves.[2] Arterial insufficiency can be caused by cholesterol deposits (atherosclerosis) or blood clots (emboli or thrombi) obstructing blood flow or by damaged, diseased, or weak vessels.[1,2] Arterial ulcers occur when there is an insufficient blood supply to the skin and subcutaneous tissues. An ulcer is usually precipitated by a combination of progressive arterial occlusion, increased external occlusive pressure (such as heel pressure in bed-bound patients), and an increase in local oxygen demand because of minor trauma.[15,16] Arterial ulcers generally do not heal unless tissue perfusion is restored.[17] If perfusion is not restored, amputation of an appendage and/or a limb is often necessary. The risk of amputation increases if the wound becomes infected

and gangrenous.[17,18] Common locations for ulcers caused by arterial insufficiency are the foot, anterior leg or tibial area, the lateral malleolus, and the tips of the toes (Fig. 29-6).[1,16]

Etiology of Arterial Insufficiency. LEAD, also known as peripheral vascular disease (PVD), peripheral arterial occlusive disease (PAOD), and PAD, is defined as "atherosclerotic disease of the aorta and arteries of the lower extremity."[19] Approximately 90% of arterial problems in the legs are caused by atherosclerosis.[10] The cause of atherosclerosis, a degenerative process of the elastic and muscular arteries, is not fully understood. Vessel injury, how vascular cells respond to lipoproteins and metabolize cholesterol, and how vascular cells multiply are all hypothesized to be related to the development of atherosclerosis.[12] Atherosclerosis causes narrowing and hardening of the arterial vessels, which then results in increased blood pressure and resistance and decreased blood flow. Narrowing may be caused by deposition of fatty streaks and plaques on the inner arterial wall. The vessels harden because material in the plaques, including lipids, cholesterol crystals, and calcium salts, are hard. The resulting impaired blood delivery leads to inadequate nutrition and oxygenation of the tissues and over time, cell death and tissue necrosis.[12] Other less common causes of PAD are thromboangiitis obliterans or Buerger's disease (common in heavy smokers), arterial trauma, entrapment syndromes, and acute embolic syndromes.[15]

Risk Factors for Arterial Ulcers. Risk factors for vascular ulcers, both arterial and venous, are listed in Table 29-1. Reversible risk factors for PAD include smoking, diabetes mellitus, hyperlipidemia, hypertension, obesity, and physical inactivity. Irreversible risk factors for PAD include male gender, advanced age, and a strong family history.[2,11,12,16,20]

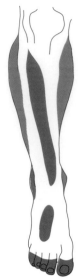

FIG. 29-6 Location of ulcers caused by arterial *(in red)* and venous *(in blue)* insufficiency.

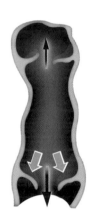 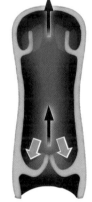

A Incompetent valve   B Normal valve

FIG. 29-7 Incompetent venous and normal valves. *Redrawn from Varicose Veins:* More Than Just a Cosmetic Issue, *Diomed Inc, Andover, Mass.*

The use of tobacco (smoked and smokeless) is the single most important preventable risk factor for arterial disease. Smoking is associated with increased rates of PAD progression, increased amputation rates, lower success rates after vascular surgeries, and increased risk of myocardial infarctions, stroke, and death.[21] Smoking contributes to atherosclerosis by promoting lipid accumulation in the vessels and by promoting plaque enlargement. Smoking also impairs circulation by reducing or preventing nitric oxide–dependent vasodilation, causing vasoconstriction, and decreasing the oxygen-carrying capacity of red blood cells by loading them with carbon monoxide.[10] There is no evidence that low tar cigarettes decrease the effect of smoking on PAD risk.[12,22]

Diabetes mellitus (DM) is associated with increased arterial plaque formation, increased blood viscosity, and hypercoagulability. Hyperinsulinemia, associated with

TABLE 29-1	Risk Factors for Vascular Ulcers
Arterial	**Venous**
Peripheral vascular disease	Thrombophilia
Smoking	Deep vein thrombosis/phlebitis
Diabetes	Trauma
Hyperlipidemia	Obesity
Hypertension	Sedentary lifestyle and occupation
Obesity	Advanced age
Physical inactivity	High number of pregnancies
Male gender	Varicose veins
Advanced age	Family history of venous disease
Strong family history	

type 2 DM, may also contribute to hypertrophy of the vascular smooth muscle. It is not uncommon to find severe PVD before the age of 40 in patients with poorly controlled DM. More than 80% of patients with diabetes have some form of arterial disease within 20 years of their diagnosis, and approximately 75% of the deaths in patients with diabetes are due to arterial disease.[12] DM increases the risk of arterial disease by a factor of four.[21]

Hyperlipidemia contributes to PAD by causing an accumulation of lipids in the arteries; this causes endothelial injury and plaque formation with eventual narrowing of the vessels and reduced blood flow. How hypertension causes vascular injury is unclear. The damage may result from increased production of vascular smooth muscle, activation of the renin-angiotensin-aldosterone system, increased production of vasoconstrictive agents, and/or increased blood coagulability.

Venous Ulcers. Venous disease or insufficiency is a compromise in the venous circulation that can impair the return of blood from the periphery to the heart and cause congestion in the lower extremities. Venous insufficiency can be caused by incompetence of the venous valves (Fig. 29-7), deep vein obstruction or thrombosis, arteriovenous fistula, and/or calf muscle pump failure (caused by paralysis, decreased ankle range of motion (ROM), or ankle joint deformity).[15,23] Common locations for ulcers caused by venous insufficiency are the medial and lateral leg (the gaiter area) and the medial malleolus (see Fig. 29-6).

Etiology of Venous Ulcers. The progression of events from venous insufficiency to soft tissue ulceration is not completely understood, although it is known that factors that cause venous insufficiency are associated with an increased risk of ulcer formation. A number of theories have been proposed to explain the association between venous insufficiency and soft tissue ulceration. Although each of these theories has its merits, the relative contribution of each is not known.

According to the white blood cell activation or white cell *rheology* theory, venous and capillary bed distention slows blood flow. This allows white blood cells to adhere to the endothelial walls of the veins and migrate out into the tissues. Reduced blood flow also allows blood to clot and plug the capillaries, further slowing blood flow. The white blood cells in the tissues then become activated, causing a release of cytokines and free radicals into the venous bed. This inflammatory reaction may injure the valves in the veins, as well as the surrounding tissue, thus predisposing to ulceration.[8,24]

According to the fibrin cuff theory, elevated pressures within the veins cause leakage of plasma, red blood cells, and fibrinogen into the tissues around the capillaries. Fibrinogen is then converted into fibrin, which causes fibrin "cuffs" to form around the capillaries.[6,8] These fibrin cuffs have been visualized by electron microscopy. It was initially thought that the fibrin cuffs blocked diffusion of oxygen and nutrients from the vessels to the tissues, causing tissue breakdown. However, a number of studies have shown that fibrin is actually permeable to oxygen and that oxygen levels are not lower in the areas around fibrin cuffs.[25-27]

According to the trap hypothesis, when venous flow is impaired, fibrin and other macromolecules leak out of the permeable capillary beds into the dermis and bind or "trap" growth factors and other substances necessary for the maintenance of normal tissue and for the healing of wounded tissue.[6,28]

Risk Factors for Venous Ulcers. The primary risk factors for venous ulcers are *thrombophilia* (a propensity to form blood clots), deep vein thrombosis/phlebitis, trauma, obesity, sedentary lifestyle and occupation, advanced age, high number of pregnancies, *varicose veins*, and a family history of venous disease (see Table 29-1).

Thrombophilia is present in as many as 41% of patients with venous ulcers.[16] Congenital conditions that cause thrombophilia include antithrombin III, protein C, or protein S deficiency; factor V Leiden; and prothrombin 20210A mutations, as well as acquired antiphospholipid and anticardiolipin antibodies. Patients with thrombophilia should generally be treated with anticoagulant drug therapy. Deep vein thrombosis (DVT) with phlebitis is associated with a 60% to 90% risk of venous ulceration that may occur up to 30 years after the DVT.[29] Trauma to the leg can initiate or exacerbate venous insufficiency in some patients.[3]

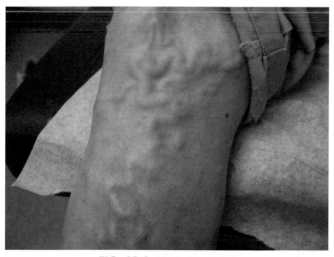

FIG. 29-8 Varicose veins.

A sedentary lifestyle and occupations that require standing or sitting with the feet dependent for long periods of time (e.g., bank tellers and cashiers) are thought to reduce oxygen supply to the skin during periods of dependency. Obesity and the sitting position also impair venous blood flow because the abdomen exerts pressure on the central vascular system.[16,30]

Advanced age (peak prevalence between 60-80 years of age) is considered to be a risk factor for venous disease. However, it must be noted that 22% of venous ulcers develop in patients under 40 years of age and 13% develop in people under 30 years of age.[3]

For women, the number of pregnancies or closeness of pregnancies increases the risk for venous disease.[9,16] It is thought that distal venous pressures may increase because of the compression of the pelvic veins and inferior vena cava.[29] If untreated, varicose veins (Fig. 29-8) are associated with a 20% to 50% risk of lower extremity ulceration.

Mixed Arterial and Venous Disease. Patients may present with ulcers caused by a combination of arterial and venous insufficiency.[16] It is estimated that 21% to 25% of patients with a venous ulcer have some degree of coexisting arterial disease.[3,31] It is challenging to establish the diagnosis and design an effective plan of care for patients with such mixed disease.

EXAMINATION

PATIENT HISTORY

A thorough examination, beginning with the patient's history, is the cornerstone of best practice, regardless of diagnosis. For the patient with a lower extremity ulcer, a thorough history may help identify factors that contributed to the etiology of the ulcer.

The patient history should include information about the patient's medical history, including risk factors (e.g., diabetes, atherosclerosis, trauma, coagulopathies, or history of DVT) and previous surgical interventions. The amount and duration of tobacco use, including tobacco products such as smokeless tobacco and nicotine patches, should also be assessed.

History of pain (amount, type, location, triggers, and reducers) and the ulcer's (or ulcers') onset and previous types of interventions used and their effects should be included. Ulcer duration and size are also important because they are indicators of healing potential. Chronic and larger ulcers are less likely to heal than more recent smaller ulcers.[9] Medications and nutritional status must also be included; the medication profile should include both prescribed and nonprescribed medications. Immunosuppressive medications, such as systemic corticosteroids, have been shown to impair the healing process in humans.[32,33] Other medications, such as pentoxifylline (Trental), which reduce platelet and white blood cell aggregation and thereby reduce capillary plugging, may improve healing of vascular ulcers.[34,35]

Laboratory results, particularly lipid profiles and indicators of blood sugar levels, should also be considered in the initial evaluation of the patient with vascular disease.

Elevated cholesterol, particularly low-density lipoprotein (LDL), is recognized as playing a part in the development of atherosclerosis, whereas high high-density lipoprotein (HDL) levels may reduce the risk of atherosclerosis.[12] Chapter 28 details other components that should be included in the history of any patient with chronic wounds.

SYSTEMS REVIEW

The systems review is used to target areas requiring further examination and to define areas that may cause complications or indicate a need for precautions during the examination and intervention processes. See Chapter 1 for details of the systems review.

For patients with vascular ulcers, a basic review of the cardiovascular and pulmonary systems should include checking for edema; measuring heart rate, respiratory rate and pattern, and blood pressure; and assessing for history of lower extremity ulcers and for indicators of peripheral vascular status (lower extremity color, temperature, and pulses).[36]

TESTS AND MEASURES
Musculoskeletal

Range of Motion. ROM of the lower extremity joints should be measured in all patients with lower extremity ulcers. A limitation in ROM of the lower extremity, especially dorsiflexion and plantarflexion at the ankle, may cause a dysfunctional gait pattern, including an ineffective foot or calf muscle pump, which may contribute to venous insufficiency.[37] ROM loss may be caused by structural or functional abnormalities, as well as by deposition of fibrotic tissue from venous insufficiency.[37,38]

Muscle Performance. A functional calf muscle pump plays a pivotal role in emptying the deep veins and reducing venous pressures, thus reducing the risk for venous ulceration and improving the prognosis for wound healing. A study comparing 49 patients with a history of venous ulcers to healthy control subjects found that those with a history of venous ulcers had statistically significantly weaker calf muscles than the control group.[39] From this study it may be postulated that improving calf muscle strength may promote healing and reduce ulcer recurrence in those with venous insufficiency.

Neuromuscular

Pain. Research has shown that many patients with wounds previously thought not to cause pain do report pain.[7,40] The pain may be constant, only occur with procedures or dressing change, or only occur when the patient is in certain positions. The clinician should ask about the onset, duration, characteristics, triggers, and reducers of pain because these can help differentiate wound etiology in patients with vascular ulcers. For example, it is common for patients with venous insufficiency to have pain that decreases with limb elevation, whereas patients with arterial insufficiency generally have less pain when their limb is in a dependent position. Box 29-1 lists questions that one should ask about a patient's

pain, and the following paragraphs describe the typical presentation of pain in patients with arterial and venous insufficiency.

Pain is typically an initial predictor of arterial disease. The location of the pain may indicate the area of arterial occlusion. More proximal involvement of the aortoiliac arteries causes pain that extends from the buttocks down the lower extremity to the calf, whereas superficial femoral artery involvement generally only causes pain in the calf. Ischemic foot pain in response to exercise generally indicates infrapopliteal artery involvement."[10] Depending on its severity, ischemia may cause IC, nocturnal pain, or rest pain. IC is pain described as "cramping" or the "leg giving out" or "leg fatigue" that occurs only with activity and that is relieved by a few minutes of rest. As arterial occlusion and ischemia worsen, nocturnal pain develops. This is an aching pain that occurs at night (or when lying down) and that is relieved by putting the legs in a dependent position. Rest pain, a sign of advanced occlusive disease, feels like a "constant deep aching" and is present regardless of position or activity.[12,16] Since the pattern of pain indicates the severity of the ischemia, it also indicates the prognosis for healing of an arterial ulcer.

Pain caused by venous insufficiency is different from that caused by arterial compromise. Arterial insufficiency, as previously noted, causes pain early, and the pain is often worsened by activity and relieved by rest and dependency. In contrast, pain from venous insufficiency comes on later in the progression of the disease, and the discomfort is described as a feeling of fullness, swelling, tightness, aching, or heaviness in the leg. Venous insufficiency can also cause skin inflammation, leading to sensations of itching, soreness, or tenderness. Pain associated with venous insufficiency is typically worst at the end of the day after the person has been upright on his or her feet for a number of hours.[9] The tightness or pressure that people feel is caused by constriction of structures by edema. These symptoms are worsened by prolonged standing or sitting, and some patients report having nocturnal leg cramps caused by irritability of the leg muscles. Since venous ulcers generally heal well, any of these types of symptoms indicate a better prognosis than the presence of symptoms associated with arterial insufficiency.

BOX 29-1	Questions to Ask about a Patient's Pain

- Do you have leg "cramping" or pain brought on by exercise and relieved by a few minutes of rest?
- Do you have pain at rest when your legs are hanging down?
- Do you have pain at night when in bed?
- Do you have pain that increases with elevation and decreases with dependency?
- What type of pain do you have (e.g., aching, shooting, sharp, dull)?
- Is your ulcer painful?
- What helps to reduce your pain?

Sensory Integrity. Paresthesia (sensations such as numbness, tingling or a "pins and needles" feeling) is one of the six "Ps" of arterial disease: Pulselessness, pain, pallor, poikilothermy (body temperature that varies with environmental temperature), paresthesia, and paralysis. Paresthesia and paralysis are signs of severe and potentially irreversible ischemia.[41]

Sensory loss is also common in patients with PAD, particularly those with neuropathy caused by diabetes. Since neuropathy and diabetes may go undiagnosed for many years, sensation should be checked in all patients with lower extremity ulcers (see Chapters 18 and 30 for more information on diabetic neuropathy and ulcers related to diabetic neuropathy). In general, sensory testing should include at least an examination of light touch in all dermatomes and a check for protective sensation on both feet with nylon monofilaments.

Cardiovascular/Pulmonary

Circulation. In the evaluation and management of vascular ulcers, the value of vascular testing by pulse palpation, Doppler ultrasound, and other tests (noninvasive and invasive) cannot be overemphasized. Testing must be done to assess the status and viability of the vascular systems, both arterial and venous, and to determine healing potential, risk of recurrence, and complications.

Examination of circulation should include the color and temperature of the involved area(s) and the effects of limb elevation and dependency. Patients with PAD typically have a blue or dusky tone to the skin, pallor with elevation, and rubor with dependency. The presence, absence, and quality of pulses; measurement of ankle-brachial index (ABI) or toe-brachial index (TBI); and measurement of transcutaneous partial pressure of oxygen ($TcPO_2$) are also included in vascular assessment. Common findings for the patient with PAD include diminished or absent pulses, reduced ABI and TBI, and reduced $TcPO_2$ levels. Measurement of TBI is frequently recommended as an alternative to ABI in patients with diabetes because calcification of vessels, which generates an artificially elevated ABI reading, is common in these patients. Measurement of both venous and capillary filling times may also help the clinician differentiate arterial from venous disease. Venous and capillary filling times are both prolonged in arterial insufficiency and shortened in venous disease.

Limb Color. Both arterial and venous insufficiency may cause changes in limb color in response to changes in position. To examine for these changes, the patient is first positioned supine with the leg horizontal. The leg is then elevated at a 45- to 60-degree angle for 15-60 seconds and the color of the plantar surface of the foot is examined. Elevational pallor of the foot (in patients with fair skin) or grey hues (in dark-skinned individuals) and rubor (purple-red discoloration) when the leg is returned to a dependent position suggest arterial insufficiency. Patients with mild disease will develop pallor within 60 seconds of elevation, those with moderately severe disease will develop pallor within 40 seconds, and those with severe occlusive disease will develop pallor within 25 seconds.[15]

Skin Temperature. Skin temperature may be a physiological indicator or precursor to the development of leg ulcers in certain diagnostic groups.[42,43] A small study (with 6 adults) compared leg skin temperature in patients with chronic venous insufficiency (CVI) to skin temperature in patients without CVI and found that the temperature in those with CVI was an average of 1.8° F higher.[43]

It is generally recommended that skin temperature measurements not be compared with typical norms, but rather that the temperature of the involved limb be compared with the temperature of the uninvolved limb (if there is one) and that temperatures be compared along the limb, from proximal to distal. It is postulated that differences in skin temperature may help identify pathology such as arterial compromise (which can cause a reduction in skin temperature distally, often with a sharp line of demarcation[43]). Temperature changes may also predict ulceration in the patient with venous pathology (temperature is increased in areas of ulceration[2]), and temperature elevation can be associated with a local inflammatory response or infection.[12] Skin temperature gradients or differences may be estimated subjectively by the sensation in the dorsum of the clinician's hands[2] or more objectively and quantitatively with an infrared thermographic scanner.

Lower Extremity Pulses. Palpation of lower extremity pulses should be performed starting proximally and moving distally, and pulses should be reported as "present" or "absent."[2] Lubdbrook and colleagues report that the dorsalis pedis (DP) pulse is congenitally absent in 4% to 12% of individuals, thus both the DP and posterior tibial pulses should be checked before concluding that pedal pulses are absent.[44,45] Many clinicians believe that palpable distal pulses indicate normal vascular status; however, some authors suggest that the presence of palpable pulses does not rule out LEAD.[16,20,46]

Ankle-Brachial Index. The most common measure of lower extremity perfusion is the ABI, which is the ratio of the systolic pressure in the ankle relative to the systolic pressure in the brachial artery in the arm. The ABI, also called ankle-arm index (AAI) and ankle pressure index (API), is a reproducible, noninvasive test that helps clinicians objectify and quantify pulse values in order to determine diagnosis and assure appropriate intervention. In the 1980s it was considered to be the most sensitive means for detecting large vessel arterial disease. Although invasive *angiography* is now considered to be a more sensitive test, ABI by Doppler is still 95% sensitive for diagnosis of PAD in comparison to the angiographic gold standard.[10,47] Therefore the ABI is still an excellent method for examining peripheral arterial circulation in most patients with lower extremity ulcers.

Toe-Brachial Index. In patients with chronic DM or renal disease, it may be necessary to use toe pressures or the TBI rather than the ABI to evaluate perfusion because the ankle pressures may be falsely elevated due to vessel calcification.[16] Toe pressures are more reliable because digital vessels are rarely calcified.

Ankle-Brachial Index Procedure and Interpretation. When measuring the ABI, the brachial artery pressure used should be the highest systolic value obtained from the patient's two arms. (See Chapter 22 for detailed descriptions of how to measure blood pressure in the arm.) The ankle pressure should be the systolic pressure in either the DP or the posterior tibial artery. Doppler ultrasound is recommended for measuring the blood pressure at the ankle.[19] The Doppler probe sends an ultrasound signal through the skin; when the signal is reflected back to the probe it changes in frequency in proportion to the rate of flow of the reflecting surface. The returning signal can be heard through a speaker and sounds like the sounds usually heard when a stethoscope is placed over a vessel (Fig. 29-9).[48]

Normally, the blood pressure at the ankle should be equal to or slightly higher than the brachial pressure, producing an ABI of 1-1.4 (Table 29-2). An ABI of less than 0.9 indicates the presence of lower extremity arterial disease.[2] An ABI of 0.5-0.8 indicates moderate arterial insufficiency, and an ABI of less than 0.4 indicates severe involvement.[8] A decrease of 0.15 or more in the ABI is considered to indicate disease progression, whereas an increase of 0.15 or more indicates clinically significant improvement or response to therapeutic intervention. In general, each major arterial blockage reduces the ABI by 0.3; thus a patient with two blockages would typically have a 0.6 reduction in ABI. ABI readings of 0.5-0.8 are generally associated with IC and an ABI of less than 0.3 is typically accompanied by rest pain and/or gangrene.[12,46]

As noted, the TBI (Fig. 29-10) is more reliable in the patient with calcified, noncompressible vessels because calcification in the toes is rare, even in advanced cases of diabetes or renal disease. The TBI is calculated in a similar manner to the ABI, substituting the systolic pressure in the great or second toe for the ankle pressure.[49] A 25-mm wide cuff should be used to obtain the pressure in the great toe. A normal TBI is greater than 0.6, and a toe pressure of less than 40 mm Hg indicates poor perfusion and a low likelihood of wound healing. Pressures of less than or equal to 30 mm Hg predict failure to heal and indicate a need for revascularization.[2,9,21]

The ABI and TBI should be rechecked periodically (every 3 months) in patients with known vascular disease because they may worsen over time.[2]

TABLE 29-2	Interpretation of Ankle-Brachial Index Pressures
ABI	**Interpretation**
1.0-1.4	Normal
<0.9	LEAD
0.5-0.8	Moderate arterial insufficiency
<0.4	Severe ischemia

ABI, Ankle-brachial index; *LEAD,* lower extremity arterial disease.

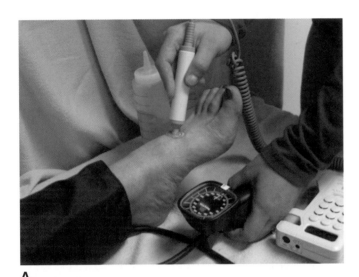

A

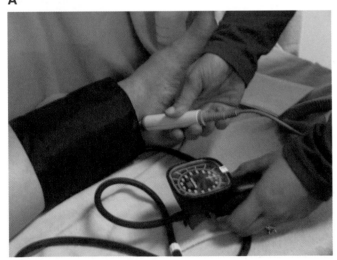

B

FIG. 29-9 Measurement of blood pressure at the ankle using Doppler ultrasound. **A,** At the dorsalis pedis; **B,** at the posterior tibial artery.

ABI = Systolic blood pressure at the ankle/Systolic blood pressure in the arm

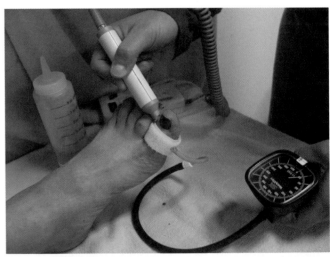

FIG. 29-10 Measurement of blood pressure at the great toe using Doppler ultrasound.

TBI = Systolic blood pressure at the great toe/Systolic blood pressure in the arm

Transcutaneous Partial Pressure of Oxygen Measurement. Another noninvasive method for assessing tissue perfusion is measurement of TcPO₂. TcPO₂ levels indicate healing potential and can be used to determine the appropriateness of aggressive debridement. TcPO₂ levels are commonly measured in the outpatient clinic or in a vascular laboratory and should be considered in the following situations:

- Nonhealing ulcer in patient with ABI <0.9 or toe pressure <30 mm Hg.
- Poorly compressible arteries at the ankle.
- Before amputation to determine the level at which healing is likely.[2]

This test is performed by placing an oxygen-sensing electrode directly on the skin of the lower extremity, often proximal to the ulcer. The electrode has a heating element that heats the skin to 41° C to facilitate oxygen transport from the capillaries to the skin. After approximately 20 minutes, a transcutaneous reading of the PO₂ is taken.[49]

A normal TcPO₂ value is 40 mm Hg, and values less than 40 mm Hg are associated with impaired healing[2] (Table 29-3). Values of less than 20 mm Hg generally indicate marked ischemia and an inability to heal.[15] Values between 20 and 40 mm Hg represent a "grey zone" where healing is likely to be slow and uncertain, and additional interventions may be needed for a good outcome. If the TcPO₂ is greater than 30 mm Hg, debridement may be considered because although healing is impaired, it is possible. However, if the TcPO₂ is less than 30 mm Hg, debridement is not recommended.[49]

Venous Filling Time. Venous filling time can also be an indicator of venous or arterial disease. To determine venous filling time, the clinician should elevate the lower extremity above the level of the heart (≈75 degrees) and then rapidly move it to a dependent position. The time it takes for the veins of the dorsum of the foot to refill with blood is the venous filling time. A tourniquet may also be placed around the thigh while the leg is elevated. This is known as the Trendelenburg test.[6]

If the venous valves are competent, the venous filling time will be longer than 20 seconds. If the valves are incompetent, indicating venous insufficiency, filling will occur much more quickly because of retrograde flow.[6,16] In addition, venous filling time will be prolonged by arterial compromise. A filling time of more than 30 seconds indicates fairly severe arterial occlusion.[2]

Capillary Refill Time. Capillary refill time is measured by pressing firmly with a finger against the toe pad to displace the contained blood and then determining how long it takes for blood to refill the area. A normal capillary refill time is 2 seconds. A delay in capillary refill (more than 3 seconds) indicates arterial insufficiency; however, capillary refill time may be normal in many patients with PAD because the emptied vessels may refill in a retrograde manner from surrounding veins.[2]

Vascular Laboratory Tests. Referral to a vascular laboratory for more detailed testing is often indicated to assess the presence, location, and severity of vascular disease (Box 29-2). Noninvasive and invasive vascular procedures are available. The noninvasive laboratory tests can provide direct images (of the vessel itself) or indirect images (changes distal to the diseased vessel).[1] Noninvasive tests include segmental systolic limb pressure, Doppler ultrasound imaging, duplex imaging (with and without color), and pulse volume recordings with air plethysmography. Invasive tests include arteriography and venography.

Segmental Systolic Limb Pressure. Segmental systolic limb pressure (SLP) uses Doppler ultrasound to determine arterial pressures at different levels of the lower extremity (high thigh, above knee, below the knee, and above the ankle). This test, which is usually performed in a vascular laboratory, provides information about the location of vascular occlusion in the lower extremity but does not produce more accurate information about distal extremity flow than a clinical assessment of ABI.[50]

Color Duplex Imaging. Color duplex imaging (CDI) is considered the most reliable noninvasive test of vascular flow and the most time-efficient tool for examination and reexamination of lower extremity vascular insufficiency.[9,32] Duplex imaging "maps out" the normal and abnormal superficial and deep venous pathways and identifies the sources of incompetence and levels of obstruction.[32] Debate continues with regard to the neces-

TABLE 29-3	Interpretation of Transcutaneous Partial Pressure of Oxygen Values
TcPO₂ Value	**Interpretation**
≥40 mm Hg	Normal cutaneous arterial supply.
20 to 40 mm Hg	Impaired cutaneous arterial supply. The patient may have problems with wound healing.
>30 mm Hg	Debridement may be considered.
<30 mm Hg	Debridement is not recommended.
<20 mm Hg	Marked ischemia

TcPO₂, Transcutaneous partial pressure of oxygen.

BOX 29-2	Indications for Consulting a Vascular Surgeon or a Vascular Laboratory

1. Absence of both dorsalis pedis and posterior tibial pulses
2. ABI <0.9 plus any one of the following
   a. Ulcer that fails to improve within 2-4 weeks of appropriate therapy
   b. Severe ischemic pain
   c. Intermittent claudication
   d. TP <30 mm Hg
   e. Ankle pressure <50 mm Hg, ABI <0.5
   f. Clinical signs of infection
3. Cellulitis, osteomyelitis
4. Urgent vascular referral if
   a. ABI <0.4
   b. Gangrene

From Bonham PA, Flemister BG: *Wound, Ostomy and Continence Nurses Society (WOCN) Clinical Practice Guideline Series: Guideline for Management of Wounds in Patients with Lower-Extremity Arterial Disease,* Glenview, Ill, 2002, WOCN.
ABI, Ankle-brachial index; *TP,* toe pressure.

sity of duplex ultrasound in every case because of the costs of the diagnostic equipment and the time required to complete the test.[32] CDI provides a safe alternative to the *arteriogram* and is offered by most hospitals in the United States.[32]

Pulse Volume Recording. The pulse volume recording test can be used to assess circulation in calcified vessels.[12,39] This test can detect vascular pathology in both the superficial and deep veins. Pulse volume recording identifies changes in venous blood volume as the blood moves in and out with each cardiac cycle.[45] However, because this test does not visualize the venous system, it is rarely used.

Magnetic Resonance Angiography. Magnetic resonance angiography (MRA) is a noninvasive alternative to arteriography that visualizes the artery, its lumen, and plaques using magnetic resonance imaging (MRI) technology. This method eliminates the risks associated with invasive arteriography but is associated with considerable expense.[12,31]

Arteriography. Arteriography is an invasive test used for evaluation of vascular disease. It is considered to be the most accurate technique for diagnosing and localizing PVD.[12,41] Arteriography, also known as angiography, is recommended for patients with diabetes and nonhealing wounds and moderate-to-severe arterial disease (ABI <0.7) before vascular surgery.[1,6,9,31] Arteriography is performed by injecting a radiopaque contrast material into the artery and then observing blood flow through the arterial system with x-ray. The risks of this invasive procedure include mechanical damage to vessels (dissection or perforation), damage at the injection site (bleeding or hematoma), or reactions to the contrast material (allergic reactions, nephrotoxicity, or cardiopulmonary toxicity).[12] Digital subtraction angiography (DSA) is a specialized type of arteriography that incorporates computerized fluoroscopy to enhance contrast visualization. This procedure is safer (because contrast is injected into a vein rather than an artery) but may produce a poorer quality image.[12]

Integumentary. Skin integrity in the lower extremities may be impaired as the result of arterial and/or venous insufficiency. The integumentary system examination and testing includes a comprehensive wound assessment. This includes the same parameters as those identified for other chronic wounds (see Chapter 28), including wound location (specified according to anatomical landmarks); dimensions (length, width, and depth in centimeters and/or surface area in square centimeters); wound bed characteristics, appearance, and color (necrosis, slough, granulation, clean but nongranulating tissue, or epithelialization); drainage (amount, odor, color, and consistency); undermining, tracts, or tunnels (location and measurements); and the status of the wound edges (open or closed). Additional parameters include the status of the surrounding skin (erythema, induration, increased warmth, local edema, sensitivity to palpation, fluctuance, boggy tissue, and trophic changes); edema (presence, type, and severity); pain (severity, characteristics, triggers, or reducers) and signs of *osteomyelitis* or gangrene.

Ulcers caused by arterial and venous insufficiency have similarities and differences. The features that most often differ between arterial and venous ulcers can be found in Table 29-4.

Ulcer location and color and the volume of drainage are the most critical for differentiating between types of lower extremity vascular ulcers. Venous ulcers are typically located in the "gaiter" or medial malleolus area, whereas arterial ulcers are usually on the toes. The wound bed of a venous ulcer has a deep red color, whereas the less-perfused arterial ulcer has a necrotic, pale, or dusky blue color. Characteristically, the ulcer caused by venous insufficiency has a moderate to copious amount of drainage, whereas the arterial ulcer is often dry with little or no drainage.

Other indicators of venous insufficiency include lower extremity edema, hemosiderosis, venous *dermatitis, ankle flare,* and *lipodermatosclerosis* (in the more advanced stages). Edema most often occurs at the site of greatest gravitational pressure, the ankle. This is also where hemosiderosis, a greyish-brown hyperpigmentation, can be seen (Fig. 29-11). This tissue discoloration is caused by blood leaking into the tissues where the subsequent breakdown of red blood cells deposits pigment. Venous dermatitis, which makes the skin itchy, erythematous, and weeping, or dry and scaly, is another common complication of venous insufficiency (Fig. 29-12). Contact dermatitis around a leg ulcer may also occur because of chemical or mechanical irritation. "Ankle flare" or "malleolar flare," a collection of small venous channels inferior to the medial malleolus and extending onto the medial foot, also often occurs in patients with a venous insufficiency (Fig. 29-13). In the later stages of the disease, lipodermatosclerosis (sclerosis of fat and dermal tissue layers) occurs as result of protein (fibrin) deposits in tissues. The leg in the "gaiter (sock) area" becomes indurated and hyperpigmented. The surrounding tissue may become very edematous, causing a "bottle leg" shape (caused by edema above and below the gaiter area in conjunction with contraction of the tissues in the gaiter area).

Indicators of arterial insufficiency include trophic changes, such as thickened toenails, loss or thinning of

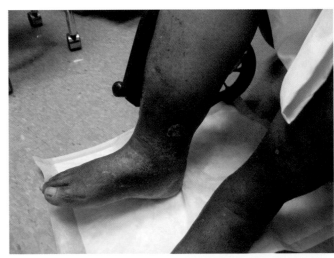

FIG. 29-11 Lower extremity hemosiderosis and edema as a result of venous insufficiency and stasis.

TABLE 29-4	Typical Characteristics of Venous and Arterial Ulcers	
Characteristic	**Arterial**	**Venous**
Location	Usually distal, in between or on tips of toes, over phalangeal heads, over lateral malleolus, areas exposed to repetitive trauma (e.g., anterior tibia) and pressure (e.g., heels).	Typically around medial malleolus and the medial and lateral leg (the gaiter area).
Wound bed color	Ulcer bed usually pale, yellow or black; ulcer typically "dry" and granulation tissue minimal or absent.	Ulcer bed ruddy in color.
Drainage	Ranges from none to scant or minimal.	Typically moderate to copious.
Edges	Typically regular and "punched-out" in appearance; margins are distinct and often indolent.	Usually irregular.
Surrounding skin	Ischemic skin changes include atrophy of subcutaneous tissue, shiny, taut, thin, dry skin, hair loss, and dystrophic nails. Color changes with position changes include elevational pallor in the fair skin, greyness in the dark-skinned patient's limb, and dependent rubor in both.	Hemosiderosis is classic indicator; defined as increased deposition of iron; presents as gray-brown pigmentation also known as "hyperpigmentation" or "tissue staining" in the gaiter area.[3] Skin tends to be shiny, leading to taut and sclerotic; dermatitis is common; may appear itchy, erythematous, and weeping or dry, crusty, and scaly. High propensity for irritant dermatitis and contact dermatitis.[24]
Pulses	Perfusion diminished as indicated by ABI of <0.8 or a TBI <0.6.	Perfusion is adequate as indicated by palpable pulses (unless edema is significant), warm feet, and ABI often 1.0.
Pain	Severe and reported as sharp; can be exacerbated by elevation of leg.	Often mild and reported as "aching" at end of day. Pain is relieved by elevation.
Infection	Infection common but may not "appear" infected since compromised blood flow results in compromised immune response (inspect for faint halo of erythema, increased pain and tenderness).	
Edema	Not characteristic of arterial insufficiency unless venous component is present. If edema is noted in these patients, it is typically a result of other co-morbid conditions, such as congestive heart failure, infections, or from long-standing dependent positioning to decrease pain.	Most often noted in site of greatest gravitational pressure, the ankle. Hemosiderosis can be seen. This tissue discoloration is the result of leakage of blood into the tissues where subsequent breakdown of red blood cells deposit pigment.

ABI, Ankle-brachial index; *TBI,* toe-brachial index.

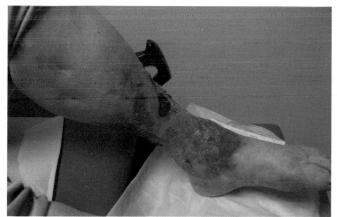

FIG. 29-12 Venous dermatitis in an area of venous insufficiency.

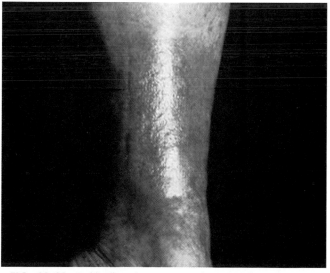

FIG. 29-13 Ankle flare in an area of venous insufficiency.

hair, and shiny skin (due to loss of cellular nourishment) and absent or diminished pulses along with a low ABI and TBI. In arterial insufficiency, Doppler examination reveals an ABI of ≤0.8 and a TBI of ≤0.6. Pain, often severe, is noted in the ischemic limb and may be less in a dependent position. Edema may be present if dependent positioning is frequently used to alleviate pain; otherwise edema is not characteristic.

Infection. Culturing of the wound bed (with sensitivity) is warranted to rule out infection if a wound fails to heal or there is deterioration and spreading erythema, an increase in the amount of drainage, onset of purulent drainage, increasing pain, or increased odor.[37] The classic signs and symptoms of invasive infection are characterized by induration, fever, erythema, and edema (IFEE).[51] Indicators of critical colonization include sudden deterioration in the quality or quantity of granulation tissue, increased volume of exudates, and increased pain but no erythema, induration, edema, or warmth in the surrounding tissue.

Infection may be difficult to identify in patients with LEAD because the typical signs of redness, warmth, and swelling may be subtle or absent when there is reduced blood flow because of arterial insufficiency. In this circumstance, infection may be indicated by no change or an increase in wound size over a 2-week period, increased drainage, increased pain, purulence, odor, or increased necrotic tissue.[2] Immediate referral to the appropriate physician (often vascular surgeons) for these infected wounds is imperative because of the potential for limb-threatening cellulitis and life-threatening sepsis.

Infection in the patient with LEVD may be confused with venous dermatitis or cellulitis. Characteristics of cellulitis include pain, edema, possible fever, and an increase in white blood cell count, whereas dermatitis typically causes a weepy, papular rash with *pruritus*.

Function

Gait. The absence of appropriate toe-off during terminal stance (see Chapter 32) often indicates poor calf muscle function. This will impair the function of the calf muscle pump and thus reduce peripheral venous return.[45]

Assistive Devices. Assistive devices may be used to assist with independence in ambulation or to reduce pressure on a lower extremity ulcer, particularly those on the soles of the feet (see Chapter 33).

Self-Care and Home Management. Current and prior functional status in self-care and home management activities (including activities of daily living [ADLs]) that should be examined in the patient with peripheral vascular disease include the patient's ability to follow care guidelines, access necessary equipment (running water, clean water source and supplies for wound cleansing, furniture to elevate an edematous leg), and the availability and nature of social supports to assist the patient.

Safety should be examined in patients with compromised lower extremity circulation because such patients are often at high risk for falls and soft tissue trauma. Any neuromusculoskeletal dysfunction (e.g., hemiparesis) may also hinder the patient's self-care and home management of a vascular ulcer. In addition, patients may adopt an unsafe compensatory gait (such as hopping on one leg) in order to decrease pressure and pain on the involved leg. These issues illustrate the importance of a comprehensive examination that includes the impact of the vascular ulcer on the patient's activities, as well as direct examination of the ulcer itself.

Work, Community, and Leisure. Patients with vascular ulcers may be incapacitated by their ulcer or by other symptoms of their underlying vascular disease (e.g., pain, edema, and drainage); because of this, many may lose work and income. In the literature, patients identify lifestyle issues and pain as their primary concerns rather than the healing of the wound.[52]

The occupation of the patient with vascular insufficiency may affect their symptoms. For example, edema caused by venous insufficiency may increase if the patient stands or sits for long periods with the legs in a dependent position. In contrast, the pain associated with arterial insufficiency will be worse if the patient has to walk long distances, particularly if this is up hills or stairs. Similarly, the patient's ulcer and associated problems, such as pain and exudate, may adversely impact leisure and/or socialization. The pain of IC or edema may also limit walking.

A draining wound takes a toll on the patient, as well as his or her family. The wound can prevent socialization because its odor and the frequency of dressing changes or clothing changes to cover the wound are awkward or embarrassing for the patient. Activities that require prolonged sitting (e.g., flying on a plane) may also be difficult because the patient will have to change positions frequently to compensate for their circulatory compromise. For patients with venous insufficiency, performing ankle pumps when sitting at work and during travel or leisure activities may facilitate venous return.

EVALUATION, DIAGNOSIS, AND PROGNOSIS

The patient's prognosis for healing is determined by the type and severity of the vascular compromise. Table 29-5 lists the common examination findings and prognosis of arterial ulcers and venous ulcers. Ulcers that rapidly increase in size, present with atypical wound margins (rolled edges [epibole], cauliflower in appearance), fail to respond to treatment, or tend to bleed should be biopsied in order to rule out squamous cell carcinoma. Approximately one third of chronic wounds are associated with malignancy.

INTERVENTION

GENERAL

All wound management interventions must start by considering the following priorities: (1) determining and correcting etiological factors, (2) addressing systemic factors, and (3) providing appropriate topical therapy.[15] In the case of vascular ulcers, wounds caused by arterial insufficiency are generally best addressed surgically by reestablishing circulation, whereas those of venous etiology are best addressed by enhancing venous return with compression. For all types of ulcers, systemic support should be pro-

TABLE 29-5	Common Examination Findings and Prognosis for Patients with Different Types of Vascular Ulcers	
	Arterial Ulcer	**Venous Ulcer**
Patient history	Cardiovascular disease, heart attack, hypertension, hyperlipidemia, diabetes mellitus,[21] stroke, increased pain with activity and/or elevation, intermittent claudication, tobacco use, traumatic injury to the extremity, vascular procedures/surgeries	Previous DVT and varicosities, thrombophlebitis, reduced mobility, sedentary lifestyle, decreased ankle mobility, obesity, traumatic injury, heart failure, orthopedic procedures, multiple pregnancies
Location	Distal, on or in area of the toes. Around the lateral malleoli. Areas exposed to pressure or trauma.	Medial aspect of the leg and ankle Superior to the medial malleoli
Edema	None	Moderate to severe
Pulses	Absent or diminished	Normal
ABI	<0.5	≥1.0
Capillary refill	>3 seconds	<3 seconds
Borders	Regular	Irregular
Wound bed	Deep	Shallow
Drainage	Scant	Copious
Surrounding skin	Shiny, scant hair, cool to touch, thickened nails	Hemosiderin staining, scarring from previous ulcers, dermatitis, lipodermatosclerosis, normal temperature or warm to touch
Pain	Early symptom, aching, better with dependency	Late symptom, tightness, worse with dependency
Prognosis	Potential for healing depends on the ability to restore perfusion. The wound will usually heal if perfusion can be reestablished. 20% of patients require surgical intervention.[21] High risk for limb loss because of ischemia.[12]	Long-standing wounds are less likely to heal. Chronic, large ulcers with a poor response to the first 3 weeks of therapy are unlikely to heal.[9] A history of vein stripping, or ligation, a total knee replacement, an ABI <0.8, fibrin on 50% or more of wound bed, and poor mobility are all indicators of a poorer prognosis.[48]

DVT, Deep vein thrombosis; *ABI,* ankle-brachial index.

vided by addressing the patient's nutritional and hydration needs, maintaining tight glucose control, and providing topical therapy, including wound bed preparation, appropriate dressings, and adjunctive therapies such as physical agents and topical medications.

Wound bed preparation for vascular ulcers is similar to that for other chronic wounds (see chapter 28) and includes cleansing, debridement of necrotic tissue, provision for moist wound healing, elimination of dead space, protection, and insulation. If the bioburden is high or infection is present, systemic antibiotics, topical antiseptics, or antimicrobial dressings are considered. If wound edges are closed but the wound is still open, the edges must be opened to allow healing to continue. General interventions for the patient with a wound may be found in Chapter 28; the selected interventions described in this chapter are specific to the vascular ulcer.

ARTERIAL ULCERS/LOWER EXTREMITY ARTERIAL DISEASE

Interventions for the patient with arterial ulcers and LEAD are based on the severity, stage, and symptoms of arterial disease; the patient's general medical status; the goals of therapy; and the expected outcome or prognosis. The primary therapeutic focus in management of LEAD is to increase arterial blood flow and diminish pain. All interventions for LEAD initially focus on improving blood supply and decreasing pain. If this cannot be achieved with conservative or pharmacological interventions, sur-

gical revascularization is considered. If surgery is not possible or would not be effective, then amputation must be considered.

Goals of nonoperative treatment focus on risk factor modification and control of disease progression, improvement of exercise tolerance, pain reduction, and prevention and/or treatment of complications. Smoking cessation, exercise, blood pressure control, dietary management, proper management of diabetes, use of physical agent modalities (e.g., hyperbaric oxygen therapy), and pharmacological therapy are the principal means to achieve these goals.[12,19] Meticulous foot care to decrease the risk of complications (e.g., trauma) is also important. Foot hygiene, daily inspection of feet and legs, and avoidance of harsh chemicals, extreme temperatures, and barefoot walking are recommended interventions for the patient with LEAD. Toenails should be trimmed by a professional health care provider because of the high risk for trauma to surrounding soft tissues.

Debridement. Debridement of an arterial ulcer is indicated only when there is adequate perfusion to support healing or when the wound is infected (in order to decrease bioburden). Debridement is recommended when an ulcer is infected, and surgical debridement is preferred in this situation[2] to minimize the risk of spreading the infection. However, debridement is contraindicated for a stable and severely ischemic wound because these wounds have poor healing potential. A stable wound is one with no induration, no erythema, no fluctuance, and no increased warmth. Thus debridement would generally be contraindicated in a patient with an ABI of <0.5 (severe ischemia) who had an ulcer with no signs of infection.[2] If the clinician's examination indicates that nonviable tissue should be debrided, a carefully monitored trial of autolytic or enzymatic debridement is typically the initial approach of choice.[2]

Dressings. Most open, dry wounds should be managed according to the principles of moist wound healing. It is recommended that intervention for an arterial ulcer includes frequent assessment for evidence of developing infection or progressive ischemia.[2] In the acute care setting the ulcer should be assessed daily; in the home health care setting, assessment is routinely done at each nursing visit, which is usually 2-3 times per week. Occlusive and adhesive semiocclusive dressings should generally be avoided because they prevent frequent visualization of the wound. Nonadherent dressings (e.g., hydrogels), which are changed daily or every other day, are usually preferred for open wounds.[15]

However, in patients with significant arterial insufficiency and dry, noninfected necrotic wounds, it is currently recommended that the area be kept dry until the nonviable tissue separates naturally from the viable tissue.[4] A clinical solution to this difficult situation is to paint a topical antiseptic (e.g., povidone iodine) over the wound and allow it to dry.[2] It should be emphasized that this recommendation only applies to the stable wound with insufficient vascular supply to allow healing.

Pain Management. Pain management is important in patients with vascular ulcers because pain can severely and adversely impact the patient's quality of life and function and because pain can cause sympathetic stimulation and vasoconstriction, which can exacerbate arterial insufficiency.[16] Pain may be controlled with systemic analgesics, transcutaneous electrical nerve stimulation (TENS), visual imagery, or relaxation. Referral to a pain management clinic may be appropriate for the patient with pain that is difficult to control and in whom pain is a predominant symptom.

Exercise and Activity. To decrease the risk of ulceration, a graduated exercise program to increase perfusion in patients with LEAD is recommended. Generally, as long as arterial insufficiency is not severe, walking is well tolerated in patients with LEAD. Walking may improve LEAD by improving oxygen use at the cellular level, decreasing resting blood pressure, decreasing stress, and improving gait efficiency. Patients with IC who participate in a regular walking program have been shown to increase their walking distance by 100% to 200%, suggesting that walking increases perfusion to the skin and soft tissues.[21]

However, walking programs are generally not effective or tolerated in patients with advanced arterial disease.[12] This includes patients who already have ulcers caused by arterial insufficiency and those who have rest pain. For these patients, initial interventions are directed toward reducing tissue metabolic demands. This may necessitate a reduction in activity until the ulcer is healed.[12,53] Therefore it is recommended that activity, including walking and other exercise, be closely monitored and modified in patients with arterial ulcers to determine if the activity is facilitating or impairing tissue healing. In addition, if the patient is allowed to ambulate, it is imperative that the area of ischemia be protected either with protective footwear or by an assistive device.[53]

Electrotherapy. Electrical stimulation (TENS) is recommended for the treatment of wounds of various etiologies. Studies show that certain types of electrical stimulation may decrease pain from ischemia,[16] augment blood flow in lower extremities with an impaired calf or foot pump, and stimulate angiogenesis. Houghton and colleagues conducted a study using sensory level high-voltage pulsed current (HVPC) on 42 patients with chronic leg ulcers (arterial and venous insufficiency included) and found that this intervention administered 3 times per week accelerated wound healing in these patients.[54] See Chapter 28 for the mechanisms underlying the effectiveness of electrical stimulation for wound healing, further evidence about the effectiveness of this approach, and details of application technique.

Growth Factors. It has been shown that topical applications of autologous-activated mononuclear cells twice per week may enhance arterial ulcer healing[2] (see Chapter 28).

Intermittent Pneumatic (Dynamic) Compression. Although compression is generally reserved for the treatment of wounds caused by venous insufficiency, the WOCN Practice Guidelines for LEAD state that there is some evidence (level of evidence: B) that patients with IC and/or limb-threatening PAD for whom surgery is not feasible may benefit from intermittent pneumatic compression (IPC) treatment. IPC consists of the alternating application and release of compression every few seconds for a total of 45 minutes to an hour for 3-4 or more hours each day.[2] This treatment is thought to increase blood flow by mimicking the calf muscle pump that occurs during ambulation.[2] The increase in arteriovenous pressure gradient results in a larger pulse pressure and thereby may enhance arterial inflow. Delis and colleagues studied 37 patients with symptomatic claudication; 25 received IPC treatments at least 4 hours per day for $4\frac{1}{2}$ months, whereas the 12 control patients received no IPC.[55] They found that after completing this treatment the patients treated with IPC had increases in claudication distances and ABIs that were greater than in the control group ($p < 0.01$). Twelve months after treatment, walking ability and ABIs in the treatment group remained elevated and significantly better than those of control subjects. They attributed these improvements to improved collateral circulation.

Although more data are necessary to determine the role of IPC in patients with LEAD, it appears that IPC may improve functional walking tolerance, blood flow, pain, and in some cases, ulcer healing.[2] It should be emphasized that this application of compression differs from the sustained, continuous compression recommended for the treatment of venous insufficiency, as described later in this chapter, and that any form of compression is contraindicated in severe arterial disease where the ABI is less than 0.5 and when there is peripheral edema caused by congestive heart failure.[2,37]

Hyperbaric Oxygen Therapy. It is proposed that hyperbaric oxygen therapy (HBOT) may help patients with ischemic ulcers by increasing soft tissue oxygenation.[2,56] It is suggested that this intervention may increase tissue oxygen perfusion, enhance wound healing, increase neovascularization and revascularization, and inhibit the growth of anaerobic bacteria. This intervention involves the patient either breathing pure oxygen at high pressure or locally exposing the wound to oxygen at high pressure and is thought to facilitate wound healing by increasing the amount of dissolved oxygen in the blood.[57,58] However, most of the oxygen in blood is carried by hemoglobin rather than being dissolved in the blood, and with a well-functioning respiratory system the hemoglobin is generally close to 100% saturated with oxygen.

HBOT is typically delivered by the patient breathing pure oxygen at 2-2$\frac{1}{2}$ times atmospheric pressure for 90-120 minutes either daily or twice daily.[59] This treatment is repeated for 10 days to 1-2 months, depending on the chronicity of the problem and the response of the wound.[56,57]

There are a number of published controlled trials on the effects of HBOT on wound healing. However, a systematic review of the literature performed in 2005 on HBOT for the treatment of chronic wounds found 6 trials meeting the authors' inclusion criteria but included no trials with patients with arterial ulcers. Five of the trials involved patients with diabetic ulcers and one involved patients with venous ulcers.[60] The authors concluded that although there is evidence that HBOT reduces the risk of major amputation in diabetic patients, there are insufficient data to support this treatment for patients with venous or arterial ulcers.

Furthermore, the overall effectiveness and cost-effectiveness of HBOT has been called into question. A retrospective study of the effects of HBOT on 54 patients with nonhealing lower extremity wounds resulting from underlying PVD or DM treated with HBOT found that the treatment was difficult to justify, given the "dismal" outcomes for most of these patients and the high cost of this intervention (the average cost for a course of 30 HBOT sessions in 2002 was $14,000).[61] Of the 54 patients, none healed completely, 6 showed some improvement, and 43 showed no improvement. In five cases, the patients required revascularization or amputation. Some recommend that HBOT be used selectively for patients in whom the TcPO$_2$ level in or around the wound is below 40 mm Hg at baseline and that increases to approximately 100 mm Hg when the patient breaths 100% pure oxygen at normobaric pressures.

Nutrition. Good nutrition is essential for patients with wounds because wound healing increases metabolic demand. Consultation by a dietitian is strongly recommended for any patient with a chronic wound with recent weight loss, low albumin or prealbumin levels, vitamin or mineral deficiencies, poorly controlled diabetes, obesity, or dehydration.[15] The dietitian will assess other essential nutritional components necessary for healing (e.g., fluids, proteins, calories, glucose levels, vitamins, minerals, and amino acids) and determine the need for supplementation.

Surgical Options. Surgical options for patients with arterial insufficiency include revascularization, angioplasty, debridement of necrotic tissue, and amputation.[2,21] Surgical revascularization to restore perfusion is preferred where possible. Surgery is indicated for patients with rest pain, tissue loss, or disabling claudication.[20,21] The vessel segment(s) to be treated are identified by angiography before surgery. Most commonly, the superficial femoral artery in the thigh is involved, although some patients have tibial or iliac artery involvement.[12] Revascularization is accomplished by bypass grafting or angioplasty.[12,16,20,21] Arterial bypass grafts may be accomplished by use of the saphenous vein, an upper extremity vein, or a synthetic graft.[4,12,16] Angioplasty is sometimes used for treatment of stenotic lesions in the iliac artery; this procedure is most effective for lesions less than 3 cm long.[12]

Surgical debridement of necrotic tissue may be necessary to rapidly remove infected tissue and reduce the risk of spreading an infection from an infected wound.[2]

Surgical amputation may be indicated if tissue loss has progressed beyond the point of salvage, if revascularization surgery cannot be performed or is too risky, if life expectancy is very low, or if functional limitations obviate the benefit of limb salvage.[20] The level of amputation is generally dictated by function and by the potential for healing at the amputation site. Generally, it is recommended that the amputation be performed at a level where preoperative TcPO$_2$ levels are greater than 20 mm Hg to ensure good potential for healing of the amputation site.[2]

Education. Education for the patient with vascular ulcers should include lifestyle modification measures to improve perfusion and minimize the risk of trauma. One of the most important "teaching points" is the negative impact of tobacco (in any form) on tissue perfusion and wound healing. Other key points to be included in patient education are included in Box 29-3. Patients with arterial insufficiency also need to maintain adequate hydration, control glucose, and see a professional for foot and nail care.

VENOUS ULCERS/LOWER EXTREMITY VENOUS DISEASE

Interventions for the patient with LEVD and venous ulcers should be based on the degree of venous insufficiency, duration of disease, and presenting complications. The desired outcome of interventions for patients with LEVD and venous ulcers is to decrease edema, prevent or resolve ulcers, return patients to an optimal level of functional activity, and educate patients and their families.

Compression Therapy. Compression is the most critical intervention for patients with venous insufficiency with and without ulceration because it supports venous return.[31] This intervention will be required for the patient's lifetime to prevent recurrence of ulcers because a compromised venous system does not recover.[8,16,29] Consistent compliance with *compression therapy* is crucial to good long-term outcomes. One study reported that in patients with lower extremity ulcers caused by venous insufficiency, 79% of those who did not adhere to compression therapy had wound recurrence as compared with

---

BOX 29-3 | **Areas of Education for Patients with Lower Extremity Arterial Disease**

- Chronic disease management (DM, HTN) and the effects of these diseases on LEAD.
- Reduction of hyperlipidemia and proper diet.
- Smoking cessation to slow progression of atherosclerosis and decrease the risk of cardiovascular events including death.
- Compliance with medications.
- Neutral or dependent position for legs.
- Avoidance of chemical, thermal and mechanical trauma.
- Routine professional nail and foot care.
- Use of properly fitting shoes and footwear.
- Wearing socks or hose with shoes.
- Pressure reduction for heels, toes, and bony prominences.
- Need for regular follow-up with healthcare provider.
- Importance of exercise.

Adapted from Bonham PA, Flemister BG: *WOCN Clinical Practice Guideline Series: Guideline for Management of Wounds in Patients with Lower-Extremity Arterial Disease,* Glenview, Ill, 2002, Wound Ostomy and Continence Nurses Society.
DM, Diabetes mellitus; *HTN,* hypertension; *LEAD,* lower extremity arterial disease.

---

only a 4% recurrence rate in those who continued with compression therapy.[62] Unfortunately, adherence to recommended compression therapy is generally poor. Jull and colleagues found that of 129 participants, 52% reported wearing stockings everyday for the first 6 months after healing of ulcer, 16% reported they wore stockings "most days," 5% reported they "occasionally" wore stockings, 22% reported they did not wear compression stockings at all once the ulcer had healed, and 4% did not report data.[63] The authors of this study concluded that the patient's belief that wearing stockings was worthwhile and the patient's belief that the stockings were comfortable to wear were the greatest determinants of adherence. Without acceptance and understanding of the importance of compression therapy, patients often do not comply with this key intervention, increasing their risk of ulcer recurrence.

Compression therapy addresses the changes caused by poor venous return and complications of venous hypertension (trophic changes, pain, edema, and venous ulceration) by providing an external support (sustained or dynamic) to the calf muscle pump. The goal of compression therapy is to augment venous return from the peripheral veins to the central circulation. Compression therapy increases interstitial tissue pressures by compressing the superficial tissues.[15] The amount of pressure underneath a bandage is governed by Laplace's law, which states that sub-bandage pressure is directly proportional to the tension and number of bandage layers and inversely proportional to leg circumference and bandage width:[64-66]

Sub-bandage pressure (mm Hg) = (tension × layers) ÷ (circumference of leg [cm] × width of bandage [cm])

$$T = P \times R$$

where
T = tension
P = pressure
R = diameter

Thus an increase in tension and/or number of layers will increase the sub-bandage pressure; whereas an increase in leg circumference and/or bandage width will decrease the sub-bandage pressure. If bandage tension is consistent along the leg, the pressure will be greatest at the level of the smallest diameter, the ankle, and gradually decrease as one moves up the leg to just below the knee[8] (Fig. 29-14). Sub-bandage or stocking compression pressure may range from less than 20 mm Hg, where the leg diameter is the greatest, to more than 60 mm Hg at the ankle, but generally 30-40 mm Hg of pressure at the ankle is recommended.[3,6,64] The current recommendation is that patients "should be offered the strongest compression with which they can comply."[9] Although adherence is better with medium compression than higher compression,[9] antiembolism stockings (e.g., TED hose), which provide approximately 13-18 mm Hg pressure compression, do not provide sufficient compression for the patient with venous insufficiency. Compression guidelines based on ABI can be found in Table 29-6; compression guidelines based on clinical presentation are given in Table 29-7.

For some patients, especially those who are skeptical of wearing compression, afraid of claustrophobic symptoms, or uncomfortable with the idea of leaving one bandage on for a number of days, a lower to mid-level amount of compression may be used at first and then advanced to a higher level of compression as the patient's tolerance increases. Compression may be sustained (static) or intermittent (dynamic). Sustained compression may be applied with an elastic or inelastic device and intermittent compression may be applied with a multichamber or single-chamber device.

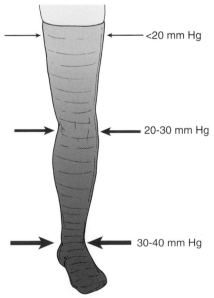

FIG. 29-14 Gradient compression from a compression bandage.

TABLE 29-6	Compression Guidelines Based on ABI
Compression	**ABI**
Standard (30-40 mm Hg)	ABI ≥0.8-1.0
Modified (23-27 mm Hg)	ABI 0.6-0.8
• Elastic, multilayered bandages are contraindicated because force is exerted with ambulation and at rest	
NO Compression	ABI <0.6

ABI, Ankle-brachial index.

TABLE 29-7	Compression Guidelines Based on Clinical Presentation
Compression Pressure (mm Hg)	**Presentation**
20-30	Varicose veins, mild edema, leg fatigue
30-40	Severe varicosities or moderate CVI
40-50 and >60	Severe CVI and its complications

CVI, Chronic venous insufficiency.

TABLE 29-8	Static Compression Bandage Categories and Examples	
Categories	**Types**	**Features and Examples**
Elastic	Multilayered (2, 3, or 4 layers)	Can maintain high compression for up to 1 week.
• Elastic bandages can change in length with edema fluctuations and can provide compression at rest and with ambulation.		Include layers for protection, absorption, and compression.
		Examples: Profore (Smith & Nephew, Largo, FL) and DynaFlex (Johnson & Johnson, New Brunswick, NJ)
	Single-layer reusable	Used for both ambulatory and nonambulatory patients.
		Cost-effective because of reuse but must have trained person to reapply.
		Offer visual guides (rectangles become squares or ovals become circles when the correct amount of stretch Is applied) to assist in accurate application.
		Examples: SurePress and Setopress (ConvaTec, Princeton, NJ) and ProGuide (Smith & Nephew, Largo, FL)
	Long-stretch	Examples: Tubigrip (ConvaTec, Princeton, NJ; 18-20 mm Hg with double layer) and ACE wraps
	Gradient elastic stockings	Many choices available: Different colors, open versus closed toe, knee-highs to chaps to full panty hose styles.
		Provide pressure both at rest and with activity in a variety of levels of compression.
Inelastic	Paste	Constructed of zinc oxide, glycerin, and gelatin impregnated into gauze with calamine added to some brands.
		Requires pleating or cutting each layer to create a smooth conformable boot (should not "give" and permit edema formation).*
		Change when loosens or soiled with wound exudate (typically changed every 3-7 days).
		Combination of inelastic and active layer (e.g., Coban wrap, 3M, St. Paul, MN) is effective in a fully ambulatory patient with a functional heel to toe gait pattern.
		Provides rigid compression (calf muscle presses against compressive force with ambulation therefore pumping effect of calf is maintained).
		Example: Unna's boot
	Short-stretch	Patient must have a functional calf muscle and a functional gait pattern.
		Example: Comprilan (Smith & Nephew, Largo, FL/Beiersdorf, Wilton, CT)
	Orthotic	Nonelastic compression device that consists of adjustable multiple Velcro straps.
		Applied over a medium-weight cotton stocking or stockinet to provide cushioning and absorption of moisture.†
		Example: CircAid Thera-Boot (Coloplast, Marietta, GA)

*Data from Wipke-Tevis DD, Sae-Sia W: *Home Health Nurse* 23(4):237-249, 2004.
†Data from Bergan JJ, Sparks SR: *J Wound Ostomy Continence Nurs* 27(2):82-83, 2000.

Static Compression (Table 29-8). Static elastic compression is generally initially applied with a multilayered bandaging system (Fig. 29-15). These are more effective than nonelastic systems in patients who are not ambulatory because they provide higher resting subbandage pressure.[16] Some multilayered wraps have visual guides to direct how much stretch should be applied (Fig. 29-16). A systematic review of 22 randomized controlled trials (RCTs) found that 3- to 4-layer compression bandage systems increased the percentage of ulcers healed more than single-layer elastic bandages or inelastic paste bandages.[34] Similarly, a Cochrane systematic review of compression with bandages or stockings for patients with venous ulcers concluded that compression

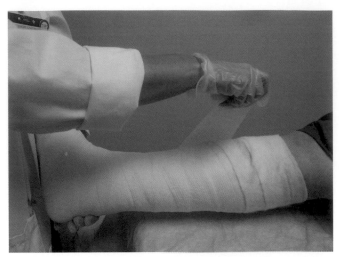

A

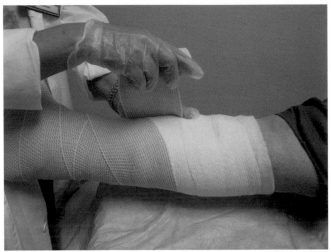

B

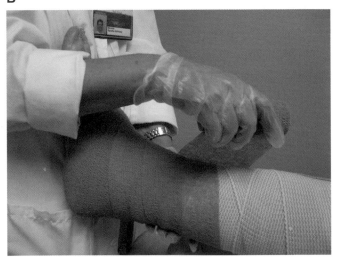

C

FIG. 29-15 Application of a 4-layer compression bandage.

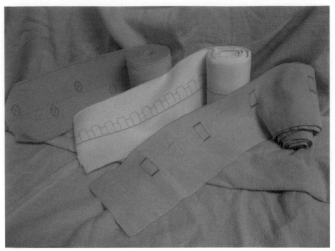

FIG. 29-16 Compression bandages with visual guides to direct how much stretch should be applied. With all of these, the bandage should be stretched until the boxes become square.

increases ulcer healing rates compared to no compression, that multilayered systems are more effective than single-layered systems, and that high compression bandages are better than moderate compression bandages.[37]

If a bandaging system is used, its application is key to safe effective therapy. Although application with too much pressure may cause ischemia,[67] more often too little pressure is used. In addition to the appropriate amount of tension, which should be based on the manufacturer's recommendations with regard to stretch, overlap, and wrapping style and be sufficient to wrap the limb snugly while maintaining palpable peripheral pulses, bony prominences should be padded and oversized footwear should be provided to accommodate the wrap.

Long-stretch elastic wraps (such as ACE bandages) are not recommended for compression in patients with venous ulcers because although they apply high resting pressure when the patient is not moving, they stretch too much when the calf muscle contracts and thus provide low compression when the patient walks.

Once the wound and the edema are stable, elastic stockings rather than bandage wraps should be used to prevent edema and ulcer recurrence. There are off-the-shelf compression stockings available for the more common sizes and custom stockings are available for the "oddly" shaped or sized leg. It is recommended that the stockings be replaced every 6 months, since washing and use decreases their elasticity over time, even with the best care. These stockings are costly, poorly reimbursed, and too hot in some areas of the country during summer seasons. Often patients think they are no longer needed once an ulcer has closed, but studies show a significant decrease in ulcer recurrence rate with continued wear.[36] However, there is no evidence that stockings that extend proximally beyond the knee are any more effective than knee-highs, and knee-highs tend to be better tolerated by patients.[8,37]

Inelastic compression may be applied with an *Unna's boot*, short-stretch bandages (SSBs), or a removable compression orthotic. Unna's boots are similar to a cast (Fig. 29-17). They can be particularly helpful during initial edema management in the ambulatory patient because they provide high pressure during walking and do not

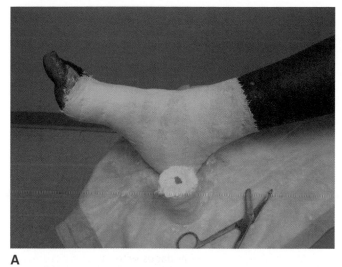

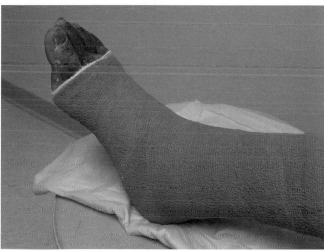

FIG. 29-17 Application of an Unna's boot.

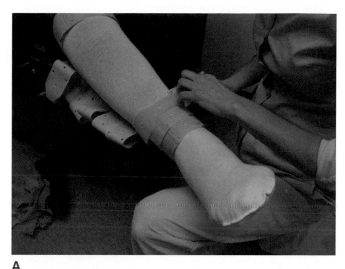

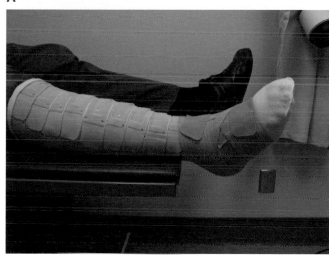

FIG. 29-18 A readily removable and adjustable Velcro-fastening compression device.

stretch out with fluctuations in edema. However, because they are not easy to remove, they should not be used in patients with large amounts of drainage and poor hygiene habits.[8] SSBs, which are bandages with little to no elasticity, also produce high pressure during walking and low resting pressures, helping to push blood proximally and allowing for deep venous filling.

Readily removable and adjustable compression devices that fasten with Velcro straps are also available (Fig. 29-18). Although this can improve patient acceptance,[64] the ease of removal can also decrease usage. A number of studies have compared these devices with Unna's boots, below-the-knee stockings, 4-layer bandages, and SSBs and found them to be a viable and low-cost option for compression therapy.[68-71] They also require fewer provider visits because patients can often change their own dressings, whereas Unna's boots must be changed at least weekly by a professional.[68]

Dynamic Compression. Intermittent pneumatic compression pumps can be used to provide additional com-

pression beyond that provided by bandages or stockings, or as an alternative to bandages or stockings in nonambulatory patients (Fig. 29-19). IPC is the application of controlled external pressure using compressed air and a pump, which cyclically inflates and deflates the chambers within a specially designed sleeve that envelops the extremity.[65] This cyclic inflation and deflation mimics calf muscle pump action and can promote venous return, reduce edema, stimulate fibrinolysis, and heal recalcitrant ulcers after other methods have failed.[65,72]

Kessler and associates found that IPC enhanced fibrinolytic activity in 86% of their subjects.[73] Chen and colleagues reported that 10 out of 21 patients with venous ulcers treated with IPC healed their wounds, whereas only 1 out of 24 healed without the use of IPC.[74] A Cochrane systematic review reported on one small trial (45 people) showing that IPC plus standard external compression increased ulcer healing as compared to compression alone, whereas two other studies (with a total of 75 subjects) found that the addition of IPC to compression did not

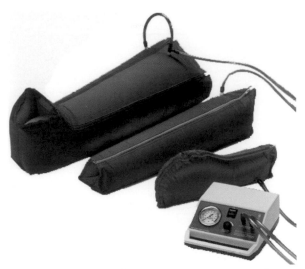

FIG. 29-19 Intermittent pneumatic compression.

provide any additional benefit, and one other small trial (16 people) found no difference in effect on ulcer healing between IPC and compression bandages alone.[75] Further research is needed to clearly determine the effect of IPC on the healing of venous leg ulcers.[72,75] Therefore patients treated with IPC should still also receive static compression with a bandage or stockings for long-term control of venous insufficiency.

Intermittent pneumatic compression devices come with either single-chamber or multichamber sleeves. The multichamber sleeve provides sequential compression that "milks" the fluid from distal to proximal, whereas the single-chamber sleeve inflates and deflates all at once. The multichamber sequential compression has been shown to be more effective in achieving venous return than the single-chamber compression.[8] For patients with venous insufficiency these devices are generally applied for 30-60 minutes twice per day at pressures of 30-50 mm Hg.

Contraindications and Precautions for Compression Therapy. All forms of compression are contraindicated in patients with symptomatic heart failure (because of the risk of system overload) and those with a thrombus (because of the risk of dislodgment) and may not be appropriate if an arterial revascularization has been performed on the involved limb.[8,57] In addition, the clinician must evaluate for the presence and severity of arterial insufficiency before compressing a limb. This is most often determined by calculating the ABI. If the ABI is less than 0.5, all forms of static compression are contraindicated. If the ABI is greater than 0.8, standard or full compression (30-40 mm Hg) may be used. When the ABI is between 0.5 and 0.8, the compression pressure should be reduced to between 23 and 27 mm Hg.[2] If the patient also has neuropathy, careful monitoring is necessary because he or she may fail to recognize symptoms of ischemia such as pain, numbness, or tingling.[2,37]

Compression Selection Guidelines. After considering contraindications and precautions, selection of compression should take into account the patient's mobility and calf muscle pump function. If the patient is actively ambulatory with a normal gait then either elastic or inelastic dressings may be used. If the patient is nonambulatory or has an ineffective gait pattern with lack of heel-to-toe and toe-off, an inelastic wrap will be ineffective because it requires the bulk of the calf muscle to push against it during gait. One should also take into account the patient's ability to don and doff the compression device. Elastic wraps should be applied by a trained professional (Figs. 29-20 and 29-21). Stockings or removable orthotic devices may be applied by the patient if they have the physical skills to apply the wrap (adequate vision and manual dexterity) and if they can reach their feet, or by a caretaker, if the patient cannot reach their feet. Assistive devices, such as the stocking butler and rubber gloves, are also available to assist with donning compression stockings (Fig. 29-22).

Additionally, the availability and cost of the product may affect selection. Not all devices are available in all geographic locations, and many of the compressive products are not covered by most health insurance. Medicare covers these products only until the ulcer is healed. The single-layered systems are generally less expensive than the multilayered systems and may be reused but may be less effective. Questions addressing these issues may include: "Can the patient return to a professional once per week for changing of the product? Is the patient cognitively intact and does he or she have sufficient sensation to be able to recognize and feel if there are problems with the bandage?" It is critical that the patient knows when to change the compression product or call for help.

Education. Box 29-4 provides guidelines for educating patients with LEVD. For the patient with venous insufficiency and resulting edema and wounds, it is important that elevation during the waking hours is emphasized and sitting with legs in a dependent position is avoided. One suggestion is to elevate the legs above the heart for 1-2 hours, 1-2 times each day, and at nighttime. Nighttime elevation can be accomplished by elevating the foot of the bed with blocks or an equivalent.[37]

Debridement. Nonviable tissue in the venous ulcer should be debrided. The type of tissue, the urgency of debridement, clinician preference, and the expected

---

BOX 29-4	Areas of Education for Patients with Lower Extremity Venous Disease

- Chronic disease management and the effects of these diseases on LEVD.
- Proper diet and weight control.
- Compliance with medications.
- Elevated position for legs.
- Avoidance of chemical, thermal, and mechanical trauma.
- Routine professional nail and foot care.
- Use of properly fitting shoes and footwear.
- Wearing socks or hose with shoes.
- Need for regular follow-up with health care provider.
- Importance of exercise.

LEVD, Lower extremity venous disease.

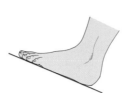

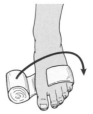 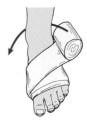

A Position the foot in a comfortable position, at a right angle to the leg.

B Begin by making two anchoring turns around the foot. Be sure to include the base of the toes.

C Next take a high turn above the heel.

FIG. 29-20 Applying an elastic bandage with a spiral wrap technique. *Redrawn from Morrison M, Moffatt C: A Colour Guide to the Assessment and Management of Leg Ulcers, ed 2, London, 1994, Mosby.*

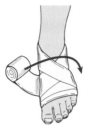 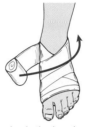 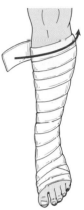

D Then fill the base of the foot with a low turn. From here, the bandage can be applied in a spiral as in this figure or in a figure of eight (Figure 29-21).

E Apply the bandage in a spiral, ensuring there is a 50% overlap.

F Ensure the bandage is applied right up to the tibial tuberosity.

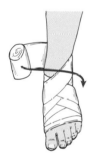 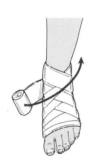 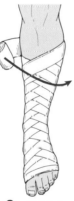

A The steep figure of eight turns aid the comformability of the bandage, accomodating contours in the leg.

B Maintain these turns.

C Finish the bandaging just below the knee.

FIG. 29-21 Applying an elastic bandage with a figure-8 wrap technique. *Redrawn from Morrison M, Moffatt C: A Colour Guide to the Assessment and Management of Leg Ulcers, ed 2, London, 1994, Mosby.*

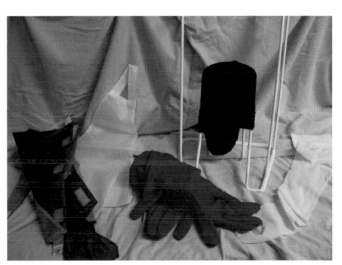

FIG. 29-22 Stocking butler and rubber gloves to assist with donning compression stockings.

outcome and prognosis determine the method of debridement. The different methods of debridement (surgical, conservative sharp, autolytic, enzymatic, and mechanical) are outlined in Chapter 28.

Dressings. Principles of moist wound healing are used with the venous ulcer in order to enhance healing and minimize complications. The venous ulcer tends to be highly exudative; therefore absorption of the excess moisture and elimination of pooled exudate will likely be the focus in dressing selection. Dressings, such as foams, alginates, or hydrofibers, should be considered because of their high absorption capacities. Protection of the surrounding skin from maceration due to excess exudate may require application of a skin sealant (e.g., Skin Prep, Smith & Nephew, Largo, FL, or AllKare, ConvaTec, Princeton, NJ) to the wound edges, especially distal to the ulcer.[15] Once exudate has been minimized, a hydrocolloid may be considered for the wound dressing. The frequency of dressing changes is determined by the volume of exudate and the absorptive capacity of the dressing; the goal is to change the dressing frequently enough to prevent maceration and dermatitis caused by pooled exudate.

Providers should avoid excessive use of topical agents because patients may become sensitized or allergic to any agent used for prolonged periods.[37] One common problem in the management of venous ulcers is the high potential for contact dermatitis. If venous dermatitis (see Fig. 29-12) is present, low-dose topical steroids may be applied for short periods of time (2-6 weeks). Barrier ointments may be effective for xerosis (abnormal dryness); good choices include plain petrolatum or dimethicone products.[15] In addition to providing a moist wound environment, the wound dressing must be compatible with the chosen compression system. The dressing must continue to absorb effectively under the force of the compression and must be able to stay in place for the same amount of time as the compression system.

Skin Substitutes—Bioengineered Skin Equivalents. Studies have shown that bioengineered tissues may promote wound healing by releasing growth factors. These factors can convert a wound from a chronic, non-healing state to actively healing[76]; however, because they are expensive, they should only be used for recalcitrant venous ulcers that fail to respond to standard therapy. Bioengineered skin equivalents, when used in conjunction with compression therapy, have been found to be an effective and cost-effective addition to compression therapy in patients with refractory venous ulcers.[6,9,77,78] A RCT with 293 patients with venous ulcers found that patients treated with a human skin equivalent (HSE) and compression therapy healed faster (63% versus 49% at 6 months, $p = 0.02$) and achieved complete wound closure sooner (61 days versus 181 days, $p = 0.003$) when compared to those treated with compression therapy alone.[79]

HSEs should not be used if the patient has associated untreated dermatitis, infection, or exposed bone or tendon.[76] The dressing over the HSE should be carefully changed once a week without forceful irrigation or debridement. If the wound is healing poorly the HSE may need to be reapplied.[76]

Growth Factors. The benefits of exogenous growth factors in the management of refractory venous ulcers remain unknown[9] (see Chapter 28 for a general discussion of the use of topical growth factors for promoting wound healing).

Exercise, Activity, and Positioning. A walking and exercise program is important for the patient with venous insufficiency because this can improve calf muscle pump function. The key elements of such a program are described in the next section.

Exercise. Exercises that activate the calf muscle pump and assist with venous blood return should be performed frequently. These include (1) isometric contraction of the quadriceps and hamstrings, (2) active and active-resistive ROM for the lower extremities, (3) ankle pumps, (4) short arc quads, and (5) standing toe and heel raises. In addition, aquatic therapy, swimming, and cycling may be encouraged.[45]

Gait Training. Gait training should focus on improving the heel-to-toe pattern during stance and toe-off in terminal stance in order to activate the foot and calf muscle pump. Patients should be encouraged to take walking and exercise breaks at work and at home.

Positioning. Lower extremity elevation is recommended for all patients with venous insufficiency and related edema. The current recommendation is to elevate the leg 6-9 inches above the level of the heart for 2-4 hours during the day and throughout the night. At night this can be accomplished by placing a 6-inch block at the foot of the bed to elevate the foot of the bed.[37]

Pain Management. As noted in the Examination section, the pain reported by the patient with venous insufficiency is different from that caused by arterial compromise. In general, these patients do not have severe pain and their pain is worse when the lower extremity is dependent. Pain caused by venous insufficiency is managed primarily by addressing the etiology—venous congestion and edema. Interventions include elevation of the lower extremity (ankle above the heart), externally applied compression, wound dressings, and changes in ADLs and work patterns (e.g., decreased amount of sitting or standing and increased number of walking breaks).[9]

Ultrasound. The WOCN *Guidelines* for LEVD state that there is some evidence that ultrasound may help venous ulcer healing.[9] A Cochrane systematic review based on seven small RCTs found that there is a possible benefit of ultrasound therapy for venous leg ulcers, but they recommended "caution" with interpretation of this finding[80] (see Chapter 28 for a general discussion of the use of ultrasound for promoting wound healing).

Electrotherapy. Electrical stimulation, particularly HVPC, may accelerate the healing of chronic wounds (see Chapter 28 and the section on Electrotherapy in this chapter).

Nutrition. Careful attention to nutrition is paramount to the wound healing process. Nutrition is as critical to healing as perfusion.[15] A dietitian consult is strongly recommended for any patient with recent weight loss, low albumin or prealbumin levels, vitamin or mineral deficiencies, poorly controlled diabetes, or obesity.[37] The dietitian will assess other nutritional components necessary for healing (e.g., fluids, proteins, calories, glucose levels, vitamins, minerals, and amino acids) and determine the need and criteria for supplementation.

Surgical Options. Surgery for the patient with venous insufficiency and ulceration is generally considered only if the ulcer shows no signs of healing after 3 months of best-practice intervention (compression and good skin care). Surgery is an option when the valvular dysfunction involves the superficial or perforator veins. The procedure most commonly recommended for these patients is *subfascial endoscopic perforator surgery* (SEPS) during which incompetent perforator veins are clipped.[16,37,81,82] It is thought that the most important factor in venous insufficiency is malfunction of perforator veins and that the SEPS procedure removes these malfunctioning veins from the circulation.[83] This surgical technique has less postoperative morbidity than open surgical procedures. For best results, compression therapy should be applied immediately after the SEPS procedure.

Other surgical interventions for patients with venous ulcers include *vein stripping* and ablative surgery, saphenectomy, and free flap. Vein stripping and ablative surgery for superficial venous insufficiency and/or perforator vein incompetence helps reduce deep venous reflux and may help prevent ulcer recurrence.[8,37] Saphenectomy is used for isolated incompetence of the greater or lesser saphenous veins.[37] Excision of the ulcer and surrounding lipodermatosclerosis and placement of a free flap of muscle and skin or omentum is also used to promote the healing of wounds caused by venous insufficiency.[8]

MIXED VENOUS AND ARTERIAL DISEASE

Management of Edema. Whether compression should be used in patients with wounds and concomitant arterial and venous insufficiency with edema depends on the patient's ABI. Compression therapy should not be instituted if the ABI is less than 0.5. However, if the patient has moderate arterial insufficiency (ABI ≥0.6 and ≤0.8) and there is edema caused by venous insufficiency or dependent positioning (used for pain control), a trial of modified- or low-pressure compression of 23-30 mm Hg at the ankle may be used. If the wound does not improve with this intervention, or the ABI is less than 0.5, a prompt consultation by a vascular surgeon is recommended.[2,9]

ADDITIONAL CONSIDERATIONS FOR VASCULAR ULCERS

If the clinician has addressed the etiology of the ulcer, provided systemic support, and implemented appropriate topical therapy and the wound does not start to heal, or if the ulcer is atypical in appearance, the clinician should consider referral for further evaluation, including biopsy.[2,8] Biopsy is considered because nonhealing chronic wounds may be caused by malignancy or may undergo malignant transformation.[2,16] Although rare, skin neoplasm (e.g., squamous or basal cell carcinoma) and certain inflammatory conditions (e.g., pyoderma gangrenosum) may also present with chronic soft tissue ulceration.[8,39]

CASE STUDY 29-1

ARTERIAL ULCER

Examination
Patient History
CV is an 85-year-old woman who has pain and two non-healing wounds on her right lower extremity (RLE). She reports that the wounds have been present for 9 months. Interventions previously used to promote wound healing include cleansing with hydrogen peroxide and application of topical antibiotic ointment twice each day.

CV has history of osteoarthritis and scoliosis and generally decreased ROM and strength in her extremities. She also has a history of atrial fibrillation, a myocardial infarction, and hypertension for 8 years. In 1996 and 1997, she underwent cardiac angioplasty. CV smoked for 22 years but has not smoked for the last 45 years. She denies alcohol use.

Systems Review
HR is 100 bpm and irregular, RR is 18 breaths per minute (breaths/min), and BP is 160/90 mm Hg.

The patient's lower extremity skin is shiny and thin bilaterally with two ulcers on the lateral aspect of the RLE. There are scattered varicosities on both lower extremities.

Tests and Measures
Musculoskeletal: Strength is approximately 3-3+/5 in both lower extremities.

Neuromuscular: CV reports a pain level of 9/10 on scale of 0-10 (0: No pain; 10: Excruciating pain) in her RLE. The pain is worse when she lies down or is walking and better when her legs are resting and dependent. Sensation is intact in both lower extremities. Her balance during transfers is fair.

Cardiovascular/Pulmonary: CV has decreased skin temperature in the RLE, worst distally, with the foot being cold to touch. Elevational pallor and dependent rubor are noted with RLE position change. ABI on the right is 0.6 and on the left is 0.8. Venous filling time is 30 seconds on the right and 22 seconds on the left. Capillary refill was 5 seconds on the right and 3 seconds on the left.

Angiogram revealed right superficial femoral and popliteal artery occlusion.

Integumentary: See Table 29-9 for characteristics of CV's open wounds.

Function

Gait/Assistive Devices The patient is using a wheelchair because of pain and generalized weakness. Until 9 months ago CV walked with a walker at home and in the community and lived independently in her own home.

TABLE 29-9	Wound Characteristics for Patient in Case Study 29-1
Location	RLE lateral aspect above the lateral malleolus.
Dimensions and depth	Wound 1: 1 × 1 cm, depth 0.5 cm. Wound 2: 2.5 × 1 cm, depth 0.5 cm.
Wound bed	Pale pink at the edges with 100% adherent slough.
Wound edges	Open.
Drainage	Minimal to scant, thin, serosanguineous.
Surrounding skin	Thin and shiny without evidence of hair.
Edema	Present at the right ankle.
Pulses	No palpable DP or posterior tibial pulse on right. No palpable DP pulse and a diminished posterior tibial pulse on left.
ABI	0.6 on right; 0.8 on left.
Pain	Generally 9/10 in RLE. 10/10 with touching of either wound.
Infection	No signs or symptoms of local or systemic infection.

RLE, Right lower extremity; *DP,* dorsalis pedis.

Self-Care and Home Management CV lives with her daughter who assists with ADLs as necessary.

Work, Community, and Leisure CV is retired. She goes to church on Sundays and has no other activity outside of the home.

Evaluation, Diagnosis, and Prognosis

CV presents with two nonhealing wounds complicated by a general decrease in function and increase in pain and significantly compromised RLE peripheral arterial circulation.

Diagnosis

CV's diagnosis is 7D: Impaired integumentary integrity associated with full-thickness skin involvement and scar formation.

Plan of Care

CV will be followed weekly for wound management, which will include cleansing and debridement of nonviable tissue as able until revascularization can be performed.

Intervention

Management included active ankle exercises in the dependent position and nutritional evaluation and intervention by a dietitian. Local wound management began with enzymatic debridement for 1 month. Once the wound bed was 50% free of adherent slough and drainage increased, the dressing was changed to calcium alginate and was replaced every other day. CV underwent surgical right popliteal to tibial bypass for revascularization of her RLE 5 weeks after first presenting for care.

Outcome

CV was seen for 7 weeks from initial examination through surgical intervention and follow-up. During this time, both wounds completely closed, the pain decreased from 9-10/10 to 0/10, and the patient was able to walk independently with a front-wheeled walker for short distances.

Please see the CD that accompanies this book for a case study describing the examination, evaluation, and interventions for a patient with a venous ulcer.

CHAPTER SUMMARY

PVD, both venous and arterial, commonly causes chronic open wounds. This chapter provides the reader with a foundation for building best practice in the management of the patient with a vascular ulcer. General anatomy and function of the lower extremity vascular system are reviewed, and pathology, examination, patient evaluation, characteristics of vascular ulceration, and interventions available for promoting healing of wounds caused by arterial and venous insufficiency are highlighted.

Examination follows these three priorities in wound management: Determining etiology, addressing systemic factors, and providing appropriate topical therapy. Interventions can be as simple as elevation or as complex as surgical procedures (e.g., revascularization of a limb). The clinician's management responsibilities also include patient and family education, physical and psychological

assessment and preparation for possible limb loss, coordination of continuity of care, monitoring for complications, and provision of emotional support.

Vascular ulcers can be challenging for the patient, the patient's family, and the clinicians involved in the management of the ulcer. Accurate examination, evaluation and management of the patient with a lower extremity vascular ulcer will lead to the most effective comprehensive care and improve the quality of life for this patient population.

ADDITIONAL RESOURCES

Books

Bonham PA, Flemister BG: *Wound, Ostomy and Continence Nurses Society (WOCN) Clinical Practice Guideline Series: Guideline for Management of Wounds in Patients with Lower-Extremity Arterial Disease,* Glenview, Ill, 2002, Wound, Ostomy and Continence Nurses Society.

Johnson J, Paustian C: *Wound, Ostomy and Continence Nurses Society (WOCN) Clinical Practice Guideline Series: Guideline for Management of Wounds in Patients with Lower-Extremity Arterial Disease,* Glenview, Ill, 2004, Wound, Ostomy and Continence Nurses Society.

Web Sites

Wound, Ostomy and Continence Nurses Society (WOCN): www.wocn.org

American Physical Therapy Association, Section on Clinical Electrotherapy and Wound Management: www.aptasce.com

GLOSSARY

Angiography: A procedure to view blood vessels by injecting a radiopaque contrast medium into them that can be seen on x-ray.

Ankle flare (malleolar flare): Visible capillaries caused by distention of small veins around the medial malleolar area.

Arterial insufficiency: Lack of sufficient blood flow in arteries to extremities. Can be caused by cholesterol deposits (atherosclerosis) or clots (emboli) or by damaged, diseased, or weak vessels.

Arteriogram: An x-ray film of an artery that has been injected with a dye.

Atherosclerosis: When plaques of cholesterol, fats, and other remains are deposited in the walls of large- and medium-sized arteries. The walls of the vessels become thick and hardened, leading to narrowing, which reduces circulation to areas normally supplied by the artery.

Claudication: Pain in the legs with cramps in the calves during walking that is relieved by rest. Caused by inadequate supply of blood to the legs.

Compression therapy: Application of sustained external pressure to the lower extremity to control edema and aid the return of venous blood to the heart, achieved by wraps, multilayer elastic compression therapy systems or a pneumatic pump.

Dermatitis: Inflammation of the skin.

Edema: A localized or generalized abnormal accumulation of fluid in body tissues.

Gangrene (dry or moist): Death of tissue, usually the result of deficient or absent blood supply.

Ischemia: Inadequate blood supply to an organ or part, often marked by pain or organ dysfunction.

Lipodermatosclerosis (hypodermitis sclerodermiformis): The induration and hyperpigmentation of the lower third of the leg that often occurs in patients who have LEVD. This frequently causes the leg to have an "apple-core" or "inverted champagne bottle" appearance.

Osteomyelitis: Inflammation of bone and marrow, usually caused by microorganisms that enter the bone at the time of injury or surgery.

Peripheral arterial disease: Narrowing of the arteries that supply the extremities.

Pruritus: Sensation of itching.

Rheology: Ease or difficulty with which a material changes shape permanently rather than temporarily.

Subfascial endoscopic perforator surgery (SEPS): A minimally invasive surgical technique for the ablation of incompetent perforator veins in the lower leg.

Thrombophilia: An increased tendency to form blood clots.

Unna's boot: Static inelastic zinc-impregnated bandage (with or without calamine) wrapped around the leg to provide compression.

Varicose veins: Swollen and twisted veins that appear blue and close to the surface of the skin. They may bulge, throb, and cause the legs to feel heavy and swell. Varicose veins may occur in almost any part of the body, but they are most often seen in the back of the calf or on the inside of the leg between the groin and the ankle.

Vein stripping: Surgical removal of varicose veins.

Venous insufficiency: Inadequate return of venous blood from periphery generally caused by poor venous valve function.

References

1. Baranoski S, Ayello EA: *Wound Care Essentials: Practice Principles,* Philadelphia, 2004, Lippincott Williams & Wilkins.
2. Bonham PA, Flemister BG: *Wound, Ostomy and Continence Nurses Society (WOCN) Clinical Practice Guideline Series: Guideline for Management of Wounds in Patients with Lower-Extremity Arterial Disease,* Glenview, Ill, 2002, WOCN.
3. de Araugo T, Valencia I, Federman D, et al: Managing the patient with venous ulcers, *Ann Int Med* 138(4):326-334, 2003.
4. Nelson EA, Bradley MD: Dressings and topical agents for arterial ulcers, *Cochrane Database Syst Rev* 1:CD001836, 2003.
5. O'Brien JF, Grace PA, Perry IJ, et al: Prevalence and aetiology of leg ulcers in Ireland, *Irish J Med Sci* 169:110-112, 2000.
6. Paquette D, Falanga V: Leg ulcers, *Clin Geriatr Med* 18(1):77-88, 2002.
7. Goncalves ML, de Gouveia Santos VLC, de Mattos Pimenta CA, et al: Pain in chronic leg ulcers, *J Wound Ostomy Continence Nurs* 31(5):275-283, 2004.
8. Weingarten MS: State-of-the-art treatment of chronic venous disease, *Clin Infect Dis* 32:949-954, 2001.
9. Johnson J, Paustian C: *Wound, Ostomy and Continence Nurses Society (WOCN) Clinical Practice Guideline Series: Guideline for Management of Wounds in Patients with Lower-Extremity Arterial Disease,* Glenview, Ill, 2004, WOCN.
10. Cimminiello C: PAD: Epidemiology and pathophysiology, *Thrombosis Res* 106(6):V295-V301, 2002.
11. Bradberry JC: Peripheral arterial disease: Pathophysiology, risk factors, and role of antithrombotic therapy, *J Am Pharm Assoc* 44(2):S37-44, 2004.
12. Lewis C: Peripheral arterial disease of the lower extremity, *J Cardiovasc Nurs* 15(4):45-63, 2001.
13. Rose S: Noninvasive vascular laboratory for evaluation of peripheral arterial occlusive disease: Part I-hemodynamic principles and tools of the trade, *J Vasc Interv Radiol* 11:1107-1114, 2000.
14. Scanlon VC, Sanders T: The vascular system. In Scanlon VC, Sanders T (eds): *Essentials of Anatomy and Physiology,* ed 3, Philadelphia, 1999, FA Davis.
15. Doughty DB, Waldrop J, Ramundo J: Lower extremity ulcers of vascular etiology. In Bryant RA (ed): *Acute and Chronic Wounds: Nursing Management,* ed 2, St. Louis, 2000, Mosby.
16. Wipke-Tevis DD, Sae-Sia W: Caring for vascular leg ulcers, *Home Healthcare Nurse* 23(4):237-249, 2004.
17. Holloway GA: Arterial ulcers: Assessment, classification and management. In Krasner D, Kane D: *Chronic Wound Care: A Clinical Source Book for Healthcare Professionals,* ed 2, Wayne, Penn, 1997, Health Management Publications.
18. Holloway GA: Lower leg ulcers: An overview. In Krasner D, Rinaldi K, Wilson D: *Chronic Wound Care: A Clinical Source Book for Healthcare Professionals,* Wayne, Penn, 1990, Health Management Publications.
19. Comerota AJ: The case for early detection and integrated intervention in patients with peripheral arterial disease and intermittent claudication, *J Endovasc Ther* 10(3):601-613, 2003.
20. Aronow WS: Management of peripheral arterial disease of the lower extremities in elderly patients, *J Gerontol A Biol Sci Med Sci* 59(2):172-177, 2004.
21. Dillavou E, Kahn MB: Peripheral vascular disease: Diagnosing and treating the three most common peripheral vasculopathies, *Geriatrics* 58(2):37-42, 2003.
22. Tobacco use—smoking and smokeless tobacco. General Health Encyclopedia. Retrieved from http://www.healthcentral.com/mhc/top/002032.cfm on 2/7/2005.
23. Sibbald G, Williamson T: Venous leg ulcers. In Krasner D, Rodeheaver GT, Sibbald G (ed): *Chronic Wound Care: A Clinical Source Book for Healthcare Professionals,* ed 3, Wayne, Penn, 2001, Health Management Publications.
24. Schmid-Schonbein GW, Takase S, Bergan JJ: New advances in the understanding of the pathophysiology of chronic venous insufficiency, *Angiology* 52:S27-34, 2001.
25. Hurley JP: Chronic venous insufficiency: Venous ulcers and other consequences. In Krasner D, Rinaldi K, Wilson D: *Chronic Wound Care: A Clinical Source Book for Healthcare Professionals,* Wayne, Penn, 1990, Health Management Publications.
26. Falanga V, Eaglstein WH: The trap hypothesis of venous ulceration, *Lancet* 341:1006-1008, 1993.
27. Falanga V, Kirsner RS, Katz MH, et al: Pericapillary fibrin cuffs in venous ulceration, *J Dermatol Surg Oncol* 18:409-414, 1992.
28. Zimmet SE: Venous leg ulcers: Evaluation and management. In Fronek HS (ed): *Fundamentals of Phlebology,* Oakland, Calif, 2004, American College of Phlebology.
29. Terry M, O'Brien SP, Kerstein MD: Lower extremity edema: Evaluation and diagnosis, *Wounds* 10(4):118-124, 1998.
30. Wipke-Tevis DD, Stotts NA: Nutrition, tissue oxygenation, and healing of venous leg ulcers, *J Vasc Nurs* 16(2):1-7, 1998.
31. Hess CT: Care tips for chronic wounds: Lower-extremity ulcers, *Adv Skin Wound Care* 16(7):338-341, 2003.
32. Min RJ, Khilnani NM, Golia P: Duplex ultrasound evaluation of lower extremity venous insufficiency, *J Vasc Intervent Radiol* 14(10):1233-1241, 2003.
33. Milne CT: Friend or foe? The role of inflammation in wound healing, The Voice of Home Healthcare: Visiting Nurse Associations of America: www.vnaa.org, 2004.
34. Bonham PA: Assessment and management of patients with venous, arterial, and diabetic/neuropathic lower extremity wounds, *AACN Clin Issues* 14(4):442-456, 2003.
35. Nelson EA, Bell-Syer SE, Cullum NA: Compression for preventing recurrence of venous ulcers, *Cochrane Database Syst Rev* 4:CD002303, 2003.
36. American Physical Therapy Association: *Guide to Physical Therapist Practice,* ed 2, Alexandria, Va, 2001, The Association.
37. Kunimoto BT: Management and prevention of venous leg ulcers: A literature-guided approach, *Ostomy Wound Manage* 47(6):36-39, 2001.
38. Phillips T, Dover J: Leg ulcers, *J Am Acad Dermatol* 25:965, 1991.
39. Yang D: Effect of exercise on calf muscles and calf muscle pump function in patients with chronic venous disease, Edith Cowan University, University of Western Australia http://www.ausport.gov.au/fulltext/2001/acsms/papers/YANG2.pdf.
40. Krasner D: Painful venous ulcers: Themes and stories about living with the pain and suffering, *J Wound Ostomy Continence Nurs* 25(3):158, 1998.
41. Navarro F: *Disease Management Project: Peripheral Arterial Disease,* Cleveland, 2003, The Cleveland Clinic.
42. Sprigle S, Linden M, McKenna D, et al: Clinical skin temperature measurement to predict incipient pressure ulcers, *Adv Skin Wound Care* 14(3):133-137, 2001.
43. Kelechi TJ, Haight BK, Herman J, et al: Skin temperature and chronic venous insufficiency, *J Wound Ostomy Continence Nurs* 30(1):17-24, 2003.
44. Lubdbrook, J. Clarke AM, McKenzie JK, et al: Significance of absent ankle pulse, *BMJ* 5492:1724-1726, 1962.
45. Orstead HL, Radke, L, Gorst R: The impact of musculoskeletal changes on the dynamics of the calf muscle pump, *Ostomy Wound Manage* 47(10):18-24, 2001.
46. Donayre C: Diagnosis and management of vascular ulcers. In Sussman C, Jensen G (eds): *Diagnosis and Management of Vascular Ulcers,* Gaithersburg, Md, 1998, Aspen Publication.
47. Logerfo FW, Coffman JD: Vascular and microvascular disease of the foot in diabetes: Implications for foot care, *N Engl J Med* 311:1615, 1984.
48. Siegel A: Noninvasive vascular testing. In Sussman C, Bates-Jensen B (eds): *Wound Care: A Collaborative Practice Manual for Physical Therapists and Nurses,* Gaithersburg, Md, 1998, Aspen Publication.
49. Bonham PA: Steps for determining the toe brachial pressure index, *Nursing* 33(9):54-55, 2003.
50. Gale SS, Scissons, RP, Salles-Cunha SX, et al: Lower extremity arterial evaluation: are segmental arterial blood pressures worthwhile? *J Vasc Surg* 27(5):831-838, 1998.
51. Alverez OL: Moist environment for healing: Matching the dressing to the wound, *Ostomy Wound Manage* 21:64-83, 1988.
52. Ryan S, Eager C, Sibbald RG: Venous leg ulcer pain, *Ostomy Wound Manage* 49(4A suppl):16-23, 2003.
53. McCulloch JM: Management of wounds secondary to vascular disease. In Kloth L, McCulloch JM (eds): *Wound Healing: Alternatives in Management*

(Contemporary Perspectives in Rehabilitation), ed 3, Philadelphia, 2002, FA Davis.

54. Houghton PE, Kincaid CB, Lovell M, et al: Effect of electrical stimulation on chronic leg ulcer size and appearance, *Phys Ther* 83(1):17-28, 2003.

55. Delis KT, Nicolaides AN, Wolfe JHN, et al: Improving walking ability and ankle brachial pressure indices in symptomatic peripheral vascular disease with intermittent pneumatic foot compression: A prospective controlled study with one-year follow-up, *J Vasc Surg* 31:650-661, 2000.

56. Van Meter K: Systemic hyperbaric oxygen therapy as an aid in resolution of selected chronic problem wounds. In Krasner D, Kane D: *Chronic Wound Care: A Clinical Source Book for Healthcare Professionals,* ed 2, Wayne, Penn, 1997, Health Management Publications, Inc.

57. Kloth LC: Adjunctive interventions for wound healing. In Kloth L, McCulloch JM (eds): *Wound Healing: Alternatives in Management* (Contemporary Perspectives in Rehabilitation), ed 3, Philadelphia, 2002, FA Davis.

58. Moon RE: Use of hyperbaric oxygen in the management of select wounds, *Adv Wound Care* 11:332, 1989.

59. Leifer G: Hyperbaric oxygen therapy: Pre- and posttreatment nursing responsibilities every staff nurse needs to know about, *Am J Nurs* 101(8):26-34, 2001.

60. Roeckl-Wiedmann I, Bennett M, Kranke P: Systematic review of hyperbaric oxygen in the management of chronic wounds, *Br J Surg* 92(1):24-32, 2005.

61. Ciaravino ME, Friedell ML, Kammerlocher TC: Is hyperbaric oxygen a useful adjunct in the management of problem lower extremity wounds? *Ann Vasc Surg* 10:558, 1996.

62. Samson RH, Showalter DP: Stockings and the prevention of recurrent venous ulcers. *Dermatol Surg* 22(4):373-376, 1996.

63. Jull AB, Mitchell N, Arroll J, et al: Factors influencing concordance with compression stockings after venous leg ulcer healing, *J Wound Care* 13(3):90-92, 2004.

64. Phillips TJ: Current approaches to venous ulcers and compression, *Derm Surg* 27:611-621, 2001.

65. Fleck CA: Putting the squeeze on: Understanding venous compression therapy, *Extended Care Product News* 80(2):4-9, 2002.

66. Thomas S: The use of the Laplace equation in the calculation of sub-bandage pressure, *World Wide Wounds,* 2003. http://www.worldwidewounds.com/2003/june/Thomas/Laplace-Bandages.html

67. Callam MJ, Ruckley CV, Dale JJ, et al: Hazards of compression treatment of the legs: an estimate from Scottish surgeons, *BMJ* 295:1382, 1987.

68. DePalma RG, Kowallek D, Spence RK: Comparison of costs and healing rates of two forms of compression in treating venous ulcers, *Vasc Surg* 33:6, 1999.

69. Spence RK, Cahall E: Inelastic versus elastic leg compression in chronic venous insufficiency: A comparison of limb size and venous hemodynamics, *J Vasc Surg* 24:783, 1996.

70. Villavicencio J: Prospective comparative trial between the conventional 4-layer elastic compression treatment and a semi-rigid orthotic compression system in patients with bilateral venous leg ulcers. Presented at the Twenty-First Annual Symposium: Current Critical Problems in Vascular Surgery, 1994, New York.

71. Partsch H, Damstra RJ, Tazelaar DJ, et al: Multicenter, randomized controlled trial of four-layer bandaging versus short-stretch bandaging in the treatment of venous leg ulcers, *Vasa* 30(2):108-113, 2001.

72. Vowden K: The use of intermittent pneumatic compression in venous ulceration, *Br J Nurs* 10(8):491-509, 2001.

73. Kessler CM, Hirsch DR, Jacobs H, et al: Intermittent pneumatic compression in chronic venous insufficiency favorably affects fibrinolytic potential and platelet activation, *Blood Coagul Fibrinolysis* 7:437, 1996.

74. Chen AH, Frangos SG, Kilaru S, Sumpio BE: Intermittent pneumatic compression devices—Physiological mechanisms of action, *Eur J Vasc Endovasc Surg* 21:383-392, 2001.

75. Mani R, Vowden K, Nelson EA: Intermittent pneumatic compression for treating venous leg ulcers, *Cochrane Database Syst Rev* 4:CD001899, 2004.

76. Dolynchuk K, Hull P, Guenther L, et al: The role of Apligraf in the treatment of venous leg ulcers, *Ostomy Wound Manage* 45(1):34-43, 1999.

77. Fivenson D, Scherschun L: Clinical and economic impact of Apligraf for the treatment of nonhealing venous leg ulcers, *Int J Derm* 42(12):960-965, 2003.

78. Omar AA, Mavor AI, Jones AM, et al: Treatment of venous leg ulcers with Dermagraft, *Eur J Vasc Endovasc Surg* 27(6):666-672, 2004.

79. Falanga V, Margolis D, Alvarez O, et al: Rapid healing of venous leg ulcers and lack of clinical rejection with an allogeneic cultured human skin equivalent, *Arch Dermatol* 134:293-300, 1998.

80. Flemming K, Cullum N: Therapeutic ultrasound for pressure sores, *Cochrane Database Syst Rev* 4:CD001180, 2004.

81. Kaha M, Gloviczki P: Surgical treatment of venous ulcers: Role of subfascial endoscopic perforator vein ligation, *Surg Clin N Am* 83:671-705, 2003.

82. Russell T, Logsdon AL: Subfascial endoscopic perforator surgery: A surgical approach to halting venous ulceration, *J Wound Ostomy Continence Nurs* 29(1):33-36, 2002.

83. Anwar S, Shrivastava V, Welch M, et al: Subfascial endoscopic perforator surgery: A review, *Hosp Med* 64(8):479-483, 2003.

Chapter 30

Neuropathic Ulcers

Rose Little Hamm, Pamela Scarborough

CHAPTER OUTLINE

OBJECTIVES

After reading this chapter, the reader will be able to:
1. Understand the pathology of neuropathic ulcers.
2. Compare and contrast normal physiology with pathological changes related to type 2 diabetes.
3. Identify causative factors for neuropathic ulcers.
4. Discuss the role of diabetes in ulcer formation.
5. Recognize key components of the physical therapy examination and evaluation of a patient with a neuropathic ulcer.
6. Develop a plan of care for a patient with a neuropathic ulcer based on etiology, tissue involvement, and comorbidities.

*N*europathic ulcers (NUs) are wounds caused by mechanical stress and sensory loss and are generally associated with *diabetes mellitus* (DM), spina bifida, Hansen's disease, and in some cases, peripheral vascular disease (PVD) or other vascular pathologies. In addition, patients with central nervous system (CNS) disorders who have limited mobility and decreased sensation are at high risk for this type of wound. NUs are not only problems in and of themselves but also predispose people to lower extremity amputation and systemic infection.

Although NUs occur in patients with a range of diseases, reports of prevalence and incidence are primarily related to the population with diabetes. The American Diabetes Association (ADA) reports that 18.2 million people, 6.3% of the total population of the United States (US), have diabetes; 13 million of these are diagnosed and 5.2 million are undiagnosed.[1] The number of Americans diagnosed with diabetes is projected to increase by 65% over the next 50 years, from 11 million in 2000 (population prevalence of 4.0%) to 29 million in 2050 (population prevalence of 7.2%).[2] The largest percentage increase in diagnosed diabetes will be among those aged 75 years or older (Fig. 30-1).[2] Among certain ethnic groups, the prevalence of diabetes among people aged 20 or older can be as high as 14.5% (Table 30-1). Fifteen percent of people with diabetes will experience a NU during their lifetime, and 14-24% of all people with foot ulcers will require a lower extremity amputation.[3] A study of 9,710 patients with diabetes in the community setting included a baseline assessment and a 2-year follow-up to determine development of foot ulcers; 291 of the patients developed new foot wounds, equivalent to a 2.2% average annual incidence.[4] Furthermore, a study of 821 patients with diabetes in Greece found that 4.75% had NUs.[5]

NUs are one of the major risk factors for lower extremity amputation in patients with diabetes.[6] In 2001 and 2002, more than 82,000 amputations per year were performed on patients with diabetes, and diabetes was the cause of more than 60% of the nontraumatic amputations in the US over this period[1] (see Chapter 12). Lavery et al studied 225 age-matched patients with diabetes (76 case patients and 149 control subjects) the factors most associated with foot ulceration are described in Box 30-1.[7] Because the majority of NUs occur in patients with type 1 or type 2 diabetes, identifying and managing factors that contribute to plantar ulceration in patients with diabetes are the focus of this chapter.

PATHOLOGY

NUs most often occur on the feet of patients with DM because the feet are generally the first areas affected

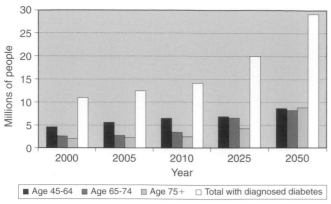

FIG. 30-1 Projections of the number of people with diagnosed diabetes by age group for selected years. *Data from American Diabetes Association:* National Diabetes Fact Sheet, *Alexandria, Va, 2005, The Association.*

TABLE 30-1	Prevalence of Diabetes by Race/Ethnicity Among People Aged 20 Years or Older in the United States in 2002

Race/Ethnicity	Number with Diabetes	Percent with Diabetes (%)
Non-Hispanic whites	12.5 million	8.4
Non-Hispanic blacks	2.7 million	11.4
Hispanic/Latino Americans	2 million	8.2
Native Americans/ Alaska natives	107,775	14.5

BOX 30-1	Factors Associated with Foot Ulcers in Patients with Diabetes

- Elevated plantar pressures (>65 N/cm^2)
- History of amputation
- Presence of diabetes >10 years
- Foot deformities (hallux rigidus or hammer toes)
- Male gender
- Poor diabetes control (glycosylated hemoglobin >9%)
- One or more subjective symptoms of neuropathy
- Elevated vibration perception threshold (>25 V)

Data from Lavery LA, Armstrong DG, Vela SA, et al: *Arch Intern Med* 158:157-162, 1998.

by peripheral neuropathy and because the feet often sustain abnormal mechanical forces or minor trauma during standing and walking. NUs usually form on the plantar surface of the foot, over the first and fifth metatarsal heads, or on the distal digits (Fig. 30-2). Bony abnormalities, diminished or absent protective sensation, decreased tissue oxygen saturation, anhidrosis caused by autonomic neuropathy, and poorly fitting shoes may initially cause blisters, calluses, or minor traumatic wounds because of direct pressure, shear, or friction. The lack of

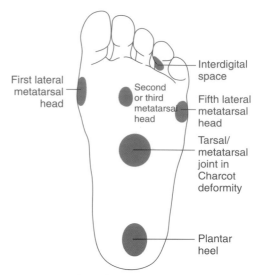

FIG. 30-2 Neuropathic ulcers usually form on the plantar surface of the foot, over the first and fifth metatarsal heads, or on the distal digits.

protective sensation then causes the patient to be unaware of the wound, and any skin break becomes a portal for bacteria to enter the subcutaneous tissue. Because the high-risk individual usually has compromised healing potential, complications from infection are common. Even a small neuropathic wound should be treated immediately to prevent increase in size, complications from infection, and the need for surgical intervention.

NEUROPATHY: SENSORY, MOTOR, AND AUTONOMIC

Diabetes and PVD are risk factors for either focal (e.g., entrapment syndromes) or diffuse somatic and autonomic neuropathies, referred to as distal symmetrical polyneuropathies (DSPN) (see Chapter 19). DSPN is a complex heterogenous syndrome that includes sensory, motor, and autonomic neuropathies, all of which may be directly involved in the formation of NUs. In addition, diminished blood flow, as a result of occluded vessels, further impairs healing and immune function.

Sensory Neuropathy. Sensory neuropathy, caused by damage to the small nerve fibers, prevents patients from feeling the pressure of a callus or foreign body, the pain of minor trauma and puncture wounds, or the friction of poorly fitting shoes. Prolonged walking and standing under such circumstances can cause subcutaneous tissue damage. Because of sensory deficits, discomfort is not perceived until the tissue damage is deep, usually as a result of infection. Damage to the small nerve fibers, associated with a deficiency of nerve growth factors and diminished blood flow to the vasa nervorum, also causes a reduction in nerve conduction velocity. Both of these conditions occur with diabetes and are exacerbated by uncontrolled *hyperglycemia.*[8]

Motor Neuropathy. Motor neuropathy, caused by damage to the large fibers, results in the following sequence of events: Intrinsic muscles of the foot atrophy and weaken; force imbalances in the foot and lower extremity cause the tendons to pull in deviated alignment; and over time, structural deformities develop. Even during normal gait, these deformities produce abnormally high peak pressures over the bony prominences of the foot, increasing the risk for blisters and callus formation. The damaged cutaneous and subcutaneous tissue is the NU.

Autonomic Neuropathy. *Autonomic neuropathy,* caused by damage to the large nerve fibers and the sympathetic ganglia, decreases the production of sweat and oil in the skin, causing it to become dry and inelastic. Plantar fissures occur because of anhidrosis (lack of perspiration from the skin) in poorly vascularized areas of the foot, especially the heel. Fissures can deepen to result in full-thickness skin loss where bacteria can enter and cause infection. The risk of ulceration and infection is increased in the presence of PVD because of reduced delivery of oxygen and nutrients, which are both needed for wound healing.

PATHOLOGY OF DIABETES MELLITUS

DM is a group of metabolic diseases characterized by hyperglycemia (elevated blood glucose) resulting from defects in *insulin* secretion and/or action. Chronic hyperglycemia is associated with long-term damage, dysfunction, and failure of various organs, especially the eyes, kidneys, nerves, heart, and blood vessels.[9] The classic signs of acute hyperglycemia are increased urination, increased thirst, and unexplained weight loss. Prolonged hyperglycemia can also cause blurred vision, fatigue, musculoskeletal changes, balance and gait impairments, and gastrointestinal abnormalities. In many instances, patients are diagnosed with diabetes only when the long-term effects of poor glucose control result in a crisis or in chronic complications.

Two of the most common complications of hyperglycemia are impaired wound healing and suppressed immune responses. Hyperglycemia impedes wound healing by inhibiting phagocytic activity of leukocytes and macrophages and by slowing the migration of fibroblasts to the wound site, thereby impairing angiogenesis and limiting the delivery of nutrients to the area. Hyperglycemia also impairs the immune response by altering chemotaxis, phagocytosis, and superoxide anion production by neutrophils and macrophages.[10] In addition, *advanced glycation end-products* (AGEs), produced as a result of hyperglycemia, are detrimental to cell structure and formation.[11] A study on nondiabetic and diabetic animals supported the concept that hyperglycemia may impede wound healing by suppressing the activity of insulin-like growth factors (IGF) in the wound microenvironment.[12] Hyperglycemia has also been shown to inhibit the effects of IGF-1 on glucose uptake and keratinocyte proliferation.[13] Another study on nondiabetic rats showed that high glucose levels had a direct inhibitory effect on angiogenesis and granulation tissue formation.[14] In another animal study using bovine aorta, Duraisamy et al found that glycation of fibroblast growth factor (FGF-2) caused a significant reduction in the ability of FGF-2 to bind to cell receptors and activate signal transduction pathways necessary for mitogenesis and capillary formation in the aorta endothelial cells. The authors postulated that this mechanism may play a part in impairing wound healing in patients with diabetes.[15]

Blood glucose levels are regulated by a balance between insulin and *glucagon* secretion and the amount and kinds of foods consumed, as well as the amount of daily activity performed by the individual. Insulin is a small protein hormone produced in the *beta cells* located in the *islets of Langerhans* of the *pancreas*.[16] Beta cells secrete insulin in response to rising levels of circulating blood glucose. Insulin binds to the insulin receptor in the plasma membrane of the responding cells (muscle, fat, and liver), causing tiny channels to open up and allow glucose into the cell. Insulin also activates transport of glucose to the cell nucleus and stimulates cells in the liver and skeletal muscle to convert glucose into *glycogen* for storage and stimulates fat cells to store fat.[17] All of these effects of insulin result in lower blood glucose levels.

Glucagon is produced by pancreatic *alpha cells* of the islets of Langerhans. It is a counter-regulatory hormone to insulin that increases circulating glucose levels. Glucagon stimulates the liver to release glucose (stored in the form of glycogen) and to produce glucose from precursors such as lactate and amino acids (known as gluconeogenesis).[18]

Type 1 Diabetes. *Type 1 diabetes,* previously termed juvenile or insulin-dependent diabetes, which has both genetic and environmental risk factors, is caused by progressive autoimmune destruction of the insulin secreting beta cells in the pancreas. Once 80% to 90% of the beta cells are destroyed, hyperglycemia results and the patient can be diagnosed with diabetes.[19] The onset of type 1 diabetes is usually during puberty but can be as early as 9 months or as late as the fifth decade. Type 1 diabetes accounts for approximately 10% of all patients with diabetes.

Type 2 Diabetes. *Type 2 diabetes,* the most common form of diabetes in older adults, is generally caused by a combination of insulin resistance and beta-cell failure (Fig. 30-3).[13] *Insulin resistance,* a decreased responsiveness of the cells to insulin, may begin years or even decades before the patient becomes hyperglycemic. Over time the beta cells also progressively produce less insulin. Diabetes results when the body cannot compensate for combined defects in insulin action and secretion, resulting in elevated blood glucose levels (Fig. 30-4 and Table 30-2). The excess circulating glucose causes tissue and organ damage and thereby induces the long-term complications commonly seen in clinical practice, including NUs.

EXAMINATION

PATIENT HISTORY

The examination of a patient with a NU begins with a complete patient history. Chapter 28 includes elements to focus on in the patient with any type of chronic wound. Special attention is directed to recent minor trauma to the affected area, footwear, foot hygiene, co-morbidities, medications, and diet. Any reported incidents may give the examiner clues as to the original etiology of the ulcer.

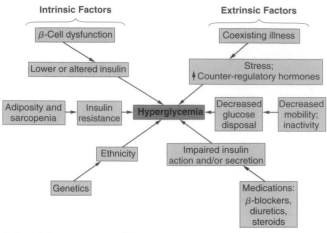

FIG. 30-3 Intrinsic and extrinsic factors contributing to hyperglycemia.

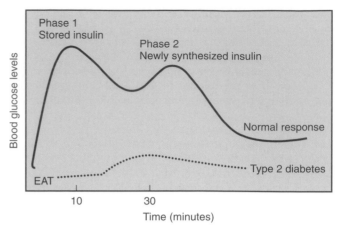

FIG. 30-4 Insulin release phases: normal and with type 2 diabetes.

TABLE 30-2	Type 2 Diabetes Diagnostic Criteria for Adults		
	Tests		
Stage	**FPG***	**Casual Plasma Glucose†**	**OGTT‡**
Normal	<100 mg/dl		2-h PG <140 mg/dl
Pre-diabetes (IGT)	≥100 and <126 mg/dl		2-h PG ≥140 and <200 mg/dl
Diabetes	≥126 mg/dl	≥200 mg/dl (plus symptoms)	2-h PG ≥200 mg/dl

FPG, Fasting plasma glucose; *OGTT,* oral glucose tolerance test; *2-h PG,* 2-hour postload glucose; *IGT,* impaired glucose tolerance.
*FPG is preferred, and one of the 3 tests must be repeated on a different day for diagnosis.
†Casual is testing any time of day without regard to time since last meal; symptoms are the classic ones of polyuria, polydipsia and unexplained weight loss.
‡Fasting is defined as no caloric intake for 8 hours.

SYSTEMS REVIEW

The systems review is used to target areas requiring further examination and to define areas that may cause complications or indicate a need for precautions during the examination and intervention processes. See Chapter 1 for details of the systems review.

Diabetes can adversely affect every system in the body and crosses all four practice pattern categories in physical therapy. The data generated from the history and systems review aid the physical therapist (PT) in determining which tests and measures are appropriate for an individual patient and specifically for the patient with a NU. The systems review also assists the PT in identifying possible problems that require consultation with, or referral to, another provider.[20]

TESTS AND MEASURES

Tests and measures should start with inspection of both feet, including the skin, nails, heels, areas between the toes, shoe fit, and inspection for foot deformities (Table 30-3).

Musculoskeletal. When assessing the patient with diabetes, it is sometimes difficult to differentiate abnormal findings caused by diabetes, aging, and other co-morbidities. Diabetes exaggerates the normal aging process and adds to the impairments and functional limitations associated with the aging musculoskeletal system. Specifically,

TABLE 30-3	Inspection of the Neuropathic Foot
Inspection	**Things to Look for**
Skin inspection	Dry skin with or without fissures
	Thick calluses and blisters
	Discoloration in the dermal layer
	Loss of toe and dorsal hair
Nail inspection	In-grown or poorly-cut toe nails
	Fungus growing beneath the nails
	Thick, cracking, malformed nails
Heel inspection	Dry skin with fissures
	Thick calluses and blisters
	Discoloration of the dermal layer
Between toes inspection	Skin maceration
Foot deformities	Pes equinus
	Hallux limitus, hallux rigidus, hallux valgus
	Hammer toes
	Cock-up deformity
	Varus deformity of the toes
	Tailor's bunion
	Charcot foot
Assessment of shoes	Fit
	Style
	Material
	Inserts
	Wear

AGEs affect joint mobility and range of motion (ROM), especially in the foot. AGEs act as "molecular glue" as a result of a chemical reaction that causes irreversible cross-linking between glucose and proteins.[17] When AGEs accumulate, they can cause tissues to become rigid and less functional. It is common for patients with diabetes to have decreased soft tissue extensibility and joint capsule mobility that cause decreased ROM and interfere with functional activities.

Patients with diabetes also frequently have multiple changes in the form and function of the foot and lower extremity. Sensory and motor neuropathies weaken the intrinsic foot muscles, causing muscle imbalances that may then result in one or more of the following deformities: Pes equinus, hallux limitus, hallux rigidus, hallux valgus, hammer toes, cock-up deformity, varus deformity of the toes, tailor's bunion, or Charcot foot (Table 30-4 and Fig. 30-5). Changes in foot muscle length and tension also

contribute to thinning or shifting of the fat pad from under the metatarsal heads leaving them unprotected.[21]

Changes in foot structure involving the joints associated with peripheral neuropathy are referred to as neuropathic arthropathy or neuroarthropathy. The most extreme example of neuroarthropathy is the Charcot foot, which is characterized by a collapsed arch with a rocker-bottom shape and shortened foot length. These changes increase peak pressures on the plantar surface of the foot during gait, particularly at the apex of the rocker bottom, which is the most common site of ulceration. Prolonged weight bearing on the insensitive Charcot foot may also result in minor trauma that can cause hyperemia, edema, joint effusion, and increased tissue warmth, which in turn can cause bone resorption and fracture, a condition referred to as an acute Charcot foot.

ROM of the foot and ankle should be measured in patients with NUs because limited joint mobility in these areas can lead to increased plantar pressures and may be a risk factor for foot ulceration.[22,23] One study of 103 patients with type 2 diabetes found that of these 33 had high mean peak pressures (>500 N/m^2), while the other 70 had lower mean peak pressures. There was a strong association between high peak pressures and the presence of sensory, motor, and autonomic neuropathies.[24]

Neuromuscular. Sensory and reflex impairments, as well as functional limitations in balance and gait, are commonly observed in patients at risk for or with NUs. Neuropathy may result in impaired joint proprioception, diminished skin sensation, paresthesias (e.g., burning, tingling), and gait and balance disturbances. Simoneau and associates found that postural instability, measured by a force plate, was associated with neuropathy but not with diabetes alone.[25] This study involved 3 groups of 17 matched subjects: One group with diabetes and significant sensory neuropathy, another group with diabetes without neuropathy, and a third group without either diabetes or sensory neuropathy. Subjects in the first group swayed as much with their eyes open and head forward as did the second group in the more challenging eyes closed, head-back condition.

TABLE 30-4	Foot Deformities Commonly Associated with Diabetes
Condition	**Characteristics**
Pes equinus	A shortening of the Achilles tendon so that there is no ankle dorsiflexion past the neutral ankle position.
Hallux limitus	Limited range of motion of the great toe MTP joint, less than the normal ROM measurement of 0-50° dorsiflexion.
Hallux rigidus	Complete loss of range of motion in the great toe MTP joint; the IP joint of the hallux may be involved as well.
Hallux valgus	Lateral deviation of the hallux in relation to the first metatarsal shaft and head that may result in exostosis, defined as a bony prominence, over the medial metatarsal head.
Hammer toes	Extension of the MTP joint of the digit combined with flexion of the PIP joint, usually resulting in corn formation over the bony prominence of the PIP joint.
Cock-up deformity	Flexion of the great toe IP joint combined with extension of the MTP joint, this may result in ulceration of the callus on the dorsum of the IP joint.
Varus deformities of the toes	Medial drifting of the third, fourth, and fifth toes that may cause nails to impinge on adjacent toes, thus producing small interdigital ulcers.
Tailor's bunion	Exostosis of the lateral fifth metatarsal heal often caused by fifth toe varus deformity.
Charcot foot	Collapse of the foot arch resulting in a rocker sole, frequently resulting in midsole ulceration.

MTP, Metatarsophalangeal; *ROM,* range of motion; *IP,* interphalangeal; *PIP,* proximal interphalangeal.

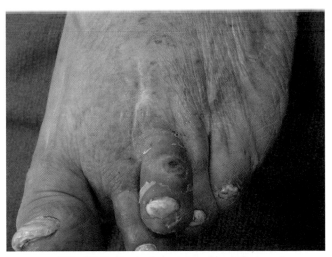

FIG. 30-5 Foot of person with diabetes.

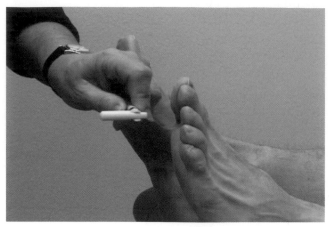

FIG. 30-6 Testing for pressure sensation with the nylon monofilaments.

TABLE 30-5	Values for the Nylon Monofilaments Used for Testing Sensation in the Neuropathic Foot
Filament Label (gm)	**Sensation**
2.83 (0.008)	The lightest pressure available
3.61 (0.4)	Normal light touch perception
3.84 (0.6)	Diminished light touch perception
4.17 (1.4)	Diminished sensation
4.31 (2.0)	Diminished protective sensation
4.56 (4.0)	Loss of protective sensation on the hand
5.07 (10)	Loss of protective sensation on the foot
6.10 (100)	Total loss of sensation

Observational gait analysis can be used to examine gait in patients with NUs (see Chapter 32). Gait changes commonly observed in patients with or at risk for NU include a wide base of support, a "marching" gait, a "slap-foot" stepping pattern, and balance disturbances during transfers and gait. Sometimes sensory "ataxia" is observed in patients with advanced neuropathy. One study compared the gait patterns of 21 healthy volunteers with gait in 61 subjects with diabetes (27 without neuropathy, 19 with neuropathy without current or prior NU, and 15 with prior NU). The evaluators determined that patients with neuropathy had significantly longer loading times in the gait cycle, and the center of pressure (COP) excursion along the mediolateral axis of the foot was decreased in all subjects with diabetes, whereas the COP excursion along the longitudinal axis was decreased in the group with previous ulceration. The combination of decreased mediolateral and longitudinal COP excursions and increased loading times suggest a predictable change in the gait patterns of patients with diabetic neuropathy.[26] Abnormal gait patterns, in addition to poorly fitting shoes, can contribute to the formation of NUs and delay the healing of existing ulcers.

Reflex Integrity. Diminished reflexes occur in patients with diabetic neuropathy because of large motor nerve involvement. These occur in a predictable pattern with the lower extremity reflexes being more involved than the upper extremity reflexes, distal reflexes more involved than proximal reflexes, and the responses being equal bilaterally. If the pattern is different from this, the deficits are probably not a result of diabetes and referral to a neurologist is recommended.[27]

Sensory Integrity. Sensation can be tested using nylon *monofilaments* (Semmes Weinstein Monofilaments [SWM]) for pressure (Fig. 30-6 and Table 30-5) and a tuning fork for vibration (Fig. 30-7). Both are useful for assessing protective sensation on the feet. The nylon monofilaments are a collection of graded filaments that apply a quantified amount of pressure to the skin. The test for protective sensation on the plantar surface of the foot uses the 5.07 filament that bends on 10 gm of pressure. This level of sensation is termed "protective sensation." The inability to

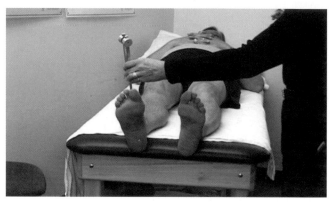

FIG. 30-7 Testing for vibratory sensation with a 128 Hz tuning fork.

feel this monofilament on the plantar aspect of the foot has been shown to predict foot ulceration in persons with type 2 diabetes.[28] However, the ability to perceive the 5.07 monofilament does not indicate normal sensation on the foot. The mean sensitivity of the foot when assessed with monofilaments on 40 healthy college-aged volunteers was found to be the 3.61 monofilament (0.4 gm pressure). Sensitivity was greatest in the lesser toes and the arch, followed by the hallux and the plantar metatarsal heads. The heel was the least sensitive at $\frac{1}{6}$ that of the toes. Based on this study, loss of protective sensation as determined by inability to feel the 5.07 monofilament represents a sensory threshold more than 50 times greater than normal, suggesting that about 98% of the sensory ability has been lost.[29]

Testing with multiple filaments at sequential examinations allows one to monitor progression of sensory loss and to determine the optimum footwear for the patient. Sensation is tested at ten sites on each foot: First, third, and fifth plantar toes; first, third, and fifth metatarsal heads; medial and lateral border of the midfoot; the heel; and the dorsum of the midfoot. The loss of protective sensation was correlated to development of NUs in a study of 358 patients with diabetes in which 20% of the subjects had loss of protective sensation by monofilament testing and these 20% accounted for 80% of the foot ulcers and 100% of the amputations that occurred during the ensuing 32 months of the study.[30]

Graded tuning forks or the 128 Hz tuning fork can be used to test vibratory sense and identify diabetic peripheral neuropathy.[31,32] The tuning fork is hit against a surface to make it vibrate and is then applied to the end of the great toe, the medial malleolus, or the tibial tuberosity. The tip of the fork handle is applied with firm pressure perpendicular to the body part being tested, and the patient answers "Yes" or "No" in response to "Do you feel the vibration?" (see Fig. 30-7). Nonvibratory stimuli should also be included to ensure that the patient is responding to vibration and not just to touch.[33] This tuning fork test only provides information about the presence or absence of vibratory sensation. This test may be quantified to some degree by timing how long the patient can continue to feel the vibration, which should be 15 seconds in the normal healthy adult. A study of 405 patients with diabetes correlated the development of NUs with abnormalities in ankle jerks, toe vibration perception thresholds, and responses to light touch with cotton. Ten-year follow-up of patients who developed lower extremity complications found that the quantitative vibratory measures were better predictors of future foot complications than the other semiquantitative tests.[34]

Both the monofilament test and the vibratory test have been correlated to the presence of diabetic neuropathy and increased risk of ulceration. In a prospective study, 248 patients with diabetes were first evaluated for neuropathy symptom score, neuropathy disability score (NDS) (see Table 30-10), vibration perception threshold (VPT), SWM perception, joint mobility, peak plantar pressures, and vascular status and then followed every 6 months for 30 months. It was found that the initial scores on these tests correlated with development of new foot ulcers. The sensitivity and positive predictive value of each risk factor were determined. Values for the most sensitive factors were: high VPT, 86%; high SWM, 91%; high NDS and VPT, 94%; high NDS and SWM, 99%, and high SWM and VPT, 98%. High NDS score and/or foot pressures combined had the best positive predictive value for ulceration (38%). The authors concluded that clinical examination (used to determine the NDS) and SWM are the most sensitive tests in identifying patients at risk for neuropathic ulcer formation.[35]

A meta analysis of evidence regarding the SWM and VPT testing in predicting NUs and amputation for patients with diabetes resulted in review of six prospective studies with the monofilaments and four with the VPT testing. The increased risk of ulceration ranged from an odds ratio of 2.2 to 2.9, and the relative risk of amputation was 2.9 when using the SWM as a predictor. The odds ratio for amputation when testing with the VPT was 4.38 to 7.99. The reviewers concluded that the SWMs are the best tool for screening for clinically significant neuropathy.[36]

Temperature. Measurement of plantar skin temperature is recommended to help locate infection, inflammation, or the fracture of an acute Charcot neuroarthropathy (Fig. 30-8). In a study of 1,588 patients with diabetes, those with Charcot neuroarthropathy had significantly higher mean plantar foot temperatures (84.8° ± 4.6°F versus 82.5° ± 4.7°F); however, there was not a significant temperature elevation in patients who developed ulcers or

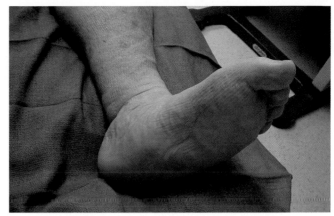

FIG. 30-8 Foot with Charcot neuroarthropathy.

infections or who had amputations.[37] There were no differences in plantar skin temperature based on neuropathy, foot laterality, foot-risk category, the presence of foot deformity, or elevated plantar foot pressures. Vascular disease was also not associated with lower skin temperatures. Baseline measurement of nonfocal mean skin temperatures are not an effective means of screening patients for future foot complications; however, using the contralateral side as a control for an individual patient may be helpful for identifying problems.[37] Thermography, in conjunction with radiography and quantitative bone scanning, may also be used to monitor the progress of Charcot neuroarthropathy.[38]

Temperature discrepancies may initially be detected qualitatively by palpation. Quantitative measures can be made with thermistors, thermocouples, or infrared scanners. Temperature should be measured at ten areas on the plantar surface of the foot. An increase of 3°F above the surrounding area or a comparable area on the opposite foot indicates a problem.[39,40] If, in addition to the skin temperature discrepancy with the surrounding tissue or the opposite foot, the examiner can probe a wound to the bone, there is a high probability of osteomyelitis.[41]

Cardiovascular

Circulation. Ulcers caused primarily by vascular disease are discussed in detail in Chapter 29. Tests of peripheral vascular circulation are discussed briefly here because PVD is 4-6 times more common in people with diabetes than in the general population.[42] PVD may cause claudication (calf pain caused by inadequate oxygen supply to muscle tissue) at rest or with activity. Intermittent activity-related claudication is a sign of mild PVD, whereas claudication at rest suggests the presence of severe PVD. During the examination, the PT should include questions about claudication, such as "Do your calves hurt during walking, when you are at rest, or during the night?" An affirmative answer to these inquiries indicates the possibility of arterial insufficiency and the need for referral for further vascular studies.

Pedal pulses are usually the first screening test for poor peripheral circulation. The dorsalis pedis and posterior tibialis pulses in the foot and ankle are palpated and graded according to the system for grading pulses in Box 30-2. If

---

BOX 30-2   System for Grading Pulses

0   Absent
1+ Faint
2+ Diminished
3+ Normal
4+ Bounding, abnormally strong

---

these are weak or absent, proximal pulses are palpated. Absence of a pulse indicates a more proximal complete or partial arterial occlusion. Faint or absent pulses are confirmed with a Doppler test; however, absent pulses audible with a Doppler are not graded but termed "positive Doppler signal."

Although pulse palpation does correlate with more objective measures of peripheral circulation, the ability to palpate a pulse has only a 40% sensitivity for detecting arterial disease defined as ankle-brachial index (ABI) ≤0.9. Therefore the clinician is advised to evaluate arterial circulation by measurement of the ABI at the first visit.[43] The ADA also recommends checking the ABI in all patients with diabetes since PVD can be asymptomatic.[44] The ABI, a ratio of the ankle systolic blood pressure to the brachial systolic blood pressure, indicates the relative blood flow to the lower extremity and the amount of peripheral arterial disease present.

In patients with diabetes the ABI may be falsely elevated with a reading of >1.3 because of calcification of the inner arterial walls. Since the digital arteries of the toes are generally not affected by calcification, great toe pressure should be checked to verify any ABI measured as >1.3.[45]

A number of other tests may also be used to evaluate peripheral circulation. These are described briefly here as they relate to the patient with a NU and in greater detail in Chapter 29.

Capillary Refill Test. During the capillary refill test the clinician observes the time required for the nail bed or toe tip to refill with blood after a blanching procedure. The clinician presses on the nail to blanch the blood out of the nail bed, removes the pressure, and notes the time it takes for the nail bed color to return to normal. The normal refill time is less than 3 seconds. Longer capillary refill may indicate microvascular insufficiency, which is common in patients with diabetes.

Venous Filling Time. To test the venous filling time, the patient is supine and the extremity passively elevated 45-60 degrees above horizontal to drain the venous blood from the limb. After 1 minute the patient is returned to sitting and the leg brought to a dependent position. The time in seconds required for the veins on the dorsal foot to fill is noted. Normal venous filling is less than 15 seconds. A 15-40 second filling time indicates moderate arterial insufficiency; greater than 40 seconds indicates severe PVD.

Rubor of Dependency Test. To perform the rubor of dependency test, the patient is positioned supine and the extremity passively elevated 45-60 degrees. After 30 seconds of elevation the foot may blanche, especially in patients with diabetes. After 60 seconds of elevation, the

foot is placed in a dependent position. Normal reperfusion is indicated by the return of pink color to the plantar surface in 15 seconds. If the color return is dark red (termed rubor) and takes 30 seconds or longer, the test is positive for arterial insufficiency.[46]

Great Toe Pressure. Great toe blood pressure is measured with a special mini-cuff designed especially to fit the great toe. The absolute toe pressure, usually 60% to 90% of the brachial systolic pressure, can be used to predict healing potential of both diabetic and nondiabetic patients (Table 30-6). The normal toe-brachial index, also considered a reliable indicator of lower extremity vascular status, is 0.8-0.99.[47] If a patient is suspected of having PVD based on the above screening tests, referral to a vascular surgeon for further testing and possible revascularization surgery is indicted.

Transcutaneous Oxygen Tension. Transcutaneous oxygen tension ($TcPO_2$), a measurement of the oxygen delivery to the cutaneous capillaries, is helpful in determining the extent of microvascular disease and wound healing potential. The $TcPO_2$ probe has an oxygen sensor composed of two parts, an inner platinum cathode and an outer silver-chloride anode. A heating element in the sensor warms the underlying tissue to 43°-45° C and dilates the cutaneous vascular bed for maximum oxygenation.

Systemic Blood Pressure. The ADA guideline for systemic arterial blood pressure in the patient with diabetes is less than 130/80 mm Hg, which is lower than that for the general population. If exercise is expected to be a part of the patient's interventions, screening for orthostatic hypotension is also recommended. The clinician can test for orthostatic hypotension by having the patient lie quietly in the supine position for approximately 5 minutes to allow the blood pressure to equalize. Blood pressure should be taken in both arms to identify the arm with the higher systolic pressure. The patient then stands and the blood pressure is taken in the arm with the higher pressure. Orthostatic hypotension is defined by a drop of more than 20 mm Hg in the systolic pressure or more than 10 mm Hg in the diastolic pressure.

Integumentary

Integumentary Integrity. Skin observation is an integral component of the examination of the patient with a

---

TABLE 30-6   Probability of Wound Healing Based on Toe Pressures

Absolute Toe Pressure (mm Hg)*		Probability of Healing (%)
With Diabetes	Without Diabetes	
<20	29	25
20-30	40	73
30-35	85	100
>55	97	100

From Carter SA: Role of pressure measurements. In Bernstein EF (ed): *Vascular Diagnosis*, ed 4, St. Louis, 1993, Mosby-Year Book.
*Absolute toe pressure <30 mm Hg indicates that a person with ischemic tissue loss will need surgical revascularization for healing to occur.

NU. Anhydrosis (lack of sweating), a common result of autonomic neuropathy, contributes to dry skin as a result of loss of sweat and oil production, two processes that normally help protect the skin. The effects of aging on the skin (e.g., thinning) make the older patient with diabetes more susceptible to complications from integumentary insults.

Problems with healing any type of wound are common in patients with NUs, especially if they have poorly controlled diabetes or diminished blood flow because of PVD. Therefore the therapist should observe traumatic wounds and incision sites for signs of complications with healing. The ADA recommends that patients with diabetes and neuropathy have a visual inspection of the feet at every visit with a health care professional. Areas of special concern include: Between the toes where maceration is common, under the metatarsal heads where callus formation is common, any areas of erythema or warmth, and cracks or fissures in the plantar heel. It is also suggested that both feet be examined during evaluation of any foot ulcer as the patient may have undetected ulcers on the other foot.

Finally, a thorough wound assessment (including measurements, location, tissue type, and drainage) should be performed and infection confirmed or ruled out (see Chapter 28). The International Diabetic Foot Working Group and the Infectious Diseases Society of America Diabetic Foot Guidelines Group have agreed on the following definition of a foot infection: "the presence of either purulent secretions or two or more signs or symptoms of inflammation suggest that a wound is infected."[47] If there are clinical signs of infection, cultures are done to determine which organisms are present and the most effective antibiotics. If an ulcer can be probed to bone, there is a high probability of osteomyelitis (Fig. 30-9). Definitive diagnosis may be made by x-ray, bone scan, bone biopsy, or magnetic resonance imaging (MRI).[48] (MRI is the most sensitive but not completely specific.)

EVALUATION, DIAGNOSIS, AND PROGNOSIS

The *Guide to Physical Therapist Practice* classification system for integumentary disorders based on patient risk and depth of tissue involvement can be used to diagnose NUs.[20] In addition, several other systems for classifying neuropathic ulcer are discussed in the literature. The Wagner and the University of Texas scales are the most frequently used to diagnose and predict outcome of NUs in patients with diabetes. The Wagner scale, developed at Rancho Los Amigos in the 1970s, is the simplest and most frequently used diagnostic scale for NUs (Table 30-7). This scale has six classifications: The first four classifications are based on the extent of tissue loss in the foot; the last two are based on the degree of perfusion loss in the foot. Because depth of tissue loss and severity of ischemia present different problems in evaluating and treating NUs, the Wagner scale has been modified to allow separate evaluation of the wound and foot perfusion (Table 30-8).[49]

The University of Texas (UT) Foot Classification System, developed by Armstrong, Lavery, and Harkless, has six categories intended to determine patient risk for ulceration and amputation (Table 30-9). In addition, treatment guidelines to lower the risk level for patients in each category are included.[50,51]

The validity of the UT classification system in predicting clinical outcomes was studied with a total of 213 patients who were classified in one of the groups 0-4 and followed for 29 months. Patients in the higher risk groups had longer duration of diabetes, worse glycemic control, vascular and neuropathic variables, and more systemic complications of diabetes. The incidence of ulceration for each group was as follows: Group 0, 5.1%; group 1, 14.3%; group 2, 18.8%; and group 3, 55.8%. The authors of this study concluded that the UT classification system predicts ulceration and amputation and is an effective tool for identifying risks, planning interventions to lower risk, and for preventing lower extremity complications of diabetes.[52]

A study comparing the Wagner system with a variation of the UT system concluded that the risk of amputation increases significantly in the higher risk groups of both systems; however, the Wagner 3 classification was found to be a heterogeneous group that required more information to make a prediction and determine appropriate interventions. The authors concluded that the Wagner

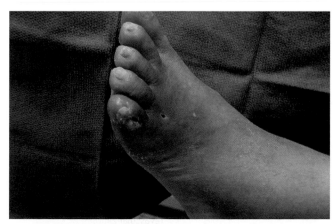

FIG. 30-9 Neuropathic ulcer with underlying osteomyelitis.

TABLE 30-7	Wagner Scale for Neuropathic Ulcers
Grade	**Characteristics**
0	Bony deformities, calluses, skin changes that are at risk for developing wounds, or postulceration that has healed.
1	Full-thickness skin loss with no infection, usually of neuropathic etiology.
2	Subcutaneous tissue involvement, infection, no bone involvement.
3	Deep ulceration, infection with cellulitis, osteomyelitis, or abscess formation.
4	Partial foot gangrene or necrosis.
5	Full foot gangrene.

TABLE 30-8	Depth-Ischemia Classification of Diabetic Foot Lesions*
Grade/Definition	**Intervention**
DEPTH CLASSIFICATION	
0: The "at-risk" foot: Previous ulcer or neuropathy with deformity that may cause new ulceration.	Patient education, regular examination, appropriate foot wear and insoles.
1: Superficial ulceration, not infected.	External pressure relief: TCC, walking brace, special foot wear, etc.
2: Deep ulceration exposing a tendon or joint (with or without superficial infection).	Surgical debridement, wound care, pressure relief if the lesion closes and converts to grade 1 (antibiotics as needed).
3: Extensive ulceration with exposed bone and/or deep infection (e.g., osteomyelitis or abscess).	Surgical debridement; ray or partial foot amputation, intravenous antibiotics, pressure relief if wound converts to grade 1.
ISCHEMIC CLASSIFICATION	
A: Not ischemic.	Observation.
B: Ischemia without gangrene.	Vascular evaluation (Doppler, TcPO$_2$, arteriogram, etc), vascular reconstruction as needed.
C: Partial (forefoot) gangrene of the foot.	Vascular evaluation, vascular reconstruction (proximal and/or distal bypass or angioplasty), partial foot amputation.
D: Complete foot gangrene.	Vascular evaluation, major extremity amputation (TTA, TFA) with possible proximal vascular reconstruction.

TCC, Total contact cast; *TTA,* transtibial amputation; *TFA,* total foot amputation.
*Modification of the original Wagner classification.

system is a "usable instrument in everyday clinical practice" but that the UT system provides more detailed information and may be preferable in multidisciplinary diabetic foot clinics and in multicenter research.[53] Another study by Oyibo et al, designed to compare the Wagner and UT systems, determined that the UT system was a better predictor of outcome than the Wagner system, based on a comparison of number of amputations and healing times of 194 patients with new foot ulcers.[54]

In a case comparison study to evaluate risk factors for ulceration among patients with diabetes, Lavery et al calculated the cumulative risk associated with neuropathy, foot deformity, and foot amputation history (the basis of the UT system). Patients with only peripheral neuropathy and no other risk factors were at 1.7 times greater risk for ulceration; patients with both neuropathy and foot deformity, 12.1 times greater; and patients with neuropathy, deformity, and a history of amputation, 36.4 times greater.[7]

Prognosis for healing may depend on the location of an ulcer and the presence of ischemia. Heel ulcers, which tend to have an ischemic component, will heal less than 50% of the time if ischemia is present, whereas heel ulcers without ischemia will heal 86% of the time. A healing probability of 74% has been reported for NUs on parts of the foot other than the heel when ischemia is present.[55] Mannari reports that while forefoot ulcers are likely to be of neuropathic origin, heel ulcers are likely to have both neuropathic and ischemic etiologies. This is because patients with diabetes and thus with neuropathy tend to have more atherosclerosis of the tibial and peroneal arteries than the dorsalis pedis and plantar arteries, putting the heel at greater risk for decreased perfusion.[56]

The North-West Diabetes Foot Care Study screened 9,710 patients with diabetes over two years to determine the incidence of, and clinically relevant risk factors for, new foot ulceration. Five different screening tools, the NDS (Table 30-10), the modified Neuropathy Symptom Score (NSS) (Table 30-11), vibration sensation using the 128 Hz tuning fork, dorsal temperature sensation, and Achilles reflex testing, were used to assess patients for peripheral neuropathy. Independent risk factors were correlated with new foot ulcer formation. The NDS was the best clinical measure for detecting patients at risk for new ulcers. In addition, the study found that insensitivity to the 10-gm monofilament force at any one of three plantar sites is sufficient to predict ulcer formation, and three or more foot deformities independently predict foot ulcer risk.[4]

The NDS involves testing both feet with a *Neurotip,* a tuning fork, hot and cold rods, and a tendon hammer, scoring one point for each incorrect answer and an extra point if the Achilles tendon reflexes are absent even with reinforcement. The maximum score for each foot is 5 points, and a score greater than 6 out of 10 suggests neuropathy.[57] The NSS uses 5 questions about pain, paresthesias, and claudication to assess the severity of symptoms associated with neuropathy.

INTERVENTION

Interventions for patients with or at risk for neuropathic foot ulcers can be divided into three stages: Prevention for the high-risk foot, treatment of the wound, and management of the foot after wound healing. During all stages, patients with diabetes should have good blood glucose control and all patients should have off-loading. Off-loading is the redistribution of foot pressures to eliminate areas of high peak pressure during weight-bearing activities.

PATIENT EDUCATION

One of the most important components for prevention of ulcers in patients with neuropathy affecting the foot is patient education. Education should cover blood glucose control, footwear, daily foot inspection, and good foot care.[58-60] One randomized controlled trial (RCT) evaluated the effectiveness of a multifaceted educational program involving 352 subjects with type 2 diabetes over a 12-month period. The program consisted of patient

TABLE 30-9	University of Texas Diabetic Foot Classification System	

Category*	Criteria	Treatment Guidelines
0: No pathology	Patient diagnosed with diabetes mellitus. Protective sensation intact. ABI >0.80 and toe systolic pressure >45 mm Hg. Foot deformity may be present. No history of ulceration.	2-3 visits per year to assess neurovascular status, dermal thermometry, and foci of stress. Possible shoe accommodations. Patient education.
1: Neuropathy, no deformity	Protective sensation absent. ABI >0.80 and toe systolic pressure >45 mm Hg. No history of ulceration. No history of diabetic neuropathic osteoarthropathy (Charcot joint). No foot deformity.	Same as Category 0 plus: Possible shoe gear accommodation (pedorthic/orthotist consultation). Quarterly visits to assess foot wear and monitor for signs of irritation.
2: Neuropathy with deformity	Protective sensation absent. ABI >0.80 and toe systolic pressure >45 mm Hg. No history of neuropathic ulceration. No history of Charcot joint. Foot deformity present (focus of stress).	Same as Category 1 plus: Pedorthic/orthotic consultation for possible custom-molded/extra-depth shoe accommodation. Possible prophylactic surgery to alleviate focus of stress (e.g., correction of hammertoe or bunion deformity).
3: History of pathology	Protective sensation absent. ABI >0.80 and toe systolic pressure >45 mm Hg. History of neuropathic ulceration. History of Charcot joint. Foot deformity present (focus of stress).	Same as Category 2 plus: Pedorthic/orthotist consultation for custom-molded/extra-depth shoe accommodation. Possible prophylactic surgery to alleviate focus of stress (e.g., correction of bunion or hammertoe). More frequent visits may be indicated for monitoring.
4A: Neuropathic ulceration	Patient diagnosed with diabetes mellitus. Sensorium may or may not be intact. ABI >0.80 and to systolic pressure of >45 mm Hg. Foot deformity normally present. No infected neuropathic ulceration. No acute diabetic neuropathic osteoarthropathy (Charcot joint) present.	Same as Category 3 plus: Off-weighting program instituted. Dressing change program instituted. Debridement program instituted. Dermal thermometric monitoring. Weekly to biweekly visits as needed. Possible prophylactic surgery.
4B: Acute Charcot joint	Patient diagnosed with diabetes mellitus. Sensorium absent. ABI >0.80 and toe systolic pressure of >45 mm Hg. Noninfected neuropathic ulceration may be present. Diabetic neuropathic osteoarthropathy (Charcot joint) present.	Same as Category 3 plus: Off-weighting program instituted; possible TCC. Weekly to biweekly visits (as per TCC regimen). Dermal thermometric and radiographic monitoring. If ulcer is present, treatment same as for category 4A.
5: Infected diabetic foot	Patient diagnosed with diabetes mellitus. Sensorium may or may not be intact. Infected wound. Charcot joint may be present.	Same as Category 4 plus: Debridement of infected necrotic tissue and bone. Possible hospitalization. Antibiotic therapy. Medical management. Contact casting generally contraindicated until diabetic category drops to 4.
6: Dysvascular foot	Patient diagnosed with diabetes mellitus. Sensorium may or may not be intact. ABI of <0.80 or toe systolic pressure of <45 mm Hg or pedal TcPO$_2$ of <40 mm Hg. Ulceration may be present.	Vascular consult, possible revascularization. If infection present, treatment same as for Category 5. Vascular consultation concomitant with control of sepsis. Contact casting generally contraindicated.

ABI, Ankle-brachial index; *TCC,* total contact cast.
*Categories 0-3 indicate risk factors for ulceration; Categories 4A-6, risk factors for amputation.

TABLE 30-10	Neuropathic Disability Score			

	Neuropathic Assessment	Right	Left	Score
Neurotip discrimination	Hallus-dorsal surface proximal to the toe nail			
Temperature discrimination	Hallus-dorsal surface proximal to the toe nail			
Reflexes	Achilles tendon			
128 Hz tuning fork	Pulp of hallux			

Score 1 point for each incorrect answer and an extra point if the Achilles tendon reflexes are absent even with reinforcement.

TABLE 30-11	Modified Neuropathy Symptom Score		
Question	**Response**		**Score**
Have you, in the past 6 months, had any pain or discomfort in your legs and feet when you are not walking?	Burning, numbness, tingling = 2 Fatigue, cramping, aching = 1 Other = 0		
Is this pain and discomfort most felt in the:	Feet = 2 Calves = 1 Thighs = 0		
Are these symptoms at their worst during the:	Night = 2 Various times of day/night = 1 Day = 0		
Have these symptoms ever kept you awake at night?	Yes = 1 No = 0		
When you get this pain or discomfort is there anything you can do to make it feel better?	Yes, walk = 2 No, or stand up = 1 All others = 0		

education on foot care, including a behavioral contract for desire to learn about self-foot care, education of health care providers on practice guidelines and informational flow sheets on foot-related risk factors for amputation, and prompters for providers to perform comprehensive foot examinations. The patients receiving the intervention were less likely to have serious foot lesions, more likely to report self-care, and more likely to receive foot care education from the providers. The physicians assigned to the intervention group were also more likely to provide patient education related to foot care. All results were statistically significant.[61]

Another study evaluated the effectiveness of a preventive foot care program in an outpatient setting for decreasing the incidence of NUs. It included 318 patients with diabetes and neuropathy. Patients were first evaluated for self-foot care, including footwear, walking, foot hygiene, callus care, nail cutting, water temperature checks, use of warming devices, foot care products, and self-inspection. Patients then attended four educational sessions about self-foot care and the lack of normal sensitivity and loss of pain perception in their feet. Patients were then placed in risk groups for ulceration according to their VPT and were further categorized as compliant (subgroup A, n = 223) or noncompliant (subgroup B, n = 95). The low-risk group developed 9 ulcers, 8 of which occurred in the noncompliant subgroup; the high-risk group developed 24 ulcers in 19 patients, 19 ulcers of which were in the noncompliant subgroup. The authors concluded that compliance with a preventive program helped reduce the incidence of NUs in patients with diabetic neuropathy.[62]

A systematic review of 8 RCTs evaluating educational programs for prevention of foot ulcers in people with diabetes concluded that although the trials were limited by poor methodological quality and conflicting results, patient education may have positive but short-lived effects on foot care knowledge and patient behavior. These posi-

tive effects may reduce foot ulceration and amputations, especially in high-risk patients.[63] This review also suggests, however, that patient education regarding care of the diabetic foot requires ongoing reinforcement and review.

BLOOD GLUCOSE CONTROL

Good blood glucose control in conjunction with lifestyle therapy (medical nutrition therapy, physical activity, and oral and insulin medication when needed) is also important for preventing complications of diabetes, including NUs. Patient education should be initiated immediately when a diagnosis of diabetes is established, although approximately 50% of patients will already have complications because of prolonged delay in diagnosis. Glycemic monitoring is used to assess the efficacy of interventions for diabetes and to adjust nutrition, exercise, and medication levels. The two techniques most frequently used are self-testing of capillary glucose levels by finger or forearm stick to obtain a measure of current blood sugar levels and laboratory or clinic testing of glycosylated hemoglobin (HbA1C) levels to indicate average blood glucose control over the preceding 2-3 months.

To optimize wound healing in patients with diabetes, blood glucose levels should be kept below 200 mg/dl. According to the ADA, the HbA1C goal to prevent complications from diabetes is 7%[64]; the American College of Endocrinologists recommends HbA1C levels below 6.5% to prevent complications.[65]

The importance of tight blood glucose control in preventing or slowing the development of diabetic neuropathy was confirmed by two landmark studies, the *Diabetes Control and Complications Trial* (DCCT) and the United Kingdom Prospective Diabetes Study (UKPDS). The DCCT was a multicenter clinical trial conducted from 1982 to 1998 to determine whether a program of intensive therapy to maintain blood glucose levels at near normal levels would affect the risk of onset and progression of diabetes complications, including retinopathy, *nephropathy,* and neuropathy. Components of the intensive therapy are listed in Box 30-3. Half of the 1,441 subjects, all with type 1 diabetes, were randomly assigned to intensive therapy and the other half to standard therapy. The intensive therapy reduced the risk of neuropathy and related complications by 60%, eye disease by 76%; and kidney disease by 50%. The researchers concluded that the increased cost of the intensive therapy was more than compensated

BOX 30-3	Components of the Intensive Therapy for Blood Glucose Control Used in the Diabetes Control and Complications Trial (DCCT)

- Testing blood glucose levels 4 or more times a day
- Four daily insulin injections or use of an insulin pump
- Adjustment of insulin doses according to food intake and exercise
- A diet and exercise plan
- Monthly visits to a health care team composed of a physician, nurse educator, dietitian, and behavioral therapist

for by the decrease in cost of medical care for the complications.[66]

The UKPDS followed 3,867 patients with type 2 diabetes for 10 years to determine if intensive blood glucose control (fasting plasma glucose of <108 mg/dl) versus conventional therapy (use of pharmacological therapy if blood sugars exceeded 270 mg/dl) could reduce the risk of renal, eye, and cardiovascular complications; however, they did not look at complications associated with neuropathy, including NUs. Median HbA1C values were 7.9% in the conventional group and 7% in the experimental group. Intensive therapy decreased diabetes-related endpoints, including retinopathy and cardiovascular complications, by 12%. An analysis of macrovascular end-points (including PVD) showed a risk reduction of 30% over the conventional therapy group.[67]

EXERCISE

Along with eating correctly, exercise or regular physical activity is a primary means of blood glucose control for people with type 2 diabetes. Findings from the Third National Health and Nutrition Examination Survey (NHANES III) indicate that most adults with type 2 diabetes did not engage in recommended levels of physical activity nor did they follow dietary guidelines.[68] Individuals with low income, over age 65, women, minority groups, or those using insulin were more likely to report engaging in no physical activity.

Exercise, even in the absence of body weight loss, helps patients with diabetes because it reduces blood glucose levels.[69] After a bout of exercise, insulin sensitivity increases so that cells are better able to take up glucose from the blood. Younger people can maintain this higher insulin sensitivity for 3-4 days after an aerobic exercise session. However, this postaerobic exercise response only lasts for 1 day in older adults.[70] Therefore, for older people seeking to prevent or control diabetes through exercise, sessions must not only be regular but frequent to take advantage of exercise's direct effect on blood glucose levels.

Exercise has been shown to prevent and reverse some microvascular muscle changes in people with diabetes.[71] One study on the effects of 9 months of endurance (cardiovascular) exercise training on decreasing glucose intolerance and skeletal muscle capillary basement membrane width found that thickening of the capillary basement membrane appears to be reversed as a result of this training, even in older individuals.[72] Progressive resistance training (PRT) is also an excellent adjunct to cardiovascular training and assists with increasing lean muscle mass, improves gait and balance, and decreases insulin resistance. Maintaining adequate microvascular circulation, reducing hyperglycemia, and avoiding gait abnormalities may reduce the risk of NU development and improve healing if a NU does occur.

Stretching exercises are recommended if the ankle ROM is limited and causing increased plantar pressures. If the patient cannot tolerate the discomfort of stretching or if ROM goals are not achieved, then the contracture deformity can be attenuated by selecting shoes with a higher heel, using heel inserts, or building up an incline on the sole of the shoe to accommodate the shortened Achilles tendon.

ORTHOSES

An ankle-foot orthosis (AFO) may be indicated for a patient with peripheral motor neuropathy sufficient to cause foot drop. ROM and structure of the foot and ankle are assessed for fitting. The typical off-the-shelf AFO is usually fixed with a 90-degree bend at the ankle, assuming that the patient can achieve a neutral ankle position. If the patient has musculoskeletal impairments or swelling that prohibit dorsiflexion of the ankle to neutral, the AFO may not fit well, and if the patient also has peripheral sensory neuropathy, insults to the foot and ankle caused by the AFO may not be perceived. The outcome of a poorly fitted AFO may be breakdown of the skin with resulting wounds (Fig. 30-10). AFOs with adjustable ankle hinges are available for the plantarflexed foot.

FOOTWEAR

Properly fitting shoes are less likely to cause blisters and calluses, thus decreasing the risk of ulceration.[73,74] The most difficult aspect of education on proper shoes may be getting the patient to accept that a good fit is more important than style or ease in putting on the shoe. Styles to avoid are platforms, high heels, pointed toes, flip-flops, stiff leather, plastic, or thin soles with no cushioning. These styles are more likely to produce mechanical friction or pressure over the bony prominences or weight-bearing surfaces of the foot. Purchasing shoes in the late afternoon when the feet are largest because of normal swelling is also advisable. Toe deformities, such as hammer or claw toes, may require extra-depth or custom-molded shoes with padded insoles to provide cushion and to improve plantar pressure distribution. See Box 30-4 for important guidelines to use in assessing shoe fit. New shoes should be gradually broken in to avoid getting blisters, using the schedule in Box 30-5.

FOOT CARE

Patients with diabetes need to be instructed in daily foot inspection. Signs of potential problems the patient should look for include red areas over bony prominences, blisters,

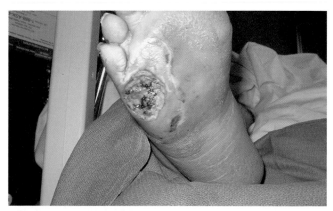

FIG. 30-10 Neuropathic ulcer on a diabetic foot as a result of a poorly fitting ankle-foot orthosis.

skin maceration between the toes, callus buildup, dry skin, cracks, subcutaneous hematomas, swelling, increased temperature, and minor cuts. The patient should be able to verbalize what he is looking for and should be able to see the plantar surface of the foot. The ability to see the plantar surface can be checked by placing a piece of tape on the bottom, writing a letter on it, and asking the patient to read the letter.[75] If the foot cannot be positioned for visualization of the plantar surface, a goose-necked mirror can be used or a mirror can be placed on the floor. If the patient is visually impaired or cannot achieve a position to see the plantar foot, a family member or caregiver needs to be instructed in how to perform the foot inspec-

tion or the patient can be instructed in tactile foot examination, feeling for calluses, maceration, or open wounds. The patient also needs to understand the importance of eliminating any source of irritation once problems arise and of seeking early medical intervention.

Proper foot care is an essential aspect of minimizing the risk of ulceration (Box 30-6). The ADA and many vendors have produced materials that can be used for patient education. Prevention is only as good as patient compliance. Good foot care should be reviewed at every foot screening and reinforced with every resource available to the health care provider. The ADA web site (www.diabetes.org) has a wealth of information for both patients and health care providers. Consultations with certified diabetic educators are recommended for patients who are newly diagnosed with diabetes or who have difficulty maintaining acceptable blood glucose levels.

TREATMENT OF THE NEUROPATHIC WOUND

The six steps of treatment of the neuropathic ulcer are (1) treat infection, (2) revascularize if needed, (3) control

BOX 30-4 Guidelines for Assessment of Proper Shoe Fit

• The shape of the shoe must conform to the shape of the foot and should be evaluated in the standing position. To demonstrate shoe fit, have the patient stand barefoot on a piece of white paper and trace the foot. When the shoe is placed on top of the drawing, the patient can see where the vulnerable spots are and how well the shoe fits. The patient can use this tracing to test for fit when shoe shopping (see Fig. 30-3).
• There should be a $3/8$-$1/2$ inch space between the end of the longest toe and the end of the shoe when the patient is standing.
• The widest part of the shoe should be at the first metatarsophalangeal joint.
• The toe box (front of the shoe that fits over the toes) should be deep enough to avoid rubbing on the joints of hammer or claw toes and wide enough to accommodate the spread of the foot in the standing and gait positions.
• The collar or back of the shoe should fit snug enough that it does not slide up and down on the heel.
• The insole should provide enough cushion that plantar abnormalities are not red or painful with the patient's maximum walking capacity.
• Laces or straps should be adjustable for a snug fit over the instep without causing friction across the top.
• There should be no areas of stitching over the forefoot of the shoe.
• The shoes should be large enough to accommodate a thick white cotton sock.

BOX 30-5 Wearing Schedule for Breaking in New Shoes

• 1 hour in the morning and 1 hour in the afternoon for the first 3 days.
• 2 hours in the morning and 2 hours in the afternoon for the next 3 days.
• 3 hours in the morning and 3 hours in the afternoon for the next 3 days.
• When a total of 8 hours is reached, the patient can feel safe wearing the shoes for a full day.
• If there is any redness that does not disappear within 15 minutes after removal of the shoes, the shoes should not be worn again until adjustments are made to alleviate the pressure.

BOX 30-6 Guidelines for Care of the Diabetic Foot

• Avoid soaking feet in water because of the risk of burns, maceration, and fungal infections. Test water with hand or thermometer before getting into bath water.
• Never walk barefoot. This includes getting up at night to go to the bathroom and is critical if the patient has loss of protective sensation.
• Keep feet away from hot surfaces (stoves, burners, heaters, etc.), chemicals, or extreme cold. Wear socks to keep feet warm; do not use heating pads or hot water bottles.
• Wash feet with non-drying soap and dry thoroughly, especially between the toes, with a clean towel.
• Lubricate skin with petroleum jelly or a non-perfumed cream at least once a day. Suggested brands include Eucerin (Beiersdorf, Inc., Wilton, CT), Sween Cream (Coloplast Corporation, Marietta, GA), or Vaseline (Kendall, Mansfield, MA).
• Do not use any adhesive on skin because removal pulls away the outer skin layer that is a natural barrier to infection and increases the chance of skin tears. This includes Band-Aids, tape, or self-adhesive pads.
• Wear thick white cotton socks. Thick is for cushion, white is for seeing signs of bleeding or drainage, and cotton is for absorbing moisture and preventing skin maceration.
• Cut nails straight across no shorter than the end of the toe, with care not to cut into nail bed or cuticle. Use a good pair of nail clippers and buff sharp edges; do not use sharp instruments. If poor eyesight makes cutting nails difficult, see a professional. Have thick nails, calluses, or corns removed by a foot care specialist who understands the complications of diabetes. Do not use chemical agents or strong antiseptic solutions on feet.
• Before donning shoes and socks, check them for foreign objects, torn linings, rough areas, or hard seams.
• Do not wear shoes without socks or stockings.
• Avoid high impact activities like jogging or aerobic exercises. Stretch the great toe and ankle to prevent friction at the end range of motion in gait.

blood sugars, (4) debride, (5) provide a moist wound dressing, and (6) off-load. If all of these components of treatment are adequately provided, NUs will heal as quickly as wounds in the normal population.[76] In addition, recent work indicates that growth factors can facilitate healing of NUs.

Treat Infection. Treatment by topical or systemic antibiotics, bone scraping, or surgical removal of infected necrotic tissue is determined on an individual basis by the medical team.[77]

Revascularize if Needed. The need for revascularization will be determined by the previously discussed vascular testing. Until the blood supply is adequate, the wound should not be debrided except to remove infected tissue or to open a pocket of purulence. Without sufficient blood supply and thus oxygen delivery, a debrided wound will become larger. Surgical revascularization may be performed using balloon angioplasty with or without stenting for focal superficial femoral artery lesions or with various by-pass procedures for iliac, long-segment superficial femoral artery, or tibial vessel lesions.[78] Controlling lower extremity edema after surgical revascularization is important for healing the NU and the surgical incision and to prevent incision dehiscence and infection.

Two interventions that may help reduce postoperative edema and facilitate healing are low compression or short-stretch bandages (these must provide less pressure than the diastolic blood pressure to avoid occluding the graft) and pneumatic foot compression. A RCT of 115 patients with diabetes who had foot infections requiring incision and drainage compared healing in 59 patients who received pneumatic compression with healing in 56 patients who received a placebo. There was a significantly higher proportion of healing in the pneumatic compression group (75%) as compared to the placebo group (51%). These findings indicate that the use of intermittent pneumatic foot compression directly after revascularization surgery for patients with NUs can facilitate healing, most likely by improving periwound edema control.[79]

Control Blood Glucose Levels. As stated previously, blood glucose levels need to be kept below 200 mg/dl to optimize protein synthesis. Blood glucose levels tend to rise with any infection in patients with diabetes, thus additional medication may be needed to maintain control until the infection is effectively managed.

Debride. Once there is adequate circulation, the NU should be debrided of all necrotic tissue and periwound callus, which is defined as hardened epithelium or hyperkeratosis. Often there will be an open wound under what appears to be a closed callus. Such a wound cannot be classified until the callus is removed. If there is discoloration under the callus, indicative of subcutaneous hemorrhage, the callus should be shaved off to prevent further complications and to explore the depth of subcutaneous damage.[62] Open areas should be explored with a sterile cotton-tipped applicator. If there is bubbly drainage, typical of synovial fluid, the wound has extended into the joint space. X-rays should be taken to detect foreign bodies, soft-tissue gas, or bony abnormalities.[80]

Debridement of callus is best performed by shaving with a sterile scalpel while the surrounding tissue is held under tension, stopping before breaching the dermal skin layer.[81] The callus on an ischemic foot will be dry, thin, glassy, and hard, whereas the callus on a well-perfused foot will be thick and soft. Because calluses can increase peak pressures during gait and cause subcutaneous tissue damage, it is important that they are removed in patients with sensory neuropathy. If a callus surrounds a NU, debridement will allow evaluation of the ulcer depth and exposure of underlying sinuses and undermining while reducing the risk of infection and transforming the chronic wound into an acute wound to facilitate healing.[82]

Debridement of the neuropathic ulcer should be performed with care to preserve the surrounding healthy tissue while removing all of the necrotic tissue. In addition to surgical and serial sharp debridement, supplemental methods (e.g., autolytic debridement with hydrogel, enzymatic debridement, and maggot therapy) may be beneficial, especially in the painful wound (see Chapter 28).[83]

Provide a Moist Wound Environment. When all of the necrotic tissue has been removed, the wound should be dressed with a moist or occlusive dressing, depending on the amount of drainage and the wound depth. Special care should be given to the interdigital spaces where skin can easily become macerated. These spaces should be dried well after cleaning and separated with lamb's wool or cotton (Fig. 30-11). If there are open areas, an appropriate dressing should be applied first and then the toes adequately separated.

Off-Load. The purpose of any off-loading device is to distribute the plantar foot pressures and reduce the stress at the wound site.

Total Contact Casts The gold standard for off-loading neuropathic wounds is the total contact cast (TCC); however, there are numerous orthotics, shoes, assistive devices, and materials that can be used if one's clinic is not equipped to do casting. It is generally accepted that even brief periods of bearing weight on a neuropathic wound, such as walking from the bed to the bathroom,

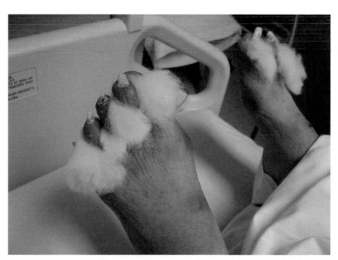

FIG. 30-11 Lamb's wool between the toes of a diabetic foot.

will delay or prevent healing; therefore, the necessity of off-loading cannot be overstressed to the patient. Several studies have reported decreases in peak pressures of up to 92% with the use of TCCs as compared to other types of shoes and barefoot walking.[84-86] Studies have also shown that the TCC is more effective in reducing forefoot pressure than midfoot pressure and is least effective in reducing pressure on the heel.[82] A RCT prospective study compared the effects of TCC (n = 21 NUs) to a control group treated with daily wound care, dressing changes, and footwear modifications (n = 19 NUs). In the TCC group, 19 of the 21 ulcers (91%) healed in a mean of 42 days; in the control group, 6 of the 19 ulcers (32%) healed in a mean of 65 days. Furthermore, no infections developed in the ulcers treated with TCC, whereas 5 of the 19 (26%) patients in the control group developed infections that required hospitalization.[87] A Cochrane review confirms that this is the only RCT for treatment of NUs with TCCs, concluding that the evidence is limited.[88]

The TCC is indicated for any Wagner grade 1 or 2 plantar ulcer in the presence of insensitivity and is absolutely contraindicated for grade 3-5 ulcers with acute or active infection, sepsis, or gangrene. Relative contraindications for the use of TCC are ulcer depth greater than ulcer width (risk of premature epithelialization), fragile skin (risk of further ulceration), and excessive leg or foot edema (poor fit of TCC if edema fluctuates; change more frequently) (Box 30-7). Patient resistance to casting as well as the patient being unable to attend therapy for cast changes, or patient being unsafe with transfers and gait while in TCC are contraindications. An ABI <0.4 is also a relative contraindication.

The procedure for performing TCC is shown in Figs. 30-12 to 30-17. The procedure illustrated is used at the Diabetic Foot Clinic at the Hershey Medical Center, Hershey, PA. There are several variations of materials and techniques for making a TCC (e.g., using plaster of Paris casting rolls, placing felt pads over the malleoli, and using a rubber walking heel); however, the principles are the same: Pad the wound, protect bony prominences, maintain even and full contact, position the knee and ankle at 90 degrees, and stabilize the walking surface. If the ulcer is on the heel, positioning the ankle in slight plantar flexion may help further off-load the heel. The first cast is usually replaced after 3-10 days to allow for inspection of the skin and to assure that there are no pressure areas. Thereafter the cast is replaced every 3-7 days (Hershey protocol) or every 1-3 weeks (Carville protocol).[89] A cast cutter is used to remove the TCC. The most common problem with the TCC is the formation of NUs over pressure points if the cast is not properly fitted and padded.[83] The cast can also be bivalved with a cast saw and held in place with Velcro straps or an elastic bandage. This permits more frequent inspection and dressing changes if infection is present, as well as removal for bathing or sleeping. The disadvantage is the patient can remove the cast, thereby reducing compliance.[90]

Cast Alternatives. Commercial or custom shoes and devices can be used to off-load a neuropathic wound and offer good alternatives when the TCC is not available (Box 30-8). Another option is to use adhesive felt padding as an adherent orthotic or accommodative dressing to off-load a plantar NU, a technique developed by James Birke.[91] The procedure for constructing the orthotic is described in Box 30-9.

One study compared the effectiveness of a wedge shoe, modified wedge shoes, a short leg walker, and a surgical shoe in reducing walking pressure over the area of previous great toe ulceration in individuals with diabetes. In-shoe walking pressures were measured on twelve subjects using a repeated-measure design with the order of treatments randomly assigned. Peak pressures over the area of the previous great toe ulceration were found to be reduced by the following percentages as compared to the traditional surgical shoe: Short leg walker, 29%; wedge shoe, 45%; wedge shoe plus soft insert, 54%; and ortho wedge shoe plus soft insert plus toe relief with adhesive felt cut out to further offload the ulcer site, 64%. The authors concluded that while the TCC is the gold standard, a wedge shoe modified with relief under the lesion may be an effective, less expensive, and less time-consuming alternative for the management of NUs.[92]

Using the same study design, great toe pressures were also compared using adhesive felt accommodative dressing, a short leg walker, a wedge-sole surgical shoe, and a surgical shoe under six different treatment conditions, which included barefoot, accommodative dressing, accommodative dressing and surgical shoe, accommodative dressing and wedge-sole surgical shoe, walker, and wedge-sole surgical shoe. Decrease in peak pressures from barefoot measurements were as follows: Wedge-sole surgical shoe, 43%; accommodative dressing, 48%; accommodative dressing and surgical shoe, 61%; walker, 61%; and accommodative dressing and wedge-sole surgical shoe, 73%. The force-time integral was also significantly reduced when the accommodative dressing was worn with the wedge-sole surgical shoe.[93]

BOX 30-7	**Indications and Contraindications for the Use of Total Contact Casting**

Indication
- Wagner grade 1 and 2 plantar ulcer with loss of protective sensation

Contraindication (Absolute)
- Wagner grade 3-5; acute or active infection, sepsis, or gangrene

Contraindication (Relative)
- Ulcer depth greater than ulcer width (risk of premature epithelialization)
- Fragile skin (risk of further ulceration)
- Excessive leg or foot edema (if edema fluctuates, TCC will fit poorly and require more frequent cast changes)
- If patient is resistant to casting or is unable to attend therapy for cast changes
- Patient unsafe with transfers and gait while in TCC
- ABI <0.4

TCC, Total contact cast; *ABI,* ankle-brachial index.

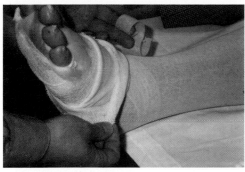

FIG. 30-12 Total contact cast procedure. The wound is cleaned, debrided, and a saline-moistened gauze dressing applied to the open area. The gauze is anchored with a gauze roll and cotton or lamb's wool is placed between the toes. A bias stockinette is placed on the extremity from the toes to above the knee.

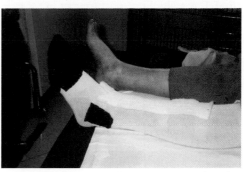

FIG. 30-13 The toes and malleoli are covered with Sci-Foam pads to protect bony prominences, and a felt pad is placed along the tibial crest.

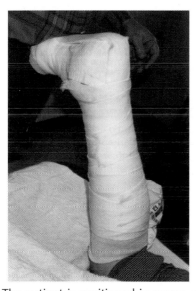

FIG. 30-14 The patient is positioned in prone and cast padding is applied from the toes to just below the knee. The toes are totally covered to prevent trauma and maintain cleanliness.

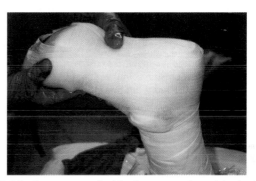

FIG. 30-15 One person holds the extremity with the knee at 90 degrees of flexion and the ankle in a neutral position. A fiberglass cast is applied, first going around the foot and then from toe to knee, being careful to maintain full contact with minimal tension throughout the process. To create a smooth edge at the top, the excess stockinette is folded down before the final layer of casting material is applied.

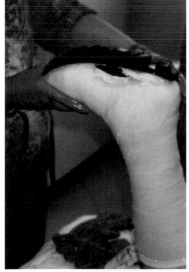

FIG. 30-16 Plaster of Paris casting strips are used to even the plantar surface, a rocker bottom sole is positioned in the center, and another roll of fiberglass casting material is used to anchor the walking sole.

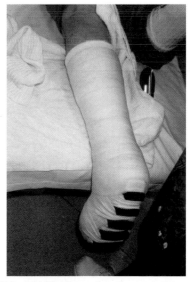

FIG. 30-17 Completed contact cast.

BOX 30-8	Commercial Alternatives to TCC for Off-Loading Neuropathic Ulcers

- The DH Walker (Royce Medical, Camarillo, CA) and Diabetic Walker (AliMed, Dedham, MA) have soles made of small octagons of Velcro foam that can be removed under the wound. Good for small wounds, however, if too much foam has to be removed, foot bottoms out and patient walks on hard surface. Boot has rocker bottom for better gait, however, it is heavy and does compromise balance. Other disadvantages are that they do not distribute weight throughout entire lower leg like boot or TCC, foam can create "do-nut" effect around small wound, thereby decreasing oxygen supply to wound and foam may be inappropriate for heavier body weights.
- Charcot Restraint Orthotic Walker (CROW) is a custom-made, bivalved AFO composed of polypropylene outer shell, Plastazote lining, total contact molding, and rocker-bottom sole. Recommended for patients who need joint stability and alignment. Advantages are ability to inspect wound and change dressings frequently, control edema, and ambulate. Risk of further skin damage is minimal. Disadvantages are decreased compliance, decreased ability to ambulate due to size and weight, vulnerability for skin breakdown, and need for frequent adjustments as edema abates.[17]
- Postoperative shoe is soft and comfortable, easy to don with Velcro straps, and will accommodate a bulky dressing. Inserts of dense moldable foam or thick felt can be used to redistribute pressure and silicone gel "plugs" can be added by cutting out a part of the foam and inserting a circle cut from the gel sheet. This device, although comfortable for patient, is not as effective at reducing pressure as the TCC or a DH Walker.
- D'Arco (D'Arco International, Huntington, WV) wedge shoe and the Integrated Prosthetic and Orthotic System (IPOS) (AliMed, Dedham, MA), used to off-load forefoot, are recommended for forefoot wounds or recent digit amputations. Will compromise balance in some patients; thus an assistive device and thick-soled shoe for the unaffected extremity are recommended.
- PRAFO (Anatomical Concepts, Boardman, OH), Multi Podus boot (AliMed, Dedham, MA), and Heel Relief Orthosis (AliMed, Dedham, MA) off-load the heel. If patient is ambulatory, an appropriate walking sole must be part of the device. If used on patient while patient is supine, brace should be on 2-hour on/2-hour off schedule to avoid prolonged pressure on Achilles tendon, which is especially important if patient has plantar flexion contracture. If off-loading heel is the only concern, pillow under calf (not heel) is effective, and use of the orthosis can be limited to when the patient is sitting or walking. If ankle stability is a concern, an alternating schedule is recommended and the Achilles tendon should be inspected with each change.

TCC, Total contact cast; *AFO,* ankle-foot orthosis.

BOX 30-9	Off-Loading Neuropathic Ulcers Using Adhesive Felt Pads

- Wound is cleansed and covered with transparent film dressing.
- Sole is cut from $\frac{1}{4}$-inch adhesive-backed felt.
- Smudge of lipstick is put on film at wound location.
- Patient stands on felt pad so that lipstick rubs off onto felt.
- Area of wound is cut from felt and edges that will be against the skin are beveled.
- Barrier film is applied to the sole of the foot.
- Position felt pad so it does not touch wound and is anchored with gauze wrap.
- Patient is instructed to wear the pad with a surgical or postoperative shoe.[1,18]

ommended to prevent bilateral foot problems. One study evaluated the peak pressures of the contralateral foot of 22 patients with diabetes who were wearing off-loading devices for active or recently healed NUs. A postsurgical sandal was worn on the contralateral foot; three different devices were tested on the affected foot (postsurgical sandal, Scotchcast boot, and Aircast). Wearing the boot or cast did not increase contralateral pressures as compared with the sandal; however, there was more contact time on the contralateral side in the groups wearing the boot and cast. The increased contact time can lead to overloading the contralateral foot.[94]

Assistive Devices. Walkers or crutches are useful for off-loading, especially in younger patients who have the balance to maintain non–weight-bearing status on the affected extremity during gait. Assistive devices are also recommended for patients with proprioception or balance deficits while adjusting to a cast or orthotic shoe. A shoe with a thick heel or sole worn on the unaffected foot is also helpful to minimize leg-length discrepancies and improve balance.

Vacuum-Assisted Closures. A retrospective study of 31 patients who were treated with subatmospheric pressure dressings, also referred to as negative pressure therapy, as provided by vacuum-assisted closure (VAC) (see Fig. 30-18) after surgical debridement of NUs (mean duration of ulcers before debridement was 25.4 ± 23.8 weeks) measured time to complete closure, proportion of patients achieving wound healing at the level of initial debridement, and complications associated with treatment. Subatmospheric pressure dressing therapy was used for a mean of 4.7 ± 4.2 weeks until 100% granulation of the wound bed was achieved. In this study, 90.3% (n = 28) of the wounds healed without further need for bony resection in a mean of 8.1 ± 5.5 weeks. The remaining 9.7% (n = 3) of patients required some level of amputation. Complications included periwound maceration (n = 6 or 19.4%), periwound cellulitis (n = 1 or 3.2%), and deep surface infection (n = 1 or 3.2%). Although the study supports the use of subatmospheric pressure dressings for indolent ulcers in patients at high risk for amputation, more RCTs are needed to establish a level of evidence.[95]

Growth Factors. The topical growth factor, becaplermin, which is recombinant human platelet-derived

During the time a patient is being treated for a NU on one foot, careful attention to the contralateral foot is imperative because of the increased demands placed on that foot during gait and because of the systemic nature of the risk factors for NUs. Proper shoes with total contact inserts, assistive devices, and meticulous skin care are rec-

growth factor, is approved by the Food and Drug Administration (FDA) for treatment of NUs and is available commercially as Regranex (Ortho-McNeil Pharmaceutical, Inc., Raritan, NJ). Several studies reported the efficacy of becaplermin for facilitating healing of NUs.[96,97] A combined analysis of 4 RCTs that evaluated the effects of daily topical use of becaplermin gel for full-thickness NUs (922 patients with ulcers of at least 8 weeks duration and ≤10 cm^2) reported a significant increase in the probability of complete healing when compared with a placebo gel. In the treated group, 50% of the wounds completely healed as compared to 35% in the placebo group, and healing time was also decreased from an average of 20.1 weeks to an average of 14.1 weeks.[98]

Another study estimated the cost-effectiveness of treating NUs with becaplermin plus good wound care compared with good wound care alone in a variety of health care settings. A 12-month Markov computer-simulation model was used to assess the cost in the two groups using information from a prospective study of 183 patients and a meta-analysis of clinical trials involving 449 patients. They found that individuals who received becaplermin plus good wound care spent 24% more time free of ulcers and had a 9% lower risk of having an amputation. Because the study was performed in Europe, there were inter-country differences in costs of treatment; however, the results suggested that becaplermin may be a cost-effective treatment for NUs.[99]

Biological Skin Substitutes. Several biological skin substitutes, also known as living skin equivalents (LSEs), are available in both autograft and allogenic form to facilitate closure of clean, granulating ulcers. One multi-centered, randomized controlled pilot study on the effectiveness of a bilayered cellular matrix in healing NUs on 40 patients with diabetes found that wounds in the treatment group epithelialized at a rate of 1.8 ± 2.5% per day, as compared to 1.1 ± 1.9% per day for a standard treatment group, defined as moist saline gauze ($p = 0.0087$). The mean rate of wound closure per day in the bilayered cellular matrix–treated wounds was 2.2 ± 2.8% per day compared to 1.1 ± 1.9% per day in those wounds treated with standard care alone ($p = 0.001$).[100] Another prospective, randomized, placebo-controlled study compared median time to wound closure and wound closure rate of NUs for 16 patients treated with LSEs with a group of 17 control patients treated with saline-moistened gauze. Patients treated with LSEs received treatment material once a week for a maximum of 4 weeks or 5 applications. The median time to complete closure for the treatment group was 38.5 days and median time for the control group was 91 days ($p < 0.01$). Complete closure was achieved in 75% of the treatment group and in 41% of the control group ($p < 0.05$ Chi-square test). Moistened saline gauze, although considered standard care for most studies, is seldom considered the recommended dressing for most NUs given the number and qualities of advanced dressings currently available.[101] Studies comparing the efficacy of advanced dressings and LSE were not found. Dressing selection is discussed further in Chapter 28.

Surgery and Amputation. Evidence thus far supports the value of conservative surgical intervention to treat both infected and noninfected NUs. A retrospective study of 58 patients hospitalized with diabetes and foot ulcers complicated by osteomyelitis evaluated the effectiveness of a conservative approach to treatment to avoid amputation or other aggressive surgery. Interventions included minimal bone resection and intravenous antibiotics during hospitalization, along with frequent dressing changes, debridement, and off-loading that was continued after discharge home. At the end of 12 months, 46 (79.3%) patients were healed with a mean healing time of 15.4 weeks, and 12 patients (20.7%) failed to heal, of whom 3 (5.2%) required a major amputation. This study supports the trend to treat NUs complicated by osteomyelitis with early conservative surgery and long-term antibiotics rather than amputation, thereby conserving bony architecture and optimizing weight-bearing foot surfaces.[102]

Another study compared surgical (n = 24) with conventional nonsurgical management (n = 22) of noninfected NUs. Surgical treatment consisted of surgical excision, eventual debridement of bone segments underlying the lesion, and surgical closure. Nonsurgical treatment consisted of relief of weight bearing and regular dressing changes. Faster healing was reported in the surgical group (46.73 days versus 128.9 days), and more of the ulcers healed with surgery (95.5% versus 79.2%). There were also fewer infections and relapses in the surgical group, as well as lower reported discomfort. This study suggests that although nonsurgical management is effective in many cases, surgical management may be more effective and facilitate faster healing.[103]

MANAGEMENT OF THE POSTAMPUTATION WOUND

The diabetic foot requires meticulous wound care after any surgical procedure. If the amputation site is left open to heal by secondary intention, the surgical dressings are removed on the first or second day postoperatively and the wound is irrigated to remove as much of the postoperative bleeding as possible. This may be accomplished with pulsed lavage using 3-6 psi pressure and gentle suction. The initial dressing can be a topical antimicrobial (e.g., ionic silver dressings or slow release cadexomer iodine) with an absorbent dressing to manage drainage, becaplermin, or collagen matrix dressings. Daily sharp debridement of devitalized tissue and dressing changes continue until the wound is granulated, at which time the dressing can be changed to one appropriate for the amount of drainage, or a negative pressure wound therapy device can be applied. Wound edges should be debrided regularly of periwound callus to prevent the epithelium from rolling under while waiting for the cavity to fill with granulation tissue. Orthoses and postoperative shoes (see Cast Alternatives section) are recommended to off-load the plantar surface of the amputation site.

Negative pressure wound therapy (NPWT), using the VAC, for closure of postsurgical lower extremity wounds has been studied with favorable results (Fig. 30-18). A controlled trial with 24 patients with nonhealing surgical wounds in the lower extremity compared the effects of NPWT with conventional saline-moistened dressing. They found that the time required for the wound to be ready

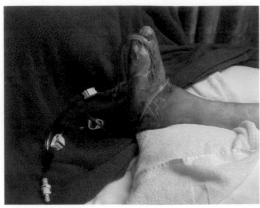

FIG. 30-18 Vacuum-assisted closure on a neuropathic ulcer after incision and debridement.

for surgical closure with a skin graft or flap procedure was shorter in the NPWT group. The mean length of treatment for the NPWT group was 11.25 days; for the control group, 15.75 days ($p = 0.05$).[104]

Another study compared treatment outcomes of foot wounds of all etiologies in 47 patients (66% with diabetes) when treated with NPWT or saline-moistened gauze. The median time for wound filling for the patients treated with NPWT was 38 days; for control patients, 80 days. Median time for wound closure for the patients treated with NPWT was 110 days; for control patients, 124 days, which was not a significant difference. The study suggests that NPWT may be more helpful for obtaining wound filling in the early postsurgical phase but would not be beneficial for full epithelialization after the cavity is filled in.[105] Other treatment options that facilitate epithelialization may be more beneficial in obtaining closure after the cavity is filled with granulation tissue (e.g., LSEs, collagen dressings, or skin grafts).

For any postsurgical patient who also received a revascularization procedure, the therapist should know the type of procedure and graft location so that graft pulses can be monitored at every postoperative visit for wound management. The patient is referred back to the vascular surgeon if the pulses are diminished or absent.

MANAGEMENT OF THE POSTHEALING FOOT

Once a NU is healed, adequate protection must be provided to prevent ulcer recurrence. The Medicare Thera-

peutic Shoe Bill[106] mandates reimbursement for 80% of the cost of footwear and orthotics for patients with diabetes and associated foot problems. Specific eligibility criteria for benefits are listed in Box 30-10. Coverage includes one pair of custom-molded shoes with inserts and two additional pairs of inserts or one pair of extra-depth shoes and three pairs of inserts. Shoe modifications may be substituted for one pair of the inserts. The patient must be under the care of a physician who is providing comprehensive diabetic care and certifies need of diabetic shoes. The physician must write the prescription for the shoes and inserts; the provider furnishes the shoes and inserts and bills Medicare.

Several kinds of custom shoes are available for the patients with diabetes. Dense moldable foam (e.g., Plastazote, American Micro Industries, Chambersburg, PA; Zotefoams, Croydon, UK) may also be custom fit for protection of the vulnerable areas of the patient's foot. Correct fit is very important. The feet should be measured, rather than depending on the patient to give a size, and the shoes should be fitted to the larger foot. If the foot is misshapen (e.g., after a digit amputation or a Charcot foot), custom-molded shoes provide more protection than diabetic shoes with inserts.

Although a Cochrane Review found that there is limited evidence (because of poor quality of research in this area) to support or refute the effectiveness of pressure-relieving interventions for prevention and treatment of NUs, most of the published studies do support the use of therapeutic shoes. For example, a study of the effectiveness of a German shoe with a rocker-shaped sole, a shock absorption insole, and soft upper construction included 92 patients with healed ulcers; 60 received therapeutic shoes, 32 did not and wore their own shoes. The patients were followed for up to 42 months until the first ulcer relapse or until the study ended. Of those who wore their own shoes, 60% had a recurrence within the first year compared to 15% of those who wore therapeutic shoes.[107]

In another study, 241 patients with diabetes who were at high risk for or had a previous neuropathic ulcer were divided into 4 groups with the following shoes: (1) sandals with microcellular rubber insoles, (2) sandals with polyurethane foam, (3) molded insoles for their own footwear, and (4) their own footwear with leather board insoles. Patients who used therapeutic footwear had lower foot pressures (6.9, 6.2, and 6.8), whereas those with non-therapeutic footwear in group 4 had increased foot pressure (40.7). The occurrence of new NUs was significantly higher in the group 4 patients (33%) than in all the other groups combined (4%).[108]

A study of patients with NUs who were provided therapeutic footwear after their ulcers healed was conducted. The patients were monitored for an average of 26 months for compliance and neuropathic ulcer recurrence. They reported ulcer recurrence in 26% of the compliant group and 83% recurrence in the noncompliant group.[55]

Therapeutic shoes need to be worn at least 60% of the time to be effective. Poor compliance is often a result of dissatisfaction with style and fit of the shoes. The patient's

---

BOX 30-10	Criteria for Eligibility for the Medicare Therapeutic Shoe Bill

- The patient must have diabetes mellitus.
- The patient must have at least one of the following conditions:
  - Previous partial or full foot amputation.
  - History of previous foot ulceration
  - History of pre-ulcerative foot calluses; peripheral neuropathy with evidence of callus formation
  - Foot deformity of either foot
  - Poor circulation of either foot

perceived value of the shoes also has more influence on compliance than does the history of ulceration.[109]

The effectiveness of extra-depth shoes and insert combinations in preventing ulceration has also been studied. This RCT included 400 patients with a history of foot ulceration and no foot deformities. The patients were followed for 2 years, during which time data was collected for physical, foot, and diabetes characteristics; footwear use; and NUs. The experimental groups received either extra-depth therapeutic shoes with or without pressure-relieving insoles, and the control group wore their own footwear. The rate of ulcer recurrence was 14% and 15% in the two treatment groups and 17% in the control group, with no statistically significant differences. One hundred percent of the NUs in the treatment groups, and 88% of the NUs in the control group, occurred in patients with sensory neuropathy. The authors concluded that therapeutic shoes with inserts may be unnecessary for patients who do not have foot deformities and that careful attention to foot care may be more important than special footwear.[110]

Several studies have looked at the effectiveness of different types of socks in reducing plantar pressures and thereby reducing the risk of recurrent ulceration. Veves et al studied the pressure-reducing effects of athletic socks. Using a pedobarograph, 27 patients were evaluated under 3 conditions: Barefoot, wearing the patient's own socks, and wearing padded hosiery. The padded hosiery designed for diabetic patients was found to be most effective in reducing plantar pressures.[111] Another study compared plantar pressures of 21 diabetic subjects who had a history of foot complications (e.g., paresthesias, ulceration, callus formation, or bunions). Pressures at the forefoot region, plantar metatarsal heads, and plantar phalanges/toes were measured during six different conditions of wearing: (1) no sock with slipper, (2) no sock with the patient's own shoe, (3) dress sock with slipper, (4) dress sock with the patient's own shoe, (5) diabetic sock with slipper, and (6) diabetic sock with the patient's own shoe. Although none of the results were statistically significant, the condition of slipper with no sock produced the highest metatarsal pressures and the lowest phalangeal pressures, both of which were reduced with shoes and socks or diabetic socks. This suggests that any socks with shoes may help distribute the plantar pressures along the plantar surface of the foot and reduce peak pressures in the metatarsal heads. No studies were done with diabetic socks with diabetic or molded shoes.[112]

Other supplies that may help protect a diabetic foot are special socks with antimicrobial fibers or silicone gel bottoms, toecaps, toe separators, tubular foam, and hammertoe splints.

The preventive measures of good blood sugar control, good foot hygiene, daily foot inspections, and immediate medical care for any skin breaks, in addition to proper off-loading footwear, as described in the section on prevention for the high risk foot, are even more important after NUs have healed because that patient has demonstrated high risk for ulcer formation and has more vulnerable tissue where the ulcer is remodeling.

CASE STUDY 30-1

PERIPHERAL VASCULAR DISEASE

Examination
Patient History

LC is a 73-year-old man with a history of PVD who presents with wounds on his left lateral foot, right heel, and right great toe. The patient is a retired insurance broker who works part-time setting up glasses displays in supermarkets. He is currently unable to work because of the drainage from the right heel wound, inability to wear regular shoes, and inability to drive. He lives with his wife in a one-story home. LC's goals are to return to independent activities at the community level and to resume his part-time job. LC's medical history includes coronary artery disease with history of coronary artery bypass graft and placement of pacemaker and defibrillator, left lower extremity bypass graft with delayed incisional wound healing, fall with a compound fracture of the right ankle requiring an open reduction with internal fixation (ORIF) and gastrocnemius flap to close the necrotic surgical wound (approximately 9 months before the current episode), and hypertension. LC is a former smoker (quit about 10 years ago) and tested negative for diabetes. Medications are clopidogrel (Plavix), ramipril (Altace), aspirin, and folic acid. LC just completed a course of systemic antibiotics (patient unable to identify which one). LC was also self-treating the wounds with bacitracin ointment.

Systems Review

Musculoskeletal: Both feet have evidence of motor neuropathy with claw toes, migrated fat pads, and dropped arches. Ankle ROM on the left: 0-50 degrees plantarflexion; on the right, 15-30 degrees plantarflexion. The right ankle has no inversion/eversion because of the ORIF. Ankle strength is grossly 3–/5 and all other muscle groups grossly 4 to 4+/5.

Neuromuscular: Sensation is intact except for slight diminished light touch over the right lateral ankle muscle flap. LC is independent with all transfers. Gait is characterized by bilateral flat-foot contact during weight acceptance phase, minimal toe push-off bilaterally, short stride length, exaggerated lateral trunk sway to compensate for lack of ankle/knee flexion. He is currently not using an assistive device. Although LC has severe foot deformities with open wounds, the patient is wearing athletic shoes without cushion inserts.

Cardiovascular: LC has no complaints of claudication with activity; however, he does exhibit shortness of breath after walking 40-50 feet, requiring brief rest stops. There is bilateral lower extremity edema, 3+ on the right, 2+ on the left.

Integumentary: Diffuse erythema with scaling skin and spotted weeping of serous fluid on both feet and ankles, right more than left. There is also a strong odor typical of fungal infection.

Tests and Measures

Neuromuscular

Reflex Integrity Absent Achilles reflexes bilaterally.

Sensation No response to the 5.07 monofilament in all 10 test areas on the feet; diminished proprioception in both great toes and ankles.

Pain No complaints of pain.

Cardiovascular

Temperature Left foot is warm to touch, right foot is slightly warmer to touch than the left.

Blood Pressure Brachial: 155/85 mm Hg.

Pulses Left: dorsalis pedis 2+, posterior tibialis 1+ with strong Doppler signal.

Right: dorsalis pedis 2+, posterior tibialis absent with no Doppler signal.

Capillary Refill Right great toe, 6 seconds; left great toe, 5 seconds

ABI Left, 0.72; right, 0.6

Integumentary

Wound Descriptions Right fourth dorsal proximal interphalangeal (PIP) joint: 0.7 × 0.5 cm, 100% granulation, min+ serous drainage, mod+ edema and erythema extending to the metatarsophalangeal (MTP) joint.

Right plantar heel: 3 × 1.5 cm, 100% dry black eschar over the calcaneus, unable to determine the depth until after debridement

Right medial heel: 1.2 cm area of soft callus with a 0.5 cm fissure.

Left plantar first metatarsal: 1.5 × 1 cm, 100% dry brown eschar.

Left lateral fifth metatarsal: 4.5 × 0.5 cm, 10% eschar, 50% eschar, 40% fibrous slough, slight serous drainage, minimal erythema along lateral foot.

Evaluation, Diagnosis, and Prognosis

Based on the information given, the patient had NUs as a result of motor, sensory, and autonomic neuropathy complicated by foot deformities and poorly fitting shoes, possible fungal infection of both feet. He has lower extremity edema because of venous insufficiency as a result of removal of saphenous vein for bypass grafts or cardiovascular problems.

The physical therapy preferred practice pattern diagnosis and the Wagner scale score of the five wounds were as follows:

Right fourth toe: 7D: Impaired integumentary integrity associated with full-thickness skin involvement and scar formation; Wagner: 2

Right plantar heel: 7E: Impaired integumentary integrity associated with skin involvement extending into fascia, muscle, or bone and scar formation; Wagner: 3

Right medial heel: 7B: Impaired integumentary integrity associated with superficial skin involvement; Wagner: 0

Left plantar first metatarsal: 7C: Impaired integumentary integrity associated with partial-thickness skin involvement and scar formation or 7D; Wagner: 1 or 2 (to be determined after debridement)

Left lateral fifth metatarsal: 7C; Wagner: 1

The feet in general were UT category 6 with the exception of the diagnosis of diabetes mellitus.

Prognosis

Prognosis for complete healing was good for the left foot, based on the ABI, with anticipated delayed healing for the right foot.

Intervention

LC was referred to an infectious disease specialist for treatment of possible fungal infection and placed on topical and systemic antifungal medications, resulting in clearing of the skin after about 3 weeks. He was also referred to an orthopedist to rule out osteomyelitis of the right heel and a cardiologist to rule out heart failure as a cause for lower extremity edema. LC was placed on a diuretic; however, he was not compliant on days that he had therapy sessions.

Selective debridement was done of all necrotic tissue. Initially, antimicrobial topical dressings were used on the right heel and the right fourth toe. A petrolatum gauze dressing was used on the left lateral foot and first metatarsal head because the wounds were superficial full thickness. Moist wound dressings were continued to full closure of all wounds.

Off-loading was achieved by using a foam reverse-wedge shoe (Darco wedge) on the right to off-load the heel and a front-wheeled walker to further decrease weight bearing. Because of diminished proprioception, the patient was uncomfortable ambulating with the wedge shoe, and he subsequently preferred non–weight-bearing gait with the walker. Total contact casting was contraindicated because of the fungal infection.

Outcome

The left foot wounds epithelialized in 3-4 weeks. The right medial heel had no open wound after debridement of the callus. The fourth toe epithelialized in 5-6 weeks. The heel wound, which extended to bone with a 1.5 cm sinus after debridement, was slower to heal and more difficult to totally off-load. After 5 months, full closure was achieved and the patient was fitted with custom-molded shoes with closed-cell foam inserts and a silicone gel plug under the calcaneus. He could ambulate for limited community distances without an assistive device and without cardiac symptoms. The patient was able to resume driving and to return to his part-time job.

CHAPTER SUMMARY

Neuropathic ulcers (NUs) occur on the foot, usually the plantar surface or the digits, because of abnormal mechanical forces or minor trauma sustained during weight-bearing activities. They occur most frequently in patients with diabetes who are at risk because of motor, sensory, and autonomic neuropathies; diminished or absent protective sensation; and decreased tissue perfusion because of peripheral vascular disease. The components of NU prevention are good blood glucose control, proper footwear, daily foot inspection, and meticulous foot care. The six steps of wound management for the NU include treatment of infection with systemic and/or topical antibiotics, revascularization for the ischemic limb, maintaining blood glucose levels below 200 mg/dl, debridement of necrotic tissue, provision of a moist wound environment, and adequate off-loading (defined as redistribution of the plantar pressures to as large an area as possible). Periodic medical inspection, adequate protection of foot abnormalities with therapeutic footwear, and comprehensive patient education are required to prevent high risk for reoccurrence. Neuropathic ulcer care includes comprehensive care of the local and systemic factors contributing to the ulcer, meticulous wound management, and extensive patient education.

ADDITIONAL RESOURCES

Books

Bowker JH, Pfeifer MA (eds): *The Diabetic Foot,* ed 6, St. Louis, 2001, Mosby

Veves A, Giurini JM, LoGerfo FW: *The Diabetic Foot: Medical and Surgical Management,* Totowa, NJ, 2002, Humana Press.

Web Sites

American Diabetes Association: www.diabetes.org

American Association of Diabetes Educators: www.aadenet.org

National Diabetes Information Clearinghouse: www.diabetes.niddk.nih.gov

GLOSSARY

Advanced glycation (or glycosylation) end-products (AGEs): Produced in the body when glucose links with protein. They play a role in damaging blood vessels and can lead to the complications commonly associated with diabetes.

Alpha cell: Pancreatic cell that releases glucagon.

Autonomic neuropathy: Disease of the nerves that control autonomic functions including sweat production, digestive function, bladder function, and cardiovascular function.

Beta cell: Pancreatic cell that releases insulin.

Blood glucose level: The amount of glucose in a given amount of blood measured in milligrams per deciliter (mg/dl).

Diabetes Control and Complications Trial (DCCT): Study by the National Institute of Diabetes and Digestive and Kidney Diseases, conducted from 1983 to 1993 in people with type 1 diabetes. The study showed that intensive therapy compared to conventional therapy significantly helped prevent or delay diabetes complications.

Diabetes mellitus (DM): A condition characterized by hyperglycemia resulting from the body's inability to use blood glucose for energy.

Glucagon: A hormone produced by the pancreatic alpha cells that increases blood glucose.

Glycogen: The form of glucose found in the liver and muscles.

Hyperglycemia: Excessive blood glucose. Fasting hyperglycemia is blood glucose above a desirable level after a person has not eaten for at least 8 hours. Postprandial hyperglycemia is blood glucose above a desirable level 1-2 hours after a person has eaten.

Insulin: A hormone that facilitates utilization of glucose for energy; produced by the pancreatic beta cells.

Insulin resistance: The inability to respond to and use the insulin. Insulin resistance may be linked to obesity, hypertension, and high levels of fat in the blood.

Islets of Langerhans: Groups of pancreatic cells that make glucagons and insulin.

Monofilament: A short piece of nylon, like a hairbrush bristle, mounted on a wand and used to check sensitivity of the nerves in the foot or hand.

Nephropathy: Disease of the kidneys.

Neuropathy: Disease of the nervous system. The three major forms associated with diabetes are peripheral neuropathy (includes motor and sensory neuropathy), autonomic neuropathy, and mononeuropathy.

Neurotip: Monofilament calibrated at 40 gm force used to assess diminished sensation to sharpness and pain. The filament is placed in a hand-held pen for sensory testing.

Pancreas: The organ that produces insulin, glucagon, and digestive enzymes. The pancreas is located behind the lower part of the stomach and is about the size of a hand.

Type 1 diabetes: A disease characterized by high blood glucose levels caused by a lack of insulin. Occurs when the body's immune system attacks and destroys the insulin-producing beta cells in the pancreas.

Type 2 diabetes: A condition characterized by high blood glucose levels caused by either a lack of insulin or the inability to use insulin efficiently.

References

1. American Diabetes Association: *National Diabetes Fact Sheet.* Retrieved from http://diabetes.org on 9/22/2004.
2. Boyle JP, Honeycutt AA, Venkat NKM, et al: Projection of diabetes burden through 2050: Impact of changing demography and disease prevalence in the US, *Diabetes Care* 24:1936-1940, 2001.
3. American Diabetes Association: Consensus development conference on diabetic foot wound care: 7-8 April 1999, Boston, Massachusetts, *Diabetes Care* 22(8):1354-1360, 1999.
4. Abbott CA, Carrington AL, Ashe H, et al: The North-West Diabetes Foot Care Study: incidence of, and risk factors for, new diabetic foot ulceration in a community-based patient cohort, *Diabetic Med* 19(5):377-384, 2002.
5. Manes C, Papazoglou N, Sossidou E, et al: Prevalence of diabetic neuropathy and foot ulceration: identification of potential risk factors—a population-based study, *Wounds* 14(1):11-15, 2002.
6. Adler A, Boyko EJ, Ahroni JH, Smith DG: Lower-extremity amputation in diabetes. The independent effects of peripheral vascular disease, sensory neuropathy, and foot ulcers, *Diabetes Care* 22(7):1029-1035, 1999.
7. Lavery LA, Armstrong DG, Vela SA, et al: Practical criteria for screening patients at high risk for diabetic foot ulceration, *Arch Intern Med* 158:157-162, 1998.
8. Vinik AI: *Diabetic neuropathy: A small-fiber disease.* Retrieved from http://www.medscape.com/viewarticle/418468 on 10/24/2004.
9. Clinical practice recommendations: Diagnosis and classification of diabetes mellitus: 2004, *Diabetes Care* 27(suppl):S5 S10, 2004.
10. McClave SA, Finney LS: Nutritional issues in the patient with diabetes and foot ulcers. In Bowker JH, Pfeifer MA (eds): *The Diabetic Foot,* ed 6, St. Louis, 2001, Mosby.
11. Soory M: Hormone mediation of immune responses in the progression of diabetes, rheumatoid arthritis and periodontal diseases, *Curr Drug Targets Immune Endocr Metabol Disord* 2(1):13 25, 2002.
12. Bitar MS: Insulin and glucocorticoid-dependent suppression of the IGF-I system in diabetic wounds, *Surgery* 127(6):687-695, 2000.
13. Spravchikov N, Sizyakov G, Gartsbein M, et al: Glucose effects on skin keratinocytes: implications for diabetes skin complications, *Diabetes* 50(7):1627-1635, 2001.
14. Teixeira AS, Andrade SP: Glucose-induced inhibition of angiogenesis in the rat sponge granuloma is prevented by aminoguanidine, *Life Sci* 64(8):655-662, 1999.
15. Duraisamy Y, Slevin M, Smith N, et al: Effect of glycation on basic fibroblast growth factor induced angiogenesis and activation of associated signal transduction pathways in vascular endothelial cells: Possible relevance to wound healing in diabetes, *Angiogenesis* 4(4):277-288, 2001.
16. Kimball JW: Hormones of the pancreas, *Kimball's Biology Pages.* Available at http://users.rcn.com/kimball.ma.ultranet/BiologyPages/P/Pancreas.html. Accessed January 28, 2004.
17. Colwell JA, Lyons TJ, Klein RL, et al: Atherosclerosis and thrombosis in diabetes mellitus: new aspects of pathogenesis. In Bowker JH, Pfeifer MA (eds): *The Diabetic Foot,* ed 6, St. Louis, 2001, Mosby.
18. Ratner RE: Pathophysiology of the diabetes disease state. In Franz MJ, Kulkarni K, Polonsky WH, et al (eds): *Diabetes and Complications: A Core Curriculum for Diabetes Education,* ed 4, Chicago, Ill, 2001, American Association of Diabetes Educators.
19. Ludwig-Beymer P, Huether SE, Zekauskus SB: Alterations of hormonal regulation. In Huether SE, McCance KL (eds): *Understanding Pathophysiology,* St. Louis, 1996, Mosby.
20. American Physical Therapy Association: *Guide to Physical Therapist Practice,* ed 2, Alexandria, Va, 2001, The Association.
21. Van Schie CH, Boulton AJ: Biomechanics of the diabetic foot: The road to foot ulceration. In Veves A, Giurini JM, LoGerfo FW: *The Diabetic Foot: Medical and Surgical Management,* Totowa, NJ, 2002, Humana Press.

22. Mueller MJ, Diamond JE, Delitto A, et al: Insensitivity, limited joint mobility, and plantar ulcers in patients with diabetes mellitus, *Phys Ther* 69:453-462, 1989.

23. Delbridge L, Perry P, Marr S, et al: Limited joint mobility in the diabetic foot: relationship to neuropathic ulceration, *Diabetic Med* 5:333-337, 1988.

24. Lobman R, Kasten G, Kasten U, et al: Association of increased plantar pressures with peripheral sensorimotor and peripheral autonomic neuropathy in Type 2 diabetic patients, *Diabetes Nutr Metab* 15(3):165-168, 2002.

25. Simoneau GG, Ulbrecht JS, Deer JA, et al: Postural instability in patients with diabetic sensory neuropathy, *Diabetes Care* 17:1411-1421, 1994.

26. Giacomozzi C, Caselli A, Macellari V, et al: Walking strategy in diabetic patients with peripheral neuropathy, *Diabetes Care* 25(8):1451-1457, 2002.

27. Tanenberg RJ, Schumer MP, Greene DA, et al: Neuropathic problems of the lower extremities in diabetic patients. In Bowker JH, Pfeifer MA (eds): *The Diabetic Foot,* ed 6, St. Louis, 2001, Mosby.

28. Olmos PR, Cataland S, O'Dorisio TM, et al: The Semmes-Weinstein monofilament as a potential predictor of foot ulceration in patients with noninsulin-dependent diabetes, *Am J Med Sci* 309(2):76-82, 1995.

29. Jeng C, Michelson J, Mizel M: Sensory thresholds of normal human feet, *Foot Ankle Int* 21(6):501 504, 2000.

30. Rith-Najarian SJ, Stolusky T, Gohdes DM: Identifying diabetic patients at high risk for lower-extremity amputation in a primary health care setting. A proposed evaluation of simple screening criteria, *Diabetes Care* 15:1386-1389, 1992.

31. Vijay V, Snehalatha C, Seena R, et al: The Rydel Seiffer tuning fork: An inexpensive device for screening diabetic patients with high-risk foot, *Pract Diabetes Int* 18:155-156, 2001.

32. Richardson JK: The clinical identification of peripheral neuropathy among older persons, *Arch Phys Med Rehabil* 83:1553-1558, 2002.

33. Jude E, Armstrong DG, Boulton AJM: Assessment of the diabetic foot. In Krasner D, Rodeheaver GT, Sibbald G (ed): *Chronic Wound Care: A Clinical Source Book for Healthcare Professionals,* ed 3, Wayne, Penn, 2001, Health Management Publications.

34. Coppini DV, Young PJ, Weng C, et al: Outcome on diabetic foot complications in relation to clinical examination and quantitative sensory testing: A case-control study, *Diabetic Med* 15(9):765-771, 1998.

35. Pham H, Armstrong DG: Screening techniques to identify people at high risk for diabetic ulceration: A prospective multicenter trial, *Diabetes Care* 23(5):606-611, 2000.

36. Mayfield JA, Sugarman JR: The use of the Semmes-Weinstein monofilament and other threshold tests for preventing foot ulceration and amputation in persons with diabetes, *J Fam Pract* 49(11 suppl):S17-29, 2000.

37. Armstrong DG, Lavery LA, Wunderlich RP, et al: 2003 William J. Stickel Silver Award: Skin temperatures as a one-time screening toll do not predict future diabetic foot complications, *J Am Podiatr Med Assoc* 9(6):443-447, 2003.

38. Nube VL, McGill M, Molyneaux L, et al: From acute to chronic: Monitoring the progress of Charcot's arthropathy, *J Am Podiatr Med Assoc* 92(7):384-389, 2002.

39. Klenerman L: The Charcot joint in diabetes, *Diabetic Med* 13:S52-S54, 1996.

40. Armstrong DG, Lavery LA: Acute Charcot's arthropathy of the foot and ankle, *Phys Ther* 78:74-80, 1998.

41. Krasner DL, Sibbald RG: Diabetic foot ulcer care: Assessment and management. In Bowker JH, Pfeifer MA (eds): *The Diabetic Foot,* ed 6, St. Louis, 2001, Mosby.

42. Vinicor F. Macrovascular disease. In Franz MJ, Kulkarni K, Polonsky WH, et al (eds): *Diabetes and Complications: A Core Curriculum for Diabetes Education,* ed 4, Chicago, 2001, American Association of Diabetes Educators.

43. Bjellerup M: Does dorsal pedal pulse palpation predict hand-held Doppler measurement of ankle-brachial index in leg ulcer patients? *Wounds* 15(7):237-240, 2003.

44. American Diabetes Association: Position statement: Preventive foot care in people with diabetes, *Diabetes Care* 27:S63-64, 2004.

45. Harris MI, Klein R, Welborn TA, et al: Onset of NIDDM occurs at least 4-7 years before clinical diagnosis, *Diabetes Care* 15:815-819, 1992.

46. Lampe KE: Methods of wound evaluation. In Kloth L, McCulloch JM (eds): *Wound Healing: Alternatives in Management* (Contemporary Perspectives in Rehabilitation), ed 3, Philadelphia, 2002, FA Davis.

47. Lipsky BL, Armstrong DG: Recognizing infections and taking appropriate cultures, *Wounds* January Supplement:S6-S7, 2003.

48. Armstrong DG, Lipsky BL, Joseph WS: Diagnosing and treating osteomyelitis, *Wounds* January Supplement:S8-S12, 2003.

49. Brodsky JW: An improved method for staging and classification of foot lesions in diabetic patients. In Bowker JH, Pfeifer MA (eds): *The Diabetic Foot,* ed 6, St. Louis, 2001, Mosby.

50. Harkless LB, Satterfield VK, Dennis KJ: Role of the podiatrist. In Bowker JH, Pfeifer MA (eds): *The Diabetic Foot,* ed 6, St. Louis, 2001, Mosby.

51. Armstrong DG: The University of Texas Diabetic Foot Classification System, *Ostomy Wound Manage* 42(8):60-61, 1996.

52. Peters EJ, Lavery LA: Effectiveness of the diabetic foot risk classification system of the International Working Group on the Diabetic Foot, *Diabetes Care* 24(8):1442-1447, 2001.

53. Van Acker K, De Block C, Abrams P, et al: The choice of diabetic foot ulcer classification in relation to the final outcome, *Wounds* 14(1):16-25, 2002.

54. Oyibo SO, Jude EB, Tarawneh I, et al: A comparison of two diabetic foot ulcer classification systems, *Diabetes Care* 24:84-88, 2001.

55. Edmonds ME, Blundell MP, Morris ME, et al: Improved survival of the diabetic foot: the role of a specialized foot clinic, *Q J Med* 60:763-771, 1986.

56. Mannari RJ, Payne WG, Ochs DE, et al: Successful treatment of recalcitrant diabetic heel ulcers with topical becaplermin (rhPDGF-BB) gel, *Wounds* 14(3):116-121, 2002.

57. Knowles EA: Painful diabetic neuropathy: Assessment and treatment, *J Diabetes Nurs,* 2002. Accessed from http://www.findarticles.com on 12/29/2004.

58. Green MF, Aliabadi Z, Green BT, et al: Diabetic foot: Evaluation and management, *South Med J* 95(1):95-101, 2002.

59. Levin ME: Management of the diabetic foot: Preventing amputation, *South Med J* 95(1):10-20, 2002.

60. Levin ME: Preventing amputation in the patient with diabetes, *Diabetes Care* 18(10):1383-1392, 1995.

61. Litzelman DK, Slemenda CW, Langefeld CD, et al: Reduction of lower extremity clinical abnormalities in patients with non-insulin-dependent diabetes mellitus: A randomized, controlled trial, *Ann Intern Med* 119(1):36-41, 1993.

62. Calle-Pascual AL, Duran A, Benedi A, et al: Reduction in foot ulcer incidence, *Diabetes Care* 24:405-407, 2001.

63. Valk GD, Kriegsman DM, Assendelft WJ: Patient education for preventing diabetic foot ulceration: a systematic review, *Endocrinol Metab Clin North Am* 31(3):633-658, 2002.

64. American Diabetes Association: Tests of glycemia, position statement, *Diabetes Care* 20(suppl 1):S91-S93, 2004.

65. American Association of Clinical Endocrinologists: The American Association of Clinical Endocrinologists medical guidelines for the management of diabetes mellitus: The AACE system of intensive diabetes self-management—2002 update, *Endocr Pract* 8(suppl 1):40-82, 2002.

66. National Diabetes Information Clearinghouse: Diabetes Control and Complications Trial (DCCT). Retrieved from http://diabetes.niddk.nih.gov/dm/pubs/control/ 9/29/2004.

67. O'Brien P: Landmark study—reducing diabetes complications. Retrieved from http://www.medicineau.net.au/clinical/medicine/medicine8.html on 9/24/2004.

68. Nelson KM, Reiber G, Boyko EJ: Diet and exercise among adults with type 2 diabetes: Findings from the Third National Health and Nutrition Examination Survey (NHANES III), *Diabetes Care* 25:1722-1728, 2002.

69. Boule N, Haddad E, Kenny GP, et al: Effects of exercise on glycemic control and body mass in type 2 diabetes mellitus: A meta-analysis of controlled clinical trials, *JAMA* 286:1218-1227, 2001.

70. Short KR, Vittone JL, Begelow ML, et al: Impact of aerobic exercise training on age-related changes in insulin sensitivity and muscle oxidative capacity, *Diabetes* 52:1888-1896, 2003.

71. Nettles AT: Diabetes in older adults. In Franz MJ et al (eds): *Diabetes in the Life Cycle and Research: A Core Curriculum for Diabetes Education,* ed 4, Chicago, 2001, American Association of Diabetes Educators.

72. Williamson JR, Hoffman PL, Kohrt WM: Endurance exercise training decreases capillary basement membrane width in older nondiabetic and diabetic adults, *J Appl Physiol* 80:747-753, 1996.

73. Levin ME: Saving the diabetic foot, *Intern Med* 5:90-103, 1997.

74. McPoil TG: Footwear, *Phys Ther* 68(12):1857-1865, 1988.

75. Birke J: Assessment of the neuropathic foot. Presented at American Physical Therapy Association Combined Sections Meeting, Boston, February, 2002.

76. Boulton AJ: Pressure and the diabetic foot: Clinical science and off-loading techniques, *Am J Surg* 187(5A):17S-24S, 2004.

77. Sumpio BE, Lee T, Blume PA: Vascular evaluation and arterial reconstruction of the diabetic foot. *Clin Podiatr Med Surg* 20(4):689-708, 2003.

78. Epstein DA, Corson JD: Surgical perspective in treatment of diabetic foot ulcers, *Wounds* 13(2):59-65, 2001.

79. Armstrong DA, Nguyen HC: Improvement in healing with aggressive edema reduction after debridement of foot infection in persons with diabetes, *Arch Surg* 135:1405-1409, 2000.

80. Caputo GM, Cavanaugh PR, Ulbrecht JS, et al: Assessment and management of foot disease in patients with diabetes, *N Engl J Med* 331(13):854-860, 1994.

81. Baker N: Debridement of the diabetic foot: A podiatric perspective, *Int J Low Extrem Wounds* 1(2):87-92, 2002.

82. Martin RL, Conti SF: Plantar pressure analysis of diabetic rocker bottom deformity in total contact casts, *Foot Ankle Int* 17:470-472, 1996.

83. Armstong DA, Attinger CE, Boulton AJ, et al: Appropriate use of NPWT in reconstructive surgery of the diabetic foot, *Ostomy Wound Manage* 50(4 suppl B):19S-23S, 2004.

84. Shaw JE, His WL, Ulbrecht JS, et al: The mechanism of plantar unloading in total contact casts: implications for design and clinical use, *Foot Ankle Int* 18:809-817, 1997.

85. Cogley D, Laing P, Crerand S, et al: Foot-cast interface vertical force measurements in casts used for healing neuropathic ulcers. Proceedings of the First International Symposium and Workshop, Noordwijkerhout, The Netherlands, May 3-4, 1991.

86. Lavery LA, Vela SA, Fleisch JG, et al: Reducing plantar pressure in the neuropathic foot: A comparison of footwear, *Diabetes Care* 20:1707-1710, 1997.

87. Mueller MJ, Diamond JE, Sinacore DR, et al: Total contact casting in treatment of diabetic plantar ulcers: Controlled clinical trial, *Diabetes Care* 12:384-388, 1989.

88. Spencer S: Pressure relieving interventions for preventing and treating diabetic foot ulcers. From *Cochrane Review Abstracts*. Posted 7/1/2004, retrieved from http://www.medscape.com/viewarticle/486169 on 1/2/2005.

89. Birke J, Patout CA: The contact cast: an update and case study report, *Wounds* 12(2):26-31, 2000.

90. Caputo GM, Ulbrecht JS, Cavanagh PR: The total contact cast: A method for treating neuropathic diabetic ulcers, *Am Fam Physician* 55(2):605-611, 1997.

91. Birke JA: Management of the insensate foot. In Kloth L, McCulloch JM (eds): *Wound Healing: Alternatives in Management* (Contemporary Perspectives in Rehabilitation), ed 3, Philadelphia, 2002, FA Davis.

92. Birke JA, Lewis K, Penton A, et al: The effectiveness of a modified wedge shoe in reducing pressure at the area of previous great toe ulceration in individuals with diabetes mellitus, *Wounds* 16(4):109-114, 2004.

93. Birke JA: The effectiveness of an accommodative dressing in offloading pressure over areas of previous metatarsal head ulceration, *Wounds* 15(2):33-39, 2003.

94. Van Schie CHM, Rowell S, Knowles A, et al: The effect of the Scotchcast boot and the Aircast device on foot pressures of the contralateral foot, *Wounds* 15(9):289-293, 2003.

95. Armstrong DG, Lavery LA, Abu-Rumman P, et al: Outcomes of subatmospheric pressure dressing therapy on wounds of the diabetic foot, *Ostomy Wound Manage* 48(4):64-68, 2002.

96. Embil JM, Papp K, Sibbald G, et al: Recombinant human platelet-derived growth factor-BB (becaplermin) for healing chronic lower extremity diabetic ulcers: An open-label clinical evaluation of efficacy, *Wound Repair Regen* 8(3):162-168, 2000.

97. Miller MS: Use of topical recombinant human platelet-derived growth factor-BB (becaplermin) in healing of chronic mixed arteriovenous lower extremity diabetic ulcers, *J Foot Ankle Surg* 38(3):227-231, 1999.

98. Smiell JM, Wieman TJ, Steed DL, et al: Efficacy and safety of becaplermin (recombinant human platelet-derived growth factor-BB) in patients with nonhealing, lower extremity diabetic ulcers: a combined analysis of four randomized studies, *Wound Repair Regen* 7(5):335-346, 1999.

99. Ghatnekar O, Persson U, Willis M, et al: Cost effectiveness of Becaplermin in the treatment of diabetic foot ulcers in four European countries, *Pharmacoeconomics* 19(7):767-778, 2001.

100. Lipkin S, Chaikof E, Isseroff Z, et al: Effectiveness of bilayered cellular matrix in healing of diabetic foot ulcers: Results of a multicenter pilot trial, *Wounds* 15(7):230-236, 2003.

101. Pham HT, Rosenblum BI, Lyons TE, et al: Evaluation of a human skin equivalent for the treatment of diabetic foot ulcers in a prospective, randomized clinical trial, *Wounds* 11(4):79-86, 1999.

102. Yadlapalli NG, Vaishnav A, Sheehan P: Conservative management of diabetic foot ulcers complicated by osteomyelitis, *Wounds* 14:31-35, 2002.

103. Piaggesi A, Schipani E, Campi F, et al: Conservative surgical approach versus non-surgical management for diabetic neuropathic foot ulcers: A randomized trial, *Diabetes Med* 15(5):412-417, 1998.

104. Etoz A, Ozgenel Y, Ozcan M: The use of negative pressure wound therapy on diabetic foot ulcers: A preliminary controlled trial, *Wounds* 16(8):264-269, 2004.

105. Page JC, Newswander B, Schwenke DC, et al: Retrospective analysis of negative pressure wound therapy in open foot wounds with significant soft tissue defects, *Adv Skin Wound Care* 17(7):354-364, 2004.

106. Medicare Therapeutic Shoe Bill. Available at www.medicare.gov/publications/pubs/pdf/10050/pdf.

107. Busch K, Chantelau E: Effectiveness of a new brand of stock "diabetic" shoes to protect against diabetic foot ulcer relapse: A prospective cohort study, *Diabetes Med* 20(8):665-669, 2003.

108. Viswanathan V, Madhavan S, Gnanasundaram S, et al: Effectiveness of different types of footwear insoles for diabetic neuropathic foot: A follow-up study, *Diabetes Care* 27(2):474-477, 2004.

109. Macfarlane DJ, Jensen JL: Factors in diabetic footwear compliance, *J Am Podiatr Med Assoc* 93(6):485-491, 2003.

110. Reiber GE, Smith DG, Wallace C, et al: Effect of therapeutic footwear on foot reulceration in patients with diabetes: A randomized controlled trial, *JAMA* 287(19):2552-2558, 2002.

111. Veves A, Masson EA, Fernando DJ, et al: Use of experimental padded hosiery to reduce abnormal foot pressures in diabetic neuropathy, *Diabetes Care* 12(9):653-655, 1989.

112. Blackwell B, Aldridge R, Jacob S: A comparison of plantar pressure in patients with diabetic foot ulcers using different hosiery, *Int J Low Extrem Wounds* 1(3):174-178, 2002.

Chapter 31

Burns

R. Scott Ward

CHAPTER OUTLINE

OBJECTIVES

After reading this chapter, the reader will be able to:
1. Describe the pathology associated with skin and soft tissue burns.
2. Examine a patient with burns considering specific factors related to burn injury such as burn etiology, burn depth, and burn size.
3. Evaluate a patient with burns in preparation for planning interventions.
4. Explain interventions for patients with burn injuries, including those directed at wound healing and rehabilitation management.
5. Describe the consequences of and interventions for scarring after burn injury.
6. Presented with a clinical case, analyze the clinical findings, propose goals of treatment, and develop a plan of care.

Burn rehabilitation programs have traditionally been designed to maximize the restoration of health and function of individuals following burn injury.[1,2] Rehabilitation of a patient with burn injury begins at the time of admission and continues through the maturation of scar tissue. During this process, patients may require ongoing surgical intervention to aid wound healing and revision of scarring, as well as rehabilitation interventions aimed at care of the burn wound, managing edema, preserving and increasing mobility and strength, improving function, and controlling scar formation.

Survival rates for patients with burns have increased steadily over the past several decades.[3] Patients are surviving because of improvements in fluid management, infection control, and emergency response, as well as more effective surgical interventions. With more patients surviving burn injury, there is a greater need for the services directed at improving their long-term outcomes. Such services often include physical therapy, occupational therapy, psychological counseling, and vocational rehabilitation. Given the many facets involved in the care of a patient with burns, from the time of injury throughout their rehabilitation, and the many problems that might result along a course of recovery, optimal treatment requires a team approach.[4]

The American Burn Association (ABA) outlines factors influencing the severity of burn injury. All of these also influence prognosis. The criteria for burn severity are based on burn depth and size, the age of the patient, the anatomical area burned, and associated injuries. Box 31-1 provides an outline of the ABA's criteria for referral to a burn center, which reflects variables that contribute to the severity of a burn injury. These and other variables associated with burn injury, including other systems affected by the burn, edema, mobility, and strength, should be considered when examining a patient after a burn injury.

PATHOLOGY

Burn injury results from exposure of the integument to excessive temperatures. Burn etiology is variable, and causes include scald, flame, contact (including friction), chemical, flash (exposure to bursts of radiant heat), electrical, and other (radioactivity, irradiation, etc).[5] Scald and flame injuries are the most common causes of burns.[5] Scald burns, caused by hot liquids (coffee, tea, water, oil, etc),[6] are the most common pediatric burns in the United States.[7] Elderly persons are also at increased risk for scald injury.[8] Flame burns result from direct contact with

BOX 31-1	American Burn Association Criteria for Referral to a Burn Center

- A patient who has partial thickness burns >10%TBSA.
- A patient with burns that involve the face, hands, feet, genitalia, perineum, or major joints.
- A patient with third-degree burns of any size in any age group.
- A patient with electrical burns, including lightning injury.
- A patient with inhalation injury.
- A patient with chemical burns.
- A patient with burn injury who has preexisting medical conditions that could complicate management, prolong recovery, or affect mortality.
- Patients with burns and concomitant trauma (such as fractures) in which the burn injury poses the greatest risk of morbidity or mortality. In such cases, if the trauma poses the greater immediate risk, the patient may be initially stabilized in a trauma center before being transferred to a burn unit. Physician judgment will be necessary in such situations and should be in concert with the regional medical control plan and triage protocols.
- Children with burns in hospitals without qualified personnel or equipment for pediatric care of such children.
- A patient with burn injury who require special social, emotional, or long-term rehabilitative interventions.

Adapted from Guidelines for the Operations of Burn Units: *Resources for Optimal Care of the Injured Patient,* 1999, Committee on Trauma, American College of Surgeons.
%TBSA, Percentage of total body surface area.

flaming objects or clothing that has been ignited with a flame. Adult men between the ages of 16 and 40 years have the highest prevalence of this type of injury.[9] Contact burns occur when contact is made with a hot object, such as a radiator, iron, curling iron, or exhaust pipe, or when contact is made with a rapidly moving object (also referred to as a friction burn) such as a treadmill.[10-12] Contact burns most commonly involve the hands and are not usually life-threatening.[10,11] Chemical burns are often related to industrial accidents and tend to be deep. The extent of a chemical injury depends on the strength and concentration of the chemical agent and the duration of its contact with the skin.[13] Electrical injuries are not classic burn injuries.[5] There may be surface burns because of an associated flash, as well as entrance and exit wounds where the current entered and exited the patient. Electrical burns can also injure deep tissues, including nerves, vessels, muscle, and bone, because resistance to current flow causes tissue heating. Electrical currents may cause cardiac arrhythmias, respiratory arrest that results from tetany of respiratory muscles, or fractures caused by skeletal muscle tetany.

Following acute burn shock, the body is in a state of hypermetabolism and protein catabolism. It is thought that protein from muscle is used to fuel gluconeogenesis for increased energy needs in healing the burn. There is evidence to suggest that much of this activity is a result of hormonal changes related to the burn injury. Alterations in both the levels of circulating hormones and

cellular hormonal receptors have been demonstrated after a burn.[14-18] All of these changes contribute to a severe catabolic state by changing or impairing metabolic activity. The hypermetabolic and catabolic state associated with burn injury causes loss of skeletal muscle and thus can impair strength. No specific data exist to indicate the trend of recovery of the muscle wasting and loss of strength associated with burns, but measurable decreases in muscle torque production, work, and power have been reported in patients several months after burn injuries.[19]

EXAMINATION

PATIENT HISTORY

The history for a patient with a burn should include standard questions such as work, social, and medical history. In addition, the patient should be asked where (e.g., home, work, etc.) and how the burn injury occurred and what caused the injury (e.g., flame, chemical, scald, etc.). The presence of an associated injury, such as an inhalation injury or fracture, may be discovered either during the history or physical examination. The history may guide the care provider to complete further testing to rule in or out suspected injuries.

SYSTEMS REVIEW

The systems review is used to target areas requiring further examination and to define areas that may cause complications or indicate a need for precautions during the examination and intervention processes. See Chapter 1 for details of the systems review. Although this chapter focuses on the injury to the integument caused by a burn injury, other systems that should be included in a systems review include the cardiovascular/pulmonary system, the musculoskeletal system, and the neuromuscular system.

Associated injuries increase the severity of a burn injury (see Box 31-1) and influence the plan of care because they generally cause additional impairments. Trauma associated with burns can have many causes, including motor vehicle accidents, escaping a fire, or falling because of electrical shock, assault, or explosion.[20] Although any type of injury can accompany a burn, the most common is inhalation injury. Other injuries associated with burns that are of particular relevance to rehabilitation are fractures and peripheral nerve damage.

TESTS AND MEASURES

Musculoskeletal. The musculoskeletal system review should include examination of the gross range of motion (ROM) and strength of unburned areas. Detailed examination of ROM and strength should be performed for any area directly affected by the burn injury. Gross anthropometric symmetry should be checked, and height and weight should be recorded. Fractures in the burn patient population are generally caused by motor vehicle accidents or falls. However, the literature suggests that fracture healing time is not significantly delayed in patients with burns, even with the additional metabolic demands of the burn injury.[20]

Anthropometric Characteristics

Edema. Edema forms immediately after burn injury. Fluid from circulating plasma shifts to the interstitium because of increased capillary permeability (caused by inflammatory mediators) and changes in oncotic and hydrostatic pressures.[21] Because of the large shift of fluid out of the vessels that occurs with large burns, patients are treated with large volumes of intravenous fluid therapy to maintain perfusion of core organs. This fluid therapy, also referred to as fluid resuscitation, has decreased the incidence of vital organ failure after burn injury but has also increased the incidence of peripheral edema. Because the fluid shifts are so great, even when the fluid shifts back into the circulation there is often a noticeable residual edema. This may be worsened if the lymphatic vessels are damaged or blocked by fibrin or debris.[22] Persistent edema may adversely affect healing by impairing oxygen and nutrient delivery[23] and can also adversely affect mobility.

Edema can be measured using any one of several standard measures such as volumetry, circumference measurements, or figure-of-eight measurements. All of these have shown good reliability in other patient populations.[24-26] These measures are commonly used in burn care settings and apply well to the measurement of burn-related edema. To avoid cross-contamination when measuring edema on a limb with an open burn wound, volumeters must be carefully cleaned after each use and measuring tapes must be disposed of or cleaned.

Range of Motion. Wound contraction, edema, and pain commonly cause restrictions of ROM in patients with burns. Wound contraction has beneficial and detrimental effects. On the positive side, it decreases wound size. On the negative side, wound contraction can impair mobility and function, and generally has poor cosmesis. If a wound heals with scarring, scar contraction creates nearly all of the late adverse sequelae of burns.[27]

Edema can limit motion because of its influence on the space within and around joints. The accumulation of exudate associated with edema may also lead to fibrosis further impeding tissue mobility.[28,29]

Pain may inhibit motion simply because of a patient's avoidance of the painful motion or their anticipation of pain with movement.

Muscle Performance. Strength testing in patients with burns can be performed similarly to other patients without burns. Manual muscle testing using standard grading (normal, good, fair, poor, trace, or the 0-5 scale) or using hand-held dynamometry should be as reliable in any age group of patients with burns as it is in patients without burns.[30-32] Other strategies for testing muscle strength, such as isokinetic testing, can also be applied in this population (see Chapter 5).[33-35] The only special caution with this population is to avoid applying excessive force to a painful burn or to a site that is healing and has fragile new tissue. Testing that requires contact over these sites should be avoided until the tissue heals sufficiently for this to be safe. There should be few restrictions in testing for at least fair grade muscle strength, which only requires movement against gravity, except for a few days when immobilization is required after surgical skin grafting.

The loss of lean body mass caused by the catabolism of muscle protein associated with burn trauma can result in decreased strength. Suman et al used many measures to study muscle strength and lean body mass in 35 children with burns.[33] Although they used dual-energy x-ray absorptiometry (DXA) to measure lean body mass, they could have used skinfold-thickness measurements, bioelectrical impedance, body mass index (BMI), and if available, even hydrostatic weighing for this measure. Although these additional measures do not appear to be as sensitive as DXA, they may be appropriate for many applications given their cost and convenience. Considerations for the use of any of these methods must include the location of burn wounds, and at later stages of healing, one should consider that skinfold measurements performed over scar tissue may not provide valid information. Research into the reliability and validity of these measurement tools for examining lean body mass, with an associated correlation to strength deficits, in patients with burns is needed.

Neuromuscular

Pain. Pain is a predictable result of a burn. The pain caused by a burn is generally described as "burning," "severe," or "acute."[36] Local pain is caused by the release of local inflammatory mediators and damage to nerve endings. Generalized pain is likely related to circulation of these inflammatory mediators, a patient's pain tolerance or perception, and anxiety about the injury or care.[37] *Superficial burns* are very painful, and any large burn, including deep burns, will provoke continuous background pain that occurs at rest as well as with activity. Certain care procedures, such as dressing changes and some exercises, can increase pain. This procedural-related pain generally declines over time.[37,38] Procedural pain is generally described as feeling different from the background pain associated with the burn wound. Procedural pain is often described as "stabbing," "severe," or "excruciating."[36]

Several common pain measures can be used to assess pain in patients with burns. A visual analog scale (VAS) for pain can be used to rate the severity of the pain on a numeric scale (e.g., 0 to 10 where 0 is no pain and 10 is unbearable pain). Children and adults may prefer a scale with visual representation of pain with tools, such as the faces pain scale (FPS) or a standardized color analog scale (see Chapter 22). In one study, patients with burns preferred the face and color scales to the numeric VAS, but the authors of this study also recommended further study.[38] Besides rating pain severity, the location of pain as related by the patient should also be documented. Furthermore, it is important to measure pain at rest, as well as during specific procedures or activities, such as wound care sessions or tissue stretching, which may worsen the pain. Knowing which activities produce more pain can help determine the type and timing of pain-relieving measures.

After the burn wound has healed, pruritus (itching) generally replaces pain as the predominant aberrant sensation in patients with burns. The severity of pruritus can be measured clinically with a VAS. The intensity of pruritus often diminishes as the remodeling phase of wound healing nears completion.

Peripheral Nerve Integrity. Peripheral neuropathy is the most common neurological complication of burn injury.[39] Mononeuropathy and peripheral neuropathy occur to varying degrees in many patients (see Chapter 18). Neuropathy is most commonly caused by electrical burns but is also more likely in patients who chronically abuse alcohol, are critically ill, severely burned, or elderly.[39] Over time, iatrogenic factors, such as improper limb positioning, improper application of compression dressings, or poorly fitted splints, can also contribute to the incidence of neuropathy.

Cardiovascular/Pulmonary. Direct cardiovascular and pulmonary responses to burn injury are mainly related to fluid moving from the blood vessels to the interstitium. This causes "burn shock" that is manifest by hypotension and relative hypothermia. Therefore blood pressure and body temperature should always be checked in patients with burns (see Chapter 22). The fluid shifts and hypotension associated with burn shock can impair perfusion of core organs, including the heart, lungs, and kidneys. Decreased perfusion of the heart and lungs, along with pulmonary edema can cause pulmonary compromise, which in conjunction with bed rest and decreased pulmonary activity can increase the risk for pneumonia and respiratory failure.

Burn shock is also associated with decreased cardiac output.[40] This cardiac compromise may be a result of the vascular fluid shifts and/or decreased efflux of calcium from myocardial sarcoplasmic reticulum.[41] Once plasma fluid volumes are regulated, cardiac function can be expected to normalize.

Inhalation injury is often associated with burns that occur in enclosed spaces such as buildings. Inhalation injury is irritation or cellular damage to lung tissue caused by toxic gases, steam vapors, or chemicals in the air coupled with a burn event. Patients with inhalation injury are at increased risk for pneumonia and respiratory failure. Patients with burns who have an associated inhalation injury have a sixfold higher mortality rate than those without inhalation injury.[42]

Aerobic Capacity. The lungs are a target of the burn-related inflammatory response even if there is no inhalation injury. The inflammatory response can cause acute pulmonary edema that decreases diffusion of oxygen from the alveoli to the vascular system.[43] This situation contributes to decreased aerobic capacity. One report suggests that although pulmonary function improves after injury, decreased pulmonary function may last as long as 5 months after the actual burn injury.[44] Inhalation injury exacerbates cardiopulmonary problems in a patient with burns because of direct damage to lung tissue.

Loss of muscle caused by increased muscle catabolism and decreased activity after an acute burn leads to decreased activity. Decreases in physical activity may contribute to decreases in aerobic capacity.

There are no published studies on specific tests of aerobic capacity or endurance for patients with burns, therefore, standard physiological measures of blood pressure, heart rate, respiratory rate, oxygen saturation, and ratings of perceived exertion (RPE) for appraising aerobic capacity are recommended (see Chapters 22 and 26). The following tests and measures could be used to examine aerobic capacity: Peak oxygen consumption ($\dot{V}O_{2max}$) and resting energy expenditure (see Chapter 23).

Integumentary

Burn Depth. The depth of a burn is related to the temperature and duration of exposure to extreme heat. The cause of the burn affects wound depth because different materials have different maximum burning temperatures, specific heats, and thermal conductivity and certain chemicals are more caustic than others. If skin is exposed to temperatures of 60° C (140° F) for more than 1 second, epidermal loss causing a *partial-thickness burn* will occur. If the temperature is increased to 70° C (158° F), a *full-thickness burn* will occur after 1 second.[45]

The depth of a burn is classified by the amount or type of tissue destroyed and can be determined by the presence of certain clinical findings.[1] The classification of depth of injury corresponds to the classifications of integumentary impairment provided in the *Guide to Physical Therapist Practice.*[46]

Superficial burns (preferred practice pattern 7B: Impaired integumentary integrity associated with superficial skin involvement, also referred to as first-degree burns) involve limited damage to the epithelial cells without exposure of dermal tissue. Sunburn is a common example of a superficial burn injury. A superficial burn is painful, dry, and erythematous and may exhibit some minor localized swelling. Superficial burns should heal in 3-5 days without scarring.[47]

Partial-thickness burns (preferred practice pattern 7C: Impaired integumentary integrity associated with partial-thickness skin involvement and scar formation, also referred to as second-degree burns) involve damage to the dermis and may be separated into subclassifications of superficial or deep partial-thickness burns (Fig. 31-1). Superficial partial-thickness burns exhibit destruction of the epidermis and minimal damage to the superficial layers of the dermis. Preservation of epidermal appendages, such as hair follicles and sweat glands, in this depth of burn allows for complete healing within 21 days with

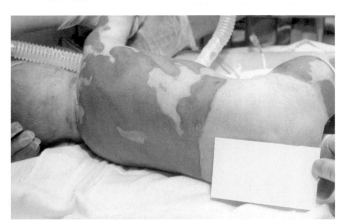

FIG. 31-1 A partial-thickness burn.

little or no scarring.[47] In deep partial-thickness burns, the epidermis and almost all of the dermis is destroyed, leaving very few epidermal appendages. Deep partial-thickness burns take longer than 21 days to heal and will heal with scarring. These wounds generally require skin grafting to close. All partial-thickness wounds are very painful, red, and weepy and have normal pliability. Blistering is associated with a partial-thickness burn.

A full-thickness burn (preferred practice pattern 7D: Impaired integumentary integrity associated with full-thickness skin involvement and scar formation, also referred to as a third-degree burn) involve complete destruction of the epidermis and dermis (Fig. 31-2). These burns require skin grafting to heal functionally. If allowed to heal on their own, they may take several weeks to heal and will scar.[47] Full-thickness burns are usually not painful with palpation because the nerves are no longer intact. They may be a tan or yellowish-brown color, and are generally leathery, with nonpliable skin.

Burn Size. The size of a burn injury is usually described as an estimate of the percentage of the total body surface area (%TBSA) that is affected. This estimate helps predict the magnitude of physiological response to the injury, including fluid loss and catabolism. The larger the burn injury, the larger the physiological responses will be. The two most common methods used to estimate burn size are the Rule of Nines and the Lund and Browder chart.[48] The Rule of Nines method estimates body surface area by dividing the body into 11 segments, each accounting for 9% of the surface area, plus another 1% for the genitals (Fig. 31-3). Charts with the body divided into these segments are often used to document and calculate burn surface area by this method. The Lund and Browder method uses a standard table for estimating surface area based on the part(s) of the body burned. Charts that include a body illustration on which the burn location is marked and a table to estimate burn size are often used for documentation when this method is used (Figure 31-4). The Lund and Browder chart was initially published in 1944 and has since been modified to take into account proportional changes in the surface area of body parts that occur during growth and development.[49] This method for estimating burn size has been shown to be reliable when completed by experienced burn care providers.[48]

Scar. Although scars do not occur immediately after a burn, scarring is one of the most problematic late morbidities associated with burn injury and wound healing. Scar assessment should be performed during reexamination of patients initially seen with acute burns whose wounds are now healing or healed, or during initial examination of a patient with healed burns. Scar assessment is performed mainly by observation and palpation. An actively maturing scar that is still forming is characterized by a rigid texture or lack of extensibility, an inflamed appearance (redness), some possible pigment changes (such as purple), and hypertrophy. It generally requires 6-18 months after the initial burn for a scar to "mature" or complete forming.[50] The most common variables used to quantify and document findings from examination of scar are the level of hypertrophy (height), the amount of redness or inflammation (vascularity), level of extensibility (pliability), and the amount of contraction.[1,51] The height of hypertrophy is generally measured with a ruler and the amount of redness is described qualitatively. Pliability is also generally described qualitatively; however, a device for quantifying pliability is available and may produce more accurate data for tracking changes over time.[52]

Two pathological types of scars can occur after burns. Burns generally cause *hypertrophic scars* (Fig. 31-5). This type of scar is excessive but stays within the boundaries of the original wound. In contrast, *keloid scars,* which are also excessive, extend beyond the boundaries of the primary wound. Both hypertrophic and keloid scars are prone to contraction.

Since 1990, the Vancouver Burn Scar Scale, or modifications of this scale, are the most commonly used assess-

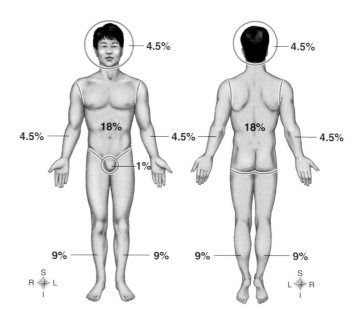

FIG. 31-3 Rule of Nines chart for estimating the surface area or size of a burn injury. The Rule of Nines divides the surface area of the body into 11 segments of 9% each, with the genitals equaling 1% of the body surface area. *From Thibodeau GA, Patton KT:* Anatomy and Physiology, *ed 6, St. Louis, 2006, Mosby.*

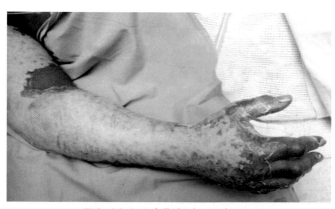

FIG. 31-2 A full-thickness burn.

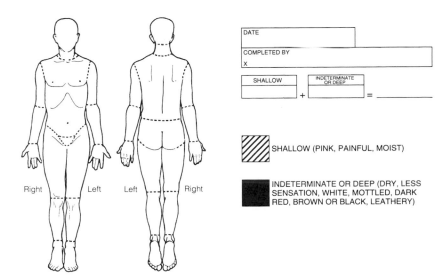

Percent surface area burned
(Berkow formula)

AREA	1 YEAR	1 to 4 YEARS	5 to 9 YEARS	10 to 14 YEARS	Y 15 YEARS	ADULT	SHALLOW	INDETERMINATE OR DEEP
Head	10	17	13	11	9	7		
Neck	2	2	2	2	2	2		
Ant. Trunk	13	13	13	13	13	13		
Post.Trunk	13	13	13	13	13	13		
R. Buttock	2½	2½	2½	2½	2½	2½		
L. Buttock	2½	2½	2½	2½	2½	2½		
Genitalia	1	1	1	1	1	1		
R. U. Arm	4	4	4	4	4	4		
L. U. Arm	4	4	4	4	4	4		
R. L. Arm	3	3	3	3	3	3		
L. L. Arm	3	3	3	3	3	3		
R. Hand	2½	2½	2½	2½	2½	2½		
L. Hand	2½	2½	2½	2½	2½	2½		
R. Thigh	5½	6½	8	8½	9	9½		
L. Thigh	5½	6½	8	8½	9	9½		
R. Leg	5	5	5½	6	6½	7		
L. Leg	5	5	5½	6	6½	7		
R. Foot	3½	3½	3½	3½	3½	3½		
L. Foot	3½	3½	3½	3½	3½	3½		
TOTAL								

FIG. 31-4 The Lund and Browder chart for estimating the surface area or size of a burn injury. The Lund and Browder chart allows for estimation of the surface area of the burn injury through growth and development. *From Goodman CC, Boissonnault WG, Fuller KS: Pathology: Implications for the Physical Therapist, ed 2, Philadelphia, 2002, Saunders.*

ment tools for burn scars[51] (Table 31-1). The reliability of the Vancouver Burn Scar Scale for the variables of height, vascularity, pigment (the color of the scar), and pliability was evaluated in 73 patients with burns. The Cohen's kappa (κ) value was approximately 0.5 for each variable for each rating pair, indicating that there is moderate interrater agreement using this scale. Height was the vertical elevation of the scar above normal skin, in millimeters. Vascularity was determined by observing the amount of redness in the scar and by blanching the scar to view the amount and rate of blood return. Pigmentation was judged by blanching the scar, comparing it to normal skin color and grading it as normally pigmented, hypopigmented or hyperpigmented. Pigmentation is the variable most frequently excluded from modified versions of the

Vancouver Burn Scar Scale. Pliability was measured by palpating the suppleness of the skin. The Vancouver Burn Scar Scale should be applied to the most severe parts of the scar being measured.

Function

Gait. Gait should be examined and evaluated in patients with lower extremity burns. Gait deviations can be related to pain, alterations in ROM, wound or scar contraction, and changes in strength. Any associated injury that might affect gait should be considered in the gait evaluation and any preexisting condition or associated injury that might affect balance and safety must also be considered when prescribing a locomotion program.

TABLE 31-1	Scores Used in the Vancouver Burn Scar Scale to Assess Burn Scar			
Score	Height	Vascularity	Pigmentation	Pliability
0	Normal; flat	Normal; color closely resembles the color over the rest of the person's body.	Normal; color closely resembles the color over the rest of the person's body.	Normal.
1	Raised <2 mm	Pink.	Hypopigmentation.	Supple; flexible with minimal resistance.
2	Raised <5 mm	Red.	Hyperpigmentation.	Yielding; gives way to pressure.
3	Raised >5 mm	Purple.		Firm; inflexible, does not move easily, resistant to manual pressure.
4				Banding; tissue is rope-like and blanches when the scar is extended.
5				Contracture; the scar is permanently shortened producing a deformity or distortion.

Adapted from Sullivan T, Smith J, Kermode J, et al: *J Burn Care Rehabil* 11(3):256-260, 1990.

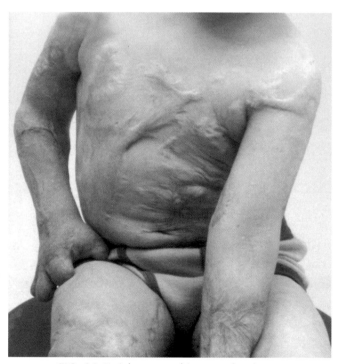

FIG. 31-5 A hypertrophic scar after burn.

Silverberg et al studied the gait of 25 adults with lower extremity burns within 5 days of discharge from an acute care facility.[53] Using an instrumented walkway to collect temporal and spatial measures of gait, this group found that cycle time and base of support were significantly greater in patients with burns than in uninjured subjects. No predictive data or information relating these gait alterations to functional activities are provided in the report of this study.

Although no further data exist regarding specific examination of gait in patients with burns, it is reasonable to consider the use of standard gait examination and assessment tools (see Chapter 32) to examine gait patterns in patients with burns.

Self-Care and Home Management. There are no specific tests for the measurement of burn-related decreases in self-care and home management. The Jebsen Hand Function Test and the Nine-Hole Peg Test have been used in studies to measure upper extremity function after burns.[54,55] Although these tests measure components of hand function and dexterity, not enough data exist to recommend their use in predicting function. The ability to carry out specific activities, such as feeding, dressing (e.g., buttoning, zipping, and tying), and hygiene activities (e.g., brushing teeth, combing hair, and toileting), are often documented and used to examine self-care in this population.

EVALUATION, DIAGNOSIS, AND PROGNOSIS

Burns over certain anatomical locations, such as joints, can cause crucial challenges in rehabilitation for the patient and the burn care provider. With increased burn size, burn-related impairments will generally also be greater, increasing the therapeutic needs of the patient. Impairments may be acute, secondary to pain or wound contraction in superficial-, partial-, and full-thickness burns. In addition, wound and scar *contracture* at a burn site can lead to chronic struggles with decreased function and disability and with certain burn locations, poor cosmesis may have implications for long-term socialization of the patient with burns.

Burn wound depth also impacts prognosis. Superficial-thickness burns will heal within a few days with little if any risk for impairment. In the absence of wound complications, partial-thickness burns generally heal without scarring within 14 days. Full-thickness burns are generally treated with skin grafting to accelerate healing and decrease the risk for complications such as infection, fluid loss, and excessive scarring. Full-thickness wounds, if not skin grafted, can take several weeks to heal and scarring can be severe. Scar contraction can occur at any time during the tissue remodeling phase, which lasts an average of 12 months, with ranges of at least 6-18 months.[50,56]

Some patients with burns may have long-term difficulties with self-care and home and work management. Cheng and Rogers found, based on interviews with ten male patients, much variability in functional outcome after severe burns.[57] Some of those interviewed returned to all their previous activities, including work, while others were independent in activities of daily living but were unable to return to full work activities and yet others had major limitations in self-care and work-related activities.

A report that included a literature review and a case series of 303 patients with burns found that patients stay off work for an average of almost 10 weeks after a burn.[58] This average time for returning to work was related to the size of the burn (larger burn → longer time off work) and the age of the patient (increased age → longer time off work). Also, in some cases, burns to the hand or upper extremity further delayed return to work. In this case series, a majority (55% to 90%) of the patients returned to some form of work by 6-24 months after the burn; however, at 24 months, only 37% of patients had returned to the same job with the same employer as before their burn. Others had taken new jobs with an old employer or simply taken different jobs altogether.

INTERVENTION

WOUND CARE

Care of burn wounds is determined primarily by the depth and location of the injury. Superficial burn wounds are typically treated with a lotion to increase moisture in the injured tissue and to enhance pliability of the damaged dry skin. Lotions without added perfume are recommended to decrease the risk of further irritating already inflamed skin.

Partial-thickness wounds are moist and should be kept moist. They can be gently cleansed using a mild soap and then dressed. Loose tissue should be debrided. Dressing should include a topical agent such as an antimicrobial ointment (e.g., bacitracin, combination bacitracin/polymyxin [Polysporin] or combination bacitracin/polymyxin/neomycin [Neosporin]) or an antimicrobial cream (e.g., silver sulfadiazine[59-61]). Chapter 28 provides general information on topical agents and dressings used in wound management.

Ointments and creams make the wound more comfortable and most include an antimicrobial agent to decrease local microbial growth. Ointments, which are typically used on partial-thickness wounds, are more lubricating and occlusive than other topical medications and are not water miscible, whereas creams are normally more soothing to the patient and are more easily washed off because they are water miscible. If an ointment is used to cover the wound, a dry gauze wrap should be used to cover the ointment. Creams should first be covered with a petroleum-impregnated gauze dressing, which is then held in place with a dry gauze wrap. Topical agents should be changed no less than once a day, with twice a day changes being optimal.

Following cleaning and any necessary debridement of loose tissue, deep-partial thickness and full-thickness burns should be covered with a topical antimicrobial agent and dressings until surgery for skin grafting can be completed. The most common dressing protocol for these wounds is to apply an antimicrobial ointment, such as silver sulfadiazine, directly to the wound and cover it with a dry gauze sheet or wrap.

Deep partial-thickness and full-thickness burns have the best outcome when treated surgically. The most common surgery to treat these deep wounds is excision of the burn eschar and coverage of the excised wound with skin grafts. Surgical coverage of the burn wound decreases the risk of sepsis. Early surgical coverage also accelerates healing, which in turn leads to less scarring and thus greater probability of good functional and cosmetic outcomes.

Following a skin graft, the graft must not be disturbed by movement or pressure until it becomes vascularized and adhered to the tissue bed. This generally takes at least 48 hours. Skin grafts to the lower extremities require caution when the leg is placed in a dependent position because of the risk of increased edema and pressure. Most clinicians therefore recommend supporting venous return in the lower extremity with some form of compression, such as elastic bandages, for the first 7-10 days after a graft procedure. If there is any concern that one wrap will not provide enough pressure support for a graft, a double wrap can be used.

Moisturizers should be used on healed wounds to decrease pruritus and skin cracking associated with dryness. Lotions without added perfumes are suggested on newly healed tissue to decrease the likelihood of developing a localized rashes or irritation.

EDEMA CONTROL

Edema control may be accomplished with various interventions. A positioning program, concentrating not only on preserving motion and proper joint position but also on elevation, is customary in the care of acutely burned extremities. Although no specific data about the most effective duration or height of extremity elevation exists, elevation of an extremity does allow gravity to assist with draining excessive interstitial fluid from the limb and decreases hydrostatic pressure in the blood vessels.[62]

Burn-related edema is also treated with compression. Compression may support tissue hydrostatic pressure and facilitate venous and lymphatic flow.[63] Elastic wraps, self-adherent stretch and static wraps, elasticized dressings, scar compression supports, and intermittent compression pumps are all used to provide compression in this population. Wraps that provide more consistent compression than intermittent pumps may better serve patients with burn-related edema. Ause-Ellias et al studied the use of intermittent compression in five patients with hand edema resulting from a burn and found no significant difference between volumetric measurements of the burned and nonburned hands before and after treatment.[64] Lowell et al published a case study describing the use of a compression wrap (Coban, 3M, St. Paul, MN) to affect edema and hand function in a patient with both hands burned. The hand that was wrapped in Coban had less edema (measured by circumferential measurements) than the unwrapped (control) hand over a 2-week course. Once the control hand was wrapped the edema in it also decreased.[55]

Many factors should be considered when applying compression wraps, including the amount of pressure, the direction of wrap, and the type of wrapping used. The amount of compression will vary with the type of material being used and the force of application of the material. It is recommended that wraps be applied with gentle firmness and wrapped in a spiral or figure-of-eight pattern (to avoid a tourniquet effect) from distal to proximal on the digit or extremity. It should also be remembered that overlapping layers of compression material will provide more pressure in the area of overlap. No data currently exist comparing the use of elastic wraps to static wraps to treat edema in patients with burns. Static wraps might be useful if chronic edema exists and more research is needed to determine whether the chronic edema in patients with burns may indeed be lymphedema and whether this persistent edema would be amenable to interventions commonly directed at clearing lymphedema such as complete decongestive therapy or manual lymphatic drainage (see Chapter 27).[65]

PAIN CONTROL

Pain experienced with wound care and other therapeutic procedures may be partially managed with pharmaceuticals. In addition, preparing the patient for the intervention (preparatory information), behavioral techniques, and cognitive techniques may also help alleviate pain during treatment sessions.[66]

Preparing a patient for the intervention should include an explanation of what will be done and how it might make the patient feel (procedural information and sensory information, respectively). For example, a patient could be told that as they sit by the side of a mat, their arm will be placed on the mat and their elbow will be stretched to try to straighten the elbow joint (procedural information). The patient can then be told that stretching the elbow may cause a feeling of tightness throughout the arm as the tissue stretches (sensory information). In a comprehensive review article related to burn pain, Everett et al described how preparatory information can decrease a patient's anxiety and pain.[36]

Reinforcement is the most common type of behavioral pain control strategy used by physical therapists (PTs). This involves encouraging the patient to focus on something other than the pain they feel and not allowing pain to become a determining factor in stopping a particular intervention. This technique requires that a preset criterion or "goal" for a specific intervention session is clearly outlined. The therapist and the patient work toward that "goal" and rewards, such as rest, are given related to the "goal" and not the amount of pain.

Distraction and reappraisal are examples of cognitive techniques frequently used to manage procedural burn pain. Distraction involves engaging the patient in thinking about something other than the painful intervention. Patients may be distracted in many ways, such as being asked to focus on a "relaxing" place, spelling words, or playing games. The therapist must be sensitive to the culture and capability of a patient to determine appropriate distraction techniques for individual patients. Reappraisal involves clarifying the purpose and benefits of an intervention. For example, when pain associated with dressing changes and stretching is interpreted by the patients as doing more harm than good, reappraisal would involve explaining to the patient that the pain caused by this procedure is not causing additional tissue injury and cannot be avoided. The patient may also accept that the pain may be a "good" sign of an appropriate, albeit possibly uncomfortable, tissue response.

Similar techniques can be used to help a patient manage pruritus. Additionally, systemic and topical medications, as well as standard moisturizers, may reduce pruritus.

STRENGTHENING EXERCISES

No evidence-based strengthening protocols exist for patients with burns. However, the indications for strengthening exercises are similar to those for any person with muscle weakness secondary to hypercatabolism and disuse. A program of progressive resistive exercise that addresses strength and mobility should be used.

Exercise activities and equipment that encourage mobilization of a joint or complex of joints should always be considered when prescribing an exercise program for the patient with burns because they are at high risk for loss of motion because of scarring. A patient may be given any set of traditional exercises using any piece of equipment. Standard recommendations for resistance training can be followed (see Chapter 5). Exercises that train major muscle groups should be included along with exercises that focus on areas of weakness found in the examination. To increase strength the exercises should be performed to the point of volitional fatigue at least twice a week through full available ROM.[67] A warm-up of up to 15 repetitions without weight with a rest period is also recommended.[67] There are no inherent contraindications to the prescription of strengthening exercises for patients with a burn injury. However, caution should be taken to avoid disrupting new skin grafts or sutures when exercising a patient after surgery, when exercising joints with associated exposed joint structure or tendons, and when exercising in the presence of a medical comorbidity such as a significant cardiac or orthopedic condition.

RANGE OF MOTION EXERCISES

Passive ROM exercises are beneficial when soft tissue restricts motion and the patient has insufficient strength or endurance to overcome the force of the soft tissue restriction for a long enough time to elongate the tissue. This is also a useful technique when patients cannot move because of sedation or critical illness or, for some other reason, cannot respond, voluntarily move or otherwise actively participate in their program. The motion should be performed slowly enough to allow for tissue elongation, the hold time should be tolerable for the patient, and the end-range should have a "leathery" or "tissue stretch" end-feel. After wound closure, this end-feel should be accompanied by visible blanching of the scar.

When end-range can be achieved actively, active-assistive and active ROM exercises are preferred to passive motion because this promotes greater patient independence. Patients should be instructed to hold the stretch for at least 30-60 seconds and should monitor their response to the stretch. Generally, a patient should feel only mild-to-moderate pain during a session and note increased mobility after stretching.

ROM exercises should be performed in anatomical planes and focus on opposing the direction of wound and scar tissue contraction forces. For example, if a wound is located over a flexor surface, the ROM exercises should emphasize extension. If joint motion is restricted and gains are not made with appropriate ROM exercises, joint mobilization can be considered. The PT should examine the tissue before hand placement and implementation of joint mobilization to determine if the tissue will tolerate hand placement and any associated sheer forces.

It is recommended that ROM exercises be started early in care, and the exercises should remain consistent through progression from passive to active so that the performance of the ROM almost becomes "habitual" for the patient. This is important because of the extended period of time it takes the scar to remodel (see Evaluation, Diagnosis, and Prognosis section).

Positioning, also mentioned under interventions for edema, can be used to help preserve gains in ROM or to achieve gains in ROM.[68] Positioning is used to counteract wound contraction. Standard anticontracture positions are outlined in Table 31-2.

Splinting can be used to prevent deformity from contracture, to maintain or increase ROM, and to protect a fragile area of tissue.[69] Three common types of splinting interventions are used in burn care: Serial, static, and dynamic splinting. Serial splinting involves making a splint that positions the involved tissue at the limit of its current ROM and then successively remolding the splint toward greater ROM as ROM is increased by exercise, passive mobilization, or positioning. Static splinting immobilizes a joint to maintain its position. Dynamic splinting applies an ongoing, generally mild, force to a body part to either mobilize it or to provide resistance for exercise.

Malleable thermoplastic material is most commonly used in burn care to fabricate individualized conforming splints for specific body parts and purposes. Splinting should be modified or discontinued if the patient develops skin or wound breakdown, pain, or other sensory impairments. Since splints frequently harbor microorganisms, they should be cleaned on a regular basis with a quaternary ammonia solution (1 fluid ounce per gallon of water).[70]

AMBULATION

Regardless of the location of the burn, patients can be prescribed a walking program to mitigate problems related to bedrest such as dependence, cardiovascular and pulmonary compromise including hypotension, and decreased ROM and diminished strength. An intervention program that includes ambulation may begin once the patient is medically stable, alert, and able to follow directions. Although burn care centers have many different protocols for ambulation after burn injury, most clinicians recommend starting ambulation as early as possible. Because of the cardiovascular consequences of the fluid shifts associated with large burns, physiological responses to ambulation should be monitored, particularly in the acute phase of care.

The effects of gravity may cause patients with lower extremity edema to feel pain and other sensations, such as tingling, when they first put their legs in a dependent position to prepare for walking. However, these sensations generally subside with ambulation as the muscle contractions help to pump fluid proximally. If the pain does not decrease with walking, supportive elastic bandage wraps that provide some vascular support will generally help decrease the pain.[71]

If there has been skin grafting of the lower extremities, the extremities should be wrapped with elastic bandage whenever they are in a dependent position for sitting or ambulation, until the graft has fully taken. This is to support the graft and prevent excessive vascular pressures that might lead to bleeding and pooling of blood between the graft and the tissue bed. Such bleeding and pooling can separate the skin graft from the vascular tissue bed to which it must adhere, causing graft disruption and failure. In burn centers, dependence of a grafted lower extremity is initiated with caution, starting with dangling the leg for a minute or two and then elevating the extremity, unwrapping it, and checking for bleeding and graft integrity. If the graft tolerated this, then the duration of dependence can be increased and the patient can try to ambulate. No standards exist for when ambulation may first be attempted after grafting, but it has been documented to occur as early as 1 day after surgery, with the average across the country being about 7 days after surgery.[72] Once the skin graft has taken, ambulation can occur without any graft-related restrictions.

Standard guarding techniques and assistive ambulation devices can be used if necessary. Open- or closed-chain

TABLE 31-2	Recommended Anticontracture Positions for Patients with Burns
Anatomical Area	**Preferred Position**
Neck	Slight hyperextension; no rotation
Shoulder	Abduction (90-110°); slight horizontal flexion
Elbow	Extension; supination
Wrist/hand	Slight wrist extension, slight MCP flexion, PIP and DIP extension, thumb abduction
Trunk	Straight postural alignment
Hip	Extension, abduction (20°), no rotation
Knee	Full extension
Ankle/foot	Neutral ankle (no planterflexion), neutral toe position (no dorsiflexion or plantarflexion)

MCP, Metacarpophalangeal; *PIP*, proximal interphalangeal; *DIP*, distal interphalangeal.

exercises directed at specific limitations in gait should be considered as part of the intervention program.

AEROBIC CONDITIONING

Patients with burns need aerobic conditioning because of the catabolic nature of the injury and the disuse frequently associated with inactivity imposed by the injury or surgical interventions. The metabolic demand of burn wound healing can affect various physiological parameters, including heart rate and blood pressure,[73] body temperature,[74-78] respiratory rate and ventilation,[73,79] and rating of perceived exertion (RPE).[73,80] Therefore these signs should be monitored with any strenuous exercise but should not preclude aerobic exercise during burn rehabilitation. To accommodate the physiological stress produced by a burn, an RPE of 12-16 has been recommended for aerobic conditioning in patients with burns.[81]

Standard protocols for aerobic conditioning can be applied to this population (see Chapter 23). The exercise intensity, duration, frequency, and mode should be selected and progressed according to the patient's tolerance. Progression should allow for adaptation to the program and take into consideration the likelihood of interruptions, or regression at times, if the patient has surgeries or other medical care needs or complications. Patients may generally begin with a program that lasts between 15 and 30 minutes 3-5 times per week and progress the exercise intensity and/or duration gradually over about a 3-6 week period. Some patients will need to start with shorter and more frequent periods of exercise.[81]

Exercise for aerobic conditioning should focus on large muscle groups and rhythmic activities such as cycling, walking, or running.[81] Standard aerobic exercise equipment, such as treadmills, upper and lower extremity ergometers, and stair steppers, can be safely used in the treatment of patients with burns. The only limiting factors for using any of these devices may be location of the burn and associated pain. Aerobic exercises may be combined with exercises intended to increase ROM. For example, cycling on an exercise bicycle may improve aerobic conditioning and increase knee flexion ROM.

SCAR MANAGEMENT

Since this chapter focuses on conservative rehabilitation management after burns, surgical and pharmacological interventions for scarring are not discussed. ROM exercises, positioning, and splinting may be used to preserve joint and soft tissue mobility that can be lost as a result of scarring. Although there is no evidence for this, it is generally assumed that lengthening scar tissue during the proliferation and remodeling phases of healing by moving it through its normal anatomic and functional range improves the alignment of the scar tissue being deposited. It is known that, during remodeling, scar tissue is deposited in a disorganized fashion without specific alignment.[82]

Pressure therapy is often recommended for hypertrophic scars because it is thought to help the scar conform to the shape of the underlying tissue.[83] Pressure may also alter scar hypertrophy by decreasing capillary flow to the fibroblasts (thereby decreasing collagen formation) or by decreasing edema or excess deposition of mucopolysaccharides in the tissue matrix.[82,84] The amount of pressure often recommended is 25 mm Hg, which is close to average capillary pressure.[85] However, Cheng et al found that although the pressure produced by custom-made pressure garments on 50 patients with burns was often below 5-15 mm Hg, as measured with an electro-pneumatic pressure transducer, they still had a positive effect on scar outcome.[86] It has also been suggested that pressure garments affect scar formation by increasing temperature and thus the activity of temperature-sensitive enzymes such as collagenase, which breaks down collagen.[87]

Pressure may be applied in a variety of ways. Standard elastic wraps and self-adherent wraps, such as Coban (3M, St. Paul, MN), and tubular cotton bandages, such as Tubigrip (SePro Healthcare, Morristown, NJ), are often used to apply pressure to control edema or prevent excessive scarring shortly after a burn injury and can also be used to apply pressure during later phases of scar treatment. Custom-fit pressure garments are most commonly used to apply pressure to areas with or at risk for hypertrophic scarring after a burn. These pressure support garments can be made to fit any extremity, the torso, the head, the face, and the hands. For optimal outcome, these garments should fit closely and apply even pressure to all areas of tissue injury. Follow-up visits should occur regularly to check and arrange for adjustment of the fit of the support if necessary.[84] These garments should be worn 23 hours a day throughout the remodeling period, which may be as long as 2 years after the initial injury. Pressure garments are available in various colors, which may help with patient self-esteem and compliance.[88] Although some patients may complain that these garments feel like they restrict movement during exercise, a study found that measured ROM at 80 burn-affected joints in 17 patients were not significantly different with the subject wearing or not wearing appropriately fitted pressure support garments.[89]

Silicone gel sheets have been used to treat scarring after burns since the 1980s.[90-92] It has been shown that this intervention decreases hypertrophy and redness of the forming scar.[90-93] It is generally recommend that this be applied during scar remodeling, since later application is unlikely to change the scar.[94] The mechanism for the effects of silicone gel on scar formation is not known. However, as with pressure garments, silicone gel may exert its effect by increasing local temperature.[95] Silicone gel sheets are thin and pliable and are applied directly over the scar to be treated. They are typically used over smaller areas of scarring or in locations where adequate pressure is difficult to administer by other means. No specific guidelines exist for how long silicone gel should be applied. Most clinicians use the intervention until the scar has flattened and the vascularity has decreased. If signs of remodeling, such as redness or hypertrophy, reappear, the gel is reapplied. Complications of this intervention may include rash or skin breakdown. Typically, a rash related to silicone gel sheeting will clear after the removal of the product and once the rash clears the product can be reapplied without reoccurrence.

Little data exist to support the use of massage for superficial scars. One study has been published that examined the effects of massage on hypertrophic scar using the outcome variables from the Vancouver Burn Scar Scale.[96] Thirty pediatric patients with burn scars were treated with friction massage to an area of the scar over a 3-month period. None of the variables of vascularity, pliability, and height showed significant progress after the friction massage, although pliability showed a trend toward improvement. However, massage may decrease pain, itching, and anxiety.[96,97]

IMPROVING FUNCTIONAL SELF-CARE AND HOME MANAGEMENT

Edema, pain, lack of mobility, and loss of strength after burn injury often combine to decrease a patient's ability to execute functional tasks. These impairments can range from simple but important self-care skills to more complex proficiency in home and work duties. Therefore exercises should address mobility and strength, as well as specific motor programming requirements for particular skills. Early in care, functional exercise may focus on basic self-care activities such as hygiene, feeding, and dressing. These activities can then be progressed to exercises that prepare the patient for jobs in the home and at work. Specific work-directed and work-hardening programs can be instituted at the judgment of the practitioner to prepare the patient to return to a particular work setting.

REHABILITATION FOR ASSOCIATED INJURIES

No specific rehabilitation intervention can be linked in the literature to inhalation injury. However, as the patient progresses through medical pulmonary care and therapy, evaluating and working to increase ventilation through a program that increases general mobility and improves endurance will likely be beneficial (see Chapters 24 and 26).[98]

The functional consequences of peripheral neuropathy in patients with burns should receive similar interventions to those applied to other patients with peripheral neuropathy (see Chapter 18). Most importantly, efforts should be taken to prevent iatrogenic neuropathy that results from pressure or poor positioning. Patients who are positioned, splinted, or bandaged should be monitored frequently to assure that no symptoms of neuropathy, such as distal numbness, pain, or weakness, are present. Areas at increased risk for neuropathy are the shoulder (brachial plexus), the elbow (ulnar nerve), and the knee (peroneal nerve).[99] Edema may also increase the risk for a pressure-related nerve compression injury.

In children and adults with burns, fractures can be successfully managed with either internal or external fixation without necessarily increasing the risk for infection.[100-102] After fracture fixation, rehabilitation of fracture-related impairments in patients with burns can proceed as it would for any other patient (see Chapter 9).

CASE STUDY 31-1

FULL-THICKNESS BURN

The following case study is presented in three sections: Immediate acute phase (presurgery), acute phase (post-surgery/inpatient), and rehabilitative phase (after discharge). This will allow the reader to appreciate the long-term nature of recovery from burn injury.

Examination
Patient History
GR is a 23-year-old female college student with no significant past medical history. She sustained an 11% TBSA full-thickness scald burn to her right anterior thigh, anterior lower leg, and dorsal foot when she spilled hot soup while cooking dinner. After evaluation of the wounds, she was scheduled for surgery to excise the burn eschar and skin graft the wound. Skin grafting surgery was performed 4 days after admission. The patient was discharged from the burn center 14 days after admission. Before the injury, she was independent in all activities.

Immediate Acute Phase (Presurgery)
Systems Review: Heart rate (HR) is 90 beats per minute (bpm), blood pressure (BP) is 145/112 mm Hg, and respiratory rate (RR) is 21 breaths per minute (breaths/min).

Tests and Measures
Musculoskeletal
Anthropometric Characteristics Patient is 5 foot 6 inches tall and weighs 125 lb. Edema noted in right lower extremity: Right midthigh 50 cm (left midthigh 43); right midcalf 41 cm (left midcalf 35 cm); right foot (figure-of-8) 54 cm (left foot 45 cm).

Muscle Performance Right hip flexion and extension 5/5; right knee flexion and extension 4/5 (test may have been affected by pain or edema, patient was hesitant). Right ankle plantarflexion and dorsiflexion 4/5 (test may have been affected by pain or edema, patient was hesitant).

Left lower extremity strength is 5/5.

Range of Motion Right hip motion in all planes within normal limits (WNL); right knee extension/flexion 0°-90°; right ankle dorsiflexion 5°, plantarflexion 20°.

Left lower extremity ROM is WNL at the hip, knee, and ankle.

Neuromuscular GR demonstrates ability to safely balance without support and transfers independently from bed to chair and is independent in sit-to-stand. No deficits in coordination noted.

Pain Pain in right lower extremity at rest 4/10, with movement 6/10.

Integumentary
Integumentary Integrity 11% TBSA, full-thickness burns to right anterior thigh, anterior lower leg, dorsal foot; potential for scarring after healing/surgery.

Function
Gait Patient able to ambulate independently 20 feet in 19.5 seconds; "step-to" gait (right to left); Tinetti Gait Assessment score 7/12.

Evaluation

GR presents with impairments of the right lower extremity: Wounds, edema, and mild pain; decreased mobility; questionable decrease in strength; and alterations of gait secondary to the burn injury.

Goals

The proposed goals of acute treatment are to manage the wounds in preparation for surgery, control edema, control pain, and improve mobility and gait.

Intervention

The burn wounds were washed with water and a mild soap twice a day followed by dressings, including application of silver sulfadiazine as a topical agent covered by gauze wrap.

Edema was controlled by positioning (elevation when resting) and movement, including ambulation to encourage activation of the muscle pump. Active ROM exercises were prescribed for the right lower extremity at every joint in every plane. Gait training was instituted to address specific gait deviations.

Acute Phase (After Surgery)

Systems Review: HR is 88 bpm, BP is 140/105 mm Hg, and RR is 19 breaths/min.

Tests and Measures

Musculoskeletal

Anthropometric Characteristics Edema noted in right lower extremity: right midthigh 46 cm (left midthigh 43); right midcalf 38 cm (left midcalf 35 cm); right foot (figure-of-8) 50 cm (left foot 45 cm)

Muscle Performance Right hip flexion and extension 5/5; right knee flexion and extension 4/5; right ankle plantarflexion and dorsiflexion 4/5.

Range of Motion Right hip motion in all planes WNL; right knee extension/flexion 0°-85°; right ankle dorsiflexion 5°, plantarflexion 15°.

Neuromuscular

Pain Pain in right lower extremity at rest 2/10, with movement 3/10; donor-site pain (before healing) with activity 7/10.

Cardiovascular

Aerobic Capacity and Endurance Measures immediately after ambulation on treadmill for 5 min: BP 155/112 mm Hg, HR 108 bpm, RR 28 breaths/min; oxygen saturation 94%; RPE 8.

Integumentary

Integumentary Integrity Split-thickness autografts to right anterior thigh, anterior lower leg, dorsal foot; potential for scarring.

Function

Gait Patient able to ambulate independently 20 feet in 14 seconds; Tinetti Gait Assessment score 9/12.

Evaluation

GRs impairments include right lower extremity edema, mild pain, healing grafts, decreased mobility, decreased strength, alterations of gait, and development of early scar.

Other impairments include the wounds at donor sites and aerobic deconditioning. Initially, functional ambulation and stair climbing were restricted.

Goals

The proposed goals of treatment acutely are to manage the donor-site wounds and the healing graft sites, control edema, control pain, improve mobility and gait, and improve aerobic capacity. The patient will be assessed for her need for scar management. The patient should be able to demonstrate independence with her physical therapy program before discharge. The patient will be measured for burn scar supports (pressure garments) for her lower extremity, which may be applied before discharge if they arrive. If not, her leg will be placed in a temporary scar support such as a tubular cotton elastic support. She will be scheduled for a follow-up appointment to evaluate her mobility, strength, aerobic capacity, and scarring.

Intervention

Donor-site wounds were treated as partial-thickness wounds and were expected to heal within 10 days to 2 weeks. Skin grafts were dressed and cared for according to the applicable postsurgical protocol.

Edema was controlled by positioning (elevation when resting) and movement, including ambulation when the grafts were sufficiently healed to allow dependent activity.

Active ROM exercises were prescribed for the right lower extremity at every joint in every plane. Since active ROM was insufficient to maintain full motion, passive and active-assisted ROM were instituted.

Gait training and specific strengthening exercises for the lower extremity were introduced to address specific gait deviations once the patient was cleared for ambulatory activity. Aerobic exercise began when the grafts healed. The intensity of each of these interventions was steadily increased as the patient prepared for discharge from the acute care hospital.

Rehabilitative Phase (After Discharge)

Systems Review: Resting BP is 125/80 mm Hg, HR is 74 bpm, and RR is 15 breaths/min.

Tests and Measures

Musculoskeletal

Anthropometric Characteristics Edema noted in right lower extremity: right midthigh 42 cm (left midthigh 43); right midcalf 37 cm (left midcalf 35 cm); right foot (figure-of-8) 47 cm (left foot 45 cm)

Muscle Performance Right hip flexion and extension 5/5; right knee flexion and extension 4/5; right ankle plantarflexion and dorsiflexion 4/5.

Range of Motion Right hip motion in all planes WNL; right knee extension/flexion 0°-140°; right ankle dorsiflexion 15°, plantarflexion 35°.

Neuromuscular

Pain Pain in right lower extremity at rest 0/10, with movement 0/10; itching at rest varies from 3/10 to 7/10.

Cardiovascular

Aerobic Capacity and Endurance Measures immediately after ambulation on treadmill for 15 min: BP 152/110 mm Hg, HR 96 bpm, RR 26 breaths/min; oxygen saturation 95%; RPE 7.

Integumentary

Integumentary Integrity Hypertrophic scarring on right anterior thigh, anterior lower leg, dorsal foot.

Function

Gait Patient able to ambulate independently 20 feet in 4 seconds; Tinetti Gait Assessment score 11/12.

Evaluation

GR's wounds are in the remodeling phase of healing. Impairments requiring attention early after discharge but which should improve with time include decreased mobility, decreased strength, alterations of gait, and aerobic deconditioning. Negotiating many stairs and ambulating distances from her dormitory to classes presented a problem for her early in this phase of care.

Goals

The proposed goals of treatment are to improve mobility and gait and improve aerobic capacity. GR should be fit with custom-fit scar supports to reduce the risk of hypertrophic scarring.

Intervention

Active ROM exercises were prescribed for the right lower extremity at every joint in every plane. Where active ROM was insufficient to maintain full motion, passive and active-assisted ROM were continued. Gait training and specific strengthening exercises for the lower extremity, as well as aerobic conditioning exercises, were continued. The intensity of each of these interventions was increased based on patient improvement. The patient was discharged from her supervised physical therapy program when normal mobility, strength, and conditioning were achieved. One set of scar supports was initially ordered and another set was ordered once it was determined that the first set fit appropriately. GR was scheduled for follow-up visits at 3-month intervals for a year to follow-up on scar management, including the maturation of the scar tissue and the fit of the pressure supports.

Please see the CD that accompanies this book for a case study describing the examination, evaluation, and interventions for a patient with a flame burn.

CHAPTER SUMMARY

Rehabilitation of patients with burns provides a diverse array of challenges and requires a broad range of practice skills. Overcoming impairments, such as pain, edema, decreased mobility, decreased strength, compromised aerobic capacity, aerobic deconditioning, and development of scar; promoting wound healing; lessening deformity; and minimizing loss of function in self-care at home and at work are examples of the many facets of burn care. This chapter provides essential information related to the pathology of burns and the rehabilitation management of patients with burns.

ADDITIONAL RESOURCES

Elastic Wraps

Ace Elastic Bandages: Becton Dickinson, Franklin Lakes, NJ

Self-Adherent Compression Wraps

Coban Self-Adherent Wrap: 3M, St. Paul, MN
Flex-Wrap: Kendall, MA
Medi-rip: International-Global Enterprises Inc, www.interglobal-ent.com/

Tubular Cotton Wraps

Tubigrip: ConvaTec, Princeton, NJ
Tubiton: Medlock Medical, Cheshire, UK
Compressogrip: AliMed, Dedham, MA

Custom Pressure Supports

Bio Concepts: Phoenix, AZ
Barton-Carey: Toledo, OH
Gottfried Medical: Toledo, OH
Medical Z Corporation: San Antonio, TX

GLOSSARY

Contracture: Permanent shortening (of muscle, tendon, or scar tissue) producing deformity or distortion.

Full-thickness burn (also third-degree burn): Severe burn characterized by destruction of the skin through the depth of the dermis and possibly into underlying tissues.

Hypertrophic scar: Connective tissue composed of fibroblasts and dense collagenous fibers that stay within the boundaries of the original wound.

Keloid scar: Scar that extends beyond the boundaries of the primary wound.

Partial-thickness burn (also second-degree burn): Burn marked by pain, blistering, and superficial destruction of dermis with edema and hyperemia of the tissues beneath the burn.

Superficial burn (also first-degree burn): Mild burn characterized by heat, pain, and reddening of the burned surface but not exhibiting blistering or charring of tissues, only affecting the epidermis.

References

1. Ward RS: The rehabilitation of burn patients, *Crit Rev Phys Rehabil Med* 2(3):121-138, 1991.
2. Petro JA, Salisbury RE: Rehabilitation of the burn patient, *Clin Plast Surg* 13(1):145-149, 1986.
3. Saffle J, Davis B, Williams P: Recent outcomes in the treatment of burn injury in the United States: A report from the American Burn Association Patient Registry, *J Burn Care Rehabil* 16(3 part 1):219-232, 1995.
4. Sproul J, Palen C: Using a team approach: Santa Clara Valley Medical Center Regional Burn Center, *Rehab Manage* 12(4):46-48, 1999.
5. van Rijn OJ, Bouter LM, Meertens RM: The aetiology of burns in developed countries: review of the literature, *Burns* 15(4):217-221, 1989.
6. Jay KM, Bartlett RH, Danet R, et al: Burn epidemiology: A basis for burn prevention, *J Trauma* 17(12):943-947, 1977.
7. Ray JG: Burns in young children: A study of the mechanism of burns in children aged 5 years and under in the Hamilton, Ontario Burn Unit, *Burns* 21(6):463-466, 1995.
8. Murray JP: A study of the prevention of hot tap water burns, *Burns Incl Therm Inj* 14(3):185-193, 1988.
9. Pruitt B Jr, Mason A Jr: Epidemiological, demographic and outcomes characteristics of burn injury. In Herndon D (ed): *Total Burn Care*, Philadelphia, 1996, WB Saunders.
10. Datubo-Brown DD, Gowar JP: Contact burns in children, *Burns* 15(5):285-286, 1989.
11. Carman C, Chang B: Treadmill injuries to the upper extremity in pediatric patients, *Ann Plast Surg* 47(1):15-19, 2001.
12. Collier ML, Ward RS, Saffle JR, et al: Home treadmill friction injuries: A five-year review, *J Burn Care Rehabil* 25(5):441-444, 2004.

13. Herbert K, Lawrence JC: Chemical burns, *Burns* 15(6):381-384, 1989.

14. Wilmore DW, Long JM, Mason AD Jr, et al: Catecholamines: Mediator of the hypermetabolic response to thermal injury, *Ann Surg* 180(4):653-669, 1974.

15. Dolecek R, AdÃ¡mkovÃ¡ M, SotornÃ¬kovÃ¡ T, et al: Endocrine response after burn, *Scand J Plast Reconstr Surg* 13(1):9-16, 1979.

16. Drost AC, Burleson DG, Cioffi WG Jr, et al: Plasma cytokines following thermal injury and their relationship with patient mortality, burn size, and time postburn, *J Trauma* 35(3):335-339, 1993.

17. Turinsky J, Gonnerman WA, Loose LD: Impaired mineral metabolism in postburn muscle, *J Trauma* 21(6):417-423, 1981.

18. Sun X, Fischer DR, Yang M, et al: Effect of burn injury on glucocorticoid receptor binding activity in rat muscle, *J Surg Res* 116(2):234-241, 2004.

19. St-Pierre D, Choiniere M, Forget R, et al: Muscle strength in individuals with healed burns, *Arch Phys Med Rehabil* 79(2):155-161, 1998.

20. Purdue GF, Hunt JL: Multiple trauma and the burn patient, *Am J Surg* 158(6):536-539, 1989.

21. Lund T, Onarheim H, Reed RK: Pathogenesis of edema formation in burn injuries, *World J Surg* 16(1):2-9, 1992.

22. Glenn W, Gilbert H, Drinker C: The flow of lymph from burned tissue with particular reference to the effects of fibrin formation upon lymph drainage and composition, *Surgery* 12:685, 1942.

23. Remensnyder JP: Topography of tissue oxygen tension changes in acute burn edema. *Arch Surg* 105(3):477-482, 1972.

24. Pani S, Vanamail P, Yuvaraj J: Limb circumference measurement for recording edema volume in patients with filarial lymphedema, *Lymphology* 28:57-63, 1995.

25. Petersen EJ, Irish SM, Lyons CL, et al: Reliability of water volumetry and the figure of eight method on subjects with ankle joint swelling, *JOSPT* 29(10):609-615, 1999.

26. Maihafer GC, Llewellyn MA, Pillar WJ Jr, et al: A comparison of the figure-of-eight method and water volumetry in measurement of hand and wrist size, *J Hand Ther* 16(4):305-310, 2003.

27. Dobbs ER, Curreri PW: Burns: Analysis of results of physical therapy in 681 patients, *J Trauma* 12(3):242-248, 1972.

28. Rempel DM, Diao E: Entrapment neuropathies: Pathophysiology and pathogenesis, *J Electromyogr Kinesiol* 14(1):71-75, 2004.

29. Casley-Smith JR, Casley-Smith JR: The pathophysiology of lymphedema and the action of benzo-pyrones in reducing it, *Lymphology* 21(3):190-194, 1988.

30. Wadsworth CT, Krishnan R, Sear M, et al: Intrarater reliability of manual muscle testing and hand-held dynametric muscle testing, *Phys Ther* 67(9):1342-1347, 1987.

31. Ottenbacher KJ, Branch LG, Ray L, et al: The reliability of upper- and lower-extremity strength testing in a community survey of older adults, *Arch Phys Med Rehabil* 83(10):1423-1427, 2002.

32. Sloan C: Review of the reliability and validity of myometry with children, *Phys Occup Ther Pediatr* 22(2):79-93, 2002.

33. Suman OE, Spies RJ, Celis MM, et al: Effects of a 12-wk resistance exercise program on skeletal muscle strength in children with burn injuries, *J Appl Physiol* 91(3):1168-1175, 2001.

34. Cucuzzo NA, Ferrando A, Herndon DN: The effects of exercise programming vs traditional outpatient therapy in the rehabilitation of severely burned children, *J Burn Care Rehabil* 22(3):214-220, 2001.

35. Cronan T, Hammond J, Ward CG: The value of isokinetic exercise and testing in burn rehabilitation and determination of back-to-work status, *J Burn Care Rehabil* 11(3):224-227, 1990.

36. Everett J, Patterson D, Chen C: Cognitive and behavioral treatments for burn pain, *Pain Clin* 3:133-145, 1990.

37. Marvin J: Management of pain and anxiety. In Carrougher GJ (ed): *Burn Care and Therapy,* St. Louis, 1998, Mosby.

38. Gordon M, Greenfield E, Marvin J, et al: Use of pain assessment tools: is there a preference? *J Burn Care Rehabil* 19(5):451-454, 1998.

39. Kowalske K, Holavanahalli R, Helm P: Neuropathy after burn injury, *J Burn Care Rehabil* 22(5):353, 2001.

40. Temples TE, Burns AH, Nance FC, et al: Effect of burn shock on myocardial function in guinea pigs, *Circ Shock* 14(2):81-92, 1984.

41. Murphy JT, Giroir B, Horton JW: Thermal injury alters myocardial sarcoplasmic reticulum calcium channel function, *J Surg Res* 82(2):244-252, 1999.

42. Rue LW 3rd, Cioffi WG, Mason AD, et al: Improved survival of burned patients with inhalation injury, *Arch Surg* 128(7):772, 1993.

43. Greenhalgh D: Preexisting factors that affect care. In Carrougher GJ (ed): *Burn Care and Therapy,* St. Louis, 1998, Mosby.

44. Whitener DR, Whitener LM, Robertson KJ, et al: Pulmonary function measurements in patients with thermal injury and smoke inhalation, *Am Rev Respir Dis* 122(5):731-739, 1980.

45. Rutan R: Physiologic response to cutaneous burn injury. In Carrougher GJ (ed): *Burn Care and Therapy,* St. Louis, 1998, Mosby.

46. American Physical Therapy Association: Guide to physical therapist practice, second edition, *Phys Ther* 81:S587, 2001.

47. Carrougher G: Burn wound assessment and topical treatment. In Carrougher GJ (ed): *Burn Care and Therapy,* St. Louis, 1998, Mosby.

48. Miller SF, Finley RK, Waltman M, et al: Burn size estimate reliability: A study, The *J Burn Care Rehabil* 12(6):546-559, 1991.

49. Lund C, Browder N: The estimation of areas of burns, *Surg Gynecol Obstet* 79:352-358, 1944.

50. Hunt TK: Disorders of wound healing, *World J Surg* 4(3):271-277, 1980.

51. Sullivan T, Smith J, Kermode J, et al: Rating the burn scar, *J Burn Care Rehabil* 11(3):256-260, 1990.

52. Boyce S, Supp A, Wickett R, et al: Assessment with the dermal torque meter of skin pliability after treatment of burns with cultured skin substitutes, *J Burn Care Rehabil* 21:55-63, 2000.

53. Silverberg R, Lombardo G, Gorga D, et al: Gait variables of patients after lower extremity burn injuries, *J Burn Care Rehabil* 21(3):259, 2000.

54. van Zuijlen PP, Kreis RW, Vloemans AF, et al: The prognostic factors regarding long-term functional outcome of full-thickness hand burns, *Burns* 25(8):709-714, 1999.

55. Lowell M, Pirc P, Ward RS, et al: Effect of 3M Coban Self-Adherent Wraps on edema and function of the burned hand: A case study, *J Burn Care Rehabil* 24(4):253, 2003.

56. Clark JA, Cheng JC, Leung KS, et al: Mechanical characterisation of human postburn hypertrophic skin during pressure therapy, *J Biomech* 20(4):397-406, 1987.

57. Cheng S, Rogers JC: Changes in occupational role performance after a severe burn: A retrospective study, *Am J Occup Ther* 43(1):17-24, 1989.

58. Brych SB, Engrav LH, Rivara FP, et al: Time off work and return to work rates after burns: Systematic review of the literature and a large two-center series, *J Burn Care Rehabil* 22(6):401-405, 2001.

59. Fox CL Jr: Silver sulfadiazine for control of burn wound infections, *Int Surg* 60(5):275-277, 1975.

60. Hadjiiski OG, Lesseva MI: Comparison of four drugs for local treatment of burn wounds. *Eur J Emerg Med* 6(1):41-47, 1999.

61. Herruzo-Cabrera R, Garcia-Torres V, Rey-Calero J, et al: Evaluation of the penetration strength, bactericidal efficacy and spectrum of action of several antimicrobial creams against isolated microorganisms in a burn centre, *Burns* 18(1):39-44, 1992.

62. Sorenson MK: The edematous hand, *Phys Ther* 69(12):1059-1064, 1989.

63. Vasudevan SV, Melvin JL: Upper extremity edema control: Rationale of the techniques, *Am J Occup Ther* 33(8):520-523, 1979.

64. Ause-Ellias KL, Richard R, Miller SF, et al: The effect of mechanical compression on chronic hand edema after burn injury: a preliminary report, *J Burn Care Rehabil* 15(1):29-33, 1994.

65. Hettrick H, Nof L, Ward S, et al: Incidence and prevalence of lymphedema in patients following burn injury: a five-year retrospective and three-month prospective study, *Lymph Res Biol* 2(1):11-24, 2004.

66. Moss B, Everett J, Patterson D: Psychologic support and pain management of the burn patient. In Richard R, Stayley M (eds): *Burn Care and Rehabilitation,* Philadelphia, 1994, FA Davis.

67. American College of Sports Medicine: *Principles of Exercise Prescription,* Baltimore, 1995, William & Wilkins.

68. Kraemer M, Jones T, Deitch E: Burn contractures: incidence, predisposing factors, and results of surgical therapy, *J Burn Care Rehabil* 9(3):261-265, 1988.

69. Lehman C: Splints and accessories following burn reconstruction, *Clin Plast Surg* 19:721-731, 1992.

70. Wright MP, Taddonio TE, Prasad JK, et al: The microbiology and cleaning of thermoplastic splints in burn care, *J Burn Care Rehabil* 10(1):79-83, 1989.

71. Helm PA, Kevorkian CG, Lushbaugh M, et al: Burn injury: rehabilitation management in 1982, *Arch Phys Med Rehabil* 63(1):6-16, 1982.

72. Burnsworth B, Krob MJ, Langer-Schnepp M: Immediate ambulation of patients with lower-extremity grafts, *J Burn Care Rehabil* 13(1):89-92, 1992.

73. Wetzel JL, Giuffrida C, Petrazzi A, et al: Comparison of measures of physiologic stress during treadmill exercise in a patient with 20% lower extremity burn injuries and healthy matched and nonmatched individuals, *J Burn Care Rehabil* 21(4):359, 2000.

74. Austin KG, Hansbrough JF, Dore C, et al: Thermoregulation in burn patients during exercise, *J Burn Care Rehabil* 24(1):9-14, 2003.

75. Ben-Simchon C, Tsur H, et al: Heat tolerance in patients with extensive healed burns, *Plast Reconstr Surg* 67(4):499-504, 1981.

76. McGibbon B, Beaumont WV, Strand J, et al: Thermal regulation in patients after the healing of large deep burns, *Plast Reconstr Surg* 52(2):164-170, 1973.

77. Roskind JL, Petrofsky J, Lind AR, et al: Quantitation of thermoregulatory impairment in patients with healed burns, *Ann Plast Surg* 1(2):172-176, 1978.

78. Shapiro Y, Epstein Y, Ben-Simchon C, et al: Thermoregulatory responses of patients with extensive healed burns, *J Appl Physiol* 53(4):1019-1022, 1982.

79. Mlcak RP, Desai MH, Robinson E, et al: Increased physiological dead space/tidal volume ratio during exercise in burned children, *Burns* 21(5):337-339, 1995.

80. Borg G: Perceived exertion as an indicator of somatic stress, *Scand J Rehabil Med* 2(2):92-98, 1970.

81. American College of Sports Medicine: *Guidelines for Exercise Testing and Prescription,* ed 5, Baltimore, 1995, Williams & Wilkins.
82. Stayley M, Richard R: Scar management. In Richard R, Stayley M (eds): *Burn Care and Rehabilitation,* Philadelphia, 1994, FA Davis.
83. Leung P, Ng M: Pressure treatment for hypertrophic scars resulting from burns, *Burns Incl Therm Inj* 6:244-250, 1980.
84. Ward R: Physical rehabilitation. In Carrougher GJ (ed): *Burn Care and Therapy,* St. Louis, 1998, Mosby.
85. Ward RS: Pressure therapy for the control of hypertrophic scar formation after burn injury. A history and review, *J Burn Care Rehabil* 12(3):257-262, 1991.
86. Cheng J, Evans J, Leung, KS, et al: Pressure therapy in the treatment of post-burn hypertrophic scar—a critical look into its usefulness and fallacies by pressure monitoring, *Burns Incl Therm Inj* 10:154-163, 1984.
87. Lee R, Capelli-Schellpfeffer M, Astumian R: A review of thermoregulation of tissue repair and remodeling, *Abstract Soc Phys Reg Biol Med* 15:23, 1995.
88. Thompson R, Summers S, Rampey-Dobbs R, et al: Color pressure garments versus traditional beige pressure garments: Perceptions from the public. *J Burn Care Rehabil* 13(5):590-596, 1992.
89. Ward RS, Hayes-Lundy C, et al: Influence of pressure supports on joint range of motion, *Burns* 18(1):60-62, 1992.
90. Quinn KJ, Evans JH, Courtney JM, et al: Non-pressure treatment of hypertrophic scars, *Burns Incl Therm Inj* 12:102-108, 1985.
91. Quinn KJ: Silicone gel in scar treatment, *Burns Incl Therm Inj* 13(suppl):S33-40, 1987.
92. Ahn ST, Monafo WW, Mustoe TA: Topical silicone gel: A new treatment for hypertrophic scars, *Surgery* 106(4):781, 1989.
93. Van den Kerckhove E, Stappaerts K, Boeckx W, et al: Silicones in the rehabilitation of burns: a review and overview, *Burns* 27(3):205-214, 2001.
94. Wittenberg GP, Fabian BG, Bogomilsky JL, et al: Prospective, single-blind, randomized, controlled study to assess the efficacy of the 585-nm flashlamp-pumped pulsed-dye laser and silicone gel sheeting in hypertrophic scar treatment, *Arch Dermatol* 135(9):1049-1055, 1999.
95. Musgrave M, Umraw N, Fish J, et al: The effect of silicone gel sheets on perfusion of hypertrophic burn scars, *J Burn Care Rehabil* 23(3):208-214, 2002.
96. Patino O, Novick C, Merlo A, et al: Massage in hypertrophic scars, *J Burn Care Rehabil* 20(3):268, 1999.
97. Field T, Peck M, Hernandez-Reif M, et al: Postburn itching, pain, and psychological symptoms are reduced with massage therapy, *J Burn Care Rehabil* 21(3):189-193, 2000.
98. Wootton R, Hodgson E: Physiotherapy in treatment of burns with inhalation injury, *Physiotherapy* 63(5):153, 1977.
99. Dutcher K, Johnson C: Neuromuscular and musculoskeletal complications. In Richard R, Stayley M (eds): *Burn Care and Rehabilitation,* Philadelphia, 1994, FA Davis.
100. Curtis MJ, Clarke JA: Skeletal injury in thermal trauma: a review of management, *Injury* 20(6):333-336, 1989.
101. English C, Carmichael KD: Management of fractures in children with thermal injuries, *J Pediatr Orthop* 22(6):725-728, 2002.
102. Saffle JR, Schnelby A, Hofmann A, et al: The management of fractures in thermally injured patients, *J Trauma* 23(10):902-910, 1983.

Chapter **32**

Gait Assessment and Training

Robert Wellmon

CHAPTER OUTLINE

OBJECTIVES

After reading this chapter, the reader will be able to:
1. Describe the components of the normal gait cycle.
2. Describe how pathological processes can affect the normal gait cycle.
3. Identify and discuss the importance of the components of the gait examination.
4. Discuss the importance of using standardized and nonstandardized measures of gait for examination and evaluation.
5. Describe common interventions for individuals with gait dysfunction.

*W*alking is an important functional skill, and mastery of this skill impacts human development. Walking provides access to the environment, which can affect cognitive, emotional, psychological, and psychomotor development. Walking also allows a vast number of behavioral goals to be achieved and provides exercise that helps maintain cardiovascular fitness and prevents adverse effects of a sedentary lifestyle.

Gait deficits are associated with significant functional limitations.[1,2] Gait deficits can make it difficult for an individual to get into and move about their home. Community access requires not only the ability to walk but also the ability to manage a variety of terrains, including uneven surfaces, elevations, curbs, and ramps.

Rehabilitation clinicians frequently treat patients who have difficulty walking. Difficulty with walking and the resultant functional limitations and disability can occur after a wide range of pathological processes. For example, after a stroke, gait disturbances are common because altered motor control can cause problems with weight bearing and balance.[3] In the elderly, gait changes often increase the risk of falling.[1] In addition, instability while walking may be the first indication of an undiagnosed disease process, particularly in the elderly.

Problems with walking can be caused by deficits in one or more body systems. Impairments in either the musculoskeletal or somatosensory systems can affect gait quality and efficiency.[4] Weakness can change the gait pattern and worsen movement quality by reducing control and stabilization of the lower limbs. Sensory deficits can alter movement quality by impairing localization of the extremity in space and the accuracy of limb placement.[5] Because inaccurate foot placement can reduce stability, the patient may try to compensate by increasing the force with which they make contact with the supporting surface to augment sensory feedback. Over time these forces can traumatize the musculoskeletal system. To improve stability in the face of weakness or sensory loss, a person may also walk more slowly, reducing walking efficiency.[6,7]

Cardiac or pulmonary dysfunction can also limit walking distance and endurance, making timely and efficient completion of activities involving gait difficult. Although cognitive deficits do not directly affect the gait pattern, they can affect the patient's ability to attend to the surrounding environment and thus impair his or her safety while walking.

Given the impact of gait-specific impairments on patient function, rehabilitation specialists have an important role in identifying and treating mobility deficits associated with walking that arise out of disease processes affecting a number of organ systems. To do this effectively, a thorough understanding of normal gait kinesiology and biomechanics and an understanding of principles of therapeutic exercise and practice promoting motor learning is needed. This chapter describes examination, evaluation, diagnosis, prognosis, and intervention for patients with gait dysfunction and provides an approach to the examination of gait that is suitable for a variety of clients, irrespective of their diagnosis.

The purposes of a gait-specific examination include: (1) determination of the impact of disease processes on a patient's ambulatory function; (2) evaluation to address gait-specific deficits that limit function and cause disability; (3) identification of the severity of the impairments, functional limitations, and disability leading to and arising out of gait dysfunction; (4) optimization of patient performance by targeting interventions to address gait-specific deficits; (5) monitoring the effectiveness of interventions on gait dysfunction; and (6) identification of when the client has achieved the maximum benefit from interventions that specifically target gait dysfunction.

PATHOLOGY

To understand and accurately diagnose and treat gait dysfunction, the clinician must first understand normal functional walking. Familiarity with the terminology used to describe gait, including sequential events related to the timing of muscle recruitment, movement of limb and joint segments, and displacement of the body's center of gravity (COG) during walking, is also essential. The terms associated with the *gait cycle,* many of which describe events that should occur during walking, help organize the examination and allow for effective communication between health care professionals and with others such as third-party payers.

FUNCTIONAL WALKING

Successful walking requires maintaining upright alignment against a number of destabilizing forces. When walking, the person's weight is constantly being transferred from limb to limb. This transition requires aligning the body weight over one limb briefly during each step. Successful walking also requires movement efficiency. Normal gait is characterized by a smooth progression of the body's COG and related limb segments as weight is shifted from one limb to the other, minimizing the associated energy demands. Gait must also be adaptable. People must be able to walk on a variety of surfaces under environmental conditions that can be destabilizing. They must be able to manage raised surfaces, such as curbs, door jambs, or steps, and be able to change their path of travel by moving sideways or walking slower or faster to accommodate other people or obstacles in the environment.

The tasks associated with successful walking are described by a number of authors. Winter suggests that the primary tasks of walking are to support the body's weight against gravity, maintain upright alignment or balance, and control the trajectory of the foot to allow the limb to clear the ground.[8] Gait can also be described and examined in terms of the functional tasks that must be achieved. Three critical functional tasks for successful walking have been identified: Acceptance of weight by the supporting limb, a period of single limb support, and advancement of the limb.[9,10] The requirements for successful walking provide a framework for gait examination because people with an atypical or nonfunctional gait pattern generally have difficulties or abnormalities in one or more of the necessary components.

THE GAIT CYCLE

The gait cycle is the fundamental unit of walking. It is defined by the events that occur between the contact of one extremity with the supporting surface and the second contact of the same extremity with the supporting surface. The gait cycle is divided into two periods or phases, which are known as stance and swing. A single gait cycle is comprised of two swing and two stance phases with associated temporal and distance characteristics (Fig. 32-1). These characteristics can be described absolutely or as a percentage of the entire gait cycle. Describing the phases as percentages of the whole cycle controls for variations in time and distance associated with gender, age, or anthropometric factors.

Stance Phase. *Stance phase* is the period of the gait cycle during which the foot or supporting limb is in contact with the ground or other supporting surface. In nondisabled adults, stance phase typically lasts less than a second and comprises approximately 60% of the gait cycle. Variations in the duration of stance phase can be due to deficits in balance, musculoskeletal changes, pain, or events associated with physical development or maturation. The amount of time spent in stance phase decreases as walking speed increases.

Swing Phase. *Swing phase* is the period of the gait cycle when the reference limb or foot is in the air or not in contact with the supporting surface. Swing phase ends just before the reference limb contacts the supporting surface. Typically, swing phase encompasses approximately 40% of the gait cycle. While one limb is in swing phase, the other (contralateral) limb is in stance phase.

Subdivisions of the Gait Cycle. Stance and swing phase can be divided into several subdivisions. One approach is to divide stance phase into three subdivisions: (1) initial *double stance,* (2) single stance, and (3) terminal double stance. Initial and terminal double stance are also referred to as the period of double support. During double support, both feet are in contact with the supporting surface. The period of double support typically comprises 20% of the gait cycle. In dysfunctional gait the period of double support often increases.

The initial double-stance period begins when the reference foot makes contact with the supporting surface. This marks the beginning of the gait cycle. During this period, weight is being transferred from one limb to the other.

The next subdivision of the stance phase, single-limb stance, begins when the nonreference leg is lifted from the supporting surface to initiate its swing phase. During single stance, the body's weight and COG are aligned over and supported by a single extremity. Achieving stable

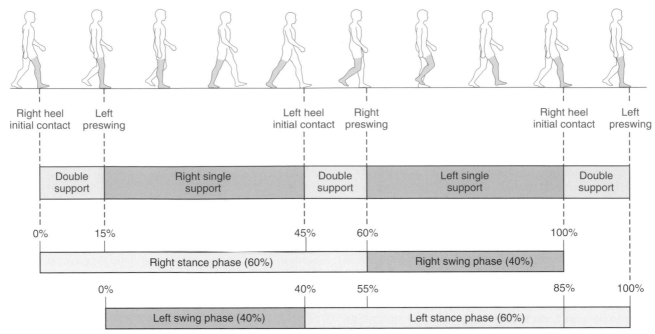

FIG. 32-1 Phases of the gait cycle. *Adapted from Inman VT, Ralston HJ, Todd F:* Human Walking, *Baltimore, 1981, Williams & Wilkins. In Magee DJ:* Orthopedic Physical Assessment, *ed 4, St. Louis, 2002, WB Saunders.*

single-limb support is a critical component of successful walking and is one of the key functional tasks that must be achieved.[9,10] Single-limb stance, which lasts less than 0.5 seconds, may be difficult for those with pathology or impairments. To increase stability, single-limb stance on the involved limb can be shortened while lengthening the duration of double stance, but this reduces gait efficiency.

Terminal double stance is the last subdivision of the stance phase. Terminal double stance starts when the nonreference extremity makes contact with the supporting surface and ends when the reference extremity is lifted from the supporting surface to initiate its swing phase.

Another approach to examining and describing gait involves dividing stance phase into five subphases and swing phase into three subphases. Two parallel sets of terms, the traditional terminology and the Rancho Los Amigos terminology, can be used to describe these subdivisions. The clinician should be familiar with both sets of terms because both are commonly used in clinical practice and in the published literature. The traditional terminology, which is based on a description of normal gait, was developed first and can be useful for describing both normal gait and many gait disturbances but is limited in some patients whose gait sequence deviates significantly from normal.

Traditional Gait Terminology. The components of stance in the traditional approach to gait are (1) heel strike, (2) foot flat, (3) midstance, (4) heel off, and (5) toe off. At *heel strike,* the reference limb makes contact with the supporting surface. *Foot flat* occurs immediately after heel strike and ends when the plantar surface of the foot makes contact with the supporting surface. The *midstance* phase of gait begins as the body's COG moves directly over the supporting limb. *Heel off* describes the period from midstance to when the heel of the reference limb leaves the supporting surface. *Toe off* describes the period from heel off to the beginning of the swing phase.

Swing phase is divided into three subphases: (1) acceleration, (2) midswing, and (3) deceleration. Acceleration begins when the toe of the reference limb leaves the supporting surface and ends when the extremity is directly under the body. *Midswing* is when the reference limb passes beneath the body. Deceleration starts after midswing when the tibia is no longer perpendicular to the ground and ends with the knee in maximum extension just before the foot contacts the supporting surface.

Rancho Los Amigos Gait Terminology. The five subphases of gait associated with stance are: (1) initial contact, (2) loading response, (3) midstance, (4) terminal stance, and (5) preswing (Table 32-1). Note that these terms do not identify which part of the foot contacts the floor. *Initial contact* begins when the foot first contacts the supporting surface and encompasses part of the period of initial double support. Typically, the heel is the first part of the foot to contact the supporting surface, and at this time the ankle is in a neutral position while the knee is extended and the hip flexed. Loading response is the part of the period of initial double support characterized by movement of the ankle into plantarflexion, allowing for gradual and controlled approximation of the foot with

TABLE 32-1	Critical Tasks and Rancho Los Amigos Terminology for the Gait Cycle						
← Stance Phase 60% →				← Swing Phase 40% →			
Weight Acceptance		Single-Limb Support		Swing-Limb Advancement			
Initial contact	Loading response	Midstance	Terminal stance	Preswing	Initial swing	Midswing	Terminal swing

the supporting surface and movement of the knee into flexion. Movements at the knee, hip, and ankle transfer weight from the contralateral extremity and help with energy conservation and shock absorption. The loading response phase of gait ends when the contralateral extremity leaves the supporting surface. Midstance begins when the contralateral limb leaves the supporting surface and ends as the body's COG moves directly over the reference or supporting limb. Terminal stance is the period when the body's COG moves anterior to the supporting limb until the opposite limb makes contact with the support surface. *Preswing* corresponds to the second period of double support. This phase begins with initial contact of the opposite limb and ends when the toes of the reference limb leave the supporting surface.

Swing phase is divided into three subphases: Initial swing, midswing, and terminal swing.[10] *Initial swing* begins when the reference limb leaves the supporting surface and ends when the knee is in maximal flexion. The period from maximal knee flexion to the point where the tibia of the reference limb is perpendicular to the supporting surface is midswing. *Terminal swing* begins with the tibia is perpendicular to the supporting surface and ends just before the foot contacting the supporting surface.

Functional Events of the Gait Cycle. Kinematic and kinetic events associated with the gait cycle can also be described by the functional tasks that must be accomplished. The three critical functional gait tasks are weight acceptance, single-limb support, and swing-limb advancement (see Table 32-1).[10] When examining gait in patients with problems walking, deficits could be classified as affecting one or more of these functional phases of gait. This approach will aid in both the diagnosis and treatment of gait dysfunction.

Weight Acceptance. Weight acceptance occurs during initial contact and the loading response of the stance phase of the gait cycle. During this time the stance-phase limb must rapidly accept the body's weight and attenuate potentially destabilizing ground reaction forces while relative movements of the various limb segments and the joints of the lower extremity and trunk smoothly move the body forward. At initial contact, ground reaction forces cause plantarflexion of the ankle and flexion of the knee and hip. Eccentric muscle activity at the ankle (pretibial), knee (quadriceps), and hip (extensors) contributes to limb stability and provides force attenuation.

Single-Limb Support. Single-limb support, which encompasses events associated with the single stance or support phase of gait, is characterized by progression of the body's COG over a single limb and includes midstance and terminal stance. The key goals of this functional task are maintaining forward momentum and stability while the body's weight is balanced on one limb.

Swing-Limb Advancement. Swing-limb advancement is the final functional task of the gait sequence and includes the events from preswing to terminal swing. The primary goal of swing limb advancement is to unload and move the reference limb forward, from behind the body to in front of the body, to prepare for the next functional phase of gait. This requires both clearing the foot and limb advancement.

Temporal and Distance Parameters of Gait. Temporal and distance parameters of gait are measured to compare an individual's performance with known norms and to track changes during rehabilitation. Normalization of walking velocity, step or stride length, increases in single-stance time, or decreases in double-support time generally indicate improvements in gait.

A single right step and a single left step (one gait cycle) make up one stride (Fig. 32-2). *Step length* is the distance between the point of initial contact of one extremity and the point of initial contact of the opposite extremity. *Stride length* is the distance between the point of initial contact of one extremity and the next point of initial contact of the same extremity.

Stride width, also called *base of support,* is the distance between the heels of the two feet during double stance. Stride width is measured either between the medial-most borders of the two heels or between lines through the midline of the two heels. Normal stride width for adults is between 1-3 inches (3-8 cm). Stride width often increases with gait instability.[11-13]

Walking velocity, also referred to as speed, is the distance covered per unit time. Walking velocity is measured in meters per second (m/sec) or miles per hour (mph). Average self-selected walking velocity in adults varies from 1.04-1.39 m/sec (Table 32-2).[14] Since height, leg length, and events associated with physical development and aging can all affect walking velocity, determining appropriate comparison norms for an individual patient can be challenging. Normalizing walking velocity to height or leg length can help control for differences in stature.

Although there are normative values for self-selected or preferred walking velocity under unchanging environmental conditions such as walking on a level surface, the capacity to walk at different speeds to meet specific

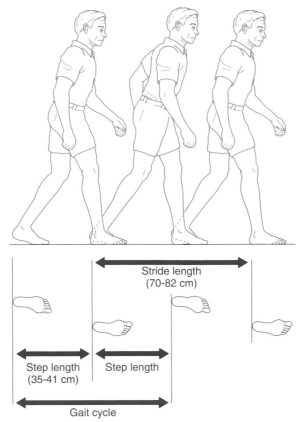

FIG. 32-2 The gait cycle: step and stride length. *In Magee DJ:* Orthopedic Physical Assessment, *ed 4, St. Louis, 2002, WB Saunders.*

TABLE 32-2	Average Walking Velocity for Young, Middle-Age, and Elderly Adults		
	Slow (m/sec)	Preferred (m/sec)	Fast (m/sec)
Young adults (20-39 years)	0.78-0.98	1.16-1.39	1.51-1.92
Middle-aged adults (40-59 years)	0.77-0.99	1.15-1.38	1.50-1.81
Elderly adults (60-79 years)	0.71-0.95	1.04-1.34	1.44-1.74

Data from Bohannon RW: *Age Ageing* 26(1):15-19, 1997; Oberg T, Karsznia A, Oberg K: *J Rehabil Res Dev* 30(2):210-223, 1993.

task and environmental demands is also important. For example, when crossing a street, one may need to walk faster to safely reach the other side, whereas when walking on a slippery surface such as ice, one may need to walk more slowly to maintain balance.

Cadence is the number of steps per unit of time. Typically, cadence is reported in steps per minute (steps/min). Cadence is fairly constant for nondisabled adults, at 100-117 steps/min when walking at preferred speeds on a level surface, but can vary with the demands of the task.[14] Once a mature pattern of gait is reached, cadence tends to be relatively stable across the adult lifespan.

Step time is the amount of time needed to complete a single step. *Stride time (stride/duration)* is the amount of time required to complete one stride. The time taken to complete a single stride should correspond to the time required to complete two steps. Swing time is the time that the foot is in the air. The amount of time when only one limb is in contact with the supporting surface is known as single-support time. The amount of time spent in *single support* is affected by a variety of factors, including limb strength,[15] balance confidence,[16] aging,[17] pain,[18-20] or the presence of pathology.[15,18,21] Single-support time decreases in the presence of weakness or pain on the support side. Step, stride, and swing time vary with gait velocity, anthropometric characteristics, and patient preference, as well as the type of task being performed. With increased gait velocity, step, swing, and stride times decrease; with decreased gait velocity, swing time increases.

Double-support time is the amount of time both lower limbs are in contact with the supporting surface and, as with the base of support, increases with instability because the phase of double support is most stable.[16,21,22] Double-support time also changes in the presence of pathology and decreases when walking velocity increases to become almost zero during running.[16,21,23]

The temporal and distance measures associated with the swing and stance phases of gait are intimately related. Nondisabled gait is generally characterized by symmetry. Step length and time and stride length and time are roughly equal for both sides, and differences between the two sides in either temporal or distance measures are indicators of gait dysfunction. For example, after a stroke, individuals often have difficulty weight bearing on the paretic or involved limb. This reduces the corresponding single-support time and the step length of the opposite extremity and increases double-support time. Other factors, such as impaired balance, loss of sensation, alterations in motor unit recruitment, and increased tone in the lower limb or trunk, can also affect temporal and distance parameters of gait and cause asymmetry.

Temporal and distance measures of gait can also be used to track patient progress. With recovery and intervention, paretic lower extremity motor control should improve, resulting in increased weight-bearing capacity and thus increased single-support time, step length on the un-involved side, and walking velocity, and decreased double-support time. Temporal and distance measures of outcomes have been shown to be valid and reliable in a wide range of populations, including patients after stroke,[24] patients with multiple sclerosis,[25] and across the lifespan.[25,26]

Limb and Trunk Kinematics During Gait. Kinematics describes movements of body parts in terms of velocity, acceleration, and displacement. Factors affecting the kinematics of gait include patient height, weight, age, balance abilities, force production capacity, flexibility, pain, speed of walking, and the presence of pathology.

Movements of the limb and trunk during gait allow a constant, rhythmic, and smooth forward progression of the body through space. As the body moves forward, the COG typically moves both vertically and laterally in a sinusoidal pattern. Limb segments primarily flex and extend to produce an average vertical displacement of about 5 cm.[27] The vertical movement upward, from the lowest point during double stance, uses metabolic energy and provides potential energy for doing work during the downward movement. When the body's COG reaches its highest point, during the midstance phase of gait, potential energy is the greatest. This potential energy is converted into kinetic energy with downward movement. Rotation and lateral listing of the pelvis, combined with knee flexion and movements of the ankle and subtalar joint, determine the vertical displacement of the COG.

When walking forward, the COG also moves laterally, an average of 2.3 cm. Lateral displacement is greatest during midstance.[9] Side-to-side excursion of the body's COG is a function of the base of support.

Interlinking of the limb segments, joint excursion, and the shape of the limb segments help to control the excursion of the COG, limiting the energy demands of walking. Normally, gait is very energy efficient. Lack of motion at one or more of the joints, as a result of soft tissue shortening, pain, increased muscle tone, or weakness, may result in excessive vertical or horizontal movement, causing instability and increased energy demands. When walking takes more energy, fatigue occurs sooner, and fatigue may further compromise motor control. Many patients with gait dysfunctions report fatigue with walking.

Tables 32-3 and 32-4 describe the expected joint excursions of the trunk, pelvis, hip, knee, ankle, and foot during stance and swing phases of gait. For example, during initial contact, the trunk is in a neutral alignment, the pelvis rotates forward 5 degrees, and the hip is in 30 degrees of flexion. The knee and ankle are in neutral positions. At loading response, the hip moves toward extension, the knee moves from neutral to 15 degrees of flexion, and the ankle moves into plantarflexion to allow approximation of the foot with the supporting surface. The subtalar joint everts during loading response.

Patterns of Muscle Recruitment During Gait. Muscles generate the force needed to initiate and control the movements of the limb segments and trunk during gait. They control the acceleration and deceleration of the limb segments to produce smooth movement and protect body structures by counteracting gravity and ground reaction forces. Most of the muscle activity during walking produces eccentric or lengthening contractions to control the moments produced by contact of the limb with the supporting surface. Muscles also provide force for upward vertical movement during gait, performing the work needed to meet the energy demands of walking.

Ground reaction forces are generated and change constantly during the stance phase of gait. These forces create a series of joint moments that are counteracted by muscle activity. For example, touching the heel to the ground creates a plantarflexion moment or force at the ankle that is controlled by the action of the ankle dorsiflexor muscles. Table 32-5 summarizes the muscles activated during stance, and Table 32-6 summarizes the muscles activated during swing.

Hip. The hip extensor muscles, including the biceps femoris, semimembranosus, semitendinosus, adductor magnus, and gluteus maximus, are active from initial contact to the end of the stance phase and from late midswing through loading response to counteract the flexor moment at the hip and trunk. The hip extensors also concentrically extend the hip after midstance.

The hip abductors, including the gluteus medius and minimus, tensor fascia lata, and a portion of the gluteus maximus, are recruited during the first half of the stance phase to stabilize the pelvis by preventing excessive vertical translation, which can increase the energy requirements for walking. These muscles control events related to swing and stance. During the later stages of stance, these muscles help to initiate forward rotation of the pelvis to assist in advancement of the swing-phase limb. The tensor fascia lata becomes active during terminal stance to resist the hip extensor moment.

The hip flexor muscles, the adductor longus, rectus femoris, gracilis, sartorius, and iliopsoas, are typically not very active after the initiation of stepping in gait. Momentum from the vertical displacement of the body's COG, along with the action of the ankle plantarflexors, provides sufficient momentum at the beginning of preswing to advance the limb through swing. Hip flexor muscles are active from late in the terminal stance phase of gait to midswing. Some muscles active at the hip also control the knee during stance.

Knee. Co-contraction of the knee extensors and flexors occurs during the first portion of stance, initial contact through a portion of midstance, in part to counteract the ground reaction forces that produce a flexion moment at the knee at initial contact. The knee moves slowly into approximately 15 degrees of flexion by loading response. In addition, muscle co-activation ensures stability at the knee as weight is being placed on the extremity during stance.

Advancement of the tibia over the pronating foot produces a force toward medial rotation of the tibia that is controlled by the biceps femoris. During midstance, the knee extensors become more active to extend the knee in preparation for swing.

Swing, in nondisabled adults, is characterized by a lack of muscle activity at the knee. Relaxation of the knee extensors allows the knee to flex for limb clearance and advancement.

Ankle. During swing the ankle dorsiflexors are active to clear the foot. At initial contact, the ankle dorsiflexors act eccentrically to control the plantarflexion moment associated with the heel of the foot contacting the supporting surface. This allows for a gradual approximation of the foot with the supporting surface and prevents the foot "slapping" the floor. After initial contact, there is a pronatory ground reaction force that is controlled by the eccentric action of the anterior and posterior tibialis.

The plantarflexors become progressively more active after initial contact to assist with shock absorption and during the later stages of stance, control advancement of the tibia over the foot.

EXAMINATION

PATIENT HISTORY

The patient history gives the therapist specific information about the person's symptoms or difficulties with

TABLE 32-3   Joint Excursion During the Stance Phase of Gait

Body Segment		Weight Acceptance		Single-Limb Support		
		Initial Contact	Loading Response	Midstance	Terminal Stance	Preswing
Trunk	Position	0° flexion/extension	0° flexion/extension	0° flexion/extension	0° flexion/extension	0° flexion/extension
Pelvis	Motion	5° forward rotation	5° forward rotation	0° rotation	5° backward rotation	5° backward rotation
Hip	Motion	Flexion	Flexion	Flexion to extension	Extension	Extension to flexion
	Angle	Positioned in 30° flexion	30 → 25° flexion	25 → 0° flexion	0 → 10° extension	20 → 0° extension
	Muscle	Gluteus maximus, hamstrings, adductor magnus	Gluteus maximus, hamstrings			Iliopsoas
Knee	Motion	Extension	Flexion	Flexion to extension	Extension	Extension to flexion
	Angle	Positioned in 0° extension	0 → 15° flexion	15 → 5° flexion	5 → 0° flexion	0 → 30° flexion
	Muscle	Quadriceps, hamstrings	Quadriceps	Quadriceps	Gastrocnemius	Gastrocnemius
Ankle	Motion	Plantarflexion	Plantarflexion	Plantarflexion to dorsiflexion	Dorsiflexion	Dorsiflexion
	Angle	Positioned in 0° dorsiflexion/plantarflexion	0 → 15° plantarflexion	15° plantarflexion to 10° dorsiflexion	5 → 0° dorsiflexion	0 → 20° plantarflexion
	Muscle	Dorsiflexors	Dorsiflexors	Plantarflexors	Plantarflexors	Plantarflexors
STJ	Position	Inversion → eversion	~5° eversion	Eversion	~2° eversion	Neutral eversion and inversion
MTP	Angle	Positioned in 0° flexion/extension	Positioned in 0° flexion/extension	Positioned in 0° flexion/extension	0 → 20° extension	30 → 60° extension

STJ, Subtalar joint; *MTP*, metatarsophalangeal.

TABLE 32-4   Joint Excursion During the Swing Phase of Gait

Body Segment		Preswing	Swing-Limb Advancement		
			Initial Swing	Midswing	Terminal Swing
Trunk	Position	0° flexion/extension	0° flexion/extension	0° flexion/extension	0° flexion/extension
Pelvis	Motion	5° backward rotation	5° backward rotation	0° rotation	5° backward rotation
Hip	Motion	Flexion	Flexion	Flexion	Flexion
	Angle	20 → 0° extension	0 → 15° flexion	15 → 25° flexion	25 → 20° flexion
	Muscle	Iliopsoas	Iliopsoas		Extensors
Knee	Motion	Extension to flexion	Flexion	Extension	Extension
	Angle	0 → 30° flexion	30 → 60° flexion	60 → 25° flexion	20 → 5° flexion
	Muscle	Gastrocnemius	Hamstrings, sartorius, gracilis	Hamstrings	Hamstrings, quadriceps
Ankle	Motion	Dorsiflexion	Dorsiflexion	Dorsiflexion	Dorsiflexion
	Angle	0 → 20° plantarflexion	20 → 5° plantarflexion	0° plantarflexion/dorsiflexion	0° plantarflexion/dorsiflexion
	Muscle	Dorsiflexors	Dorsiflexors	Dorsiflexors	Dorsiflexors
STJ	Position	Neutral inversion and eversion	Neutral inversion and eversion	Inversion	Inversion
MTP	Angle	30 → 60° extension	Positioned in 0° flexion/extension	Positioned in 0° flexion/extension	Positioned in 0° flexion/extension

STJ, Subtalar joint; *MTP*, metatarsophalangeal.

TABLE 32-5	Muscle Activity during the Stance Phase of Gait*					

	Weight Acceptance		Single-Limb Support		
Muscle	IC	LR	MSt	TSt	PSw
Gluteus maximus					
Gluteus medius					
Hip flexors					
Adductors					
Quadriceps femoris					
Hamstrings					
Pretibial/dorsiflexors†					
Plantarflexors‡					

IC, Initial contact; *LR,* loading response; *MSt,* midstance; *TSt,* terminal stance; *PSw,* preswing.
*Shaded areas of the table indicate when muscles groups are most active during the stance phase of gait.
†Pretibial/dorsiflexors: Tibialis anterior, extensor hallucis longus, extensor digitorum longus.
‡Plantarflexors: Gastrocnemius, soleus, tibialis posterior, flexor hallucis longus, flexor digitorum longus, peroneus longus and brevis.

TABLE 32-6	Muscle Activity during the Swing Phase of Gait*				

	Swing Limb Advancement			
Muscle	PSw	ISw	MSw	TSw
Gluteus maximus				
Gluteus medius				
Hip flexors				
Adductors				
Quadriceps femoris				
Hamstrings				
Pretibial/dorsiflexors†				
Plantarflexors†				

PSw, preswing; *ISw,* initial swing; *MSw,* midswing; *TSw,* terminal swing.
*Shaded areas of the table indicate when muscles groups are most active during the swing phase of gait.
†Pretibial/dorsiflexors: Tibialis anterior, extensor hallucis longus, extensor digitorum longus.
‡Plantarflexors: Gastrocnemius, soleus, tibialis posterior, flexor hallucis longus, flexor digitorum longus, peroneus longus and brevis.

walking such as pain with walking, loss of balance when ambulating on an uneven surface, or weakness or fatigue with walking.[28]

After gathering and recording patient demographics, one should determine the patient's primary reason for seeking rehabilitative services. The next step is to ascertain the time course or progression of the symptoms. Finding out when the problem with walking first occurred begins to identify the historical progression of the symptoms and provides information about the stability of the gait changes. Changes in gait may reflect the progression of various disease processes.[29-34] For example, more frequent falls may be the first sign of Parkinson's disease or a consequence of a recent stroke.[30,35] Walking instability and falling are not an inevitable part of aging and both can be due to modifiable impairments.[29,36] Progressive worsening of gait also indicates a poor prognosis for rehabilitation.[37,38]

The next steps in the interview process are to determine when the problem is at its worst, how often the person experiences difficulty with walking, the specific functional activities that are limited, the degree of participation in the functional activity that makes the problem worse, and how the patient compensates for the identified problem with walking.

When and how often the person experiences difficulty with walking is related to the severity of the problem, the activity pattern of the symptoms, and how much the person's participation in usual and expected roles is disrupted. To establish when the problem is at its worst, one could ask "Does the problem occur more frequently at a particular time during the day, week, or month?" or "Tell me about your typical day."

How long or how far the patient can walk before experiencing the symptoms may help to identify the cause(s) of the problem and give a baseline against which progress can be evaluated. The specific type of walking activities that cause symptoms and limitations in different environments and with different tasks should be addressed to get a sense of the patient's functional status and activity level.

How the patient compensates for problems with walking helps to identify factors that ease the problem or reduce symptoms. A variety of context-specific strategies may be used to compensate for difficulties with walking. For example, if the primary problem is endurance, the patient may compensate by limiting the distance walked or by resting frequently during activities. Depending on the patient's expected roles, this strategy may or may not be effective. Frequently, patients are discharged from rehabilitation unable to walk far enough to access community resources and will therefore either not have access to these resources or require assistance to access areas outside the home.[39]

Assistive devices may also be used to offset lower extremity weakness, problems with balance, or pain (see Chapter 33). The type of assistive device may vary with the environment. For example, a patient may use a walker for increased support in the community, but while at home, he or she may use a cane or no device.

The impact of a gait dysfunction on the person's ability to fulfill expected roles establishes the purpose and need for rehabilitative services. Weakness or limitations that do not impact function are generally not considered sufficient justification for physical therapy or other rehabilitative services.[40]

Information about the available social support may influence interventions and prognosis. The availability of someone to help at home and to bring the patient to therapy may determine whether a patient can go home to receive further care as an outpatient or must go to a facility where help is provided. After discharge from rehabilitation, patients will frequently require some level of assistance with activities of daily living (ADLs) that depend on ambulation. For some patients, although fully independent walking may not be a realistic goal, walking at home with assistance may be achievable. The clinician should determine if assistance is available and if so, what the caregiver is able to do. Interventions may include teaching the caregiver how to help the patient.

Questions about the home, community, and work environment should also be included in the patient history (see Chapter 35). At home, the location of bathrooms and sleeping quarters, the number steps to enter and within the home, and the presence of rails to provide support when walking on steps may all be important. In the community, function may depend on the patient's ability to manage curbs, walk on uneven surfaces, or ascend and descend ramps. At work, function may depend on the physical structure and layout of that environment. Many patients need to walk at work or to access the job site. The patient's work and hobbies provide a context for understanding the level of disability being imposed by the impairments and functional limitations reported by the patient.

The patient history for a patient with a gait dysfunction should also include relevant information about the patient's past medical history, the effects of previous interventions for the current problem, social and health habits, and in some cases, information about the patient's family history. It is also helpful to ask the patient about his or her goals and expectations for the episode of care. Achieving consensus about realistic goals before starting therapy is likely to optimize patient satisfaction.

SYSTEMS REVIEW

The systems review is used to target areas requiring further examination and to define areas that may cause complications or indicate a need for precautions during the examination and intervention processes. See Chapter 1 for details of the system review. The systems review for a patient with gait disturbances will depend on their underlying problems.

TESTS AND MEASURES

The selection of tests and measures should be based on ruling in or out hypotheses about possible sources of symptoms as derived from the patient history. The following section discusses tests and measures commonly applied to patients with gait dysfunction. Since abnormal gait patterns can arise from range of motion (ROM) restrictions,[41-44] weakness,[45-48] pain as a result of short- or long-term changes in the musculoskeletal system,[44,49] and postural alterations,[50] these aspects are the focus of this section. This is followed by a detailed discussion of gait-specific tests and measures.

Musculoskeletal

Anthropometric Characteristics. Increased joint girth, particularly from inflammation, can cause pain that limits the patient's desire to either move or bear weight on an extremity. Reduced limb girth is generally caused by muscle atrophy, which correlates with weakness.

Range of Motion. Excessive or limited ROM can adversely affect gait.[51-53] ROM may be altered by changes in ligamentous stability, loss of joint capsule integrity, or changes in the articular surfaces of the joint, as well as by alterations in muscle and tendon length or involvement of a neural structure crossing the joint. The length of muscles crossing the hip, knee, and ankle should also be tested, as shortening can limit the excursion available for gait and can make movement into the range required for gait painful by pulling on the involved structure. Such pain can limit the patient's willingness or desire to move the joint. For example, iliopsoas tightness can limit the available hip extension ROM and alter the phases of the gait cycle when the supporting limb should be behind the body.[51] Increased tone can also contribute to restrictions of joint motion during gait. Table 32-7 summarizes the ROM required in the pelvis and lower extremities for normal gait.

Muscle Performance. Lower extremity strength affects gait in a variety of patient populations,[54-61] and weakness has been shown to impair motor performance and control during walking.[45,54,62-66] Therefore all patients with gait

TABLE 32-7	Pelvis and Joint Range of Motion Required for Normal Gait	
Joint	**Stance Phase**	**Swing Phase**
Pelvis	0-5° forward and backward rotation	0-5° forward and backward rotation
Hip	0-30° flexion 0-10° extension	20-30° flexion
Knee	0-40° flexion	0-60° flexion
Ankle	0-10° dorsiflexion	0° dorsiflexion/ plantarflexion
	0-20° plantarflexion	
STJ	0-5° eversion	

STJ, Subtalar joint.

dysfunctions should be screened for weakness of the muscles involved in gait.

Manual muscle testing (MMT) may be used to screen for weakness in patients with gait dysfunction. However, MMT focuses on isometric strength when muscle recruitment during gait is typically eccentric.[9] MMT also does not reliably detect small changes in strength. Thus its clinical application for ongoing assessment of patients with gait dysfunction caused by weakness is limited. MMT may also fail to detect problems with the speed of recruitment needed for gait and has limited application in patients who cannot perform isolated volitional movements, such as those with central nervous system (CNS) lesions that result in synergistic movement patterns or mass limb movements. When using the MMT grading scale, 5/5 strength is typically not required for gait. Walking at preferred speeds or slightly faster usually requires the ability to produce muscle force at a grade of 3 to 3+/5.

A hand-held dynamometer can also be used to measure the strength of muscles used for gait. A hand-held dynamometer provides a reliable,[67-71] valid,[69,72,73] and easy-to-use alternative to isokinetic and manual muscle testing.[74] A hand-held dynamometer can detect small changes over time but is limited to isometric testing at limited points in the available range of motion.[75,76] As with MMT, the force that can be measured by a hand-held dynamometer is limited by the force the tester can exert.

Isokinetic testing, which allows dynamic measurement of the strength, speed, and endurance of eccentric, concentric, and isometric contractions at any point in a joint's available ROM, can be a more precise and accurate indicator of force production problems related to gait than MMT. However, such testing is time consuming and may limit the number of muscles that are tested and the frequency of retesting. Isokinetic testing may also be inappropriate for patients with poor isolated control. Force deficits detected by isokinetic testing have been found to correlate with gait dysfunction[57,77-79] and with the risk for falls when walking.[56,57,80] The precision of isokinetic testing makes it suitable for monitoring the effectiveness of interventions designed to address gait-related weakness.[79,81]

Joint Integrity and Mobility. Joint stability may be assessed by selective application of varus, valgus, compressive, or distractive forces to the joint. These techniques can implicate potential hypomobile, hypermobile, painful, or inflamed structures that can limit the motion available at a joint for gait.

Neuromuscular

Pain. Pain may be assessed from the patient's report and by palpation of muscles, joints, and other superficial soft tissue structures. Pain elicited with palpation can indicate a problem with one or more underlying soft tissue and/or osseous structures and can affect the pattern of movement during gait. Pain elicited with weight bearing is often a result of dysfunction in intraarticular structures.

Sensory Integrity. The intactness of light touch sensibility, sharp-dull discrimination, and joint position sense should be examined in all patients with gait dysfunction.

In addition, monofilament testing should be considered to predict the risk for skin breakdown and quantify the severity of the sensory deficit (see Chapter 18).

Sensory loss can alter gait biomechanics. Individuals with sensory loss are at greater risk for falling and for damage to the feet when walking.[5,31,82-85] When sensation is impaired, the patient often exerts more force during the weight-acceptance phase of gait, increasing the risk for skin breakdown and damage to joint structures.[5] Impaired sensation may also limit the types of orthotic or prosthetic interventions that may be implemented to address gait dysfunction.

Highly coordinated movements, including gait, can occur in the absence of sensory feedback because much of the programming of muscle recruitment for gait occurs within the spinal cord. There is evidence that humans and other organisms can produce gaitlike movement, although of a different quality, in the absence of sensory feedback from peripheral limb and joint receptors.[8,86-88]

Cranial and Peripheral Nerve Integrity. Central factors or structures responsible for acquiring information from the environment and programming motor output residing within the CNS will also contribute to overall quality of movement during gait. Gait function can be affected by impairments of the cranial nerves (CNs) and/or spinal nerve segments. CNs II, III, IV, and VI have a role in vision and should be examined whenever a patient reports difficulty with walking. The integrity of CNs III, IV, and VI, which are responsible for eye movements, affect the patient's ability to acquire information about the environment that is used to guide and plan motor output. CNs II and III affect the quality of the visual information gathered. The vestibular component of CN VIII affects balance while walking. The vestibular system provides feedback on the position of the head in space and movement of the body as it is being translated during walking. The functioning of peripheral sensory receptors, the visual system, and the vestibular system all affect balance during walking (see Chapter 13).

Although vision and the vestibular system provide a great deal of the information needed to control motor output for gait, the peripheral nervous system must also provide feedback about the position of the extremities and provide input to the muscles to produce muscle contractions. Peripheral nerve integrity can be examined with motor and sensory tests, as described previously, and with electrophysiological testing.

Motor Function—Control and Learning. Several simple tests of motor control can provide useful information about the patient with gait dysfunction. Reaching for and touching a target with the foot or performing rapidly alternating movements of the ankle or knee that require the recruitment and relaxation of agonist and antagonist muscle groups can provide insight into problems with motor control. Difficulties with these activities may indicate difficulty coordinating movement when walking, since walking requires the capacity to reciprocally and sequentially recruit and relax muscles.

The presence of atypical movement patterns should be noted and explored. Atypical movement patterns can be caused by pain, weakness, dyscoordination, or the inability to move independently of synergistic influences. Atypical movement patterns reduce gait efficiency by altering the translation of the body's COG. Lesions in the brain, such as those caused by stroke, traumatic brain injury, multiple sclerosis, or Parkinson's disease, may disrupt supraspinal input and make muscles overactive, underactive, or recruited out of sequence, resulting in atypical movements during gait.[84,85,89,90] The atypical movement patterns and their impact on gait are often most readily examined in a gait analysis laboratory equipped to perform gait-specific examination tests and measures as described later.

Surface or needle electromyography performed while the patient is walking may provide information about the timing of muscle recruitment during the gait cycle.[91] Fig. 32-3 demonstrates normal and atypical patterns of recruitment of lower extremity muscles during gait.

Abnormal tone can also affect movement control and adversely affect movement quality during gait. Tone may be measured with the Modified Ashworth Scale (see Chapter 16).

Cardiovascular/Pulmonary

Ventilation and Respiration/Gas Exchange. Respiratory rate at rest and during and after exercise will give an indication of the patient's activity tolerance. Monitoring

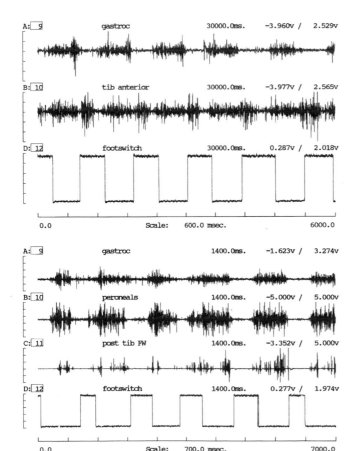

FIG. 32-3 Electromyographic profile of walking (*top*, atypical; *bottom*, normal). *From Craik R, Oatis CA: Gait Analysis: Theory and Application, St. Louis, 1994, Mosby.*

of oxygen saturation with pulse oximetry is also recommended initially during gait training of patients with cardiovascular or pulmonary dysfunction. Oxygen saturation levels should generally be kept above 95% during gait training.

Aerobic Capacity and Endurance. Walking places a demand on the cardiovascular and pulmonary systems. Checking heart rate and blood pressure at rest, while the patient walks, and immediately after the patient stops walking will provide the therapist with information on how the patient's cardiovascular and pulmonary systems respond to functional ambulation (see Chapter 22). An increase in heart rate and blood pressure in response to ambulation is normal, but this increase will be more pronounced in deconditioned patients. A decrease in heart rate or blood pressure in response to walking is a sign of poor activity tolerance. Additional cardiovascular monitoring with telemetry is recommended for patients with more severe impairments in cardiac and pulmonary function such as those who have recently undergone cardiac surgery or those with a recent myocardial infarction.

Integumentary

Integumentary Integrity. The feet should be inspected for signs of skin breakdown such as open wounds, areas of redness, and other indications of excessive of pressure such as callus formation. Individuals with impaired sensory integrity, particularly those with diabetes, are at increased risk for skin breakdown and soft tissue ulceration on the plantar surface of the foot if they walk or increase their walking.[11] This occurs primarily because loss of sensation limits the person's ability to perceive trauma to the feet from walking (see Chapter 30).

Gait-Specific Tests and Measures. A variety of gait-specific tests and measures have been developed to examine, evaluate, and diagnose gait dysfunction. Gait-specific tests and measures are generally designed to either examine impairment or functional limitations. At a minimum, the therapist should observe the patient walking from multiple perspectives and determine if the patient needs an assistive device and if the patient needs personal assistance with ambulation. Walking should be observed in a variety of environments such as on a level surface; up and down a curb, ramp, or steps; and on uneven surfaces.

Selection of additional gait-specific tests and measures depends on the purpose of the test and its reliability and validity, sensitivity and specificity, responsiveness or capacity to detect change, and appropriateness for a particular population, as well as its ease of use. Each of the tests and measures discussed in this section was developed for a specific purpose. Some tests and measures were developed to identify individuals at increased risk for falling when walking (see Chapter 13), whereas others, such as the Wisconsin Gait Scale, were developed for identification and description of gait dysfunction in a specific population. Certain measures primarily quantify the degree of functional limitation and focus less on quantifying the degree of impairment. For example, two items on the Functional Independence Measure (FIM), a tool used to predict burden of care, examine the level of functional independence for gait on level surfaces and when ascending stairs. The test indirectly captures impairments affecting gait.

Observational Gait Analysis. Observational gait analysis (OGA) is an approach frequently used for the examination and quantification of gait dysfunction in the clinical setting. OGA can be used to identify patients who would benefit from a more detailed examination, possibly in a gait laboratory and to qualitatively or quantitatively classify the degree of gait impairment. OGA is popular because it is relatively quick and easy to use, requires no equipment, and can be performed in any setting.

Observational Gait Analysis Procedure. Several published sources provide guidelines for performing OGA.[9,10,92] The history and the results of impairment-specific tests and measures should guide the focus of OGA. The patient should wear a minimal amount of clothing so the clinician can see the joints and limb segments of the upper and lower extremities. The clinician should observe from the right and left sides to focus on kinematic changes in the sagittal plane, including step and stride length; single- and double-stance times; vertical displacements of the body's COG; flexion and extension movements of the hip, knee, and ankle; and the position of the head and trunk. This should be followed by observation from the front and back to appreciate kinematic changes in the frontal plane, including base of support during double stance, foot angle, lateral or horizontal displacements of the body's COG, varus and valgus deformities at the knee, alterations in normal hip abduction and adduction, and the position and movements of the subtalar joints. The examiner should monitor changes in limb and joint segments from each perspective during each phase of gait. This generally requires multiple observations from each side.

During OGA the examiner should also monitor the movements of the various limb segments (tibia-foot complex, femur-tibia, femur-trunk). Observe one joint at a time, starting where the patient reports symptoms or where earlier testing suggests that there are deficits. For example, if the patient reports one knee giving out or buckling during the single stance phase of gait or if weakness was previously found in muscles crossing the knee, then start the examination at the knee and move proximally to the hip and trunk and distally to the ankle.

If the patient history and prior testing do not localize a source for the gait impairment, then start OGA at the ankle and systematically move up the kinetic chain, observing movements of each joint and related limb segments from all directions. First, examine movements of the ankle joint and the tibia relative to the foot and ankle complex and then look at the knee.

The primary goal of OGA is to identify primary and secondary gait changes caused by specific impairments. Secondary changes are those caused by a primary gait deviation. For example, decreased ankle dorsiflexion ROM will cause the primary gait deviation of reduced anterior movement of the tibia on the ankle-foot complex during weight acceptance. To compensate, there may be secondary changes such as increased knee extension or hip flexion during weight acceptance (initial contact and loading response).

Gait should be observed at a variety of speeds. Although it is easiest to start with the patient's preferred walking speed, faster and slower walking speeds should also be observed. Some gait deviations may only be apparent at faster speeds because the patient's preferred speed is likely to be one that minimizes gait deviations. With patients who report difficulty with prolonged walking, the OGA may also need to include longer distances or durations for gait deviations to occur. Various speeds and inclines, as well as distances and durations of walking, may be simulated in the clinic using a treadmill.

Community ambulation may also need to be observed to see how the patient manages uneven surfaces and obstacles such as other pedestrians, traffic, and curbs. Negotiation of environmental obstacles requires step-length alteration and predictive motor planning to avoid contact with an obstacle in the path of travel.[93-95] McFadyen and Prince examined obstacle avoidance and accommodation strategies during gait in healthy, community-dwelling, and young and elderly males.[96] Both age groups used the same general sagittal plane movement strategies to avoid and accommodate the obstacle; however, the elderly group demonstrated significantly reduced and riskier lead toe clearance that was believed to be a result of limited frontal plane pelvic motion, shorter stride lengths, and differences in the interplay of lower limb movement patterns.

OGA should also include observation of how the patient starts and stops walking and changes direction, since these tasks are problematic for some patients.[97,98] Walking while performing functional tasks, such as scanning the environment or carrying objects in the upper extremities, may also be observed if the patient history indicates that these cause difficulties. One cannot assume that performance while walking on a level surface in a straight line in a controlled environment necessarily predicts performance in other environments. OGA can also be extended to examining patient function during various activities such as ascending and descending stairs.

Reliability and Validity of Observations Gait Analysis. A number of studies have examined the reliability of OGA.[99-104] Although experience is thought to improve the reliability of OGA and it does help the observer become familiar with the normal variability of gait and the gait dysfunctions typical with certain diagnoses, such as stroke, multiple sclerosis, or amputation, research has not clearly demonstrated improved OGA reliability with increased experience.[101,102] Krebs and colleagues reported only moderate intrarater reliability for expert raters using OGA to examine gait in a sample of pediatric patients with lower limb disability wearing an orthotic device. The authors concluded that inadequate rater training, personal bias, and the limitations of using human sight may contribute to measurement error and reduced reliability.[101,105]

McGinley et al reported that physical therapists (PTs) using OGA could consistently identify and grade deficits in push-off of patients diagnosed with a stroke.[100,106] The therapists watched a videotape of the subject walking and rated their plantarflexion force during push-off/terminal stance with a score of 0-10, 0 denoting no force and 10 denoting normal or near-normal force. Both intrarater and interrater reliability for these scores were high. These findings suggest that a scoring scale may help clinicians focus on specific aspects of gait during OGA and thereby help them produce consistent reliable ratings.

Only a few studies have attempted to examine the validity of OGA and these have had conflicting findings.[99,100,103] In the study described, McGinley et al also found that therapists' ratings of ankle force production correlated strongly with force data gathered from an instrumented walkway, giving OGA in this context good criterion validity.[100] However, another study found that observers using OGA to examine the gait of individuals with a unilateral below-knee amputation identified only 22.2% of the gait deviations detected with an alternative quantitative analysis procedure.[103]

Although OGA has many limitations, the simplicity and ready availability of the approach will likely result in its ongoing use in a variety of clinical and research settings. The findings may be used to direct care or to screen for dysfunction and direct the selection of other more reliable and specific tests and measures that can implicate specific system involvement, localize the impairments, and quantify functional gait deficits. The use of standardized instruments in conjunction with OGA can improve reliability and therefore provide better tracking of patient progress during an episode of care.

Videotaping of Observational Gait Analysis. Videotaping may enhance the reliability of OGA, particularly when a standardized measurement tool is used.[102,106,107] Videotaping also creates a permanent record of the client's walking, allowing for comparison of preintervention and postintervention performance and for repeated viewing of a walking trial, avoiding patient fatigue with repetition.

Standardized Tests and Measures That Rely on Observational Gait Analysis. A number of standardized tests and measures have been developed to quantify the findings from OGA. These tests and measures include decision rules and standardized scoring systems for OGA. There is evidence that raters can reliably identify gait impairments in patients with cerebral palsy,[99] stroke,[107] and spinal cord injury[104] when using standardized scoring systems in conjunction with OGA.

Rancho Los Amigos Observational Gait Analysis System. A form was developed at Rancho Los Amigos Hospital to document the findings from OGA, and this form has since been used in a variety of settings and been refined many times over the years.[10] This instrument allows for consistent documentation of OGA; however, its reliability, sensitivity, specificity, and its capacity for detecting change, have not been studied.

Wisconsin Gait Scale. The Wisconsin Gait Scale (WGS), developed in 1996, is a 14-item scale intended to measure clinically relevant components of gait in persons after stroke.[107] Asymmetries in step length and single-stance time, capacity for weight bearing on the involved extremity, base of support during double stance, and changes in joint excursions frequently occur after a stroke.[108] The WGS uses an ordinal scale to categorize the findings from OGA. The scale appears to possess face and content valid-

ity and has been shown to have high interrater and intrarater reliability when used by trained experts and novices to rate patients after a stroke.[105,107,109] Turani and colleagues also reported improvements in WGS scores in patients after rehabilitation for stroke-related gait deficits, with improvements correlating positively with increased gait velocity.[110]

Gait Abnormality Rating Scale. The Gait Abnormality Rating Scale (GARS) is a scale for evaluating gait that was specifically developed to identify elderly adults at risk for falling in a nursing home environment, although it can be used to quantify various aspects of gait in a variety of populations.[111] A 0-3 ordinal scale is used to rate 16 aspects of gait noted during OGA. When scoring the items, 0 = normal, 1 = mildly impaired, 2 = moderately impaired, and 3 = severely impaired. The total score is the sum of scores for all items, with a higher score indicating greater impairment and fall risk. The 16 scored items are: (1) variability in the rhythm of the stepping and arm movements, (2) guardedness, (3) weaving or an irregular line of forward progression, (4) excessive side-to-side movements of the trunk, (5) staggering or lateral deviations from the path of travel, (6) percentage of time spent in stance phase, (7) heel strike at initial contact, (8) hip ROM, (9) knee ROM, (10) elbow extension ROM, (11-12) shoulder abduction and extension ROM, (13) arm-heel strike synchrony, (14) forward-head positioning, (15) shoulder elevation, and (16) upper trunk flexion. GARS scores have been shown to correlate negatively with gait velocity and step length and positively with a history of falling, but this test's ability to predict falls or detect changes in response to rehabilitative interventions has not been established.[111]

Modified Gait Abnormality Rating Scale. The Modified Gait Abnormality Rating Scale (GARS-M), a variant of the GARS, is a 7-item scale developed to predict fall risk among community-dwelling, frail elderly adults.[112] The items are scored with the same 0-3 scale as the GARS but only the following qualities of gait are evaluated: (1) variability, (2) guardedness, (3) staggering, (4) initial contact, (5) hip ROM, (6) shoulder extension, and (7) arm-heel strike synchrony. These items were selected as they were found to be the most reliable of the original GARS.[112] Using the Kappa statistic, VanSwearingen and colleagues reported high intrarater and interrater reliability ($\kappa = 0.97$) for this scale.[112] Scores on the GARS-M correlate negatively with gait speed and stride length and positively with step variability.[16] In a sample of community-dwelling, frail elderly males, the sensitivity and specificity of the GARS-M for predicting fall risk were 62.3% and 87.1%, respectively, when using a cut-off score of 9.[113] The instrument's ability to detect change has not been evaluated.

Tinetti's Performance-Oriented Mobility Assessment. Tinetti's Performance-Oriented Mobility Assessment (POMA) is a commonly used clinical measure of both gait and balance that was developed specifically for use with older adults.[114] This instrument consists of 16 items, 7 related to gait and 9 related to balance (see Chapter 13). The POMA examines step length and height, gait initiation, step symmetry and continuity, straightness of the path of travel while trying to walk in a straight line, trunk position, and base of support during the period of double support. Performance on all items is scored from 0-1 or 2 for a maximum score of 28, with a higher score indicating better gait and balance. Low scores on the instrument have been shown to correlate with fall risk in elderly adults.[115,116] A total score of 19 or less indicates a high risk for falling and a score between 19 and 24 indicates a moderate risk.[114,117]

Dynamic Gait Index. The Dynamic Gait Index (DGI) is a gait-related tool developed to identify elderly adults at risk for falls (see Chapter 13). It rates the following eight tasks on a 0-3 scale: (1) walking on a level surface, (2) capacity for changing gait speed, (3-4) ability to walk and turn the head in a horizontal and vertical direction, (5) balance for rapid directional changes, (6-7) capacity for stepping over and around an obstacle, and (8) stair performance. Lower scores indicate greater impairment. A score of 19 or less has been shown to be related to increased risk for falling, and scores have been shown to increase in adults undergoing rehabilitation for balance disorders because of central and peripheral nerve impairments.[118-121]

Standardized Tests and Measures Related to Gait That Do Not Rely on Observational Gait Analysis

Timed Up and Go Test. The Timed Up and Go (TUG) test is a performance-based measure of functional mobility that was initially developed to identify mobility and balance impairments in older adults.[122,123] The test requires the subject to rise from a chair, walk 3.0 m at a comfortable pace to a mark placed on the floor, turn around at the 3.0 m mark, walk back to the starting point, and return to sitting in the chair. The test's score is the time it takes the subject takes to complete the test (see Chapter 13).[123]

The TUG has demonstrated high interrater and intrarater reliability when used to examine elderly adults.[123] It has also demonstrated validity for assessing functional mobility. Individuals who take longer than 30 seconds to complete the test need physical assistance with transfers and generally cannot manage steps.[122] Individuals who can complete the test in less than 20 seconds will likely be independently mobile and most can manage steps and walk outside the home.[122] Table 32-8 provides a summary of the time required for nondisabled elderly adults to complete the TUG.

The TUG has been used to examine and document mobility in patients with osteoarthritis,[124-126] dementia,[127] Parkinson's disease,[120,121] low back pain,[128] amputation,[129,130] Alzheimer's disease,[131] cerebral palsy,[132] and stroke[133-135] and patients at risk for falling.[136-138] To monitor the effectiveness of rehabilitation, it is recommended that the TUG be combined with other tests and measures to ensure examination of all of the dimensions of functional gait performance.[124] A variant of the TUG, a timed ascent and descent of 10 steps, can be used to examine patient performance on steps.

Emory Functional Ambulation Profile. The Emory Functional Ambulation Profile (E-FAP) is a scale that combines performance on the TUG test with the time required to walk 5 m on a level surface (7 m on carpet), to negotiate an obstacle course, and to ascend and descend 4 steps using a handrail.[139] Scores on the five tasks are summed. The instrument can be administered in 20 minutes or less, is inexpensive, and provides quantitative information about the patient's ability to ambulate under a variety of environmental constraints. For each of the items, interrater reliability for participants with and without disability was high (ICC ≥0.997) and test-retest reliability for patients after a stroke was high (ICC = 0.998).[140] For the patients after a stroke, increased times on the E-FAP correlated with poor performance on the Berg Balance Scale and the TUG, supporting concurrent validity of the E-FAP.[139] This tool is also sensitive to changes in gait.[140]

Berg Balance Scale. The Berg Balance Scale (BBS) is a performance-oriented measure of balance for use with elderly adults. It consists of 14 items scored on a 0-4 scale. The tool measures balance during mobility tasks that form the basis for walking together with a number of other measures such as strength, integrative balance, flexibility, and cognition (see Chapter 13 for further details of the BBS).

Activities-Specific Balance Confidence Scale. The Activities-Specific Balance Confidence (ABC) Scale is a 16-item questionnaire used to rate self-perceptions of mobility confidence for a variety of walking and standing activities. Each item is scored from 0%-100% in 10% increments, with higher scores indicating greater confidence in mobility.[141,142] A score of 0% to 10% indicates no confidence in performing the activity, whereas 90% to 100% indicates complete confidence when performing the listed activity. Some of the items contained in the tool assess the client's ability to walk under a variety of task conditions. The scale has been shown to be a reliable and valid indicator of self-efficacy for mobility skills among elderly individuals.[141-143] The instrument captures the individual's perception of his or her abilities when performing a variety of functional tasks involving standing and walking.[142,143] Poor performance on this measure may indicate that the patient would benefit from interventions that increase their confidence in walking.

Lack of confidence in walking has been shown to be related to changes in gait performance.[16,144] Maki reported that elderly adults who were concerned about falling had reduced stride length and gait speed and increased base of support and double-support time.[16] Elderly adults with low balance confidence were also more disabled, had lower self-efficacy, and lower scores on the BBS.[145]

Although the ABC allows the clinician to examine the effects of affective factors on walking, the literature provides little evidence that gait-related interventions can

TABLE 32-8	Mean Time for Elderly Nondisabled Adults to Complete the Timed Up and Go Test		
Age (Years)	**Gender**	**Mean (sec)**	**Range (sec)**
60-69	Male	9.93 ± 1.40	4-12
	Female	10.15 ± 2.91	4-12
70-74	Male	10.45 ± 1.85	3-15
	Female	10.37 ± 2.23	5-13
75-79	Male	10.48 ± 1.59	8-12
	Female	10.98 ± 2.68	5-17

lead to improvements in mobility confidence. There is also no published research using the ABC to examine individuals with known pathology. The existing literature describes use of the ABC for elderly adults who are functioning at a fairly high level. One study has used the tool to examine balance confidence in adults with dizziness.[146]

Functional Independence Measure. The Functional Independence Measure (FIM) is an instrument that was developed as a measure of disability for a variety of populations.[147] The instrument includes measures of independence for self-care, including sphincter control, transfers, locomotion, communication, and social cognition. The locomotion scale examines walking ability on steps and level surfaces. Walking is scored according to the observed distance walked and the level of assistance required. The FIM, with proper rater training, is highly reliable,[148] valid,[149] and demonstrates high internal consistency.[149] The tool as a whole can detect changes in dependence occurring during rehabilitation. However, the capacity for detecting change in a single item of the instrument has not been reported.

Stride Analysis, Gait Velocity, and Footfall Measurement Technologies. Various tools and devices can be used to measure temporal and distance parameters of gait. These range from simple, inexpensive, and easy-to-use tools, such as a stopwatch and tape measure, to complex but more expensive devices, such as instrumented walkways specifically designed to measure gait. The more complex devices provide more detailed and precise information allowing for closer monitoring of patient progress over time.

Hand-Held Stopwatch. The simplest way to determine gait velocity is to time the patient walking a measured distance. High interrater, intrarater, and test-retest reliability has been reported for timing a 25 foot (approximately 8 m) walk with a stopwatch.[25] A few feet should be allowed at the beginning and end of the timing walkway to allow for acceleration and deceleration. Gait velocity can be determined on various surfaces, with or without obstacles.[150]

Gait velocity is an excellent global indicator of walking capacity.[151-154] Gait velocity can discriminate between different levels of functional community ambulation.[152,154] Elderly adults who walk more slowly are more disabled, have lower self-efficacy or balance confidence, and have lower scores on the BBS.[145] Gait velocity, along with distance covered, is also related to perception of general health in elderly adults.[155] Changes in gait velocity can also predict functional dependence in elderly adults.[156]

During ADLs, people need to be able to walk at different velocities, thus walking velocity should be measured at an individual's preferred pace and at slow and fast speeds. Various impairments and pathologies are associated with reduced walking velocity.[54,63-65,157-160] For example, after a stroke, gait velocity may be reduced because of impaired motor control in the affected lower extremity.[45,54] This may slow or delay initiation of hip flexion during preswing and delay or decrease hip extension during stance, both of which contribute to reduced

walking velocity. Atypical movement patterns can also affect distance parameters gait such as stride length, cadence, and the duration of the swing and stance phases of gait.[45,161] Improvements in motor control are associated with increased gait velocity, and gait velocity can be an indicator of the effectiveness of interventions.[45,153]

Decreased gait velocity has also been linked to an increased risk of falling.[162,163] Individuals who walk at a speed of 0.57 m/sec or less have an increased fall risk (sensitivity = 72%; specificity = 74%)[113] and may benefit from rehabilitation services.[164]

Six-Minute Walk Test. The 6-minute walk test (6MWT) requires the patient to walk for 6 minutes at their preferred pace. The patient is instructed to walk as long and as far as possible in the prescribed amount of time, and the test is scored by measuring the total distance walked. Rest breaks may be taken as needed. The test is stopped when the 6-minute time limit is reached or when vital signs or patient fatigue indicate a need to stop. The test can be completed in as little space as a 100-foot walkway and requires minimal rater training. Self-ratings of perceived exertion, heart rate, and/or oxygen saturation may be recorded before, during, and after the test is completed. These measures can be used to monitor and track intervention effectiveness and to set safe guidelines for aerobic conditioning activities that involve walking. Observational gait analysis can be completed during the 6MWT, and this test also allows for examination of the effects of fatigue on gait.

The 6MWT can be used to examine functional exercise capacity in patients with a wide range of conditions.[165-168] In patients with mild-to-moderate heart failure, covering a distance of less than 300 m in 6 minutes is a marker of subsequent cardiac death.[166] The 6MWT has also been used to examine functional mobility in elderly adults,[169,170] monitor the effects of peripheral vascular disease,[171] track the functional performance of patients with fibromyalgia,[172,173] and monitor the effectiveness of interventions to improve fitness and walking abilities in patients with neurological diseases such as stroke and Parkinson's disease.[174,175]

Harada and colleagues found the test-retest reliability of the 6MWT to be excellent when used in nondisabled healthy older adults.[169] Their research also supported the validity of this test, finding that the distance covered by active elderly adults was significantly greater than for inactive older adults. Moderate correlation with transfer function, standing balance, and gait speed were also found, whereas correlation with self-reported physical functioning and general health perceptions was low.

Inked Footprint Methods. Temporal and distance measures of gait can also be examined by applying inked moleskin to a patient's feet and then having him or her walk on a roll of paper.[176] The moleskin is first applied to the heel and toe of the patient's shoes (Fig. 32-4) and then ink is applied to the moleskin. The patient then walks on paper, leaving marks as they go (Fig. 32-5). Step length, stride length, base of support during double stance, and angle of *toe out* can then be measured. The inked footprint method provides a reliable, valid, and low-cost means to quantify gait function.[176] An even simpler alternative to

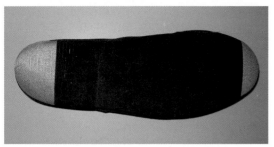

FIG. 32-4 Moleskin attached to the heel and toe of the shoe.

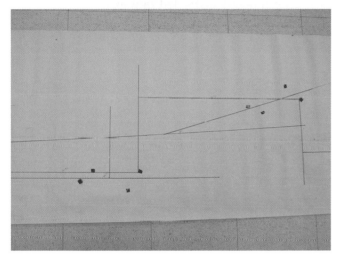

FIG. 32-5 Measurement of selected gait parameters from footprints made with moleskin attached to the heel and toe of shoes.

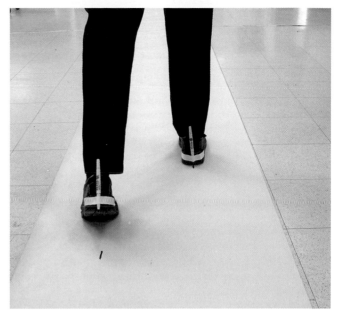

FIG. 32-6 Felt-tipped markers attached to the back of the shoes.

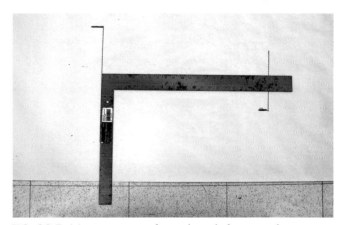

FIG. 32-7 Measurement of step length from marks generated by the felt-tipped marker method.

using moleskin involves the attachment of felt-tipped markers to the heel of the shoe (Fig. 32-6). As the subject walks, marks made on the paper can be used to measure step and stride length (Fig. 32-7).

The Gait Grid Gait Mat is a device that works similarly to using inked moleskin and paper to record gait measures (Fig. 32-8). The Gait Grid Gait Mat is a 7.62 × 0.762 m naugahyde mat with lines on it 4 cm apart. Marks are made on it by applying powder to the soles of the patient's shoes (Fig. 32-9). The mat is reusable and can be cleaned with water between gait trials. Interrater, intrarater, and test-retest reliability and concurrent validity have been demonstrated for this method in a nondisabled sample of young and middle-aged adults, and this procedure generally takes less time to complete than the inked footprint method.[177]

Instrumented Walkways. Instrumented walkways automate the process of collecting temporal and distance gait measures. The GAITRite Gait Mat is an example of the many available instrumented walkway products (Fig. 32-10). It consists of a mat 4.6 m long by 0.9 m wide with six sensor pads that contain 2,304 pressure sensors each, arranged in a 48 × 48 grid pattern.[163] The sensor pads send information to a computer every 26-31 ms, and this information is processed by the GAITRite software program (Fig. 32-11). The software records the time and number of

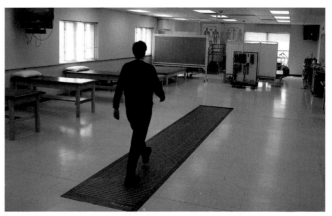

FIG. 32-8 Gait Grid Gait Mat. *Courtesy Gait Rite, Tustin, CA.*

switches activated and deactivated with each step and from this information can compute a wide range of temporal and distance gait parameters, including step and stride length, single- and double-stance time, swing time, step ratio (step length/leg length), and gait velocity. The program's software contains several algorithms to identify known footfall pattern abnormalities. This system has been shown to produce reliable and valid measures of selected temporal and distance parameters of gait, with an accuracy of ±0.6 cm.[178]

The major advantages of automated walkways are the ease of data collection and analysis. These systems are also generally easy to use with minimal training. The GAITRite system can measure up to 70 gait parameters within minutes, and this information can readily be kept as a record of performance. Performance can be tracked over time to demonstrate changes during an episode of care. As with many advanced technologies, the primary disadvantage of this system is cost, which is approximately $10,000-$15,000.

Stride Analyzers and In-Shoe Microprocessor Systems. Stride analyzers use data collected from pressure-activated microprocessor switches on an insole placed in the patient's shoes. Pressure-activated switches are located in four areas of each foot: Heel, first and fifth metatarsal heads, and the great toe (Fig. 32-12). Data generated from up to 4 walking trials are initially stored in a recorder worn in a small pack around the patient's waist (Fig. 32-13) and are later downloaded to a computer for analysis. Stride analyzers can record and calculate gait velocity, cadence, stride length, single- and double-support time, swing and stance time, and total gait cycle time (Fig. 32-14). This type of system has the advantage of allowing the patient to move about freely rather than being restricted to a straight walkway. However, these systems are expensive and for a similar cost to an automated walkway, provide less information about gait pattern.

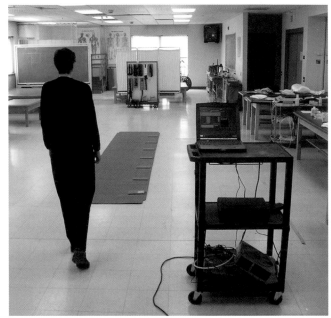

FIG. 32-10 GAITRite Gait Mat. *Courtesy Gait Rite, Tustin, CA.*

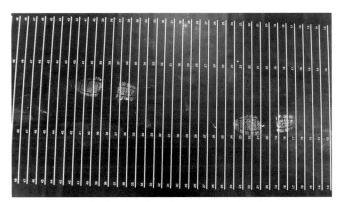

FIG. 32-9 Marks left by powder on the sole of the shoe on the Gait Grid Gait Mat.

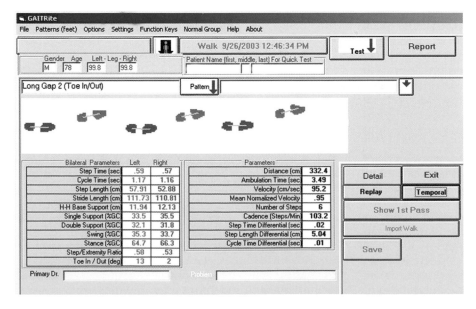

FIG. 32-11 GAITRite Gait Mat screen shot of selected temporal and distance gait measures. *Courtesy GaitRite, Tustin, CA.*

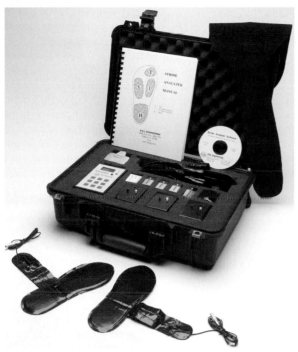

FIG. 32-12 Stride analysis system components. *Courtesy GaitRite, Tustin, CA.*

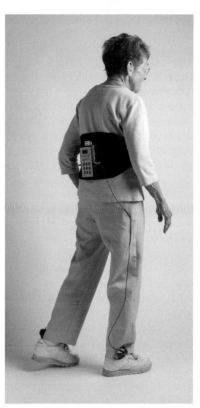

FIG. 32-13 Stride analysis system on model. *Courtesy B & L Engineering, Tustin, CA.*

FIG. 32-14 Stride analysis system computer screen shot. *Courtesy B & L Engineering, Tustin, CA.*

Stride Analyzer - John Smith (JS01)

File Edit View Activities Help

Your Department's Name
Your Institution's Name
Gait Analysis Report - Walking

Name:	SMITH, JOHN	Trial Name:	JS01
Number:	1234	Trial Length:	5.97 seconds
Date:	05/13/93	Conditions:	WALK
Diagnosis:	Sprained Right Ankle	Strides:	4
Age:	29 years 0 months	Trial Type:	Walking Trial
Gender:	Male	Distance:	6.000 meters

Stride Characteristics

	Actual	%Normal
Velocity (M/MIN):	60.3	74.0
Cadence (STEPS/MIN):	100.7	93.0
Stride Length (M):	1.197	79.6
Gait Cycle (SEC):	1.19	106.4

	-R-	-L-
Single Limb Support		
(SEC):	0.411	0.400
(%NORMAL):	82.9	80.6
(%GC):	34.7	33.4
Swing (%GC):	33.5	34.5
Stance (%GC):	66.5	65.5
Double Support		
Initial (%GC):	15.2	15.4
Terminal (%GC):	16.5	15.2
Total (%GC):	31.7	30.6

Ready   NUM

EVALUATION, DIAGNOSIS, AND PROGNOSIS

Evaluation of the data from all components of the examination should lead the clinician to a preferred practice pattern and prognosis. For example, data may implicate force production problems localized to the knee extensors and limitations in aerobic capacity and endurance as being responsible for an observed gait dysfunction and the associated functional limitations and disability.

When evaluating the underlying causes of gait dysfunction, the clinical decision-making skill lies in the ability to classify the importance of and causal links between the problems observed during the examination. Primary problems are those that have the greatest impact on patient function and that are thought to be the cause of other observed problems. These are the most appropriate target of procedural interventions. Secondary problems are problems that arise out of, or are a consequence of, the primary problems. Targeting a procedural intervention toward a secondary problem will generally be less effective in ameliorating the patient's problems with walking.

An example of identifying primary and secondary problems involves the appearance of genu recurvatum during the stance phase of gait. Observational gait analysis may reveal the following gait changes: Excessive displacement or forward leaning of the trunk in the sagittal plane as weight is placed on the involved limb during the loading response; loss of tibial advancement over the foot from loading response to the midstance phase; and rapid, early, and excessive knee extension as the midstance phase is approached. Step-length asymmetry will arise as the patient will have difficulty advancing the uninvolved limb during swing because of alterations in the normally smooth forward trajectory of the body, and gait velocity will decrease as the typical forward progression is disrupted. Dysfunctions at the trunk (hip extensor weakness), the knee (excessive knee extensor tone or weakness), or the ankle (loss of ROM for dorsiflexion) can be causing the observed gait changes, but to be effective, the clinician must identify which of these is occurring and direct interventions at this primary cause.

Diagnosis is the process of assigning meaning to the findings of the examination.[28,167] The *Guide* recommends assigning the patient to one or more of the preferred practice patterns within the broad categories of musculoskeletal, neuromuscular, cardiopulmonary, and integumentary.[28]

Another way to categorize information from the examination to guide selection of procedural interventions for gait dysfunction is presented in Table 32-9. This table identifies impairment level causes of observed gait changes. Impairment level tests can thus be used to confirm or rule out a cause of an observed gait change and to direct procedural interventions. Information in Fig. 32-1 and Table 32-1 and Tables 32-10 and 32-11 can be used to make a final diagnosis.

Although the *Guide* can be used to predict the expected length of treatment and expected outcomes for different preferred practice patterns,[28] the expected level of recovery and the time frames for recovery listed are very broad.

After a stroke, between 50% to 80% of patients regain some degree of walking ability, although the rate of recovery may vary.[168,179] Baer and Smith, in examining a group of patients after stroke of varying severity, found that the median time for taking 10 steps was 5 days and for walking 10 m was 8 days.[151] Mayo and colleagues found that getting out of bed and walking a short distance was a strong predictor of the potential for discharge home among patients after stroke.[3] Rabadi and Blau, in a sample of 373 patients admitted for acute rehabilitation after stroke, found that ambulation speed at admission was a strong predictor of length of stay and discharge disposition.[180] Mean length of stay was 17 ± 19 days, and the sensitivity and specificity of gait speed as a predictor of home discharge in patients ambulating at more than 0.15 m/sec were 0.5 and 0.87, respectively. The location of a stroke may also affect the prognosis for recovery from gait dysfunction. Patients with strokes caused by partial anterior circulation infarcts, lacunar infarcts, or infarcts affecting the posterior circulation had a quicker recovery of gait function than patients with infarcts in other areas.[151,181]

Miki and colleagues examined the recovery of walking in a sample of patients who underwent total hip arthroplasty.[182] Walking speed reached values expected for healthy adults 12 months after surgery and correlated with gains in hip ROM and peak force of hip extension.

Predicting the level of functional outcome based solely on gait data remains difficult.[183] Patient self-efficacy, premorbid capacity for ambulation, severity of disease, the presence of comorbidities, and age may all affect outcome and the recovery of ambulatory function.

INTERVENTION

A number of interventions have been proposed to address deficits in gait function.[36,184-188] Neurodevelopmental treatment (NDT) approaches advocate the use of tactile and verbal feedback in the context of task-specific and non–task-specific practice paradigms.[184] Task-specific interventions emphasize practicing the actual task of walking under a variety of environmental conditions. Non–task-specific practice would include performing activities that either strengthen or enhance the recruitment of muscles contributing to gait[184,188] or repetitively practicing the problematic elements of walking outside the context of the actual task.[36,184] Although continuing to be popular clinically, there is little evidence to support the effectiveness of NDT approaches in improving measurable parameters of gait.[189] A number of randomized control trials (RCTs) supports the effectiveness of gait-specific interventions in a number of populations. A systematic review of the effectiveness of physical therapy interventions on functional outcomes reported that there is strong evidence to support the use of task-oriented training approaches to restore balance and gait.[190] Non–gait-specific interventions that combine strengthening activities,

TABLE 32-9   Impairment Level Causes of Observed Gait Changes

Body Segment	Period	Observed Gait Problem	Phase of the Gait Cycle	Evaluation and Diagnosis
Trunk	Stance	Lateral lean	IC through PSw	Weak hip abductors Hip joint pain Leg-length discrepancy
		Backward lean	IC through PSw	Hip extensor weakness
		Forward lean	IC through PSw	Hip extensor weakness Inadequate lumbar flexibility Hip flexor or joint contracture
	Swing	Lateral lean	ISw through TSw	Compensation for weak hip abductors on the contralateral stance-phase limb
		Backward lean	ISw through MSw	Compensation to advance the involved limb through swing
Pelvis	Stance	Posterior tilt	Stance and/or swing	Inadequate lumbar flexibility Back pain Postural malalignment Tonal increases
		Anterior tilt	Stance and/or swing	Inadequate lumbar flexibility Hip flexor or joint contracture Back pain Impaired abdominal force production Postural malalignment
		Retraction	Stance and/or swing	Inadequate hip flexor or joint flexibility
		Pelvic drop	Stance	Force production deficit: Abductors
Hip	Swing Stance	Inadequate flexion	IC to LR	Impaired force production: Hip flexors Decreased ambulation velocity Impaired motor control: Synergistic movement patterns Pain
		Excessive flexion	IC through PSw	Hip flexor contracture Joint contracture
		Inadequate extension	IC through PSw	Hip flexor contracture Joint contracture Pain
		Abduction	IC through PSw	Varus deformity Leg length discrepancy Joint contracture Pain
		Adduction	IC through PSw	Valgus deformity Adductor contracture Increased adductor tone/hypertonicity Impaired motor control associated with CNS impairments
	Swing	Excessive flexion	ISw through TSw in conjunction with increased knee flexion	Compensation for decreased dorsiflexion due to impaired force production of the ankle dorsiflexors
Knee	Stance	Inadequate flexion	During any of the stance phases, less than the expected of amount of knee flexion is observed	Inadequate knee extensor strength Contracture at the knee: Joint or muscle Pain Knee extensor hyperactivity Co-contraction: Knee flexor and extensor Inadequate ankle dorsiflexion Impaired proprioception
		Excessive flexion	During any of the stance phases, more than the expected of amount of knee flexion is observed	Inadequate knee extensor strength Contracture: Joint capsule, ligaments or muscle Knee flexor hypertonicity or hyperactivity Co-contraction: Knee flexors and extensors secondary to CNS dysfunction Pain

Continued

TABLE 32-9 Impairment Level Causes of Observed Gait Changes—cont'd

Body Segment	Period	Observed Gait Problem	Phase of the Gait Cycle	Evaluation and Diagnosis
				Leg-length discrepancy on the contralateral side: Osseous changes or joint contracture (hip, knee, or ankle)
				Excessive ankle dorsiflexion Impaired proprioception
		Hyperextension or rapid movement of the knee into extension	IC to MSt	Inadequate knee extensor strength
				Contracture: Decreased dorsiflexion at the ankle
				Knee extensor hypertonicity or hyperactivity
				Contracture at the ankle: Limited dorsiflexion
				Impaired proprioception
				Mechanism for increasing limb stability
		Varus/valgus posture	IC through PSw	Knee joint or ligamentous instability
				Bone deformity or erosion
				Varus or valgus deformity at the hip
		Rapid knee flexion/ buckling	LR through TSt	Knee extensor weakness
				Poor eccentric control of the gastrocnemius-soleus muscle group (See Chapters 12 and 33 for the effects of orthotics and prosthetics)
	Swing	Inadequate flexion		Contracture: Joint or muscle
				Knee extensor hypertonicity or hyperactivity
				Co-contraction: Knee flexor and extensor
		Excessive flexion		Limited dorsiflexion at the ankle
Ankle	Stance	Forefoot first contact	IC occurs with the ball of the foot.	Plantar flexion contracture
				Heel pain
				Excessive knee flexion at the end of swing
		Flat foot contact	IC occurs with the whole plantar surface of the foot.	Ankle joint contracture
				Limitations in force production at the knee
				Pain
		Foot slap	At IC leading into loading response, foot rapidly plantarflexes when contacting the supporting surface.	Weakness of ankle dorsiflexors
				Impaired proprioception
		Increased plantar flexion/decreased dorsiflexion	At LR, lack of mobility into dorsiflexion.	Plantar flexion contracture
				Increased tone in the plantarflexors
				Impaired proprioception
		Excessive inversion	At IC, foots lands on the lateral border in excessive inversion.	Overactivity of the tibialis anterior, tibialis posterior, or gastrocnemius-soleus muscles
				Plantarflexor contracture
				Internal tibial torsion
				Calcaneovarus deformity
		Lack of heel off	TSt	Gastrocnemius: Soleus weakness
		Early/rapid heel rise	MSt through PSw	Lack of dorsiflexion: Joint or plantarflexor contracture
		Delayed heel rise	MSt through PSw	Impaired force production: Plantarflexors
		Medial heel whip	Lateral movement of heel at terminal stance.	Lack of dorsiflexion: Joint or plantarflexor contracture
	Swing	Foot or toe drag	Contact of the toes or ball of the foot with the supporting for either a portion of or throughout swing phase.	Lack of dorsiflexion: Joint or plantarflexor contracture
				Increased tone in the plantarflexors
				Weakness of ankle dorsiflexors
				Inadequate hip flexion
				Inadequate knee flexion
				Somatosensory deficits: lack of awareness of the position of the foot in space

TABLE 32-9		Impairment Level Causes of Observed Gait Changes—cont'd		
Body Segment	**Period**	**Observed Gait Problem**	**Phase of the Gait Cycle**	**Evaluation and Diagnosis**
Foot	Stance	Excessive eversion or pronation	IC through PSw	Ligamentous laxity; compromised osseous integrity: Long-term musculoskeletal trauma
				Leg-length discrepancy
				Tibialis anterior weakness
		Excessive inversion or supination	IC through TSt	Overactive invertor muscles
				Overactive gastrocnemius-soleus
				Leg-length discrepancy
		Toe clawing	LR through PSw	Overactive toe flexors
				Increased toe flexor tone
				Reduced length of the toe flexors
	Swing	Excessive inversion	Swing	Overactive invertor muscles
				Underactive evertor muscles
				Overactive gastrocnemius-soleus

IC, Initial contact; *PSw,* preswing; *ISw,* initial swing; *TSw,* terminal swing; *LR,* loading response; *MSt,* midstance; *TSt,* terminal stance.

balance training, and endurance training have also been shown to be effective in some cases.

TASK-SPECIFIC TRAINING

Currently, the evidence supports a task-specific approach to gait training that involves practicing walking within the context that it must be performed. Richards et al examined the effects of early, intensive, gait-focused physical therapy on ambulatory ability in patients after stroke.[191] Twenty-seven patients were randomly assigned to either an experimental group or one of two control groups. All participants received conventional physical therapy. The experimental group and one of the control groups received early intensive physical therapy and had a similar intensity of treatment. The second control group received later and thus less intensive standard care. The experimental group participated in additional therapeutic activities that were gait specific. Overall, the findings support the importance of early gait-specific therapy. Gait velocity was significantly faster in the experimental group than in either of the other two groups and the improvement correlated with the time dedicated to gait training.

Dean et al examined the short- and long-term effects of task-specific gait training in a sample of patients with chronic stroke.[192] A convenience sample of 12 adults was randomly assigned to either a treatment or control group. The treatment group practiced a variety of gait-related functional tasks, such as walking on a variety of level surfaces, sit-to-stand transfer training, and lower extremity strengthening exercises, for 1 hour, 3 times per week for 4 weeks. The control group participated in an exercise class designed to improve upper extremity function for a similar amount of time. Immediately and 2 months after treatment, patients in the experimental group were able to walk significantly faster and further than the control group.

BODY WEIGHT–SUPPORTED TRAINING

Treadmill (Fig. 32-15) and overground body weight–supported training (Fig. 32-16) are promising interventions that can accelerate the return to walking and improve ambulation in a variety of patients with gait dysfunction.[193-196] Body weight supported training involves partially supporting the patient's body weight with a harness during walking. The harness is suspended from a ceiling, a supporting structure, or a mobile device with wheels. Supported walking is intended to increase the strength of muscles used for standing or walking, improve balance, allow for task-specific practice to facilitate the relearning of movement patterns, and enhance patterns of muscle activation or recruitment for standing and walking tasks. Gradually decreasing the amount of support and increasing the amount of weight being managed by the patient, while controlling the speed of walking, is thought to most effectively improve gait performance.

Much of the literature on supported ambulation focuses on patients with impairments and functional limitations as a result of CNS pathology, although unweighting during gait training may also help patients with pain as a result of arthritis to exercise at a sufficient intensity to improve aerobic conditioning.[197] Support by the harness reduces joint loading and ensures patient safety when walking, allowing those who otherwise need a substantial amount of assistance from another person or a device to walk unassisted. This approach to training is task-specific and utilizes a whole task practice paradigm. Feedback via tactile cues or physical assistance with lower extremity placement can also be provided by the treating therapist.

In subjects with spinal cord injury, walking with partial body weight support produces functional patterns of muscle activation that vary with the speed of walking (see Chapter 20).[196] The rhythmic weight bearing and proprioceptive input, combined with progressive lower extremity loading, are thought to enhance recovery by stimulating activity of central pattern generators (CPG) in the spinal cord responsible for walking.[196] In addition, supported walking can strengthen paretic lower extremity muscles and improve aerobic conditioning.

TABLE 32-10	Terms Used to Describe Gait Pathology		
Term	**Description**	**Phase of Gait Cycle**	**Evaluation and Diagnosis**
Antalgic	Difficulty or decrease in weight bearing on a limb during stance phase due to the presence of pain.	Stance	Pain caused by the compression of a joint or soft tissue structure when bearing weight.
Crouch-knee gait	Pattern of gait characterized by excessive flexion affecting both knees.	Stance	Tonal increases associated with CNS involvement; contracture involving either the joint and/or soft tissue structure crossing the joint
Early heel rise/ premature heel rise	Premature rise of the heel during the stance phase of gait.	Stance	Ankle joint or soft tissue structure contracture; hyperactivity of the plantarflexors.
Gluteus maximus lurch	Posterior inclination of the trunk during the stance phase of gait as a compensation for weakness.	Stance	Gluteus maximus weakness.
Quadriceps avoidance pattern	A decrease in the typical amount of flexion seen during stance to prevent excessive anterior tibial translation.	Stance	ACL injury.*
Trendelenburg	Lateral inclination of the trunk during stance phase.	Stance	Weakness of the hip abductions.
Circumduction	Circular movement of the lower extremity into increased abduction.	Swing	Leg-length discrepancy arising from a hip, knee, or ankle joint or soft tissue structure contracture; osseous shortening or lengthening.
Hip hiking	Increased vertical translation of the pelvis.	Swing	Compensation for a leg-length discrepancy.
Scissoring gait	A gait pattern characterized excessive hip adduction.	Swing	Increased adductor tone or recruitment; synergistic pattern of recruitment.
Steppage gait	Excessive hip and knee flexion during the swing phase to allow increased clearance.	Swing	Excessive plantarflexion at the ankle because of a lack of recruitment or excessive tone.
Toe drag	Contact of the foot with the supporting surface throughout swing.	Swing	Impaired dorsiflexor force production; plantarflexor hypertonicity; ankle joint contracture; loss of sensation.
Ataxic	An uncoordinated pattern of gait that can be characterized by difficulty with stability the trunk or achieving a smooth trajectory with the limb during swing.	Stance and swing	CNS dysfunction; impaired lower extremity sensation.
Stiff-knee gait	Decreased knee flexion	Stance and swing	Compensation for weak knee extensors; pain; increased knee extensor tone; synergistic pattern of recruitment.
Vaulting	Increased vertical translation of the body's center of gravity by plantarflexing at the ankle and increasing knee extension during stance.	Stance and swing	Leg-length difference caused by osseous tissue structure changes; inadequate hip or knee flexion during swing.

CNS, Central nervous system; *ACL,* anterior cruciate ligament.
*Data from Ferber R, Osternig LR, Woollacott MH, et al: *Clin Biomech* (Bristol) 17(4):274-285, 2002; Georgoulis AD, Papadonikolakis A, Papageorgiou CD, et al: *Am J Sports Med* 31(1):75-79, 2003.

For stroke patients, body weight–supported training on a treadmill has been found to improve overground walking speed, endurance, and balance.[194] These benefits were found to persist for at least 3 months after the intervention, and this type of training was found to be more effective than treadmill training alone.[194]

NON–TASK-SPECIFIC TRAINING

Strength Training. Since weakness has been shown to affect gait, strength training has been used with the goal of improving gait.[54,198-200] Strength training has been associated with improvements in gait function for patients with a variety of diagnoses,[11,17,192,198-209] and is frequently a component of interventions designed to improve walking performance.

Huang and colleagues found that increased knee extensor strength resulting from an isokinetic exercise program improved walking velocity and endurance in a sample of 132 patients diagnosed with osteoarthritis.[158] Study participants also had less pain and disability after strength training.

A RCT comparing a 4-week home-based exercise program emphasizing strength training with no intervention in adults with hip fracture found that only the exer-

TABLE 32-11	Gait Dysfunctions and Possible Causes
Gait Dysfunction	**Evaluation and Diagnosis**
Decreased ambulation velocity	Lower extremity weakness
	Tonal increases
	Balance deficits
	Decreased mobility confidence
Asymmetrical step length	Lower extremity weakness
	Tonal increases
Reduced step length	Decreased ambulation velocity
	Reduced capacity for weight bearing on an involved limb
	Impaired lower extremity motor control
Asymmetrical stance and swing phase times	Lower extremity weakness
	Tonal increases
Increased base of support during double stance	Tonal increases
	Osseous changes at the hip or knee
	Valgus deformity at the knee
	Balance deficits
Increase toe in/toe out	Femoral or tibial medial or lateral torsion
	Retroversion or introversion of the hip
	Inadequate dorsiflexion: Joint contracture, gastrocnemius-soleus shortening

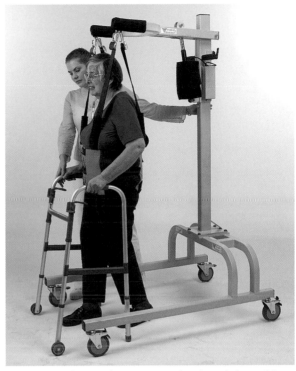

FIG. 32-16 Body weight–supported gait training with walker. *Courtesy LiteGait System, Mobility Research, Tempe, AZ.*

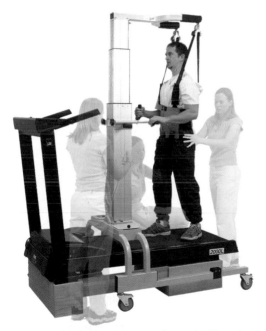

FIG. 32-15 Body weight–supported treadmill ambulation. *Courtesy LiteGait System, Mobility Research, Tempe, AZ.*

cise group had improved quadriceps strength and that this gain was associated with faster walking velocity.[65] Hip extensor strengthening has also been recommended to improve walking capacity in elderly adults,[210] and lower extremity strengthening programs have been shown to improve gait function[211] and reduce fall risk in elderly adults.[212,213]

Additional studies on the effects of strength training, either alone or in conjunction with other interventions such as aerobic conditioning activities or balance exercises, are summarized in Table 32-12. The importance of strengthening exercises as an intervention to address gait dysfunction arises out of its confirmed impact on walking velocity. Interventions leading to an increase in walking velocity can positively impact function.

Neurodevelopmental Treatment Approaches. NDT approaches were developed for patients with CNS impairments such as stroke or cerebral palsy.[214] NDT emphasizes the use of verbal and tactile feedback in conjunction with functional retraining to help promote motor skill acquisition. Feedback can be provided either within the context of walking (task-specific training) or as a therapeutic pre-gait activity (non–task-specific training). The theoretical rationale to support the effectiveness of NDT is based on concepts of motor control from the 1950s, and the rationale has recently been updated to reflect a modern understanding of neurophysiology and principles of motor control and motor learning.[212,215]

There are no published RCTs supporting the effectiveness of NDT in treating individuals with gait dysfunction

TABLE 32-12	Summary of Non–Task-Specific Interventions on Gait

Subjects (No.)	Intervention	Outcome
Elderly adults with disability[11] (130)	Lower extremity strengthening using resistive bands 3 × week; control group no exercise	Improved gait stability, lower extremity strength, and decreased base of support in treatment group compared to control.
Community dwelling elderly adults with mild strength and balance deficits[212] (105)	Three groups participated in a supervised program of strength training on weight machines, endurance training using a stationary cycle or strength and endurance training for 1 hour, 3 × week for 24-26 weeks; control group received no treatment.	Training effect demonstrated in the treatment groups for strength and endurance. No effects noted on gait and balance. Positive effects shown for a reduction in fall risk in the exercise groups.
Elderly adults[209] (31)	12 weeks of strength and balance training; control group performed sitting flexibility exercises.	Significant increases in lower extremity strength in the trained group; significant improvements in preferred and a trend indicating an improvement in maximal gait speed; no change noted in control group.
Deconditioned males residing in a nursing home* (14)	Exercise group participated in a 12 week program of strengthening and conditioning exercises	Significant improvements in preintervention and postintervention measures of lower extremity strength, balance, gait velocity, and stride length.
Chronic stroke† (13)	10 week lower extremity exercise and aerobic conditioning program implemented 3 × week; control group: no intervention.	Significant between and within group increases in lower strength, gait speed, and stair climbing ability for the intervention group; significant improvements in gait kinematic and kinetics for intervention group.
Hip arthritis, hip arthroplasty[68] (28)	Preoperative and postoperative supervised exercise program consisting of stationary cycling and lower extremity resistive exercises; control group: Typical postoperative care.	Improved the rate of recovery in ambulatory function as evidenced by significantly better gait performance, 25 m and 6MWT, in the first 6-months postoperative for exercise group.

*Sauvage LR, Jr., Myklebust BM, Crow-Pan J, et al: *Am J Phys Med Rehabil* 71(6):333-342, 1992.
†Teixeira-Salmela LF, Nadeau S, McBride I, et al: *J Rehabil Med* 33(2):53-60, 2001.

and non-RCTs have had mixed results. Adams and colleagues reported improvements in stride and step length, foot angle, and velocity in a homogenous sample of children diagnosed with cerebral palsy after a 6-week course of NDT-based intervention. The American Academy of Cerebral Palsy and Developmental Medicine (AACPDM) in its systematic review of the evidence on the effectiveness of NDT concluded that there is no clear evidence to support the approach.[189] Despite the lack of supporting evidence, NDT approaches continue to be used clinically.

Motor Relearning Programme Approach. The Motor Relearning Programme (MRP) involves practicing the most difficult components of gait.[216] For example, if the patient has difficulty shifting weight onto a paretic limb when walking, then one would work on that element outside the context of gait. For example, in standing, the patient works on shifting weight from the noninvolved limb to the paretic limb. Work by Winstein has questioned the validity of interventions that use this part-whole approach, and there is no specific evidence regarding the effects of the MRP on gait.[217]

Balance Training. Balance training has been proposed as an intervention for improving walking; however, Winstein and colleagues found that adding balance training alone to conventional therapy did not improve gait velocity, cadence, stride length, or cycle time any more than conventional therapy alone in patients after stroke.[218] Similarly, Walker and colleagues found that adding standing weight-shifting activities with either visual or verbal and tactile feedback to conventional therapy for patients after stroke did not augment improvements in balance or gait.[219] Although the intuitively appealing part-whole training paradigm that would suggest that practicing a problematic element of gait, such as balance, would improve gait as a whole, there are no studies that indicate that practicing standing balance actually improves gait. This may be because balance control for walking is different from balance control for other activities such as standing.[220] During gait, large muscle groups must counteract the forces generated by movements of the body's COG, whereas in standing, only small muscles around the ankle and knee need to act to control small anterior-posterior perturbations.[220]

In contrast, working on balance within the context of walking may improve walking performance. Activities that may improve walking balance include walking on uneven surfaces, stepping up on to curbs, practicing directional changes, stepping over and around obstacles, and performing multiple tasks such as carrying objects in the upper extremities. Stepping over obstacles has been shown to improve walking speed, stride length, performance on the 6MWT, and the capacity for clearing obstacles, as well as improving the mechanics of walking and thereby reducing its energy demand.[221] Tai chi, which consists of slow, rhythmic movements that emphasize trunk rotation and weight shifting, has been reported to improve gait and reduce fall risk in elderly adults, although its reported effects on gait in healthy adults are mixed.[17,222-225]

Aerobic Conditioning. Cardiopulmonary impairments can affect gait performance.[226] Kelly and colleagues examined the cardiorespiratory fitness of 17 patients less than 7 weeks after stroke to determine if a reduction in fitness is associated with reduced gait performance. They found that cardiorespiratory fitness and walking velocity and endurance were less than 50% of predicted for nondisabled age-matched adults. Fitness, as well as gait performance, can be improved by participation in task-specific gait training.[222]

CASE STUDY 32-1

GAIT DYSFUNCTION AFTER STROKE

Examination
Patient History
MM is a 40-year-old right-handed woman who reports difficulty walking outside of her home, managing steps, and using her right upper extremity for ADLs. She was diagnosed with Hodgkin's lymphoma approximately 2 years ago and was treated with radiation therapy that resulted in stenosis of the left carotid artery that subsequently caused a left-sided stroke 1 year ago. MM reports fatigue when walking more than one-half block, occasional tripping but no falls to date when walking on uneven surfaces, and difficulty managing steps, particularly when leading up or down with the right lower extremity. MM feels unstable managing steps without a rail, and her maximum reported ambulation distance is one block. The patient lives alone in a 2-story home and is currently employed in sales on a part-time basis. The only medication she takes is aspirin.

Systems Review
Heart rate is 70 bpm, and blood pressure is 100/70 mm Hg.

Tests and Measures
Musculoskeletal
Posture In standing without her ankle-foot orthosis (AFO) but with her assistive device, the right ankle is maintained in a supinated position with increased lateral weight bearing and the right toes are curled with a hammertoe deformity of the great toe. MM has a posterior pelvic tilt and holds her right elbow flexed approximately 20 degrees.

Range of Motion Active and passive ROM of the left upper and lower extremity are within normal limits (WNL). Passive ROM of the right upper and lower extremity are WNL except for slight limitations of right shoulder passive external rotation, flexion, and abduction and elbow supination.

Muscle Performance MMT: Left upper and lower extremity are 4/5 throughout. Testing of the right upper and lower extremity were deferred.

Neuromuscular
Attention, Arousal, and Cognition Alert and oriented ×3. MM has no memory deficits and is able to follow multistep verbal directions. She has occasional word-finding difficulty because of mild expressive aphasia.

Pain Patient denies pain.

Sensory Integrity Intact throughout both upper and lower extremities to light touch, sharp/dull discrimination, and proprioception.

Cranial Nerve and Peripheral Nerve Integrity CN II-XII are intact.

Motor Function Right upper extremity: Volitional control was characterized by a predominance of non functional synergistic movements consisting of shoulder elevation and abduction (0-45 degrees) with elbow flexion and pronation or shoulder adduction and internal rotation with elbow extension. No active movement could be elicited at the hand. No isolated movement was noted. Velocity-dependent tonal increases noted for the following: Shoulder external rotation and elbow extension and flexion.

Right lower extremity: Synergistic movements noted, which consisted of hip flexion and abduction, with knee extension and ankle dorsiflexion, or hip and knee extension with ankle plantarflexion. No isolated volitional movement was noted at any joint. Velocity-dependent tonal increases noted for the knee flexors and extensors. Tonal increases noted for the toe flexors of first digit. Motor functions of the left upper and lower extremities were WNL.

Cardiovascular/Pulmonary
Ventilation and Respiration/Gas Exchange Lungs are clear to auscultation bilaterally.

Aerobic Capacity and Endurance Blood pressure after ambulating 150 feet was 112/90 mm Hg and heart rate was 90 bpm without shortness of breath. Two minutes after ambulation blood pressure was 100/70 mm Hg and HR was 72 bpm.

Integumentary
Integumentary Integrity Skin is dry and intact.

Function
Orthotic, Protective, and Supportive Devices A molded AFO (MAFO) is used when walking outside the home and in the community. The patient does not consistently use the orthosis within the home.

Assistive and Adaptive Devices MM states she occasionally will use a straight cane when walking outside of her home.

Gait, Locomotion, and Balance
Balance Sitting balance was good. Standing: Unsupported static and dynamic balance were both good. The patient could reach to the floor and retrieve a pen without loss of balance (LOB). Increased postural sway noted with the eyes closed while standing, no LOB.

Ambulation No LOB noted with any of the following: Ambulation on level surfaces, directional changes, walking backward and sideways, sudden starts and stops, and at changing velocities.

Observational Gait Analysis: The following changes were observed (without the use of the MAFO):

1. Unequal step length: Right greater than left.
2. Unequal single stance time: Left greater than right.
3. Decreased knee flexion during both swing and stance phase on the right.
4. Decreased hip extension during stance phase from midstance to preswing on the right.
5. Initial contact on the right occurs with a flat foot at the start of weight acceptance.
6. Increased right ankle inversion at initial contact with rapid pronation at loading response and decreased supination at terminal swing and preswing on the right.
7. Increased toe out and hip external rotation on the right during stance.
8. Delayed initiation of swing phase on the right.
9. Posterior pelvic tilt maintained throughout all phases of gait.
10. No LOB.

With the MAFO, MM's pattern of gait was consistent with these observations except that ambulation velocity, step and stride length, and single-stance times were increased. There was also no loss of balance under this condition.

3-Meter ambulation velocity: 0.7 m/sec without the MAFO

TUG: 10 seconds
Wisconsin Gait Scale SCORE (Table 32-13)
GAITRite Gait Mat data (Table 32-14)

Evaluation, Diagnosis, and Prognosis

Based on the examination, MM has limitations in function because of altered patterns of muscle recruitment at the hip, knee, and ankle, leading to alterations in a variety of gait parameters. Altered patterns of recruitment, primarily related to delayed muscle relaxation, result in limitations in normal joint excursions at the hip and knee during ambulation. Without the MAFO, MM's ankle is positioned in excessive inversion and plantarflexion creating an unstable foot for walking. Recruitment of the ankle dorsiflexors is either limited or overpowered by the ankle plantarflexors, leading to circumduction and a steppage pattern of gait. The patient also presents with minor musculoskeletal limitations involving the toe flexors that result in a hammertoe deformity and creates discomfort during the preswing phase of gait, which requires the toes to extend. The patient currently wears a MAFO that provides adequate ankle control for inversion and eversion but cannot completely influence the genu recurvatum that begins with the loading response phase of gait. This is attributable to the amount of plantarflexion built into the ankle. MM's preferred practice pattern is 5D: Impaired motor function and sensory integrity associated with nonprogressive disorders of the central nervous system—acquired in adolescence or adulthood.

Goals

Given the present pattern of motor control, MM is stable for walking but could benefit from outpatient rehabilitation to improve gait efficiency and prevent repetitive stress to the musculoskeletal system resulting from her current pattern of gait. The following items will be assessed at 3 and 6 weeks as indicators of progress toward a more efficient pattern of gait:

1. GAITRite Gait Mat: velocity, step length and step-length symmetry, and single-stance time and symmetry.
2. Wisconsin Gait Scale score.

TABLE 32-13	Wisconsin Gait Scale Score for Patient in Case Study 32-1
Item	**Score**
1. Uses assistive device	1
2. Stance time	2
3. Step length	1
4. Weight shift	1
5. Stance width	2
6. Guardedness	2
7. Hip extension	2
8. External rotation in initial swing	2
9. Circumduction	1
10. Hip hiking	2
11. Knee flexion toe off to midswing	2
12. Toe clearance	3
13. Pelvic rotation	1
14. Initial foot contact	2
TOTAL	26

TABLE 32-14	GAITRite Gait Mat Data for Patient in Case Study 32-1			
Parameter	**Without MAFO**		**With MAFO**	
	Left	Right	Left	Right
Step time (sec)	0.48	0.68	0.42	0.67
Cycle time (sec)	1.16	1.16	1.11	1.09
Step length (cm)	36.08	37.90	48.87	60.24
Stride length (cm)	73.37	73.06	110.74	109.18
Base of support (cm)	11.59	11.55	16.55	17.52
Single support (% gait cycle)	42.2	28.6	43.9	32.6
Double support (% gait cycle)	29.0	28.9	22.1	20.3
Swing (% gait cycle)	28.6	42.4	32.1	44.6
Toe in/toe out (deg)	8	16	1	4
Velocity (m/sec)	0.625		1.001	
Cadence (steps/min)	101.0		110.1	

3. Observational gait analysis: Monitor joint kinematics at the knee and hip for increases in excursion and disappearance of genu recurvatum.

Prognosis

MM's prognosis is good.

Plan of Care

MM will be seen 3 times per week for 4-6 weeks.

Interventions

1. Task-specific gait training utilizing verbal feedback and tactile feedback at the knee and hip to improve swing and stance phase knee control, increase hip extension at terminal stance, and increase step length; walking in an outdoor environment on a variety of surfaces to improve anticipatory control of gait that will minimize the potential for tripping; progress ambulation velocity from 0.6-1.5 m/sec in response to observed improvements in hip and knee kinematics; and step management with and without using a rail.

2. Wearing the MAFO, gait training on the treadmill with verbal feedback to emphasize longer step lengths, enhance motor recruitment and relaxation across a range of velocities, and promote improvements in endurance; ambulation velocity between 0.8-1.5 m/sec; target heart rate = 120-140 bpm × 10-20 minutes per trial.

3. Request consultation or referral for further modification to the MAFO to reduce the amount of plantarflexion in the orthosis. If insurance coverage is available, have patient fitted for a hinged ankle AFO to enhance biomechanics of the lower extremity for gait and incorporate plantarflexion stops that limit the potential for genu recurvatum.

CHAPTER SUMMARY

Gait dysfunction, a common problem for patients in rehabilitation, can result from impairments in a variety of diagnostic categories. Systematic gait examination is used to identify the underlying source or cause of gait dysfunction so interventions can be directed to ameliorate the effects of impairment on function and disability. The patient history provides information for the selection of tests and measures. Findings from impairment level tests and measures are combined with information from qualitative or quantitative gait-specific tests and measures to determine a patient diagnosis.

Observational gait analysis is one of the most commonly used qualitative methods of screening for gait dysfunction. Quantitative information can be obtained with simple tools such as stop watch and a measured walkway. Gait velocity, a reliable and valid indicator of gait dysfunction and rehabilitation effectiveness, can easily be calculated and is a widely recognized indicator of performance and level of independence. Gait velocity may be the best measure of function given the ease of measurement, its capacity to objectively document progress, and the link to functional performance and outcomes in a variety of populations with disability. A variety of standardized tests, including the TUG, the WGS, the E-FAP, the FIM, and the GARS-M, are reliable and valid measures of functional walking and may provide indicators of rehabilitation effectiveness.

A number of interventions may be used to address gait dysfunction. Intervention selection is determined in part by patient diagnosis and the experience and training of the clinician. Few RCTs exist to support the effectiveness of gait-directed interventions; however, task-specific gait training and interventions designed to improve lower extremity strength, balance, and cardiovascular endurance are most likely to be helpful. Body weight–supported training can also be effective, although at a greater cost than is possible in many settings.

ADDITIONAL RESOURCES

Useful Forms

Activities-Specific Balance Confidence (ABC) Scale
Berg Balance Scale (BBS)
Dynamic Gait Index (DGI)
Rancho Los Amigos Observational Gait Analysis System
Tinetti's Performance-Oriented Mobility Assessment (POMA)
Wisconsin Gait Scale (WGS)

Books

Craik R, Oatis CA (eds): *Gait Analysis: Theory and Application,* St. Louis, 1994, Mosby.
Inman VT, Ralston HJ, Todd F, et al: *Human Walking,* Baltimore, 1981, Williams & Wilkins.
Perry J: *Gait Analysis: Normal and Pathological Function,* Thorofare, NJ, 1982, SLACK.
Winter DA: *ABC of Balance during Standing and Walking,* Waterloo, Ontario, 1985, Waterloo Biomechanics.

Web Sites

Alfred I duPont Gait Lab Online Clinical Cases: http://gait.aidi.udel.edu/res695/homepage/pd_ortho/gait_lab/cases/casehome.htm#top
Clinical Biomechanics: www.ispgr.org/index.html
Clinical Gait Analysis: http://guardian.curtin.edu.au/cga/
Gait and Clinical Movement Analysis Society: www.gcmas.org/
Journal of Biomechanic: www.jbiomech.com/issues
The Journal of Gait and Posture: www.ispgr.org/index.html
International Society for Posture and Gait Research: www.ispgr.org/index.html

Interactive CD-ROM and Videos

Gait: An Interactive Tutorial CD-ROM: www.slackbooks.com/view.asp?SlackCode=47220
Gillette Children's Normal and Pathological Gait Analysis CD-ROM and Videos: www.gillettechildrens.org/default.cfm/PID=1.3.9.1
Medical College of Ohio Observational Gait Analysis CD-ROM: www.mco.edu/cci/projects/gait.html

GLOSSARY

Base of support: The distance between midpoint of the heel of one foot to the same point of the other foot.
Cadence: Number of steps taken in a minute (steps/min).
Double stance: Period of time when both feet are in contact with the supporting surface.

TABLE 33-1	Number of People in the United States (Ages 18-64) Using a Wheelchair or Scooter According to Diagnosis

Diagnosis	Number
Multiple sclerosis	58,000
Paraplegia	48,000
Cerebrovascular disease	45,000
Quadriplegia	44,000
Osteoarthritis	32,000
Loss of lower extremity	31,000
Cerebral palsy	29,000
Rheumatoid arthritis or polyarthropathies	21,000
Diabetes	21,000
Orthopedic impairment of back/neck	21,000
All conditions	635,000

From Kaye HS, Kang T, LaPlante MP: *Disability Statistics Report—Mobility Device Use in the United States,* Washington, DC, 2000, US Department of Education, National Institute of Disability and Rehabilitation Research.

than 65, osteoarthritis and cerebrovascular disease are the most common diagnoses related to the provision of wheeled devices.

EXAMINATION

PATIENT HISTORY

The patient history helps the clinician develop a broad understanding of the physical impairments causing the need for an assistive device and the internal and external factors that influence the person's mobility needs. The history can be obtained through a direct interview, interview of a family member or caregiver, review of medical records, or verbal reports from colleagues. Areas to be addressed include the following:

Demographics What is the patient's age? Will an assistive device need to accommodate physical growth? Does the person attend school, work, or live in an institution?

Health/medical history What primary diagnosis has resulted in the patient's requiring a device? When did the disorder start, and what is the expected progression? Does the patient have any pertinent secondary diagnoses; how may these affect mobility needs? What surgery has the patient undergone, and what future procedures may affect the need for devices?

Psychosocial and cognitive status How important is the appearance of the device to the patient? The behavioral status of a patient influences device selection. The patient may need to understand safety precautions, the gait sequence, weight-bearing precautions, and the possible sequencing of device selection.

Self-management skills Can the patient conduct activities of daily living (ADLs) independently? Does the patient require a device to complete ADLs?

Current mobility equipment What is the patient currently using? Is the device effective? Is the patient satisfied? Should the patient change to a different device, or should the current device be modified? For example, modifying the grip portion of a cane may decrease hypertonic grip responses.

Home and environmental demands Is the device needed for indoor and/or outdoor use? Is the home environment suitable for the device, particularly floor surfaces, stairs, and width of doorways? Is a caregiver present to assist with use of the device?

Transportation What are the transportation needs of the patient? Does the patient need to disassemble the device to place it in a car? Does the patient have assistance with transportation?

Vocational demands What mobility requirements are imposed by the patient's vocational and avocational activities?

Ability to maintain the device Does the patient have the physical and cognitive ability to keep the device in safe working order? Is a caregiver able to maintain the device?

Funding Does the patient's insurance pay for durable medical equipment? Does the patient require assistance to locate funding sources? Recent Medicare regulations governing payment for powered wheelchairs specify that the candidate must be examined by the physician or treating practitioner and that pertinent parts of the medical record kept by the durable medical equipment supplier must be made available to the Centers for Medicare and Medicaid Services.[48]

SYSTEMS REVIEW

The systems review is used to target areas requiring further examination and to define areas that may cause complications or indicate a need for precautions during the examination and intervention processes. According to the *Guide to Physical Therapist Practice,* the systems review should include a review of the cardiopulmonary, integumentary, musculoskeletal, and neuromuscular systems.[49] See Chapter 1 for details of the systems review.

TESTS AND MEASURES
Musculoskeletal

Posture. An assistive device should be selected and fit to optimize patient function. Optimal patient function will usually be achieved by promoting a more symmetrical, erect posture, although in some cases incorporating or accommodating an abnormal posture may allow the patient to be more independent. Examine the patient's posture, as described in detail in Chapter 4, and determine if observed deformities are fixed or flexible. Fixed deformities should be accommodated by any device selected. With flexible deformities, the device may help reduce the deformity or accommodate it.

Anthropometric Characteristics. When selecting and fitting an ambulatory assistive device, measure the patient's height and arm length. For wheeled mobility devices, also measure the patient's sitting breadth, thigh length (from buttock to popliteal crease), leg length (from popliteal crease to heel), and note their general body composition.

Range of Motion. Passive and active range of motion (ROM), as well as the assumed positions of the joints, should be measured. This component of the examination may be performed with the patient supine or sitting on a mat. ROM affects the selection, fitting, and modification of devices. For example, an individual with a fixed elbow flexion contracture who needs to use a cane, crutch, or walker will need a forearm platform. The position of the patient's joints when sitting on the mat may also give an indication of functional sitting ability to sit and the need for support in a wheelchair. For example, an individual with limited hip flexion who requires a wheelchair will need a back-to-seat angle of more than 90 degrees to accommodate this loss of range.

Muscle Performance. Strength, power, and endurance should be measured as described in detail in Chapter 5. Impairments of strength, power, or endurance are often major factors contributing to a patient's need for an assistive mobility device and will affect which device is most suitable for an individual. Patients may need a variety of devices if their strength and endurance vary over time or are expected to worsen.

Joint Integrity and Mobility. Quantitative and qualitative changes in joint integrity and mobility can have substantial bearing on the clinician's final recommendation for a specific device. Impairments of joint integrity or mobility may exclude the use of certain devices or may require the clinician to balance the potential benefits of the device against the injury risk associated with its use. For example, a manually propelled wheelchair may not be suitable for the patient with shoulder joint dysfunction because of the stresses its use places on the shoulder complex.

Neuromuscular

Arousal, Attention, and Cognition. The level of arousal, attention, and cognitive ability affect the individual's ability to use an assistive device. This is particularly important when improper handling of the device may lead to injury to the user or others. Cognition and attention influence the patient's ability to solve logistical problems and learn to negotiate the environment with a new piece of equipment. Various members of the rehabilitation team, including the physical therapist (PT), occupational therapist, speech therapist, physician, and psychologist, may be involved in examining the patient's cognitive abilities.

Pain. Information regarding the location, quality, and intensity of pain can aid in the selection of an assistive device. Baseline data about pain from the initial examination can also be used to assess the effectiveness of a device.

Cranial Nerve Integrity. The cranial nerves (CNs) involved in vision and eye movements (i.e., CN II, III, IV, and VI) should be tested because visual perception can impact the safe operation of an assistive device. In addition, the function of CN VIII should be examined (see Chapter 13) because this may affect balance and thus the need for and choice of a device.

Peripheral Nerve Integrity. Any history that might indicate an upper extremity neuropathy should be investigated, since weakness or sensory loss in the upper extremity may prevent safe or effective use of many assistive devices.

Sensory Integrity. If the patient's history or systems review reveals sensory loss or dysfunction, then sensation should be tested thoroughly (see Chapter 18). Sensory modalities that may need to be examined include pain, temperature, touch, proprioception, and vision.

Cardiovascular/Pulmonary. A basic review of the cardiovascular and pulmonary systems, including checking for edema, monitoring heart rate, respiratory rate and pattern, and blood pressure (see Chapter 22) and assessing aerobic capacity and endurance (see Chapter 23), should be performed as the use of most assistive devices increases energy demand.

Integumentary. The examination should include inspection of the skin, looking particularly for scars, open or healing wounds, grafts, and areas of pressure and any other potential sites of skin and soft tissue breakdown (see Chapter 28).

EVALUATION, DIAGNOSIS, AND PROGNOSIS

Most patients needing assistive devices for mobility have a range of abnormal examination findings, often including pain, weakness, restricted ROM, and edema from musculoskeletal disorders, and abnormal tone, weakness, and insensitivity from neuromuscular disorders.

Studies evaluating the effectiveness of assistive devices for patients with musculoskeletal and neuromuscular disorders have yielded varied results. People with osteoarthritis or arthroplasty of the hip or knee report that using a cane, particularly when held in the contralateral hand, helps to relieve pain.[5,12] This is in part because the cane reduces forces through the hip joint by lessening the pull of the abductor muscle on the femur[50] and because the cane reduces stress on the tibia and knee joint.[51] One study reported that people with arthritis walk faster when using crutches than without assistance,[13] but another study found that although adults with hip arthroplasty who used forearm crutches took longer strides and had more symmetrical gait, they walked with a slower cadence than when walking without crutches.[11] Although studies have shown that assistive devices help reduce pain and improve function, a survey of individuals with rheumatoid arthritis and osteoarthritis found that 30% of respondents did not use prescribed assistive devices.[7] This survey and another large-scale study found that those who were older or in poorer health and those with greater pain or disability were more apt to use their prescribed devices.[4] In patients with hemiparesis, use of a cane on the uninvolved side has been shown to reduce mediolateral and anteroposterior sway and increase walking speed and stability, as well as stance time on the affected leg.[23] Similarly, individuals with peripheral neuropathy affecting the lower extremities have been found to have better balance and more hip and knee excursion when walking with a cane,[36] and children with spina bifida have less pelvic motion with forearm crutches than without them.[35] People with vestibular disorders have reduced sway when using a cane,[39] and those with Parkinson's disease have less difficulty initiating gait and walk somewhat faster with a wheeled walker.[40] Assistive devices can also improve safety, reduce falls, and thus reduce health-care costs in the frail, elderly population.[52]

Despite the documented improvements in function achieved with assistive devices, adults who walk with a cane are apt to be less active than adults of the same age who do not use assistive devices,[44,46] and hospitalized older people who require a cane or walker at the time of discharge have been found to have a higher risk of functional decline than those who were able to walk unaided.[53]

INTERVENTION

SELECTION OF ASSISTIVE DEVICES FOR AMBULATION

Assistive devices for ambulation include canes, crutches, and walkers. Selection is based on the ability of the patient to use the device safely and for the desired function. Additional factors to consider in device selection are short- and long-term prognosis and comorbidities. One or more of the following functions may be served by assistive devices for ambulation:

- Improve balance.
- Assist propulsion.
- Reduce load on one or both lower extremities.
- Transmit sensory cues through the hand(s).
- Enable the individual to obtain the physiological and psychological benefits of upright posture and to maneuver in places inaccessible to a wheelchair.
- Provide a safe environment for patients with cognitive impairment.
- Notify passersby that the user requires special considerations, such as additional time when crossing streets or a seat on the bus.

At any stage in the rehabilitation process the clinician must consider the level of stabilization the patient requires for safe mobility. For example, immediately after lower extremity amputation, the patient may require maximal assistance to maintain standing balance because the loss of the limb deprives the person of weight bearing on the amputated side and shifts the center of gravity toward the intact side. Before gait training, the clinician may choose to initiate standing and weight-shifting activities in parallel bars, which provide more stability than crutches or walkers. As the patient gains stability and is able to walk in a protected environment, the clinician may then choose a walker. Later, the clinician may progress the patient to a large-base quadruped cane, then a single-point cane, and eventually walking with no assistive device if the patient can proceed safely. Some patients continue using a cane outdoors to signal others that they need extra time or assistance. When walking long distances, they may also use a cane to reduce load on the amputated side.

Canes. The simplest assistive device for ambulation is the cane. It offers balance or light support, as well as sensory feedback, from the walking surface. Canes are made from a variety of sturdy materials, such as walnut, oak, and other woods; metal, especially aluminum; and plastics, such as acrylics (e.g., Lucite), as well as fiberglass and carbon fiber. Canes can be decorated in many colors and patterns.

There are several kinds of cane handles (Fig. 33-1). The basic handle is an inverted U, which permits one to hang the cane over the forearm or the back of a chair when not walking with it. Other handle options include a pistol grip, handles designed to contact more of the hand to increase comfort, and a handle designed to keep the wrist in a neutral rather than an extended position.

Cane shafts may be solid, straight, offset, folding, or height adjustable (Fig. 33-2). Solid straight shafts are the least expensive and most durable. The SuperCane has an offset shaft with a higher hand grip for walking and a lower hand grip for coming to stand from sitting. Folding canes are easier to store; an adult-sized cane can be folded to approximately 1 foot in length. One type of cane has a force measuring device in the shaft and a feedback mechanism in the handle to let the user know how much weight they are transferring to the cane. This can be

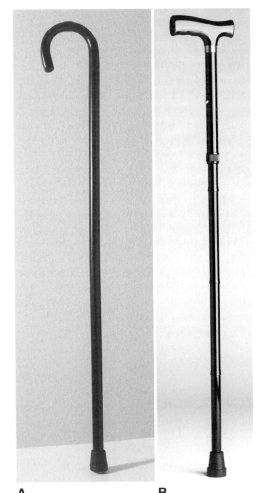

A   **B**

FIG. 33-1 Cane handles. **A,** Inverted U; **B,** pistol grip.

FIG. 33-2 Cane shafts. **A**, Offset; **B**, SuperCane; **C**, folding.

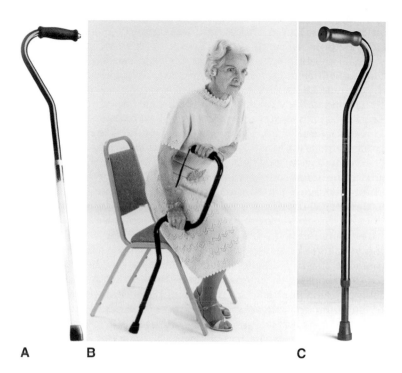

A   B   C

helpful for patients who need to limit loading on an affected lower extremity.

The base of the cane is usually a single rubber tip (Fig. 33-3). It should be broad with deep grooves and kept clean to provide maximum traction. Other designs include the standard or wide-based quadruped (quad) base, made of a rectangle with tips off each corner. Having these four tips increases the base of support; however, patients with hemiplegia may not find this type of cane base any more effective than a standard single tip.[54,55] More novel designs include the side walker/cane, which has four widely spaced rubber tips to increase stability, especially when used unilaterally by a patient with hemiplegia. Another base has a spring-loaded tip to absorb shock at initial contact. The AbleTripod has a flexible triangular tip that maintains floor contact at a wide range of shaft angles; this tip also absorbs shock. To increase stability when the user walks on ice or snow, the cane may have a retractable metal spike. The Pilot Rolling Cane has an L-shaped base fitted with three *casters*, providing the user with the support of a *quad cane* without the need to lift the cane with each step. It also has a brake in the handle for added stability. The Pilot Step-Up Cane has a broad base with a flip-up platform that allows patients to maneuver over curbs and stairs without losing cane support. The user pushes a button on the handle to flip the hinged platform open to enable stepping half the distance of the conventional 8-inch step. With the step retracted, the cane functions as a standard quad cane. The cane also has a second handle farther down on the shaft to facilitate rising from toilets and other bench-type seats.

Several canes are specifically designed to allow adults with unilateral lower extremity amputation to ambulate without a prosthesis (Fig. 33-4). The iWALKFree has a platform on a vertical shaft to support the transtibial amputation limb; the patient supports weight through the thigh and knee. The iWALKFree can also be used in place of standard crutches for patients with non–weight-bearing lower leg injuries, including fractures, sprains, tendon damage, foot ulcers, or amputations. The ED Walker has a bicycle seat mounted on top of a vertical shaft and a second curved shaft with a platform for the amputation limb. Both of these devices have a stationary base. The Roll-A-Bout has four wheels. This folding device has a cushioned platform for the lower leg and a handle that the user holds while propelling with the opposite foot.

Most patients who use a cane to assist with ambulation use one cane, usually on the side opposite the affected lower extremity, although some people use a pair of canes for added stability. A few individuals may refuse to use a cane, regarding it as a sign of disability or senility. Some people with visual impairment use a long cane to transmit sensory cues through the hand. The lower portion of the shaft is painted red to alert passersby not to impede them (Fig. 33-5).[56-60]

Crutches. The four major types of crutches are the underarm, triceps, forearm (Lofstrand), and platform crutches. Crutches, regardless of design, are usually used in pairs.

Underarm Crutches. Underarm crutches, also known as *axillary crutches*, are made of wood, aluminum, or titanium (Fig. 33-6). Although called underarm or axillary crutches, the patient should never support themselves on the crutch through the axilla because the crutch may impinge on superficial nerves and blood vessels. The top of the crutch should be held firmly against the side of the chest. The top of the crutch is usually covered with sponge rubber to increase friction and cushion stress against the user's chest. One crutch design has a top considerably longer than the basic top to provide a larger support area on the

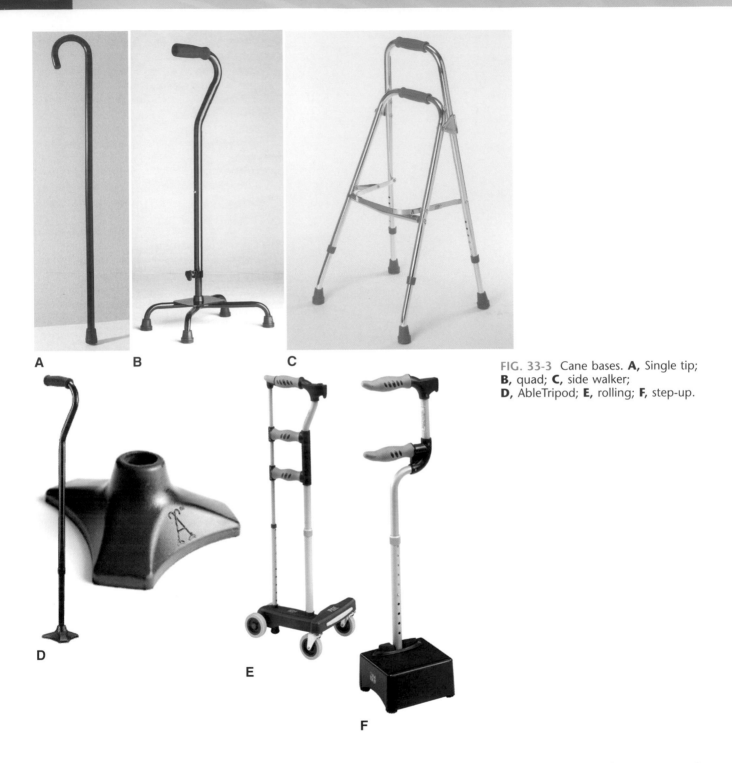

FIG. 33-3 Cane bases. **A,** Single tip; **B,** quad; **C,** side walker; **D,** AbleTripod; **E,** rolling; **F,** step-up.

chest. This has been found to reduce energy consumption during the first few minutes of walking but has not been found to alter energy consumption when walking for longer periods.[61] The Easy Strutter Functional Orthosis System has a crutch top that includes, in addition to the underarm piece, a cushioned strap intended to go over the shoulder to distribute weight over a broad, pressure-tolerant area. This crutch also has two parallel struts that terminate in a broad, spring-loaded shock-absorbing base. When three-point gait with regular axillary crutches was compared to performance with the Easy Strutter Func-

tional Orthosis System, the latter put less stress on the palms and subjects also reported feeling more secure on level surfaces and stairs with the novel crutches.[62]

The shape of the crutch handle does not appear to affect function or comfort.[63] The handle should have a resilient cover to cushion compressive stress on the palm. The shaft of a metal crutch has several spring-loaded detents to expedite adjusting length and hand-grip height. The traditional shaft bifurcates partway up from the base; however, streamlined single-shaft crutches are available. The usual crutch tip is rubber; however, many tips

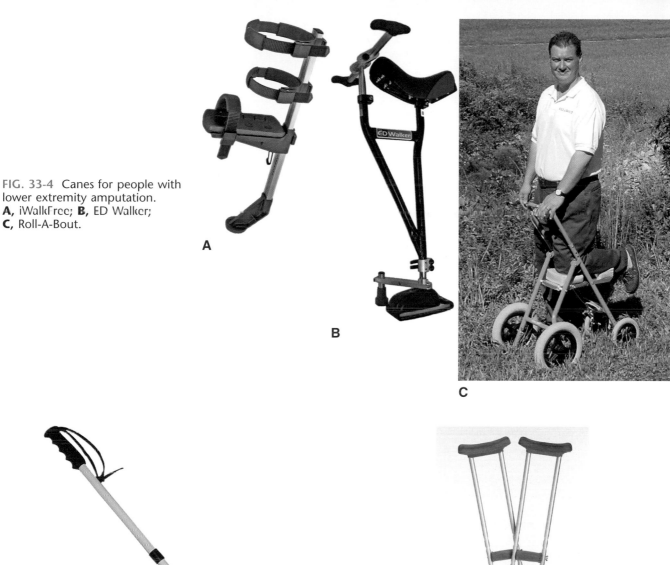

FIG. 33-4 Canes for people with
lower extremity amputation.
A, iWalkFree; **B,** ED Walker;
C, Roll-A-Bout.

A

B

C

FIG. 33-5 Long cane for people with visual impairment.

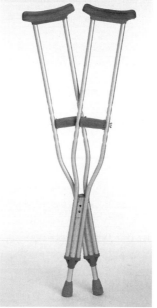

FIG. 33-6 Underarm crutches.

described for canes can also be used on crutches. A novel
design is the Safe Walk Titanium Crutch. It has two distal
shafts and both end with rubber tips; regardless of the
angle of the crutch, one tip is always on the floor. Crutches
can also have a spring-loaded mechanism at the distal end
to absorb shock at impact. This type of mechanism was
found in a limited trial to reduce shock waves and peak
stresses.[64] Rocker-bottom crutches are also available.

Studies conflict on whether this does[65,66] or does not[67]
reduce energy consumption as compared with single-tip
crutches.

Triceps Crutches. *Triceps crutches* are always made of
aluminum (Fig. 33-7). Triceps crutches, sometimes known
as Warm Springs crutches, were popularized at the
Roosevelt Institute for Rehabilitation in Warm Springs,
Georgia, during the poliomyelitis epidemic in the

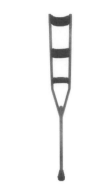

FIG. 33-7 Triceps crutch.

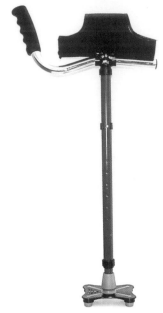

FIG. 33-9 Platform crutch.

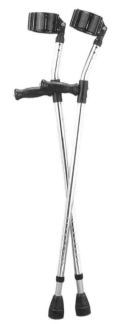

FIG. 33-8 Forearm crutches.

twentieth century. The crutch is intended for use by patients with paralyzed shoulder muscles. The proximal portion of each crutch has medial and lateral uprights joined by a pair of posterior bands that keep the elbow extended, mimicking the action of the triceps muscle. The distal part of the crutch is a single shaft with a rubber tip at the base.

Forearm (Lofstrand) Crutches. Forearm *(Lofstrand)* crutches are made of aluminum or titanium with a vinyl-covered steel forearm cuff (Fig. 33-8). European model cuffs are more streamlined than those generally available in the United States. Forearm crutches are available in many colors and allow adjustment of length and cuff position. A folding model convenient for storage is also available. The Kenny Armband, named after Sister Kenny, a pioneering clinician who treated patients with poliomyelitis, is less restrictive than the rigid cuff and is used by some individuals with post-polio syndrome and by some people with cerebral palsy. A forearm crutch

made of compliant composite plastic with an S-curve shaft has also been designed to absorb shock.[68]

Platform Crutches. Platform crutches have a horizontal support for bearing weight on the forearm (Fig. 33-9). These crutches are used by patients who cannot tolerate weight transmission through the hand, wrist, or forearm.

Walkers. Walkers are frames, usually made of aluminum, designed to provide support through both arms without the control needed to use a pair of canes or crutches. Walkers come in a variety of styles. The base may be fixed, requiring the patient to pick up the walker to move it, or wheeled, so it can be advanced by rolling. The uprights may be rigid, folding, reciprocating, or stair climbing. In addition, various hand grips and platforms, as well as accessories, such as a seat or a basket, can be added to many walkers.

Pickup Walkers. Pickup walkers are the simplest walkers (Fig. 33-10), with four legs ending in rubber tips. They are stable and sturdy but must be lifted with each step. They are appropriate for patients with poor balance and for use on high-friction surfaces, such as carpet, grass, and gravel. Walker uprights may be height adjustable. The front uprights of the Rising Star SuperWalker are angled with upper and lower handles for the patient to use when rising from a chair and to provide stability when the patient is upright.

Rolling Walkers. Rolling walkers have two or more wheels at the base (Fig. 33-11). They can be pushed forward and provide moderate stability and are suitable for use on smooth surfaces, such as hardwood flooring and vinyl tiles. Many rolling walkers have two front wheels and two rubber tips on the rear uprights. Tennis balls or other glides on the rear uprights reduce friction and may ease ambulation. The Strider and Wenzelite walkers have adjustable wheels and handles. The foldable Red Dot Walker has front swivel 5-inch wheels and rear glide

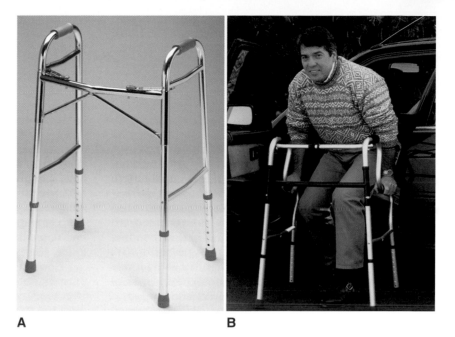

FIG. 33-10 Pickup walkers. **A,** Standard. **B,** Rising Star.

A   B

brakes. The Walkabout has an upper portion that encircles the user's shoulders. It also has a built-in seat with a basket.[69] Other walkers with seats include the folding steel Merry Walker and the polyvinylchloride Dura-Walker, both designed to provide a secure environment for patients with cognitive impairment; their bulkiness impedes passage through narrow doorways. The steel U-Step Walker has a padded seat, hand brakes, folding mechanism, and an optional laser light intended to encourage patients with Parkinson's disease to step forward. Some walkers have a reciprocating mechanism to facilitate stepping. The Universal Stair Climbing Walker is intended to aid the patient when climbing a staircase.

Three-Wheeled Walkers. Three-wheeled walkers have three angled uprights, each ending in a wheel; they are easier to maneuver in narrow corridors than traditional walkers with four uprights (Fig. 33-12).

Basic wheeled and pickup walkers are available in various sizes to accommodate a range of patient heights and trunk girths. Adaptations can be added to many walkers. For example, direct-forming thermoplastic can be added to the handles to improve conformation to the user's hand and reduce the risk of compression trauma. The child with cerebral palsy may walk with more erect posture with a walker fitted with hip guards or with the walker used posteriorly.[33,34,70] A motorized robotic walker is being developed by the Veterans Affairs Personal Adaptive Mobility Aid Laboratory for use by the elderly or adults with visual impairments.[71]

FITTING OF ASSISTIVE DEVICES FOR AMBULATION

An assistive device must fit properly for the patient to walk most comfortably and with the least effort.[47,72] A properly adjusted and positioned device keeps the patient's line of gravity within the base of support created by the device and the patient's feet.

The height of any device and the position of the handles should be assessed when all accessories, such as rubber tips, hand cushions, and top pad, are installed and with the patient wearing the type of shoes they would usually wear when using the device. Measurements should be performed with the patient standing erect in a secure environment, such as in parallel bars. The following guidelines apply for most circumstances but may need to be modified, depending on the patient's size, available joint excursion, and strength, as well as expected gait pattern.

Canes. When holding a cane by its handle, its height should allow the elbow to be slightly flexed, at less than 30 degrees, and the tip of the cane should be 5-10 cm lateral and 15 cm anterior to the shoe.[73,74] If the cane is too long, the user may bend backward or place insufficient weight on the cane. If it is too short, the user will tend to bend too far forward. Canes with a broad base, rather than a single tip, should be positioned so that the edge that flares laterally faces away from the shoe to avoid the base hitting the ankle during the swing phase of gait.

Crutches

Underarm Crutches. A crutch should extend from a point approximately 4-5 cm (2 finger breadths) below the axilla to a point on the floor 5 cm lateral and 15 cm anterior to the shoe.[75] The hand piece should generally be placed so that the elbows flex about 30 degrees.[76] The elbows should be flexed a little more if the patient will use a gait that requires raising both feet from the floor simultaneously, such as the drag-to, swing-to, or swing-through patterns. A double-blind repeated measures study of healthy subjects found that as long as the length of the crutch was within 1 inch (2.5 cm) of the recommended length, the respiratory-exchange ratio, walking speed, and perceived exertion were not affected.[77]

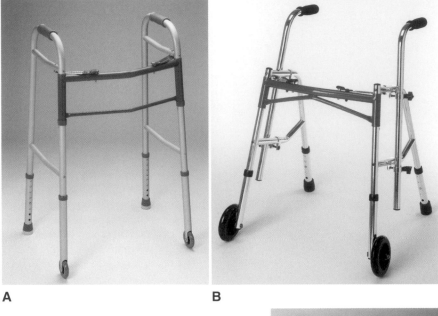

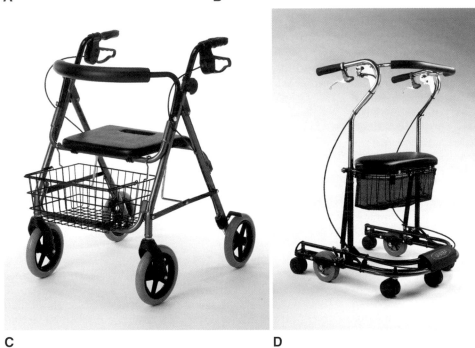

FIG. 33-11 Rolling walkers.
A, Fixed front wheels;
B, adjustable; **C,** four wheels;
D, U step.

Forearm Crutches. The forearm cuff should lie on the proximal third of the forearm. The crutch tip should be 5-10 cm lateral and 15 cm anterior to the shoe when the patient is standing with the crutch hand piece adjusted to provide 15-30 degrees of elbow flexion.

Triceps Crutches. The upper cuff should contact the proximal third of the upper arm, approximately 5 cm below the anterior fold of the axilla. The lower cuff should lie 1-4 cm below the olecranon process, avoiding bony contact, yet providing adequate stability.[78]

Platform Crutches. The platform should be angled so that the forearm rests at a 90-degree angle to the upper arm, affording the greatest comfort and control of the crutch. The height should allow the person to stand

upright with the shoulders relaxed. If platform crutches are too short, the user will have to lean forward. If they are too long, they can force the shoulders up and cause compression of the radial or suprascapular nerve.

Walkers. When holding a walker, the elbows should be flexed approximately 15 degrees.[39] Slight elbow flexion allows for some downward push on the walker, allowing the patient to bear some weight through the upper extremities. If the handles are too low, the patient may keep their elbows extended or bend too far forward, and if using a front wheeled walker, they may push harder and hinder wheel rotation. Forward bending of the trunk can also inhibit hip extension during the stance phase of gait and, by moving the center of gravity forward, can

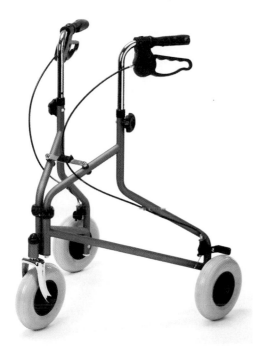

FIG. 33-12 3-wheeled walker.

interfere with forward weight shifting, making it difficult to achieve adequate propulsion during terminal stance. If the handles are too high, the patient may need to flex the elbows more and lean excessively on the walker or push the walker farther forward from the trunk, increasing the risk of falling if this places the person's center of gravity behind the walker's base of support.

Complications of Assistive Device Use. It is not uncommon for musculoskeletal and neurovascular complications to develop when canes, walkers, and crutches are adjusted improperly or used incorrectly.[79] Problems can occur in the hand, arm, shoulder, or axilla. Injury to the radial,[80-82] ulnar,[83] median,[84,85] radial palmar,[86] and suprascapular[87] nerves have all been reported. Improperly fitted or used underarm crutches can cause axillary artery thrombosis.[88-90] Even when using properly adjusted crutches, some people develop painful abrasions of the lateral chest, shoulder pain, tenderness or bruising over the medial aspect of the arm, cramping of the triceps, or wrist osteoarthritis[91] or exert undue stress on the ulna.[92] Misuse of walkers has also been implicated in falls among some patients.[93]

WHEELCHAIR SELECTION

Although wheeled mobility can be achieved with many devices, such as scooters, adult tricycles, golf carts, hand-controlled cycles, sports wheelchairs, and standing motorized wheeled platforms, manual and powered wheelchairs are the most commonly used wheeled mobility devices. All wheelchairs enable the seated occupant to move or be moved about in the environment. Seated mobility is generally selected when the patient cannot ambulate safely or when the energy demands of ambulation limit functional ambulation distance. Many patients use a cane or a walker to assist with walking short distances and have someone push them in a wheelchair for longer distances. Wheelchairs can thus improve safety and participation.

Selection of a wheelchair should be based on a thorough examination of the patient's current and anticipated needs, as well as environmental, activity, and financial constraints. Although environmental constraints such as narrow doorways or carpeted floor can often be modified, an alternative wheelchair design or component may be more cost-effective. For example, wheelchair wheels with less camber or a narrowing device installed on the wheelchair may allow the chair to pass through a narrow doorway. A wheelchair with solid or semi-pneumatic tires is easier to propel over carpeted floors than one with pneumatic tires. Negotiating stairs and hoisting the wheelchair into an automobile require less strength and effort with a lightweight wheelchair, and a folding wheelchair can be transported more easily than one with a rigid frame.[94]

Goals of wheelchair selection include the following:
- Providing comfort
- Supporting postural alignment to address:
  - Balance
  - Prevention or correction of flexible deformities
  - Accommodation of fixed deformity
  - Normalizing tone
  - Protecting skin integrity
- Facilitating function of:
  - Respiration
  - Swallowing and digestion
  - Circulation
  - Communication
  - Seated activities
  - Mobility

In addition to these goals, the wheelchair must allow for weight shifting and transfers. Patients must shift weight periodically while seated to avoid debilitating and sometimes life-threatening skin breakdown. This is usually done by transferring weight onto the patient's arms despite the fact that this places high loads on the shoulder and elbow joints,[95] especially for those with tetraplegia.[96] A firm cushion makes this type of weight shifting easier. In addition, the chair may have a seat-back tilt and recline mechanism to allow for weight shifting without weight bearing through the arms. How a patient is expected to transfer into and out of the wheelchair influences wheelchair selection and fitting, particularly seat height and angle, wheel and footrest placement, and armrest position.

WHEELCHAIR FEATURES

The basic wheelchair prescription should specify the following:
- Mode of propulsion
- Frame
- Seat, including seat cushion
- Backrest, including insert
- Armrests, including lapboard
- *Front rigging* (i.e., footrests and leg rests)
- Wheels, including tires, casters, hand rims, and brakes
- Support accessories

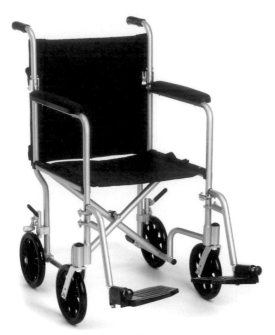

FIG. 33-13 Dependent propulsion wheelchair. *Courtesy Sunrise Medical.*

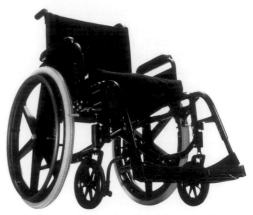

FIG. 33-14 Manual propulsion wheelchair.

When feasible, the clinician should test wheelchair options by simulating various choices with a highly adjustable wheelchair. Many long-term users of manual and electrically powered wheelchairs have customized wheelchairs to optimize function, including posture and reach.[97] However, since customizing adds to cost, persons with limited funds, particularly the elderly, often do not have customizable wheelchairs.[98]

Mode of Propulsion

Dependent Propulsion. Dependent mobility is when the chair is propelled by someone other than the occupant (Fig. 33-13). Shower chairs, standing and seating systems, recliners, and tilt-in-space systems are often pushed by a caregiver. The frame of this type of chair usually does not fold, making it sturdy and relatively inexpensive but cumbersome to transport and store. One should always consider the physical capabilities of the caregiver who will assist the occupant of a wheelchair when selecting a chair for dependent propulsion. Caregiver training can improve use and safety, and as little as 50 minutes of wheelchair-handling skills training has been shown to carry over into skills that are retained for at least 6 months.[99]

Independent Manual Propulsion. Manual wheelchairs can be propelled by the patient independently using upper and/or lower extremity power (Fig. 33-14). Wheelchairs intended for independent manual propulsion have a folding or rigid frame and can be made of steel or other more lightweight materials. Aluminum, titanium, graphite, or magnesium wheelchairs weigh about half as much as a steel wheelchair.[100] Among able-bodied subjects, using a lightweight wheelchair reduces the frequency of collisions but increases the frequency of the front casters leaving the ground, as compared with using a standard-weight wheelchair.[101] It is recommended that patients

with spinal cord injury use lightweight adjustable wheelchairs as these are associated with a lower incidence of upper extremity pain and injury.[102] The lightweight wheelchair is also easier for the patient and caregiver to lift when placing it in a car. Although a folding frame makes a wheelchair easier to transport, a rigid frame increases strength and durability while reducing weight and vibration.

The position and camber (angle) of the rear wheels, the size of the wheels or casters, and the type of hand rim can all affect the ease and efficiency of wheelchair propulsion. For most patients, positioning the rear axle as far forward as possible without compromising stability optimizes upper extremity propulsion. Using cambered wheels, which are closer together at the top than at the bottom, makes it easier to reach the top of the wheel while also increasing the stability of the wheelchair. But the greater overall width of the chair imposed by cambered wheels can limit access in narrow areas. Larger wheels and casters make it easier to propel the wheelchairs on carpet or rough ground. A hand rim with two driving rings can be placed on one of the wheels to allow for independent propulsion of the two rear wheels by the patient who can only use one hand.

A manual wheelchair may be propelled using the upper and/or lower extremities, depending on the individual's strength, ROM, and coordination, as well as his or her cardiopulmonary fitness. A manually propelled wheelchair is usually pushed by holding the hand rims on the wheels. Arm cranks and arm levers are also available, but these have not been shown to improve energy efficiency during wheelchair propulsion.[103]

The pectoralis major and anterior deltoid muscles are the primary muscles used for wheelchair propulsion.[104] They work together with the supraspinatus, infraspinatus, and the long head of the biceps to move the wheels and thus the wheelchair forward. The middle and posterior deltoid and the supraspinatus muscles contract to extend the arm during the recovery phase of propulsion.[105] Upper body strength training can improve wheelchair propulsion skill.[106] When using the lower extremities for wheelchair propulsion, using both legs is more energy efficient and quicker than using one leg, even in people with hemiplegia.[107]

Independent Powered Propulsion. When a patient does not have the physical capability to propel a manual wheelchair, an electrically powered wheelchair or scooter may be used to provide independent propulsion (Fig. 33-15). Changing from a manual to a powered wheelchair can often increase independence and improve occupational performance in patients with mobility limitations.[108] An electric wheelchair can be controlled and steered with a joystick if the user has good hand function. For those with limited manual dexterity, the chair can be adapted for control with virtually any other type of volitional action, such as chin or head movement, sip-and-puff breathing, or visual scanning. Electrically powered wheelchairs vary greatly in their stability, braking, the user's energy consumption,[109] and durability.[110] Most powered wheelchair users consider reaching, moving in confined spaces, and avoiding collisions more important than speed and avoiding the need to drive backward.[111] Therefore patients with powered wheelchairs should be taught maneuvering skills as part of wheelchair training.

Combination Manual and Powered Wheelchairs. Hybrid manual and electrically powered wheelchairs usually have a motor on the rear wheels to supplement the force the user exerts on the hand rims of the chair's rear wheels. This decreases the workload for the user and may allow weaker patients to propel themselves independently.[112]

Frame. The basic wheelchair has a frame with vertical posterior uprights with push handles attached for a caregiver to use when the occupant is not propelling the wheelchair. Wheelchairs intended for patients with lower extremity amputations have the posterior uprights angled to position the rear wheels farther back than usual to increase stability, particularly when ascending ramps.

Seat. Most people who depend on a wheelchair for mobility are seated for extended periods every day. The basic leatherette sling seat typically found in a transportation wheelchair intended for occasional brief use is inexpensive and easy to fold but is not suitable for long-term use because it does not distribute pressure evenly and tends to maximize pressure on the tissue overlying the ischial tuberosities. Augmenting this sling seat with a solid, firm base with a cushion may be sufficient for patients who intend to use the wheelchair for short periods.

Seat Cushion. For patients expected to spend many hours each day in a wheelchair for months or years, a specialized seat cushion should be used. The cushion lies under the patient's buttocks and thighs and should distribute pressure widely while also dissipating moisture and heat and reducing shear. This improves comfort, reduces the risk of tissue breakdown, and contributes to postural control and stability. A wide range of wheelchair cushions are available and made of different materials and with different designs.

The cushion may be made of plastic or rubber foam. Foam cushions vary in density, thickness, memory (ability to return to their original shape), and cell type (open or closed). Thicker foam cushions have been found to decrease subcutaneous pressure more than thinner cushions, but they can also increase subcutaneous shear stress.[113] Because foam is solid, it generally provides a fairly stable surface for postural control. It can also easily be carved or molded specifically for the individual to accommodate postural variation. Foam is flammable, which may be hazardous if the patient smokes.[114] In general, foam is relatively inexpensive and requires little maintenance except for changing and laundering the cloth cover when it becomes soiled.

Wheelchair cushions may also be made of a vinyl-covered viscous synthetic gel. This type of cushion can be used alone over a flat wheelchair seat or in combination with a rigid contoured seating surface if more stability is desired. *Gel cushions* require little maintenance, but the vinyl cover of the pack can tear, causing the gel to leak out. They are also heavier than foam cushions.

Cushions made of multiple air or fluid cells are also available. These types of cushions do not provide as much postural control and stability as solid cushions, but they distribute pressure very effectively. The air or liquid conforms to the bony prominences, equalizing pressure over the entire sitting surface. Air pressure between 17 and 42 mm Hg provides optimal reduction in interface pressure at the ischial tuberosities for patients with spinal cord injury.[115] This type of cushion needs to be looked after carefully because it is easily punctured.

Hybrid cushions made of more than one type of material are also available. These are intended to provide the desirable characteristics of each material. For example, a contoured foam cushion with a cut-out for placement of air cells under the buttocks may be used to give postural support while also distributing pressure at bony prominences.

Backrest. The backrest of a wheelchair is usually made of leatherette and attached to the frame. Backrests are available in various heights; for example, a patient with poor neck control may benefit from an extended high backrest (Fig. 33-16). Someone who needs to transfer backward from the wheelchair may require a backrest with a vertical zipper or snap fasteners. Backrest tilt-and-recline mechanisms can reduce fatigue by enabling the user to breathe more efficiently, improve pressure

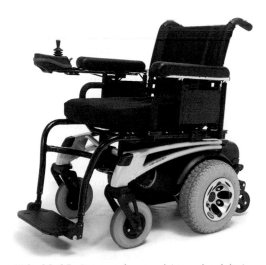
FIG. 33-15 Powered propulsion wheelchair.

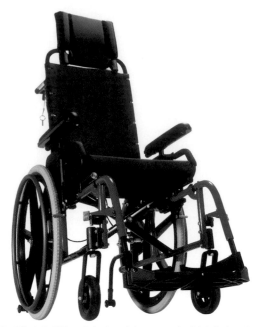

FIG. 33-16 Wheelchair with extended high backrest.

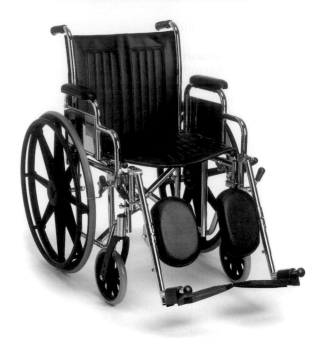

FIG. 33-17 Wheelchair with desk armrests and elevating leg rests.

distribution to increase comfort and postural stability, and can enhance visual orientation. Backrest support may be increased by adding a solid insert with cushioning, although functional evaluation of 27 subjects with recent spinal cord injury tested with four different back supports found that for most activities, the type of back support did not affect activity participation.[116]

Armrests. Wheelchair armrests may be fixed or removable, with the latter facilitating transfers in and out of the wheelchair. The front of the armrests may be straight or desk style to allow them to fit under a desk (Fig. 33-17). Some armrests are adjustable to accommodate elbow flexion contractures. A tray may be added to the armrests to allow the user to eat and engage in other manual activities while sitting in the wheelchair. The tray can make it harder to get out of the chair, which may be cumbersome but may also improve safety in patients with poor safety awareness and standing balance who might otherwise try to stand up from the chair without assistance.

Front Rigging. There are many different types of footrests and leg rests. Footrests are used to keep the feet off the floor and support the legs to reduce stress on the posterior thighs. Most footrests flip up to facilitate transfers. The foot rests usually have a heel strap to prevent the feet from sliding backward. Leg rests may be fixed, swing away, or elevating (see Fig. 33-17). Swing-away leg rests allow the patient to get close to the transfer destination. Leg rests are usually detachable to reduce the wheelchair size when necessary for maneuvering in confined spaces. Elevating leg rests with a cushioned calf pad should be used if the patient would otherwise develop edema with the lower extremities in a dependent position.

Wheels. Wheel selection is largely influenced by the physical environment in which the wheelchair will be

used, whether indoors or outdoors, with firm or resilient surfaces, and whether one needs to traverse curbs or stairs.

Generally, the front and rear wheels are different sizes, with large wheels at the rear to facilitate transfers and foster more erect sitting posture when the occupant propels the wheelchair. However, putting large wheels in the front makes it is easier to turn in confined spaces. In addition, moving the seat closer to the rear wheels reduces rolling resistance, making the wheelchair easier to propel.[117]

Large wheels have pneumatic or semi-pneumatic tires. Semi-pneumatic tires are recommended if the wheelchair will only be used indoors. Pneumatic tires are recommended if one wants to traverse soft or rough terrain. They should be inflated to 100 lb per square inch (psi) of pressure. Lower tire pressures will increase energy expenditure during wheeling.[118,119] The large wheels should have toggle or lever type brakes that should be engaged whenever the patient transfers to or from the wheelchair.

Smaller wheels are known as casters. Larger diameter casters make the ride smoother. Casters have solid rubber tires.

Hand rims are attached to the large wheels to allow the user to turn the wheels without soiling the hands. The hand rims are usually chrome plated, but vinyl coating, knobs, and projections are available to facilitate use by those with poor grip. Although hand-rim design was found in one study not to affect submaximal task performance by able-bodied subjects, different designs may have more impact on experienced wheelchair users, those with limited upper extremity or trunk function, or those who need to perform more difficult tasks such as negotiating slopes.[120] The patient with unilateral upper extremity amputation or paralysis may benefit from a one-arm drive mechanism, in which both hand rims are placed on one side.

Support Accessories. Patients with poor trunk control, such as some individuals with cerebral palsy, muscular dystrophy, amyotrophic lateral sclerosis, or tetraplegia, may be more secure in a wheelchair equipped with supportive pads or other accessories. A medial thigh support (synonyms: Hip abductor, *pommel,* anti-adductor pad, abductor post, abduction wedge, knee abductor) maintains the hips in the prescribed amount of abduction and prevents hip adduction. Lateral thigh supports (synonyms: Lateral knee adductor, adduction pads) prevent excessive or unwanted hip abduction and control hip external rotation. Lateral pelvic supports (synonyms: Hip support pads, lateral hip blocks, pelvic support, side cushions, hip guides) maintain the lower trunk centered in the seat and provide counterforce to help control pelvic obliquity in conjunction with lateral thoracic supports. An anterior pelvic support (synonym: seat belt) prevents the occupant from sliding forward on the seat. Seat belts are particularly important to prevent falls from electrically powered wheelchairs.[121]

WHEELCHAIR FITTING

Ideally, during wheelchair fitting, the patient is seated in an adjustable wheelchair in the most erect posture obtainable and wearing the shoes and orthoses he or she will use in the final wheelchair. If the person has extensive paralysis or very poor trunk control, then two or more people may need to support the patient while the lead clinician measures the person. Fig. 33-18 and the next section provide general guidelines for wheelchair dimensions. These may need to be modified for patients with special needs, such as trunk deformity or unusual proportions.

Seat

Width. The width of the seat affects the occupant's comfort and posture, as well as which doorways and other narrow areas the wheelchair can pass through. The seat

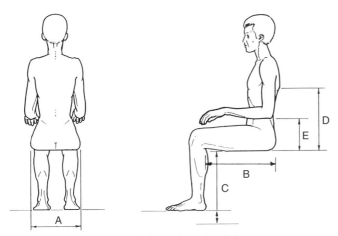

FIG. 33-18 General guidelines for wheelchair measurement. **A,** Seat width; **B,** seat depth; **C,** seat height; **D,** backrest height; **E,** armrest height. *Adapted from Wilson AB Jr.:* Wheelchairs: A Prescription Guide, *New York, 1992, Demos Publications.*

should be 1-2 inches wider than the widest part of the trunk in the frontal plane. The widest trunk measurement is usually the distance between the hips near the level of the greater trochanters in sitting. If the seat is too narrow, there will be too much pressure on the trochanters and lateral aspects of the thighs, and squeezing the tissue will also be uncomfortable. It is also difficult to transfer into and out of an unduly narrow seat. If the seat is too wide, it will be hard for the patient to reach the hand rims of a manually propelled wheelchair, and the wheelchair may not pass through narrow doorways. The patient may also develop postural asymmetry if they lean to one side to support one forearm on an armrest. Asymmetrical posture can also interfere with respiration, speech, and swallowing and may lead to high pressure concentration on the portion of the trunk in greatest contact with the backrest.

Depth. To ensure that the depth of the seat is correct, measure the longest body segment in a lateral view, usually from the back of the lower trunk to the popliteal fossa. Children should have seat depth approximately 1-inch shorter than this length. For adults, the seat depth should be approximately 2-inches shorter than this length. This will allow the seat to support the buttocks and thighs and avoid the front edge compressing the neurovascular structures in the popliteal fossa. Patients with significant kyphosis or who wear trunk orthoses may need extra seat depth. For patients with leg-length discrepancy, the depth of a sling seat should accommodate the length of the shorter leg. A solid seat can be modified to a different depth on each side; initially, the seat should suit the length of the longer leg.

A shallower seat should be used if the patient has tight hamstrings or intends to propel the wheelchair with the legs. However, in general, a shallow seat should be avoided because it reduces the area for pressure distribution and thus increases pressure on the ischial tuberosities and sacrum, increasing discomfort and the risk for tissue breakdown. A shallow seat also does not provide optimal distal lateral thigh stabilization and can cause the patient to sit with excessive hip abduction and external rotation. A seat that is too deep may impose excessive pressure on the popliteal fossa. The patient may compensate for this by tilting the pelvis posteriorly and adopting a kyphotic posture to prevent sliding forward. A wheelchair with excessive seat depth also reduces maneuverability in crowded areas.

Height. The distance from the footrests to the top of the seat cushion should equal the distance from the popliteal fossa to the base of the heel with the patient wearing typical footwear. For patients with plantarflexion contractures, use the distance from the popliteal fossa to the base of the toes. The height of the seat from the floor should allow the patient to place both feet completely on the floor when transferring and propelling the wheelchair with the feet when the leg rests are removed. With the leg rests installed, the footrests should be far enough off the floor to keep the feet from dragging.

If the seat is too low, the footrests may scrape the floor. Also, increased pressure will be placed on the ischial tuberosities because of inadequate lower extremity support. If the seat is too high, the patient may have difficulty transferring and may not be able to reach the ground for foot propulsion. A high seat can also lead to compensatory sliding into a posterior pelvic tilt. Seat height also affects wrist motion during wheelchair propulsion.[119]

Backrest

Width. For most patients, the width of the back of the chair should equal the width of the widest part of the patient's body in a frontal plane (facing the person). Patients with scoliosis may require a wider back to accommodate their spinal curvature. A wider backed chair may also be needed if lateral thoracic supports are going to be placed in the chair. If the chair back is too narrow, there may be more pressure on sides of the trunk from the back canes and the patient may have inadequate trunk support. If the chair back is too wide, the patient may not be able to reach the wheels as readily and may have inadequate trunk support, which can lead to postural asymmetry.

Height. The backrest height should be determined with the seat cushion in place. The height of the backrest depends on the size of the patient and the amount of support needed. For full back support, the backrest height should equal the distance from the ischial tuberosities to top of the shoulders. If the patient does not require full back support, the backrest should extend from the ischial tuberosities only to the inferior angle of the scapulae to allow for greater upper extremity mobility. A backrest that is too low will not provide adequate support and may lead to compensatory kyphosis, which can contribute to fatigue or pain. If the backrest is too high, it may impede shoulder girdle mobility.

Armrests. Armrest height should be set to allow the patient to sit with the forearms supported and the elbows flexed 90 degrees. If the armrests are too low, the upper extremity may not be supported adequately, which may lead to shoulder subluxation and pain, particularly if the patient has a flaccid or hypotonic upper extremity. Unduly high armrests interfere with upper extremity function.

Complications of Wheelchair Use. Using a wheelchair can be associated with pain and injuries to the neck, back, shoulder, and buttocks.[122] The frequent and sustained extension of the neck caused by trying to look at the face of people standing and the frequent rotation required to look around when turning the body are both thought to contribute to neck and back discomfort.[123] Shoulder injuries because of overuse are common, particularly in those who began using a wheelchair in adulthood and did not develop the necessary strength and flexibility early on.[124] Buttock pain and pressure ulcers commonly result from the sustained pressure that occurs with prolonged sitting. The risk for pressure ulcers is greatest in patients, such as those with spinal cord injuries, who have reduced sensation and muscle mass in areas of pressure. Training in pressure relief, as well as scheduled periodic inspections of the wheelchair, can reduce the incidence of pressure ulcers.[125] Wheelchair inspections help with maintenance of safety features and can thus also contribute to injury risk reduction through accident prevention.

CASE STUDY 33-1

ELECTRIC WHEELCHAIR FOR A PATIENT WITH CEREBRAL PALSY AND RECENT CERVICAL SPINE DECOMPRESSION

Examination
Patient History

MT is a 68-year-old woman who was transferred to a skilled nursing facility from an acute care hospital after having cervical spine decompression. MT had this surgery to treat cervical stenosis, which was causing progressive weakness of her upper and lower extremities. MT also has cerebral palsy with spastic tetraplegia since birth. She has used a wheelchair for mobility for the past 20 years. She had functional use of her left upper extremity, enabling self-feeding, and her left lower extremity, permitting foot propulsion of her wheelchair for short distances. Before the decompression surgery, she had lost most of the functional movement in her extremities and had limited trunk control. MT also has chronic back pain. The decompression surgery provided no significant improvement in function, and the prognosis for improved physical function was poor.

Test and Measures
Musculoskeletal

Posture MT has spastic quadriplegia with bilateral upper extremities in flexor pattern and lower extremities in extensor synergy with fixed bilateral foot drop. She has poor postural control.

Range of Motion Upper extremity ROM: Elbows in 110 degrees of flexion with soft tissue contractures forming. Lower extremity ROM: Knees with 40-degree flexion contractures and ankles 30 degrees from neutral in plantarflexion.

Strength MT has trace contraction (MMT 1/5) of the finger flexors bilaterally. Trunk and extremities grossly nonfunctional with no volitional movement.

Neuromuscular

Arousal, Attention, and Cognition MT is alert and has good insight into her condition, as well as good safety awareness and judgment.

Pain MT has moderate-to-severe back and extremity pain on passive motion of the upper or lower extremities or when in a supported seated position for longer than 1 hour. Pain in sitting varies from 0-7/10, depending on position. Pain is usually localized in the neck or sacral region.

Sensory Integrity Reduced sensation below the C7 dermatome. Proprioception and light touch were fair-to-poor below the neck.

Motor Function No functional movement below the neck with increased tone in all extremities.

Cardiovascular/Pulmonary

Circulation Although she has had episodes of orthostatic hypotension, MT currently tolerates being transferred to a sitting position without any cardiovascular instability.

Integumentary

Integumentary Integrity Skin is intact. Because of her low weight (92% of ideal body weight), inability to shift weight, and impaired sensory function, MT is at risk for developing pressure ulcers.

Function

Self-Care and Home Management MT is dependent in all ADLs. She has a pressure-sensitive switch call light, which she operates by head turning. MT can verbally express her wants and needs.

Evaluation, Diagnosis, and Prognosis

Prognosis for regaining enough functional extremity movement to allow ambulation or enable the operation of a manual wheelchair is poor. MT is at risk for skin breakdown because of her inability to conduct independent pressure relief and poor nutritional status (see Chapters 20 and 28). Seating interventions are indicated to increase mobility so she can interact with her environment more safely.

Short-Term Goals

1. Seating system that will allow MT to sit upright for 4 hours without pain or signs of skin breakdown.
2. Ability to conduct independent weight shifts in the seating system.
3. Ability to operate an electric wheelchair using head movement.

Long-term Goal

MT will demonstrate safe, independent operation of her electric wheelchair within 4 weeks of receiving it.

Meeting these goals would allow MT to have increased independence in her residence for socialization, pressure relief management to decrease the risk of skin breakdown, and decrease her reliance on staff for her functional mobility needs.

Intervention

To test MT's tolerance of various seating options, an adjustable trial wheelchair was provided by the wheelchair vendor. An appropriate electric wheelchair was unavailable, thus a manual wheelchair with reclining backrest was used as a trial device. A solid, padded high-back backrest was added to this wheelchair to support the patient's trunk. A deep contoured foam base with a gel pad overlay cushion was added to distribute pressure more effectively on the buttocks. The patient could tolerate sitting in this wheelchair for 4 hours without pain. She could request to be tilted and reclined as her comfort level dictated. She preferred the chair to be tilted because this more effectively reduced sacral loading. Simulation of a chin-control wheelchair interface was also conducted, and MT demonstrated sufficient head and neck control to access this control interface. Positioning the lower extremities in the trial wheelchair was complicated by her foot drop that, with standard footrests, caused her to bear weight only on her forefeet and was painful.

Incorporating the findings of the evaluation, anatomical measurements, and the data and observations obtained from the trial wheelchair, the following wheelchair recommendations were generated:

Mode of Propulsion and Frame

Electric-powered wheelchair with chin control. The system has an upright LCD screen display to allow the patient to scroll through a controller menu to independently operate the propulsion and backrest tilting systems.

Seat

The seat was 16-inch square with a deep contoured foam base and gel pad overlay cushion. Given MT's risk of skin breakdown, an air-cell cushion was considered but not selected because it requires more maintenance, and the foam and gel hybrid cushion trial was successful.

Backrest

Powered tilt backrest with a contoured, padded, and solid high-back backrest was selected. Lateral supports were used to assist with trunk alignment and compensate for the patient's poor trunk control. The high back allowed for mounting of a headrest as required for the tilting system.

Armrests

Adjustable padded armrests to accommodate MT's elbow flexion contractures and to accommodate possible future positioning needs.

Front Rigging

Swing-away leg rests with adjustable foot plates to accommodate the bilateral foot drop.

Wheels

Semi-pneumatic tires because wheelchair will be used almost exclusively indoors.

Pelvic and Thigh Accessories

Medial thigh support to prevent hip adduction.

Outcome

MT's wheelchair was delivered, and fitting and adjustments were made by the wheelchair vendor with the therapist providing oversight assistance. The treating therapist was familiarized with the control interface and positioning features of the wheelchair. She trained MT and her caregivers in the operation of the wheelchair. Two weeks later, MT needed two additional treatment sessions for further adjustments to the chin control interface, as well as patient and nurses' aide training in the use and maintenance of the wheelchair. After 2 weeks of trials, the treating therapist reassessed MT's mobility and recommended to her physician that she be allowed to use her wheelchair independently throughout the skilled nursing facility. All short-term and long-term goals were met, and therapy was discontinued.

Please see the CD that accompanies this book for a case study describing the examination, evaluation, and interventions for a patient needing assistive devices for ambulation and a wheelchair after a transtibial amputation.

CHAPTER SUMMARY

Interacting with people and the environment is fundamental to quality of life. Assistive devices can increase, maintain, or improve the functional capabilities of individuals with disabilities. More people than ever are using assistive devices for mobility, particularly canes, walkers, and wheelchairs. Examination of the candidate for an assistive device should include medical history; demographics; psychosocial factors; self-management skills; current mobility equipment; home, environmental, and vocational demands; transportation requirements; and funding. Review of the musculoskeletal, neuromuscular, cardiopulmonary, and integumentary systems should focus on ROM, strength, and endurance.

Assistive devices for ambulation can improve balance, assist propulsion, reduce load on one or both lower extremities, transmit sensory cues through the hand(s), allow the individual to obtain the physiological and psychological benefits of upright posture and maneuver in places not accessible with a wheelchair, provide a safe environment for patients with cognitive impairment, and notify passersby that the user requires special considerations, such as additional time when crossing streets. Canes, the simplest assistive device for mobility, offer a choice of handle, shaft, and base. Crutch designs include underarm, triceps, forearm, and platform. Walkers have various types of bases, uprights, hand grips and platforms, and accessories.

Wheelchairs can increase the user's comfort, support postural alignment, protect the skin, reduce energy consumption, improve safety, and facilitate function. The basic wheelchair prescription should specify the mode of propulsion, whether dependent, independent manual, or independent powered; frame; seat, including seat cushion; backrest, including insert; armrests, including lapboard; front rigging (i.e., footrests and leg rests); wheels, including tires, casters, hand rims, and brakes; and pelvic and thigh control accessories. Fitting assistive devices properly can prevent neurovascular compression and other complications of device misfit or misuse.

ADDITIONAL RESOURCES

Books

ANSI/RESNA: *Wheelchair Standards.* Arlington, Va, 1998, RESNA.

Axelson P, Chesney DY, Minkel J, et al: *The Manual Wheelchair Training Guide,* Minden, Nev, 1998, PAX Press.

Axelson P, Minkel J, Perr A, et al: *The Powered Wheelchair Training Guide,* Minden, Nev, 2002, PAX Press.

Cook A, Hussey S: *Assistive Technologies: Principles and Practice,* ed 2, Arlington, Va, 2002, RESNA.

Cooper RA: *Wheelchair Selection and Configuration,* New York, 1998, Demos Medical Publishing.

Croteau C: *Wheelchair Mobility: A Handbook,* Worcester, Mass, 1998, Park Press.

Furumasu J (ed): *Pediatric Powered Mobility,* Arlington, Va, 1997, RESNA.

Karp G: *Choosing a Wheelchair: A Guide to Optimal Independence,* Sebastopol, Calif, 1998, O'Reilly & Associates.

RESNA: *Resource Guide for Assistive Technology Outcomes,* Arlington, Va, 1998, RESNA.

Web Sites

ABLEDATA: www.abledata.com (Sponsored by National Institute on Disability and Rehabilitation Research)

Adaptive Device Locator System: www.AdaptWorld.com

Assistive Technology Industry Association: www.atia.org

Rehabilitation and Assistive Technology Society of North America (RESNA): www.resna.org

Devices

Rising Star SuperCane: Momentum Medical Corporation: 800-644-2263

AbleTripod Cane: Walking Cane Company: www.walkingcanedepot.com

Pilot Walker, Pilot Rolling Cane, Pilot Step-Up Cane: www.FullLifeProducts.com

Merry Walker: Merry Walker Corporation: www.merrywalker.com

Wenzelite Safety Roller: Wenzelite Rehab Supplies: www.wenzelite.com

U-Step Walking Stabilizer: In-Step Mobility Products Corporation: www.ustep.com

Roll-A-Bout: Roll-A-Bout Corporation: www.roll-a-bout.com

GLOSSARY

Axillary crutches: Underarm crutches.

Casters: Small wheelchair wheels, usually 5 or 8 inches in diameter.

Front rigging: Wheelchair leg rests and footrests.

Gel cushions: Wheelchair cushions filled with synthetic viscous material.

Lofstrand crutches: Forearm crutches.

Mobility device: Device which improves the user's ability to move within the environment, including canes, walkers, crutches, and wheelchairs; sometimes the term is used also to encompass adapted automobiles.

Pickup walker: Walking frame with four metal posts each ending in a rubber high-traction tip.

Pommel: Wheelchair accessory located between the thighs to provide medial thigh support.

Quad cane: Also known as quadruped cane. A cane with a base with four distal projections, each ending in a rubber high-traction tip.

Triceps crutches: Also known as Warm Springs crutches. Top cuff rests on the middle third of upper arm.

References

1. Laplante MP, Hendershot GE, Moss AJ: *Assistive Technology Devices and Home Accessibility Features: Prevalence, Payment, Needs, and Trends,* Hyattsville, Md, 1992, National Center for Health Statistics.
2. Kaye HS, Kang T, LaPlante MP: *Disability Statistics Report—Mobility Device Use in the United States,* Washington, DC: 2000, US Department of Education, National Institute of Disability and Rehabilitation Research.
3. Bateni H, Maki BE: Assistive devices for balance and mobility: Benefits, demands, and adverse consequences, *Arch Phys Med Rehabil* 86:134-145, 2005.
4. Blount WP: Don't throw away the cane, *J Bone Joint Surg Am* 38:695-708, 1956.
5. Brand RA, Crowninshield RD: The effect of cane use on hip contact force, *Clin Orthop Relat Res* 147:181-184, 1980.
6. McGibbon CA, Krebs DE, Mann RW: In vivo hip pressures during cane and load-carrying gait, *Arthritis Care Res* 10:300-307, 1997.
7. Van der Esch M, Heijmans M, Dekker J: Factors contributing to possession and use of walking aids among persons with rheumatoid arthritis and osteoarthritis, *Arthritis Rheum* 49:838-842, 2003.
8. Ajemian S, Thon D, Clare P, Kaul L, et al: Cane-assisted gait biomechanics and electromyography after total hip arthroplasty, *Arch Phys Med Rehabil* 85:1966-1971, 2004.
9. Ely DD, Smidt GL: Effect of cane on variables of gait for patients with hip disorders, *Phys Ther* 57:507-512, 1977.
10. Neumann DA: An electromyographic study of the hip abductor muscles as subjects with a hip prosthesis walked with different methods of using a cane and carrying a load, *Phys Ther* 79:1163-1173, 1999.

11. Sonntag D, Uhlenbrock D, Bardeleben A: Gait with and without forearm crutches in patients with total hip arthroplasty, *Int J Rehabil Res* 23:233-243, 2000.
12. Chan GN, Smith AW, Kirtley C, et al: Changes in knee moments with contralateral versus ipsilateral cane usage in females with knee osteoarthritis, *Clin Biomech* 20:396-404, 2005.
13. Crosbie WJ, Nicol AC: Aided gait in rheumatoid arthritis following knee arthroplasty, *Arch Phys Med Rehabil* 71:299-303, 1990.
14. Edwards BG: Contralateral and ipsilateral cane usage by patients with total knee or hip replacement, *Arch Phys Med Rehabil* 67:734-740, 1986.
15. Imms FJ, MacDonald IC, Prestidge SP: Energy expenditure during walking in patients recovering from fractures of the leg, *Scand J Rehabil Med* 8:1-9, 1976.
16. Waters RL, Campbell J, Perry J: Energy cost of three-point crutch ambulation in fracture patients, *J Orthop Trauma* 1:170-173, 1987.
17. Kirby RL, Tsai HY, Graham MM: Ambulation aid use during the rehabilitation of people with lower limb amputations, *Assist Technol* 14:112-117, 2002.
18. Buurke JH, Mermens JH, Erren-Wolters CV, Nene AV: The effect of walking aids on muscle activation patterns during walking in stroke patients, *Gait Posture* 22:164-170, 2005.
19. Chen CL, Chen HC, Wong MK, et al: Temporal stride and force analysis of cane-assisted gait in people with hemiplegic stroke, *Arch Phys Med Rehabil* 82:43-48, 2001.
20. Hesse S, Jahnke MT, Schaffrin A, et al: Immediate effects of therapeutic facilitation on the gait of hemiparetic patients as compared with walking with and without a cane, *Electroencephalogr Clin Neurophysiol* 109:515-522, 1998.
21. Kuan TS, Tsou JY, Su FC: Hemiplegic gait of stroke patients: The effect on using a cane, *Arch Phys Med Rehabil* 80:777-784, 1999.
22. Laufer Y: The effect of walking aids on balance and weight-bearing patterns on patients with hemiparesis in various stance positions, *Phys Ther* 83:112-122, 2003.
23. Lu CL, Yu B, Basford JR, et al: Influences of cane length on the stability of stroke patients, *J Rehabil Res Dev* 34:91-100, 1997.
24. Maeda A, Nakamura K, Higuchi S, et al: Postural sway during cane use by patients with stroke, *Am J Phys Med Rehabil* 80:903-908, 2001.
25. Tyson SF: The support taken through walking aids during hemiplegic gait, *Clin Rehabil* 12:395-401, 1998.
26. Biering-Sorensen F, Hansen RB, Biering-Sorensen J: Mobility aids and transport possibilities 10-45 years after spinal cord injury, *Spinal Cord* 42:699-706, 2004.
27. Ijzerman MJ, Baardman G, van't Hof MA, et al: Validity and reproducibility of crutch force and heart rate measurements to assess energy expenditure of paraplegic gait, *Arch Phys Med Rehabil* 80:1017-1023, 1999.
28. Jaeger RJ, Yarkony Roth EJ: Rehabilitation technology for standing and walking after spinal cord injury, *Am J Phys Med Rehabil* 68:128-133, 1989.
29. Melis EH, Torres-Moreno R, Barbeau H, et al: Analysis of assisted-gait characteristics in persons with incomplete spinal cord injury, *Spinal Cord* 37:430-439, 1999.
30. Noreau L, Richards CL, Comeau F, et al: Biomechanical analysis of swing-through gait in paraplegic and non-disabled individuals, *J Biomech* 28:689-700, 1995.
31. Rovic JS, Childress DS: Pendular model of paraplegic swing-through crutch ambulation, *J Rehabil Res Dev* 25:1-16, 1988.
32. Ulkar B, Yavuzer G, Guner R, et al: Energy expenditure of the paraplegic gait: Comparison between different walking aids and normal subjects, *Int J Rehabil Res* 26:213-217, 2003.
33. Greiner BM, Czerniecki JM, Deitz JC: Gait parameters of children with spastic diplegia: A comparison of effects of posterior and anterior walkers, *Arch Phys Med Rehabil* 74:381-385, 1993.
34. Levangie PK, Guihan MF, Meyer P, et al: Effects of altering handle position of a rolling walker on gait in children with cerebral palsy, *Phys Ther* 69:130-134, 1989.
35. Vankoski SJ, Moore C, Statler KD, et al: The influence of forearm crutches on pelvic and hip kinematics in children with myelomeningocele: Don't throw away the crutches, *Dev Med Child Neurol* 39:614-619, 1997.
36. Aston-Miller JA, Yeh MW, Richardson JK, et al: A cane reduces loss of balance in patients with peripheral neuropathy: Results from a challenging unipedal balance test, *Arch Phys Med Rehabil* 77:446-452, 1996.
37. Kling C, Persson A, Gardulf A: The ADL ability and use of technical aids in persons with late effects of polio, *Am J Occup Ther* 56:457-461, 2002.
38. Wilson DJ: Braces, wheelchairs, and iron lungs: The paralyzed body and the machinery of rehabilitation in the polio epidemics, *J Med Humanit* 26:173-190, 2005.
39. Nandapalan V, Smith CA, Jones AS, et al: Objective measurement of the benefit of walking sticks in peripheral vestibular balance disorders, using the Sway Weigh balance platform, *J Laryngol Otol* 109:836-840, 1995.
40. Cubo E, Moore CG, Leurgans S, et al: Wheeled and standard walkers in Parkinson's disease patients with gait freezing, *Parkinsonism Relat Disord* 10:9-14, 2003.
41. Fay BT, Boninger ML: The science behind mobility devices for individuals with multiple sclerosis, *Med Eng Phys* 24:375-383, 2002.
42. Aminzadeh F, Edwards N: Factors associated with cane use among community dwelling older adults, *Pub Health Nurs* 17:474-483, 2000.
43. Brooks LL, Wertsch JJ, Duthie EH: Use of devices for mobility by the elderly, *Wis Med J* 93:16-20, 1994.
44. Mann WC: Aging, disability, and independence: Trends and perspectives. In Mann WC (ed): *Smart Technology for Aging, Disability, and Independence,* Hoboken, NJ, 2005, John Wiley.
45. Mathieson KM, Kronenfeld JJ, Keith VM: Maintaining functional independence in elderly adults: The roles of health status and financial resources in predicting home modifications and use of mobility equipment, *Gerontologist* 42:24-31, 2002.
46. Pine Z, Gurland B, Chen MM: Use of a cane for ambulation: Marker and mitigator of impairment in older people who report no difficulty walking, *J Am Geriatr Soc* 50:263-268, 2002.
47. Van Hook FW, Demonbreun D, Weiss BD: Ambulatory devices for chronic gait disorders in he elderly. *Am Fam Physician* 67:1717-1724, 2003.
48. Wolff JL, Agree EM, Kasper JD: Wheelchairs, walkers, and canes: What does Medicare pay for, and who benefits? *Health Aff* 24:1140-1149, 2005.
49. American Physical Therapy Association: *Guide to Physical Therapist Practice,* ed 2, Alexandria Va, 1998, The Association.
50. Vargo MM, Robinson LR, Nicholas JJ: Contralateral vs ipsilateral cane use: Effects on muscles crossing the knee joint, *Am J Phys Med Rehabil* 71:170-176, 1992.
51. Mendelson S, Milgrom C, Finestone A, et al: Effect of cane use on tibial strain and strain rates, *Am J Phys Med Rehabil* 77:333-338, 1998.
52. Mann WC, Ottenbacher KJ, Fraas L, et al: Effectiveness of assistive technology and environmental interventions in maintaining independence and reducing home care costs for the frail elderly: A randomized controlled trial, *Arch Fam Med* 8:210-217, 1999.
53. Mahoney JE, Sager MA, Jalaluddin M: Use of an ambulation assistive device predicts functional decline associated with hospitalization, *J Gerontol A Biol Sci Med Sci* 54:M83-88, 1999.
54. Milczarek JJ, Kirby RL, Harrison ER, et al: Standard and four-footed canes, their effect on the standing balance of patients with hemiparesis, *Arch Phys Med Rehabil* 74:281-285, 1993.
55. Laufer Y: Effects of one-point and four-point canes on balance and weight distribution in patients with hemiparesis, *Clin Rehabil* 16:141-148, 2002.
56. Johnson JT, Johnson BF, Blasch BB, et al: Gait and long cane kinematics: A comparison of sighted and visually impaired subjects, *JOSPT* 27:162-166, 1998.
57. Maeda A, Nakamura K, Otomo A, et al: Body support effect on standing balance in the visually impaired elderly, *Arch Phys Med Rehabil* 79:994-997, 1998.
58. Mount J, Howard PF, Dalla Palu AL, et al: Postures and repetitive movements during use of a long cane by individual with visual impairment, *JOSPT* 31:375-383, 2001.
59. Ramsey VK, Blasch BB, Kita A, et al: A biomechanical evaluation of visually impaired persons' gait and long-cane mechanics, *J Rehabil Res Dev* 36:323-332, 1999.
60. Schellingerhout R, Bongers RM, van Grinsven R, et al: Improving obstacle detection by redesign of walking canes for blind persons, *Ergonomics* 44:513-526, 2001.
61. Hinton CA, Cullen KE: Energy expenditure during ambulation with Ortho crutches and axillary crutches, *Phys Ther* 62:813-819, 1982.
62. Nyland J, Bernasek T, Markee B, et al: Comparison of the Easy Strutter Functional Orthosis System and axillary crutches during modified 3-point gait, *J Rehabil Res Dev* 41:195-206, 2004.
63. Sala DA, Leva LM, Kummer FJ, et al: Crutch handle design: Effect on palmar loads during ambulation, *Arch Phys Med Rehabil* 79:1473-1476, 1998.
64. Parziale JR, Daniels JD: The mechanical performance of ambulation using spring-loaded axillary crutches: A preliminary report, *Am J Phys Med Rehabil* 68:192-195, 1989.
65. Annesley AL, Almada-Norfleet M, Arnall DA, Cornwall MW: Energy expenditure of ambulation using the Sure-Gait crutch and the standard axillary crutch, *Phys Ther* 70:18-23. 1990.
66. Basford JR, Rhetta HL, Schleusner MP: Clinical evaluation of the rocker bottom crutch, *Orthopaedics* 13:457-460, 1990.
67. Nielsen DH, Harris JM, Minton YM, et al: Energy cost, exercise intensity, and gait efficiency of standard versus rocker-bottom axillary crutch walking, *Phys Ther* 70:487-493, 1990.
68. Shortell D, Kucer J, Neeley WL, et al: The design of a compliant composite crutch, *J Rehabil Res Dev* 38:23-32, 2001.
69. Wolfe RR, Jordan D, Wolfe ML: The Walkabout: A new solution for preventing falls in the elderly and disabled, *Arch Phys Med Rehabil* 85:2067-2069, 2004.
70. Logan L, Byers-Kinkley K, Ciccone C: Anterior vs. posterior walkers: A gait analysis study, *Dev Med Child Neurol* 32:1044-1048, 1990.

71. Rentschler AJ, Cooper RA, Blasch B, et al: Intelligent walkers for the elderly: Performance and safety testing of VA-PAMAID robotic walker, *J Rehabil Res Dev* 40:423-431, 2003.

72. Ross DE: Relationships among cane fitting, function, and falls, *Phys Ther* 73:494, 1993.

73. Dean E, Ross J: Relationships among cane fitting, function, and falls, *Phys Ther* 73:94-500, 1993.

74. Kumar R, Roe MC, Scremin OU: Methods for estimating the proper length of a cane, *Arch Phys Med Rehabil* 76:1173-1175, 1995.

75. Pardo RD, Deathe AB, Winter DA: Walker use risk index: A method for quantifying stability in walker users, *Am J Phys Med Rehabil* 72:301-305, 1993.

76. Reisman M, Burkett RG, Simon SK, et al: Elbow moments and forces at the hands during swing through axillary crutch gait, *Phys Ther* 65:601-605, 1985.

77. Mullis R, Dent RM: Crutch length: Effect on energy cost and activity intensity in non-weight-bearing ambulation, *Arch Phys Med Rehabil* 81:569-572, 2000.

78. Schmitz TJ: Preambulation and gait training. In O'Sullivan SB, Schmitz TJ (eds): *Physical Rehabilitation: Assessment and Treatment,* ed 4, Philadelphia, 2001, FA Davis.

79. Karpman RR: Problems and pitfalls with assistive devices, *Top Geriatr Rehabil* 8:1-5, 1992.

80. Ball NA, Stempien LM, Pasupuleti DV, et al: Radial nerve palsy: A complication of walker usage, *Arch Phys Med Rehabil* 70:236, 1989.

81. Brooks AL, Fowler SB: Axillary artery thrombosis after prolonged use of crutches, *J Bone Joint Surg Am* 46:863-864, 1964.

82. Rudin LN, Levine L: Bilateral compression of radial nerve (crutch paralysis), *Phys Ther Rev* 31:229, 1951.

83. Veerendrakumar M, Taly AB, Nagaraja D: Ulnar nerve palsy due to axillary crutch, *Neurol India* 49:67-70, 2001.

84. Kellner WS, Felsenthal G, Anderson JM, et al: Carpal tunnel syndrome in the nonparetic hands of hemiplegics: Stress-induced by ambulatory assistive devices, *Orthop Rev* 15:608-611, 1986.

85. Werner R, Waring W, Davidoff G: Risk factors for median mononeuropathy of the wrist in postpoliomyelitis patients, *Arch Phys Med Rehabil* 70:464-467, 1989.

86. Hug U, Burg D, Baldi SV, et al: Compression neuropathy of the radial palmar thumb nerve, *Chir Main* 23:49-51, 2004.

87. Shabes D, Scheiber M: Suprascapular neuropathy related to the use of crutches, *Am J Phys Med* 65:298-299, 1986.

88. Feldman DR, Vujic I, McKay D, et al: Crutch-induced axillary artery injury, *Cardiovasc Intervent Radiol* 18:296-299, 1995.

89. McFall B, Arya N, Soong C, et al: Crutch induced axillary artery injury, *Ulster Med J* 73:50-52, 2004.

90. Platt H: Occlusion of the axillary artery due to pressure by a crutch, *Arch Surg* 20:314-316, 1930.

91. Werner RA, Waring W, Maynard F: Osteoarthritis of the hand and wrist in the post poliomyelitis population, *Arch Phys Med Rehabil* 73:1069-1072, 1992.

92. Amin A, Singh V, Saifuddin A, et al: Ulnar stress reaction from crutch use following amputation for tibial osteosarcoma, *Skel Radiol* 33:541-544, 2004.

93. Charron PM, Kirby RL, MacLeod DA: Epidemiology of walker-related injuries and deaths in the United States, *Am J Phys Med Rehabil* 74:237-239, 1995.

94. van Drongelen S, van der Woude LH, Janssen TW, et al: Glenohumeral contact forces and muscle forces evaluated in wheelchair-related activities of daily living in able-bodied subjects versus subjects with paraplegia and tetraplegia, *Arch Phys Med Rehabil* 86:1434-1440, 2005.

95. Behrman AL: Factors in functional assessment, *J Rehabil Res Dev Clin* Suppl 17-30, 1998.

96. van Drongelen S, van der Woude LH, Janssen TW, et al: Mechanical load on the upper extremity during wheelchair activities, *Arch Phys Med Rehabil* 86:1214-1220, 2005.

97. Hastings JD, Fanucchi ER, Burns SP: Wheelchair configuration and postural alignment in persons with spinal cord injury, *Arch Phys Med Rehabil* 84:528-534, 2003.

98. Hunt PC, Boninger ML, Cooper RA, et al: Demographic and socioeconomic factors associated with disparity in wheelchair customizability among people with traumatic spinal cord injury, *Arch Phys Med Rehabil* 85:1859-1866, 2004.

99. Kirby RLO, Mifflen NJ, Thibault DL, et al: The manual wheelchair-handling skills of caregivers and the effect of training, *Arch Phys Med Rehabil* 85:2011-2019, 2004.

100. Ragnarsson KT: Prescription considerations and a comparison of conventional and lightweight wheelchairs, *J Rehabil Res Dev Clin* Suppl 8-16, 1998.

101. Rogers H, Berman S, Fails D, et al: A comparison of functional mobility in standard vs. ultralight wheelchairs as measured by performance on a community obstacle course. *Disabil Rehabil* 25:1083-1088, 2003.

102. Boninger ML, Koontz AM, Sisto SA, et al: Push rim biomechanics and injury prevention in spinal cord injury: Recommendations based on CULP-SCI investigations, *J Rehabil Res Dev* 42:9-20, 2005.

103. Mukherjee G, Bhowmik P, Samanta A: Effect of chronic use of different propulsion systems in wheelchair design on the aerobic capacity of Indian users, *Indian J Med Res* 121:747-758, 2005.

104. Gutierrez DD, Mulroy SJ, Newsam CJ, et al: Effect of fore-aft seat position on shoulder demands during wheelchair propulsion: Part 2. An electromyographic analysis, *J Spinal Cord Med* 28:222-229, 2005.

105. Lin HT, Su FC, Wu HW, et al: Muscle force analysis in the shoulder mechanism during wheelchair propulsion, *Proc Inst Mech Eng* (H) 218:213-221, 2004.

106. Kilkens OJ, Dallmeijer AJ, Nene AV, et al: The longitudinal relation between physical capacity and wheelchair skill performance during inpatient rehabilitation of people with spinal cord injury, *Arch Phys Med Rehabil* 86:1575-1581, 2005.

107. Makino K, Wada F, Hachisuka K, et al: Speed and physiological cost index of hemiplegic patients pedaling a wheelchair with both legs, *J Rehabil Med* 37:83-86, 2005.

108. Buning ME, Angelo JA, Schmeler MR: Occupational performance and the transition to powered mobility: A pilot study, *Am J Occup Ther* 55:339-344, 2001.

109. Rentschler AJ, Cooper RA, Fitzgerald SG, et al: Evaluation of selected electric-powered wheelchairs using the ANSI/RESNA standards, *Arch Phys Med Rehabil* 85:611-619, 2004.

110. Fass MV, Cooper RA, Fitzgerald SG, et al: Durability, value, and reliability of selected electric powered wheelchairs, *Arch Phys Med Rehabil* 85:805-814, 2004.

111. Holliday PJ, Mihailidis A, Rolfson R, et al: Understanding and measuring powered wheelchair mobility and maneuverability. Part I. Reach in confined spaces, *Disabil Rehabil* 27:939-949, 2005.

112. Corfman TA, Cooper RA, Boninger ML, et al: Range of motion and stroke frequency differences between manual wheelchair propulsion and push rim-activated power-assisted wheelchair propulsion, *J Spinal Cord Med* 26:135-140, 2003.

113. Ragan R, Kernozek TW, Bidar M, et al: Seat-interface pressures on various thicknesses of foam wheelchair cushions: A finite modeling approach, *Arch Phys Med Rehabil* 83:872-875, 2002.

114. Ferguson-Pell MW: Seat cushion selection, *J Rehabil Res Dev Clin* Suppl:49-73, 1998.

115. Hamanami K, Tokuhiro A, Inoue H: Finding the optimal setting of inflated air pressure for a multi-cell air cushion for wheelchair patients with spinal cord injury, *Acta Med Okayama* 58:37-44, 2004.

116. May LA, Butt C, Kolbinson K, et al: Wheelchair back-support options: Functional outcomes for persons with recent spinal cord injury, *Arch Phys Med Rehabil* 85:1146-1150, 2004.

117. Brubaker C: Ergonometric considerations, *J Rehabil Res Dev Clin* Suppl:37-48, 1998.

118. Sawatzky BJ, Miller WC, Denison I: Measuring energy expenditure using heart rate to assess the effects of wheelchair tire pressure, *Clin Rehabil* 19:182-187, 2005.

119. Wei SH, Huang S, Jiang CJ, Chiu JC: Wrist kinematic characterization of wheelchair propulsion in various seating positions: Implication to wrist pain, *Clin Biomech* 18:S46-S52, 2003.

120. van der Woude LH, Formanoy M, de Groot S: Hand rim configuration: Effects on physical strain and technique in unimpaired subjects? *Med En Phys* 25:765-774, 2003.

121. Corfman TA, Cooper RA, Fitzgerald SG, et al: Tips and falls during electric-powered wheelchair driving: Effects of seatbelt use, leg rests, and driving speed, *Arch Phys Med Rehabil* 84:1797-1802, 2003.

122. Gibson J, Frank A: Pain experienced by electric-powered chair users: A pilot exploration using pain drawings, *Physiother Res Int* 10:110-115, 2005.

123. Kirby RL, Fahie CL, Smith C, et al: Neck discomfort of wheelchair users: Effect of neck position, *Disabil Rehabil* 26:9-15, 2004.

124. Sawatzky BJ, Slobogean GP, Reilly CW: Prevalence of shoulder pain in adult-versus childhood-onset wheelchair users: A pilot study, *J Rehabil Res Dev* 42:1-8, 2005.

125. Hansen R, Tresse S, Gunnarsson RK: Fewer accidents and better maintenance with active wheelchair check-ups: A randomized controlled clinical trial, *Clin Rehabil* 18:631-639, 2004.

Chapter 34

Orthotics

Joan E. Edelstein

CHAPTER OUTLINE

Objectives
Pathology
   Design Factors
   Materials
   Orthoses
Case Study
Chapter Summary
Additional Resources
Glossary
References

OBJECTIVES

After reading this chapter, the reader will be able to:
1. Identify the biomechanical principles underlying the design and prescription of orthoses.
2. Compare the characteristics of materials used in the construction of orthoses.
3. Describe the main components of lower extremity, trunk, and upper extremity orthoses.
4. Identify the principal features of lower extremity, trunk, and upper extremity orthoses assessed during the examination and evaluation process.
5. Recognize the role of the rehabilitation clinician in management of clients fitted with lower extremity, trunk, and upper extremity orthoses.

The word *orthosis* derives from the Greek expression "making straight." An orthosis is an orthopedic appliance used to support, align, prevent, or correct deformities of a body part or improve the function of movable parts of the body. The term *brace* is synonymous with orthosis. A *splint* is a temporary orthosis. Although "orthotic" is an adjective, the term is sometimes used to designate a foot orthosis. An *orthotist* is the health care practitioner who designs, fabricates, and fits patients with orthoses for any portion of the body. A *pedorthist* designs, fabricates, and fits patients with foot orthoses. Orthotics refers to the field of knowledge relating to orthoses and their use.

Physical therapists (PTs) should have an integral role in patient management that includes orthotic prescription. Therapists evaluate the *strength,* range of joint motion, skin condition, and functional status of their patients. PTs must also be knowledgeable about the patient's risk of developing contractures. They set short- and long-term goals for patients as part of treatment planning. This information, combined with familiarity regarding contemporary orthoses, equips the therapist to recommend specific designs. Once the patient receives the orthosis, the therapist is responsible for evaluating its fit, function, and appearance, as well as training the patient in its use.

This chapter describes the common orthoses used by patients in multiple practice patterns. The examination and evaluation of patients may indicate that an orthosis is part of the overall intervention plan.

PATHOLOGY

Orthoses may be part of the treatment plan for patients who fall into a wide range of preferred practice patterns. These patients may have musculoskeletal disorders, such as fractures, metatarsalgia, and scoliosis; neuromuscular disorders, including poliomyelitis, stroke, and Charcot-Marie-Tooth disease; integumentary disorders, particularly burns; and cardiopulmonary disorders, such as limitation in vital capacity after spinal cord injury. Orthoses are often helpful for patients with weakness, postural abnormalities, and poor control of motion; and lower extremity orthoses are commonly indicated for individuals with gait deviations.

DESIGN FACTORS

Orthosis Function. Orthoses apply forces to the body to resist motion, assist motion or transfer force from one area to another. For example, a trunk orthosis with pads strategically placed to resist motion may be used to prevent a thoracic scoliosis from increasing. A person with quadriceps paralysis may wear a knee-ankle-foot orthosis (KAFO) that has a mechanical lock to resist knee flexion and maintain knee extension. Motion resistance is sometimes referred to as support. Two closely related functions are maintaining a particular alignment and protecting a body part from unwanted motion. For example, a KAFO may prevent the knee of an older adult with post-polio syndrome from hyperextending and a wrist-hand orthosis (WHO) may protect the joints of a patient with rheumatoid arthritis from pain and development of deformity.

The use of an orthosis to assist motion is illustrated by an ankle-foot orthosis (AFO) that assists dorsiflexion in the patient with foot drop. This orthosis may have a plastic or metal spring at the ankle area that compensates for the impairment by assisting ankle dorsiflexion during swing phase of gait. A foot orthosis that shifts load from subluxed metatarsal heads to the heel is an example of an orthosis that transfers force.

Comfort. Regardless of its purpose, an orthosis must be comfortable. An uncomfortable orthosis will probably not be worn and, if it is worn, it may cause skin irritation or breakdown, and may injure underlying structures. A major element in ensuring comfort is minimizing *pressure* by maximizing the area covered by the orthosis. The amount of subcutaneous fat and muscle tissue also influences orthotic fit and comfort. Therefore the individual with atrophy will need an orthosis that covers a wider area than the person who has a normal amount of soft tissue. Covering a large portion of the body can also cause some discomfort because the skin under the orthosis cannot readily dissipate heat or perspiration. Another way to improve comfort is to make the orthosis longer to provide greater leverage for the longitudinal segments of the orthosis to apply force through, but the orthosis must not be so long that it impinges on adjacent joints.

Some portion of an orthosis always touches the body. This contact should be snug but not constricting. An overly tight *band* will compress superficial blood vessels, causing pain and potentially tissue breakdown. Equally important, the contact should not be too loose, as this will likely result in friction with movement and may thus also cause skin irritation and breakdown. For example, a loose calf band on an AFO will rub on the calf and irritate the skin as the individual passes through the stance phase of gait.

Pressure Systems. Supportive systems involve a series of forces and counterforces, known as pressure systems. The basic pressure system for an orthosis is the three-point force system. A principal force acts in one direction, and two counterforces located proximal and distal to the principal force act in the opposite direction. For example, a man with genu valgum will have the deformity controlled by wearing an orthosis that exerts laterally directed force on the medial aspect of the knee and medially directed counterforces on the lateral aspect of the thigh and leg (Fig. 34-1).

The ground-reaction force may also be used strategically to help an orthosis perform its function. The ground-reaction force is the force exerted on the body by the floor in response to the force that the person exerts on the floor. All lower extremity orthoses interact with ground-reaction forces when the wearer stands or is in the stance phase of gait.

MATERIALS

Many materials are used to make contemporary orthoses. These materials differ in strength, flexibility, ease of forming, weight, and appearance. Certain principles should be used when selecting a material to achieve the purpose of the orthosis. The thicker a material, the less flexible, heavier, and bulkier it will generally be. Materials can be strengthened by corrugation, curving, rolling the edges, or by reinforcement with a stronger material such as carbon fiber. A given material shaped with an acute

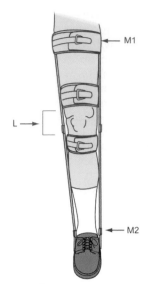

FIG. 34-1 Three-point force system to control genu valgum. *From Edelstein JE, Bruckner J:* Orthotics: A Comprehensive Clinical Approach, *Thorofare, NJ, 2002, Slack.*

angle will bend and break more readily than will the same material with a wider angled curve. Thus breakage is more apt to occur at the site of a nick or hammer mark than in a smooth portion.

Material Properties—Stress, Strain, Stiffness, and Elasticity. The ability of a material to resist forces is known as its strength. Strength is measured by *stress* resistance, which is the amount of force that can be resisted per unit area. Pressure refers to the amount of force applied per unit surface area. When a high force is applied over a small area, as occurs with a narrow band, particularly with a heavy patient, high local pressure and high stress occur. To avoid breakage, either the contact area must be increased or a very strong material must be used.

Compressive stress occurs when force squeezes a material; for example, the patient compresses the shoe heel during the early stance phase of walking. Tensile stress involves pulling the material, as in the case of a coiled spring in an AFO that pulls the shoe upward during the swing phase of gait. The third type of stress is *shear,* which occurs when planes of the material slide over each other; the components of an overlapping joint in a WHO exert shear stress on one another.

Strain is the change in shape of a material as a result of stress. *Stiffness* is the amount of stress that must be applied to a material to cause strain, whether for intentionally shaping or unintentionally deforming or breaking the material. A brittle material breaks when relatively low force is applied. Metal becomes more brittle when cold, thus the patient is more likely to damage a brace in the winter than in the summer. Fatigue resistance is the ability of the material to withstand cyclic loading. An active child, for example, subjects his orthoses to frequent repetitive loading that may cause the joints to eventually fail because of material fatigue.

Elasticity is the ratio of stress to strain and thus represents the ability of a material to recover its original dimensions. *Plasticity* characterizes a material that changes shape without cracking; a malleable material reshapes under compression, whereas a ductile material alters under *tension*. Corrosion resistance refers to the extent to which materials deteriorate when exposed to chemicals. Some materials, particularly certain metals, are vulnerable to corrosion by urine and perspiration.

Specific Materials—Plastics, Metals, and Others. Plastic and metal components predominate in contemporary orthoses, although some orthoses have leather, rubber, wood, or cloth elements. The physical and aesthetic properties of each material influence orthotic design, durability, and cost, as well as the patient's acceptance of the device.

Plastics are synthetic, organic (carbon-containing) materials. The enormous variety of plastics results from the myriad ways in which molecules can be combined. Molecular arrangement dictates the properties of the plastic. As a group, plastics are relatively lightweight, easily shaped, strong, easily cleaned, corrosion resistant, and available in many colors.

Thermoplastics are popular materials for orthoses. When heated, thermoplastics become malleable and can be reshaped and then retain the new shape upon cooling. Usually, thermoplastics can be reheated and reshaped indefinitely, allowing the orthotist to alter the fit of the appliance by heating the plastic, as well as by removing or adding material. The temperature at which thermoplastics become malleable varies. Many WHOs are formed from plastics that become malleable when immersed in warm water. The warm plastic is then molded directly on the patient. Unfortunately, if the person who wears a WHO made of such plastic washes dishes in hot water, the orthosis may also change shape. Thermoplastics that require a high temperature to become malleable are usually formed over a plaster model of the body part. Many thermoplastics are relatively weak, stain easily, and are flammable.

Alternate molecular arrangements produce *thermosetting plastics* such as polyester. Under most circumstances, thermosetting plastics cannot be reshaped after they are molded and the chemical reaction is complete. An orthosis made of thermosetting plastic cannot be reshaped by heating but can be altered by removing plastic or by adding pads or other material.

A metal is a chemical element that is lustrous, opaque, fusible, and ductile. Most metals used in orthoses are alloys, which are a combination of elements at least one of which is a metal. Combining a metal with other elements usually improves strength, wear resistance, and corrosion resistance. The mechanical properties of metals depend on their chemical structure. As a group, metals are strong, stiff, fatigue resistant, and impervious to the effects of environmental heat.

When steel is used in an orthosis, it is usually stainless steel, which is an alloy of iron, nickel, and chromium. Nickel increases corrosion resistance, while chromium improves *ductility*. Stainless steel is heavier, stiffer, and stronger than most other materials. Because it is radiopaque, steel is undesirable if the patient requires radiographs to assess alignment while wearing the orthosis,

for example, when a trunk orthosis is worn by someone with scoliosis.

Aluminum alloys that have copper, manganese, or other elements added to the aluminum are often used in orthoses. Aluminum is radiolucent, more malleable, and much lighter than steel. To achieve the same rigidity as steel the aluminum components of an orthosis need to be thicker but are still lighter than steel parts. Aluminum is not suitable for hinges in orthoses because it is subject to fatigue failure.

Titanium is as strong as steel but is much lighter and corrosion resistant. However, it is much more expensive than steel or aluminum.

Some elements, such as carbon and silicone, have properties that are similar to both metals and nonmetals and are known as metalloids. Silicone is not malleable or ductile and is a poor conductor of heat but offers little friction resistance. Thus silicone is an excellent interface between an orthosis and tender portions of skin. Carbon is considered both a metal and a metalloid; it is stiff, light, and strong but not very malleable and is often used to reinforce an orthosis made primarily of other weaker materials.

Leather is animal skin that has been chemically treated by tanning to toughen the skin and make it more flexible, stronger, and more porous. The specific skin and the type of tanning determine the flexibility, durability, and appearance of the leather. The chemicals used for tanning can cause skin allergies in some patients, but a patient who is allergic to one particular type of leather may not react to another type of leather. Alternatively, a fabric or plastic interface may be placed between the patient's skin and the leather to prevent an allergic reaction caused by contact. Leather is porous and incompressible and can be molded over a model of a body part.

Cowhide is an exceptionally strong type of leather and is therefore frequently used for straps and the upper portion of shoes. Horsehide frequently lines bands, such as a calf band or thigh band, because its texture is particularly comfortable next to the skin. Kidskin and deerskin are very soft and may be used in shoe *uppers* for patients who have hammertoes and other tender areas on the dorsum of the foot.

Cork, which is made of the bark of the cork oak tree, is the most common wood used in orthoses. Cork is exceptionally lightweight and resilient and is used primarily for shoe lifts and arch supports. Sometimes cork is ground and mixed with rubber or other materials to achieve greater flexibility or reduce cost. Cushion cork is a combination of cork and rubber. Cork may also be combined with polyolefin to create a material that is easy to mold. Cork mixed with ethyl vinyl acetate is flexible and an excellent shock absorber. Other woods are occasionally used in shoe construction. For example, balsa is sometimes used for shoe elevations because it is appreciably lighter than cork, yet has comparable strength and resilience.

Rubber is the sap of rubber trees that has been cured. Rubber has considerable elasticity, shock absorbency, and toughness. Synthetic rubber, such as neoprene, is less expensive and more resistant to corrosion but may be less elastic than natural rubber. Whether natural or synthetic, rubber provides excellent traction on shoe soles and is a good padding material. Rubber strands may be woven with cotton or other fabric to create elastic straps and *inserts*. Open-cell (sponge) rubber is made by adding sodium bicarbonate to the rubber to make carbon dioxide bubbles that create the open-cell structure. Sponge rubber recovers quickly when compressive stress is removed and is washable, soft, and very resilient. The cells, however, compress permanently after a relatively brief period of use. Closed-cell (expanded) rubber is manufactured by forcing nitrogen into rubber. It has excellent shear force and moisture resistance and responds more slowly than open-cell rubber to compressive stress.

Cotton, wool, and various synthetic fabrics are also commonly used in the manufacture of orthoses. The properties of the fabric depend on the material itself and the way it is formed. Cotton is strong, absorbs perspiration readily, and is hypoallergenic. Consequently, cotton canvas is often used for sturdy abdominal fronts on trunk orthoses. Cotton flannel is a good padding material, particularly for the metal components of a trunk orthosis. Knitted cotton conforms readily to the body and is often used as a liner worn under an orthosis.

Wool has excellent resilience. Wool felt is used in certain foot orthoses and cervical orthoses. Felt is a fabric made of wool and other fibers matted together by steam and pressure. The higher the wool content the more durable the felt. Felt is lightweight and porous but compresses readily.

Polyester and nylon are synthetic fabrics that can be used in orthoses. Polyester fibers may be combined with cotton to create a relatively inexpensive material that is strong and dries easily. A *corset* made of polyester and cotton will not retain perspiration as much as one made entirely of cotton; cotton, however, is more absorbent. A very popular use of nylon is hook and pile fasteners (Velcro) that are easier to engage than buckles, snaps, buttons, or laces.

In some orthoses, a combination of materials is used. The materials may be sewn, riveted, or glued to one another. Adhesion by gluing depends on the chemical characteristics of the surfaces to be joined because no universal adhesive exists. Synthetic resin glues, whether thermoplastic or thermosetting, are widely used because they bond many surfaces. Rubber-based adhesives resist impact loads, making them suitable for many foot orthoses.

ORTHOSES

Lower Extremity Orthoses. Lower extremity orthoses include foot orthoses (FOs), which may be an insert worn inside the shoe, an *internal modification* glued inside the shoe, or an *external modification* secured to the shoe sole or heel. AFOs cover some portion of the foot and leg. Knee orthoses (KOs) extend from the distal thigh to the proximal leg. KAFOs encompass the thigh, leg, and foot. Hip orthoses (HOs) surround the hip. A hip-knee-ankle-foot orthosis (HKAFO) originates on the pelvis and terminates at the foot. A trunk-hip-knee-ankle-foot orthosis (THKAFO) encircles the trunk, both thighs and legs, and ends at the feet.

Shoes and Foot Orthoses. The foundation for nearly all lower extremity orthoses is the shoe. Each part of the shoe contributes to the efficacy of orthotic management and offers many options for selection. Shoes transfer body weight to the ground and protect the wearer from the bearing surface and the weather. The ideal shoe should distribute bearing forces to preserve optimum comfort, function, and appearance of the foot. For the individual with a musculoskeletal or neurological disorder, footwear may serve two additional purposes: (1) reducing pressure on sensitive deformed structures by redistributing weight toward pain-free areas and (2) being the foundation of AFOs or other more extensive bracing. Unless the shoe is correctly fitted and appropriately modified, the alignment of any attached orthosis will not provide the intended pattern of weight bearing. The major parts of the shoe are the upper, sole, heel, and reinforcements (Fig. 34-2). These features are found in both the traditional leather shoe and the contemporary athletic sneaker.

The upper is the portion of the shoe over the dorsum of the foot. If the shoe is to be used with an AFO that has an insert as its distal attachment, then the upper should extend to the proximal portion of the dorsum to secure the orthosis high onto the foot. For most orthotic purposes, an upper in the *Blucher* pattern is preferable. This type of upper has a separation at the distal margin of the lace stay. The Blucher opening has substantial adjustability, an important feature for the patient with edema. It also offers a large inlet into the shoe, useful for ensuring that paralyzed toes lie flat within the shoe. The alternate upper design is the *Bal*, or Balmoral. This type of upper does not have a separation at the distal margin of the lace stay; consequently, it is less adjustable and cannot be opened as widely as a shoe with a Blucher upper. An extra-depth shoe is one with an upper contoured to have extra vertical space. Extra-depth shoes are manufactured with a second inner sole that can be removed to accommodate an insert or surgical dressing.

The sole is the bottom portion of the shoe. If the shoe is intended to accommodate a riveted metal attachment from an orthosis, it should have an outer and an inner sole, both made of leather with a metal reinforcement between them to receive the rivets. This type of shoe is heavier than one with a single sole. Rubber soles are often

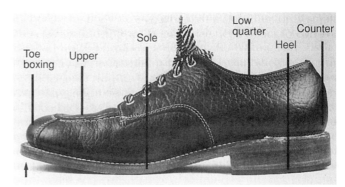

FIG. 34-2 Parts of a shoe. *From O'Sullivan S, Schmitz T (eds): Physical Rehabilitation: Assessment and Treatment, ed 4, Philadelphia, 2001, FA Davis.*

used because they absorb more impact shock and provide better traction than leather. If a riveted orthotic attachment is to be used, the rubber sole must be reinforced with metal. Except for a slight upward curve at the distal end, the outer sole is usually flat. The sole may be modified with a convex rocker bar to facilitate late stance or a *metatarsal bar* to transfer force posteriorly from painful metatarsal heads and reduce irritative motion.

The heel is the portion of the shoe adjacent to the outer sole and under the anatomical heel. A broad low heel provides the greatest stability and distributes force evenly between the back and front of the foot. For adults, a 2.5-cm (1-inch) heel tilts the center of gravity slightly forward, which aids transition through stance phase, while not disturbing knee and hip alignment significantly. A higher heel places the ankle in greater plantarflexion and forces the tibia forward. The wearer compensates either by retaining slight knee and hip flexion or by extending the knee and exaggerating the lumbar lordosis. The high heel also transmits more stress to the metatarsals while reducing tension on the Achilles tendon and other posterior structures and accommodating a rigid pes equinus. Most heels are made of firm material with a rubber plantar surface; however, a compressible heel is indicated to permit slight plantar flexion if the ankle cannot move because of orthotic or anatomical limitation.

Reinforcements preserve the shape of the shoe. *Toe boxing* in the upper also protects the toes from horizontal trauma (e.g., stubbing) and vertical trauma and should be high enough to accommodate hammertoes or similar deformities. The *shank piece* is a longitudinal plate that reinforces the sole under the midfoot, between the anterior border of the heel and the widest part of the sole at the metatarsal heads. A corrugated steel shank is necessary if a riveted orthotic attachment is to be used. The *counter* stiffens the posterior portion of the upper and usually terminates at the anterior border of the heel. The patient with pes valgus should have a shoe with a longer medial counter to reinforce the medial border of the shoe to the head of the first metatarsal to resist the tendency of the foot to collapse medially.

FOs are appliances that apply forces to the foot. The shoe itself may serve a foot orthosis. Other FOs include an insert placed in the shoe, an internal modification affixed inside the shoe, or an external modification attached to the sole or heel of the shoe. FOs can enhance function by relieving pain and improving the wearer's transition during stance phase.[1] Pain may be lessened by modifications that transfer weight-bearing stresses to pressure-tolerant sites and by protecting painful areas from contact with the shoe and with adjacent portions of the foot. FOs may also improve gait and lessen back pain by equalizing foot and leg lengths[2] and by altering the rollover point in late stance.[3-5] Comfort and mobility can also be improved by correcting alignment of a flexible segment[6] or by accommodating a fixed deformity. In many instances, a particular therapeutic aim can be achieved by various devices.

Inserts and internal modifications are widely used because they are inconspicuous and may have a more direct effect on the foot than external modifications. Mass-produced inserts are also relatively inexpensive. Biomechanically, inserts and internal shoe modifications are identical. An insert can be transferred from one shoe to another, as long as the shoes have the same heel height, whereas internal shoe modifications are fixed to the specific shoe. Most inserts terminate anteriorly just behind the metatarsal heads; thus they may slip forward, particularly if the shoe has a relatively high heel. Some inserts extend the full length of the sole, preventing slippage, but occupying the often-limited space in the anterior portion of the shoe. A heel insert (also known as a heel cup) extends from the back of the shoe to the midfoot (Fig. 34-3). This type of orthosis may be made of viscoelastic plastic or rubber. In either case, the orthosis will slope anteriorly to reduce load on the painful heel and will have a concave relief to minimize pressure on the tender area.

Internal modifications are fixed to the shoe's interior, guaranteeing the desired placement, but limiting the patient to the single pair of modified shoes. Both inserts and internal modifications reduce shoe volume, so proper shoe fit must be judged with these components in place. Inserts made of soft materials, such as the viscoelastic plastics, reduce shear and impact shock, thus protecting painful or sensitive feet.[7-9] A randomized controlled trial (RCT) on the effects of flexible inserts issued to military recruits found that those who wore these orthoses had less leg pain and no training injuries.[10] Inserts can also be constructed of semirigid or rigid plastics, rubber, or metal, often with a resilient overlay. These more rigid inserts can exert greater force and thus provide more support than compressible orthoses. Obese patients may need rigid inserts to provide support when weight bearing.

Longitudinal arch supports are intended to prevent depression of the subtalar joint. Different designs provide different amounts of support. A rubber scaphoid pad positioned at the medial border of the insole, with the apex between the sustentaculum tali and the navicular tuberosity, provides the least amount of support. A wedge (post) may be added to this orthosis to alter foot alignment. Medially wedged orthoses decrease rearfoot pronation during stance phase[11] but do not exert a consistent effect

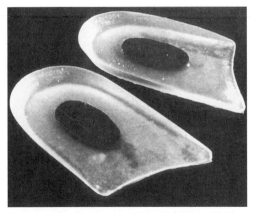

FIG. 34-3 Insert for heel spur. *From Edelstein JE, Bruckner J: Orthotics: A Comprehensive Clinical Approach, Thorofare, NJ, 2002, Slack.*

on metatarsophalangeal movement.[12] A flexible flat arch can be realigned with a semirigid plastic University of California Biomechanics Laboratory (UCBL) insert (Fig. 34-4). This orthosis is molded over a plaster model of the foot made with the foot placed in maximum correction. The orthosis encompasses the heel and midfoot, applying a medial force to the calcaneus, and a lateral and upward force to the medial portion of the midfoot. Kinematic and kinetic analyses have demonstrated that the *UCBL insert* significantly affects the orientation and movement of the subtalar, ankle, and knee joints.[13]

Longitudinal arch supports may alter muscle activation and joint strain during gait. One study reported that subjects with pes planus had greater activation of the tibialis posterior when wearing an orthosis than when barefoot,[14] although other investigators did not find that orthoses affected tibialis anterior, peroneus longus, and gastrocnemius activity.[15] Among young adults with no foot disorders, lateral wedges were associated with earlier onset of erector spinae activity, while a unilateral heel lift delayed onset of ipsilateral gluteus medius contraction.[16] A wedged insert was also found to significantly decrease lateral thrust at the knee in patients with anterior cruciate ligament insufficiency,[17] and arch supports have been found to reduce patellofemoral pain.[18,19] Foot orthoses may also have a role in management of plantar fasciitis, although RCTs comparing different orthoses are lacking.[20]

Recent evidence is equivocal regarding the effectiveness of foot orthoses in improving athletic performance. Orthoses may help limit abnormal pronation, reduce injurious torque on the leg and knee in runners,[21] and affect rearfoot kinetics in runners using either forefoot or rearfoot strike pattern.[22] Sixteen of a sample of 20 elite athletes who wore foot orthoses for 6 months reported disappearance of leg pain and demonstrated significantly increased contact duration, surface, and pressure.[23] However, other recent research involving foot orthotic use by runners showed inconsistent kinematic and kinetic effects.[24] In addition, foot orthoses were found to have little effect on leg movement in five healthy male subjects who had intracortical pins inserted in the calcaneus and tibia and ran in the gait laboratory.[25]

The *metatarsal pad* is intended to transfer stress from the metatarsal heads to the metatarsal shafts. The pad has a convexity with its apex under the metatarsal shafts, and it may either be incorporated into the design of an insert or be a separate component that is glued to the inner sole of the shoe.

An external modification has advantages and disadvantages when compared with an insert or internal modification. An external modification will not reduce internal shoe volume and ensures that the patient wears the appropriate shoes, but it will be eroded by external elements as the patient walks and is somewhat conspicuous. In addition, the client is limited to wearing the modified shoe, rather than being able to choose from a wider selection of shoes. A heel wedge is a frequently prescribed external modification. A medial heel wedge (Fig. 34-5) applies laterally directed force and can aid in realigning flexible pes valgus or can accommodate rigid pes varus by filling the void between the sole and the floor on the medial side. A cushion heel is made of resilient material to absorb shock at heel contact. Because it allows the ankle to plantar flex slightly, the cushion heel should be used when the patient wears an orthosis with a rigid ankle. Sole wedges alter mediolateral metatarsal alignment. A lateral wedge shifts weight bearing to the medial side of the front of the foot and compensates for fixed forefoot valgus, allowing the entire front of the foot to contact the floor.

A metatarsal bar is a flat strip of leather or other firm material placed on the sole posterior to the metatarsal heads. At late stance the bar transfers stress from the metatarsophalangeal joints to the metatarsal shafts. A rocker bar is a convex strip affixed to the sole proximal to the metatarsal heads. It shifts load from the metatarsophalangeal joints to the metatarsal shafts. The rocker bar also improves late stance by transferring the point of heel-off posteriorly; thus the wearer can substitute trunk momentum for triceps surae contraction to generate propulsive force.

Ankle-Foot Orthoses. The components of an AFO are a foundation, ankle control, and a superstructure, and in some cases, foot control.

The foundation consists of the shoe and a plastic or metal component. An insert foundation is most frequently used today because it facilitates donning the orthosis as the shoe can be separated from the rest of the brace[26] and it can be used with various shoes, as long as they have the same heel height. Sneakers can be worn

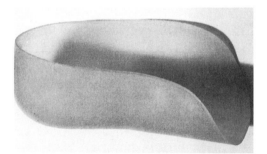

FIG. 34-4 University of California Biomechanics Laboratory (UCBL) insert. *From Edelstein JE, Bruckner J:* Orthotics: A Comprehensive Clinical Approach, *Thorofare, NJ, 2002, Slack.*

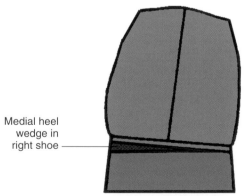

Medial heel wedge in right shoe

FIG. 34-5 Medial heel wedge. *From Edelstein JE, Bruckner J:* Orthotics: A Comprehensive Clinical Approach, *Thorofare, NJ, 2002, Slack.*

because the insert foundation is not riveted to the shoe. The orthosis with an insert is relatively lightweight because the insert is usually made of a thermoplastic such as polyethylene or polypropylene. Internal modifications can be incorporated into the insert.

An insert foundation should not be used if the patient cannot be relied upon to consistently wear the orthosis with a shoe of appropriate heel height. If the orthosis is placed in a shoe with too low a heel, the *uprights* will incline posteriorly, increasing the tendency of the wearer's knee to extend. Conversely, if the orthosis is worn with too high a heel, the knee may not extend sufficiently and may be unstable. Inserts reduce interior shoe volume and thus must be used with a suitably spacious shoe. Custom-molded foot plates may be more expensive than other types of foundations. If the orthosis is to be used by a very obese or exceptionally active individual, a metal or rigid plastic foot plate should be considered because an ordinary plastic foot plate may not provide adequate support. Some insurance policies deny reimbursement for the shoe unless the shoe is physically attached to the remainder of the brace.

The older style of AFO foundation is a steel stirrup, a U-shaped fixture, the center portion of which is riveted to the shoe through the shank. The arms of the stirrup join the brace uprights at the level of the anatomical ankle, providing congruency between the orthotic and the anatomical joints. The stirrup can be solid or split. A *solid stirrup* is made of one piece of steel and provides maximum stability of the orthosis on the shoe. The *split stirrup* is made of three segments: A central portion, riveted to the sole, with a transverse rectangular opening into which the medial and lateral angled side pieces fit. The split stirrup simplifies donning the orthosis because the wearer can detach the uprights from the central portion of the stirrup. Additionally, if a central piece is riveted to other shoes, then the orthosis can also be worn with these shoes. Disadvantages of the split stirrup are that an extremely active client may dislodge a side piece from its receptacle unintentionally, and it is bulkier and heavier than a solid stirrup.

Ankle control involves limiting plantarflexion and/or dorsiflexion or assisting ankle motion. The patient with dorsiflexor weakness or paralysis is likely to drag the toes during the swing phase of gait. An AFO can help in this circumstance, either by assisting dorsiflexion with a spring or by resisting plantar flexion with a rigid *stop*. Assistance can be provided by a posterior leaf spring that arises from a plastic or carbon fiber insert. With this type of AFO the upright is bent backward slightly during stance phase, and when the patient progresses into swing phase, the upright recoils forward to lift the foot. The thin, narrow upright permits relatively greater motion. An AFO with a stirrup can assist motion with a steel dorsiflexion spring incorporated into the stirrup. The coil spring compresses in stance and rebounds during swing phase to prevent the foot from dragging. This type of orthosis has the advantage of adjustability, but it is bulkier than the posterior leaf spring model. Both types of springs yield slightly into plantarflexion at heel contact, protecting the wearer from inadvertent knee flexion. A plantar flexion stop can also

be used to prevent toe drag, but this is generally not recommended because an AFO with a stop imposes a flexion force at the knee during early stance, potentially causing instability at the knee.

An anterior stop limits dorsiflexion, aiding the individual with paralysis of the triceps surae.[27] The anterior stop functions during stance phase, preventing the wearer from lurching forward at the ankle. The stop also improves late stance by transferring the point of heel-off posteriorly so that the wearer can substitute trunk momentum for muscular contraction to generate propulsive force. A limited motion stop is a metal joint that resists both plantarflexion and dorsiflexion. The plastic solid-ankle AFO limits all foot and ankle motion. Its border, known as the trimline, is anterior to the malleoli. To compensate for lack of plantarflexion in early stance, the shoe should have a resilient heel. Similarly, to facilitate early rollover in late stance, the shoe sole should have a rocker bar. The solid-ankle AFO may be hinged at the ankle to provide slight sagittal motion, fostering achievement of the foot-flat position in early stance. The joint at the hinge may be a plastic overlap or a plastic rod. A versatile option is a pair of metal hinges that can be adjusted to alter the amount of ankle motion.

Foot control involves limiting mediolateral motion. Both *solid-ankle* and *hinged* AFOs have rigid sides that restrict transverse, sagittal and frontal plane motions of the foot. A metal-leather orthosis with a leather valgus or varus correction strap can also be used to control foot motion. The *valgus correction strap* is sewn to the medial portion of the shoe-upper, near the sole, and buckles around the lateral upright, exerting a laterally directed force to restrain pronation (Fig. 34-6). The varus correction strap has opposite attachments and force application. Either strap, although adjustable, complicates donning.

The superstructure of an AFO is the proximal portion, consisting of uprights and a *shell*, band, or brim. Plastic AFOs usually have a single upright or shell. Solid-ankle and hinged AFOs both have a posterior shell extending from the medial to the lateral midline of the leg to maximize mediolateral control. The broad surface of the shell minimizes pressure. The *posterior leaf spring AFO* has a single posterior upright that therefore does not contribute to frontal or transverse plane control. The spiral AFO is made of nylon acrylic or polypropylene with a single upright that spirals from the medial aspect of the foot plate around the leg, terminating medially in a proximal band. The spiral orthosis controls but does not eliminate motion in all planes. Orthoses with plastic shells or uprights are molded over a cast of the patient's leg and should fit snugly for maximal control and minimal conspicuousness. Such AFOs are contraindicated for the individual whose ankle and leg volume fluctuates markedly because the orthosis cannot be readily adjusted.

Metal-leather orthoses usually have medial and lateral uprights to maximize structural stability. Occasionally, a single side-upright will suffice when a less conspicuous orthosis is required, and the wearer is not expected to exert much force. Aluminum uprights are lighter than steel; to increase the rigidity of the orthosis, a broader bar

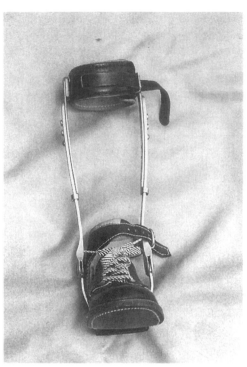

FIG. 34-6 Valgus correction strap. *From Edelstein JE, Bruckner J:* Orthotics: A Comprehensive Clinical Approach, *Thorofare, NJ, 2002, Slack.*

of aluminum can be used. Carbon graphite uprights weigh appreciably less than aluminum and rival the strength of steel; however, orthoses made of this material are more expensive.

A posterior calf band made of plastic or leather-upholstered metal is used to secure the orthosis to the patient's leg. The band has an anterior buckled or pressure-closure strap. The farther the band is from the ankle joint, the greater the leverage of the orthosis on the ankle joint; but the band must not be so proximal that it compresses the peroneal nerve. An anterior band that is part of a solid-ankle AFO imposes a posteriorly directed force near the knee, enabling the AFO to resist knee flexion and assist ankle dorsiflexion. This type of orthosis is sometimes known as a *floor reaction orthosis*, although all lower extremity orthoses are influenced by the *floor reaction* when the wearer stands or is in the stance phase of gait. If the AFO is intended to reduce the amount of weight transmitted through the foot, it may have a brim resembling a transtibial (below-knee) prosthetic socket (see Chapter 12). This plastic brim has a slight indentation over the patellar ligament (tendon) and may be hinged to facilitate donning. The brim must be used with a solid-ankle or limited-motion orthotic ankle joint.

Recent research involving adults with hemiparesis indicates that subjects walk faster at less energy cost[28-31] and feel more confident[29] when wearing an AFO. They also have more dorsiflexion in early stance,[32] longer single-stance time on the paretic foot and greater quadriceps activity.[33] A metal AFO has been found to provide better ankle control than a plastic one.[34] Despite all the advantages of AFOs, patients needing an AFO on discharge from rehabilitation still generally perform more poorly on functional tests than those who do not need any type of brace.[35]

The effect of AFOs in children with cerebral palsy has also been extensively studied. The posterior leaf spring AFO reduced excessive equinus in swing while allowing ankle dorsiflexion in midstance.[36] Comparison of posterior leaf spring AFO use with hinged and solid-ankle AFOs indicated that all three orthotic designs altered dorsiflexion but had no effect on velocity, cadence, stride length, or energy consumption; no subjects chose the solid-ankle AFO, and the others were almost equally divided in their preference for the other two designs.[37] Other research demonstrated that the solid-ankle AFO increased the dorsiflexion angle at heel strike and reduced muscle activity significantly more than a supramalleolar orthosis.[38,39] A hinged AFO is associated with better control of late stance[40] and swing phase plantarflexion,[41] as well as improved sit-to-stand maneuvering[42] and stair climbing.[43] The hinged AFO, however, increases peak knee extensor moment in early stance and can result in excessive dorsiflexion, decreased velocity, and increased energy cost, as compared with a posterior leaf spring AFO or a solid-ankle AFO.[44]

Among children with spina bifida, walking with AFOs increases gait speed and reduces oxygen cost as compared with barefoot gait.[45] Those with L4 and L5 level spina bifida had significant reduction in ankle dorsiflexion, increased plantarflexor moment, and reduction in knee extensor moment.[46]

There is also a published case study of a 40-year-old man with Charcot-Marie-Tooth disease who had less stance-phase hip and knee flexion and swing-phase ankle plantarflexion when wearing either bilateral posterior leaf spring AFOs or solid-ankle AFOs. He preferred to wear the solid-ankle AFOs when bicycling because they provided more control during pedal downstroke.[47]

Knee-Ankle-Foot Orthoses. KAFOs consist of a shoe, foundation, ankle control, knee control, and superstructure (Fig. 34-7). They often also include a foot control. The shoe, foundation, ankle control, and foot control of the KAFO may be selected from the components already described for AFOs. Donning a plastic-metal KAFO is appreciably faster than putting on a metal-leather orthosis.[27]

A hinge is the simplest type of orthotic knee joint. Hinges attached to the uprights on either side of the knee provide mediolateral, rotational, and hyperextension restriction while permitting knee flexion. An offset joint is a hinge placed posterior to the midline of the leg so that the patient's weight line falls anterior to the joint. This stabilizes the knee during the early stance phase of gait when the wearer is on a level surface and does not hamper knee flexion during swing or sitting. The joint may, however, flex inadvertently when the wearer walks down a steep ramp. An offset joint should not be used by the patient with a knee flexion contracture because the contracture will make the floor reaction force pass posterior to the knee.

The most common knee control is the *drop ring lock*. When the client stands with the knee fully extended, the

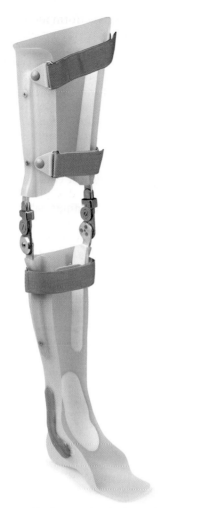

FIG. 34-7 Knee-ankle-foot orthosis (KAFO). *Courtesy Becker Orthopedic, Beaverton, OR.*

ring drops, preventing the uprights from bending. Both medial and lateral joints should be locked for maximum stability. A pair of drop ring locks is inconvenient because the user has to hold both rings up at the same time to be able to flex the knee. If two drop ring locks are used, the uprights should be equipped with a spring-loaded retention button that keeps one ring up after the wearer lifts it, allowing one to then attend to the other ring without having the first one drop.

An alternative to the drop ring lock is the *pawl lock* with bail release. This mechanism simultaneously locks both uprights. The pawl is a spring-loaded projection that fits into a notched disk. The patient unlocks the brace by pulling upward on the posterior bail. Some people can nudge the bail by pressing it against a chair. Disadvantages of this type of lock are that it is bulky and may release the locks unexpectedly if the wearer is jostled against a rigid object.

The basic drop ring and pawl locks should not be used by a patient with a knee flexion contracture because the contracture would prevent aligning the orthotic uprights straight for either type of lock to engage. If full passive

knee extension cannot be achieved, an adjustable knee joint with a drop ring lock that locks in partial flexion is required for stability.

An anterior band or a *knee cap* is needed to augment sagittal stability provided by the drop ring or pawl locks. The band or cap produces a three-point pressure system to optimize stability by applying a posteriorly directed force to complement the anteriorly directed forces from the back of the shoe and the thigh band. A rigid plastic anterior band, placed either slightly above or slightly below the knee, applies a posteriorly directed force on the knee without interfering with sitting and makes the KAFO easier to don. The leather knee cap is the more traditional component for delivering a posteriorly directed stabilizing force. It has four straps buckled to both uprights above and below the knee. Two straps remain buckled to the medial thigh and leg uprights, and the patient buckles the other two straps when donning the orthosis. When the straps are tight enough to stabilize the knee, the pad is likely to restrict flexion when the wearer sits.

Frontal plane control may be achieved with a plastic calf shell shaped to apply corrective force. To reduce genu valgum, the medial portion of the shell extends proximally to apply a laterally directed force at the knee. A semirigid shell is more effective for this than a valgum correction strap, which is a knee cap with an extra strap buckled around the lateral upright. Application of force in the opposite direction can be used to reduce genu varum. The shell does not add to donning time; it applies force over a broad area without impinging on the popliteal fossa and provides control in the transverse plane.

Thigh bands provide structural stability to the orthosis. If the distal portion of the extremity cannot tolerate full weight bearing, then the proximal thigh band may be shaped to form a weight-bearing brim similar to a quadrilateral transfemoral (above-knee) prosthetic socket (see Chapter 12). To eliminate all weight bearing through the leg, the orthosis must include a weight-bearing brim, a locked knee joint, and a patten bottom as a distal extension of the KAFO. The shoe on the braced side is also fitted with medial and lateral "D" rings attached to the orthotic uprights to keep the shoe and thus the patient's foot off the floor. To maintain a level pelvis the patient must wear a lift on the opposite shoe with height equal to the height of the patten.

Several new developments have the potential to improve the function of patients who wear KAFOs. Rather than steel or aluminum uprights, some KAFOs have carbon fiber or titanium uprights that reduce the weight but not the strength of the orthosis. A trial with 55 patients with poliomyelitis who used carbon fiber KAFOs found that nearly half of the subjects increased their maximum walking distance significantly, and virtually all preferred the lighter orthosis.[48] Another innovation is the stance-phase knee lock. This locks in late swing phase, just before heel contact, unlocks at the heel-off phase, and stays unlocked through the remainder of the gait cycle. Some versions have mechanical linkages, while others have computerized control that makes gait kinematics more normal.[49-51] This lock allows free swinging of the knee during swing phase and stability during stance phase but it is more mechanically complex and expensive than other types of orthotic knee joints.

Hip-Knee-Ankle-Foot Orthoses. A HKAFO is a KAFO with a *pelvic band* and hip joints (Fig. 34-8). The usual hip joint is a metal hinge that connects the lateral upright of the KAFO to a pelvic band. The joint prevents hip abduction, adduction, and rotation. If the patient wears HKAFOs bilaterally and only needs control of hip rotation, a simpler alternative to the hip joint and pelvic band is a webbing strap that attaches to the lateral uprights of both KAFOs. To reduce internal rotation, the strap extends from the lateral uprights to the posterior center point of a webbing waist belt. To reduce external rotation, the strap joins the lateral uprights and passes anteriorly at the level of the groin. If flexion control is required, a drop ring lock is added to the hip joint. A two-position lock stabilizes the patient in hip extension for standing and walking and at 90 degrees of hip flexion for sitting.

An upholstered metal band is used to anchor the HKAFO to the trunk. This band should lodge between the greater trochanter and the iliac crest on each side. HKAFOs are not used very often because they are much more difficult to don than KAFOs, and if the hip joints are locked, they restrict gait to the swing-to or swing-through pattern. The pelvic band is also often uncomfortable when the wearer sits.

Trunk-Hip-Knee-Ankle-Foot Orthoses. A THKAFO incorporates a lumbosacral orthosis attached to a KAFO (Fig. 34-9). The pelvic band of the trunk orthosis serves as the pelvic band used on HKAFOs. A THKAFO may be used by a patient with spinal cord injury to allow them to experience orthotically assisted ambulation. Because the THKAFO is very difficult to don and is heavy and

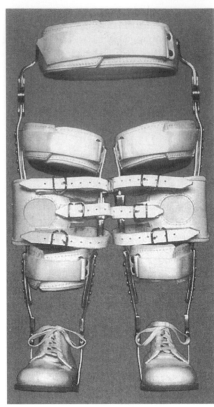

FIG. 34-8 Hip-knee-ankle-foot orthosis (HKAFO). *From Edelstein JE, Bruckner J:* Orthotics: A Comprehensive Clinical Approach, *Thorofare, NJ, 2002, Slack.*

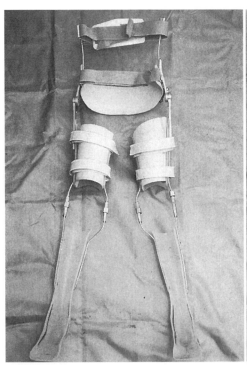
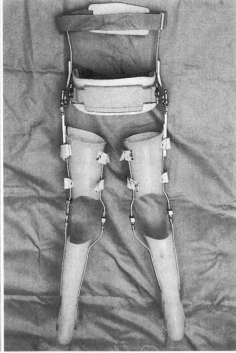

A   **B**

FIG. 34-9 Trunk-hip-knee-ankle-foot orthosis (THKAFO). **A,** Anterior view; **B,** posterior view. *From Edelstein JE, Bruckner J:* Orthotics: A Comprehensive Clinical Approach, *Thorofare, NJ, 2002, Slack.*

cumbersome, it is seldom worn after the client is discharged from the rehabilitation program.

The functional capacity of patients fitted with KAFOs and more extensive bracing is limited. Among boys with Duchenne muscular dystrophy, wearing KAFOs prolongs assisted walking but does not seem to extend the time the child can walk functionally.[52] A comprehensive review of energy consumption confirms that patients who wear KAFOs and higher orthoses walk 66% or more slower and require 230% or more energy expenditure than nondisabled peers.[53] A limited study of patients with paraplegia who walked with stance-control KAFOs demonstrated that although the subjects walked slightly faster with the new orthoses, their energy consumption per distance walked remained high.[54] Even when THKAFOs are combined with functional electrical stimulation, walking speed is much slower than that of able-bodied adults.[55-57] A longitudinal study of THKAFO use demonstrated a positive effect of bracing[28]; patients with spina bifida averaged 9.7 years of brace wear, during which time none of them incurred a pressure ulcer or fracture.[58]

Trunk Orthoses. Trunk orthoses are usually named for the section of the torso encircled, as well as the type of control provided. They may be worn with lower extremity orthoses or may be prescribed to reduce the disability caused by low-back pain, neck sprain, scoliosis, or other musculoskeletal or neuromuscular disorders. These orthoses support the trunk, thereby assisting in the control of spinal motion; however, forces that the orthosis exerts are modified by the skin, subcutaneous tissue, and musculature that surround the vertebral column and, in the case of higher orthoses, by the thoracic cage. Patients with spinal cord injury benefit from trunk orthoses in two ways: (1) the orthoses control motion of the lumbar region,[59] with or without thoracic control, and (2) they compress the abdomen to improve respiration.[60,61] Individuals with cervical spinal cord lesions may need to wear an orthosis that restrains neck motion until stability is achieved by surgery or spontaneous healing. A special group of trunk orthoses is designed for children and adolescents with scoliosis.

Corsets. A corset is a fabric orthosis with no horizontal rigid structures, although it may have vertical rigid reinforcements (Fig. 34-10). The corset may cover only the sacroiliac or lumbosacral regions or may extend superiorly as a thoracolumbosacral corset. The primary effect of a corset is to compress the abdomen to increase intraabdominal pressure. Greater pressure increases spinal stability[62,63] and reduces stress on posterior spinal musculature,[64] but the effect of corset wear on trunk muscle activity is variable.[65,66] Although temporary reduction of abdominal and erector spinae muscular activity may be therapeutic,[67] long-term reliance on a corset is apt to promote muscle atrophy and contracture, as well as psychological dependence on the orthosis.

Rigid Lumbosacral and Thoracolumbosacral Orthoses. Most lumbosacral (LS) and thoracolumbosacral (TLS) orthoses include a corset or a fabric abdominal front that compresses the abdomen. Rigid orthoses have horizontal and vertical, rigid plastic, or metal components. Motion restriction is accomplished by a series of three-point pres-

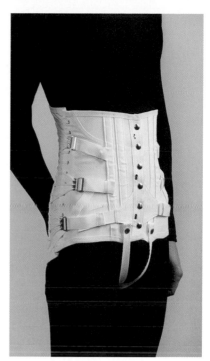

FIG. 34-10 Lumbosacral (LS) corset. *From Edelstein JE, Bruckner J: Orthotics: A Comprehensive Clinical Approach, Thorofare, NJ, 2002, Slack.*

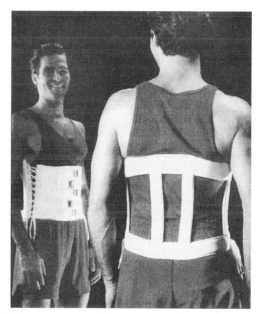

FIG. 34-11 Lumbosacral flexion-extension lateral-control (LS FEL) orthosis. *Courtesy Becker Orthopaedics.*

sure systems, in which force in one direction is counteracted by two forces in the opposite direction.

The LS flexion-extension lateral-control (LS FEL) orthosis, also known as a Knight spinal orthosis, has pelvic and thoracic bands, vertical posterior uprights, an abdominal front, and a pair of lateral uprights at the lateral midline of the torso that resist lateral flexion (Fig. 34-11). A LS extension lateral-control (LS EL) orthosis, also known as a Williams orthosis, has oblique, rather than vertical, posterior uprights from the lateral uprights to the pelvic band; the orthosis restricts lateral flexion and extension but permits trunk flexion.

The TLS flexion-extension control (TLS FE) orthosis, originally known as the Taylor brace, consists of a pelvic band, posterior uprights terminating at midscapular level, an abdominal front or corset, and axillary straps attached to an interscapular band. This orthosis reduces flexion by a three-point system consisting of posteriorly directed force from the axillary straps and the bottom of the abdominal front or corset and anteriorly directed force from the midportion of the posterior uprights. Extension resistance is provided by posteriorly directed force from the midsection of the abdominal front or corset and anteriorly directed force from the pelvic and interscapular bands. Addition of lateral uprights provides lateral control and converts the orthosis to a TLS FE lateral-control (TLS FEL) orthosis (Fig. 34-12). The TLS flexion-control orthosis consists of a sternal and suprapubic plate anteriorly and a dorsolumbar plate posteriorly; the plates are held in place by a rigid plastic or metal frame. Biomechanical investigation with healthy subjects confirms that the orthosis significantly reduces segmental and gross spinal movements.[68] A plastic TLS jacket provides maximum support to the lower torso by limiting trunk motion in the frontal, sagittal, and transverse planes.

The clinical efficacy of rigid orthoses is controversial with few published randomized trials evaluating their effects. A meta-analysis of 13 preventive and therapeutic trials of back orthoses provides moderate evidence that lumbar supports are not effective for primary prevention of low back pain, although limited evidence suggests that lumbar supports are more effective than no intervention in the treatment of low back pain.[69] Recent evidence indicates that LS orthoses may reduce muscle activity in patients with low back pain.[70]

A new TLS orthosis intended for wear by postmenopausal women with one or more osteoporotic vertebral fractures has been found to allow the wearers to increase the strength of their back extensor and abdominal muscles substantially, with modest increase in vital capacity and decrease in pain.[71]

Cervical Orthoses. Cervical orthoses are classified as collars or post orthoses. Collars encircle the neck with fabric, resilient material, or rigid plastic. A few collars also encompass the chin and posterior head for slightly greater restraint. The most common collar is made of soft material and provides minimal restraint (Fig. 34-13). When used by patients with soft tissue injuries of the neck, collars have not been found to hasten recovery.[72,73] The Philadelphia collar is intended for use by patients with cervical fractures. This collar surrounds the neck and covers the lower portion of the jaw and the occipital area of the skull with foamed polyethylene reinforced with a rigid anterior strut. Nineteen patients with upper cervical fractures who were treated with the Philadelphia collar obtained stable fracture healing.[74] Wearing a rigid cervical orthosis interferes with driving and other activities by decreasing axial rotation, thereby limiting the ability to see to the side or rear.[75]

For moderate control a two-, three-, or four-post cervical orthosis can be used (Fig. 34-14). Usually these orthoses have one or two anterior adjustable posts joining a sternal plate to a mandibular plate and one or two posterior uprights connecting a thoracic plate to an occipital plate. The sternal plate is strapped to the thoracic plate and the occipital plate is strapped to the mandibular plate. Of this group of orthoses, the four-post version is the most restrictive, particularly to neck extension.[76,77]

Maximum orthotic control of the neck is achieved either with a *Minerva,* or a *halo vest,* orthosis. The Minerva orthosis is a noninvasive appliance with a rigid plastic posterior section extending from the head to the mid trunk;

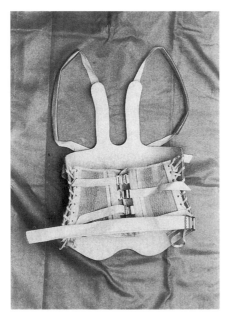

FIG. 34-12 Thoracolumbosacral flexion-extension lateral-control (TLS FEL) orthosis. *From Edelstein JE, Bruckner J: Orthotics: A Comprehensive Clinical Approach,* Thorofare, *NJ, 2002, Slack.*

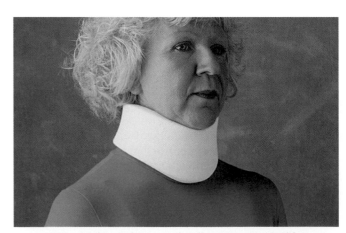

FIG. 34-13 Soft cervical collar. *Courtesy Trulife.*

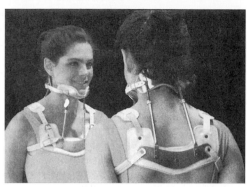

FIG. 34-14 Four-post cervical orthosis. *From Edelstein JE, Bruckner J: Orthotics: A Comprehensive Clinical Approach, Thorofare, NJ, 2002, Slack.*

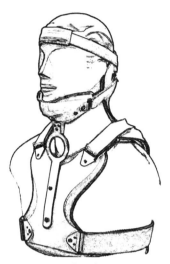

FIG. 34-15 Minerva cervical orthosis. *From Edelstein JE, Bruckner J: Orthotics: A Comprehensive Clinical Approach, Thorofare, NJ, 2002, Slack.*

the superior portion is held in place by a forehead band (Fig. 34-15). The Minerva orthosis is named for the Roman goddess of war and wisdom who is traditionally depicted wearing a forehead band. This orthosis provides good neck control below the first cervical vertebra.[78,79] The halo vest orthosis has a circular band of metal that is fixed to the skull by four screws. Uprights connect the halo to a vest-like thoracic orthosis. The relative effectiveness of the halo vest as compared with the Minerva for patients with unstable cervical spine injuries is controversial.[80,81]

Orthoses for Patients with Scoliosis. Children and adolescents with thoracic, thoracolumbar, or lumbar scolioses or kyphoses may be fitted with a TLS orthosis that applies forces intended to maintain alignment of or realign the vertebral column and thoracic cage. While substantial improvement is evident when the orthosis is worn, long-term follow-up indicates that the orthosis usually only prevents the curve from increasing beyond its original contour.[82-84] Decreased effectiveness of scoliosis orthoses is associated with failure to fasten the orthosis snugly[85] and the presence of obesity.[86]

The *Milwaukee orthosis* is one type of TLSO often prescribed for patients with scoliosis. This orthosis consists of a frame composed of a pelvic girdle, two posterior uprights, an anterior upright, and a superior ring. Unlike the original Milwaukee orthosis, the current version features a superior ring that lies on the upper chest rather than just below or on the chin as with older models; the current design can be hidden by most clothing. Various pads are strapped to the frame to apply corrective forces. The *Boston orthosis* is an alternative to the Milwaukee. It usually does not extend as high as the Milwaukee, and its foundation is a mass-produced plastic module that the orthotist alters to meet the needs of the individual patient (Fig. 34-16). A retrospective study of 151 patients who wore the Boston brace confirms that this orthosis can prevent curve progression.[87] It is most effective if worn for at least 18 hours a day,[88,89] and when the strap tension is between 20 and 40 N.[90]

The *Wilmington orthosis* is another contemporary design of TLSO used to treat scoliosis. It consists of a custom-made TLSO jacket intended to guide the trunk to straighter alignment and thereby avoid exaggeration of the scoliotic curve.[91] The *Charleston bending brace* and the *Providence orthosis* provide overcorrection of the spinal curve and have also been shown to control relatively slight scoliotic curves (Fig. 34-17).[92-95]

Orthoses for patients with scoliosis are most effective when the patient has an immature spine and moderate vertebral curves in the midthoracic or more inferior portions of the trunk.[96] The classic protocol required the youngster to wear the orthosis 23 hours each day; part-time wearing produces results somewhat less favorable in terms of maintaining trunk alignment but is better tolerated.[86] Another approach is for the patient to wear an orthosis only at night in bed when the effects of gravity are minimized.

Upper Extremity Orthoses. Orthoses for the upper extremity include appliances for the shoulder, including slings and rigid orthoses, elbow orthoses, and a very wide variety of wrist-hand appliances. Splints are orthoses

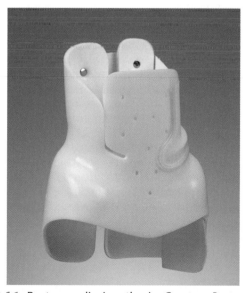

FIG. 34-16 Boston scoliosis orthosis. *Courtesy Boston Brace International, www.bostonbrace.com.*

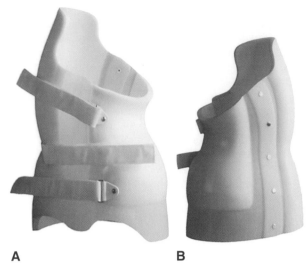

A   **B**

FIG. 34-17 Charleston bending brace. **A,** Anterior view; **B,** posterior view. *Courtesy Spinal Technology, Inc, www.spinetech.com.*

intended for relatively short-term use. In addition to considering orthoses according to the portion of the upper extremity that is braced, one may also classify devices with regard to primary function, namely assistive or substitutive, protective, or corrective. Assistive and substitutive orthoses are indicated for patients with paralysis; the devices augment residual motor power or substitute mechanical joint motion and stabilization for absent anatomical function. Protective orthoses either shield the affected joint from developing contracture, as is the case with burns, or reduce painful motion, often required with patients with arthritis or overuse injuries. Corrective orthoses are used to increase joint range of motion (ROM) in the presence of dermal or capsular contracture.

Wrist-Hand Orthoses

Assistive and Substitutive Wrist-Hand Orthoses. Assistive and substitutive WHOs are widely used. Although many designs were developed in the first half of the twentieth century for patients with poliomyelitis, current orthoses are prescribed primarily for those with central and peripheral neuropathies. Assistive orthoses position the hand so that the patient can make maximum use of the residual motor power. Substitutive orthoses enable the patient to achieve prehension by moving the wrist or a more proximal body segment to cause finger movement.

The *basic opponens orthosis* is one of the simplest assistive WHOs. Formerly called the short opponens splint, it keeps the thumb pad beneath the palmar surfaces of the index and middle fingers, helping the patient use residual motor power to achieve palmar prehension. Its dorsal and palmar bars support the transverse palmar arch, protecting it from flattening. The abduction bar keeps the thumb abducted, preventing thenar web contracture and placing the thumb in a suitable position for opposition. The opponens bar prevents the first metatarsal from migrating to the plane of the other fingers. This orthosis is useful for the patient with median neuropathy who is in jeopardy of developing thenar contracture and a flat

hand posture and who needs assistance for prehension (see Chapter 18).

A forearm bar added to the basic opponens orthosis creates the opponens WHO with wrist control, also known as the long opponens splint (Fig. 34-18). The forearm bar may be located on the palmar, dorsal, radial, or ulnar aspect of the wrist and forearm. The forearm bar maintains the wrist in a fixed position, preventing the hand from dropping into palmar flexion.

A *metacarpophalangeal-extension stop* is another possible addition to the basic opponens orthosis. The stop, sometimes called a lumbrical bar, is secured to the palmar bar and applies palmar-ward force to the proximal phalanges to resist metacarpophalangeal hyperextension. This component aids prehension by protecting the hand from forming a claw hand deformity, which is a risk with ulnar or combined median and ulnar neuropathy, and thereby aids prehension.

The wrist flexion control WHO, also called a cock-up splint, is another assistive orthosis. This design features a palmar hand bar and forearm bar with straps to secure the orthosis to the extremity. The orthosis prevents the wrist from dropping into palmar flexion, thereby assisting the median- and ulnar-innervated muscles by placing them in a more functional position. The same orthosis is often used to protect the wrist from repetitive motion stress, as experienced by keyboard operators.

Prehension orthoses are examples of substitutive appliances. They are especially suited to the patient with tetraparesis or tetraplegia. The orthoses enable the wearer to grasp an object, hold it, and release it voluntarily. The wrist-driven prehension WHO was originally called the flexor hinge orthosis because it has a hinge between the forearm bar and the finger stabilizer (Fig. 34-19). The orthosis includes a bar and a band to stabilize the first interphalangeal joint and a separate bar and band unit to prevent motion of the second and third proximal and distal interphalangeal joints. The two stabilizers pivot on a palmar and dorsal hand-bar assembly, and there is a second pivot at the junction between the hand and forearm bar. Wrist dorsiflexion causes the finger stabilizers to approach the thumb stabilizer, enabling grasp. The user

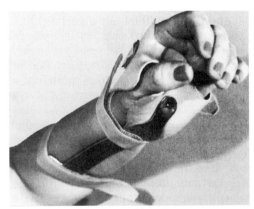

FIG. 34-18 Opponens orthosis with wrist control. *From American Academy of Orthopaedic Surgeons:* Atlas of Orthotics: Biomechanical Principles and Application, *ed 2, Philadelphia, 1985, WB Saunders, p. 165.*

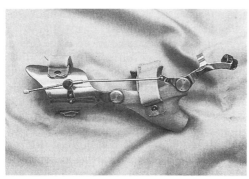

FIG. 34-19 Wrist-driven prehension orthosis. *From Edelstein JE, Bruckner J: Orthotics. A Comprehensive Clinical Approach, Thorofare, NJ, 2002, Slack.*

must maintain active dorsiflexion to retain the held object. Some prehension orthoses have a locking mechanism to relieve stress on the dorsiflexors. Most also have a mechanism to allow the wearer to select the size of grasp relative to the angle of wrist dorsiflexion. For grasping a piece of paper, the wearer would adjust the mechanism so that a small arc of wrist motion achieved finger closure. For grasping a thicker object, the wearer would adjust the mechanism so that the same small arc of wrist dorsiflexion achieved closure. The object is released when the wearer relaxes the dorsiflexors, allowing the wrist to passively palmar flex. The patient with C6 tetraplegia can use this type of orthosis only with the forearm pronated. If the forearm is supinated, the wearer could achieve grasp and holding but could not release the object voluntarily because of lack of control of the palmar flexors. Despite these limitations, the wrist-driven prehension WHO is a relatively useful device, facilitating hygiene, writing, and feeding.

The person with C4 or C5 tetraplegia lacks sufficient control of the wrist dorsiflexors to use a wrist-drive prehension WHO and therefore requires a different type of orthosis. The electrically driven prehension WHO is sometimes prescribed for these patients. The rigid parts of this orthosis are similar to those of the wrist-driven model but instead of a linkage between the hand and forearm components, the electrically driven orthosis has a steel cable secured to the finger stabilizer. The proximal end of the cable terminates in a rod linked to a battery-operated motor. To achieve grasp, the patient moves an actuator, usually located over the contralateral shoulder. Shoulder elevation triggers a microswitch, which turns on the motor that pulls the cable proximally. Cable movement causes the finger stabilizer to approach the thumb stabilizer. Holding occurs when the patient keeps the motor in the neutral position. Release is attained by voluntary shoulder pressure on a second microswitch in the actuator that reverses the direction of the motor, relieving tension on the cable. A spring located on the finger stabilizer is then able to recoil, opening the fingers. Usually a relatively large arc of shoulder elevation causes grasp and a smaller arc triggers the releasing microswitch. The battery and motor for this device are relatively heavy and bulky, making the orthosis awkward for an ambulatory

patient but practical for transport on a wheelchair for a wheelchair user. As with all battery-powered motors, the battery in the orthosis must be recharged periodically. Many patients eventually opt for a much simpler lighter orthosis, such as those described the next section, to perform grasp functions.

The *utensil holder,* sometimes called a universal cuff, is an orthosis that is usually mass-produced and consists of a spring clip or elastic webbing that wraps around the hand, across palm (Fig. 34-20). The palmar side of the clip has a pocket into which one may place a pen, spoon handle, or other objects of appropriate size. This orthosis may have a forearm bar to prevent unwanted wrist motion and keep the hand in a more functional position. Grasping is achieved by inserting an object or a handle into the pocket. Patients often accomplish this by holding the object with the teeth and directing it into the pocket. Alternatively, an attendant may place an object in the pocket. Holding occurs by means of friction from the pocket. If the object is too slender it will wobble in the pocket and if it is too large it will not fit into the pocket. Therefore the object will need an adapter with an appropriately-sized flange to fit snugly in the pocket. Release requires removing the object from the pocket with the teeth or by other means.

Protective Wrist-Hand Orthoses. There are many mass-produced protective WHOs available, although nearly all the designs can be custom made of plaster or plastic sheeting. The wrist-hand stabilizing orthosis, also termed a resting splint, is a molded sheet of semirigid plastic formed to fit the palmar surface of the hand and forearm. The sheet extends from the distal tips of the fingers to the middle third of the forearm and is curved to support the palmar arch and cradle the forearm. Straps secure the plastic to the hand and forearm. Some wrist stabilizers also include a thumb component for thumb stabilization. Patients with inflammatory arthritis have been shown to have significantly less pain after 4 weeks of wearing a protective WHO, regardless of whether the orthosis was a custom leather version or a commercial plastic design.[97,98] Two RCTs concluded that patients with carpal tunnel syndrome who wore a protective WHO only at night reported improvement.[99] However, the results of another RCT indicate that wearing a protective WHO full-time more

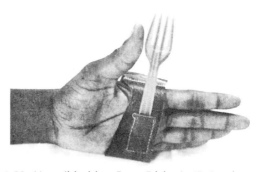

FIG. 34-20 Utensil holder. *From Edelstein JE, Bruckner J: Orthotics: A Comprehensive Clinical Approach, Thorofare, NJ, 2002, Slack.*

effectively improves median nerve sensory and motor function than part-time wear.[100] In contrast, a meta-analysis of 19 studies of protective WHOs for adults with upper extremity hemiplegia after stroke concluded that there was insufficient evidence to support or refute the effectiveness of hand splinting for this population.[101]

Thumb and Finger Orthoses. A thumb-stabilizing orthosis without a wrist-stabilizing component can also be used to prevent movement of the first interphalangeal and metacarpophalangeal joints in patients with exacerbation of arthritis and in those with burns who are vulnerable to flexion contractures. This orthosis has a longitudinal bar along the length of the thumb, with stabilizing straps or a sleeve on the thumb and a strap around the hand.

Finger stabilizers are used by some patients to stabilize or correct a boutonniere deformity (hyperflexion of the proximal interphalangeal joint). This orthosis includes a band that applies palmar-directed force at the proximal interphalangeal joint. This force is opposed by two bands that apply dorsally directed forces to the proximal and middle phalanges.

A corrective WHO that applies a low, constant force with appropriate counterforces to reduce contracture can be used to correct extension contractures of the metacarpophalangeal joints. This device, known as a *finger flexor WHO* or a knuckle bender, has a dorsal plate over the metacarpals and another plate over the proximal phalanges linked to a palmar rod. Springs or rubber bands apply tensile force to the orthosis. If worn for a sufficient period of time, the orthosis will cause the metacarpophalangeal joints to yield. Care must be taken, however, to avoid skin breakdown and ulceration from undue pressure. The finger extensor hand orthosis, also called the reverse knuckle bender, has an opposite force system to the knuckle bender. It has a palmar-located bar linked to two dorsal bars. Tension is exerted by rubber bands or springs. Versions of these corrective orthoses are also available to correct extension and flexion deformities of the interphalangeal joints. Corrective WHOs were associated with improved grip strength and finger mobility in patients with rheumatoid arthritis and finger flexion contractures.[102] Among patients with traumatic upper extremity injury, those who wore a corrective WHO for 6-12 hours per day achieved significantly greater joint excursion than those who wore the orthosis for less than 6 hours daily.[103]

Forearm and Elbow Orthoses. A few patients benefit from protective or corrective elbow orthoses and a very few tolerate assistive or substitutive elbow orthoses. Forearm cuffs are readily available orthoses intended to reduce stress on the forearm extensor muscles and tendons in patients with lateral epicondylitis. The typical cuff is made of sturdy fabric with hook and pile closure. Some cuffs have reinforcing bars. No definitive evidence indicates the relative merit of wide or narrow cuffs nor the optimum site of cuff placement.[104-106]

The elbow extensor orthosis is a device intended to increase elbow extension in the presence of an elbow flexion contracture. This type of device is intended for continuous wear. Both mass-produced and custom-made elbow extension orthoses are available. All of these orthoses have the same three-point pressure system, with anteriorly directed force in the vicinity of the olecranon and posteriorly directed counterforces at the distal forearm and proximal upper arm. Most models allow the clinician to increase the angle between the forearm and upper arm as the flexion contracture reduces. Others have a spring mechanism that is designed to maintain maximum separation between the cuffs. In the absence of an adjustable joint or spring, the orthosis is designed to be remolded periodically as the contracture reduces. A clinical study of 22 patients with elbow contracture showed that most achieved a functional arc of movement after wearing an elbow extensor orthosis for 2-6 months.[107]

Elbow assistive and substitutive orthoses are intended for patients with paralyzed elbow flexors or extensors. Lacking voluntary control of the elbow, the individual would have a limited work area in which to use the naturally or orthotically powered hand. The simplest orthosis is the elbow stabilizing orthosis that maintains the elbow at 90 degrees of flexion and the forearm in moderate pronation. This orthosis places the hand in a position to perform tabletop functions. The orthosis has no moving parts, making it durable and relatively inexpensive. However, the elbow is kept flexed, which is awkward when the individual walks or dons a jacket.

Shoulder Orthoses. Most shoulder orthoses (SOs) are intended to protect the glenohumeral joint from subluxation caused by flaccid hemiplegia or injury to the shoulder joint capsule. The simplest and most widely used SO is a sling. Although there are many sling designs, the most common are single-strap, multiple-strap, and humeral-cuff slings. The typical single-strap sling has a canvas forearm support to which is sewn a strap that is worn over the contralateral shoulder. The forearm support may be a continuous piece of fabric or may be divided into proximal and distal forearm sections. The single-strap sling supports the weight of the forearm, wrist, and hand. The sling reduces the risk of shoulder subluxation in patients with shoulder muscle flaccidity and can protect the upper extremity from swinging and inadvertently bumping into objects. The single-strap sling is easier to don than other models.

Multiple-strap slings have two or more straps. The forearm support has proximal and distal straps. The proximal strap passes over the ipsilateral shoulder, while the distal strap goes over the opposite shoulder. In the back, the two straps may be sewn to another oblique strap that maintains the appropriate distance between the two vertical straps. Because this sling has a strap lying vertically over the ipsilateral shoulder, it directly resists downward shoulder subluxation. As with single-strap slings, multiple-strap slings also support the weight of the forearm and hand to prevent the extremity from swinging into objects. Biomechanical analysis demonstrated that single- and multiple-strap slings were more effective than an axillary roll or a lap tray in supporting the flaccid shoulder.[108]

Humeral cuff slings do not support the forearm. Instead, they have a broad cuff that encircles the upper arm. Vertical straps extend from the anterior and posterior proximal margins of this cuff to a horizontal strap that encircles the chest. Some models have a pad over the shoulder to disperse pressure. Humeral cuff slings prevent shoulder subluxation without encumbering the elbow or forearm. Consequently, the wearer can conceal the sling under a shirt. One version of a humeral cuff sling has cuffs on both upper arms. The cuffs are joined posteriorly by a strap. Tightening the strap pulls both upper arms posteriorly, helping the humeral heads to lodge firmly in their respective glenohumeral fossae. Radiographic evidence confirms that the humeral cuff is significantly more effective than the single-strap sling in reducing subluxation.[109] However, a meta-analysis of RCTs involving the use of slings in hemiplegic patients with shoulder subluxation did not find any particular sling design to be significantly more effective than any other in reducing subluxation or related pain.[110]

Other SOs include appliances with a jointed metal frame with cuffs and straps. Depending on the type of metal joint, these orthoses may either correct an existing axillary contracture or substitute motion if the patient has shoulder paralysis and distal weakness. SOs intended to stabilize the shoulder after trauma usually restrict motion to the limits of pain-free excursion. Proper fit of this type of device is essential for patient compliance and clinical success.[111] The shoulder abductor orthosis is designed to correct an axillary contracture by positioning the arm in the maximum-tolerated degree of abduction. The orthosis has a trough to support the forearm. The trough is secured to a frame that encircles the upper torso. An adjustable joint lies at the junction between the trough and the body frame. The orthosis is sometimes referred to as the "Statue of Liberty" because the patient's arm is held in an upright position, similar to the posture of the torch-holding extremity of the famous statue.

Patients with good hand and elbow function who have lost shoulder control can make better use of the hand if the shoulder is stabilized. A shoulder stabilizing orthosis with a metal or rigid plastic frame for the upper arm joined to a trunk orthosis is often used for this purpose. The most common shoulder joint in this type of orthosis is a friction joint that keeps the shoulder where the wearer moves it.

The *balanced forearm orthosis* (BFO) is a practical orthosis to assist shoulder and elbow motion (Fig. 34-21). The BFO is sometimes referred to as a feeder because it facilitates the shoulder and elbow motions needed for feeding. This is a mass-produced appliance that is usually bolted to a person's wheelchair. The BFO consists of a proximal arm that fits into a ball-bearing receptacle attached to the wheelchair or other support and a distal arm that fits into a second ball-bearing receptacle between the proximal and distal arm. The distal arm is attached to a pivoting rocker arm mechanism to which the forearm trough is screwed. By adjusting the tilt and rotational position of the proximal and distal arms, one can assist or resist shoulder flexion, extension, and rotation. The first mechanical principle governing the BFO is that objects move down a slope. The second principle is that of the first-class lever exemplified by the action of the forearm trough. If the proximal portion of trough is screwed into the pivoting mechanism, elbow extension is aided. Locating the screws toward the distal end of the trough assists elbow flexion.

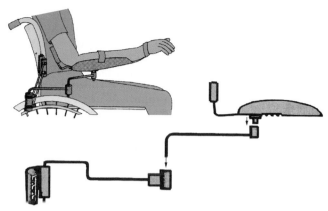

FIG. 34-21 Balanced forearm orthosis. *From Edelstein JE, Bruckner J: Orthotics: A Comprehensive Clinical Approach, Thorofare, NJ, 2002, Slack.*

The BFO is a relatively inexpensive orthosis that enables the user to move the arm horizontally and vertically. It is usually employed with a wheelchair to enable the patient with tetraparesis to accomplish many daily activities, such as feeding, facial hygiene, writing, keyboard operation, and painting, if the patient retains natural or orthotically assisted prehension.

CASE STUDY 34-1

ANKLE-FOOT ORTHOSES FOR A PATIENT WITH MULTIPLE SCLEROSIS

Examination
Patient History
EA is a 48-year-old mail delivery clerk in a large medical center. He lives with his wife in an apartment. Two years ago, EA started to have difficulty focusing on the television and noticed tingling in both his feet, as well as increasing discomfort when wearing leather shoes. Some days he was so fatigued that he had to rest while delivering mail to the various departments in the medical center. At other times, he could drive to see his grandchildren and engage them in vigorous play. After he stumbled twice in the same week and then dropped a sack of mail in front of his supervisor, he sought medical attention. He was diagnosed with multiple sclerosis (MS) after undergoing magnetic resonance imaging (MRI), cerebrospinal fluid examination, and evoked potential testing. Immunosuppressants and other medications were partially effective in controlling his symptoms.

Tests and Measures
Musculoskeletal
Anthropometric Characteristics EA is a well-developed, well-nourished man of average height and weight. Both lower extremities and upper extremities were symmetrical in size and posture.

Range of Motion Ankle dorsiflexion is limited to the neutral position bilaterally. Both feet exhibit mild pes varus. No restriction of knee, hip, trunk, or upper extremity ROM.

Muscle Performance Bilaterally, dorsiflexors 3/5; plantar flexors 4/5; invertors 4/5; evertors 2/5; quadriceps 3/5; hip extensors 3/5; hip flexors 4/5. Trunk and upper extremity strength within normal limits (WNL).

Neuromuscular

Reflex Integrity Mild clonus elicited in both ankles.

Sensory Integrity EA complains of numbness on the plantar surface of both feet.

Cardiovascular/Pulmonary

Circulation Skin temperature is normal to touch bilaterally.

Integumentary

Integumentary Integrity EA has bruises from recent falls on both lateral thighs. Feet show abrasions on the medial portion of the dorsum where the feet have been rubbing on the margin of the shoes.

Evaluation, Diagnosis, and Prognosis

EA's medical diagnosis is MS, with mild exacerbations. The examination findings would classify EA under preferred practice pattern 5E: Impaired motor function and sensory integrity associated with progressive disorders of the central nervous system. It is expected that EA will have an immediate reduction in falls with use of appropriate orthoses and a cane; however, as his disease progresses, he will need reevaluation for additional interventions to enable continued safe walking.

Intervention

1. Hinged AFOs fitted bilaterally to control pes varus and drop foot.
2. Shoes with rubber soles to increase traction and pliable leather uppers to minimize irritation on medial aspect of feet.
3. Cane to assist with balance; trial with cane in either hand to determine best use.
4. Orthosis donning, balance, and gait training with emphasis on safe performance and increased endurance.
5. Home evaluation to assess for extrinsic fall risk factors.
6. At work, request wheeled cart to reduce need to carry mail sacks.

Outcome

Wearing his AFOs, EA walks 50 yards in 3 minutes. He walks without a cane in the home and uses a cane outdoors. Fall hazards have been removed from inside the home. He has no new abrasions on his feet. He also uses a wheeled cart at work to eliminate the need for rest periods during work.

Please see the CD that accompanies this book for case studies describing the examination, evaluation, and interventions for a thoracolumbosacral orthosis for a child with scoliosis and for upper extremity orthoses for a patient with a cervical spinal cord injury.

CHAPTER SUMMARY

Orthoses are orthopedic appliances that apply force to support, align, prevent, or correct deformities of a body part or that improve the function of a movable part of the body. Comfortable orthotic fit is achieved through minimizing pressure by maximizing the area covered by the orthosis, as well as increasing the leverage through which the longitudinal segments of the orthosis apply force. Orthotic support involves force systems, usually a three-point system consisting of a principal force and two counterforces. The materials from which the orthosis is constructed influence its function. There are orthoses designed for the lower extremities, upper extremities, trunk, and cervical spine. Orthosis selection depends on the function of the orthosis (motion control or assistance or prevention of joint contractures), the affected joint(s), patient preference, and patient function while wearing the orthosis.

ADDITIONAL RESOURCES

Books

Aisens ML: *Orthotics in Neurologic Rehabilitation,* New York, 1992, Demos.

Bowker P, Condie DN, Bader DL, et al (eds): *Biomechanical Basis of Orthotic Management,* Oxford, 1993, Butterworth-Heinemann.

Coppard BM, Lohman H: *Introduction to Splinting,* St. Louis, 2001, Mosby.

Edelstein JE, Bruckner J: *Orthotics: A Comprehensive Clinical Approach,* Thorofare, NJ, 2002, Slack.

Edelstein JE, Bruckner J: *Orthotics: A Comprehensive Interactive Tutorial CD ROM,* Thorofare, NJ, 2003, Slack.

Goldberg B, Hsu JD (eds): *Atlas of Orthoses: Rehabilitation Principles and Application of Orthotic and Assistive Devices,* ed 3, St. Louis, 1996, Mosby.

Lusardi MM, Nielsen CC (eds): *Orthotics and Prosthetics in Rehabilitation,* Boston, 2000, Butterworth Heinemann.

McKee P, Morgan L: *Orthotics in Rehabilitation: Splinting and Hand and Body,* Philadelphia, 1998, FA Davis.

Redford JB, Basmajian JV, Trautman P (eds): *Orthotics: Clinical Practice and Rehabilitation Technology,* New York, 1995, Churchill Livingstone.

Seymour R: *Prosthetics and Orthotics: Lower Limb and Spinal,* Philadelphia, 2002, Lippincott Williams & Wilkins.

Shurr DG, Michael JW: *Prosthetics and Orthotics,* ed 2, Upper Saddle River, NJ, 2002, Prentice Hall.

Periodicals

O&P Almanac: www.aopanet.org/op_almanac/index.php

Journal of Rehabilitation Research and Development: www.vard.org/jour/jourindx.htm

O&P (Orthotics and Prosthetics) Business News: www.oandpbiznews.com

Web Sites

ABLEDATA: www.abledata.com

Adaptive Device Locator System: www.adaptworld.com

American Academy of Orthotists and Prosthetists: www.oandp.org

American Board for Certification in Orthotics & Prosthetics, Inc: www.abcop.org

American Orthotic and Prosthetic Association: www.aopanet.org

Association of Children's Prosthetic-Orthotic Clinics: www.acpoc.org

Family Center on Technology and Disability: www.fctd.info/

Interdisciplinary Society for the Advancement of Rehabilitative and Assistive Technology (RESNA): www.resna.org

Pedorthic Footwear Association: www.pedorthics.org

GLOSSARY

Bal (Balmoral): Shoe upper design in which the distal margin of the lace stay does not have a separation.

Band: Rigid horizontal component in a lower extremity or trunk orthosis.

Basic opponens orthosis: Hand orthosis that includes an opponens bar, thumb abduction bar, and dorsal and palmar hand bands; maintains the thumb in opposition.

Balanced forearm orthosis: Mass-produced orthosis that assists shoulder and elbow motion, usually mounted on a wheelchair.

Blucher: Shoe upper design in which the distal margins of the lace stays are separate.

Boston orthosis: Plastic thoracolumbosacral orthosis that controls scoliosis. Made of a mass-produced module custom fitted to the patient.

Brace: Orthosis.

Charleston bending brace: Plastic thoracolumbosacral orthosis that controls scoliosis; intended to be worn by a recumbent patient, usually at night.

Corset: Trunk orthosis that has no rigid horizontal components but may have rigid vertical components.

Counter: Posterior reinforcement of a shoe upper.

Drop ring lock: Metal rectangle that, when engaged, prevents movement of orthotic uprights.

Ductility: Property of a material that can be shaped by tension.

Elasticity: Ratio of stress to strain in a material, the ability of a material to recover its original dimensions.

External modification: FO consisting of material added to the exterior of the shoe, usually the sole.

Finger flexor WHO: Orthosis that applies forces to flex the metacarpophalangeal joints.

Floor reaction: Force exerted by the floor, affects the tendency of the ankle, knee, and hip to move in the direction of the floor reaction. Also known as ground reaction.

Halo vest: Rigid circular ring secured to the skull by four screws. Provides superior attachment points for posts in a cervicothoracic orthosis.

Hinged ankle-foot orthosis: AFO with trimlines anterior to the malleoli in which the leg portion of the orthosis is attached to the foot portion by a pair of hinges.

Insert: Removable foot orthosis that fits inside the shoe.

Internal modification: Foot orthosis that is attached to the interior of the shoe.

Knee cap: Leather pad fitted to a KAFO, usually has 4 straps, one buckled to the medial thigh upright, one buckled to the lateral thigh upright, one buckled to the medial leg upright, and one buckled to the lateral leg upright.

Metacarpophalangeal-extension stop: Band on a WHO that resists extension of the metacarpophalangeal joints.

Metatarsal bar: External foot orthosis located on the sole posterior to the metatarsal heads.

Metatarsal pad: Internal foot orthosis with apex located posterior to the metatarsal heads.

Milwaukee orthosis: Plastic cervicothoracolumbosacral orthosis that controls scoliosis. Pelvic girdle connected to neck ring by one anterior and two posterior uprights; control pads are attached to the uprights.

Minerva: Cervical orthosis that includes a forehead band.

Orthosis: Orthopedic appliance used to support, align, prevent, or correct deformities of a body part or to improve the function of movable parts of the body.

Orthotist: Health care practitioner who designs, fabricates, and fits patients with orthoses.

Pawl lock: Knee lock including a spring-loaded projection that fits into a notched disk.

Pedorthist: Health-care practitioner who designs, fabricates, and fits patients with foot orthoses and shoes.

Pelvic band: Rigid portion of a lower extremity or trunk orthosis that fits over the posterior portion of the lower trunk.

Plasticity: Property of a material that changes shape without cracking.

Posterior leaf spring AFO: Plastic or carbon fiber orthosis consisting of a foot plate to which is attached a posterior upright terminating in a calf band and anterior strap.

Pressure: Force applied per unit surface area.

Providence orthosis: Plastic thoracolumbosacral orthosis that controls scoliosis; intended to be worn by a recumbent patient, usually at night.

Shank piece: Shoe reinforcement located beneath the midfoot.

Shear: Stress occurring when force causes planes of a material to slide over each other.

Shell: Rigid plastic posterior portion of an AFO or KAFO.

Solid-ankle AFO: AFO with trimlines anterior to the malleoli.

Solid stirrup: One-piece steel U-shaped AFO attachment to a shoe.

Splint: Temporary orthosis.

Split stirrup: Three-piece steel AFO attachment to a shoe; center portion is riveted to the shoe; two L-shaped side portions fit into the center portion.

Stiffness: Amount of stress that must be applied to a material to cause strain.

Stop: Rigid restraint in an orthotic ankle joint that resists dorsiflexion.

Strain: Change in shape of a material as a result of stress.

Strength: Ability of a material to resist forces.

Stress: Force applied per unit of area.

Tension: Stress occurring when force pulls on a material.

Thermoplastic: Plastics that become malleable when heated and retain the new shape on cooling.

Thermosetting plastics: Plastics that retain their shape upon completion of the original chemical reaction.

Toe boxing: Anterior reinforcement of a shoe upper.

UCBL insert: Custom-made plastic 3/4 length foot orthosis that controls pes valgus.

Upper: Portion of a shoe located above the sole.

Upright: Rigid vertical component of a lower extremity or trunk orthosis.

Utensil holder: WHO that includes a pocket on the palm; utensils can be inserted into the pocket.

Valgus (varus) correction strap: Leather strap attached to the medial (lateral) portion of the shoe; strap buckles around the lateral (medial) upright of the AFO.

Wilmington orthosis: Plastic thoracolumbosacral orthosis that controls scoliosis.

References

1. Jannink MJ, Ijzerman MJ, Groothuis-Oudshoorn K, et al: Use of orthopedic shoes in patients with degenerative disorders of the foot, *Arch Phys Med Rehabil* 86.687-692, 2005.
2. Defrin R, Ben Benyamin S, Aldubi RD, et al: Conservative correction of leg-length discrepancies of 10 mm or less for the relief of chronic low back pain, *Arch Phys Med Rehabil* 86:2075-2080, 2005.
3. Frykberg RG, Bailey LF, Matz A, et al: Off-loading properties of a rocker insole, *J Am Podiatr Med Assoc* 92:48-53, 2002.
4. Hsi WL, Chai HM, Lai JS: Evaluation of rocker sole by pressure-time curves in insensate forefoot during gait, *Am J Phys Med Rehabil* 83:500-506, 2004.
5. Wu WL, Rosenbaum D, Su FC: The effects of rocker sole and SACH heel on kinematics in gait, *Med Eng Phys* 26:639-646, 2004.
6. Rome K, Brown CL: Randomized clinical trial into the impact of rigid foot orthoses on balance parameters in excessively pronated feet, *Clin Rehabil* 18:624-630, 2004.
7. Branthwaite HR, Payton CJ, Chockalingam N: The effect of simple insoles on three-dimensional foot motion during normal walking, *Clin Biomech* 19:972-977, 2004.
8. Mohamed O, Cerny K, Rojek L, et al: The effects of Plastazote and Aliplast/Plastazote orthoses on plantar pressures in elderly persons with diabetic neuropathy, *J Prosthet Orthot* 16:55-63, 2004.
9. Seligman DA, Dawson DR: Customized heel pads and soft orthotics to treat heel pain and plantar fasciitis, *Arch Phys Med Rehabil* 84:1564-1567, 2003.
10. Esterman A, Pilotto L: Foot shape and its effect on functioning in Royal Australian Air Force recruits. Part 2: Pilot, randomized, controlled trial of orthotics in recruits with flat feet, *Mil Med* 170:629-633, 2005.
11. Nester CJ, van der Linden ML, Bowker P: Effect of foot orthoses on the kinematics and kinetics of normal walking gait, *Gait Posture* 17:180-187, 2003.

12. Nawoczenski DA, Ludewig PM: The effect of forefoot and arch posting orthotic designs on first metatarsophalangeal joint kinematics during gait, *JOSPT* 34:317-327, 2004.

13. Leung AK, Mak AF, Evans JH: Biomechanical gait evaluation of the immediate effect of orthotic treatment of flexible flat foot, *Prosthet Orthot Int* 22:25-34, 1998.

14. Kulig K, Burnfield JM, Reischl S, et al: Effect of foot orthoses on tibialis posterior activation in persons with pes planus, *Med Sci Sports Exerc* 37:24-29, 2005.

15. Tomaro J, Burdett RG: The effects of foot orthotics on the EMG activity of selected leg muscles during gait, *JOSPT* 18:532-536, 1993.

16. Bird AR, Bendrups AP, Payne CB: The effect of foot wedging on electromyographic activity in the erector spinae and gluteus medius muscles during walking, *Gait Posture* 18:81-91, 2003.

17. Yoshimura I, Naito M, Hara M, et al: The effect of wedged insoles on the lateral thrust of anterior cruciate ligament-insufficiency knees, *Am J Sports Med* 31:909-1002, 2003.

18. Gross MT, Foxworth JL: The role of foot orthoses as an intervention for patellofemoral pain, *JOSPT* 33:661-670, 2003.

19. Saxena A, Haddad J: The effect of foot orthoses on patellofemoral pain syndrome, *J Am Podiatr Med Assoc* 93:264-271, 2003.

20. Landorf KB, Keenan AM, Herbert RD: Effectiveness of different types of foot orthoses for the treatment of plantar fasciitis, *J Am Podiatr Med Assoc* 94:542-549, 2004.

21. Arendse RE: A biomechanical basis for the prescription of orthoses in the treatment of common running injuries, *Med Hypotheses* 62:119-120, 2004.

22. Stackhouse CL, Davis IM, Hamill J: Orthotic intervention in forefoot and rearfoot strike running patterns, *Clin Biomech* 19:64-70, 2004.

23. Bandettini MP, Innocenti G, Contini M, et al: Postural control in order to prevent chronic locomotion injuries in top level athletes. *Ital J Anat Embryol* 108:189-194, 2003.

24. Nigg BM, Stergiou P, Cole G, et al: Effect of shoe inserts on kinematics, center of pressure, and leg joint moments during running, *Med Sci Sports Exerc* 35:314-319, 2003.

25. Stacoff A, Reinschmidt C, Nigg BM, et al: Effects of foot orthoses on skeletal motion during running, *Clin Biomech* 15:54-64, 2000.

26. Krebs D, Edelstein J, Fishman S: Comparison of plastic/metal and leather/metal knee-ankle-foot orthoses, *Am J Phys Med Rehabil* 67:175-185, 1988.

27. Lehmann JF: Push-off and propulsion of the body in normal and abnormal gait: correction by ankle-foot orthoses, *Clin Orthop* 288:97-108, 1993.

28. de Wit DC, Burke JH, Nijlant JM, et al: The effect of an ankle-foot orthosis on walking ability in chronic stroke patients: A randomized controlled trial, *Clin Rehabil* 18:550-557, 2004.

29. Wang RY, Yen L, Lee CC, et al: Effects of an ankle-foot orthosis on balance performance in patients with hemiparesis of different durations, *Clin Rehabil* 19:37-44, 2005.

30. Danielsson A, Sunnerhagen KS: Energy expenditure in stroke subjects walking with a carbon composite ankle foot orthosis, *J Rehabil Med* 36:165-168, 2004.

31. Tyson SF, Thornton HA: The effect of a hinged ankle foot orthosis on hemiplegic gait: Objective measures and users' opinions, *Clin Rehabil* 15:53-58, 2001.

32. Miyazaki S, Yamamoto S, Kubota T: Effect of ankle-foot orthosis on active ankle moment in patients with hemiparesis, *Med Biol Eng Comput* 35:381-385, 1997.

33. Hesse S, Werner C, Matthias K, et al: Non-velocity related effects of a rigid double-stopped ankle-foot orthosis on gait and lower limb muscle activity of hemiparetic subjects with an equinovarus deformity, *Stroke* 30:1855-1861, 1999.

34. Gok H, Kucukdeveci A, Altinkaynak H, et al: Effects of ankle-foot orthoses on hemiparetic gait, *Clin Rehabil* 17:137-139, 2003.

35. Teasell RW, McRae MP, Foley N, et al: Physical and functional correlations of ankle-foot orthosis use in the rehabilitation of stroke patients, *Arch Phys Med Rehabil* 82:1047-1049, 2001.

36. Ounpuu S, Bell KH, Davis RB, et al: An evaluation of the posterior leaf spring orthosis using joint kinematics and kinetics, *J Pediatr Orthop* 16:378-384, 1996.

37. Smiley SJ, Jacobsen FS, Mielke C, et al: A comparison of the effects of solid, articulated, and posterior leaf spring ankle-foot orthoses and shoes alone on gait and energy expenditure in children with spastic diplegic cerebral palsy, *Orthopaedics* 25:411-415, 2002.

38. Carlson WE, Vaughan CL, Damiano DL, et al: Orthotic management of gait in spastic diplegia, *Am J Phys Med Rehabil* 76:219-225, 1997.

39. Lam WK, Leong JCY, Li YH, et al: Biomechanical and electromyographic evaluation of ankle foot orthosis and dynamic ankle foot orthosis in spastic cerebral palsy, *Gait Posture* 22:189-197, 2005.

40. Radtka SA, Skinner SR, Johanson ME: A comparison of gait with solid and hinged ankle-foot orthoses in children with spastic diplegic cerebral palsy, *Gait Posture* 21:303-310, 2001.

41. Romkes J, Brunner R: Comparison of a dynamic and a hinged ankle-foot orthosis by gait analysis in patients with hemiplegic cerebral palsy, *Gait Posture* 15:18-24, 2002.

42. Park ES, Park CI, Chang HJ, et al: The effect of hinged ankle-foot orthoses on sit-to-stand transfer in children with spastic cerebral palsy, *Arch Phys Med Rehabil* 85:2053-2057, 2004.

43. Sienko Thomas S, Buckon CE, Jakobson-Huston S, et al: Stair locomotion in children with spastic hemiplegia: The impact of three different AFO configurations, *Gait Posture* 16:180-187, 2002.

44. Buckon CE, Thomas SS, Jakobson-Huston S, et al: Comparison of three ankle-foot orthosis configurations for children with spastic diplegia, *Dev Med Child Neurol* 46:590-598, 2004.

45. Duffy CM, Graham HK, Cosgrove AP: The influence of ankle-foot orthoses on gait and energy expenditure in spina bifida, *J Pediatr Orthop* 20:356-361, 2000.

46. Thomson JD, Ounpuu S, Davis RB, et al: The effect of ankle-foot orthoses on the ankle and knee in persons with myelomeningocele: An evaluation using three-dimensional gait analysis, *J Pediatr Orthop* 19: 27-33, 1999.

47. Burdett RG, Hassell G: Effects of three types of ankle-foot orthoses on the gait and bicycling of a patient with Charcot-Marie-Tooth disease, *J Prosthet Orthot* 16:25-30, 2004.

48. Steinfeldt F, Seifert W, Gunther KP: Modern carbon fiber orthoses in the management of polio patients: A critical evaluation of the functional aspects, *Z Orthop Ihre Grenzgeb* 141:357-361, 2003.

49. Hebert JS, Liggins AB: Gait evaluation of an automatic stance-control knee orthosis in a patient with postpoliomyelitis, *Arch Phys Med Rehabil* 86:1676-1680, 2005.

50. McMillan AG, Kendrick K, Michael JW, et al: Preliminary evidence for effectiveness of a stance control orthosis, *J Prosthet Orthot* 16:6-13, 2004.

51. Suga T, Kameyama O, Ogawa R, et al: Newly designed computer controlled knee-ankle-foot orthosis (Intelligent Orthosis), *Prosthet Orthot Int* 22:230-239, 1998.

52. Bakker JP, de Groot IJ, Beckerman H, et al: The effects of knee-ankle-foot orthoses in the treatment of Duchenne muscular dystrophy: Review of the literature, *Clin Rehabil* 14:343-359, 2000.

53. Gonzalez E, Edelstein J: Energy expenditure in ambulation. In Gonzalez E, Myers S, Edelstein JE, et al (eds): *Downey and Darling's Physiological Basis of Rehabilitation Medicine*, ed 3, Boston, 2001, Butterworth-Heinemann.

54. Kawashima N, Sone Y, Nakazawa K, et al: Energy expenditure during walking with weight-bearing control (WBC) orthosis in thoracic level of paraplegic patients, *Spinal Cord* 41:506-510, 2003.

55. Beillot J, Carre F, Le Claire G, et al: Energy consumption of paraplegic locomotion using reciprocating gait orthosis, *Eur J Appl Physiol Occup Physiol* 73:376-381, 1996.

56. Spadone R, Merati G, Bertocchi E, et al: Energy consumption of locomotion with orthosis versus Parastep-assisted gait: A single case study, *Spinal Cord* 41:97-104, 2003.

57. Merati G, Sarchi P, Ferrarin M, et al: Paraplegic adaptation to assisted-walking: Energy expenditure during wheelchair versus orthosis use, *Spinal Cord* 38:37-44, 2000.

58. Roussos N, Patrick JH, Hodnett C, et al: A long-term review of severely disabled spina bifida patients using a reciprocal walking system, *Disabil Rehabil* 23:239-244, 2001.

59. Puckree T, Amy Lauten V, Moodley S, et al: Thoracolumbar corsets alter breathing pattern in normal individuals, *Int J Rehabil Res* 28:81-85, 2005.

60. Maloney FP: Pulmonary function in quadriplegia: Effects of a corset, *Arch Phys Med Rehabil* 60:261-265, 1979.

61. Vogt L, Pfeifer K, Portscher M, et al: Lumbar corsets: Their effect on three-dimensional kinematics of the pelvis, *J Rehabil Res Dev* 37:495-499, 2000.

62. Cholewicki J, Ivancic PC, Radebold A: Can increased intra-abdominal pressure in humans be decoupled from trunk muscle co-contraction during steady state isometric exertions? *Eur J Appl Physiol* 87:127-133, 2002.

63. Norton PL, Brown T: The immobilizing efficiency of back braces: Their effect on the posture and motion of the lumbosacral spine, *J Bone Joint Surg Am* 39:111-139, 1957.

64. White AA, Panjabi MM: *Clinical Biomechanics of the Spine*, Philadelphia, 1978, JB Lippincott.

65. Waters RL, Morris JM: Effects of spinal supports on the electrical activity of the muscles of the trunk, *J Bone Joint Surg Am* 52: 51-60, 1970.

66. Calmels P, Fayolle-Minon I: An update on orthotic devices 1996; for the lumbar spine based on a review of the literature, *Rev Rheum Engl Ed* 63:285-291, 1996.

67. Lahad A, Malter AD, Berg AO, et al: The effectiveness of four interventions for the prevention of low back pain, *JAMA* 272:1286-1291, 1994.

68. Van Leeuwen PJ, Bos RP, Derksen JC, et al: Assessment of spinal movement reduction by thoraco-lumbar-sacral orthoses, *J Rehabil Res Dev* 37:35-403, 2000.

69. Jellema P, van Tulder MW, van Poppel MN, et al: Lumbar supports for prevention and treatment of low back pain: A systematic review within

the framework of the Cochrane Back Review Group, *Spine* 26:377-386, 2001.

70. Cholewicki J: The effects of lumbosacral orthoses on spine stability: What changes in EMG can be expected? *J Orthop Res* 22:1150-1155, 2004.

71. Pfeifer M, Begerow B, Minne HW: Effects of a new spinal orthosis on posture, trunk strength, and quality of life in women with postmenopausal osteoporosis: A randomized trial, *Am J Phys Med Rehabil* 83:177-186, 2004.

72. Gennis P, Miller L, Gallagher EJ, et al: The effect of soft cervical collars on persistent neck pain in patients with whiplash injury, *Acad Emerg Med* 3:568-573, 1996.

73. Crawford JR, Khan RJ, Varley GW: Early management and outcome following soft tissue injuries of the neck: A randomised controlled trial, *Injury* 35:891-895, 2004.

74. Cosan TE, Tel E, Arslantas A, et al: Indications of Philadelphia collar in the treatment of upper cervical injuries, *Eur J Emerg Med* 8:33-37, 2001.

75. Barry CJ, Smith D, Lennarson P, et al: The effect of wearing a restrict neck brace on driver performance, *Neurosurgery* 53:98-101, 2003.

76. Gavin TM, Carandang G, Havey R, et al: Biomechanical analysis of cervical orthoses in flexion and extension: A comparison of cervical collars and cervical thoracic orthoses, *J Rehabil Res Dev* 40:527-537, 2003.

77. Sandler AJ, Dvorak J, Humke T, et al: The effectiveness of several cervical orthoses: An in vivo comparison of the mechanical stability provided by several widely used models, *Spine* 21:1624-1629, 1996.

78. Sharpe KP, Rao S, Ziogas A: Evaluation of the effectiveness of the Minerva cervicothoracic orthosis, *Spine* 20:1475-1479, 1995.

79. Benzel EC, Larson SJ, Kerk JJ, et al: The thermoplastic Minerva body jacket: A clinical comparison with other cervical spine splinting techniques, *J Spinal Disord* 5:311-319, 1992.

80. Richter D, Latta LL, Milne EL, et al: The stabilizing effects of different orthoses in the intact and unstable upper cervical spine: A cadaver study, *J Trauma* 50:848-854, 2001.

81. Vieweg U, Schultheiss R: A review of halo vest treatment of upper cervical spine injuries, *Arch Orthop Trauma Surg* 121:50-55, 2001.

82. Bullmann V, Halm HF, Lerner T, et al: Prospective evaluation of braces as treatment in idiopathic scoliosis, *Z Orthop Ihre Grenzgeb* 142:403-409, 2004.

83. Danielsson AJ, Nachemson AL: Radiologic findings and curve progression 22 years after treatment for adolescent idiopathic scoliosis: Comparison of brace and surgical treatment with matching control group of straight individuals, *Spine* 26:516-525, 2001.

84. Rowe DE, Bernstein SM, Riddick MF, et al: A meta-analysis of the efficacy of nonoperative treatments for idiopathic scoliosis, *J Bone Joint Surg Am* 79:664-674, 1997.

85. Wong MS, Mak AF, Luk KD, et al: Effectiveness and biomechanics of spinal orthoses in the treatment of adolescent idiopathic scoliosis (AIS), *Prosthet Orthot Int* 24:148-162, 2000.

86. O'Neill PJ, Karol LA, Shindle MK, et al: Decreased orthotic effectiveness in overweight patients with adolescent idiopathic scoliosis, *J Bone Joint Surg Am* 87:1069-1074, 2005.

87. Vijvermans V, Fabry G, Nijs J: Factors determining the final outcome of treatment of idiopathic scoliosis with the Boston brace: A longitudinal study, *J Pediatr Orthop* 13:143-149, 2004.

88. Katz DE, Durrani AA: Factors that influence outcome in bracing large curves in patients with adolescent idiopathic scoliosis, *Spine* 26:2354-2361, 2001.

89. Lou E, Raso JV, Hill DL, et al: Correlation between quantity and quality of orthosis wear and treatment outcomes in adolescent idiopathic scoliosis, *Prosthet Orthot Int* 28:49-54, 2004.

90. Mac-Thiong JM, Petit Y, Aubin CE, et al: Biomechanical evaluation of the Boston brace system for the treatment of adolescent idiopathic scoliosis: Relationship between strap tension and brace interface forces, *Spine* 29:26-32, 2004.

91. Gabos PG, Bojescul JA, Bowen JR, et al: Long-term follow-up of female patients with idiopathic scoliosis treated with the Wilmington orthosis, *J Bone Joint Surg Am* 86:1891-1899, 2004.

92. Katz DE, Richards BS, Browne RH, et al: A comparison between the Boston brace and the Charleston bending brace in adolescent idiopathic scoliosis, *Spine* 22:1302-1312, 1997.

93. Howard A, Wright JG, Hedden D: A comparative study of TLSO, Charleston, and Milwaukee braces for idiopathic scoliosis, *Spine* 23:2404-2411, 1998.

94. Gepstein R, Leitner Y, Zohar E, et al: Effectiveness of the Charleston bending brace in the treatment of single-curve idiopathic scoliosis, *J Pediatr Orthop* 22:84-87, 2002.

95. D'Amato CR, Griggs S, McCoy B: Nighttime bracing with the Providence brace in adolescent girls with idiopathic scoliosis, *Spine* 26:2006-2012, 2001.

96. van Rhijn LW, Varaart BE, Plasmans CM: Application of a lumbar brace for thoracic and double thoracic lumbar scoliosis: A comparative study, *J Pediatr Orthop B* 12:178-182, 2003.

97. Gerritsen AA, Korthals-de Bos IB, Laboyrie PM, et al: Splinting for carpal tunnel syndrome: Prognostic indicators of success, *J Neurol Neurosurg Psychiatry* 74:1342-1344, 2003.

98. Werner RA, Franzblau A, Gell N: Randomized controlled trial of nocturnal splinting for active workers with symptoms of carpal tunnel syndrome, *Arch Phys Med Rehabil* 86:1-7, 2005.

99. Haskett S, Backman C, Porter B, et al: A crossover trial of custom-made and commercially available wrist splints in adults with inflammatory arthritis, *Arthritis Rheum* 51:792-799, 2004.

100. Walker WC, Metzler M, Cifu DX, et al: Neutral wrist splinting in carpal tunnel syndrome: a comparison of night-one versus full-time wear instructions, *Arch Phys Med Rehabil* 81:424-429, 2000.

101. Lannin NA, Herbert RD: Is hand splinting effective for adults following stroke? A systematic review and methodologic critique of published research, *Clin Rehabil* 17:807-816, 2003.

102. Li-Tsang CW, Hung LK, Mak AF: The effect of corrective splinting on flexion contracture of rheumatoid fingers, *J Hand Ther* 15:185-191, 2002.

103. Glasgow C, Wilton J: Tooth: Optimal daily total end range time for contracture: Resolution in hand splinting, *J Hand Ther* 16:207-218, 2003.

104. Hijmans JM, Postema K, Geertzen JHB: Elbow orthoses: A review of literature, *Prosthet Orthot Int* 28:263-272, 2004.

105. Wuori JL, Overend TJ, Kramer JF, et al: Strength and pain measures associated with lateral epicondylitis bracing, *Arch Phys Med Rehabil* 79:832-837, 1998.

106. Borkholder CD, Hill VA, Fess EE: The efficacy of splinting for lateral epicondylitis: A systematic review, *J Hand Ther* 17:181-199, 2004.

107. Gelinas JJ, Faber KJ, Patterson SD, et al: The effectiveness of turnbuckle splinting for elbow contractures, *J Bone Joint Surg Br* 82:74-78, 2000.

108. Spaulding SJ: Biomechanical analysis of four supports for the subluxed hemiparetic shoulder, *Can J Occup Ther* 66:169-175, 1999.

109. Zorowitz RD, Idank D, Ikai T, et al: Shoulder subluxation after stroke: a comparison of four supports, *Arch Phys Med Rehabil* 76:763-771, 1995.

110. Foongchomcheay A, Ada L, Canning C: Use of devices to prevent subluxation of the shoulder after stroke, *Physiother Res Int* 10:134-145, 2005.

111. Reuss BL, Harding WB, Nowicki KD: Managing anterior shoulder instability with bracing: An expanded update, *Orthopedics* 27:614-618, 2004.

Chapter 35

Environmental Assessment: Home, Community, and Work

Martha Paterson, Tom Mets

OBJECTIVES

After reading this chapter, the reader will be able to:
1. Examine environmental barriers in a patient's home, the community, and the work place.
2. Identify risks and abatements to maximize safety and function.
3. Examine reach barriers and provide basic solutions to reducing such barriers.
4. Reduce environmental barriers and make recommendations for cost-effective environmental modifications.

Environmental barriers are the physical impediments that keep people from functioning optimally in their surroundings.[1] Environmental barriers may include safety hazards, difficult access, and poor home or office design. This chapter provides a basic template for examining patients and their environments and presents interventions to reduce environmental barriers that can be customized for the patient in home, community, and *work environments*. This chapter particularly focuses on examination, evaluation, and interventions for patients needing to use an *assistive device* or a wheelchair for mobility.

EXAMINATION

A comprehensive analysis of environmental barriers begins with a thorough examination of the patient as well as his or her home, community, and work place. The goal of this analysis is to maximize functional independence by eliminating barriers and creating a plan for interventions that support preferred movement patterns and optimal *function*.

PATIENT HISTORY

The first part of the examination is the patient history, which should include the following:

1. The patient's prior level of function in self-care, home management, community involvement, and essential job tasks.
2. Resources and support systems, including where and with whom the patient lives.
3. Transportation, specifying type, frequency, and destination (e.g., doctor's visits, work, restaurants, sporting events, or shopping).
4. The patient's expected occupational roles and tasks.
5. How the patient and their family are coping with the patient's condition at this time.
6. The patient's current functional limitations.
7. Whether the patient's limitations are expected to be permanent or temporary and if they are likely to progress?
8. The assistive devices needed for this person to function in their environments.
9. The patient's goals for home, work, and leisure.

This information can be obtained by a combination of interviewing the patient and family members, having them complete questionnaires, and completing a chart review. Detailed information about the patient's work history and available resources at the worksite may also be obtained from the company representative responsible for implementing change on the worker's behalf. This representative may be able to provide information on available resources for accommodations and on how these resources will be integrated into the overall plan. An accurate and comprehensive patient history is essential to establishing realistic and meaningful goals.

SYSTEMS REVIEW

The systems review is used to target areas requiring further examination and to define areas that may cause complications or indicate a need for precautions during the examination and intervention processes. See Chapter 1 for details of the systems review.

TESTS AND MEASURES

Although tests and measures related to environmental barriers generally focus on the environment, the examination should also include relevant components related to the patient.

The therapist gathers information about environmental barriers using one or more of these test and measure techniques: Observation, measurement of patient and environmental features, patient report, functional performance testing, and/or caregiver interview. Videotape and photographs can sometimes substitute for direct observation. Photographs document the environmental barrier and can facilitate communication between people contributing to the design and implementation of interventions.

The tests and measures component of the examination of a patient's environment should be carried out systematically. When planning to examine a patient in a community setting, prepare a list of locations to be examined and have an accessible vehicle with driver available. It is also important to have the appropriate equipment. A digital camera, tape measure, and worksheets are essential for an on-site examination. A transfer bench, stethoscope, and blood pressure cuff may also be helpful. To prepare for an examination of the patient's work place, a profile of work expectations should be obtained from the patient or from the manager or human resources representative at the work place. A job description provided by the patient's employer may also be helpful, but this generally does not provide much information about the specific physical demands of a job.

Musculoskeletal

Posture. The postural examination should include the patient's posture while performing functional tasks in the home, community, and work place. Ideally, prolonged postures should keep all joints in midrange, also known as neutral position (see Chapter 4). This maximizes muscle leverage, efficiency, and performance while minimizing strain on soft tissues and joints. Posture should generally be observed with the patient standing, sitting in a chair, and manipulating objects as needed. One should check if the patient maintains neutral postures, leans to one side, leans on a bony prominence, or props himself or herself up with items in the environment. Also, check if any environmental barriers, such as low hanging lights, a high or low seat, or a high or low work surface, compromise the patient's ability to maintain neutral positioning.

Anthropometric Characteristics. Average anthropometric measurements, including height, reach depth, hip, shoulder, and hand width, are often used to design furniture, countertops, appliances, chairs, and vehicles.[2] Most products are designed to work well for people within the 5th to 95th percentile of the general population of nondisabled individuals (Table 35-1). For example, most products are designed to accommodate a 34-cm (14-inch) range in

TABLE 35-1	Stature and Functional Reach of American Population				
	Stature in Inches/Percentile				
	1st	**5th**	**50th**	**95th**	**99th**
Men	63.1	64.8	69.1	73.5	75.2
Women	58.4	60.2	64.1	68.4	70.1
	Functional Reach in Inches/Percentile				
	1st	**5th**	**50th**	**95th**	**99th**
Men	28.4	29.1	31.5	34.1	35.3
Women	25.9	26.7	28.9	31.4	32.4

Data from FAA Human Factors Design Guide: http://hf.tc.faa.gov/hfds/.

height. Therapists should measure patients' height, reach depth, hip, shoulder, and hand width to identify individuals who do not fit within the typical range.[3] The presence of a disability may also alter an individual's anthropometric characteristics, necessitating change of the environment for successful integration of function.

Range of Motion. Functional range of motion (ROM) rather than individual joint motion is generally most relevant to the examination of environmental barriers. The multidirectional reach test (MDRT), an expanded version of the functional reach test (FRT), is an effective test of functional ROM.[4] The FRT measures the distance an individual is willing or able to lean in a forward direction, and the MDRT assesses reach distance in forward, backward, and lateral directions.

Another measure of functional ROM is a map of the patient's reach zones (Fig. 35-1). Reach zones look like semicircles extending in front of and to the side of the patient. These zones can be classified as primary, secondary, or tertiary. Objects are then placed in the zones according to frequency of use. Frequently used objects should be placed in the primary zone, closest to the body. In this zone the elbows can be kept at the side of the body and the hands move from side to side like windshield wipers to reach objects. Objects that are used four to ten times an hour should be placed in the secondary zone, where the hands can reach without the elbow moving further forward than the anterior portion of the rib cage. Occasionally used objects should be placed in the tertiary zone, where they can still be reached without exceeding full elbow extension or 90 degrees of shoulder flexion. Setting up activities according to the patient's reach zones reduces strain on joints and the physiological cost of movement, optimizes muscle performance, and improves movement speed and accuracy.[5]

Muscle Performance. Muscle power, strength, and endurance will influence a patient's ability to achieve leverage and operate or handle tools and environmental controls. *Functional muscle testing,* such as whether the individual has the strength to handle tools, operate levers, and lift, carry, push, and pull objects as required by their expected roles, can be more useful than examination of strength by measurement of individual muscle performance with manual muscle tests or other approaches. When measuring functional strength, one should note if

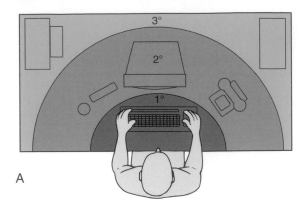

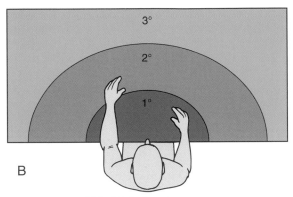

FIG. 35-1 Reach zones.

there are movement variations or muscle substitutions that may increase the risk of injury. Handling tools requires dexterity, power, and control. The patient's method of handling tools should be safe and when work-related, adhere to company guidelines.

Joint Integrity and Mobility. Compromised joint integrity and mobility affects an individual's ability to access the environment freely and safely. Examination of mobility limitations assists in identifying positions and forces that block freedom of movement and trigger discomfort or alter muscle performance.

Neuromuscular

Arousal, Attention, and Cognition. Arousal, attention, and cognition should be examined because these can impact task completion and safety. Many people with cognitive impairments perform better if the activity is familiar to them and if the objects are within their visual field. One should also consider the effects of medication and time of day on a patient's arousal, attention, and cognition when critical tasks are performed.

Pain. Environmental barriers are often first noticed when a person develops pain as a result of assuming awkward postures, working at surfaces that are too high or too low, or moving objects that are too heavy. Close attention should be paid to tasks that require whole body coordination, such as getting in and out of a car, other vehicles, equipment, or a bathtub; turning knobs or levers to open doors or control equipment; and transporting objects from one place to another.

Sensation. Sensation should be examined because sensory impairments can increase the risk of thermal and mechanical injury, including burns, cuts, and bruises. See Chapter 18 for detailed descriptions of tests and measures that can be used to examine sensation.

Cardiovascular. Particular attention should be paid to endurance and response to exertion in all patients with cardiovascular and pulmonary problems. Note the patient's response to climbing a flight of stairs, how many times the patient needs to sit or lean against a wall, the speed of ascending and descending, and requests for breaks. Since patients may have endurance limitations, one should be sure to offer and plan for possible breaks during the environmental examination. A variety of tools for examining cardiovascular responses to activity, including heart rate response and rate of perceived exertion, are described in Chapter 23.

Function

Gait, Locomotion, and Balance. The patient's movement patterns and balance should be observed throughout the environmental assessment, including how the patient moves in and out of a vehicle or other equipment, climbs steps, traverses uneven surfaces, anticipates and maneuvers trip hazards, stands and sits while talking, and balances when sitting and standing, as well as how fatigue impacts these motions. Balance recovery strategies, including which objects are used for stabilization (wall, door frame, towel bar), as well as how much force is applied to a contact point to aid recovery, should also be noted. Throughout the examination, note how the patient adjusts to moving between surfaces (weight shift, lean, foot drag) and the stability of the landing.

Self-Care and Home Management. The patient should perform a variety of functional tasks (Box 35-1) in the appropriate setting for a complete examination of self-care and home management.

Assistive, Adaptive, Orthotic, Protective, and Prosthetic Devices. Ask the patient to use their recommended ambulatory assistive devices, wear prescribed orthoses, and any other required protective or supportive device during the examination. List all devices used and identify any that may risk the patient's safety.[6] It is important for the patient to understand what equipment is recommended as well as where and how it will be used in the environment that is being examined. Ask the patient: "Are you comfortable in handling the equipment?" and "Do you feel more or less stable or safe when using the device?" and "Does the device pose potential safety risks, such as making it difficult to feel or grip objects or achieve necessary positions, when using certain equipment or performing certain tasks?"

Ergonomics and Body Mechanics. Examination of *ergonomics* and body mechanics should include examination of the efficiency of task performance, the impact of environmental variables, and how the task challenges maintenance of neutral postures. Certain anthropometric measures may also be included in this part of the examination, particularly the distance from the floor to eye level, shoulder height, waist height, and elbow height in sitting and standing, and floor to knee height in sitting.

BOX 35-1	Functional Tasks to Be Included in the Examination

Self-Care at Home
Shower transfers
Toilet transfers
Hygiene at the sink, toilet and shower
Access to medicine and contents of medicine cabinet
Access in bedroom
Light switch control
Bed transfers
Access clothing

Home Management
Mobility throughout home
Carrying, lifting, pushing, and pulling
Refrigerator access
Oven operation
Telephone operation
Alarm clock operation
Response to door bell
Chair and sofa transfers
Appliance and electronics operation (heaters, lamps, microwave, stovetop, dishwasher)
Send and retrieve mail
Change bed linens and make bed
Access pots, pans, dishes, glasses, and utensils

Work
Mobility through work environment
Operate job tools
Perform job functions
Operate communication systems

Community
Negotiate ramps, curbs, uneven ground, and stairways
Car transfers and fasten seat belt
Street crossing: Time and safely
Mobility with packages
Management of money
Public transportation: Plan route, transfers, payment

Determine if the patient wears glasses, and if so, for what types of tasks.

The efficiency of task performance is influenced by the demands of the task and the abilities and dimensions of the patient, as well as the way a patient chooses to perform the task.[7] The demands of the task may be determined by asking the patient about what they do but is often best accomplished by watching them perform tasks in the setting in which they are usually performed, at home, in the community or at work. Jobs may be categorized from sedentary to very heavy according their physical demands (Table 35-2). Inefficiencies at work have been found to add as much as 2% to 22% to task performance times and increase the risk for injury.[8,9]

Environmental Barriers. Environmental barriers may be encountered in and around the home, community, or work place. A systematic approach to examining these barriers is recommended. Examination should start with the exterior access routes and then proceed to the interior. The interior examination should include examination of the interior access routes, doors, and evaluation of whether there is sufficient space to turn in the rooms. If the interior has more than one story, or if the entry is not at ground level, one should examine stairs and ramps and their railings, elevators, and escalators if present. After a general examination of environmental accessibility, one should also examine task specific barriers and unique barriers that may be encountered in specific rooms.

Exterior Barriers

Exterior Access Routes. When examining exterior access routes, the therapist should consider the mode of transportation typically used to reach the destination, whether the patient can use this mode of transportation, how often they go to the destination, and whether there is parking near an accessible building entrance. Identify problems the patient may have with parking, lighting in the parking area, and safely traveling to the entrance. Can the patient identify signage indicating handicap accessibility? Do not assume that the predetermined routes as indicated by posted signs will be appropriate for the patient. Handicap signs are posted to indicate accessibility, an elevator, or a handicap bathroom but not necessarily an accessible route

TABLE 35-2	Lifting and Energy Consumption Associated with Different Levels of Occupational Physical Demands			
Physical Demand Level	Occasional (0%-33% of Workday) Lifting Weight	Frequent (34%-66% of Workday) Lifting Weight	Constant (67%-100% of Workday) Lifting Weight	Typical Energy Requirement (METs)
Sedentary	10 lb	Negligible	Negligible	1.5-2.1
Light	20 lb	10 lb and/or walk/ stand/push/pull of arm/leg controls	Negligible and/or push/pull of arm/leg controls while seated	2.2-3.5
Medium	20-50 lb	10-25 lb	10 lb	3.6-6.3
Heavy	50-100 lb	25-50 lb	10-20 lb	6.4-7.5
Very heavy	>100 lb	>50 lb	>20 lb	>7.5

From Dictionary of Occupational Titles: www.occupationalinfo.org/front_148.html.
METs, Metabolic equivalents: 1 MET = energy consumption at rest.

for your patient's specific needs. Note the path surface (cement, asphalt, grass, or gravel), width, slope (gentle, moderate, or steep), condition (e.g., level, cracked, or uneven), and the adequacy of path lighting.[10] Can the patient manage curbs, cross the street in a timely manner, open doors, navigate electronic doors, and comply with security measures?

Stairs. Stairs can be unavoidable obstacles to entering and moving through a building. Note the number of steps, dimensions (i.e., step height, width, and depth), general stair condition, and the presence or absence of handrails. Steps should have a maximum height of 7 inches and depth of at least 11 inches and should not have tread lip projections.[11] Tread and risings should be consistent in size and not have tripping surfaces (e.g., projecting screws or nails). Note if the top and bottom stairs are different sizes. If so, they should be marked to avoid a misstep.

Ramps. If the patient cannot manage stairs, measure the space available for a ramp or stair lift. If an elevator is indicated, a licensed elevator technician should measure the space unless the therapist has had specific training in this area. If the patient currently has a ramped home entrance, ensure that they can safely ascend and descend it and that it is soundly built. Measure the height, width, and length of the ramp. For safety and ease of use, ramps should ideally have an incline of at least 1-foot length for each inch of rise (slope of 1:12). Thus a 6-inch step leading into the home/building would require a 6-foot ramp. Building codes allow steeper inclines where such slopes are necessary because of space limitations or if the step height is less than 3 inches, but a slope steeper than 1:8 is prohibited. Note if there are handrails and edge protection and if there is a sufficient landing at the top and bottom of the ramp. Can the patient propel the wheelchair or ambulate up and down the ramp?

Handrails. Handrails within the house may be helpful for wheelchair users, for those who walk with difficulty, and for those with impaired balance. Handrails are particularly important on stairs and ramps. Edge protection is also essential on ramps used by wheelchair users. If there are no handrails on stairs or ramps, check if there is enough space to install them. Note where rails are or should be (right, left, or both sides), the rail height, the security of the attachment, and the condition of the rails (are they free of splinters, blemishes, slippery when wet, etc?) According to the American Association of Retired Persons (AARP), one out of three older adults falls each year and many of these falls could have been prevented if these individuals used properly installed handrails on stairs.[12]

Elevators. Where there are elevators, check if the patient can get into the elevator. There may be a rise or gap between the floor outside the elevator and inside the elevator. Check if the patient can make adjustments to enter and exit safely and in a timely manner, whether the door opens wide enough for access, and whether the patient can reach the buttons.

Escalators. Escalators are not uncommon in community environments and can pose a barrier to people with mobility limitations. Escalators cannot be used by a person in a wheelchair and require considerable speed and coordination for people with other mobility limitations. If escalator use appears possible, examine how the patient manages getting on and off the escalator, including timing, foot clearance, and hand-rail grasp.

Interior Barriers

Interior Access Routes. Paths and flooring from the entry of a building leading to and through various rooms should be examined to ensure that there is enough space for basic mobility in and out of rooms with any assistive device the patient requires (Figs. 35-2 and 35-3). Also consider the type and resistance of the floor covering. Is the floor covered with tile or low pile carpet? Does it have a variety of textures or surface area rugs? Be aware that smooth tile may be too slippery for safe ambulation, whereas high-pile carpeting with soft padding may make wheelchair mobility difficult and increase foot drag during gait. Uneven floor boards, bumps in the surfaces, holes or rips in carpeting, and items on the floor, including cords, wires, and throw rugs, should also be identified and corrected or removed because any of these can be hazardous.

Doorways. Examination of environmental barriers for a wheelchair-bound patient should always include measurement of doorway width since narrow doorways are the most frequent obstacles preventing full access in a residence or in the community. Bathroom doors are generally the narrowest doors in the home setting. A door must be at least 32 inches wide for a standard wheelchair to pass and ideally 1-2 inches wider than this to account for inaccurate maneuvering and the usual oblique approach to doors. One should also observe the patient's ability to open, close, lock, and unlock doors and whether they can

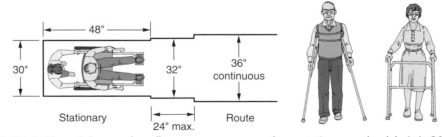

FIG. 35-2 The minimum clear floor space necessary for a stationary wheelchair is 30 inches wide by 48 inches long. The minimum path width for a standard wheelchair or for ambulating with an assistive device is 36 inches to allow for passing space. A corridor can narrow to widths of 32 inches for distances less than 24 inches in length (i.e., to pass through doorways). *Redrawn from ADA Build it Right, 2004, Vancouver, WA.*

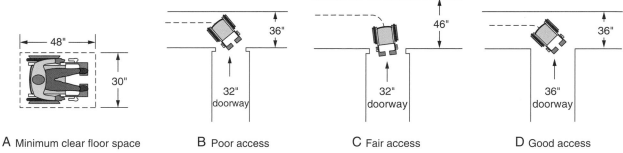

FIG. 35-3 Access for a 90-degree turn to enter a room based on the width of the hallway and door. **A,** Minimum clear floor space required for a standard wheelchair. **B,** Poor room access. **C,** Fair room access. **D,** Good room access. *A Redrawn from ADA Build it Right, 2004, Vancouver, WA. B, C, D Redrawn from Department of Justice, ADA Accessibility Guidelines for Buildings and Facilities, 2002.*

FIG. 35-4 The minimum wheelchair floor space requirements for door management. **A,** When pulling a door open the necessary floor space is 60 inches perpendicular to door and 18 inches parallel to the latch side of the door. **B,** When pushing a door open, only 48 inches perpendicular to the door is required. *Redrawn from Department of Justice, ADA Accessibility Guidelines for Buildings and Facilities, 2002.*

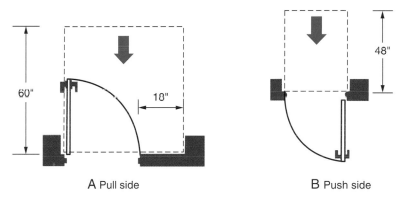

A Pull side

B Push side

manage screen doors and sliding glass doors, as well as regular hinged doors if needed.

If a doorway is located in a hallway that requires a 90-degree turn to enter, measure both the width of the doorway and the width of the hall. Check if there is enough open floor space on either side of the door for the patient to approach the door and how much force is needed to open and close it. If the door opens toward the wheelchair, a floor space of at least 5 feet × 5 feet perpendicular to the doorway will be required to open the door. Another 18 inches of open floor space to the side of the door where the lock and lever are will allow the individual to park and swing the door past them to the fully open position (Fig. 35-4).

Turning. A standard wheelchair user will need at least a 60 inch × 60 inch area to make a 180-degree turn, and this can only be accomplished if the patient can pull back on one wheelchair wheel while simultaneously pushing forward on the other. If the patient can only push one wheel at a time, they will need an area measuring 60 inches × 72 inches to complete a 180-degree turn (Fig. 35-5).

Lighting. Different tasks require different amounts of light. Check that lighting in all areas is bright enough for safe task performance and that light switches can be reached by the patient or that lights come on automatically as the patient enters the environment. Each room should have multiple light sources to provide diffuse lighting to reveal any safety hazards such as furniture edges

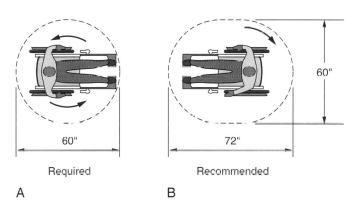

Required

Recommended

A

B

FIG. 35-5 Turning radius of a standard wheelchair. **A,** The minimum space requirement to make 180-degree turn with a standard wheelchair when utilizing two hands (i.e., one hand pushing forward as the other pulls backward). **B,** The minimum space recommended when only utilizing one arm to turn the wheelchair. *Redrawn from ADA Build it Right, 2004, Vancouver, WA.*

and stairs. There should also be lighting on all accessible paths, doorways, and porches. Ideally, emergency lights should be provided in multiple rooms of the residence and the work place. Note any deficiencies in task lighting and their cause, for example, light from windows or overhead lights casting shadows that limit vision and affect positioning or light switches that are too high for the patient to reach from his or her wheelchair. Also, note any tasks that have to be performed with vision occluded such as reaching under the sink, in the back of a drawer or closet, or patting the wall for a light switch.

Seating. Examine the height, width, depth, and stability of all seating. The height should be measured from the top of the seat pan to the floor. The width should be measured as the distance between armrests from one side of the seat pan to the other. Compare these measurements to those of the patient to determine if a change is needed. Note the condition of the seat cushion and padding and placement of the armrests. Do the armrests aid or interfere with sitting down in the chair? Does the seat provide enough back and seat support (firm not sagging)? Note type of fabric and how it affects mobility. Chairs with leather or fabrics "breathe" better and provide traction that reduces slippage.

Optimal seating depends on the tasks that will be performed while sitting in the chair. For most tasks a chair should have the following features: A five-point pedestal for a sturdy foundation; casters; adequate seat cushion to avoid pressure points; forward seat tilt to assist with neutral spine posture; chair depth sufficient to support two-thirds of the thigh length; an adjustable back rest for neutral spine support; and adjustable armrests (Fig. 35-6). See Chapter 4 for more information on selecting and adjusting seating to optimize posture and Chapter 33 for specific recommendations for wheelchair seating.

Countertops/Tables/Work Surfaces. Measure the height and depth of all work surfaces. The height should be measured from the floor to both the top and the underside of the work surface to determine if the patient will be able to reach and use items on the surface and clear their legs under the surface. Also note if the surface height is adjustable, and if so, if the adjustment is manual or electric. Although the ideal surface height for many tasks is around 29 inches, a surface for typing or mousing should ideally be lower, at or 1 inch below the height of the elbow (tip of the olecranon) when the elbows are at the patient's side.

Certain adaptations may be needed for the patient in a wheelchair. Average horizontal forward reach from a wheelchair is 24 inches from the patient's shoulder. This reach generally puts the patient's hand directly above the footrests of the chair (Fig. 35-7, *A*). If a patient cannot fit their legs under a work surface, they will have very limited ability to reach over that surface. A surface must be at least 27 inches high (from the floor to the undersurface) and 32 inches wide and 24 inches deep for the legs of a patient in a standard wheelchair to pass under it and at least 30 inches high for the armrests of a standard wheelchair to pass under it. This will allow a functional reach over the countertop of 17-19 inches (Fig. 35-7, *B*). Most work sur-

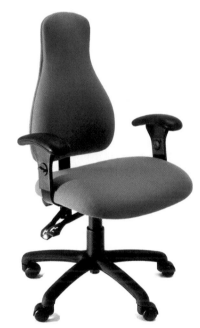

FIG. 35-6 Chair for computer work. *Courtesy Soma Ergonomics, Berkeley, CA.*

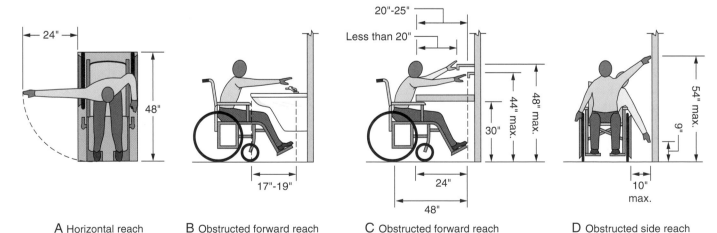

A Horizontal reach   B Obstructed forward reach   C Obstructed forward reach   D Obstructed side reach

FIG. 35-7 Forward reach from a wheelchair. **A,** Unobstructed forward reach is 24 inches. **B,** Forward reach when leg space is allowed is 17-19 inches. **C,** Forward reach when the arm rests and legs are allowed to pass under objects is 24 inches. **D,** Unobstructed high and low reach of 54 inches and 9 inches. *Redrawn from ADA Build it Right, 2004, Vancouver, WA.*

faces are 29 inches high and 24 inches deep, and most countertops are 29½ inches deep (Fig. 35-7, *C*).

Reach Zones. Examine the three reach zones discussed previously in the section on ROM (see Fig. 35-1). Look for obstacles that prevent getting close to frequently used objects. Check if there are environmental barriers limiting the patient's ability to grasp frequently used objects while keeping the elbows by their side. Are objects that are used less frequently but at least hourly in the second reach zone? Are objects in the third reach zone beyond reach with the elbows fully extended?

Check where objects can be placed, as well as where they are placed. Moving things closer can often improve movement safety and efficiency.

Sinks. There are often sinks in various rooms in the home, community, and work place. Check if the sink faucets are accessible and easy to use, and if the patient is a wheelchair user, if the wheelchair will fit underneath the sink. Is there enough clearance to avoid the patient's knees hitting cabinet doors, drawers and pipes? For a wheelchair user, the faucet should be no more than 22 inches from the edge of the counter, and the sink should be no higher than 34 inches from the floor and no more than 5-6 inches deep.

Environmental Barriers in Specific Rooms

Kitchen. The extent of the kitchen examination will depend in part on how your client plans to use the kitchen. If your client is not the primary cook and only performs light meal preparation (e.g., making sandwiches and snacks), then a cursory examination focusing on safety is sufficient. However, if the client lives alone or is the primary cook for the family, a more extensive examination is recommended. Examination may include checking if the patient can lift one or more glasses, dishes, pots, and pans and if they can open and close the refrigerator, oven, and cabinets. Surface heights should also be examined to check if they can be reached and if so, to what degree. Also, examine the area for fire risks, including grease, towels, and aerosols close to heat sources and check if there is a working fire extinguisher and smoke detector in the area. Check if the patient can reach and use the fire extinguisher.

Bathroom. In the bathroom, check the door width, as well as the safety and accessibility of the sink(s), toilet, and bath and/or shower. Sinks should be examined as noted in the kitchen section.

Toilet. For the toilet, measure the seat height (ideally 17-19 inches), location of toilet paper, presence or absence of grab bars, and the distance from the toilet to the side-wall. Check if there is enough clearance for the patient and any needed assistive device to be positioned near the toilet. Depending on the level of assistance required, is there space for a caregiver? Note if there are difficulties or limitations during transfers on and off of the toilet.

Bath/Shower. For the bath and/or shower, depending on the needs of the patient, check for accessibility of the faucets, the presence of a bath or shower seat and grab bars, and if the patient is able to transfer in and out of the bath and/or shower safely. Soap dishes and towel racks should never be used as grab bars to assist with transfers as they pull out of the wall too easily. Measure the dimen-

sions of the bath or shower, especially in older homes, and identify the material of the interior of the bath or shower. A shower stall must be at least 36 inches × 60 inches with a 36-inch door opening to allow access by a wheelchair user. Also check if the floor in and around the bath or shower is slip resistant. For the seated patient, check that the height of the shower hose is adjustable. The use of assistive devices in a bath or shower is generally not safe because the floor surfaces become slippery when wet.

Bedroom. Examine the width of the bedroom door opening, as well as lighting, flooring, and accessibility to bed and clothing. Also check if the bedroom has enough space for the patient to safely maneuver and if the bed, closet, and dresser are accessible. Can clothing be accessed readily without the patient losing balance, grasping the closet rod, or falling backward when opening a drawer? Does the closet door open far enough to allow the patient to reach items in the closet when using an ambulation aide? Measure the height of rods and shelves. Can clothes and shoes be reached and transported safely? Removing or rearranging items may improve access and reduce fall risk. Where necessary, check if there is enough space for a hospital bed or bedside commode if these are needed now or are likely to be needed in the future.[13]

Measure the height of the bed relative to the patient. Ideally, when the patient is sitting on the edge of the bed with their feet on the ground, their thighs will be tilted so that the knees are slightly below the hips. This makes it easiest to move from sitting to standing. It is also important that the edge of the mattress is firm so the patient does not slip off the mattress edge.

Laundry Room. Access to and operation of a washer and dryer can be challenging to patients with mobility impairments. Check if the patient can enter the laundry room with any needed mobility device and can access the appliances safely. Success in using the washer and dryer are often determined by the space available next to the machine, the location of the controls, whether the machine is front-loading or top-loading, and the direction the doors open. Measure how far one needs to reach to operate the controls, the height that clothes need to be lifted to be placed into the machines, and the reach required for retrieving clothes from the machines. If the user is seated (wheelchair/chair), his or her maximum side reach will be 24 inches, maximum reach up will be 54 inches, and unobstructed low reach will be 9 inches from the floor (Fig. 35-7, *D*). Bottom-hinged front doors should be avoided because they reduce the patient's ability to get clothes from the bottom of the machine.

Determine if the ironing board is accessible. If so, can the patient set-up and break down the ironing board, plug and unplug the iron, and handle the iron safely? Factors influencing success in ironing include ironing board height, weight of the iron, and the patient's grip strength.

Communication

Telephone. Check what type of phone the patient has and see if they can hold it, dial numbers, access emergency contacts, and connect with 911 in case of an emergency. Can the patient handle the phone and don the earpiece for hands-free use? Can they see the numbers on the display clearly? Can their fingers depress one key at a time? Can the patient write or take messages while on the phone? Can the patient hear the phone ring, see who is calling, and pick up the call in a timely manner? Can the patient hear someone talking on the phone?

Writing. Writing can be difficult if the surface is too high or unstable, particularly if writing for a prolonged period. Therefore measure the height of the writing surface and test the surfaces for stability. Also check if writing instruments are within easy reach and if the angle of the surface affects the patient's ability to maintain a neutral spine.

Computer Use. People use computers for a wide range of functions, including entertainment, accounting, correspondence, and shopping. In the community, people also use computers when banking or at point-of-sale transactions. At work, even if a patient does not use a computer to perform work-related tasks, they may use a time clock or other electronic device. If computer use is frequent and/or prolonged, the set-up should be optimized. Box 35-2 lists areas for examination of a computer set-up. (This list is also available on the CD that accompanies this book.)

Unique Work Place Considerations. In the work place, patients need to perform a variety of tasks that extend beyond their activities of daily living (ADLs) and home management. These tasks can be summarized as essential job functions (EJFs). EJFs are the tasks and performance expectations for a job, for example, lifting and handling boxes of merchandise and sweeping the showroom floor. During an examination of environmental barriers in the work place, one should note the nature, frequency, duration, and strength demands of EJFs and observe the patient performing or attempting to perform these activities. If the patient is unable to perform the activities, observing others perform the same job may provide valuable information about the barriers that may be encountered in performing specific tasks. One should consider if

the patient can achieve the positions needed to perform the tasks, can sequence the tasks, and has the dexterity and strength to perform the tasks and how the tasks may be modified if needed. During the examination, also observe for risk factors for injury, including highly repetitive tasks, forceful exertions, awkward postures, sustained postures, and vibration.[14]

EVALUATION, DIAGNOSIS, AND PROGNOSIS

Evaluation is the process of integrating information from all components of the examination to determine a plan of care. In the case of evaluating environmental barriers, findings from the examination of the patient's musculoskeletal, neuromuscular, cardiovascular, pulmonary, and functional performance should be integrated with findings of environmental barriers. The evaluation and plan of care should take into account not only current limitations but also the patient's prognosis for change so that interventions address expected needs over time.

LEGISLATION

Some countries have adopted legislation regarding safety in the work place and environmental barriers in the work place and the community. In the United States, there are two primary areas of national legislation designed to improve accessibility for people with disabilities:[15-17] the Americans with Disabilities Act (ADA)[18] and the Ergonomics Program Rule from the *Occupational Safety and Health Administration* (OSHA).[19]

The ADA was enacted in 1990 to provide a clear and comprehensive national mandate for the elimination of discrimination against individuals with disabilities and to provide guidance for reasonable accommodations. The ADA prohibits discrimination against people with disabilities in employment (Title I), public services (Title II), in places of public accommodation and commercial facilities (Title III), and telecommunications (Title IV).[20] According to the ADA, employers must make reasonable accommodations to allow disabled employees to perform their jobs, and public and commercial places must make reasonable accommodations to make places accessible to people with disabilities. Therapists can assist patients by providing justification for ADA-prescribed reasonable accommodations to employers, insurance companies, and others. The ADA requires employers to make accommodations for an employee if this would not impose an "undue hardship" on the operation of the employer's business. Undue hardship is an action requiring significant difficulty or expense when considered in light of factors such as an employer's size, financial resources, and the nature and structure of its operation.[21] An employer is not required to lower quality or production standards to make an accommodation nor is an employer required to provide personal use items such as glasses or hearing aids.

Complaints about violations of Title I (employment) of the ADA may be filed with the Equal Employment Opportunity Commission. Call 800-669-4000 (voice) or 800-669-6820 (TTY) to reach the field office in your area. Complaints about violations of Title II by units of state and local government or violations of Title III by public

BOX 35-2	**Examination of the Computer Set-Up**

What type of computer: Desktop or laptop?
Is the computer on a secure surface?
Is the work surface adjustable?
Is the work height ideal for the person and the task?
Is the leg and foot clearance under the work surface ample?
Is the chair design and size appropriate?
Does the keyboard surface slide or elevate and lower?
Is the monitor directly in front of the keyboard?
Is the lighting appropriate?
Is the ventilation adequate?

Computer Set-Up Measurements
Floor to elbow with feet on the floor _____ inches
Floor to top of the work surface _____ inches
Floor to the top of a keyboard tray _____ inches
Floor to the top of the monitor screen _____ inches

accommodations and commercial facilities (private businesses and nonprofit service providers) should be filed with the Department of Justice.

OSHA also has directives to minimize risk for work-related musculoskeletal disorders (WMSDs).[19] Because WMSDs are so common among American workers, OSHA requires that companies with frequent WMSD's have ergonomic programs intended to reduce musculoskeletal risks. It is estimated that currently approximately 16% of employers nationwide have developed such ergonomics programs.[22] OSHA has pledged to become more involved in this process and to ensure its effectiveness by promoting a culture of safety and health.[22] As of 2006, the states of Washington and California have passed additional regulations intended to specifically control risks for overexertion and repetitive motion injuries (RMI).[23]

INTERVENTION

Interventions related to environmental barriers are generally in the form of recommendations for modifying the environment. The recommended modifications should improve safety, maximize functional independence, and be acceptable to the patient. Recommendations should be customized to each individual based on findings from the examination. The following interventions are sequenced to parallel the sequence of the examination presented earlier in this chapter.

MUSCULOSKELETAL

Posture. Posture can be optimized by selection and adjustment of furniture to allow the patient to maintain a neutral posture for most activities and to optimize mechanical advantage for power and balance. Changes may be recommended for the height of counters, the type and adjustment of seating, and the position and height of lighting. All seating and work surfaces should be accessible by the patient. The American National Standards Institute (ANSI) and Human Factors and Ergonomics Society (HFES) published initial recommendations for work place seating in 1988 and revised recommendations in 2005.[3] The initial recommendations were that the work place be designed so that the individual could assume an upright posture with the hips, knees and elbows flexed to approximately 90 degrees. The later recommendations were that the individual should be able to work from reclined sitting, declined sitting, standing, and from an upright sitting position so that positioning can be varied throughout the day (Fig. 35-8).

Anthropometric Characteristics. As most products are designed for people whose anthropometric characteristics fall within the 5th to 95th percentile of the general population of nondisabled individuals,[17] environmental modifications are often required for people shorter than 5 foot 1 inch or taller than 6 foot 1 inch, lighter than 100 lb or heavier than 300 lb, and for those with disproportionate trunk to leg length. A standing ambulatory individual will require 25 inches × 15 inches of floor space, a 16- to 26-inch aisle width, and no additional space for turning.[17] Wheelchair users have an eye-level that is generally 15-16 inches below that of most standing people, and they require at least 48 inches × 30 inches of open

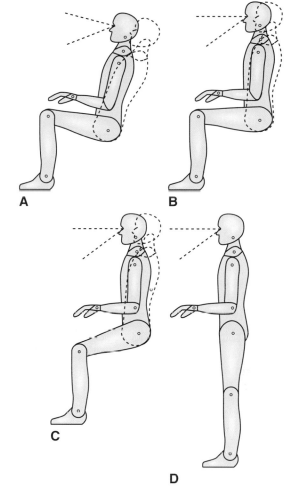

FIG. 35-8 Reference postures. **A,** Reclined sitting. The torso and neck are at 105-120 degrees to the horizontal. **B,** Upright sitting. The torso and neck are approximately vertical and in line, the thighs are approximately horizontal, and the lower legs vertical. **C,** Declined sitting. The thighs are inclined below the horizontal, the torso is vertical or slightly reclined behind the vertical, and the angle between the thighs and the torso is greater than 90 degrees. **D,** Standing. The legs, torso, neck, and head are approximately in line and vertical. *Redrawn from Department of Labor, Occupational Safety and Health Administration: Computer Workstations: Good Working Positions, 2006.*

floor space for mobility, aisle clearance of 31.5 inches, and a turning circle of between 60 and 72 inches.

Range of Motion. ROM limitations are among the most common disabilities. For patients with limited ROM, objects may be moved closer and retractable cables, extended handles, and reachers may be helpful.

Muscle Performance. When muscle weakness is identified in the examination, environmental changes can be made to reduce the force demands from the environment. Examples of such changes include using lighter-weight dishes; replacing door knobs with levers to allow use of larger muscles; providing powered tools such as can openers, carving knives, door openers, and construction tools as appropriate to the individual's goals; providing voice recognition software where strength or endurance limit writing; and installing smooth flooring or low-pile carpeting where wheelchair propulsion is needed. In addition, manually or electrically powered carts may be helpful for moving items in and around an environment, and suspended tools can compensate for reduced grip strength and limited lifting strength or endurance.

Joint Integrity. The recommendations described to optimize posture and for patients with reduced ROM or muscle performance may also be applied to patients with impaired joint integrity. Interventions that support good alignment, limit reach, and avoid overloading muscles will also help preserve joint integrity.

NEUROMUSCULAR

Cognition. In patients with cognitive impairments the environment should be simplified sufficiently to allow maximal safe participation in activities. Recommended modifications include providing single number dialing for emergency medical service access; limiting access to dangerous items, such as power tools, cook surfaces, guns, and flames; and providing simple pictorial instructions for daily activities.

Pain. If pain is caused by pressure, consider padding, changing the height of a surface, or changing the patient's posture to avoid such contact. If leg, foot, or back pain is triggered with standing, consider a floor mat for cushioning or alternative positioning.

Coordination. If impaired dexterity limits safe access to an environment, then consider ways to simplify or power the activity, such as using a food processor to cut food, keyless controlled entry for doors, and voice recognition software for writing.

Sensory Integrity. Textured surfaces can help compensate for sensory impairments. For patients with loss of temperature discrimination, hot water should not be hotter than 54° C (130° F).[24]

CARDIOVASCULAR/PULMONARY

For patients with cardiovascular or pulmonary performance limitations, demands can be reduced by placing commonly used objects close by and at waist level, and access to the environment may be improved by use of a motorized wheelchair or scooter.

FUNCTION

Assistive, Adaptive, Orthotic, Protective, and Prosthetic Devices. Assistive, adaptive, orthotic, protective, and prosthetic devices should be recommended with caution as they can give a false sense of safety. Although they can limit extremes of motion and provide some support, no brace is a substitute for good body mechanics and a workload appropriate to the individual's abilities.

Ergonomics and Body Mechanics. Ideally, tasks can be modified in all settings to match the patient's abilities. However, even with the best task adaptations, to optimize safety and efficiency, the patient should be educated in the ideal way to work within these different settings. Such education may include instruction and practice of ideal ways for performing tasks and instruc-

tion on pacing by taking short breaks, rotating tasks, and stretching.

Environmental Barriers. Interventions that address environmental barriers are generally in the form of recommendations that may range from simple changes of habits, routines, and behaviors to structural changes requiring a skilled contractor. One should try to provide the patient with options and choices so they can select modifications that most fit their needs and abilities.

Exterior Barriers

External Access Routes. Behavioral changes may include encouraging the patient to park within designated handicap parking closest to building entrances and recommending they carry a flashlight if path lighting is compromised. Structural recommendations will vary according to the specific needs of the patient. For a patient in a wheelchair, access routes should be at least 36 inches wide (see Fig. 35-2). For any patient with limited mobility, access routes should have a smooth slip-resistant surface clear of obstacles, have a maximum grade of 8% with no sudden elevations, and good lighting.[11] Surface blemishes, uneven surfaces, and damaged or cracked concrete that impair the ease of mobility or increase fall risk should be repaired. In public places where changes cannot be made at the patient's request the patient should seek alternative routes. In addition, the patient can seek out community areas with sidewalks with accessible curbs.

Stairs. It is recommended that steps that are in poor condition, with broken concrete, wood planks, or uneven areas, be repaired and that tread lips that can become a trip hazard be removed. Stairs should be lighted so that each step, particularly the step edges, can be seen clearly. The lighting should not produce glare or shadows along the stairway. For the visually impaired patient, placing red, orange, or yellow tape on the border of each stair is helpful.[11] To clearly identify the top and bottom stair, place a wider strip of tape on the edge of the stair and/or a corresponding circular band of tape on the handrail. For an entry step to accommodate a walker safely, it should be at least 30 inches wide by 22 inches deep.

Ramps. If a patient cannot manage exterior stairs safely, stairs may be replaced or supplemented by a ramp. The ramp should be wide enough to accommodate the patient and their mobility device, have appropriate landings, and a nonskid surface. For safety and ease of use, ramps should have an incline of between 1:8 and 1:12 (Table 35-3). There should be a level landing at the top

TABLE 35-3	Maximum Ramp Slope and Rise for Existing Sites, Buildings, and Facilities	
Slope	**Rise**
Steeper than 1:12 but not steeper than 1:10	6 inches (150 mm)
Steeper than 1:10 but not steeper than 1:8	3 inches (75 mm)
A slope steeper than 1:8 is prohibited.	

From ADA and ABA Accessibility Guidelines: www.access-board.gov/ada-aba/final.htm.

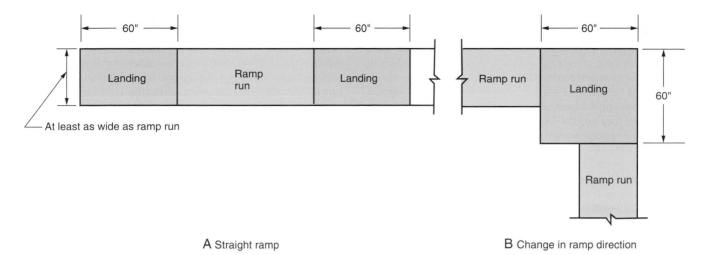

A Straight ramp   **B** Change in ramp direction

FIG. 35-9 Landings are required at the top and bottom of ramps. **A,** When the ramp is straight the landing must be at least 60 inches long and at least as wide as the ramp run. **B,** When the ramp changes direction the landing must have a minimum dimension of 60 inches wide by 60 inches long. *Redrawn from Department of Justice, ADA Accessibility Guidelines for Buildings and Facilities, 2002.*

and bottom of the ramp. If the ramp is over 30 feet long, the landing should be 5 feet long and as wide as the ramp. If the ramp has a right angle, it should have a 5 foot × 5 foot landing between segments (Fig. 35-9).

Edge Protection and Handrails. To prevent a wheelchair wheel or assistive device from falling off a ramp, it should have edge protection. This must be at least 2 inches high and be placed less than 4 inches above the top of the ramp.[11] Handrails should be installed by a professional and secured on each side of a stairwell and on any ramp that is more than 6 feet long or any step that is more than 6 inches high (Fig. 35-10). Handrails should be installed between 34-38 inches above the walking surface for ambulatory adults, 28 inches for children, and extend approximately 12 inches onto the landing.[10] The diameter of the rail can range from $1\frac{1}{4}$-$1\frac{1}{2}$ inches and should be set $1\frac{1}{2}$ inches from the wall to allow for gripping without scraping knuckles against the wall. Handrails need to support 250 lb of weight and must therefore be anchored securely to the wall. Stainless steel handrails require less maintenance and last longer than wood in extreme weather conditions.

Elevators. Reinforce the need to pay attention when using an elevator. Remind the patient that the doors may open between floors and that the elevator floor may not be flush with the outside. A reacher or dowel can be used by a person in a wheelchair to reach elevator buttons that are too high.

Escalators. Practice use of escalators in the community with the patient if this is an important task for him or her. Use of escalators should only be attempted with the patient who has at least fair plus dynamic standing balance.

Interior Barriers

Interior Access Routes. When an inside area has poor access because the path is too narrow, try to rearrange furniture or select an alternative pathway. For the patient in a wheelchair a path width of 36 inches that is clear of any

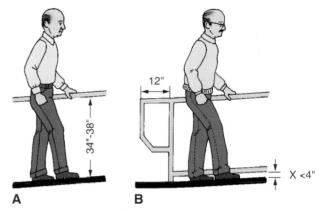

FIG. 35-10 A, Handrail should be placed parallel to the slope of the ramp and 34-38 inches above it. **B,** Ramp edging is required to prevent 4-inch objects from rolling off the edge. *Redrawn from Department of Justice, ADA Accessibility Guidelines for Buildings and Facilities, 2002.*

hazards or sudden elevation changes is needed (see Fig. 35-2). For patients with decreased balance, difficulties with ambulation or those in a wheelchair, remove obstacles that narrow the path width and items on the floor, including cords, wires, throw rugs, and clutter that can be a safety hazard. Recommend using a cordless telephone to eliminate the telephone cord. A stair lift or elevator can be installed for nonambulatory patients who need to move between stories.

Flooring. Patients with difficulties ambulating generally walk or wheel more readily on high-density low-pile carpeting, indoor/outdoor carpeting, nonskid ceramic tile, or brushed cement. For the visually impaired patient, light-colored flooring with low reflectance (reduces glare) and in colors that contrast with other objects in the room can be helpful. Recommend that any flooring that is ripped or has holes in it, throw rugs, and runners or mats that slide, be removed. Placing double-faced adhesive carpet tape or rubber matting on the backs of rugs and runners or replacing current rugs with ones with slip-resistant backing can also improve safety. The flooring in the kitchen and bathroom should be nonslip and easy to clean.

Doorways. Although the clinician may recommend that a door be widened, the doorway should always be examined by a building contractor to check that this is structurally safe and feasible.

Doorways are the most frequent obstacles preventing full access to and around buildings. For patients in a wheelchair, bathroom doors should ideally open outward and be 32-36 inches wide. If the door opening is too narrow, consider the suggestions listed in Box 35-3 or the purchase of a narrower transport chair for use in the bathroom.

Turning. For the patient in a wheelchair who can use both hands to manipulate the wheelchair assure that areas for turning are at least 60 inches by 60 inches. If the patient can only use one hand to push the wheelchair, a 60-inch by 72-inch area is needed (see Fig. 35-5). Suggest moving pieces of furniture to accommodate these needs before considering structural changes.

Lighting. Adequate lighting in and around the home is important for safety, particularly for the elderly. Changes in vision accelerate after the age of 50 and increase in severity after age 65, and 1 in 20 individuals over 85 years of age is legally blind.[25] It is estimated that for the older eye to function adequately, it needs approximately three times the amount of light as the eye of a younger person.[26] Changes in vision and impaired dark adaptation in the aging eye may also cause an older person to be virtually blind for a minute or more on moving from a bright to a darker area.[27]

To reduce fall risk, lighting should be sufficient to allow depth perception and perception of edges of walking surfaces, and light switches should be readily accessible from the doorway.[27] Box 35-4 lists a number of recommendations to improve lighting effectiveness.

Seating. Routinely used furniture should be reasonably firm for support and comfort and stable to ensure function and safety. A piece of $^1/_2$-inch or $^3/_4$-inch plywood cut to fit under the seat surface can improve seat firmness, and removing casters, rockers, and swivel-bases will improve stability.

For most seats the seat height should allow the individual's feet to easily touch the floor with the knees approximately level with the hips.[28] If the seating surface is too low, it may be difficult for the person to rise from sitting to standing. The height may be increased by having the seat cushion replaced or restuffed, by adding 3-5 inch

---

BOX 35-3	**Door and Doorway Modifications to Improve Access**

Increasing Door Width
- Install offset, fold-back or swing-clear hinges. These hinges will allow the door to be swung flush with the hinge-side jamb, and increases opening $1^1/_2$-$1^3/_4$ inches.
- Remove the door stop on the door frame, and reinstall 3 feet above the floor (adds $^3/_4$ inch to opening).
- Remove interior door and/or replace with an inexpensive rod and curtain if privacy is desired. This will increase door opening $1^1/_2$-2 inches.
- Remove door and doorstop (increases door opening $2^1/_4$-$2^3/_4$ inches).

Limited Floor Space
If floor space is limited, and/or the patient has difficulty opening and passing through the doorway, the following recommendations can be made:
- Install a double-action hinge. These hinges will allow the door to be pushed open from either direction.
- Reverse the door hinges so that the door will open toward the larger room.
- Install lever-type latch handles. These handles are preferred over the standard doorknob, which requires greater hand function and strength.
- Install pull handles on the front of doors that open inward. These handles, installed horizontally 36-39 inches from the floor, aide in pulling the door shut from outside of the room.
- Doorway thresholds should be removed or lowered to no greater than $^1/_2$ inch in height and have beveled edges. Kick plate installation near the bottom of each door will protect doors from being marred by the wheelchair footrests. Kick plates should extend from the floor up to a height of at least 10 inches and preferably 16 inches.
- Build an outside shelf near the door. This shelf will allow patient to store packages while fishing for keys.
- Recommend a keyless door lock system for patients who have difficulty turning a stiff lock, or lack the dexterity to manage keys.

BOX 35-4	**Home Lighting Recommendations**

- Daylight fluorescent lights (preferred as they use a broader light spectrum).
- Replace old light bulbs with the highest wattage light bulbs accepted by the fixture (some fixtures will only accept a maximum 60 watt bulb).
- The level of light should be consistent between rooms (i.e., bedroom and bathroom).
- Emergency night lights should illuminate commonly used pathways in the home.
- Replacing the existing light switches with a "glow switch," or surrounding the switch with glow-in-the-dark tape will help identify its location in the dark.
- Lamps should be placed near main seating areas.
- Patients should be able to turn lights on and off easily. Often, a tabletop pad switch, touch turn-on adaptor for lamps, and rheostat switches for wall switches are easiest.
- Wall switches should be placed to allow turning on and off before entering and exiting the room.
- Clearly mark changes in floor levels with colored or reflecting tape.
- Avoid using similar colors together. Use contrasting colors between doorways and walls, the risers and flat surfaces of steps, dishes and tablecloths, etc. Yellow-orange and reds are more easily distinguished by the older adult than blue or green.

leg extenders to chairs and sofas that will accept them, or by placing the sofa or chair on a platform.[28] A platform lip should be attached to prevent the chair or sofa slipping off the edge. If the patient still cannot rise from the seat, manual or electric lift seats or chairs that tilt or lift the patient forward to assist with standing can be used.

Chairs for the home or work place should be selected to meet the needs of the patient when performing their expected tasks. It is usually best to acquire a chair that fits the patient and that can be adjusted to meet various needs. In addition, the chair should have a five-point pedestal for a sturdy foundation, casters to reduce friction, enough seat cushion to avoid pressure points, enough depth to support two-thirds of the length of the thighs, and an adjustable back rest and armrests (see Fig. 35-6). Adjustable seat tilt may also assist with spine positioning. Most people do not need a headrest on a task chair. Recommend a chair that has a warranty for the patient's weight. Most chairs have a warranty for up to 250 lb, but chairs that accommodate heavier people are available. Petite chairs are available to accommodate people shorter than 5 foot 1 inch, and large chairs are available to accommodate people taller than 6 foot 1 inch.

Countertops/Tables/Work Surfaces. Recommend raising or replacing tables that are too low or that do not have enough space to allow for easy access. Leg extenders can be purchased to raise tables by 3-5 inches. A platform, as described in the previous seating section, can also be made to elevate pedestal-type tables. Typically, a work surface for a seated task is 29 inches high. Raising the height of the underside of a work surface to 30 inches will allow the armrest of a wheelchair to pass under a workspace and thus allow the patient in a wheelchair to reach forward up to 24 inches, which is the usual width of most countertops (see Fig. 35-7, *C*). Surfaces that are too high may be lowered, or a higher chair with a footrest may be used.

Reach Zones. Move objects around according to the reach zones described previously (see Fig. 35-1 and section on Range of Motion). A lazy Susan or a rotating book caddy can reduce the need for reaching and save space. Long-handled reachers can also eliminate an extended reach that can cause strain and compromise balance.

Work Area Triangles. Rearrange space according to frequency of use. Consider the most efficient design for the patient, such as a triangle, U-shaped, or L-shaped design, for tool or appliance placement (Fig. 35-11). Table 35-4 outlines recommended work triangle dimensions for a kitchen according to the assistive device used.

Sink. For patients with strength or ROM restrictions in the upper extremities, sink faucets can be modified to have a single-lever handle allowing the patient to use large rather than small muscle groups to turn the water on and off. For wheelchair users the sink should be no higher than 34 inches from the floor, and to allow for knee clearance, the space under the sink should be open and at least 27 inches high, 30 inches wide, and 19 inches deep.[29] The leg space under a sink can be increased by removing cabinet doors, central rail, and toe board and by cutting back the cabinet floor. Also, pad sharp edges and insulate hot water pipes under the sink.

Environmental Barriers in Specific Rooms

Kitchen. Kitchens have inherent dangers, including risk of food spillage, container breakage, slip and fall injuries, and burns from foods or stoves. To reduce the risk of burns from reaching over burners, a range with the control knobs along the front edge is recommended. A horizontal or staggered burner arrangement is also better than a symmetrical layout because it reduces the chance of the patient leaning on the front burners to reach a back burner. A mirror placed over the stove will also allow the burners to be seen from a seated position. An eye-level oven with a drop front will be safer than a traditional lower oven.[30] A wheeled trolley may help with food transportation, and a dishwasher can save time and energy and reduce strain on the distal extremities. When considering appliances, a side-by-side refrigerator with slide-out

TABLE 35-4	Recommended Kitchen Work Triangle Dimensions		
Appliance/ Fixture	Standard (ft)	Wheelchair (ft)	Walker/ Crutches (ft)
Total distance connecting refrigerator, range, and sink	12-22	14-24	10-20
Refrigerator to sink	4-7	6-9	2-5
Sink to range	4-6	6-8	2-4
Range to refrigerator	4-9	6-11	2-7

From The Accessible Kitchen: WSU Rehabilitation Engineering Accessible Kitchen: www.cs.wright.edu/bie/rehabengr/kitchens/kitchint.htm.

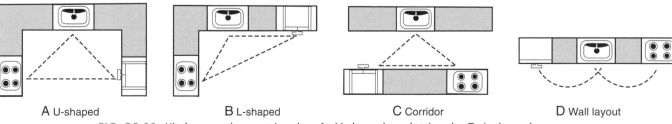

A U-shaped   **B** L-shaped   **C** Corridor   **D** Wall layout

FIG. 35-11 Kitchen work area triangles. **A,** U-shaped work triangle. **B,** L-shaped triangle. **C,** Corridor layout. **D,** Wall layout work area.

drawers and a water and ice dispenser will optimize access for the wheelchair user.

Storing and retrieving needed items can be made easier by using lazy Susan-type rotating trays on countertops and in cabinets. Heavy items should be placed at waist level for easiest access.

Bathroom

Toilet. Toilet seat height should be adjusted to maximize independence and safety. The ideal seat height is 17-19 inches for most adults and 11-17 inches for most children.[10] However, individuals with weakness or ROM restrictions may find it easier to use a higher seat. For patients using a wheelchair or assistive ambulation device, floor space in front and to the side of the toilet should be maximized to allow for transfers and maneuverability. A side transfer from a wheelchair requires a 42-inch space on one side of the toilet. A stand-pivot transfer from a wheelchair to the front of the toilet requires at least 18 inches of transfer space.[31] If the patient has weakness or balance problems, a 42-inch long grab bar should be installed at a height of 33 inches from the floor at the side of the toilet projecting 24 inches beyond the front of the toilet seat. A 36-inch grab bar placed behind the toilet can also be helpful (Fig. 35-12).[11] If there are no walls close to the toilet, floor mounted bars, a toilet safety frame, a raised toilet with armrests, or a commode can be used.

Bath/Shower. Consider faucet extensions and adjustable hand-held shower hoses for both standing and sitting individuals. If the patient will sit during bathing or showering, recommend a shower chair or bath bench that has four legs positioned in the shower or tub or a transfer bench with two legs on the outside of the tub and a seat that straddles the edge of the tub. A transfer bench is ideal for an individual at increased risk for falls because of poor balance or hemiparesis. Check that the recommended seat has a weight limit appropriate for the patient. Weight limits range from 285-350 lb. Whether the patient will be sitting or standing to bathe, ensure that the flooring of the bath and shower is nonslip.

Grab bars may be installed to assist with transfers and safety. According to the ADA guidelines, grab bars for adults should be easy to grasp, be $1\frac{1}{4}$-$1\frac{1}{2}$ inches in diameter, have a $1\frac{1}{2}$-inch clearance between the bar and the wall, and be mounted 33-36 inches up from the floor. For children ages 3-12, grab bars should be mounted between 18-27 inches up from the floor.[11] If the shower door is too narrow or the glass door of a combination tub-shower interferes with transfers, then the door and its housing can be removed and replaced with a shower curtain and rod. A shower stall that is at least 30 inches wide by 60 inches long can be converted into a roll-in-shower, which is more convenient for many wheelchair users.[31]

Bedroom. The bed height should be adjusted to make transfers as easy as possible. A bed can be raised using bed elevators attached to the legs (raises the bed 3-5 inches), by standing the bed on concrete blocks or boards, or by adding an additional box spring or mattress. Whichever method is used, check that the bed is stable before the patient uses it. A bed can be lowered by removing the casters, exchanging a typical 7-inch high metal frame for a 3-inch high frame, or by cutting the legs of a wooden frame. A bed rail may also help with transfers. If trips from the bed to the bathroom will be difficult or unsafe, recommend a bedside commode.

To improve access to clothing, closet doors may be removed, clothes rearranged, or the clothes rod lowered. For the wheelchair user, the clothes rod should be located 36-46 inches from the floor. Shelves should be placed no lower than 9 inches from the floor and no higher than 54 inches from the floor, and they should be no more than 16 inches deep.[13,32]

Laundry Room. Washers and dryers are easiest to use when they are front loading and have side-hinged rather than bottom-hinged doors. For the patient with limited lifting strength and endurance, recommend washing smaller loads and transporting laundry in a wheeled hamper or cart. Also recommend installing a shelf for soap accessories that is within the patient's reach.

Ironing. If setting up a standard ironing board and iron are difficult for the patient, suggest a wall-mounted ironing board and a lightweight iron. Cordless irons also reduce the fall risk associated with cords. A compact travel iron or a clothing steamer is a lightweight option for those with upper extremity weakness.

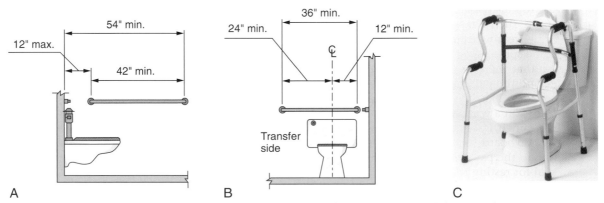

FIG. 35-12 Toilet transfer aides. **A,** Recommended placement of grab bars on the sidewalls. **B,** Recommended placement of grab bars on the back wall. **C,** A 3-in-1 commode often utilized in place of grab-bar installation. *Redrawn from Department of Justice, ADA Accessibility Guidelines for Buildings and Facilities, 2002. C Courtesy Momentum Medical, Idaho Falls, ID.*

Communication

Telephone. Post-emergency telephone numbers for a nearby neighbor, the police, the fire department, and the local poison control center clearly near the phone, and if possible, program these into the patient's phone for ease of use. A telephone or emergency medical alert system may also be appropriate for patients at risk for falling or for being unable to reach the phone. If the patient is going to be home alone, a cordless or wireless phone carried in a fanny pack can ensure access at all times. Telephones with hands-free headsets, larger buttons, lighted keypads, larger visual display, speakers, and pager features may also be helpful for some patients.

Writing. Changing the height and angle of the writing surface and writing tools can make writing easier and safer. Ideally, a writing or working surface should be 2 inches higher than elbow height. If the surface cannot be raised or lowered, try tilting materials by placing them on a tilt board or ring binder to simulate the angle of a drafting table. This brings materials closer to the user and reduces hip, thoracic, and cervical spine flexion. Larger diameter grip pens and pencils can also help reduce the required holding force and require less fine motor control to use.

Computer Use. When using a computer, ideally the elbows should be flexed between 70 and 135 degrees,[33-36] the shoulders abducted less than 20 degrees[37,38] and flexed less than 25 degrees,[37] the wrists held between 30 degrees of flexion and 10 degrees of extension,[39-41] and the torso-to-thigh angle should be at least 90 degrees.[37] A desk with a fixed keyboard height that is a few inches lower than the desk surface generally works well for people who use a computer for less than 2 hours per day. For people who use computers for 4 or more hours per day, an adjustable keyboard platform is recommended for optimal keyboard positioning.

When adjusting items at a computer desk, adjust the chair first so that the patient is sitting with a neutral spine and their feet supported. If the chair height can be adjusted, but the work surface height is fixed, adjust the chair height so that the patient's hands lie comfortably on the keyboard and then place a support under the feet if necessary to avoid dangling.[3] Then adjust the monitor height so that the top of the screen is at eye level and the monitor distance is such that the patient can see the screen clearly while wearing needed corrective lenses and maintaining neutral spine posture. Finally, adjust the keyboard position so that the f-g-h keys are in line with the patient's midline and the patient can glide the hands and fingers over the keys, like playing the piano, without anchoring the wrists on a wrist rest. The keyboard should be approximately 1-inch lower than the patient's elbow. The monitor and keyboard should be in line with each other and midline to the patient (Fig. 35-13). A soft wrist rest can be helpful for resting the hands briefly when not typing, but patients should not rest on these for prolonged periods because this can lead to excessive compression of the median nerve at the wrist.[42,43]

For patients with or at risk for musculoskeletal injuries, a variety of specialized computer *input devices* can reduce strain and allow for safer pain-free computer use. Key-

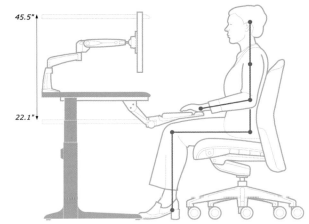

FIG. 35-13 Recommended computer station set-up. *Courtesy Work Rite Ergonomics, Inc, Petaluma, CA.*

boards may be split with or without adjustability. *Pointing and navigation devices* include the mouse, trackball, touch pads, and tablets. Selection among these devices is generally based on patient comfort. In addition, a wide variety of adaptive computer equipment is available through specialized rehabilitation centers.

Laptop Computers. If the patient will be using a laptop computer consistently for more than 2 hours per day, advise that the laptop display be elevated and used as the monitor, and an external keyboard and mouse placed at an appropriate height be used. Monitor risers are commercially available in 1-2 inch increments.

Community. Community access can be improved through patient education. Many stores, restaurants, and other community buildings are accessible by patients with mobility limitations. Furthermore, many stores will carry customers' purchases to the car and deliver to the home. Most hotels have rooms designed for wheelchair accessibility, and most car rental companies will provide cars with hand controls at no extra cost. Patients in a wheelchair may find a 12-inch length of dowel helpful for reaching elevator buttons in many community settings.

CASE STUDY 35-1

SPINAL CORD INJURY WITH RESULTING PARAPLEGIA

Examination

Patient History

MS is a 45-year-old man who fell from a ladder while trimming a tree on his property. The fall resulted in a T12 burst fracture and a spinal cord injury with complete paralysis below the level of the injury. The patient underwent surgical decompression and fusion of T10 to L3 segments bilaterally. After stabilization of his acute medical condition, the patient was transferred to an inpatient rehabilitation facility to address his functional limitations, initiate patient and family training and education, and begin planning for his return home. He was hospitalized and received inpatient therapy for a total of 4 weeks. MS's past medical history is unremarkable. Before his accident he ambulated and performed all ADLs independently. He lived with his wife and 2 children, worked full-time as a high school English teacher, enjoyed playing golf and dancing, and walked 1-2 miles 3-4 days per week. House-hold activities were yard work, some laundry and kitchen tasks, and taking out the trash.

MS now presents at the end of his 4 weeks of inpatient treatment shortly before his planned return home when the treatment team scheduled an evaluation of his home for environmental barriers.

Systems Review
Heart rate was 76 bpm. Blood pressure was 134/85 mm Hg.

Tests and Measures
Only abnormalities are noted. All other measures were within normal limits (WNLs).

Musculoskeletal
Muscle Performance Strength was functionally suffi-cient for the patient to independently perform transfers needed to get from the hospital to his home by car and to get in and out of the vehicle. His upper extremity strength was 5/5 throughout by manual muscle test, while his lower extremity strength was 0/5 throughout bilaterally.

Neuromuscular
Sensory Integrity Sensation was completely intact above the T12 dermatome, decreased but present at the T 12 dermatome, and absent to all modalities below this level.

Integumentary: MS had an epithelialized scar on his low back in the area of the surgical incision.

Function
Locomotion and Balance MS used a manually powered wheelchair comfortably on level surfaces but with decreased confidence and hesitation on ramps and curbs. MS required no assistance to balance in sitting. Standing balance was not tested.

Assistive and Adaptive Devices MS has a manually powered wheelchair with the following dimensions: 27.5 inches wide, 48 inches long, and 18-inch seat height.

Environmental Barriers
Home MS lives in a single-story home with 2 bedrooms, 1½ bathrooms, and a detached garage. There are 2 steps up to the front door, each 6 inches high, 10 inches deep, and 48 inches wide. The rooms have the following barriers:

Living Room Shag carpet with soft pad, throw rug without nonskid backing, sofa and chair height are 15 inches from floor to seat. MS needs a higher seat to be able to transfer independently.

Bedroom Bed height is 24 inches, which is too high for MS to transfer to independently. There is no bed rail, no telephone easily accessible from the bed, and the bedside lamp has a standard switch that MS cannot use. The door to the bedroom closet is 27 inches wide, which is too narrow for wheelchair access, the clothes hang at 72 inches from the floor and are out of reach for MS, and neither the uppermost nor the lower-most storage areas can be reached from the wheelchair.

Bathroom The bathroom door is 27 inches wide, which is too narrow for wheelchair access, and the toilet height is 15 inches, which is too low for transfers. The shower has no seat or grab bars, the shower head is at a fixed height, the shampoo and soap are too high to reach from a seated position, and the shower floor surface is slippery.

Kitchen The lighting is poor. There is an area floor rug without nonskid backing. The cabinets and freezer are too high to reach from a seated position. Only the front two burners of the counter-top stove can be reached from a seated position. The sink can be reached.

Laundry Room There is insufficient space to fit a wheel-chair next to the washer and dryer, and the controls cannot be reached from a seated position.

Self-Care and Home Management MS required minimal assistance to roll in bed and minimal-to-moderate assistance to scoot in bed, mostly needing help to move his legs. He required minimal assistance to move from supine to sitting and only stand-by assistance to transfer in sitting from one surface to an adjacent surface at the same level. MS could feed himself while seated at the kitchen table and perform grooming activities from his wheelchair as long as items were placed on a surface within his reach. He can also dress his upper body independently but needs assistance with lower body dressing.

Community Some curbs in MS's neighborhood have ramps, but many do not. MS is not interested in playing golf at this time.

Work In the staff room: The mailbox cannot be reached from a seated position.

In the classroom: The desk is too high for typing but does allow the wheelchair arms to clear. MS finds his desk comfortable for writing and for counseling students. The white board is too high for MS to reach all areas.

Transportation MS requires moderate assistance with transferring in and out of his vehicle with his wheelchair. He has been trained to drive with hand controls, and his vehicle has been adapted.

Evaluation, Diagnosis, and Prognosis
After the examination, the findings were evaluated and recommendations were made to MS and his wife. The evaluation focused on resolution of environmental barri-ers in the home and on planning for return to optimal participation in the home, community, and work place. It was determined that most of the patient's home could be accessed and managed independently from a wheelchair level except for the exterior stairway and narrow doorways to the bathroom and bedroom closet. Addressing these before MS returns home will allow him access to all areas of the home. It is expected that MS will be able to con-tinue his home activities of paying bills and assisting with kitchen and laundry tasks and return to his job teaching.

Intervention
Interventions consisted of recommendations for changes to the environment. The recommendations were as follows.

Home

Exterior: Because MS cannot independently go up or down stairs, a ramp with handrails and edge protection should be installed to access the front door. This should be accomplished before MS returns home since his wife cannot pull or push him up the stairs into the home.

Living Room: Current flooring should be replaced with material that is easier for wheelchair propulsion. This may include high-density, low-pile carpeting, linoleum, wood, or other smooth surface materials. Throw rugs should be removed, fixed to the floor with double-faced adhesive carpet tape, or replaced with rugs with slip-resistant backing. Leg extenders should be used to raise the sofa and chair by 3-4 inches.

Bedroom: The bed height should be lowered by removing the wheels from the bed frame or replacing the frame with a lower one. A rail should be added to the bed and a telephone placed on the bedside table. An accessible switch should be added to the bedside lamp. To widen access to the closet the closet doors may be removed or off-set hinges installed. The clothes hanging rod should be reinstalled at 36-46 inches high, shelves should be lower than 54 inches, and a reacher may be used to reach objects placed on the floor.

Bathroom: Initially, a narrow transport chair may be used to access the bathroom. Ideally, a wider door and accessible shower will be installed. The toilet seat height should be increased by using a raised seat or for greater safety, replacing it with one with a seat 18 inches high. L-shaped grab bars should also be installed next to the toilet. A tub transfer bench, grab bars, a hand-held shower, and a lower shower organizer should be installed in the shower.

Kitchen: To optimize lighting the highest power bulbs that are safe for the fixtures should be used in all fixtures. The area floor rug should be removed. All frequently used utensils and kitchen wares should be placed at counter-top level or below. A side-by-side refrigerator may be purchased to allow MS access to both the refrigerator and the freezer.

Laundry Room: A reacher should be purchased to help with unloading items from the washer and dryer. Ideally, front-loading units should be purchased.

Community

Since ramped curbs are not likely to be installed in all community areas, MS worked on learning to manage curbs and steps in his wheelchair (see Chapter 20), as well as transferring in and out of his vehicle during his remaining therapy. Since he was not playing golf, MS was encouraged to participate in wheelchair sports to maintain fitness and resume a competitive sport.

Work

MS's mailbox should be placed lower. A keyboard tray that can be placed on the wheelchair arm rests should be purchased. A white board that raises and lowers on vertical tracks should be installed in MS's classroom.

CHAPTER SUMMARY

This chapter describes the examination of environmental barriers in a patient's home, community, school, and work-place. Environmental barriers may be safety hazards or may reduce access. These barriers affect people of all ages with a wide variety of limitations. The examination of environmental barriers is different from a traditional patient examination because it takes place in the patient's environment and elements of the examination, such as the tests and measures, may be performed on the environment, as well as on the patient. Interventions are generally in the form of recommendations for modifying the environment. Recommendations for adaptations and modifications of environmental barriers are described in this chapter with a focus on access and function for individuals who use assistive devices or wheelchairs for mobility. A case study is provided to demonstrate the application of the concepts to an individual. The aim of environmental barrier modification is the integration or reintegration of a patient to his or her roles and function in the home, school, and community, as well as to improve safety and reduce injury risk.

ADDITIONAL RESOURCES

Useful Forms

Outcome Assessment Information Set (OASIS)
VDT Checklist: OSHA screening tool
Computer Set-Up Examination (see Box 35-2)

Web Sites

Americans With Disabilities Act: www.eeoc.gov/ada/adatext.html
Occupational Safety and Health Administration: www.osha.gov
California Code of Regulations—Repetitive Motion Injuries: www.dir.ca.gov/Title8/5110.html
National Institute for Occupational Safety and Health (NIOSH) site concerning work-related musculoskeletal disorders: www.cdc.gov/niosh/muskdsfs.html
Job Accommodation Network's Searchable Online Accommodation Resource (SOAR): www.jan.wvu.edu/soar
FAA Human Factors Model training program: www.hf.faa.gov/webtraining/HFModel/Variance/anthropometrics1.htm
Cornell University Ergonomics web site: www.ergo.human.cornell.edu/
Typing Injury. A web site containing a wide variety of information about repetitive strain injuries: www.tifaq.org/
Healthy Computing: www.healthycomputing.com/
Board of Certification in Professional Ergonomics: www.bcpe.org

GLOSSARY

Assistive device: A variety of implements or equipment used to aid the performance of an action, activity, movement, or task.

Environmental barriers: The physical impediments that keep people from functioning optimally in their surroundings.

Ergonomics: The relationships between the worker, the work activities, and the environment in which the work is performed.

Function: Those activities identified by an individual as essential to support physical and psychological well being.

Functional muscle testing: Performance-based muscle strength assessment in particular positions simulating functional tasks and activities and usually under specific test conditions.

Input devices: Tools used to input data and access a computer system. Typically, these devices are the keyboard and mouse.

Occupational Safety and Health Administration (OSHA):
United States governmental agency that regulates work place safety.

Pointing and navigation devices: Specific tools used to move the cursor on a computer (e.g., mouse, trackball, touch pad, stylus, tablet, hands-free mouse).

Work environment: Macroenvironment that refers to the place of employment. The work environment extends beyond the *workstation* and includes any surrounding areas associated with the place of employment.

Workstation: Microenvironment where the worker is assigned to perform their essential job functions.

References

1. American Physical Therapy Association: *Guide to Physical Therapist Practice,* ed 2, Alexandria, Va, 2001, American Physical Therapy Association.
2. Chandler Sutherlund R: *Ergonomics for Therapists,* New York, 1995, Butterworth-Heinemann.
3. HFES 100: *Human Factors Engineering of Computer Workstations,* Human Factors and Ergonomics Society.
4. Duncan PW, Weiner DK, Chandler J, et al: Functional reach: A new clinical measure of balance? *J Gerontol Med Sci* 45:192-197, 1990.
5. Konz S, Johnson S: *Work Design: Industrial Ergonomics,* Scottsdale, Ariz, 2000, Holcomb Hathaway Publishing.
6. Allen CK, Earhart CA, Blue T: *Understanding Cognitive Performance Modes,* Ormond Beach, Fla, 1997, Allen Conferences Inc.
7. Chaffin DB, Andres R, Garg A: Volitional postures during maximal push pull exertions in the sagittal plane, *Hum Factors* 25(5):541-550, 1983.
8. ErgoDynamix: The economics of ergonomics page. Available at: http://www.ergodmx.com/articles/article_1.html. Accessed July 13th 2005.
9. Enscore E, Emory K, Knott B, et al: A comparison of alternative time slotting systems for indirect time standards. In Shell RL (ed): *Work Measurement: Principles and Practice,* Atlanta, 1986, Institute of Industrial Engineers.
10. 69 FR 44084, Rules and Regulations, Architectural and Transportation Barriers Compliance Board, 36 CFR Parts 1190 and 1191, [Docket No. 99-1] RIN 3014-AA20: *Americans with Disabilities Act (ADA) Accessibility Guidelines for Buildings and Facilities; Architectural Barriers Act (ABA) Accessibility Guidelines,* Part II, Friday, July 23, 2004. Action: Final rule. Federal Register, 69(141).
11. Schmitz TJ: Environmental assessment. In O'Sullivan SB, Schmitz TJ: *Physical Rehabilitation: Assessment and Treatment,* ed 3, Philadelphia, 1994, FA Davis.
12. http://www.aarp.org/life/homedesign/doors/Articles/a2004-03-02-d-handrails.html
13. Consumer Product Safety Alert: *Tap Water Scalds,* Document #5098: US Consumer Product Safety Commission, Washington, DC, Office of Information and Public Affairs.
14. http://www.cdc.gov/niosh/muskdsfs.html
15. http://factfinder.census.gov/servlet/DTTable?_bm=y&-geo_id=04000US03&-ds_name=ACS_2003_EST_G00_&-redoLog=false&-mt_name=ACS_2003_EST_G2000_P058
16. http://www.census.gov/ipc/www/usinterimproj/natprojtab02a.pdf
17. http://ergo.human.cornell.edu/DEA325notes/anthrodesign.html
18. http://www.eeoc.gov/ada/adatext.html
19. Occupational Safety and Health Administration (OSHA): *Ergonomics Program,* Final rule:29 CFR Part 1910, Department of Labor, Federal register 64:68261-68870.
20. US Equal Employment Opportunity Commission: *The Americans with Disabilities Act of 1990,* (Pub. L. 101-336) (ADA), Vol 42 of US Code, Section 12101.
21. http://www.eeoc.gov/facts/fs-ada.html
22. Heller-Ono A: WorksiteInternational.com
23. Subchapter 7. General Industry Safety Orders Group 15: *Occupational Noise Article 106,* Ergonomics 5110. Repetitive Motion Injuries: www.dir.ca.gov'oshsa/5110.html
24. www.waterheaterrescue.com
25. Lewis CB, Bottomley JM: *Geriatric Physical Therapy: A Clinical Approach,* Norwalk, Conn, 1994, Appleton & Lange.
26. Sharpe DT: *The Psychology of Color and Design,* Chicago, 1974, Nelson-Hall.
27. Lord SR, Dayhew J: Visual risk factors for falls in older people, *J Am Geriatr Soc* 49(5):676-677, 2001.
28. The Accessible Home: *Remodeling Concerns for the Disabled,* Remodeling Ideas, Fall 1981.
29. Architectural and Transportation Barriers Compliance Board Agency: Architectural and Transportation Barriers Compliance Board. 36 CFR Part 1191: *Americans With Disabilities Act (ADA) Accessibility Guidelines for Buildings and Facilities,* [Docket No. 90-2] RIN 3014-AA09, 56 FR 35408, July 26, 1991 [Part 1 of 2], Action: Final guidelines.
30. Trombly CA, Versluys HP: Environmental evaluation and community reintegration. In Trombly CA (ed): *Occupational Therapy for Physical Dysfunction,* ed 3, Baltimore, 1989, Williams & Wilkins.
31. Assistive Technology Quick Reference Series: *Bathroom Accommodations: Activities of Daily Living,* Collaborative project of the United Cerebral Palsy Associations, the Center for Assistive Technology and Environmental Access at Georgia Tech and Southeast Disability and Business Technical Assistance Center. Available from: Http://www.techconnections.org. June 2003.
32. Maguire GH: The changing realm of the senses. In Lewis CB (ed): *Aging: The Health Care Challenge,* ed 2, Philadelphia, 1990, FA Davis.
33. Cushman WH: Data-entry performance and operator preferences for various keyboard heights. In Grandjean E (ed): *Ergonomics and Health in Modern Offices,* Philadelphia, 1984, Taylor & Francis.
34. Grandjean E, Hunting W, Pidermann M: VDT workstation design: preferred settings and their effects, *Hum Factors* 25:161-175, 1983.
35. Miller I, Suther TW: Preferred height and angle settings of CRT and keyboard for a display station input task. In Proceedings of the Human Factors Society 25th annual meeting. Santa Monica, Calif, 1981, Human Factors and Ergonomics Society.
36. Weber A, Sancin E, Grandjean E: The effects of various keyboard heights on EMG and physical discomfort. In Grandjean E (ed): *Ergonomics and Health in Modern Offices,* Philadelphia, 1984, Taylor & Francis.
37. Chaffin DB, Andersson G: *Occupational Biomechanics,* New York, 1984, Wiley Interscience.
38. Karlqvist LK, Hagberg M, Köster M, et al: Musculoskeletal symptoms among computer-assisted design (CAD) operators and evaluation of a self-assessment questionnaire, *Int J Occup Environ Health* 2:185-192, 1996.
39. Hedge A, McCrobie D, Morimoto D: Beneficial effects of a preset tilt-down keyboard system on posture and comfort in offices (monograph), Ithaca, NY, 1995, Cornell University.
40. Rempel D, Horie S: Effect of wrist posture during typing on carpal tunnel pressure. In Proceedings of Working with Display Units 1994, Milan, 1994, University of Milan.
41. Weiss ND, Gordon L, Bloom T, et al: Wrist position of lowest carpal tunnel pressure and implications for splint design, *J Bone Joint Surg Am* 77:1695-1699, 1995.
42. Armstrong TJ, Chaffin DB: An investigation of the relationship between displacements of the finger and wrist joints and the extrinsic finger flexor tendons, *J Biomechanics* 11:119-128, 1978.
43. Lundborg G, Gelberman R, Minteer-Convery M, et al: Median nerve compression in the carpal tunnel-functional response to experimentally induced controlled pressure, *J Hand Surg* 7:252-258, 1982.

Index

Page numbers followed by f refer to figures; t to tables; b to boxes.

Use the enclosed CD-ROM to improve your practical knowledge of physical rehabilitation!

Take your understanding beyond the book with the assortment of helpful review tools, study aids, and resources provided on CD-ROM. Specifically developed to complement the material presented in the book, you'll find:

- ⮕ Useful forms
- ⮕ Study questions
- ⮕ Additional case studies
- ⮕ Links to web sites mentioned in the chapters
- ⮕ References with Medline links
- ⮕ Vocabulary-building exercises based on the chapter glossaries
- ⮕ Realistic, 3-D animations

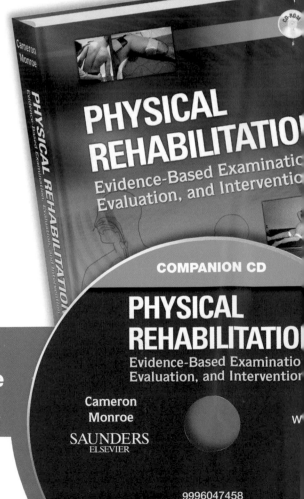

Cameron
Monroe

PHYSICAL REHABILITATION
Evidence-Based Examination
Evaluation, and Intervention

COMPANION CD

PHYSICAL REHABILITATION
Evidence-Based Examinatio
Evaluation, and Intervention

Cameron
Monroe

SAUNDERS
ELSEVIER

9996047458

Simply insert the CD-ROM into any computer to begin using these valuable resources now!